Miller and Evans' Anatomy of the Dog
Fifth Edition

Miller and Evans' Anatomy of the Dog

John W. Hermanson, PhD

Associate Professor
Department of Biomedical Sciences
College of Veterinary Medicine
Cornell University
Ithaca, New York

Alexander de Lahunta, DVM, PhD

James Law Professor of Anatomy, Emeritus
Department of Biomedical Sciences
College of Veterinary Medicine
Cornell University
Ithaca, New York

Howard E. Evans, PhD

Professor of Veterinary and Comparative Anatomy, Emeritus
Department of Biomedical Sciences
College of Veterinary Medicine
Cornell University
Ithaca, New York

ELSEVIER

ELSEVIER

3251 Riverport Lane
St. Louis, Missouri 63043

MILLER AND EVANS' ANATOMY OF THE DOG, FIFTH EDITION   ISBN: 978-0-323-54601-0
Copyright © 2020, Elsevier Inc. All rights reserved.
Previous editions copyrighted 2013, 1993, 1979 and 1964.

No part of this publication may be reproduced or transmitted in any form or by any means, electronic or mechanical, including photocopying, recording, or any information storage and retrieval system, without permission in writing from the publisher. Details on how to seek permission, further information about the Publisher's permissions policies and our arrangements with organizations such as the Copyright Clearance Center and the Copyright Licensing Agency, can be found at our website: www.elsevier.com/permissions.

This book and the individual contributions contained in it are protected under copyright by the Publisher (other than as may be noted herein).

Notices

Practitioners and researchers must always rely on their own experience and knowledge in evaluating and using any information, methods, compounds, or experiments described herein. Because of rapid advances in the medical sciences, in particular, independent verification of diagnoses and drug dosages should be made. To the fullest extent of the law, neither the Publisher nor the authors, contributors, or editors, assume any liability for any injury and/or damage to persons or property as a matter of products liability, negligence or otherwise, or from any use or operation of any methods, products, instructions, or ideas contained in the material herein.

978-0-323-54601-0

Content Strategist: Jennifer Flynn-Briggs
Content Development Management: Ellen Wurm-Cutter
Content Development Specialist: Melissa Rawe
Publishing Services Manager: Shereen Jameel
Project Manager: Aparna Venkatachalam
Designer: Ryan Cook

Printed in Canada

Last digit is the print number: 9 8 7 6 5 4 3

Sandy de Lahunta and Howard Evans collectively were on the anatomy faculty from 1950 to 2005 at Cornell University. This represents a remarkable span of time during which they mentored a multitude of students and worked together as colleagues. With this fifth edition, we recognize the contribution of Professor Evans in the title:

Miller and Evans' Anatomy of the Dog.

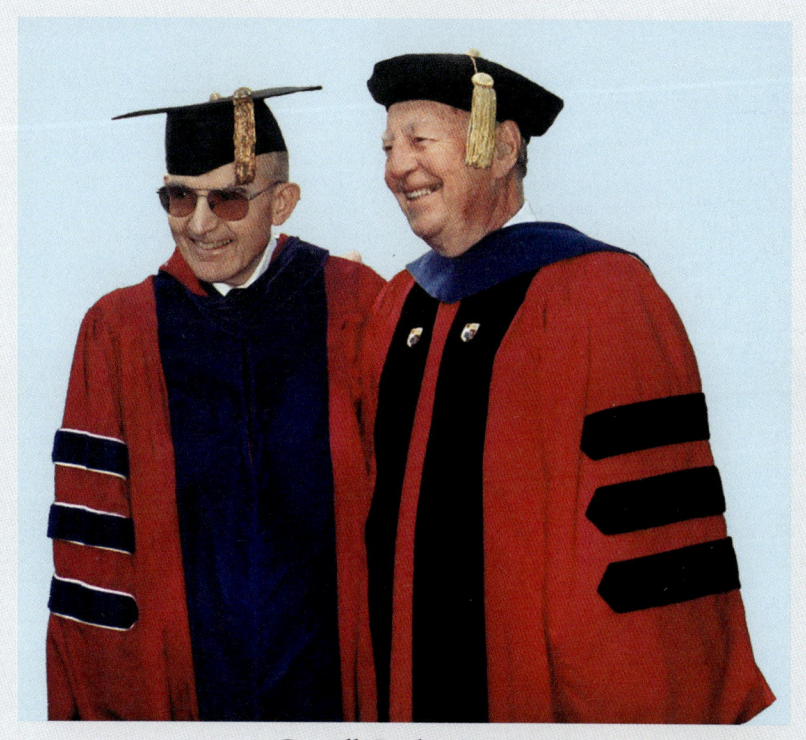

Cornell Graduation, 2005

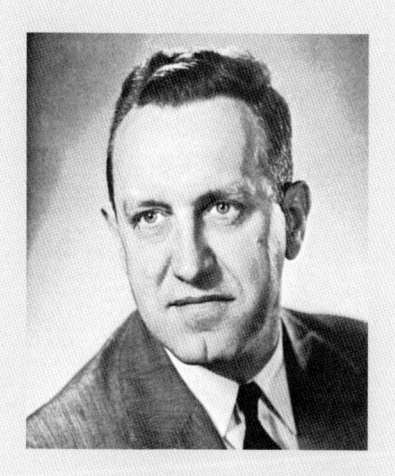

Malcolm E. Miller, BS, DVM, MS, PhD (1909–1960). Dr. Malcolm E. Miller was born on a farm in Durrell, Pennsylvania; studied for two years at Pennsylvania State University; and then earned his BS and DVM (1934), MS (1936), and PhD (1940) degrees from Cornell University. He was appointed Instructor in 1935 and, at the time of his death, was Professor and Head of the Department of Anatomy and Secretary of the New York State Veterinary College at Cornell University. His zest for life, devotion to his family, and his enjoyment of teaching and anatomical research sustained his spirit through several brain operations which provided only temporary relief from epileptic attacks.

This volume was envisioned by Dr. Miller in 1944 as a comprehensive treatise documenting the morphology of the dog. His efforts were aided considerably by the encouragement of Dean W.A. Hagan and the appointment of a medical illustrator in 1946. Preliminary work with the help of his wife, Mary, resulted in the 1947 publication by Edwards Brothers Press of *Miller's Guide to the Dissection of the Dog*, which now appears as *Guide to the Dissection of the Dog*, eighth edition (2017) by Evans and de Lahunta.

About the Authors

Howard Evans was an undergraduate student in Entomology at Cornell University when he was called to active duty in the Army during World War II in 1943. Upon completion of 3 years of service as a Second Lieutenant and graduation from Cornell *in absentia*, he returned as a graduate teaching assistant in Comparative Anatomy. He received a PhD in 1950, with a thesis on the anatomy of Cyprinid fishes. That same year he was hired by Dr. Malcolm Miller as an Assistant Professor in the Veterinary College. He taught Veterinary Anatomy for 36 years until his retirement in 1986. During his tenure, he taught Dog Anatomy, Horse and Cow Anatomy, and the Anatomy of Fish and Birds. As an emeritus professor, he has taught a course on Natural History to veterinary students at Cornell for 12 years. For 2 or 3 weeks each year since 2002, he has taught Fish and Bird Anatomy and Natural History at St. George's University Veterinary College in Grenada, West Indies.

He was a co-author of the first and second editions of *Miller's Anatomy of the Dog* and the sole author of the third edition. The fourth edition with Dr. de Lahunta was the first to have all illustrations in color. He is co-author with Dr. de Lahunta of *Guide to the Dissection of the Dog*, which is in its eighth edition. Evans has written chapters in other texts on tropical fish anatomy, bird anatomy, ferret anatomy, and woodchuck anatomy. His research has concerned fetal development of Beagle dogs, cyclopia in sheep, and the replacement of teeth in fishes. His sabbaticals were spent at the Veterinary College in Davis, California, learning surgical techniques for fetal studies of dog development; the University of Hawaii, teaching Comparative Anatomy; the Medical School of the University of Pennsylvania, studying fetal development of sheep; and the Marine Station of the University of Georgia, studying the anatomy of the Spotted Sea trout.

His interest in natural history led to giving courses to veterinary students at Cornell and at St. George's University in Grenada, West Indies. He and his wife Erica have led many Cornell University trips to Africa, Hawaii, New Guinea, and Antarctica. He has continued to enjoy his interactions with students and sharing the anatomical collections in his office almost daily since his retirement in 1986.

Alexander de Lahunta ("Sandy" to his colleagues, or "Dr. D." as he was known to his students) received his DVM from the College of Veterinary Medicine at Cornell University in 1958. After 2 years of mixed practice in Concord, New Hampshire, he returned to the Department of Anatomy at Cornell where he obtained his PhD. For the next 42 years he taught gross anatomy of the dog, veterinary neuroanatomy and clinical neurology, applied anatomy, embryology, and neuropathology.

He established a consultation service in clinical neurology in the Teaching Hospital and was a founding member of the Neurology Specialty of the American College of Veterinary Internal Medicine (ACVIM).

He was chairperson of the newly developed Department of Clinical Sciences. He received numerous awards for his teaching and the Robert W. Kirk Distinguished Service Award of the ACVIM. He retired in 2005 and has been active in textbook writing since that time.

In addition to this text, he has authored or co-authored a fourth edition of *Veterinary Neuroanatomy and Clinical Neurology*, an eighth edition of *Miller's Guide to the Dissection of the Dog*, *The Embryology of Domestic Animals: Developmental Mechanisms and Malformations*, *Veterinary Neuropathology*, and *Applied Anatomy*.

John Hermanson was an undergraduate at the University of Massachusetts, Amherst, where he first became interested in comparative vertebrate anatomy as a student of the late David Klingener. He received an MS from Northern Arizona University in 1978, and a PhD from the University of Florida in 1983. It was at Florida where he first engaged in teaching veterinary anatomy at the College of Veterinary Medicine in Gainesville. After postdoctoral studies at Emory University (neuroscience) and at the University of Pittsburgh School of Medicine (muscle regeneration), he began his career at Cornell University in 1987. He has taught anatomy of "whatever is in the barnyard" since that time, including Horse Anatomy, Ruminant Anatomy, Bird Anatomy, and comparative anatomy that caters to lab animal, zoo animal, and wildlife conservation interests. His research has spanned bat biology, equine biomechanics, and paleontology.

Preface

The first edition of this text was based on an unfinished manuscript with illustrations that Professor Miller had been working on for many years prior to his death in 1960. At the request of his wife, Mary Miller (Ewing), the manuscript was completed by Howard E. Evans and George C. Christensen. The first edition of *Anatomy of the Dog* by Miller, Christensen, and Evans appeared in 1964. "Mac" Miller had supervised the preparation and completion of almost all of the illustrations by Pat Barrow and Marion Newson that appeared in the first edition.

The second edition, entitled *Miller's Anatomy of the Dog*, by Evans and Christensen, was published in 1979. It incorporated the most recent nomenclature of *Nomina Anatomica Veterinaria* and had new chapters on fetal development, the endocrine system, the spinal cord, and the eye. There were also many new drawings by Marion Newson, Lewis Sadler, and William Hamilton.

The third edition of *Miller's Anatomy of the Dog*, by Evans, updated the literature, added new material, and incorporated nomenclatorial changes that appeared in *Nomina Anatomica Veterinaria 1983*. Many figures were modified structurally or relabeled, and several were replaced. There were chapters by eight new contributors, and the introductory chapter was expanded to include the phylogenetic relationships of canids to other carnivores and the history of domestication of the dog. The chapter on muscles was augmented to include current histochemical and electrophysiologic evidence of muscle function. The material on the nervous system was amplified by new chapters on the brain and cranial nerves.

Miller's Anatomy of the Dog attempts to meet the varied needs of anatomists, veterinary students, clinicians, and experimentalists. Throughout the text, the intent is to describe and illustrate the specific morphology of the dog, with reference to older literature. Although there are many similarities between species, it is often surprising how different anatomical specifics can be. What is a functional structure in one may be only a vestige or absent in another, and care is required when extrapolating to other species.

The fourth edition was the first fully colorized version, and it required removal of all former labels (which were made with LeRoy lettering stencils, something unknown to new generations of students) and dotted lead-lines. Some of these illustrations appeared in the eighth edition of *Guide to the Dissection of the Dog* (2017, Elsevier/Saunders) by Evans and de Lahunta.

This fifth edition includes many new radiographs and computed tomography (CT) scans that were kindly provided by Dr. Peter Scrivani, supplementing a number of radiographs from earlier editions that were contributed by Dr. Vic Rendano. New digital imaging technology allows an ever-improving insight into the structure of the dog's body. Michael Simmons provided new illustrative interpretations of a number of images of the lymphatic system, replacing images that had grown darker with each subsequent printing. Illustrations were added or updated in Chapter 21. Nomenclatural revisions were included as appropriate, and we attempted to retain some synonyms where their use would clarify discrepancies with human medical anatomy texts and other veterinary anatomy texts. New research was referenced throughout the text to enhance our interpretations of anatomic structures.

We appreciated correspondence received and offer our thanks to the many people who pointed out errors or suggested improvements. The illustrations have been particularly well received, and requests for their reuse in books and journals stand as a tribute to the dissectors and illustrators whose combined efforts produced them.

Anatomical Terms

The terms used for structures of the body are numerous, and, in the course of medical history, about 50,000 names have been given to some 5000 structures. This has led to considerable ambiguity.

The history of anatomical terminology shows gradual regional changes from the Arabic to the Greek of Hippocrates, Aristotle, and Galen to the Latin of Vesalius, Fallopius, Eustachius, Fabricius, and Malphighi, when the center of medical education shifted to Italy. Some Arabic terms, such as "saphena" and "nucha," remain, as do several Greek terms, some with Latin endings. Each country often used different endings for Latin terms, and later vernacular terms made the medical vocabulary unusable internationally. (For example, the hypophysis, or pituitary gland, had at least 30 names in Greek, Latin, German, French, and English.)

For any meaningful communication, it is necessary that anatomical terms be clear and precise. With this in mind, international anatomical nomenclature committees sponsored by various anatomical societies have published Nomina for humans (*Nomina Anatomica* [NA], 1989 and *Terminologia Anatomica* [TA], 1998), and Nomina for domestic animals (*Nomina Anatomica Veterinaria* [NAV], 2005), and (*Nomina Anatomica Avium* [NAA], 1993) to promote international communication and facilitate learning. There are lists of Nomina for gross, histologic, and embryologic terms.

Several anatomists, including Burt Green Wilder, MD, Professor of Physiology, Vertebrate Zoology, and Neurology at Cornell and Secretary of the Committee on Anatomical Nomenclature of the Association of American Anatomists, tried (between 1880 and 1890) to standardize anatomical nomenclature, but their results lacked international agreement. In 1887, the German Anatomical Society undertook the task and assembled an international committee that worked for 6 years before issuing a final list in 1895. This *Basel Nomina Anatomica* (BNA) for the human included about 5000 terms from approximately 30,000 proposed by the subcommittee (O'Rahilly, 1989, "Anatomical terminology, then and now." *Acta Anat. 134*:291–300). This BNA formed the basis for subsequent revisions in Birmingham (BR) in 1933, Jena (JNA) in 1936, and Paris in 1955. The latter was published as the first edition of the NA. In 1977, the fourth edition of the NA included *Nomina Histologica* (NH) and *Nomina Embryologica* (NE). The current NA for the human is in its sixth edition. In 1989, the International Federation of Associations of Anatomists created a new committee to write *Terminologica Anatomica* (TA), which was published in 1998 by Thieme. Both the NA and the TA are only for human anatomy.

A committee on veterinary anatomical nomenclature was established in 1895, at the Sixth International Veterinary Congress in Bern because the BNA was not applicable to domestic animals. At the next Veterinary Congress in Baden-Baden in 1899, a nomenclature for domestic animals was approved but not printed or distributed internationally, although the terms were used in several textbooks. In 1923, the American Veterinary Medical Association published the *Nomina Anatomica Veterinaria* (NAV) based on the BNA, but it was not widely known or used. In 1957, the International Association of Veterinary Anatomists established a nomenclature committee that incorporated the earlier unpublished lists of the American Association of Veterinary Anatomists with terms in current use. After several preliminary lists and many meetings in different countries, the first edition of the internationally approved NAV was published by the World Association of Veterinary Anatomists in 1968. This Nomina is currently in a sixth edition (2017) and is available for free on the worldwide web.

Although anatomical structures are quite stable, our understanding and interpretation of what we see will continue to require changes at all levels: gross, microscopic, and ultrastructural. Formal procedures exist for making changes in anatomical terms, and the International Committee for Veterinary Anatomical Nomenclature of the World Association of Veterinary Anatomists welcomes suggestions and help.

The terminology used in this text follows NAV 2005, with subsequent recommendations (NAV 2017). We also consulted Constantinescu and Schaller's *Illustrated Veterinary Anatomical Nomenclature* (2012) as we considered terminology used in this edition. The following constraints serve as guidelines in the work of anatomical nomenclature committees:

1. Each anatomical concept should be designated by a single term. Synonyms have been used in rare exceptions, usually as transitional terms, but in some cases both terms may be used such as: peroneus = fibularis.
2. Each term should be in Latin (Greek remains in some terms: ischiadic [G.] = sciatic [L.]; splen [G.] = lien [L.]).
3. Each term should be as short and simple as possible.
4. The terms should be easy to remember and should have instructive and descriptive value.
5. Structures that are closely related topographically should have similar names (e.g., femur: femoral artery, vein, and nerve).
6. Differentiating adjectives should generally be opposites (major/minor; superficial/deep).
7. Terms derived from proper names (eponyms) should not be used because the choice of the eponym has varied by country and was not descriptive of the structure (e.g., Eustachian tube = auditory tube; canal of Schlemm = scleral venous sinus; foramen of Monro = interventricular foramen).

Directional terms as applied to quadrupeds are different from those applied to humans. The anatomical position of a standing dog is with four paws on the supporting surface and the abdomen ventral. For a human, the standing position is with the forelimbs hanging by the side, palms held forward: the palms and the abdomen are thus considered to be anterior. For the dog, the terms *cranial* and *caudal* apply to the neck, trunk, and tail as well as to the limbs as far distally as the end of the antebrachium and crus. The terms for the forepaw or manus are *dorsal* and *palmar*; those for the hindpaw or pes are *dorsal* and *plantar*. On the head the terms *rostral*, *caudal*, *dorsal*, and *ventral* are preferred. Only in a few locations, such as the jaws, eye, and inner ear, are such terms as *anterior, posterior, superior,* and *inferior* used. *Medialis* and *lateralis* apply to the whole body except on the digits, where *axialis* and *abaxialis* refer to the sides of the digit toward the axis of the limb or away from the axis of the limb, respectively. The axis of the limb passes between the third and the fourth digits.

Planes of the Body

The planes of the body are formed by any two points that can be connected by a straight line.

Median Plane: Divides the head, body, or limb longitudinally into equal right and left halves.
Sagittal Plane: Passes through the head, body, or limb parallel to the median plane.
Transverse Plane: Cuts across the head, body, or limb at a right angle to its long axis or across the long axis of an organ or a part.

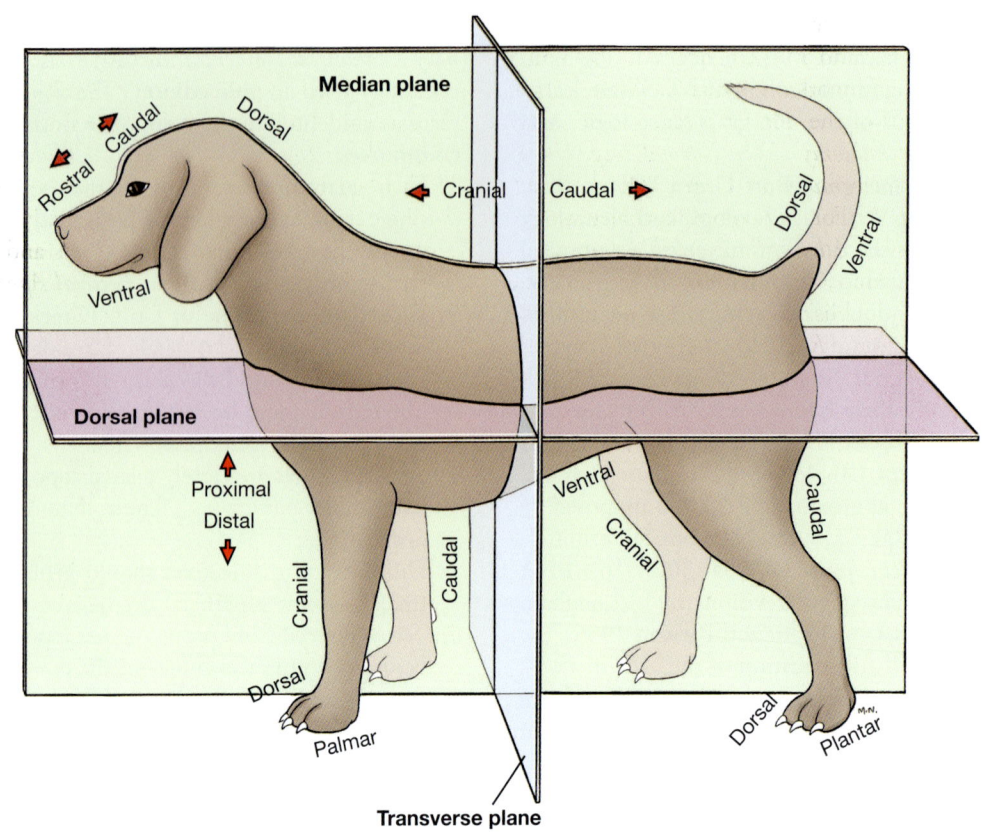

• Fig. PF1.1 (From *Guide to the Dissection of the Dog*, by Evans and de Lahunta, Elsevier, 2017.)

Dorsal Plane: Runs at right angles to the median and transverse planes and divides the body or head into dorsal and ventral portions (see Fig. PF1.1).

Movement

Parts of the body can move relative to one another primarily because of muscular action on bones articulated with each other by joints. *Flexion* is the movement of one bone on another so that the angle between them is reduced; thus, the limb, digit, or vertebral column is bent, folded, retracted, or arched. *Extension* is the lengthening of a part by increasing the angle between bones, straightening the limb, digit, or vertebral column. Extension beyond 180 degrees is *overextension* (sometimes referred to as *dorsiflexion*).

Abduction is the moving of a part away from the median plane; *adduction* is the moving of a part toward the median plane. *Rotation* is the movement of a part around its long axis (action of the radius when using a screwdriver). *Supination* (lying on the back = supine) is lateral rotation of the paw so that the palmar or plantar surface faces medially or dorsally. *Pronation* (lying on the belly = prone) is medial rotation so that the palmar or plantar surface of the paw faces ventrally.

On radiographs the view is described in relation to the direction of penetration by the x-ray: from the point of entrance to the point of exit before striking the film. A radiograph of the carpus in the standing position with the film under the palmar surface of the paw would be a *dorsopalmar* view.

In the text that follows, structures are generally designated by their anglicized terms in common use unless none exists. Each term, when introduced for the first time, is followed by its Latin equivalent.

Literature

Much anatomical information is published in several thousand scientific journals, of which about 100 frequently contain anatomical articles in one of several languages. Language differences and the accessibility of periodicals are still considerable barriers to the dissemination of anatomical information, although abstracting services and electronic retrieval systems have eased the burden of keeping current.

Literature on anatomy of the dog is not always easy to categorize by system, and, as a result, there are many old as well as recent monographs and books that are not cited by abstracting systems or in the chapters that follow. Some are little known: for example, the extensively illustrated doctoral thesis of Madeleine A. Hamon "Atlas de la Tete du Chien: Coupes Series-Radioanatomie-Tomographies" (1977) presented at the University Paul Sabatier of Toulouse. This study includes serial transverse, sagittal, and horizontal sections and has a bibliography of 997 references relating to structures of the head of the dog. Current interest in multiplanar imaging, such as CT scans, ultrasonography (sonograms), and nuclear magnetic resonance (NMR) scans make such works invaluable. A book that compares body sections of the dog with scans is the *Atlas of Correlative Imaging Anatomy of the Normal Dog: Ultrasound and Computed Tomography*, by Feeney, Fletcher, and Hardy (Saunders, 1991). For radiographic anatomy, the most detailed source is the *Atlas of Radiographic Anatomy of the Dog and Cat*, by Schebitz, Wilkens, and Waibl (Elsevier, 2011). Thrall's recently published seventh edition of *Textbook of Veterinary Diagnostic Radiology* (Saunders, 2018) is also highly useful.

Dated but still useful and authoritative anatomical information on the dog can be found in the out-of-print *Handbuch der Vergleichenden Anatomie der Haustiere*, by Ellenberger and Baum (1943). Dissection guides for the dog include *Atlas der Anatomie des Hundes*, by Budras (Hannover: Schluter, 2010); *Canine Anatomy: A Systemic Study*, by Adams (Ames, Iowa State University Press, 2004); *Dog and Cat Dissection Guide*, by Susan and Chris Pasquini (Pilot Point Texas, 2009); *A Regional Approach to the Dissection of the Dog* by M.S.A. Kumar (Linus Learning, 2017); and *Guide to the Dissection of the Dog*, by Evans and de Lahunta (Elsevier 2017).

Acknowledgments

Contributors

The cooperation of contributing authors was essential for this revision, and we thank them as colleagues and friends.

Fakhri Al-Bagdadi, BVMS, Diploma, MS, PhD
Professor
Department of Veterinary Comparative Biomedical Sciences
School of Veterinary Medicine
Louisiana State University
Baton Rouge, Louisiana
The Integument

Marnie FitzMaurice, VMD, PhD
Senior Lecturer
Biomedical Sciences
Cornell University College of Veterinary Medicine
Ithaca, New York
Introduction to the Nervous System, The Autonomic Nervous System

J. Claudio Gutierrez, DVM, PhD
Assistant Professor
Department of Anatomy, Physiology and Cell Biology
School of Veterinary Medicine, University of California-Davis
Davis, California
The Eye

Ronald L. Hullinger, DVM, PhD
Professor *Emeritus*
Department of Basic Medical Sciences
College of Veterinary Medicine
Purdue University
West Lafayette, Indiana
The Endocrine System

Linda Mizer, DVM, MSc, PhD
Senior Lecturer
Biomedical Sciences
Cornell University of Veterinary Medicine
Ithaca, New York
The Digestive Apparatus and Abdomen

Christopher J. Murphy, DVM, PhD
Professor
Department of Surgical and Radiological Sciences
School of Veterinary Medicine, University of California-Davis
Davis, California
The Eye

Peter V. Scrivani, DVM
Associate Professor
Department of Clinical Sciences, College of Veterinary Medicine
Cornell University
Ithaca, New York
Radiographs and CT images

Most of the illustrations were made by Marion Newson, RN, medical illustrator in the Department of Anatomy from 1951 to 1972. Her skill as an illustrator, her knowledge of anatomy, and her concern for accuracy proved invaluable. Other illustrators from the Department of Anatomy include Pat Barrow (who worked with us from 1947 to 1950), Lewis Sadler (1973–76), William Hamilton IV (1977–83), and Michael Simmons (1983–2010), each of whom had different techniques that they used to make their work distinctive. Other illustrations were produced for the first edition by Algernon R. Allen and Neil Harris (*Nervous System* and *The Autonomic Nervous System*), Robert R. Billiar, Dan J. Hillmann, and Santiago B. Plurad (*Sense Organs* and *The Integument*). The few illustrations borrowed from other works are credited in the figures' legends. The conversion of black-and-white illustrations to color and the removal and replacement of all labels and lead-lines was a major undertaking for Jeanne Robertson and the other people involved with the fourth edition. Michael Simmons provided revisions of several illustrations for this fifth edition. Talia Coppens, currently a veterinary student at Cornell University, contributed a revision of one illustration in Chapter 6. Chrisoula Toupadakis Skouritakis, at the University of California, Davis, provided several new illustrations and greatly improved the presentation of several other illustrations in Chapter 21.

Specimen preparation by Pam Schenck and library assistance from Susanne Whitaker was much appreciated, as were the suggestions for corrections and additions made by our many students and colleagues. Jen Patterson provided clerical support and helped update and edit many of the illustrations for submission to the publisher. We offer our heartfelt thanks to her.

Several colleagues provided critical review of individual chapters, and we wish to thank them for their insights. Specifically we are grateful to James Ryan and Adam Boyko (Chapter 1), Soon Hon Cheong (Chapter 2), Peter Scrivani (Chapter 4), Santiago Peralta (Chapter 7), and Bradley Njaa and Andrew Miller (Chapter 20).

We also wish to thank several people at Elsevier who have helped us revise this volume. Penny Rudolph, Content Strategy Director, understood our needs, listened to our concerns, and made wise decisions. She initiated the development of the fifth edition prior to her retirement. Jennifer Flynn-Briggs, a Senior Content Strategist at Elsevier, assumed leadership of the project. We are most grateful to Laurel Shea and Melissa Rawe, Content Development Specialists at Elsevier. Laurel and Melissa kept loose ends together and kept the project on target while we made revisions in the illustrations and text, and especially while one of us (JWH) was learning the ropes in a large-scale endeavor such as this book.

To readers of this text, we urge that you not hesitate to write about any errors, omissions, or addenda that come to your notice.

Former Contributors in Past Editions

Alvin Beitz, PhD
The Brain

Abraham J. Bezuidenhout, BVSc, DVSc (Pret), DTE (Pret)
The Heart and Arteries
Veins
The Lymphatic System

John Bowne, DVM, PhD
Taste

Gregory Chibuzo, DVM, MS, PhD
The Tongue

George C. Christensen, DVM, PhD
Coauthor of first and second edition

Juliet Clutton-Brock, DSc, FSA
Origin and Domestication of the Dog

Thomas F. Fletcher, DVM, PhD
The Brain
Spinal Cord and Meninges

Peter Jewell, BSc, MA, PhD, FI Biol
Origin and Domestication of the Dog

Robert Getty, DVM, PhD
Sense Organs

Robert Hadek, DVM, PhD
Nasal Cavity

Ralph L. Kitchell, DVM, PhD
Introduction to the Nervous System
Spinal Nerves
Cranial Nerves and Cutaneous Innervation of the Head

James Lovell, DVM, MS, PhD
The Integument

Robert McClure, DVM, PhD
Spinal Cord and Meninges
Cranial Nerves

Hermann Meyer, DVM, PhD
The Brain

Roy V.H. Pollock, DVM, PhD
The Eye

Victor Rendano, VMD
Contributed radiographs to various chapters

Donald Samuelson, PhD
The Eye

J.F. Smithcors, DVM, PhD
The Endocrine System

Melvin W. Stromberg, DVM, PhD
The Autonomic Nervous System

Robert K. Wayne, PhD
Phylogenetic Relationships of Canids to Other Carnivores

John W. Hermanson
Alexander de Lahunta
Howard E. Evans

Contents

1 The Dog and Its Relatives, 1
The Order Carnivora, 1
The Family Canidae, 2
   Hybrids, 2
Breeds of Dogs, 5

2 Prenatal Development, 13
Early Development, 13
Length of Gestation, 13
Prenatal Periods, 15
Oocyte–Embryo, 15
Embryo, 17
Age Determination, 21
   Measurements and Growth Plots, 23
   Size Index, 26
Fetus, 26
   Skeletal Age Criteria, 27
   Skull, 27
   Vertebral Column, 35
   Ribs, 44
   Sternum, 44
   Limbs and Girdles, 44
   Carpus, 51

3 The Integument, 64
Epidermis, 65
Dermis, 65
Structure of the Dermis and Changes with Age, 65
Pigmentation, 66
Nasal Skin, 67
Digital Pads, 67
Hairy Skin, 69
   Growth Rate of the Hair Shaft, 69
   Embryology of Hair Follicles, 69
   Development of Complex Follicle, 71
   Complex Hair Follicle, 73
   Hair Types, 74
   Variability in Hair Coat, 74
   Coat Color, 74
   Hair Length, 75
   Implantation of Hair, 75
   Hair Follicle Cycle and Seasonal Shedding, 75
   Surface Contour of Hairy Skin and Histologic Characteristics of Epidermis, 78
Muscles of the Skin, 79
Glands of the Skin, 79
   Tail Gland Area (*gll. caudae*), 81
Blood Supply to the Skin, 81
Nerve Supply to the Skin, 82
Skin Grafting, 82
Claw, 82

4 The Skeleton, 86
General, 86
   Classification of Skeletal Elements, 86
Axial Skeleton, 91
   Skull, 91
   Vertebral Column, 125
   Thoracic Skeleton, 139
Appendicular Skeleton, 140
   Bones of the Thoracic Limb, 140
   Bones of the Pelvic Limb, 156

5 Arthrology, 176
General, 176
   Fibrous Joints, 176
   Cartilaginous Joints, 176
   Synovial Joints, 177
Ligaments and Joints of the Skull, 179
   Temporomandibular Joint, 179
   Intermandibular Joint, 180
   Joints of Auditory Ossicles, 180
   Joints of Hyoid Apparatus, 180
   Synchondroses of the Skull, 180
   Sutures of the Skull, 181
Ligaments and Joints of the Vertebral Column, 181
   Atlantooccipital Articulation, 181
   Atlantoaxial Articulation, 182
   Other Synovial Joints of the Vertebral Column, 183
   Long Ligaments of the Vertebral Column, 184
   Intervertebral Discs and Short Ligaments of the Vertebral Column, 185
Ligaments and Joints of the Ribs and Sternum, 186
Ligaments and Joints of the Thoracic Limb, 188
   Shoulder Joint, 188
   Elbow Joint, 189
   Radioulnar Joints, 191
   Carpal, Metacarpal, and Phalangeal Joints (*Articulationes Manus*), 192

xvii

Ligaments and Joints of the Pelvic Limb, 196
  Joints of Pelvic Girdle (*Articulationes Cinguli Membri Pelvinae*), 196
  Hip Joint, 197
  Stifle Joint, 198
  Tibiofibular Joints, 202
  Tarsal, Metatarsal, and Phalangeal Joints (*Articulationes Pedis*), 202

6 The Muscular System, 207
Introduction, 207
Skeletal Muscles, 210
  Origin and Insertion, 211
  Function, 212
  Accessory Structures, 213
  Connective Tissue, 213
  Blood and Nerve Supply, 213
  Regeneration, 214
Muscle Description, 214
Muscles of the Head, 214
  Muscles of Facial Expression, 214
  Muscles of Mastication, 222
  Muscles of Bulbus Oculi: Extrinsic, 225
  Muscles of the Tongue, 227
  Muscles of the Pharynx, 229
  Muscles of the Soft Palate, 230
  Muscles of the Larynx, 231
  Muscles of the Hyoid Apparatus, 233
  Muscles of the Cervical Vertebrae, 235
  Fasciae of the Head, 236
Muscles of the Neck, 237
  Fasciae of the Neck, 240
Muscles of the Dorsum, 241
  Extrinsic Thoracic Limb Muscles, 241
  Erector Spinae Muscles, 242
  Transversospinalis Muscle, 245
  Interspinal Muscles, 247
  Intertransverse Muscles, 247
Muscles of the Thoracic Wall (*Musculi Thoracis*), 248
  Diaphragm, 250
Muscles of the Abdominal Wall (*Musculi Abdominis*), 252
Muscles of the Tail (*Musculi Caudae*), 258
Fasciae of the Trunk and Tail, 262
Muscles of the Thoracic Limb, 263
  Extrinsic Muscles, 263
  Intrinsic Muscles, 265
  Brachial Muscles, 269
  Antebrachial Muscles, 273
  Muscles of the Forepaw, 285
  Fasciae of the Thoracic Limb, 286
Muscles of the Pelvic Limb, 287
  Muscles of the Pelvis and Thigh, 287
  The Femoral Triangle and Associated Structures, 302
  Muscles of the Crus, 303
  Muscles of the Pes, 311
  Fasciae of the Pelvic Limb, 312

7 The Digestive Apparatus and Abdomen, 319
Oral Cavity, 319
  Vestibule, 319
  Lips, 319
  Cheeks, 320
  Oral Cavity Proper, 320
Pharynx, 344
The Alimentary Canal, 346
  Esophagus, 346
  Abdomen, 349
  Stomach, 359
  Small Intestine, 364
  Large Intestine, 368
  Perineum, 374
Liver, 375
Pancreas, 381

8 The Respiratory System, 388
External Nose, 388
  Cartilages of the Nose, 388
  Vomeronasal Organ, 390
  Ligaments of the Nose, 391
Nasal Cavity, 391
  Nasal Conchae, 392
  Nasal Meatuses, 393
  Paranasal Sinuses, 394
  Nasal Mucosa, 394
  Glands of the Nose, 395
  Functional Considerations, 395
  Nasal Portion of the Pharynx, 396
Larynx, 396
  Cartilages of the Larynx, 397
  Muscles of the Larynx, 400
  Cavity of Larynx and Laryngeal Mucosa, 400
  Innervation of the Larynx, 401
Trachea, 402
Bronchi, 402
Thoracic Cavity and Pleurae, 404
  Thoracic Cavity, 404
  Mediastinum, 405
  Pleurae, 407
Lungs, 408
  Shape of Lobes and Position of Interlobar Fissures, 409
  Relationship of Lungs to Other Organs, 411
  Pulmonary Vessels, 411
  Bronchial Vessels, 412
  Pulmonary Lymphatics, 413

9 The Urogenital System, 416
Urinary Organs, 416
  Kidneys, 416
  Ureters, 420
  Urinary Bladder, 421

Reproductive Organs, 423
   Male Genital Organs, 423
   Female Genital Organs, 445
   Mammae, 458
Embryologic Characteristics of the Urogenital System, 462

10 The Endocrine System, 469
General Features of the Endocrine Glands, 469
The Hypophysis, 470
   Macroscopic Features, 471
   Mesoscopic Features, 473
   Developmental Anatomy, 473
   Microscopic Features, 474
   Vascularization, 475
   Innervation, 476
Thyroid Gland, 476
   Macroscopic Features, 476
   Mesoscopic Features, 477
   Developmental Anatomy, 478
   Microscopic Features, 479
   Vascularization, 479
   Innervation, 480
Parathyroid Glands, 480
   Mesoscopic Features, 480
   Developmental Anatomy, 481
   Microscopic Anatomy, 481
   Vascularization and Innervation, 481
Pineal Gland, 481
   Mesoscopic Features, 481
   Developmental Anatomy, 482
   Microscopic Anatomy, 482
   Vascularization and Innervation, 482
Adrenal Gland, 482
   Macroscopic Features, 482
   Developmental Anatomy, 483
   Mesoscopic Features, 484
   Microscopic Features, 485
   Vascularization, 486
   Innervation, 486
Pars Endocrina Pancreatis, 487
   Developmental and Mesoscopic Anatomy, 487
   Microscopic Features, 487
Enteroendocrine Cells, 488
Endocrine Tissues of the Ovary, 488
Fetal Membrane Endocrine Tissues, 488
Endocrine Tissues of the Testis, 489
Endocrine Cells of the Kidney, 489

11 The Heart and Arteries, 495
Pericardium and Heart, 495
   Pericardium, 495
   Heart, 495
Pulmonary Arteries and Veins, 509
   Pulmonary Trunk, 509
   Pulmonary Veins, 509

Systemic Arteries, 510
   Aorta, 510
   Aortic Arch, 510
   Thoracic Aorta, 548
   Abdominal Aorta, 551
   Median Sacral Artery, 578

12 The Veins, 582
General Considerations, 582
Cranial Vena Cava, 582
   Azygos System of Veins, 590
Veins of the Thoracic Limb, 591
   Superficial Veins of the Thoracic Limb, 591
   Deep Veins of the Thoracic Limb, 593
   Veins of the Forepaw, 594
Caudal Vena Cava, 595
Portal Vein, 598
Veins of the Pelvic Limb, 599
   Superficial Veins of the Pelvic Limb, 599
   Deep Veins of the Pelvic Limb, 600
   Veins of the Pelvis, 603
   Veins of the Hindpaw, 605
Veins of the Central Nervous System, 606
   Venous Sinuses of the Cranial Dura Mater, 606
   Veins of the Brain, 610
   Veins of the Diploë, 611
   Meningeal Veins, 611
   Veins of the Spinal Cord and Vertebrae, 611

13 The Lymphatic System, 616
General Considerations, 616
Ontogenesis of the Lymphatic System, 616
Lymph Drainage, 617
Lymph Vessels, 619
Innervation of Lymph Vessels and Lymph Nodes, 620
Lymphoid Tissue, 620
Lymph Nodes, 621
Hemal Nodes, 621
Lymph Nodules, 621
Regional Anatomy of the Lymphatic System, 621
   Large Lymph Vessels, 622
   Lymph Nodes and Vessels of the Head and Neck, 624
   Lymph Nodes and Vessels of the Thoracic Limb, 628
   Lymph Nodes and Vessels of the Thorax, 628
   Lymph Nodes and Vessels of the Abdominal and Pelvic Walls, 633
   Lymph Nodes and Vessels of the Abdominal and Pelvic Viscera, 636
   Lymph Nodes and Vessels of the Pelvic Limb, 640
Spleen, 642
Thymus, 644

14 Introduction to the Nervous System, 650
General, 650
- Structure of Neurons, 650
- Functional Segments of Neurons, 652
- Groups of Neurons, 654
- Supporting Cells, 657
- The Central Nervous System (CNS), 657
- The Peripheral Nervous System, 659

Functional Components of Nerves, 659
Reflexes, 661

15 The Autonomic Nervous System, 663
General Visceral Efferent System, 663
- Parasympathetic Division, 664
- Sympathetic Division, 671

Enteric Nervous System, 675

16 The Spinal Cord and Meninges, 679
The Spinal Cord, 679
Morphologic Features of the Spinal Cord, 679
Spinal Cord Segments, 681
Segmental Relationships to Vertebrae, 683
Gray Matter of the Spinal Cord, 685
- Gray Matter Organization, 686
- Gray Matter Nuclei, 687
- Gray Matter Laminae, 687

White Matter of the Spinal Cord, 688
- Spinal Cord Cranial Projecting Tracts, 689
- Spinal Cord Caudal Projecting Tracts, 693

Spinal Reflexes, 695
Transverse Sections of the Spinal Cord, 696
Meninges, Brain Ventricles, and Cerebrospinal Fluid, 696
- The Meninges, 699
- The Ventricular System, 700
- Cerebrospinal Fluid, 701

17 The Spinal Nerves, 704
Initial or Primary Branches of a Typical Spinal Nerve, 705
General Features of Spinal Nerves, 706
Cervical Nerves, 708
Nerves to the Diaphragm, 711
Brachial Plexus, 712
- Nerves of the Brachial Plexus That Supply Intrinsic Muscles of the Thoracic Limb, 715
- Nerves of the Forepaw (Manus), 723
- Nerves of the Brachial Plexus That Supply Extrinsic Muscles of the Thoracic Limb, 727

Thoracic Nerves, 728
Lumbar Nerves, 731
Sacral Nerves, 743
- Nerves of the Plantar Surface of the Hindpaw (Pes), 752

Caudal Nerves, 754

18 The Brain, 757
THE BRAINSTEM, 757
- Cranial Nerve Nuclei Overview, 757
- Reticular Formation Overview, 758
- The Medulla Oblongata, 759
- The Pons, 766
- Neuromodulation Overview, 767
- The Midbrain, 767
- The Diencephalon, 771

The Subthalamus, 778
THE CEREBRUM, 778
- Cerebral Hemisphere, 778
- The Rhinencephalon, 781
- Olfactory Pathways, 783
- Hippocampal Formation, 785
- The Limbic System, 786
- Cerebral Neocortex, 787

Basal Nuclei, 789
THE CEREBELLUM, 792
- Cerebellar Nuclei, 792
- Cerebellar Peduncles, 794
- The Cerebellar Cortex, 795

Brain Atlas, 796

19 Cranial Nerves, 814
Olfactory Nerve (Cranial Nerve I), 815
Optic Nerve (Cranial Nerve II), 816
Oculomotor Nerve (Cranial Nerve III), 816
Trochlear Nerve (Cranial Nerve IV), 817
Trigeminal Nerve (Cranial Nerve V), 818
- The Ophthalmic Nerve, 819
- The Maxillary Nerve, 819
- The Mandibular Nerve, 824

Abducent Nerve (Cranial Nerve VI), 828
Facial Nerve (Cranial Nerve VII), 829
Vestibulocochlear Nerve (Cranial Nerve VIII), 832
Glossopharyngeal Nerve (Cranial Nerve IX), 832
Vagus Nerve (Cranial Nerve X), 833
Accessory Nerve (Cranial Nerve XI), 836
Hypoglossal Nerve (Cranial Nerve XII), 837
Cutaneous Innervation of the Head by Noncranial Nerves, 837

20 The Ear, 839
The Internal Ear, 839
- Bony Labyrinth, 839
- Membranous Labyrinth, 842

The Middle Ear, 846
- Tympanic Membrane, 846
- Tympanic Cavity, 847
- Bones and Articulations of the Middle Ear, 849

The External Ear, 850
- External Acoustic Meatus, 850
- Auricle, 850
- Muscles of the Ear, 852

21 The Eye, 858
    Development, 858
    The Eyeball, 861
        Fibrous Tunic, 861
        Vascular Tunic, 866
        Internal Tunic, 873
        Lens, 876
        Chambers of the Eye, 878
    The Eye as an Optical Device, 879
    Orbit, 880
        Zygomatic Gland, 883
        Orbital Fasciae (*Fasciae Orbitales*), 884
    Eyelids, 885
        Conjunctiva, 887
        Third Eyelid, 887
    Lacrimal Apparatus, 888
        Lacrimal Gland, 889
        Superficial Gland of the Third Eyelid, 890
        Conjunctiva, 890
        Nasolacrimal Duct System, 890
    Muscles, 891
        Intraocular Muscles, 891
        Extraocular Muscles, 891
        Palpebral, 894
    Innervation, 896
        Optic Nerve, 896
        Oculomotor Nerve, 897
        Trochlear Nerve, 898
        Trigeminal Nerve, 898
        Abducent Nerve, 900
        Facial Nerve, 900
    Vasculature, 901
        Arteries, 901
        Veins, 903
    Comparative Ophthalmology, 904

Index, 912

1

The Dog and Its Relatives

This text is based on anatomic studies of many dogs of diverse and usually unknown ancestry commonly referred to as *mongrels.* Domestic dogs are probably the most polymorphic mammals referred to as a single species, *Canis familiaris,* and some workers have suggested that no domestic animal be given species designation (Groves, 1971). The alternatives are the use of subspecific names or breed designations. Because all members of the family Canidae are interfertile and human interaction has affected their hybridization and distribution throughout the world, it appears simplest to adopt one term for all purebreds, mongrels, and feral dogs. While the complete genome of the domestic dog was published in 2005 (Lindblad-Toh et al., 2005), subsequent analyses have revealed the importance of feral dogs, or the "village dogs" around the world, in developing an understanding of the origins of the domestic breeds (Boyko, 2011). The village dogs are descendants of ancient village-dog populations with little inflow of genes from modern breeds of dog (Boyko et al., 2009) and provided the genetic foundation for modern domesticated breeds (Boyko, 2011). Domestication may have preceded human agricultural practices (Clutton-Brock, 1995) and may have had several origins, one in Europe and another in central Asia (Shannon et al., 2015; Frantz et al., 2016). While Shannon et al. (2015) placed the domestication of dogs at least 15,00 years before present, others suggest a single domestication path starting between 20,000 to 40,000 years before present (Botigué et al., 2017). Parker et al. (2017) investigated the relationships of breeds within functional groups (herding dogs, for example) and elucidated how some physical traits may have arisen in separate breed lineages. For historical considerations of the world's wild and domestic dogs, see Smith (1845–1846) *Mammalia: Dogs,* vols. I and II (with color plates), in *The Naturalist's Library,* vol. 18, by W. Jardine; Darwin (1868); *Animals and Plants under Domestication,* Ash (1972); Fiennes and Fiennes (1968); Titcomb (1969); Epstein (1971); American Kennel Club (AKC) *The Complete Dog Book* (2006) and *The New Complete Dog Book* (2017); and Fogle and Morgan (2009) *Encyclopedia of the Dog,* which covers 420 breeds.

The Order Carnivora

The domestic dog, gray wolf, red wolf, coyote, dingo, jackals, dhole, and others are interfertile and frequently cross in their native habitats all over the world. They have been assigned to various genera over the years depending on the criteria used and will probably continue to be a problem for systematists for many years to come. It is not possible to assign the domestic dog with certainty to any one progenitor, but it is clear that the dog and the wolf are closely related and evolved together.

Order Carnivora
Family Canidae
   Genus *Canis*
      Species familiaris

The order Carnivora is worldwide in distribution and is an assemblage of intelligent, mostly flesh-eating mammals with prominent canine teeth; molars adapted for crushing, cutting, and grinding; and a relatively short alimentary canal. Members of the order have digits provided with claws and sometimes with interdigital webs. Behavioral characteristics identify most of them as predators with strong family ties and devoted to the care of their young. Many of the species adapt readily to domestication (Clutton-Brock & Jewell, 1993; Ewer, 1973).

Since the time of Linnaeus the levels of classification have become more accurate and useful, and we can now also consider genomic evidence for relationships between animals.

Wayne and Ostrander (2007) have investigated the dog genome sequence and associated genomic resources and declared that these studies "will revolutionize the study of dog evolution, population structure and genetics." They presented a chart of canid relationships that shows the major groupings of species. A more accurate phylogeny of the Dog family, Canidae, is in the making, and molecular markers that identify gene pools now allow the assignment of mixed "breeds" to specific gene pools. The WISDOM Panel MX of Mars Veterinary, Inc., has a DNA-based test that is said to identify 134 breeds registered by the American Kennel Club (AKC) that may be present in a mixed-breed dog (Giger et al., 2007). A newer entry in the pool for consumer genomics—or, in this case, canine genetic testing—is EMBARK (www.embarkvet.com), whose testing platform aims to provide information related to a dog's risk for inherited diseases, as one example.

The most complete treatment of fossil and living families and genera of mammals can be found in *Classification of*

Mammals above the Species Level, by Malcolm McKenna and Susan Bell (1997) with contributions from George G. Simpson. This classification project was begun by Simpson (1945) in 1927, at the American Museum of Natural History in New York City. Many people cooperated in assembling this tome, which includes all mammals of the world. The number of extinct taxa is much greater than living forms, and many fossil animals are known only from a few bones or teeth.

Wozencraft (2005) revised the order Carnivora in Wilson and Reeder's (2005) *Mammalian Species of the World.* He raised the Giant Panda, the Madagascan Carnivores, the African Palm Civet, the Skunks, and the Walrus each to family rank. While Wozencraft recognized 273 species, Nyakatura and Bininda-Emonds (2012) proposed recognition of 286 species based on changes in taxonomic opinion and new discoveries.

This pictorial family tree (Fig. 1.1A) is an approximation of how animals in the order Carnivora are related to each other according to prior classifications. The major divisions are the Feliformia (cats) and the Caniformia (dogs), which may have arisen from Miacid stock between the Eocene and the Paleocene approximately 40 to 60 million years ago. This time frame witnessed the evolution of modern mammals and birds. Every year new fossils are found (as well as extant forms), and we are able to improve our understanding of animal phylogeny. For photographs of various mammals see Nowak (1991).

Cat Families
  Felidae
   Lion, Leopard, Snow Leopard, Cheetah, Tiger, Lynx, Bobcat, Domestic Cat, Marble Cat, Flat-Headed Cat, Golden Cat, Black-Footed Cat, Roaring Cats, Caracal, Ocelot, Puma, Jaguarundi, Serval, Jaguar, Eyra
  Herpestidae
   Mongooses, Ichneumon, Cusimanses
  Hyaenidae
   Hyaena, Aardwolf
  Viverridae
   Oriental Civet, Genets, African Civet, Palm Civets, Water Civet, Linsangs, Binturong, Bornean Mongoose, Suricate, Meerkat
  Eupleridae
   Fanaloka, Fossa (Madagascan Carnivores)
  Nandinidae
   African Palm Civet
Dog Families
  Canidae
   Dogs, Wolves, Coyote, Foxes, Dhole, African Hunting Dog, Culpeo, Guara, Crab-Eating Fox, Raccoon Dog, Dingo, Bush Dog, Jackals, Dire Wolf
  Ursidae
   Bears
  Ailuridae
   Giant Panda
  Otariidae
   Eared Seals, Fur Seals, Sea Lions
  Odobenidae
   Walrus
  Phocidae
   Harbor Seal, Ringed Seal, Ribbon Seal, Harp Seal, Hair Seals, Earless Seal, Bearded Seal, Gray Seal, Hooded Seal, Elephant Seal, Monk Seal, Ross Seal, Leopard Seal, Weddell Seal
  Mustelidae
   Minks, Otters, Stink Badger, Marten, Sable, Fisher, Pine Marten, Weasels, Stoat, Ferret, Polecat, Badgers, Grison, Zorille, Taira, Ratel, Wolverine
  Mephitidae
   Skunks
  Procyonidae
   Ring-Tailed Cat, Olingo, Kinkajou, Coatis, Raccoon, Lesser Red Panda

The Family Canidae

The family Canidae is a distinct group of dog- and foxlike animals distributed throughout the world (Gittleman, 1989; Mivart, 1890; Sheldon, 1992). Although there is general agreement about which genera are included in the family, there has been disagreement about the generic status of several species and their groupings into subfamilies. Clutton-Brock et al. (1976) reviewed the family Canidae using numeric methods and suggested a classification at the generic level based on 90 characters of the skeleton, pelage, internal anatomy, and behavior. Their results indicated that the three largest genera—*Canis* (dog, wolf, coyote, jackal), *Vulpes* (foxes), and *Dusicyon* (South American foxes and foxlike animals)—all are closely related but merit the separate designations they now have.

Wayne (1993) Wayne & Ostrander (1999, 2007), and Wayne et al. (1989) have investigated the evolutionary relationships of carnivores using karyologic and molecular procedures. Their techniques, such as DNA hybridization, protein electrophoresis, albumin immunologic distance, and high-resolution G-banding of karyotypes, have helped define relationships. Our current understanding of the taxonomy of carnivores and dogs, in particular, is discussed by Wayne and Ostrander (2007) and Boyko et al. (2010).

Behavior is a feature that is sometimes characteristic of a breed. Takeuchi and Mori (2006) compared the behavior of purebred dogs in Japan with those in the United States and the United Kingdom. Stockard (1941) also took note of behavior in the purebred crosses he was producing.

Hybrids

Because all dogs are interfertile, many intermediate physiognomies are not assignable to any particular breed (Stockard, 1941; Van Gelder, 1977). Even first-generation hybrids of purebred parents may exhibit bizarre combinations of body characteristics (Figs. 1.2 and 1.3).

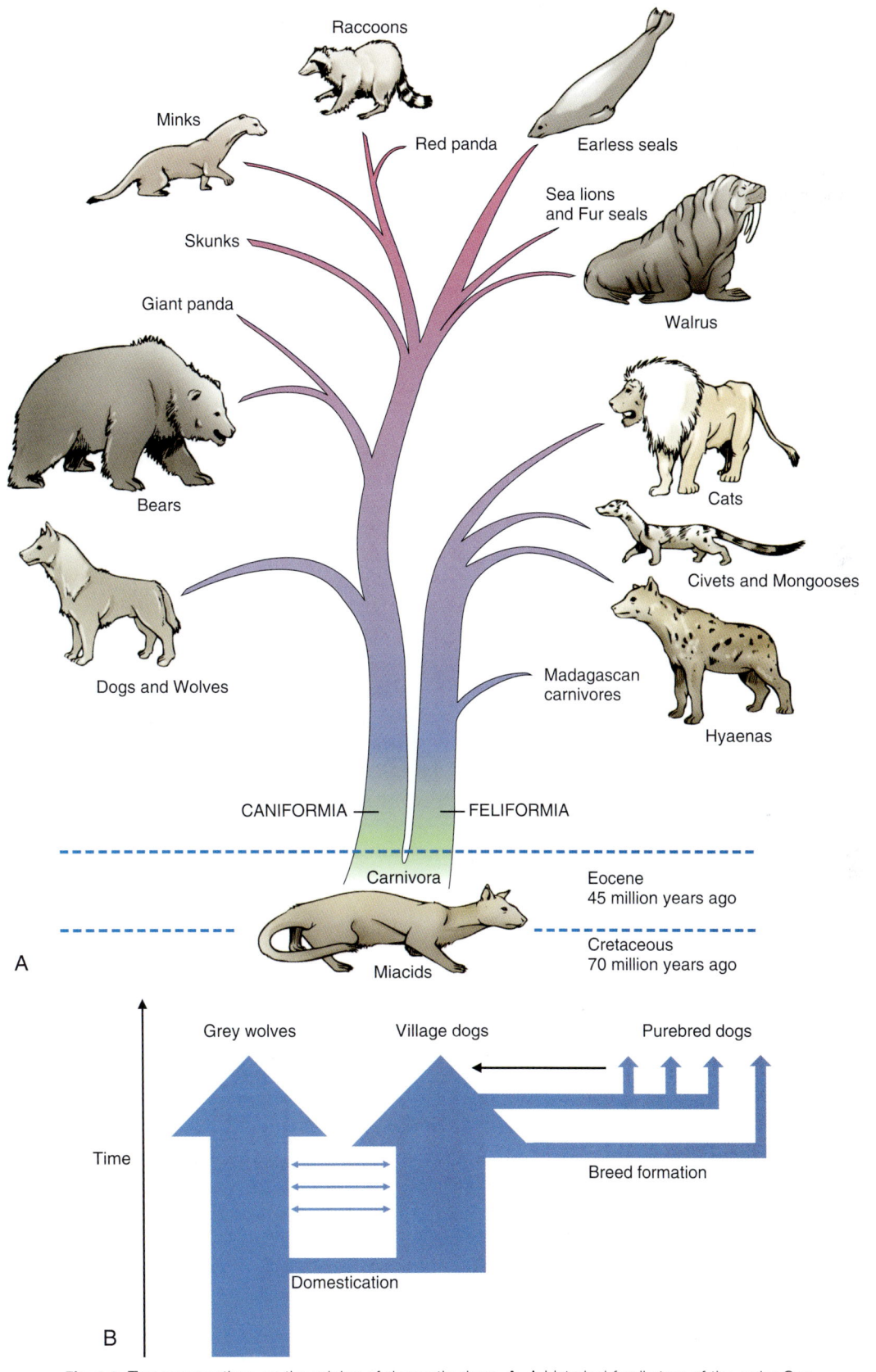

• **Fig. 1.1** Two perspectives on the origins of domestic dogs. **A,** A historical family tree of the order Carnivora. In addition to the domestic dog and cat, Madagascan carnivores include three species of civets (Viverridae): fosa (Cryptoprocta), striped civet (Fossa), and falanouc (Eupleres) and five species of mongooses (Herpestidae). **B,** The relation of dogs as descendants of the Gray Wolf with a founding population of various village dogs giving rise to the multiple breeds of living domestic dogs. (Modified with permission from Boyko, 2011.)

Differences in the conformation of the body or its parts are common and are considered as malformations only when extreme. Susceptibility of the developing embryo or fetus to malformation varies with developmental stage or age, and malformation may affect only one part or organ of the body. Malformations may be due to genetic, endocrine, metabolic, infectious, or mutagenic influences.

Charles R. Stockard of the Cornell Medical College undertook an investigation, starting about 1926, of the genetic and endocrinic basis for differences in form and behavior in dogs. He made crosses between many purebred dogs of various breeds and their F_1 and F_2 generations to study the physiognomy, skeleton, and endocrine organs of the resulting litters. Unfortunately, like Malcolm E. Miller, who started *Anatomy of the Dog*, Stockard died before his work was completed, but, from his extensive notes, photographs, and specimens, his colleagues were able to publish many of his findings as a monograph of the Wistar Institute (Stockard, 1941). What remains of the records and the extensive skeletal collection is now housed and cataloged in the Museum of Natural History on the campus of the University of Georgia in Athens and can be examined by appointment. Stockard's monumental study has left a legacy of numerical comparisons of body and skeletal parts, documented photographs of parents and hybrids, and many disarticulated skeletons. The purebred crosses he produced raise many questions as to the interactions of a large number of breed factors on external features and deformations of the skeleton.

Cartilage growth distortion (achondroplasia) in the skeleton may be restricted to the appendicular or the axial skeleton, or it may affect both. For example, the lower jaw is developmentally independent of the upper jaw. Thus brachygnathic, prognathic, and normal-muzzled pups may appear in the same litter. Such a disharmony between the superior (upper) and the inferior (lower) jaws usually results in malocclusion, difficulty in eating, uneven wear, and loss of teeth.

In many instances Stockard was able to produce and examine F_2 generations from back-crosses to parent stocks. These back-crosses indicated that reversions were common and that the head and tail ends of the axial skeleton often act independently. For example, the very extreme type of Bulldog head may be present in a dog with a long straight tail, or a dog with a normal long muzzle may have a short screw-tail. All F_1 hybrids of the screw-tailed Bulldog × straight-tailed Basset Hound develop long, straight tails. However, in the F_2 generation, the tail deformity reappears in several different patterns.

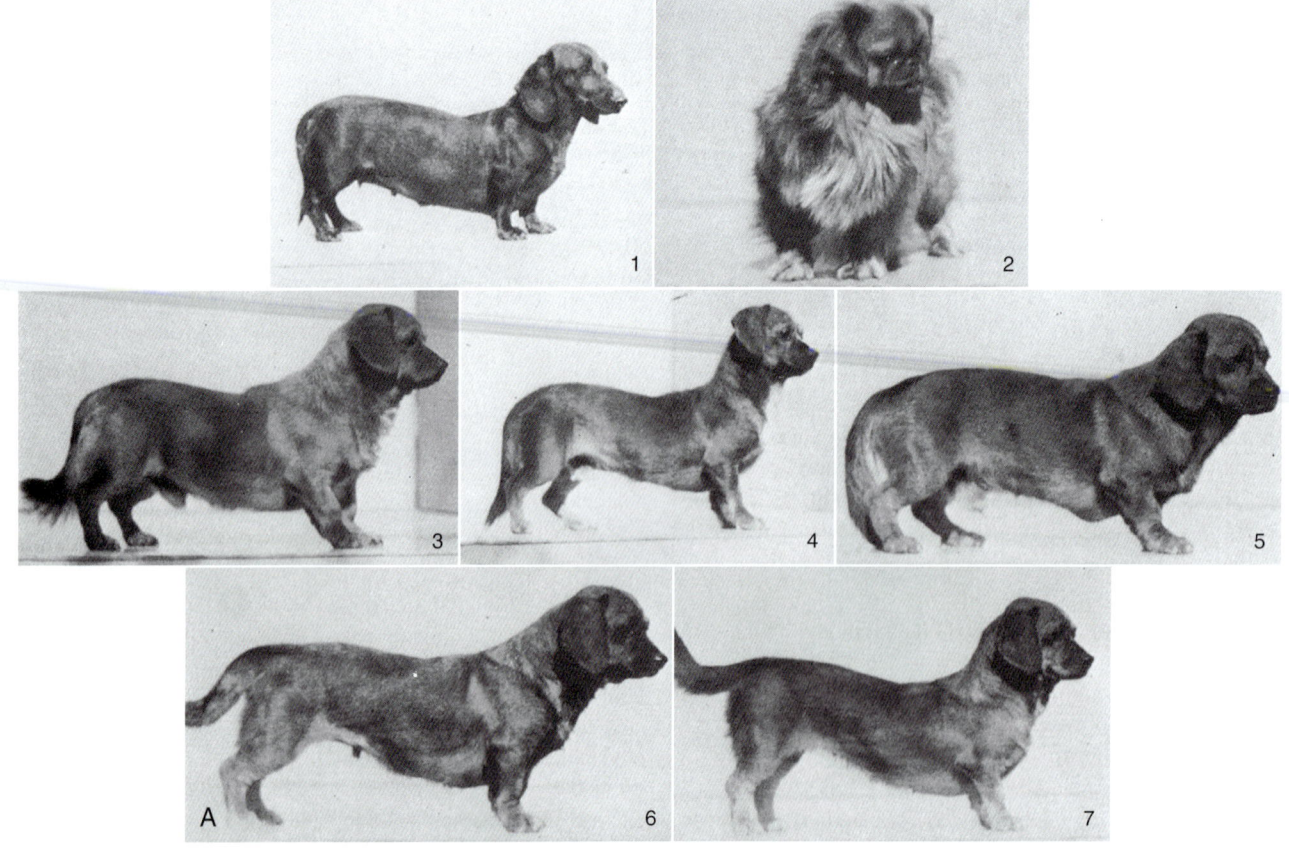

- **Fig. 1.2** A, Cross between the long-muzzled Dachshund and the short-muzzled Pekingese to show inheritance of head type. Dachshund female (1), Pekingese male (2), F1 hybrids (3 to 7). This Dachshund bitch was actually larger and heavier than the Pekingese stud.

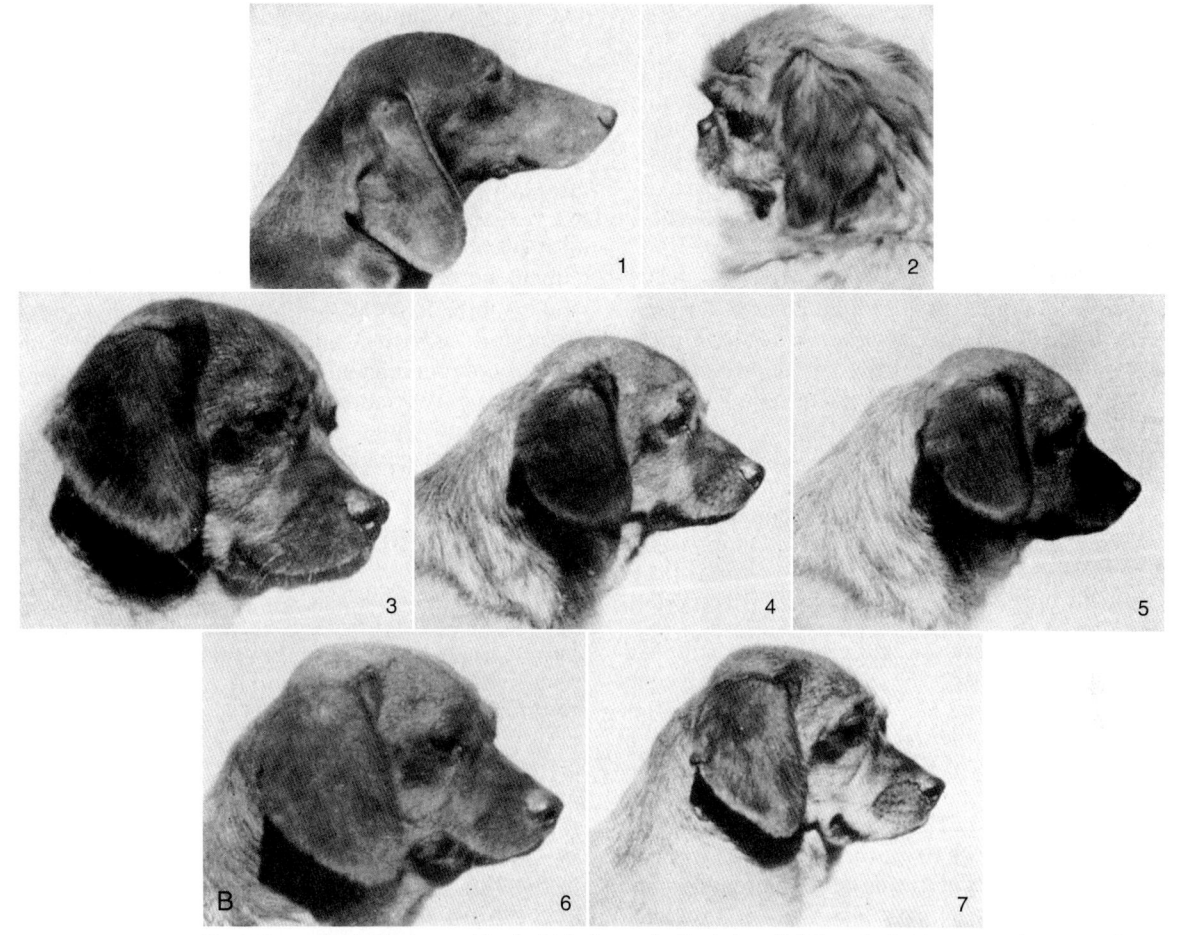

• **Fig. 1.2, cont'd** B, Close-up of the facial features of a Dachshund bitch and a Pekingese stud compared with the same first-generation hybrids as shown in Fig. 1.2A. Of the 22 F1 hybrids produced by several bitches, all were uniform in size and type irrespective of whether they were whelped from Dachshund or Pekingese dams. The hybrids were larger and more vigorous than either parent stock. (From Stockard CR, Johnson AL. The contrasted patterns and modifications of head types and forms in the pure breeds of dogs and their hybrids as the result of genetic and endocrinic reactions. In CR Stockard, editor, *The genetic and endocrinic basis for differences in form and behavior: American anatomical memoirs*, vol. 19, Philadelphia, 1941, Wistar Institute of Anatomy and Biology.)

Dachshund-Pekingese hybrids are good examples of genetic influences on variations in skull form (see Figs. 1.2 and 1.3). The Pekingese dog has a greatly reduced muzzle and a bulging forehead. This is probably a result of achondroplasia of the basicranium and the cartilaginous forerunner of the upper (superior) jaws, a condition similar to that seen in the Bulldog. The Asiatic origin of the Pekingese suggests descent from Chow-Chow ancestors, whereas the Bulldog was developed at a later date from European stock. Thus very different breeds of dog can have very similar mutations in various parts of the world, and, if selected, these mutations can be enhanced.

Because the dominant factor for achondroplasia in the appendicular skeleton results in a more severe shortening of the bones in Bulldog types than in Hounds, Stockard suggested that the "breed quality" of bone may depend on a large number of factors in the genetic constitution of the animal. Thus "Bulldog bone" and "Hound bone" may be more complex entities than we currently imagine.

Breeds of Dogs

The result of human intervention for more than two centuries has established genetic lines that kennel clubs have agreed to recognize as breeds. New breeds will continue to be developed and granted registry according to the rules of national kennel clubs. Not all breeds are granted recognition in all countries, and breed standards are changed from time to time. There were 153 breeds recognized by the American Kennel Club in the 20th edition of *The Complete Dog Book* (2006). This was revised to more than 200 breeds in *The New Complete Dog Book* (2017) and as listed online (akc.org). There are more than 300 breeds of dogs in the world, and each country has some distinctive breeds, as well as introduced breeds.

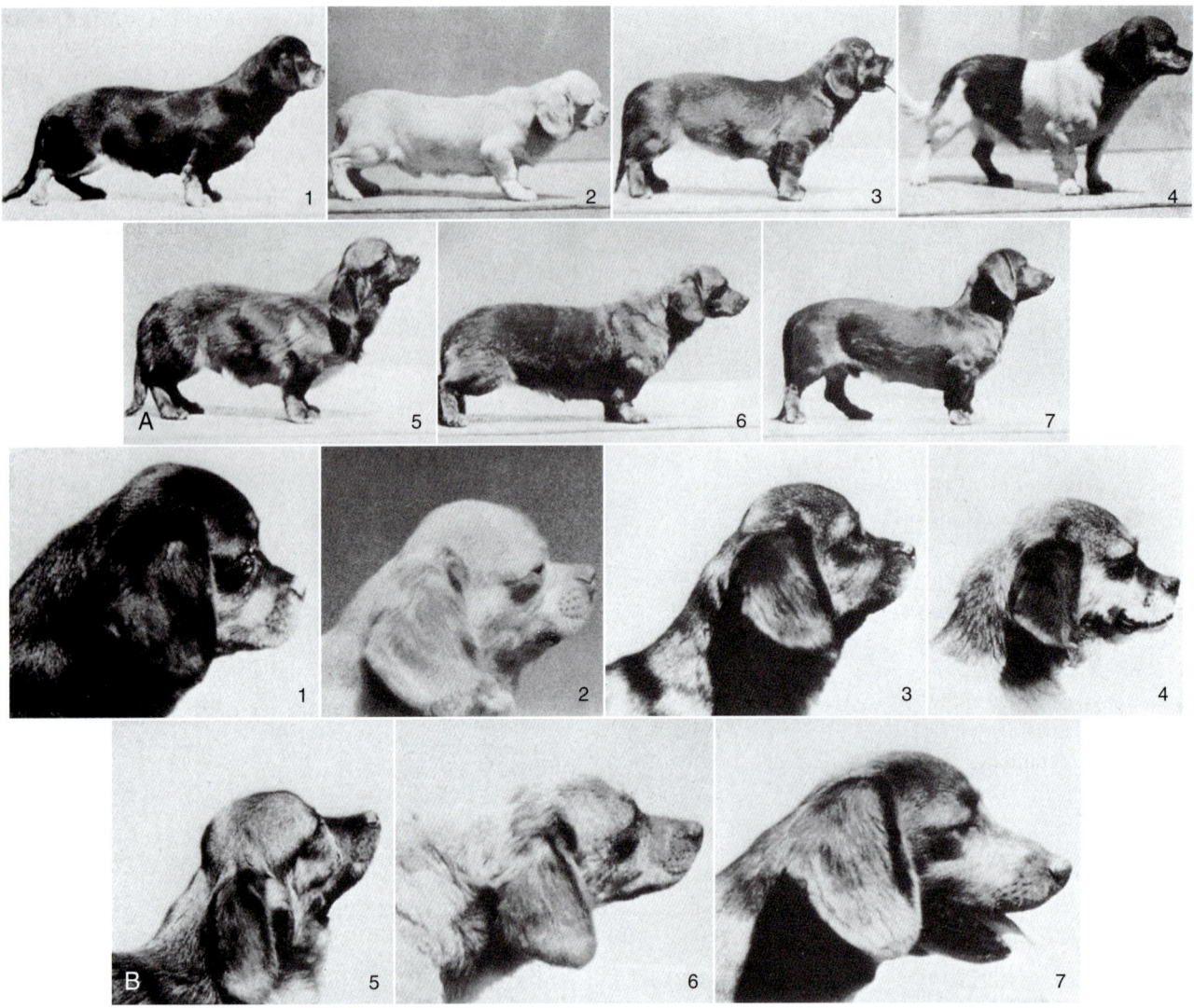

• **Fig. 1.3 A**, Second-generation Dachshund-Pekingese hybrids. Four F_1 bitches were mated with four F_1 studs and produced 47 pups. The F_2 hybrids varied considerably in size and color. None had a typical Pekingese coat, and none held the tail curled over the rump, which is characteristic of the Pekingese and other Asiatic dogs. All of the F_2 animals had short limbs. The large ears of the Dachshund were dominant. **B**, Close-up of the facial features of the same F_2 Dachshund-Pekingese hybrids as shown in Fig. 1.3A. None of the F_2 hybrids had the very short face of the Pekingese. The dental occlusion of F_2 hybrids varied greatly: a few showed superior and inferior jaws of about the same length with normal occlusion, approximately the same number were slightly undershot (mandibular incisors closing ahead of the superior incisors), and the most frequent condition was prognathism of the superior jaws and malocclusion. The long superior (maxilloincisive) jaw of the Dachshund was inherited independently of the short mandibular jaw of the Pekingese, resulting in a disharmony, which, in the extreme, allowed the tongue to hang out rostral to the chin and made feeding from shallow pans difficult. (From Stockard CR, Johnson AL. The contrasted patterns and modifications of head types and forms in the pure breeds of dogs and their hybrids as the results of genetic and endocrinic reactions. In CR Stockard, editor, *The genetic and endocrinic basis for differences in form and behavior: American anatomical memoirs,* vol. 19, Philadelphia, 1941, Wistar Institute of Anatomy and Biology.)

Australia still has a large population of wild Dingoes in the central and northern regions that often cross with domestic dogs (Corbett, 1995). New Guinea has an unknown number of wild "singing dogs," and, on various isolated Pacific Ocean islands, there are dogs that resemble Dingoes (Titcomb, 1969).

The Chinese were probably the earliest breeders of pure-bred dogs, several of which are still popular. Often there are several names for the same breed because the name may change when the dog is introduced into another country; thus the Borzoi is also known as the Russian Wolfhound, the German Shepherd Dog as the Alsatian, the Vizsla as the

Hungarian Pointer, the Scottish Deerhound as the Irish Wolfhound, the Great Dane as the German Mastiff, the Chow-Chow as the Canton Dog, and so on. Several breeds are well known in one country and almost unheard of in another, such as the Canaan Dog of Israel and the Swedish Vallhund.

A *breed* is any group of animals derived from a common stock and bred for their distinctive features, which are then codified as the standard for the breed by those willing to recognize the breed. The French Bulldog, for instance (Fig. 1.4), was probably derived from the English Bulldog, which it resembles in most features.

In the United States more than half the breeds are of English ancestry, and the AKC recognizes seven groups of dogs plus a miscellaneous class, for a total of more than 200 breeds. For a summary of all breeds with illustrations, see the 20th edition (or later) of *The Complete Dog Book* (online at akc.org), published by the American Kennel Club.

The seven categories of dog breeds recognized by the AKC are grouped (Figs. 1.5 to 1.11) for show purposes and do not necessarily represent genetic closeness or ancestry. Several breeds have been moved from one group to another at the request of breed clubs. Each club originates its own standards and revisions and submits them to the AKC for approval. The standard for each breed is therefore a composite of the desired features for each breed. Rarely are all the desired features found in any one dog. There may be several varieties within a breed, and often features acceptable in one breed are unacceptable in another.

The external appearance of the various breeds of dogs may be misleading as concerns skeletal conformation and is further compounded by differences in muscle development. It would be useful to have anatomic documentation

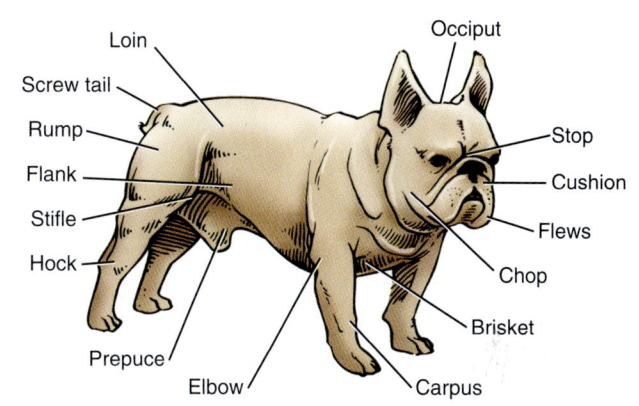

• **Fig. 1.4** External topography of a French Bulldog. This alert, short-limbed muscular dog shows the facial features of a brachycephalic breed.

**Group I
Sporting dogs**

Golden Retriever

Irish Setter

Pointer

Cocker Spaniel

American Water Spaniel	English Setter	Irish Red and White Setter	Spinone Italiano
Boykin Spaniel	English Springer Spaniel	Irish Setter	Sussex Spaniel
Brittany	Field Spaniel	Irish Water Spaniel	Vizsla
Chesapeake Bay Retriever	Flat-Coated Retriever	Labrador Retriever	Weimaraner
Clumber Spaniel	German Shorthaired Pointer	Lagotto Romagnolo	Welsh Springer Spaniel
Cocker Spaniel	German Wirehaired Pointer	Nova Scotia Duck Tolling Retriever	Wirehaired Pointing Griffon
Curly-Coated Retriever	Golden Retriever	Pointer	Wirehaired Vizsla
English Cocker Spaniel	Gordon Setter		

• **Fig. 1.5** There are 30 sporting breeds recognized by the American Kennel Club.

**Group II
Hound Breeds**

Afghan Hound	Bluetick Coonhound	Irish Wolfhound	Redbone Coonhound
American English Coonhound	Borzoi	Norwegian Elkhound	Rhodesian Ridgeback
American Foxhound	Cirneco Dell 'etna	Otterhound	Saluki
Basenji	Dachshund	Petit Basset Griffon Vendeen	Scottish Deerhound
Basset Hound	English Foxhound	Pharaoh Hound	Sloughi
Beagle	Greyhound	Plott	Treeing Walker Coonhound
Black and Tan Coonhound	Harrier	Portuguese Podengo Pequeno	Whippet
Bloodhound	Ibizan Hound		

• **Fig. 1.6** There are 28 hound breeds recognized by the American Kennel Club.

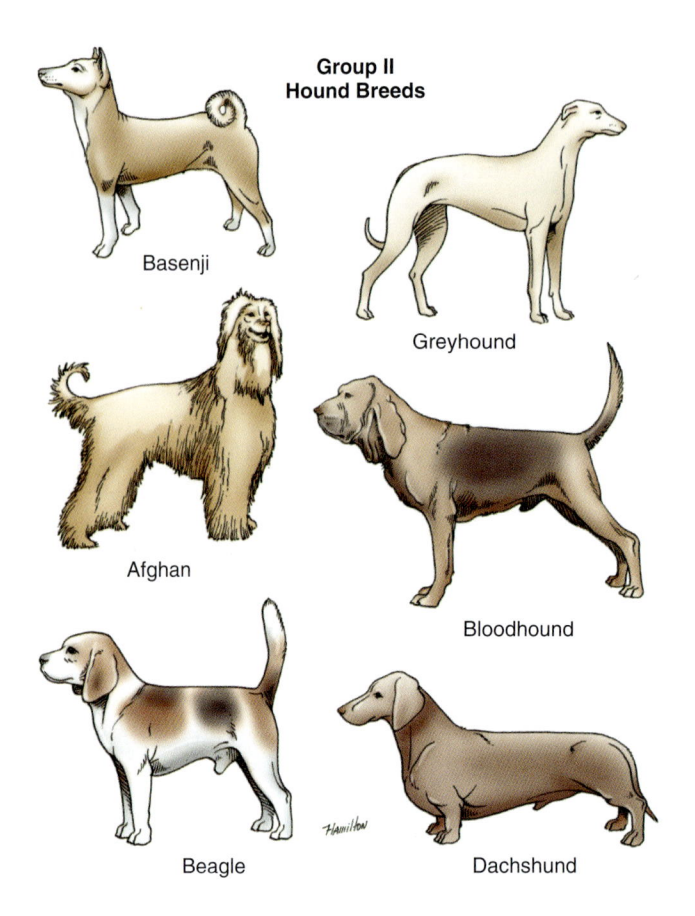

for the standards of breed conformation as established by each club.

Kleinman (1990) radiographed four standard Smooth-Haired Dachshunds standing in show-pose to answer some of the questions regarding the anatomic basis for soundness. Three of the four dogs in this study were champions with good angulation, lay-back, ribbing, and keel. He compared two previously published drawings of the Dachshund skeleton with his radiographs and suggested changes in the drawings. The Dachshund was bred as a field dog for its ability to flush small game out of burrows. Its short chondrodystrophic limbs, pointed head, and elongated trunk were an advantage in such pursuits. Kleinman found that the skeleton did not conform with surface contours and that the muscles have a greater role in determining the appearance of the dog than has been previously thought. There were curvatures of the vertebral column in the midback and pelvis; the spine of the scapula was at approximately 23 degrees from the vertical, not 45 degrees as commonly stated; and the long axis of the pelvis was in line with the vertebral column.

For the many breeds not officially recognized by the AKC, the first step for registry is acceptance into the "miscellaneous class." This requires proof that a substantial nationwide interest in the breed exists, as shown by an active club, breed registry, and expanding breeding activity. When the AKC is satisfied that a breed is continuing to grow in number and sponsorship, it may admit the breed to registration in the Stud Book and grant the opportunity to compete in shows.

The following breeds were in the miscellaneous class and were being considered for recognition at the time this chapter was written:

Azawakh
Barbet
Belgian Laekenois
Dogo Argentino

Group III Working Breeds

Boxer
Alaskan Malamute
Saint Bernard
Akita
Standard Schnauzer
Doberman Pinscher

Akita	Great Pyrenees
Alaskan Malamute	Greater Swiss Mountain Dog
Anatolian Shepherd Dog	Komondor
Bernese Mountain Dog	Kuvasz
Black Russian Terrier	Leonberger
Boerboel	Mastiff
Boxer	Neapolitan Mastiff
Bullmastiff	Newfoundland
Cane Corso	Portuguese Water Dog
Chinook	Rottweiler
Doberman Pinscher	Saint Bernard
Dogue de Bordeaux	Samoyed
German Pinscher	Siberian Husky
Giant Schnauzer	Standard Schnauzer
Great Dane	Tibetan Mastiff

• **Fig. 1.7** There are 30 working breeds.

Group IV Terrier Breeds

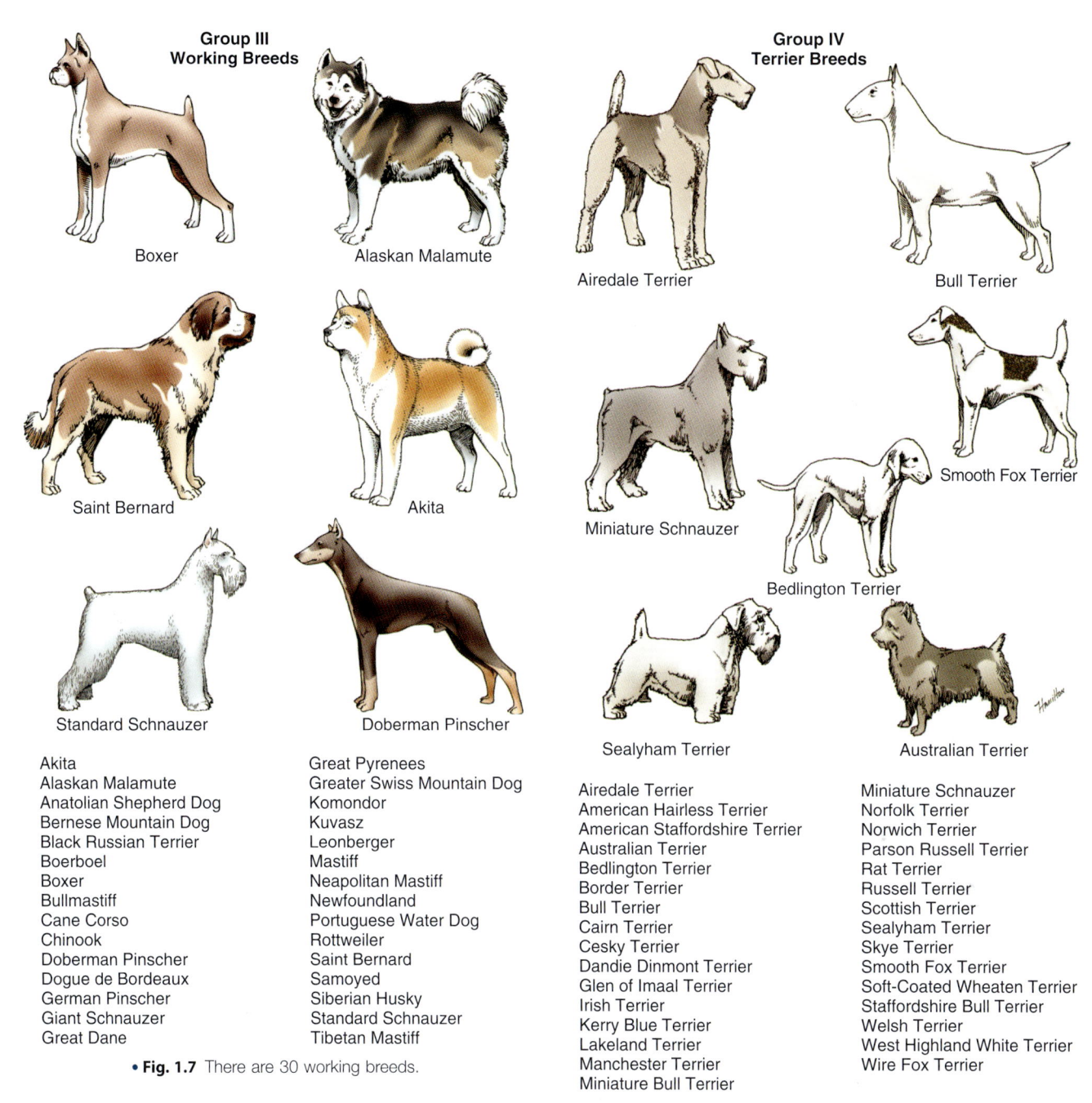

Airedale Terrier
Bull Terrier
Miniature Schnauzer
Smooth Fox Terrier
Bedlington Terrier
Sealyham Terrier
Australian Terrier

Airedale Terrier	Miniature Schnauzer
American Hairless Terrier	Norfolk Terrier
American Staffordshire Terrier	Norwich Terrier
Australian Terrier	Parson Russell Terrier
Bedlington Terrier	Rat Terrier
Border Terrier	Russell Terrier
Bull Terrier	Scottish Terrier
Cairn Terrier	Sealyham Terrier
Cesky Terrier	Skye Terrier
Dandie Dinmont Terrier	Smooth Fox Terrier
Glen of Imaal Terrier	Soft-Coated Wheaten Terrier
Irish Terrier	Staffordshire Bull Terrier
Kerry Blue Terrier	Welsh Terrier
Lakeland Terrier	West Highland White Terrier
Manchester Terrier	Wire Fox Terrier
Miniature Bull Terrier	

• **Fig. 1.8** There are 31 terrier breeds.

Dutch Shepherd
Grand Bassett Griffon Vendeen
Nederlandse Kooikerhondje
Norrbottenspets
Peruvian Inca Orchid
Portuguese Podengo

The relative popularity of a breed may vary from time to time and from country to country. As a result, the mongrel population also changes owing to the prevalence of a particular breed's acting as a sire or dam, although the change is gradual. Because there are specific characteristics associated with each breed, one can expect to see subtle changes in the anatomic features of the mongrel population. As an example, one may cite the tendency toward reduction of the stylohyoid muscle in the Beagle (Evans, 1959) and the loss of teeth in brachycephalic breeds like the Bulldog. There are several specific pathologic conditions more prevalent in some breeds than in others. For reference to these conditions, see Earl (1978); de Lahunta, Glass, and Kent (2015); and Noden and de Lahunta (1985).

An extensive collection of reference materials on dogs (more than 3000 titles) is housed in the library of the College of William and Mary in Williamsburg, Virginia, as the Peter Chapin Collection of Books on Dogs (Chapin, 1938). The library of the AKC, at 51 Madison Avenue, New York, is open to the public and also houses many books and journals about dogs.

CHAPTER 1 The Dog and Its Relatives

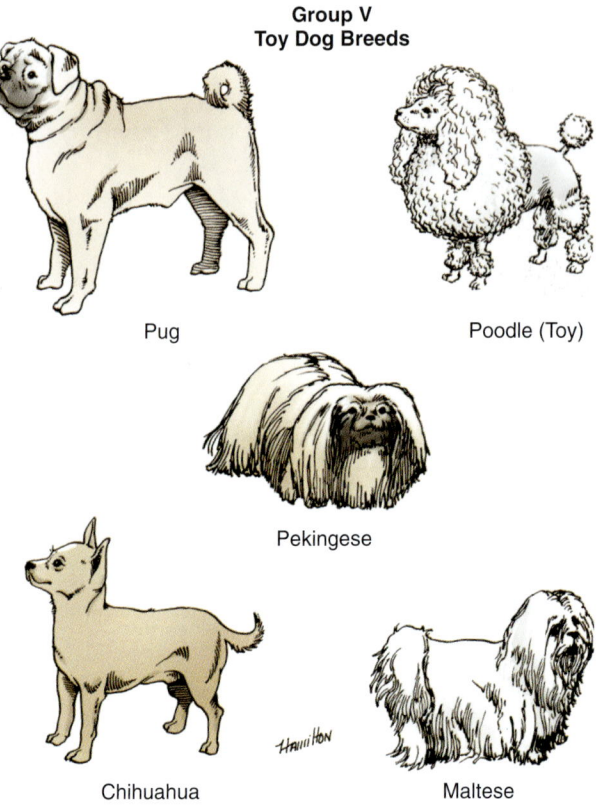

Group V
Toy Dog Breeds

Pug

Poodle (Toy)

Pekingese

Chihuahua

Maltese

Affenpinscher	Havanese	Papillon	Silky Terrier
Brussels Griffon	Italian Greyhound	Pekingese	Toy Fox Terrier
Cavalier King Charles Spaniel	Japanese Chin	Pomeranian	Yorkshire Terrier
Chihuahua	Maltese	Poodle (Toy)	
Chinese Crested	Manchester Terrier (Toy)	Pug	
English Toy Spaniel	Miniature Pinscher	Shih Tzu	

• **Fig. 1.9** There are 21 breeds in the toy group.

Group VI
Non-Sporting Breeds

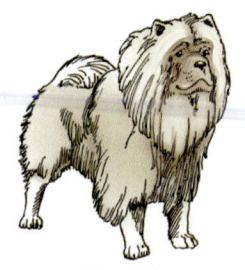

Chow Chow

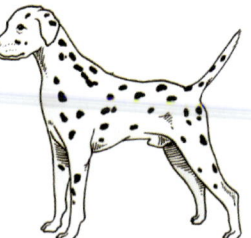

Dalmation

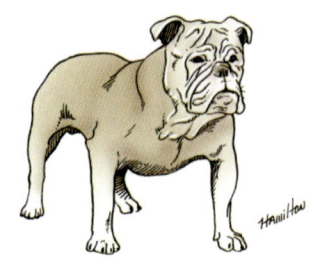

English Bulldog

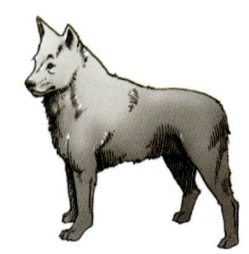

Schipperke

American Eskimo Dog	Chow-Chow	Keeshond	Schipperke
Bichon Frise	Coton de Tulear	Lhasa Apso	Shiba Inu
Boston Terrier	Dalmation	Löwchen	Tibetan Spaniel
Bulldog	Finnish Spitz	Norwegian Lundehund	Tibetan Terrier
Chinese Shar-Pei	French Bulldog	Poodle (Miniature and Standard)	Xoloitzcuintli

• **Fig. 1.10** There are 19 non-sporting breeds.

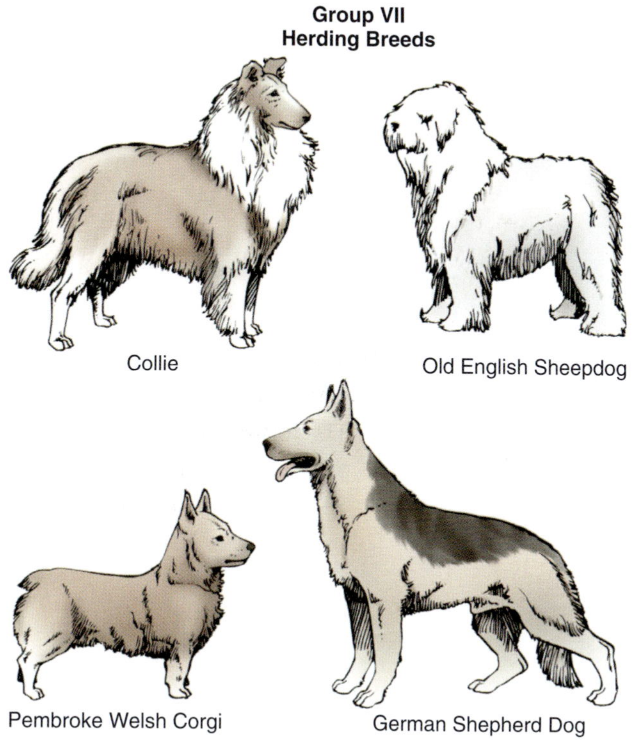

**Group VII
Herding Breeds**

Collie

Old English Sheepdog

Pembroke Welsh Corgi

German Shepherd Dog

Australian Cattle Dog	Berger Picard	Finnish Lapphund	Polish Lowland Sheepdog
Australian Shepherd	Border Collie	German Shepherd Dog	Puli
Bearded Collie	Bouvier des Flandres	Icelandic Sheepdog	Pumi
Beauceron	Briard	Miniature American Shepherd	Pyrenean Shepherd
Belgian Malinois	Canaan Dog	Norwegian Buhund	Shetland Sheepdog
Belgian Sheepdog	Cardigan Welsh Corgi	Old English Sheepdog	Spanish Water Dog
Belgian Tervuren	Collie	Pembroke Welsh Corgi	Swedish Vallhund
Bergamasco Sheepdog	Entlebucher Mountain Dog		

• **Fig. 1.11** There are 30 herding breeds

Bibliography

American Kennel Club (2006). *The complete dog book: The photograph, history and official standard of every breed admitted to AKC registration, and the selection, training, breeding, care and feeding of pure-bred dogs* (20th ed.). New York: American Kennel Club.

American Kennel Club (2017). *The new complete dog book: The photograph, history and official standard of every breed admitted to AKC registration, and the selection, training, breeding, care and feeding of pure-bred dogs* (22nd ed.). New York: American Kennel Club.

Ash, E. C. (1972). *Dogs: Their history and development* (Vol. 2). London. Reprinted New York: Benjamin Blom.

Boyko, A. R. (2011). The domestic dog: man's best friend in the genomic era. *Genome Biol, 12*, 216. doi:10.1186/gb-2011-12-2-216.

Boyko, A. R., Boyko, R. H., Boyko, C. M., et al. (2009). Complex population structure in African village dogs and its implications for inferring dog domestication history. *PNAS, 106*, 13903–13908.

Boyko, A. R., et al. (2010). A simple genetic architecture underlies morphological variation in dogs. *PLoS Biol, 8*(8), 1–13.

Botigué, L. R., Song, S., Scheu, A., et al. (2017). Ancient European dog genomes reveal continuity since the early Neolithic. *Nat Comm, 8*, 16082.

Chapin, H. M. (1938). The Peter Chapin collection of books on dogs. *Bull Coll William and Mary, 32*(7).

Clutton-Brock, J. (1995). Origins of the dog: domestication and early history. In J. Serpell (Ed.), *The domestic dog: Its evolution, behaviour, and interactions with people*. Cambridge, UK: Cambridge University Press.

Clutton-Brock, J., Corbet, G. B., & Hills, M. (1976). A review of the family canidae with a classification by numerical methods. *Bull Br Mus Zool, 29*(3), 1–99.

Clutton-Brock, J., & Jewell, P. (1993). Origin and domestication of the dog. In H. E. Evans (Ed.), *Miller's anatomy of the dog* (3rd ed.). Philadelphia: Saunders.

Corbett, L. K. (1995). *The dingo in Australia and Asia*. Ithaca, NY: Comstock.

Darwin, C. (1868). *The variation of animals and plants under domestication* (2nd ed., Vol. 1). New York: Appleton.

de Lahunta, A., Glass, E., & Kent, M. (2015). *Veterinary neuroanatomy and clinical neurology* (4th ed.). Philadelphia: Elsevier.

Earl, F. L. (1978). Developmental malformations: dogs. In K. Benirschke, F. M. Garner, & T. C. Jones (Eds.), *Pathology of laboratory animals* (Vol. 2). New York: Springer-Verlag.

Epstein, H. (1971). *The origin of the domestic animals of Africa* (Vol. 1). New York: Africana.

Evans, H. E. (1959). Hyoid muscle anomalies in the dog (canis familiaris). *Anat Rec, 133*, 145–162.

Ewer, R. (1973). *The carnivores*. Ithaca, NY: Cornell University Press.

Fiennes, R., & Fiennes, A. (1968). *The natural history of the dog.* London: Weidenfeld and Nicolson.

Fogle, B., & Morgan, T. (2009). *Encyclopedia of the dog.* Verona Italy: Dorling Kindersley, USA and GRB Editrice.

Frantz, L. A. F., Mullin, V. F., Pionnier-Capitan, M., et al. (2016). Genomic and archaeological evidence suggests a dual origin of domestic dogs. *Science, 352,* 1228–1231. doi:10.1126/science.aaf3161.

Giger, U., Ostrander, E. A., Markwell, P., et al. (2007). A novel breed-detection test for mixed breed dogs: breed identification and implications for veterinary practice. *Mars Veterinary Symposium,* 1–13.

Gittleman, J. L. (1989). *Carnivore behavior, ecology, and evolution.* Ithaca, NY: Cornell University Press.

Groves, C. P. (1971). Request for a declaration modifying article so as to exclude names proposed for domestic animals from zoological nomenclature. *Bull Zool Nom, 27,* 269–272.

Kleinman, G. M. (1990). Anatomy of the dachshund: x-ray studies. *Newsletter Dachshund Club of America, 14,* 62–70.

McKenna, M. C., & Bell, S. K. (1997). *Classification of mammals above the species level.* New York: Columbia University Press.

Lindblad-Toh, K., Wade, C. M., Mikkelsen, T. S., et al. (2005). Genome sequence, comparative analysis and haplotype structure of the domestic dog. *Nature, 438,* 803–819.

Mivart St, G. (1890). *A monograph of the Canidae.* London: RH Porter: Dulau & Co.

Noden, D. M., & de Lahunta, A. (1985). *The embryology of domestic animals: Developmental mechanisms and malformations.* Baltimore: Williams & Wilkins.

Nowak, R. M. (1991). *Walker's mammals of the world* (5th ed., Vol. 2). Baltimore: Johns Hopkins University Press.

Nyakatura, K., & Bininda-Emonds, O. R. P. (2012). Updating the evolutionary history of Carnivora (Mammalia): a new species-level supertree complete with divergence time estimates. *BMC Biol, 10,* 12.

Parker, H. G., Dreger, D. L., Rimbault, M., et al. (2017). Genomic analyses reveal the influence of geographic origin, migration, and hybridization on modern dog breed development. *Cell Rep, 19,* 697–708. doi:10.1016/j.celrep.2017.03.079.

Shannon, L. M., Boyko, R. M., Castelhano, M., et al. (2015). Genetic structure in village dogs reveals a central Asian domestication origin. *PNAS, 112,* 13639–13644. doi:10.1073/pnas.1516215112.

Sheldon, J. W. (1992). *The natural history of the nondomestic Canidae.* Orlando, FL: Academic Press.

Simpson, G. G. (1945). The principles of classification and a classification of mammals. *Bull Am Mus Nat Hist, 85,* 1–350.

Smith, C. H. (1845–1846). Dogs. In W. Jardine (Ed.), The Naturalist's Library (Vol. 1–2). Edinburgh: W. Lizar Publ.

Stockard, C. R. (1941). *The genetic and endocrinic basis for differences in form and behavior: The American anatomical memoirs* (Vol. 19). Philadelphia: Wistar Institute of Anatomy and Biology.

Stockard, C. R., & Johnson, A. L. (1941). The contrasted patterns and modifications of head types and forms in the pure breeds of dogs and their hybrids as the results of genetic and endocrinic reactions. In C. R. Stockard (Ed.), *The genetic and endocrinic basis for differences in form and behavior: The American anatomical memoirs* (Vol. 19, pp. 149–376). Philadelphia: Wistar Institute of Anatomy and Biology.

Takeuchi, Y., & Mori, Y. (2006). A comparison of the behavioral profiles of purebred dogs in Japan to profiles of those in the United States and the United Kingdom. *J Vet Med Sci, 68,* 789–796.

Titcomb, M. (1969). Dog and man in the ancient pacific. *Bernice P. Bishop Museum Special Publication (Honolulu), 59,* 1–91.

Van Gelder, R. G. (1977). Mammalian hybrids and generic limits. *Am Mus Novitates, 2635,* 1–25.

Wayne, R. K. (1993). Phylogenetic relationships of canids to other carnivores. In H. E. Evans (Ed.), *Miller's anatomy of the dog* (3rd ed., pp. 15–21). Philadelphia: Saunders.

Wayne, R. K., Benveniste, R. E., Janczewski, D. N., & O'Brien, S. J. (1989). Molecular and biochemical evolution of the Carnivora. In J. L. Gittleman (Ed.), *Carnivore behavior, ecology, and evolution* (pp. 465–494). Ithaca, NY: Cornell University Press.

Wayne, R. K., & Ostrander, E. A. (1999). Origin, genetic diversity, and genomic structure of the domestic dog. *Bioessays, 21,* 247–257.

Wayne, R. K., & Ostrander, E. A. (2007). Lessons learned from the dog genome. *Science Direct. Trends Genet, 23*(11), 557–567.

Wozencraft, W. C. (2005). Order Carnivora. In D. E. Wilson & D. M. Reeder (Eds.), *Mammal species of the world* (3rd ed., Vol. 2). Washington, DC: Smithsonian Institute.

2

Prenatal Development

Early Development

Ovulation in the dog occurs spontaneously early in estrus, as was shown by Bischoff in 1844. The germ cell of the dog at this time (unlike most other mammals) is a primary oocyte, may be ovulated at immature stages, and may require up to 72 hours postovulation to complete its nuclear maturation (Reynaud et al., 2005). A recently ovulated oocyte with its covering of corona radiata cells can be seen with the unaided eye and is approximately 230 μm in diameter. Photographs of preimplantation ova have been published by Holst and Phemister (1971). The induction of estrus and fertile ovulations was studied by Concannon et al. (1997). A study of ovulation, fertilization, and early development in the dog was reported by Renton et al. (1991).

At the time of ovulation, the fimbria of the infundibulum are swollen and help to engulf ovulated oocytes. They effectively block the slitlike opening of the ovarian bursa and thus prevent transperitoneal migration of oocytes or their loss into the peritoneal cavity.

Passage of spermatozoa through the uterus and tubouterine junction and within the uterine tube can be rapid in the dog. Bischoff (1844) noted that it takes 6, 18, or 20 hours for sperm to enter the uterine tube. Doak et al. (1967) found motile spermatozoa in high concentration in all parts of the dog's uterus for 6 days after copulation, and some were present for as long as 11 days. Holst and Phemister (1974) confirmed at least a 7-day life span of dog spermatozoa.

Uterine glands and the uterotubal junction may function as sperm reservoirs as these regions contain high numbers of sperm after artificial insemination not coincident with ovulation in bitches (Rijsselaere et al., 2004).

The nuclear chromosomes of the sperm become the male pronucleus, which fuses with the female pronucleus of the zygote to determine the genetic constitution of the zygote. The dog has a great number of small chromosomes, which makes it difficult to demonstrate all of them in a single preparation even after cell culture. Moore and Lambert (1963) illustrated and described the karyotype of the Beagle from an analysis of several metaphase plates taken from cultured kidney cells. They confirmed the findings of Minouchi (1928) and Ahmed (1941) that the diploid number in somatic cells of the dog was 78 in both sexes. The chromosomes appear to be aligned into 38 homologous pairs of autosomes and two sex chromosomes. All of the autosomes have acrocentric or terminal centromeres. The X chromosome is one of the largest, whereas the Y chromosome is equal to the smallest. The X chromosomes have metacentric centromeres. For a discussion of genetics in the dog, see Asdell (1966).

For a wealth of information on the genetic basis of breed characteristics in purebred dogs, see the monograph of Stockard (1941) who noted striking reproductive peculiarities during the course of his cross-breeding program. Certain of the giant breeds were poor producers, either failing to whelp or producing only one to three pups. In contrast, closely related dogs produced from 10 to 17 puppies at a whelp, and one of his bitches produced 50 puppies within 2 years.

Songsasen, Spindler, and Wildt (2007) studied in vitro cultivation of dog oocytes and pointed out that, although intraovarian oocytes can be recovered, matured, and fertilized in vitro (Rodriques & Rodriques 2006), embryo transfer or other assisted reproductive techniques have been difficult in the dog (Abe et al., 2011). New protocols for in vitro fertilization in dogs were reported by Nagashima et al. (2015), who confirmed the first live births resulting from in vitro fertilization. Such methods will allow the rescue of genetic material from valuable genotypes of domestic and wild canids. Songsasen and Wildt (2005) showed that the size of the donor follicle was most important in determining meiotic competency during follicular development. Hewitt and England (1999) studied the maturation of oocytes in vitro.

Length of Gestation

The extensive endocrinologic investigations of Concannon (1975), Phemister (1974), Phemister et al. (1973), Concannon and Lein (1989), summarized by Concannon (1991), have shown that the average onset of estrus in the dog is 1 day after the luteinizing hormone (LH) surge, which can be identified by a rise in serum progesterone in the blood (Fig. 2.1). They reported increases of 20 to 40 times in the level of LH (8 to 50 ng/mg with an average of 20 ng/mg) during the 1- to 2-day preovulatory surge. The average time of ovulation was day 2 of estrus. However, there were ovulations before behavioral estrus, early in estrus, and in late estrus. The peak of fertility for natural matings ranged from 1 day before the preovulatory LH surge until 5 or 6 days after the LH surge.

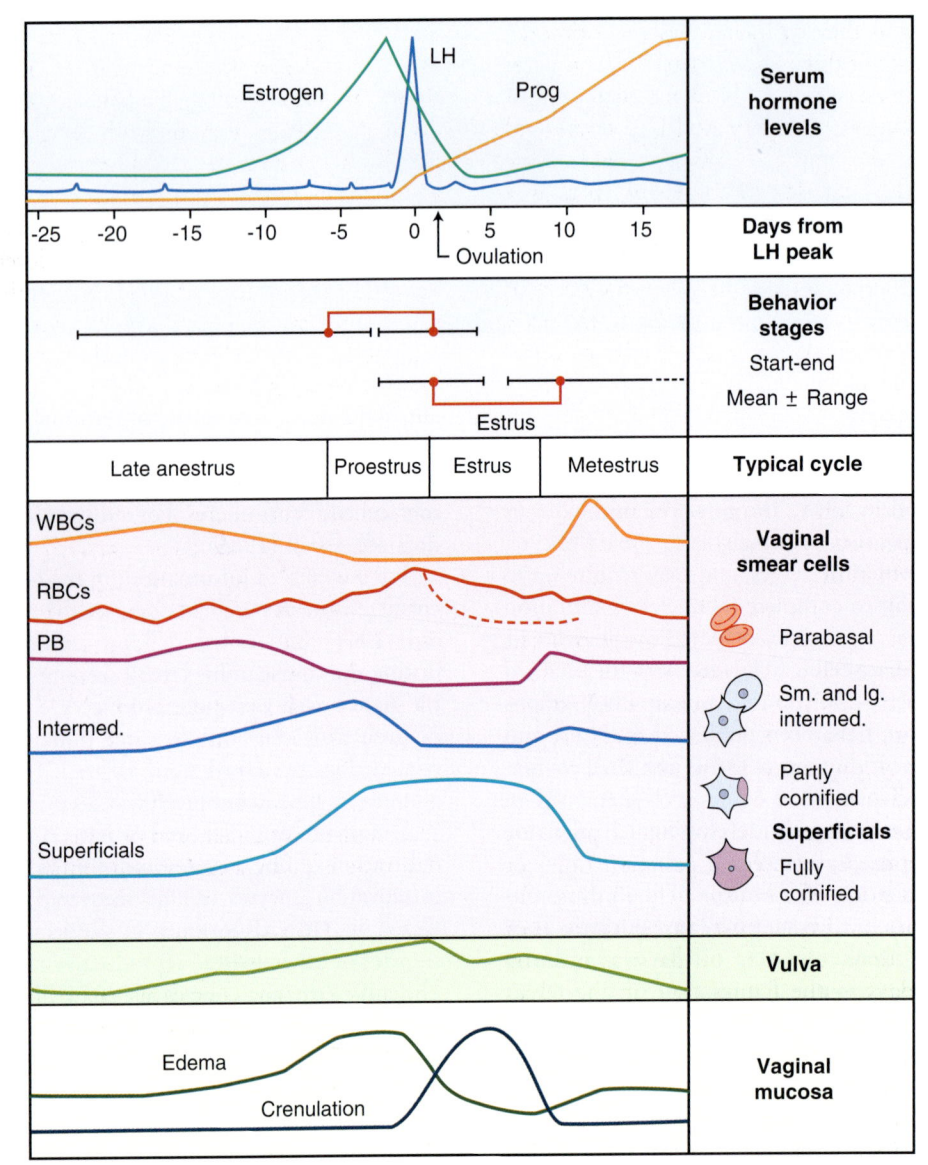

- **Fig. 2.1** Temporal relationships of periovulatory endocrine events. Note the luteinizing hormone peak and its relationship to ovulation in early estrus. (With permission from Concannon PW, Lein DH: Hormonal and clinical correlates of ovarian cycles, ovulation, pseudopregnancy, and pregnancy in dogs. In Kirk RW, editor: *Current veterinary therapy X*. Philadelphia, 1989, Saunders.)

When Evans (1956) was breeding Beagles for the collection of the embryos and fetuses used in prior versions of this chapter, the method of using the LH surge as the most fixed point in the estrous cycle had not been described. The method used to determine gestation times, as cited in the accompanying tables and figures, was to examine the bitches daily for signs of estrus and to test how they reacted to the stud. When the bitch would stand for the stud without snapping or sitting down, she was isolated and bred 24 hours later. Using this system of a single mating for each estrus in a colony of 19 purebred Beagles, all single matings in the first year were successful. From these matings, 24 hours after first acceptance, embryos or fetuses were surgically removed singly or in groups at various intervals for study. A single stud was used for 6 years, and the average litter size from this inbred colony of 20 Beagles was 6.7 pups. Bitches came into heat at all times of the year, although there was a peak in the spring and summer period. Some of the largest litters were from the youngest bitches.

According to Concannon (1991) maximum receptivity of the bitch is seen at the peak of the LH surge, and ovulation usually occurs 2 or 3 days later. Using his system of timing gestation, day "0" is the day of the LH surge, and birth occurs 65 days later, which would be 62 to 63 days after ovulation.

Because gestation per se (development of the embryo) cannot begin until after fertilization, and fertilization (fusion of gametes) occurs at variable periods after ovulation, there is always a question about the exact age of an embryo.

Holst and Phemister (1974) observed that the diestrous period (now called *metestrus*) was closely correlated with the length of gestation, and they calculated gestation time by backdating to the onset of this period. Metestrus is the last period of the luteal phase, when the bitch no longer stands for the stud. The beginning of this period is characterized by a marked shift in the epithelial cell type seen in the vaginal smear. On the first day of metestrus there is a decrease in the number of cornified cells and an increase (often more than 50 percent) in noncornified cells from the deeper layers of the vaginal epithelium. When the onset of metestrus was used as a fixed point to backdate the early stages of embryonic development, Holst and Phemister (1971) made the following correlations:

Metestrus minus 1 day = the two-cell cleavage stage
M minus 3 days = fertilization
M minus 4 days = formation of secondary oocyte
M minus 5 days = beginning of meiosis
M minus 6 days = ovulation

They suggested that if the day of fertilization is counted as "day 1," then the Beagle has a gestation period of 60 days, and whelping takes place on day 57 of metestrus. Holst and Phemister (1974) found that the highest conception rate could be attained by two matings: one at the time of first acceptance and the other on the third day or later.

Evans's method for timing gestation, from a point 24 hours after first acceptance, resulted in gestation times of 59 to 63 days, with a mean of approximately 60 days. (To convert gestation times, as cited in this chapter, to the post LH peak "gestation" times of 64 to 66 days, as used by Concannon, add 5 days to the figures cited in the tables and graphs.)

Doppler and A-mode or B-mode ultrasound for pregnancy diagnosis in the dog is a highly useful, noninvasive technique that is approximately 99 percent accurate (Bondestam, et al., 1984; Cartee & Rowles, 1984; Shille and Gontarek, 1985; Taverne & van Oord, 1989; Toal et al., 1986). With B-mode ultrasound many features of the conceptus, embryo, and fetus can be recognized in greater detail (England and Allen, 1990; England et al., 1990; Yeager et al., 1992). Yeager and Concannon (1990), using ultrasonography for detection of early pregnancy, cited the embryonic heartbeat as the earliest detectable sign of a viable pregnancy. They first detected the heartbeat at 23 to 25 days after the LH surge, at which time the embryonic mass was 1 to 4 mm in length. They found that the correlation of first breeding and ultrasonic detection of pregnancy was more variable than the correlation between LH surge and the ultrasonic detection of pregnancy.

Yeager et al. (1992) summarized the ultrasonic appearance of the uterus, placenta, fetus, and fetal membranes throughout gestation in the Beagle. For timing gestation they used the day of the LH surge as "day 0," as described earlier. Their investigations showed the earliest detection of the chorionic cavity at day 20; embryo and heartbeat at day 23 to 25; yolk sac membrane at days 25 to 28 (see Figs. 2.5 and 2.6); allantoic membrane at days 27 to 31; and skeleton at days 33 to 39. Of the fetal structures, head diameter was the best indicator for estimation of gestational age. The timing of breeding using the behavior of the bitch, vaginal cytologic examination, or both as guides, although less precise than timing from an LH assay, can also result in good correlations with gestation age judging from the similarity of development of embryos and fetuses at any given date and their stages of skeletal development (Evans, 1958–1974). By surgically removing embryos or fetuses at various intervals during gestation, it was possible to measure individuals or entire litters from the same dog. Knowing the interval between removals allowed for the calculation of growth rates.

The data and specimens collected for this study are available in the Cornell Embryo Collection, Department of Biomedical Sciences at the College of Veterinary Medicine. As an example of incremental growth changes that can be seen, a bitch with 10 conceptuses was operated at 35 days postinsemination, and five fetuses were removed from the right horn that averaged 41 mm in crown-rump (C-R) length. On day 40, five fetuses were removed from the left horn that averaged 70 mm in C-R length. This average increase of 29 mm in 5 days indicated a growth rate of approximately 6 mm a day (Evans, 1959). Thus there can be a considerable discrepancy in the size or morphologic characteristics of an embryo or fetus if the estimated gestation time is off by a day or two (Table 2.1).

Prenatal Periods

The successive stages of cleavage, gastrulation, implantation, and early somite formation are completed before day 20 of gestation. The length of time required for the entire development of a fertilized oocyte into a newborn puppy is approximately 60 days, and it is no wonder that marked changes in development can be seen at daily intervals. Phemister (1974) divided prenatal development in the dog into three periods: (1) *the period of the ovum*, following fertilization, which is characterized by a blastocyst (Fig. 2.2) that lies free in the uterine tube and migrates to the uterus (days 2 to 17); (2) *the period of the embryo*, which begins with implantation of the blastocyst (Fig. 2.3) and ends with the completion of major organogenesis (days 19 to 35); (3) *the period of the fetus*, the time during which the characteristic features of the dog appear and most of the growth occurs (day 35 to birth).

Oocyte–Embryo

Fertilization takes place in the cranial part of the uterine tube (oviduct), and the fertilized oocyte (zygote) begins to divide within a few hours. Tubal transport of oocytes/embryos takes longer in the dog (7 to 10 days) than in most other mammals (3 to 4 days), although some embryos reach the region of the tubouterine junction in approximately 5 days. Holst and Phemister (1971) found that developing embryos may enter the uterus as early as the 16-cell stage

CHAPTER 2 Prenatal Development

TABLE 2.1 Transuterine Migration of Blastocysts In 13 Beagles

Number of Oocytes Ovulated from Each Ovary		Number of Implantations in Each Uterine Horn		Probable Number That Migrated	Number of Blastocysts or Early Embryos Lost
Left	Right	Left	Right		
7	1	4	3	2 Left to Right	1
1	6	4	3	3 Right to Left	0
7	3	4	3	None	3
3	6	4	3	1 Right to Left	2
4	2	2	4	2 Left to Right	0
2	4	3	3	1 Right to Left	0
3	4	2	4	None	1
4	6	6	4	2 Right to Left	0
5	3	3	5	2 Left to Right	0
3	6	3	6	None	0
0	7	3	4	3 Right to Left	0
2	3	2	1	None	2
3	4	3	4	None	0
44	55	43	47		9
99		90		6 Left to Right 10 Right to Left	

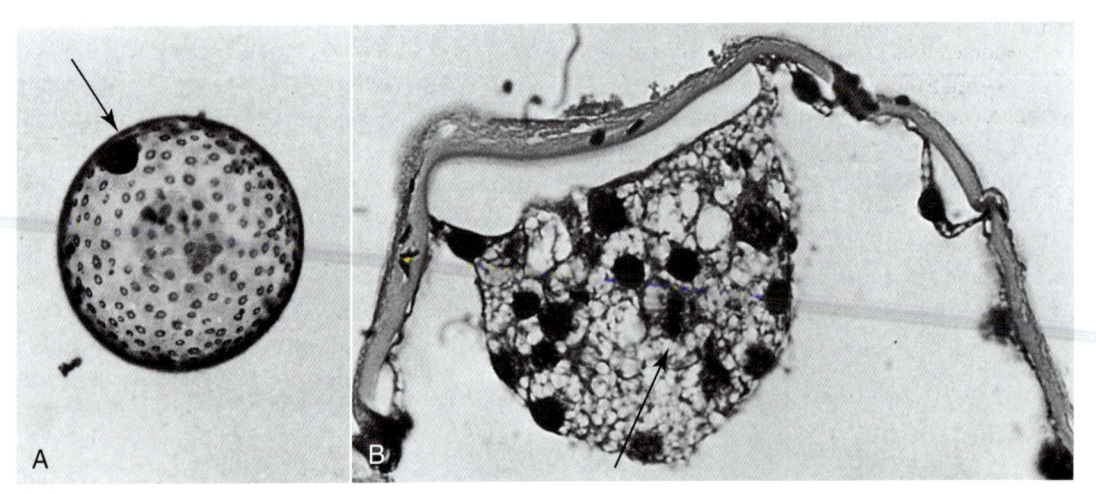

• **Fig. 2.2 A,** Dog blastocyst approximately 600 μm in diameter, 11 days after breeding. The inner cell mass is dense and globular in form (*arrow*). Note the trophoblast cells. (Unstained, 90×). **B,** Section of a 500 μm dog blastocyst showing the inner cell mass. Note mitotic figure (*at the arrow*) and several spermatozoan heads embedded in the zona pellucida. Eleven days after breeding. (Stained with hematoxylin and eosin, 460×.) (**A** and **B** with permission from Holst PA, Phemister RD: The prenatal development of the dog: preimplantation events, *Biol Reprod* 5:194–206, 1971.)

but more commonly as morulae or even early blastocysts. This agrees with the observations of Anderson (1927) and Van der Stricht (1923). Estrogen inhibits the transport of developing embryos into the uterus, whereas progesterone enhances it.

Within the uterus the morula develops into the rather spherical blastocyst, with an inner cell mass and a thin surface trophoblast surrounded by a zona pellucida (see Fig. 2.2). Unattached blastocysts range in size from 250 μm to 3 mm as they pass along the uterine lumen prior to

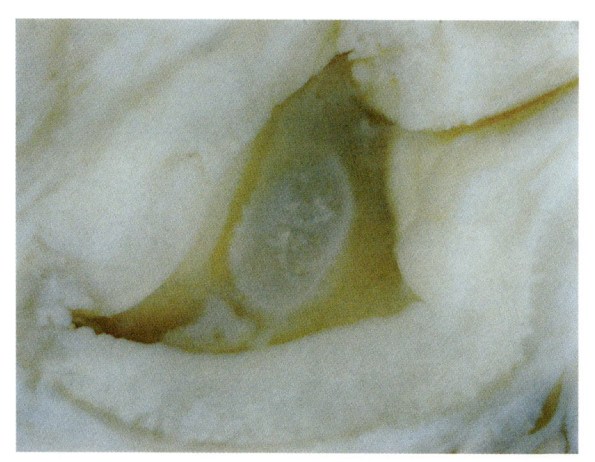

• **Fig. 2.3** Blastocyst within the implantation chamber on the 18th day in the Beagle.

• **BOX 2.1** **Summary of Morphologic Events During the First Trimester of Development (Based on a 60-Day Gestation)**

1 to 7 days	Formation of the zygote and cleavage in the uterine tube.
8 days	8- to 16-cell morula.
9 days	16- to 32-cell morula.
11 days	32- to 64-cell morula.
12 to 16 days	Blastocyst enters the uterus and increases in size while migrating to a receptive site. Inner cell mass distinct.
17 to 18 days	Implantation by the trophoblast, zona pellucida shed, formation of the neural plate and primitive streak.
19 to 20 days	Formation of the first somites.

implantation on about day 17 after breeding. The free-floating blastocyst stage lasts approximately 7 days (Gier, 1950; Holst & Phemister, 1971; Tietz & Selinger, 1967). There is usually an even spacing of blastocysts in each uterine horn, but there is often a marked difference in the number of oocytes ovulated from each ovary, as ascertained by the number of corpora lutea seen. Thus oocytes ovulated by one ovary and fertilized in the cranial end of the uterine tube on that side may migrate through the body of the uterus and traverse the opposite uterine horn to implant.

The path taken by ovulated oocytes from one ovary to the opposite uterine horn in the mammal depends on the morphologic characteristics of the genital tract. External, or transperitoneal, migration is possible in those species that lack an ovarian bursa and have ovaries in close proximity to one another. The process involves ovulation into the peritoneal cavity in close proximity to the ostia of both uterine tubes, thus allowing either to engulf and transport the oocyte. The distance traveled within the peritoneal cavity is short and aided by ciliary action in the region of the infundibulum. Internal or transuterine migration is the more common phenomenon in mammals. It frequently occurs even in species that are anatomically capable of transperitoneal migration and always occurs in those species that have an ovarian bursa surrounding the ovary. In animals with duplex uteri, such as the rabbit, in which each uterine horn enters the vagina separately, transuterine migration is not possible.

The early studies of Bischoff (1844) on the dog called attention to the phenomenon of transuterine migration, as did later studies in the cat by Hill and Tribe (1924) and other carnivores by Boyd et al. (1944). Evans (1956) examined the ovaries and uterine horns of 13 bred Beagles for evidence of transuterine migration and found that in 8 dogs a total of 16 morulae or blastocysts had crossed from one uterine horn to the other. There was no way of telling how many others had changed sides without affecting the final balance because no marker was used to distinguish right from left ovulations (see Table 2.1).

The spacing of blastocysts along the uterine horn is the result of ciliary action, muscular contraction, and unoccupied sites of uterine receptivity. Irregularities in spacing caused by the early death of a blastocyst or embryo are adjusted by differential hypertrophy of the uterus and resorption of the dead conceptus.

See Box 2.1 for a summary of the morphologic events during the first trimester of development.

Embryo

The implanting blastocyst on day 18 of gestation lies in a pear-shaped cavity of the uterus that is hardly discernible on external examination (see Fig. 2.3). The uterine lumen between successive implantations is very narrow, and therefore implantation sites can be readily identified on dissection. Fluid that collects within the blastocyst causes it to expand and fill the small uterine cavity. The attachment process, referred to as *central implantation,* is a superficial apposition of trophoblast to the antimesometrial surface of the uterine endometrium. The trophoblast cells are responsible for initiating formation of the placenta, and, in the dog, they elaborate the enzymes that erode the maternal tissues to form the definitive endotheliochorial deciduate zonary placenta.

Barrau et al. (1975) studied early implantation in the dog and found the invasive form of trophoblast to be syncytial, as did Schoenfeld (1903), rather than cellular, as reported by Amoroso (1952). Three types of trophoblast are ultimately recognizable: (1) syncytial trophoblast around maternal blood vessels, (2) cytotrophoblast in the necrotic zone, and (3) phagocytic cytotrophoblast around the hematomata. In addition to the variety of absorptive cells present in the dog's placenta, there are occasional decidual cells associated with the trophoblast of the labyrinth (Anderson, 1969). In some species the trophoblast is primarily nutritive and hormone-producing, whereas in others it is very

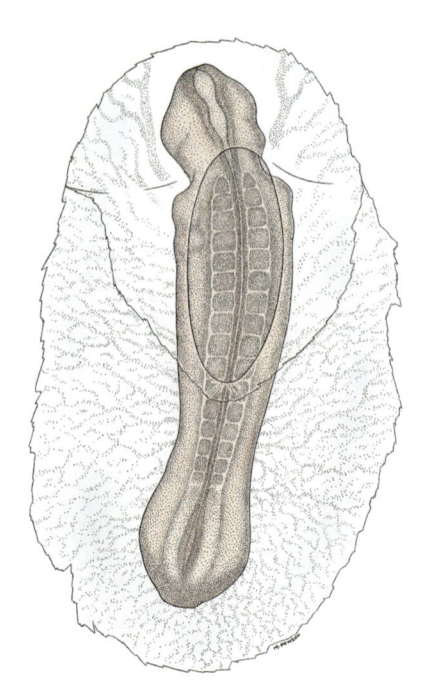

• **Fig. 2.4** Dorsal view of a 16-somite, 5-mm-long dog embryo being enclosed by the amniotic fold.

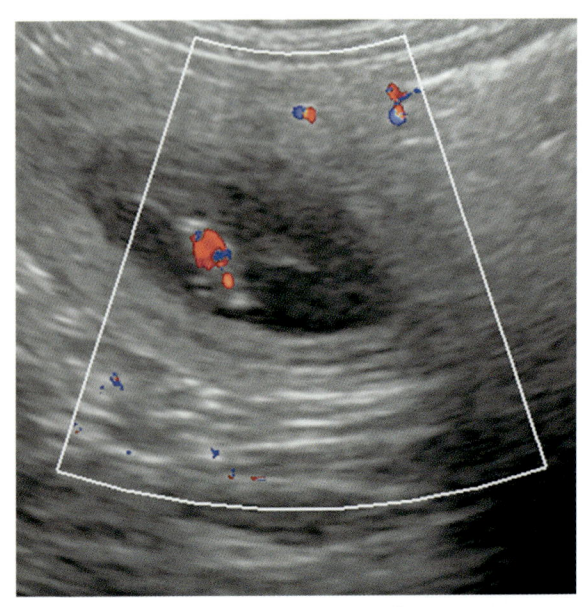

• **Fig. 2.5** Ultrasound image of a 4-mm embryo in a uterine swelling 13 mm in diameter (25 days after the luteinizing hormone surge).

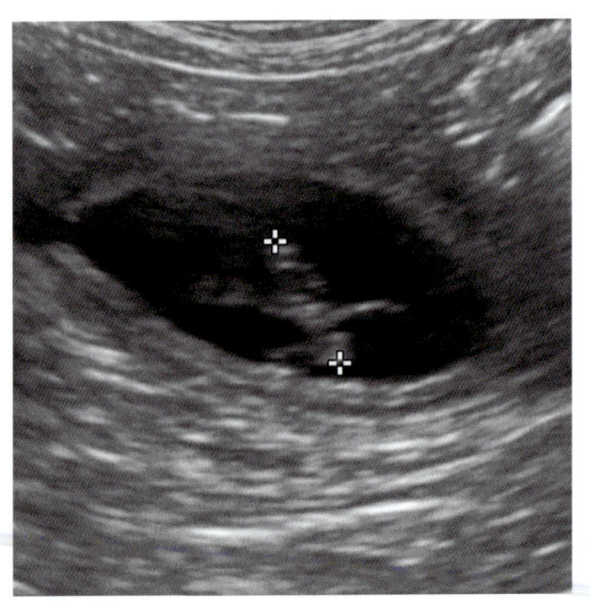

• **Fig. 2.6** Ultrasound image of a 7-mm embryo in a uterine swelling 18 mm in diameter. Length of the chamber was 30 mm (27 days after the luteinizing hormone surge). (Courtesy Dr. Amy Yeager.)

invasive. In the dog it is invasive and syncytial (see Miglino et al., 2006; Sandoval et al., 2001).

The embryo develops in a cephalocaudal sequence, beginning with head folds, then neural tube closure, followed by somite formation, appearance of branchial clefts, lens placode, otic placode, cardiac bulge, and the growth of limb buds. For specifics on domestic animal embryologic development, including the dog, see Noden and de Lahunta *The Embryology of Domestic Animals* (1985); McGeady et al., *Veterinary Embryology* (2017); and Hyttel et al., *Essentials of Domestic Animal Embryology* (2010).

Several days after implantation, the developing embryo is enveloped by amniotic folds that grow across its dorsal surface (Fig. 2.4). At the 21-day stage (16 somites, 4.5 mm), the embryo is crescent-shaped, and the yolk sac, which is continuous with the midgut, rapidly fills the chorionic vesicle (Figs. 2.5 to 2.7). Where the trophoblastic ectoderm and yolk sac endoderm are in apposition on the mesometrial wall of the uterus, it is called the *bilaminar omphalopleure*. Closer to the embryo, where the extraembryonic mesoderm and its vitelline vessels extend between the trophoblast and the yolk sac endoderm, a trilaminar omphalopleure or choriovitelline membrane is formed that serves as a transitory placenta.

The embryonic membranes of the dog include a chorion, yolk sac, amnion, and allantois, which grow and change their relationships to each other during the early embryonic period.

The amnion of the dog develops by outfolding after the embryo is well organized. This is unlike the process in the human, in whom the amnion develops by cavitation of the inner cell mass in the presomite embryo prior to the establishment of germ layers. By day 21 in the dog, the amniotic folds are well developed over the dorsum of the embryo, and the vitelline vessels are extensive (Fig. 2.8). The amnion fills with fluid as the embryo grows and, in later fetal stages, becomes a sizable sac. By day 23, when the uterine swellings are almost spherical (Fig. 2.9A), the embryo has approximately 32 somites and is approximately 5 mm long. The yolk sac is very extensive, closely applied to the chorion, and well vascularized (see Fig. 2.9B). The vascularity, as well as the size of the yolk sac, increases throughout gestation, although it is superseded functionally by the allantois on about day 25 of gestation.

CHAPTER 2　Prenatal Development　19

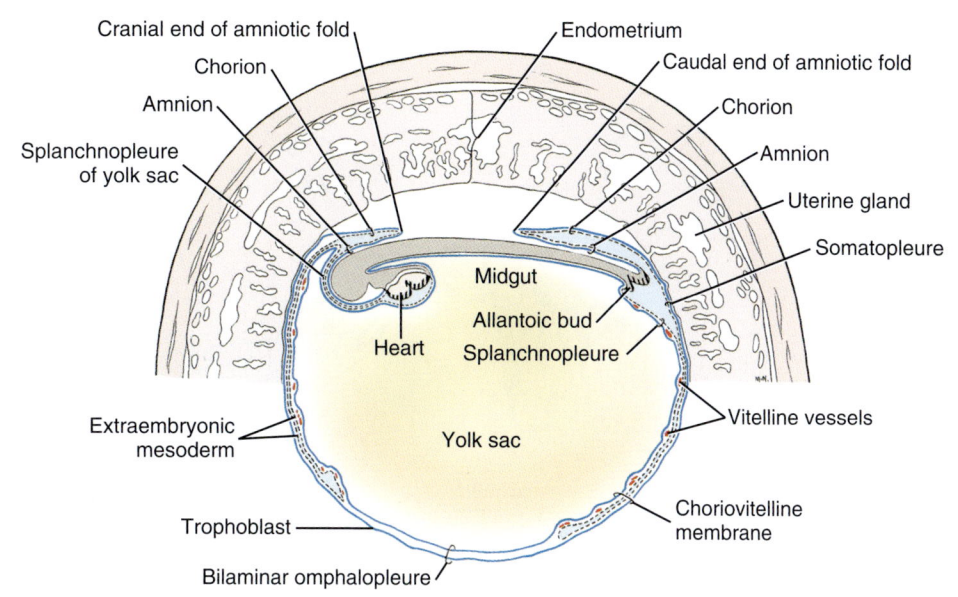

• **Fig. 2.7** Early somite dog embryo, approximately 16 somites, 4.5 mm, 21 days. A diagrammatic transverse section of a portion of the uterus and placenta that passes through the longitudinal axis of the embryo. The large yolk sac fills the uterine cavity, and extensions of extraembryonic mesoderm are seen between the yolk sac and the chorion. The amnion forms by the folding of somatopleure over the dorsum of the embryo, and the allantoic bud in the hindgut region makes its appearance. (From Evans HE: *Prenatal development of the dog*. Ithaca, NY, 1974, 24th Gaines Veterinary Symposium.)

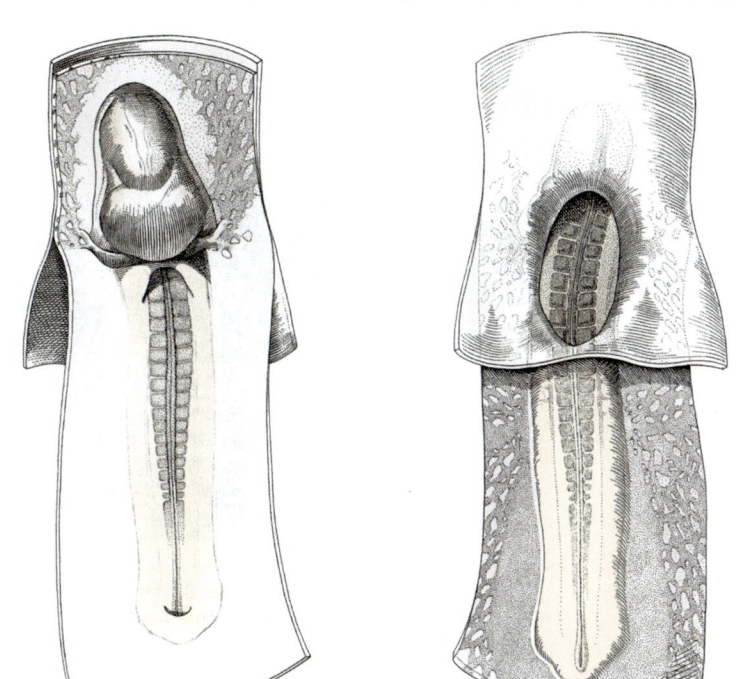

• **Fig. 2.8** A 19-somite dog embryo showing closure of the amniotic fold and development of the vitelline circulation. **A**, Ventral view. **B**, Dorsal view. **C**, Sagittal section.

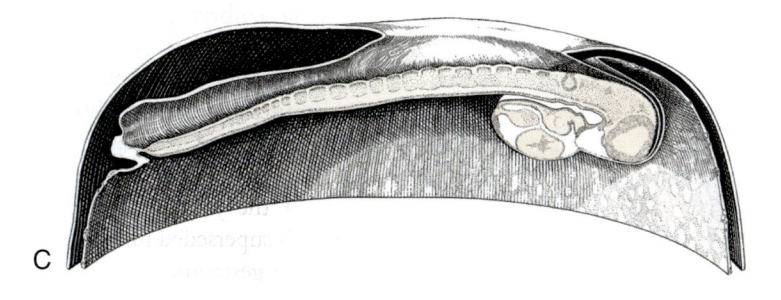

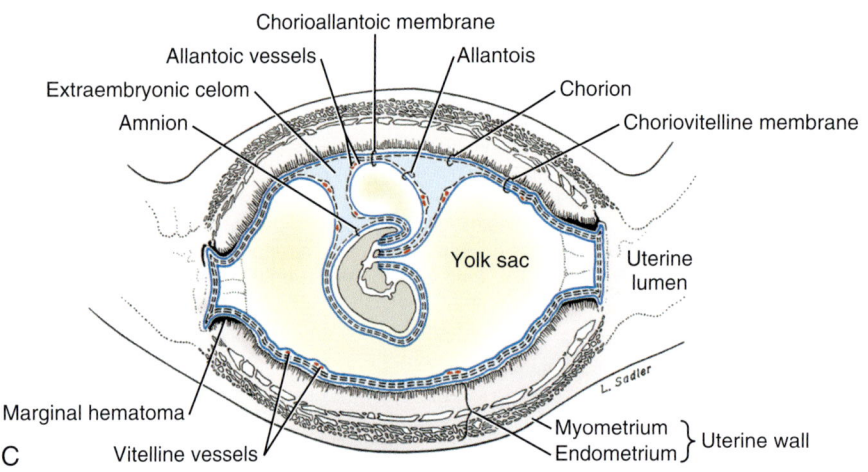

• **Fig. 2.9** Uterus and early limb-bud embryo at 23 days of gestation. **A**, External view. **B**, Longitudinal section with a 32-somite, 5-mm embryo in situ. **C**, Schematic section of **B** showing fetal membranes and placenta. (From Evans HE: *Prenatal development of the dog.* Ithaca, NY, 1974, 24th Gaines Veterinary Symposium.)

The allantois, a diverticulum of the hindgut, is first visible as a bud on day 21, and, by day 23, it is a spherical sac located ventral to the caudal end of the embryo and projecting into the exocoelom (see Fig. 2.9C). As it progressively expands, the allantois contacts the chorion (somatopleure) over most of the exocelomic surface, and allantoic blood vessels can be seen on its surface. By day 25 the allantois has intercalated itself between the chorion and the body of the yolk sac, thus completing the formation of the definitive chorioallantoic membrane. The enveloped yolk sac is separated from the chorion except at the poles, where it remains attached.

The choriovitelline placenta that exists from days 21 to 23 has simple villi that project into the openings of the endometrial glands. The villi are avascular and thus likely serve a histiotrophic function, as suggested by Wimsatt (1974), who studied the 23-somite black bear.

As the placenta grows, the uterine swelling changes from pear-shaped (20 days) (see Fig. 2.3) to spherical (25 days) to ovoid (30 days) (see Figs. 2.9 and 2.10). During this time the thickening of the uterine glands and the rapid expansion of the allantoic sac result in a change from a primary choriovitelline (yolk sac) placentation to the definitive chorioallantoic placentation. Embryos appear most vulnerable to physiologic stress during this period of rapid growth and placental change. Pressures within the uterus are greatest when the allantoic sac has expanded and the uterine swellings are spherical or beginning to elongate on day 25 of gestation. Death of the embryo prior to day 25 usually results in complete resorption with little or no visual evidence at term on the placental site. Death of early embryos is manifested by a reduced litter size but can be confirmed only by examination of the interior of the uterus.

Most carnivores have marginal or central blood sinuses or hematomata associated with the placenta (Creed, 1963). The dog has a marginal "green band," which can first be recognized in early limb-bud stages as a slightly thickened region between the choriovitelline membrane and the endometrium at the constricted ends of each uterine loculus (see Fig. 2.9C). This incipient marginal hematoma thus appears simultaneously with the expansion of the allantoic sac but prior to allantoic contact in the marginal region. The green band at each end of the zonular placenta increases in size throughout gestation (see Fig. 2.9C). Occasionally, there

TABLE 2.2 Summary of Morphologic Events During the Second Trimester of Development

	Bitch	Embryo
17 to 18 days	Uterus same size as in a pseudopregnant dog.	Blastocysts evenly spaced from one another, trophoblastic attachment, zona pellucida shed, primitive streak visible, *caudal to* neural plate.
20 days	Implantation chamber of the uterus is a pear-shaped cavity.	8 somites; 4 mm long; neural tube closing.
21 days	Uterus slightly enlarged at placental sites.	16 somites; 5 mm long and crescent-shaped; longitudinal axis of embryo transverse to uterine horn; head flexed invaginating yolk sac; cardiac bulge prominent; allantoic bud developing; amniotic folds closing; yolk sac fills uterine cavity and is widely confluent with the midgut; branchial arches I and II present.
23 days	Uterine swellings distinct; vascular and glandular layers of the uterus hypertrophied (see Fig. 2.9A to C).	32 somites; 10 mm long; twisted with cranial end invaginated into yolk sac; forelimb bud prominent; otic placode and lens placode present; mandibular and maxillary processes distinct; branchial arches I, II, and III present; liver bulge marked; allantoic sac spherical and beneath tail (Fig. 2.10).
25 days	Corpora lutea completely fill the ovary; uterine swelling almost spherical, 30 × 35 mm; width of placenta approximately 29 mm (Fig. 2.11A and B).	14 mm; cephalic flexure prominent; otic pit and eye well formed; mammary ridge present (see Fig. 2.11C); limb buds at plate stage; vertebral elements chondrify; dental lamina forms.
28 days		17 mm; first ossification seen in mandible, maxilla, frontal bone, and clavicle.
30 days	Uterine swellings 33 × 50 mm; width of placenta is greater than length of embryo (Fig. 2.12A).	19 mm; eyelids and external ear forming; sensory hairs on snout, chin, and eyelid; intestine herniated into umbilical stalk; five pairs of nipples; digits on forelimbs distinct; genital tubercle prominent (see Fig. 2.12B).
33 days		27 mm; ossification of nasal, incisive, palatine, zygomatic, and parietal bones; midshaft of ribs 4 through 10; midshaft of humerus, radius, and ulna; femur, tibia, and fibula; canine teeth in early cap stage; palatal shelves fuse; digits on hindpaws distinct (see Fig. 2.12C).

are isolated hematomatous patches in the central area of a normal dog placenta. These structures have been called *hemophagous organs* by Creed and Biggers (1963). Hematomata form by necrosis of both the maternal and the fetal tissues. Maternal vessels hemorrhage into the necrotic area and form pools of blood with a greenish color. These hematomata are surrounded by trophoblasts rather than being between cytotrophoblast and maternal endometrium (Barrau et al., 1975).

Duke (1946) described developing monozygotic twins (10 mm C-R) in a dog that had eight other normal conceptuses. The embryos were in a limb-bud stage. Although monozygotic twins occur commonly in some species, they are rare in carnivores, and this was the first description of such embryos in the dog. (Evans examined more than 400 pregnant uterine horns and never found more than one embryo or fetus in a single loculus.) The two embryos described by Duke shared a placenta, were enclosed by a single chorion, and had a common yolk sac. Each embryo had its own amnion, indicating that the twinning process had occurred before amniogenesis.

See Table 2.2 for a summary of the morphologic events during the second trimester of development.

Age Determination

Various external and internal features have been used as criteria for determining chronologic age. External features include somite count; branchial arch development; eye, ear, and nose formation; limb-bud development; and linear measurements. Internal features include maturation of various organs, stages of tooth development, and, most commonly, the appearance of ossification centers.

Streeter (1951) divided the human embryonic period into 23 "horizons" based on both external and internal features. Following the 23rd horizon was the fetal period, characterized in the human by the appearance of bone marrow in the humerus. This occurred in the 28- to 30-mm embryo at approximately 7 weeks of age. During the fetal period, linear dimensions are used for the assessment of age, the commonest being C-R, or sitting height, and crown-heel, or total length, for man.

• **Fig. 2.10** Early limb-bud embryo at 23 days of gestation. **A**, Lateral view. **B**, Dorsal view. (From Evans HE: *Prenatal development of the dog.* Ithaca, NY, 1974, 24th Gaines Veterinary Symposium.)

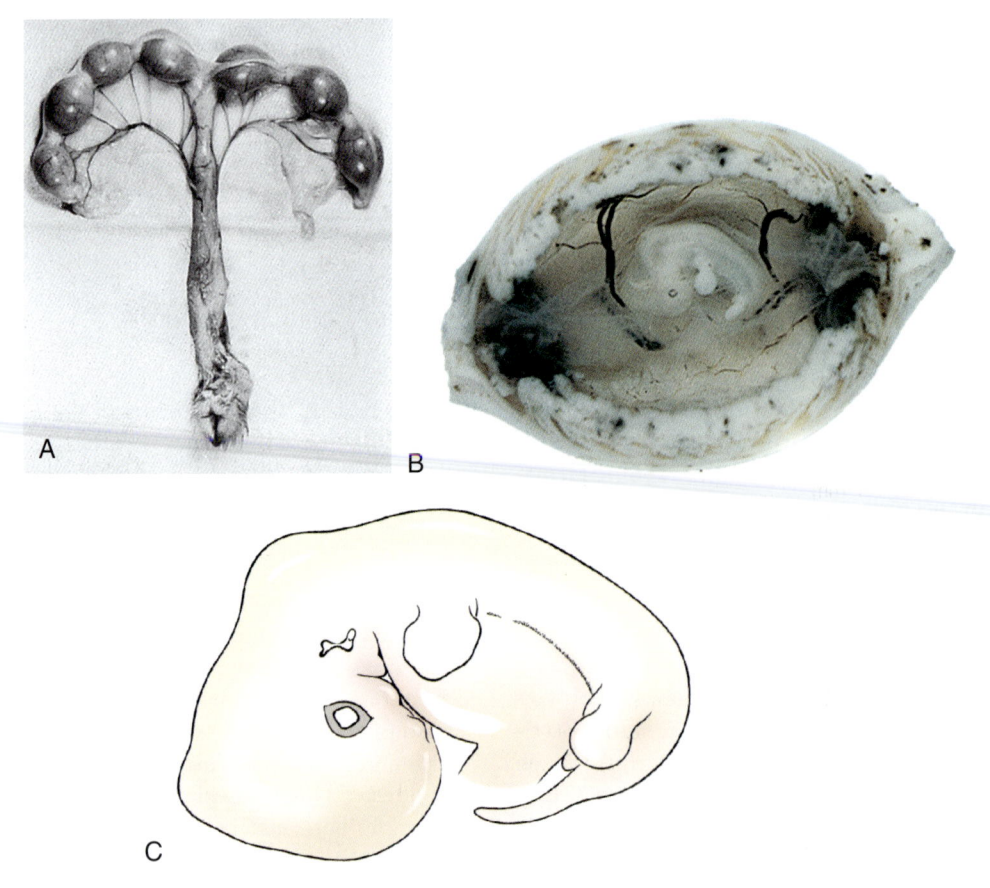

• **Fig. 2.11** A, Uterine horns at 25 days of gestation. B, Longitudinal section of a uterine swelling on the 25th day of gestation. C, Beagle embryo at 25 days of gestation, 14 mm, crown-rump length. (B and C from Evans HE: A dog comes into being. *Gaines Dog Research Progress,* Fall 1956.)

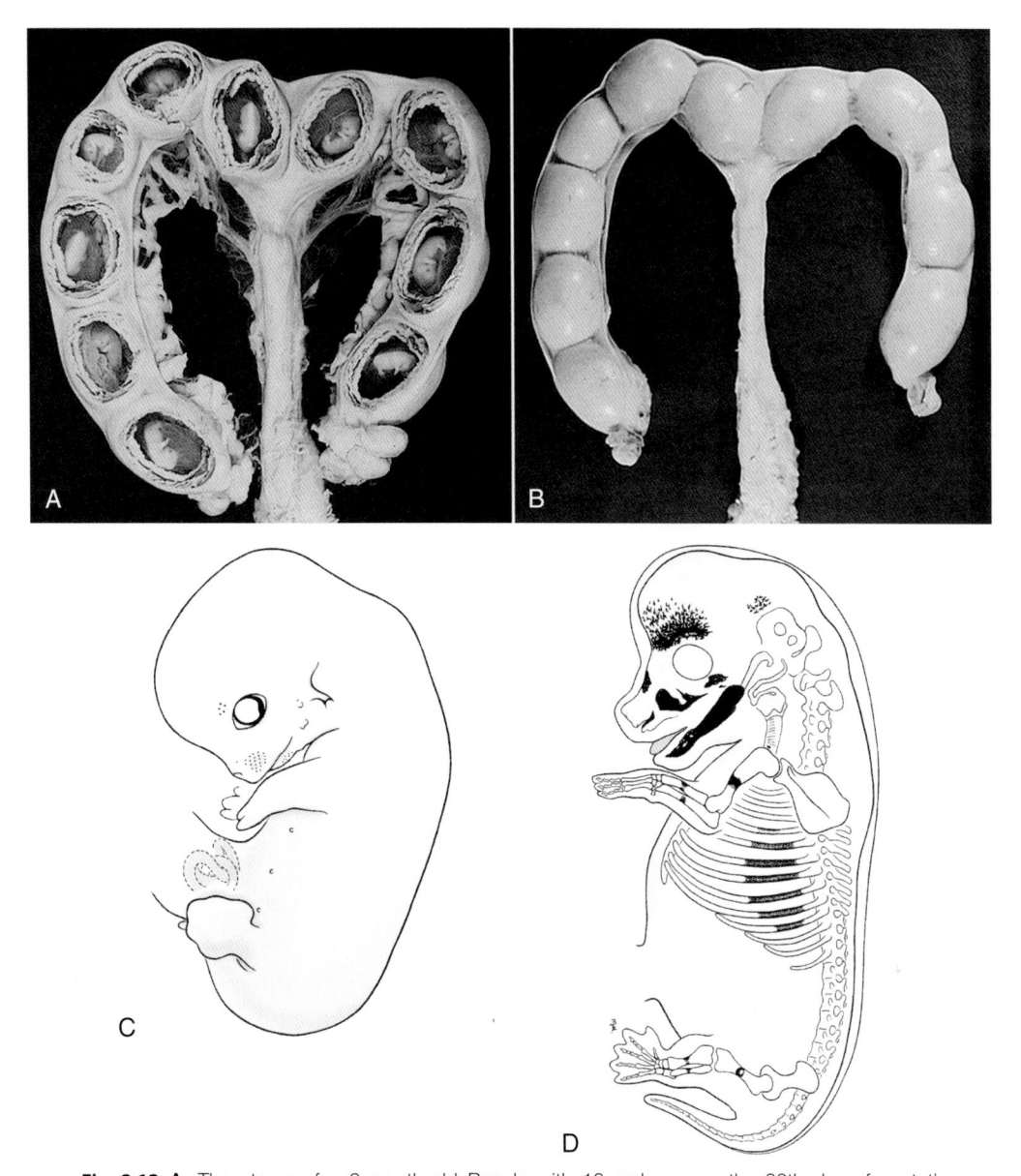

• **Fig. 2.12 A,** The uterus of a 9-month-old Beagle with 10 embryos on the 30th day of gestation. **B,** Outer surface of uterus. **C,** External features of a 30-day, 9-mm Beagle fetus. **D,** Ossifications in a 33-day, 27-mm Beagle embryo. (**A** and **B** from Evans HE: A dog comes into being. *Gaines Dog Research Progress,* Fall 1956.)

In domestic animal embryos and fetuses the most widely used measurement is the straight line C-R length, which allows for continuous measurement during most of the prenatal period (Table 2.3). Evans and Sack (1973) plotted prenatal growth in several domestic animals, including the dog, and considered the fetal stage of the dog to begin on day 35, when the digits on both limbs were fully formed and the external features were clearly those of a dog (Fig. 2.13).

The weights of individual embryos or fetuses within a litter often vary considerably, and there may be a great disparity between the smallest and the largest individual within an age class or within a litter (Fig. 2.14). When the litter is small, each individual tends to be heavier in the later stages of gestation, and, conversely, in large litters individual weights are often below average for their age class.

Measurements and Growth Plots

For recording standard linear measurements of fetal growth it is necessary to take straight-line as well as curvilinear measurements, as indicated in Fig. 2.15. For a discussion of the coefficients of variation for various fetal measurements, see Cloete (1939), who worked with sheep.

CHAPTER 2 Prenatal Development

TABLE 2.3 Crown-Rump Length Estimates for Each Day of Gestation in the Beagle

Day	Total Length	Day	Total Length
18	1 to 2 mm	40	65 mm
19	2.3 mm	41	67 mm
20	4 mm	42	70 mm
21	4.5 mm	43	75 mm
22	4.5 to 5 mm	44	78 mm
23	5 to 6 mm	45	86 mm
24	10 mm	46	90 mm
25	14 mm	47	95 mm
26	15 mm	48	97 mm
27	16 mm	49	100 mm
28	17 mm	50	107 mm
29	18 mm	51	120 mm
30	19 mm	52	130 mm
31	20 mm	53	138 mm
32	25 mm	54	142 mm
33	30 mm	55	144 mm
34	32 mm	56	145 mm
35	35 mm	57	150 mm
36	41 mm	58	155 mm
37	47 mm	59	157 mm
38	53 mm	60	158 mm
39	59 mm	63	165 mm

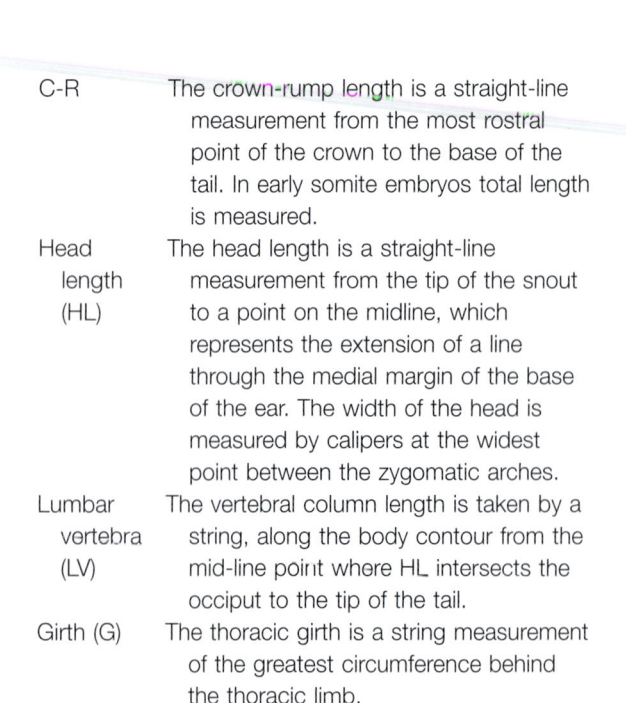

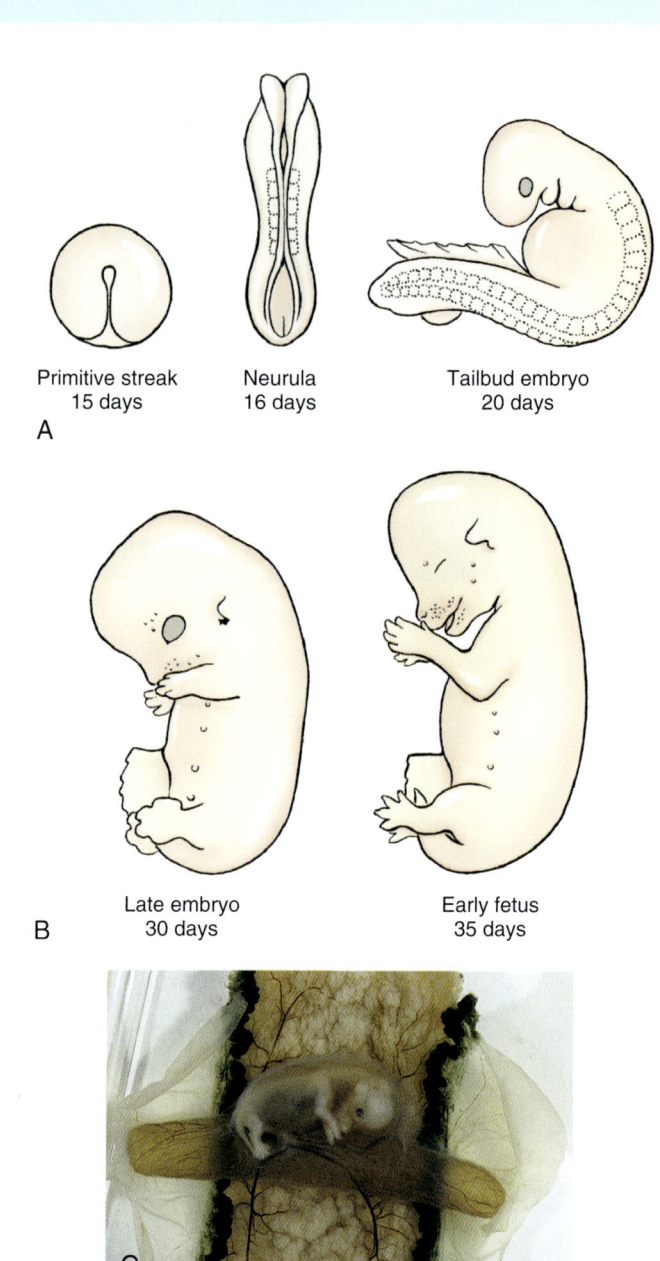

C-R The crown-rump length is a straight-line measurement from the most rostral point of the crown to the base of the tail. In early somite embryos total length is measured.

Head length (HL) The head length is a straight-line measurement from the tip of the snout to a point on the midline, which represents the extension of a line through the medial margin of the base of the ear. The width of the head is measured by calipers at the widest point between the zygomatic arches.

Lumbar vertebra (LV) The vertebral column length is taken by a string, along the body contour from the mid-line point where HL intersects the occiput to the tip of the tail.

Girth (G) The thoracic girth is a string measurement of the greatest circumference behind the thoracic limb.

• **Fig. 2.13** A, B, Representative developmental stages of the dog based on more than 457 embryos and fetuses from many sources. C, Beagle placenta opened at 35 days of gestation. Note that the yolk sac is twice as long as the fetus. (With permission from Evans HE, Sack WO: Prenatal development of domestic and laboratory mammals: growth curves, external features, and selected references, *Anat Histol Embryol* 2:11–45, 1973.)

Successive removals of embryos and fetuses during gestation allow comparisons to be made between litters and provides data for calculating incremental growth (Evans, 1956, 1974, 1979). The average increase in length between days 35 and 40 is approximately 30.5 mm, which indicates growth of 6.1 mm per day for the Beagle fetus (Fig. 2.16 and Table 2.4).

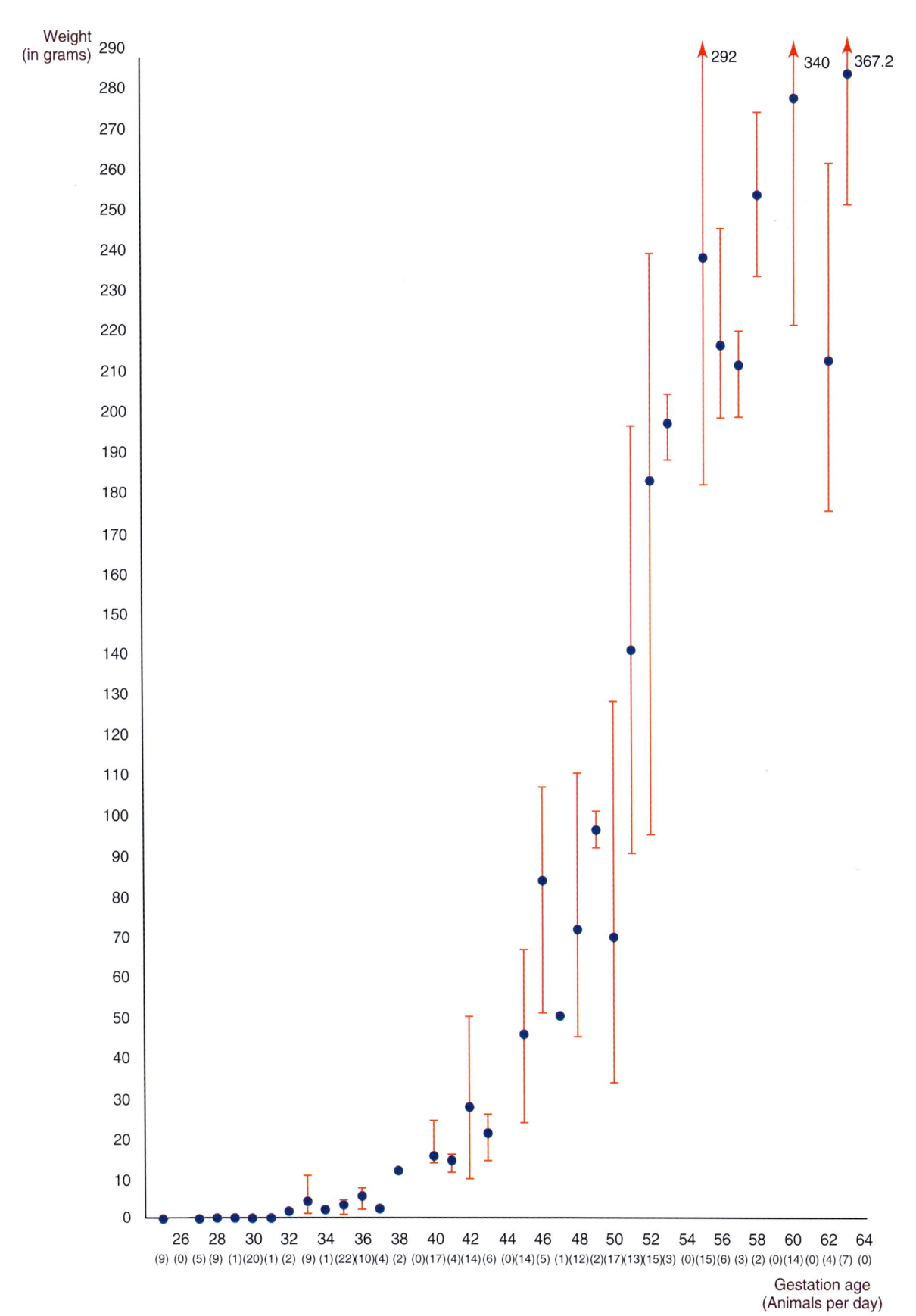

- **Fig. 2.14** Weight in grams versus gestation age in days. The vertical bar indicates the minimum and maximum weights of individuals within the age class. (From Evans HE: *Prenatal development of the dog.* Ithaca, NY, 1974, 24th Gaines Veterinary Symposium.)

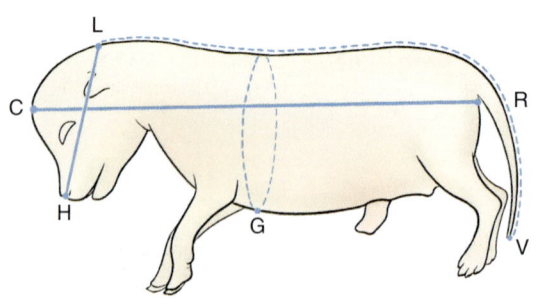

Fig. 2.15 Standard measurements taken for plotting fetal growth. The most reliable fetal measurements are thoracic girth (G) and vertebral column length (LV) taken with a thread, head width between the zygomatic arches, head length (HL), and crown-rump (C-R). (From Evans HE: *Prenatal development of the dog,* Ithaca, NY, 1974, 24th Gaines Veterinary Symposium.)

Size Index

The size index is a combined figure that is an average of the sum of the five most reliable measurements: C-R length, HL, head width, vertebral column length, and chest girth (Fig. 2.17). By combining the most reliable measurements, any variation caused by fixation or manner of taking the measurement is minimized. (All measurements were taken three times and the average was used.)

Fetus

By the time the dog embryo is a little more than halfway through gestation (35 days of the 60-day mean), it has completed the embryonic period of major organ formation. The external features enable one to recognize it as a dog,

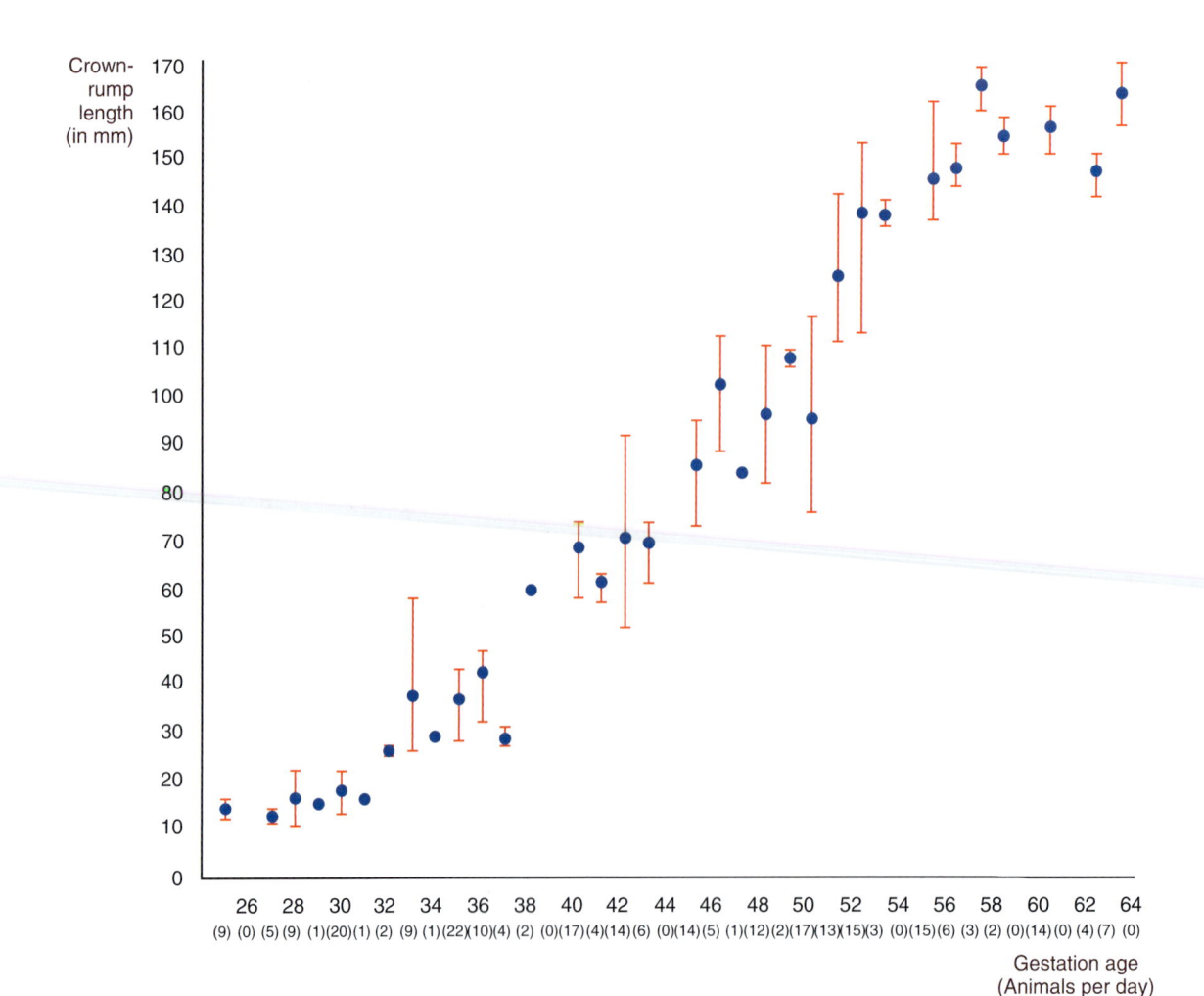

Fig. 2.16 Crown-rump length in millimeters versus gestation age in days for the Beagle. The smallest and largest fetus for each age is indicated by the *vertical bar,* and the *spot* indicates the mean crown-rump length. (From Evans HE: *Prenatal development of the dog,* Ithaca, NY, 1974, 24th Gaines Veterinary Symposium.)

TABLE 2.4 Percentage Increments of Growth in Crown-Rump (C-R) Length of Beagle Fetuses Removed from the Uterus at 5-Day Intervals in Six Dogs

Age in Days	C-R Length	C-R Growth Increment
28	13 mm	
		→ 107.6%
33	27 mm	
27	14 mm	
		→ 85.7%
32	26 mm	
28	14 mm	
		→ 142.8%
33	34 mm	321.4%
		→ 83.5%
38	59 mm	
29	15 mm	
		→ 93.3%
34	29 mm	
28	19 mm	
		→ 152.6%
33	48 mm	
30	21 mm	
		→ 104.7%
35	43 mm	247.6%
		→ 69.7%
40	73 mm	

and, from this point on, it can be referred to as a *fetus*. A Beagle fetus of 35 days postcoitus is approximately 35 mm in C-R length. Larger dogs have somewhat larger fetuses, but in either case the length of the fetus is equal to the width of the placental band.

Successive removals of fetuses at intervals from the same dog midway through gestation show the gradual increase in the size of the uterus and the marked increase in the size of the embryo and fetus. Fig. 2.18A to F show changes at 5-day intervals for purebred Beagles.

External features characteristic of fetal stages are development of pigmentation, growth of hair and claws, closure and fusion of the eyelids, growth of the external ear, elongation of the trunk, and sexual differentiation. At 30 days of gestation (19 mm), the genital tubercles of the male and female appear similar (Fig. 2.19). As the genital area develops in the male, the mammary primordia in the vicinity involute and regress as the prepuce forms around the growing phallus. In the female, the vulva grows caudally as it envelops the genital tubercle, which becomes the clitoris (Figs. 2.20 to 2.25).

Skeletal Age Criteria

Although the weight or size of embryos and fetuses may vary within a litter, the sequence of ossification is rather uniform within the litter.

To see the cartilaginous structures and incipient ossifications in three dimensions, it is possible to stain the cartilage and bone preferentially, clear the entire embryo in hydroxide and glycerin, and examine it under a dissecting microscope. For staining embryonic cartilage, in toto, the Alcian blue technique is ideal and can be applied to fixed or fresh material (Simons & Van Horn, 1971; Watson, 1977). When calcified cartilage or bone is present, it can be stained with alizarin red stain. Both techniques may be combined (Dingerkus & Uhler, 1977), resulting in a differentially stained specimen that leaves no doubt as to the morphologic stage of the cartilage or bone in question.

Ossification centers can be seen at an earlier stage using alizarin-stained clearings than by using radiographic techniques. When staining and clearing is preceded by the injection of contrast media into the vessels or organs (Evans, 1948), the resulting specimen is ideal for studying developing vessels and organs in relation to the skeleton (Fig. 2.26).

Skull

The earliest indication of the skull is seen as parachordal, trabecular, and branchial cartilages, which are of neural crest origin. A well-illustrated study of the early development of the vertebrate skull was made by de Beer (1937). As the parachordal and trabecular cartilages enlarge and fuse with one another beneath the brain, they incorporate the sense capsules (olfactory, optic, and otic) and form a troughlike cartilaginous skull called the **chondrocranium** (Figs. 2.27 to 2.29). This cartilaginous forerunner of the definitive skull, which has been studied in the dog by Olmstead (1911) and Schliemann (1966), is destined to ossify endochondrally ventral to the brain (Figs. 2.30 and 2.31) and combine with the membrane-formed bone of the **desmocranium** dorsal to the brain (Fig. 2.32). Drews (1933) using mongrel dog fetuses, Schliemann (1966) studying Whippet embryos and fetuses, and Evans (1956, 1974, 1979) studying Beagle embryos and fetuses have described several stages of skull ossification. The cartilages of the jaws, hyoid, and middle ear, constituting the **viscerocranium** (see Fig. 2.31), form bone in both membrane and cartilage, which is incorporated or attached to the adult skull, or **cranium**. The jaw is formed by the maxillary and mandibular bones and their articulation at the temporomandibular joints. Movement at this joint opens and closes the mouth. Evans (1958) found the sequence of fetal skull ossification to be first facial at

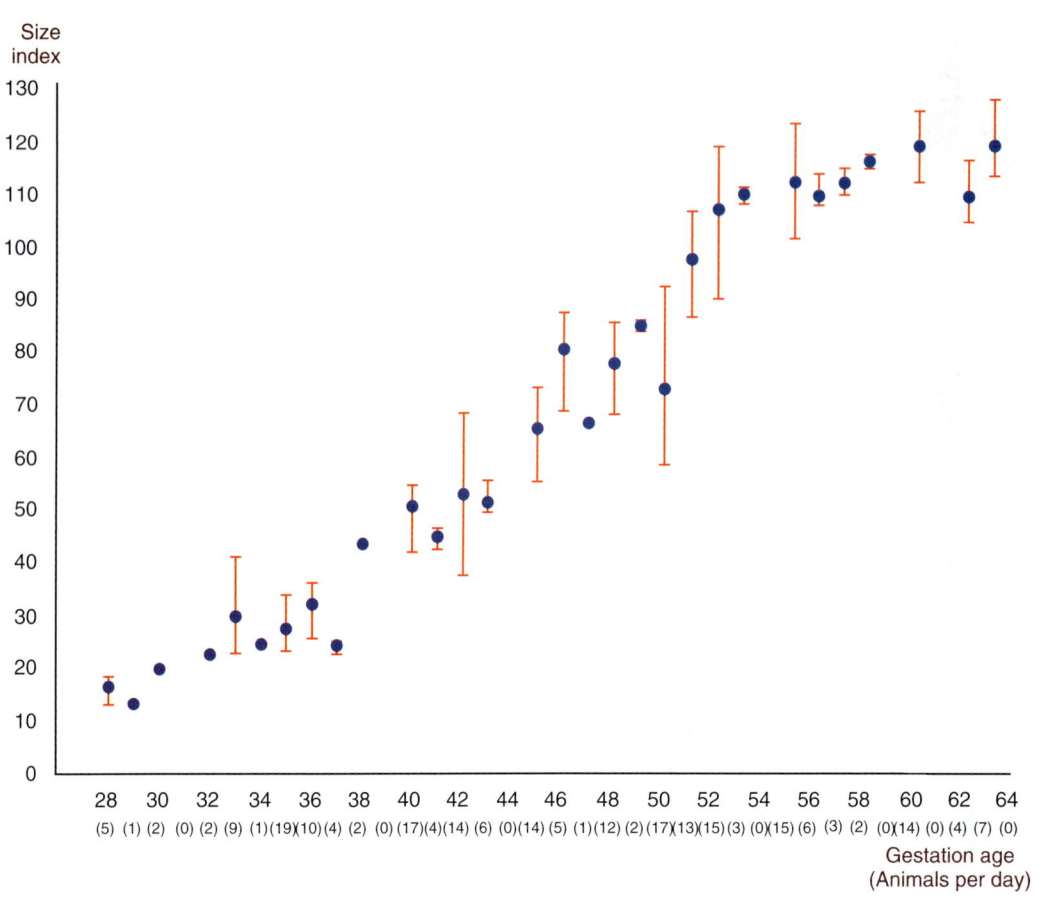

• **Fig. 2.17** Size index versus gestation age in days based on 229 Beagle fetuses. (From Evans HE: *Prenatal development of the dog,* Ithaca, NY, 1974, 24th Gaines Veterinary Symposium.)

34 mm/35 days (maxilla, mandible), palatal (palatine, pterygoid), and calvarial (frontal, parietal) centers, followed by basicranial centers at 54 mm (basisphenoid, basioccipital) and finally the otic capsule (89 mm) and hyoid apparatus (93 mm) (see Fig. 2.32).

Regardless of whether the bones are formed in cartilage or membrane, there may be one or more centers of ossification, and the structure of the definitive bone is the same. Bones developed in membrane ossify earlier than those developed in cartilage.

Thus the sheathing bone of the mandibular cartilage (dentary) and the sheathing bone of the palatoquadrate cartilage (maxilla) begin to ossify on day 28 in the 19-mm embryo, at the same time as the frontal bone of the skull roof and the membranous portion of the clavicle. Other membrane-formed bones of the skull, which develop early, are the nasal, incisive, palatine, zygomatic, and parietal, which form by day 32 in the 27-mm embryo.

The branchial arches give rise to the cartilages of the jaws, the auditory ossicles, the hyoid apparatus, and the larynx. The lower jaw, which is part of the first branchial arch, is present as a rodlike mandibular cartilage (Meckel's cartilage) on each side by day 25 of gestation, when the embryo is 13 to 16 mm in length. The mandibular cartilages join rostrally, whereas caudally each lies within a middle ear cavity, where its hook-shaped articular cartilage is destined to become the malleus of the middle ear (see Fig. 2.31 and Fig. 2.33). By day 28 of gestation (19 mm) membrane bone begins to form around the mandibular cartilage as the dentary. The cartilage itself at a later stage will undergo endochondral ossification (Fig. 2.34) in the region of the canine tooth, and thus the lower jaw is formed by both perichondral membrane bone and endochondral cartilage bone. On the dorsocaudal border of the dentary bone a condyle develops as secondary cartilage, which then ossifies and fuses with the body of the mandible to become part of the temporomandibular joint.

Later developmental stages of the skull show that the sequence of primary ossification centers shifts from facial and calvarial centers to basicranial and otic centers, followed by hyoid centers (Figs. 2.35 to 2.37). In some instances bone is being formed in both membrane and cartilage simultaneously, as in the supraoccipital, mandible, pterygoid, and temporal bones.

Calvarial Centers

The skull roof, or calvaria (see Fig. 2.32 and Fig. 2.38), is composed of bones that develop in membrane as paired frontal and parietal centers. Each bone shows a central trabecular network that spreads to cover the brain. In

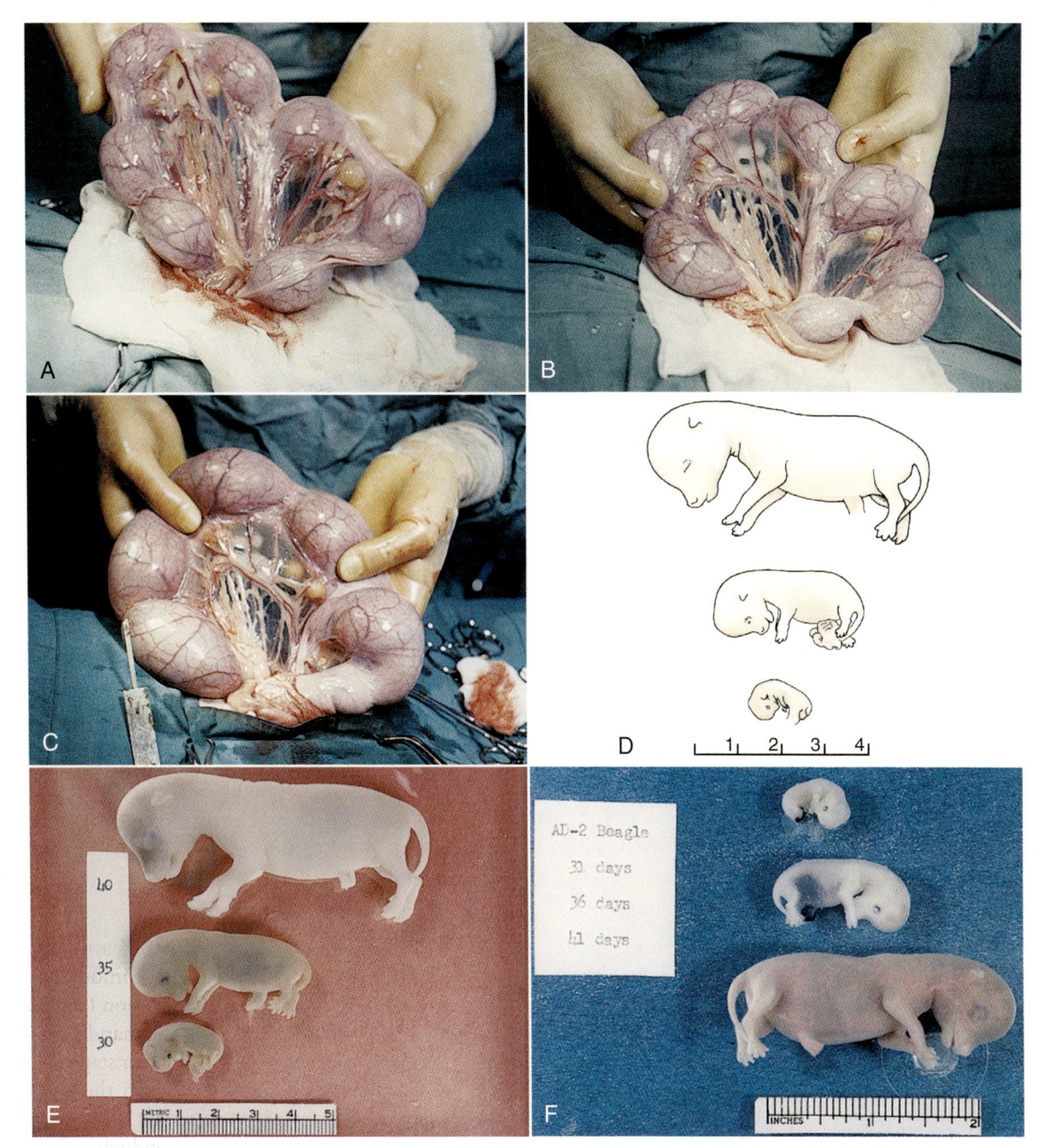

• **Fig. 2.18** Serial removals from the same Beagle in one gestation. **A**, Uterus at 28 days. **B**, Uterus at 33 days. **C**, Uterus at 38 days. **D**, 28-, 33-, and 38-day embryos removed from **A**, **B**, and **C**. (**E** and **F** are serial removals at 5-day intervals from another Beagle.) Scale bar in **C** is in cm.

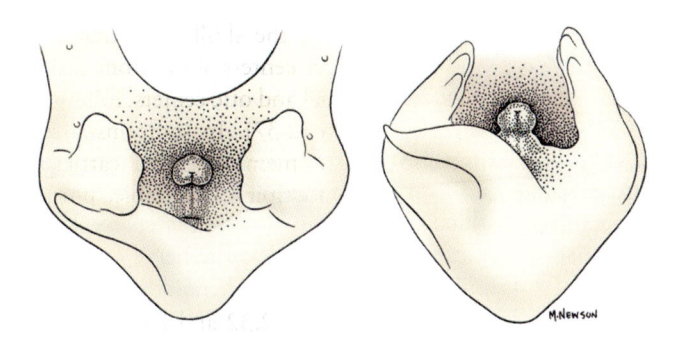

• **Fig. 2.19** Undifferentiated genital tubercle of a 30-day Beagle embryo.

addition to these primary roofing bones, there is an unpaired interparietal bone lying more superficially (overlapping the edges of the parietal and supraoccipital bones), which fuses with the supraoccipital bone on day 45 of gestation and only rarely maintains its separate identity (Fig. 2.39).

Basicranial Centers

The chondrocranium ossifies to form the bones of the floor, walls, and sense capsules of the braincase. The process is gradual, as can be seen from Figs. 2.40 to 2.47, and involves endochondral loci that spread to predetermined borders of homogeneous cartilaginous anlagen. Thus the basicranial axis is formed by a central ossification for the basioccipital

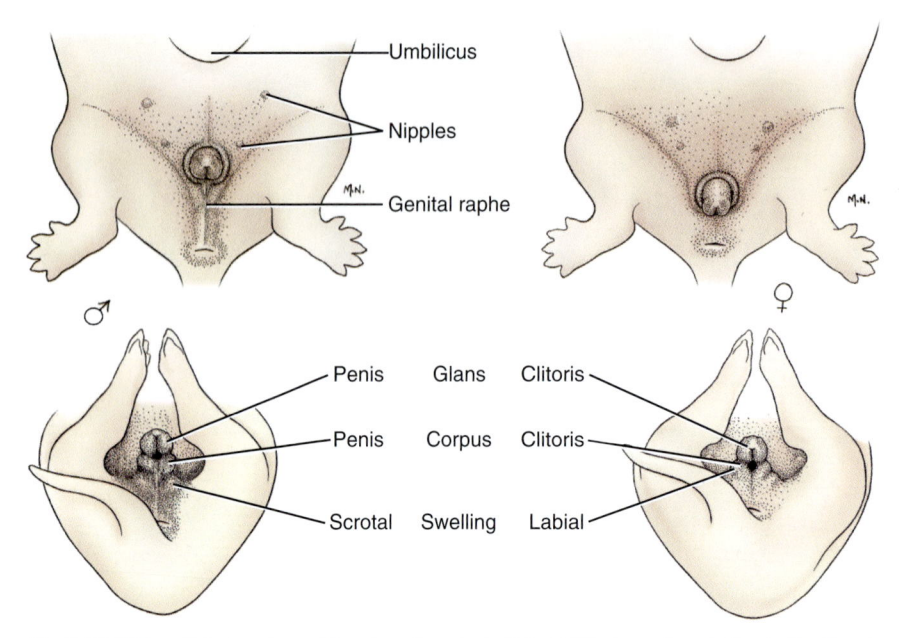

• **Fig. 2.20** Differentiated male and female external genitalia at 35 days of gestation in the Beagle.

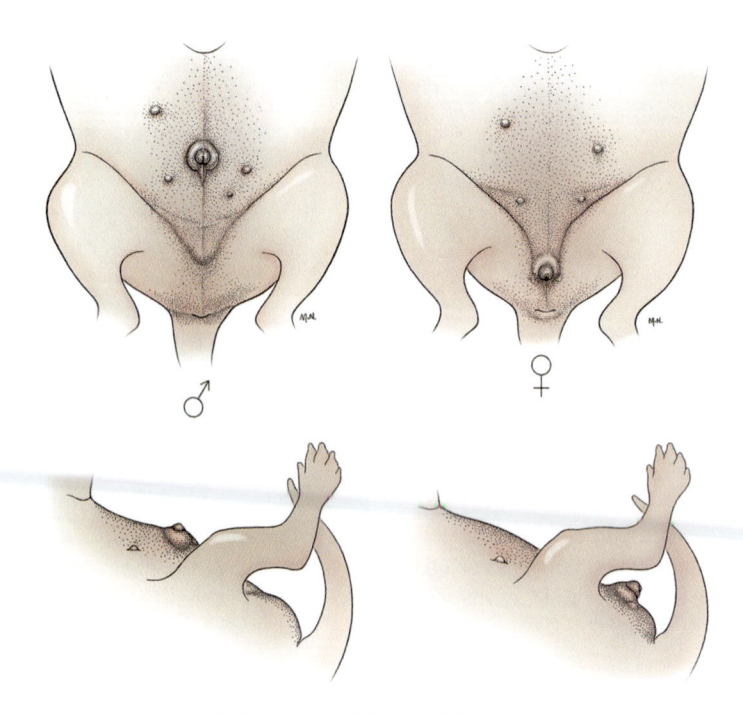

• **Fig. 2.21** External genitalia of 40-day fetal Beagles.

bone, a similar one for the basisphenoid bone, and paired ossifications for the presphenoid and ethmoid bones. These median elements fuse with their lateral component wings to form a sphenoidal complex. The presphenoid fuses with the orbitosphenoids on each side to form a presphenoid with orbital wings, whereas the basisphenoid fuses with the alisphenoids on each side to form a basisphenoid with temporal wings. Both of these sphenoids fuse with each other (never completely in the dog) to form the sphenoidal complex.

Ossification centers for the orbital wings appear first in the preoptic root and later in the metoptic roots of the chondrocranial ala orbitalis. Expansion of these centers results in a C-shaped ossification around each optic nerve (see Figs. 2.44 and 2.45). The body of the basisphenoid first appears as diffuse ossifications on the midline. The temporal wings are the earliest portion of the sphenoid complex to ossify. They form as a single plaque in each ala temporalis of the chondrocranium, and, as growth proceeds, they fuse with the

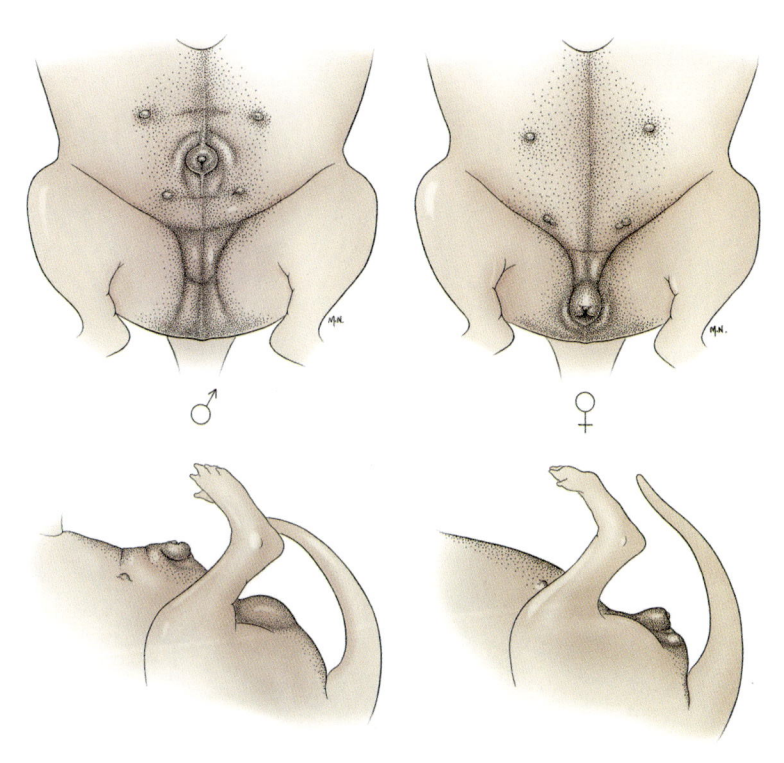

- **Fig. 2.22** External genitalia of 45-day fetal Beagles.

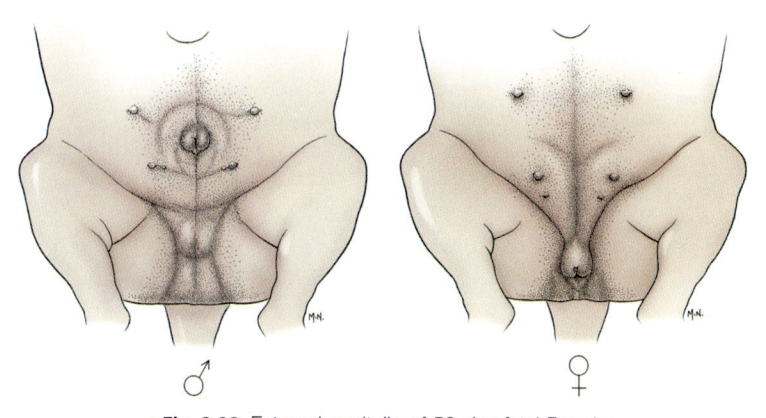

- **Fig. 2.23** External genitalia of 50-day fetal Beagles.

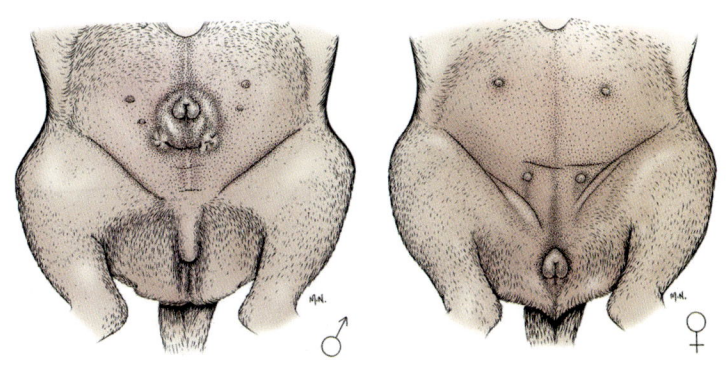

- **Fig. 2.24** External genitalia of 55-day fetal Beagles.

32 CHAPTER 2 Prenatal Development

• **Fig. 2.25** The external genitalia of male and female newborn Beagles (60 days).

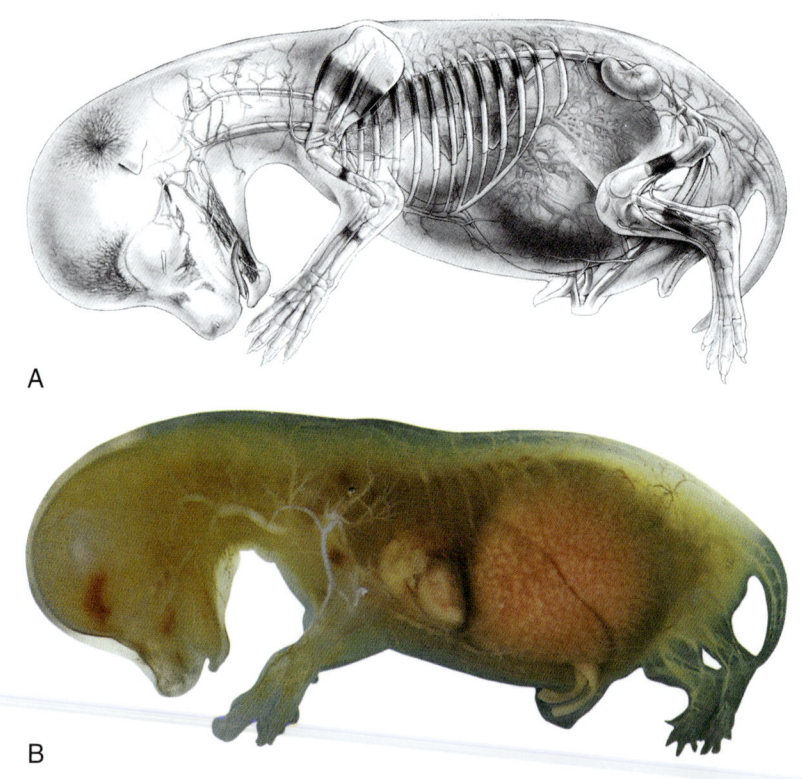

• **Fig. 2.26** Developing vessels and organs in relation to the skeleton of a 40-day Beagle fetus. **A**, Drawing by Lewis Sadler. **B**, Injected, cleared, and stained fetus used for the drawing.

median basisphenoid. There is no indication in the chondrocranium as to where joints will form with neighboring bones. The sequence of sphenoidal ossification centers is temporal wing at 35 days (41 mm C-R), body of basisphenoid at 40 days (59 mm C-R), preoptic root of orbital wing at 42 days (71 mm C-R), and metoptic root and body of presphenoid at 43 days (76 mm C-R). The presphenoid and their orbital wings fuse when the fetus is approximately 108 mm C-R or at 50 days of gestation. The pituitary or hypophysis rests in the sella turcica, formed by the basisphenoid with the help of late ossifications called *clinoid processes*. On the rostral end of this complex the lateral ethmoids fuse to form the sphenethmoids below the cribriform plate, and the mesethmoid forms a median perpendicular plate.

The joint between the basisphenoid and the basioccipital is known as the *sphenooccipital synchondrosis* and that between the basisphenoid and presphenoid is the intersphenoidal synchondrosis. Premature fusion of either of these joints, as is seen in brachycephalic animals, limits growth and shortens the basicranial axis. When this occurs, the lower jaw continues to grow in length but, being unopposed rostrally, will arch dorsally.

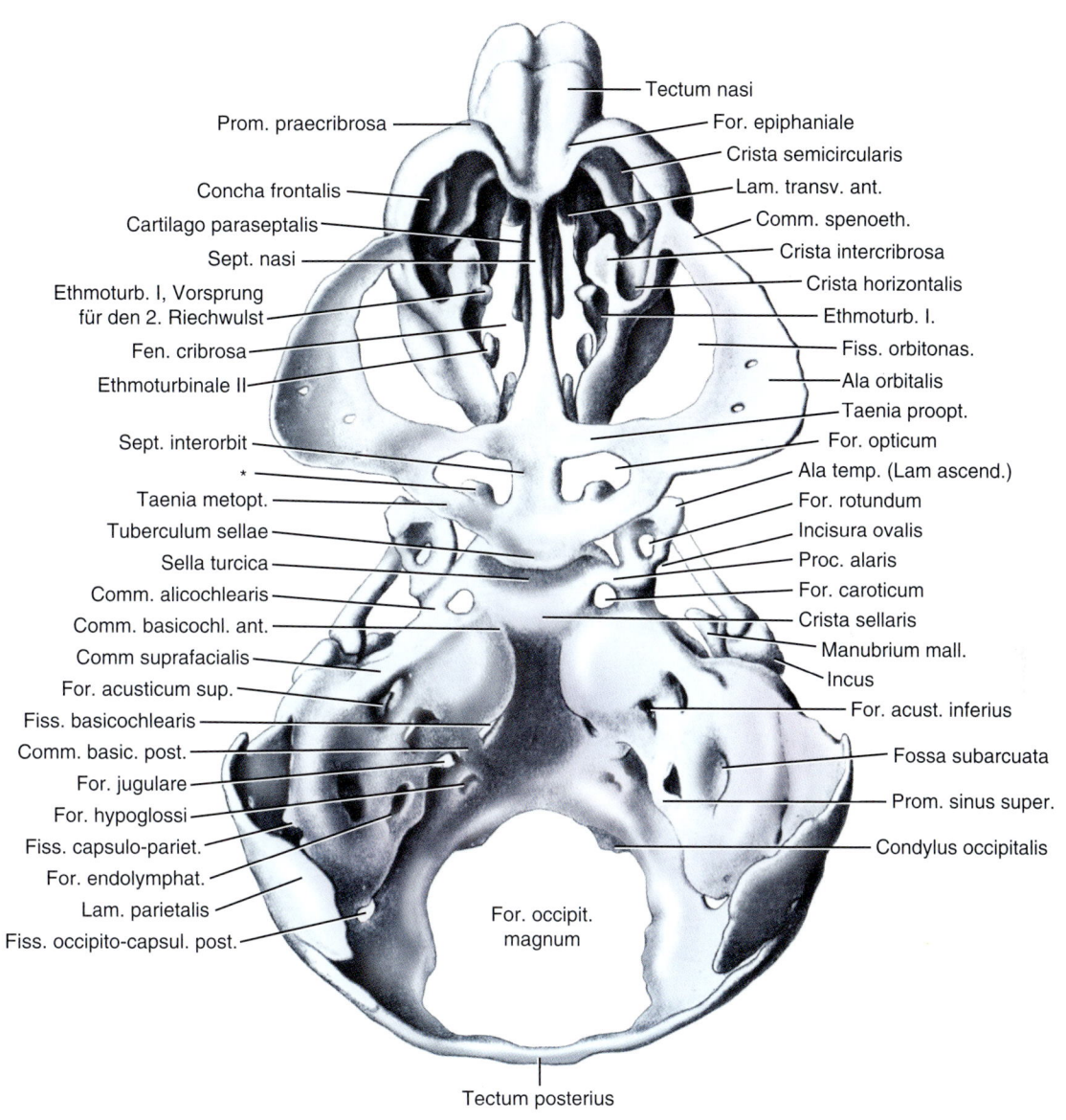

• Fig. 2.27 The chondrocranium of the dog. Dorsal view. (From Olmstead MP: Das Primordialcranium eines Hundembryo, *Anat Hefte* 130:339–375, 1911.)

Otic Centers

The otic region consists of a cartilaginous **otic capsule** containing the **membranous labyrinth** (see Fig. 2.36A). Numerous ossification centers develop around the membranous labyrinth of the inner ear to form the petrosal bone. The latter fuses with the squamous temporal bone and the tympanic ring to form the temporal complex. As the tympanic cavity develops, the **middle ear ossicles** (of branchial arch origin) are enclosed in a tympanic bulla of tympanic ring origin. The sequence of ossification for the ossicles is malleus (38 days), incus (50 days), and stapes (55 days).

Hyoid Apparatus

The **stylohyoid** cartilage (Figs. 2.37 and 2.48) ossifies by 47 days (93 mm) followed by the **thyrohyoid** at 53 days (138 mm) and the **epihyoid** on day 54 (141 mm). The **basihyoid** ossifies 1 month after birth and the **ceratohyoid** 2 months after birth. The **tympanohyoid** does not ossify.

Teeth

The development of the dentition has been studied by Williams (1961), who found that calcification of all deciduous teeth was initiated by day 55 of gestation and completed by day 20 postpartum for the crowns or day 45 postpartum for the roots. The only tooth of the permanent dentition to calcify prenatally is the mandibular first molar, which appears on day 55 of gestation.

Williams and Evans (1978) examined sectioned dog embryos and fetuses as well as whole-mounts to determine the time sequence of standard morphologic stages of dental

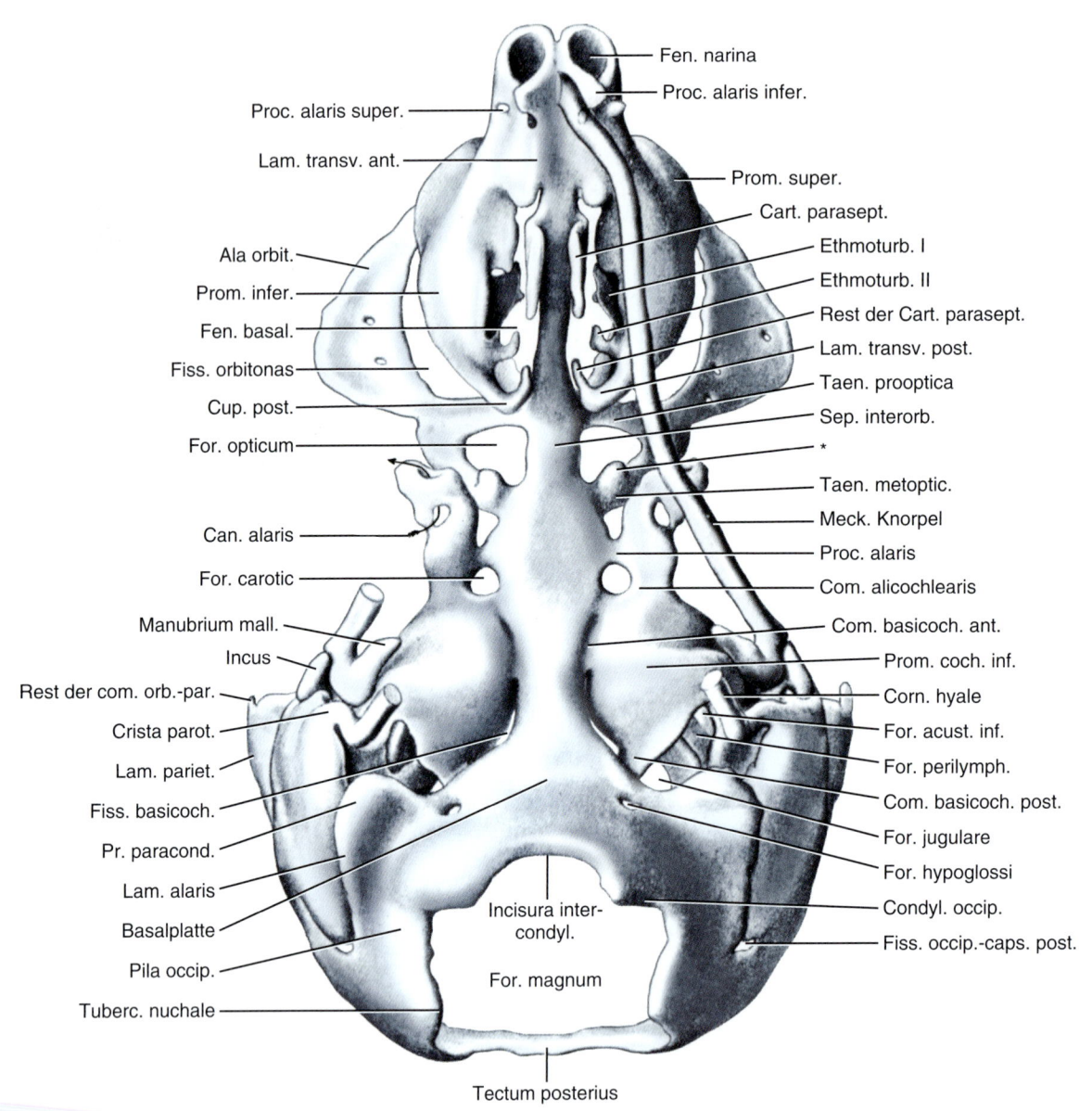

• **Fig. 2.28** Chondrocranium of the dog. Ventral view with the mandibular (Meckel) cartilage partially removed on one side, and the hyoid cornu (Reichert cartilage) cut on both sides. (From Olmstead MP: Das Primordialcranium eines Hundembryo, *Anat Hefte* 130:339–375, 1911.)

development. The **dental lamina** first appeared at 25 days of gestation (14 mm), and, by 30 days, the right and left laminae joined across the midline, forming a continuous dental arch. The **vestibular lamina**, which separates the gums from the lips and cheeks, first arises as a distinct invagination lateral to the dental lamina. It is recognizable in the incisor region of the 30-day embryo.

Differentiation of the deciduous enamel organs in the dog begins on about day 30 of gestation and exhibits the following typical sequence: bud, early cap, cap, advanced cap, early bell, and advanced bell stages. The relationship of the enamel organ to the dentary bone and mandibular cartilage can be seen in Fig. 2.49A to C.

The sequence of calcification of the teeth in the Beagle is:

Teeth	Days (size)
Third mandibular premolars Fourth mandibular premolars	42 days (70 mm)
Maxillary and mandibular canines	45 days (86 mm)
Third Maxillary premolars Dorsal incisors	45 to 48 days (86-97 mm)
Ventral incisors Fourth maxillary premolars Second maxillary and mandibular premolars	49 to 51 days (100-120 mm)

CHAPTER 2 Prenatal Development 35

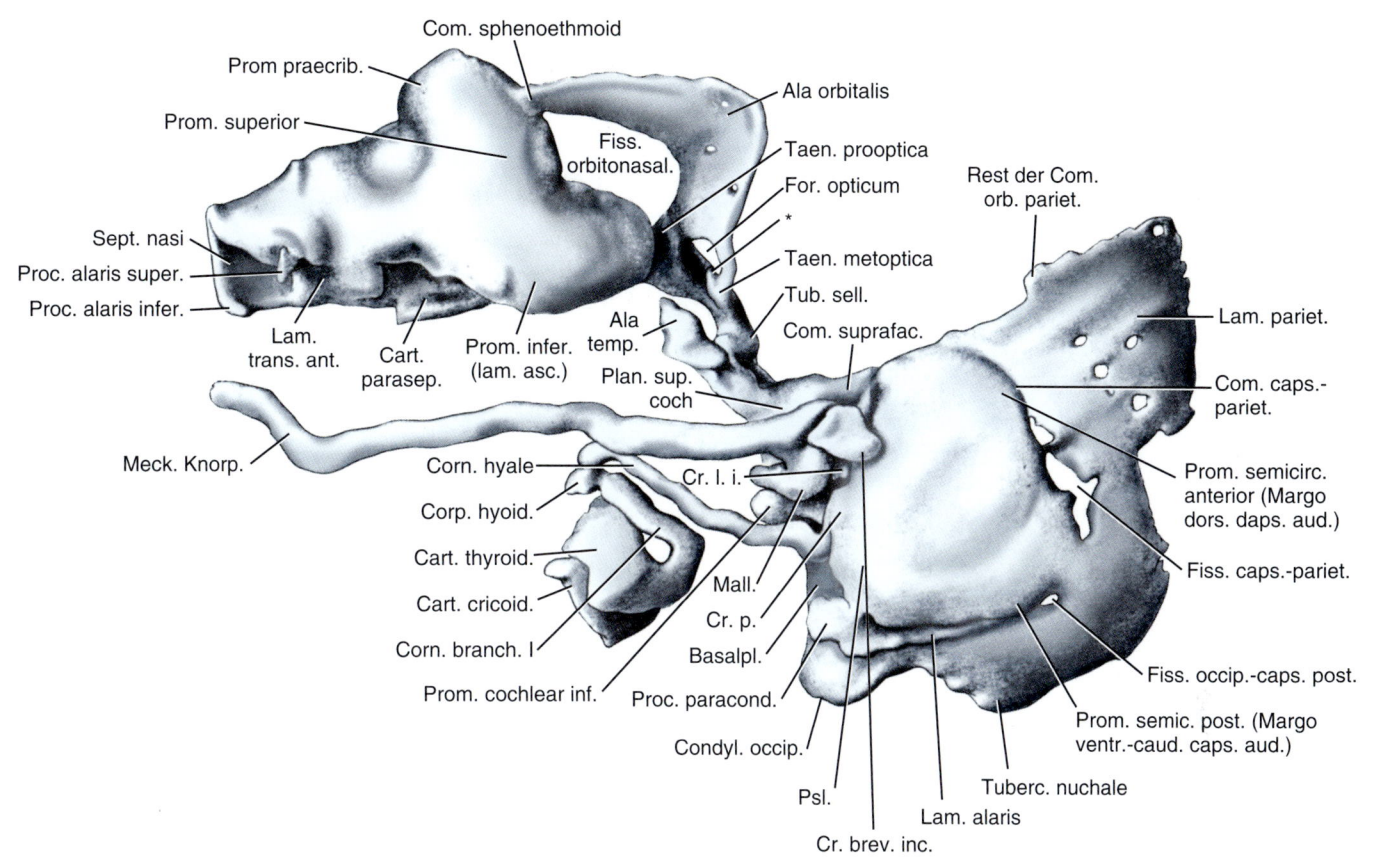

• **Fig. 2.29** Chondrocranium of the dog. Left lateral view with the hyoid cornu and larynx. (From Olmstead MP: Das Primordialcranium eines Hundembryo, *Anat. Hefte* 130:339–375, 1911.)

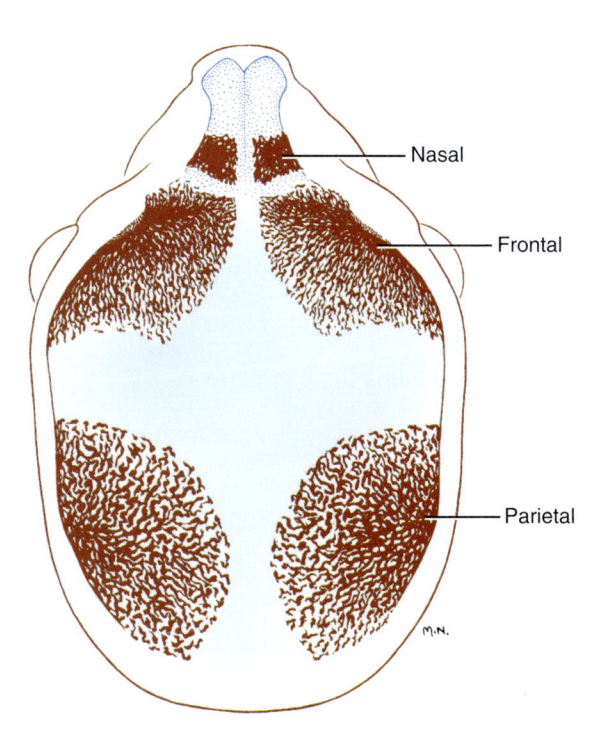

• **Fig. 2.30** Ossification of the membrane bones (desmocranium) in a 40-day Beagle fetus calvaria.

By day 55 (141 mm) all deciduous teeth show calcification, as does the lower [mandibular] first molar of the permanent dentition.

Williams and Evans (1978) were unable to determine with certainty whether the first premolar tooth is a member of the deciduous or permanent dentition. Tooth buds for the first premolars did not appear until 47 days (95 mm), which is long after all of the other deciduous tooth primordia have made their appearance.

Vertebral Column

The notochord is the forerunner of the vertebral column, and, in the early embryo, it is present as a solid rod of cells surrounded by a sheath of paraxial mesoderm. Condensations within the somites form the sclerotomes that surround the notochord and partially enclose the neural tube. When chondrification takes place in the sclerotome, the notochord is almost completely obliterated within the centrum. The notochord persists as a soft central core, the nucleus pulposus, within the intervertebral disc. The intervertebral disc is a remnant of the intercentral portion of the early chondrification.

The lateral portions of the vertebral condensation chondrify and grow dorsally to form the neural arches and

Prenatal Development

• **Fig. 2.31** Dorsal view of the skull of a 40-day Beagle fetus with the roof removed to show the cartilaginous chondrocranium. Several membrane bones of the jaws, palate, and face are ossified, as are the membrane bones of the roof (see Fig. 2.28).

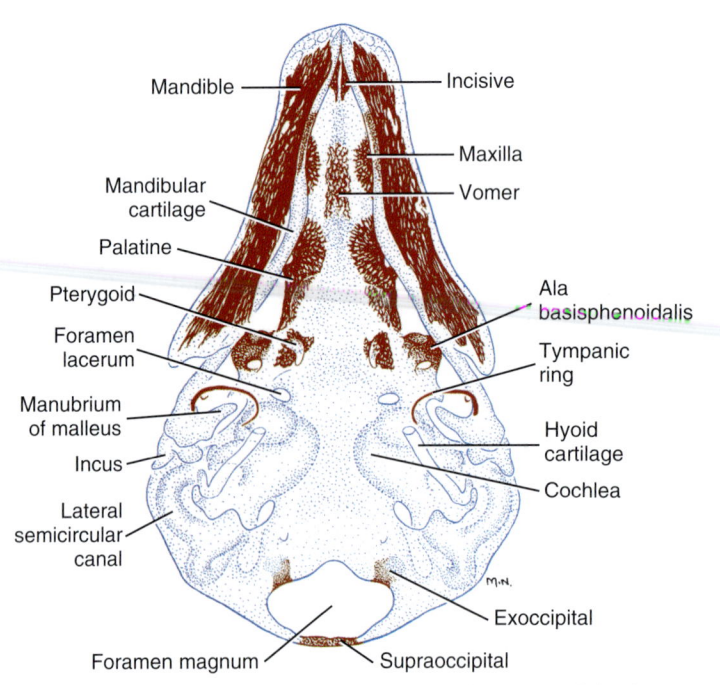

• **Fig. 2.32** The skull of a 40-day Beagle fetus in ventral view to show parts of the viscerocranium: mandibular cartilages, middle ear cartilages, and hyoid apparatus (Reichert cartilage).

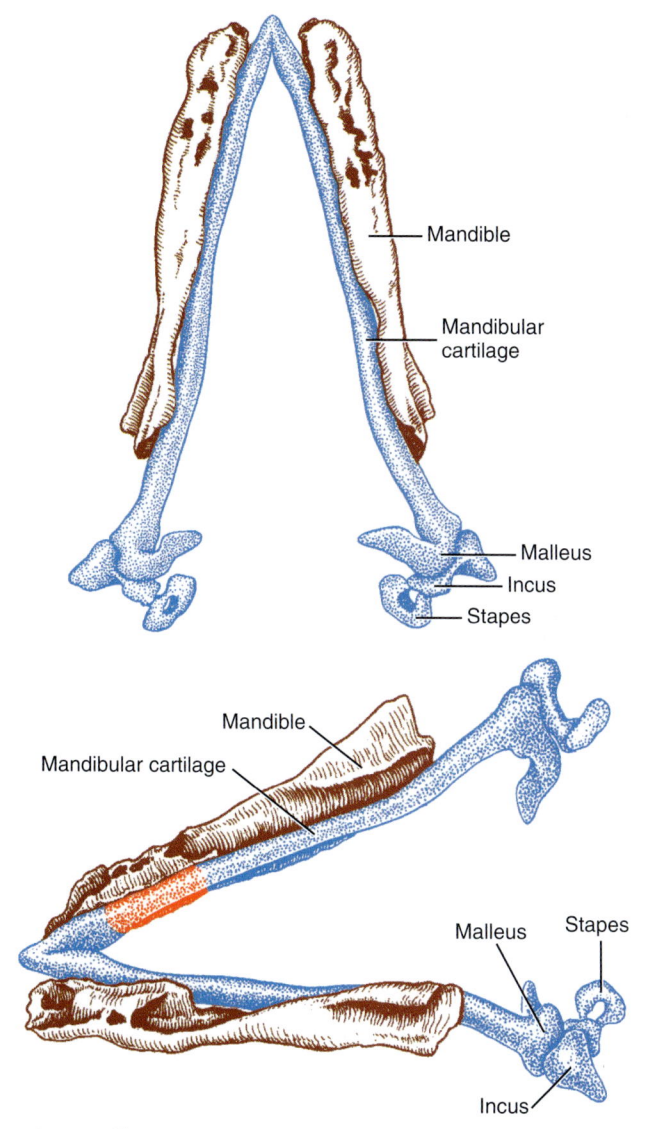

Fig. 2.33 The developing mandible and middle-ear ossicle cartilages of a 35-mm Beagle. The mandible is beginning to cover the mandibular cartilage.

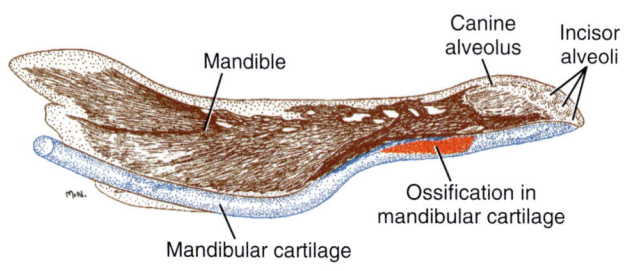

Fig. 2.34 Medial view of the developing mandible of a 40-day Beagle fetus. Note the ossification within the mandibular cartilage in the region of the canine alveolus and the lack of any articular condyle at this stage.

ventrolaterally to form the transverse and costal processes and part of the body. The spinous process of the neural arch develops after the arches meet and fuse. Failure of the neural arches to close dorsally results in rachischisis or spina bifida.

By day 25 of gestation the vertebral column consists of individual chondrified elements resembling definitive vertebrae. Each vertebra (except the atlas and axis) is ossified from three primary centers, one for the centrum and one for each neural arch. The centra first appear as endochondral nodular condensations, whereas the neural arches form as perichondral collars around the base of the cartilaginous arch (Fig. 2.50). Although the manner of formation of centra and neural arches differs in the early stages, later growth and ossification involves simultaneous perichondral as well as endochondral ossification.

Centra

The first endochondral ossifications of the Beagle vertebral column appear at 38 days (54 mm) in thoracic and lumbar regions. These are closely followed by ossifications of C2, C6, and T4 to T6. Intervening centra are ossified rapidly in both directions, resulting in a continuous series from C2 through L6 by 55 mm (Fig. 2.51).

The composition of the body (corpus) of the atlas and also that of the axis is different from that of all other vertebrae because, developmentally, part of the atlas centrum fuses with that of the axis (Figs. 2.52 and 2.53). The atlas is left with only intercentrum I as a body (Fig. 2.54), whereas the axis has centrum I, intercentrum II, and centrum II as its body (Fig. 2.55).

Watson and Evans (1976) and Watson (1981) studied a series of known-age Beagle fetuses and newborns to determine the time of initial ossification and the number of elements that fuse to form the atlas and axis.

At birth the atlas is composed of three ossifications: a pair of arches and a body that is only its intercentrum (see Fig. 2.54). Thus seven bony elements form the axis and three bony elements form the atlas, a total of ten bones. The appearance and fusion times of these elements varies even within litters (Watson et al., 1986).

The body of the atlas (intercentrum I) first appears as an ossification in the 42-day (73-mm) fetus and is always present after 46 days (92 mm). The earliest appearance of an ossified dens is on day 42 (71 mm), although it may still be lacking in some individuals as old as 46 days (89 mm). Between the dens and the centrum of the axis after birth there is an ossified intercentrum II. All elements of the axis fuse with one another by the fourth month postpartum.

Lumbar centra and the first sacral centrum are all present by day 40 (59 mm). Sacral vertebrae are slow to ossify, but by 43 days (73 mm) all three sacral centra are present (see Fig. 2.58). Additional ossifications in the sacral region are located lateral to S1 and S2 and represent sacral "ribs" of ancestral forms. Subsequent growth and fusion result in a combined sacrum dominated by S1, with its large auricular surface for articulation with the ilium.

Caudal centra are the last to appear. They exhibit typical endochondral ossifications from Cd1 to Cd4 but have perichondral plus endochondral ossifications from Cd5 to

Text continued on p. 44

• **Fig. 2.35** Ventral view of the skull of a 45-day Beagle fetus with the mandible removed to show the extent of the palate and alveolar surface.

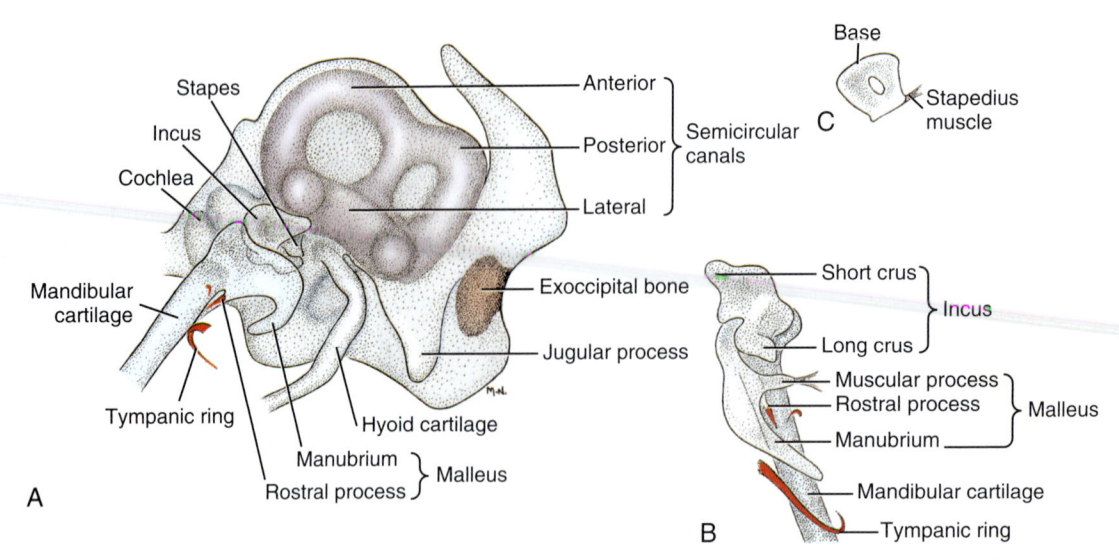

• **Fig. 2.36** The otic region. **A**, The labyrinth of the inner ear, the developing middle ear ossicles, and the attachment of the hyoid apparatus in lateral view. **B**, Ventral view of the middle ear cartilages. **C**, The stapes prior to ossification.

CHAPTER 2 Prenatal Development 39

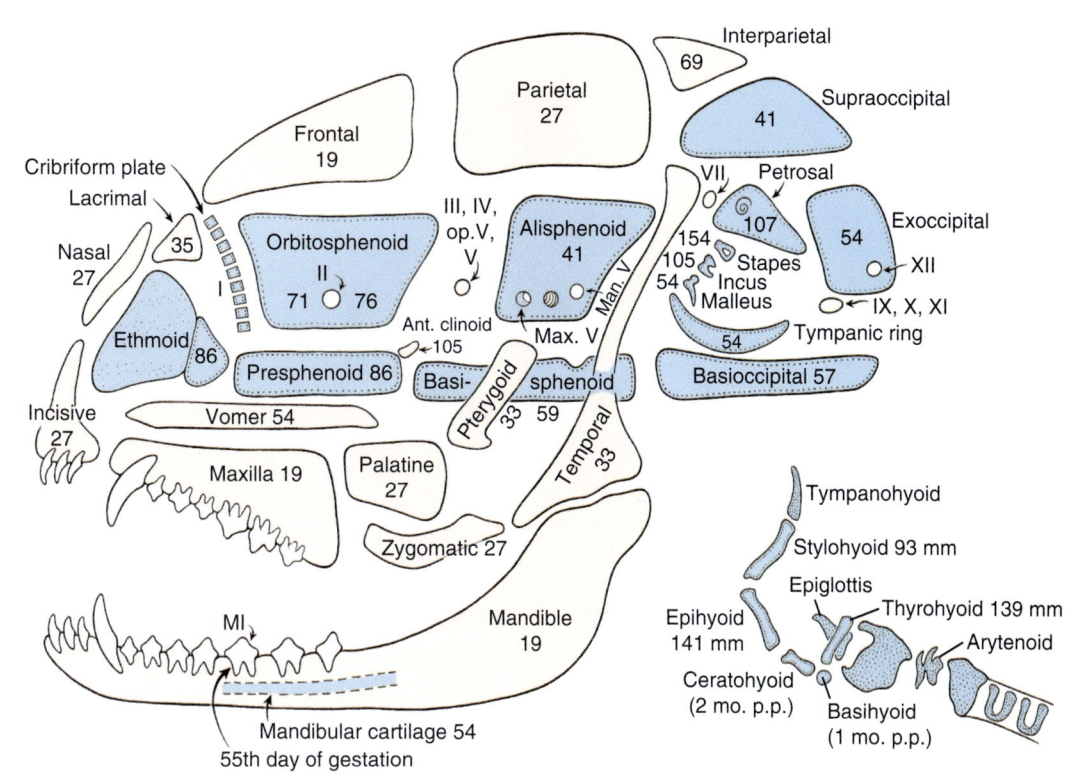

• **Fig. 2.37** Diagrammatic dog skull showing the sequence of initial ossifications. The numerals indicate the fetal size in millimeters at which time each of the bones begins to ossify. Blue bones with a dotted outline are formed in cartilage. Tympanohyoid, thyrohyoid and arytenoid do not ossify. (From Evans HE: *Prenatal development of the dog,* Ithaca, NY, 1974, 24th Gaines Veterinary Symposium.)

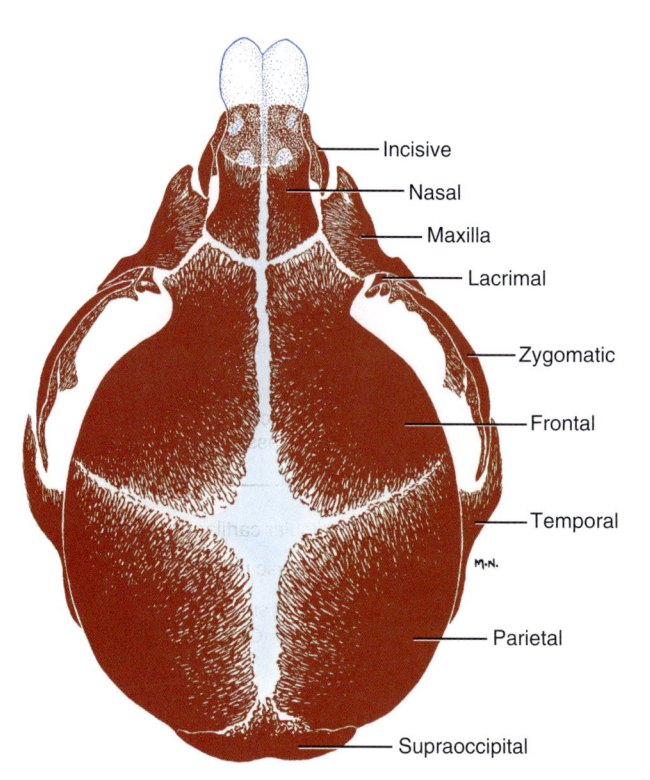

• **Fig. 2.38** Dorsal view of the skull in a 45-day Beagle fetus. The fontanel between the frontal and parietal bones will close before birth.

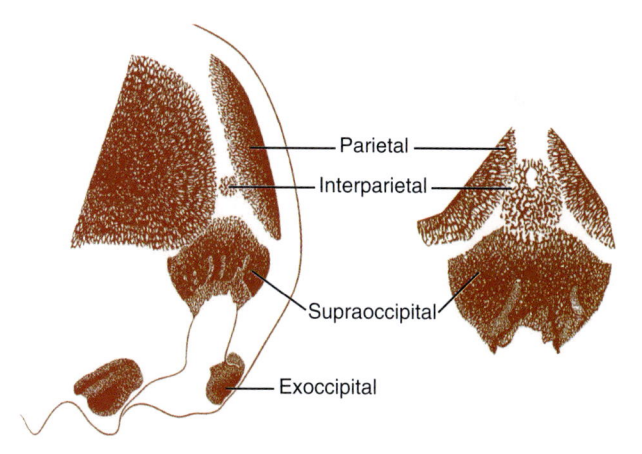

• **Fig. 2.39** The interparietal bone makes a transitory appearance on about the 45th day of gestation. It soon fuses with the supraoccipital bone and becomes indistinguishable from it. On rare occasions it remains as a separate bone in the adult. Note that its position is more superficial than that of the supraoccipital and parietal.

40 CHAPTER 2 Prenatal Development

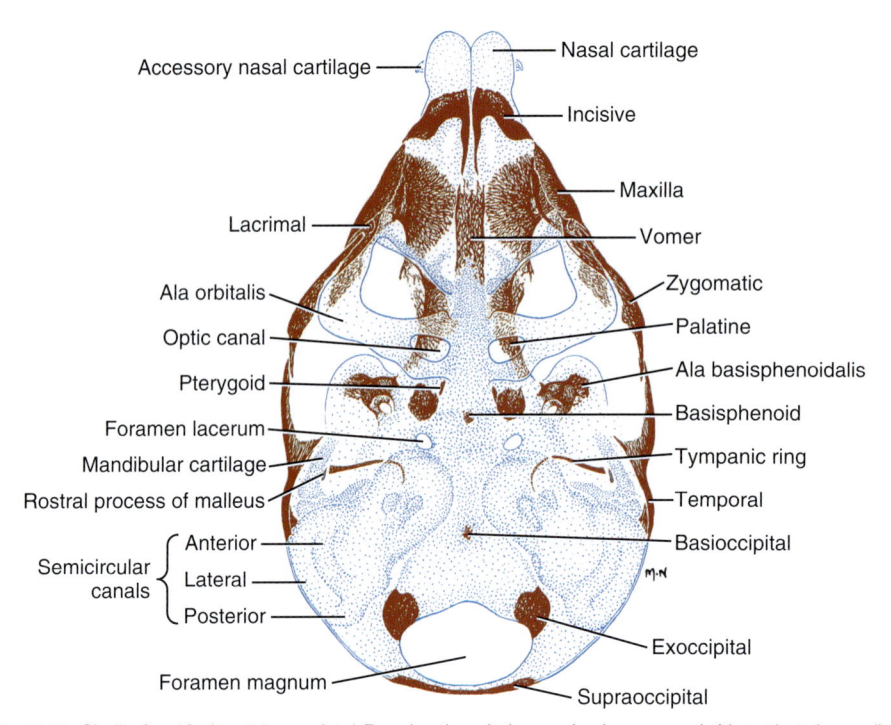

• **Fig. 2.40** Skull of a 40-day, 59-mm fetal Beagle, dorsal view, calvaria removed. Note that the earliest ossifications of the basicranial axis are in the basisphenoid and basioccipital bones.

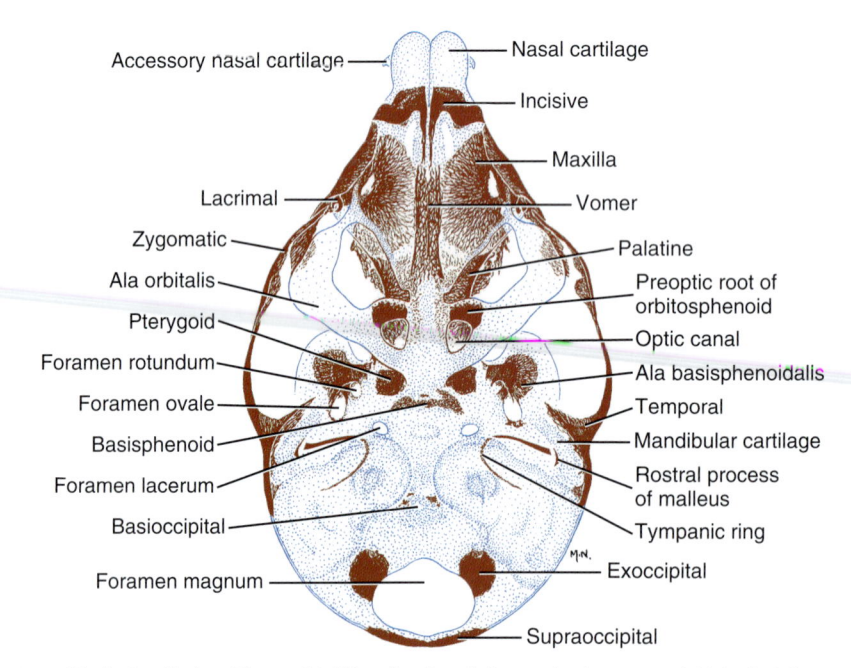

• **Fig. 2.41** Skull of a 40-day, 71-mm fetal Beagle, dorsal view, calvaria removed. Note that the preoptic root of the orbitosphenoid wing has ossified.

CHAPTER 2 Prenatal Development 41

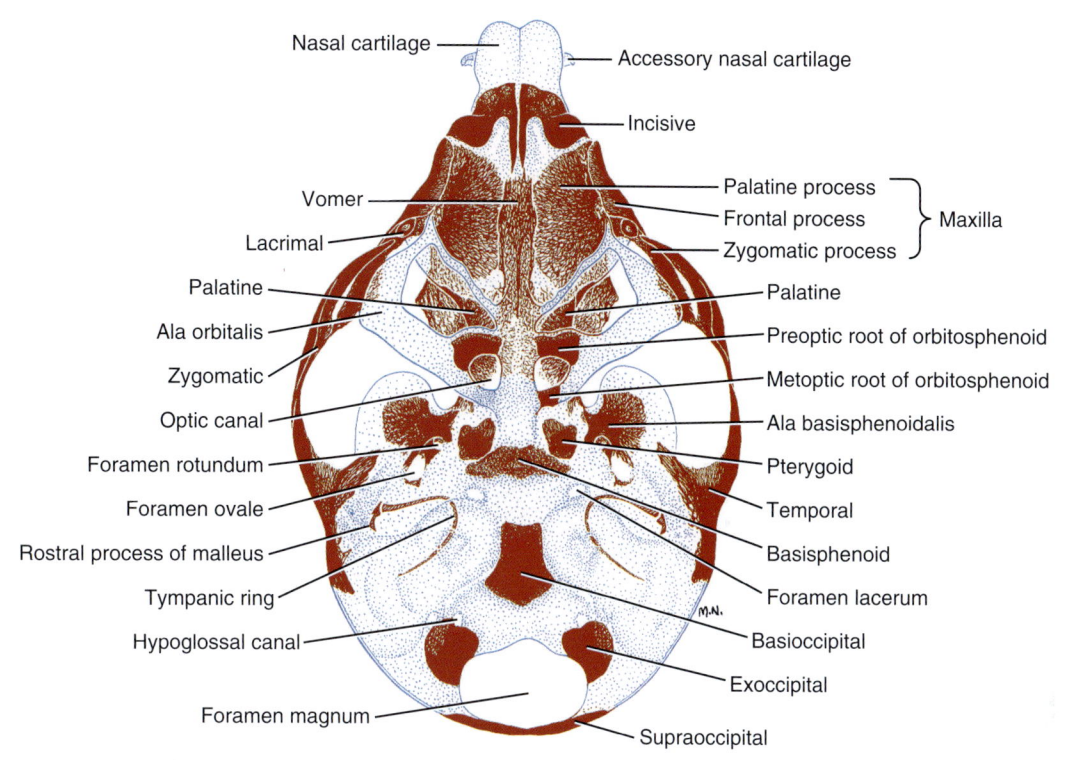

• **Fig. 2.42** Dorsal view of the skull of a 45-day, 73-mm Beagle fetus, calvaria removed. Note the metopic root of the orbitosphenoid on one side.

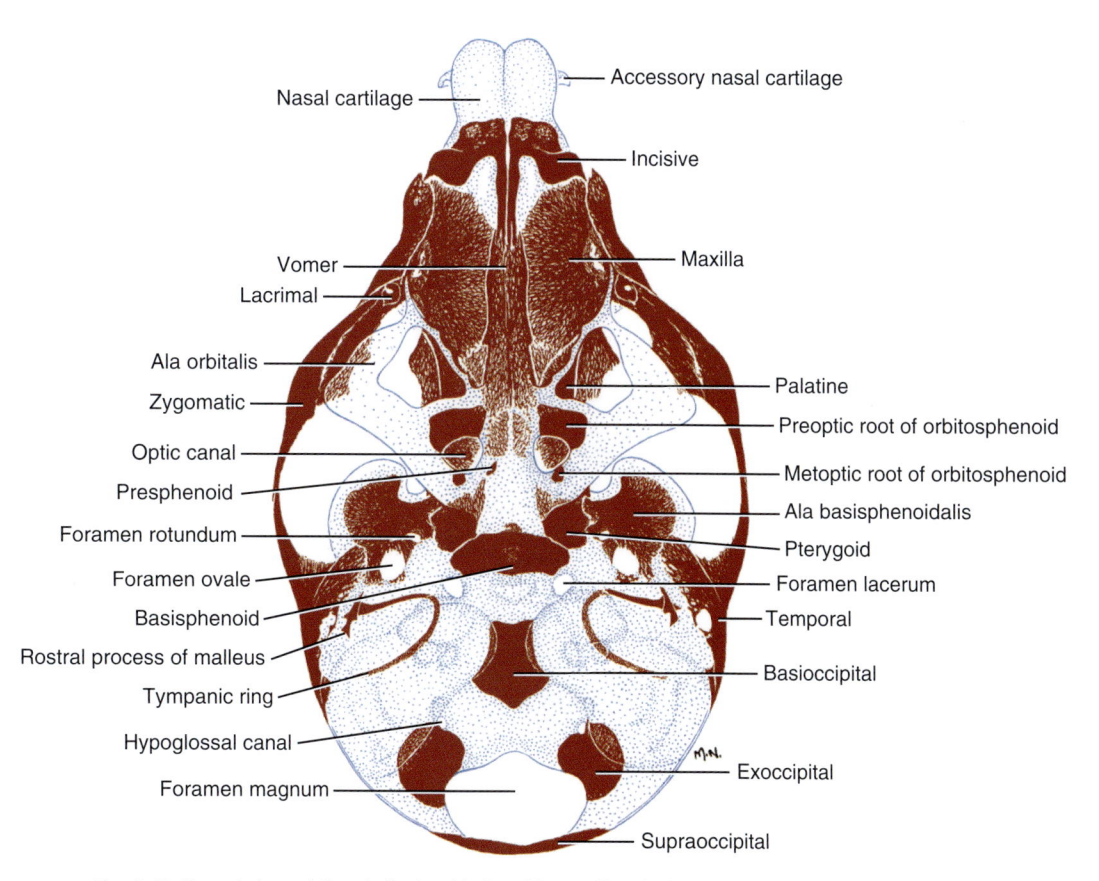

• **Fig. 2.43** Dorsal view of the skull of a 42-day, 88-mm Beagle fetus, calvaria removed. Note the presphenoid on the left side.

42 CHAPTER 2 Prenatal Development

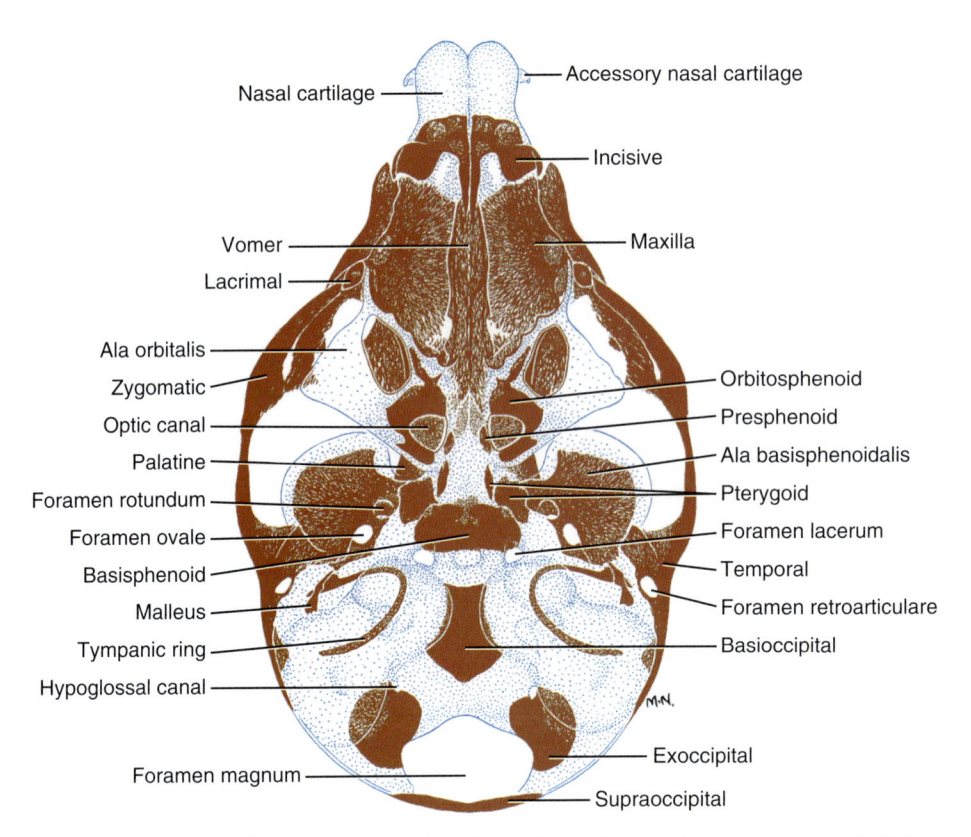

• **Fig. 2.44** Dorsal view of the skull of a 45-day, 92-mm Beagle fetus, calvaria removed. Note that the preoptic and metoptic roots *have fused*, that both presphenoids are present, and that each pterygoid has two ossification centers.

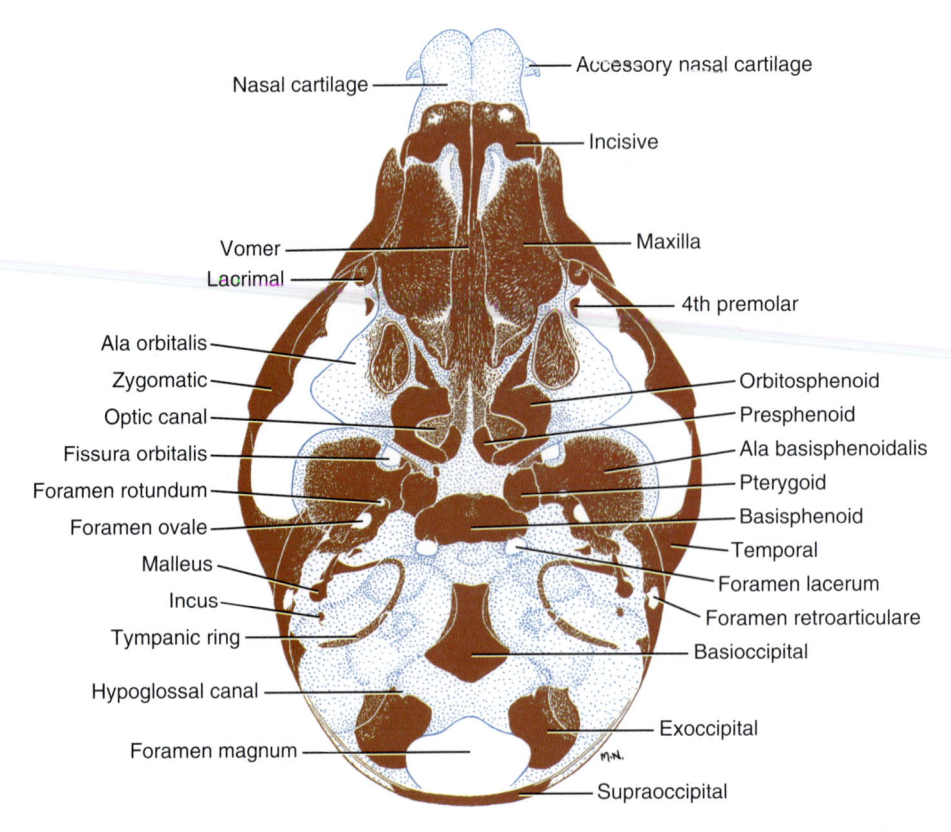

• **Fig. 2.45** Dorsal view of the skull of a 50-day, 105-mm Beagle fetus, calvaria removed. Note that the incus and fourth superior premolar are ossified.

CHAPTER 2 Prenatal Development 43

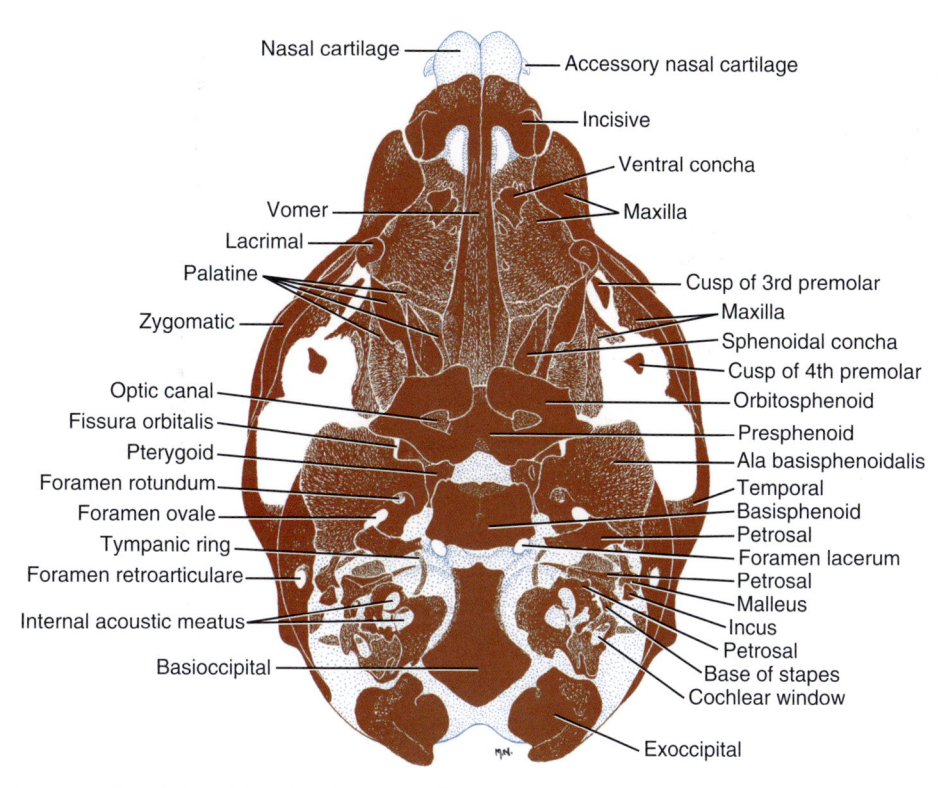

• **Fig. 2.46** Dorsal view of the skull of a 55-day Beagle fetus, calvaria removed. Note the ossifications of the inner ear region. The *ventral nasal* concha is beginning to ossify.

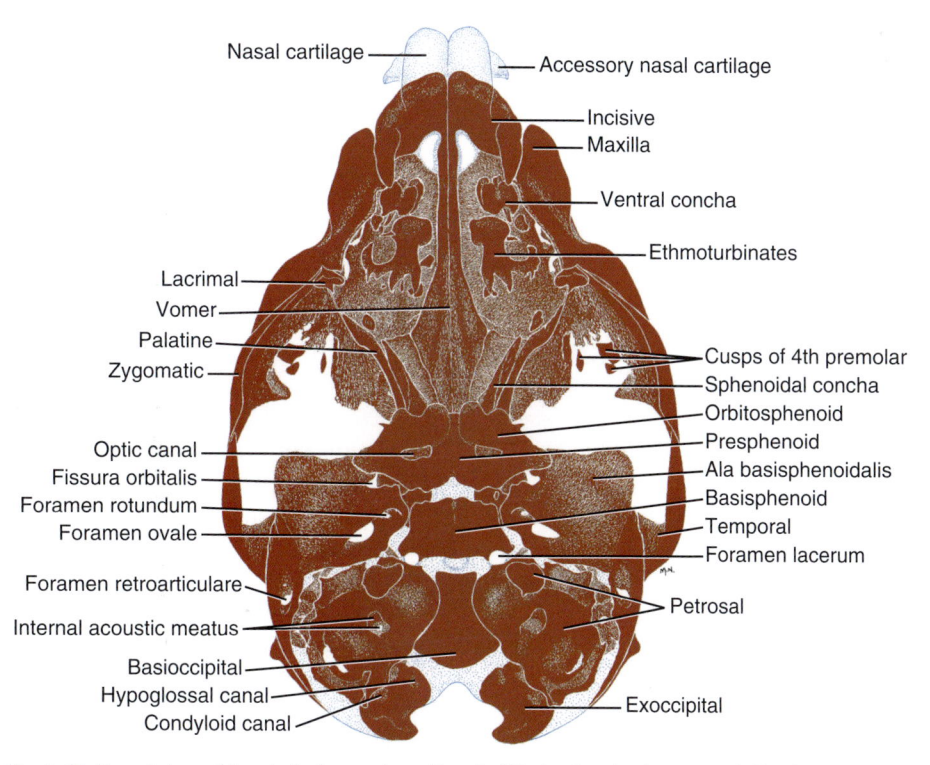

• **Fig. 2.47** Dorsal view of the skull of a newborn Beagle (60 days), calvaria removed. The intersphenoidal synchondrosis and the sphenooccipital synchondrosis are very prominent.

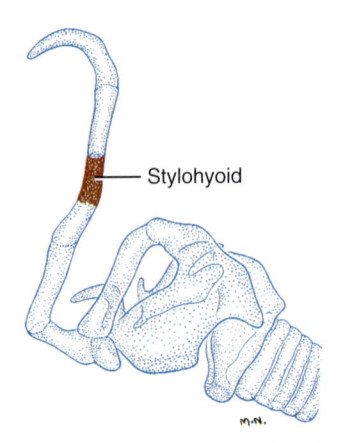

• **Fig. 2.48** The larynx and hyoid apparatus of a 47-day Beagle fetus. Only the stylohyoid is ossified, and only at the midbelly, at this stage of development.

Cd20. The number of caudal vertebrae was a constant 20 in the Beagles studied.

Neural Arches

Neural arch ossification was seen in fetuses from 48 to 58 mm C-R length. The initial bilateral perichondral plaques become bony collars before ossification spreads into the pedicles and laminae prior to birth. Bone forms a little sooner in the axis than in the atlas (see Fig. 2.51).

Paired perichondral neural arch ossifications first appear in the cervical region and increase in a craniocaudal sequence. Their earliest appearance at 38 days (54 mm) shows them to be present from C1 through T7. Rarely do the right or left ossification centers differ in their time of formation. By day 42 (72 mm) the sequence of neural arch ossifications becomes discontinuous because caudal neural arches 5 through 8 show premature ossification before sacrals 1 and 2 or caudals 1 to 4 ossify (see Fig. 2.51). The precocious development of these caudal vertebrae in fetuses between 42 and 45 days may be a response to the developing rectococcygeus muscle, which attaches to the fifth and sixth caudal vertebrae.

The extent of vertebral ossification at 40 days and at birth is shown for each of the regions in Figs. 2.54 to 2.59.

Ribs

All ribs are cartilaginous until day 31, when ribs 3 through 9 begin to ossify at midshaft as perichondral collars. By 40 days the shafts of all ribs are ossified dorsally (see Fig. 2.77B).

Sternum

Evans (1960a, 1960b) investigated the development of the sternum in 67 embryos and fetuses from 18 purebred Beagles.

The sternum consists of eight sternebrae with intervening cartilages to which the ribs attach. In the early embryo (15 mm) a longitudinal mesodermal bar develops on each side in the lateral body wall independent of the ribs and clavicle. As the body wall grows and encloses the pericardial sac, the sternal bars migrate toward the ventral midline, followed closely by the ventral ends of the ribs. By 18 mm (25 days) the sternal bars almost meet at the manubrium but are widely separated caudally (Fig. 2.60). Subsequent growth and fusion of the sternal bars is followed by hypertrophy of the chondroblasts and initiation of ossification in sternal regions between the attachments of the costal cartilages.

The ventral ends of ribs 2 through 7 fuse homogeneously with the sternal bars, whereas the first, eighth, and ninth ribs remain independent of the sternum for a short period. Growth of the body wall allows the sternal bars to unite progressively caudalward with each other on the midline (Fig. 2.61). All evidence of the bilateral nature of the sternal bars is usually lost after fusion of the cartilages occurs and prior to ossification. However, nonunion of the sternal bars in the xiphoid region can result in the presence of a xiphisternal foramen (Figs. 2.61 and 2.62) or widely separated terminal ends (Fig. 2.63) that will never fuse.

The earliest ossifications of the sternum are seen in 40-day (73-mm) fetuses as endochondral centers (Fig. 2.64). Later ossifications (Fig. 2.65) may be either endochondral or perichondral. There is considerable interlitter and intralitter variation in both the manner of ossification and the number of sternebrae ossified at any particular time, even in closely related dogs. Occasionally, the ossification center for the first sternebra is lacking, although the second through sixth are present. The seventh and eighth sternebrae often exhibit eccentric ossification centers in early development (Figs. 2.64 and 2.65). The xiphisternum is the most variable element and may have a foramen, a fissure, or a cleft, depending on the manner of final fusion of the sternal bars.

Chen (1953) demonstrated experimentally that hypertrophy of the chondroblasts and subsequent ossification are inhibited where sternal ribs are attached. Evidence of this phenomenon can be seen in Figs. 2.66 and 2.67, which represents atypical development of the first sternebra caused by the inhibitory effect of an atypical sternal rib. All ossification centers of the sternebrae bear a constant relationship to the attachment of ribs, although a very wide sternum may minimize the inhibitory effect and result in variable fusions of adjacent sternebrae to form a sternal bar or irregular plates.

Limbs and Girdles

The thoracic limb-bud is the first to develop, on about day 23 of gestation, when the embryo is about 5 mm long. It appears as an oval paddle closely attached at midbody (see Fig. 2.10A). The pelvic limb-bud develops about a day later.

On gestational day 25 (14 mm) the thoracic limb shows incipient digit formation in the form of a crenulated

CHAPTER 2 Prenatal Development 45

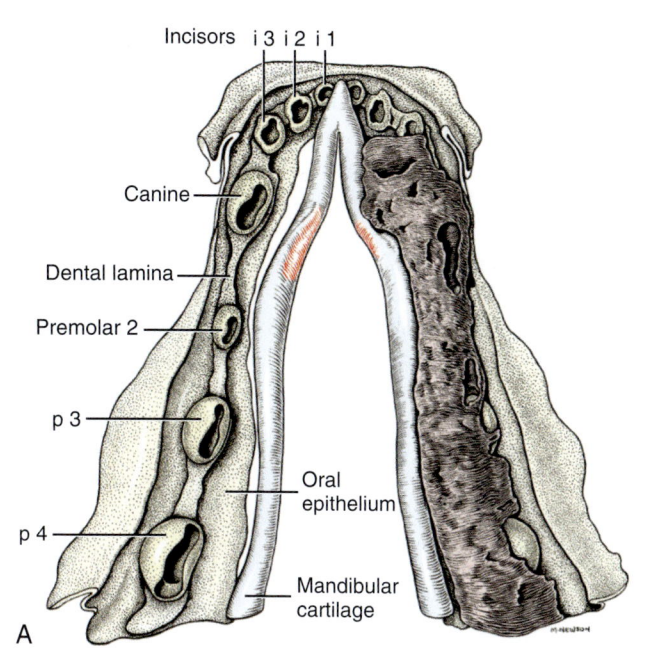

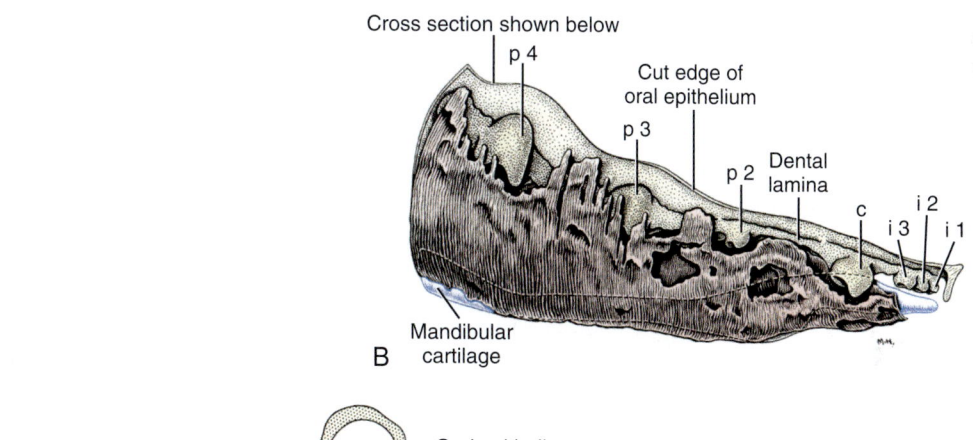

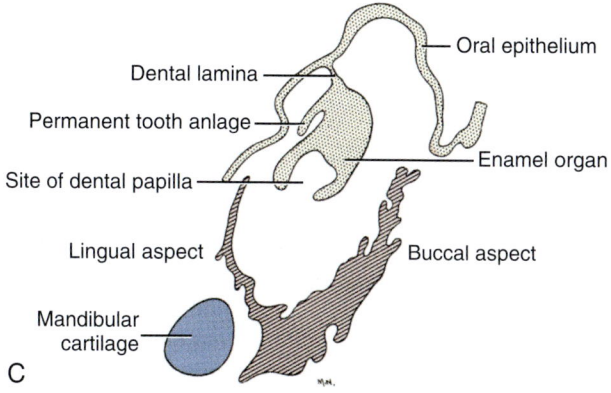

• **Fig. 2.49** The relationship of the enamel organs to the dentary bone and mandibular cartilage. Based on a reconstruction of a 71-mm Beagle fetus. **A**, Ventral view—dentary bone removed on the right side of the fetus. **B**, Lateral view. **C**, Transverse view. (With permission from Williams RC, Evans HE: Prenatal dental development in the dog, *Canis familiaris:* chronology of tooth germ formation and calcification of deciduous teeth, *Zbl Vet Med C Anat Histol Embryol* 7:152–163, 1978.)

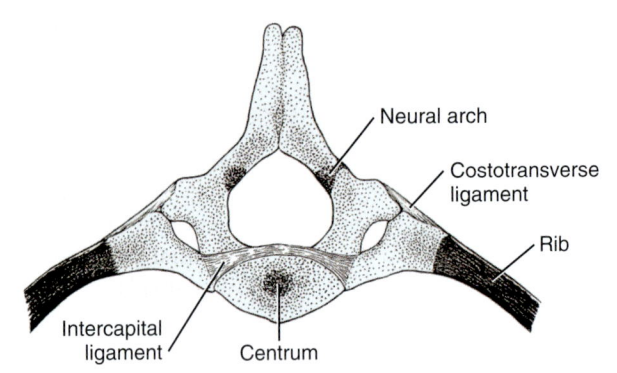

Fig. 2.50 Cranial view of the eighth thoracic vertebra and rib of a 40-day Beagle fetus.

margin of the apical ridge (see Fig. 2.11C). On day 28 the clavicle ossifies as one of the first four bones to appear in the embryo. (The others are the mandible, maxilla, and frontal.)

By gestational day 30 the thoracic limb has lengthened and pronated, and its digits are distinct. The pelvic limb at 30 days resembles the thoracic limb of 5 days earlier (see Fig. 2.12B). A further increase in the size and length of the limbs by day 35 (35 mm) delimits the joints and produces well-formed digits with developing claws. At this time perichondral ossification of the long bones begins at midshaft in both limbs and results in primary bone

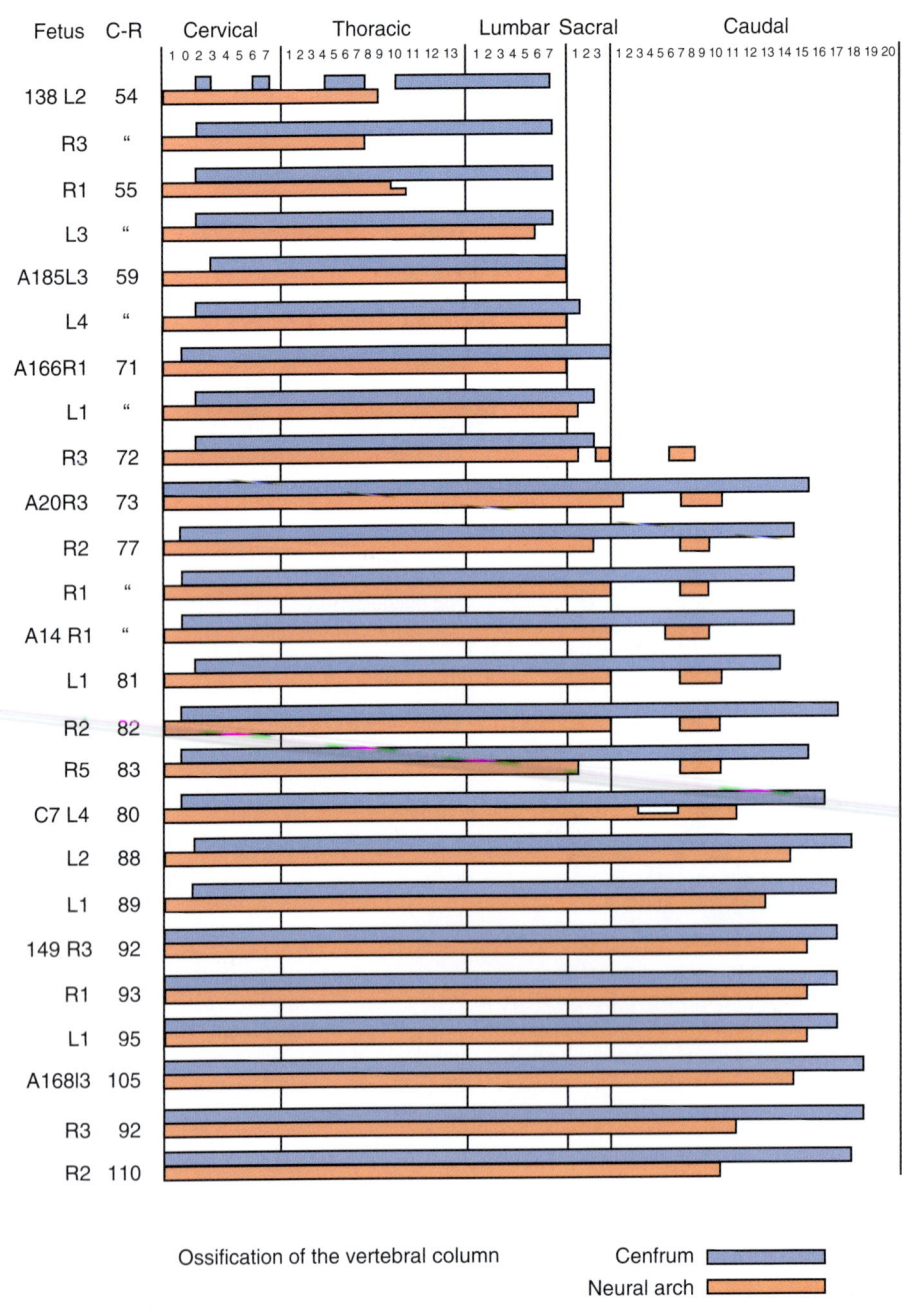

Fig. 2.51 Histogram of vertebral ossifications within several litters of purebred Beagles. (From Evans HE: *Prenatal development of the dog*, Ithaca, NY, 1974, 24th Gaines Veterinary Symposium.)

CHAPTER 2 Prenatal Development 47

collars without endochondral involvement (Fig. 2.68A to H).

The scapula at 35 days has three perichondral ossification centers: (1) a triangular area on the cranial margin of the supraspinous fossa, (2) a short bar at the midpoint of the scapula spine, and (3) a plaque in the central area of the infraspinous fossa. All three ossification centers join by day 40 and form a continuous perichondral collar around the scapula, although there is a distinct triangular region on the cranial edge of the supraspinous fossa that persists until birth (Figs. 2.69 and 2.70).

The clavicle (Figs. 2.68 to 2.71) originates as a comma-shaped "membrane" bone in the tendinous intersection of the brachiocephalicus muscle on day 28 and increases in size by the addition of bone formed in secondary cartilage. It continues to grow in size after birth as a thin plaque rather than as the hooklike nodule of earlier stages.

The humerus, radius, and ulna do not form epiphyses prior to birth. Although all of the metacarpals and

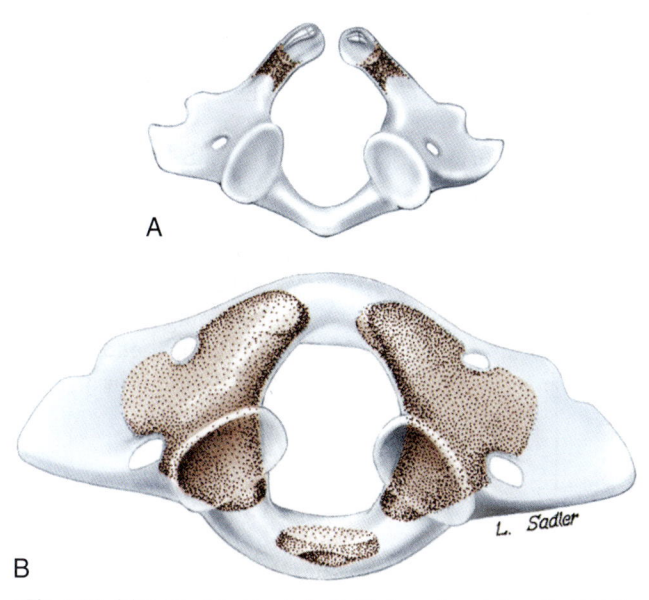

• **Fig. 2.52** Atlas, caudal aspect. **A,** At 40 days of gestation. **B,** At birth.

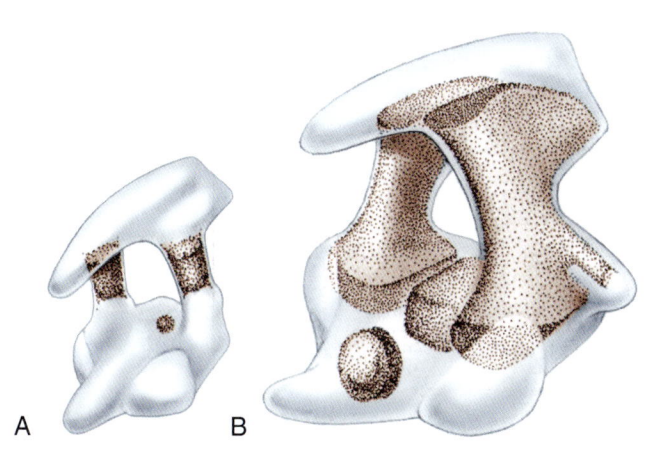

• **Fig. 2.53** Axis, craniolateral aspect. **A,** At 40 days of gestation. **B,** At birth.

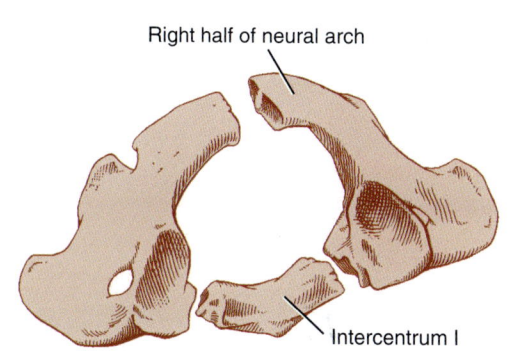

• **Fig. 2.54** The three components of the atlas of an 80-day-old Beagle pup. Intercentrum I will become the body of the atlas. (From Watson AG: *The phylogeny and development of the atlas-axis complex in the dog,* Thesis, Ithaca, NY, 1981, Cornell University.)

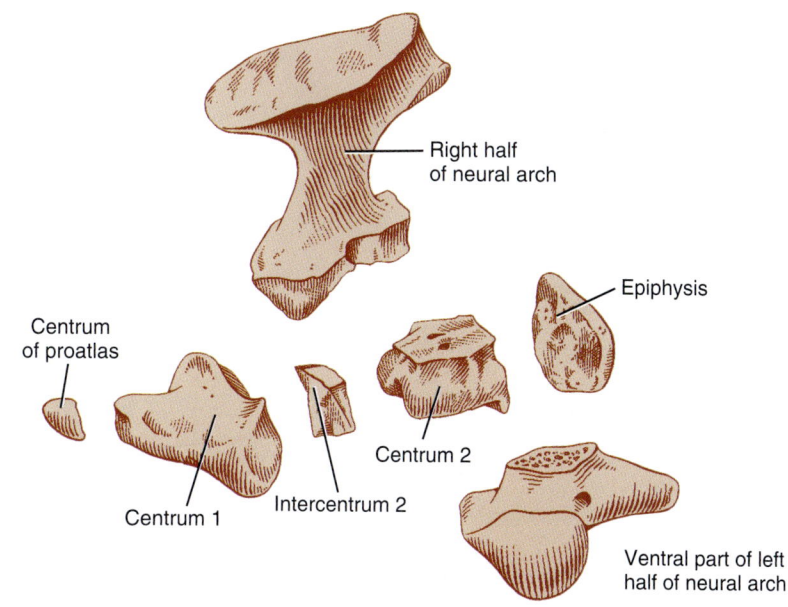

• **Fig. 2.55** The seven components of the axis of an 80-day-old Beagle pup. (From Watson AG: *The phylogeny and development of the atlas-axis complex in the dog,* Thesis, Ithaca, NY, 1981, Cornell University.)

48 CHAPTER 2 Prenatal Development

• **Fig. 2.56** Third cervical vertebra, cranial aspect. **A**, At 40 days of gestation. **B**, At birth.

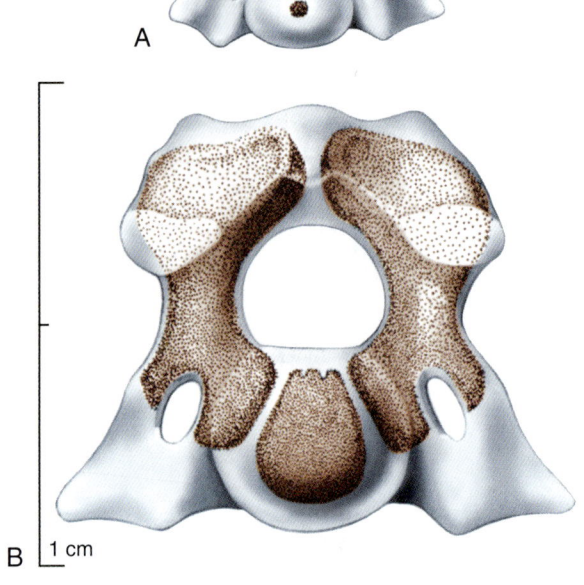

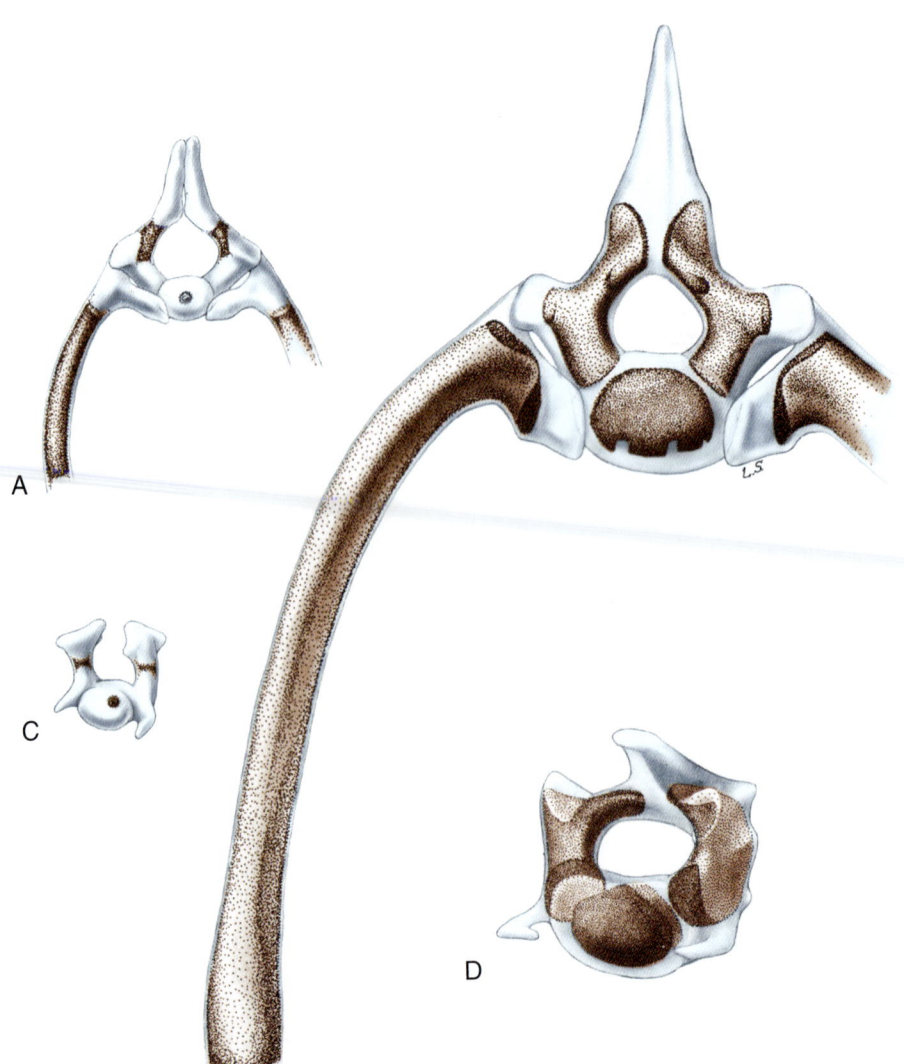

• **Fig. 2.57** Cranial aspect of fourth thoracic vertebra. **A**, At 40 days of gestation. **B**, At birth. Craniolateral aspect of fourth lumbar vertebra. **C**, At 40 days. **D**, At birth.

CHAPTER 2 Prenatal Development 49

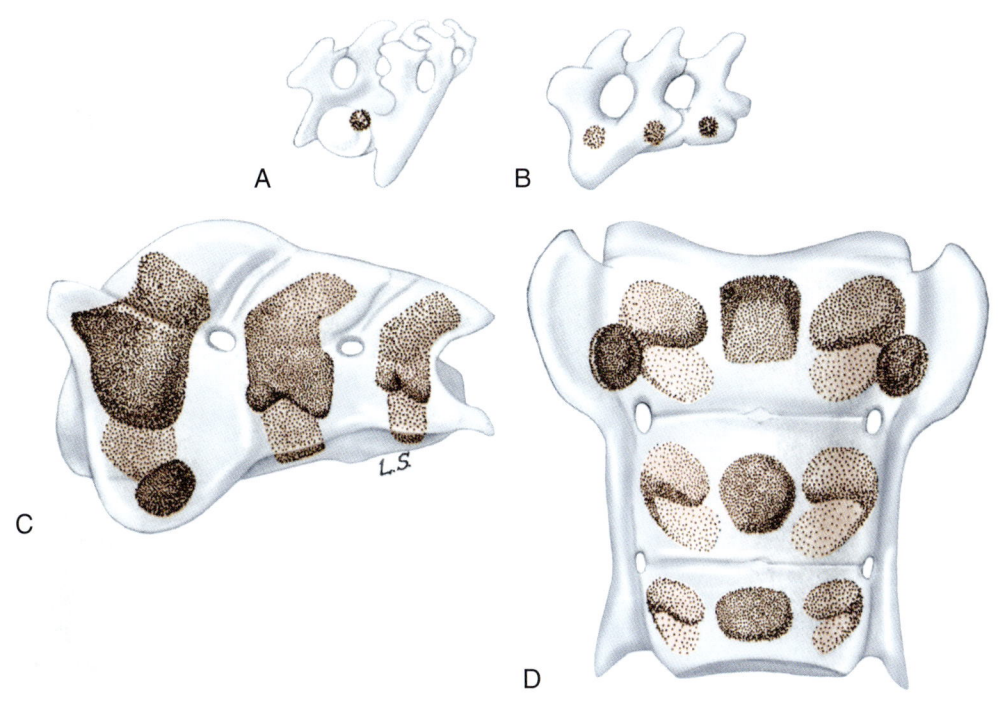

• **Fig. 2.58** The sacrum at 40 days. **A,** Craniolateral aspect. **B,** Left lateral aspect. The sacrum at birth. **C,** Left lateral aspect. **D,** Ventral aspect. (Note the ossified nodule on each side of the first sacral vertebra. This is a remnant sacral "rib.")

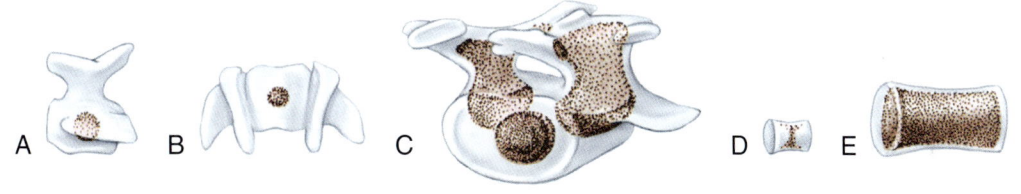

• **Fig. 2.59** Caudal vertebrae. **A,** First caudal vertebra, 40 days, lateral aspect. **B,** First caudal vertebra, 40 days, dorsal aspect. **C,** First caudal vertebra at birth, craniolateral aspect. **D,** Fifth caudal vertebra, 40 days, craniolateral aspect. **E,** Tenth caudal vertebra, at birth, craniolateral aspect.

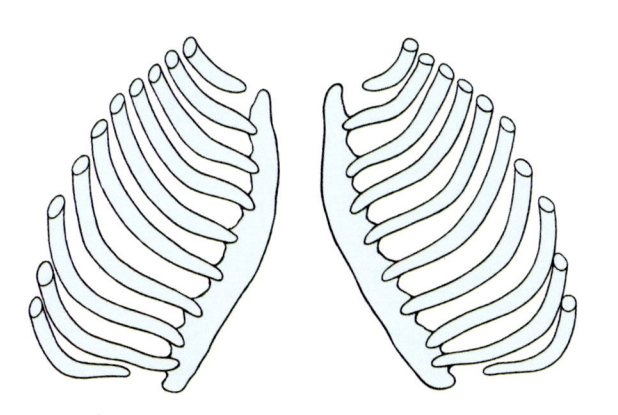

• **Fig. 2.60** Sternal bars and ribs of a 25-day Beagle fetus. Dorsal view.

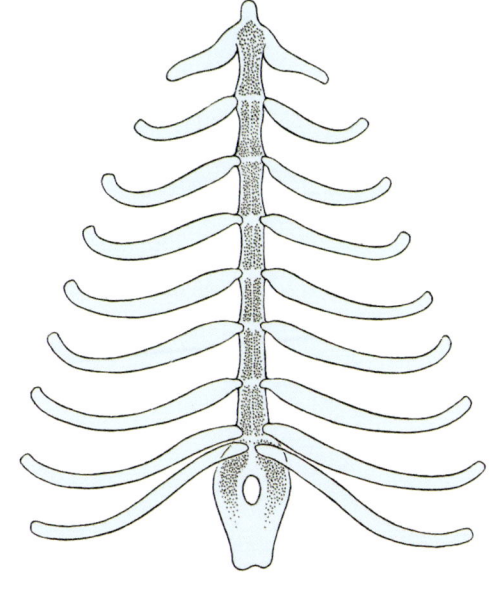

• **Fig. 2.61** Evidence of the bilateral origin of the sternum can still be seen after fusion of right and left sternal bars.

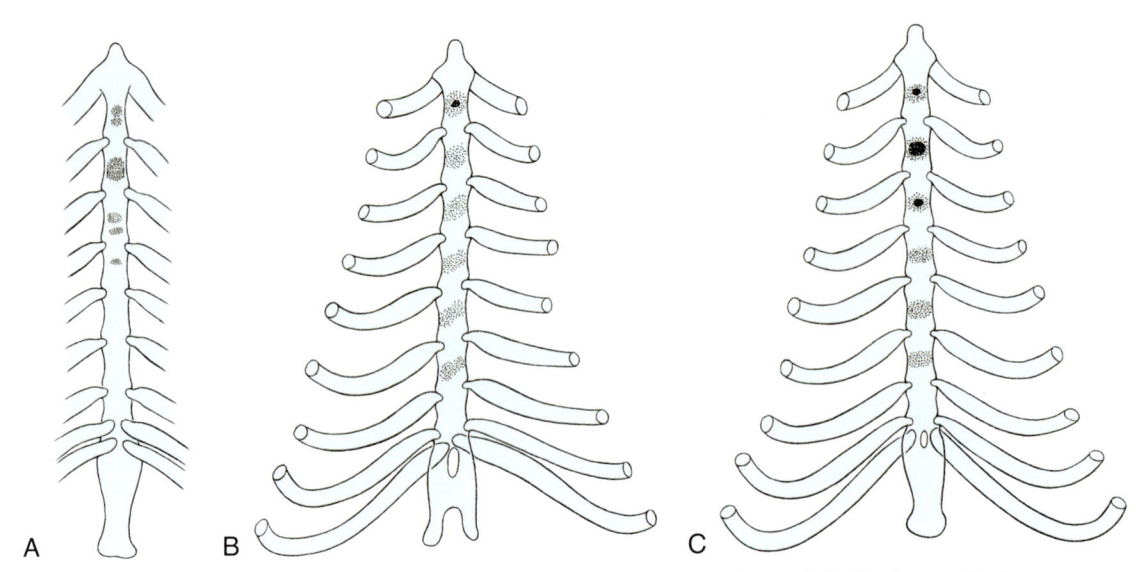

Fig. 2.62 Ossification of sternebrae at about 40 days of gestation (72 mm). **A,** The first ossifications may be single or in tandem. **B** and **C** are fetal-mates showing endochondral ossifications. In **B**, the sternal ossifications are oblique owing to the uneven placement of the ribs, which inhibit ossification. In **C**, the ossification centers are normal, as are the ribs.

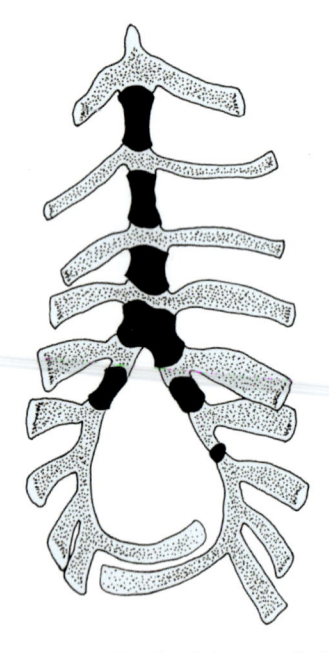

Fig. 2.63 Widely separated ends of the nonunited sternal bars can result in an anomalous infracostal arch.

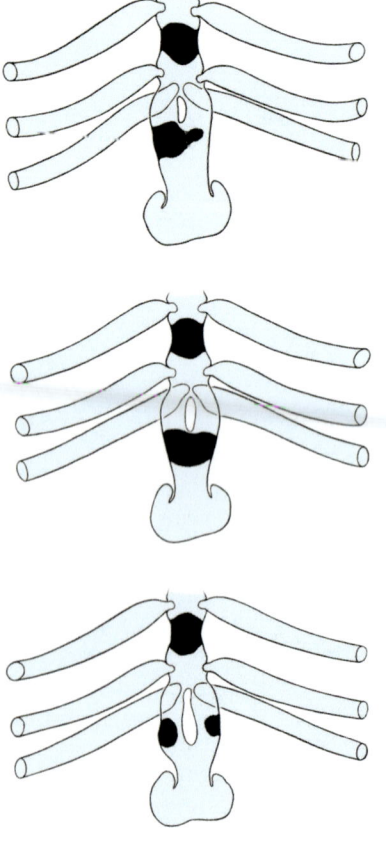

Fig. 2.64 Fetal-mates at 55 days of gestation (138 to 150 mm crown-rump length) showing differences in the pattern of ossification of the xiphisternum.

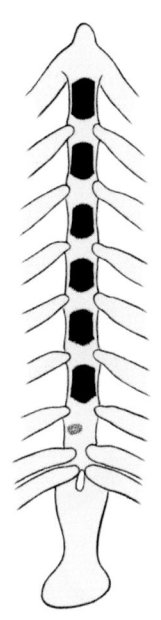

• **Fig. 2.65** The endochondral ossification center for the seventh sternebra in this 50-day Beagle fetus (110 mm) is eccentric.

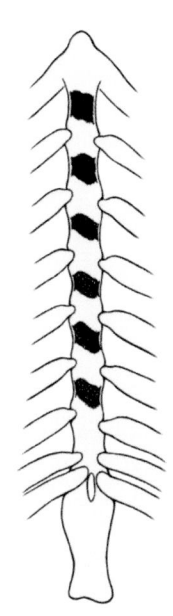

• **Fig. 2.67** Diagonal ossification centers due to uneven apposition of ribs.

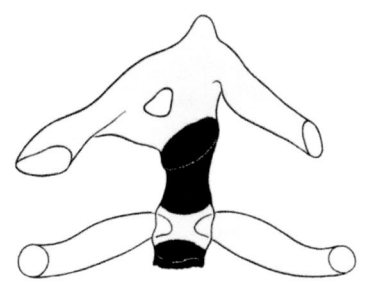

• **Fig. 2.66** Inhibition of ossification of the first sternebra due to an anomalous first rib.

phalanges are ossified by the end of gestation, none of the carpals ossifies fully prior to birth (see Figs. 2.69 to 2.71).

The pelvic girdle is completely cartilaginous until day 40, when a perichondral bone collar develops around the ilium (Fig. 2.72). Several days later (day 45) the ischium ossifies (Fig. 2.73), and, shortly before or at birth (day 55 to 60), pubic centers appear (Fig. 2.74; see also Smith, 1964). An analysis of small-sized dogs suggest that the pubis may ossify relatively later, perhaps during the third week postnatally (Modina et al., 2017). The acetabular bone does not appear until several weeks after birth.

The femur, tibia, and fibula ossify perichondrally at first, as do the metatarsals and phalanges. A cartilaginous patella is present in the tendon of the quadriceps muscle throughout the second half of gestation. Only the talus and calcaneus ossify before birth in the tarsus.

The forepaw and hindpaw show intra- and interlitter variations of the metapodials as to their presence, duplication, and time of ossification. Metapodials 3 and 4 are followed closely by 2, 5, and 1. All of the phalanges ossify in the typical mammalian sequence of distal, then proximal, then middle phalanx (Figs. 2.70, 2.71, and 2.73 through 2.75). Digits 2 and 3 are the first to ossify.

Carpus

Reconstructed serial sections of the carpus of a 35-mm C-R length Beagle fetus showed that the radiale and intermedium of the embryonic carpus had fused to form an intermedioradial carpal cartilage (see Fig. 2.69), but the central carpal was still distinct. At some later stage the central carpal fuses with the combined radial carpal plus the intermediate carpal. Thus by 55-mm C-R length (42 days of gestation), if not before, there are only seven carpal cartilages: a proximal row consisting of intermedioradial, ulnar, and accessory; and a distal row of carpals 1 to 4. By 55 mm the only bones in the forepaw are metacarpals 2, 3, 4, and 5, which have perichondral ossifications at midshaft (see Fig. 2.69). The next ossifications to be seen are distal phalanges by 59 mm, followed by proximal phalanges at 71 mm, and middle phalanges at 80 mm (see Fig. 2.75).

See Table 2.5 for a summary of the morphologic events during the third trimester of development.

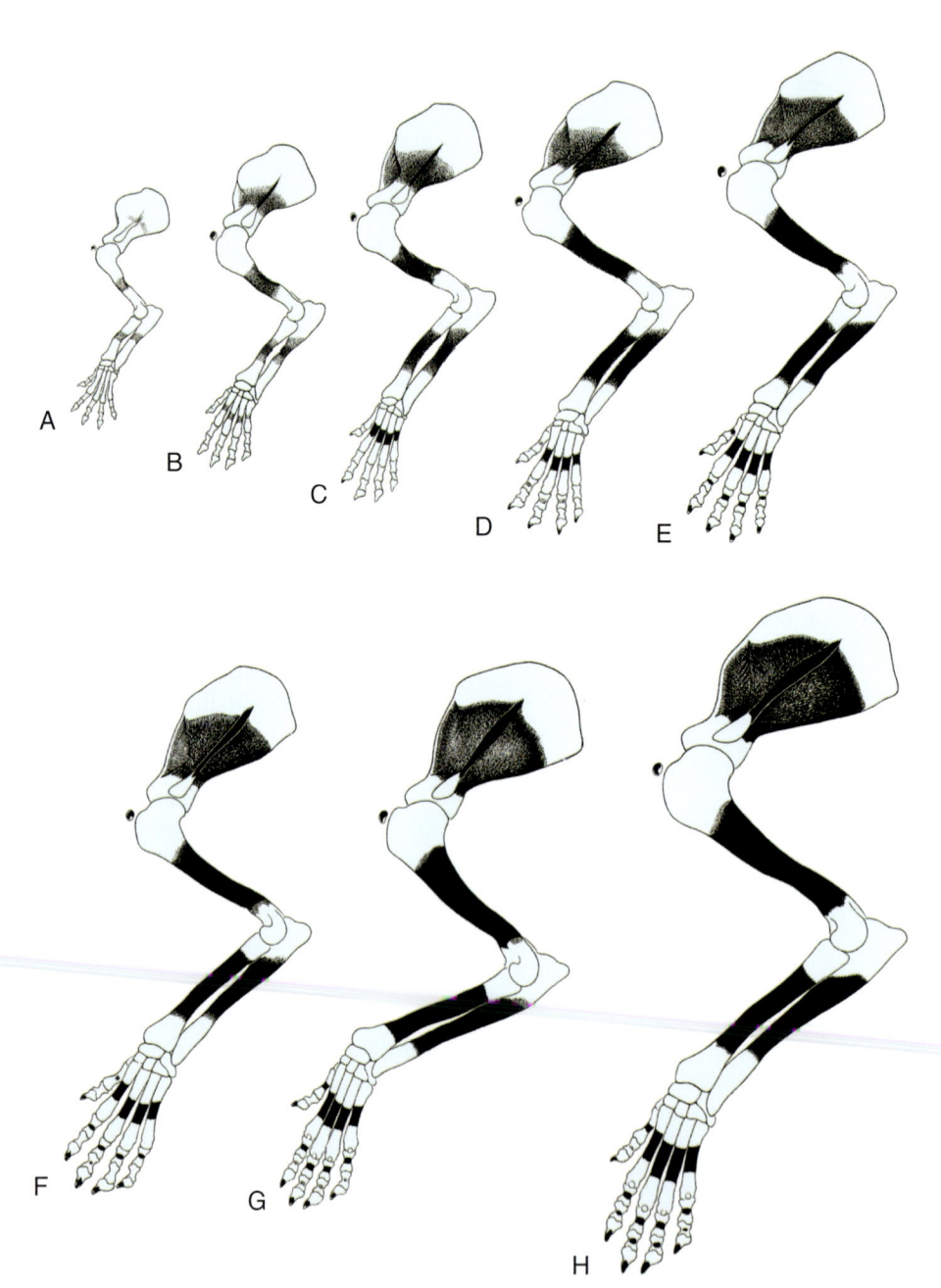

• **Fig. 2.68** A to H, Progressive ossification (dark shading) of the thoracic limb and girdle.

CHAPTER 2 Prenatal Development 53

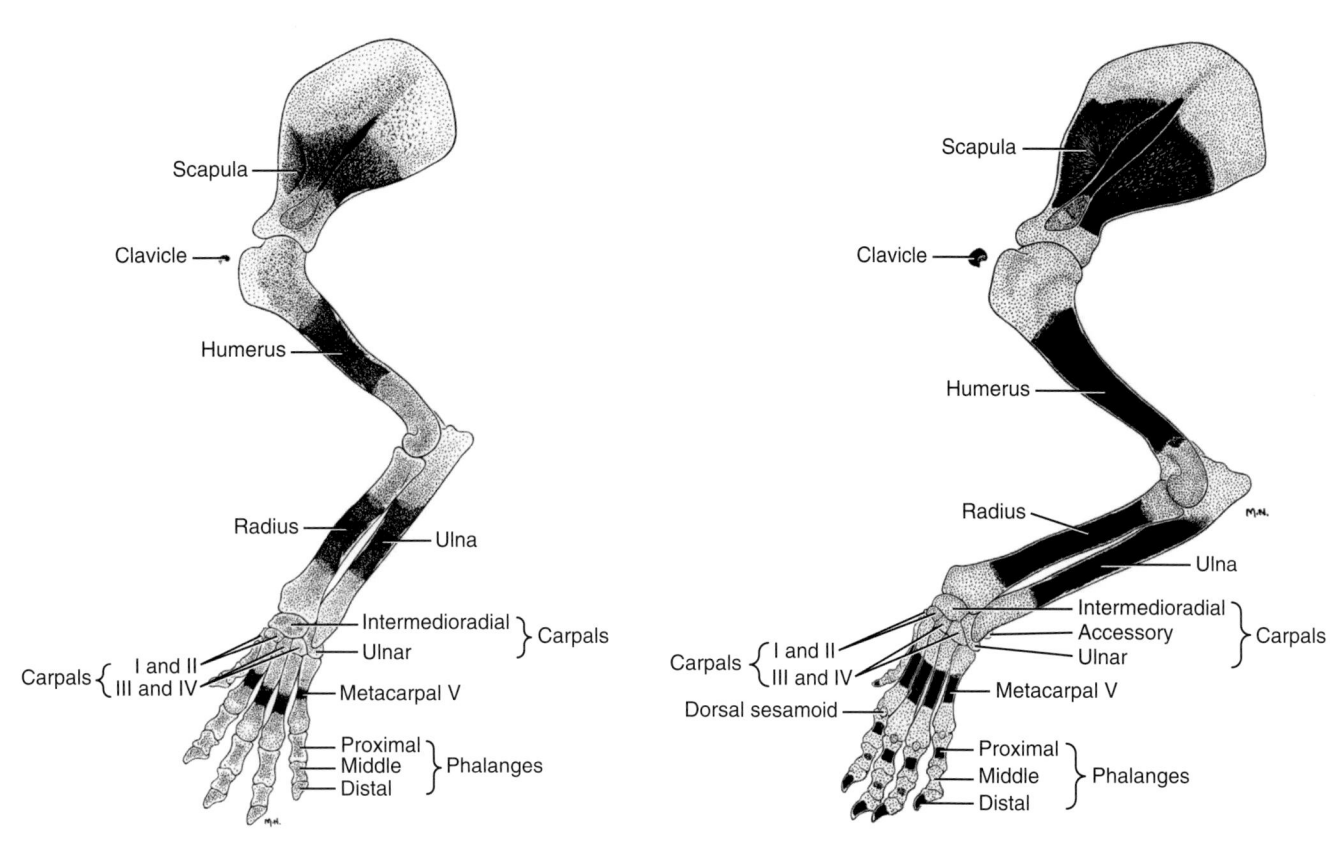

- **Fig. 2.69** The pectoral girdle and limb of a 55-mm (42-day) Beagle fetus. There are no ossifications in the carpus or digits.

- **Fig. 2.70** The pectoral girdle and limb of a 93-mm (45-day) Beagle fetus. The distal phalanges of all digits are ossified as well as the proximal phalanges of digits 2 through 5. Of the middle phalanges, only 2, 3, and 4 show small endochondral centers.

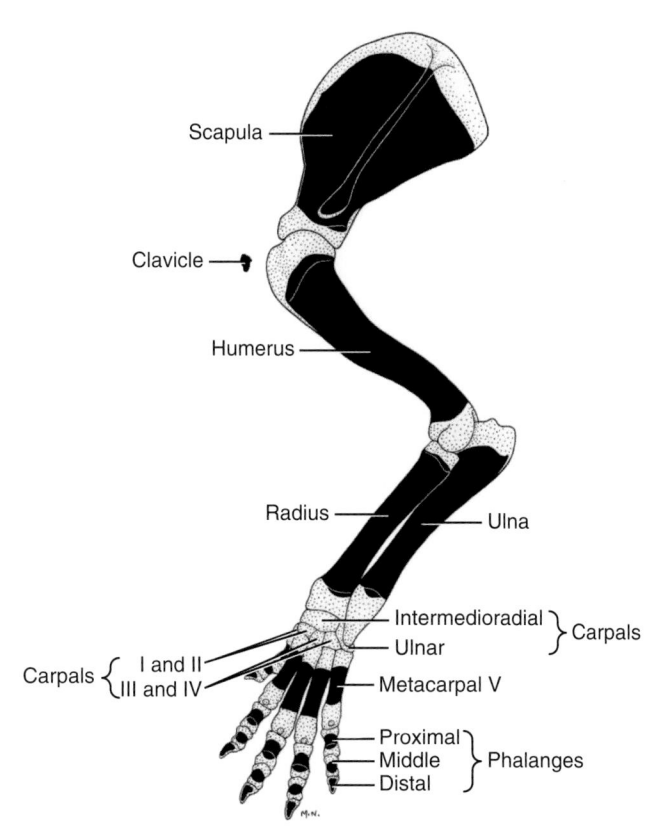

- **Fig. 2.71** The thoracic limb and girdle at birth (60 days).

54 CHAPTER 2 **Prenatal Development**

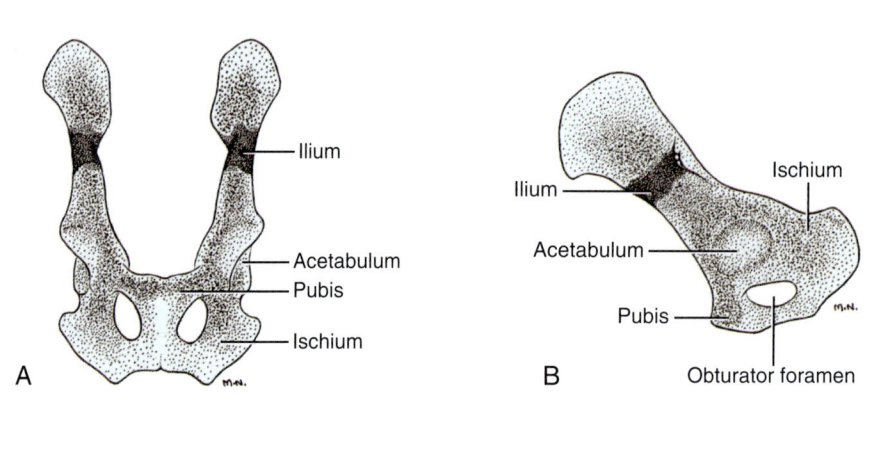

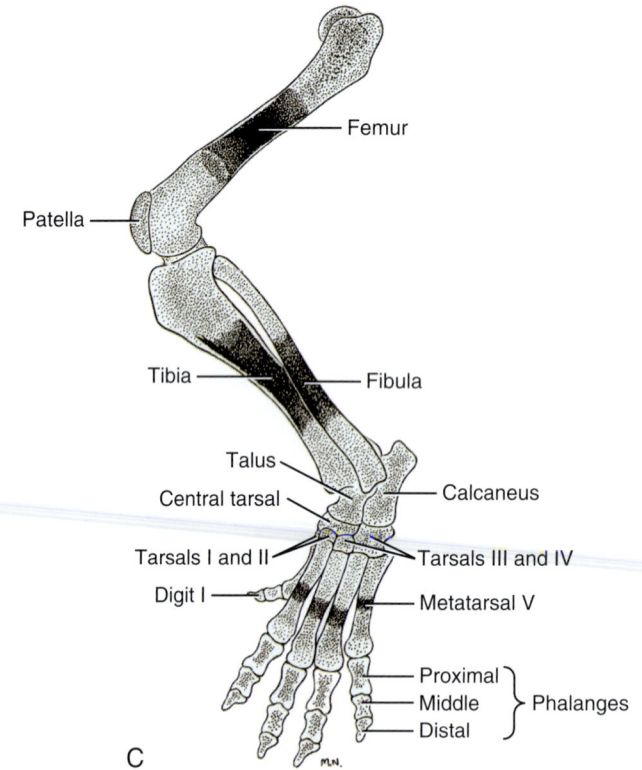

• **Fig. 2.72** Ossification of the pelvic limb and girdle on the fortieth day of gestation in the Beagle. **A**, Ventral view of pelvis. **B**, Lateral view of pelvis. **C**, Laterodorsal view of pelvic limb.

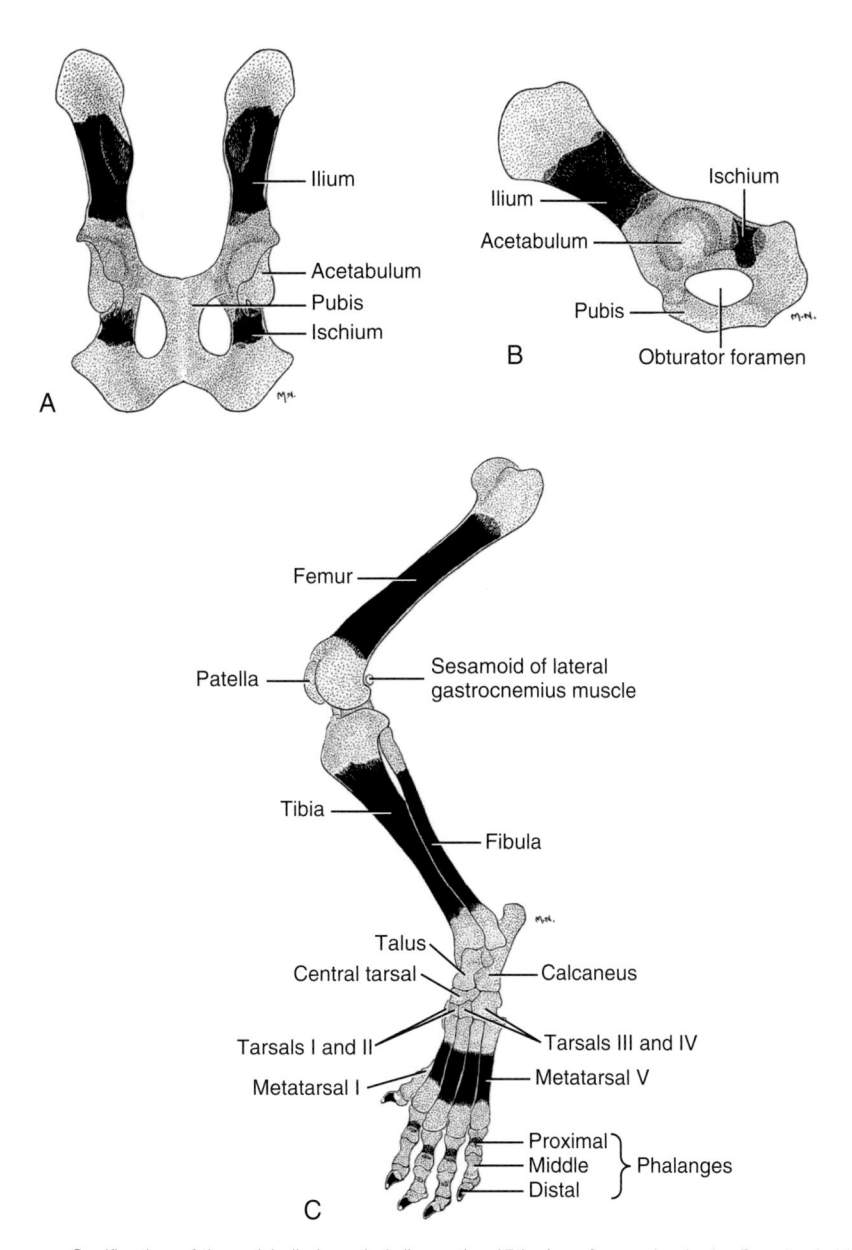

• **Fig. 2.73** Ossification of the pelvic limb and girdle on the 45th day of gestation in the Beagle. **A,** Ventral view of pelvis. **B,** Lateral view of pelvis. **C,** Laterodorsal view of pelvic limb.

56 CHAPTER 2　Prenatal Development

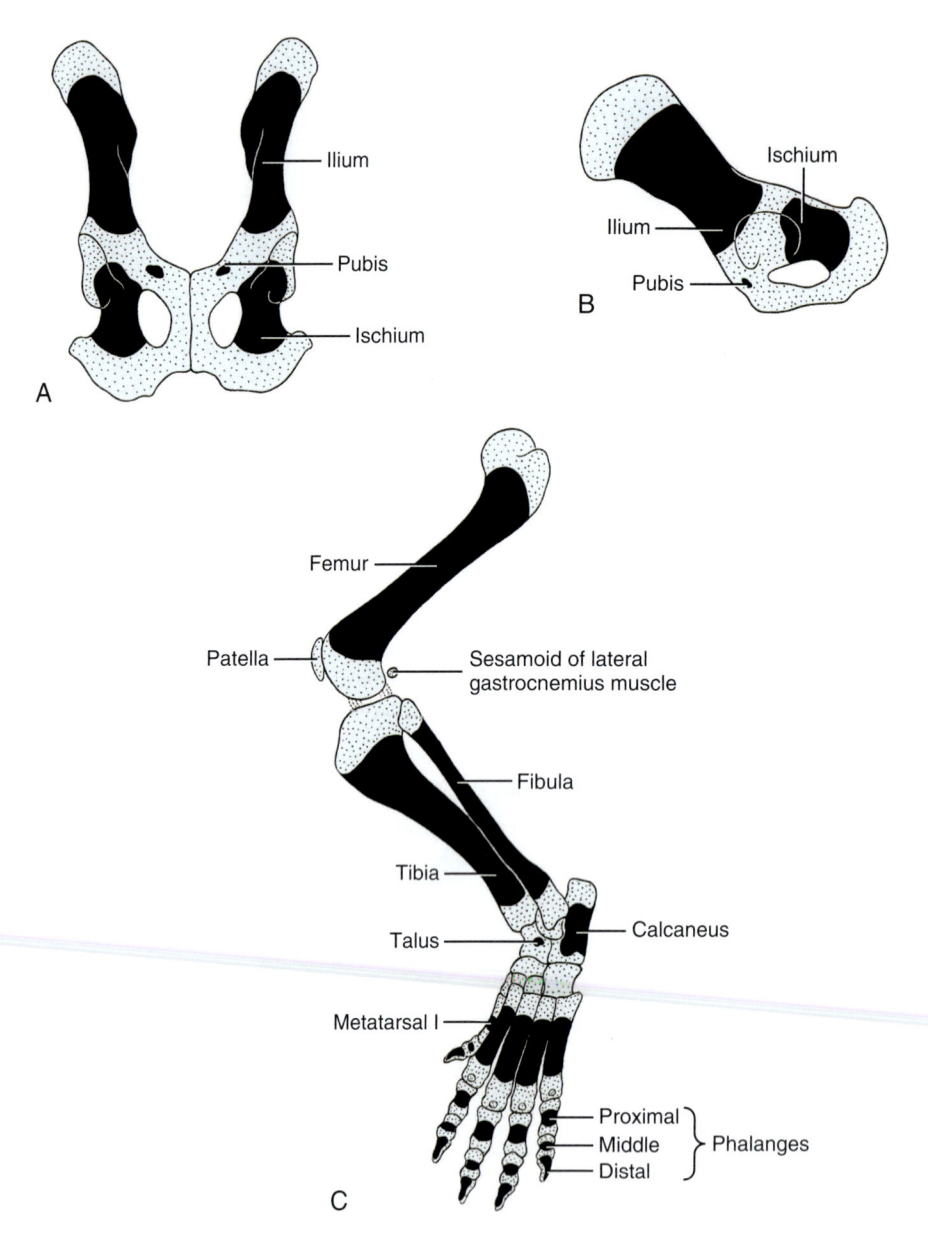

• **Fig. 2.74** Ossification of the pelvic limb and girdle in the Beagle, at birth (60 days). **A**, Ventral view of the pelvis. **B**, Lateral view of the pelvis. **C**, Laterodorsal view of the pelvic limb.

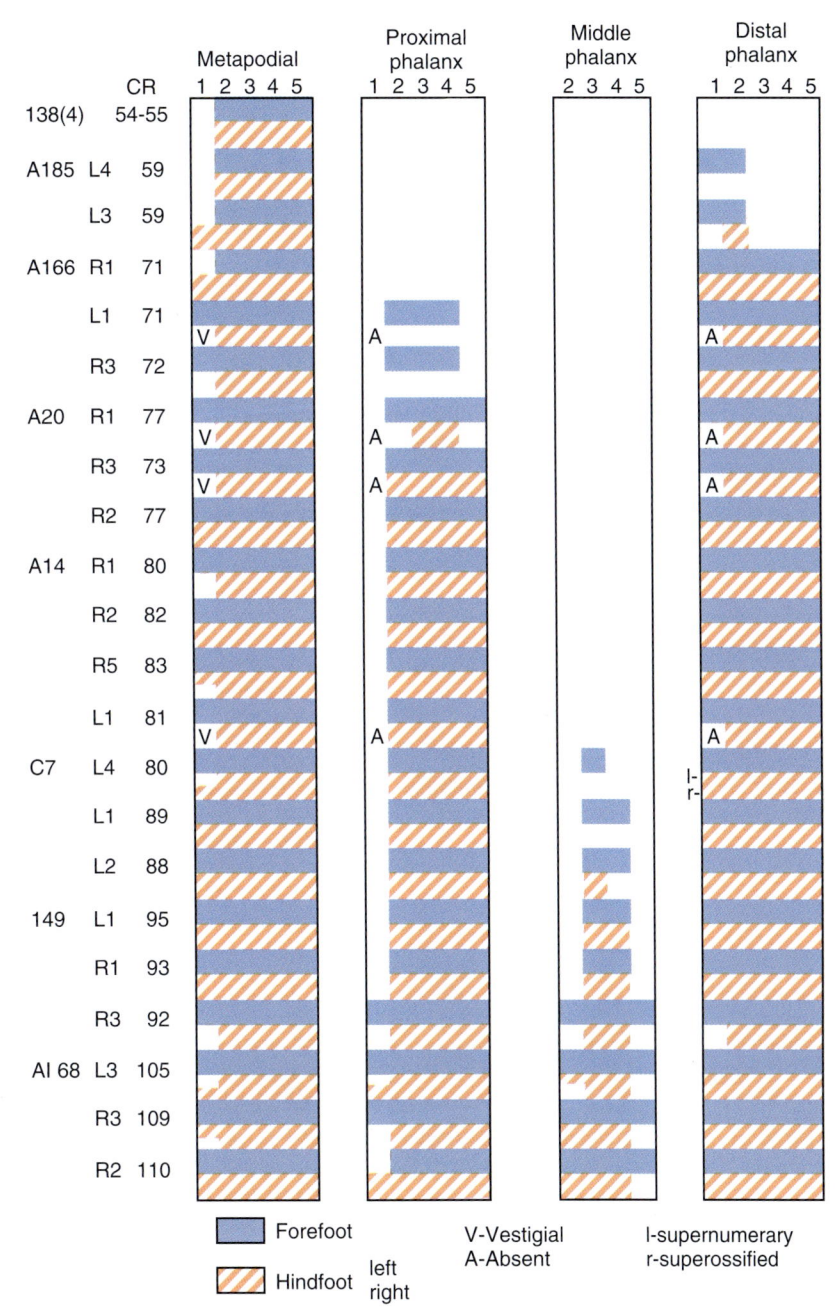

- **Fig. 2.75** Histogram of the sequence of ossification in the metapodials and phalanges. Increasing crown-rump length is indicated from top (youngest) to bottom (oldest). (From Evans HE: *Prenatal development of the dog,* Ithaca, NY, 1974, 24th Gaines Veterinary Symposium.)

TABLE 2.5 Summary of Morphologic Events During the Third Trimester of Development

	Bitch	Fetus
35 Days (Fig. 2.76)	Uterine swellings 43 × 74 mm, width of placenta equal to length of fetus.	35 mm; eyelids developing so that eye is almost covered; pinna covers ear opening; sex determination possible externally; sternal bars united on midline; ossification of temporal, pterygoid, and lacrimal bones; scapula and ribs 2 through 13 are ossified at midshaft.
37 Days		47 mm; ossification of supraoccipital and temporal wing of basisphenoid; first rib neural arches C1 through C4; metacarpals 2, 3, and 4; ilium at midshaft.
38 Days		53 mm; ossification of exoccipital, vomer, tympanic ring, malleus, and midportion of mandibular cartilage; vertebral centra C2 through L6; vertebral arches C1 through T8; metacarpals 1 through 5 and metatarsals 2 through 5.
39 Days		60 mm; ossification of orbital wing of presphenoid; basisphenoid; and basioccipital; central C2 through S1, arches C1 through S1; distal phalanges of digits 1 and 2 of forepaw and digit 2 of hindpaw.
40 Days (Fig. 2.77)	Uterine swellings 54 × 81 mm; width of placenta approximately equal to the length of fetus; a firm cervical plug is formed.	65 mm; eyes closed and lids fused; umbilical hernia eliminated; claws formed on all digits.
42 Days		70 mm; ossification of dens of axis; caudal vertebral centra 6 through 11; sternebrae 1 through 5; distal phalanges 1 through 5 in both paws; proximal phalanges 3 and 4 in both paws.
43 Days		76 mm; ossification of body of atlas (intercentrum 1); caudal vertebral centra 1 through 14, arches 6 through 8; sternebrae 1 through 7; proximal phalanges 1 through 5 in forepaw, 2 through 5 in hindpaw.
45 Days (Fig. 2.78)	Uterine swellings less distinct from one another; uterus bent upon itself to conform with available space in the abdomen; width of placenta less than the length of fetus.	86 mm; color markings appear, and body hair begins to grow; scrotal swellings are large, and labia are prominent; calcification of mandibular premolars; interparietal bone ossifies independently and then fuses with the supraoccipital; ossification of presphenoid; vertebral centra C1 through Cd17, arches C1 through S3, Cd2 through Cd4, Cd9 through Cd13; middle phalanges 3 and 4 of forepaw; phalanx 3 of hindpaw; ischium.
50 Days (Figs. 2.79 2.81)	The uterus has enlarged to such a degree that individual swellings are no longer apparent; adjacent fetuses are in contact.	107 mm; body well proportioned; caudal nipples of male involute as penile structures grow cranially; ossification of lateral ethmoid, petrosal, incus, stylohyoid; vertebral centra and arches C1 through Cd18; sternebrae 1 through 8; all metacarpals and phalanges of forepaw.
55 Days	The uterus is very large, and the fetuses can move freely within the placental band.	144 mm; all deciduous teeth show calcification, and mandibular first molar calcifies (a permanent tooth); ossification of thyrohyoid and epihyoid; sacral "ribs" 1 and 2; all vertebral arches and centra; all metapodials and phalanges; pubis; calcaneus. 150 mm; ossification of basihyoid; sacral wing of S1; talus.

TABLE 2.5	Summary of Morphologic Events During the Third Trimester of Development—cont'd	
	Bitch	**Fetus**
60–63 Days: Whelping (Parturition)	Restless, prepares bed, cervix dilates, fetal movement apparent. Corpora lutea are the source of progesterone and are required for the maintenance of pregnancy throughout gestation in the dog. Concannon et al. (1977) and Concannon (1991) found that progesterone levels of more than 5 ng/mL prevent normal parturition. The levels in pregnant bitches decline rapidly 36 to 48 hours prior to parturition, and no pups are born until levels are less than 2 ng/mL. Kim et al. (2007) reviewed the methods used for timing canine gestational age. Their study evaluated pregnancies of 63 bitches from 19 breeds. The most reliable key was the preovulatory luteinizing hormone (LH) surge and concomitant increase in serum progesterone concentration. The peak in serum LH (Day 0) is followed by ovulation in approximately 2 days (Day 2) as shown by Concannon et al. (1983).	158 to 175 mm long. Well haired; eyelids closed. Carpals and tarsals not ossified except for calcaneus and talus. The only tooth of the permanent dentition to be ossified at birth (but not erupted) is the first mandibular molar (Evans, 1956).

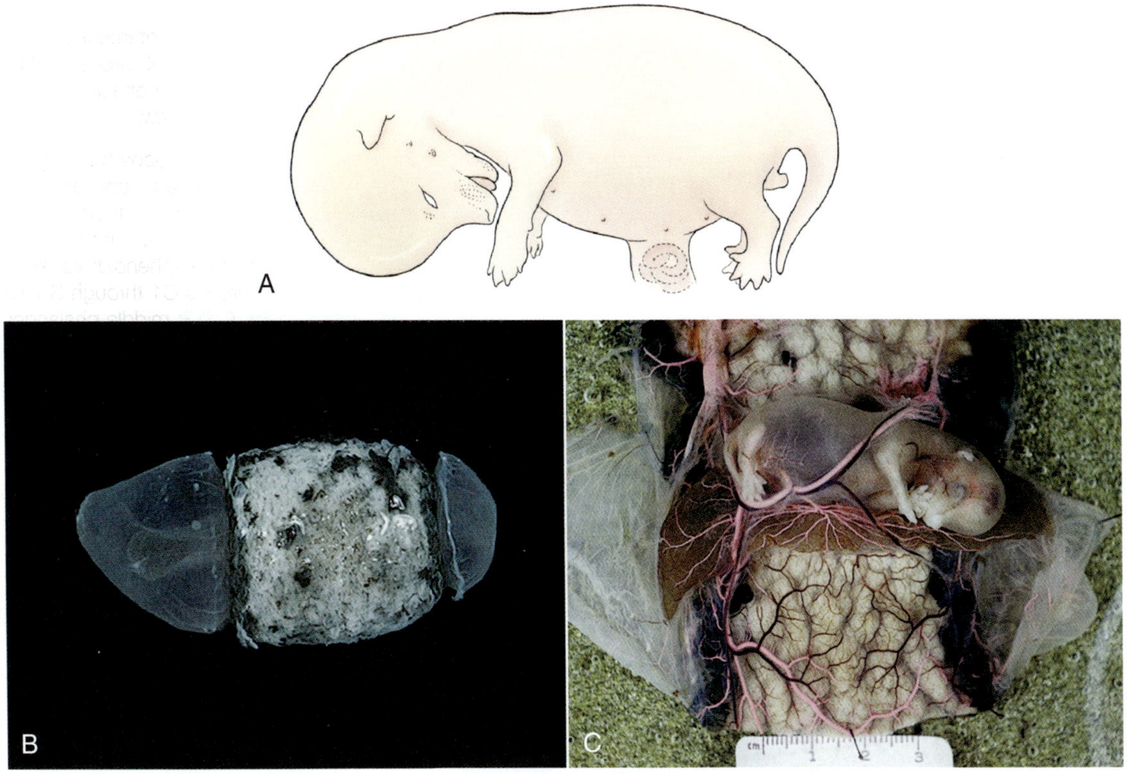

• **Fig. 2.76** Developmental status on the 35th day of gestation. **A,** External features. Note the normal occurrence of umbilical hernia of the intestine shown in pink. **B,** Fetus within its membranes and placenta. Note the faint outline of the yolk sac. **C,** A mongrel fetus and placenta of about 35 days of gestation. The placenta has been opened, and the vessels injected with latex. (Note vascularization of yolk sac.)

60 CHAPTER 2 Prenatal Development

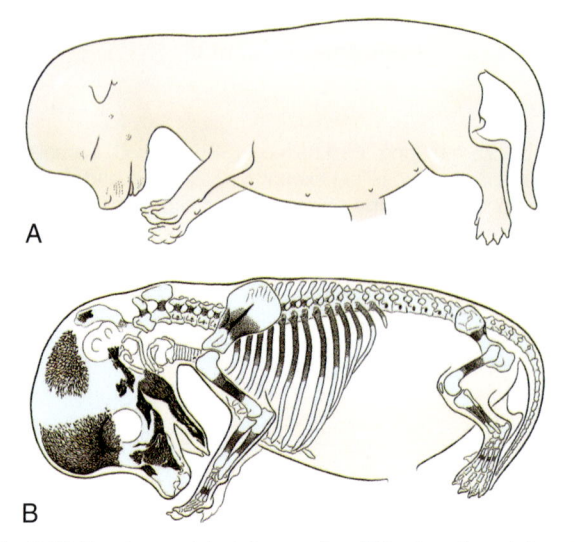

• **Fig. 2.77** Developmental status on the 40th day of gestation. **A**, External features. **B**, The skeleton.

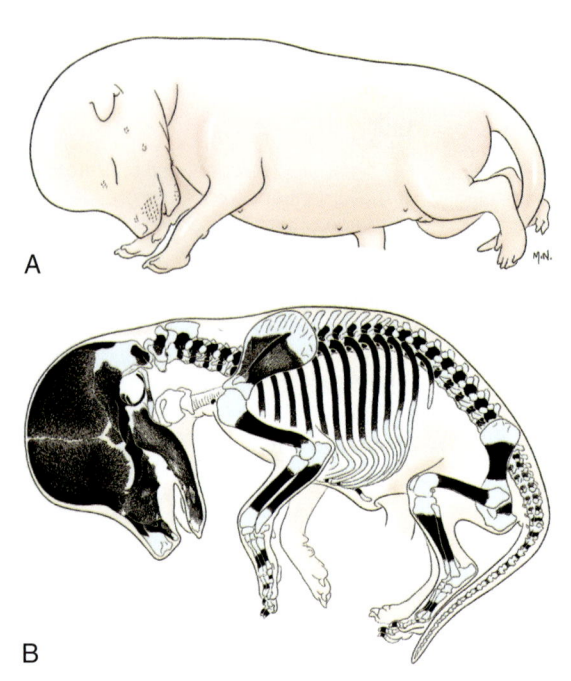

• **Fig. 2.78** Developmental status on the 45th day of gestation. **A**, External features. **B**, The skeleton.

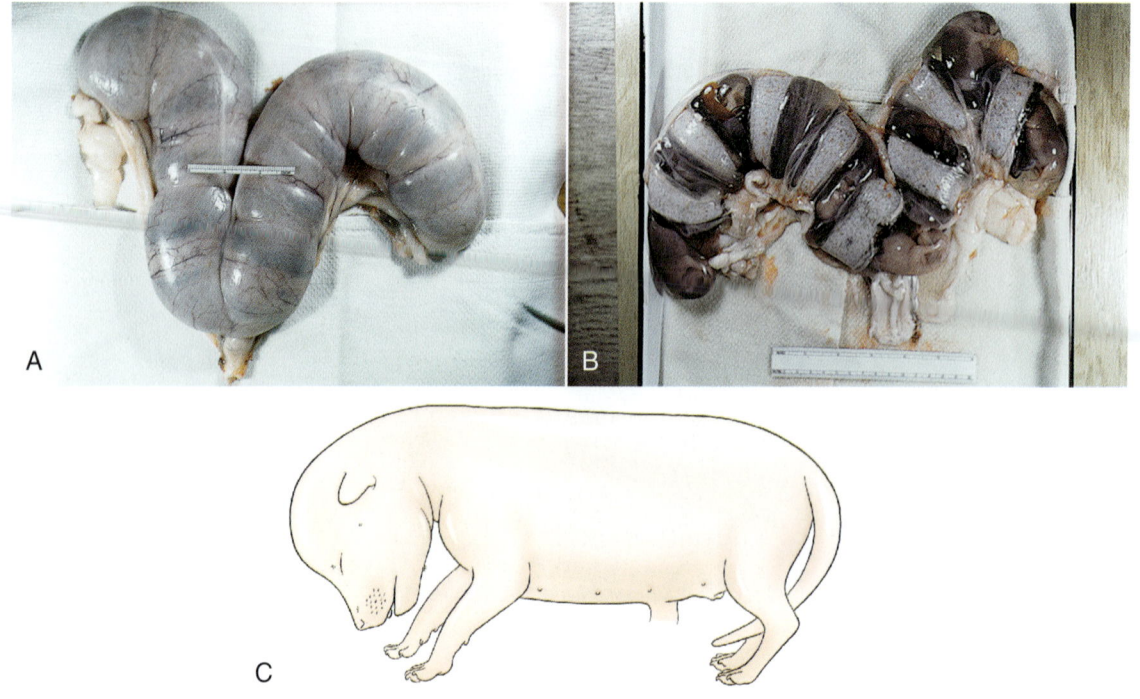

• **Fig. 2.79** Developmental status on the 50th day of gestation. **A**, Exterior of the uterus. **B**, Placental bands, myometrium removed. **C**, External features of the fetus.

CHAPTER 2 Prenatal Development 61

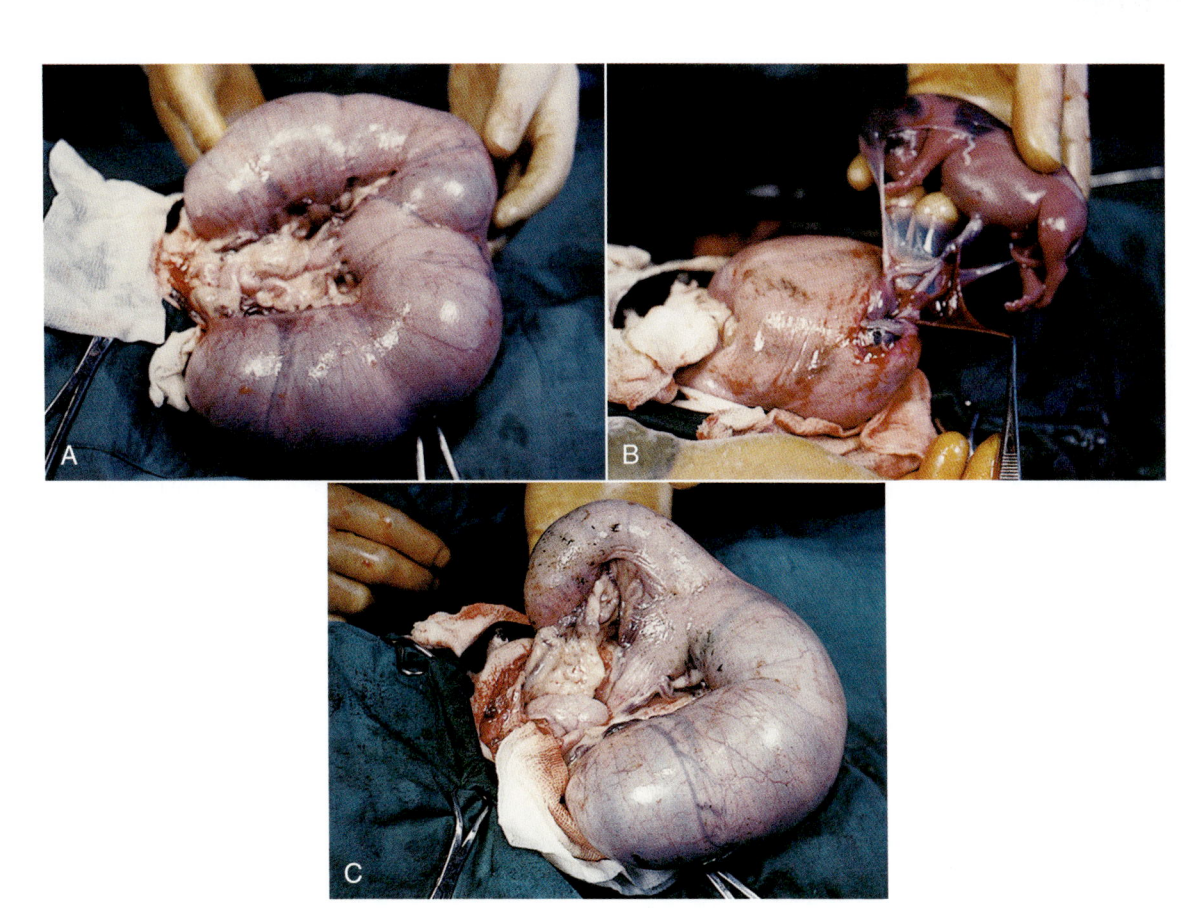

• **Fig. 2.80** A, exteriorized uterus of a Beagle at 50 days of gestation. **B**, Removal of fetuses from the left horn. **C**, exteriorized uterus at 55 days prior to the removal of fetuses from the other uterine horn. Note the shrinkage of the left horn of the uterus after a 5-day interval.

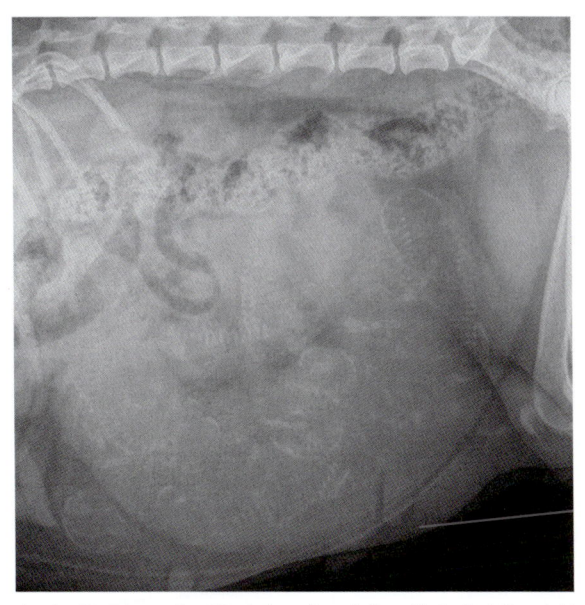

• **Fig. 2.81** Radiograph of a Beagle on the 52nd day of gestation. Note that the eight pups are distributed throughout the abdominal cavity, indicating the folded nature of the enlarged uterine horns.

Bibliography

Abe, Y., Suwa, Y., Asano, T., et al. (2011). Cryopreservation of canine embryos. *Biol Rep, 84*, 363–368.

Ahmed, I. A. (1941). Cytological analysis of chromosome behavior in three breeds of dogs. *Proc R Soc Edinburgh, 61*, 107–118.

Amoroso, E. C. (1952). Placentation. In A. S. Parkes (Ed.), *Marshall's physiology of reproduction* (Vol. 2). Boston: Little, Brown & Co.

Anderson, D. (1927). The rate of passage of the mammalian ovum through various portions of the fallopian tube. *Am J Physiol, 82*, 557–569.

Anderson, J. W. (1969). Ultrastructure of the placenta and fetal membranes of the dog. 1. The placental labyrinth. *Anat Rec, 165*, 15–36.

Asdell, S. A. (1966). *Dog breeding. Reproduction and genetics*. Boston: Little, Brown & Co.

Barrau, M. D., Abel, J. H., Torbit, C. A., et al. (1975). Development of the implantation chamber in the pregnant bitch. *Am J Anat, 143*, 115–130.

Bischoff, T. L. W. (1844). *Beweis der von der begattung unabhängigen periodischen reifung und loslösung der eier der säugetiere und des menschen als die erste bedingung ihrer fortpflanzung*. Giessen.

Bondestam, S., Karkkainen, M., Alitalo, I., et al. (1984). Evaluating the accuracy of canine pregnancy diagnosis and litter size using real-time ultrasound. *Acta Vet Scand, 25*, 327–332.

Boyd, J. D., Hamilton, W. J., & Hammond, J., Jr. (1944). Transuterine (internal) migration of the ovum in sheep and other mammals. *J Anat, 78*, 5–14.

Cartee, R. E., & Rowles, T. (1984). Preliminary study of the ultrasonographic diagnosis of pregnancy and foetal development in the dog. *Am J Vet Res, 45*, 1259–1265.

Chen, J. M. (1953). Studies on the morphogenesis of the mouse sternum. III. Experiments on the closure and segmentation of the sternal bars. *J Anat, 87*, 130–149.

Cloete, J. H. L. (1939). Prenatal growth in the merino sheep. *Onder J Vet Sci Anim Indust, 13*, 417–564.

Concannon, P. W. (1991). Reproduction in the dog and cat. In P. T. Cupps (Ed.), *Reproduction in domestic animals* (4th ed.). New York: Academic Press.

Concannon, P. W., Hansel, W., & McEntee, K. (1977). Changes in LH, progesterone and sexual behavior associated with preovulatory luteinization in the bitch. *Biol Reprod, 17*, 604–613.

Concannon, P. W., Hansel, W., & Visek, W. J. (1975). The ovarian cycle of the bitch: plasma estrogen, LH and progesterone. *Biol Reprod, 13*, 112–121.

Concannon, P. W., Powers, M. E., Holder, W., et al. (1977). Pregnancy and parturition in the bitch. *Biol Reprod, 16*, 517–526.

Concannon, P., Lasley, B., & Vanderlip, S. (1997). LH release, induction of estrus, and fertile ovulation in response to pulsatile administration of gnRH to anestrus dogs. *J Reprod Fertil, 51*, 41–54.

Concannon, P. W., & Lein, D. H. (1989). Hormonal and clinical correlates of ovarian cycles, ovulation, pseudopregnancy, and pregnancy in dogs. In R. W. Kirk (Ed.), *Current veterinary therapy X*. Philadelphia: WB Saunders Co.

Concannon, P. W., Whaley, S., Lein, D., et al. (1983). Canine gestation length: variation related to time of mating and fertile life of sperm. *Am J Vet Res, 44*, 1819–1821.

Creed, R. F. S. (1963). Haemophagocytic structures in the placenta of some carnivora. *J Physiol, 170*, 44–45.

Creed, R. F. S., & Biggers, J. D. (1963). Development of the raccoon placenta. *Am J Anat, 113*, 417–445.

de Beer, G. R. (1937). *The development of the vertebrate skull*. Oxford: Oxford University Press.

Dingerkus, G., & Uhler, L. D. (1977). Enzyme clearing of alcian blue stained whole small vertebrates for demonstration of cartilage. *Stain Technol, 52*, 229–232.

Doak, R. L., Hall, A., & Dale, H. E. (1967). Longevity of spermatozoa in the reproductive tract of the bitch. *J Reprod Fertil, 13*, 51–58.

Drews, M. (1933). Über ossifikationsvorgange am katzen und hundeschädel. *Gegenbaurs Morphol Jahrb, 73*, 185–237.

Duke, K. L. (1946). Monozygotic twins in the dog. *Anat Rec, 94*, 35–42.

England, G. C. W., & Allen, W. E. (1990). Studies on canine pregnancy using B-mode ultrasound: diagnosis of early pregnancy and the number of conceptuses. *J Small Anim Pract, 31*, 321–323.

England, G. C. W., Allen, W. E., & Porter, D. J. (1990). Studies on canine pregnancy using B-mode ultrasound: development of the conceptus and determination of gestational age. *J Small Anim Pract, 31*, 324–329.

Evans, H. E. (1948). Clearing and staining small vertebrates, in toto, for demonstrating ossification. *Turtox News, 26*, 42.47.

Evans, H. E. (1956). *A dog comes into being, Gaines dog research progress*. Gaines Dog Research Center.

Evans, H. E. (1958). Prenatal ossification in the dog. *Anat Rec, 130*, 406.

Evans, H. E. (1959). Prenatal skeletal development in the dog. *Rept NY State Vet College, 1958-59*, 23.

Evans, H. E. (1960a). Prenatal skeletal development in the dog. *Rept NY State Vet College, 1959-60*, 17–18.

Evans, H. E. (1960b). Development and ossification of the sternum in the dog. *Anat Rec, 136*, 190.

Evans, H. E. (1961). Prenatal growth and development of the dog. *Rept NY State Vet College, 1960-61*, 23–24.

Evans, H. E. (1962). Fetal growth and skeletal development in the dog. *Am Zool, 2*, 521.

Evans, H. E. (1974). *Prenatal development of the dog*. Ithaca, NY: 24th Gaines Veterinary Symposium.

Evans, H. E. (1979). Reproduction and prenatal development. In H. E. Evans & G. C. Christensen (Eds.), *Miller's anatomy of the dog* (2nd ed.). Philadelphia: Saunders.

Evans, H. E., & Sack, W. O. (1973). Prenatal development of domestic and laboratory mammals. *Zbl Vet Med C Anat Histol Embryol, 2*, 11–45.

Gier, H. T. (1950). Early embryology of the dog. *Anat Rec, 108*, 561–562.

Hewitt, D. A., & England, G. C. W. (1999). Influence of gonadotrophin supplementation on the in vitro maturation of bitch oocytes. *Vet Rec, 144*, 237–239.

Hill, J. P., & Tribe, M. (1924). The early development of the cat (*Felis domestica*). *Q J Microscop Sci, 68*, 513–602.

Holst, P. A., & Phemister, R. D. (1971). The prenatal development of the dog: preimplantation events. *Biol Reprod, 5*, 194–206.

Holst, P. A., & Phemister, R. D. (1974). Onset of diestrus in the beagle bitch: definition and significance. *Am J Vet Res, 35*, 401–406.

Hyttel, P., Sinowatz, F., & Vejlsted, M. (2010). *Essentials of domestic animal embryology*. Philadelphia: Saunders.

Kim, Y. H., Travis, A. J., & Meyers-Wallen, V. N. (2007). Parturition prediction and timing of canine pregnancy. *Theriogenology, 68*, 1177–1182.

McGeady, T. A., Quinn, P. J., Fitzpatrick, E. S., et al. (2017). *Veterinary embryology* (2nd ed.). Blackwell.

Minouchi, O. (1928). The spermatogenesis of the dog, with special reference to meiosis. *Jap J Zool, 1*, 255–268.

Miglino, M. A., Ambrósio, C. E., dos Santos Martins, D., et al. (2006). The carnivore pregnancy: the development of the embryo and fetal membranes. *Theriogenology, 66*, 1699–1702.

Modina, S. C., Veronesi, M. C., Moioli, M., et al. (2017). Small-sized newborn dogs skeletal development: radiologic, morphometric, and histological findings obtained from spontaneously dead animals. *BMC Vet Res*, doi:10.1186/s12917-017-1092.6.

Moore, W., Jr., & Lambert, P. D. (1963). The chromosomes of the beagle dog. *J Heredity, 54*, 273–276.

Nagashima, J. B., Sylvester, S. R., Nelson, J. L., et al. (2015). Live births from domestic dog (*Canis familiaris*) embryos produced by *in vitro* fertilization. *PLoS ONE, 10*, e0143930. doi:10.1371/journal.pone.0143930.

Noden, D., & de Lahunta, A. (1985). *The embryology of domestic animals: developmental mechanisms and malformations.* Baltimore: Williams & Wilkins.

Olmstead, M. P. (1911). Das primordial cranium eines hundembryo. *Anat Hefte, 130*, 339–375.

Phemister, R. D. (1974). Nonneurogenic reproductive failure in the bitch. *Vet Clin North Am, 4*, 573–586.

Phemister, R. D., Holst, P. A., Spano, J. S., et al. (1973). Time of ovulation in the beagle bitch. *Biol Reprod, 8*, 74–82.

Renton, J. P., Boyd, J. S., Eckersall, P. D., et al. (1991). Ovulation, fertilization, and early embryonic development in the bitch (*Canis familiaris*). *J Reprod Fertil, 93*, 221–231.

Reynaud, K., Fotnbonne, A., Marseloo, N., et al. (2005). *In vivo* meiotic resumption, fertilization and early embryonic development in the bitch. *Reproduction, 130*, 193–201. doi:10.1530/rep.1.00500.

Rijsselaere, T., Van Soom, A., Van Cruchten, S., et al. (2004). Sperm distribution in the genital tract of the bitch following artificial insemination in relation to the time of ovulation. *Reproduction, 128*, 801–811. doi:10.1530/rep.1.00273.

Rodriques, B. A., & Rodriques, J. (2006). Responses of canine oocytes to in vitro maturation and in vitro fertilization outcome. *Theirogenology, 66*, 1667–1672.

Sandoval, C., Fisher, P. J., & Schlafer, D. H. (2001). Characterization of trophoblast cell populations by lectin histochemistry in canine placenta during development. *J Reprod Fertil Suppl, 57*, 199–206.

Schliemann, H. (1966). Zur morphologie und entwicklung des craniums von *Canis lupus familiaris*. *Gegenbaurs Morphol Jahrb, 109*, 501–603.

Schoenfeld, H. (1903). Contributions à l'étude de la fixation de l'oeuf des mammifères dans la cavité uterine des premiers stades de la placentation. *Arch Biol, 19*, 701–830.

Shille, V. M., & Gontarek, J. (1985). The use of ultrasonography for pregnancy diagnosis in the bitch. *J Am Vet Med Assoc, 187*, 1021–1025.

Simons, E. V., & Van Horn, J. R. (1971). A new procedure for wholemount alcian blue staining of the cartilaginous skeleton of chicken embryos, adapted to the clearing procedure in potassium hydroxide. *Acta Morphol Neerl Scand, 8*, 281–292.

Smith, R. N. (1964). The pelvis of the young dog. *Vet Rec, 76*, 975–980.

Songsasen, N., & Wildt, D. E. (2005). Size of the donor follicle, but not stage of reproductive cycle or seasonality, influences meiotic competency of selected domestic dog oocytes. *Mol Rep Dev, 72*, 113–119.

Songsasen, N., Spindler, R. E., & Wildt, D. E. (2007). Requirement for, and patterns of, pyruvate and glutamine metabolism in the domestic dog oocyte in vitro. *Mol Reprod Dev, 74*, 870–877.

Stockard, C. R. (1941). The genetic and endocrinic basis for differences in form and behaviour. *Am Anat Mem, 19*, 1–775.

Streeter, G. L. (1951). Developmental horizons in human embryos. Carnegie institute wash publ 592. *Contrib Embryol, 34*, 165–196.

Taverne, M. A. M., & van Oord, H. A. (1989). Accuracy of pregnancy diagnosis in dogs by means of linear-array ultrasound scanning. In M. A. Taverne & A. H. Willemse (Eds.), *Diagnostic ultrasound and animal reproduction*. Norwell, MA: Kluwer.

Tietz, W. J., & Selinger, W. G. (1967). Temporal relationship in early canine embryogenesis. *Anat Rec, 157*, 333–334.

Toal, R. L., Walker, M. A., & Henry, G. A. (1986). A comparison of real time ultrasound, palpation, and radiography in pregnancy detection and litter size determination in the bitch. *Vet Radiol, 27*.

Van der Stricht, O. (1923). The blastocyst of the dog. *J Anat, 58*, 52–53.

Watson, A. G. (1977). In toto alcian blue staining of the cartilaginous skeleton in mammalian embryos. *Anat Rec, 187*, 743.

Watson, A. G. (1981). *The phylogeny and development of the occipito-atlas-axis complex in the dog, Thesis*. Ithaca, NY: Cornell University.

Watson, A. G., & Evans, H. E. (1976). The development of the atlas-axis complex in the dog. *Anat Rec, 184*, 558.

Watson, A. G., Evans, H. E., & de Lahunta, A. (1986). Ossification of the atlas-axis complex in the dog. *Zbl Vet Med C Anat Hist Embryol, 15*, 122.138.

Williams, R. C. (1961). *Observations on the chronology of deciduous dental development in the dog, Thesis*. Ithaca, NY: Cornell University.

Williams, R. C., & Evans, H. E. (1978). Prenatal dental development in the dog, *Canis fumitiuris*: chronology of tooth germ formation and calcification of deciduous teeth. *Zbl Vet Med C Anat Histol Embryol, 7*, 152.163.

Wimsatt, W. A. (1974). Morphogenesis of the fetal membranes and placenta of the black bear, *Ursus americanus* (Pallas). *Am J Anat, 140*, 471–496.

Yeager, A. E., & Concannon, P. W. (1990). Association between the preovulatory luteinizing hormone surge and the early ultrasonic detection of pregnancy and fetal heartbeats in beagle dogs. *Theriogenology, 34*, 655–665.

Yeager, A. E., Mohammed, H. O., Meyers-Wallen, V., et al. (1992). Ultrasonic appearance of the uterus, placenta, fetus, and fetal membranes throughout accurately timed pregnancy in beagle dogs. *Am J Vet Res, 53*, 342–351.

3

The Integument

FAKHRI AL-BAGDADI

The common integument (*integumentum commune*) includes the skin, hair, claws, pads, and skin glands, including the glands of the paranal sinus and the mammary glands (Bereiter-Hahn et al., 1986). It is the largest and most visible organ of the dog's body (Miller et al., 2013).

The **skin** (cutis) consists of a superficial **epidermis** of stratified squamous epithelium and an underlying connective tissue, the **dermis**. The interface between the epidermis and the dermis is formed by a functional basement membrane made up of matrix proteins (Ghohestani et al., 2001). The skin is underlain by a **subcutis** (tela subcutanea or hypodermis), which is not part of the skin. The subcutis functions as a moveable support for the skin, allowing it to glide over underlying tissues. It connects the dermis with the fascia and the various forms of hair (pili) that compose the coat. The skin prevents desiccation and contains nerve endings that inform the central nervous system of its contacts and condition. The skin of puppies is more permeable than that of adult dogs.

As a sensory organ, the skin is the receptor for the perception of touch, pressure, vibration, tension, noxious stimuli, heat, cold, and harmful chemicals (Iggo, 1962, 1977). It prevents trauma, protects the body from the invasion of microorganisms and noxious chemicals, and contributes to temperature regulation. In regard to heat regulation, however, the skin of the dog serves only a limited role via sweat glands (Iwabuchi, 1967) and superficial capillary beds because of the important role of thermal panting (Blatt et al., 1972). The skin lacks superficial arteriovenous shunts (Thoday & Friedman, 1986), and the hairy skin is devoid of atrichial sweat glands (Miller et al., 2013). The skin acts as the site of vitamin D synthesis (How et al., 1994), and the subcutaneous tissues serve as a reservoir for fat, electrolytes, water, carbohydrates, and proteins. Secretions of skin glands not only waterproof and lubricate the skin but also function as pheromones for recognition (Parks & Bruce, 1961) and, in the case of the mammary glands, as nourishment for the young.

The skin has an immunosurveillance potential and is often subject to allergic reactions, dermatitis, and parasitic invasion. Immunologic events are modulated by the production of a cytosine, an epidermal cell–derived thymocyte-activating factor (Choi & Sander, 1986). The skin may reflect the state of health of the animal as well as indicate cutaneous manifestations of internal disease, such as icterus, cyanosis, and edema. After injury or surgery the edges of skin wounds gape owing to continuous tension of the skin.

The **dermis** (corium) consists of a connective tissue bed containing blood vessels, lymphatics, muscles, and nerve endings covered by stratified squamous epithelium. The skin is continuous at the natural body openings with the mucous membranes of the digestive, respiratory, and urogenital tracts as well as with the conjunctivae of the eyelids, the lacrimal duct, and the tympanic membrane.

The **hair coat** (*pili*), consisting of **cover hairs** (*capilli*) and **wool hairs** (*pili lanei*), is densest on the dorsal and lateral portions of the body, whereas the abdomen, the flanks, the inside of the ears, and the underside of the tail are sparsely haired. The **claws** (*unguicula*) are horny coverings of the third phalanges of the digits.

There are large **tactile hairs** (*pili tactiles*) on the muzzle (*pili tactiles labiales superiores*), mandible (*pili tactiles mentalis*), and dorsal to the eyes (*pili tactiles supraorbitales*). There are usually two genal tubercles on each side of the face, from which long hairs grow. The specialized hairs of the eyelids, or **eyelashes** (*cilia*), are stiff and larger than other hairs. The ventral body surface (Fig. 3.1) is characterized by hairless areas, such as the **median raphe of the linea alba**, the umbilicus, nipples, and the sparsely haired **mammary glands** (*glandula mammaria*). The hairy skin is thickest over the neck, dorsal thorax, rump, and base of the tail. The skin of the pinna of the ear, axilla, and inguinal and perianal regions is thinnest.

All skin areas are composed of epidermis and dermis (*corium*) and are underlined by the **subcutis** (hypodermis, tela subcutanea). The skin is thicker on the dorsal part of the neck, trunk, and tail than on the belly, the flanks, or medial side of the limbs. The skin, hair, and subcutis of the newborn puppy represent approximately 24% of the total body weight. Owing to differential growth of various body parts, this percentage is reduced to 12% by 6 months of age. Additional information concerning canine skin may be

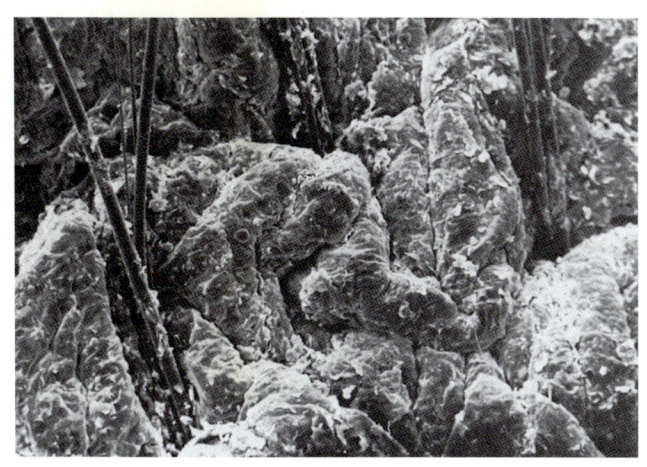

• Fig. 3.1 Scanning electron micrograph shows the folded skin and sparsely scattered complex hair follicles on the abdomen, near the linea alba by the umbilicus of an adult male Fox Terrier.

found in Webb and Calhoun (1954); Lovell and Getty (1957); Blackburn (1965); Warner and McFarland (1970); Calhoun and Stinson (1976); Sokolov (1982); Miller, Griffin, and Campbell (2013); and Singh (2017). The skin surfaces of a haired dog have an acidic pH to help protect the skin from microbial invasion (Rippke et al., 2002).

Epidermis

The thickness of the hairy skin ranges from 0.5 to 5 mm (Miller et al., 2013). Processing skin samples obtained from dogs for histologic evaluation caused changes in sample dimensions; the samples decreased in length and width 32% and increased in thickness 75%, compared with their original dimensions (Reiner et al., 2005). The thicker portions of the skin are found near the hair follicle orifices and the hairy margins of the mucocutaneous junctions. According to Lloyd and Garthwaite (1982) the canine stratum corneum has a mean thickness of 13 μm and consists of 50 cell layers. The epidermis of nonhairy skin varies in thickness owing to the system of ridges that occur at the dermal–epidermal junction. The nonhairy margins are of the lip, eyelid, prepuce, vulva, and anus. The thickest epidermis occurs on the nasal skin and digital and metapodial pads. The epidermis of the planum nasale is 200 μm at the time of birth and 600 μm at 6 months of age. The epidermis of the foot pads is 200 μm at birth and increases to 1800 μm at 6 months of age. The thickness of various cutaneous sites in the live dog in relation to hydration status and fluid distribution has been recorded by the use of high-frequency ultrasonography. The skin thickness (epidermis plus dermis) ranged from 2.211 to 3.249 mm. The greatest thickness is in the sacral, frontal, flank, and metatarsal regions (in decreasing order). Ultrasonography is a noninvasive tool in the evaluation of skin hydration in healthy dogs and in dogs with skin edema (Diana et al., 2008) and can be used instead of the current evaluation of skin hydration in dogs, which relies on clinical palpation by picking up the skin with the fingers (Chesney, 1995; Hester et al., 2004; Welzel

et al., 2001). The greatest skin thickness is found in the Shar Pei breed and the least skin thickness in the Miniature Pinscher and the Toy Poodle breeds. There was no correlation between body weight and skin thickness of dogs according to Diana et al. (2004). A positive correlation in vivo was detected between cutaneous thickness measured by the use of ultrasonography and measurements obtained by the use of histologic examination, which is invasive, time-consuming, and costly (Diana et al., 2004).

Dermis

The thickness of the **dermis**, or corium, varies in different body areas and at different ages. The dermis of the planum nasale and foot pads is 300 μm at birth and increases to 800 μm at 6 months of age. The differences in thickness of the hairy skin that can be observed by comparing the dorsal area with the abdominal area are due to the difference in thickness of the dermis. Dermal papillae of the hairy skin are not present in the dog owing to the lack of the epidermal rete ridges (Miller et al., 2013). The dermis of the skin of the dorsal region is 700 μm at birth and increases to 1500 μm at 6 months of age. The dermis in the abdominal region is 300 μm at birth and increases to 800 μm at 6 months of age.

Structure of the Dermis and Changes with Age

The dermis is composed of fibroblasts, fibers, and various structures such as blood vessels, nerves, cells of blood or tissue origin, and tissue fluid. According to Miller, Griffin, and Campbell (2013), the dermis of the Chinese Shar-Pei, a breed with excessive skin folds, contains a considerable amount of mucin. Fibronectin released by fibroblasts, endothelial cells, and histiocytes (Clark, 1983; Quaissi & Capron, 1985) regulates vascular permeability, wound healing, and cytoskeletal orientation (Miller et al., 2013). Skin glands and hair follicles are embedded in the dermal tissue. Fibers of smaller diameter are found in the superficial dermis adjacent to the epidermis. The larger collagenous fibers are in the deeper layer of the dermis. The size of the fibers, the population density of fibroblast nuclei, and the plasma cell content of the dermis undergo developmental changes with the increase in thickness that occurs between birth and 6 months of age.

At the time of birth, there are many reticular fibers throughout the dermis. By 3 weeks most of them have been replaced by collagen fibers. A few reticular fibers remain just deep to the epidermis, around hair follicles, and surrounding sebaceous and sweat glands. Collagen fiber bundles increase in size and number as the dermis thickens with age. Collagen fibers account for 90% of the fiber component of the dermis (Thomsett, 1986). At birth, the collagen fiber bundles measure 3 or 4 μm in diameter, and at 6 months they measure 19 to 20 μm. Concurrent with this gradual increase is a corresponding decrease in the size of the spaces between the fiber bundles. There is also an increase in the size and number of elastic fibers. At birth, elastic fibers are small, branching, and filamentous, less than 0.5 μm in diameter. By 6 months they are thick, undulating fibers of 1.5 to 2 μm in diameter. Irwin (1966) illustrated tension lines in dog skin that are determined by the orientation of connective tissue, gravity, and physical forces. Subsequent determination of tension lines was produced by Oiki, Nishida, Ichihara and colleagues (2003) and yields slightly different patterns useful for dermoplasty.

Senile changes in dog skin were noted by Baker (1967). A skin incision made across the tension line produces maximum gape, takes a longer time to heal, requires more sutures, and results in a wider scar. A skin incision made parallel to the tension lines requires fewer sutures and heals better with minimum or no scarring (Fig. 3.2).

Fibroblast nuclei in the dermis are more densely distributed at birth than at 6 months of age. Per unit area, there are twice as many nuclei at birth as at 6 months. Mast cells occur in all parts of the dermis and subcutaneous fat tissue (Emerson & Cross, 1965). They are present in greatest numbers in the reticular layer of the dermis, with fewer in the papillary layer and subcutis. They are usually most numerous around the walls of small blood vessels (Sokolov, 1982) and frequently surround sebaceous glands and apocrine or eccrine glands. They are most numerous in the skin of the ears and appear in decreasing numbers in the skin of the vulva, prepuce, medial thigh, foot pad, and external nares. The subcutis consists of panniculus adiposus and fibrous connective tissue. The subcutis anchors the dermis to the bone periosteum, muscle epimysium, and cartilage perichondrium. Subcutis fat is characteristic of the carpal, metacarpal, metatarsal, and digital pads; it acts as a shock absorber. The adipose layer varies according to breed and individual variations for body regions (Schwarz et al., 1979). The histologic examination of various regions of aged dogs showed atrophy of the epidermis, appendages, and dermis with decrease in hair numbers (Baker, 1967). Normal-haired skin of dogs does not have epidermal rete ridges or dermal papillae (Miller et al., 2013). The dermis contains about 87% type I collagen, 87% type III collagen, and 3% type V collagen (Miller et al., 2013). Dermal melanocytes are present in dark-skinned dogs such as Doberman pinschers and Black Labrador retrievers (Miller et al., 2013).

Pigmentation

Conroy and Beamer (1970) studied the development of melanoblasts and melanocytes in the skin of Labrador Retriever fetuses. The earliest melanoblasts were demonstrable in the primordial dermis of the head, thorax, and abdomen of 29-day fetuses. The melanoblasts were most numerous in the deeper two-thirds of the primordial dermis in contact with or near blood vessels. The frequent contact or close association of melanoblasts with blood vessels suggests that the cells migrate along blood vessels in their journey from the neural crest to their destination in the epidermis. Dendritic dermal melanocytes first appeared in the 37-day fetus, and scattered epidermal melanocytes appeared in 29-day fetuses. Their numerical distribution in various regions of the body conformed to a dorsoventral gradient. Melanocytes were present in primordial and differentiating hair follicles, atrichial sweat glands, and sebaceous glands.

Skin pigment is not visible in Labrador Retriever fetuses of less than 33 days but is readily observed in a 37-day fetus. In 40-day fetuses, cutaneous pigmentation is prominent on the muzzle, eyelids, and ears. A fetus of 46 days is heavily pigmented except for parts of the digital pads, the central part of the planum nasale, the metapodial pads, the median dorsal and ventral lips, the chin, the hard palate, and the tongue. Skin pigmentation is most prominent on the dorsal and lateral aspects of the head and body. A nearly full-term fetus of 55 days has abundant hair and is completely pigmented externally including digital pads and claws, although the claws are somewhat less pigmented than the integument. The oral cavity is not pigmented except for the lips.

According to Schmutz and Berryere (2007) seven genes that cause specific coat colors and/or patterns in dogs have been identified: melanocortin 1 receptor, tyrosinase-related protein 1, agouti signal peptide, melanophilin, SILV (formerly PMEL17), microphthalmia-associated transcription factor, and beta-defensin 103. Although not all alleles have been identified at each locus, DNA tests are available for

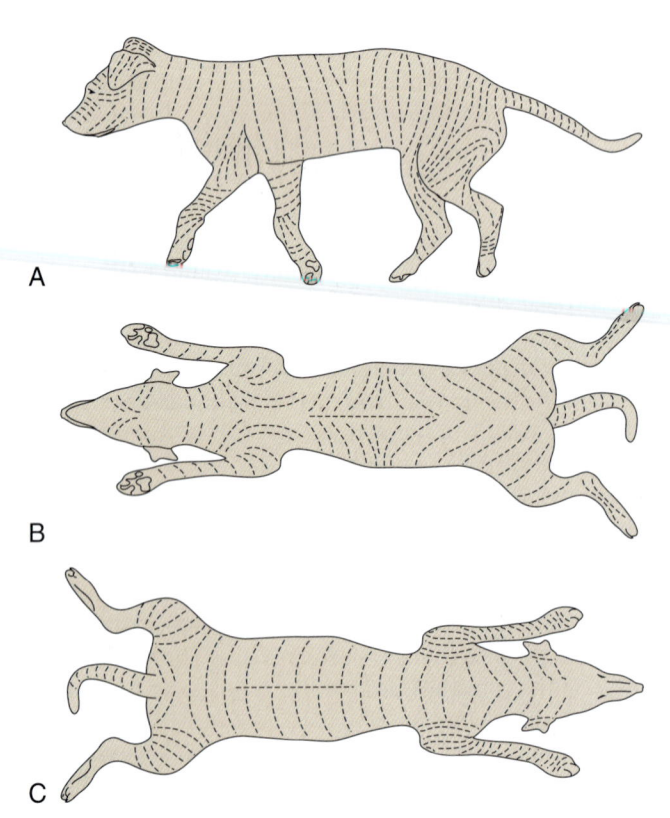

• **Fig. 3.2** Composite drawings of three dogs to show tension lines in the skin. **A**, Lateral. **B**, Ventral. **C**, Dorsal. (Courtesy Irwin DHG: Tension lines in the skin of the dog, *J Sm An Pract* 7:593–598, 1966.)

many. The identification of these alleles has provided information on interactions in this complex set of genes involved in both pigmentation and neurological development. There are pleiotropic effects of some coat color genes as they relate to disease. The alleles found in various breeds shed light on some potential breed developmental histories and phylogenetic relationships. The information is of value to dog breeders who have selected for and against specific colors since breed standards and dog showing began in the late 1800s.

Nasal Skin

The nasal skin is usually heavily pigmented, tough, and moist. On close examination of the surface of the planum nasale, polygonal plaque-like areas are observed that give the nasal skin an irregular appearance (Fig. 3.3A and B).

On histologic examination, no glands can be demonstrated in the epidermis or dermis of nasal skin. The moisture that appears on the nasal surface is derived primarily from serous gland secretions of the lateral nasal gland and other glands that drain into the vestibule (Blatt et al., 1972).

The **dermis** of nasal skin is composed of reticular, collagenous, and elastic fibers, together with fibroblasts, blood vessels, and nerves. The blood vessels and nerves are larger in the deeper layers of the dermis than in the more superficial layers. Adjacent to the epidermis, the dermal papillae interdigitate with epidermal projections to form an irregular line of attachment between the dermis and epidermis (Fig. 3.3C and D).

The **epidermis** of the nasal skin, which averages 630 μm in thickness in adult dogs, is composed of three layers: stratum basale, stratum spinosum, and stratum corneum. The stratum basale of the epidermis rests on a basement membrane underlined by the condensed thickened superficial portion of the dermis and consists of one layer of cylindrical cells. The stratum spinosum is made up of 10 to 20 layers of diamond-shaped, dome-shaped, or flattened polygonal cells that have a lighter staining cytoplasm than that of the cylindrical cells. In heavily pigmented nasal skin there are many pigment granules in the cytoplasm. There is no stratum granulosum or stratum lucidum in the epidermis of the nasal skin. The more peripheral spinosum cells apparently do not undergo keratinization, as they do in other regions of epidermis. Their cytoplasm becomes weakly acidophilic, and the nuclei become pyknotic with the cells flattening out into a squamous type. As they approach the surface, they remain as a thin, atypical nucleated stratum corneum, four to eight cell layers thick. Nose prints, similar to finger prints, can be used to distinguish between individuals (Horning et al., 1926; Schummer et al., 1981).

Digital Pads

The skin of the digital pads, the torus digitalis, is usually heavily pigmented and is the thickest region of canine skin. The surface of the pads is smooth in cats and rough in dogs, owing to the presence of numerous conical projections that are heavily keratinized and are readily seen with the naked eye (Fig. 3.4A and B). When dogs are kept on concrete or

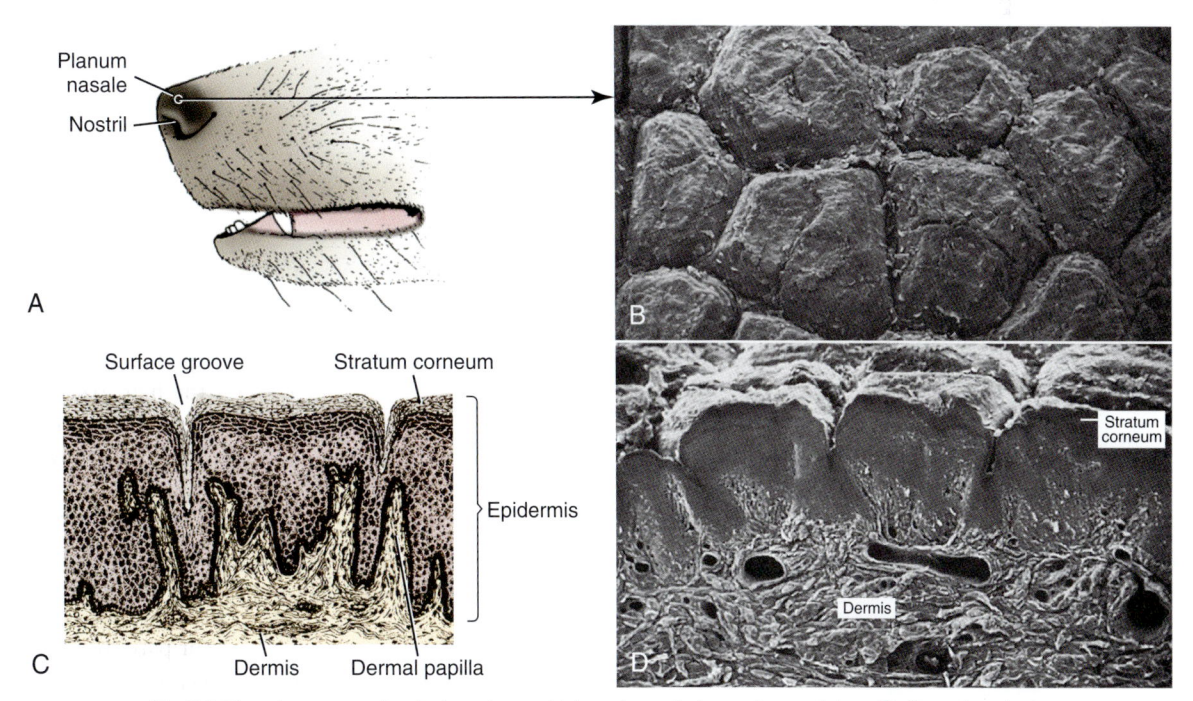

• **Fig. 3.3** The planum nasale. **A**, Area from which surface photograph was taken. **B**, Scanning electron micrograph shows polygonal plaques of varied shapes separated by grooves. **C**, Section of epidermis and dermis. **D**, Scanning electron micrograph of a section of the planum nasale of a 2-year-old Doberman Pinscher. The stratum corneum is thick and has grooves separating the individual plaques. The dermis has coarse collagen fibers and a rich blood supply.

68 CHAPTER 3 The Integument

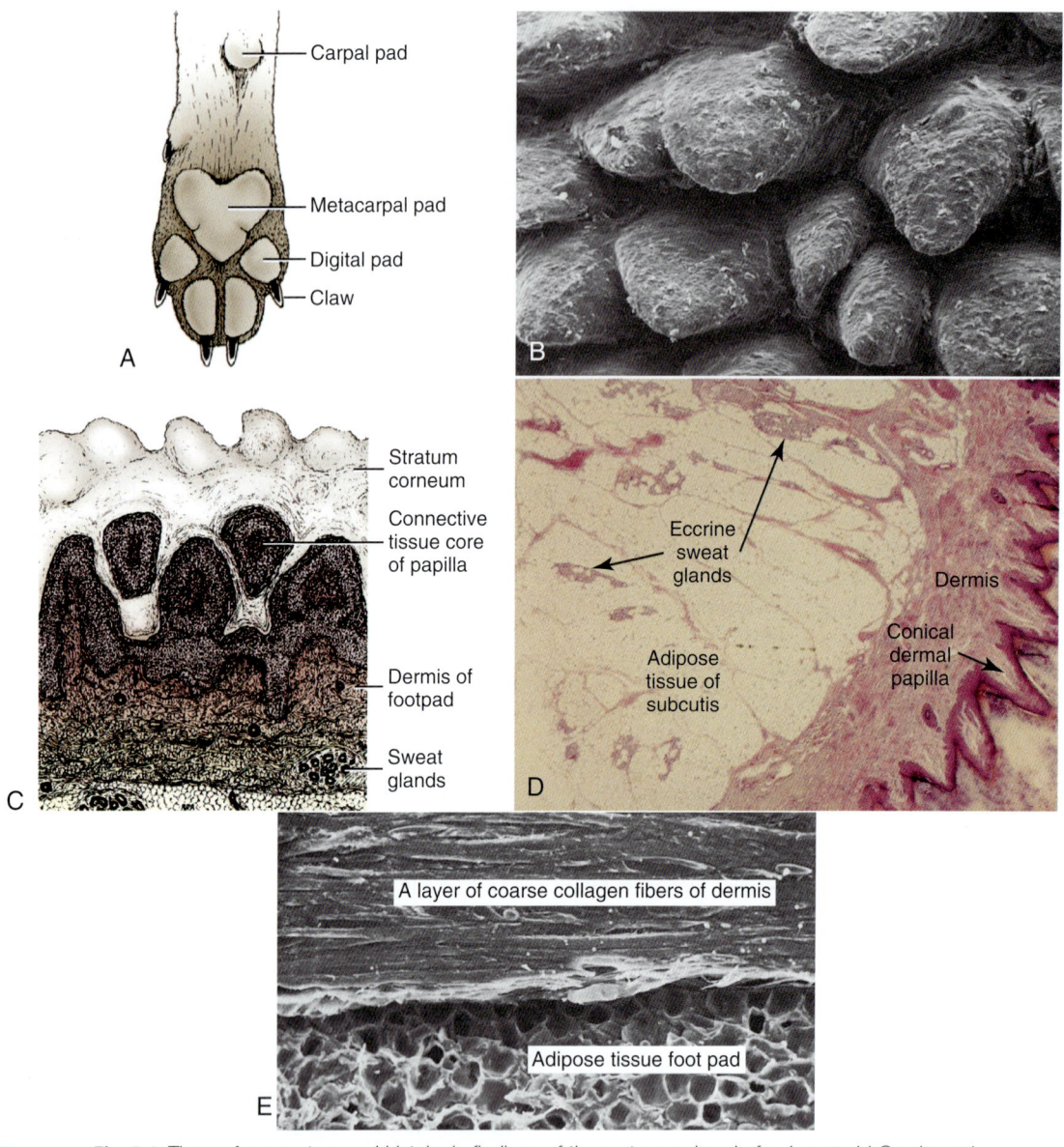

• **Fig. 3.4** The surface contour and histologic findings of the metacarpal pad of a 4-year-old Greyhound. **A**, Gross appearance of pads of manus. **B**, Scanning electron micrograph of conical projections on the surface of the metacarpal pad. **C**, Diagram of the surface layers of a foot pad. **D**, Histologic section of a foot pad. **E**, Scanning electron micrograph of a vertical section of the deeper part of the dermis of a foot pad. Note many layers of coarse collagen fibers cushioned by a thick pad of adipose tissue below. (**D** with permission from Lovell J, Getty R: The hair follicle, epidermis, dermis, and skin glands of the dog, *Am J Vet Res* 18:873–885, 1957.)

rough surfaces, the projections sometimes become worn smooth so that they are rounded instead of conical in shape.

The **digital cushion**, or base of the foot pad, is made up of subcutaneous adipose tissue that is partitioned by reticular, collagenous, and elastic fibers. Many elastic fibers are present in the deeper layers. Atrichial sweat glands and lamellar corpuscles are embedded in the adipose tissue (Fig. 3.4C and D). The long excretory ducts of the eccrine glands are found deep in the dermis, through which they carry secretions to the surface of the epidermis. Adjacent to the epidermis, the dermal connective tissue is dense and papillate, forming conical dermal cores for the epidermis.

There are also secondary dermal papillae within the conical structure.

The epidermis of the digital pad, which averages 1800 μm in thickness in the adult dog, is composed of five layers: stratum basale, stratum spinosum, stratum granulosum, stratum lucidum, and stratum corneum. The *stratum basale* is made up of a single layer of basal cells resting on the basement membrane. The *stratum spinosum* is composed of 10 to 15 layers of diamond- or dome-shaped cells. In both the digital pads and the planum nasale, cell outlines and intercellular bridges (desmosomal attachments) may be observed on the spinous cells. The *stratum granulosum* is made up of four to seven layers of flattened cells that contain basophilic keratohyalin granules in their cytoplasm. The *stratum lucidum* is a completely keratinized layer of dead cells (Miller et al., 2013) and appears as a shiny, acidophilic layer of homogenous substance with refractile droplets called *eleidin*. The *stratum corneum* of the digital pads consists of a thick layer of keratinized nonnucleated material, thicker than all the cellular layers combined. The excretory ducts of the atrichial sweat glands of the digital pad become continuous with the epidermis, where their epithelium joins with the stratum basale of the epidermis. The lumen of the excretory duct follows a tortuous path through the epidermal cells to the surface, where the glandular secretion is expelled.

Hairy Skin

The dog has a compound type of hair follicle arrangement (Meyer, 2009). The basic unit of hair production is the individual **hair follicle** (*folliculus pili*). The follicle wall, which is continuous with the surface epithelium, is divided into two layers, the external and internal root sheaths. The follicle attains its greatest diameter at the base, where it is dilated to form a bulb in which the hair-producing matrix is contained. Invaginating the bulb is the dermal papilla, which supplies by diffusion the germinative epithelium as long as the hair is growing. The **hair shaft** (Fig. 3.5) consists of a central medulla; a thick cortex containing the pigment that gives the hair its color (Miller et al., 2013), which forms the bulk of the hair; and a single-layered cuticle of flat, cornified anuclear cells arranged like slates on a roof with their free edges facing the tip of the hair follicle. Computer evaluation of the cuticular hair pattern by scanning electron microscopy can be used to differentiate between mammalian species (Meyer et al., 1997a,b, Meyer, 2009). The keratin shaft of the hair is formed by the germinative epithelium of the bulb region, which is active only during the time of hair growth. It has been reported that immunohistochemical evaluation indicated that the bulge-like (hair bulb) region of the dog hair follicle contains stem cells (Mercati et al., 2008). There are periods during which the growth of the hair is arrested. At this time there is a regression of the hair root, and the dead club hair is held in the follicle completely disconnected from the inactive germinal matrix. After a variable period, the dormant germinal cells become active and enter a period of organogenesis in which a new hair root is regenerated and production of hair is resumed. At this time the old dead hair will be shed and replaced by the new hair. Growing hair follicles are said to be in **anagen** and quiescent ones in **telogen**; the period of transition between the two is called **catagen**.

Growth Rate of the Hair Shaft

Differences may be observed in hair growth rates in various breeds and during certain seasons of the year. Al-Bagdadi (1975) found that the average rate of daily hair growth in male Beagle dogs was 0.4 mm/day in the winter and 0.34 mm/day in the summer. Butler and Wright (1981) reported determinations from male Greyhounds to be 0.04 mm/day in the summer and 0.18 mm/day in the fall. Although the two observers found widely different values, which may reflect strain differences, they agreed that the daily growth rate of the hair shaft was greater during the colder season than it was during the warmer time of the year. The rate of hair growth in mongrel dogs varies individually and by region of the body (Gunaratnam & Wilkinson, 1983). The pattern of regrowth of the clipped hair coat of a Beagle dog is illustrated in Figs. 3.6 and 3.7 (Al-Bagdadi, 1975). According to Diaz et al. (2006), the hairs in the lumbosacral region of the Siberian Husky breed were proportionally shorter than the lateral thigh hairs 2 months after clipping. Miller, Griffin, and Campbell (2013) reported that a short hair coat takes 3 to 4 months to regrow after shaving, and a long hair coat takes about 18 months. Brushing had no effect on hair regrowth after clipping the normal dog.

Embryology of Hair Follicles

The terms *pregerm, hair germ, hair peg,* and *bulbous peg* are used to designate progressive developmental stages of the canine hair follicle. In a study of the development of cutaneous pigment, Conroy and Beamer (1970) described the embryologic development of the canine hair follicle.

The first evidence of a follicle in the embryo is seen as a thickening of the epidermis (pregerm stage). The pregerm stage passes rapidly into the hair-germ stage as the basal cells become taller and the entire structure sinks into the dermis. From its point of origin the hair germ grows obliquely, deep into the mesenchyme, in the form of a solid column. This is called the *hair-peg stage*. The advancing border enlarges, becomes bulbous, and envelops part of the mesenchymal

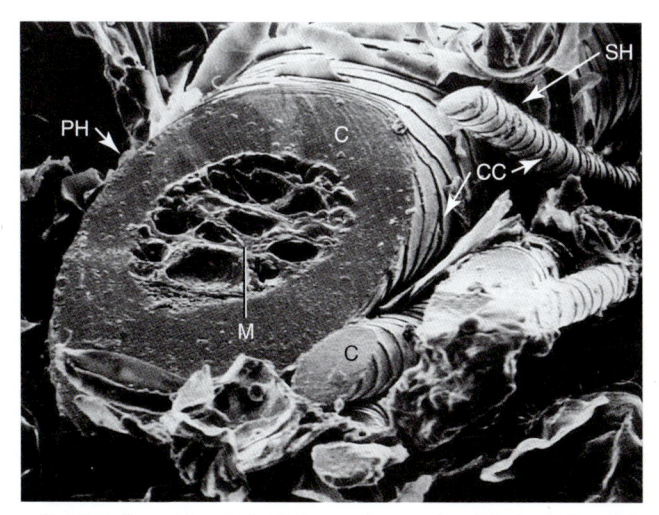

• **Fig. 3.5** Scanning photoelectron micrograph of hair shafts. *CC,* Cuticle cells; *M,* medulla; *PH,* primary hair; *SH,* secondary hair; *C,* cortex.

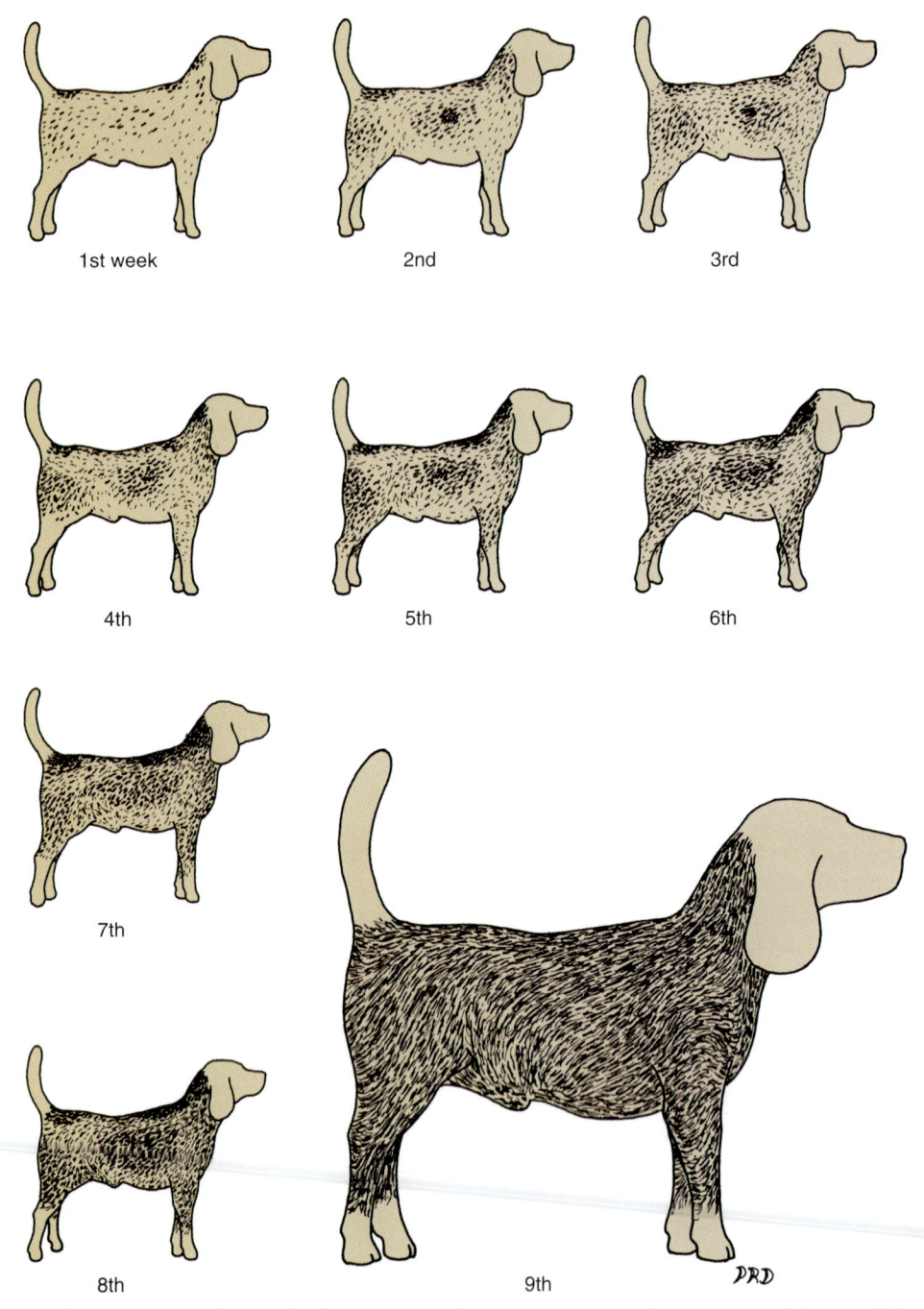

• **Fig. 3.6** Lateral view of regrowth of the hair coat after clipping a 1-year-old male. (From Al-Bagdadi FK: *The hair cycle in male Beagle dogs*, Ph.D. thesis, Champaign, 1975, University of Illinois.)

material ahead of it, thus entering the bulbous-peg stage. Later the hair bulb and the dermal papilla become differentiated into the productive hair follicle, complete with glandular and muscular accessories. As the dermis increases in thickness between birth and 6 months of age, the length of the hair follicles increases. In 40-day fetuses, all stages of follicles have developed. Secondary hair follicles (Fig. 3.8) begin development before birth but usually have no external hair shaft until after birth.

The first hairs to appear in the 29-day fetal dog are in the region of the eyelids, dorsal lip, and rostral portion of the mandible (see Chapter 2). These develop into large tactile hairs of the face, which will become specialized sinus hairs. The follicles of the general hairy skin appear in the pregerm stage on the head and neck as early as 30 days. They reach the hair-germ stage at 32 days and hair-peg stage at 37 days of gestation. In the general development of the pelage, the hairs are farthest advanced near the head, and development spreads caudally and ventrally. The primary hair germs form more or less simultaneously at fairly even distances. As the skin grows, increasing the surface area, new primary germs develop among the earlier ones. This results

1st week 2nd 3rd
4th 5th 6th
7th
8th 9th

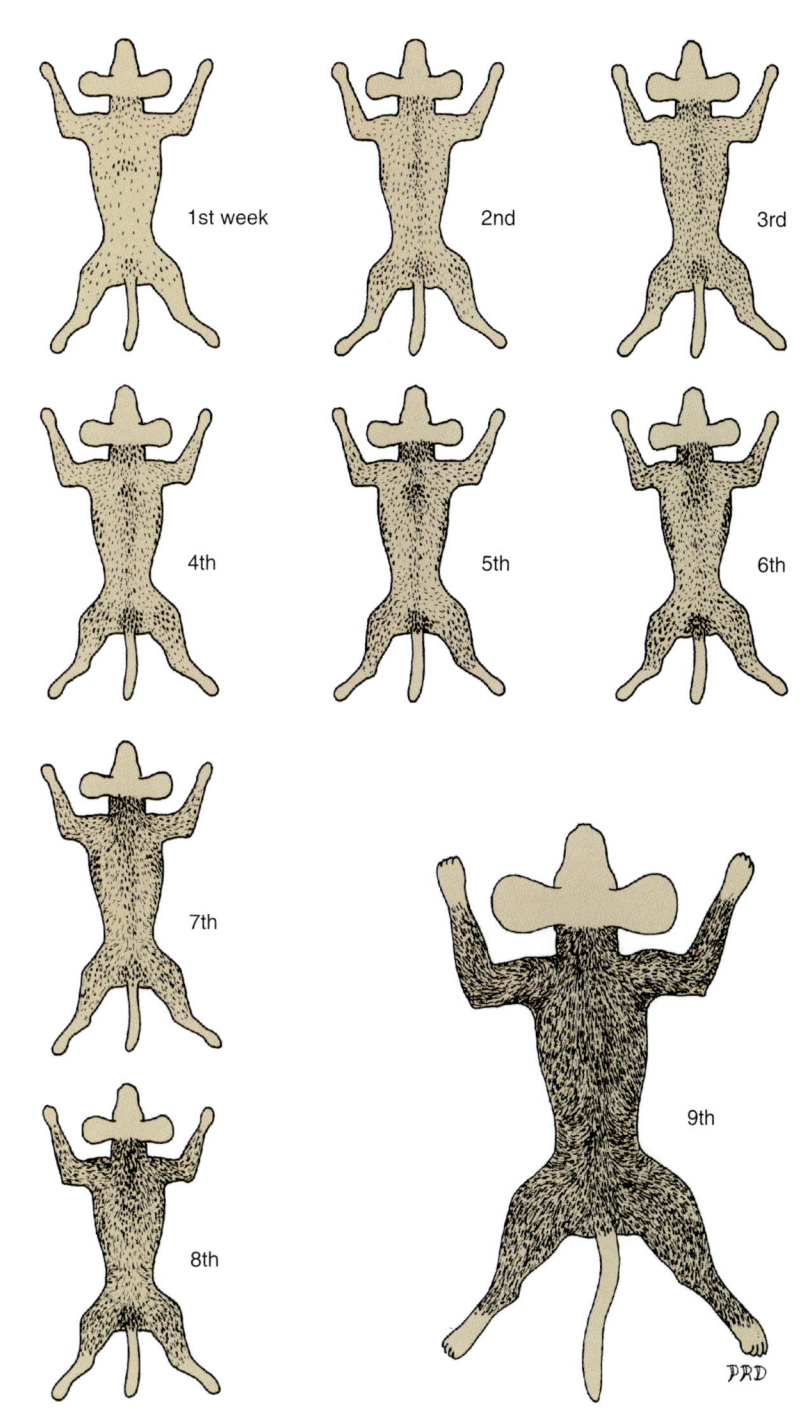

- **Fig. 3.7** Dorsal view of regrowth of the hair coat after clipping a 1-year-old male. (From Al-Bagdadi FK: *The hair cycle in male Beagle dogs,* Ph.D. thesis, Champaign, 1975, University of Illinois.)

in two, three, or four groups of follicles being clustered together. Later, the secondary germs develop close to the primary ones and form the complex follicle arrangement. This process starts before birth and is completed after birth (see Fig. 3.8).

Development of Complex Follicle

The embryologic development of hair was described by Pinkus (1958). Observations on the development of the hair follicle in the dog have been reported by Al-Bagdadi et al. (1977b). It can be observed by examining the hair coat of a puppy during the first few days after birth when there is usually only a single hair emerging from each external follicle orifice of the skin. At birth the majority of hair follicles of dogs are primary hairs. Secondary hairs develop caudal to the primary hairs during the first 12 to 28 weeks of life (Dunstan, 1995). On microscopic examination it can be observed that secondary follicles form as strands of intensely basophilic cells running deeply into the dermis

72 CHAPTER 3 The Integument

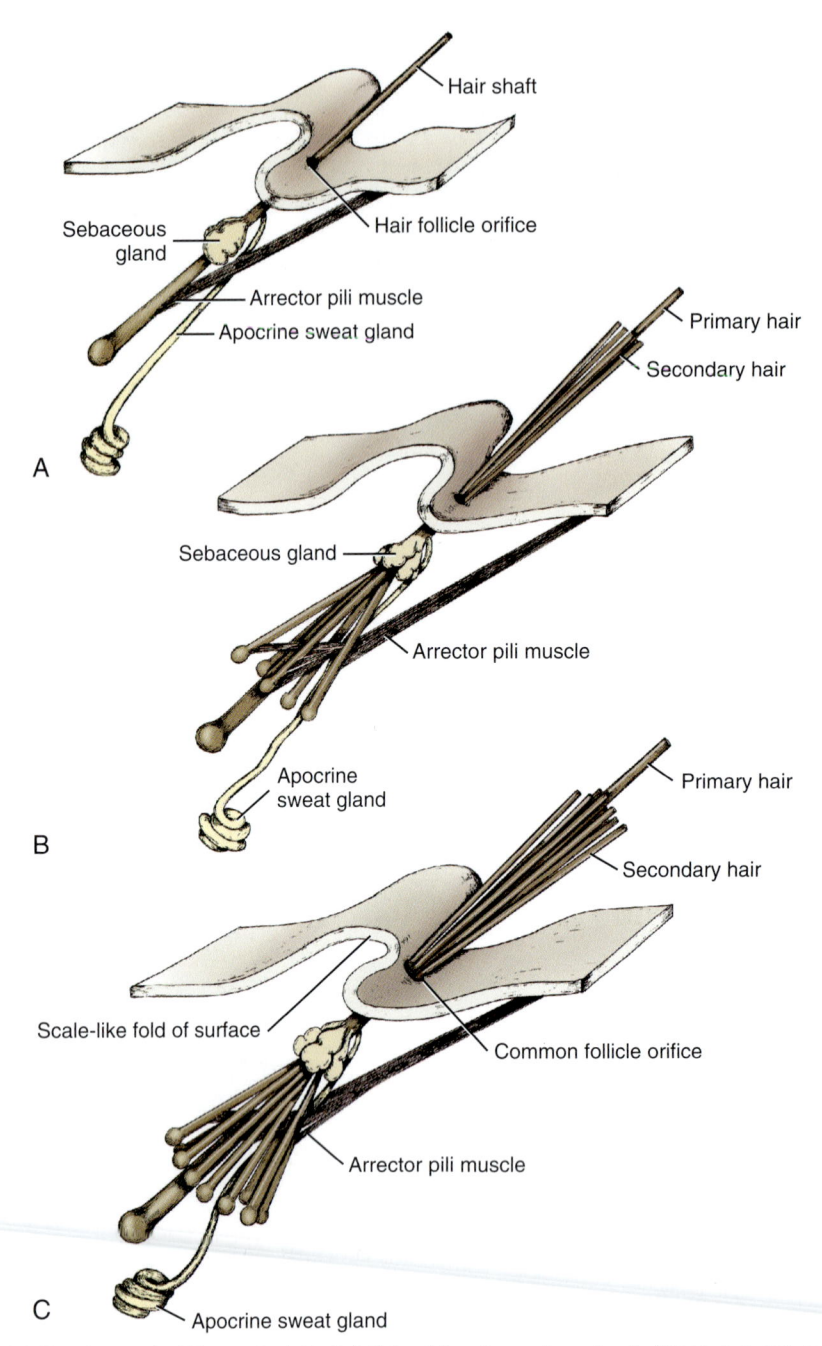

- **Fig. 3.8** Development of the postnatal hair follicle of the dog, schematic. **A**, Simple hair follicle during the first postnatal week. **B**, Complex hair follicle during the 12th postnatal week with secondary hair shafts. **C**, More elaborate complex hair follicle during the 28th postnatal week.

from their point of origin adjacent to the sebaceous gland of the primary follicle. These satellite, or accessory, hairs appear externally at 3 or 4 weeks of age, when each primary follicle can be seen to be giving rise to two or three secondary hairs. At 8 to 10 weeks of age the secondary follicles are arranged in a crescent around the central and lateral primary hairs. They are on the same side as the apocrine gland. Subsequently, secondary follicle formation continues until puberty, when from 6 to 10 or more hairs may emerge from a single follicle orifice. The larger primary hairs have a well-developed honeycomb-like medulla (Al-Bagdadi et al., 1988). Their nerve and blood supply is better developed than that of the secondary hair follicles. As a general rule, the coarser guard hairs appear earlier than these secondary hairs. In the development of the dog, the nature of the puppy's hair changes, and, in the young adult, the fine, fluffy hair of the pup is replaced by a coarser hair. In a young adult dog, the hair growth is profuse and abundant. In old dogs the hair covering is thinner, the hairs are not as long, and frequently the coloring fades to gray. As the hair becomes more brittle, the flexibility of the skin and subcutaneous tissue decreases.

Complex Hair Follicle

The hairy skin of an adult dog contains complex hair follicles that are bundles of hairs that share common openings on the surface. These complex hair follicles are usually arranged in groups of two or three oriented in rows. The typical complex group consists of a group of secondary, or underhairs, and a single longer and stiffer primary or cover hair. The primary hair of a three-bundle group is coarser than the thinner secondary hairs (Fig. 3.9).

The hair shafts that share a common opening in the skin are enclosed in a common follicle down to the level of the sebaceous glands. Deep to this point the hair shafts have their own individual hair follicle and bulb. In this way, as many as 15 hairs may share a single external follicle orifice. The individual follicle and hair bulb of the primary hair are larger and penetrate more deeply into the subcutaneous tissue than those of the secondary hairs. There are breed variations in the number of follicle groups per square centimeter and also in the number of hairs in each complex hair follicle (Brusch, 1956). The Smooth-Haired Dachshunds, Smooth-Haired Terriers, and Toy Poodles have 400 to 600 hair groups per square centimeter. German Shepherd Dogs, Airedales, and Rottweilers have only 100 to 300 hair groups per square centimeter. Other breeds have numbers somewhere in between. The number of hairs per group complex vary from 9 to 15 in the Rottweiler to 2 to 5 in the Dachshund. In general, the hair of those breeds that have many hair groups is finer. Miniature animals of all breeds have a greater number of hair groups with fewer and finer hairs. Dogs produce 60 to 180 g/kg of hair growth per year, depending on the breed (Mundt & Stafforst, 1987).

The dog's hair follicle is part of a pilosebaceous arrector muscle complex. The sebaceous glands of individual hair follicles appear in clusters and sometimes fuse. The arrector pili muscles originate from the external root sheath of each hair follicle and then join as a common muscle bundle that is inserted into the dermis. When the arrector pili muscle

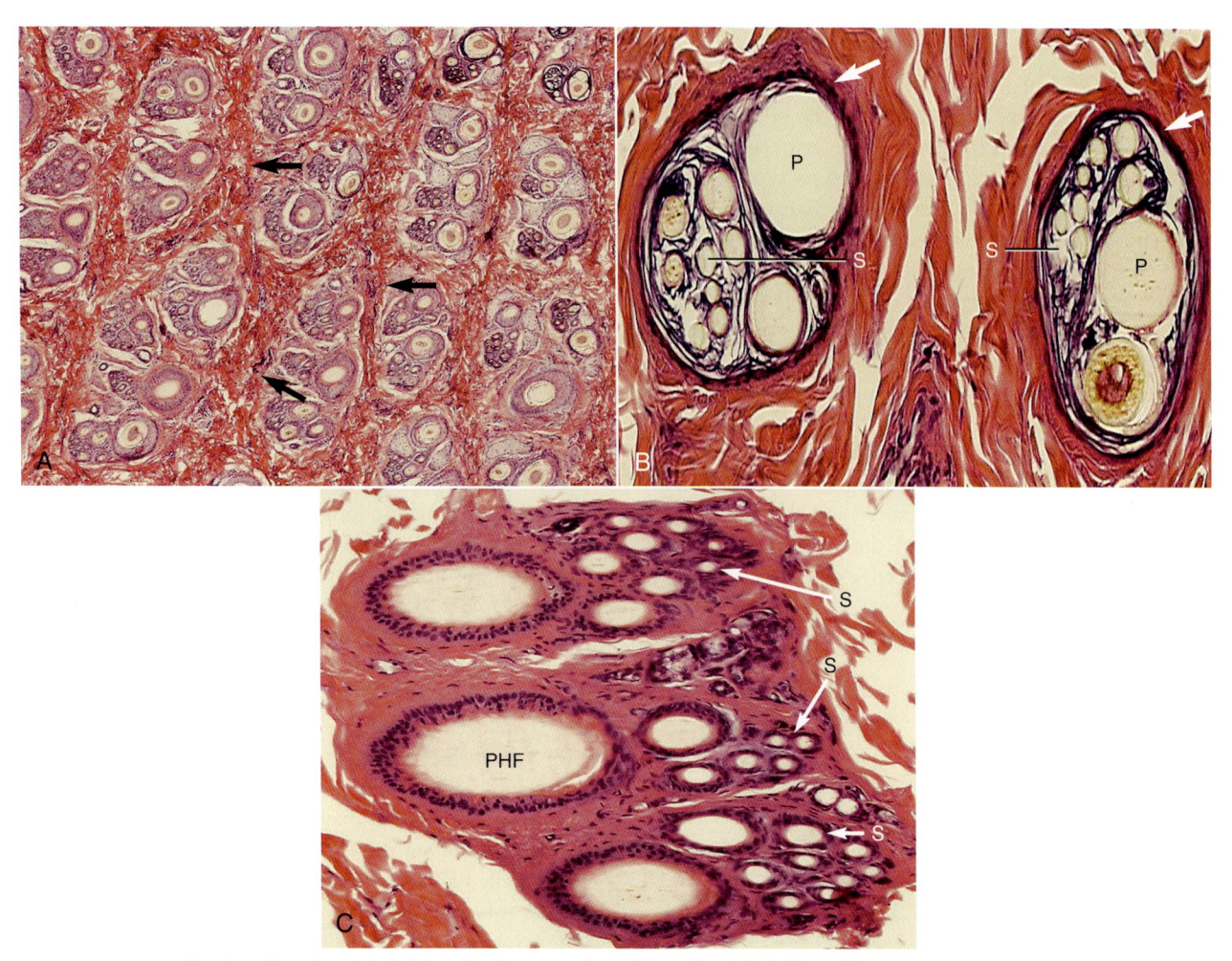

• **Fig. 3.9** Complex hair follicles. **A**, Cross-section of complex hair follicles. Fibrous connective tissue trabeculae (*arrows*) separate the complex hair follicles into groups of two and three. **B**, Two complex hair follicles, separated by connective tissue trabeculae, exit from the epidermal orifices (*arrow*). Primary hair shaft (*P*). Secondary hair shaft (*S*). **C**, Cross-section of a group of three complex hair follicles. Each has one primary hair follicle (*PHF*) and multiple secondary hair follicles (*S*). Stained with hematoxylin and eosin. (From Al-Bagdadi FK: *The hair cycle in male Beagle dogs,* Ph.D. thesis, Champaign, 1975, University of Illinois.)

contracts, the entire complex of follicles is elevated, and the sebaceous gland material empties into a common follicle sleeve that is shared by all the hairs. A single apocrine gland is associated with each follicle complex. The coiled secretory tubule lies deep in the subcutaneous tissue. A direct extension of this tubule becomes the excretory duct for the apocrine secretion, which extends into the dermis along the follicle complex and empties into the common part of the follicle superficial to the opening of the sebaceous glands. The epitrichial glands are sweat glands but do not play a major role in the heat-regulating mechanism of the dog. They are comparable to the atrichial sweat glands associated with hair follicles of the axillary and pubic regions of humans. The oily secretion from the glands associated with the hair follicles tends to keep the skin soft and pliable and spreads out over the hair shafts. This gives the coat a glossy sheen. During periods of sickness, malnutrition, or parasitism, the hair coat frequently becomes dull and dry as a result of inadequate functioning of the skin glands.

Hair Types

There is a great deal of variability in hair length, color, diameter, and transverse contour among the various breeds of dogs and between individuals of the same breed (Fig. 3.10). The canine hairs are classified into six types:

1. **Straight hair** is a bristly, firm primary hair often deeply pigmented. It is sometimes called a *protective hair* or *cover hair*. This is the largest hair and is the chief hair in the compound hair follicles. It is also usually the longest hair, and the shaft is either straight or bowed. It has a thick medulla and a thin cortex.
2. **Bristle hair** is a bristle with a spinelike tip, but thinner and softer near the base. The distal third is similar to type 1, but the proximal two-thirds may be slightly wavy. In the hair coat it is difficult to distinguish this from type 1. The medulla is slightly smaller than that of type 1. The bristle hair is shorter than the straight hair but is regarded as an overhair or protective hair. This type may be the primary hair in a group but is usually a secondary hair to type 1.
3. **Wavy bristle hair** is finer and shorter than type 2. It is wavy with a well-developed bristle. These are the larger secondary hairs but are usually included with the cover hairs or protective hairs. The medulla and cortex are smaller than in type 2, but the cortex is relatively heavier.
4. **Bristled wavy hair** is a long, soft hair that is shorter and finer than type 3, with a poorly developed bristle and a smaller medulla. It is wavy in the lower two-thirds of the shaft. This type represents the largest hairs of the undercoat.
5. **Large wavy hair** is shorter and finer than type 4, and the shaft is very wavy with a small bristle on the tip. The medulla is very small and may be discontinuous. The cortex is relatively thick. This type gives a fur- or wool-like feel to the undercoat.
6. **Fine wavy hair** is shorter and finer than type 5 and is sometimes described as *vellus hair, fuzz, down,* or *lanugo hair*. The medulla is discontinuous or absent. This type represents the finest and smallest hairs of the undercoat and is usually wavy with a small and poorly developed bristle on the tip.

Variability in Hair Coat

The formation of bristles at the tips of some hair shafts suggests that the early part of the hair growth cycle is the most productive because the tips of these shafts have a greater diameter than the shaft. Follicles with a rich blood supply as a source of metabolites will synthesize more hair shaft.

There are three hair-coat types based on hair length. The normal coat, which resembles the hair covering of wild canids (wolf, jackal) is typified by the German Shepherd Dog. The short-hair coat is represented by the Boxer, and the long-hair coat by the Chow-Chow. There are many variations among the long-haired types, such as wire hair, tight, curly, and flat. Hilton and Kutscha (1978) described the distinguishing characteristics of the hair of the coyote, dog, red fox, and bobcat.

The various coats observed in domestic breeds of dogs are made up of the six types of hair with some exceptions, described by Brusch (1956). The wirehaired breeds, such as the Schnauzer, have a preponderance of bristle-type hairs, with a seventh type not found in other breeds. The Cocker Spaniel and the Setter have fine, long, silky hair with less obvious bristle development. The Poodle has extremely long hair that resembles the wool hair type. The medullary canal of a Poodle hair is greatly reduced or absent. Bristle formation in this breed is characterized by a rhythmic pattern of differences in the thickness of the hair, thus suggesting continuous growth with variation in growth intensity.

Coat Color

The color of the hair shaft is produced by pigment cells in the bulb of the hair follicle. From these cells granules of

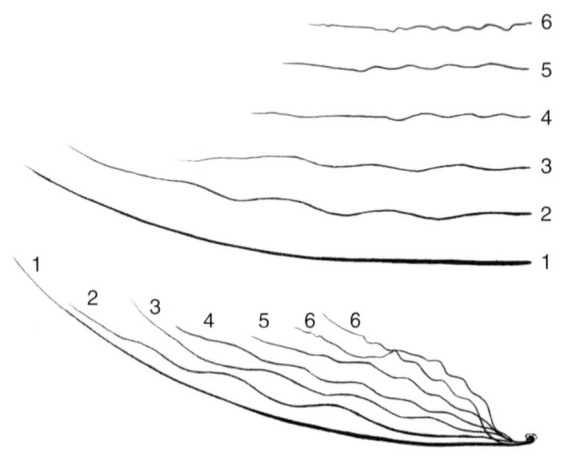

• Fig. 3.10 Hair types in the dog (see text for description).

pigment enter cortical and medullary cells during development. The granules may remain between the cells, as is the case in the medulla, but most of them are engulfed by the cells. The amount of pigment and variations in location produce different optical effects. The pigmentation may be uniform through the entire length of the hair, or it may vary. Hair color ranges from all black to all white, with variations of banding, spotting, blazes, tricolors, and blended grays. In the agouti type of hair, which is found in wolves and in some breeds of dog (German Shepherd Dog and Norwegian Elkhound), the tip of the hair is white and the thick part of the bristle is heavily pigmented (black or dark brown), with the proximal two-thirds of the hair having lighter pigmentation (yellow or red).

Despite the wide range of colors that are possible in the coat, microscopic examination has revealed only black, brown, and yellow pigment granules. The black-brown pigment (eumelanin) is designated as "tyrosine-melanin" because it is formed by enzyme oxidation of tyrosine to melanin. The yellow-red pigment is designated as "pheomelanin." DaFonsica and Cabral (1945) classified the dog's coat according to color and pattern into three types: simple, compound, and mixed. The studies of inheritance and genetic control of color and coat patterns have been summarized by Little (1957), Burns (1966), and Miller, Griffin, and Campbell (2013). Gobello et al. (2003) found that the color of the hair coat of the dog can be altered through the inhibition of the secretion of melanocyte-stimulating hormone.

Hair Length

The length of the hair is controlled to a large extent by the genetic makeup of the individual. A short coat is dominant to long. Straight or wavy types are recessive or partially recessive to wire coat types. Temperature and climate also stimulate seasonal variation in hair length in most breeds of dogs.

The short-haired breeds show a definite reduction in the undercoat. This process has gone farthest in the Poodle, in which the outer coat has been reduced, thus increasing the proportion of the undercoat. In such a manner, selective breeding has succeeded in altering the characteristics of the coat of dogs from that found in foxes and wolves.

Implantation of Hair

Some of the differences seen in the coat of various types of dogs are due to the variation in the implantation angle of the hair follicle. The Chow-Chow, Airedale, and Scottish Terrier have an implantation angle of 45 degrees. Other breeds, such as the Long-Haired Dachshund, Cocker Spaniel, and Irish Setter, have an implantation angle of less than 30 degrees. The majority of all breeds examined by Brusch (1956) had an angle between 30 and 40 degrees. There is a tendency for long-haired dogs to have a higher implantation angle. Generally, the hairs slant in a caudal direction from the nose toward the tip of the tail.

Wakuri et al. (1987) described the streams of convergent and divergent whorls and the points where streams of different directions join. The patterns are subject to great variation. Some of the more obvious features that can be easily observed on short-haired dogs are the center of nasal divergence, cheek whorls, ear center, ventral cervical stream, neck diverging line, diverging mammary gland whorls, ventral center line (division of hair cover on both sides of the body), thoracic whorls from the ventral cervical stream, a whorl in the region of the elbow, and rump whorls.

Hair Follicle Cycle and Seasonal Shedding

The process of shedding is gradual, and the coat of one season merges into that of the next so the dog is normally never without a protective covering. Shedding is genetically controlled to some extent, but environment is certainly a factor in expression of genetic potential. The ovarian hormonal influence on the hair cycle (Butler & Wright, 1981) supersedes the influence of the photoperiod and seasonal changes of temperature (Hale, 1982). There is said to be little shedding of hair in Poodles, Old English Sheepdogs, and Schnauzers, but, according to Miller, Griffin, and Campbell (2013), this is yet to be documented.

It has been observed by dog owners that short-haired breeds of house dogs may shed a little all year long and that long-haired outdoor dogs may be seasonal shedders twice a year. Blackburn (1965) found in confined dogs with hair of normal length that there is shedding in spring and autumn. In the spring the shedding of the hair in a dog that is groomed daily lasts about 5 weeks. During the first 10 to 14 days, the majority of the hairs shed are bristle hairs and bristle-lanugo hairs. After this it is mainly the lead hairs and lanugo hairs that are shed.

Al-Bagdadi et al. (1977a) correlated the stages of the hair follicle cycle as observed from microscopic examination of monthly skin biopsies to the mean weight of monthly hair samples collected by combing male Beagle dogs each week. A definite correlation was found between the highest percentage of telogen hair follicles and the greatest amount of shedding that occurred in the spring and autumn. Hair shedding in Beagle dogs is greatest in the spring and the fall. A comparison of the temperature changes with the amount of material combed from Beagle dogs indicates that the hair does not shed only during or just before the period of high temperatures, but is shed in a seasonal pattern.

The hair follicle cycle as observed in the Beagle by Al-Bagdadi et al. (1977a) was described in three stages: the anagen, catagen, and telogen (Figs. 3.11 and 3.12). Miller, Griffin, and Campbell (2013) have illustrated five stages: catagen, telogen, anagen, exogen, and anagen. Their exogen stage is a shedding stage.

The **anagen** stage is characterized by a well-developed flame-shaped dermal papilla, which is completely capped by the hair matrix of the bulb of the hair follicle. Ultrastructural studies of the basement membrane between the

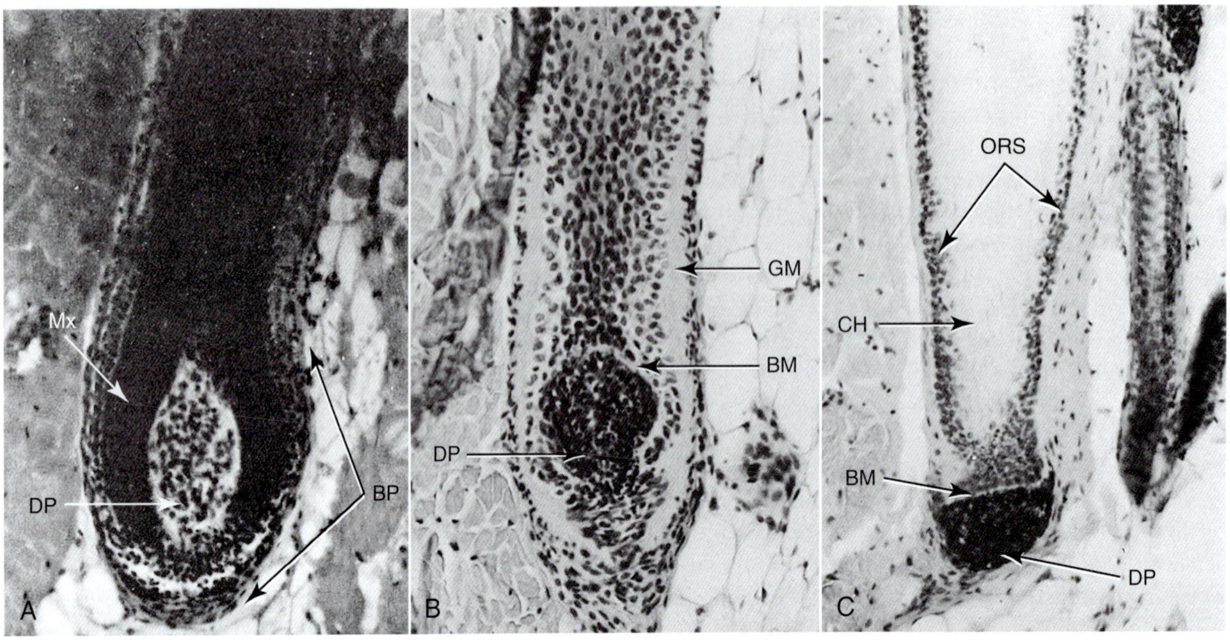

Fig. 3.11 Stages of the hair follicle. **A,** Anagen. Longitudinal section of a primary follicle from the saddle region of a 6-month-old Beagle dog. This is an example of the anagen stage, and it illustrates a well-developed dermal papilla (*DP*), which is completely bordered by the matrix cells (*Mx*). The bulb of the hair follicle is labeled (*BP*). (Magnification 240×. Stained with hematoxylin and eosin.) **B,** Catagen. Longitudinal section of a primary hair follicle from the saddle region of a 2-week-old Beagle dog. This is an example of a catagen hair follicle. It has a rounded dermal papilla (*DP*). The glassy membrane (*GM*) is thick and somewhat irregular above the bulb region. The basement membrane (*BM*) can be observed. (Magnification 265×. Stained with hematoxylin and eosin.) **C,** Telogen. Longitudinal section of a primary hair follicle from a 9-month-old Beagle dog. This is an example of a telogen hair follicle. The dermal papilla (*DP*) is outside the bulb, separated from the matrix cells by a basement membrane (*BM*). The external root sheath (*ORS*) borders the club hair (*CH*) directly, owing to lack of internal root sheath. (Magnification 190×. Stained with hematoxylin and eosin.)

matrix cells and dermal papilla cells suggest that granular ground substance diffuses from the dermal papilla cells to the matrix cells to furnish metabolites and materials that are needed for the rapid synthesis of keratin. Hair follicles of the anagen stage are the longest, with the bulb extending deep into the dermis or even into the subcutis, where they are surrounded by adipose tissue. In the larger primary hair follicles, blood vessels have been demonstrated entering the dermal papilla at the hair bulb. The smaller hair follicles of lanugo hair seem to have dermal papillae that are devoid of blood vessels.

The **catagen** stage is identified by the presence of a thick, glassy membrane on the outside of the follicle (see Figs. 3.12B and 3.13B). This glassy membrane is irregular and has an undulated appearance in the deeper third of the hair follicle. Thickening of the glassy membrane is accompanied by a thickening of the basement membrane between the dermal papilla and the bulb matrix. The follicle bulb becomes smaller, and the dermal papilla more rounded. The entire follicle becomes shorter, and the rounded bulb is not as deep in the dermis as the spindle-shaped bulb of the anagen hair follicle.

Hair follicles during the **telogen** stage have a smaller dermal papilla, which is separated from the bulb and is no longer capped by matrix cells, which have decreased in number (see Fig. 3.12). The hair follicle of the telogen stage is very short; it contains a club hair, and the internal root sheath disappears. A club hair is the reduced hair shaft just prior to its loss from the follicle.

The rate of growth varies in different follicles and in different regions of the body. A club hair that has been shed naturally is differentiated from one that has been broken or shorn by the slightly bulbous proximal end, which is frayed out into fibrillae. When club hairs are plucked during the resting phase (telogen), new hairs begin to grow at once, whereas new hair growth occurs much later if the resting hair is allowed to shed naturally. This may influence the development of coats of Wire-Haired Fox Terriers, which are customarily plucked when being groomed for show purposes. When a growing hair is plucked during anagen, nearly all of the deeper half of the follicle is pulled out with it.

Dogs shed more cover hairs in the spring than in the summer, and the number of hairs in each bundle increases in the winter. There is a great deal of variation in the manner in which dogs shed their hair, even among individuals of the same breed kept under similar environmental conditions and fed the same diet.

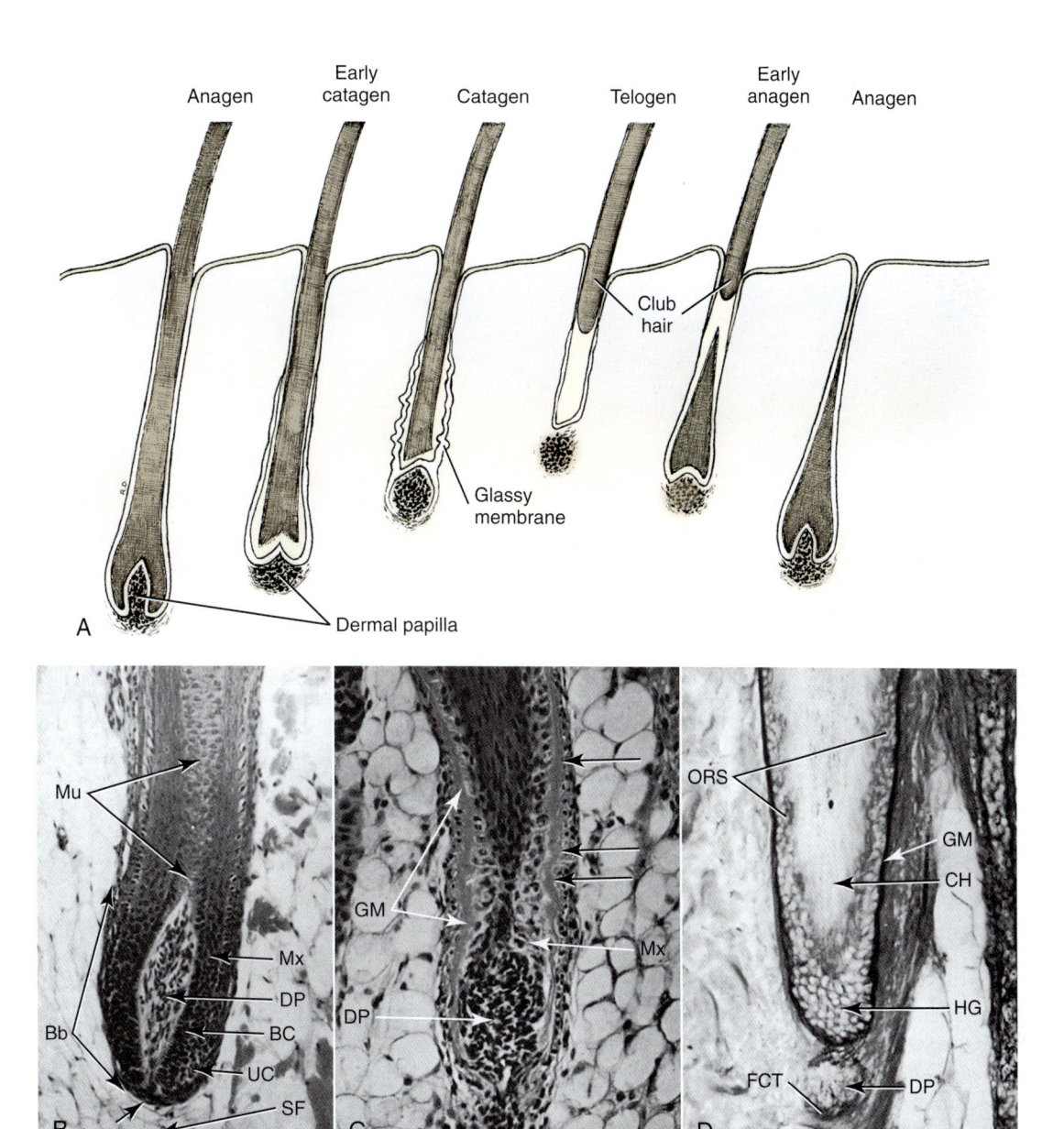

• **Fig. 3.12** Schematic representation of changes observed in a primary hair follicle of the saddle region of Beagle dogs during the hair cycle. **A**, Drawings of the stages of the hair cycle. **B–D**, Histologic sections of three hair cycle stages. **B**, Anagen hair follicle. Longitudinal section of a secondary hair follicle in the anagen stage from the saddle region of a 28-month-old Beagle. The bulb (*Bb*) extends into the subcutaneous fat (*SF*). The spindle-shaped dermal papilla (*DP*) extends toward the medulla of the hair (*Mu*), and the base of the dermal papilla is continuous with the connective tissue (*CT*) of the hair follicle. The dermal papilla is surrounded by the matrix cells (*Mx*) of the bulb (*Bb*). The basal cells of the matrix are columnar (*BC*). The deeper part of the bulb contains undifferentiated matrix cells (*UC*). (Magnification 350×. Stained with hematoxylin and eosin.) **C**, Catagen. Longitudinal section of a hair follicle in the catagen stage from the saddle region of a 2-week-old Beagle. The dermal papilla (*DP*) is oval in shape. The nuclei are crowded closely together, and the matrix cells (*Mx*) that border the dermal papilla have lost their orientation. The glassy membrane (*GM*) is thick and straight at the superficial part of the hair follicle (*single black unlabeled arrow in the upper part of the picture*), while superficial to the bulb the glassy membrane is undulating (*two black unlabeled arrows in the lower part of the picture*). (Magnification 395×. Stained with hematoxylin and eosin.) **D**, Telogen. Longitudinal section of a primary hair follicle in the telogen stage from the saddle region of a 3.month-old Beagle. The dermal papilla (*DP*) is separated from the matrix cells of the hair follicle. It is surrounded by fibrous connective tissue (*FCT*) and appears to contact the base of the follicle at one point. The hair germ cells (*HG*) are located at the base of the club hair (*CH*). The cells of the external root sheath (*ORS*) lack glycogen granules. The glassy membrane (*GM*) is thick and periodic acid Schiff positive. The hair follicle at this stage is surrounded by connective tissue that separates the follicle from the adipose tissue. (Prepared with periodic acid Schiff reaction of McManus [1968] without diastase treatment. Magnification 400×.)

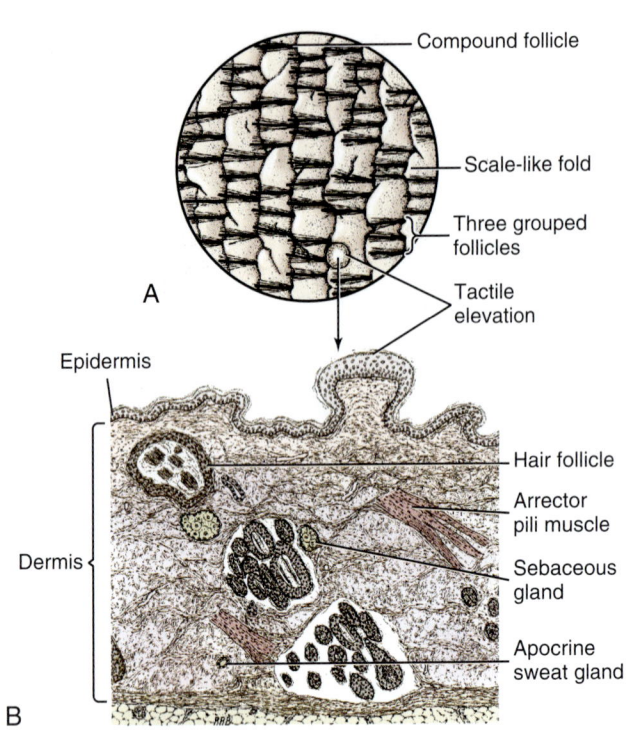

• **Fig. 3.13** Surface contour, hair arrangement, and histologic section of the hairy skin. **A**, View of scalelike folds and arrangement of hair follicles. **B**, Histologic section of hairy skin. (Lovell JE, Getty R: The hair follicle, epidermis, dermis, and skin glands of the dog, *Am J Vet Res* 18:873–885, 1957.)

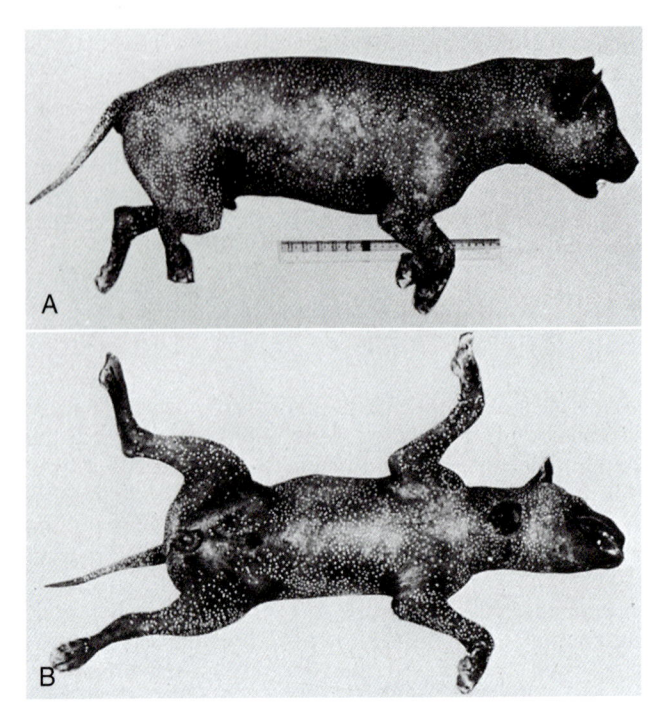

• **Fig. 3.14** A male mongrel dog prepared to show the location of toruli tactiles. Lateral (**A**) and ventral (**B**) views. (With permission from Wakuri H, Mutoh K, Narita M: Density of toruli tactiles in the dog, *Okajimas Folia Anat Jpn* 64:71–80, 1987.)

Surface Contour of Hairy Skin and Histologic Characteristics of Epidermis

The surface of the hairy skin is irregular because of scale-like folds that form depressions into which the complex hair follicles invaginate. The surface of the skin is slightly wavy on the dorsal neck and trunk and becomes heavily folded on the abdomen and especially in the area of the inguinal fold (Lloyd & Garthwaite, 1982). The pattern of skin folds is occasionally interrupted by the presence of knoblike enlargements 0.33 to 0.35 mm in diameter, which are sensory tactile elevations of the skin, known as tactile toruli (*torulus tactilis*) (Figs. 3.13 and 3.14). Various terms have been used to describe these structures: *epidermal papillae* (Lovell & Getty, 1957), *integumentary papillae* (Strickland & Calhoun, 1963), *Haarscheiben* (Mann, 1965; Smith, 1967; Straile, 1961), and *toruli tactiles* or *touch spots* (Iggo, 1977). The primary tactile hair that is associated with the tactile elevations is referred to as a **tylotrich hair** by many authors (Mann, 1965; Smith, 1967; Straile, 1960, 1961). The tactile elevations are more pedunculated in the dog and cat than in other species and may lie medial, lateral, cranial, or caudal to the tactile hair. This positional relationship is of importance in sensory functions. Montagna (1967) stated that all animals have tactile hairs (*Haarscheiben*). Adam et al. (1970) illustrate the epidermal pad of the tactile hair follicle in the dog. It was observed that the tactile elevation is a dome-shaped enlargement of the epidermis at birth and becomes more pedunculated by 6 months of age. English et al. (1983) stated that, after chronic denervation of the skin, the cutaneous type I receptor sites—tactile toruli—degenerate but do not disappear entirely. Wakuri and Narita (1986) have published color micrographs and an electron scan of a tactile torulus of a dog. According to Wakuri et al. (1987) the tactile toruli of a female dog are twice as numerous (10 to 13 per 2 cm^2) as those of a male (6 to 9 per 2 cm^2). They found the density of toruli greatest on temporal and buccal areas, on the dorsum of the trunk, on the lateral surfaces of the forearms, in the gluteal area, and on the lateral surfaces of the thigh. There were few on the face, ears, axilla, and external genitals.

Histologic findings reveal that the epidermis of the hairy skin ranges in thickness from 25 to 40 μm and usually consists of three layers: stratum basale, stratum spinosum, and stratum corneum. In a few areas the stratum granulosum and stratum lucidum are evident, but these are infrequent and are in areas where keratinization is retarded (i.e., around hair follicle orifices). The number of layers of epidermal cells varies between three and six. In regions where the stratum granulosum and stratum lucidum are evident, there are as many as eight layers of cells. The mean number of cell layers of stratum corneum is 47.5 (Lloyd & Garthwaite, 1982). The aged epidermis becomes thinner, the dermoepidermal junction becomes flattened, and the melanocytes and Langerhans cells decrease in number (Fenske & Lober, 1986). The tactile elevations are covered by a thickened epidermis that is usually 6 to 12 cell layers thick, approximately twice as thick as the surrounding epidermis.

The dermis in the tactile elevations is composed of very fine, closely packed connective tissue fibers that lie deep to the thickened epidermis to form the elevation. Schwarz et al. (1979) reviewed the micromorphologic characteristics of the skin of the dog.

Muscles of the Skin

The **arrector pili muscles** (*mm. arrectores pilorum*) are smooth muscles that are best developed on the dorsal line of the neck, trunk, and tail (Figs. 3.8, 3.15, and 3.16). They are very small or absent in the ventral surface of the body. During the first 8 weeks of life in pups, the arrector pili muscles of the interscapular area range from 10 to 40 μm in diameter. At the ages of 4 to 6 months they ranged from 30 to 40 μm in the same region (Lovell, 1955). Smooth muscles are also present in the dermis of the scrotum, teat, and penis.

Striated cutaneous muscle fibers occur in the superficial fascia deep to the skin, closely associated with the subcutis. In the cranial region they consist of the *sphincter colli superficialis, platysma,* and *sphincter colli profundus* (see Chapter 6). These primary muscle sheets delaminate and divide into many slips, which are associated with the lips, eyelids, face, and external ears. Around the muzzle region some fibers are associated with the sinus hair follicles.

A large skin muscle called the *cutaneous trunci* covers a great portion of the thorax and abdomen. It extends from the gluteal region to the thoracic region. Some fibers from the cutaneous trunci form the preputial muscle in the male and supramammary muscle (m. supramammaricus) in the female (St. Clair, 1975). The cutaneous muscles are attached to the dermis of the skin and are anchored to the subcutaneous fascia rather than to bone. Contraction of cutaneous muscles causes wrinkling of the skin and erection of the hair.

Glands of the Skin

Atrichial sweat glands (*glandula sudorifera merocrina*) are found only in the foot pads (Nielsen, 1953) (see Fig. 3.4D). These were formerly called *eccrine sweat glands*. They are placed deeply in the fat and fibrous tissue of the foot pad cushion. They are small (25 to 35 μm in diameter), tightly coiled, tubular glands, with minute lumina that are lined with cuboidal cells. They contain coarse granules scattered in the clear cytoplasm. Myoepithelial cells may be demonstrated peripheral to the secretory tubules. The excretory ducts follow a tortuous path through the dermis and epidermis and empty in the crevices between the conical projections of the foot pads. The eccrine secretion is watery. Atrichial sweat glands are innervated by cholinesterase-positive nerves (Winkelmann & Schmit, 1959).

Epitricheal sweat glands (*glandula sudorifera apocrina*) are found mainly in connection with hair follicles (see Figs. 3.8 and 3.16). These were formerly called the *apocrine sweat glands*. The secretory parts of the glandular tubules are situated in the dermis of the skin and the subcutis. The excretory duct passes through the dermis and empties into the hair follicles superficial to the ducts of the sebaceous glands. The tubules and individual cells attain sizes of 30 to 90 μm, depending on the secretory phase. In some sections there are huge, dilated, cystlike tubules, 90 μm in diameter, lined with flattened, elongated cells. In others the tubules are small, with high, cylindrical epithelium 30 to 45 μm in diameter. Secretory vesicles in the apocrine

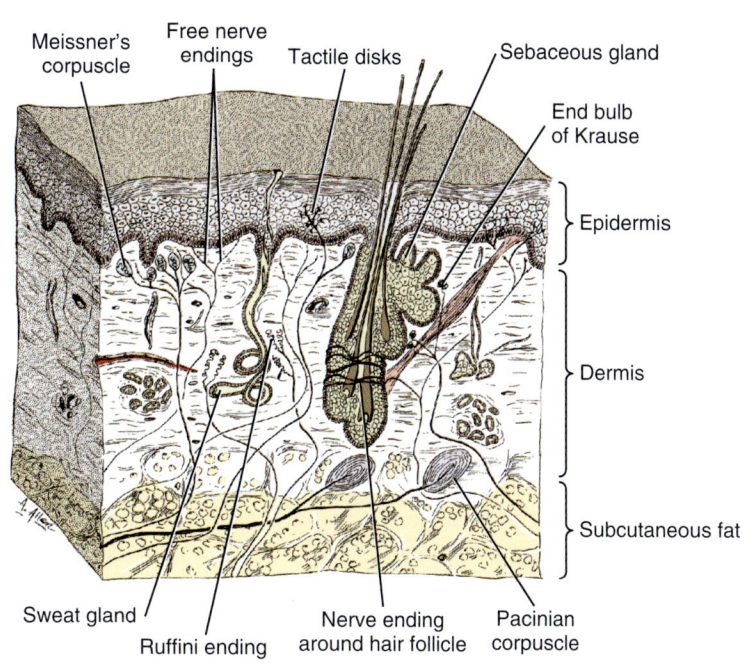

• **Fig. 3.15** Schematic representation of the nerve supply to human skin, illustrating receptor morphologic characteristics.

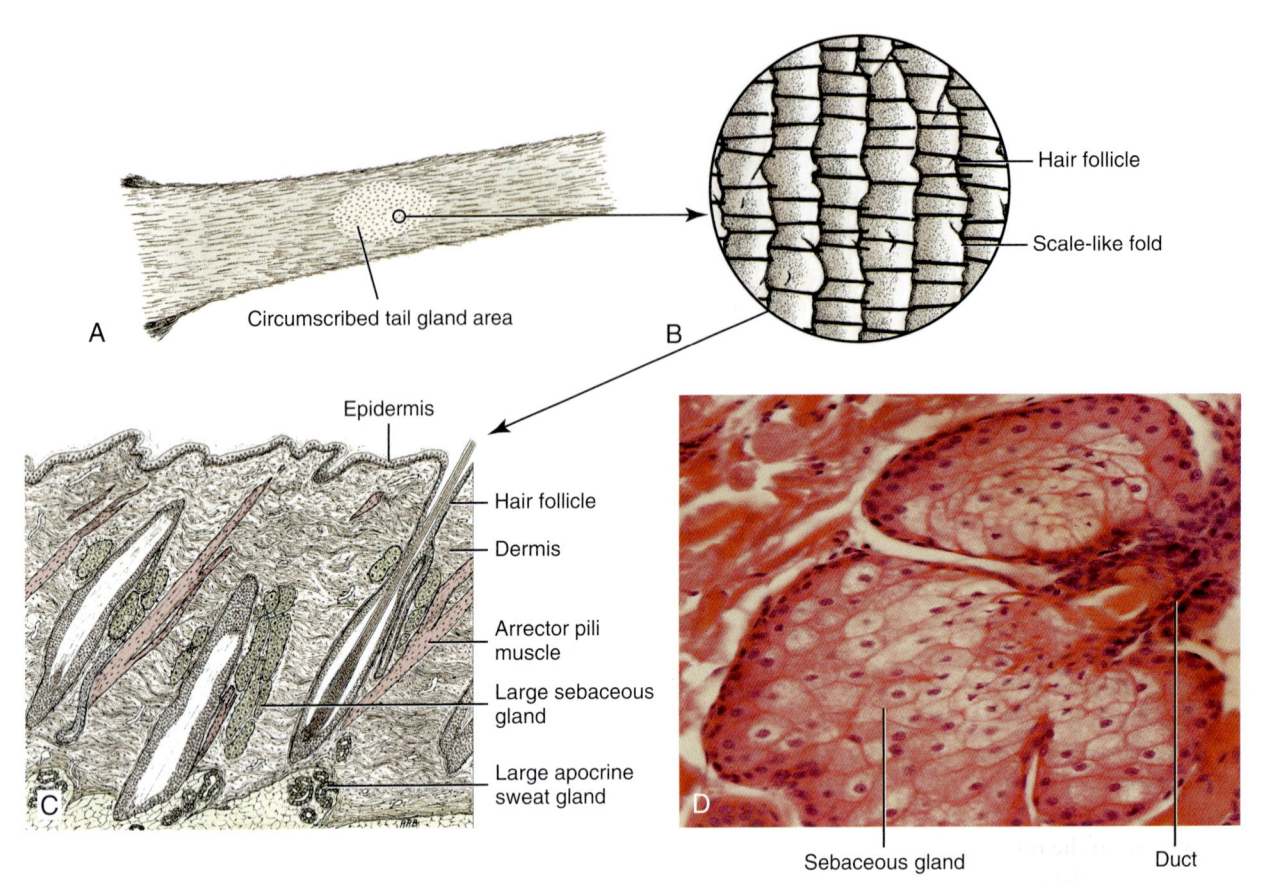

• **Fig. 3.16** Surface contour, hair arrangement, and histologic section of tail gland area. (After Lovell JE, Getty R: The hair follicle, epidermis, dermis, and skin glands of the dog, *Am J Vet Res* 18:873–885, 1957.)

sweat gland develop from the Golgi apparatus and discharge into the lumen by exocytosis and micro-apocrine and macro-apocrine secretion (Iwasaki, 1981). Thomsett (1986) reported apocrine gland sweating in the axilla and groin and along the ventral abdomen in the German Shepherd Dog, Labrador Retriever, and other large breeds. The epitrichial sweat glands have no identified innervation (Miller et al., 2013).

Sebaceous glands (*gll. sebacea*) are holocrine in secretion (see Figs. 3.8 and 3.16) and are distributed over the integument in association with hair follicles. They are largest along the dorsal part of the neck, trunk, and tail, particularly in the specialized tail gland area. The **tarsal glands** (Meibomian glands) of the eyelids are also specialized sebaceous glands.

The size of the sebaceous glands in the skin of the dorsal neck and trunk at birth is 30 to 50 μm in diameter. There is a gradual increase from 80 to 250 μm at 6 months of age. The largest sebaceous glands are present at the mucocutaneous junctions of the lips, anus, vulva, and eyelids. Sebaceous secretion gives the skin and hair hydrophobic protection and plays a role in thermoregulation by providing insulation (Smith & Thiboutot, 2008; Zouboulis et al, 2008).

The **glands of the ear canal** (*gll. ceruminosae*) are apocrine and sebaceous. Cerumen is a product of both glandular types and appears as a fairly dry, dark brownish substance. Fernando (1966) reported that long-haired breeds have more sebaceous and apocrine glandular tissue in the external auditory canal than do short-haired breeds.

The **circumanal glands** (*gll. circumanales*) are most numerous in the vicinity of the anal orifice (Isitor & Weinman, 1979; Parks, 1950). They are associated with the sebaceous glands located in the cutaneous zone of the anal canal and consist of solid masses of large polygonal hepatoid-like cells with no excretory ducts. They are derived from the sebaceous glands located here but have no excretory ducts. Konig et al. (1985) investigated both the circumanal glands and the tail glands of dogs and found similar cells. They denote only the deeper hepatoid lobules as circumanal glands, contrary to other authors. They never observed bursting of "retention" cysts or emptying of contents; thus these nonvacuolated hepatoid glands are not exocrine. Vacuolated hepatoid cells were found only in the circumanal glands of newborn and young puppies, and they do not have ducts. Isitor and Weinman (1979) reported that the hepatocyte-like cell of the circumanal glands develops from hair follicle sheath cells. The transitional hepatocyte-like cells develop within the deep poles of sebaceous glands. They are involved in metabolism of steroid hormones and are the site of canine tumors. These hepatocyte-like cells are positive for cytokeratin (Vos et al., 1993).

The paired **paranalis sinuses** (anal sacs) are spherical and average approximately 1 cm in diameter. One lies on each side of the anal canal between internal and external anal

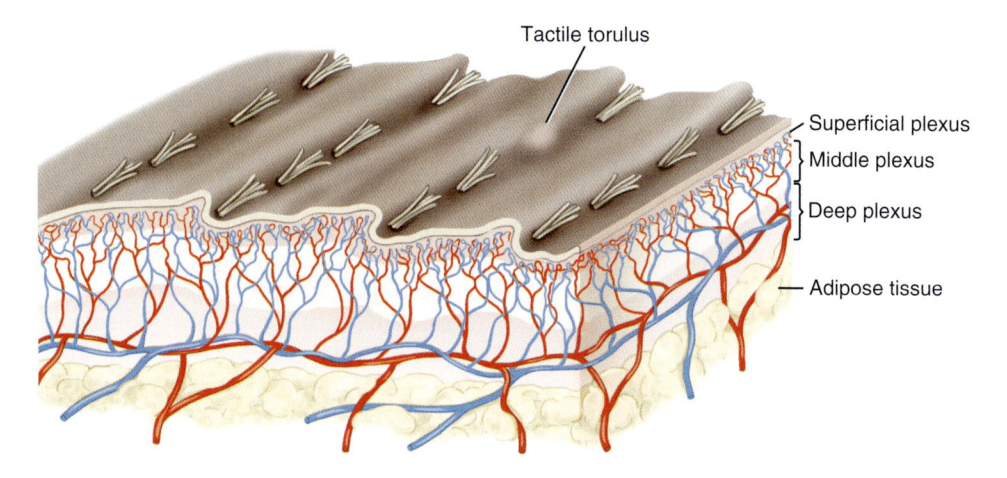

• Fig. 3.17 Schematic section of the skin of the dog showing tactile torulus and blood vessels.

sphincter muscles. Each sinus opens onto the lateral margin of the anus by a single duct. The sacs form pockets that function as a reservoir into which apocrine and sebaceous glands open. They are lined by a thin, stratified squamous epithelium supported by connective tissue containing many sebaceous and apocrine glands (*gll. sinus paranalis*). The sebaceous glands line the neck of the sinus, whereas the apocrine glands are concentrated in the fundus. The combined secretions of the tubules of the apocrine glands of the sinus wall and the sebaceous glands associated with its excretory duct form a viscous, putrescent liquid or paste. Gerisch and Neurand (1973) found only tubular apocrine glands in the sinus.

Therapeutic administration of female steroids has been reported to affect sinus gland secretions (Donovan, 1969). The paranalis sinuses function in scent marking. According to Pappalardo et al. (2002), seven bacterial species were isolated from the sinuses of normal dogs. The same bacterial strains were isolated from their paranalis sinuses and from their abdominal skin and hair.

Tail Gland Area (*gll. caudae*)

An oval to elongated rudimentary area of the tail glands (*glandulae caudae*), known as the *Viole* in some literature, is located on the dorsum of the tail, at the level of the seventh to ninth caudal vertebrae in almost all dogs (see Fig. 3.16A). The gland area is 2.5 to 5 cm long. The hair shafts in the area are larger in diameter and differ in appearance from the surrounding hair. They emerge from the hair follicle singly (see Fig. 3.16C), whereas surrounding hair is of the complex follicle type, supporting 6 to 11 hairs. The single hairs of this specialized area are very stiff and coarse, and the surface of the skin has a yellow, waxy appearance probably owing to an abundance of sebaceous secretion. The sebaceous and apocrine glands of the area are large, extending deep into the dermis and subcutaneous tissue. Hildebrand (1952) suggested that secretions of the tail glands in wild canids function in species recognition. Kristensen (1975) believed that the tail glands play a role in sexual activity. Meyer (1971) studied the tail gland of 134 pedigreed dogs from 35 different breeds and found that it was similar to that described in wild canids and mongrel dogs. Meyer and Wilkens (1971) found a seasonal dimorphism in the activity of the glands in the fox. Konig et al. (1985) described the tail gland complex as modified sebaceous glands with both vacuolated and nonvacuolated hepatoid cells. They believe that this indicates some connection with steroid metabolism.

Blood Supply to the Skin

The arteries to the skin include simple cutaneous arteries, which reach the skin by running between muscles while supplying small branches to the muscles, and mixed cutaneous arteries, which run through muscles and supply large muscular branches before terminating in the skin. The arteries are arranged in a general segmental pattern that is not as regular as that of spinal cutaneous nerves. Hughes and Dransfield (1959) have listed 23 mixed cutaneous arteries and 16 simple cutaneous arteries. For additional information on regional blood supply to the skin refer to Chapters 11 and 12. The vessels anastomose extensively with one another.

Microscopic examination has revealed that the arterial supply to the skin of the dog is divided into three distinct plexuses, all lying parallel to the surface. These are the deep, or subcutaneous, plexus; the middle, or cutaneous plexus; and the superficial, or subpapillary, plexus (Fig. 3.17).

The *subcutaneous plexus* (deep plexus) is made up of the terminal branches of the cutaneous arteries. Branches from this plexus form the *cutaneous plexus*, which is associated with the hair follicles and epitrichial sweat glands (Miller et al., 2013). There is a *middle plexus* that supplies the middle portion of the hair follicles and some sebaceous glands, as well as middle portions of hair follicles.

The *subpapillary plexus* (superficial plexus) is formed by the union of small vessels arising from the middle plexus. The skin dermal papillae contain numerous capillary loops that come from the superficial plexus. The superficial plexus supplies epidermis and superficial portions of hair follicles (Miller et al., 2013). In general the veins and arteries parallel one another. Arteriovenous anastomoses have been observed in the deeper layers. Variations in the circulatory pattern have been noted in the various modified skin areas. Information concerning the blood supply to the skin of the dog is reviewed by Pavletic (1985). Arteriovenous anastomoses occur in all areas of the skin and are common in and over the ears and limbs of the dog (Miller et al., 2013).

The lymphatics arise from capillary nets that lie in the superficial part of the dermis or surround the hair follicles and glands. The vessels arising from these nets drain into a subcutaneous lymphatic plexus (Baum, 1917). For a description of the lymph vessels and nodes associated with the skin see Chapter 13.

Nerve Supply to the Skin

Small nerve branches are generally distributed in a segmental pattern to the subcutis in all areas of the body. On the head they originate from cutaneous components of cranial nerves, mainly the trigeminal and facial nerves. Along the body, cutaneous nerves are branches of cervical, thoracic, lumbar, sacral, and caudal spinal nerves. The segmental order is altered somewhat in the region of the limbs, where the cutaneous nerves arise from the axillary, radial, ulnar, and median nerves from the brachial plexus, and from the gluteal, sciatic, tibial, fibular, and femoral nerves from the lumbosacral plexus. For information on cutaneous innervation, refer to Chapters 17 and 19 and the references cited therein.

Microscopic examination reveals that large nerve trunks enter the dermis from the subcutis, where they branch and give rise to nerves that ramify alongside the blood vessels, forming a branching plexus that supplies the blood vessels, hair follicles, skin glands, and epidermis (see Fig. 3.17). Nerve fibers have not been demonstrated in the apocrine sweat glands of the general body surface of the dog. Iwabuchi (1983) presented evidence that catecholamines of the adrenal medulla provoke general sweating on the hairy skin of dogs and suggests that these sweat glands receive adrenergic innervation from the sympathetic nerves. The eccrine sweat glands of the foot pad are innervated. Nerve fibers innervate the sebaceous glands of both primary and secondary hairs. In the dog there are connections between the nerves associated with the hair follicle and those in the arrector pili muscle.

Iggo and Muir (1963) investigated cutaneous sense organs in the hairy skin of cats. Iggo (1977) summarized somesthetic sensory mechanisms. The regional cutaneous innervation of the head of the dog was documented by Whalen and Kitchell in 1983 (see Chapter 19), and the cutaneous innervation of the thorax and abdomen of the dog was reported by Bailey et al. (1984) using electrophysiologic techniques that provide information on autonomous and overlapping zones of skin innervation. These innervation "maps" have been most helpful clinically for the diagnosis of lesions.

Skin Grafting

Autogenous skin grafts (Jensen, 1959), homografts (Puza & Gombos, 1958), and allografts (Rehfeld et al., 1970) have been performed on dogs. For information on different techniques of using grafts and skin flaps see Converse et al. (1977), Pavletic (1981, 1985), and Probst and Peyton (1983).

Histopathologic studies of transplants indicated that degenerative changes involve the epidermis and the superficial layers of the dermis during the first 8 to 10 postoperative days, at which time regenerative processes equalize the degenerative changes.

The combination of the ultrasonographic and color-flow Doppler as noninvasive methods is used to identify the cutaneous arteries (superficial cervical, thoracodorsal, deep circumflex iliac, and caudal superficial epigastric arteries) for axial pattern skin flaps in dogs (Reetz et al., 2006). The ultrasonographic assessment of direct cutaneous arteries is used for axial pattern skin flaps in dogs. The blood supply to the transplant is adequate by the 12th day and completely normal by the 24th day. According to Wells and Gottfried (2010), a full-thickness scrotal skin graft used as a meshed skin graft to the dorsal aspect of the left pes was successful.

Claw

The superficial layers of the epidermis are modified to form the **horny claw** (*unguiculus*) (see Fig. 3.18). Gross examination shows that the claw consists of a sole, two walls, and a central dorsal ridge (*margo dorsalis*). The claw is frequently strongly pigmented and is curved and compressed laterally. The dorsal ridge is made up of thicker horny material than

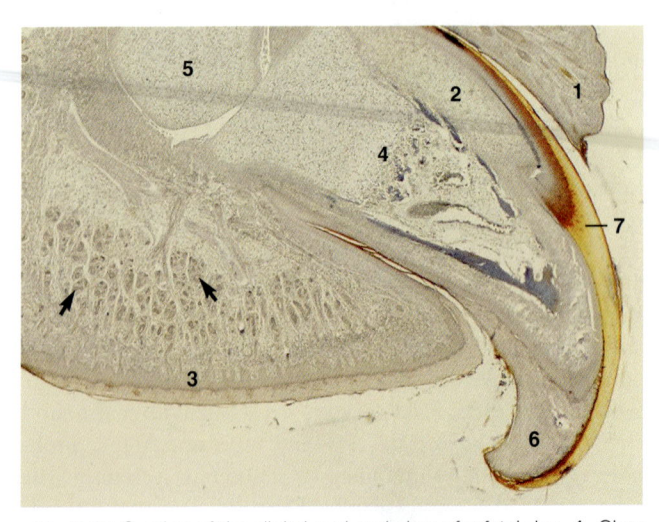

• Fig. 3.18 Section of the digital pad and claw of a fetal dog. **1**, Claw fold, **2**, dermis, **3**, digital pad, **4**, distal phalanx, **5**, middle phalanx, **6**, sole, **7**, wall. The digital pad contains eccrine sweat glands (*arrows*) ×20. Stained with hematoxylin and eosin. (Courtesy F. Al-Bagdadi collections.)

are the walls and sole, which maintains the pointed appearance of the claw. The coronary border of the claw fits into the space beneath the ungual crest of the third phalanx. This relationship is hidden by the skin of the claw fold (vallum). Dorsally, this fold is a modification of the hairy skin, which is free from hair on one side and fused to the horn of the claw. As the horny material is produced and grows out, it is covered by a thin stratum tectorium that adheres to the proximal part of the claw. A furrow along the palmar or plantar surface of the claw separates it from the digital pad in a similar manner.

The periosteum of the third phalanx and dermis of the claw are continuous and fill the space between the bony and epidermal structures. The vascularity of this tissue is well demonstrated by the hemorrhage that follows trimming the canine claw into the connective tissue. On microscopic examination, the dermis of the coronary and dorsal ridge areas has been described as having a papillated structure.

The stratum basale, which is the epidermal layer supported by the dermis, is most active in the coronary and dorsal ridge areas, where most of the horny claw is formed. The inner surface of the claw wall bears small epidermal lamellae. The epidermis of the claw is composed largely of the horny stratum corneum, which consists of flat, cornified epidermal cells. The epidermis of the sole has a well-developed stratum granulosum and stratum lucidum.

The claw grows at a rapid rate and, if not worn off or trimmed, may continue to grow in a circular fashion until the point of the claw invades the palmar/plantar furrow between the base of the claw and the foot pad or the foot pad itself (Fig. 3.19).

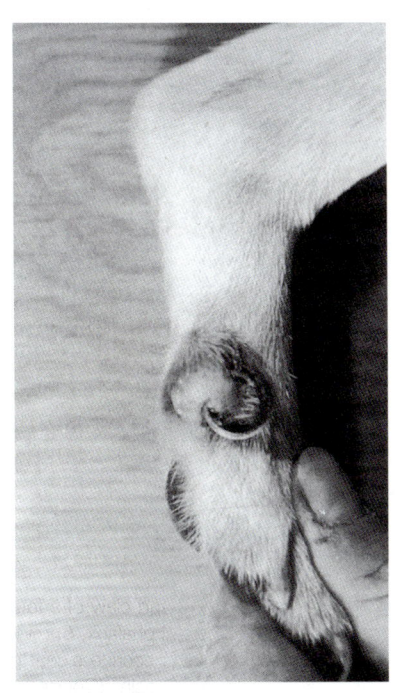

• **Fig. 3.19** An in-grown dewclaw of a Beagle.

Bibliography

Adam, W. S., Calhoun, M. L., Smith, E. M., et al. (1970). *Microscopic anatomy of the dog: a photographic atlas*. Springfield, IL: C. C. Thomas.

Al-Bagdadi, F. K. (1975). *The hair cycle in male beagle dogs*, Ph.D. thesis, Champaign, IL: University of Illinois.

Al-Bagdadi, F. K., Titkemeyer, C. S., & Lovell, J. E. (1977a). Hair follicle cycle and shedding in male beagle dogs. *Am J Vet Res, 38*, 611–616.

Al-Bagdadi, F. K., Titkemeyer, C. W., & Lovell, J. E. (1977b). Ultrastructural morphology of the anagen stage hair follicle of male beagle dogs. *Proc Electron Microsc Soc Am, 35*, 652–653.

Al-Bagdadi, F. K., Titkemeyer, C. W., & Lovell, J. E. (1978). Alkaline phosphatase reaction in hair follicles of male beagle dogs during hair cycle stages. *Anat Hist Embryol, 7*, 245–252.

Al-Bagdadi, F. K., Ruhr, L. P., Archibald, L. F., et al. (1988). Hair dye effects on the hair coat and the skin of the dog: a scanning electronmicroscopic study. *Anat Histol Embryol, 17*, 349–359.

Bailey, C. S., Kitchell, R. L., & Haghighi, S. S. (1984). Cutaneous innervation of the thorax and abdomen of the dog. *Am J Vet Res, 45*, 1689–1698.

Baker, K. P. (1967). Senile changes of dog skin. *J Small Anim Pract, 8*, 49–54.

Baum, H. (1917). Die lymphgefasse der haut des hundes. *Anat Anz, 50*, 1–15.

Bereiter-Hahn, J., Matoltsy, A. G., & Richards, K. S. (1986). *Biology of the integument, 2: vertebrates*. New York: Springer-Verlag.

Blackburn, P. S. (1965). The hair of cattle, horse, dog and cat. In A. J. Rook & G. S. Walton (Eds.), *Comparative physiology and pathology of skin*. Philadelphia: FA Davis.

Blatt, C. M., Taylor, C. R., & Habal, M. B. (1972). Thermal panting in dogs: the lateral nasal gland, a source of water for evaporate cooling. *Science, 177*, 804–805.

Brusch, A. (1956). Vergleichende untersuchungen am haarkleid von wildcaniden und haushunden. A. tierzunchtung und zuchtungs. *Biologie, 67*, 205–240.

Burns, M. (1966). *Genetics of the dog—inheritance of color and hair type*. Philadelphia: JB Lippincott.

Butler, W. F., & Wright, A. I. (1981). Hair growth in the greyhound. *J Small Anim Pract, 22*, 655–661.

Calhoun, M. L., & Stinson, A. W. (1976). Integument. In H. D. Dellmann & E. M. Brown (Eds.), *Textbook of veterinary histology*. Philadelphia: Lea & Febiger.

Chesney, C. J. (1995). Measurement of skin hydration in normal dogs and in dogs with atopy or scaling dermatosis. *J Small Anim Pract, 36*, 305–309.

Choi, K. L., & Sander, D. N. (1986). The role of langerhans cells and keratinocytes in epidermal immunity. *J Leukocyte Biol, 39*, 343–358.

Clark, R. A. (1983). Fibronectin and the skin. *J Invest Dermatol, 81*, 475.

Conroy, J. D., & Beamer, P. D. (1970). The development of cutaneous and oral pigmentation in Labrador Retriever fetuses (*Canis familiaris*). *J Invest Dermatol, 54*, 304–315.

Converse, J. M., McCarthy, J. G., Brauer, R. O., et al. (1977). Transplantation of skin: grafts and flaps. In J. M. Converse (Ed.), *Reconstructive plastic surgery: principles and procedures in correction, reconstruction, and transplantation*. Philadelphia: Saunders.

DaFonsica, P., & Cabral, A. (1945). Pelagnes dos caes. *Rev Med Vet, 40*, 187–191.

Diana, A., Guglielmini, C., Federico, F., et al. (2008). Use of high-frequency ultrasonography for evaluation of skin thickness in relation to hydration status and fluid distribution at various cutaneous sites in dogs. *J Am Vet Res, 69*(9).

Diana, A., Apreziosi, R., Gugleilmini, C., et al. (2004). High-frequency ultrasonography of the skin of clinically normal dogs. *J Am Vet Res, 65*(12).

Diaz, S. F., Torres, S. M., Nogueira, S. A., et al. (2006). The impact of body site, topical melatonin and brushing on hair regrowth after clipping normal Siberian Husky. *Vet Dermatol, 17*(1), 45–50.

Donovan, C. A. (1969). Canine anal glands and chemical signals (pheromones). *J Am Vet Med Assoc, 155*, 1995–1996.

Dunstan, R. W. (1995). A pathomechanistic approach to diseases of the hair follicle. *Br Vet Dermatol Study Group, 17*, 37.

Emerson, J. L., & Cross, R. F. (1965). The distribution of mast cells in normal canine skin. *Am J Vet Res, 26*, 1379–1382.

English, K., Norman, D., & Horch, K. (1983). Effects of chronic denervation in type I cutaneous mechanoreceptors (Haarscheiben). *Anat Rec, 207*, 79–88.

Fenske, N. A., & Lober, C. W. (1986). Structural and functional changes of normal aging skin. *J Am Acad Dermatol, 15*, 571–585.

Fernando, S. D. A. (1966). A histological and histochemical study of the glands of the external auditory canal of the dog. *Res Vet Sci, 7*, 16–119.

Gerisch, D., & Neurand, K. (1973). Topographic und histologie der drusen der regio analis des hundes. *Anat Hist Embryol, 2*, 280–294.

Ghohestani, R. F., Li, K., Rouselle, P. R., et al. (2001). Molecular organization of cutaneous basement membrane zone. *Clin Dermatol, 19*, 551–562.

Gobello, C., Caster, G., Broglia, G., et al. (2003). Coat colour changes associated with cabergoline administration in bitches. *J Small Anim Pract, 44*, 352–354.

Gunaratnam, P., & Wilkinson, G. (1983). A study of normal hair growth in the dog. *J Small Anim Pract, 24*, 445–453.

Hale, P. A. (1982). Periodic hair shedding by a normal bitch. *J Small Anim Pract, 23*, 345.

Hester, S. L., Rees, C. A., Kennis, R. A., et al. (2004). Evaluation of corneometry (skin hydration) and transepidermal water-loss measurement in two canine breeds. *J Nutr, 134*(8 Suppl.), 2110S–2113S.

Hildebrand, M. (1952). The integument in canidae. *J Mammal, 33*, 419–428.

Hilton, H., & Kutscha, N. P. (1978). Distinguishing characteristics of the hairs of eastern coyote, domestic dog, red fox, and bobcat in Maine. *Am Mid Nat, 100*, 223–227.

Horning, J. G., McKee, A. J., Keller, H. E., et al. (1926). Nose printing your cat and dog patient. *Vet Med, 21*, 432–453.

How, K. L., Hazewinkel, H. A., & Mol, J. A. (1994). Dietary vitamin D dependence of cat and dog due to inadequate cutaneous synthesis of vitamin D. *Gen Comp Endrocrinol, 96*, 12–18. doi:10.1006/gcen.1994.1154.

Hughes, H. V., & Dransfield, J. W. (1959). The blood supply to the skin of the dog. *Br Vet J, 115*, 1–12.

Iggo, A. (1962). New specific sensory structures in hairy skin. *Acta Neuroveg, 24*, 175–180.

Iggo, A. (1977). Somesthetic sensory mechanisms. In M. J. Swenson (Ed.), *Dukes' physiology of domestic animals* (9th ed.). Ithaca, NY: Cornell University Press.

Iggo, A., & Muir, A. R. (1963). A cutaneous sense organ in the hairy skin of cats. *J Anat, 97*, 151.

Irwin, D. H. (1966). Tension lines in the skin of the dog. *J Small Anim Pract, 7*, 593–598.

Isitor, G. A., & Weinman, D. E. (1979). Origin and early development of canine circumanal glands. *Am J Vet Res, 40*, 487–492.

Iwabuchi, T. (1967). General sweating on the hairy skin of the dog and its mechanisms. *J Invest Dermatol, 49*, 61–70.

Iwabuchi, T. (1983). Electron microscopy of the canine apocrine sweat duct. *Jpn J Vet Sci, 45*, 739–746.

Iwasaki, T. (1981). An electron microscopic study on secretory process in canine apocrine sweat gland. *Jpn J Vet Sci, 43*, 733–740.

Jensen, E. C. (1959). Canine autogenous skin grafting. *Am J Vet Res, 20*, 898–908.

Konig, M., Mosimann, W., & Devaux, R. E. (1985). Micromorphology of the circumanal glands and the tail gland area of dogs. *Vlaams Diergeneeskd Tijdschr, 54*, 278–286.

Kristensen, S. (1975). A study of skin diseases in dogs and cats. I. histology of the hairy skin of dogs and cats. *Nord Veterinaermed, 27*, 593–603.

Little, C. C. (1957). *The inheritance of coat color in dogs*. Ithaca, NY: Comstock.

Lloyd, D. H., & Garthwaite, G. (1982). Epidermal structure and surface topography of canine skin. *Res Vet Sci, 33*, 99–104.

Lovell, J. E. (1955). *Histological and histochemical studies of canine skin, Masters thesis*. Ames: Iowa State University.

Lovell, J. E., & Getty, R. (1957). The hair follicle, epidermis dermis, and skin glands of the dog. *Am J Vet Res, 18*, 873–885.

Mann, S. J. (1965). Haarscheiben in the skin of sheep. *Nature, 205*, 1228–1229.

Mercati, F., Pascucci, L., Gargiulo, A. M., et al. (2008). Immunohistochemical evaluation of intermediate filament nestin in dog hair follicle. *Histol Histopathol, 23*(9), 1035–1041.

Meyer, P. (1971). Das dorsale shwanzorgan des hundes (canis familiaris). *Zbl Vet Med, 18*, 541–557.

Meyer, P., & Wilkens, H. (1971). Die "viole" des rot fuchses (vulpes vulpes l.). *Zbl Vet Med, 18*, 353–364.

Meyer, W. (2009). Hair follicles in domesticated mammals with comparison to laboratory animals and humans. In L. Mecklenburg, M. Link, & D. J. Tobin (Eds.), *Hair loss disorders in domestic animals*. Ames Iowa.

Meyer, W., Seger, H., Hulmann, G., & Nuerand, K. (1997a). A computer assisted method for the determination of the hair cuticula patterns in mammals. *Berl Munch Tierarzt Wochenschr, 110*, 81–85.

Meyer, W., Seger, H. (Hulmann, G., & Neurand, K. (1997b). Species determination of mammals based on their hair cuticle pattern – a comparison of domestic mammals and their wild ancestors from the forensic viewpoint. *Arch Kriminol, 200*, 45–55.

Miller, W. H., Jr., Griffin, C. E., & Campbell, K. L. (2013). *Muller and Kirk's small animal dermatology* (7th ed.). St. Louis: Elsevier.

Montagna, W. (1967). Comparative anatomy and physiology of the skin. *Arch Dermatol, 96*, 357–363.

Mundt, H. C., & Stafforst, C. (1987). Production and composition of dog hair. In A. T. P. Edney (Ed.), *Nutrition, malnutrition and dietetics on the dog and cat*. London: British Veterinary Association and Waltham Centre for Pet Nutrition.

Nielsen, S. W. (1953). Glands of canine skin: morphology and distribution. *Am J Vet Res, 14*, 448–454.

Oiki, N., Nishida, T., Ichihara, N., et al. (2003). Cleavage line patterns in beagle dogs:as a guideline for use in dermatoplasty. *Anat Histol Embryol, 32*, 65–69.

Pappalardo, E., Mario, P. A., & Noli, C. (2002). Macroscopic, cytological and bacteriological evaluation of anal sac content in normal dogs and in dogs with selected dermatological diseases. *Vet Dermatol, 13*, 315–322.

Parks, H. (1950). *Morphological and cytochemical observations on the circumanal glands of the dog,* Ph.D thesis. Ithaca, NY: Cornell University.

Parks, A. S., & Bruce, H. M. (1961). Olfactory stimuli in mammalian reproduction. *Science, 134*, 1049–1054.

Pavletic, M. M. (1981). Canine axial pattern flaps, using the omocervical, thoracodorsal, and deep circumflex iliac direct cutaneous arteries. *Am J Vet Res, 42*, 391.

Pavletic, M. M. (1985). The integument. In D. Slatter (Ed.), *Small animal surgery*. Philadelphia: Saunders.

Pinkus, H. (1958). Embryology of hair. In W. Montagna & R. A. Ellis (Eds.), *The biology of hair growth*. New York: Academic Press.

Probst, C. W., & Peyton, L. C. (1983). Split-thickness skin grafting. In M. J. Bojrab (Ed.), *Current techniques in small animal surgery* (2nd ed.). Philadelphia: Lea & Febiger.

Puza, A., & Gombos, A. (1958). Acquired tolerance of skin homografts in dogs. *Transplant Bull, 5*, 30–32.

Quaissi, M. A., & Capron, A. (1985). Fibronectins: structure et functions. *Am Inst Pasteur Immunol, 136*, 12.

Reetz, J. A., Gabriela, S., Mayhew, P. D., et al. (2006). Ultrasonographic and color-flow doppler ultrasonographic assessment of direct cutaneous arteries used for axial pattern skin flaps in dogs. *JAVMA, 228*(9), 1361–1365.

Rehfeld, C. E., Dammin, G. J., & Hester, W. J. (1970). Skin graft survival in partially in-bred beagles. *Am J Vet Res, 31*, 733–745.

Reiner, S. B., Seguin, B., DeCock, H. E., et al. (2005). Evaluation of the effect of routine histologic processing on the size of skin samples obtained from dogs. *Am J Vet Res, 66*, 500–505.

Rippke, F., Schreiner, V., & Schwanitz, H.-J. (2002). The acidic milieu of horny layer: new findings on the physiology and pathophysiology of skin pH. *Am J Clin Dermatol, 3*, 261–272.

Schummer, A., Wilkens, H., Vollmerhaus, B., & Habermehl, K.-H. (1981). *The circulatory system, the skin, and the cutaneous organs of the domestic mammals*. Berlin: Springer-Verlag.

Schmutz, S. M., & Berryere, T. G. (2007). Genes affecting coat colour and pattern in domestic dogs: a review. *Anim Genet, 38*, 539–549. doi:10.1111/j.1365-2052.2007.01664.x.

Schwarz, R., LeRoux, J. M. W., Schaller, R., et al. (1979). Micromorphology of the skin (epidermis, dermis, subcutis) of the dog. *Onderstepoort J Vet Res, 46*, 105–109.

Singh, B. (2017). *Dyce, Sack, and Wensing's Textbook of veterinary anatomy* (4th ed.). Philadelphia: Elsevier.

Smith, K. R. (1967). The structure and function of the haarscheibe. *J Comp Neurol, 131*, 459–474.

Smith, K. R., & Thiboutot, D. M. (2008). Sebaceous gland lipids: friend or foe? *J Lipid Res, 49*, 272–281. doi:10.1194/jlr.R700015-JLR200.

Sokolov, V. E. (1982). *Mammal skin*. Berkeley: University of California Press.

St. Clair, L. E. (1975). Carnivore myology. In R. Getty (Ed.), *Sisson and Grossman's anatomy of the domestic animals* (5th ed., Vol. 2). Philadelphia: Saunders.

Straile, W. E. (1960). Sensory hair follicles in mammalian skin: the tylotrich follicle. *Am J Anat, 106*, 133–147.

Straile, W. E. (1961). Morphology of tylotrich follicles in the skin of the rabbit. *Am J Anat, 109*, 1–13.

Strickland, J. H., & Calhoun, M. L. (1963). The integumentary system of the cat. *Am J Vet Res, 24*, 1018–1029.

Thoday, A. J., & Friedman, P. S. (1986). *Scientific basis of dermatology: a physiological approach*. New York: Churchill Livingstone.

Thomsett, L. R. (1986). Structure of canine skin. *Br Vet J, 142*, 116–123.

Vos, J. H., van den Ingh, T. S., Ramaekers, F. C., et al. (1993). The expression of keratins, vimentin, neurofilament proteins, smooth muscle actin, neuron-specific enolase and synaptophysin in tumors of the specific glands in the canine anal region. *Vet Pathol, 30*, 352–361. doi:10.1177/030098589303000404.

Wakuri, H., Mutoh, K., & Narita, M. (1987). Density of toruli tactiles in the dog. *Okajimas Folia Anat Jpn, 64*, 71–80.

Wakuri, H., & Narita, M. (1986). The microscopic anatomy of the torulus tactilis of the dog. *Kitasato Arch Exp Med, 59*, 115–127.

Warner, R. L., & McFarland, L. Z. (1970). Integument. In A. Anderson & L. S. Good (Eds.), *The beagle as an experimental dog*. Ames: Iowa State University Press.

Webb, A. J., & Calhoun, M. L. (1954). The microscopic anatomy of the skin of mongrel dogs. *Am J Vet Res, 15*, 274–280.

Wells, S., & Gottfried, S. D. (2010). Utilization of the scrotum as a full thickness skin graft in a dog. *Canadian Vet J, 51*(11), 1269–1273.

Welzel, J., Reinhardt, C., Lankenau, E., et al. (2001). Changes in function and morphology of normal human skin: evaluation using optical coherence tomography. *Br J Dermatol, 150*, 220–225.

Whalen, L. R., & Kitchell, R. L. (1983). Electrophysiologic studies of the cutaneous nerves of the head of the dog. *Am J Vet Res, 44*, 615–627.

Winkelmann, R. K., & Schmit, R. W. (1959). Cholinesterase in the skin of the rat, dog, cat, Guinea pig and rabbit. *J Invest Dermatol, 35*, 185–190.

Zouboulis, C. C., Baron, J. M., Bohm, M., et al. (2008). Frontiers in sebaceous gland biology and pathology. *Exp Dermatol, 17*, 542–551. doi:10.1111/j.1600-0625.2008.00725.x.

4

The Skeleton

General

The skeleton serves as support and protection while providing levers for muscular action. It functions as a storehouse for minerals and as a site for fat storage and blood cell formation. In the living body the skeleton is composed of a changing, actively metabolizing tissue that may be altered in shape, size, and position by mechanical or biochemical demands. For a consideration of various aspects of development, maintenance, and repair of the skeleton, reference can be made to Kimmel and Jee (1982), Kincaid and Van Sickle (1983), Jurvelin et al. (1988), and Marks and Popoff (1988). The process of bone repair and the incorporation of heavy metals and rare earths (including radioisotopes) in the adult skeleton attest to its dynamic nature. Bone responds in a variety of ways to vitamin, mineral, and hormone deficiencies or excesses. Inherent in these responses are changes in the physiognomy, construction, and mechanical function of the body.

For a review of the history of the vertebrate skeleton and the bones that constitute it, reference may be made to comparative anatomy texts, such as *The Vertebrate Body* by Romer and Parsons (1986) or *Hyman's Comparative Vertebrate Anatomy* by Wake (1979). Much useful information on the skeleton can be found in such older works as Owen (1866), on all vertebrates, and Flower (1870), on mammals. Specific information and references on the skeleton of the dog and other domestic animals can be found in current veterinary anatomy texts and the classic out-of-print *Handbuch der Vergleichenden Anatomie der Haustiere* by Ellenberger and Baum (1943). For a helpful atlas of radiographic anatomy, see Schebitz and Wilkins (1986).

For a discussion of the structure and function of bone in health and disease, reference may be made to *The Biochemistry and Physiology of Bone* by Bourne (1972, 1976), *The Biology of Bone* by Hancox (1972), *Biological Mineralization* by Zipkin (1973), *The Physiological and Cellular Basis of Metabolic Bone Disease* by Rasmussen and Bordier (1974), and *Bone: A Treatise* by Hall (1989–1992). For more recent reviews of bone and cartilage biology, see Buckwalter et al. (1995), Hall (2015), and Pourquie (2009).

Various aspects of skeletal morphology in the dog have been considered by multiple authors: Lumer (1940) has studied evolutionary allometry; Stockard (1941), genetic and endocrine effects; Haag (1948), osteometric analysis of aboriginal dogs; Hildebrand (1954), Clutton-Brock et al. (1976), and Wayne (1984, 1985, 1986) studied comparative skeletal morphology in canids; and Huja and Beck (2007) described bone remodeling of the maxilla, mandible, and femur in young dogs.

Classification of Skeletal Elements

Bones may be grouped according to shape, structure, function, origin, or position. Heterotopic bones are defined by position and may be located anywhere in the body. The os penis or baculum is an example of such a bone. It is located in the glans of the penis and can be found in all mammals except humans, whales, and some others (Chaine 1926). It functions to stiffen the glans and dilate the fundus of the vagina. Its homolog in the female is the os clitoris, which is more restricted in occurrence and usually absent in the dog (see Chapter 9, Urogenital System). The total average number of bones in each division of the skeletal system, as found in an adult dog (Figs. 4.1 and 4.2), is given in Table 4.1. (Sesamoid bones associated with the limbs are included.) In this enumeration, the bones of the dewclaw (the first digit of the hindpaw) are not included because this digit is absent in many breeds of dogs, and, in other breeds, a single or double first digit is required for show purposes (American Kennel Club, 2017). Because dewclaws are nonfunctional, but are frequently injured or ingrown and require treatment, they are often removed.

Classification of Bones According to Shape

Bones may be classified in various ways. Anatomists have long grouped bones according to shape, although borderline forms exist. For descriptive purposes five general divisions on this basis are recognized: long bones, short bones, sesamoid bones, flat bones, and irregular bones. Long, short, and sesamoid bones are found in the limbs, whereas the flat and irregular bones are characteristic of the skull and vertebral column. The terms are readily understandable, except possibly **sesamoid**, which is derived from the Greek word for a seed that is small, flat, and ovate. Sesamoid bones vary from tiny spheres to the slightly bent, ovoid patella that is 2 cm or longer in a large dog. Some sesamoid elements never ossify but remain as cartilages throughout life, such as those of the distal interphalangeal joints.

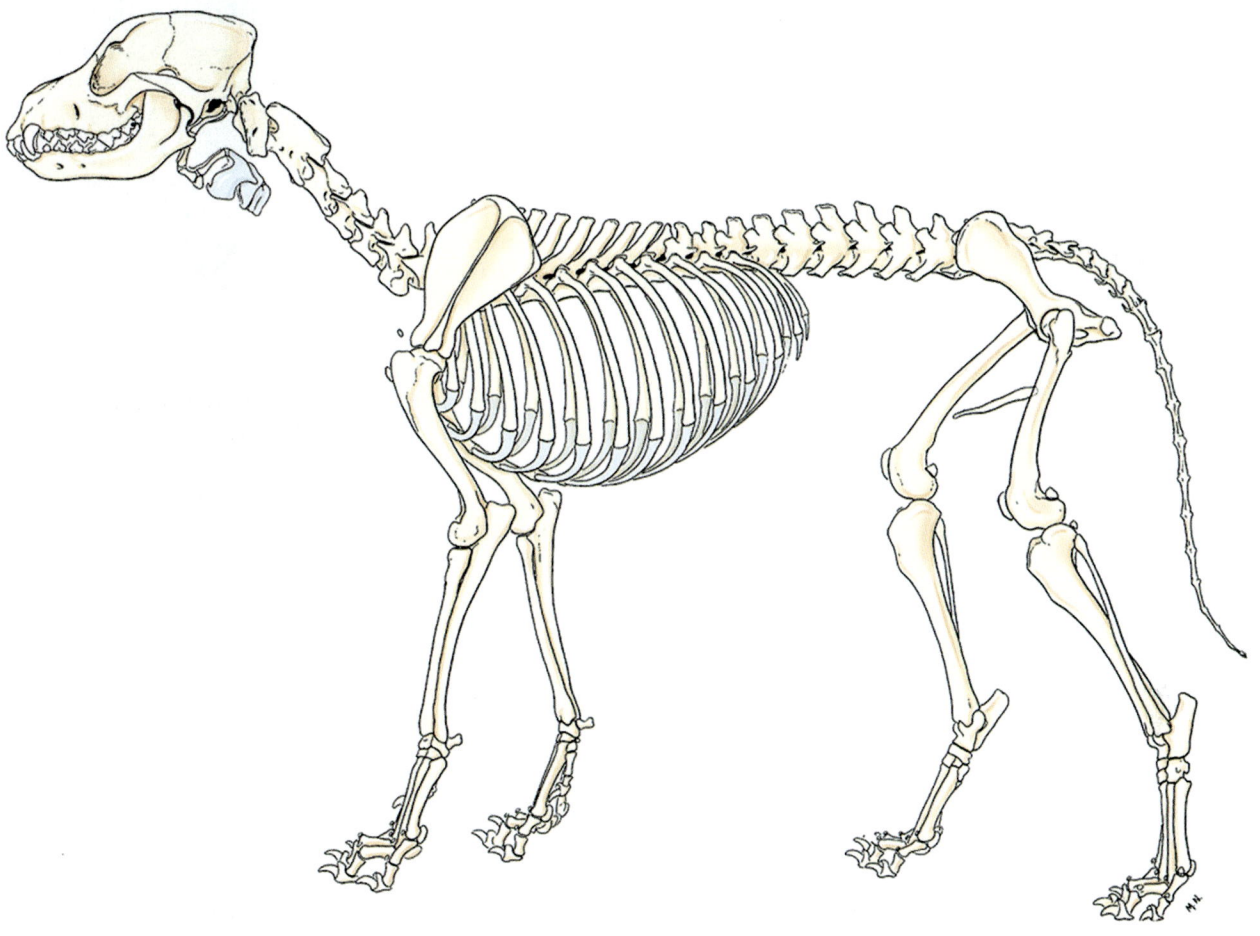

• Fig. 4.1 Skeleton of a male dog, left lateral view.

TABLE 4.1 Bones of Skeletal System

Division	Total Average Number
Axial Skeleton	
Vertebral column	50
Skull and hyoid	50
Ribs and sternum	34
Appendicular Skeleton	
Thoracic limbs	90
Pelvic limbs	96
Heterotopic Skeleton	
Os penis	1
Total	321

Long bones (*ossa longa*) are characteristic of the limbs. The bones of the thigh and arm, that is, the femur and humerus, are good examples. Typically a long bone, during its growth, possesses a shaft, or **diaphysis**, and two ends, the **epiphyses** (Haines, 1942). During development each end is separated from the shaft by a **plate** of growing cartilage, the **physeal cartilage**.

The epiphysial cartilage (*cartilago epiphysialis*) is the cartilage on the articular surface of the epiphysis. The rapidly growing, flared end of the bone between the shaft and the epiphysis is called the **metaphysis**. At maturity the physeal cartilage ceases to grow, and the epiphysis fuses with the shaft as both share in the bony replacement of the physeal cartilage. Farnum and Wilsman (1989) and Farnum et al. (1990) have studied chondrocytes of the growth plate cartilage in situ using differential interference contrast microscopy and time-lapse cinematography. They were able to visualize living hypertrophic chondrocytes as they pass through a sequence of phases, including proliferation, hypertrophy, and death at the chondroosseous junction. Fractures sometimes occur at the physis. Usually, after maturity, no distinguishable division exists between epiphysis and diaphysis. The ends of most long bones enter into the formation of freely movable joints. Long bones form levers and possess great tensile strength. They are capable of resisting many times the stress to which they are normally subjected. The stress on long bones is both through their long axes, as in standing, and at angles to these axes, as exemplified by the pull of muscles that attach to them. Although bones appear to be rigid and not easily influenced

The Skeleton

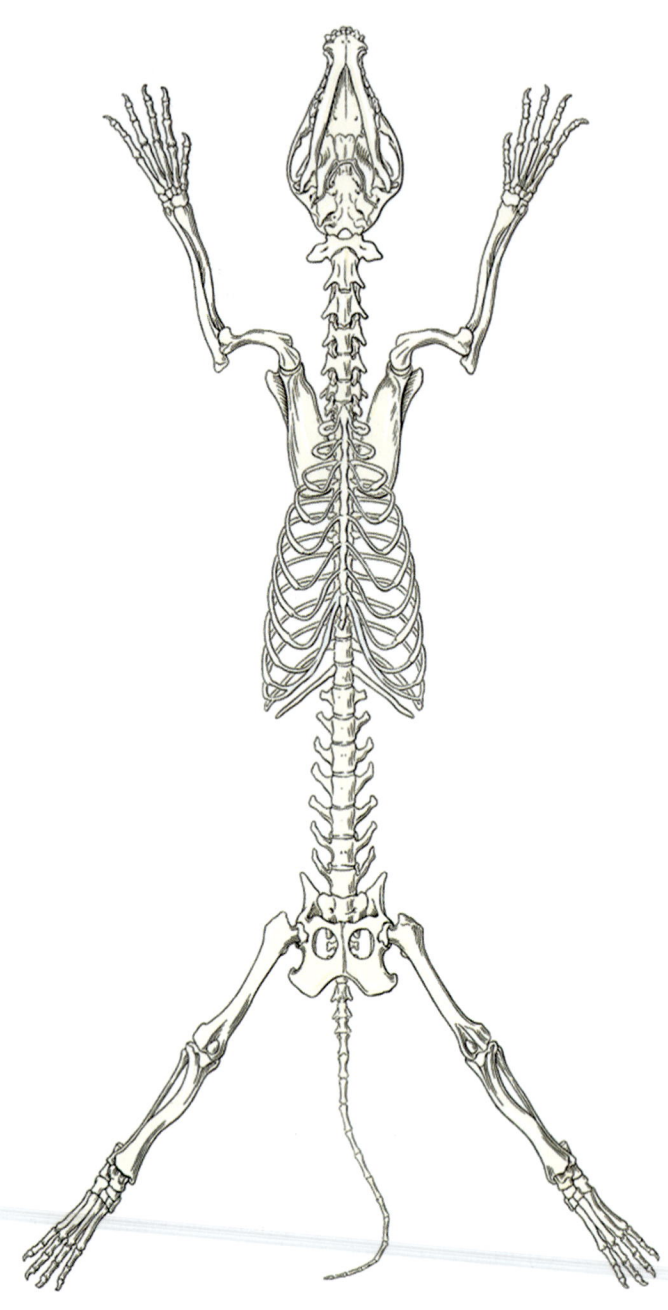

• **Fig. 4.2** Skeleton of dog, ventral view.

by the soft tissues that surround them, soft tissues actually do contour the bones. Indentations in the form of grooves are produced by blood vessels, nerves, tendons, and ligaments that lie adjacent to them, whereas roughened elevations or depressions are produced by the attachments of tendons and ligaments. The ends of all long bones are enlarged and smooth. In life, these smooth surfaces are covered by a layer of hyaline cartilage, as they enter into the formation of joints. The enlargement of each extremity of a long bone serves a dual purpose. It diminishes the risk of dislocation and provides a large bearing surface for the articulation. The distal end of the terminal phalanx of each digit is an exception to the stated rule. Because it is covered by horn and is not articular, it is neither enlarged nor smooth.

Short bones (*ossa brevis*) are confined to the carpal and tarsal regions, which contain seven bones each. They vary in shape from the typical cuboidal shape with six surfaces to irregularly compressed rods with only one flat, articular surface. In those bones having many surfaces, at least one surface is nonarticular. This surface provides an area where ligaments may attach and blood vessels may enter and leave the bone.

Sesamoid bones (*ossa sesamoidea*) are present near freely moving joints. They are usually formed in tendons, but they may be developed in the ligamentous tissue over which tendons pass. They usually possess only one articular surface, which glides on a flat or convex surface of one or more of the long bones of the extremities. Their chief function is to protect tendons at the places where greatest friction is developed.

Flat bones (*ossa plana*) are found in the limb girdles, where they serve for muscle attachment, and in the head, where they surround and protect the sense organs and brain as well as serve for muscle attachment. The bones of the face are flat, providing maximum shielding without undue weight, and streamlining the head. Furthermore, the heads of all quadrupeds overhang their centers of gravity; a heavy head would be a handicap in locomotion. The flat bones of the cranium consist of outer and inner tables of compact bone and an intermediate uniting spongy bone, called *diploë*. In certain bones of the head the diploë is progressively invaded during growth by extensions from the nasal cavity that displace the diploë and cause a greater separation of the tables than would otherwise occur. The intraosseous air spaces of the skull formed in this way are known as the *paranasal sinuses*. Bones that contain air cavities are called **pneumatic bones** (*ossa pneumatica*).

Irregular bones (*ossa irregulata*) are those of the vertebral column, but the term also includes all bones of the skull not of the flat type, and the three parts of the hip bone (*os coxae*). Jutting processes are the characteristic features of irregular bones. Most of these processes are for muscular and ligamentous attachments; some are for articulation. The vertebrae of quadrupeds protect the spinal cord and furnish a relatively incompressible bony column through which the propelling force generated by the pelvic limbs is transmitted to the trunk. The vertebrae also partly support and protect the abdominal and thoracic viscera, and give rigidity and shape to the body in general. The amount of movement between any two vertebrae is small, but the combined movement permitted in all the intervertebral articulations is sufficient to allow considerable mobility of the whole body in any direction (Slijper, 1946).

Development of Bone

Bone consists of cells in a specialized intercellular organic matrix called **osteoid**, which is mineralized primarily by hydroxyapatite. The cells that direct the formation of cartilage and bone may be derived either from mesoderm or from neural crest (Hall, 1988; Noden & de Lahunta, 1985). The most abundant protein of the organic matrix of bone is type I collagen, which gives bone its structural support and strength. However, bone matrix contains numerous other matrix macromolecules, including collagen types III and V, proteoglycans, lipids, morphogenetic proteins, and enzymes as well as phosphoproteins and glycoproteins specific to bone, such as osteocalcin, osteonectin, and osteopontin. The function of these bone-specific proteins is a major area of current research, and, in the future, many new noncollagenous proteins of bone will undoubtedly be discovered.

Cartilage, often a precursor of bone, has been reviewed in books by Hall (1977) and Hall and Newman (1991), who considered developmental and molecular aspects of cartilage (see Chapter 2 for a discussion of fetal bone development and illustrations of ossification sequences in various bones). Another review of cartilage development with an emphasis on molecular components and signaling pathways may be found in Grässel and Aszódi (2016).

Bone-forming cells, or **osteoblasts**, are capable of synthesizing extracellular collagenous and noncollagenous proteins and proteoglycans, the building blocks of bone matrix. They also respond to circulating hormones and produce growth factors that mobilize osteoclast precursor cells. Osteoblasts on the bone surface become osteocytes as they are surrounded by mineralized matrix (Bonewald, 2008). Each bone cell or osteocyte rests in a lacuna and has long branching processes that extend through canaliculi in the mineralized matrix to lacunae of neighboring cells. All bone-lining cells are interconnected and appear capable of maintaining active transport in calcium homeostasis.

The formation of bone by osteoblasts and the resorption of bone by osteoclasts are linked, or "coupled," in ways that are not completely understood. However, the controlling cell for bone remodeling, which goes on throughout life, is the osteoblast. Mechanical stress via muscle attachment, nutrition, vitamin D, calcitonin, parathormone, and sex hormones play a great role in bone remodeling throughout life. In old age some bone cells die, whereas some become "uncoupled" and are not replaced, thus disrupting bone metabolism. This results in the thinning of cortical as well as trabecular bone. Resorption or deposition may be excessive and result in clinical problems, some of which still defy treatment. For a consideration of overnutrition and skeletal disease, see Wu (1973).

For an excellent review of bone cell biology, which the authors contend is still in its infancy, see Marks and Popoff (1988). Recent books on the osteoblast and osteocyte and the osteoclast are part of a seven-volume series titled *Bone: A Treatise*, edited by B. K. Hall (1989–1992). This is a timely update for the still useful four-volume, second edition of *The Biochemistry and Physiology of Bone* by Bourne (1972, 1976).

The fetal skeleton (see Chapter 2) is characterized by bones formed in membrane (intramembranous) that precede or accompany bones formed in cartilage (endochondral). Both intramembranous bone and endochondral bone are remodeled during development and form lamellar bone with haversian systems indistinguishable from each other. The terms *membrane bone* and *cartilage bone* refer to the primary tissue being mineralized. Almost all so-called cartilage bones begin their ossification beneath a perichondral membrane, followed by vascular invasion and endochondral ossification. Several membrane bones develop secondary cartilage after membranous ossification has begun. This secondary cartilage ossifies to form compact bone indistinguishable from the remainder of the structure.

For further information, see *Calcified Tissue Research*, an international journal founded in 1967 and devoted to the structure and function of bone and other mineralized systems, and *Developmental and Cellular Skeletal Biology* by Hall (1978).

The bones of the face and dorsum of the cranium develop in sheets of connective tissue, not in cartilage. This type of bone formation is known as intramembranous ossification. Osteoblasts and osteoclasts continue to be the laborers in this activity. The compact bone formed by the periosteum is identical with membrane bone in its elaboration. Bony tissue of either type is capable of growing in any direction. The jaws and hyoid arches are preceded by cartilages, which are derived from the neural crest. In the proceedings of the Third International Conference on Bone (Dixon et al., 1991), more than 50 papers consider present methods for studying the growth of cartilage and bone. A common technique for studying developing cartilages and bones in the fetus is the use of color stains and the subsequent clearing of tissues. For cartilage, Alcian blue or toluidine blue is used to stain the mucopolysaccharide and for bone, alizarine red, combined with calcium to stain them red. Subsequent maceration of tissues with sodium or potassium hydroxide followed by clearing in glycerine, benzyl benzoate, or ethylene glycol make cartilage and bone formation visible. Examples of such staining can be seen in Chapter 2 (Evans 1948, Orsini 1962, Crary 1962, Dingerkus & Uhler 1977, Kelly & Bryden 1983, Taylor & VanDyke 1985).

Structure of Bone

The gross structure of a dried, macerated bone is best revealed if the bone is sectioned in various planes. Two types of bone structure are seen. One is compact, or dense, which forms the outer shell of all skeletal parts. The other is spongy, or cancellous, which occupies the interior of the extremities of all long bones and the entire interior of most other bones except certain of the skull bones and the bones of the thoracic and pelvic girdles. Spongy bone is not found in the girdles, where the two compact plates are fused.

Compact bone (*substantia compacta* and *substantia corticalis*) is developed in direct ratio to the stress to which the bone is subjected. It is thicker in the shafts of long bones than in their extremities. It attains its greatest uniform thickness where the circumference of the bone is least. The maximum thickness of the compact bone found in the femur and humerus of an adult Great Dane is 3 mm. Local areas of increased thickness are present at places where there is increased tension from muscles or ligaments.

Spongy bone (*substantia spongiosa*) is elaborated in the extremities of long bones, forms the internal substance of short and irregular bones, and is interposed between the two compact layers of most flat bones. Spongy bone consists of a complicated maze of crossing and connecting osseous leaves and spicules that vary in shape and direction. The spongy bone of the skull is known as **diploë**.

The shafts of long bones in the adult are filled largely with **yellow bone marrow** (*medulla ossium flava*). This substance is chiefly fat. In the fetus and the newborn, **red bone marrow** (*medulla ossium rubra*) occupies this cavity and functions in forming red blood cells. No spongy bone is present in the middle of the shaft of a long bone, and the marrow-filled space thus formed is known as a **medullary cavity** (*cavum medullare*).

Spongy bone is developed where greatest stress occurs. The leaves or lamellae and bars are arranged in planes where pressure and tension are greatest, this structural development for functional purposes being best seen in the proximal end of the femur. The interstices between the leaves and the bars of spongy bone are occupied by red marrow. The spongy bone of ribs and vertebrae and of many other short and flat bones is filled with red marrow throughout life. In the emaciated or the extremely aged, red marrow gives way to fatty infiltration.

The **periosteum** is an investing layer of connective tissue that covers the nonarticular surfaces of all bones in the fresh state. The connective tissue covering of cartilage, known as **perichondrium**, does not differ histologically from periosteum. Perichondrium covers only the articular margins of articular cartilages but invests cartilages in all other locations. Periosteum blends imperceptibly with tendons and ligaments at their attachments. Muscles do not actually have the fleshy attachment to bone that they are said to have since a certain amount of connective tissue, periosteum, intervenes between the two. At places where there are not tendinous or ligamentous attachments it is not difficult, when bone is in the fresh state, to scrape away the periosteum.

The **endosteum** is similar in structure to periosteum but is thinner. It lines the large medullary cavities, being the condensed peripheral layer of the bone marrow. Both periosteum and endosteum, under emergency conditions such as occur in fracture of bone, provide cells (osteoblasts) that aid in repair of the injury. Sometimes the fractured part is overrepaired with bone of poor quality. Such osseous bulges at the site of injury are known as **exostoses**.

Mucoperiosteum is the name given to the covering of bones that participate in forming boundaries of the respiratory or digestive system. It lines all of the paranasal sinuses and contains mucous cells.

Physical Properties of Bone

Bone is about one-third organic and two-thirds inorganic material. The inorganic matrix of bone has a microcrystalline structure composed principally of calcium phosphate. The exact constitution of the crystal lattice is still under study, but it is generally agreed that bone mineral is largely a hydroxyapatite with adsorbed carbonate. Some consider that it may exist as tricalcium phosphate hydrate with adsorbed calcium carbonate (Dixon & Perkins, 1956). The organic framework of bone can be preserved while the inorganic part is dissolved. A 20% aqueous solution of hydrochloric acid will decalcify any of the long bones of a dog in approximately 1 day. Such bones retain their shape but are pliable. A slender bone, such as the fibula, can be tied into a knot after decalcification. The organic material is essentially connective tissue, which on boiling yields gelatin.

Surface Contour of Bone

Much can be learned about the role in life of a specific bone by studying its eminences and depressions. There is a functional, an embryologic, or a pathologic reason for the existence of almost every irregularity. For age-related changes, see Simon et al. (1988).

Most eminences serve for muscular and ligamentous attachments. Grooves and fossae, in some instances, serve a similar function. Facets are small articular surfaces that may be flat, concave, or convex. Trochleas and condyles are usually large articular features of bone. The roughened, enlarged parts that lie proximal to the condyles on the humerus and femur are known as *epicondyles*.

Vessels and Nerves of Bone

Bone, unlike cartilage, has both a nerve and a blood supply. Long bones and many flat and irregular bones have a conspicuous **nutrient** (medullary) **artery** and **vein** passing through the compact substance to serve the marrow within. Such arteries pass through a **nutrient foramen** (*foramen nutricium*) and **canal** (*canalis nutricius*) of a bone and, on reaching the marrow cavity, divide into proximal and distal branches that repeatedly subdivide and supply the bone marrow and the adjacent cortical bone. In the long and short bones, terminal branches reach the physeal plate of cartilage, where, in young animals, they end in capillaries. In adults it is likely that many twigs nearest the epiphyses anastomose with twigs arising from vessels in the periosteum. Nutrient veins pursue the reverse course. Not all of the blood supplied by the nutrient artery is returned by the nutrient vein or veins; much of it, after traversing the capillary bed, returns through veins that perforate the compact bone adjacent to the articular surfaces at the extremities of these bones. The **periosteal arteries** and **veins** are numerous but small; these arteries supply the extremities of long bones and much of the compact bone also. They enter minute canals that lead in from the surface and ramify proximally and distally in the microscopic tubes that tunnel the compact and spongy bone. The arterioles of the nutrient artery anastomose with those of the periosteal arteries deep within the compact bone. It is chiefly through enlargement of the periosteal arteries and veins that an increased blood supply and increased drainage are obtained at the site of a fracture. Veins within bone are devoid of valves, the capillaries are large, and the endothelium from the arterial to the venous side is continuous. **Lymph vessels** are present in the periosteum as perivascular sheaths and probably also as unaccompanied vessels within the bone marrow.

The **nerves** in bone are principally sensory, and evidence has been accumulating that the nervous system plays a crucial role in remodeling of bone and the maintenance of bone mass (Martin & Sims, 2009). It is thought that approximately 10% of the human skeleton is replaced each year by remodeling. Both the central and sympathetic part of the peripheral nervous systems are believed to be involved in such regulation. Neuroendocrine controls include leptin, which inhibits bone formation. Sensory nerves carry impulses that may result in pain. Kuntz and Richins (1945) state that both the afferent and the sympathetic efferent fibers probably play a role in reflex vasomotor responses in the bone marrow.

Function of Bone

The skeleton of the vertebrate body serves four functions.
1. Bone forms the supporting and, in many instances, the protecting framework of the body.
2. Many bones serve as first-, second-, or third-class levers, owing to the action of different muscles at different times and to changes in the positions of force and fulcrum. Nearly all muscles act at a mechanical disadvantage. The speed at which the weight travels is in direct proportion to the shortness of the force arm, and this is determined by the distance of the insertion of the muscle from the joint, or fulcrum.
3. Bone serves as a storehouse for calcium and phosphorus and for many other elements in small amounts. The greatest drain occurs during pregnancy; conversely, the greatest deposition takes place during growth. In the large breeds, such as the Great Dane and St. Bernard, the skeleton is the system most likely to show the effects of a nutritional deficiency. Undermineralization of the skeleton is a common manifestation of underfeeding, improper feeding, or inability of the individual to assimilate food adequately. Overnutrition can result in a variety of skeletal diseases (Hedhammer et al., 1974; Nap and Hazewinkel 1994; Debarekeleer et al., 2010; Richardson et al., 2010).
4. Bone serves as a factory for red blood cells and for several kinds of white blood cells: blood cell progenitors are found within the marrow of adult bone. In the normal adult it also stores fat.

Axial Skeleton

Skull

The axial skeleton is composed of the skull, hyoid bones, vertebral column, ribs, and sternum. The bones of the head compose the skull. It is divided into the bones of the cranium that surround the brain and the bones of the face that surround the eyes and respiratory and digestive passageways (Figs. 4.3 to 4.5).

The facial region, consisting of 36 bones, is specialized to provide a large surface area subserving respiratory and olfactory functions and a long surface for the implantation of the teeth. This elongation results in a pointed rostral end, or apex, and a wide, deep base that imperceptibly blends with the cranium. Indices of size, described later, are shown in Figs. 4.6 to 4.8.

The **cranial cavity** (*cavum cranii*), is separated from the **cavity of the nose** (*cavum nasi*) by a perforated plate of bone, the cribriform plate (see Fig. 4.9). Caudally the large opening through the occipital region, the *foramen magnum*, allows for the medulla oblongata to continue into the spinal cord along with its associated vessels.

The ventral part of the cranium has a number of foramina and canals for the passage of nerves and blood vessels. At the junction of the facial and cranial parts, on each side, are the orbital cavities, in which are located the globes of the eyes and accessory structures.

The bones of the ventral part (see Fig. 4.5) of the cranium, or basicranial axis, are preformed in cartilage, whereas those of the dorsum, or calvaria, are formed in membrane.

A classic treatment of the development of the vertebrate skull by de Beer (1937) considers the homologies of skull components, compares chondrocrania, and discusses modes of ossification. *The Mammalian Skull* by Moore (1981)

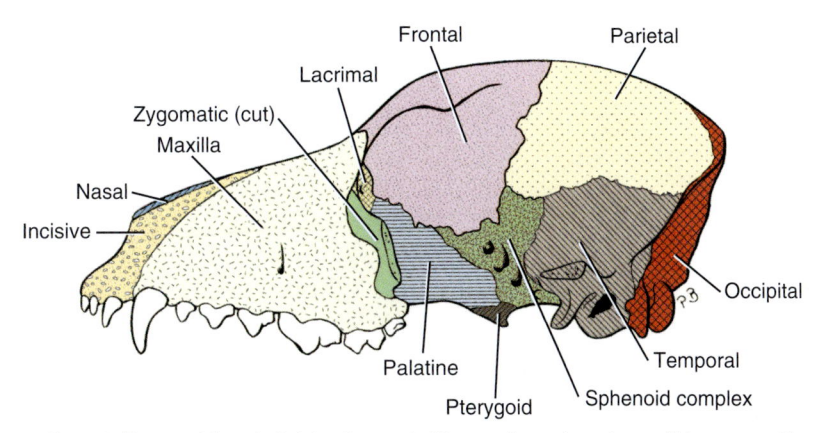

• Fig. 4.3 Bones of the skull, lateral aspect. (Zygomatic arch and mandible removed.)

92 CHAPTER 4 The Skeleton

• **Fig. 4.4** Bones of the skull, dorsal aspect.

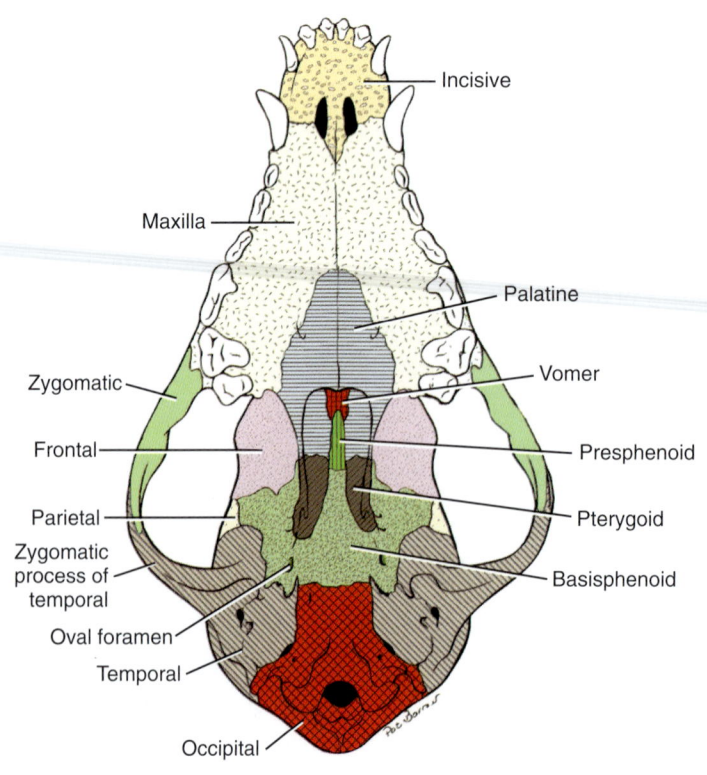

• **Fig. 4.5** Bones of the skull, ventral aspect.

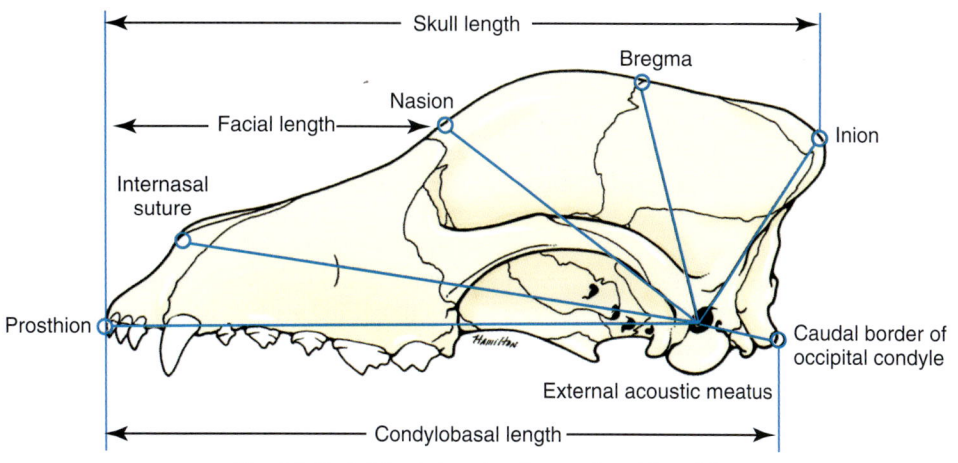

- **Fig. 4.6** Skull, lateral view showing craniometric points.

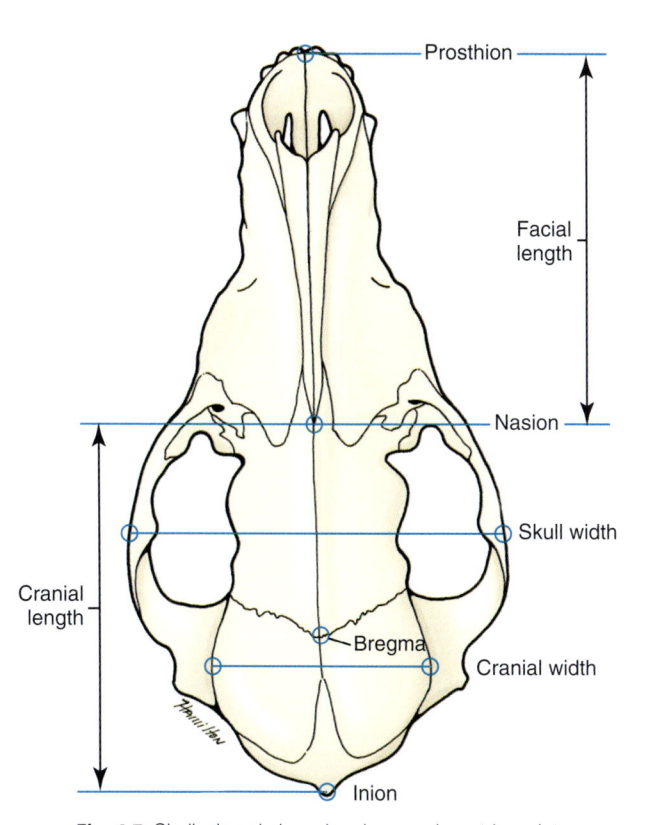

- **Fig. 4.7** Skull, dorsal view showing craniometric points.

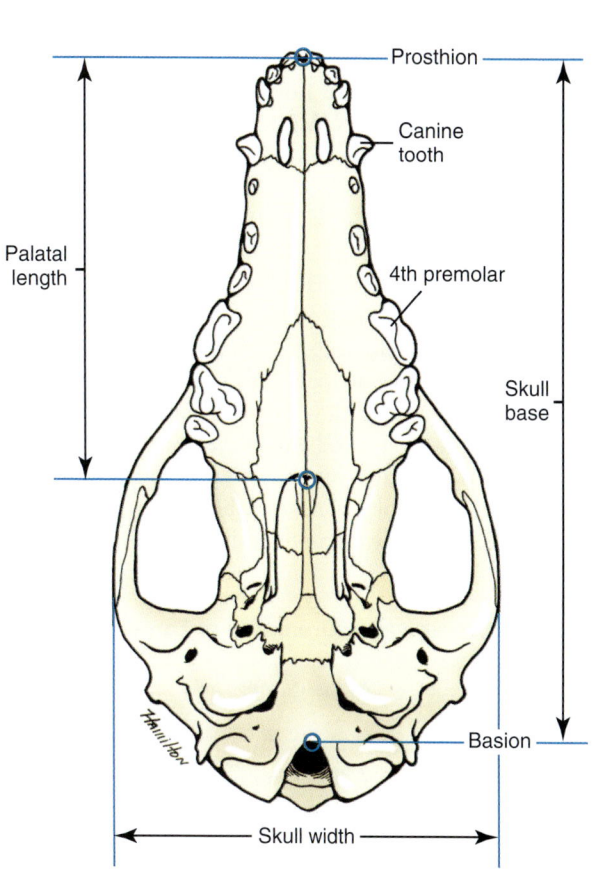

- **Fig. 4.8** Skull, ventral view showing craniometric points.

includes detailed descriptions of skull components, evolutionary changes, functional adaptations, and developmental anatomy. The bibliography is extensive. Hamon (1977) published a very detailed radiographic atlas of the dog skull.

Skulls differ more in size and shape among domestic dogs than in any other mammalian species. For this reason, craniometry in dogs takes on added significance when characterizing specific breeds and crosses. Certain points and landmarks on the skull are recognized in making linear measurements and have been used by Stockard (1941) and others. The more important of these are (Figs. 4.6 to 4.8):

Inion: Central surface point on the external occipital protuberance

Bregma: Junction on the median plane of the right and left frontoparietal sutures, or the point of crossing of the coronal and sagittal sutures

Nasion: Junction on the median plane of the right and left nasofrontal sutures

Prosthion: Rostral end of the interincisive suture, located between the roots of the dorsal central incisor teeth

Pogonion: Most rostral part of the mandible, at the intermandibular articulation, located between the roots of the ventral (mandibular) central incisor teeth

Basion: Middle of the ventral margin of the foramen magnum

The center of the external acoustic meatus: Although unnamed, this spot also serves as a reference point.

Three terms are frequently used to designate head shapes (see Fig. 4.49):

Dolichocephalic means "long, narrow-headed." Breed examples are Collie and Russian Wolfhound.

Mesaticephalic means a head of medium proportions. Breed examples are German Shepherd Dog, Beagle, and Setter.

Brachycephalic means "short, wide-headed." Breed examples are Boston Terrier and Pekingese.

Although these terms are not referenced in the *Nomina Anatomica Veterinaria* (NAV), they have achieved popular and clinical utility. Other studies have developed criteria for head shapes using radiologic analyses, including Regodon et al. (1993) and Koch et al. (2012).

The face of the dog varies more in shape and size than does any other part of the skeleton. In brachycephalic breeds the facial skeleton is shortened and broadened. In some brachycephalic breeds, the English Bulldog, for example, the ventral jaw protrudes rostral to the dorsal jaw, producing the undershot condition known as **prognathism** of the mandible. Most other breed types have **brachygnathic** mandibles, that is, receding ventral jaws. Although brachygnathism of the mandibles is relative, both the Collie and the Dachshund frequently exemplify this condition to a marked extent. Stockard (1941) demonstrated that discrepancies in the pattern between the dorsal and the ventral jaws in the dog are inherited and develop as separate and independent characters. This can lead to marked disharmonies in facial features and dental occlusion, as was shown by the many crosses he made between purebred dogs. In the cross between the Basset Hound and the Saluki, two dogs with different skull proportions but without abnormally dissimilar jaws, some of the F_2 hybrids showed the independent inheritance of dorsal and ventral jaw features. When one pup can inherit the muzzle and dorsal jaw of one parent and the ventral jaw from the other, it can have serious effects on dental occlusion and thus mastication, tooth loss, prehension, and so on. Occasionally, breed-specific features are accentuated in the crossbred dog so that minor aberrations become major features. Photographs of a variety of crosses of purebred dogs can be found in Stockard's memoir (1941). Included are such crosses as Basset Hound–Shepherd, Basset Hound–Saluki, Basset Hound–English Bulldog, Dachshund–Boston Terrier, Dachshund–French Bulldog, Dachshund–Brussels Griffon, Pekingese–Saluki, Dachshund–Basset Hound, and Dachshund–Pekingese.

Table 4.2 shows average measurements in millimeters taken from randomly selected adult skulls of the three basic types. From these data it can be seen that the greatest variation in skull shape occurs in the facial part. In making comparisons of skull measurements it is essential that the overall size of the individuals measured is taken into consideration. As a rule the dolichocephalic breeds are larger than the brachycephalic, whereas the working breeds fall in the mesaticephalic group, and these as a division have the greatest body size. The only measurement in which the brachycephalic type exceeds the others, in the small sampling shown, is facial width. To obviate the size factor

TABLE 4.2 Average Measurements of Three Skull Types

	Measurement	Brachycephalic	Mesaticephalic	Dolichocephalic
Facial length	Nasion to prosthion	48 mm	89 mm	114 mm
Facial width	Widest interzygomatic distance	103 mm	99 mm	92 mm
Cranial length	Inion to nasion	99 mm	100 mm	124 mm
Cranial width	Widest interparietal distance	56 mm	56 mm	59 mm
Cranial height	Middle of external acoustic meatus to bregma	54 mm	60 mm	61 mm
Mandibular length	Caudal border of condyle to pogonion	85 mm	134 mm	163 mm
Skull length	Inion to prosthion	127 mm	189 mm	238 mm
Skull width	Widest interzygomatic distance	103 mm	99 mm	92 mm
Indices				
Skull base length	Basion to prosthion	107 mm	170 mm	216 mm
Skull index		81	52	39
Cranial index		57	56	48
Facial index		215	111	81

among the breed types, indices are computed (Table 4.3). These indicate relative size and are expressed by a single term representing a two-dimensional relationship. The cranial index is computed by multiplying the cranial width by 100 and dividing the product by the cranial length. Skull and facial indices are computed in the same manner. Stockard (1941) found rather consistent differences between the sexes in most breeds, suggesting an endocrine influence for the differential structural expression.

Trouth et al. (1977) have devised a morphometric index for determining the sex of a dog from the skull. On the ventral surface, in the basioccipital region there is a triangular area that extends from the basion to a line joining the medial points of the two tympanooccipital fissures. In the male it appears narrow and elevated. In the female skull the rostral half of the basioccipital area is wider and flat. Their formula for the sex index is

(Breadth × 100)/Length
 = Male if less than 123; or female if more than 136

where breadth is the distance between the two tympanooccipital fissures at their most lateral points, and length is the distance between the basion (ventral midline of foramen magnum) and the midpoint of a line drawn between the two most medial points of the tympanooccipital fissures.

Values not within these ranges may indicate an immature or castrated dog and require other criteria to determine sex. (The terminology used here is from the NAV and differs from the authors' original.)

Differences among the breeds in facial skeletal development are the most salient features revealed by craniometry. The face is not only short in the brachycephalic breeds but also is actually wider than in the heavier, longer-headed breeds. These data do not show that appreciable asymmetry exists, especially in the round-headed types. Even though the cranium varies least in size, it frequently develops asymmetrically. The caudal part of the skull is particularly prone to showing uneven development. The further a breed digresses from the ancestral wolf type (Suminski 1975 compares the wolf and dog skulls), the more likely are distortions to be found. This is particularly true of the round-headed breeds. The appearance of the English Bulldog is produced by the prognathic condition of the ventral jaw as well as the brachygnathic condition of the dorsal jaw. This structural disharmony results in poor occlusion of the teeth. Stockard (1941) found that the formation of the Bulldog type of skull results from a defective growth reaction of the basicranial physeal cartilages. This defective growth is foreshadowed by a deficiency in the cartilaginous matrix that is the precursor of the basioccipital and basisphenoid bones themselves. An early ankylosis of these growth cartilages (chondrodystrophy) causes the shortening of the basicranial axis. On sagittal section (Fig. 4.9) the limits of the cranial and facial portions of the skull are clearly demarcated by the cribriform plate of the ethmoid.

Cranial capacity may vary between breeds and has been measured by filling the crania with mustard seed after the foramina have been closed with modeling clay and then determining the volume of seed used. Average Boston Terrier skulls held 82 cc. A sampling of skulls of medium size and medium length showed an average capacity of 92 cc; the average skull capacity of the crania of the Russian Wolfhound and of the Collie was 104 cc. Wayne (1984) studied the morphologic similarity of skulls in wild and domestic canids.

Bones of the Cranium

The names of the individual bones making up the 50 that compose the skull are listed in Box 4.1. Lateral and ventral views of an "exploded skull" showing the individual bones in relation to one another appear as Figs. 4.42 and 4.45.

Occipital Bone

The occipital bone (Figs. 4.5, 4.10, 4.11, 4.44, and 4.48) forms a ring, the foramen magnum, around the junction of

TABLE 4.3 A Comparison of Indices

	German Shepherd Dog	Saluki	English Bulldog	Pekingese	Brussels Griffon
Cranial index	51	64	69	84	84
Skull index	56	56	107	107	103
Palatal index	60	57	122	122	125
Snout index	60	53	171	179	183
Groups of Breeds Having Similar Types of Skulls					
I. German shepherd dog	II. St. Bernard	III. English Bulldog			
Foxhound	Great Dane	French Bulldog			
Saluki	Dachshund	Boston Terrier			

From Stockard CR: The genetic and endocrinic basis for differences in form and behavior, *American Anatomy Memoir* 19, Philadelphia, 1941, Wistar Institute of Anatomy and Biology.

Fig. 4.9 Bones of the skull, medial aspect of sagittal section.

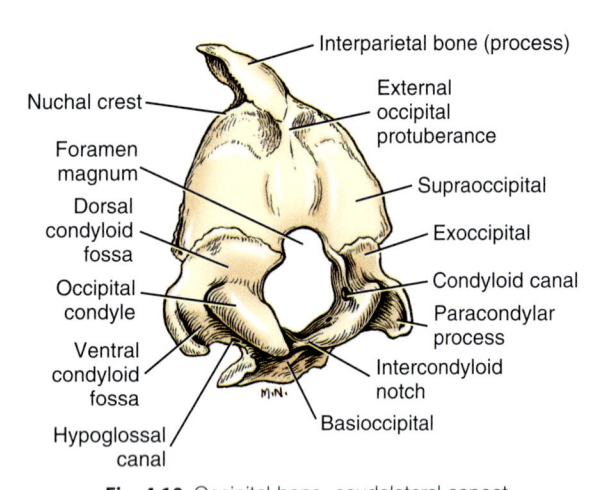

Fig. 4.10 Occipital bone, caudolateral aspect.

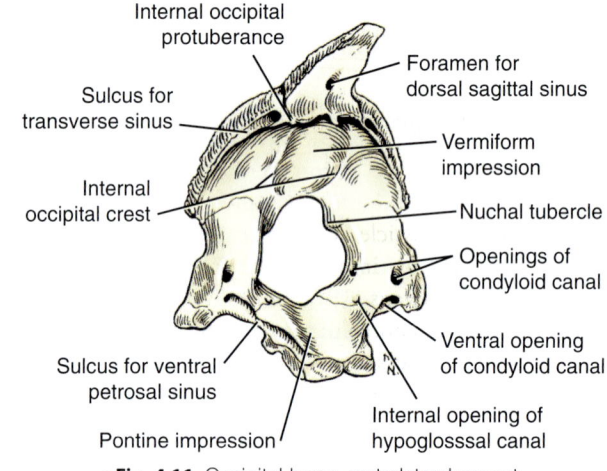

Fig. 4.11 Occipital bone, rostrolateral aspect.

• **BOX 4.1 Individual Bones of the Skull**

BONES OF THE CRANIUM

Paired	1. Exoccipital	3. Frontal	
	2. Parietal	4. Temporal	
Unpaired	1. Supraoccipital	4. Basisphenoid	
	2. Interparietal	5. Presphenoid	
	3. Basioccipital	6. Ethmoid	

BONES OF THE FACE

Paired	1. Incisive	6. Zygomatic	
	2. Nasal	7. Palatine	
	3. Maxilla	8. Lacrimal	
	4. Dorsal concha	9. Pterygoid	
	5. Ventral concha	10. Mandible	
Unpaired	1. Vomer		

BONES OF THE HYOID APPARATUS AND MIDDLE EAR

Paired	1. Stylohyoid	5. Malleus	
	2. Epihyoid	6. Incus	
	3. Ceratohyoid	7. Stapes	
	4. Thyrohyoid		
Unpaired	1. Basihyoid		

the medulla oblongata and the spinal cord. The ring develops from four centers: a squamous part dorsally, two lateral condylar parts, and a basilar part ventrally. A keyhole-shaped notch may be present dorsally (Fig. 4.12). This normal feature is common in the brachycephalic toy breeds (Watson, 1981).

The **squamous part** (*squama occipitalis*), also known as the supraoccipital, is the largest division. This bone forms the dorsal border of the foramen magnum and hides the cerebellum. An unpaired, median, interparietal bone (Fig. 2.39) makes its appearance on about the 45th day of gestation. It is superficial to the paired parietal bones and to the supraoccipital bone. Usually, it fuses with the dorsorostral border of the supraoccipital bone forming part of the sagittal crest, but, in some dogs, it remains as a separate entity, the *os interparietale*. Occasionally an unfused interparietal bone is found in an adult dog. It may be more apparent inside the cranium than externally. Erhart (1943) examined 127 dog skulls for the presence of a separate interparietal bone, and he found 17 examples in 33 brachycephalic skulls, 9 in 30 mesaticephalic skulls, and none in 64 dolichocephalic skulls. Of the 14 brachycephalic fetuses studied,

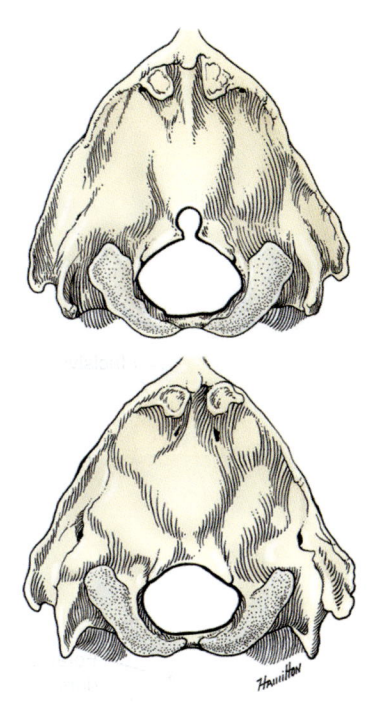

• **Fig. 4.12** Occipital region of mongrel mesocephalic dogs showing a "keyhole" notch compared with a rather circular foramen magnum.

12 had a distinct ossicle, whereas only 1 of 5 dolichocephalic fetuses had an independent ossicle. In the Beagle fetuses studied by Evans (1974) there was always a separate median interparietal bone for a brief period that fused indistinguishably with the squamous part of the supraoccipital bone before birth. From the **interparietal process** arises the mid-dorsal **external sagittal crest** (*crista sagittalis externa*), which, in some specimens, is confined to this bone. The rostral end of the interparietal process is narrower and thinner than the caudal part, which turns ventrally to form a part of the caudal surface of the skull. The **nuchal crest** (*crista nuchae*) marks the division between the dorsal and the caudal surfaces of the skull. It is an unpaired, sharp-edged crest of bone that reaches its most dorsal point at the external occipital protuberance. On each side it arches ventrally before ending on a small eminence located dorsocaudal to the external acoustic meatus. The **external occipital protuberance** (*protuberantia occipitalis externa*) is the median, triangular projection forming the most dorsocaudal portion of the skull. The **external occipital crest** (*crista occipitalis externa*) is a smooth median ridge extending from the external occipital protuberance to the foramen magnum. It is poorly developed in some specimens.

Within the dorsal part of the occipital bone and opening bilaterally on the cerebral surface is the **transverse canal** (*canalis transversus*), which, in life, contains the venous transverse sinus. The transverse canal is continued laterally, on each side, by the **sulcus for the transverse sinus** (*sulcus sinus transversi*). Mid-dorsally, or to one side, the dorsal sagittal sinus enters the transverse sinus via **the foramen for the dorsal sagittal sinus** (*foramen sinus sagittalis dorsalis*). Between the laterally located sulci the skull protrudes rostroventrally to form the **internal occipital protuberance** (*protuberantia occipitalis internus*). Extending rostrally from the internal occipital protuberance is the variably developed, usually paramedian, and always small **internal sagittal crest** (*crista sagittalis interna*). The **vermiform impression** (*impressio vermialis*), forming the thinnest part of the caudal wall of the skull, is an irregular excavation of the median portion on the cerebellar surface of the squamous part of the occipital bone that houses a part of the vermis of the cerebellum. The vermiform impression is bounded laterally by the paired **internal occipital crest** (*crista occipitalis interna*), which is usually asymmetric and convex laterally. Lateral to the internal occipital crest, as well as on the ventral surface of the interparietal process, there are elevations, *juga cerebralia et cerebellaria*, and depressions, *impressiones digitatae*. Ventrally the squamous part is either curved or notched to form the dorsal part of the foramen magnum. On either side the squamous part is fused with the lateral part. This union represents the former articulation (*synchondrosis intraoccipitalis squamolateralis*), which extends from the foramen magnum to the temporal bone.

The paired **lateral parts** (*partes laterales*), also known as *exoccipital parts*, bear the **occipital condyles** (*condyli occipitales*), which are convex and, with the atlas, form the atlantooccipital joints. The **paracondylar process** (*processus paracondylaris*) is located, one on either side, lateral to the condyle and ends in a rounded knob ventrally, usually on a level with the ventral portion of the rostrally located tympanic bulla. Between the paracondylar process and the occipital condyle is the **ventral condyloid fossa** (*fossa condylaris ventralis*). On a ridge of bone rostral to this fossa is the **hypoglossal canal** (*canalis n. hypoglossi*), which is a direct passage through the ventral part of the occipital bone for the hypoglossal nerve. The **dorsal condyloid fossa** (*fossa condylaris dorsalis*) is located dorsal to the occipital condyle. The rather large **condyloid canal** (*canalis condylaris*) that contains the basilar sinus runs through the medial part of the lateral part of the occipital bone. There is an intraosseous passage between the condyloid canal and the hypoglossal canal. Usually there is also a small passage between the condyloid canal and the petrobasilar fissure.

The **basilar part** (*pars basilaris*), also referred to as the *basioccipital part*, is unpaired and forms the caudal third of the cranial base. The central dorsal surface of the basioccipital part is concave to form the pontine impression (*impressio pontina*) rostrally and the impression for the medulla oblongata (*impressio medullaris*) caudally. It is roughly rectangular, although caudally it tapers to a narrow, concave end that forms the central portion of the **intercondyloid notch** (*incisura intercondyloidea*). The adjacent occipital condyles on each side deepen the incisure as they contribute to its formation. The incisure bounds the ventral part of the foramen magnum. The *foramen magnum* is a large, transversely oval opening in the caudoventral portion of the skull through which the medulla is continuous with the spinal cord and their associated structures: the meninges, vertebral venous sinuses, the spinal portion of the accessory nerve, and the various arteries associated with the spinal cord. In brachycephalic breeds the foramen is more circular than oval, and it is frequently asymmetric or notched. The dorsal boundary of the foramen magnum is featured by the caudally flared ventral part of the squamous part of the occipital bone. The caudal extension is increased by the paired **nuchal tubercles** (*tubercula nuchalia*). The lateral surfaces of the caudal half of the basioccipital part fuse with the lateral parts along the former **ventral intraoccipital synchondrosis** (*synchondrosis intraoccipitalis basilateralis*). The ventral surface of the basioccipital part adjacent to the petrotympanic synchondrosis possesses **muscular tubercles** (*tubercula muscularia*). These are rough, sagittally elongated areas, located medial to the smooth, rounded tympanic bullae. The longus capitis muscles attach here. The **pharyngeal tubercle** (*tuberculum pharyngeum*) is a single triangular rough area rostral to the intercondyloid incisure. Laterally the basioccipital bone is grooved to form the **sulcus for the ventral petrosal sinus** (*sulcus sinus petrosi ventralis*), which concurs with the pyramid of the temporal bone to form the **petrooccipital canal** (*canalis petrooccipitalis*), which contains the ventral petrosal sinus.

Ventrally the rostral end of the basioccipital part articulates with the body of the basisphenoid bone at the cartilaginous **sphenooccipital joint** (*synchondrosis sphenooccipitalis*). Ventrolaterally the occipital bone articulates with the tympanic part of the temporal bone to form the cartilaginous **occipitotympanic joint** (*sutura occipitotympanica*). Dorsal to this joint is the important **petrooccipital suture** (*sutura petrooccipitalis*), in which the jugular foramen opens. The joint between the petrosal part of the temporal bone and the occipital bones that forms the petrooccipital suture is the *synchondrosis petrooccipitalis*. Laterally, and proceeding dorsally, the occipital bone first articulates with the squamous part of the temporal bone superficially, the **occipitosquamous suture** (*sutura occipitosquamosa*), and with the mastoid process of the petrous part of the temporal bone deeply, the **occipitomastoid suture** (*sutura occipitomastoidea*); further dorsally it articulates with the parietal bone, the **lambdoid suture** (*sutura lambdoidea*). Where the squamous and lateral parts of the occipital bone articulate with each other and with the mastoid process of the temporal bone, the **mastoid foramen** (*foramen mastoideum*) is formed. This foramen contains the caudal meningeal vessels.

Variations in the occipital bone are numerous. The foramen magnum varies in shape and is not always bilaterally symmetric (Figs. 4.12 and 4.13) (Simoens et al., 1994; Watson et al., 1989). The condyloid canal may be absent on one or both sides. Even when both canals are present, connections between the hypoglossal and the condyloid canals may fail to develop. The paracondylar processes may extend several millimeters ventral to the tympanic bullae so that they will support a skull without the mandibles when it is placed on a horizontal surface; conversely, they may be short, retaining the embryonic condition. The vermiform impression may be deep, causing a caudomedian rounded, thin protuberance on the caudal surface of the skull. The

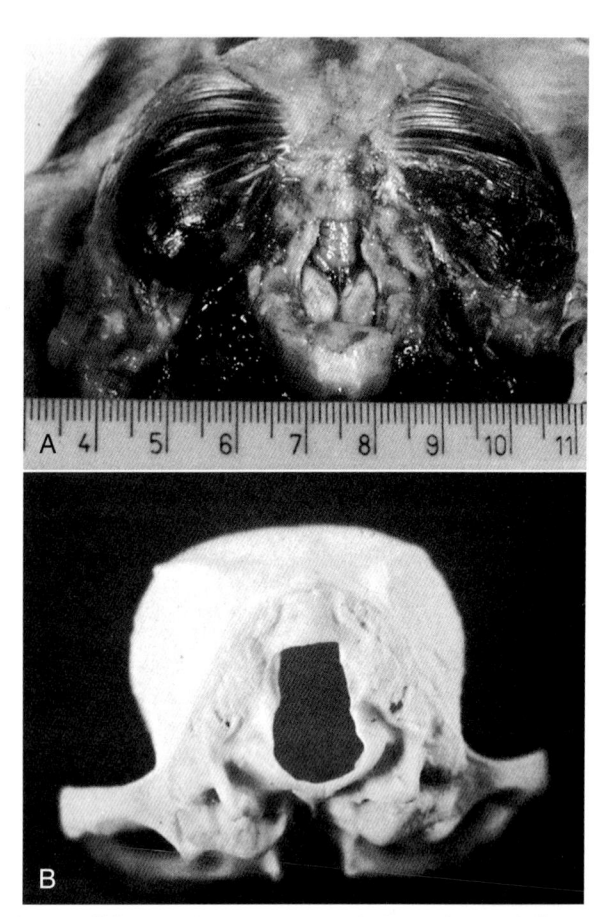

• **Fig. 4.13** When the foramen magnum is large, the cerebellum can be seen after removal of the overlying muscles. (Courtesy of Prof. Simoens.)

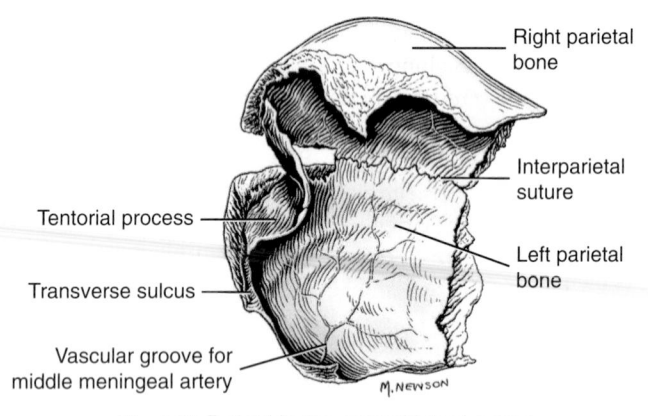

• **Fig. 4.14** Parietal bones, ventral lateral aspect.

foramen for the dorsal sagittal sinus may be double. It is rarely median in position. A sutural bone may be present at the rostral end of the interparietal bone.

Parietal Bone

The parietal bone (*os parietale*) (Fig. 4.3 to 4.5, 4.9, 4.14) is paired and forms most of the dorsolateral part of the calvarial portion of the cranium. It articulates dorsally with its fellow and with the interparietal bone, an unpaired bone in the fetus that fuses with the occipital bone (thus referenced as the interparietal process of the occipital bone in previous editions). Each parietal bone lies directly rostral to the squamous part of the occipital bone and dorsal to the squamous part of the temporal bone. In the newborn no elevation is present at the sagittal interparietal suture or on the interparietal bone, but soon thereafter in the heavily muscled breeds, particularly in the male, the mid-dorsal external sagittal crest is developed. This crest, which increases in size with age, forms the medial boundary of the **temporal fossa** (*fossa temporalis*), a large area on the external surface (*facies externa*) of the cranium from which the temporal muscle originates. In dolichocephalic breeds with heavy temporal muscles, the external sagittal crest may reach a height of more than 1 cm and extend from the external occipital protuberance to the parietofrontal suture. Rostrally, it continues as the diverging frontal crests. In most brachycephalic skulls the external sagittal crest is confined to the interparietal part of the occipital bone and is continued rostrally as the diverging **temporal lines** (*lineae temporales*). The temporal lines at first are convex laterally, then become concave as they cross the parietofrontal, or coronal, suture and are continued as the external frontal crests to the zygomatic processes. The temporal lines replace the external sagittal crest in forming the medial boundaries of the temporal fossae in most brachycephalic skulls.

The **internal surface** (*facies interna*) of the parietal bone presents *digital impressions* and *intermediate ridges* corresponding, respectively, with the cerebral gyri and sulci. A well-defined vascular groove, the **sulcus for the middle meningeal artery** (*sulcus arteriae meningeae mediae*), starts at the ventrocaudal angle of the bone and arborizes over its internal surface. The groove runs dorsally toward the sagittal margin (*margo sagittalis*) of the bone, giving off smaller branched grooves along its course. A leaf of bone, the **tentorial process** (*processus tentoricus*), projects rostromedially from the dorsal part of the caudal border. This leaf concurs with its fellow and with the internal occipital protuberance to form the curved *tentoriumcerebelli osseum*. On the internal surface of the parietal bone near its caudal border is a portion of the **transverse sulcus**, which leads dorsally into the transverse canal of the occipital bone and ventrally into the temporal meatus. The transverse sinus is located in these passageways.

The borders of the parietal bone are rostral, dorsal, and ventral in position because the bone is essentially a curved, square plate. The rostral, or **frontal**, **border** (*margo frontalis*) overlaps the frontal bone, forming the frontoparietal, or **coronal**, **suture** (*sutura coronalis*). The caudal, or **occipital**, **border** (*margo occipitalis*) meets the occipital bone to form the **occipitoparietal suture** (*sutura occipitoparietalis*). The rostral half of the dorsal, or **sagittal**, **border** (*margo sagittalis*) articulates with its fellow on the midline to form the **sagittal suture** (*sutura sagittalis*). The caudal half of the dorsal border articulates with the interparietal bone and the occipital bone to form the **parietointerparietal suture** (*sutura parietointerparietalis*). The ventral, or **squamous**, **border** (*margo squamosus*) is overlaid by the squamous part of the temporal bone in forming the **squamous suture** (*sutura squamosa*). A small area of the squamous border at its rostral end articulates with the wing of the basisphenoid bone to form the **parietosphenoidal suture** (*sutura parietosphenoidalis*). Overlapping of the bones at the squamous and coronal sutures allows for cranial compression of the fetal skull during its passage through the pelvic canal.

Frontal Bone

The **frontal bone** (*os frontale*) (Figs. 4.3, 4.4, 4.9, 4.15, and 4.16) is irregular in shape, being broad caudally and somewhat narrower rostrally. Laterally, the rostral part is concave and forms the medial wall of the orbit. Caudal to this concavity, it flares laterally to form part of the temporal fossa. The **frontal sinus** (*sinus frontalis*) is an air cavity located between the inner and the outer tables of the rostral end of the frontal bone and is divided into two or three compartments. It is discussed in greater detail in the section on paranasal sinuses.

For descriptive purposes the frontal bone is divided into an orbital part, a temporal surface, a frontal squama, and a nasal part.

The **orbital part** (*pars orbitalis*) is a segment of a cone with the apex directed at the optic canal and the base forming the medial border of the **infraorbital margin** (*margo infraorbitalis*). Lateral to the most dorsal part of the **frontomaxillary suture** (*sutura frontomaxillaris*) the orbital margin is slightly flattened for the passage of the vena angularis oculi. Ventrally, a long, distinct, dorsally arched muscular line marks the approximate ventral boundary of the bone. The **ethmoidal foramina** (*foramina ethmoidalia*) are

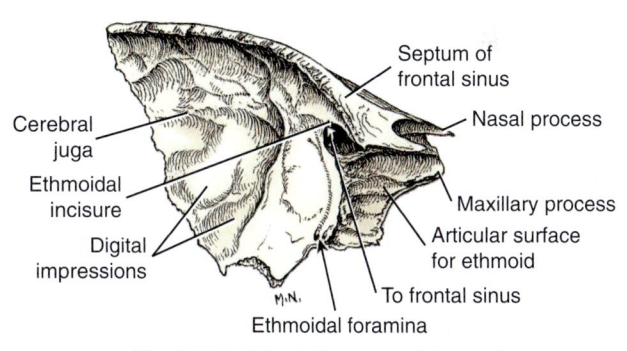

• Fig. 4.15 Left frontal bone, medial aspect.

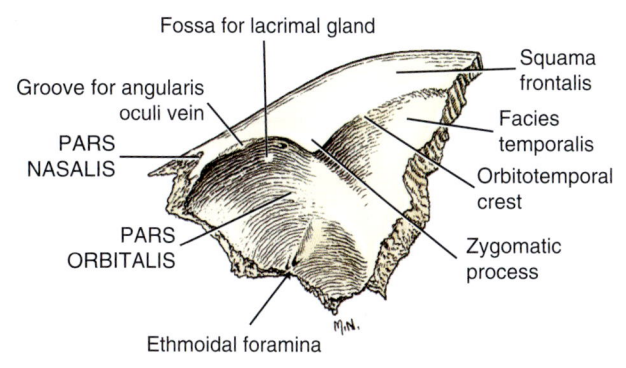

• Fig. 4.16 Left frontal bone, lateral aspect.

two small openings approximately 1 cm rostral to the optic canal. The smaller opening is in the frontosphenoidal suture; the larger foramen, located dorsocaudal to the smaller, passes obliquely through the orbital part of the frontal bone. Sometimes the two ethmoidal foramina are confluent. These foramina contain the external ethmoidal vessels and the ethmoidal nerve. At the orbital margin, the frontal and orbital surfaces meet, forming an acute angle. The **zygomatic process** (*processus zygomaticus*) is formed where the orbital margin meets the **temporal line** (formerly orbitotemporal crest).

The **temporal surface** (*facies temporalis*) forms that part of the frontal bone caudal to the orbital part. Dorsally the two tables of the frontal bone are separated to form the frontal sinus, whereas ventrally and caudally the two tables are fused or united by a small amount of diploë where the bone articulates with the parietal and basisphenoid bones and contributes to the calvaria.

The **frontal squama** (*squama frontalis*) is roughly triangular, with its base facing medially and articulating with that of the opposite bone. It is gently rounded externally and is largely subcutaneous in life. Its caudal boundary is the temporal line and the lateral part of its rostral boundary is the orbital margin.

The **nasal part** (*pars nasalis*) is the rostral extension of the frontal bone. Its sharp, pointed **nasal process** (*processus nasalis*) lies partly ventral to and partly between the caudal parts of the nasal and maxillary bones. The **septum of the frontal sinus** (*septum sinuum frontalium*) is a vertical median partition that closely articulates with its fellow in separating right and left frontal sinuses. It is widest near its middle, which is opposite the cribriform plate. Rostrally it is continuous with the septal process of the nasal bone. The ventral part of the septum of the frontal sinus is the **internal frontal crest** (*crista frontalis interna*). The conjoined right and left crests articulate with the perpendicular plate of the ethmoid bone ventrally and with the conjoined right and left septal processes of the nasal bones rostrally. The **ethmoid incisure** (*incisura ethmoidalis*), which lies dorsal and lateral to the cribriform plate of the ethmoid bone, is formed by the smooth concave edge of the internal table of the nasal part of the frontal bone.

The **internal surface** (*facies interna*) of the frontal bone forms a part of the calvaria caudally and a small portion of the nasal cavity rostrally. The salient ethmoidal incisure separates the two parts. The caudal part is deeply concave and divided into many shallow grooves called **digital impressions** and ridges called **cerebral juga**. Fine, dorso-caudally running vascular grooves indicate the position occupied in life by the rostral meningeal vessels. The large **aperture to the frontal sinus** is located dorsal to the ethmoidal incisure. The nasal part of the internal surface of the frontal bone is marked by many longitudinal lines of attachment for the ethmoturbinates.

The mid-dorsal articulation of the frontal bones forms the **frontal suture** (*sutura interfrontalis*). This suture is a rostral continuation of the sagittal suture between the parietal bones. Caudally the frontal bone is overlapped by the parietal bone, forming the **frontoparietal suture** (*sutura frontoparietalis*). Ventrally the rather firm **sphenofrontal suture** (*sutura sphenofrontalis*) is formed. Rostrally the frontal bone articulates with the nasal, maxillary, and lacrimal bones to form the **frontonasal suture** (*sutura frontonasalis*), the **frontomaxillary suture** (*sutura frontomaxillaris*), and the **frontolacrimal suture** (*sutura frontolacrimalis*). Deep in the orbit, the frontal bone articulates with the palatine bone to form the **frontopalatine suture** (*sutura frontopalatina*). Medially, hidden from external view, the frontal bone articulates with the ethmoid bone in forming the **frontoethmoidal suture** (*sutura frontoethmoidalis*).

Sphenoid Bones

The **sphenoid bones** (*ossa sphenoidales*) (Figs. 4.3, 4.5, 4.17 to 4.19, and 4.44) form the rostral two-thirds of the base of the cranial cavity between the basioccipital caudally and the ethmoid rostrally. Each consists of a pair of wings and a median body. The more rostral bone with orbital wings is

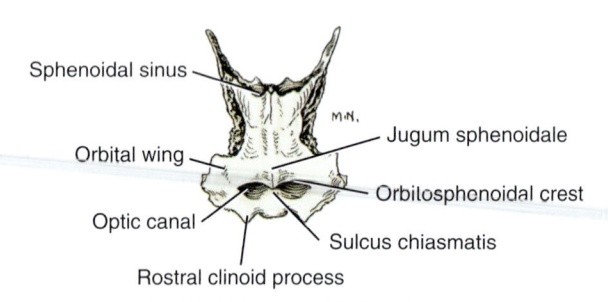

• **Fig. 4.17** Presphenoid, dorsal aspect.

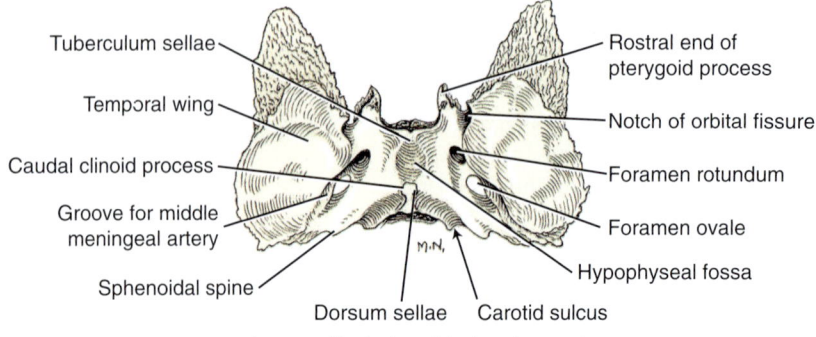

• **Fig. 4.18** Basisphenoid, dorsal aspect.

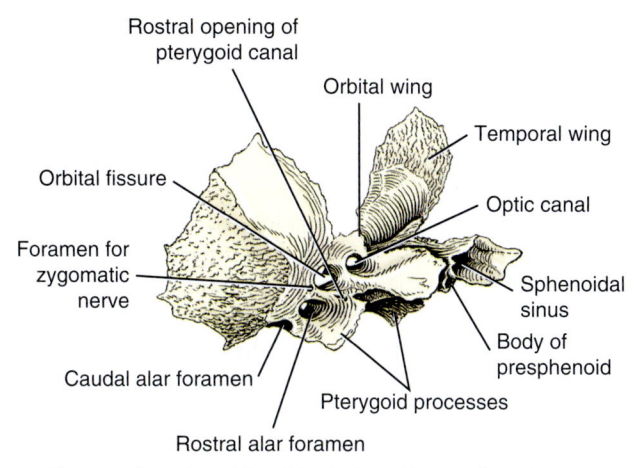

Fig. 4.19 Presphenoid and basisphenoid, rostrolateral aspect.

the **presphenoid** (*os presphenoidale*); the caudal bone with the larger wings is the **basisphenoid** (*os basisphenoidale*).

Presphenoid. The dorsal part of the **body** (*corpus*) of the presphenoid is roofed over by the fusion of right and left **wings** (*alae*) to form the **yoke** (*jugum sphenoidale*). The yoke forms the base of the rostral cranial fossa. A small median tubercle, the **rostrum** (*rostrum sphenoidale*), divided in the newborn, projects from the rostral border of the yoke. Caudally, the yoke forms a shelf, the **orbitosphenoidal crest** (*crista orbitosphenoidalis*). Ventral to this lie the diverging **optic canals** (*canales optici*) for the optic nerves and internal ophthalmic arteries. On each side of the caudal end of the presphenoid is a **rostral clinoid process** (*processus clinoideus rostralis*) that projects caudally. On the dorsum of the body, caudal to the optic canals, is the unpaired *sulcus chiasmatis*, in which lies the optic chiasma. The sphenoid sinus is a cavity between the inner and outer tables of the body of the presphenoid. It is divided by a **longitudinal sphenoidal septum** (*septum sinuum sphenoidalis*). Endoturbinate IV of the ethmoid occupies this sinus.

Basisphenoid. The **body** (*corpus*) of the basisphenoid (see Fig. 4.18) forms the base of the middle cranial fossa. The middle of its dorsal surface is slightly dished to form the oval **hypophyseal fossa** (*fossa hypophysialis*). This fossa is limited rostrally by the *tuberculum sellae*, a dorsally sloping ridge of bone formed at the junction of the presphenoid and basisphenoid and the laterally positioned **rostral clinoid processes** (*processus clinoideus rostralis*) on the caudal border of the wings of the presphenoid. The hypophyseal fossa is limited caudally by a bony process, the *dorsum sellae*, which, in adult skulls, is flattened and expanded at its free end. Projecting rostrally on each side of the dorsum sellae is a **caudal clinoid process** (*processus clinoideus*). This complex of bony structures, consisting of the tuberculum sellae with the rostral clinoid processes, the hypophyseal fossa, and the dorsum sellae with its two caudal clinoid processes, is called the *sella turcica*, or "Turkish saddle." In life it contains the hypophysis. Occasionally the small **craniopharyngeal canal** (*canalis craniopharyngeus*) persists in the adult, particularly in English Bulldogs. This canal is a remnant of the pharyngeal diverticulum to the hypophyseal fossa from which the pars glandularis (adenohypophysis) of the hypophysis develops.

The large **wing** (*ala*) of the basisphenoid curves dorsally and laterally. It has an internal **cerebral surface** (*facies cerebralis*) that faces the brain with a **piriform fossa** (*fossa piriformis*) for the piriform lobe. The lateral **temporal surface** (*facies temporalis*) articulates with the palatine bone ventrally at the **sphenopalatine suture** (*sutura sphenopalatina*), the frontal bone rostrodorsally at the **sphenofrontal suture** (*sutura sphenofrontalis*), and the parietal bone caudodorsally at the **sphenoparietal suture** (*sutura sphenoparietalis*). The caudal two-thirds of the temporal surface of the wing of the basisphenoid are covered laterally by the squamous part of the temporal bone to form the broad **squamosal suture** (*sutura squamosa*). The **orbital fissure** (*fissura orbitalis*) is formed in the suture between the wings of the presphenoid and basisphenoid bones. This large opening is slightly ventral and caudolateral to the optic canals and contains the oculomotor, trochlear, abducent, and ophthalmic nerves and the venous communication between the ophthalmic plexus and cavernous sinus.

At the base of each wing, near its junction with the body, are a series of foramina. The **oval foramen** (*foramen ovale*) is a large opening that leads directly through the wall of the cranial cavity. It is located approximately 0.5 cm medial to the temporomandibular joint and contains the mandibular nerve. A small notch or even a foramen, *foramen spinosum*, may be present in its caudolateral border for the middle meningeal artery to enter the cranial cavity. A ventrolateral extension of the basisphenoid is the **pterygoid process** (*processus pterygoideus*). The **alar canal** (*canalis alaris*) runs through the rostral part of the base of the pterygoid process with its maxillary artery and vein. Its smaller opening is the **caudal alar foramen** (*foramen alare caudalis*), and its larger one is the **rostral alar foramen** (*foramen alare rostralis*). Opening into the canal from the cranial cavity is the **round foramen** (*foramen rotundum*) for the maxillary nerve. It can be seen by viewing the medial wall of the alar canal through the rostral alar foramen. Dorsorostral to the alar canal is the orbital fissure. A small *foramen alare parvum* may be present as the dorsal opening of a small canal that leaves the alar canal. It is located on the ridge of bone separating the orbital fissure from the rostral alar foramen. When present it conducts the zygomatic nerve branch from the maxillary nerve. Two pairs of grooves are present on the basisphenoid bone. The extremely small **pterygoid groove** (*sulcus nervi pterygoidei*) leads into the minute **pterygoid canal** (*canalis pterygoideus*) for the nerve of the pterygoid canal. This begins rostral to the small, pointed, muscular process of the temporal bone, where it is located in the suture between the pterygoid and the basisphenoid bones. It ends in the caudal part of the pterygopalatine fossa. Probing with a horse hair will reveal that it runs medial to the pterygoid process of the sphenoid in the suture between this process and the pterygoid bone. The second groove of the basisphenoid is the **sulcus for the middle meningeal artery** (*sulcus arteriae* *meningeae mediae*). This groove runs obliquely dorsolaterally from the oval foramen on the cerebral surface of the wing and continues mainly on the temporal and parietal bones. Two notches indent the caudal border of the wing. The medial notch is the **carotid incisure** (*incisura carotica*), which concurs with the temporal bone to form the **foramen lacerum**. The lateral notch, with its counterpart on the temporal bone, forms the **sulcus for the short auditory tube** (*sulcus tubae auditivae*), which transmits the tendon of the m. tensor veli palatini and the **auditory tube** (*tuba auditiva*). A low ridge of bone, the **sphenoidal spine** (*spina ossis sphenoidalis*), ending in a process, separates the two openings.

The **pterygoid processes** (*processi pterygoidei*) are the only ventral projections of the basisphenoid. They are thin, sagittal plates approximately 1 cm wide, 1 cm long, and a little more than 1 cm apart. The alar canal passes through each process. Attached to their medial surfaces are the caudally hooked, approximately square pterygoid bones. The processes and pterygoid bones separate the caudal parts of the pterygopalatine fossae from the nasal pharynx.

The body of the basisphenoid articulates caudally with the basioccipital, forming the **sphenooccipital synchondrosis** (*synchondrosis spheno-occipitalis*), and rostrally with the presphenoid, forming the **intersphenoidal synchondrosis** (*synchondrosis intersphenoidalis*). Rostrally, the presphenoid contacts the vomer, forming the **vomerosphenoidal suture** (*sutura vomerosphenoidalis*). The ethmoid also contacts the body of the presphenoid, forming the **sphenoethmoidal suture** (*sutura sphenoethmoidalis*). As the wing of the presphenoid bone extends dorsorostrally, the **sphenopalatine suture** (*sutura sphenopalatina*) is formed ventrally and the **sphenofrontal suture** (*sutura sphenofrontalis*) dorsally. Caudodorsally, the temporal surface of the wing is overlapped by the squamous temporal bone, forming the **sphenosquamous suture** (*sutura sphenosquamosa*). The dorsal end of the wing overlaps the parietal bone, forming the **sphenoparietal suture** (*sutura sphenoparietalis*). The medial surface of the pterygoid process, with the pterygoid bone, forms the **pterygosphenoid suture** (*sutura pterygosphenoidalis*).

Temporal Bone

The **temporal bone** (*os temporale*) (Figs. 4.3 to 4.5, 4.20 to 4.23, and 4.44) forms a large part of the ventrolateral wall of the calvaria. Its structure is intricate owing to the presence of the cochlea and the semicircular canals and an extension of the nasal pharynx into the middle ear. In a young skull the temporal bone can be separated into petrosal, tympanic, and squamous parts. The petrosal part has a mastoid process caudally, with an external surface. The petrosal part houses the cochlea and the semicircular canals and is the last to fuse with the other parts in development. It is located completely within the skull. The tympanic part includes a sac-shaped protuberance, roughly as large as the end of one's finger, which lies ventral to the mastoid process, the tympanic bulla (*bulla tympanica*). The squamous part consists of two basic divisions, an expanded plate that lies dorsal to the bulla and the rostrally projecting zygomatic process that forms the caudal half of the zygomatic arch.

The **petrosal part** (*pars petrosa*), also known as the *pyramid* or *petrosum* (see Fig. 4.21), is fused around its periphery laterally to the medial surfaces of the tympanic and squamous parts. It is roughly pyramidal in shape and

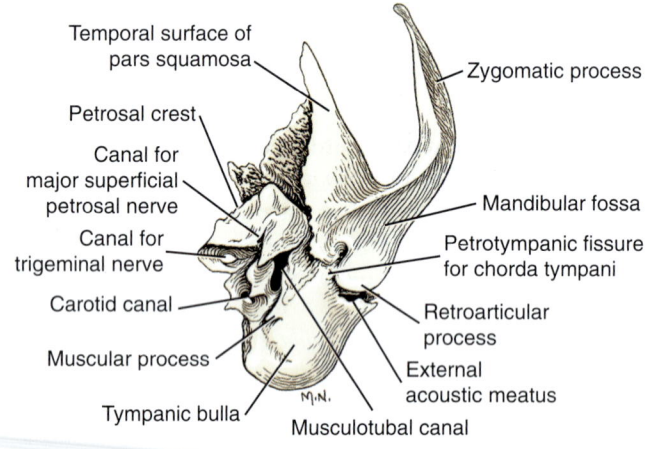

• **Fig. 4.20** Left temporal bone, rostral aspect.

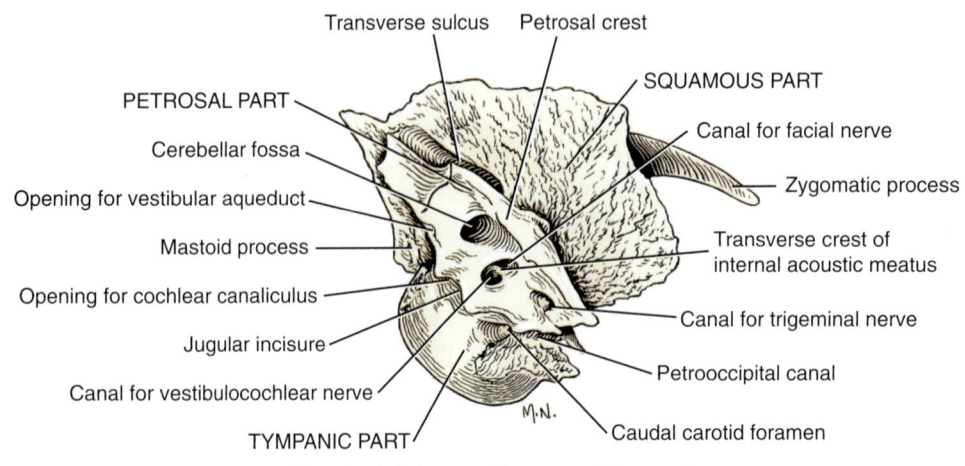

• **Fig. 4.21** Left temporal bone, medial aspect.

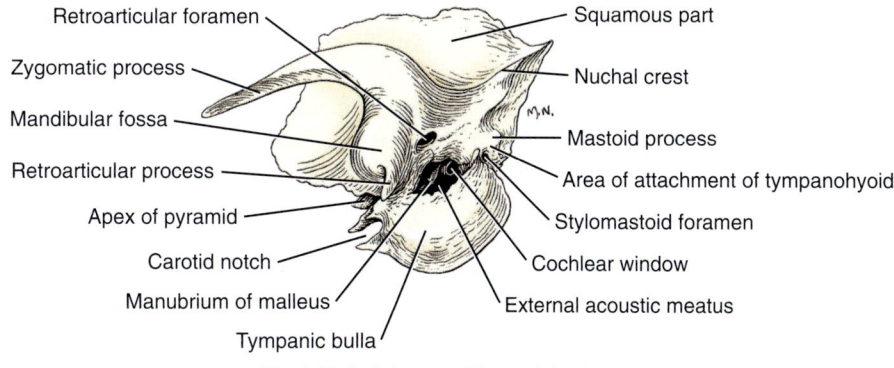

- **Fig. 4.22** Left temporal bone, lateral aspect.

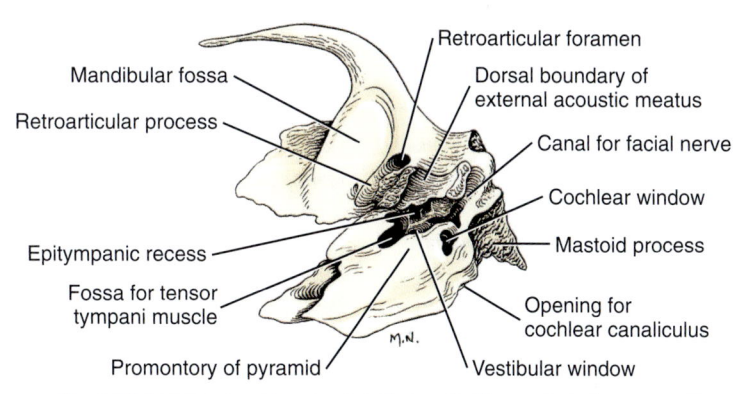

- **Fig. 4.23** Left temporal bone, ventral aspect. (Tympanic bulla removed.)

is called the *pyramid* for this reason. The part immediately surrounding the membranous labyrinth ossifies first and is composed of dense bone. The cartilage that surrounds the inner ear, known as the **otic capsule**, is a conspicuous feature of early embryos. Its sharp **petrosal crest** (*crista petrosa*) extends rostroventrally; its axis forms an angle of approximately 45 degrees caudally with a longitudinal axis through the skull. It nearly meets the tentorium osseum dorsally to form a partial partition between the cerebral and the cerebellar parts of the brain; rostrally it ends in a sharp point, the **petrosal apex** (*apex partis petrosae*). Its surface is divided by the petrosal crest into rostrodorsal and caudomedial parts. The ventral surface faces the **tympanic cavity**.

The caudomedial surface presents several features. The most dorsal of these is the **cerebellar fossa** (*fossa cerebellaris*), which attains its greatest relative size in puppies and houses the paraflocculus of the cerebellum. Ventral to the cerebellar fossa is a recess, the **internal acoustic meatus** (*meatus acusticus internus*). The opening into this recess is the *porus acusticus internus*. The meatus is an irregularly elliptical depression that is divided deeply by the **transverse crest** (*crista transversa*). Dorsal to the crest is the opening of the facial canal, which contains the facial nerve as well as the cribriform **superior vestibular area** (*area vestibularis superior*) for the passage of nerve bundles from the membranous labyrinth. Ventral to the crest is the **inferior vestibular area** (*area vestibularis inferior*), through which pass additional vestibular nerve bundles that come from a deep, minute depression, the *foramen singulare*. The cochlear area (*area cochleae*) is also ventral to this crest, on which lies the **spiral cribriform tract** (*tractus spiralis foraminosus*) which is formed by the wall of the hollow modiolus of the cochlea. The perforations contain the fascicles of the cochlear nerve that arise from the spiral ganglion on the external surface of the modiolus. The cochlea and semicircular canals can be seen by removing a portion of the petrosal part of the temporal bone. Ventrorostral to the internal acoustic meatus is the short **canal** through the petrosal part for the passage of the **trigeminal nerve** (*canalis trigemini*). The caudoventral part of the petrosal part articulates with the occipital bone. On the cerebral surface, or on the border between the cerebral surface and the suture for the occipital bone, is the **external opening of the cochlear canaliculus** (*apertura externa canaliculi cochleae*). This opening is in the rostral edge of the jugular foramen and is large enough to be probed with a horse hair. This canaliculus contains the perilymphatic duct. A smaller opening for the vestibular aqueduct (*apertura externa aqueductus vestibuli*) is located caudodorsal to the opening of the cochlear canaliculus in a small but deep cleft in the bone. The **jugular foramen** (*foramen jugulare*) is located between the petrosal part of the temporal and the occipital bones. It contains the glossopharyngeal, vagus, and accessory nerves and the sigmoid sinus.

The rostrodorsal part of the cerebral surface of the petrosal part is gently undulating, its only features being the digital impressions and jugal elevations corresponding to the gyri and sulci of the cerebrum. Its lateral border is usually grooved by the small middle meningeal artery.

The **ventral surface** of the petrosal part forms much of the dorsal wall of the **tympanic cavity** (*cavum tympani*). At its periphery it articulates with the squamous part of the temporal bone dorsally and the tympanic part of the temporal bone ventrally. It can be seen from the outside through the external acoustic meatus. An eminence, two openings (windows), and three fossae are the prominent features of this surface. The barrel-shaped eminence, or **promontory** (*promontorium*), has at its larger caudolateral end the **cochlear window** (*fenestra cochleae*), formerly called the *round window*. In life, this is closed by the secondary tympanic membrane. Just rostral and slightly dorsolateral to the cochlear window is the **vestibular window** (*fenestra vestibuli*), formerly called the *oval window*, which is occluded by the footplate of the stapes. The fossae lie at the angles of a triangle located rostrolateral to the windows. The smallest fossa is a curved groove with its concavity facing the vestibular window; it is the open part of the canal for the facial nerve peripheral to the genu and rostral to the stylomastoid foramen. The largest is the **fossa for the tensor tympani muscle** (*fossa m. tensor tympani*), which is a spherical depression that lies rostral to the vestibular window. A thin scale of bone with a point extending caudally forms part of its ventral wall. The **epitympanic recess** (*recessus epitympanicus*), the third fossa, lies caudolateral to the fossa m. tensor tympani and at a more dorsal level. The incus and the head of the malleus lie in this recess.

The petrosal part contains the **osseous labyrinth**, which is divided into three parts: the cochlea, semicircular canals, and vestibule. The basal turn of the cochlea is located lateral to the ventral part of the internal acoustic meatus, its initial turn producing the bulk of the promontory. The **semicircular canals** (*canales semicirculares ossei*) are three in number, each located in a different plane caudal to the cochlea. The bony **vestibule** (*vestibulum*) is the osseous common chamber where the three semicircular canals and the cochlea join. The vestibular and cochlear windows communicate with the tympanic cavity in well-cleaned skulls. (For details of the labyrinth, see Chapter 20, The Ear.)

The **facial canal** (*canalis facialis*) carries the seventh cranial, or facial, nerve (see Figs. 4.21 and 4.23). It enters the petrosal part in the dorsal part of the internal acoustic meatus and, after pursuing a sigmoid course through the temporal bone, emerges at the stylomastoid foramen. The initial 3 mm of the canal, starting at the internal acoustic meatus, is straight. The canal makes its first turn on arriving at the thin medial wall of the fossa m. tensor tympani. At this turn, or **genu of the facial canal** (*geniculum canalis facialis*), there is an indistinct enlargement for the sensory geniculate ganglion of the facial nerve. In the concavity of this bend is the rostral half of the vestibule. As the facial canal straightens after the first turn, and before the second turn begins, it opens into the cavity of the middle ear lateral to the vestibular window. The direction of the second bend of the canal is the reverse of that of the first so that the whole passage is S-shaped but does not lie in one plane. The **fossa for the stapedius muscle** (*fossa m. stapedius*) is located on the dorsal wall of the facial canal just before the canal opens into the middle ear cavity. After completing its second arch the facial canal opens to the outside by the deeply placed **stylomastoid foramen** (*foramen stylomastoideum*). The small **canal for the major petrosal nerve** (*canalis petrosi majoris*) leaves the facial canal at the genu and extends rostrally, dorsal to the fossa m. tensor tympani. It runs rostroventrally just within the wall of the fossa to a small opening near the distal end of the petrosquamous suture and lateral to the canal for the trigeminal nerve. If a dark bristle is inserted in the canal, its path can be seen through the wall of the fossa. The major petrosal nerve passes through this canal. The *canaliculus chordae tympani* carries the chorda tympani nerve from the facial canal to the cavity of the middle ear. It arises from the peripheral turn of the facial canal. After the nerve has crossed the medial surface of the handle of the malleus, it passes under a fine bridge of bone of the tympanic ring to continue in the direction of the auditory tube. The chorda tympani usually passes through a small canal in the rostrodorsal wall of the bulla tympanica and emerges through the **petrotympanic fissure** (*fissura petrotympanica*) by a small opening medial to the retroarticular process. When the canal fails to develop, the opening is through the rostrolateral wall of the tympanic bulla. Both the canal for the major petrosal nerve and the canaliculus chordae tympani leave the facial canal at an acute angle. In the rostral wall of the ventral surface of the petrosal part of the temporal bone is a small **canal for the minor petrosal nerve** (*canalis n. petrosi minoris*), which is a branch from the tympanic plexus of the glossopharyngeal nerve. This canal opens into the osseous part of the auditory tube.

Two minute canals run from the labyrinth to the medial surface of the petrosal part of the temporal bone. The **perilymphatic duct** (*ductus perilymphaticus*) runs in the cochlear canaliculus ventrally from a point on the ventral wall of the scala tympani near the cochlear window to the border of the jugular foramen. This duct connects the scala tympani to the subarachnoid space. The **vestibular aqueduct** (*aqueductus vestibuli*) from the vestibule passes caudoventrally to the caudal part of the medial surface of the petrosal part approximately 3 mm dorsorostral to the cochlear opening. This bony duct is too small to be probed easily. It contains the membranous endolymphatic duct, which extends from the saccule to the dura mater.

The **mastoid process** (*processus mastoideus*) of the petrosal part is the only part to have an external surface. This surface lies between the **mastoid foramen** (*foramen mastoideum*) dorsally and the **stylomastoid foramen** (*foramen stylomastoideum*) ventrally, both of which it helps to form. It articulates with the lateral part of the occipital medially and the squamous part laterally. The ventral part is slightly enlarged and serves for the attachment of the tympanohyoid cartilage. The facial canal, as it leaves the stylomastoid foramen, grooves the ventral surface of the mastoid process.

The stylomastoid foramen is dorsal to the caudal part of the tympanic bulla.

The **tympanic part** (*pars tympanica*) of the temporal bone, or **tympanicum**, is the ventral portion and is easily identified by its largest component, the smooth bulbous enlargement, or *bulla tympanica*, which lies between the retroarticular and paracondylar processes. In puppies its walls are not thicker than the shell of a hen's egg. The cavity it encloses is the fundic part of the tympanic cavity, which is delimited from the dorsal part of the tympanic cavity proper by a thin edge of bone. In old animals this bony ledge has fine, knobbed spicules protruding from its free border. The osseous **external acoustic meatus** (*meatus acusticus externus*) is the canal from the cartilaginous external ear to the tympanic membrane. Its length increases with age but rarely exceeds 1 cm even in old, large skulls. It is piriform, with its greatest dimension dorsoventrally and its smallest dimension transversely. In carefully prepared skulls the malleus can be seen through the meatus, somewhat displaced but articulated with the incus. All but the dorsal part of the osseous external acoustic meatus is formed by the tympanicum. The **tympanic membrane** (*membrana tympani*), or eardrum, is a membranous diaphragm attached to the **tympanic ring** (*anulus tympanicus*). If planes are drawn through the tympanic membranes, they meet at the rostral end of the cranial cavity. At the rostral margin of the bulla, lateral to the occipitosphenoidal suture, there are paired notches and two large openings. The more medial of the two openings is the **foramen lacerum** (*foramen lacerum*), formerly called the *external carotid foramen*. It contains a loop of the internal carotid artery and is flanked on the medial and lateral sides by sharp, pointed processes of bone from the bulla wall. The medial process meets the spine of the sphenoid bone in separating the foramen from the lateral opening, the **musculotubal canal** (*canalis musculotubarius*). The musculotubal canal contains the auditory tube. By means of the auditory tube, the tympanic cavity communicates with the nasal pharynx. The **carotid canal** (*canalis caroticus*) runs longitudinally through the medial wall of the osseous bulla where it articulates with the basioccipital bone. It begins at the **caudal carotid foramen** (*foramen caroticum caudalis*), which is hidden in the depths of the petrobasilar fissure. It runs rostrally, makes a ventral turn at a little more than a right angle, and opens to the outside at the foramen lacerum. At its sharp turn ventrally it concurs with the caudal part of the sphenoid bone, which here forms not only the rostral boundary of the vertical parts of the carotid canal but also the rostral boundary of an opening in the cranial cavity, the **internal carotid foramen** (*foramen caroticum internum*). The carotid canal transmits the internal carotid artery and postganglionic sympathetic axons. The lateral boundary of the **petrooccipital canal** (*canalis petrooccipitalis*) is formed by the tympanic bulla and petrosal part of the temporal bone. Medially the basioccipital bone bounds it. The petrooccipital canal contains the ventral petrosal sinus, which parallels the horizontal part of the carotid canal and lies medial to it.

The **tympanic cavity** (*cavum tympani*) is the cavity of the middle ear. It can be divided into three parts: The largest, most ventral part is located entirely within the tympanic bulla and is the fundic part. The smaller, middle compartment, which is located opposite the tympanic membrane, is the tympanic cavity proper, and its most dorsal extension, for the incus, part of the stapes, and head of the malleus, is the **epitympanic recess** (*recessus epitympanicus*).

The **squamous part** (*pars squamosa*) of the temporal bone possesses a long, curved, **zygomatic process** (*processus zygomaticus*) (see Figs. 4.21 and 4.22), which extends rostrolaterally and overlies the caudal half of the zygomatic bone in forming the **zygomatic arch** (*arcus zygomaticus*). The ventral part of the base of the zygomatic process expands to form a transversely elongated, smooth area, the **mandibular fossa** (*fossa mandibularis*), which receives the condyle of the mandible to form the **temporomandibular joint** (*articulatio temporomandibularis*). The **retroarticular process** (*processus retroarticulare*) is a ventral extension of the squamous temporal bone. Its rostral surface forms part of the mandibular fossa, and its caudal surface is grooved by an extension of the **retroarticular foramen** (*foramen retroarticulare*). The temporal sinus emerges from this foramen as the emissary vein of the retroarticular foramen (*v. emissaria foraminis retroarticularis*), which joins with the maxillary vein. The dorsal part of the squamous part of the temporal bone is a laterally arched, convex plate of bone that articulates with the parietal bone dorsally, the wing of the basisphenoid bone rostrally, the tympanicum ventrally, and the mastoid process and the squamous occipital caudally. Near the caudolateral border of the bone is the ventral part of the **nuchal crest**. This crest is continued rostrally dorsal to the external acoustic meatus on to the zygomatic process as the **supramastoid crest** (*crista supramastoidea*). The smooth, rounded outer surface dorsal to the root of the zygomatic process is the *facies temporalis*. The **temporal canal**, seen on the inner surface, between the squamous and the petrous parts, forms a passage for the temporal sinus, which exits by means of the retroarticular foramen as the emissary vein of the retroarticular foramen.

The squamous part of the temporal bone overlaps the parietal bone, forming a **squamosal suture** (*sutura squamosa*). It also extends over the caudal margin of the wing of the sphenoid bone, forming the **sphenosquamosal suture** (*sutura sphenosquamosa*). Rostrally, the zygomatic process of the squamosum meets the zygomatic bone at the **temporozygomatic suture** (*sutura temporozygomatica*). Ventrally, the tympanic part of the temporal bone meets the basioccipital to form the rostral part of the **tympanooccipital fissure** (*fissura tympanooccipitalis*). This fissure contains the glossopharyngeal, vagus, and accessory nerves; postganglionic sympathetic axons; the internal carotid artery; and the origins of the vertebral and internal jugular veins. Caudally, the tympanicum articulates with the paracondylar process of the lateral part of the occipital bone to form the caudal part of this joint. The **petrooccipital fissure** (*fissura petrooccipitalis*) is formed between these articulations. At the depth of this fissure the petrous part of the temporal bone articulates with the occipital bone in forming the **petrooccipital synchondrosis** (*synchondrosis petrooccipitalis*).

Ethmoid Bone

The **ethmoid bone** (*os ethmoidale*) (Figs. 4.9, 4.24 to 4.29, and 4.47) is located between the cranial and the facial parts of the skull, both of which it helps to form. It is completely hidden from view in the intact skull. Its complicated structure is best studied from sections and disarticulated specimens. Although unpaired, it develops from paired anlagen. It is situated between the walls of the orbits and is bounded dorsally by the frontal, laterally by the maxillary, and ventrally by the vomer and palatine bones. It consists of four parts: a median perpendicular plate, or lamina; two ethmoid labyrinths covered by external laminae; and a cribriform plate, to which the ethmoturbinates of the labyrinths attach.

The **perpendicular plate** (*lamina perpendicularis*), formerly mesethmoid, is a median vertical sheet of bone that, by articulating with the vomer ventrally and the septal processes of the frontal and nasal bones dorsally, forms the **osseous nasal septum** (*septum nasi osseum*). This bony septum is prolonged rostrally by the cartilaginous nasal septum. Caudally, it fuses with the cribriform plate but usually does not extend through it to form a *crista galli*. It forms only the ventral half of the nasal septum as the septal plates of the frontal and nasal bones extend ventrally halfway and fuse with it. The perpendicular plate is roughly rectangular in outline, with a rounded rostral border and an inclined caudal one so that it is longer ventrally than it is dorsally. The turbinates of the ethmoid labyrinths fill the nasal cavities so completely that an inappreciable **common nasal meatus** (*meatus nasi communis*) remains between each ethmoid labyrinth and the lateral surface of the septum. The dorsal border does not follow the contour of the face but parallels the hard palate. The dorsal lamina tectoria arises from the dorsal part of the perpendicular plate.

An external lamina of the ethmoid bone is developmentally the osseous lining of the nasal fundus. It is extremely thin and in places it is deficient, as it coats the inner surfaces of the heavier bones that form this part of the face. This lamina is divided into dorsal, lateral, and ventral parts, commonly called the roof (*lamina tectoria*), side (*lamina orbitalis*), and floor (*lamina basalis*) plates, respectively, of the ethmoid labyrinths. From its origin on the perpendicular plate the external lamina runs dorsally in contact with frontal and nasal parts of the septum, swings laterally over the top of the ethmoidal labyrinth, forming the **roof plate** (*lamina tectoria*), and continues ventrally on each lateral side (lamina orbitalis) as the lateral plate. It partly covers the side of the ethmoturbinates. This portion of the lamina is exceedingly thin, incomplete in places, and porous throughout. Its rostrodorsolateral part is channeled to form the **uncinate process** (*processus uncinatus*), which is a part of the first endoturbinate as well as of the orbital (lateral) lamina. The **uncinate notch** (*incisura uncinata*), in the meatus between the first two endoturbinates, is located dorsocaudal to the uncinate process. A depressed area of the orbital lamina forms the medial wall of the **maxillary recess** (*recessus maxillaris*). The external lamina is deficient caudally, occurring only as paper-thin, irregular plaques that remain attached to the basal laminae of the scrolls of bone. The individual turbinates arise from the roof and lateral portions of this delicate covering. The ventral lamina (*lamina basalis*), which forms the floor plate, can be isolated

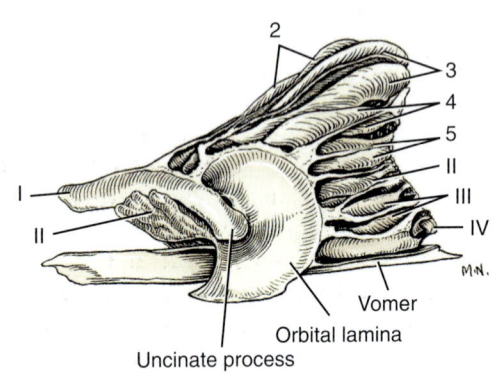

• **Fig. 4.24** Vomer and left ethmoid, lateral aspect. Roman numerals indicate endoturbinates. Arabic numerals indicate ectoturbinates.

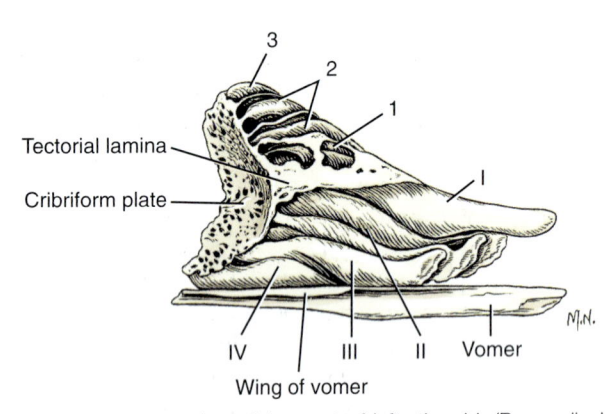

• **Fig. 4.25** Vomer and medial aspect of left ethmoid. (Perpendicular plate removed.) Roman numerals indicate endoturbinates. Arabic numerals indicate ectoturbinates.

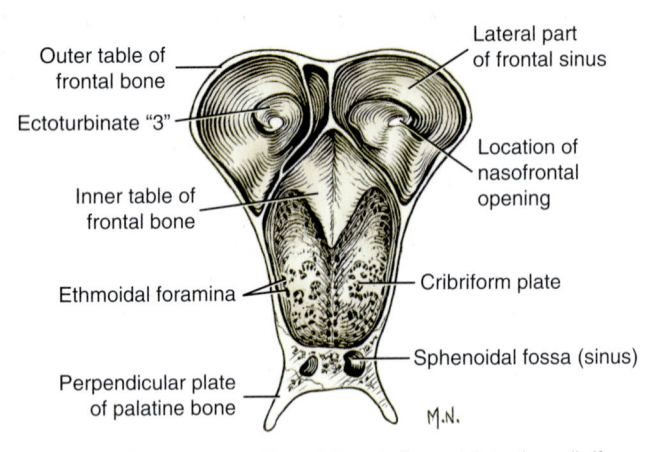

• **Fig. 4.26** Transverse section of the skull caudal to the cribriform plate. The sphenoid fossa is the rostral part of an excavation within the presphenoid bone occupied by ethmoturbinates IV and can be considered part of a sinus.

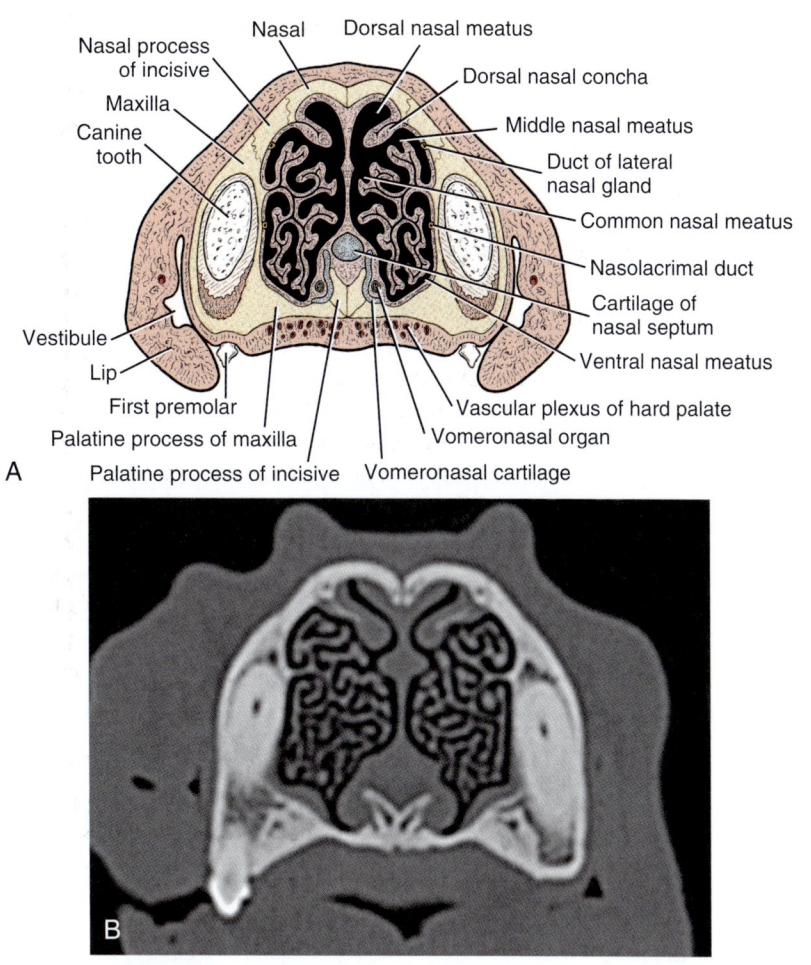

• **Fig. 4.27** **A**, Transverse section of nasal cavity. **B**, A computed tomography (CT) scan taken from a comparable transverse plane.

as a thin, smooth leaf fused to the medial surfaces of the maxillae. It continues from the ventral part of the orbital plate medially to the vomer in a transverse, dorsally convex arch. It is closely applied to the horizontal part of the vomer. The two conjoined sheets in this manner form a partition that separates the ethmoturbinates in the nasal fundus from the nasopharynx.

The **cribriform plate** (*lamina cribrosa*) (see Figs. 4.25 and 4.26) is a deeply concave partition, protruding rostrally, that articulates with the ethmoidal notches of the frontal bones dorsally and with the presphenoid ventrally and laterally. It is the sievelike partition between the nasal and the cranial cavities. Approximately 300 foramina, some as large as 1.5 mm in diameter, perforate the plate and serve for the transmission of olfactory nerve bundles. These **cribriform foramina** (*foramina laminae cribrosae*) are grouped into tracts that surround the attachments of the turbinates, the larger foramina being adjacent to these attachments as well as around the periphery of the bone. Extending rostromedially from the middle of the lateral border is a slightly raised, foramen-free ridge of bone that is surrounded by large foramina. Caudal to this low ridge, the ethmoid concurs with the presphenoid to form one of the double **ethmoidal foramina** (*foramina ethmoidalia*) on each side. These two foramina carry the external ethmoidal vessels and the ethmoidal nerve. A *crista galli*, dividing the caudal surface of the cribriform plate into right and left fossae for the olfactory bulbs of the brain, is present only in old specimens. The most rostral limit of the fossae for the olfactory bulbs reaches a transverse plane passing through the middle of the orbital openings. The cribriform plate is not transverse in position. The right and left halves lie in nearly sagittal planes and meet rostrally at an angle of approximately 45 degrees. Its cerebral surface forms the inside of a laterally compressed cone that is curved in all directions.

The **ethmoidal labyrinths** (*labyrinthus ethmoidalis*) form the bulk of the ethmoid bone. Each is composed largely of delicate bony scrolls, or **ethmoturbinates** (*ethmoturbinalia*), which attach ventrally to the basal laminae and attach caudally to the cribriform plate. Because the cribriform plate does not extend to the body of the presphenoid, but only to its inner table, a space extends caudally into the body of the presphenoid. Likewise, the cribriform plate attaches dorsally to the inner table of the frontal bone, which in old, long skulls is separated from the outer table by more than 2 cm. The ethmoturbinates extend into these spaces. So completely is the cavity of the presphenoid filled by the ethmoturbinates that the dog is usually regarded

108 CHAPTER 4 The Skeleton

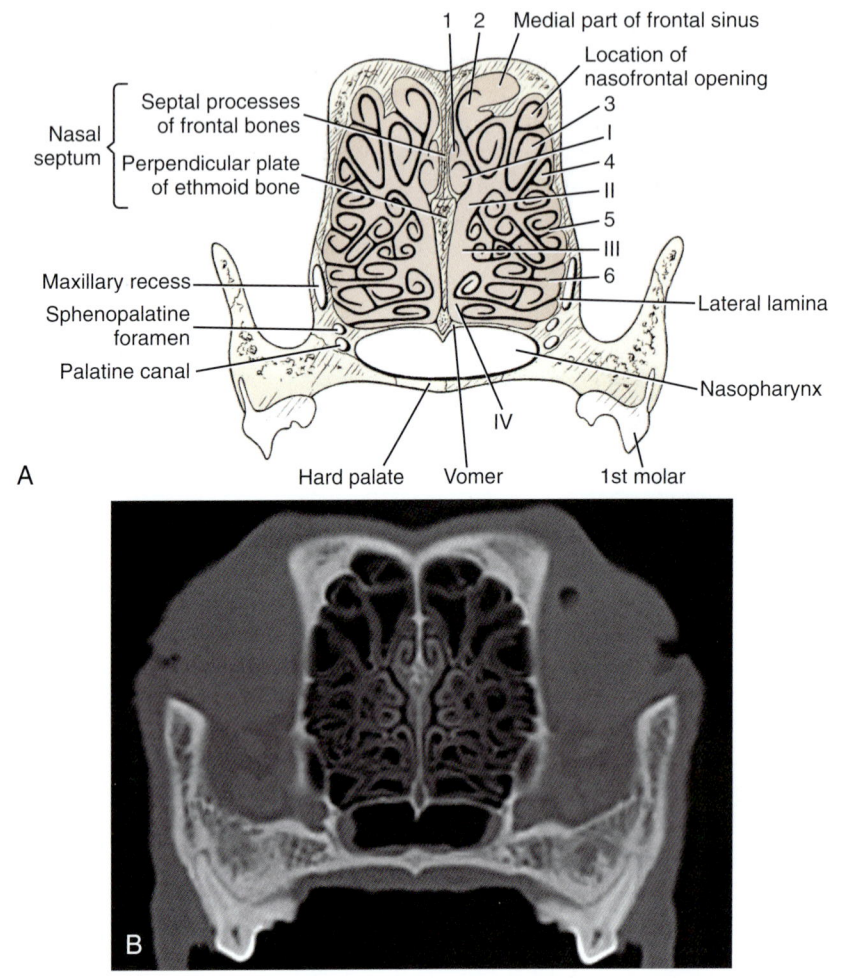

• **Fig. 4.28** **A**, Scheme of the ethmoturbinates in transverse section immediately rostral to cribriform plate. Roman numerals indicate endoturbinates. Arabic numerals indicate ectoturbinates. **B**, A computed tomography (CT) scan at about this same transverse plane.

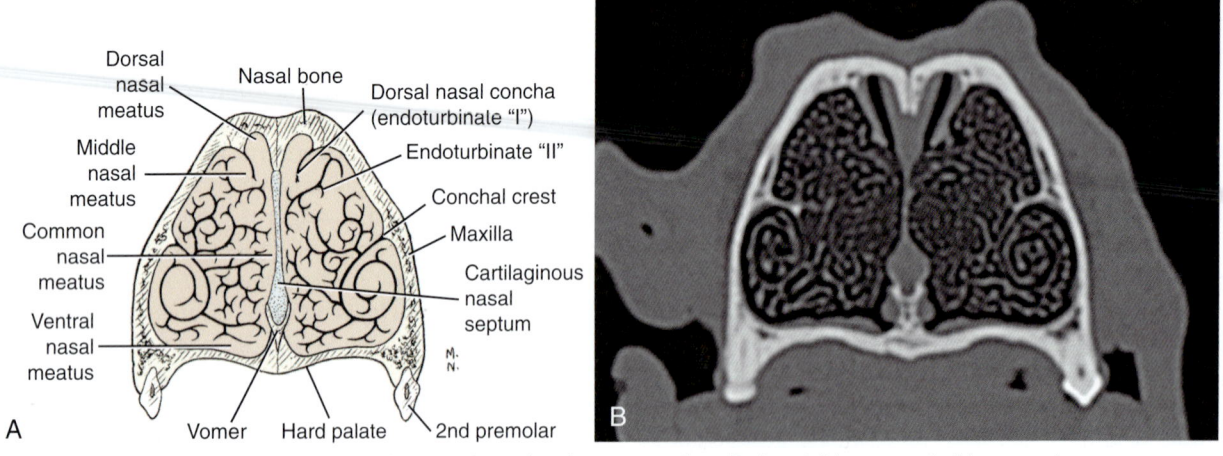

• **Fig. 4.29** **A**, Scheme of the ventral conchae in cross-section. **B**, A matching computed tomography (CT) scan from a transverse level similar to A.

as not possessing a **sphenoidal sinus** (*sinus sphenoidalis*), although in every other respect a sinus does exist. The most dorsal turbinates grow dorsally and caudally from the cribriform plate into the cavity of the **frontal sinus**. Usually all compartments of the medial part of the frontal sinus have secondary linings formed by ethmoturbinates. The rostral end of the large lateral compartment contains the end of an ethmoturbinal scroll that is always open, allowing free interchange of air between the nasal fossa and the sinus. The ethmoturbinates are surprisingly alike in different specimens. They may be divided into four long, ventrally lying **endoturbinates** (*endoturbinalia I to IV*) and six smaller, more dorsally lying **ectoturbinates** (*ectoturbinalia 1 to 6*). The difference between these two groups of turbinates is in their location and not in their form. Each ethmoidal element (turbinate) possesses a basal leaf that attaches to the external lamina. Most of these scrolls come from the lateral part of this lamina, but some arise from the roof plate proper, and others from the septal part. Most turbinates also attach to the cribriform plate caudally. Each ethmoturbinate is rolled into one or more delicate scrolls of one and a half and two and a half turns. Those turbinates with a single scroll turn ventrally, with the exception of the first endoturbinate, which turns dorsally. The elements with two scrolls usually turn toward each other, and thus toward their attachments. Variations are common, as the illustrations show. The endoturbinates nearly reach the nasal septum medially. The **first endoturbinate** is the longest and arises from the dorsal part of the cribriform plate caudally as well as from the medial part of the roof plate. In the region dorsal to the infraorbital foramen it passes from the roof plate to the medial surface of the maxilla. Further rostrally it attaches to the medial wall of the nasal bone as the **dorsal nasal concha**, formerly the *nasal turbinate*. The uncinate process is formed at the attachment of the basal lamina to the nasal bone. This process is coextensive with the orbital lamina and extends caudoventrally into the maxillary recess. The caudal part of the first endoturbinate is represented by a dorsomedially rolled plate. The small, ventrally infolded first endoturbinate is located dorsally. The **second endoturbinate** arises from its basal lamina near the middle of the orbital lamina. It divides into two or more scrolls, which become widened and flattened in a sagittal plane rostrally and rest against the caudodorsal part of the **ventral nasal concha**, formerly the *maxilloturbinate*. Viewed from the medial side, the **third** and **fourth endoturbinates** have the same general form as the second. They are progressively shorter than the second so that the wide rostral free end of the second overlaps the third as do shingles on a roof. The fourth element is the smallest and lies dorsal to the wing of the vomer. Caudally it invades the sphenoid sinus.

The **ectoturbinates** are squeezed in between the basal laminae of the endoturbinates and do not approach the nasal septum as closely as do the endoturbinates. The first two protrude through the floor of the frontal sinus. According to Maier (1928), the second ectoturbinate pushes up into the medial compartment of the frontal sinus, whereas the third ectoturbinate pushes up into the lateral compartment. Because the form of any one turbinate changes so drastically from level to level, these delicate bones can best be studied from sagittally sectioned heads that have been decalcified.

The **cribriform plate** of the ethmoid articulates ventrally with the presphenoid to form the **sphenoethmoid suture** (*sutura sphenoethmoidalis*) and with the vomer to form the **vomeroethmoid suture** (*sutura vomeroethmoidalis*). Laterally and dorsally the **frontoethmoidal suture** (*sutura frontoethmoidalis*) is formed by the union of the cribriform plate with the medial surface of the frontal bone. The basal lamina and the rostral part of the orbital lamina attach to the maxilla, forming the **ethmoidomaxillary suture** (*sutura ethmoidomaxillaris*). The caudal part of the orbital lamina as it meets the basal lamina attaches to the palatine bone, forming the **palatoethmoid suture** (*sutura palatoethmoidalis*). The orbital lamina attaches to the small lacrimal bone to form the **lacrimoethmoidal suture** (*sutura lacrimoethmoidalis*). Dorsally the tectorial lamina of the ethmoid articulates with the nasal bones to form the **nasoethmoidal suture** (*sutura nasoethmoidalis*). These laminae intimately fuse with the bones against which they lie so that, in a young disarticulated skull, lines and crests are present on the inner surfaces of the bones against which the ethmoidal labyrinth articulates. The more salient lines are for the attachment of the endoturbinates and the smaller ones for the attachment of the ectoturbinates because these laminae have largely fused to the bones against which they lie.

Bones of the Face and Palate

Incisive Bone

Each **incisive bone** (*os incisivum*), formerly premaxilla (Figs. 4.3 to 4.5, 4.30) has a small **body** (*corpus ossis incisivum*) rostrally with three processes. The **alveolar process** (*processus alveolaris*) has three alveoli for the three dorsal incisor teeth. These teeth are anchored in deep, conical sockets called **alveoli** (*alveoli dentales*) that increase in size from the medial to the lateral position. The bony partitions between the alveoli are the **interalveolar septa** (*septa interalveolaria*). A laterally facing concavity on the caudal alveolar surface forms the rostromedial wall of the alveolus for the canine tooth. The dorsocaudal part of the incisive bone is the curved, tapering **nasal process** (*processus nasalis*), the free rostral border of which bounds the **bony nasal aperture** (*apertura nasi ossea*). A minute groove on the medial surface of each incisive bone concurs with its fellow to form the **interincisive canal** (*canalis interincisivus*) in the **interincisive suture** (*sutura interincisiva*) for blood vessels. This canal varies in size and position and occasionally is absent. Extending caudally from the body is the laterally compressed, pointed **palatine process** (*processus palatinus*). This process, with that of the opposite bone, forms a **dorsal sulcus** (*sulcus septi nasi*) in which the rostral part of the cartilaginous nasal septum fits. The oval space formed by the articulation of the palatine process of the incisive bone

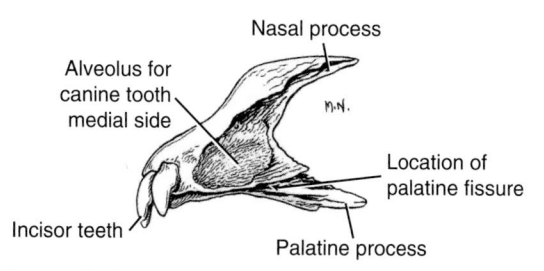

• **Fig. 4.30** Left incisive bone (premaxilla), ventral lateral aspect.

with the palatine process of the maxilla is the **palatine fissure** (*fissura palatina*), which is the only large opening in each half of the bony palate. This fissure contains small blood vessels and the incisive duct from which the vomeronasal organ arises. The incisive bone articulates caudally with the maxilla to form the **incisivomaxillary suture** (*sutura incisivomaxillaris*). The caudodorsal parts of the right and left palatine processes form the **vomeroincisive suture** (*sutura vomeroincisiva*) as they articulate with the vomer. The medial surface of each nasal process articulates with the nasal bone to form the **nasoincisive suture** (*sutura nasoincisiva*).

Nasal Bone

The **nasal bone** (*os nasale*) (Figs. 4.3, 4.4, 4.31) is long, slender, and narrow caudally but, in large dogs, is almost 1 cm wide rostrally. The **dorsal**, or **external**, **surface** (*facies externa*) of the nasal bone varies in size and shape, depending on the breed. In brachycephalic types the nasal bone is very short, whereas in dolichocephalic breeds of the same weight, its length may exceed its width by 15 times. The external surface usually presents a small foramen at its midlength for the transmission of a vein.

The **ventral**, or **internal**, **surface** (*facies interna*) in life is covered by mucous membrane. It is deeply channeled throughout its rostral half, where it forms the **dorsal nasal meatus** (*meatus nasi dorsalis*) and ventral to this meatus bears the **dorsal nasal concha** (*concha nasalis dorsalis*), which is a rostral extension from the ethmoturbinates. The caudal half of the nasal surface is widened to form the shallow **ethmoidal fossa**, which bounds the dorsal part of the ethmoid labyrinth of the ethmoid. The **ethmoidal crest** (*crista ethmoidalis*) is a thin shelf of bone that serves for the attachment of the dorsal nasal concha throughout its rostral half and to the first endoturbinate in its caudal half. The division between the two parts of this concha is arbitrary. The nasal bone ends rostrally in a concave border that, with that of its fellow, forms the dorsal boundary of the bony nasal aperture. The lateral pointed part is more prominent than the medial and is called the **nasal process**. The caudal extremity of the bone is usually pointed near the median plane and is known as the **frontal process**.

The nasal bone articulates extensively with its fellow on the median plane, forming the **internasal suture** (*sutura internasalis*) externally and the **nasoethmoidal suture** (*sutura nasoethmoidalis*) internally. Caudally it articulates with the frontal bone, forming the **frontonasal suture** (*sutura frontonasalis*). Laterally the nasal bone articulates with the maxilla and the incisive bone, forming the **nasomaxillary suture** (*sutura nasomaxillaris*) and the **nasoincisive suture** (*sutura nasoincisiva*), respectively.

Maxilla

The **maxilla** (Figs. 4.3 to 4.5, 4.32, 4.43, 4.44, 4.48) and the incisive bone of each side form the dorsal jaw. The maxilla is divided grossly into a body and four processes: the frontal, zygomatic, palatine, and alveolar. It is the largest bone of the face and bears all of the dorsal cheek teeth. It is roughly pyramidal in form, with its apex rostrally and its wide base caudally. Like the other facial bones, it shows great variation in size and form, depending on the skull type.

The smooth **external surface** (*facies facialis*) of the maxilla has as its most prominent feature an elliptical **infraorbital foramen** (*foramen infraorbitale*) for the passage of the infraorbital nerve and vessels. The ventrolateral surface of the bone that bears the teeth is the **alveolar process** (*processus alveolaris*). The partitions between adjacent teeth are the **interalveolar septa** (*septa interalveolaria*), and the septa between the roots of an individual tooth are the **interradicular septa** (*septa interradicularia*). The smooth elevations on the ventrolateral facial surface of the maxilla caused by the roots of the teeth are the **alveolar juga** (*juga alveolaria*). The juga for the canine and the lateral roots of the shearing tooth (fourth maxillary premolar) are the most

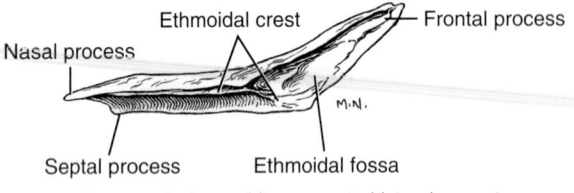

• Fig. 4.31 Left nasal bone, ventral lateral aspect.

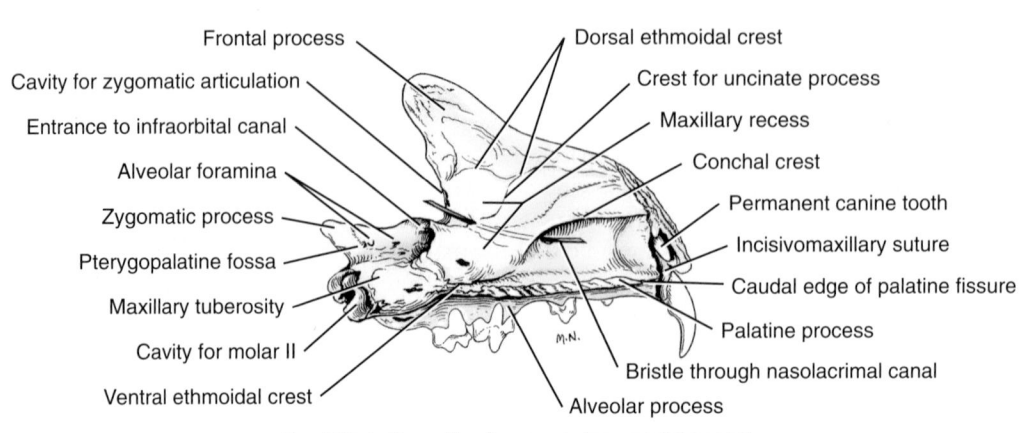

• Fig. 4.32 Left maxilla of a young dog, medial aspect.

prominent. The alveolar process contains 15 **alveoli** (*alveoli dentales*) for the roots of the seven teeth that it contains. Where the teeth are far apart the spaces between them are known as **interdental spaces**, and the margin of the maxilla at such places is called the **interalveolar margin**. Interdental spaces are found between each of the four premolar teeth and caudal to the canine tooth. The **lateral border** of the alveolar process (*margo alveolaris*) is scalloped as a result of the presence of the tooth alveoli, with their interalveolar and interradicular septa. There are three alveoli for each of the last three cheek teeth, two each for the next two rostrally, and one for the first cheek tooth. In addition to these alveoli the large caudally curved alveolus for the canine tooth lies dorsal to those for the first two cheek teeth, or premolars I and II. Lying dorsal to the three alveoli for the shearing tooth is the short **infraorbital canal** (*canalis infraorbitalis*). This canal begins caudally at the **maxillary foramen** (*foramen maxillare*) where the infraorbital vessels and nerve enter the canal. Leading from the infraorbital canal to the individual roots of the premolar teeth (first four cheek teeth) are the **alveolar canals** (*canales alveolares*), which open by numerous **alveolar foramina** (*foramina alveolaria*) at the apex of each alveolus. The special **incisivomaxillary canal** (*canalis maxilloincisivus*) carries the nerves and blood vessels to the first three premolar and the canine and incisor teeth. It leaves the medial wall of the infraorbital canal within the infraorbital foramen, passes dorsal to the apex of the canine alveolus with which it communicates, and enters the incisive bone. It continues rostrally and medially in the incisive bone, giving off branches to the incisor alveoli.

The **frontal process** (*processus frontalis*) arches dorsally between the nasal bone and the orbit to overlap the frontal bone in a squamous suture. The **zygomatic process** (*processus zygomaticus*) is largely hidden, in an articulated skull, by the laterally lying zygomatic bone, which is mitered into the maxilla both dorsal and ventral to the bulk of the process. This type of articulation prevents dislocation at a place where injury frequently occurs. The **palatine process** (*processus palatinus*) is a transverse shelf of bone that, with its fellow, forms most of the **hard palate** (*palatum osseum*) and separates the respiratory from the digestive passageway. The dorsal surface of the palatine process forms part of the floor of the ventral nasal meatus. Its **ventral surface** (*facies palatina*) is grooved on each side by the **palatine sulcus** (*sulcus palatinus*) and forms part of the roof of the oral cavity. Each sulcus extends rostrally from the **major palatine foramen** (*foramen palatinum majus*), which is an oval, oblique opening in the suture between the palatine process of the maxilla and the palatine bone. It contains the major palatine vessels and nerve. In some specimens the palatine sulcus may reach the **palatine fissure** (*fissura palatina*), which is a large, sagittally directed oval opening formed caudally by the rostral border of the palatine process of the maxilla. The most caudal process of the maxilla is a small pointed spur, the **alveolar process of the maxilla** (*processus alveolaris*), located caudomedial to the alveolus for the last molar tooth.

This process and the palatine bone form a notch, rarely a foramen, through which the minor palatine vessels pass.

The **nasal surface** (*facies nasalis*) of the maxilla is its medial surface and bears several crests. The **conchal crest** (*crista conchalis*) begins at or near the incisivomaxillary suture, runs caudally, inclines ventrally, and terminates rostral to the opening of the maxillary recess. A small sagittofrontal crest serves for the attachment of the basal lamina of the ethmoid bone. Another small crest limits the maxillary recess dorsally and marks the line of attachment of the orbital lamina of the ethmoid to the maxilla. An oblique line passes from the nasoturbinate crest caudoventrally and laterally to the mouth of the maxillary recess to which the uncinate process of the ethmoid is attached. The **lacrimal canal** (*canalis lacrimalis*) continues from the lacrimal bone into the maxilla, where it opens ventral to the conchal crest. The medial wall of the canal is thin and may be incomplete. The **maxillary recess** (*recessus maxillaris*) lies medial to the infraorbital and lacrimal canals, both of which protrude slightly into it. The lateral wall of the maxillary recess is formed largely by the maxilla with the addition of the palatine bone caudally. The floor of the **pterygopalatine fossa** (*fossa pterygopalatina*) lies caudal to the maxillary foramen. The shelf of bone that forms it is thicker rostrally and contains many alveolar foramina that lead to the alveoli for the last two cheek teeth. The thin caudal part, barely thick enough to cover the roots of the last molar tooth, is the **maxillary tuberosity** (*tuber maxillae*).

The maxilla articulates with the incisive bone rostrally, forming the **maxilloincisive suture** (*sutura maxilloincisiva*). Dorsomedially, the nasal bone meets the maxilla at the **nasomaxillary suture** (*sutura nasomaxillaris*). Dorsocaudally, the maxilla articulates with the frontal bone, forming the **frontomaxillary suture** (*sutura frontotmaxillaris*) at its dorsocaudal angle. Ventral to this suture the lacrimal bone and maxilla form the short **lacrimomaxillary suture** (*sutura lacrimomaxillaris*). The ventrolateral part of the maxilla forms the unusually stable **zygomaticomaxillary suture** (*sutura zygomaticomaxillaris*) as it articulates with the zygomatic bone. Ventrocaudally, the maxilla forms the extensive **palatomaxillary suture** (*sutura palatomaxillaris*) with the palatine bone. The **median palatine suture** (*sutura palatina mediana*) is formed by the two palatine processes. The transitory joint between the ethmoid and the maxilla is the **ethmoidomaxillary suture** (*sutura ethmoidomaxillaris*). The **vomeromaxillary suture** (*sutura vomeromaxillaris*) is formed in the median plane, within the nasal cavity.

Dorsal Nasal Concha

The **dorsal nasal concha** (*concha nasalis dorsalis*) was formerly called the *nasal turbinate*. It is the continuation of endoturbinate I of the ethmoid, which attaches by means of an ethmoidal crest (see Fig. 4.31) to the nasal bone. Baum and Zietzschmann (1936) regarded the first endoturbinate and the dorsal nasal concha as one structure. The uncinate process and the caudally extending scroll constitute endoturbinate I of the ethmoid. The dorsal nasal concha, unlike the ethmoturbinates and ventral nasal concha, is a simple curved shelf of bone that is separated from the ventrally lying ventral nasal concha by a small cleft, the **middle nasal meatus** (*meatus nasi medius*). In life, the scroll is continued rostral to the ethmoidal crest by a plica of mucosa that diminishes and disappears in the vestibule of the nose.

Ventral Nasal Concha

The **ventral nasal concha** (*os conchae nasalis ventralis*) (see Figs. 4.27 and 4.29) was formerly called the *maxilloturbinate*. It is attached to the medial wall of the maxilla by a single basal lamina, the conchal crest. The **common nasal meatus** (*meatus nasi communis*) is a small sagittal space between the conchae and the nasal septum. The space between the two conchae is the **middle nasal meatus** (*meatus nasi medius*), and the space ventral to the ventral nasal concha is the **ventral nasal meatus** (*meatus nasi ventralis*). The osseous plates of the concha are continued as soft tissue folds that converge rostrally to form a single medially protruding ridge that ends in a clublike eminence in the vestibule called the **alar fold**. The direction of the bony scrolls is caudoventral. Usually five primary scrolls can be identified, and they are numbered, dorsoventrally, from 1 to 5. The first primary unit leaves the dorsal surface of the basal lamina and runs toward the dorsal concha. It is displaced laterally in its caudal part by endoturbinates I and II. The second primary unit arises several millimeters peripheral to the first, and some of its subsequent leaves reach nearly to the nasal septum. The third unit and its secondary and tertiary scrolls largely fill the space formed by the union of the nasal septum with the hard palate. The fourth unit at first runs ventrally nearly to the palate and then inclines medially, ventral to the third unit. The fifth, or terminal, unit curves dorsally as a simple caudally closed scroll that runs ventral to the conchal crest. It has fewer secondary scrolls than do the others. The secondary scrolls divide further so that the whole nasal fossa is nearly filled with a labyrinthine mass of delicately porous, bony plates. The larger the nasal cavity, the more numerous the bony scrolls.

Zygomatic Bone

The **zygomatic bone** (*os zygomaticum*) (Figs. 4.4, 4.33), formerly called *jugal* or *malar bone*, forms the rostral half of the **zygomatic arch** (*arcus zygomaticus*). It is divided into two surfaces and two processes. The **lateral surface** (*facies lateralis*) is convex longitudinally and transversely, although it is slightly dished ventral to the orbit. Usually a nutrient foramen is present near its middle. The **medial**, or **orbital**, **surface** (*facies orbitalis*) is concave in all directions. Rostrally the zygomatic bone articulates broadly with the maxilla and is recessed to form an unusually stable foliate type of sutural joint. At the middle of this articular border the zygomatic bone receives the zygomatic process of the maxilla, which it partly overlays. Caudally the zygomatic bone forms a long harmonial suture with the zygomatic process of the temporal bone. This suture is one of the last to close. The **infraorbital margin** (*margo infraorbitalis*) forms the ventral margin of the orbit. It is thick and beveled medially. The ventral margin is also thick but is beveled laterally. Both the thickness of the border and the degree to which it is beveled decrease caudally. This border provides the origin for the large masseter muscle. The caudoventral margin of the zygomatic bone is turned down and pointed; it is the **temporal process** (*processus temporalis*). The **frontal process** (*processus frontalis*), smaller than the others, is located between the orbital and the temporal borders. It is joined to the zygomatic process of the frontal bone by the **orbital ligament**.

The zygomatic bone articulates with the maxilla in forming the mitered **zygomaticomaxillary suture** (*sutura zygomaticomaxillaris*). At the rostral edge of the orbit the **lacrimozygomatic suture** (*sutura lacrimozygomatica*) is formed by the zygomatic joining the lacrimal bone. The **temporozygomatic suture** (*sutura temporozygomatica*) is an oblique, late-closing suture between the zygomatic process of the temporal bone and the temporal process of the zygomatic bone.

Palatine Bone

The **palatine bone** (*os palatinum*) (Figs. 4.3 to 4.5, 4.34, 4.43 and 4.44) is located caudomedial to the maxilla, where it forms the caudal part of the hard palate, the rostromedial wall of the pterygopalatine fossa, and the lateral wall of the nasopharynx. It is divided into horizontal and perpendicular laminae. The **horizontal lamina** (*lamina horizontalis*) forms, with its fellow, the caudal third of the **hard palate** (*palatum osseum*). Each horizontal lamina has a **palatine surface** (*facies palatina*), a **nasal surface** (*facies nasalis*), and a free concave caudal border. The nasal surface of the bone adjacent to the median palatine suture is raised to form the **nasal crest** (*crista nasalis*). The rostral part of this crest articulates with the vomer. The nasal crest ends caudally in the unpaired, but occasionally bifid, **caudal nasal spine** (*spina nasalis caudalis*). Sometimes a notch in the lateral, sutural margin of the horizontal part concurs with a similar, but always deeper, notch in the maxilla to form the **major palatine foramen** (*foramen palatinum majus*), which opens on the hard palate for the major palatine vessels and nerve. Caudal to this foramen there is usually one or, occasionally, two or more **minor palatine foramina** (*foramina palatina minora*) also for the major palatine vessels and nerve. All of these openings lead into the **palatine canal** (*canalis*

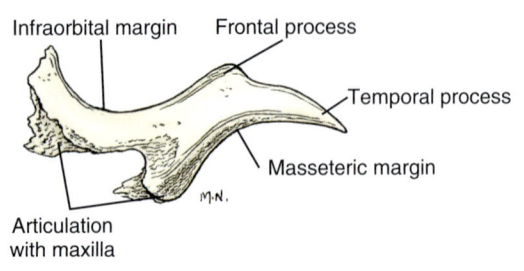

• Fig. 4.33 Left zygomatic bone, lateral aspect.

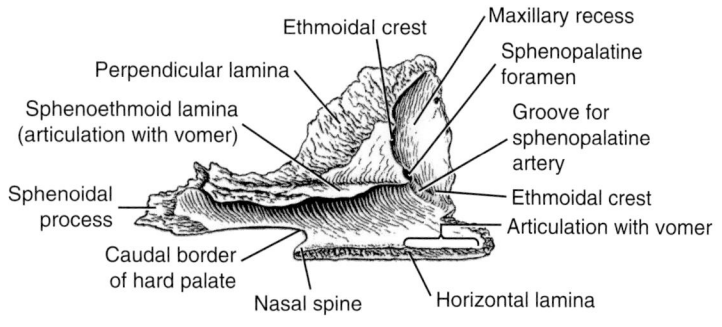

Fig. 4.34 Left palatine bone, dorsal medial aspect.

palatinus), which runs through the palatine bone from the pterygopalatine fossa. This canal transmits the major palatine artery, vein, and nerve.

The **perpendicular lamina** (*lamina perpendicularis*) of the palatine bone leaves the caudolateral border of the horizontal lamina at nearly a right angle. Medially it forms the lateral wall (*facies nasalis*) of the nasopharyngeal meatus, and laterally it forms the medial wall (*facies maxillaris*) of the pterygopalatine fossa. The nasal surface is partly divided by a frontally protruding shelf, the **sphenoethmoid lamina** (*lamina sphenoethmoidalis*). This shelf parallels the horizontal part of the bone as it lies dorsal to it and extends approximately half its length caudal to it. Dorsal to the rostral end of the sphenoethmoid lamina is the **sphenopalatine foramen** (*foramen sphenopalatinum*), which lies dorsal to the caudal palatine foramen and extends from the pterygopalatine fossa to the nasal cavity. The sphenopalatine vessels and caudal nasal nerve traverse the sphenopalatine foramen and follow the groove in the rostral end of the lamina sphenoethmoidalis. The area dorsal to this lamina is articular for the orbital wing of the sphenoid and the orbital lamina of the ethmoid bones. The rostral part of the nasal surface forms the caudolateral part of the **maxillary recess**. The small ventral ethmoidal crest, located at the caudoventral margin of the maxillary recess, marks the line along which the lateral lamina of the ethmoid articulates with the palatine bone to form the medial wall of the maxillary recess. The part of the palatine bone ventral to the sphenoethmoid crest is smooth, slightly concave, and faces medially to form the rostral part of the lateral wall of the nasopharyngeal meatus. The caudal border of the hard palate provides attachment for the soft palate. The perpendicular lamina of the palatine bone has two processes. The caudal part between the pterygoid bone medially and the sphenoid bone laterally is the **sphenoidal process** (*processus sphenoidalis*). The **orbital process** (*processus orbitalis*) articulates with the frontal bone on the medial wall of the orbit. Rostrally the palatine bone articulates with the maxilla at the rostroventrolateral extremity of the perpendicular part. The thin, irregularly convex border of the most dorsal part of the palatine bone is the **ethmoidal crest** (*crista ethmoidalis*), which conceals the medially lying ethmoid bone. The medial wall of the **pterygopalatine fossa** is formed by the palatine bone. The round dorsal opening is the **sphenopalatine foramen**, and the oblong ventral one, approximately 1 mm distant, is the **caudal palatine foramen** (*foramen palatinum caudalis*). The latter contains the major palatine vessels and nerve. The palatine bone articulates caudally with the sphenoid and pterygoid bones, rostrally with the maxilla and ethmoid, dorsolaterally with the lacrimal and frontal bones, dorsomedially with the vomer, and ventromedially with its fellow at the **median palatine suture** (*sutura palatina mediana*). Rostrally the palatine bones articulate with the maxillae by a suture that crosses the midline, the **transverse palatine suture** (*sutura palatina transversa*). Dorsally, at the rostral end of the median palatine suture, the vomer articulates with the palatine bones, forming the **vomeropalatine suture** (*sutura vomeropalatina*). In the medial part of the pterygopalatine fossa the palatine bone articulates with the maxilla, forming the **palatomaxillary suture** (*sutura palatomaxillaris*), which is a continuation of the transverse palatine suture. Where the palatine bone articulates with the pterygoid process of the sphenoid bone, as well as with its orbital wing, the **sphenopalatine suture** (*sutura sphenopalatina*) is formed. The **pterygopalatine suture** (*sutura pterygopalatina*) is formed by the small pterygoid bone articulating with the medial surfaces of the caudal part of the palatine bone as it unites with the pterygoid process of the sphenoid. On the medial side of the orbit the **frontopalatine suture** (*sutura frontopalatina*) runs dorsorostrally. The deep surface of the palatine bone joins rostrally with the ethmoid bone to form the **palatoethmoidal suture** (*sutura palatoethmoidalis*).

Lacrimal Bone

The **lacrimal bone** (*os lacrimale*) (Figs. 4.3, 4.4, 4.35), located in the rostral margin of the orbit, is roughly triangular in outline and pyramidal in shape. Its **orbital face** (*facies orbitalis*) is concave and free. Located in its center is the **fossa for the lacrimal sac** (*fossa sacci lacrimalis*), which is approximately 6 mm in diameter. (The two lacrimal ducts, one from each eyelid, unite in a slight dilation to form the lacrimal sac. From the lacrimal sac the soft nasolacrimal duct courses to the vestibule of the nose.) The osseous **lacrimal canal** (*canalis lacrimalis*), containing the nasolacrimal duct, begins in the lacrimal bone at the fossa for the lacrimal sac, runs ventrorostrally through the lacrimal bone, and leaves at the apex of the bone. It continues

• **Fig. 4.35** Left lacrimal bone, lateral aspect.

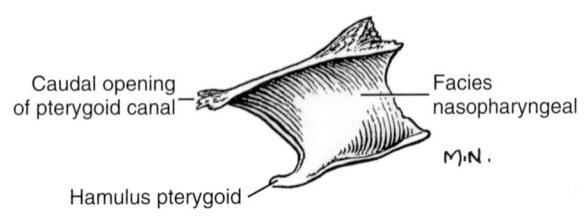

• **Fig. 4.36** Left pterygoid bone, medial aspect.

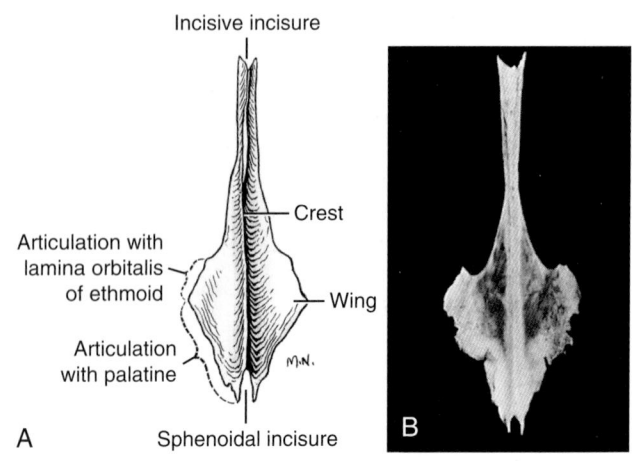

• **Fig. 4.37** Drawing (*A*) and radiograph (*B*) of the vomer, ventral aspect.

in a dorsally concave groove in the maxilla and opens ventral to the caudal end of the conchal crest. The lacrimal bone forms part of the margin of the orbit. The **frontal process** (*processus frontalis*) is a narrow strip of the orbital margin that projects dorsally. The **facial surface** (*facies facialis*) meets the orbital surface at an acute angle. Only a small part of the facial surface is free; most of it is covered by the maxilla and zygomatic bones. In some specimens a free facial surface is lacking. The **nasal surface** (*facies nasalis*) forms a small portion of the nasal cavity.

The lacrimal bone articulates dorsocaudally with the frontal bone, forming the **frontolacrimal suture** (*sutura frontolacrimalis*); rostrally with the maxilla, forming the **lacrimomaxillary suture** (*sutura lacrimomaxillaris*); and rostroventrally with the zygomatic bone, forming the **lacrimozygomatic suture** (*sutura lacrimozygomatic*). Caudoventrally the **palatolacrimal suture** (*sutura palatolacrimalis*) is formed by the articulation between the palatine and the lacrimal bones. Medially, the ethmoid bone articulates with the lacrimal bone.

Pterygoid Bone

The **pterygoid bone** (*os pterygoideum*) (Figs. 4.3, 4.5, 4.36) is a small, thin, slightly curved, nearly four-sided plate of bone that articulates with the bodies of both the presphenoid and the basisphenoid bones, but particularly with the medial surface of the pterygoid process of the basisphenoid. It extends ventrally beyond this process, to form the caudal part of the osseous lateral wall of the nasopharynx. The **pterygoid hamulus** (*hamulus pterygoideus*) extends from the caudoventral angle in the form of a caudally protruding hook. The tendon of the m. tensor veli palatini crosses its surface here. The smooth concave medial surface forms the **pterygoid fossa** (*fossa pterygoidea*), which is in the lateral wall of the nasopharynx. Running in the suture between the pterygoid bone and the pterygoid process of the sphenoid is the minute **pterygoid canal** (*canalis pterygoideus*), which carries the autonomic (parasympathetic) nerve of the pterygoid canal. The pterygoid bone forms an extensive squamous suture with the pterygoid process of the sphenoid bone caudally, the **pterygosphenoid suture** (*sutura pterygosphenoidalis*), and with the palatine bone rostrally, the **pterygopalatine suture** (*sutura pterygopalatina*).

Vomer

The **vomer** (Figs. 4.9, 4.37, 4.45) is an unpaired bone that forms the caudoventral part of the nasal septum. It contributes to the roof of the choana. Because this bone runs obliquely from the base of the cranial cavity to the nasal surface of the hard palate, the choanae are located in oblique planes in such a way that the ventral parts of the choanae are rostral to a transverse plane through the caudal border of the hard palate. The choanae are the openings whereby the right and left nasal cavities are continued as the single nasopharyngeal meatus. The vomer has sagittal and horizontal parts.

The sagittal part is formed of two thin, bony leaves that unite ventrally to form a sulcus (*sulcus vomeris*) that in turn receives the cartilaginous nasal septum rostrally and the bony nasal septum, or perpendicular plate of the ethmoid caudally. It articulates ventrally with the palatine processes of the maxillae, with the caudal parts of the palatine processes of the incisive bones, and with the rostral parts of the horizontal portions of the palatine bones. This caudal articulation is at the palatine suture and the ventrorostral half of the vomer. The sagittal part of the vomer is sharply forked at each end.

The horizontal part of the vomer is composed of the **wings** (*alae vomeris*), which are located caudally and at right angles to the sagittal part. They flare laterally and articulate with the sphenoid, ethmoid, and palatine bones. The wings, with the transverse lamina of the ethmoid, form a thin septum that separates the dorsally lying nasal fundus, in which lie the ethmoturbinates, from the ventrally lying nasopharynx.

The vomer articulates dorsally with the sphenoid bone, forming the **vomerosphenoid suture** (*sutura vomerosphenoidalis*). Rostral to this suture and hidden from external

...moid suture (*sutura vomeroethmoida*...
...ation with the ethmoid bone. Laterally the ...of the vomer articulate with the palatine bones, forming the **dorsal vomeropalatine sutures** (*sutura vomeropalatina dorsalis*). The vomer articulates with the conjoined palatine crests to form the **ventral vomeropalatine suture** (*sutura vomeropalatina ventralis*). Rostral to this suture the vomer articulates with the palatine processes of the maxillae and incisive bones to form the **vomeromaxillary suture** (*sutura vomeromaxillaris*) and the **vomeroincisive suture** (*sutura vomeroincisiva*), respectively.

Mandible

The ventral part of the jaw of the dog consists of right and left mandibles (*mandibula*) (Figs. 4.38 and 4.39) firmly united in life at the **intermandibular suture** (*sutura intermandibularis*), which is a strong, rough-surfaced, fibrous joint. Each mandible is divided into a horizontal part, or body, and a vertical part, or ramus. Scapino (1965, 1981) has investigated the morphologic characteristics and function of the intermandibular suture in the dog and other carnivores. He described four types of sutures, ranging from flexible to synostosed. He considers the dog to have a flexible joint that permits a moderate amount of independent movement of the two mandibles and says that this is the most common type of union in carnivores. When the mandibles of such a joint are separated, the articular plates are flat or have low rugosities. A smooth area can be seen rostrodorsally, and the articular space is usually wider caudally than rostrally. The joint is characterized by a single fibrocartilage pad, cruciate ligaments, and a venous plexus. The **body of the mandible** (*corpus mandibulae*) can be further divided into the part that bears the incisor teeth (*pars incisiva*) and the part that contains the molar teeth (*pars molaris*). The alveoli (*alveoli dentales*), which are conical cavities for the roots of the teeth, indent the **alveolar border** (*arcus alveolaris*) of the body of the mandible. There are single alveoli for the roots of the three incisor teeth, the canine, and the first and last cheek teeth. The five middle cheek teeth have two alveoli each, with those for the first molar, or fifth cheek tooth, being the largest, as this is the shearing tooth of the mandible. The alveolar-free dorsal border of the mandible between the canine and the first cheek tooth (first premolar) is larger than the others and is known as the **interalveolar margin** (*margo interalveolaris*). Similar but smaller spaces are usually present between adjacent premolar teeth, where the **interalveolar septa** (*septa interalveolaria*) end in narrow borders. From the intermandibular suture, the bodies of each mandible diverge from each other, forming a space in which lies the tongue. The body of each mandible presents a lateral surface. Caudally this faces the cheek and is the **buccal surface** (*facies buccalis*). Rostrally this faces the lips and is the **labial surface** (*facies labialis*). The medial side of each body faces the tongue and is the **lingual surface** (*facies lingualis*). The lingual surface may present a wide, smooth, longitudinal ridge, **the mylohyoid line** (*linea mylohyoidea*), for the attachment of the mylohyoid muscle. The lateral surface is long, smooth, and of a uniform width caudal to the symphysis. It ends in the thick, convex **ventral border** (*margo ventralis*), with which the lateral and lingual surfaces are confluent. Rostrally it turns medially and presents a **mental foramen** (*foramen mentale*) near the suture, ventral to the alveolus of the central incisor tooth. The largest of the mental foramina, the **middle mental foramen**, is located ventral to the septum between the first two cheek teeth. A small mental foramen or several foramina are present caudal to the middle opening. Mental vessels and nerves emerge from these foramina.

The **ramus of the mandible** (*ramus mandibulae*) is the caudal non–tooth-bearing, vertical part of the bone. It contains three salient processes. The **coronoid process** (*processus coronoideus*), which forms the most dorsal part of the mandible, extends dorsally and laterally. It is a large, thin plate of bone with a thickened rostral border. The **condylar process** (*processus condylaris*) is a transversely elongated, sagittally convex articular process that forms the temporomandibular joint by articulating with the mandibular fossa of the squamous temporal bone. The **mandibular notch** (*incisura mandibulae*) is located between the condyloid and the coronoid processes. The **angle of the mandible** (*angulus mandibulae*) is the caudoventral part of the bone. It contains a salient hooked process in the dog, the **angular process** (*processus angularis*), which serves for the attachment of the pterygoids medially and the masseter laterally. The lateral

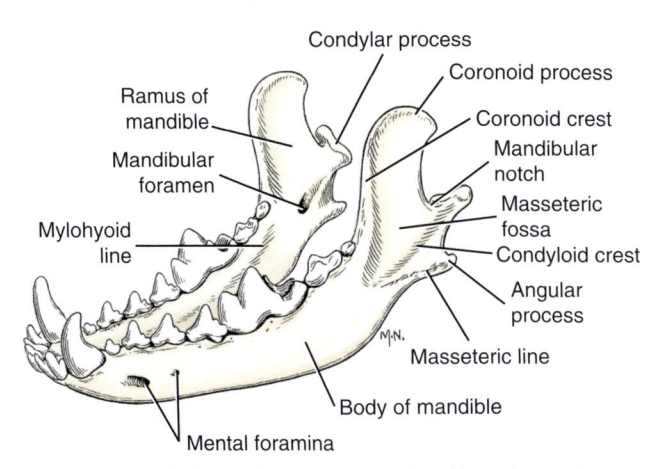

• **Fig. 4.38** Left and right mandibles, dorsal lateral aspect.

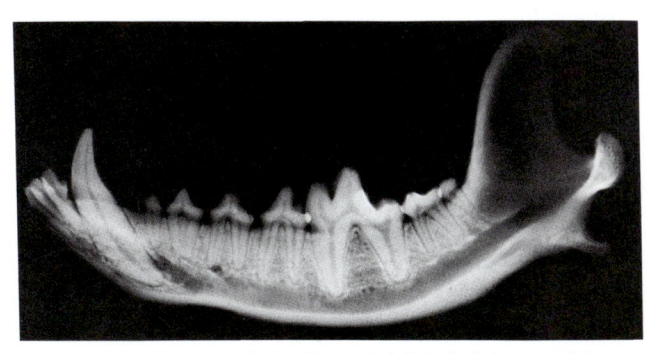

• **Fig. 4.39** Lateromedial radiograph, left half of the mandible.

surface of the ramus contains a prominent, three-sided depression, the **masseteric fossa** (*fossa masseterica*), for the insertion of the masseter muscle. This muscle attachment is limited rostrally by the rostral border of the ramus and ventrocaudally by the neck of the condylar process. The medial surface of the ramus is slightly dished for the insertion of the temporal muscle. Directly ventral to this insertion is the **mandibular foramen** (*foramen mandibulae*). It is the caudal opening of the **mandibular canal** (*canalis mandibulae*), which opens rostrally by means of the mental foramina. The mandibular canal contains the inferior alveolar nerve and vessels, which supply the mandibular teeth and mandibular soft tissues. The mandible articulates with the temporal bone at the temporomandibular joint.

By closing the jaw the force of the teeth are brought to bear on whatever is between them. This is called the *bite*. Cranial dimensions affect the forces of biting and have been analyzed for their predictive value and use by the pet food industry. Force transducers were used to measure bite forces in dogs: bite forces had a maximum of 1394 N (Lindner et al. 1995). Using dry skull measurements, Ellis et al. (2009), predicted bite forces for two-lever models. The effect of skull shape on bite force was significant in medium and large dogs. Nine size–shape groups were developed based on three skull-shape categories and three skull-size categories. Their results may be of use to paleontologists interested in estimating the bite of fossil mammals.

Bones of the Hyoid Apparatus

The **hyoid apparatus** (*apparatus hyoideus*) (Figs. 4.40 and 4.41) acts as a suspensory mechanism for the tongue and larynx. It attaches to the skull dorsally and to the larynx and base of the tongue ventrally, suspending these structures in the caudal part of the space between the bodies of the mandible. The component parts, united by synchondroses, consist of the single basihyoid and paired thyrohyoid, ceratohyoid, epihyoid, and stylohyoid bones and tympanohyoid cartilages.

Basihyoid
The **basihyoid body** (*basihyoideum*) is a transverse, unpaired bone in the musculature of the base of the tongue as a ventrally bowed, dorsoventrally compressed rod. Its extremities articulate with both the thyrohyoid and the ceratohyoid bones.

Thyrohyoid
The **thyrohyoid** (*thyrohyoideum*) is a laterally bowed, sagittally compressed, slender bone that extends dorsocaudally from the basihyoid to articulate with the cranial cornu of the thyroid cartilage of the larynx.

Ceratohyoid
The **ceratohyoid** (*ceratohyoideum*) is a small, short, tapered rod having a distal extremity that is approximately twice as large as its proximal extremity. It articulates with the

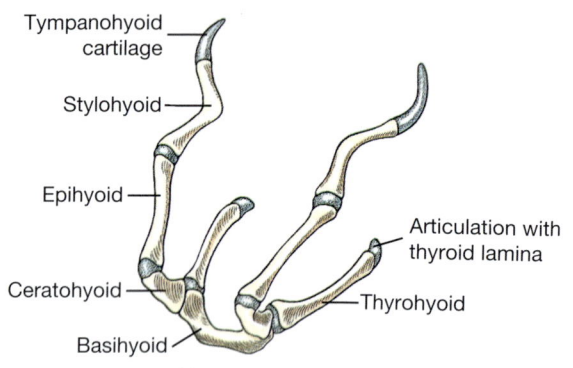

• **Fig. 4.40** Hyoid bones, rostrolateral aspect.

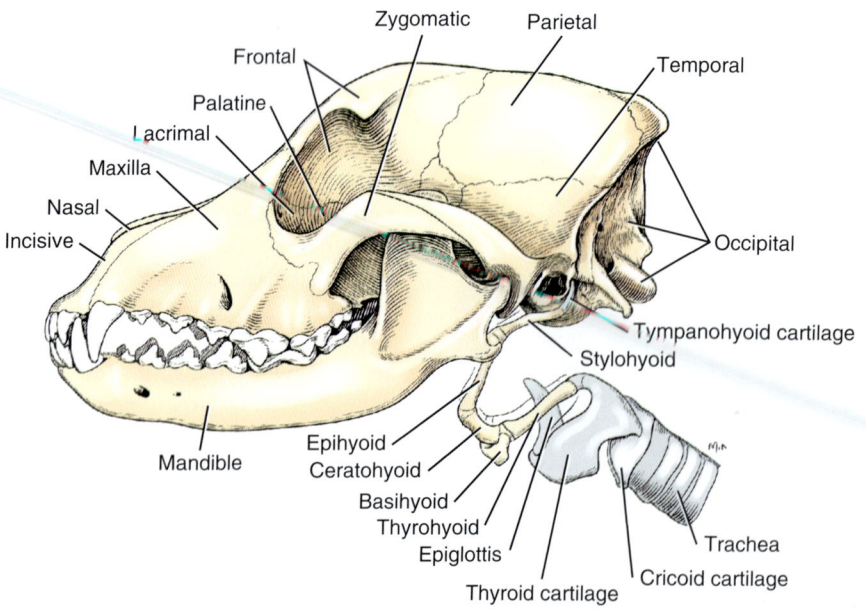

• **Fig. 4.41** Bones of the skull, hyoid apparatus, and laryngeal cartilages, lateral aspect.

...yrohyoid. The proximal extremity, ...nearly rostrally in life, articulates with the ...oid at a right angle.

Epihyoid
The **epihyoid** (*epihyoideum*) is approximately parallel to the thyrohyoid bone. It articulates with the ceratohyoid at nearly a right angle cranially and with the stylohyoid caudally without any angulation.

Stylohyoid
The **stylohyoid** (*stylohyoideum*) is slightly longer than the epihyoid, with which it articulates. It is flattened slightly craniocaudally and is distinctly bowed toward the median plane. It gradually increases in size from its proximal to its distal end. Both ends are slightly enlarged.

Tympanohyoid Cartilage
The **tympanohyoid cartilage** (*cartilago tympanohyoideum*) is a small cartilaginous bar that continues the proximal end of the stylohyoid to the inconspicuous mastoid process of the skull.

The Skull as a Whole
Dorsal Surface of the Skull
See Figs. 4.4 and 4.7.

Cranial Part. The calvaria is the dorsal surface of the cranial, or neural, part of the skull (neurocranium). It is nearly hemispherical in the newborn and is devoid of prominent markings. On the other hand, a skull from a heavily muscled adult possesses a prominent external sagittal crest, a median longitudinal projection that is the most prominent feature of the dorsal surface of the skull. Caudally, the dorsal surface is limited by the nuchal crest, a transverse, variably developed crest that marks the transition between the dorsal and the caudal surfaces of the skull. The right and left temporal lines diverge from the sagittal crest and continue rostrally to the zygomatic processes of the frontal bones. The convex surface on each side of the dorsum of the skull is the temporal fossa, from which the temporal muscle arises. It is bounded medially by the external sagittal crest or, in brachycephalic breeds, by the temporal lines, and by the nuchal crest caudally in all breeds. This surface of the skull is the parietal plane (*planum parietale*).

Facial Part. The dorsal surface of the facial part of the skull is extremely variable, depending on the breed, and is greatly foreshortened in brachycephalic dogs. It is formed by the dorsal surfaces of the nasal, incisive, and maxillary bones and the nasal processes of the frontal bones. Its most prominent feature is the unpaired external bony nasal aperture (apertura nasi ossea) formerly called the *piriform aperture*. In brachycephalic skulls this opening is not piriform because its transverse dimension is greater than its dorsoventral one.

The **stop**, or **glabella**, prominent only in brachycephalic skulls, is a wide, smooth, transverse ridge that lies directly dorsal to the dish of the face or in a transverse plane through the caudodorsal parts of the frontomaxillary sutures. An unpaired midsagittal depression, the **frontal fossa** (*fossa frontalis*) extends rostrally on the nasal bones from the frontal bones.

Lateral Surface of the Skull
See Figs. 4.3, 4.41, 4.42, and 4.43.

Cranial Part. The salient features of the lateral surface of the cranial part of the skull are the prominent zygomatic

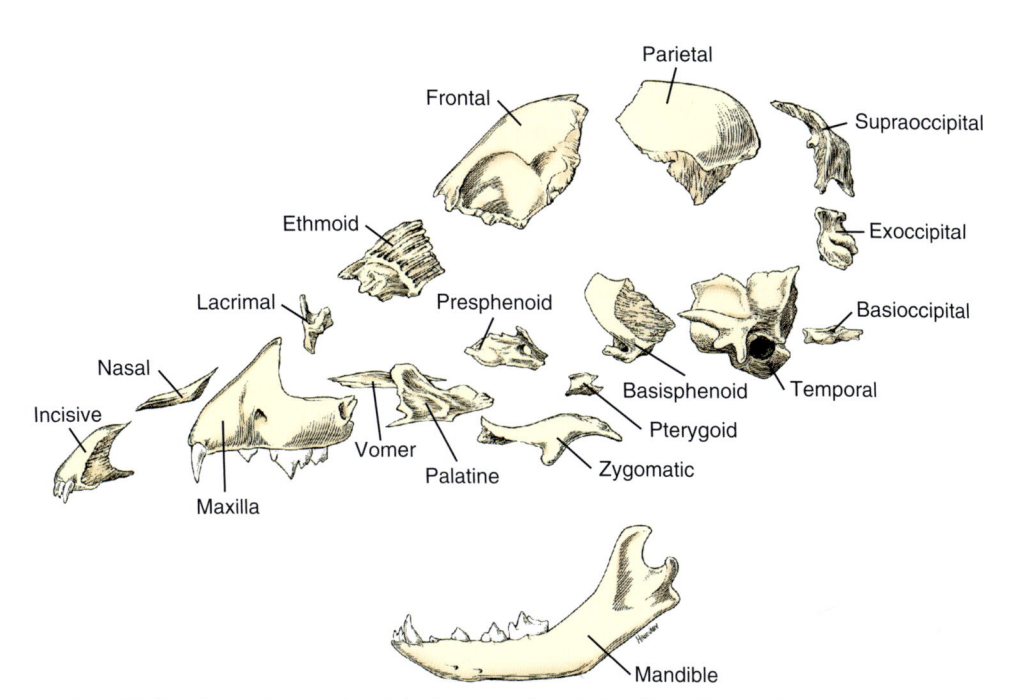

- **Fig. 4.42** Disarticulated expanded skull of a puppy, lateral view. (From Evans HE, de Lahunta A: *Guide to the Dissection of the Dog*, ed. 8, Philadelphia, 2017, Elsevier.)

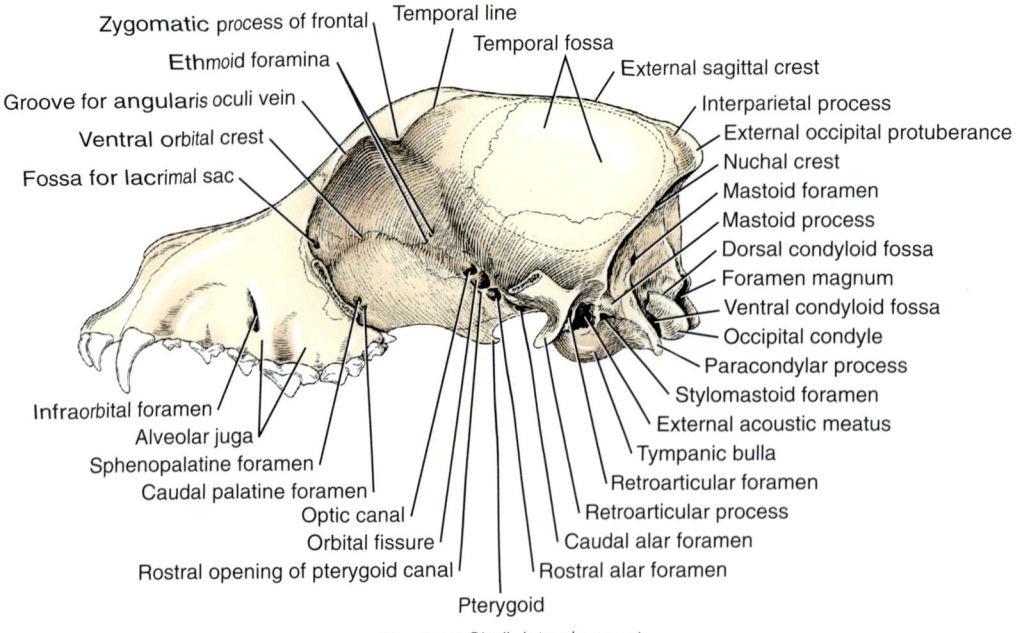

• Fig. 4.43 Skull, lateral aspect.

arch and the orbit. The zygomatic arch (*arcus zygomaticus*) is a heavy, laterodorsally convex bridge of bone located between the facial and the cranial parts of the skull; it is laterally compressed rostrally and laterally and dorsoventrally compressed caudally. It is composed of the zygomatic bone and the zygomatic processes of the temporal bone. It serves three important functions: to protect the eye, to give origin to the masseter and a part of the temporal muscle, and to provide an articulation for the mandible. The osseous external acoustic meatus is the opening to which the external ear is attached. Ventral and medial to the external acoustic meatus is the bulla tympanica, which can be seen best from the ventral aspect. The paracondylar process is a sturdy ventral projection caudal to the bulla tympanica and lateral to the occipital condyle.

The **orbital region** is formed by the **orbit** and the ventrally lying **pterygopalatine fossa**. The orbital opening faces rostrolaterally and is nearly circular in the brachycephalic breeds and irregularly oval in the dolichocephalic breeds. Approximately the caudal fourth of the orbital margin is formed by the **orbital ligament**. A line from the center of the optic canal to the center of the orbital opening is the axis of the orbit. The eyeball and its associated muscles, nerves, vessels, glands, and fascia are the structures of the orbit. Only the medial wall of the orbit is entirely osseous. Its caudal part is marked by three large openings that are named, from rostrodorsal to caudoventral, the **optic canal**, **orbital fissure**, and **rostral alar foramen**. In addition to these there are usually two **ethmoidal foramina**, which are located rostrodorsal to the optic canal. Within the rostral orbital margin is the **fossa for the lacrimal sac**. The **lacrimal canal** leaves the fossa and extends rostroventrally. Ventral to the medial surface of the orbit, and separated

from it by the dorsally arched **ventral orbital crest** (*crista orbitalis ventralis*), is the **pterygopalatine fossa**. The rostral end of this fossa funnels down to the maxillary foramen, which is located dorsal to the caudal end of the fourth maxillary premolar, the shearing tooth. In prepared skulls a small part of the medial wall of the fossa just caudal to the maxillary foramen frequently presents a defect. This is where the ventral oblique eye muscle is attached to the skull. Still farther caudally are the more ventrally located **sphenopalatine foramen** and the **caudal palatine foramen**. The more dorsally located sphenopalatine foramen is separated from the caudal palatine foramen by a narrow septum of bone. The ventral orbital crest marks the dorsal boundary of the origin of the medial pterygoid muscle. The crest ends caudally in the septum between the orbital fissure and the rostral alar foramen. The caudal border of the pterygoid bone also forms the caudal border of the pterygopalatine fossa.

Facial Part. The lateral surface of the facial part of the skull is formed primarily by the maxilla. It is gently convex dorsoventrally and has as its most prominent feature the vertically oval **infraorbital foramen**, which lies dorsal to the septum between the third and the fourth cheek teeth. The **alveolar juga** of the shearing and canine teeth are features of this surface.

Ventral Surface of the Skull

See Figs. 4.5, 4.44, 4.45, and 4.46.

Cranial Part. The ventral surface of the cranial part of the skull extends from the foramen magnum to the hard palate. Caudally, it presents the rounded occipital condyles with the intercondyloid notch and the median basioccipital, which extends rostrally between the hemispherical tympanic

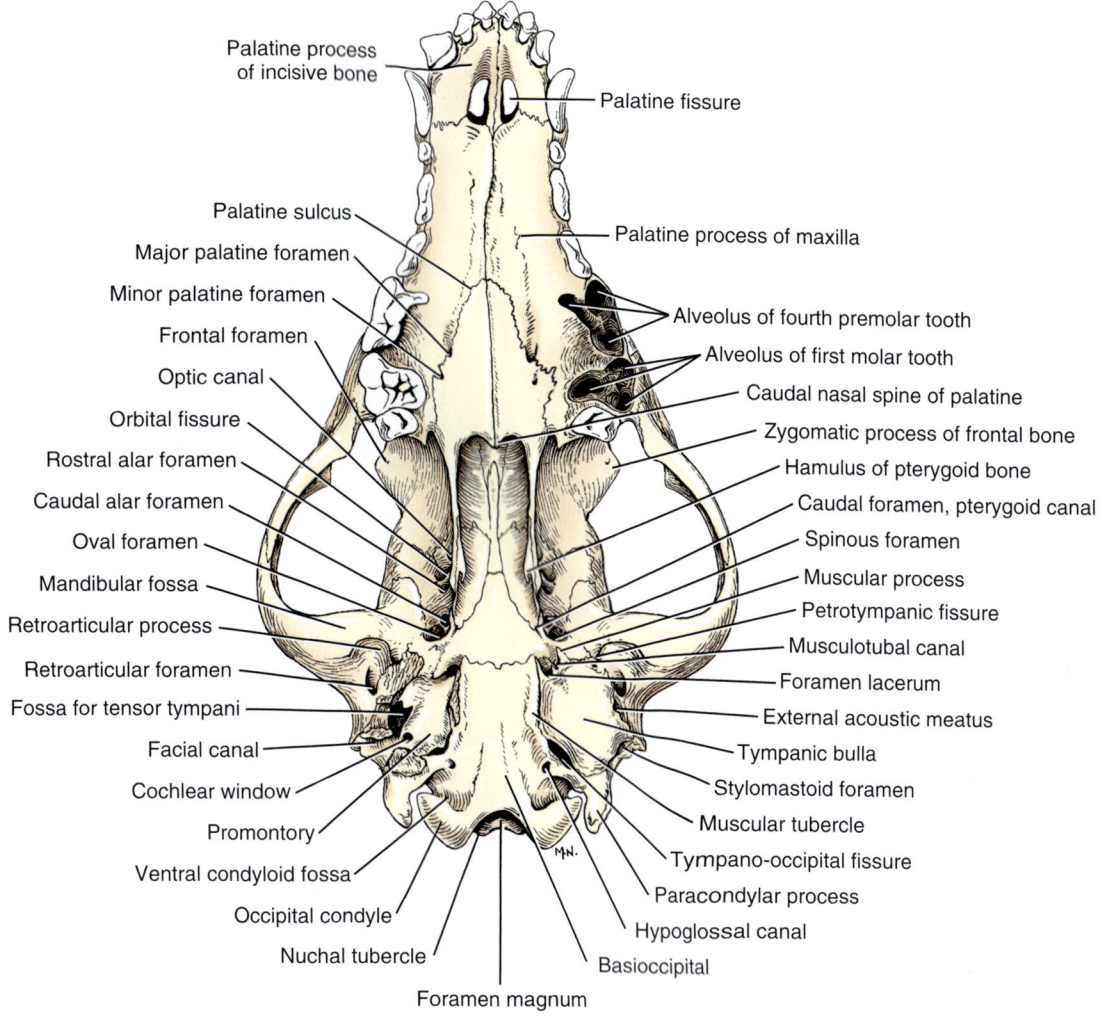

• **Fig. 4.44** Skull, ventral aspect. (Right tympanic bulla removed. Left fourth premolar and left first molar removed.)

bullae. The muscular tubercles are low, rough, sagittally elongated ridges of the basioccipital bone that articulate with the medial surfaces of the bullae. Between the bullae and the occipital condyle is the ventral condyloid fossa, in which opens the small circular hypoglossal canal. Between this small, round opening and the tympanic bulla (in the petrooccipital suture) is the obliquely placed, oblong tympanooccipital fissure, into which open the jugular foramen and carotid canal. Fused to the caudal surface of the bulla is the paracondylar process. Immediately rostral to the bulla and guarded ventrally by the sharp-pointed muscular process of the temporal bone is the musculotubal canal for the auditory tube. The foramen lacerum lies medial to the musculotubal canal and lateral to the rostral part of the basioccipital, where it is flanked by small bony processes from the tympanic bulla. The largest foramen of this region is the oval foramen, which lies medial to the mandibular fossa. The mandibular fossa is the smooth concave articular area on the transverse caudal part of the zygomatic arch. This fossa is on the ventral surface of the zygomatic process of the squamous part of the temporal bone. Caudal dislocation of the mandible, which articulates in the mandibular fossa, is prevented by the curved, spadelike retroarticular process. The caudal surface of this process contains a groove that helps form the retroarticular foramen. The minute opening medial to the retroarticular process is the petrotympanic fissure, through which passes the chorda tympani nerve.

The osseous part of the nasopharynx extends from the choanae to the caudal borders of the pterygoid bones. It is twice as long as it is wide, and its width approximates its depth. Jayne (1898) referred to this area as the *basipharyngeal canal*. The palatine and pterygoid bones form its lateral walls and part of the roof. The median portion of its roof is formed by the vomer, presphenoid, and basisphenoid. In young skulls a small space exists between the presphenoid and the vomer, which is later closed by a caudal growth of the vomer. In the living animal the soft palate completes the nasopharynx by forming a tube which starts rostrally at the choanae and ends caudally at the **intrapharyngeal ostium** (*ostium intrapharyngeum*).

At the junction of the wing with the body of the basisphenoid is the short **alar canal**. Running in the suture

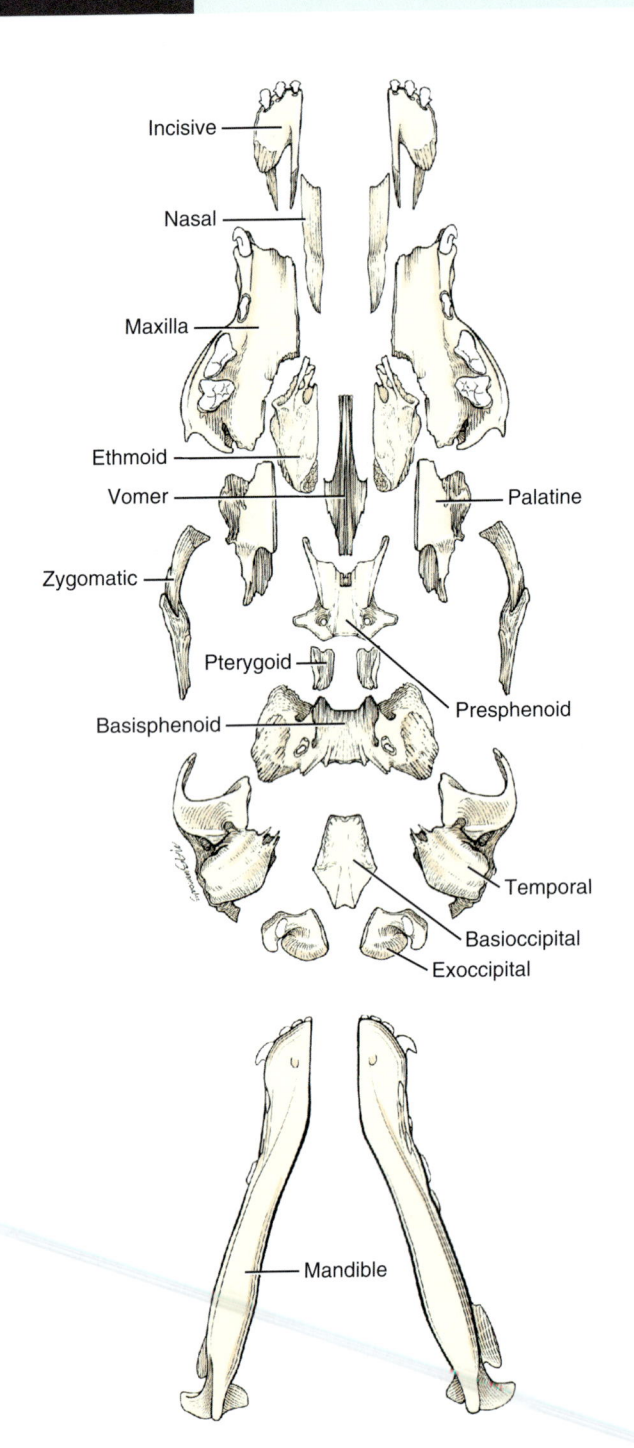

120 CHAPTER 4 The Skeleton

- Fig. 4.45 Disarticulated, expanded skull of a puppy, ventral view.

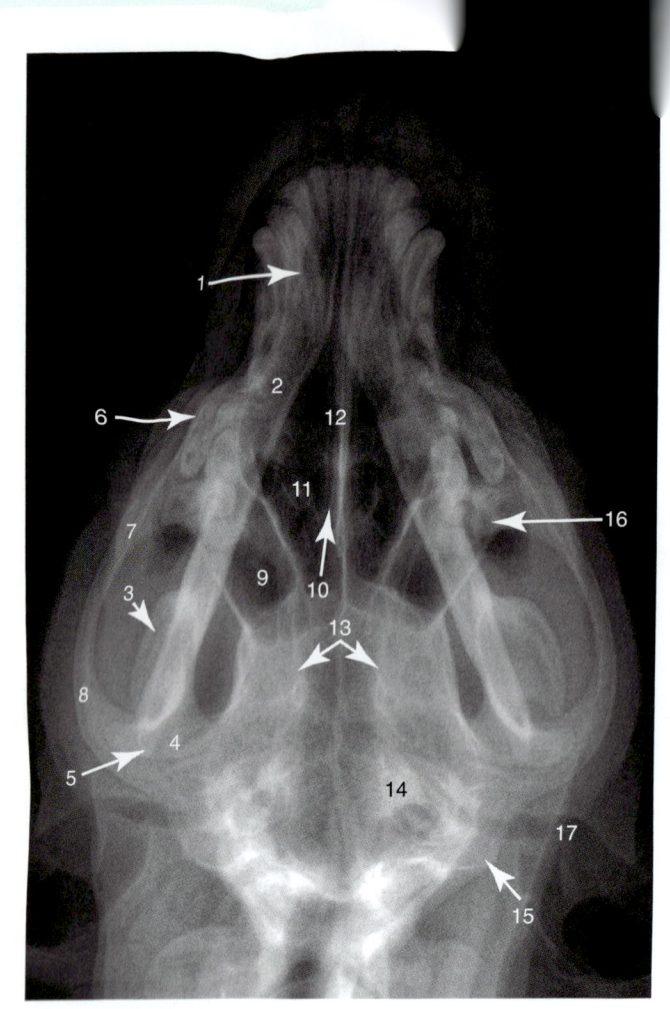

1. Dorsal canine tooth
2. Body of mandible
3. Coronoid process of mandible
4. Condylar process of mandible
5. Angular process of mandible
6. Dorsal (maxillary) fourth premolar tooth
7. Zygomatic bone
8. Zygomatic process of squamous temporal bone
9. Frontal sinus
10. Cribriform plate of ethmoid bone
11. Ethmoid labyrinth
12. Nasal septum
13. Palatine bones
14. Apex of petrosal part of temporal bone
15. Mastoid process of petrosal part of temporal bone
16. Zygomatic process of frontal bone
17. External acoustic meatus

- Fig. 4.46 Dorsoventral radiograph of the skull.

between the pterygoid process of the sphenoid bone and the pterygoid bone is the **pterygoid canal**. The minute **pterygoid groove** leading to the caudal opening of the canal will be seen in large skulls lying dorsal to and in the same direction as the muscular process of the temporal bone. The rostral opening of the canal is in the caudal part of the pterygopalatine fossa in the vicinity of the septum between the orbital fissure and the optic canal. It conducts the nerve of the pterygoid canal.

Facial Part. The ventral surface of the facial part of the skull is formed largely by the horizontal parts of the palatine, maxillary, and incisive bones, which form the **hard palate**. Lateral to the hard palate on each side lie the teeth in their alveoli. There are three alveoli for each of the last three cheek teeth, two for each of the next two, rostrally, and one for the first cheek tooth. The largest alveolus is at the rostral end of the maxilla, for the canine tooth. At the rostral end of the hard palate, in the incisive bones, are the six incisor teeth in individual alveoli. In the puppy skull only nine alveoli are present in each maxilla. There is one for the canine tooth, two for the first cheek tooth, and three for each of the last two deciduous premolar teeth. The first permanent premolar has no deciduous predecessor. The medial alveoli for the last three cheek teeth diverge from the lateral ones, and the lateral alveoli of the shearing tooth diverge from each other.

The features of the hard palate vary with age. The palatine sulcus extends to the **palatine fissure** only in adult skulls. In old skulls, transverse ridges and depressions may be present on the hard palate. The **major palatine foramina** medial to the carnassial teeth lie rostral to the **minor palatine foramina**. The minor palatine foramina are usually two in number, located close together ventral to the palatine canal. The major palatine vessels and a nerve leave the palatine foramina, run rostrally in the palatine sulcus, and supply the hard palate and adjacent soft structures. The caudal border of the hard palate exhibits a median eminence, the **caudal nasal spine**, which may be inconspicuous. The lateral caudal part of the hard palate presents a distinct notch, which follows the palatomaxillary suture and is located between the palatine bone and the pterygoid process of the maxilla. The minor palatine vessels and nerve pass through it. The sagittal parts of the palatine bones and the pterygoid bones project ventrally to a frontal plane through the hard palate. The oval **palatine fissures** between the canine teeth are separated by the palatine processes of the incisive bones. Through them the palatine vessels anastomose with the infraorbital and nasal vessels. On the midline the two halves of the hard palate join to form the **palatine suture**. On the incisive part of this suture is located the small ventral opening of the **interincisive canal**.

Caudal Surface of the Skull

The caudal surface of the skull (*planum nuchale*) is three-sided and irregular. It is formed laterally by the lateral parts of the occipital bone, formerly called the *exoccipitals*, with their condyles and paracondylar processes, dorsally by the squamous part of the occipital bone, formerly called the *supraoccipitals*, and midventrally by the basal part called the *basioccipital*. The lateral sides of the caudal surface are separated from the temporal fossae by the **nuchal crest**. The **external occipital protuberance** is the mid-dorsal caudal end of the external sagittal crest. Lateral to the external occipital protuberance is a rough area for the attachment of the m. semispinalis capitis. Between the external occipital protuberance and the foramen magnum is the **external occipital crest**, which is frequently bulged in its middle by the **vermiform impression**. The **foramen magnum** is the large, frequently asymmetric, ventral, median opening for the junction of the medulla oblongata and the spinal cord and associated structures. Lateral to the foramen magnum are the smooth, convex occipital condyles. Each is separated from the paracondylar process by the ventral condyloid fossa, in the rostral part of which is the hypoglossal canal. In the young skull the occipitomastoid suture is present lateral to the paracondylar process. This suture fails to close dorsally, forming the **mastoid foramen**. The mastoid process is that part of the temporal bone dorsal to the **stylomastoid foramen**.

Apex of the Skull

The apex of the skull is formed by the rostral ends of the incisive bones and mandibles, each of which bears six incisor teeth. Its most prominent feature is the nearly circular **osseus nasal aperture**.

Cavities of the Skull

Cranial Cavity

The **cranial cavity** (*cavum cranii*) (Figs. 4.9, 4.47, and 4.48) contains the brain, with its coverings and vessels. Its capacity varies more with body size than with head shape. The smallest crania have capacities of approximately 40 cc and are known as *microcephalic*; the largest have capacities of approximately 140 cc and are known as *megacephalic*. The boundaries of the cranial cavity may be considered as the roof, base, caudal wall, rostral wall, and the side walls. The roof of the skull (cranial vault, or skull cap) is the **calvaria**. It is formed by the parietal and frontal bones, although caudally the interparietal process of the occipital bone contributes to its formation. The rostral two-thirds of the base of the cranium is formed by the sphenoid bones and the caudal third by the basioccipital. The caudal wall is formed by the occipitals and the rostral wall by the cribriform plate of the ethmoid. The lateral wall on each side is formed by the temporal, parietal, and frontal bones, although ventrally the sphenoid and caudally the occipital bones contribute to its formation. The base of the cranial cavity is divided into rostral, middle, and caudal cranial fossae. The interior of the cranial cavity contains smooth digital impressions bounded by irregular elevations, the cerebral and cerebellar juga. These markings are formed by the gyri and sulci, respectively, of the brain.

The **rostral cranial fossa** (*fossa cranii rostralis*) supports the olfactory bulbs and tracts and the remaining parts of the frontal lobes of the brain. It lies at a higher level and is much narrower than the part of the cranial floor caudal to it. It is continued rostrally by the concave **cribriform plate**. Only in old dogs is a *crista galli* present, and this vertical median crest is confined usually to the ventral half of the cribriform plate. In most specimens a line indicates the caudal edge of the perpendicular plate of the ethmoid, which takes the place of the crest. The cribriform plate is so deeply indented that its lateral walls are located more nearly in sagittal planes than in a transverse plane. It is perforated by the numerous **cribriform foramina**. At the junction of the ethmoid with the frontal and sphenoid bones are located the double ethmoidal foramina. The transversely concave **body** of the presphenoid bone forms most of the floor of this fossa. The right and left optic canals diverge as they run rostrally through the presphenoid bone. The *sulcus chiasmatis* lies between the caudal ends of the optic canals, and in young specimens its middle part forms a transverse groove connecting the internal portions of the two canals. The shelf of bone located above the rostral part of the sulcus chiasmatis is the **sphenoidal crest**.

The **middle cranial fossa** (*fossa cranii media*) is situated at a more ventral level than the rostral fossa. The body of

122 CHAPTER 4 The Skeleton

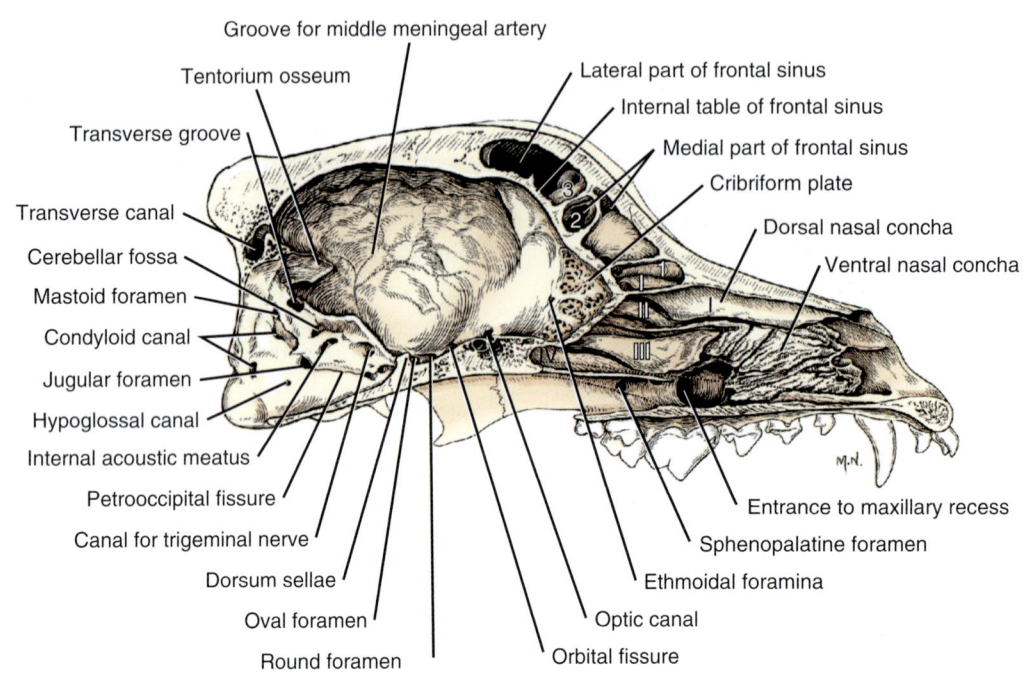

• **Fig. 4.47** Sagittal section of skull. The position of the vomer is indicated by a dotted line. Roman numerals indicate endoturbinates. Arabic numerals indicate ectoturbinates.

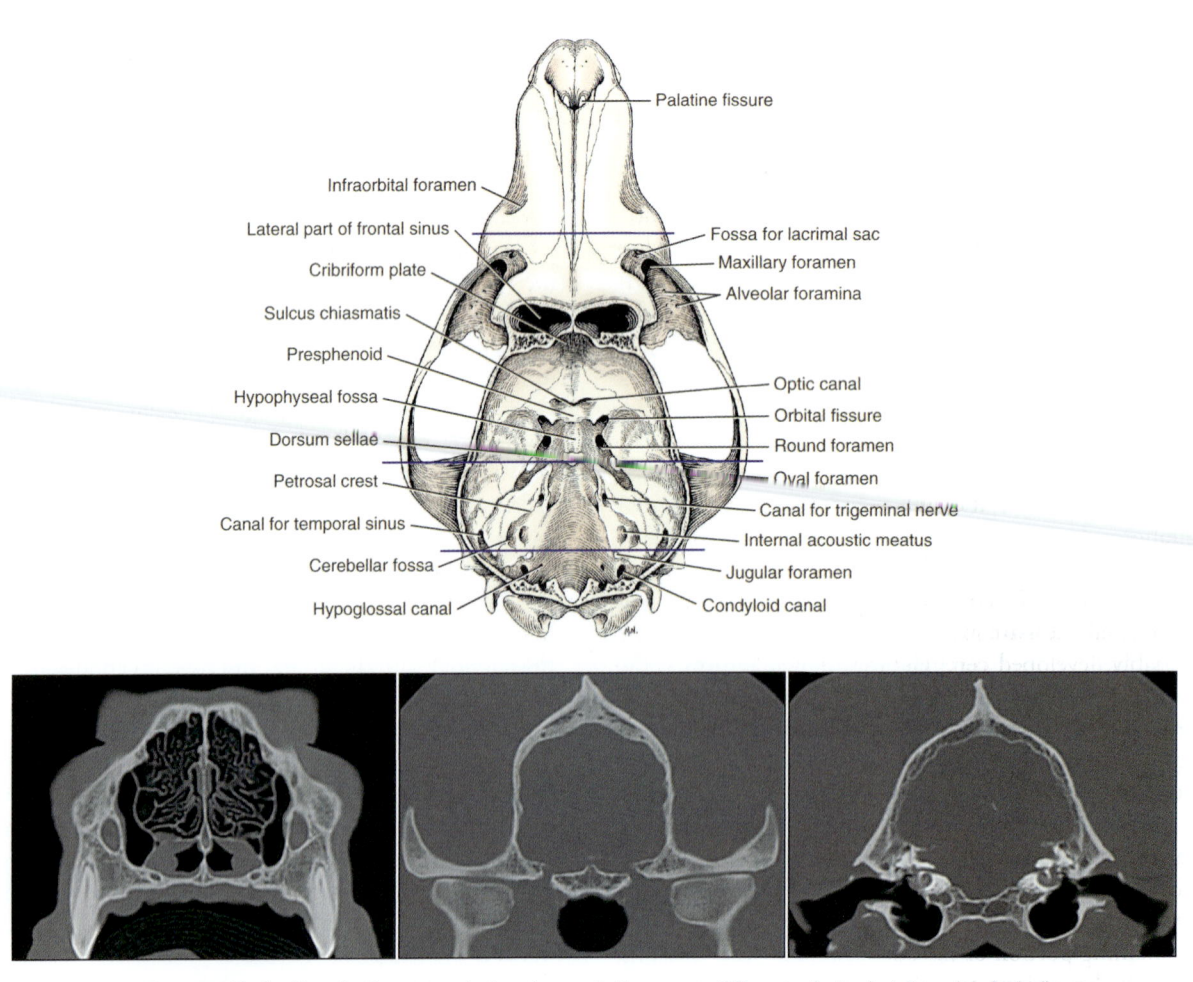

• **Fig. 4.48** Skull with calvaria removed, dorsal aspect. Transverse CT scans (below) at three levels, indicated by the blue lines on the skull (above).

the basisphenoid forms its floor. Caudally, it is limited by the rostrodorsal surfaces of the petrosal parts of the temporal bones, which end medially in the sharp petrosal crests. The **orbital fissures** are large, diverging openings on the lateral sides of the rostral clinoid processes. Caudal and slightly lateral to the orbital fissures are the **round foramina**, which open into the alar canals. Caudolateral to the round foramina are the larger **oval foramina**. The complex of structures on the dorsal surface of the basisphenoid that surround the hypophysis is called the *sella turcica*. It consists of the *tuberculum sellae*, a presphenoid shelf between the rostral clinoid processes, and a caudal elevation, or *dorsum sellae*. The **caudal clinoid processes**, which are irregular in outline, form the sides of the flat but irregular top of the dorsum sellae. The **hypophyseal fossa**, in which the pituitary gland lies, is a shallow oval depression of the basisphenoid bone, located between the presphenoid and the dorsum sellae. The temporal lobes of the brain largely fill the lateral parts of the middle cranial fossa.

The **caudal cranial fossa** (*fossa cranii caudalis*) is formed by the dorsal surface of the basioccipital bone and is located caudal to the middle cranial fossa. It is bounded rostrally by the dorsum sellae; caudally, it ends at the *foramen magnum*. Its dorsal surface is concave where the pons, medulla oblongata, and vessels rest on it. Laterally a considerable cleft exists between the apical part of the petrous part of the temporal and the basioccipital bones. At the caudomedial part of this cleft is located the **petrooccipital fissure** (*fissura petrooccipitalis*). The **petrooccipital canal** opens at the rostral end of this fissure. This opening is continued toward the dorsum sellae by a groove. This canal conducts the ventral petrosal venous sinus. The **carotid canal** is located lateral to the petrooccipital canal, which it resembles in size and shape. Its rostral opening lies directly ventral to the apex of the petrous part of the temporal bone, where it is located ventral to the canal for the trigeminal nerve and dorsal to the foramen lacerum. The carotid canal conducts the internal carotid artery and a vein and nerve. The **canal for the trigeminal nerve** is located in the rostral end of the petrosal part of the temporal bone and is nearly horizontal in direction. It contains the trigeminal nerve and ganglion.

Caudolateral to the canal for the trigeminal nerve is located the **internal acoustic pore**, which leads into the short **internal acoustic meatus**. Dorsolateral to the pore is the variably developed **cerebellar fossa**. At the caudal end of the petrooccipital fissure is the **jugular foramen**. Caudomedial to this opening is the small internal opening of the **hypoglossal canal**. Located within the medial portion of the lateral part of the occipital bone is the large **condyloid canal** for the transmission of the basilar sinus. The rostral part of the canal frequently bends dorsally so that its opening faces rostrodorsally.

The cranial fossae form the floor of the cranial cavity. The remaining portion of the cranium is marked internally by smooth depressions and elevations that are formed by the gyri and sulci of the brain. The impressions are called **digital impressions**. The elevations are formed by the sulci of the cerebellum as well as those of the cerebrum and are called *juga*. The **vascular groove** (*sulcus vasculosus arteriae meningeae mediae*), for the middle meningeal artery and vein, begins at the oval foramen and ramifies dorsally. Its branches vary greatly in their course and tortuosity, and in old specimens parts of the groove may be bridged by bone.

The edges of the **petrosal crests** and the *tentorium ossium* serve for the attachment of the *tentorium cerebelli*, which separates the cerebrum from the cerebellum. Extending from the tentorium ossium to the suture between the petrosal and squamous parts of the temporal bone is the **groove of the transverse sinus** (*sulcus sinus transversi*). The **canal for the transverse sinus** (*canalis sinus transversi*) is in the dorsomedial portion of the occipital bone. It opens into the groove for the transverse sinus, which continues ventrolaterally to the **temporal meatus** (*meatus temporalis*), which leads to the outside by the **retroglenoid foramen**. The **foramen for the dorsal sagittal sinus** (*foramen sinus sagittalis dorsalis*) is usually a single opening, not necessarily median in position, which is located on the rostral surface of the internal occipital protuberance dorsal to the tentorium ossium. The small **internal sagittal crest** (*crista sagittalis interna*) is a median, low, smooth ridge that runs a short distance rostrally from the internal occipital protuberance and provides attachment for the falx cerebri. No constant sulcus for the dorsal sagittal sinus exists. Ventral to the internal occipital protuberance is the **vermiform impression** (*impressio verminalis*) for the vermis of the cerebellum. The divided **internal occipital crest** flanks it.

Nasal Cavity

The **nasal cavity** (*cavum nasi*) is the facial part of the respiratory tract. It is composed of two symmetric halves separated from each other by the **nasal septum** (*septum nasi*). This median partition is formed rostrally by the septal cartilage and caudally by the septal processes of the frontal and nasal bones, the perpendicular plate of the ethmoid, and the sagittal portion of the vomer. The **osseous nasal opening** (*apertura nasi ossea*) was formerly known as the *piriform aperture*. Each nasal cavity is filled largely by the ventral nasal conchae rostrally and the ethmoturbinates caudally.

The **dorsal nasal concha** (*concha nasalis dorsalis*), formerly called the *nasoturbinate* (see Fig. 4.29), is a curved shelf of bone that protrudes medially from the ethmoidal crest into the dorsal part of the nasal cavity. It separates the relatively large, unobstructed **dorsal nasal meatus** from the **middle nasal meatus**, which is located between the dorsal and ventral nasal conchae (see Fig. 4.29).

The **ventral nasal concha** (*concha nasalis ventralis*), formerly called the *maxilloturbinate* (see Figs. 4.27 and 4.29), protrudes into the nasal cavity from a single leaf of attachment, the **conchal crest** (*crista conchalis*). The basal lamina of the ventral nasal concha curves medially and ventrally from this crest. From the convex surface of the lamina arise five or six accessory leaves that divide several times, forming a complicated but relatively constant pattern of delicate bony scrolls. The greatest number of subdivisions leaves the first accessory leaf. Subsequent accessory leaves have fewer subdivisions. The free ends of the bony plates are flattened near the floor of the nasal septum and dorsal nasal concha.

In each nasal cavity the conchae divide the nasal cavity into four primary passages, known as *meatuses* (see Fig. 4.29). The **dorsal nasal meatus** (*meatus nasi dorsalis*) is located between the dorsal nasal concha and the nasal bone. The **middle nasal meatus** (*meatus nasi medius*) is located between the dorsal concha and the ventral concha. The **ventral nasal meatus** (*meatus nasi ventralis*) is located between the ventral concha and the dorsum of the hard palate. The **common nasal meatus** (*meatus nasi communis*) is the median longitudinal space located between the conchae and the nasal septum.

The **nasopharyngeal meatus** (*meatus nasopharyngeus*) is the air passage extending from the caudal ends of the ventral and common nasal meatuses to the choana. In the fresh state, it is continued by the nasopharynx. It is bounded by the sagittal part of the vomer medially and by the maxillary and palatine bones laterally and ventrally. The dorsal part is bounded by the basal plate of the ethmoid bone. The entire mass of bony scrolls of the ventral conchae are so formed that numerous ventrocaudally directed air passages exist. The caudal portion of the ventral conchae is overlapped medially by endoturbinates II and III. Incoming air is directed by the conchae scrolls toward the maxillary recess and the nasopharyngeal meatus.

The **ethmoidal labyrinth** (*labyrinthus ethmoidalis*) (see Figs. 4.24 and 4.25) forms the scrolls that lie largely in the nasal fundus. Each ethmoidal labyrinth is composed of four ventrally lying **endoturbinates** and six smaller, dorsally lying **ectoturbinates**. The ectoturbinates are interdigitated between the basal laminae of the endoturbinates. The endoturbinates attach caudally to the cribriform plate. By means of basal laminae both the endoturbinates and the ectoturbinates attach to the **orbital lamina** of the ethmoid bone. The orbital lamina is a thin, imperfect, papyraceous osseous lateral coating of the ethmoidal labyrinth. It is fused largely to adjacent bones around its periphery. The most ventrocaudal extension of the ethmoturbinates is endoturbinate IV, which fills the body of the presphenoid so that what would otherwise be a **sphenoidal sinus** (*sinus sphenoidalis*) is largely obliterated. The most dorsocaudal extensions of the ethmoturbinates are the first two ectoturbinates, which invade the **frontal sinus**, completely lining the medial part and also, to some extent, the rostral portion of the lateral part. A caudoventrally running canal exists between the ventral nasal concha and the ethmoturbinates. This canal lies against the maxilla and directs incoming air past the opening of the maxillary recess into the nasopharyngeal meatus. The ethmoturbinates occupy the most caudal portion of the nasal cavity. This area is separated from the nasopharyngeal meatus by the basal plate of the ethmoid bone and the wings of the vomer. Rostrally, the floor of each nasal cavity contains the oblong palatine fissure. The nasolacrimal canal arises from the rostral part of the orbit and courses to the concavity of the conchal crest, where it opens. Its medial wall may be deficient in part. The **sphenopalatine foramen** (*foramen sphenopalatinum*) is an opening into the nasopharyngeal meatus from the rostral part of the pterygopalatine fossa.

Paranasal Sinuses

The **maxillary recess** (*recessus maxillaris*) (Figs. 4.47, 4.49) is a large, lateral diverticulum of the nasal cavity bounded by the ethmoid, maxillary, palatine, and lacrimal bones. Other species have a maxillary sinus confined to that bone. The opening into the recess usually lies in a transverse plane through the rostral roots of the maxillary fourth premolar tooth; the recess runs caudally to a similar plane through the last cheek tooth. The caudal part of the recess forms a rounded fundus by a convergence of its walls. The medial wall of the maxillary recess is formed by the orbital lamina of the ethmoid bone, and the lateral wall is formed by the maxillary, palatine, and lacrimal bones. The medial and lateral walls meet dorsally and ventrally at acute angles.

Although this diverticulum of the nasal cavity may appear as a large recess in the prepared dry skull, it is reduced in size and has a restricted opening in the fresh state. The lateral nasal gland lies against the medial wall of the maxilla within the maxillary recess.

The **frontal sinus** (see Figs. 4.47 to 4.49) is located chiefly between the outer and the inner tables of the frontal bone. It varies more in size than any other cavity of the skull. It is divided into lateral, medial, and rostral parts. The **lateral part** occupies the whole truncated enlargement of the frontal bone that forms the zygomatic process. It may be partly divided by osseous septa that extend into the cavity from its periphery. Rostrally an uneven transverse partition unites the two tables of the frontal bone. This partition is deficient medially, resulting in formation of the **nasofrontal opening** (*apertura sinus frontalis*) into the nasal cavity. Through the opening extends the delicate scroll of ectoturbinate 3, the caudal extremity of which flares peripherally and ends as a delicate free end closely applied to the heavier frontal bone. Not only is the ectoturbinate covered by mucosa, but the whole sinus is also lined with mucosa because it is an open cavity in free communication with the nasal cavity in and around ectoturbinate 3. The **medial part** of the frontal sinus is more irregular and subject to greater variations in size than is the lateral. The inner table of the frontal bone here is largely deficient so that the ethmoturbinates completely invade this compartment. Ectoturbinates 1 and 2 are the scrolls that are located in this compartment. They are usually separated by a lateral shelf of bone, to which ectoturbinate 2 is attached in such a way that ectoturbinate 1 lies rostral to 2, although many variations occur. The **rostral part** of the frontal sinus is small. The size and form of the frontal sinus depend on skull form and age. In heavily muscled, dolichocephalic breeds, the lateral compartment is particularly large. In brachycephalic breeds, the medial compartment is much reduced in size or absent, and the lateral part is small. All paranasal sinuses

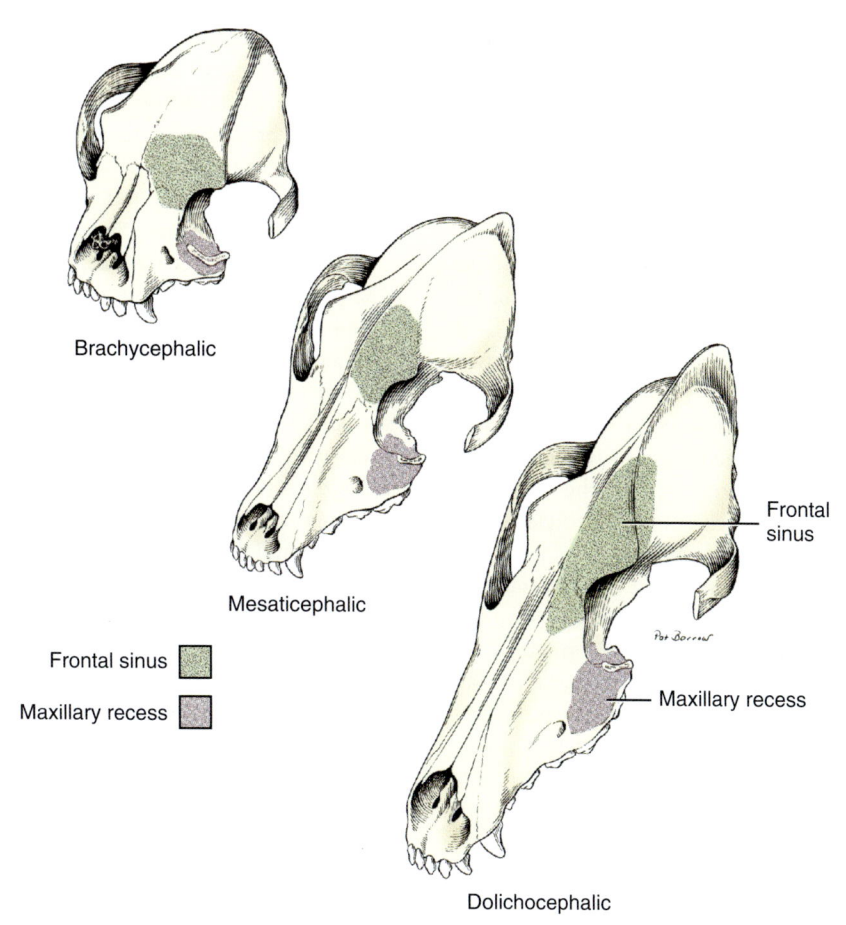

• Fig. 4.49 Paranasal sinuses in three types of skull.

enlarge with age, and only the largest definitive diverticula are present at birth.

The **sphenoid sinus** (*sinus sphenoidalis*) lies within the presphenoid bone and is occupied largely by endoturbinate IV (see Fig. 4.47). Thus, it has not been regarded as a sinus or has not been included in the lists of paranasal sinuses found in dogs (see Kumar, 2015; König & Liebich 2004; Singh, 2017, for example). The ethmoturbinate IV protrudes into the presphenoid, occupying a space described as a sphenoid fossa (in prior editions of this book). It is important to recognize that there is a respiratory epithelium-lined excavation in the presphenoid that the ethmoturbinates occupy.

Vertebral Column

The **vertebral column** (*columna vertebralis*) consists of approximately 50 irregular bones, the **vertebrae**. (The three separate hemal arches to be described later are not included in this number.) The vertebrae are arranged in five groups: **cervical**, **thoracic**, **lumbar**, **sacral**, and **caudal** (formerly coccygeal). The first letter (or abbreviation) of the word designating each group, followed by a digit designating the number of vertebrae in the specific group, constitutes the vertebral formula. That of the dog is $C_7 T_{13} L_7 S_3 Cd_{20}$. The number 20 for the caudal vertebrae may be rather constant for the Beagle, but many dogs have fewer, and a few have more. All vertebrae except the sacral vertebrae remain separate and articulate with contiguous vertebrae in forming movable joints. The three sacral vertebrae are fused to form a single bone, the **sacrum** (*os sacrum*). The vertebrae protect the spinal cord and roots of the spinal nerves, aid in the support of the head, and furnish attachment for the muscles governing body movements. Although the amount of movement between any two vertebrae is limited, the vertebral column as a whole possesses considerable flexibility (Badoux, 1969, 1975; Slijper, 1946).

A typical vertebra consists of a **body** (*corpus vertebrae*); a **vertebral arch** (*arcus vertebrae*) consisting of right and left **pedicles** and **laminae**; and various processes for muscular or articular connections, which may include **transverse**, **spinous**, **articular**, **accessory**, and **mamillary processes**.

The **body** (*corpus vertebrae*) of a typical vertebra is constricted centrally. It has a slightly convex cranial articular surface and a centrally depressed caudal articular surface. Developmentally, a typical vertebra is formed from three ossification centers: a body and two laminae. Postnatally epiphyses form on each end of the body and fuse with it. (In some carnivores, such as the bear, bony epiphyses remain separate throughout life.) Hare (1961a) determined the time at which the epiphyses of the vertebrae of the dog appear radiographically and later fuse with the vertebral body. He found that epiphyseal centers appeared from the second to the eighth weeks and that union was complete by the fourteenth month. In life, the **intervertebral disc** (*discus intervertebralis*) consists of fibrocartilage located between adjacent vertebrae. Its center consists of a gel-like material, the **nucleus pulposus,** which is surrounded by multiple laminae of highly organized fibrous tissue, the **anulus fibrosus**. The thick anulus fibrosus of the disc attaches firmly to adjacent vertebrae, forming a formidable retaining wall for the amorphous, gelatinous center (Hansen, 1952).

The **vertebral arch** (*arcus vertebralis*) consists of two **pedicles** (*pediculi arcus vertebrae*) and two **laminae** (*laminae arcus vertebrae*). Together with the body, the arch forms a short tube, the **vertebral foramen** (*foramen vertebrale*). All the **vertebral foramina** converge to form the **vertebral canal** (*canalis vertebralis*). On each side the pedicle of the vertebra extends dorsally from the dorsolateral surface of the body, presenting smooth-surfaced notches. The **cranial vertebral notch** (*incisura vertebralis cranialis*) is shallow; the **caudal vertebral notch** (*incisura vertebralis caudalis*) is deep. When the vertebral column is articulated in the natural state, the notches on either side of adjacent vertebrae, with the intervening fibrocartilage, form the right and left **intervertebral foramina** (*foramina intervertebralia*). Through these pass the spinal nerves, arteries, and veins. The dorsal part of the vertebral arch is composed of right and left laminae, which unite at the mid-dorsal line to form a single **spinous process** (*processus spinosus*), without leaving any trace of its paired origin. Most processes arise from the vertebral arch. Each typical vertebra has, in addition to the single, unpaired, dorsally located spinous process, on either side an irregularly shaped **transverse process** (*processus transversus*), which projects laterally from the region where the pedicle joins the vertebral body. At the root of each transverse process, in the cervical region except C7, is the **transverse foramen** (*foramen transversarium*), which divides the process into dorsal and ventral parts. The dorsal part is an intrinsic part of the transverse process. It is comparable to the whole transverse process found in a thoracic vertebra. The part ventral to the transverse foramen is serially homologous with a rib, a costal element that has become incorporated into the transverse process. It is usual in the dog for this costal element to be free from the seventh cervical vertebra on one or both sides. In such instances the separate bone is known as a *cervical rib* and there is no transverse foramen.

Paired **articular processes** are present at both the cranial and the caudal surfaces of a vertebra, at the junction of the pedicle and lamina. The **cranial process** (*processus articularis cranialis*), or prezygapophysis, faces craniodorsally or medially, whereas the **caudal process** (*processus articularis caudalis*), or postzygapophysis, faces caudoventrally or laterally. In the articulated vertebral column, the interval between adjacent arches is the **interarcuate space** (*spatium interarcuale*) where the yellow ligament is located dorsally.

Cervical Vertebrae

The **cervical vertebrae** (*vertebrae cervicales*) (Figs. 4.50 to 4.63) are seven in number in most mammals. The first two, differing greatly from each other and also from all the other vertebrae, can be readily recognized. The third, fourth, and fifth differ only slightly and are difficult to differentiate. The

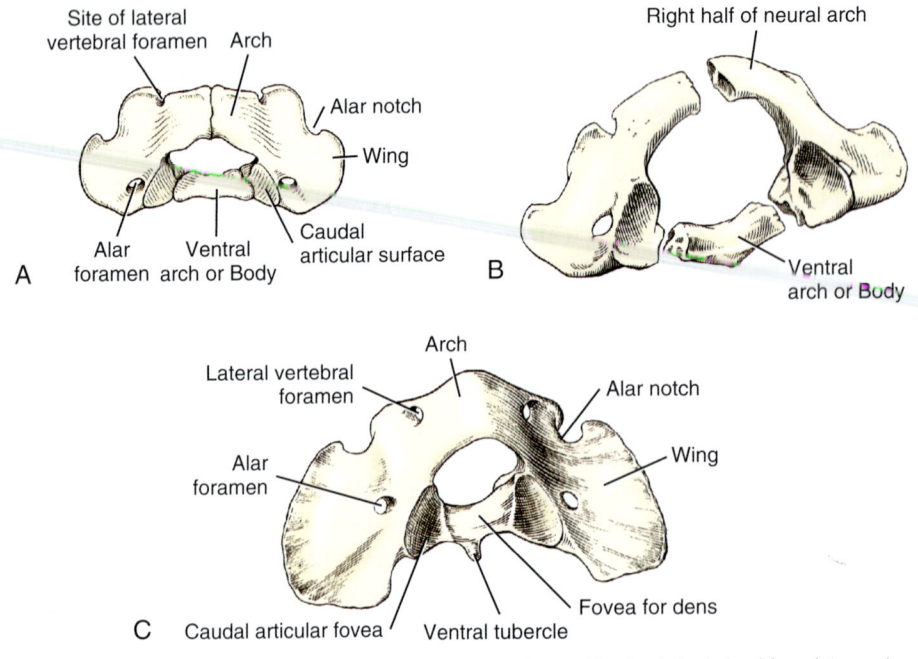

• **Fig. 4.50** A, Atlas of a 3½-month-old Beagle, caudodorsal view. The body is derived from intercentrum 1. **B**, Developmental ossific components of the atlas. **C**, Atlas of an adult dog, caudodorsal view. (With permission from Watson AG: *The phylogeny and development of the occipito-atlas-axis complex in the dog*, Thesis, Ithaca, NY, 1981, Cornell University.)

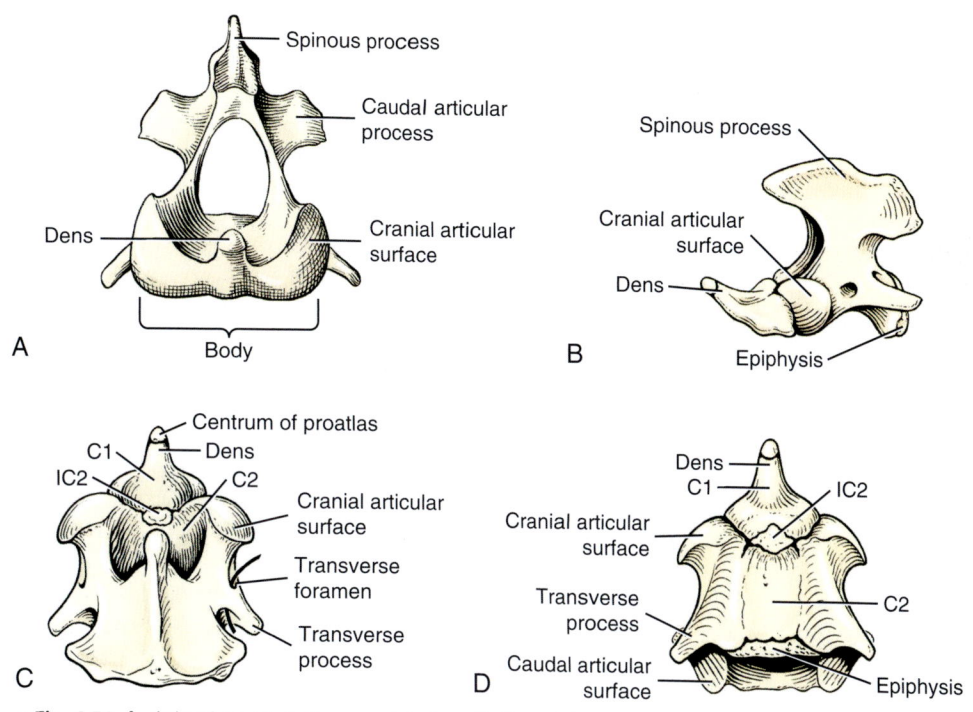

• **Fig. 4.51** **A**, Axis of an adult dog, cranial view. **B**, **C**, and **D**, Lateral, dorsal, and ventral views of the axis of a 3.5-month-old Beagle. C = centrum; IC = intercentrum.

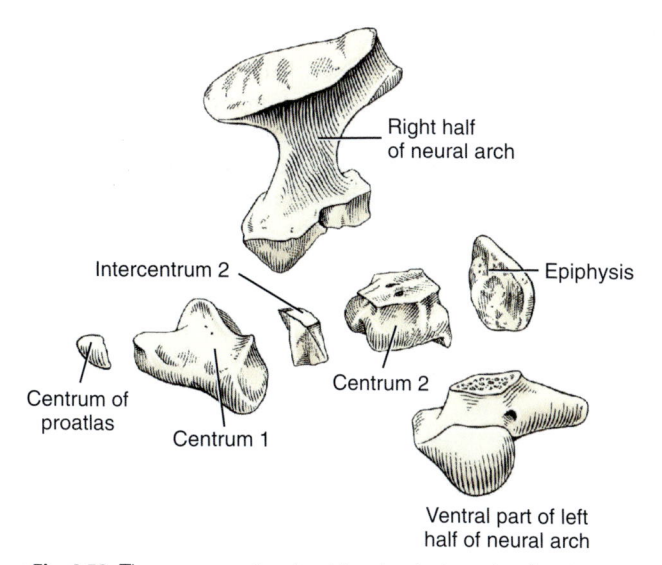

• **Fig. 4.52** The component parts of the developing axis, disarticulated. (With permission from Watson AG: *The phylogeny and development of the occipito-atlas-axis complex in the dog*, Thesis, Ithaca, NY, 1981, Cornell University.)

sixth and seventh cervical vertebrae present differences distinct enough to make their identification possible. Hare (1961b) documented the ossification of cervical vertebrae radiographically.

The **atlas** (see Fig. 4.50), or first cervical vertebra, is atypical in both structure and function. It articulates with the skull cranially and with the axis caudally. Its chief peculiarities are the modified articular processes that "cup" the occipital condyles, the winglike lateral expansions, the lack of a spinous process, and reduction of its body to form a ventral arch (Watson et al., 1986). The thick lateral portion of the atlas is known as the **lateral mass** (*massa lateralis*). They unite the **dorsal arch** (*arcus dorsalis*) with the **ventral arch** (*arcus ventralis*), also known as the *body* of the atlas formed by intercentrum I. The elliptical space between the dorsal arch of the atlas and the occipital bone is the *spatium interarcuale atlantooccipitale*. The shelflike transverse processes, or **wings** (*alae atlantis*), project from the lateral masses. Other eminences of the atlas are the **dorsal tubercle** (*tuberculum dorsale*), located on the cranial end of the dorsal arch and the **ventral tubercle** (*tuberculum ventrale*), which projects from the caudal end of the ventral arch. Frequently the dorsal tubercle is bifid, and the ventral tubercle may take the form of a conical process. The **cranial articular fovea** (*fovea articularis cranialis*) consists of two cotyloid cavities that sometimes meet ventrally. They articulate with the occipital condyles of the skull, forming a joint of which the main movements are flexion and extension. Because the atlantooccipital joint allows rather free up-and-down movement of the head, it may be remembered as the "yes joint." The **caudal articular fovea** (*fovea articularis caudalis*) consists of two shallow glenoid cavities that form a freely movable articulation with the second cervical vertebra. This is sometimes spoken of as the "no joint," because rotary movement of the head occurs at this articulation. The dorsal surface of the ventral arch of the atlas contains the **fovea of the dens** (*fovea dentis*) (see Fig. 4.50C), which is concave from side to side and articulates with the dens of the second cervical vertebra. This articular area of the fovea of the dens blends with the articular areas on the caudal surface of the lateral masses, which are the **caudal articular foveae** (*fovea articularis caudalis*). In addition to the large **vertebral**

128 CHAPTER 4 The Skeleton

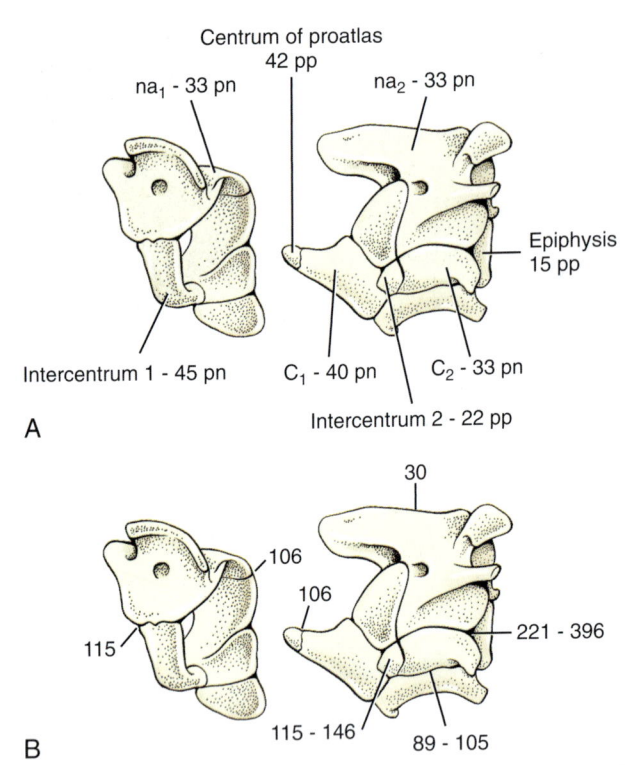

• **Fig. 4.53** **A,** Summary illustration of the ages in days (*pn,* prenatal; *pp,* post-partum) of the initial ossification of the 10 bony elements in the atlas-axis complex of 200 known-age Beagles (Table 4.1). Initial ossification was determined by examining specimens prepared as alizarin-clearings (148 specimens), cleaned bones (16), and histologic sections (16). *na₁, na₂,* first and second pairs of neural arch elements; *C₁, C₂,* centrum 1 and centrum 2. **B,** Summary illustration of the post-natal ages in days of the fusion of the 10 bony elements in the atlas-axis complex of known-age Beagles. Fusion was determined by the examination of alizarin-clearings (53), cleaned bones (36), and histologic sections (16). There were only 24 dogs, aged between 80 days and 13 months (396 days), during which time most of the fusions occurred, and thus the ages given must be interpreted with caution. (With permission from Watson AG, Evans HE, de Lahunta A: Ossification of the atlas-axis complex in the dog, *Zbl Vet Med C Anat Histol Embryol* 15:122–138, 1986.)

foramen, through which the spinal cord passes, there are two pairs of foramina in the atlas (see Fig. 4.50C). The **alar foramen** (*foramen alare*) is a short canal passing obliquely through the transverse process, or wing, of the atlas for the vertebral artery and vein. The **lateral vertebral foramen** (*foramen vertebrale laterale*) perforates the craniodorsal part of the vertebral arch for the first cervical spinal nerve and vertebral artery. Richards and Watson (1991) described a variation of the lateral vertebral foramen of the atlas that remained open as a notch on the cranial border of the atlas in a Miniature Schnauzer. The **alar notch** (*incisura alaris*) is located on the cranial border of the base of the transverse process for the vertebral artery. The **atlantal fossae** (*fossae atlantis*) are depressions ventral to the wings. In some specimens there is an intraosseous canal running from the atlantal fossa into the lateral mass. The vertebral vein and artery traverse the atlantal fossa. The vein extends through the alar foramen caudally and anastomoses with the internal jugular

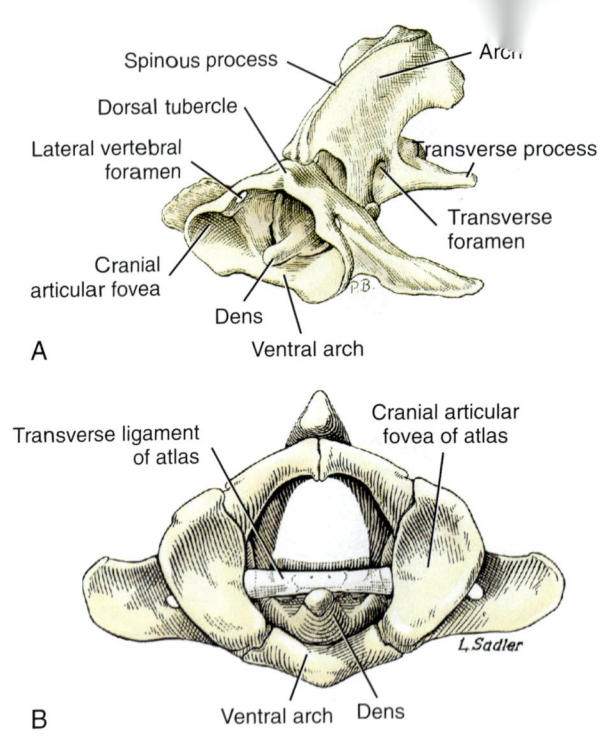

• **Fig. 4.54 A,** Atlas and axis of an adult dog, cranial lateral aspect. (The transverse ligament over the dens has been removed.) **B,** Atlas and axis of a 6-month-old Beagle, cranial view. (With permission from Watson AG: *The phylogeny and development of the occipito-atlas-axis complex in the dog,* Thesis, Ithaca, NY, 1981, Cornell University.)

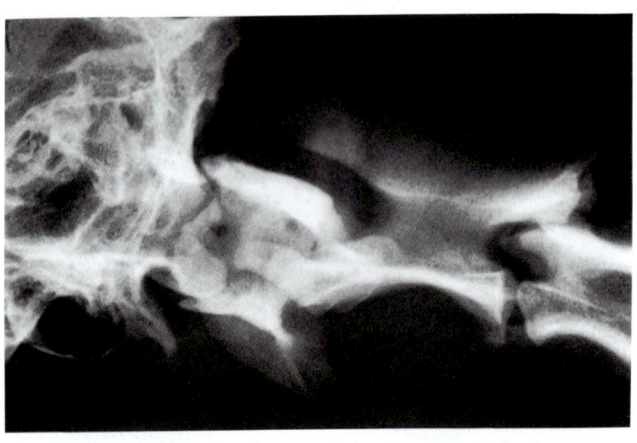

1. Dens
2. Arch of the atlas
3. Spinous process of axis

• **Fig. 4.55** Radiograph. Occipitoatlantoaxial region. Occipital condyles and atlas have been rotated to show the dens.

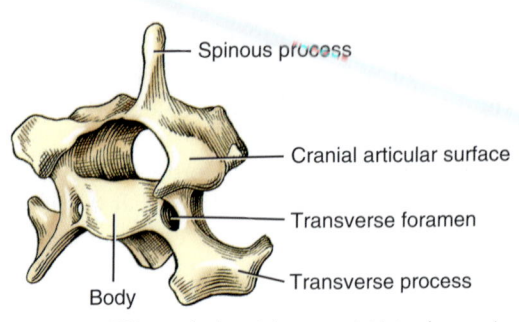

• **Fig. 4.56** Fifth cervical vertebra, cranial lateral aspect.

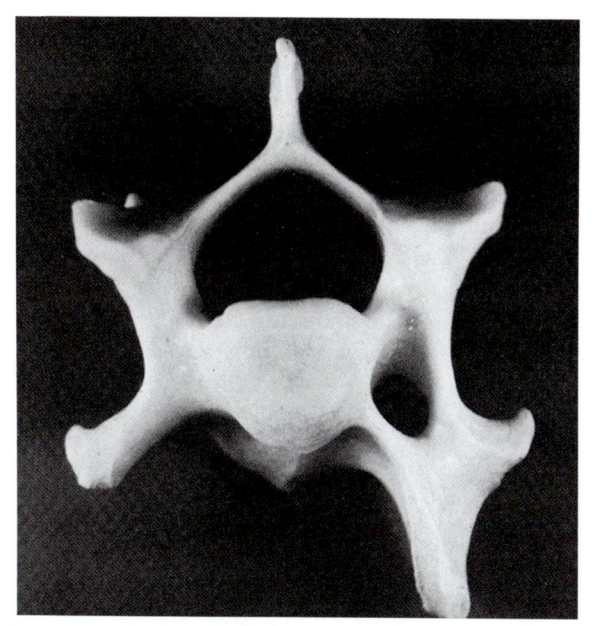

CHAPTER 4 The Skeleton 129

• **Fig. 4.57** An anomalous sixth cervical vertebra of a mongrel dog, cranial view. The left side has a transverse foramen, which is normal for C6, whereas the right side lacks it and resembles C7.

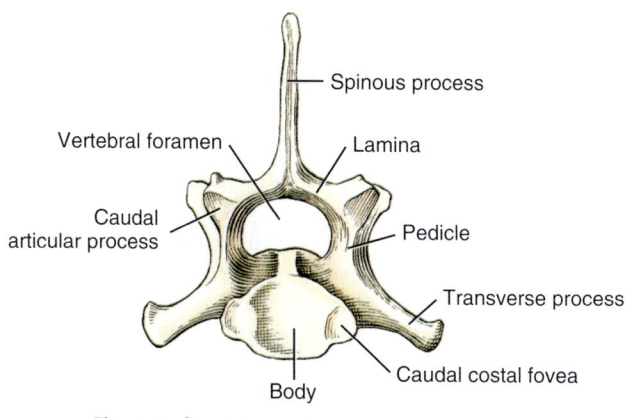

• **Fig. 4.58** Seventh cervical vertebra, caudal aspect.

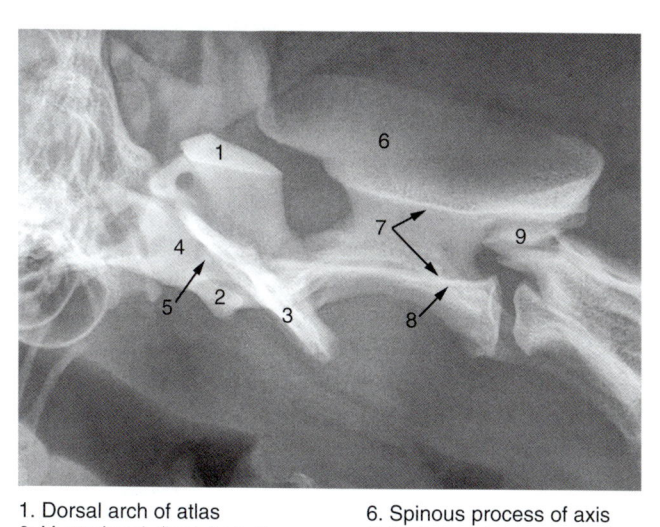

- Spinous process
- Vertebral foramen
- Lamina
- Caudal articular process
- Pedicle
- Transverse process
- Caudal costal fovea
- Body

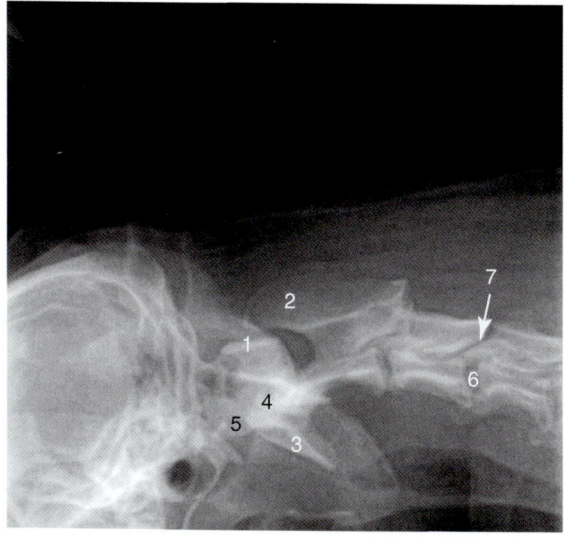

1. Dorsal arch of atlas
2. Spinous process of axis
3. Transverse process (wing) of atlas
4. Dens
5. Occipital condyle
6. Intervertebral disc between C3 and C4
7. Synovial articulation between caudal articular processes of C3 and cranial articular processes of C4

• **Fig. 4.60** Lateral radiograph of cranial cervical vertebrae with head rotated.

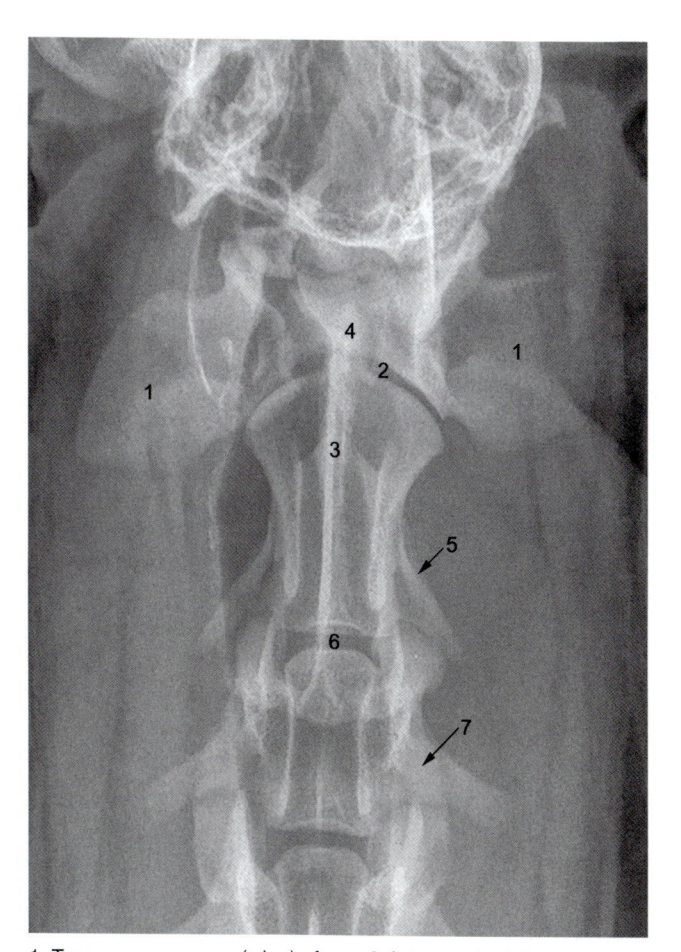

1. Dorsal arch of atlas
2. Ventral arch (body) of atlas
3. Transverse process (wing) of atlas
4. Occipital condyle
5. Dens
6. Spinous process of axis
7. Vertebral foramen of axis
8. Transverse process of axis
9. Caudal articular process of axis

• **Fig. 4.59** Lateral radiograph of cranial cervical vertebrae.

1. Transverse process (wing) of atlas (C1)
2. Atlantoaxial joint
3. Spinous process of axis (C2)
4. Dens of axis
5. Transverse process of axis
6. Intervertebral disc between C2 and C3
7. Overlapping caudal articular process of C3 and cranial articular process of C4

• **Fig. 4.61** Ventrodorsal radiograph of cranial cervical vertebrae.

1. Spinous process of C3
2. Vertebral foramen of C3
3. Vertebral arch of C3
4. Caudal articular processes of C3
5. Cranial articular processes of C4
6. Intervertebral synovial joints
7. Intervertebral disc
8. Transverse processes of C3
9. Transverse processes of C4

• **Fig. 4.62** Lateral radiograph of middle cervical vertebrae.

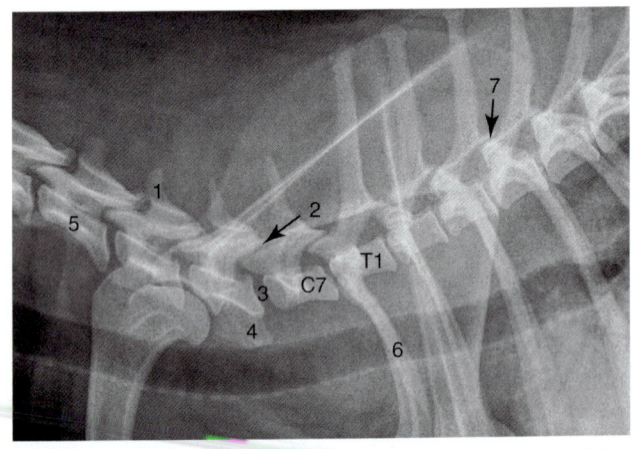

1. Spinous process of fifth cervical vertebra
2. Synovial joints between the caudal articular processes of C6 and the cranial articular processes of C7
3. Intervertebral disc between the vertebral bodies of C6 and C7
4. Transverse processes of C6
5. Transverse processes of C4
6. First rib
7. Synovial joints between the caudal articular processes of T3 and the cranial articular processes of T4

• **Fig. 4.63** Lateral radiograph of cervicothoracic vertebral junction.

overhangs the cranial and caudal articular surfaces of the vertebra. The axis is further characterized by a cranioventral peglike eminence, the **dens** (*dens*), also known as the *odontoid process*. This process and the cranial part of the cranial articular surface of the axis are morphologically the centrum of the atlas (centrum 1), which developmentally attaches to the axis. The dens lies within the vertebral foramen of the atlas, held down by the transverse ligament. The cranial articular surfaces of the axis are located laterally on the expanded cranial end of the vertebral body. Atlantoaxial subluxation with absence of the dens has been reported frequently, particularly in toy breeds, and ascribed to either degenerative or congenital causes. In almost all instances there is a tilting or dorsal displacement of the axis into the vertebral canal, with resultant compression of the spinal cord (Oliver & Lewis, 1973). The caudal articular processes are ventrolateral extensions of the vertebral arch and spinous process that face ventrally. Through the pedicles of the vertebra extends the short transverse foramen. Two deep fossae, separated by a median crest, mark the ventral surface of the body. The cranial vertebral notches converge on either side with those of the atlas to form the large intervertebral foramina for the transmission of the second pair of cervical spinal nerves and the spinal vessels. The caudal notches converge with those of the third cervical vertebra to form the third pair of intervertebral foramina, through which pass the third pair of cervical spinal nerves and the spinal vessels.

A review of the history of tetrapod vertebrae by Williams (1959) summarized the developmental theories of the most influential workers in the field. It appears that three elements—a neurapophysis, a pleurocentrum, and a hypocentrum (with its associated rib and ventral arch)—can be traced with clarity from the Paleozoic amphibia through reptiles to mammals. The pleurocentrum has become the centrum of mammals, and the hypocentrum has been reduced to a remnant intercentrum.

On the apical tip of the dens there is a transient ossification seen in almost all mammals that has been known for a long time as the *proatlas*. The significance of the proatlas as part of the atlas–axis complex has always been a puzzle, and several explanations have been advanced to account for it (Albrecht, 1880; Evans, 1939). The proatlas is most likely a remnant vertebra interposed between the skull and the atlas. As would be expected from the phylogenetic development of mammals, the proatlas is best represented in ancient reptiles such as *Dimetrodon* and mammal-like reptiles such as the cynodonts. The presence of large proatlas arches in these forms limited the mobility of the head. Various elements of the proatlas are typically present in some living reptiles (proatlas arches in alligators) and are a regular feature in many mammals at some stage of their skeletal development. The proatlas centrum in the dog forms as a nodule, and then appears as a cap on the cranial end of the dens. It fuses imperceptibly with the dens (see Figs. 4.52 and 4.53A and B). A radiograph of an un-united proatlas centrum could be interpreted as a fracture of the dens rather than as the separate element it represents. There are many

vein in the ventral condyloid fossa rostrally. A venous branch runs dorsally through the alar notch in the wing and aids in forming the external vertebral venous plexus. The vertebral artery enters the vertebral canal through the lateral vertebral foramen, after first having run through the alar foramen of the atlas.

The **axis** (see Fig. 4.51), or second cervical vertebra, presents an elongated, dorsal **spinous process** that is bladelike cranially and expanded caudally. The spinous process

...rts of fractures of the dens and the apparent absence of the dens in dogs and humans. Although fractures are often asymptomatic, there are reports of accompanying neurologic signs including death. For discussions of the phenomenon in dogs, see Geary et al. (1967) and Gage and Smallwood (1970). In humans, see Wollin (1963), Freiberger et al. (1965), and Schatzker et al. (1971). Watson (1981) found the earliest ossification of the proatlas centrum in the Beagle to occur 42 days postpartum, as an apical nodule in the cartilage of the dens. By approximately 106 days the proatlas is fused with the dens.

Sawin et al. (1962), when studying chondrodystrophy (dachs gene) in rabbits, found that this gene (DaDa) induced bizarre changes in the occipitovertebral region that may help elucidate the phylogenetic changes that have taken place in mammals. They found and illustrated remnants of both the proatlas centrum and the proatlas arches in their rabbits.

Watson and Evans (1976) and Watson (1981) confirmed that the adult atlas develops from three bony elements: a pair of neural arches that become the dorsal arch and transverse processes, and a ventral arch (body) that develops from intercentrum 1 (see Fig. 4.50). The axis develops from seven bony elements (see Fig. 4.52): a pair of neural arches; centrum 2 and a caudal epiphysis; intercentrum 2; centrum 1 (from the atlas), which forms the dens; and an apical element on the dens that represents the centrum of the proatlas. The latter is distinct for only a short time in the puppy. The appearance and fusion times of these elements vary even within litters. Watson and Stewart (1990) examined the atlas and axis of 62 pups and 4 adult Miniature Schnauzers of various ages to see whether there were characteristic differences in the ossification pattern of a miniature breed. They found 10 ossification centers in the atlas–axis complex, as has been reported in other breeds. In all dogs the dens developed from two distinct centers: the centrum of the proatlas and centrum 1. There did not appear to be any significant developmental differences in this breed from others that have been studied.

The **third**, **fourth**, and **fifth cervical vertebrae** (see Fig. 4.56) differ slightly from each other. The spinous processes increase in length from the third to the fifth vertebrae. The laminae are particularly large on the third cervical vertebra but gradually become shorter and narrower on the remaining vertebrae of the series. Tubercles are present on the caudal articular processes, decreasing in prominence from the third to seventh cervical segment. The transverse processes are two-pronged and slightly twisted in such a manner that the caudal prong lies at a more dorsal level than the cranial. The transverse processes of the fifth cervical vertebra are the shortest. On each vertebra there is a pair of **transverse foramina**, which extend through where the transverse processes attach to the junction of the body and the pedicle. These foramina contain the vertebral vessels and nerve. The latter consists of postganglionic sympathetic axons.

The **sixth cervical vertebra** possesses a higher spinous process than the third, fourth, or fifth, but its main peculiarity is the expanded sagittal platelike transverse processes, a **lamina ventralis**. These plates, which extend ventrally and laterally, represent only the caudal portion of the transverse processes. The remaining cranial portion is in the form of a conical projection ventrolateral to the transverse foramen.

In contrast with all other vertebrae, the first six cervical vertebrae are characterized by transverse foramina. Occasionally one side differs from the other (see Fig. 4.57).

The **seventh**, or **last**, **cervical vertebra** (see Fig. 4.58) lacks transverse foramina. Cervical ribs, when these are present, articulate with the ends of the single-pronged transverse processes of this vertebra. The spinous process of this vertebra is the highest of all those on the cervical vertebrae. Sometimes costal foveae appear caudoventral to the caudal vertebral notches. In these instances the heads of the first pair of true ribs articulate here.

The transverse processes of cervical vertebrae represent, in part, fused ribs and are sometimes referred to as *pleurapophyses*. In a well-reasoned paper, Cave (1975) reviewed the terms applied by various authors to the parts of a cervical transverse process.

Thoracic Vertebrae

There are 13 **thoracic vertebrae** (*vertebrae thoracicae*) (Figs. 4.64 to 4.69). The first nine are similar; the last four present minor differences from each other and from the preceding nine. The bodies of the thoracic vertebrae are shorter than those of the cervical or lumbar region. Although there are approximately twice as many thoracic as lumbar vertebrae, the thoracic region is slightly less than one-third longer than the lumbar region. The body of each thoracic vertebra possesses a cranial and a caudal **costal fovea** (*fovea costalis cranialis et caudalis*) on each side as far caudally as the eleventh. The body of the eleventh frequently lacks the caudal costal fovea and the twelfth and thirteenth thoracic vertebrae always have only a complete cranial fovea on each side. The foveae on the bodies of the thoracic vertebrae are for articulation with the heads of the ribs. The bodies of most of the thoracic vertebrae have a pair of nutrient foramina entering the middle of the ventral surface. All show paired vascular foramina on the flattened dorsal surface of the body. The **pedicles** of the vertebral arches are short. The caudal vertebral notches are deep, but the cranial notches are frequently absent. The **laminae** give rise to a **spinous process**, which is the most conspicuous feature of the first nine thoracic vertebrae. The spinous process of the first thoracic vertebra is more massive than the others but is of approximately the same length. The massiveness gradually decreases with successive vertebrae, but there is little change in the length and direction of the spinous processes until the seventh or eighth thoracic is reached. These then become progressively shorter and are inclined increasingly caudally through the ninth and tenth segments. The spinous process of the eleventh thoracic vertebra is nearly perpendicular to the long axis of that bone. This vertebra, the **anticlinal vertebra** (*vertebra anticlinalis*), is the transitional segment of the thoracolumbar region. All spinous processes caudal to those of the twelfth and thirteenth thoracic vertebrae are directed cranially, whereas those of all vertebrae cranial to the eleventh thoracic are directed caudally. In an articulated vertebral column the palpable tips of the spinous processes of the sixth and seventh thoracic vertebrae lie dorsal to the cranial parts of the bodies of the eighth and ninth; the tips of the spinous processes of the eighth to tenth thoracic vertebrae lie dorsal to the bodies of the vertebrae caudal to them.

The heads of the first pair of ribs articulate with the first thoracic and sometimes with the last cervical vertebra. The first ribs therefore articulate usually with the cranial part of the body of the first thoracic vertebra and with the fibrocartilage that forms the joint between the last cervical and the first thoracic segment. The heads of ribs 2 through 10 articulate with the cranial costal fovea of the thoracic vertebra of the same number and the caudal costal fovea of the vertebra cranial to it. The tubercles of the ribs articulate with the costal fovea of the transverse processes of the thoracic vertebrae of the same number in all instances. The last three thoracic vertebrae usually possess only one pair of costal fovea on their bodies, owing to a gradual caudal shifting of the heads of each successive pair of ribs.

The **transverse processes** are short, blunt, and irregular. All contain **foveae** (*foveae costales transversales*) for articulation with the tubercles of the ribs. These foveae decrease in size and convexity from the first to the last thoracic vertebra.

The **mamillary processes** (*processus mamillaris*), or metapophyses, start at the second or third thoracic vertebra and continue as paired projections through the remaining part

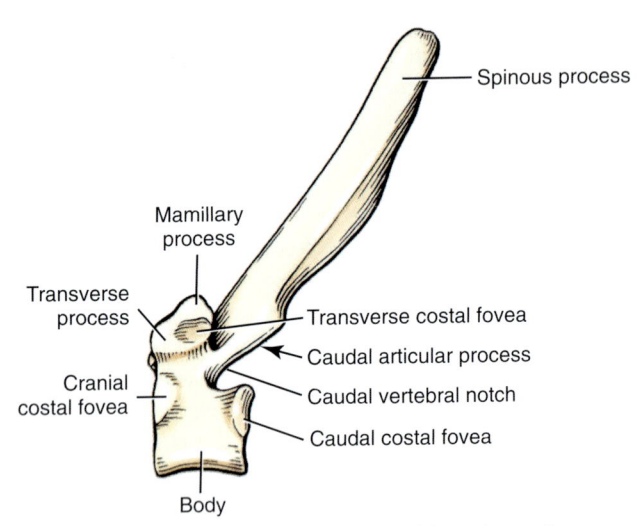

• **Fig. 4.64** First thoracic vertebra, left lateral aspect.

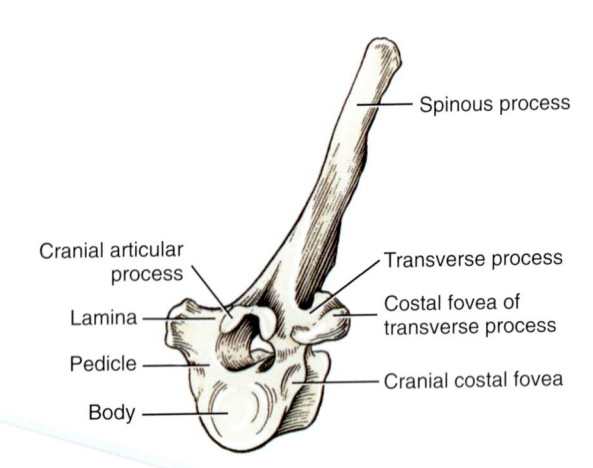

• **Fig. 4.65** Sixth thoracic vertebra, cranial lateral aspect.

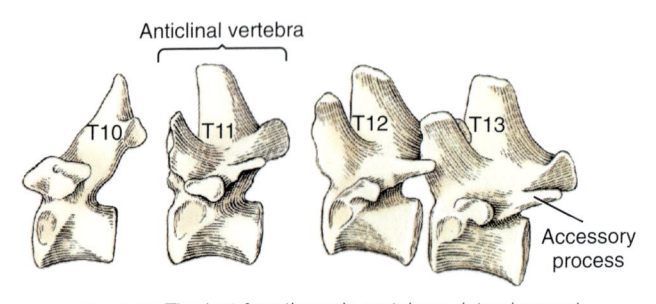

• **Fig. 4.66** The last four thoracic vertebrae, lateral aspect.

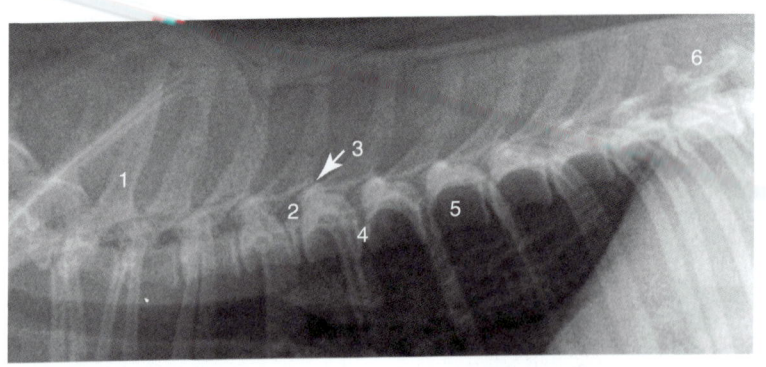

1. Spinous process of T1
2. Intervertebral foramina between T4 and T5
3. Synovial articulations between the caudal articular processes of T4 and the cranial articular processes of T5
4. Intervertebral disc between the bodies of T5 and T6
5. Body of T7
6. Anticlinal vertebra-T11

• **Fig. 4.67** Lateral radiograph of thoracic vertebrae.

of the thoracic and through the lumbar, sacral, and caudal regions. They are small, knoblike eminences that project dorsally from the transverse processes. At the eleventh thoracic vertebra they become associated with the cranial articular processes and continue as laterally compressed tubercles throughout the remaining vertebrae of the thoracic and those of the lumbar region.

The **accessory processes** (*processus accessorii*), or anapophyses, appear first in the midthoracic region and are located on succeeding segments as far caudally as the fifth or sixth lumbar vertebra. They extend caudally from the caudal borders of the pedicles and, when well developed, form a notch lateral to the caudal articular process that articulates with the cranial articular process of the vertebra caudal to it.

The **articular processes** are located at the junctions of the pedicles and the laminae. The cranial pairs of processes are widely separated on the first and second thoracic vertebrae and nearly confluent at the median plane on thoracic vertebrae 3 to 10. On thoracic vertebrae 11, 12, and 13, the right and left processes face each other across the median plane and are located at the base of the mamillary processes. The cranial articular processes, with the exception of those on the last three thoracic vertebrae, face cranially and dorsally. The caudal articular processes articulate with the cranial ones of the vertebra caudal to it, are similar in shape, and face ventrally and caudally on thoracic vertebrae 1 to 9. The joints between thoracic vertebrae 10 to 13 are conspicuously modified because the articular surfaces of the caudal articular processes are located on the lateral surfaces of dorsocaudally projecting processes. This type of interlocking articulation allows flexion and extension of the caudal thoracic and the lumbar regions while limiting sagittal movement. Foveae on the transverse processes and on the vertebral bodies for articulation with the ribs characterize the thoracic vertebrae.

Dabanoglu et al. (2004) presented computed tomographic (CT) images of the thoracic vertebrae of 13 German Shepherd Dogs to determine the cross-sectional area of the vertebral canal. The canal was largest at the level of T1.

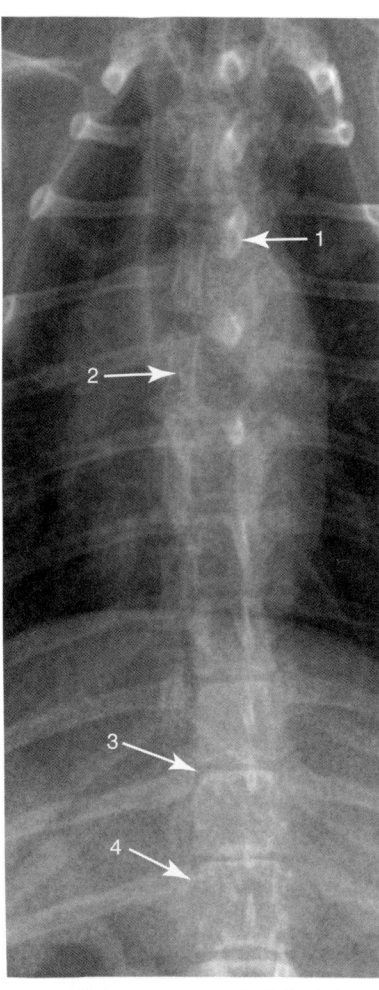

Lumbar Vertebrae

The **lumbar vertebrae** (*vertebrae lumbares*) (Figs. 4.70 to 4.77), seven in number, have longer bodies than those of the thoracic vertebrae. They gradually increase in width

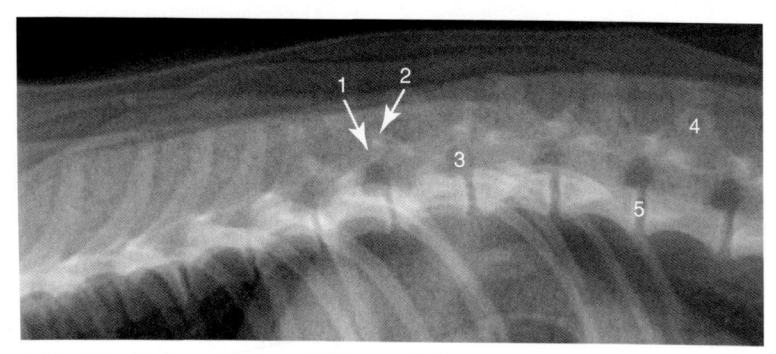

1. Spinous process of T3
2. A sternebra
3. Articulation of the head of rib 10 with the bodies of T10 and T11
4. Articulation of the head of rib 11 with the body of T11

• **Fig. 4.68** Ventrodorsal radiograph of thoracic vertebrae.

1. Caudal articular processes of T11
2. Cranial articular processes of T12
3. Intervertebral foramina between T12 and T13
4. Spinous process of L2
5. Intervertebral disc between L1 and L2

• **Fig. 4.69** Lateral radiograph of thoracolumbar vertebral junction.

throughout the series and in length through the first five or six segments. The body of the seventh lumbar vertebra is approximately the same length as the first. The ventral foramina of each body are not always paired or present. The dorsal foramina are paired and resemble those of the thoracic vertebrae. Although longer and more massive, the pedicles and laminae of the lumbar vertebrae resemble those of typical vertebrae of the other regions.

The **spinous processes** are highest and most massive in the midlumbar region. These processes are about half as long, and the dorsal borders are approximately twice as wide as those of the vertebrae at the cranial end of the thoracic region. They have a slight cranial inclination.

The **transverse processes** are directed cranially and slightly ventrally. They are longest in the midlumbar region. In emaciated animals the broad extremities of the transverse processes can be palpated.

The **accessory processes** are well developed on the first three or four lumbar vertebrae, and absent on the fifth or sixth. They overlie the caudal vertebral notches and extend caudally lateral to the articular processes of the succeeding vertebrae.

The **articular processes** lie mainly in sagittal planes. The caudal processes lie between the cranial processes of succeeding vertebrae and restrict lateral flexion. All cranial articular processes bear **mamillary processes**.

There are 20 vertebrae in the thoracolumbar region. This number is quite constant. Iwanoff (1935) found only one specimen out of 300 with 21 thoracolumbar vertebrae; all of the remaining had 20. Among the specimens he studied, the last lumbar segment was sacralized (fused to the sacrum) in three, and the first sacral vertebra was free in two.

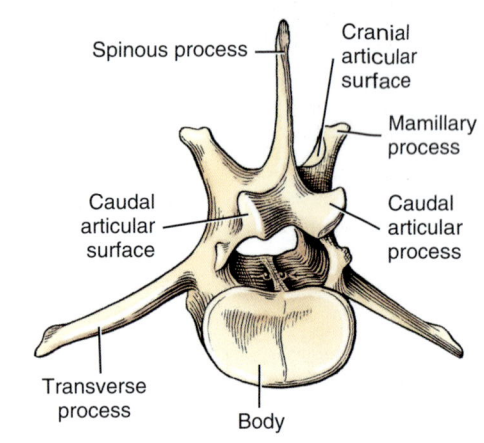

• **Fig. 4.71** Fifth lumbar vertebra, caudal lateral aspect.

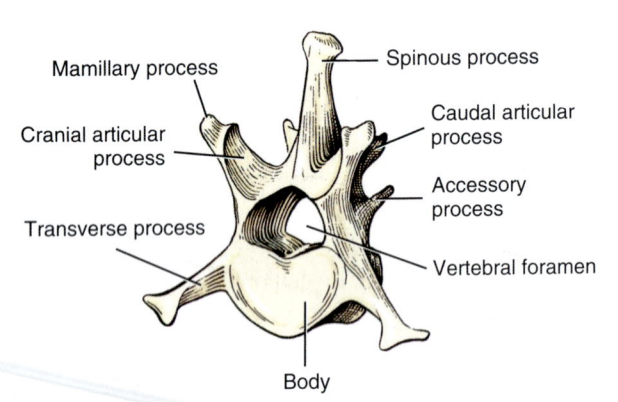

• **Fig. 4.70** First lumbar vertebra, cranial lateral aspect.

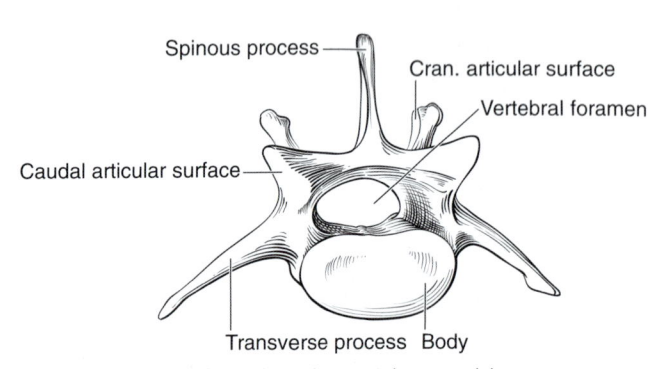

• **Fig. 4.72** Seventh lumbar vertebra, caudal aspect.

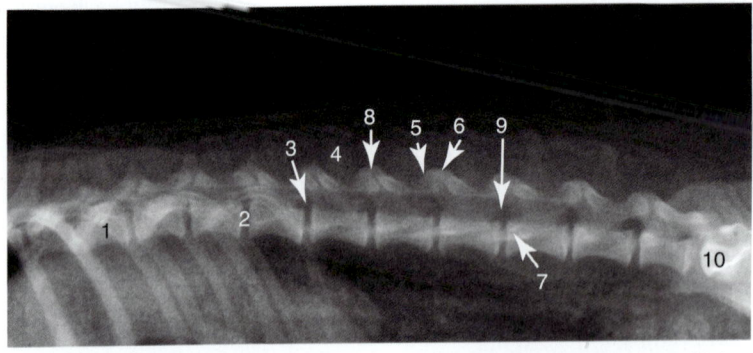

1. T11: the anticlinal vertebra
2. Intervertebral disc between T13 and L1
3. Intervertebral foramina between L1 and L2
4. Spinous process of L2
5. Caudal articular processes of L3
6. Cranial articular processes of L4
7. Transverse processes of L5
8. Mamillary processes on the cranial articular processes of L3
9. Accessory processes on the laminae of L4
10. Sacrum

• **Fig. 4.73** Lateral radiograph of lumbar vertebrae.

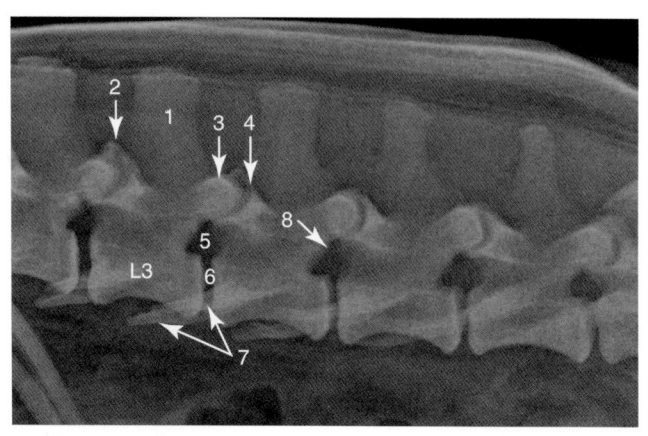

1. Spinous process of L3
2. Mamillary processes on the cranial articular processes of L3
3. Caudal articular processes of L3
4. Cranial articular processes of L4
5. Intervertebral foramina between L3 and L4
6. Intervertebral disc between L3 and L4
7. Transverse processes of L4
8. Accessory processes of L4

• **Fig. 4.74** Lateral radiograph of middle lumbar vertebrae.

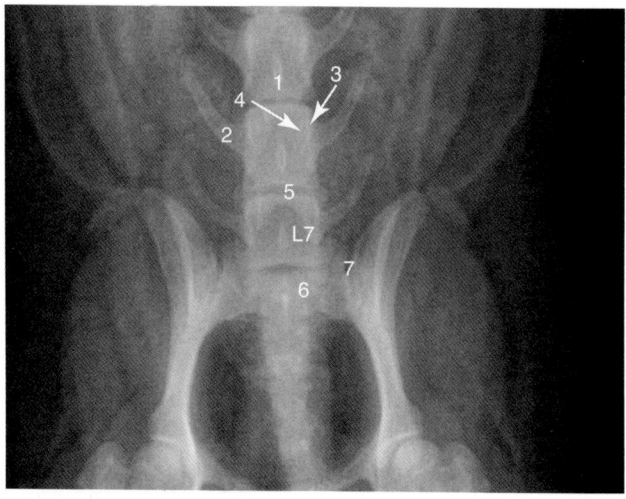

1. Spinous process of L5
2. Transverse process of L6
3. Cranial articular process of L6
4. Caudal articular process of L5
5. Intervertebral disc between L6 and L7
6. Sacrum
7. Sacroiliac articulation

• **Fig. 4.76** Ventrodorsal radiograph of lumbosacral vertebrae.

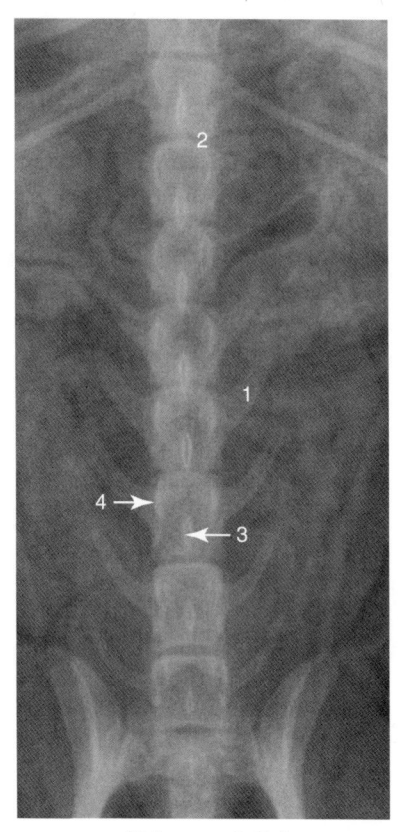

1. Transverse process of L4
2. Intervertebral disc between T13 and L1
3. Spinous process of L5
4. Cranial articular process of L5

• **Fig. 4.75** Dorsoventral radiograph of lumbar vertebrae.

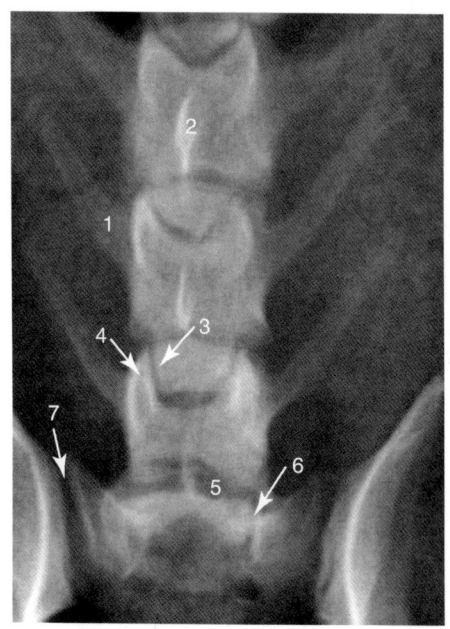

1. Transverse process of L6
2. Spinous process of L5
3. Caudal articular process of L6
4. Cranial articular process of L7
5. Lumbosacral intervertebral disc
6. Caudal articular process of L7 articulating with the cranial articular process of the sacrum
7. Sacroiliac joint

• **Fig. 4.77** Ventrodorsal radiograph of lumbosacral vertebrae.

Sacral Vertebrae

The bodies and processes of the three **sacral vertebrae** (*vertebrae sacrales*) fuse in the adult to form the **sacrum** (*os sacrum*) (Figs. 4.78 to 4.81). The bulk of this four-sided, wedge-shaped complex lies between the ilia and articulates with them. The body of the first segment is larger than the bodies of the other two segments combined. The three are united to form an arched, bony mass with a concave ventral, or pelvic surface, a feature of obstetric importance.

The **dorsal surface** (*facies dorsalis*) (see Figs. 4.78 and 4.79) presents the **median sacral crest** (*crista sacralis mediana*), which represents the fusion of the three spinous processes. Two indentations on the crest indicate the areas

136 CHAPTER 4 The Skeleton

• **Fig. 4.78** Sacrum, caudal lateral aspect.

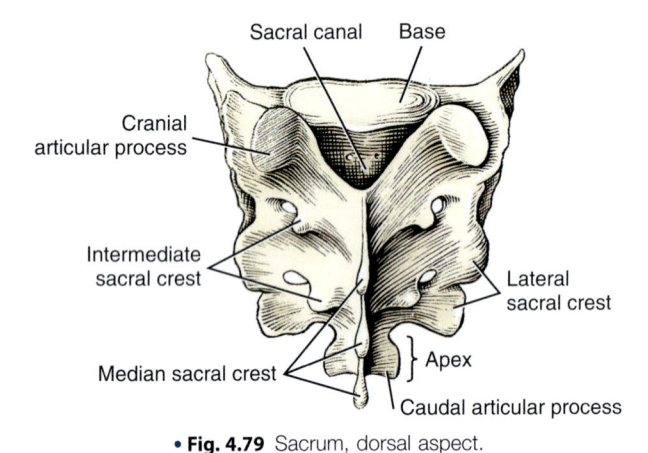

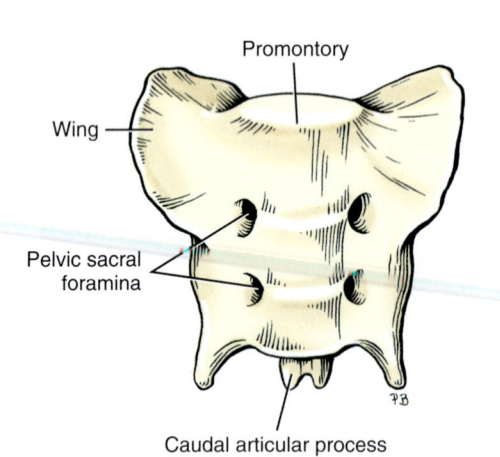

• **Fig. 4.79** Sacrum, dorsal aspect.

• **Fig. 4.80** Sacrum, ventral aspect.

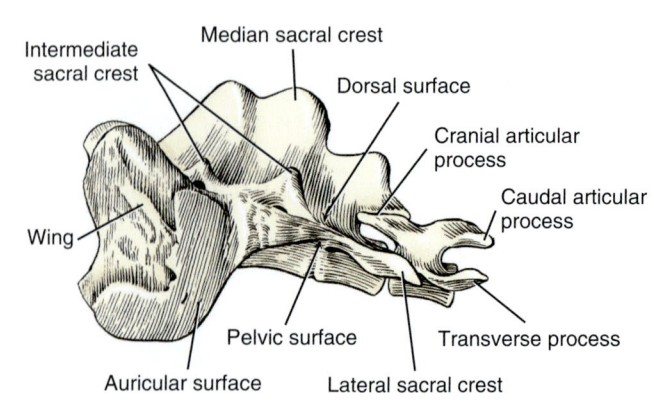

• **Fig. 4.81** Sacrum and first caudal vertebra, lateral aspect.

of fusion. The dorsal surface also bears two pairs of **dorsal sacral foramina** (*foramina sacralia dorsalia*), which transmit the dorsal divisions of the sacral spinal nerves and spinal vessels. Medial to these foramina are low projections representing the fused mamilloarticular processes of adjacent segments. In some specimens the three mamilloarticular processes on each side are united by intervening ridges. The aggregate of the processes and the connecting ridges then forms the **intermediate sacral crest** (*crista sacralis intermedia*). The **caudal articular processes** are small and articulate with the first caudal vertebra. The **cranial articular processes** are large, face dorsomedially, and form joints with the seventh lumbar vertebra.

The **pelvic surface** (*facies pelvina*) (see Fig. 4.80) of the sacrum is variable in its degree of concavity. During the first 6 postnatal months, two intervertebral fibrocartilages mark the separation of the vertebral bodies. These persist in the adult as two **transverse lines** (*lineae transversae*). Two pairs of **pelvic sacral foramina** (*foramina sacralia pelvina*), situated just lateral to the fused sacral bodies, are larger than the corresponding dorsal foramina. In addition to blood vessels, they transmit the ventral branches of the first two sacral nerves. Lateral to the pelvic sacral foramina are the fused transverse processes. Those of the first and part of the second segment are greatly enlarged and modified for articulation with the ilium. The transverse processes of the third segment and part of the second form the narrow, thin **lateral sacral crest** (*crista sacralis lateralis*), which terminates caudally in a flattened, pointed process, the caudolateral angle. This angle frequently articulates with the adjacent transverse process of the first caudal vertebra.

The **wing of the sacrum** (*ala ossis sacri*) is the enlarged **lateral part** (*pars lateralis*), which has a large, rough **auricular surface** (*facies auricularis*), which articulates with the ilium. (A fetal "sacral rib" is incorporated in this wing of the sacrum [see Fig. 2.58].)

The **base of the sacrum** (*basis ossis sacri*) faces cranially. Above its slightly convex articular surface is the beginning of the wide **sacral canal** (*canalis sacralis*), which traverses the bone and is formed by the coalescence of the three vertebral foramina. The dorsal and ventral parts of the base are clinically important. The cranioventral part of the base has a transverse ridge, the **promontory** (*promontorium*). This slight ventral projection, along with the ilia, forms the dorsal boundary of the smallest part of the bony ring, or **pelvic inlet** (*inlet pelvina*), through which the fetuses pass during birth. The laminae of the first sacral vertebra dorsal to the entrance to the sacral canal extend caudally and leave a concave caudal recession in the osseous dorsal wall of the sacral canal, which is covered only by soft tissue. The caudal extremity of the sacrum, although broad transversely, is known as the **apex** (*apex ossis sacri*) and articulates with the

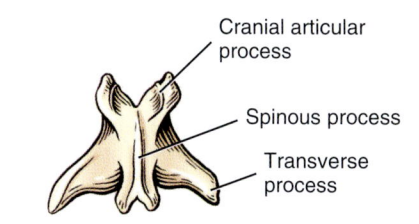

• **Fig. 4.82** First caudal vertebra, dorsal aspect.

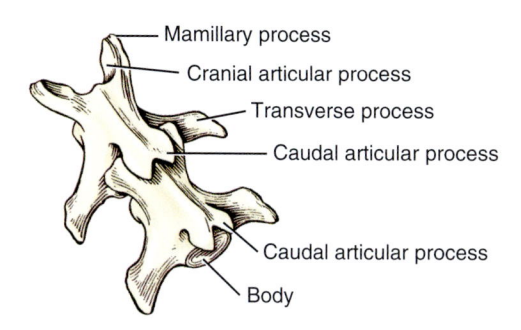

• **Fig. 4.83** Second and third caudal vertebrae, dorsolateral aspect.

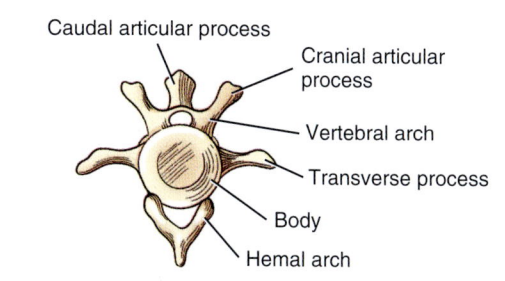

• **Fig. 4.84** Fourth caudal vertebra, cranial aspect. (Note the hemal arch, which in life encloses vessels.)

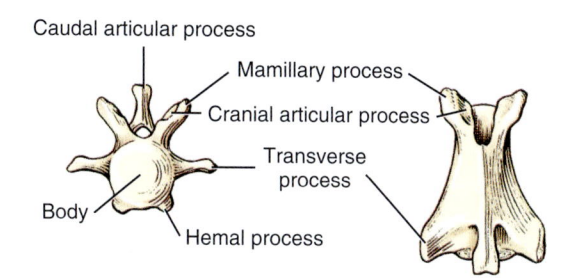

• **Fig. 4.85** Fifth caudal vertebra, cranial and dorsal aspects.

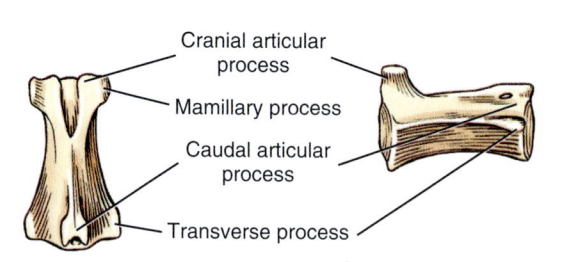

• **Fig. 4.86** Sixth caudal vertebra, dorsal and lateral aspects.

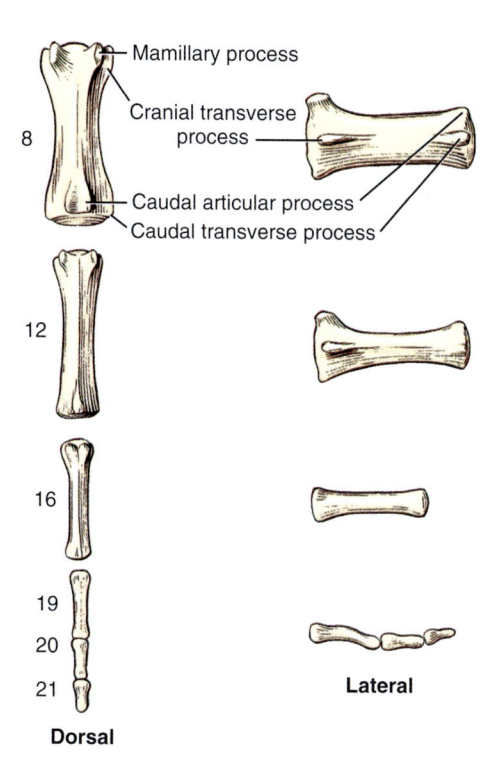

• **Fig. 4.87** Representative caudal vertebrae.

first caudal vertebra. Its base, in a similar manner, articulates with the last lumbar vertebra. Occasionally the first caudal vertebra is fused to the sacrum.

Caudal Vertebrae

The average number of **caudal vertebrae** (*vertebrae caudales*) (Figs. 4.82 to 4.87) is usually 20, although the number may vary from 6 to 23. The caudal vertebrae, formerly referred to as *coccygeal vertebrae*, are subject to greater variation than are the vertebrae of any other region, although they may be constant within a breed. The cranial members of the series conform most typically to the representative type, whereas the caudal segments are gradually reduced to simple rods.

The **body** of the first caudal vertebra is as wide as it is long. Succeeding segments gradually lengthen, as far as the middle of the series, after which they become progressively shorter. The segments decrease in width from the sacrum caudally. The last segment is minute and ends as a tapering process.

The **vertebral arch** is best developed in the first caudal segment. The lumen, which the consecutive arches enclose, becomes progressively smaller until in the sixth or seventh caudal vertebra only a groove remains to continue the vertebral canal. The caudal part of the vertebral canal contains the caudal spinal nerves, which supply the structures of the tail (the spinal cord usually ends at the articulation between the last two lumbar vertebrae). The **cranial articular processes** exist, although they have lost their articular function. Each vertebra bears a **mamillary process**, which persists caudally in the series until all trace of the articular process has vanished. The **caudal articular processes** project from the caudal border of the arch and are frequently asymmetric. They gradually disappear in a craniocaudal sequence. The spinous processes are small and disappear early in the series, at approximately the seventh caudal vertebra. The first four or five pairs of transverse processes are well developed and typical. Caudal to the fifth caudal vertebra they are reduced in size, and they disappear at about the fifteenth segment.

Hemal arches (*arcus hemales*) (see Fig. 4.84) are present as separate bones that articulate with the ventral surfaces of the caudal ends of the bodies of the fourth, fifth, and sixth caudal vertebrae. They slope caudally and are shaped like a V or Y. In life, they protect the median caudal artery, which passes through them. Caudal to the hemal arches, and in corresponding positions on succeeding vertebrae, are the paired **hemal processes** (*processus hemales*). Hemal processes are the last processes to disappear, and remnants of them can still be identified as far caudally as the seventeenth or eighteenth caudal vertebra.

The Vertebral Column as a Whole

The vertebral column protects, supports, and acts as a flexible, slightly compressible rod through which the propelling force generated by the pelvic limbs is transmitted to the rest of the body. It is also used by the axial and abdominal muscles in locomotion. The basic movements of the vertebral column are flexion or dorsal arching of the vertebral column so that the head and pelvic region move ventrally, closer to the ground surface; extension, straightening, or ventral arching of the vertebral column so that the head and pelvic region move dorsally, away from the ground surface; lateral flexion; and rotation.

In the support of the viscera of the trunk, Slijper (1946) compares the vertebral column to a bow and the abdominal muscles and linea alba to a string. As the string, the abdominal muscles, particularly the recti, do not attach to the ends of the bow, but at some distance from them. Cranially, the attachment is to the rib cage; caudally it is to the ventral cranial edge of the pelvis. This variance does not alter the aptness of the comparison because the abdominal muscles and the vertebral column form a functional unit that is supported by the four limbs. The intrinsic architecture of the vertebral column would not support the abdominal viscera without the powerful abdominal muscles, which act for this purpose as a complete elastic apron. Badoux (1975) explains the support of the body axis as a compromise between the requirements of meeting the forces of gravity and the requirements of propulsion for locomotion. The modern view is represented by a modified "bow and string" concept by which the vertebral column forms a bow with a variable curvature stabilized by its ligaments and muscles. Changes in the curvature are effected by the action of three muscular "strings" with adjustable tension: (1) a dorsal string of epaxial muscles, (2) an interrupted ventral string of hypaxial muscles including the psoas muscles, and (3) an uninterrupted abdominal muscle group.

In the fetus the vertebral column is uniformly flexed from the head to the tip of the tail. In the adult standing position the head is elevated, resulting in a secondary cervical curvature, which extends the joints between the caudal cervical vertebrae. It is interesting to note that the greatest movement of the vertebral column takes place near one or both ends of the several regions into which it is divided: at both ends of the cervical region, near the caudal end of the thoracic region, at the lumbosacral junction, and in the cranial part of the caudal region.

The total length of a freshly isolated vertebral column of a Shepherd-type, medium-proportioned mongrel dog weighing 45 pounds was found to be 109 cm. The lengths of the various regions as measured along the ventral surface of the articulated vertebral column are shown in Table 4.4.

The size of the vertebral canal reflects quite accurately the size and shape of the contained spinal cord because there is only a small amount of epidural fat in the dog. The spinal cord is largest in the atlas, where its diameter is approximately 1 cm. It tapers to approximately half this size in the spinal cord caudal end of the axis. The canal in the first three cervical vertebrae is nearly circular. In the fourth cervical vertebra the canal enlarges and becomes slightly oval transversely. This shape and enlargement continues through the second thoracic vertebra. The increased size of the spinal cord in this region, the cervical intumescence, is caused by the need to innervate the thoracic limbs via the brachial plexus of nerves and accounts for the larger size and oval shape of the vertebral canal. From the second thoracic to the anticlinal segment, or eleventh thoracic vertebra, the vertebral canal is nearly circular in cross-section and is of a uniform diameter. From the eleventh thoracic vertebra through the lumbar region the height of the canal remains approximately the same, but the width increases so that the canal becomes transversely oval. The shape of the canal does not grossly change in the last two lumbar vertebrae, where it is larger than in any other vertebra caudal to the first thoracic. The lumbar enlargement of the vertebral canal accommodates the lumbosacral enlargement, intumescence, of the spinal cord. Possibly the small lumbar subarachnoid cistern and epidural fat in addition to the cauda equina contribute to this enlargement as the spinal cord usually ends opposite the fibrocartilage between the last two lumbar vertebrae.

Ueshima (1961) studied the pathology of vertebral deformity in the short-spine dog and found more cartilage than normal. The nucleus pulposus was invaded by cartilage shortly after birth, the articular cartilages were degenerate,

TABLE 4.4 Length of Various Regions of a Freshly Isolated Vertebral Column

Region	With Intervertebral Fibrocartilages	Without Intervertebral Fibrocartilages
Cervical	19 cm	16.5 cm
Thoracic	25.5 cm	23.0 cm
Lumbar	20.0 cm	17.5 cm
Sacral	4.5 cm	4.0 cm
Caudal	40.0 cm	36.0 cm

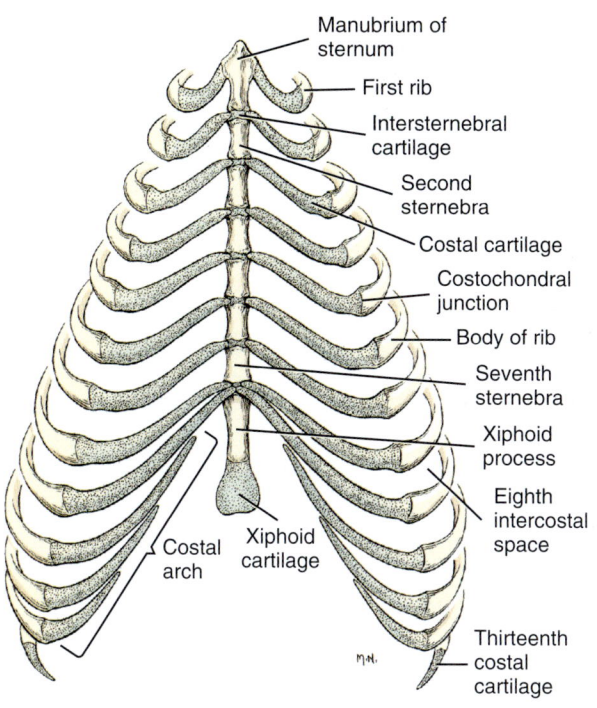

• Fig. 4.88 Ribs and sternum, ventral aspect.

and there was fusion of the vertebrae. There was faulty ossification during gestation.

Thoracic Skeleton

Ribs

The **ribs** (*costae*) (Figs. 4.88 and 4.89) form the largest part of the **thoracic skeleton**, which includes the mid-dorsal and midventral strips formed by the vertebral column and the sternum, respectively. There are usually 13 pairs of ribs in the dog. Each rib is divided into a laterally and caudally convex dorsal bony part, the *os costale*, and a ventral cartilaginous part, the **costal cartilage** (*cartilago costalis*). The first nine ribs articulate with the sternum and are called the **sternal** or **true ribs** (*costae verae*); the last four are called the **asternal** or **false ribs** (*costae spuriae*). The costal cartilages of the tenth, eleventh, and twelfth ribs unite with the cartilage of the last sternal rib (the ninth) to form the **costal arch** (*arcus costalis*) on each side. Because the cartilages of the last (thirteenth) pair of ribs end freely in the musculature, these ribs are sometimes called **floating ribs**. The ninth ribs are the longest, with the longest costal cartilages. Passing both caudally and cranially from the ninth rib, both the bony and the cartilaginous parts of the other ribs become progressively shorter. The costochondral junctions of the third through eighth ribs lie nearly in the same horizontal plane. Because the sternum and thoracic vertebral column diverge from the thoracic inlet and the successive ribs become progressively more laterally arched, the caudal part of the thorax is much more capacious than the cranial part. The space between adjacent ribs is known as the **intercostal space** (*spatium intercostale*). These spaces are two or three times as wide as the adjacent ribs.

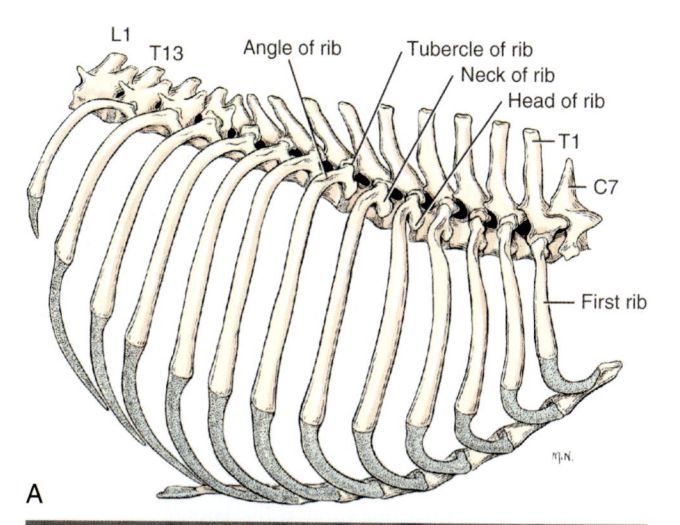

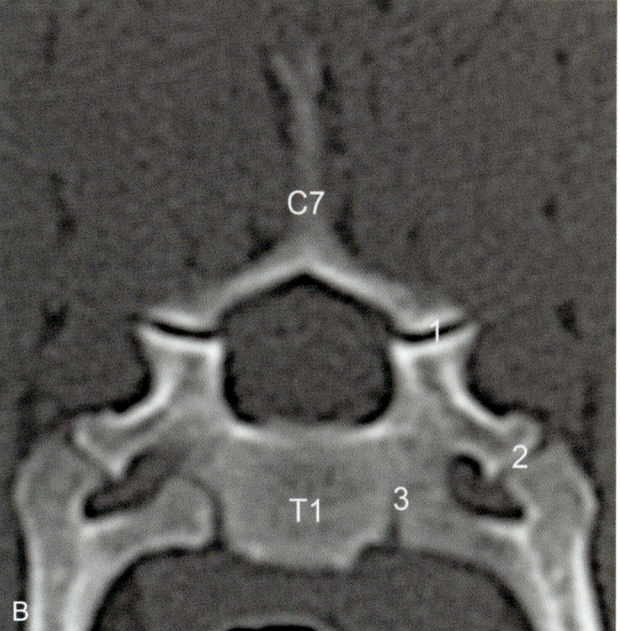

• Fig. 4.89 A, Ribs and sternum, right lateral aspect. B, Transverse computed tomography (CT) scan at the level of T1 showing articulation of the rib with C7 and T1.

A typical rib (*os costale*) as exemplified by the seventh, presents a vertebral extremity, a sternal extremity, and an intermediate shaft, or body. The vertebral extremity consists of a **head** (*caput costae*), a **neck** (*collum costae*), and a **tubercle** (*tuberculum costae*). The head of the rib has a wedge-shaped **articular surface** that articulates with adjacent costal foveae of contiguous vertebral bodies and the intervening fibrocartilage. The rib articular surfaces (*facies articularis capitis costae*), corresponding to those of the vertebrae with which they articulate, are of approximately equal size, convex, and face cranially and caudally, separated by a **crest** (*crista capitic costae*) or transverse ridge. In the thoracic region T1–T10 the head of each rib (*caput costae*) articulates over the intervertebral disc with the costal fovea formed by parapophyses of adjacent vertebrae. At the eleventh or twelfth thoracic vertebra the caudal pair of costal fovea disappear as the last two or three ribs articulate only with their corresponding vertebrae. The heads of these ribs are modified accordingly, and each lacks the crest that separates the two articular surfaces when they are present. The tubercle of the rib bears an **articular surface** (*facies articularis tuberculi costae*) for articulation with the transverse process of the vertebra of the same number. The space between the neck and tubercle of the rib and the body of the vertebra is known as the **costotransverse foramen,** which is homologous to the transverse foramen of a cervical vertebra. In the last two or three ribs the articular surfaces of the head and that of the tubercle become confluent, but the tubercle remains for muscular attachment.

The **body** of the rib (*corpus costae*), in general, is cylindrical and slightly enlarged at the costochondral junction. The third, fourth, and fifth ribs show some lateral compression of the distal halves of the bony parts. In the large breeds the ribs are flatter than they are in the small breeds. In all breeds the vertebral portions of the ribs are slightly thicker from lateral to medial than they are from cranial to caudal. The **angle** (*angulus costae*) is the accentuated curvature of the rib approximately 2 cm distal to the tubercle. The **costal groove** (*sulcus costae*) on the inner surface, for the intercostal vessels and nerve, is not distinct on any of the ribs.

The **costal cartilage** is the cartilaginous cylindrical distal continuation of the bony rib. It is smaller in diameter than the bony rib and, in mature dogs, may be calcified. Near the costochondral junctions the cartilages incline cranially. This is most marked in the first and twelfth ribs. The first rib articulates with the **first sternebra** (*manubrium sterni*). Succeeding true rib cartilages articulate with successive intersternebral cartilages. However, the eighth and ninth costal cartilages articulate with the cartilage between the seventh sternebra and the last sternebra, or xiphoid process. The costal cartilages of the tenth, eleventh, and twelfth ribs are long, slender rods with each joined to the one above by connective tissue to form the costal arch. The costal cartilage of the thirteenth rib, shorter and more rudimentary than those of the adjacent ribs, enters the musculature of the flank, in which it terminates.

Sternum

The **sternum** (see Figs. 4.88 and 4.89) is an unpaired segmental series of eight bones, *sternebrae*, that form the ventral boundary of the thorax. It is slightly turned dorsally cranially and turned ventrally caudally. The consecutive sternebrae are joined by short blocks of cartilage, the **intersternebral cartilage** (*cartilago intersternebralis*). The sternal ends of the ribs articulate with the intersternebral cartilages, with the exception of the first pair, which articulate with the first sternebra. The first and last sternebrae are specialized. The cranial half of the first sternebra is expanded and bears lateral projections for the attachment of the first costal cartilages. The first sternebra is longer than the others and is known as the **manubrium** (*manubrium sterni*).

The last sternebra, called the **xiphoid process** (*processus xiphoideus*), is wide and flat. Its length is approximately three times its width. It is roughly rectangular and may have an elliptical foramen in its caudal half. A thin cartilaginous plate, the **xiphoid cartilage** (*cartilago xiphoidea*), prolongs the xiphoid process caudally. In rare instances the xiphoid cartilage may appear as a "fork" or a perforated plate because of a failure of the sternal bars to unite completely in the fetus (see Figs. 2.60 to 2.63).

The cartilaginous joints between the sternebrae (*synchondroses sternales*) may ossify in old individuals.

Appendicular Skeleton

The development of the limbs and epiphyseal fusion in the dog have been studied by Schaeffer (1934), Pomriaskinsky-Kobozieff and Kobozieff (1954), Bressou et al. (1957), Hare (1960, 1961c), and Smith and Allcock (1960). Smith (1960) documented the fusion of all epiphyses on the appendicular skeleton of normal Greyhounds from the age of 3 months to the time of fusion. By 1 year of age, all epiphyses of the forelimb have completely united except for the proximal epiphysis of the humerus. In the hindlimb the only place where there is incomplete fusion is the tibial tuberosity. Wayne (1986) investigated the extent to which similarities in morphologic characteristics of the limb between domestic and wild canids are a consequence of a developmental pattern common to all domestic dogs. He used bivariate and discriminate function analyses to compare limb morphologic characteristics of adult dogs and wild canid species. Many wolflike canids cannot be distinguished from domestic dogs of equivalent size, but all dogs can be separated from fox-sized wild canids proximally by subtle differences of olecranon, metapodial, and scapular morphology. Casinos et al. (1986) have made a similar analysis of 63 different breeds of dogs and 12 wolves. They found that the morphologic characteristics of the long bones of the limbs do not differentiate dogs from wolves.

Bones of the Thoracic Limb

Each thoracic limb (*membrum thoracicum*) consists of its half of the shoulder girdle (*cingulum membri thoracici*), composed of the **clavicle** and **scapula**; the arm, or brachium, represented by the **humerus**; the forearm, or antebrachium, consisting of the **radius** and **ulna**; and the forepaw, or manus. The manus includes the **carpal** bones, the **metacarpals**, the **phalanges** of the digits and dorsal as well as palmar **sesamoid** bones.

Clavicle

The **clavicle** (*clavicula*) (Fig. 4.90) is not articulated with the skeleton in the dog. It is located at the tendinous intersection of the brachiocephalicus muscle, and its medial end is attached to the sternal fascia by a distinct ligamentous band. A large clavicle may be more than 1 cm long and a third as wide. It is thin and slightly concave both longitudinally and transversely. Its medial half may be twice as wide as its lateral half. The clavicle is more closely united to the

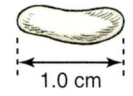

• **Fig. 4.90** Left clavicle, cranial aspect.

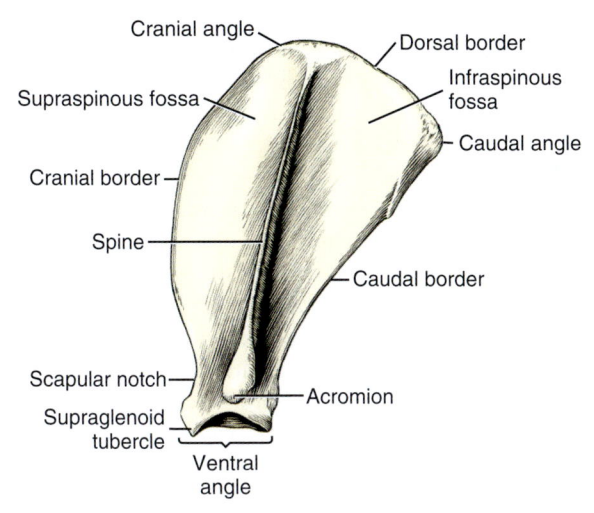

• **Fig. 4.91** Left scapula, lateral aspect.

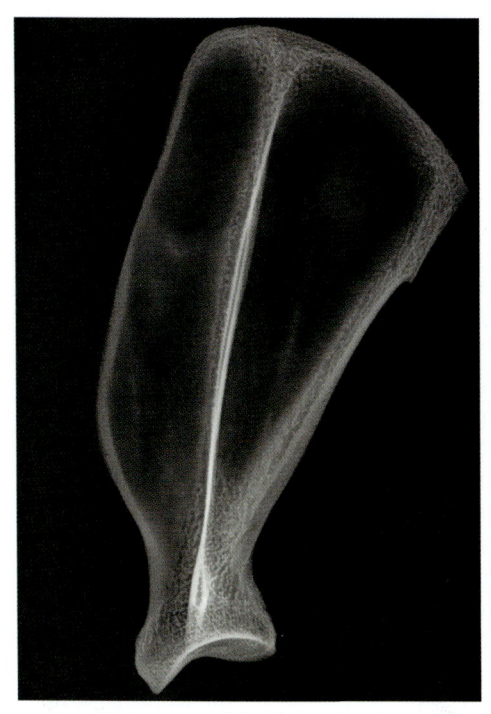

• **Fig. 4.92** Lateromedial radiograph, left scapula.

clavicular tendon between the cleidocephalicus muscle and the cleidobrachialis muscle than to the underlying axillary fascia to which it is related. The clavicle of the dog does not usually appear on lateral radiographs, although it is always present. It is commonly seen on dorsoventral or ventrodorsal radiographs of the neck and cranial thorax. (The clavicle is one of the first bones to ossify in the dog fetus.)

McCarthy and Wood (1988) examined 50 dogs of 10 breeds and found the clavicle ossified in 86% of the specimens. Evans (1958, 1962, 1974) always found an ossified clavicle in fetal Beagles by 30 to 35 days (see Fig. 2.68), at which time it was the only bone in the appendicular skeleton to be ossified. Cerny and Čižinauskas (1995) examined the histology of the clavicle and noted that half of the 42 dogs they studied had separate cartilaginous elements at the sternal end of the rudimentary clavicle, with ossification found in the distal part of the clavicle. Unlike the progressive degeneration of the fetal clavicle in ruminants, the dog's clavicle remains ossified throughout the fetal period.

Scapula

The scapula (Figs. 4.91 to 4.94) is the large, flat bone of the shoulder joint. Its most dorsal part lies just ventral to the level of the free end of the spinous process of the first or second thoracic vertebra. Longitudinally, it extends from a transverse plane cranial to the manubrium sterni to one through the body of the fourth or fifth thoracic vertebra. Because the thoracic limb has no articulation with the axial skeleton and supports the trunk by muscles only, the normal position of the scapula may vary by the length of one vertebra. In outline it forms an imperfect triangle having two surfaces, three borders, and three angles.

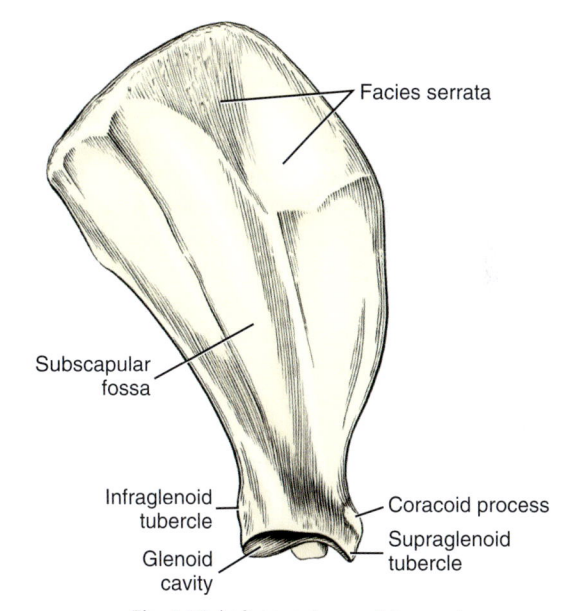

• **Fig. 4.93** Left scapula, medial aspect.

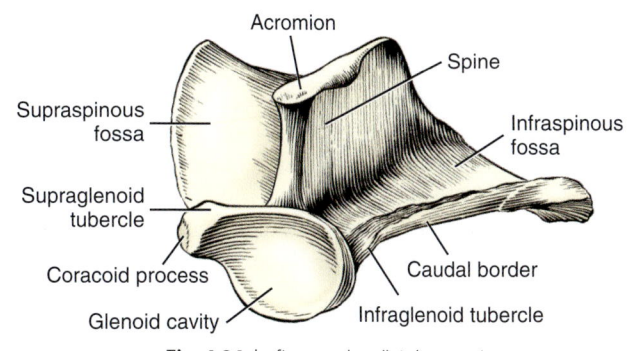

• **Fig. 4.94** Left scapula, distal aspect.

The **lateral surface** (*facies lateralis*) (see Fig. 4.91) is divided into two nearly equal fossae by a shelf of bone, the **spine of the scapula** (*spina scapulae*). The spine is the most prominent feature of the lateral surface of the bone. It begins proximally at the junction of the cranial and middle thirds of the dorsal border as a thick, low ridge, which gradually becomes wider but thinner as it is traced distally so that it presents definite cranial and caudal surfaces throughout most of its length, and near its distal end there is a definite caudal protrusion. The free border, or crest, of the spine is slightly thickened and rolled caudally in heavily muscled specimens. The widened truncate distal end of the spine of the scapula is called the **acromion**. Its broadened superficial portion is subcutaneous and easily palpated in the living animal. A nutrient foramen is frequently present at the junction of the distal extent of the spine and the scapula proper. The acromial part of the deltoideus muscle arises from the acromion and extends distally (see Fig. 6.46). The omotransversarius muscle arises from the distal end of the spine adjacent to the acromion and extends cranially. The trapezius muscle inserts on, and the spinous part of the deltoideus muscle arises from, the whole crest of the spine proximal to the origin of the omotransversarius muscle.

The **supraspinous fossa** (*fossa supraspinata*) is bounded by the cranial surface of the scapular spine and the adjacent lateral surface of the scapula. It is widest in the middle because the cranial border of the scapula extends in an arc from the cranial angle proximally to the scapular notch distally. The whole thin plate of bone that forms the supraspinous fossa is sinuous, possessing at its greatest undulation a lateral projection involving the middle of the fossa. The m. supraspinatus arises from all but the distal part of the supraspinous fossa.

The **infraspinous fossa** (*fossa infraspinata*) is in general triangular. Because the caudal and dorsal borders are thick and the spine leaves the lateral surface at nearly a right angle, this fossa is well defined. The m. infraspinatus arises from the infraspinous fossa.

The **medial**, or **costal**, **surface** (*facies costalis*) (see Fig. 4.93) of the scapula lies opposite the first five ribs and the adjacent four or five thoracic vertebrae. Two areas are recognized: a small dorsocranial rectangular area, *facies serrata*, from which arises the thick m. serratus ventralis, and the large remaining part of the costal surface, or the **subscapular fossa** (*fossa subscapularis*). It is nearly flat and usually presents three relatively straight muscular lines that converge toward the ventral angle at the distal end of the bone. Between the lines the bone is smooth, and in some places it is concave. The largest concavity lies opposite the spine. The m. subscapularis arises from the whole subscapular fossa and particularly from the muscular lines.

The **cranial border** (*margo cranialis*) is thin except at its extremities. Distally, it forms a concavity, the **scapular notch** (*incisura scapulae*), which marks the position of the constricted part of the bone. The border undulates as it reflects the warped nature of the supraspinous fossa. In the working breeds, the cranial border forms an arc, whereas in dogs with slender extremities, the border is nearly straight. Distally, the border becomes smoother and thicker; proximally, it becomes rougher and thicker as it runs into the dorsal border at the cranial angle.

The **dorsal border** (*margo dorsalis*), sometimes called the *vertebral border* or *base*, extends between the cranial and the caudal angles. In life it is capped by a narrow band of **scapular cartilage** (*cartilago scapulae*), which represents the unossified part of the bone. The m. rhomboideus attaches to the dorsal border of the scapula.

The **caudal border** (*margo caudalis*) (see Fig. 4.94) is the thickest of the three borders and bears, just dorsal to the ventral angle, the **infraglenoid tubercle** (*tuberculum infraglenoidale*). This tuberosity is much thicker than the border and is located largely on the costal surface of the bone. Parts of the mm. triceps–caput longum and teres minor arise from the infraglenoid tuberosity. The distal third of the thick caudal border contains two muscular lines that diverge distally; the more cranially located line extends nearly to the lip of the glenoid cavity, and the more caudal one ends in the infraglenoid tubercle. The more cranial line and adjacent caudal border of the scapula give origin to the m. teres minor; the more caudal line and adjacent caudal border give origin to the mm. triceps–caput longum. The middle third of the caudal border of the scapula is broad and smooth; the m. subscapularis curves laterally from the medial side and arises from it here. Approximately the proximal fourth of the caudal border is surrounded by a lip in the heavily muscled breeds. From this part arises the m. teres major.

The **caudal angle** (*angulus caudalis*) is obtuse as it unites the adjacent thick caudal border with the thinner, rougher, gently convex dorsal border. The m. teres major arises from the caudal angle and the adjacent caudal border of the scapula.

The **cranial angle** (*angulus cranialis*) imperceptibly unites the thin, convex cranial border to the rough, convex, thick dorsal border. No muscles attach directly to the cranial angle.

The **ventral angle** (*angulus ventralis*)—formerly called the *articular*, *glenoid*, or *lateral angle*—forms the expanded distal end of the scapula. Clinically, the ventral angle is the most important part of the bone because it contains the **glenoid cavity** (*cavitas glenoidalis*), which receives the head of the humerus in forming the shoulder joint. The glenoid cavity is very shallow; its lateral border is flattened, and cranially it extends out on the articular surface of the supraglenoid tuberosity. The medial border forms a larger arc than does the caudal border.

The **supraglenoid tuberosity** (*tuberculum supraglenoidale*) is the largest tuberosity of the scapula. For the most part it projects cranially, with a medial inclination. From it arises the single tendon of the m. biceps brachii. The small beaklike process that leaves the medial side of the scapular tuberosity is the **coracoid process** (*processus coracoideus*), from which the m. coracobrachialis arises. The coracoid process is a remnant of the coracoid bone, which is still

Humerus

The **humerus** (Figs. 4.95 to 4.100) is the bone of the brachium (arm). Proximally it articulates with the scapula in forming the shoulder joint; distally it articulates with the radius and ulna in forming the elbow joint. Developmentally it is divided into a shaft and two extremities; definitively it is divided into a head, neck, body, and condyle.

The **head** (*caput humeri*) is oval, being elongated in a sagittal plane. The articular area it presents is approximately twice the size of that of the glenoid cavity of the scapula with which it articulates. Although it is rounded in all planes, it does not form a perfect arc in any plane as the cranial part is much flatter than the caudal part. The articular surface of the head is continued distally by the **intertubercular groove** (*sulcus intertubercularis*), which ridges the craniomedial part of the proximal extremity of the bone. The extension of the shoulder joint capsule into the groove lubricates the bicipital tendon that lies in it (see Figs. 5.14, 5.16, and 5.17).

The **greater tubercle** (*tuberculum majus*) is the large craniolateral projection of the proximal extremity of the humerus. It has a smooth, convex summit that in most breeds extends proximal to the head. It serves for the total insertion of the m. supraspinatus and the partial insertion

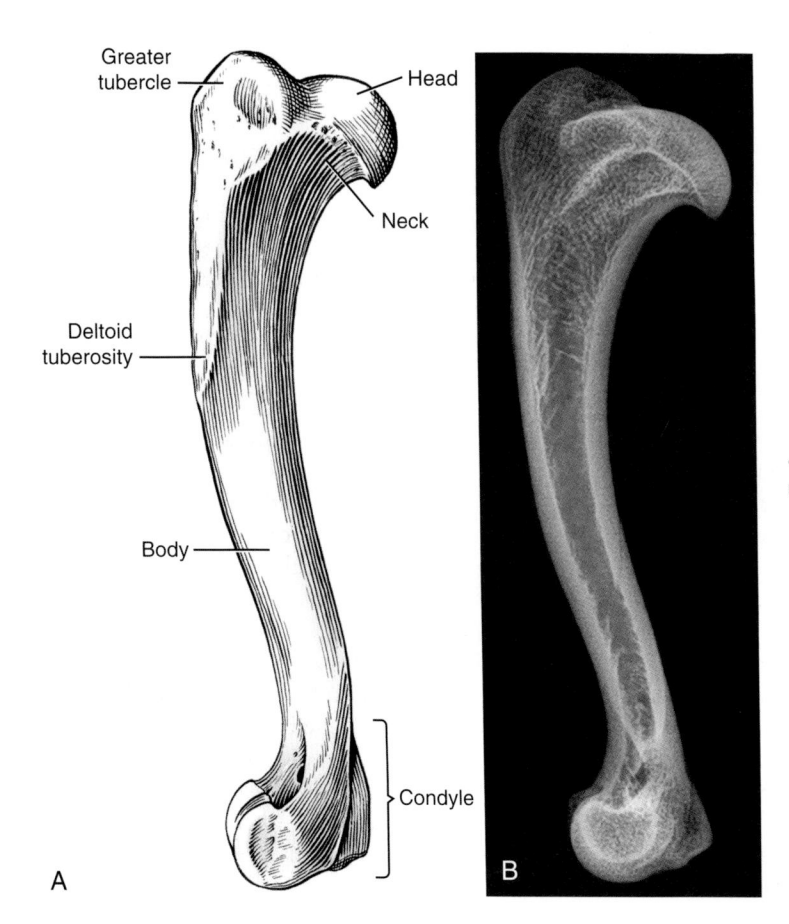

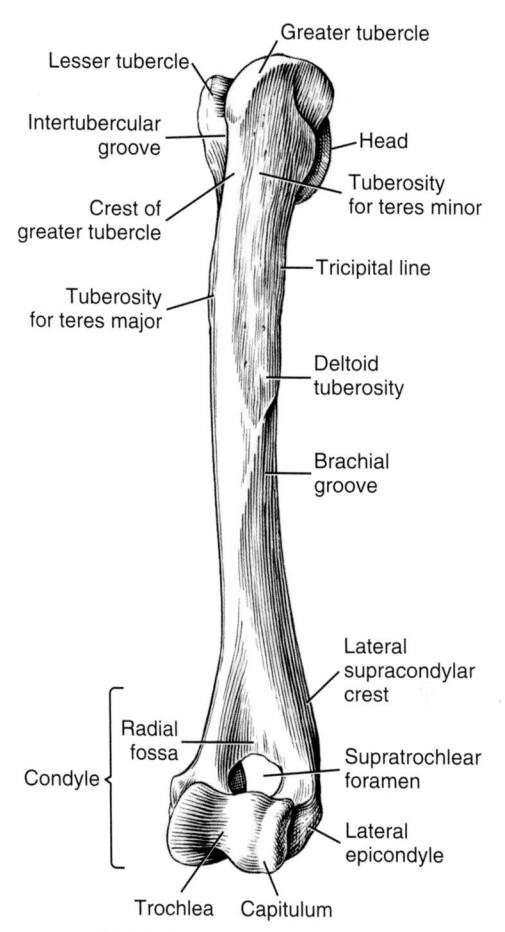

• **Fig. 4.95** Left humerus, cranial lateral aspect.

• **Fig. 4.96** A, Left humerus, lateral aspect. B, Lateromedial radiograph, left humerus.

144 CHAPTER 4 The Skeleton

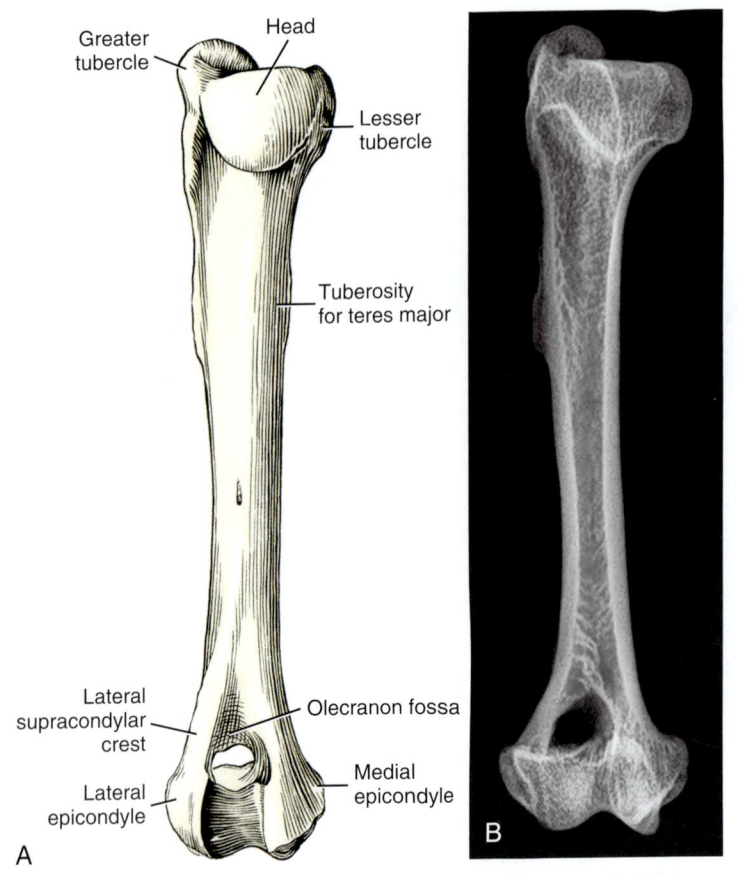

• **Fig. 4.97** A, Left humerus, caudal aspect. B, Caudocranial radiograph, left humerus.

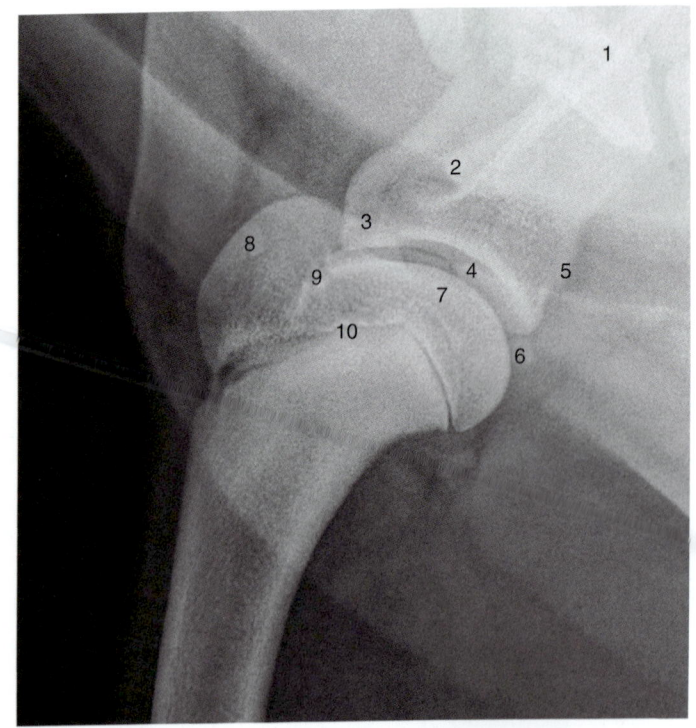

1. Spine
2. Acromion
3. Supraglenoid tubercle
4. Glenoid cavity
5. Infraglenoid tubercle
6. Scapulohumeral joint
7. Humeral head
8. Greater tubercle
9. Lesser tubercle
10. Proximal humeral physis

• **Fig. 4.98** Lateral radiograph of the shoulder.

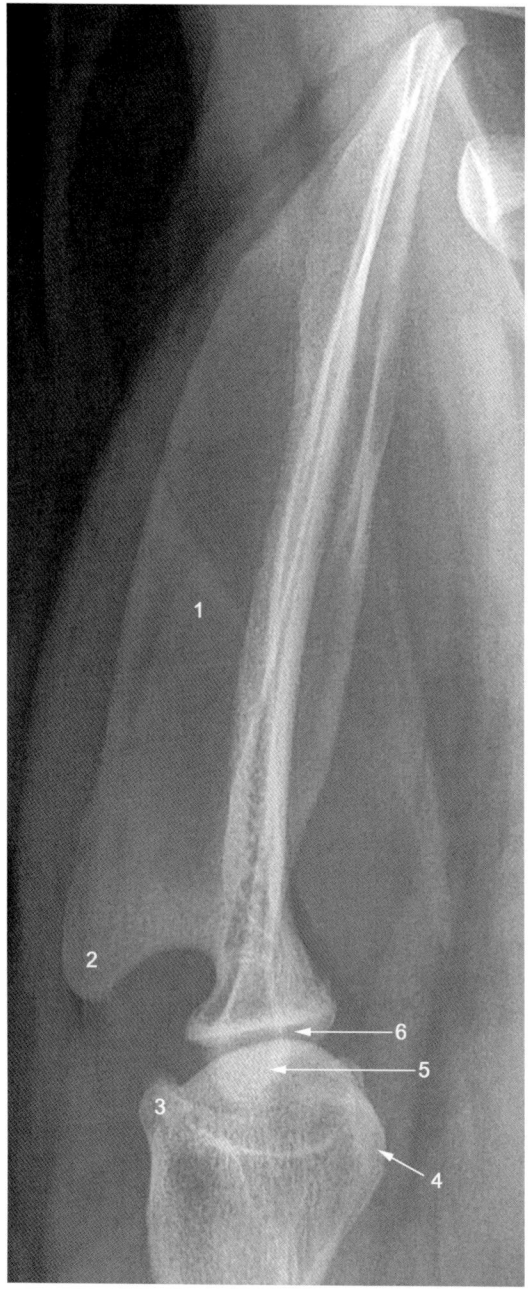

1. Spine of scapula
2. Acromion
3. Greater tubercle of humerus
4. Lesser tubercle of humerus
5. Supraglenoid tubercle
6. Glenoid cavity of scapula

• **Fig. 4.99** Caudocranial radiograph of shoulder.

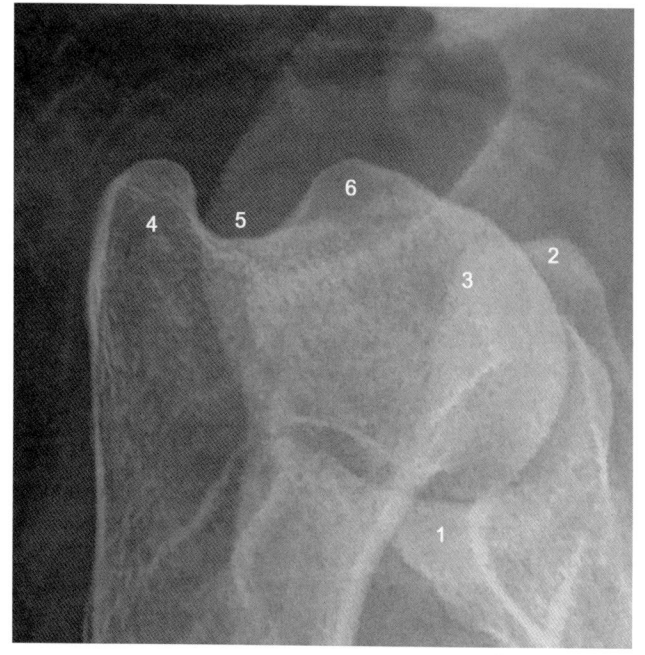

1. Spine of scapula
2. Acromion
3. Supraglenoid tubercle
4. Greater tubercle of humerus
5. Intertubercular groove
6. Lesser tubercle of humerus

• **Fig. 4.100** Caudocranial radiograph of the flexed shoulder.

of the m. pectoralis profundus. Between the head and the greater tubercle are several small foramina for the transmission of veins. The relatively smooth facet distal to the summit of the greater tubercle serves for the insertion of the m. infraspinatus. The **lesser tubercle** (*tuberculum minus*) is a medially flattened enlargement of the proximal medial part of the humerus, the convex border of which does not extend as far proximal as the head. To this convex border attaches the m. subscapularis. Planes through the lesser and the greater tubercle meet at about a right angle cranially. The two tubercles are separated craniomedially by the intertubercular groove (*sulcus intertubercularis*) and caudolaterally by the head of the humerus.

The **neck** of the humerus (*collum humeri*) is distinct only caudally and laterally. It indicates the line along which the head and parts of the tubercles have fused with the shaft.

The **body** of the humerus (*corpus humeri*), or shaft, is the long, slightly sigmoid-shaped part of the humerus that unites the head and neck with the condyle. It varies greatly in shape and size, depending on the breed. Usually it is laterally compressed and consists of four surfaces.

The **lateral surface** (*facies lateralis*) (see Fig. 4.96) is marked proximally by the **tricipital line** (*linea m. tricipitis*), formerly called the *anconeal line*, and the deltoid tuberosity that divides it into a narrow, slightly convex area, which faces craniolaterally, and a wider, smoother surface, which is slightly concave and faces caudolaterally. The tricipital line begins at the head of the humerus caudal to the greater tubercle and, in an uneven, cranially protruding arc, extends distally in the shape of a crest to the elongated **deltoid tuberosity** (*tuberositas deltoides*). On the tricipital line just distal to the head is a small enlargement for the insertion of the m. teres minor. The remaining distal part of the line serves for the origin of the mm. triceps–caput laterale. The deltoid tuberosity is the most prominent feature of the lateral surface of the humerus and serves for the insertion of the m. deltoideus.

The **brachialis groove** (*sulcus m. brachialis*), or musculospiral groove (Hughes & Dransfield, 1953), forms the smooth, flat to convex, lateral surface of most of the humerus. It begins at the neck caudally and extends laterally and finally cranially as it twists to the distal extremity of the bone. Although the m. brachialis lies in the whole groove, it arises from the proximal part only. Both the proximal and the distal parts of the lateral surface incline cranially. The proximal part lies between the **crest of the greater tubercle** (*crista tuberculi majoris*) medially and the tricipital line laterally.

The **medial surface** (*facies medialis*) is rounded transversely, except for a nearly flat triangular area in its proximal fourth. Caudally, this area is bounded by the **crest of the lesser tubercle** (*crista tuberculi minoris*), which ends distally in an inconspicuous eminence, and the **tuberosity for the teres major** (*tuberositas teres major*), which lies in the same transverse plane as the laterally located deltoid tuberosity. The m. coracobrachialis inserts on the crest of the lesser tubercle adjacent to the teres tuberosity. Cranial to this insertion the mm. triceps–caput mediale arises from the crest of the lesser tubercle by a small aponeurosis. The mm. teres major and the latissimus dorsi insert on the teres tuberosity. The medial surface of the humerus is loosely covered by the m. biceps brachii.

The **cranial surface** (*facies cranialis*) of the humerus is narrow and begins proximally at the crest of the greater tubercle. This crest passes just medial to the deltoid tuberosity, where it reaches the cranial edge of the brachialis groove. The entire m. pectoralis superficialis attaches to the crest of the greater tubercle, and a portion of the m. pectoralis profundus attaches to its proximal part.

The **caudal surface** (*facies caudalis*) (see Fig. 4.97) begins at the neck of the humerus where the mm. triceps–caput accessorium arises. As a transversely rounded margin, it extends to the distal fourth of the bone, where it is continued by the **lateral supracondylar crest** (*crista supracondylaris lateralis*). The mm. brachioradialis, extensor carpi radials, and anconeus attach to this crest. The caudal border is perforated below its middle by the distally directed **nutrient foramen**.

The **humeral condyle** (*condylus humeri*) is the entire sagittally rounded distal end of the humerus exclusive of the epicondyles. It may be divided into a small, lateral articular surface, the **capitulum humeri**, for articulation with the head of the radius, and the **trochlea humeri**, a much larger medially located, pulley-shaped part that extends proximally into the adjacent fossae (see Figs. 4.95 and 4.96). The trochlea articulates extensively with the trochlear notch of the ulna in forming one of the most stable hinge joints in the body. Laterally it also articulates with a portion of the fovea of the radius.

The **olecranon fossa** (*fossa olecrani*) (Fig. 4.97) is a deep excavation of the caudal part of the humeral condyle. It receives the anconeal process of the ulna when the elbow joint is extended. The olecranon fossa, in life, is covered by the m. anconeus, which arises from its margin. Opposite the olecranon fossa is the **radial fossa** (*fossa radialis*) on the cranial surface of the condyle (Fig. 4.101). This has also been called the *coronoid fossa* (*fossa coronoidea*) by Getty (1975), Baum and Zietzschmann (1936), and Hughes and Dransfield (1953). The dog has no coronoid fossa because

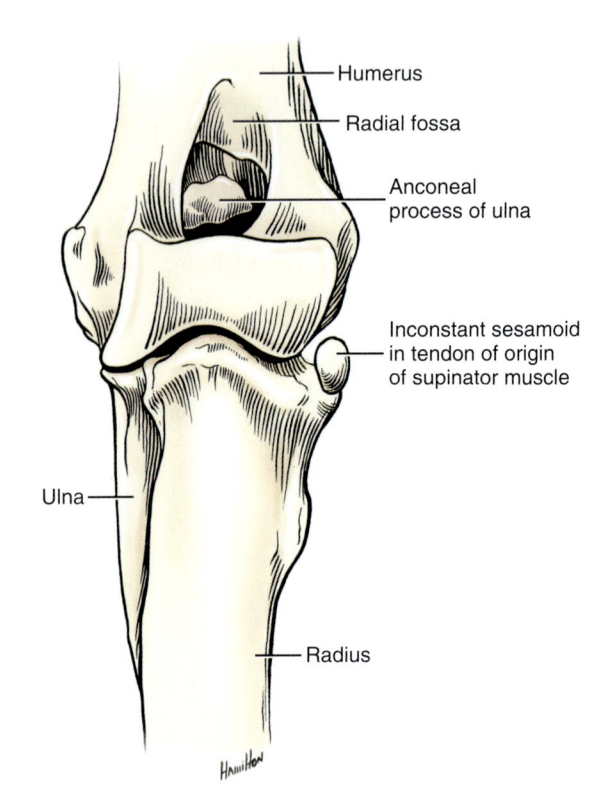

• **Fig. 4.101** Left elbow joint of a coy-dog, cranial view.

only the head of the radius enters this depression when the elbow joint is flexed, and not the coronoid process of the ulna. The radial and olecranon fossae communicate with each other by means of the **supratrochlear foramen** (*foramen supratrochleare*). No structures pass through this foramen. The foramen may be absent when the humerus is small.

The **lateral epicondyle** (*epicondylus lateralis*) (see Figs. 4.95 and 4.97) is a lateral prominence on the humeral condyle. It lies caudoproximal to the lateral articular margin of the capitulum. It gives origin to the mm. extensor digitorum communis, extensor digitorum lateralis, and the ulnaris lateralis. Functionally, it is known as the extensor epicondyle of the humerus. The proximal end of the lateral ligament of the elbow joint attaches to the articular margin and adjacent surface of the lateral epicondyle. The lateral supracondylar crest (*crista supracondylaris lateralis*) extends proximally from the lateral epicondyle. It is a thick, rounded crest that ends by blending with the caudal border at the beginning of the distal fourth of the humeral body. The m. brachioradialis arises from the proximal part of the crest, and the m. extensor carpi radialis arises from the remaining part.

The **medial epicondyle** (*epicondylus medialis*) (see Fig. 4.97) is a prominence on the medial side of the condyle just proximal to the medial border of the articular surface of the trochlea. It is functionally known as the *flexor epicondyle*. Larger than the lateral epicondyle, it gives origin to the m. flexor carpi radialis, m. flexor digitorum superficialis, and the humeral heads of the mm. flexor digitorum profundus and flexor carpi ulnaris. The proximal end of the medial ligament of the elbow joint attaches to the articular margin and adjacent surface of the medial epicondyle.

Radius

The **radius** (Fig. 4.102 through 4.108) is the main weight-supporting bone of the forearm; it is shorter than the ulna, which parallels it and serves primarily for muscle attachment. The radius articulates with the humerus proximally in forming the elbow joint and with the carpal bones distally in forming the antebrachiocarpal joint, which is the main joint for motion in the carpus. It also articulates with the ulna proximally by its caudal surface and distally by its lateral border. The radius is divided into a proximal head and neck, a body and a trochlear distally.

The **head** (*caput radii*) is irregularly oval in outline as it extends transversely across the proximal end of the bone. Its concave **articular fovea** (*fovea capitis radii*) articulates with the capitulum and lateral part of the trochlea of the humerus and bears practically all the weight transmitted from the arm to the forearm. The **articular circumference** (*circumferentia articularis*) is a caudal, smooth, osseous band on the head for articulation with the radial notch of the ulna (Fig. 4.102). The articular circumference is longer than the corresponding notch in the ulna so that a limited amount of rotation of the forearm is possible. The bulbous eminence on the lateral surface of the head does not serve for muscular attachment. The m. supinator passes over it in its course to a more distal attachment. A sesamoid bone is frequently associated with the supinator muscle at this site.

The **neck** (*collum radii*) is the constricted segment of the radius that joins the head to the body. The constriction is more distinct laterally and cranially than it is elsewhere. The **radial tuberosity** (*tuberositas radii*) is a small projection that lies distally on the neck on the medial border and adjacent caudal surface of the bone. It is particularly variable in development, depending on the breed. This tuberosity serves for the lesser insertion of the mm. biceps brachii. A large eminence lies proximal to the radial tuberosity on the lateral border of the radius and serves for the distal attachment of the cranial crus of the lateral collateral ligament of the elbow joint (see Fig. 5.22).

The **body** (*corpus radii*), or shaft, is compressed so that it presents two surfaces and two borders. Its width is two or three times its thickness. The **cranial surface** (*facies cranialis*) (see Fig. 4.103) is convex both transversely and vertically. At the junction of the proximal and middle thirds, on the medial border, there frequently is an obliquely placed rough line or ridge to which the m. pronator teres attaches. The m. supinator originates from the lateral epicondyle of the humerus and inserts on most of the cranial surface of

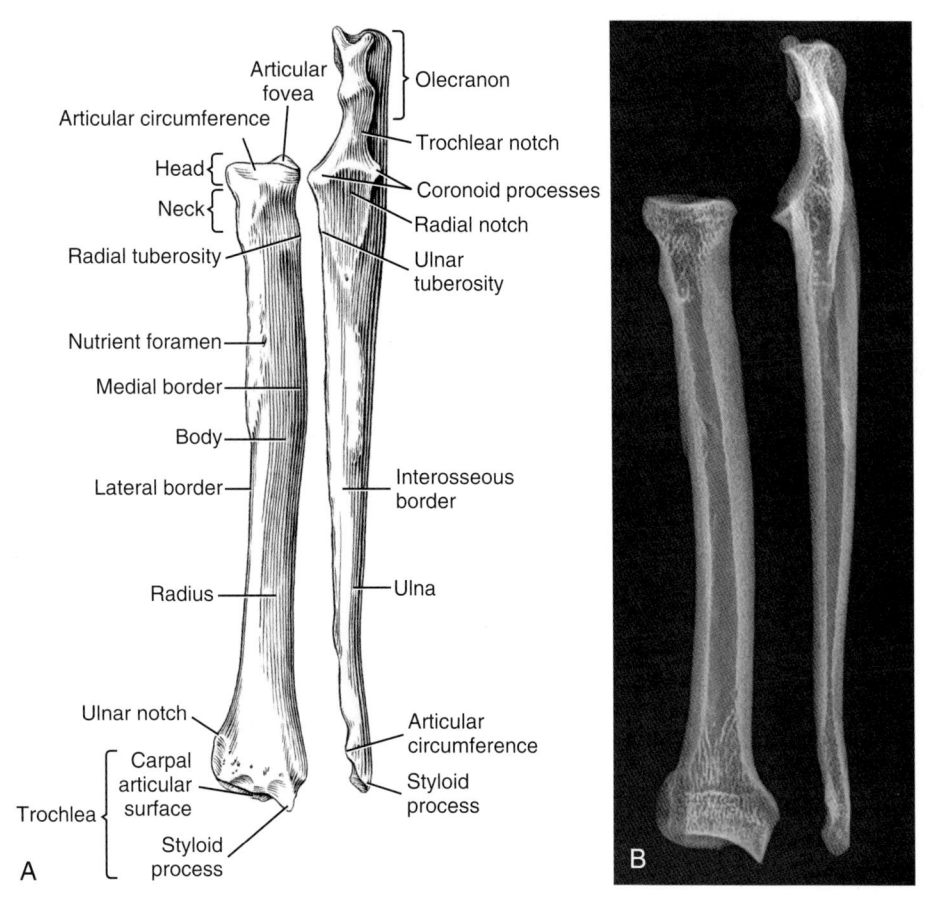

• **Fig. 4.102** A, Left radius, caudal surface. Left ulna, cranial surface. B, Craniocaudal radiograph, left radius and ulna disarticulated.

148 CHAPTER 4 The Skeleton

- **Fig. 4.103 A,** Left radius and ulna articulated, cranial aspect. **B,** Left radius and ulna articulated, caudal aspect. **C,** Craniocaudal radiograph, left radius and ulna articulated. **D,** Lateromedial radiograph, left radius and ulna articulated.

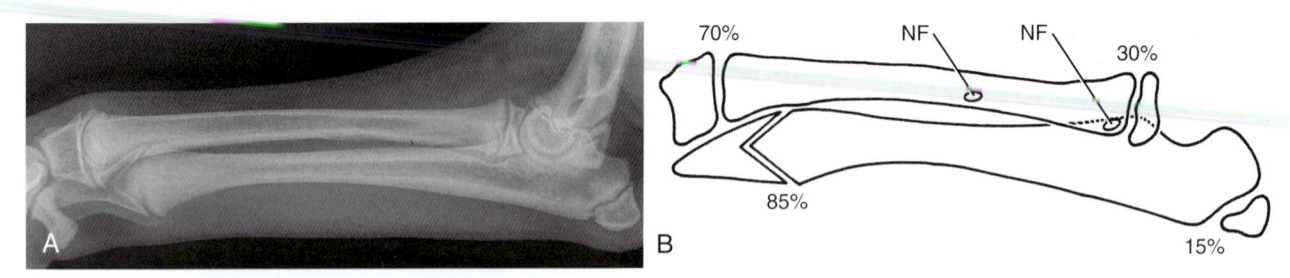

- **Fig. 4.104 A,** Radiograph of a 4-month-old dog. Note that the ulna is larger in the diameter than the radius at this age. Because of the more rapid growth of the distal end of the radius, it tends to bow. **B,** Drawing of the radius and ulna, depicting the percentage of growth each growth plate contributes to its bone length and the location of the nutrient artery for each bone. NF = nutrient foramen. (With permission from Riser WH: The dog: His varied biological make-up and its relationship to orthopaedic diseases, *Am Anim Hosp Assoc Monograph* 1985.)

the radius proximal to the insertion of the m. pronator teres. In large specimens, starting at the middle of the lateral border, and continuing distally from this border, there are alternating smooth ridges and grooves that run across the cranial surface of the radius; these markings converge toward a short but distinct, oblique groove on the medial part of the distal extremity of the bone. The m. abductor digiti I longus, which arises on the ulna as it courses distally, crosses the cranial surface of the radius obliquely and accounts for these markings (see Figs. 6.55 and 6.58).

• **Fig. 4.105** Lateral radiograph of the elbow.

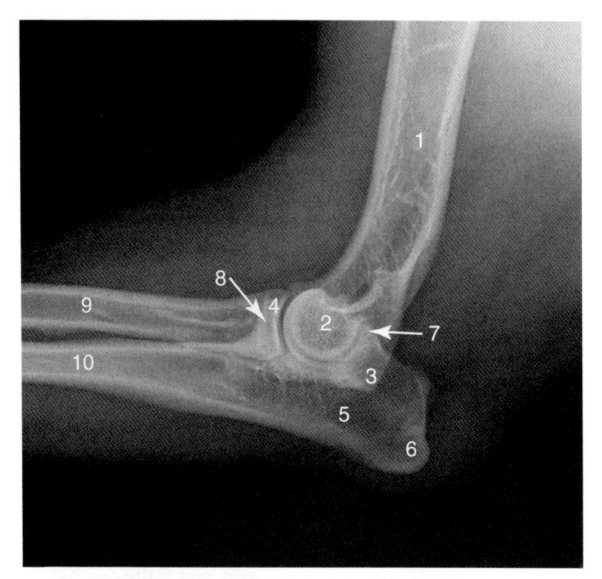

1. Body of humerus
2. Humeral condyle
3. Medial epicondyle of humerus
4. Head of radius
5. Olecranon of ulna
6. Olecranon tuber
7. Anconeal process of olecranon
8. Medial coronoid process of ulna
9. Body of radius
10. Body of ulna

• **Fig. 4.106** Lateral radiograph of a young dog's elbow.;

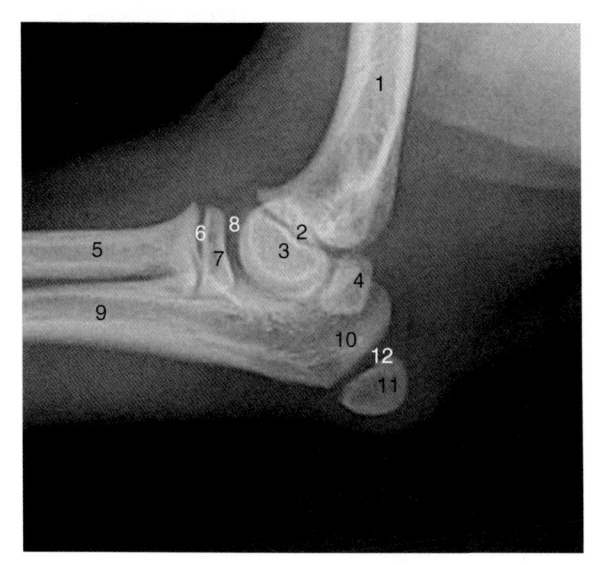

1. Humerus
2. Distal humeral physis
3. Humeral condyle (distal epiphysis)
4. Medial epicondyle (apophysis)
5. Radius
6. Proximal radial physis
7. Head of radius (proximal epiphysis)
8. Radiohumeral joint
9. Ulna
10. Olecranon
11. Olecranon tuber (apophysis)
12. Physis for olecranon tuber

• **Fig. 4.107** Craniocaudal radiograph of the elbow:

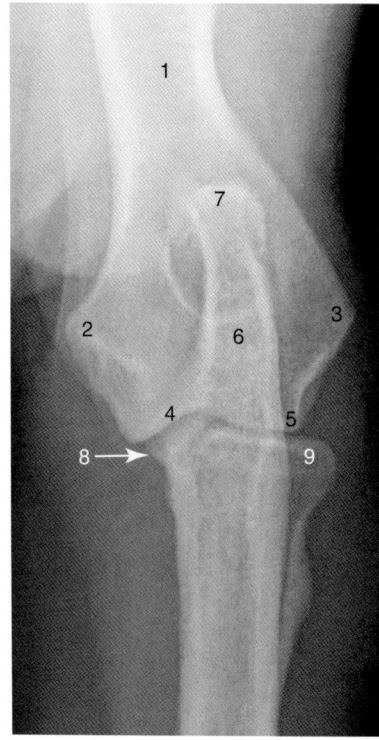

1. Body of humerus
2. Medial epicondyle
3. Lateral epicondyle
4. Trochlea of humerus
5. Capitulum of humerus
6. Olecranon
7. Olecranon tuber
8. Medial coronoid process
9. Head of radius

The **caudal surface** (*facies caudalis*) is divided into two flat to concave areas by a vertical interosseous border, which does not extend to either extremity of the radius (see Fig. 4.102). It divides the caudal surface into a medial two-thirds and a lateral one-third. The interosseous membrane attaches to it. The larger, flat, rough area medial to the border gives attachment to the m. pronator quadratus (Fig. 6.53). A prominent rough area extends from the proximal part of the interosseous border distally to the lateral border. The heavy, short, interosseous ligament that unites the radius and ulna attaches to this raised, roughened area. Slightly proximal to the middle of the caudal surface of the radius is the proximally directed nutrient foramen. Distally, the caudal surface becomes smoother, wider, and more convex as it blends with the caudal surface of the distal extremity of the bone.

The **medial** and **lateral borders** of the body of the radius present no special features. They are smooth and acutely rounded as they form the margins of the two surfaces of the bone. In large specimens, the rough area just proximal to the middle of the bone on the caudal surface encroaches on the lateral border. This serves for the attachment of the interosseous ligament.

The **trochlea** (trochlear radii) is the distal extremity of the radius and the most massive part of the bone. Its distal articular surface (*facies articularis carpea*) articulates primarily with the intermedioradial carpal bone (see Fig. 4.108) and to a lesser extent with the ulnar carpal. This surface is concave, both transversely and longitudinally, except for a caudomedial projection that lies in the groove of the intermedioradial carpal bone. The lateral surface of the trochlea is slightly concave and lipped, forming the **ulnar notch** (*incisura ulnaris*), which articulates with the **articular circumference** (*circumferential articularis*) near the distal end

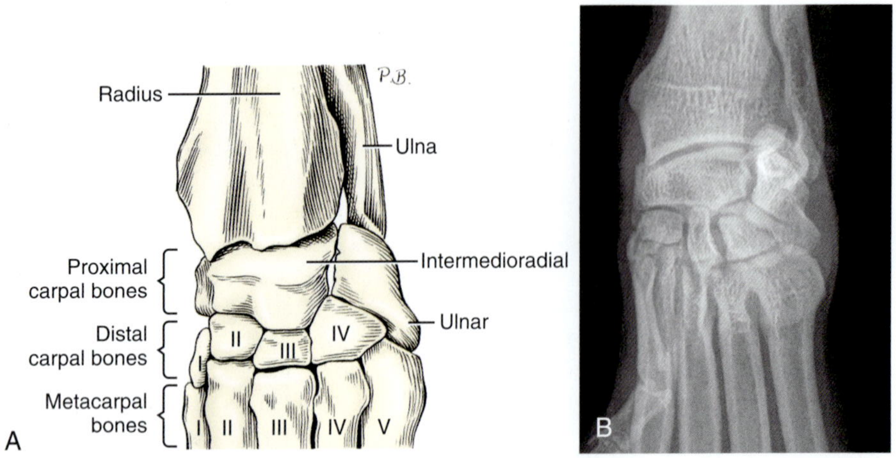

• **Fig. 4.108** **A**, Left carpus, articulated, dorsal aspect. **B**, Dorsopalmar radiograph of left carpus.

of the ulna head. Medially, the **radial styloid process** (*processus styloideus*) extends distal to the main carpal articular surface in the form of a sharp, wedge-shaped projection. The lateral surface of the styloid process enters into the formation of the carpal articular surface. The medial portion is somewhat flattened for the proximal attachment of the medial ligament of the carpal joint. The cranial surface of the trochlea of the radius presents three distinct grooves (Fig. 4.103). The most medial groove, which is short, distinct, and obliquely placed, lodges the tendon of the m. abductor digiti I longus. The middle groove, which is the largest, contains the tendon of the m. extensor carpi radialis. The most lateral groove, which is wider but occasionally less distinct than the others, contains the tendon of the m. extensor digitorum communis. The extensor retinaculum blends with the periosteum on the lip of the carpal articular surface. The caudal surface of the distal extremity is rough-ended and tuberculate. It contains many foramina for the passage of veins from the bone. The flexor retinaculum blends with the periosteum on this surface.

Ulna

The **ulna** (Figs. 4.102 to 4.108), for descriptive purposes, is divided into a body, or shaft, and two extremities. The proximal extremity is the olecranon and the distal extremity is the head. Located largely in the postaxial part of the forearm, it exceeds the radius in length and is, in fact, the longest bone in the body. Proximally it articulates with the humerus by the **trochlear notch** (*incisura trochlearis*) and with the articular circumference of the radius by the **radial notch** (*incisura radialis*). Distally it articulates with the ulnar notch of the radius and with the ulnar carpal and accessory carpal bones by means of two confluent articular surfaces on the knoblike head.

The proximal extremity of the ulna includes the olecranon and the articulation of the ulna with the humerus and radius. The **olecranon** includes the olecranon tuber, the anconeal process and the proximal part of the trochlear notch. It serves as a lever arm, or tension process, for the powerful extensor muscles of the elbow joint. It is four-sided, laterally compressed, and medially inclined; its proximal end is grooved cranially and enlarged and rounded caudally. The mm. triceps brachii, anconeus, and tensor fasciae antebrachii attach to the caudal part of the olecranon; the mm. flexor carpi ulnaris–caput ulnare and the flexor digitorum profundus–caput ulnare arise from the medial and caudal surfaces of the olecranon (see Figs. 6.53 and 6.54).

The **trochlear notch** (*incisura trochlearis*) is known in some texts as the *semilunar notch*. It is a smooth, vertical, half-moon–shaped concavity that faces cranially. The semilunar outline of this salient notch is formed by a sagittally placed ridge that divides its articular area into two nearly equal parts. The whole trochlear notch articulates with the trochlea of the humerus so that the sharp-edged, slightly hooked **anconeal process** (*processus anconeus*), at its proximal end, fits in the olecranon fossa of the humerus when the elbow is extended.

Van Sickle (1966) made a radiographic study of the osseous development of the elbow in the German Shepherd Dog and Greyhound. By comparison of radiographs of both breeds it was observed that bone development was similar. At 11 to 12 weeks of age several small ossific centers appeared in the cartilage of the anconeal process. Fusion of the small centers formed a single nodule that for a time was separated from the ulna by a plate of cartilage. The first fusion of the anconeal center to the ulna took place at the margin of the semilunar notch. Fusion of the anconeal process with the ulna was complete by 14 to 15 weeks in the Greyhound and 16 to 20 weeks of age in the German Shepherd Dog (see Fig. 4.104).

At the distal end of the trochlear notch are the medial coronoid process (*processus coronoideus medialis*) and the lateral coronoid process (*processus coronoideus lateralis*) that form a notch that articulates with the articular circumference of the radius. The medial coronoid process is considerably larger than the lateral process and projects on the medial surface of the elbow joint. Both of these eminences are articular, facing cranially and proximally, where they articulate with the radius and humerus, respectively. They area of the elbow joint without contributing materially to its weight-bearing function.

The **body** (*corpus ulnae*), or shaft, in the larger working breeds is typically compressed laterally in its proximal third, three-sided throughout its middle third, and cylindrical in its distal third. Great variation exists, however, and, in long-limbed breeds, the body is somewhat flattened throughout its length. The **cranial surface** (*facies cranialis*) is rough and convex, both longitudinally and transversely. Its most prominent feature is a slightly raised, oval, rough area on the middle third of the bone. It serves for the ulnar attachment of the short, but thick, interosseous ligament that attaches to the radius. The **interosseous border** (*margo interosseous*) extends proximally from the notch that separates the distal extremity, the head, from the body of the ulna. The interosseous membrane attaches to the interosseous border. Medial to the border a faint vascular groove indicates the position, in life, of the caudal interosseous artery. The largest nutrient foramen is directed proximally and is usually located proximal to the rough area for the attachment of the interosseous ligament, near the interosseous border. Other smaller nutrient foramina are located along the course of the vascular groove in the middle third of the body. The m. pronator quadratus attaches to the cranial surface of the ulna medial and adjacent to the interosseous border. The mm. abductor digiti I longus, extensor digiti I, and extensor digiti II arise in that order from the cranial surface of the body of the ulna, progressing from the interosseous border to the lateral border (Fig. 6.58). The **caudal border** (*margo caudalis*) of the ulna body, unlike the cranial surface, is smooth and concave throughout. It gradually tapers toward the head. The m. flexor digitorum profundus–caput ulnare arises largely from this surface lateral to the radius. The mm. biceps brachii and brachialis insert mainly on the roughened area formerly called the **ulnar tuberosity** (*tuberositas ulnae*), which is located near the proximal end of the medial border just distal to the medial coronoid process. The **medial border** (*margo medialis*) is sharper and straighter than the lateral one. The **lateral border** (*margo lateralis*) continues the wide, rounded, caudal border of the olecranon distally and laterally to the distal extremity of the bone.

The foregoing description of the body of the ulna does not apply to some specimens, in which the middle third is more prismatic than flat. When the middle third is definitely three-sided, this feature continues distally, transforming the usually rodlike distal third to one that is three-sided.

The distal extremity of the ulna is the head of the ulna. It is separated from the body of the bone by a notch in its cranial border. An oval, slightly raised articular surface, the **articular circumference** (*circumferentia articularis*) is located in the distal part of the notch for articulation with the ulnar notch of the radius. The pointed, enlarged distal extremity of the head is the **styloid process** (*processus styloideus*). On its distomedial part there are two confluent surfaces. The one that faces cranially is concave and articulates with the ulnar carpal bone; the smaller, convex, medial surface articulates with the accessory carpal bone. The styloid process of the ulna projects slightly farther distally than the styloid process of the radius. Johnson (1981) reported retardation of endochondral ossification at the distal ulna growth plate.

Carrig and Morgan (1975) studied the asynchronous growth of the radius and ulna. They documented early radiographic changes following experimental retardation of longitudinal growth of the ulna.

Forepaw

The skeleton of the **forepaw** (*manus*) (Figs. 4.108 to 4.117) includes the bones of the carpus, metacarpus, phalanges, and certain sesamoid bones associated with them. The **carpus** is composed of seven bones arranged in two transverse rows, plus a small medial sesamoid bone. Articulating with the distal row of carpal bones are the five metacarpal bones that lie alongside one another and are enclosed in a common integument. Each of the lateral four metacarpal bones bears three phalanges that, with their associated sesamoid bones, form the skeleton of the four main digits. The small, medially located, first metacarpal bone bears only two phalanges, which form the skeleton of the rudimentary first digit. The bones of a typical tetrapod manus are serially homologous with those of the pes. In the lower vertebrate forms, three groupings of the carpal and tarsal bones are

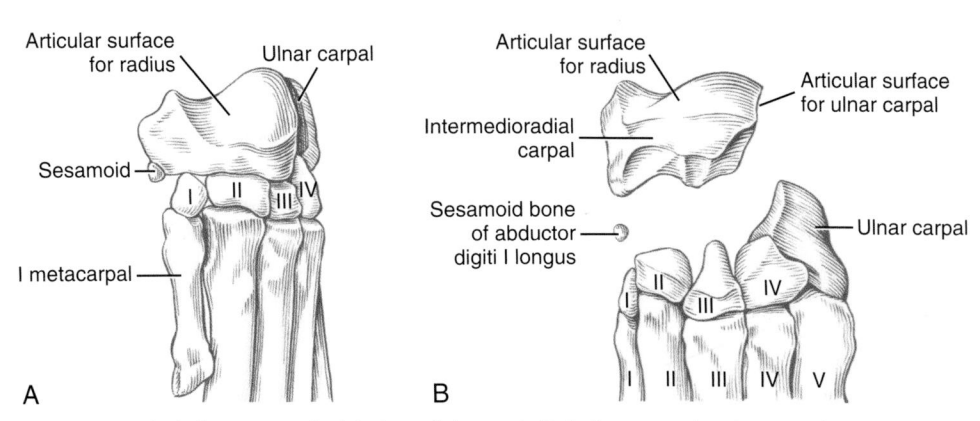

• **Fig. 4.109** A, Left carpus, articulated, medial aspect. B, Left carpus, dorsal aspect. Intermedioradial carpal disarticulated.

152 CHAPTER 4 The Skeleton

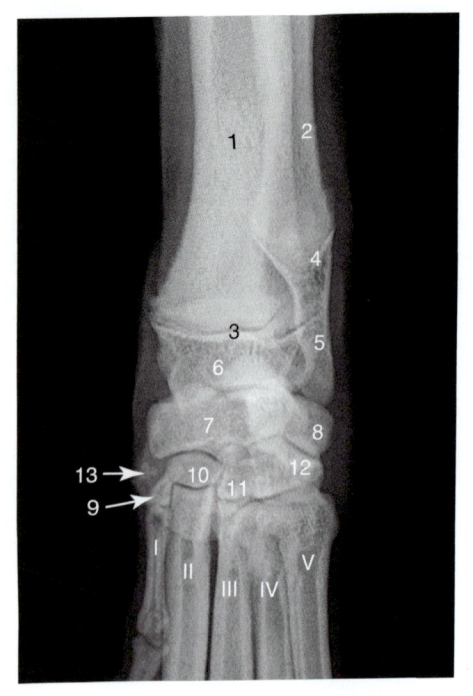

1. Radius
2. Ulna
3. Distal radial physis
4. Distal ulnar physis
5. Styloid process
6. Radial trochlea (distal epiphysis)
7. Intermedioradial carpal bone
8. Ulnar carpal bone
9. First carpal bone
10. Second carpal bone
11. Third carpal bone
12. Fourth carpal bone
13. Sesamoid bone in abductor digiti 1 longus
14. I-V Metacarpal bones

• **Fig. 4.110** Dorsopalmar radiograph of the carpus.

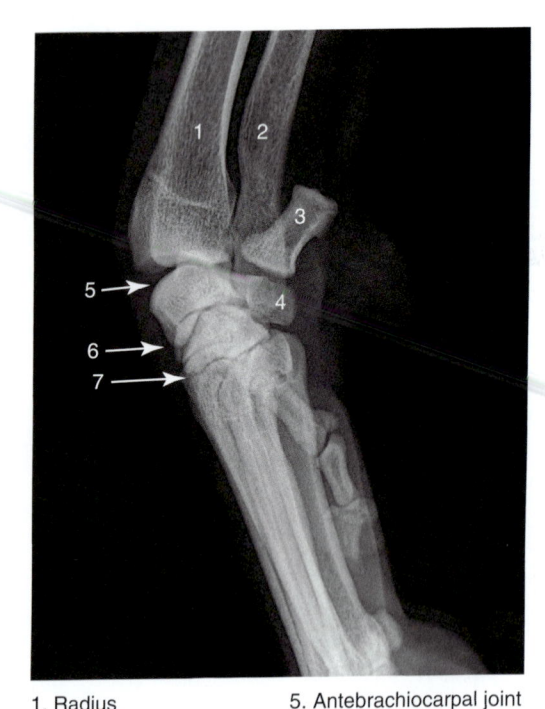

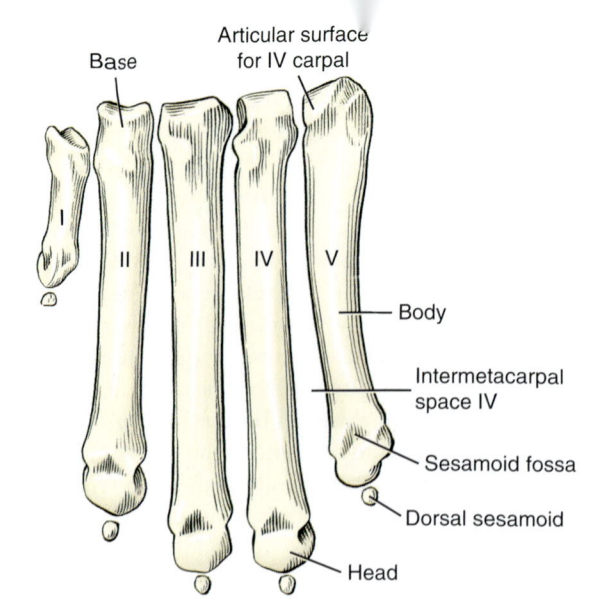

• **Fig. 4.112** Left metacarpal and sesamoid bones, disarticulated, dorsal aspect.

1. Radius
2. Ulna
3. Accessory carpal
4. Ulnar carpal
5. Antebrachiocarpal joint
6. Middle carpal joint
7. Carpometacarpal joint

• **Fig. 4.111** Lateral radiograph of the flexed carpus.

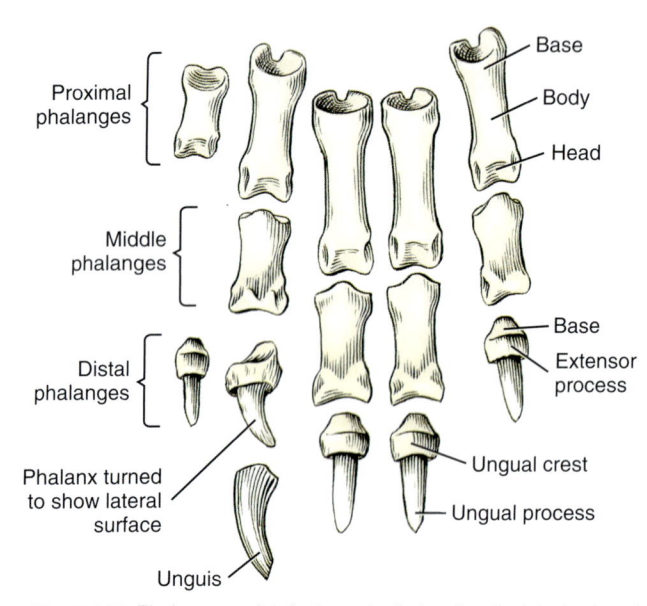

• **Fig. 4.113** Phalanges of left thoracic limb, disarticulated, dorsal aspect.

made. The proximal grouping includes the radial, intermediate, and ulnar carpal bones for the manus, and the tibial, intermediate, and fibular tarsal bones for the pes. The middle grouping includes the central elements, of which there are three or four in each extremity. The distal grouping comprises a row of five small bones that articulate distally with the five metacarpal or metatarsal bones. There has been considerable modification of this primitive arrangement in mammals with the fusion or loss of various elements.

Carpus

The **carpus** (Figs. 4.108 to 4.111, 4.115, and 4.116) includes the **carpal bones** (*ossa carpi*) and the associated sesamoid bones. The term *carpus* also designates the

CHAPTER 4 The Skeleton 153

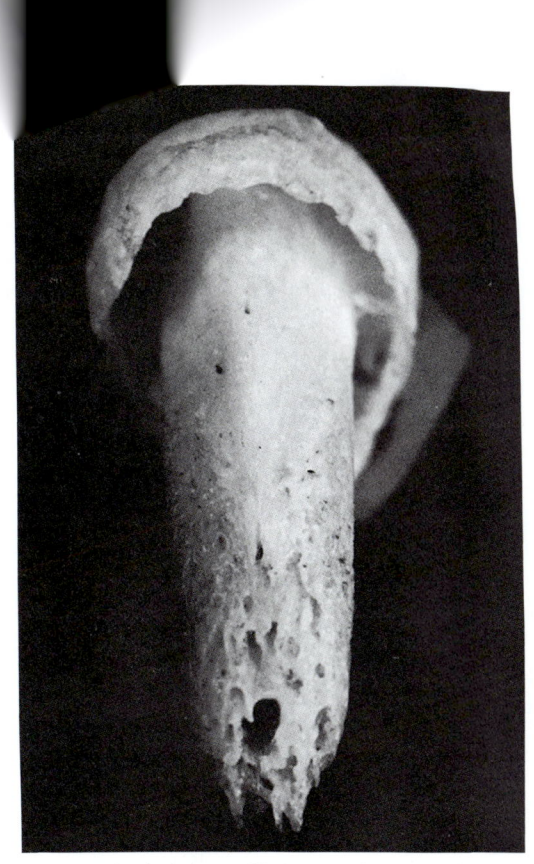

• Fig. 4.114 A distal phalanx with the unguis removed, dorsal view.

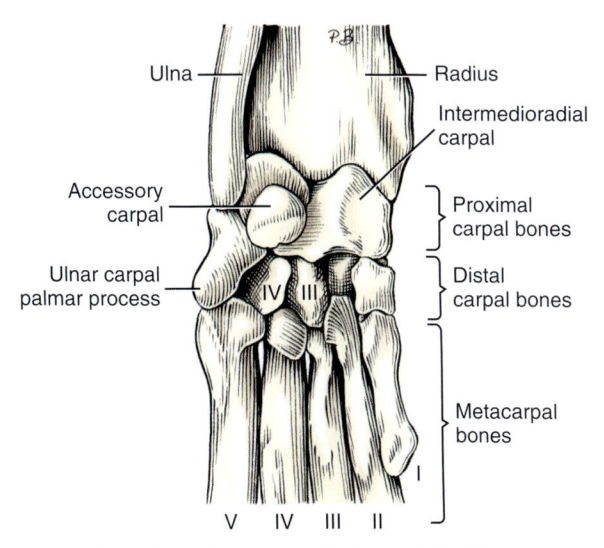

• Fig. 4.115 Left carpus, articulated, palmar aspect.

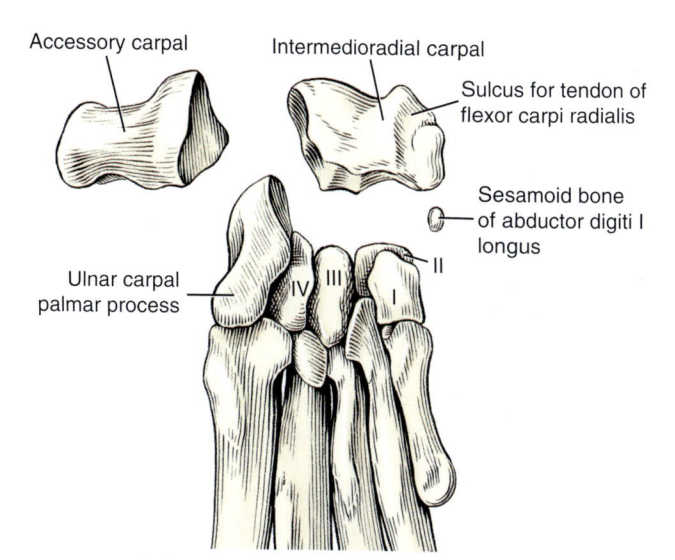

• Fig. 4.116 Left carpal and metacarpal bones, palmar aspect. Intermedioradial and accessory carpals disarticulated.

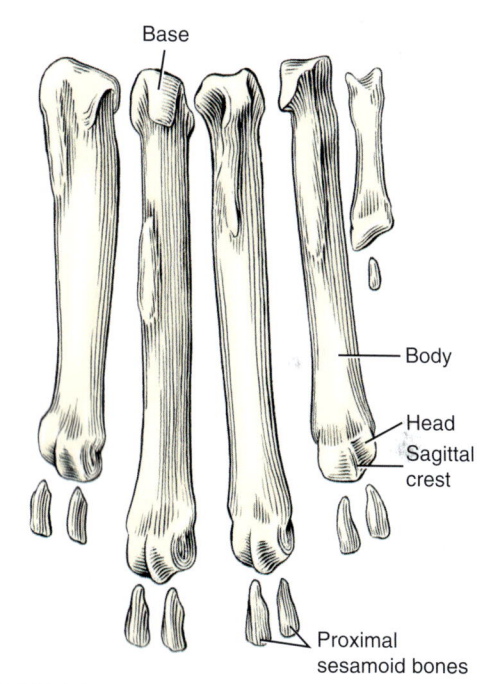

• Fig. 4.117 Left metacarpal and sesamoid bones, disarticulated, palmar aspect.

compound joint formed by these bones, as well as the region between the forearm and the metacarpus. The carpal bones of the dog are arranged in a proximal and a distal row so that they form a transversely convex dorsal outline and a concave palmar one. The bones of the proximal row are the intermedioradial, ulnar, and accessory carpal bones. Those of the distal row are the first, second, third, and fourth carpal bones.

The **intermedioradial carpal bone** (*os carpi intermedioradiale*) located on the medial side of the proximal row, is the largest of the carpal elements. It represents a fusion of the primitive radial carpal bone with the central and intermediate carpal bones. The proximal surface of the bone is largely articular for the trochlea of the radius. The distal surface of the intermedioradial carpal bone articulates with all four distal carpal bones. Laterally it articulates extensively with the ulnar carpal. Its transverse dimension is about twice its width.

The **ulnar carpal bone** (*os carpi ulnare*) is the lateral bone of the proximal row. It is shaped somewhat like the intermedioradial carpal but is smaller. It articulates proximally with the ulna and radius, distally with the fourth carpal and the fifth metacarpal, medially with the intermedioradial carpal, and on the palmar side with the accessory carpal. It possesses a small lateral process and a larger palmar one for articulation with the accessory carpal and metacarpal V. This latter process is separated from the main part of the bone on the lateral side by a concave articular area for articulation with the styloid process of the ulna.

The **accessory carpal bone** (*os carpi accessorium*) is a truncated rod of bone located on the palmar side of the ulnar carpal. Both ends of this bone are enlarged. The basal enlargement bears a slightly saddle-shaped articular surface for the ulnar carpal, which is separated by an acute angle from a smaller, transversely concave, proximally directed articular area for the styloid process of the ulna. The free end is thickened and overhangs slightly. The accessory carpal bone is not a true carpal bone phylogenetically but is rather a relatively new acquisition found in reptiles and mammals (Romer & Parsons, 1986). The mm. flexor carpi ulnaris and ulnaris lateralis insert on it.

The **first carpal bone** (*os carpale primum*) is the smallest carpal bone. It is somewhat flattened as it articulates with the palmaromedial surfaces of the second carpal and the base of metacarpal II. It articulates proximally with the intermedioradial carpal and distally with metacarpal I.

The **second carpal bone** (*os carpale secundum*) is a small, wedge-shaped, proximodistally compressed bone that articulates proximally with the intermedioradial carpal, distally with metacarpal II, laterally with the third carpal, and medially with the first carpal.

The **third carpal bone** (*os carpale tertium*) is larger than the second carpal. It has a large palmar projection, which articulates with the three middle metacarpal bones (see Fig. 4.115). It articulates medially with the second carpal, laterally with the fourth carpal, proximally with the intermedioradial carpal, and distally with metacarpal III.

The **fourth carpal bone** (*os carpale quartum*) is the largest bone of the distal row. It presents a caudal enlargement and is wedge-shaped in both dorsal and proximal views. It articulates distally with metacarpals IV and V, medially with the third carpal, proximomedially with the intermedioradial carpal, and proximolaterally with the ulnar carpal bone.

Each carpal element chondrifies independently before losing its identity. The intermediate carpal element fuses with the radial carpal and then the two, in turn, fuse with the central carpal. The accessory carpal bone has an apophyseal center of ossification that elaborates the cap of the enlarged palmar end of the bone.

The smallest bone of the carpus is a spherical sesamoid bone, about the size of a radish seed, that is located in the tendon of insertion of the m. abductor digiti I longus on the medial side of the proximal end of the first metacarpal.

Metacarpus

The term metacarpus refers to the region of the manus, or forepaw, located between the carpus and the digits. The **metacarpal bones** (*ossa metacarpalia I to V*) (Figs. 4.108 to 4.112, Figs. 4.115 to 4.117, and Fig. 4.119) are typically five in number in primitive mammals, although supernumerary metacarpal bones and digits may appear. In many mammals some of the metacarpal bones accompanying digits have been lost. Like the distal row bones, the metacarpal bones are numbered from the medial to the lateral side. The five metacarpal bones are each cylindrically shaped and enlarged at each end, proximally to form the **base**, and distally to form the **head**. The middle portion, or shaft, of each metacarpal bone is known as the **body**. Unlike the first metatarsal bone of the hindpaw, the **first metacarpal bone** of the forepaw is usually present, although it is by far the shortest and most slender of the metacarpal bones. It bears the first digit, which does not quite reach the level of the second metacarpophalangeal joint. Metacarpal I articulates proximally with the first carpal and laterally with the second metacarpal. Distally, its laterally enlarged head articulates with the proximal phalanx of the first digit and a single palmar sesamoid bone.

Metacarpal bones II to V are the main metacarpal bones. They are irregular rods with a uniform diameter. Metacarpals II and V are shorter than III and IV and are four-sided, particularly at their base whereas metacarpals III and IV are more triangular at their base. Distally, the bones diverge, forming the intermetacarpal spaces. The heads of the main metacarpal bones possess roller-like dorsal parts that are undivided and are separated from the bodies dorsally by **sesamoid fossae** (*fossae sesamoidales*). Between the heads and the bodies of the metacarpal bones on the palmar side are the **sesamoid impressions** (*impressiones sesamoidales*). The palmar parts of the heads possess prominent, sharp-edged **sagittal crests** (*cristae sagittales*), which effectively prevent lateral luxation of the two crescent-shaped sesamoid bones that articulate with these heads. The base of metacarpal II extends farther proximally than do the other metacarpal bones. It articulates with the first, second, and third carpals as well as with metacarpals I and III. In addition to articulating with adjacent metacarpals, the base of metacarpal III articulates with the third and fourth carpals; the base of metacarpal IV articulates with the fourth carpal; the base of metacarpal V articulates with the fourth carpal and the distopalmar extension of the ulnar carpal. The interosseous muscles arise from the palmar surfaces of the bases of all of the main metacarpal bones. The proximal palmar surfaces of the bodies of metacarpals II and III provide insertion for the m. flexor carpi radialis, and the dorsal surfaces of the bases provide insertion for the m. extensor carpi radialis. The m. ulnaris lateralis inserts on the lateral surface of the base of metacarpal V. The small m. adductor digiti V inserts on the medial surfaces of the distal parts of metacarpals IV and V and on the lateral surface of metacarpal V near the base of the bone. The m. abductor digiti I longus inserts on the proximal medial part of metacarpal I, and the m. extensor digiti I inserts on the proximal medial part of metacarpal I.

The middle parts of the bodies of the metacarpal bones have particularly dense walls. These walls become thinner toward the extremities so that the articular cartilages lie on thin cortical bases. During development, the main metacarpal bones have only distal epiphyses. According to Schaeffer has only a proximal epiphysis. On the ... of the palmar surface of each of the four ... metacarpal bones there is a nutrient foramen.

Shively (1978) has drawn attention to what several investigators have pointed out in the past regarding an inconsistency in the ossification pattern of the first metacarpal and metatarsal bones compared with those of digits II to V. The so-called first metapodials have an ossified growth plate on their proximal end, whereas the growth plate is on the distal end of ossa metacarpalia II to V and ossa metatarsalia II to V. If homologic development is the deciding factor, then the implication of this difference is that what is generally regarded as a first metapodial is really a first phalanx, and what is missing is a distal carpal element. Perhaps the sesamoid in the m. abductor digiti I longus is really the first metacarpal bone? There is fossil evidence, as Shively points out, of a mammalian ancestor, *Oudenodon*, that had elongated first carpal and first tarsal bones that could have served as metapodials, and there are three phalanges on each of the five digits.

Phalanges

The **digital skeleton** (*ossa digitorum manus*) (Figs. 4.113, 4.117, and 4.118) of the forepaw consists of five units, of which four are fully developed and one is rudimentary. The rudimentary first digit is called the *dewclaw* and in some breeds such as the St. Bernard it may be double (Alberch, 1985). Each main digit consists of a proximal phalanx, middle phalanx, and distal phalanx, and two large palmar sesamoid bones at the metacarpophalangeal joint. A small osseous nodule is also located in the dorsal part of the joint capsule of each of the metacarpophalangeal joints, and a small cartilaginous nodule is located in a like place on each of the distal interphalangeal joints.

The **proximal**, or **first**, **phalanx** (*phalanx proximalis*) of each of the main digits, II to V, is a medium-length rod with enlarged extremities. Proximally, at its base, it bears a transversely concave articular surface with a sharp dorsal border and a bituberculate palmar border. The palmar tubercles are separated by a deep groove that receives the sagittal crest of the head of a metacarpal bone when the joint is flexed. The palmar tubercles articulate with the distal end of the palmar sesamoid bones. The joint surface of the distal head is saddle-shaped, sagittally convex, and transversely concave. It extends more proximally on the palmar surface than on the dorsal one. As if to prevent undue spreading of the main abaxial digits, the m. adductor digiti V inserts on the medial surface of the proximal phalanx of digit V, and the m. adductor digiti II inserts on the lateral surface of the proximal phalanx of digit II. The proximal phalanx of digit I receives the insertions of mm. abductor digiti I brevis and adductor digiti I.

The **middle**, or **second**, **phalanx** (*phalanx media*) is present only in each of the main digits, there being none in digit I. Each middle phalanx is a rod approximately one-third shorter than the corresponding proximal phalanx with which it articulates. A palmar angle of approximately 135 degrees is formed by the proximal interphalangeal joint, whereas distally an obtuse palmar angle is formed as the distal phalanx butts against the middle phalanx, forming nearly a right angle dorsally. Each middle phalanx, like the proximal ones, is divided into a proximal **base**, a middle **body**, and a distal **head**. The base of each middle phalanx possesses an intermediate sagittal ridge, with palmar tubercles that are smaller and a palmar groove between these

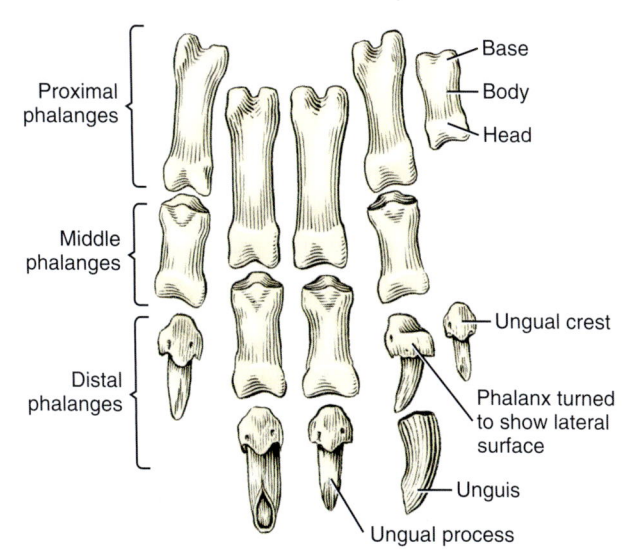

• **Fig. 4.118** Phalanges of left thoracic limb, disarticulated, palmar aspect.

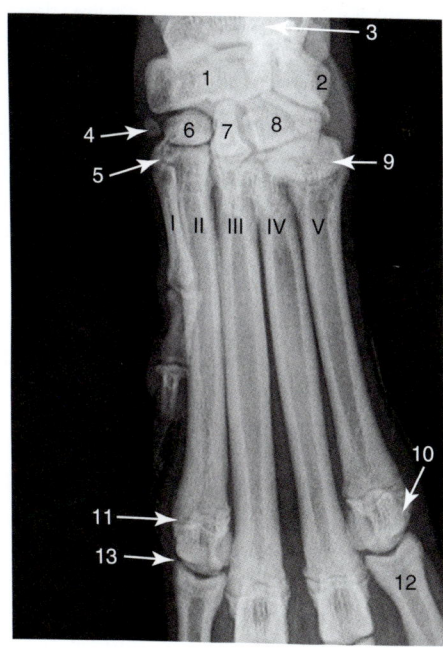

1. Intermedioradial carpal
2. Ulnar carpal
3. Accessory carpal
4. Sesamoid bone in abductor digiti I longus
5. Carpal I
6. Carpal II
7. Carpal III
8. Carpal IV
9. Base of metacarpal V
10. Head of metacarpal V
11. Distal physis of metacarpal II
12. Proximal phalanx of digit V
13. Metacarpophalangeal joint between metacarpal II and the first phalanx of digit II

• **Fig. 4.119** Dorsopalmar radiograph of the manus.

tubercles that is shallower than are those of the proximal phalanges. The m. flexor digitorum superficialis attaches to the palmar surface of the base of the four middle phalanges by means of its four tendons of insertion.

The **distal**, or **third**, **phalanx** (*phalanx distalis*) is approximately the same size in all four main digits. The distal phalanx of digit I is similar to the others in form but is smaller. The proximal part of the distal phalanx is enlarged. It has a shallow, sagittally concave articular area for contact with the middle phalanx (proximal phalanx of digit I), to form the distal interphalangeal joint. A rounded, broad, low tubercle on the palmar side serves for the insertion of one of the five parts into which the tendon of the m. flexor digitorum profundus divides. Each side of this tubercle is perforated by a foramen, the opening of a vascular canal that transversely perforates the bone. The dorsal part of the bone is also perforated by a vascular canal. The dorsal parts of the four main distal phalanges have a small extensor process to serve for the insertions of the four branches into which the tendon of the m. extensor digitorum communis divides. Joining the branches of the tendon of the m. extensor digitorum communis over the proximal phalanges is the tendon of the mm. extensor digiti I and extensor digiti II and the tendons of the m. extensor digitorum lateralis to digits III, IV, and V. The distal part of the distal phalanx is a laterally compressed cone, the **ungual process** (*processus unguicularis*), that is shielded by the horny claw (see Figs. 4.113, 4.114, and 4.118). It is porous and has ridges on its proximal dorsal part that fade distally. The wall of the claw attaches to this surface. The sole of the claw attaches to the flattened palmar surface. The lateral and dorsal parts of the base of the ungual process are overhung by a crescent-shaped shelf of bone, the **ungual crest** (*crista unguicularis*), under which the root of the claw is located (Fig. 4.118).

Sesamoid Bones

On the palmar surface of each metacarpophalangeal joint of the main digits are two elongated, slightly curved **sesamoid bones** (*ossa sesamoidea*) (see Fig. 4.117) that are located in the tendons of insertion of the interosseus muscles. They articulate primarily with the head of each metacarpal bone and secondarily with the palmar tubercles of the base of each proximal phalanx. Their truncated distal ends articulate by small facets with the palmar tubercles of the corresponding proximal phalanges. Only a single osseous bead is located on the palmar side of the metacarpophalangeal joint of digit I.

Small bony nodules are located in the dorsal parts of the extensor tendons of the four main digits at the metacarpophalangeal joints (see Fig. 4.112), whereas cartilaginous nodules are found at both the dorsal and the palmar sides of the distal interphalangeal joints.

Bones of the Pelvic Limb

Each pelvic limb (*membrum pelvinum*) consists of its half of the pelvic girdle (*cingulum membri pelvini*), composed of the **ilium**, **ischium**, **pubis**, and **acetabular** the hip bone (*os coxae*); the thigh, represented by the and the **sesamoids** associated with the stifle, the crus, or leg, consisting of the **tibia** and **fibula**; and the hindpaw, or pes. The pes includes the **tarsal bones**, **metatarsals**, and digits consisting of three **phalanges** in each, and the **sesamoid bones** associated with the phalanges.

The bony **pelvis** (see Fig. 4.120) is formed by the ossa coxarum and the sacrum.

Os Coxae

The *os coxae*, or **hip bone** (Figs. 4.120 to 4.126), is composed of four distinct bones developmentally. These are the ilium, ischium, pubis, and acetabular bone. They fuse during the twelfth postnatal week, forming the socket that receives the head of the femur in creation of the hip joint. This socket is a deep, cotyloid cavity called the **acetabulum**. The acetabulum in a medium-sized dog is 1 cm deep and 2 cm in diameter. The **lunate surface** (*facies lunata*) (Figs. 4.124 and 4.125) is the smooth articular circumference that is deficient over the medial portion of the acetabulum. The cranial part of the lunate surface is widest as it extends from the acetabular margin three fourths of the distance to the depth of the acetabulum. The lunate surface is narrowest midlaterally, being approximately one-half its maximum width. The cranial portion ends medially in a rounded border. Medially the acetabulum is indented by a **notch**, the *incisura acetabuli*. The caudal part of the acetabular margin, or lip, which forms the caudal boundary of the notch, is indented by a fissure 2 to 4 mm deep. The quadrangular, nonarticular, thin, depressed area that extends laterally from the acetabular notch is the **acetabular fossa** (*fossa acetabuli*). During the seventh postnatal week, a small osseous element, the **acetabular bone** (*os acetabuli*) (see Fig. 4.122A), located in the floor of the acetabulum between the ilium and the ischium, becomes incorporated with these larger bones. The **pelvic cavity** is of considerable obstetric importance because, for survival of the species in nature, it must be large enough to allow for the passage of the young during parturition. The **cranial pelvic aperture** (*apertura pelvis cranialis*), or **pelvic inlet**, is formed by the **promontory** of the sacrum dorsally, the **cranial border of the pubis**, or **pecten**, ventrally, and the **arcuate line** (*linea arcuata*) bilaterally. The arcuate line is the ventromedial border of the body of the ilium. It extends from the auricular surface to the **iliopubic eminence** (*eminentia pubica*). The **terminal line** (*linea terminalis*) is a circular line that outlines the cranial pelvic aperture by passing along the sacral promontory, the wing of the sacrum, the arcuate line and the pecten of the pubis. The following conventional measurements of the pelvis are useful in obstetrics: the **transverse diameter** (*diameter transversa*) is the greatest transverse measurement of the bony pelvic cavity. According to Roberts (1986), only in the achondroplastic types of dogs, such as the Sealyham and Pekingese, are the transverse diameters greater than the conjugate or sacropubic diameters. The **conjugate** (*conjugata*) measurement is the

CHAPTER 4 The Skeleton 157

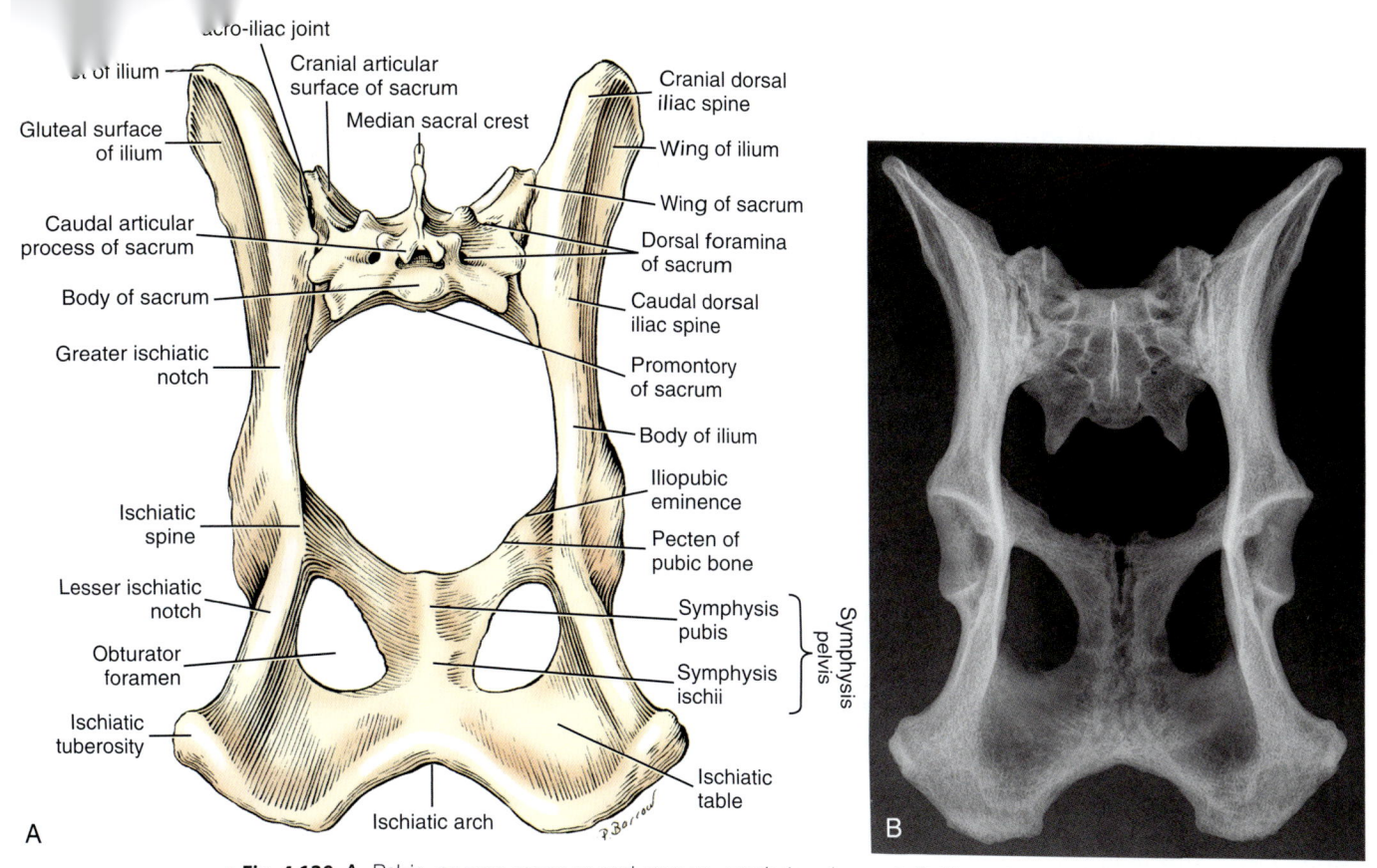

• **Fig. 4.120** **A**, Pelvis, or ossa coxarum and sacrum, caudodorsal aspect. **B**, Ventrodorsal radiograph, ossa coxarum and sacrum.

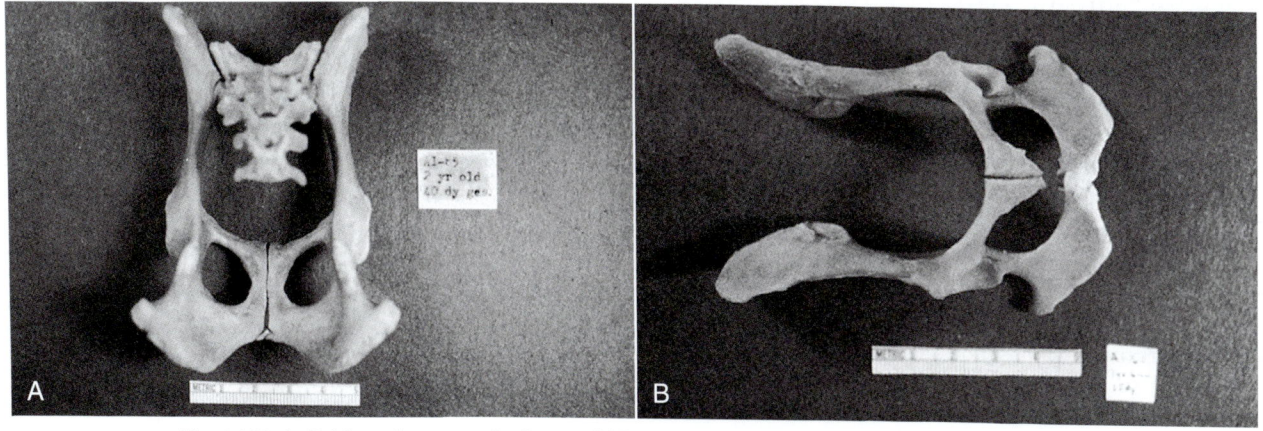

• **Fig. 4.121** **A**, Pelvis and sacrum of a 2-year-old Beagle. Note that only the caudal portion of the pelvic symphysis is fused. (Dermestid beetle preparation.) **B**, Pelvis of a Beagle 1 year and 6 months old with an incomplete fusion of the pelvic symphysis.

distance from the sacral promontory to the cranial border of the symphysis pubis. The **oblique diameter** (*diameter obliqua*) is measured from the sacroiliac articulation of one side to the iliopubic eminence of the other. The **pelvic axis** (*axis pelvis*) is an imaginary, slightly curved line drawn through the middle of the pelvic cavity from the pelvic inlet to the pelvic outlet. The **caudal pelvic aperture** (*apertura pelvis caudalis*), or **pelvic outlet**, is bounded dorsally by the first caudal vertebra, bilaterally by the sacrotuberous ligament, and ventrally by the caudolateral border of the tuber ischiadicum on each side and the ischiatic arch located between them. The sacral part of the roof of the pelvic canal is approximately as long as its floor but is offset to the extent that a transverse plane touching the caudal part of the sacrum also touches the cranial border of the pubis. The lateral osseous wall of the pelvic canal is formed largely by the body of the ilium and caudally, to a small extent, by the bodies of the ischium and pubis as these fuse to form the acetabulum. The floor of the bony pelvis is formed by the sacropelvic surfaces of the rami of the pubes and ischia. Between these rami and the body of the ischium is the large, oval to triangular **obturator foramen** (*foramen obturatum*). The **symphysis pelvis** is the median synostosis formed by the right and left pubic and ischial bones. It is therefore composed of the **symphysis pubis** cranially and the **symphysis ischii** caudally. Occasionally, in young specimens, there is in the caudal part of the symphysis a separate triangular bone that is widest and thickest caudally.

The **ilium** (*os ilium*) is the largest and most cranial of the bones that compose the os coxae. It is basically divided into a cranial, nearly sagittal, laterally concave part, the **wing** (*ala ossis ilii*), and a narrow, more irregular caudal part, the **body** (*corpus ossis ilii*). The body, at its expanded caudal end, forms the cranial two-fifths of the acetabulum. In this cavity it fuses with the ischium and acetabular bone caudally and the pubis medially.

The **iliac crest** (*crista iliaca*) is composed of the tuber sacrale and tuber coxae and forms the cranial border of the ilium between these two tubera. Fagin et al. (1992) found radiographically that the secondary ossification center that develops on the cranial border of the iliac crest does not always fuse completely with the ilium even in adult dogs. Of 750 dogs examined, most had a fused iliac crest by 2 years of age. However, 18% of dogs 10 years or older and 10% of dogs 14 years or older had incompletely fused iliac crests. They concluded that the prevalence of this incomplete union at the iliac crest, which can be misdiagnosed as a fracture fragment, is more common than previously thought. The iliac crest forms a cranially protruding arc that is thin in its ventral half. The dorsal half gradually increases in thickness until it reaches a width of nearly 1 cm dorsally in the large working breeds. The iliac crest, in heavily muscled breeds, presents a slight lateral eversion. The dorsal border of this crest is thicker in its cranial half than in its caudal half. The eminence of the iliac crest located dorsal to the iliosacral joint between the thick parts of this border is the **caudal dorsal iliac spine** (*spina iliaca dorsalis caudalis*). The obtuse angle located between the cranial and the dorsal borders is the **cranial dorsal iliac spine** (*spina iliaca dorsalis cranialis*). These two spines and the intermediate border constitute what is known as the **tuber sacrale** in the dog and in the large herbivores, in which it is more salient than it is in the dog. The ventral margin begins at the **cranial ventral iliac spine** (*spina iliaca ventralis cranialis*). This spine and the adjacent lateroventral projection of the wing of the ilium is the **tuber coxae**. Approximately 1 cm caudal to this spine is a small eminence on the thin ventral border that is known as the **alar spine** (*spina alaris*). Grooving the ventral border just caudal to the tuber coxae and extending on the lateral surface of the ilium in old specimens is the vascular groove for the iliolumbar artery and vein. Caudal to the tuber sacrale the dorsal border of the body of the ilium is gently concave, forming the **greater ischiatic notch** (*incisura ischiadica major*). The dorsal border of the body of the ilium is continuous with the dorsal border of the ischium as a slight convexity dorsal to the acetabulum. This is the **ischiatic spine**. Caudoventrally on the lateral surface of the body of the ilium is a fa.. **origin of the rectus femoris** (*area lateralis m. rect..*) This is just cranial to the acetabulum.

The **gluteal surface** (*facies glutea*) of the iliac wing faces laterally and slightly dorsally. It embodies the whole external surface of the bone. An intermediate fossa that parallels the axis of the bone divides the surface into a strong ridge dorsally and a triangular, moderately rough area ventrally. The medial, or **sacropelvic surface** (*facies sacropelvina*) of the iliac wing articulates with the wing of the sacrum by a synchondrosis that forms the ear-shaped **auricular surface** (*facies auricularis*). The **iliac tuberosity** (*tuberositas iliaca*) is the rough, slightly protruding eminence of the sacropelvic surface (*facies sacropelvina*) located dorsal to the auricular surface. The **iliac surface** (*facies iliaca*) is a nearly square, smooth flat portion of the sacropelvic surface cranial to the auricular surface. The **arcuate line** is the ventromedial border of the ilium, which extends from the auricular surface to the iliopubic eminence. It divides the sacropelvic surface of the body of the ilium into a medial two-thirds and a ventromedial one-third. The caudally directed nutrient foramen is located near the middle of this surface adjacent to the ventral border. The mm. sartorius and tensor fasciae latae arise from the tuber coxae and alar spine. The mm. iliacus attaches adjacent to the arcuate line. The mm. longissimus lumborum and iliocostalis lumborum attach to the iliac surface and portions of the mm. coccygeus and levator ani attach to the caudal portion of the sacropelvic surface (see Fig. 6.70). The mm. gluteus medius, gluteus

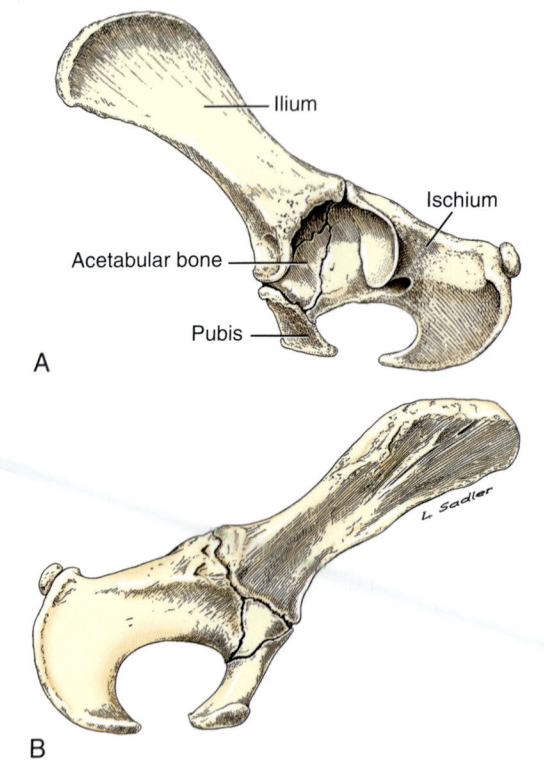

• **Fig. 4.122** A, Left os coxae of a 15-week-old Beagle, lateral (A) and medial (B) aspects. Continued on next page. Left os coxae of an adult dog, lateral (C) and medial (D) aspect.

CHAPTER 4 The Skeleton 159

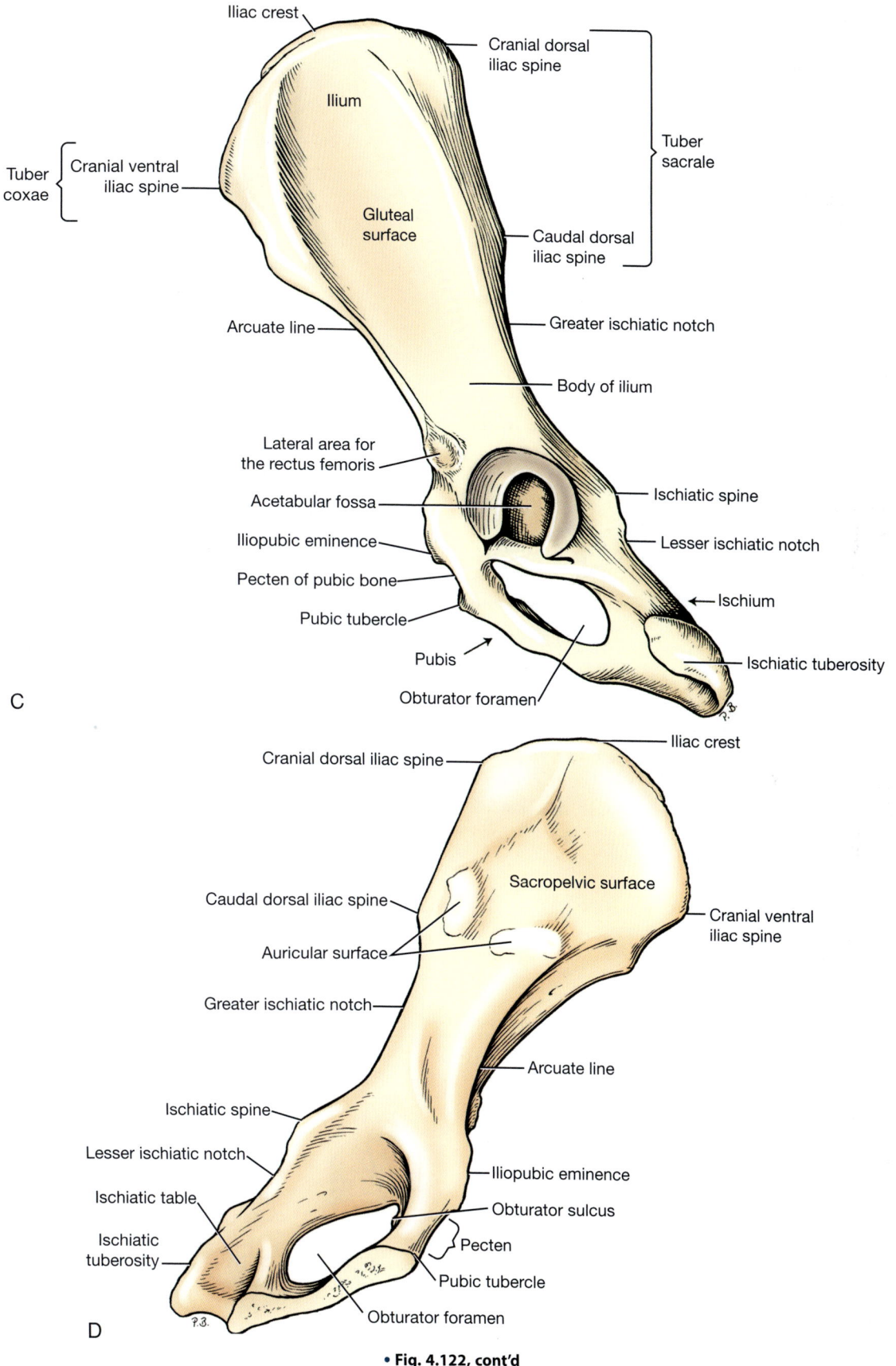

• Fig. 4.122, cont'd

160 CHAPTER 4 The Skeleton

profundus, and articularis coxae arise from the gluteal surface of the ilium. The mm. psoas minor attaches to the ventral portion of the arcuate line. The rectus abdominis and pectineus attach to the iliopubic eminence.

The **ischium** (*os ischii*) consists of a body, ramus, table, and tuberosity. It forms the caudal third of the os coxae and enters into the formation of the acetabulum, obturator foramen, and symphysis pelvis.

The **body of the ischium** (*corpus ossis ischii*) is the cranial part of the bone that lies lateral to the obturator foramen and, at its cranial end, forms about two-fifths of the acetabulum. Its thick dorsal border is lateral and continues with the dorsal border of the ilium in a slight convexity, forming the **ischiatic spine** (*spina ischiadica*). Caudal to the spine the dorsal border is flattened and creased by approximately five shallow grooves, in which lie the multiple tendons of the m. obturatorius internus. In life the **lesser**

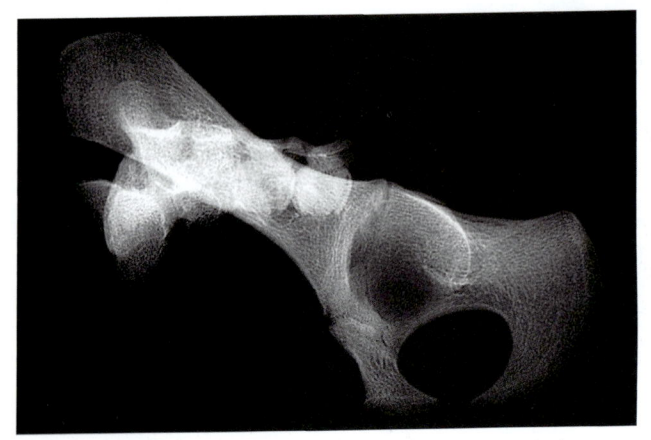

• **Fig. 4.123** Lateromedial radiograph, left ossa coxarum and sacrum of a young dog.

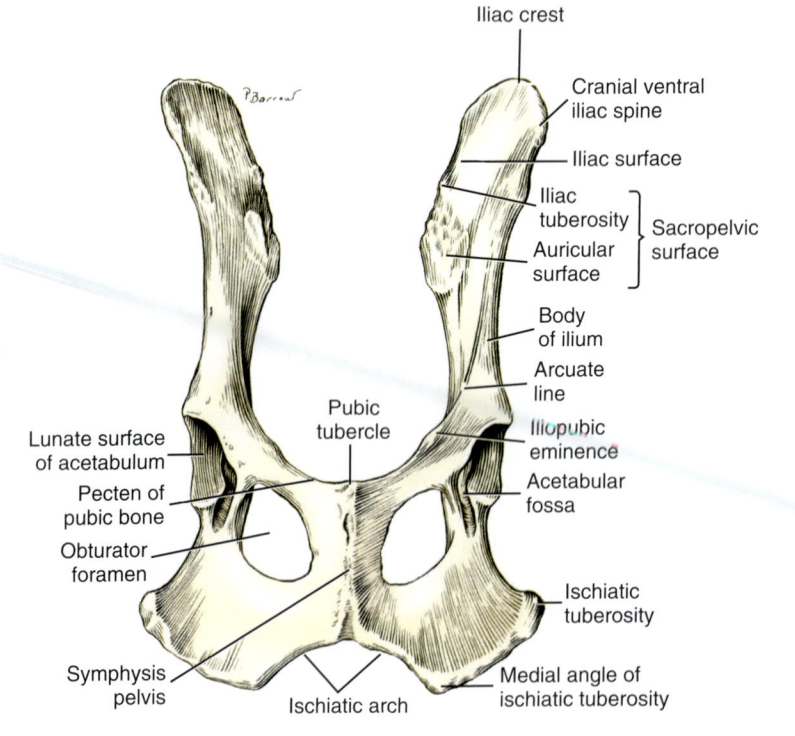

• **Fig. 4.124** Ventral aspect of ossa coxarum. Note the fused symphysis pelvis.

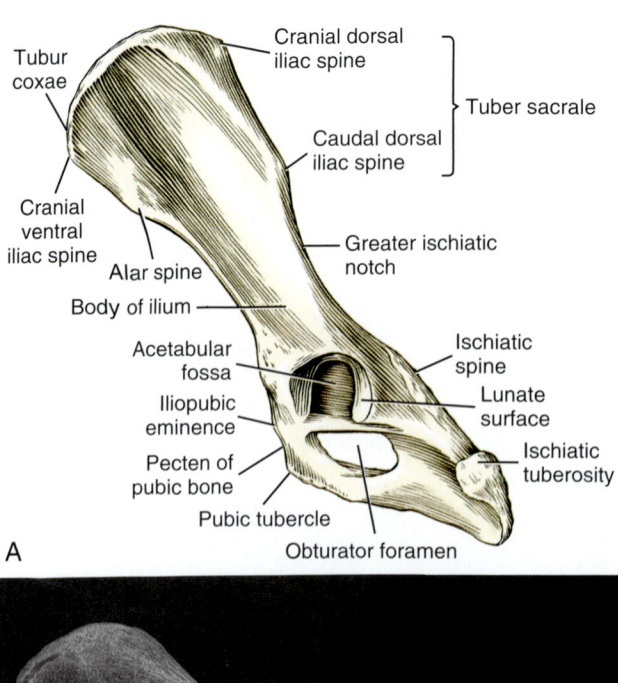

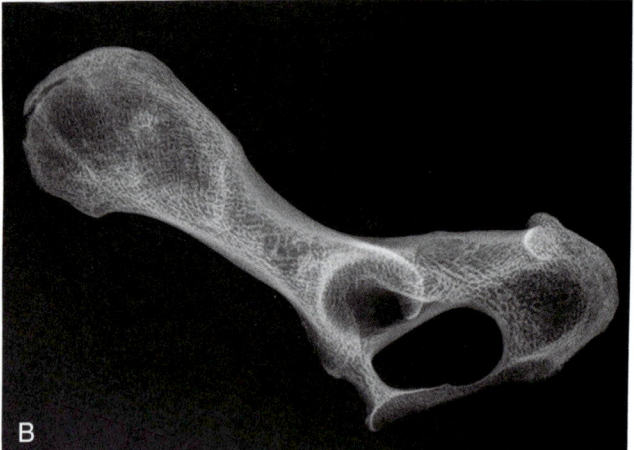

• **Fig. 4.125** A, Left os coxae of an adult dog, lateral aspect. B, Lateromedial radiograph, left os coxae.

Fig. 4.126 Ventrodorsal radiograph of the pelvic region:

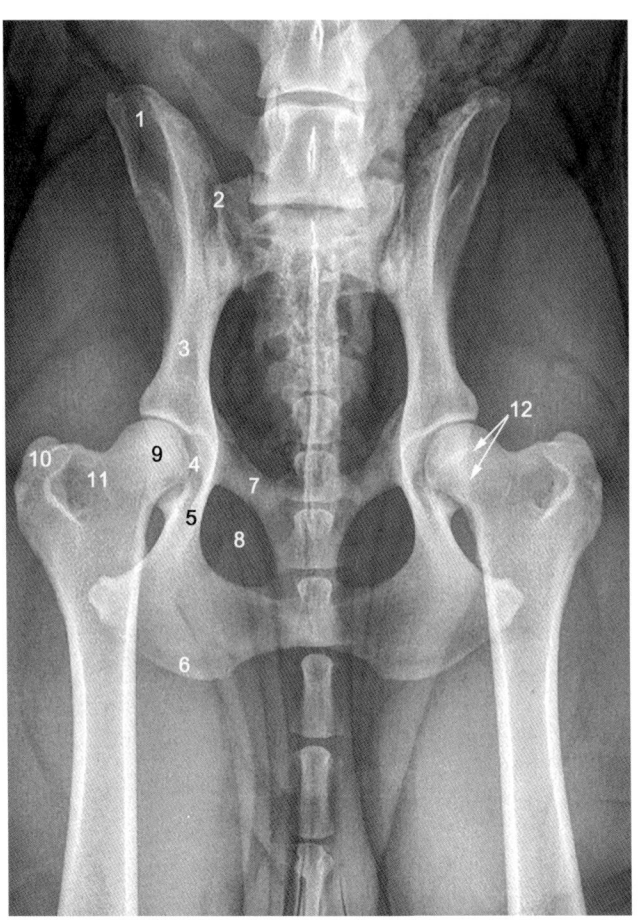

1. Iliac crest
2. Sacroiliac joint
3. Body of ilium
4. Acetabulum
5. Ischium
6. Ischiatic tuberosity
7. Pubis
8. Obturator foramen
9. Femoral head
10. Greater trochanter
11. Intertrochanteric crest
12. Dorsal rim of acetabulum

ischiatic notch (*incisura ischiadica minor*) is converted into a large opening, the **lesser ischiatic foramen** (*foramen ischiaticus minus*), by the sacrotuberous ligament. The **ramus of the ischium** (*ramus ossis ischii*) is medial to the obturator foramen and is continuous caudally with the table of the ischium. The medial border of the ramus forms the **ischiatic symphysis** (*symphysis ischiatica*) with the opposite ischiatic ramus. The **ischiatic table** (*tabula ossis ischii*) is the largest component of the ischium. It is curved so that its dorsomedial aspect faces dorsally and its dorsolateral aspect faces medially and along with the body forms the caudal part of the lateral boundary of the pelvic cavity. The m. obturatorius internus arises from the shallow fossa of the ischiatic table that lies cranial to the ischiatic tuberosity, as well as from the medial and cranial edges of the obturator foramen and the adjacent pelvic surface of the os coxae. The caudomedial border of the ischiatic table forms the deep **ischial arch** (*arcus ischiadicus*), with the opposite ischiatic table. The **ischiatic tuberosity** (*tuber ischiadicum*) is the caudolateral part of the ischium caudolateral to the ischiatic table and lateral to the ischial arch. It is wide and gradually thickens, from the medial to the lateral side, where it ends in a pronounced rough hemispherical eminence. The caudal end of the sacrotuberous ligament attaches to the dorsal surface of this eminence. The ventral surface of the ischiatic tuberosity gives rise to the largest muscles of the thigh, the hamstring muscles: mm. biceps femoris, semitendinosus, and semimembranosus. The adjacent ventral surface of the table gives rise to the m. quadratus femoris, and a zone next to the caudal and medial borders of the obturator foramen gives rise to the m. obturatorius externus. The m. adductor arises from the ischiatic symphysis and the ventral surface of the ischium adjacent to it. The mm. gemelli arise from the lateral surface of the ischium ventral to the lesser ischiatic notch. Each root (*crus*) of the penis, with its covering muscle, m. ischiocavernosus, attaches to the medial angle of the ischiatic tuberosity. (For a discussion of the os penis, the bone within the penis, see Chapter 9.)

The **pubis** (*os pubis*) is a dorsoventrally compressed, curved bar of bone that extends from the ilium and ischium laterally to the symphysis pubis medially. Its caudal border bounds the cranial part of the obturator foramen, which is particularly smooth and partly grooved by the obturator nerve and vessels. It is divided into a body and two rami. The **body** (*corpus ossis pubis*) is the central flat triangular part of the bone, forming the craniomedial border of the obturator foramen. It fuses with the ilium and contributes to the formation of the acetabulum. The **cranial ramus** (*ramus cranialis ossis pubis*) fuses with the ilium and enters into the formation of the acetabulum. The **iliopubic eminence** (*eminentia iliopubica*) is located on the cranial border of the cranial ramus as it joins the ilium. The **caudal ramus** (*ramus caudalis ossis pubis*) forms the medial border of the obturator foramen and fuses with the opposite side to form the symphysis pubis. The ventral surface of the pubis gives origin to the mm. gracilis, adductor, and obturatorius externus. The dorsal, or pelvic, surface gives rise to the m. levator ani and a part of the m. obturatorius internus. The **ventral pubic tubercle** (*tuberculum pubicum ventrale*) is located on the cranioventral surface of the pubis adjacent to the pubic symphysis. The cranial border of the pubis, stretching from the iliopubic eminence to the symphysis pubis, is also called the **pecten** (*pecten ossis pubis*), or the ventromedial part of the terminal line. The pubic tubercle and pecten serve for the attachment of the prepubic tendon, whereby all of the abdominal muscles, except for the m. transversus abdominis, attach wholly or in part. The m. pectineus also arises here.

Femur

The **femur** (*os femoris*) (Figs. 4.127 to 4.131) is the heaviest bone in the skeleton. In well-proportioned breeds it is slightly shorter than the tibia and ulna but is about one-fifth longer than the humerus. It articulates with the os coxae proximally, forming a flexor angle of 110 degrees cranially. Distally, it articulates with the tibia, forming a flexor angle of 110 degrees caudally (Rumph & Hathcock 1990). Right

162 CHAPTER 4 The Skeleton

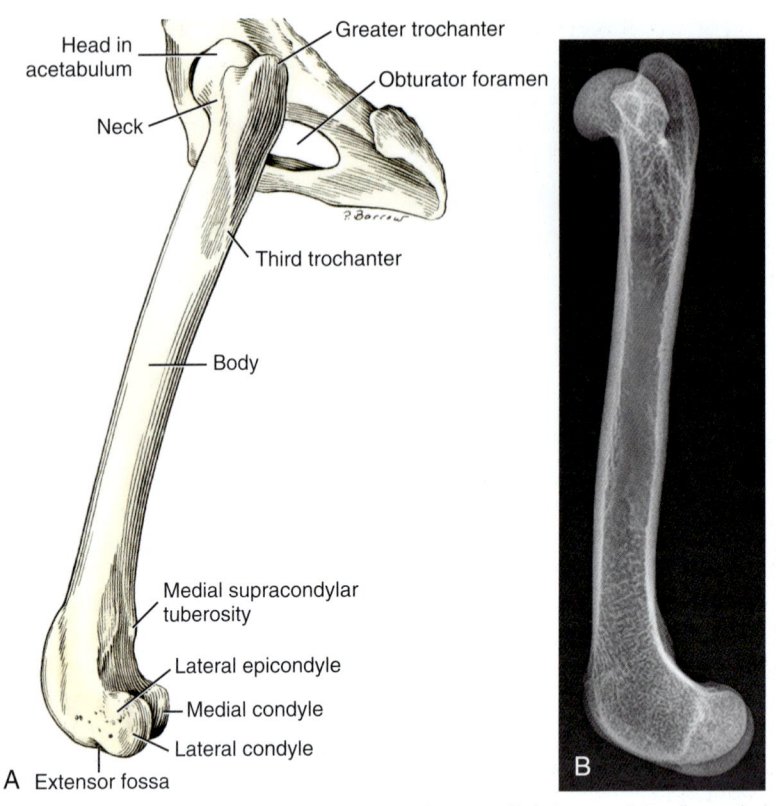

- **Fig. 4.127** A, Left femur and os coxae articulated, lateral aspect. B, Lateromedial radiograph, left femur.

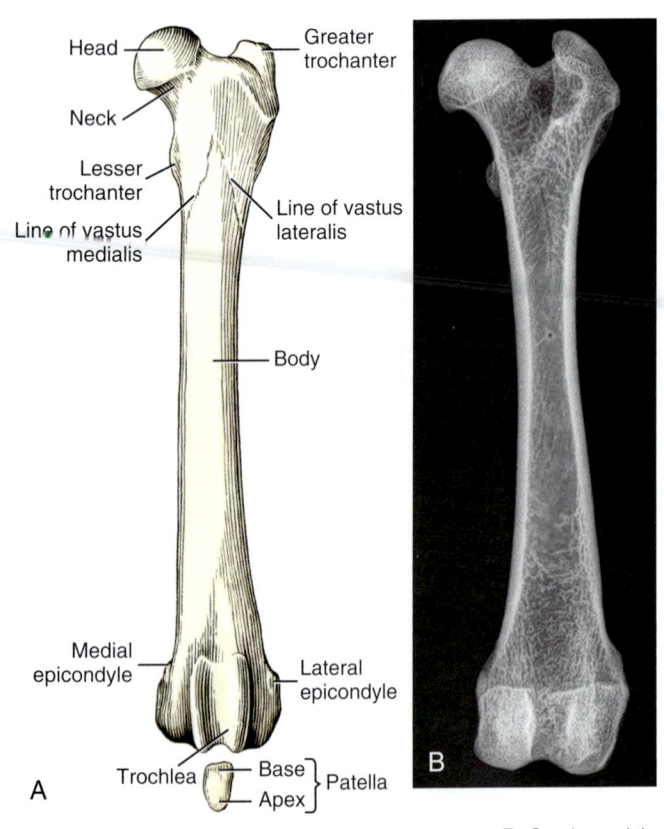

- **Fig. 4.128** A, Left femur with patella, cranial aspect. B, Craniocaudal radiograph, left femur.

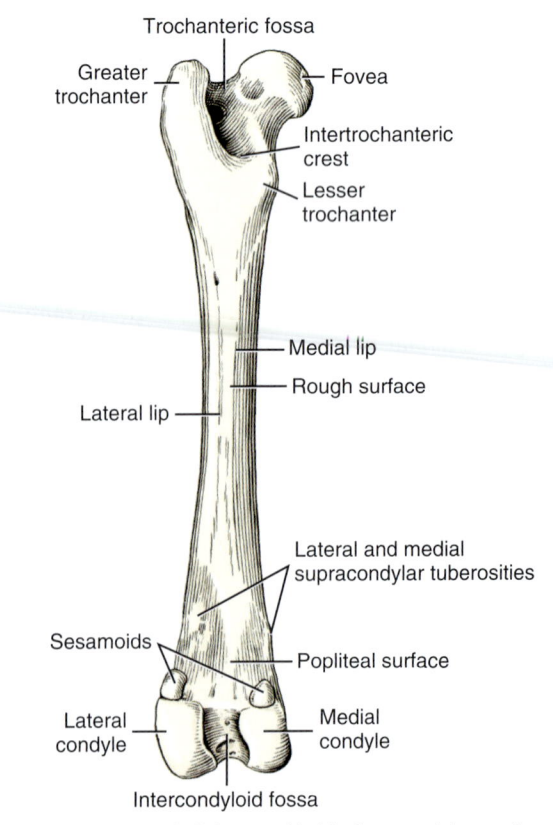

- **Fig. 4.129** Left femur with fabellae, caudal aspect.

CHAPTER 4 The Skeleton   163

• Fig. 4.130 Lateral radiograph of the femur.

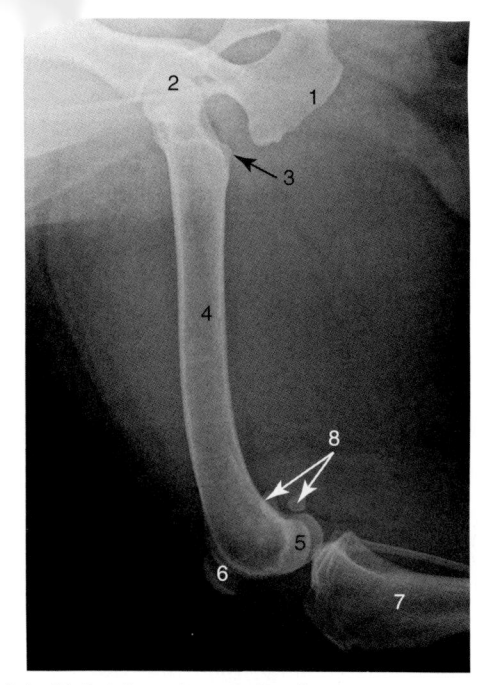

1. Ischiatic tuberosity
2. Femoral head
3. Lesser trochanter
4. Body of femur
5. Femoral condyles
6. Patella
7. Tibia
8. Sesamoid bones in medial and lateral heads of gastrocnemius muscle

• Fig. 4.131 Craniocaudal radiograph of the femur.

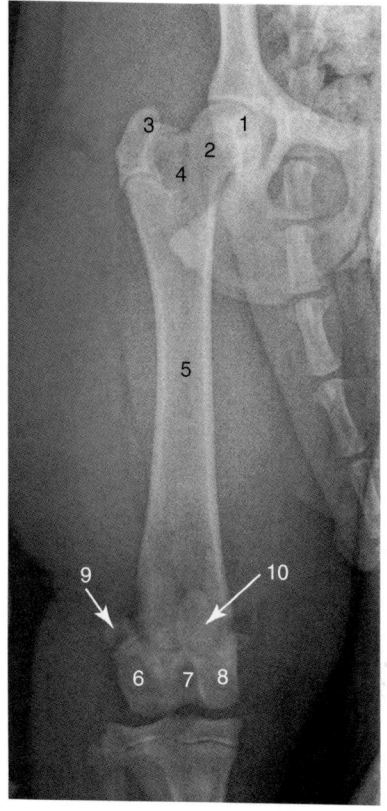

1. Femoral head
2. Femoral neck
3. Greater trochanter
4. Trochanteric fossa
5. Body of femur
6. Lateral condyle
7. Intercondylar fossa
8. Medial condyle
9. Lateral gastrocnemius sesamoid bone
10. Patella

and left femurs lie in parallel sagittal planes when the animal is standing. In fact, all the main bones of the pelvic limb are in about the same sagittal plane as those of the ipsilateral thoracic limb, but the flexor angles of the first two joints of each limb face in opposite directions.

The proximal end of the femur consists of a head, neck, and two processes or trochanters. The smooth nearly hemispherical **head** (*caput ossis femoris*) caps the dorsocaudal and medial parts of the neck. The **fovea** (*fovea capitis*) is a small, rather indistinct, circular pit on the medial part of the head. Occasionally a depressed, moderately rough, nonarticular strip extends from the fovea to the nearest caudoventral nonarticular margin. The fovea serves for the attachment of the **ligament of the head of the femur** (*ligamentum capitis ossis femoris*), formerly called the *round ligament*. The **neck** (*collum femoris*) unites the head with the rest of the proximal extremity. It is about as long as the diameter of the head, slightly compressed craniocaudally, and it is reinforced by a ridge of bone that extends from the head to the large, laterally located greater trochanter.

The **greater trochanter** (*trochanter major*), the largest tuber of the proximal extremity of the bone, is located directly lateral to the head and neck. Its free, pyramid-shaped apex usually extends nearly to a dorsal plane lying on the head. Between the femoral neck and the greater trochanter, caudal to the ridge of bone connecting the two, is the deep **trochanteric fossa** (*fossa trochanterica*). The mm. glutei medius, gluteus profundus, and piriformis insert on the greater trochanter. The mm. gemelli, obturatorius internus, and obturatorius externus insert in the trochanteric fossa. The **lesser trochanter** (*trochanter minor*) is a distinct, pyramid-shaped eminence that projects from the caudomedial surface of the proximal extremity near its junction with the body of the femur. It is connected with the greater trochanter by a low but wide arciform crest, the **intertrochanteric crest** (*crista intertrochanterica*). The m. quadratus femoris inserts distal to the intertrochanteric crest adjacent to the lesser trochanter. The m. iliopsoas attaches to the lesser trochanter.

The **body** (*corpus femoris*) is nearly cylindrical and is straight proximally and cranially arched distally. Its cranial, lateral, and medial surfaces are not demarcated from each other, but the caudal surface is flatter than the others. The **third trochanter** (*trochanter tertius*) is a small lateral eminence of the proximal body approximately 2 cm distal to the apex of the greater trochanter at approximately the same level as the lesser trochanter. The m. gluteus superficialis inserts on the third trochanter. A small proximal nutrient foramen pierces the cranial surface of the cortex in a distal direction. Covering all but the caudal surface of the femur is the large m. quadriceps femoris. All except the rectus femoris division of this muscle arise from the proximal part of the body of the femur, where occasionally indistinct lines indicate the most proximal attachments for the m. vastus lateralis and the m. vastus medialis. The caudal surface of the body is marked by a finely roughened surface, the *facies aspera*, which is narrow in the middle and wider at both ends. This slightly roughened face is bounded by the **medial and lateral lips** (*labium mediate et laterale*), which diverge proximally, running into the lesser and greater trochanters, and, distally, becoming obscured in the medial and lateral epicondyles, respectively. The sagittally concave, transversely flat area enclosed distally by these lips is the **popliteal surface** (*facies poplitea*). The relatively flat surface proximally, which is flanked by the diverging femoral lips, is called the *trochanteric surface* by Nickel et al. (1977). The largest nutrient foramen to enter the femur is found on the caudal surface at approximately the junction of the proximal and middle thirds of the bone. The m. adductor longus inserts on the lateral lip distal to the third trochanter, whereas the m. adductor magnus et brevis inserts on the whole lateral lip from the third trochanter to the popliteal surface. The m. pectineus inserts on the distal end of the medial femoral lip just proximal to the cranial insertion of the m. semimembranosus.

At the proximal edge of the popliteal surface of the femoral body are located tubercles that are known as the **medial and lateral supracondylar tuberosities** (*tuberositas supracondylaris medialis et lateralis*). These are just proximal to the articular surfaces for the gastrocnemius sesamoid bones on the femoral condyles and are described with the condyles. The m. gastrocnemius arises from both tuberosities. The m. flexor digitorum superficialis also arises from the lateral supracondylar tuberosity.

The distal end of the femur is quadrangular and protrudes caudally. It contains three main articular surfaces. Two of these are on the medial and lateral condyles, and the third is the trochlea, an articular groove on the cranial surface. The **lateral condyle** (*condylus lateralis*) is convex in both the sagittal and the transverse planes. The **medial condyle** (*condylus medialis*) is smaller and less convex in both the transverse and the sagittal planes. Each condyle articulates medially directly with the tibia. The remainder of each condyle articulates extensively with the menisci of the tibia. The condyles are separated by the **intercondylar fossa** (*fossa intercondylaris*), which is slightly oblique in direction as the caudal part of the intercondyloid fossa is located farther laterally than is the cranial part. The articular surfaces of the condyles are continuous proximocaudally with small articular surfaces for the sesamoid bones (*fabellae*) associated with the medial and lateral heads of m. gastrocnemius. The articular surface on the lateral condyle is larger than that on the medial one. The **femoral trochlea** (*trochlea ossis femoris*), or patellar surface, is the smooth, wide articular groove on the cranial surface of the distal extremity that is continuous with the articular surfaces of the condyles. It is bounded by medial and lateral ridges. Proximally, the limiting ridges diverge slightly. The medial ridge is somewhat thicker than the lateral one. The **patella** articulates with the articular surface of the trochlea of the femur. This is the sesamoid bone associated with the of the m. quadriceps femoris. Proximal and cranial to the articular surfaces of the medial and lateral condyles are the **medial and lateral epicondyles** (*epicondylus medialis et lateralis*). These serve for the proximal attachments of the medial and lateral collateral ligaments of the stifle joint. The **extensor fossa** (*fossa extensoria*) is a small pit located at the epicondylar border of the lateral condyle at its junction with the lateral ridge of the trochlea. From it arises the m. extensor digitorum longus. The m. popliteus arises from the lateral condyle of the femur deep to the lateral collateral ligament. Kuhn et al. (1990) described morphometric and anisotropic symmetries of the distal femur.

Sesamoid Bones of the Stifle Joint

The **patella** (see Fig. 4.128A) is the largest sesamoid bone in the body. It is ovate in shape and curved to articulate with the trochlear of the femur. The **base** (*basis patellae*) is blunt and faces proximally. It may extend beyond the adjacent articular surface. The distally located **apex** (*apex patellae*) is slightly more pointed than the base and does not extend beyond the articular surface. The **articular surface** (*facies articularis*) is smooth, convex in all directions, and in some specimens shows longitudinal striations. Several nutrient foramina enter the bone from the medial side. The patella is an ossification in the tendon of insertion of the large extensor of the stifle, the m. quadriceps femoris. That part of the tendon between its insertion on the tibial tuberosity and the patella is also known as the *patellar ligament*. The patella alters the direction of pull of the tendon of the quadriceps; it protects the tendon, and it provides a greater bearing surface for the tendon to play on the trochlea of the femur than would be possible without it.

The articular surface of the trochlea is greatly increased by the presence of two or three **cartilaginous processes** (*processus cartilagineus*) referred to as *parapatellar fibrocartilages*. These are grooved cartilages, one on each side of the patella, that articulate with the ridges of the femoral trochlea. Proximally, the two cartilages may extend far enough proximal to the patella to curve toward each other and meet, or a third cartilage may be located at this site. For a more complete description of these cartilages refer to Chapter 5, Arthrology.

There are three sesamoid bones in the stifle region. Two of these, often referred to as *fabellae* (Latin, "little bean"), are located in the heads of the m. gastrocnemius caudal to the stifle joint on the medial and lateral condyles (see Figs. 4.127 and 4.129), and the third is intercalated in the tendon of origin of the m. popliteus (see Fig. 4.134). The sesamoid located in the lateral head of origin of the m. gastrocnemius is the largest. It is globular in shape, except for a truncated end, which faces distally and has a nearly flat articular surface for articulation with the articular surface on the caudal part of the lateral femoral condyle. The sesamoid in the medial head of origin of the m. gastrocnemius is smaller than the lateral one and is angular in form. It may not have a distinct articular surface on the medial condyle. The smallest sesamoid bone of the stifle region is the sesamoid located in the tendon of origin of the m. popliteus, adjacent to its muscle fibers. It articulates with the lateral condyle of the tibia.

Tibia

The **tibia** (Figs. 4.132 to 4.136) is a long, thick bone that lies in the medial part of the crus (the anatomic leg). The tibia articulates proximally with the femur, distally with the tarsus, and on its lateral side both proximally and distally with the companion bone of the crus, the fibula. The proximal half of the tibia is triangular in cross-section and more massive than its distal half, which is nearly cylindrical.

The proximal end of the tibia is relatively flat and triangular, with its apex cranial. It consists of two condyles that provide a **proximal articular surface** (*facies articularis proximalis*) and an **intercondylar eminence** (*tuberculum intercondylaris*) for ligamentous attachments that lie between the condyles. The divided proximal articular surface lies on the **lateral and medial condyles** (*condylus lateralis et medialis*). The articular surfaces of the condyles are separated by a sagittal, nonarticular intercondylar eminence with two intercondylar tubercles. Although the surface area of the two is approximately the same, the medial condyle is oval and the lateral condyle is nearly circular. Both are convex in the sagittal plane, and concave transversely. In the fresh state they are covered by articular cartilage and have only a small area of contact with the articular cartilage of the femoral condyles. The larger area of contact is with the menisci. Functionally the medial and lateral tibial condyles are separated from the medial and lateral femoral condyles by the **medial and lateral menisci** (*meniscus medialis et lateralis*). These fibrocartilages are biconcave, incomplete discs that are open toward the axis of the bone. The central edges of these C-shaped cartilages are thin and concave, and their peripheral margins are thick and convex. The **intercondylar eminence** is a low but stout divided eminence between the medial and the lateral tibial condyles. The two spurs that are articular on their abaxial sides are known as the **medial and lateral intercondylar tubercles** (*tuberculum intercondylare mediale et laterale*). The medial tubercle is cranial to the lateral tubercle. The oval, depressed area cranial to the intercondyloid eminence is the *area intercondylaris cranialis*; the smaller, depressed area caudal to it is the *area intercondylaris caudalis*. The meniscal ligaments attach to these areas. The condyles are more expansive than the articular areas located on their proximal surfaces. Between the condyles caudally is the large **popliteal notch** (*incisura poplitea*). The **extensor groove** (*sulcus extensorius*) of the tibia is a smaller notch that cuts into the lateral condyle as far as the articular surface. The tendon of the m. extensor digitorum longus arises from the extensor fossa of

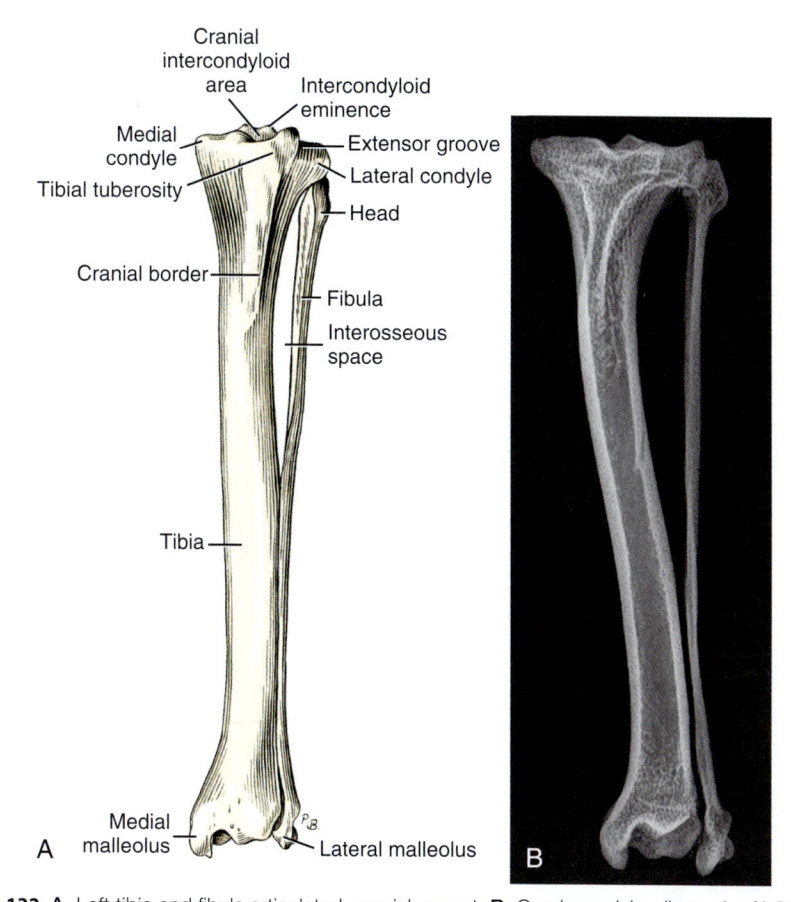

• **Fig. 4.132** A, Left tibia and fibula articulated, cranial aspect. B, Craniocaudal radiograph of left tibia and fibula, articulated.

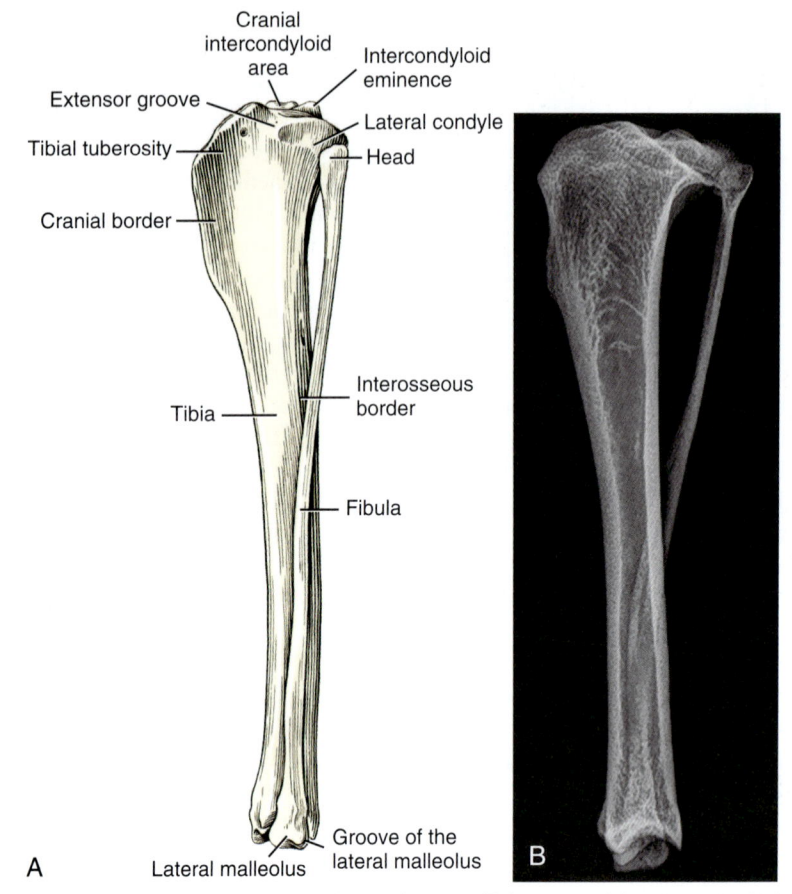

166 CHAPTER 4 The Skeleton

Fig. 4.133 A, Left tibia and fibula articulated, lateral aspect. B, Lateromedial radiograph of left tibia and fibula, articulated.

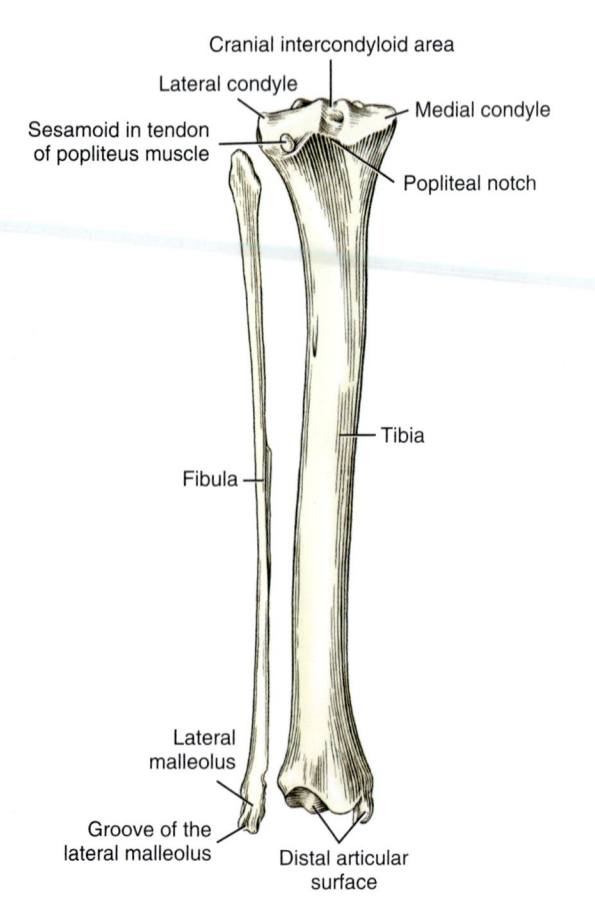

Fig. 4.134 Left tibia and fibula disarticulated, caudal aspect.

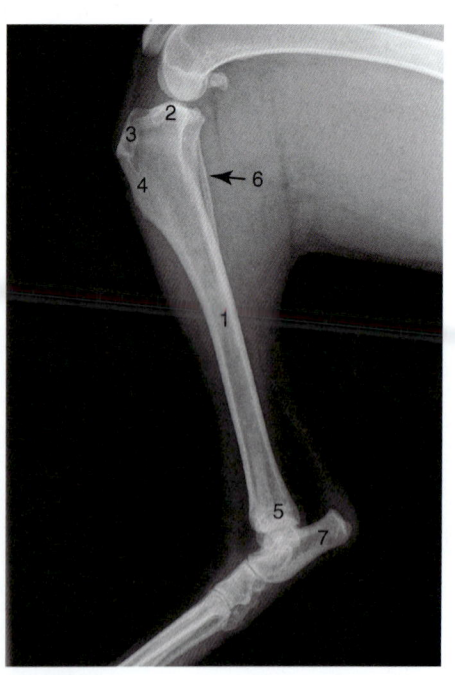

1. Body of tibia
2. Tibial condyles
3. Tibial tuberosity
4. Cranial border of tibia
5. Tibial cochlea-tarsocrural joint
6. Fibula
7. Calcaneus

Fig. 4.135 Lateral radiograph of the tibia.

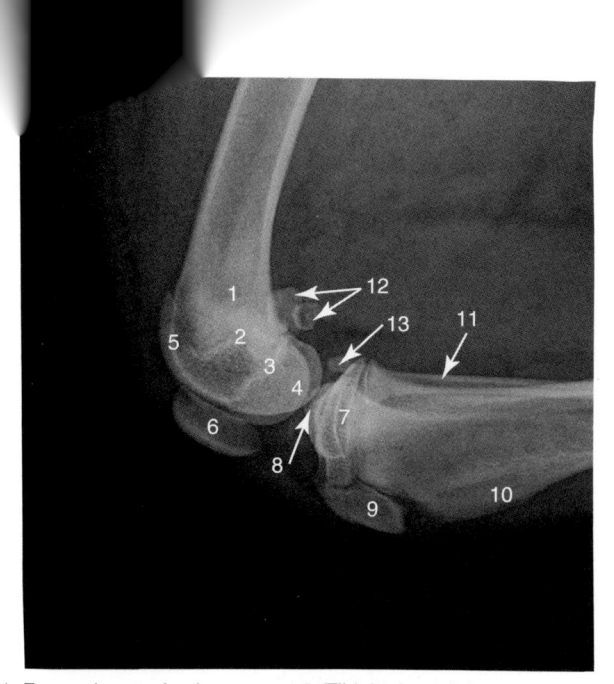

1. Femoral metaphysis
2. Distal femoral physis
3. Intercondylar fossa
4. Femoral condyles
5. Trochlea
6. Patella
7. Tibial condyles
8. Intercondylar eminence
9. Tibial tuberosity
10. Cranial border of tibia
11. Fibula
12. Sesamoid bones in medial and lateral heads of gastrocnemius muscle
13. Popliteus sesamoid bone

• **Fig. 4.136** Lateral radiograph of the stifle.

the lateral femoral condyle and passes through this extensor groove. On the caudolateral surface of the lateral condyle is an obliquely placed **articular surface for the head of the fibula** (*facies articularis fibularis*). The **tibial tuberosity** (*tuberositas tibiae*) is the large, quadrangular, proximocranial process that provides insertion for the powerful m. quadriceps femoris and parts of the mm. biceps femoris and sartorius. Extending distally from the tibial tuberosity is the **cranial border** (*margo cranialis*) of the tibia, formerly called the *tibial crest*. To it insert the mm. gracilis and semitendinosus and parts of the mm. sartorius and biceps femoris. The m. semimembranosus inserts on the caudal part of the medial condyle, and the proximal part of the origin of the m. tibialis cranialis arises from the lateral condyle.

The **body** (*corpus tibiae*) is three-sided throughout its proximal half, whereas the distal half is essentially quadrilateral or cylindrical. Three surfaces and three borders are recognized in the proximal half of the tibia. These are the caudal, medial, and lateral surfaces and the medial, lateral and cranial borders. The **lateral border** (*margo lateralis*) or interosseous border is replaced in the distal half of the tibia by a narrow, flat surface apposed to the adjacent, closely lying fibula.

The **caudal surface** (*facies caudalis*) presents an oblique popliteal line (*linea m. popliteii*) that courses from the proximal part of the lateral border to the middle of the medial border. At the junction of the proximal and middle thirds of the lateral border is the distally directed nutrient foramen of the bone. The m. popliteus inserts on the proximal medial part of the caudal surface, the proximal part of the medial border, and the adjacent medial surface of the tibia proximal to the popliteal line. The mm. flexor digitorum lateralis, tibialis caudalis, and flexor digitorum medialis arise from the proximal half of the caudal surface in lateral to medial sequence. Running obliquely distolaterally across the distal part of the caudal surface may be a vascular groove that extends to the distal end of the bone adjacent to the lateral malleolus.

The **medial surface** (*facies medialis*) of the tibia is wide and nearly flat proximally as it is partly formed by the cranial border of the tibia. Near this cranial border in large specimens is a low but wide muscular line for the insertions of the mm. semitendinosus, gracilis, and sartorius. The medial surface of the tibia is relatively smooth throughout as it is largely subcutaneous in life.

The **lateral surface** (*facies lateralis*) of the tibia is smooth, wide, and concave proximally; flat in the middle; and narrow and convex distally. Part of the m. biceps femoris inserts on the medial surface of the cranial border of the tibia, and, just caudal to this attachment, the m. tibialis cranialis arises. This muscle intimately covers the lateral surface of the tibia. The m. flexor digitorum lateralis arises from the proximal three-fourths of the lateral border of the tibia. The m. fibularis brevis arises from the lateral surfaces of the distal two-thirds of the fibula and tibia.

The **distal end** of the tibia is quadrilateral and slightly more massive than the adjacent part of the body. The distal articular surface is in the form of two nearly sagittal, arciform grooves, the **cochlea tibiae**, which receive the ridges of the trochlea of the talus. The grooves are separated by an intermediate ridge. A transversely located synovial fossa extends from one groove to the other across the intermediate ridge. The whole medial part of the distal extremity of the tibia is the **medial malleolus** (*malleolus medialis*). Its cranial part is formed by a stout, pyramid-shaped process. Caudal to this is a semilunar notch. The small but distinct sulcus for the tendon of the m. flexor digitorum medialis grooves the lip of the medial malleolus at the center of the semilunar notch. On the caudal side of the distal extremity is a much wider sulcus for the tendon of the m. flexor digitorum lateralis. The lateral surface of the distal extremity of the tibia is in an oblique plane as it slopes caudolaterally. It is slightly flattened by the fibula. At the distal end of the fibular surface is a small articular surface the *facies articularis malleoli*, for articulation with the distal end of the fibula. No muscles attach to the distal half of the tibia except for a small portion of m. fibularis brevis on the lateral side.

Fibula

The fibula (see Figs. 4.132 to 4.134) is a long, thin, laterally compressed bone located in the lateral part of the crus. It articulates with the caudolateral part of the lateral condyle of the tibia proximally and with the tibia and talus distally. It serves mainly for muscle attachment as it supports little weight. It is divided into a proximal head, a neck, a body, and distally a lateral malleolus.

The **head of the fibula** (*caput fibulae*) is flattened transversely, being expanded beyond the planes through the borders of the body both cranially and caudally. A small tubercle, which is articular, projects from its medial surface, facing proximomedially. This small articular surface (*the facies articularis capitis fibulae*) articulates with a similar one on the caudolateral part of the lateral condyle of the tibia.

A short **neck** (*collum fibulae*) blends with the body with no specific demarcation.

The **body of the fibula** (*corpus fibulae*) is slender and irregular. Its distal half is flattened transversely; its proximal half is also thin transversely but is slightly concave facing medially. Near its middle it is roughly triangular in cross-section. The proximal half of the body of the fibula is separated from the tibia by a considerable interosseous space. The cranial margin of the fibula is the **interosseous border** (*margo interosseus*). It runs straight distally and disappears at about the middle of the fibula, where the bone widens as it contacts the tibia. The interosseous membrane, which in life stretches across the interosseous space, attaches to this border or to the rounded ridge of bone that lies adjacent to it, facing the tibia. The proximal half of the fibula may be twisted; the distal half is wider, thinner, and more regular than the proximal half. The **medial surface** (*facies medialis*) is rough as it lies closely applied to the tibia. A fine, proximally directed nutrient foramen pierces the middle of its medial surface. The **lateral surface** (*facies lateralis*) is smooth as it lies embedded in the muscles of the crus.

The distal end of the fibula is known as the **lateral malleolus**. Medially, it contains the **articular surface** (*facies articularis malleoli*), which articulates with the distal lateral surface of the tibia as well as the lateral surface of the trochlea of the talus and the craniolateral surface of the calcaneus (Fig. 4.141). The distal border of the lateral malleolus is thin and flat. Its caudal angle contains a distinct groove, the *sulcus tendinum mm. extensoris digitorum lateralis et fibularis brevis*, through which run the tendons of the mm. extensor digitorum lateralis and fibularis brevis. Cranial to this sulcus is another groove on the lateral side of the malleolus. This *sulcus tendinum m. fibularis longus* contains the tendon of the fibularis longus. The muscles that attach to various parts of the fibula include the head of fibula (the m. flexor digitorum medialis), the head and adjacent shaft (mm. extensor digitorum lateralis and fibularis longus), the medial part of the proximal end (m. tibialis caudalis), the caudal surface of the proximal three-fifths (m. flexor digitorum lateralis), the cranial border between the proximal and middle thirds (m. extensor digiti I longus), and the distal two-thirds (m. fibularis brevis).

Hindpaw

The skeleton of the hindpaw (*pes*) (Figs. 4.137 to 4.146) is composed of the tarsal and metatarsal bones, the phalanges, and the sesamoid bones associated with the phalanges. The tarsus is composed of bones basically arranged in two transverse rows. Articulating with the distal surfaces of the most distally located tarsal bones are the four (sometimes five)

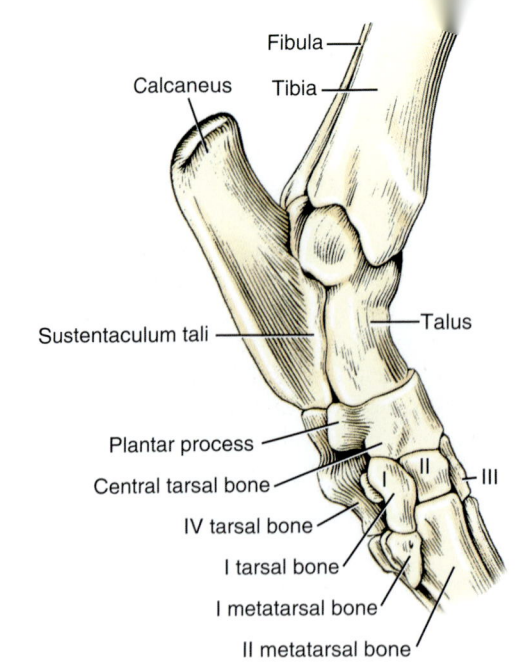

• **Fig. 4.137** Left tarsus, articulated, medial aspect.

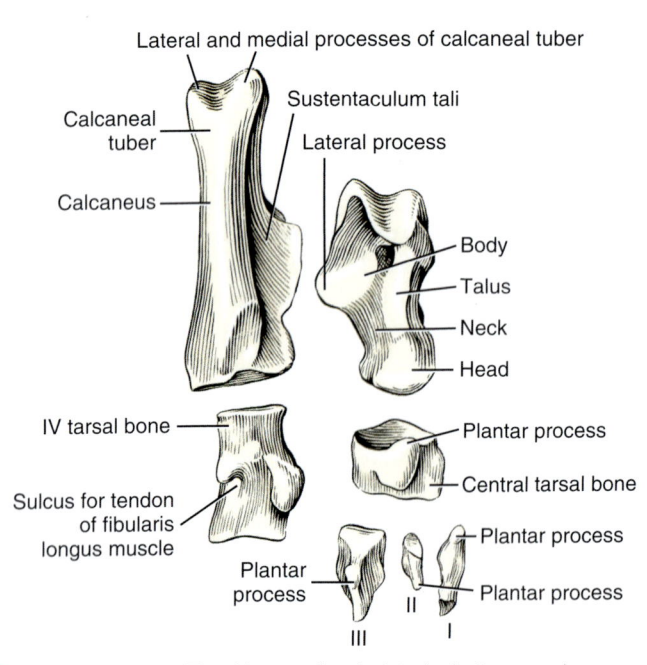

• **Fig. 4.138** Tarsal bones disarticulated, plantar aspect.

metatarsal bones. Each of the four main metatarsal bones bears three phalanges that, with their associated sesamoid bones, form the skeleton of each of the four digits. The first digit, or *hallux*, is usually absent in the dog. When it is fully developed, as it is in some breeds, it contains only two phalanges. The first digit of the hindpaw is known as the **dewclaw**, regardless of its degree of development. Except for the first digit, the skeleton of the hindpaw distal to the tarsus closely resembles the comparable part of the forepaw.

Tarsus

The tarsus, or hock, consists of seven **tarsal bones** (*ossa tarsi*). The term also applies collectively to the several joints between the tarsal bones, as well as to the region between the crus and the metatarsus. The tarsal bones of the dog are arranged in such a way that the tibia and fibula articulate essentially with only the talus. The tarsus is more than three times as long as the carpus, and the distance between its most proximal and its most distal articulation may be 9 cm. The long, laterally located calcaneus and the shorter, medially located talus make up the proximal row. The distal row consists of four bones. Three small bones, the first, second, and third tarsal bones, are located side by side and are separated from the proximal row by the central tarsal bone. The large fourth tarsal bone, which completes the distal row laterally, is as long as the combined lengths of the third and central tarsal bones against which it lies.

The **talus** is the second largest of the tarsal bones. It articulates proximally with the tibia and fibula, distally with the central tarsal, and on the plantar side with the calcaneus. The talus may be divided for descriptive purposes into a head, neck, and body. The **body** (*corpus tali*) forms the proximal half of the bone. The most prominent feature of the body is the **trochlea** (*trochlea tali*) with its two parallel semicircular ridges and a central groove. This trochlea articulates with the sagittal grooves and the intermediate ridge of the cochlea of the tibia. The sides of the trochlea have articular surfaces that articulate with the medial and lateral malleoli and are known as the *facies malleolaris medialis* and *facies malleolaris lateralis*, respectively. The plantar surface of

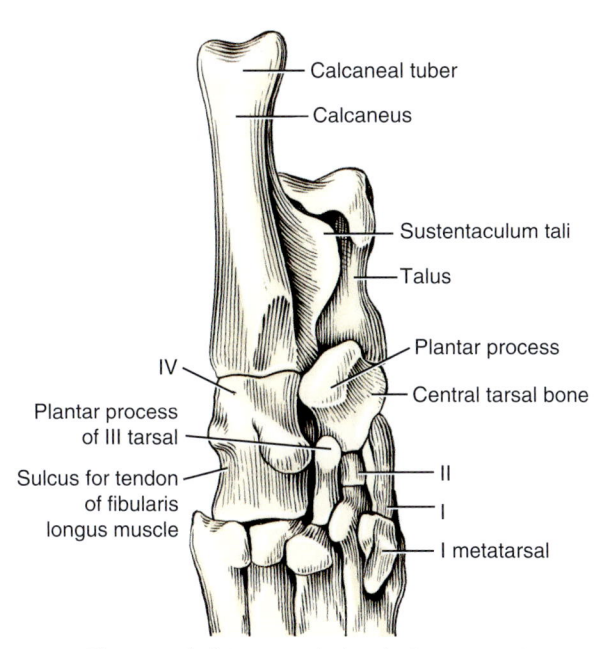

• **Fig. 4.139** Left tarsus, articulated, plantar aspect.

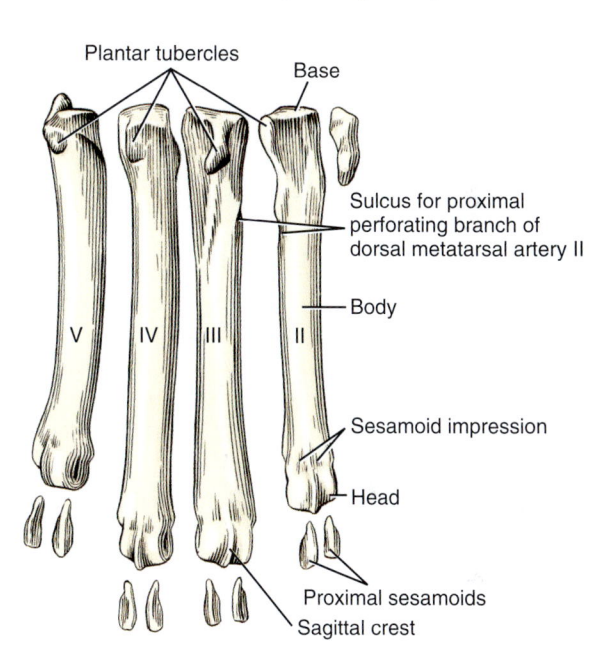

• **Fig. 4.140** Left metatarsal and sesamoid bones, disarticulated, plantar aspect.

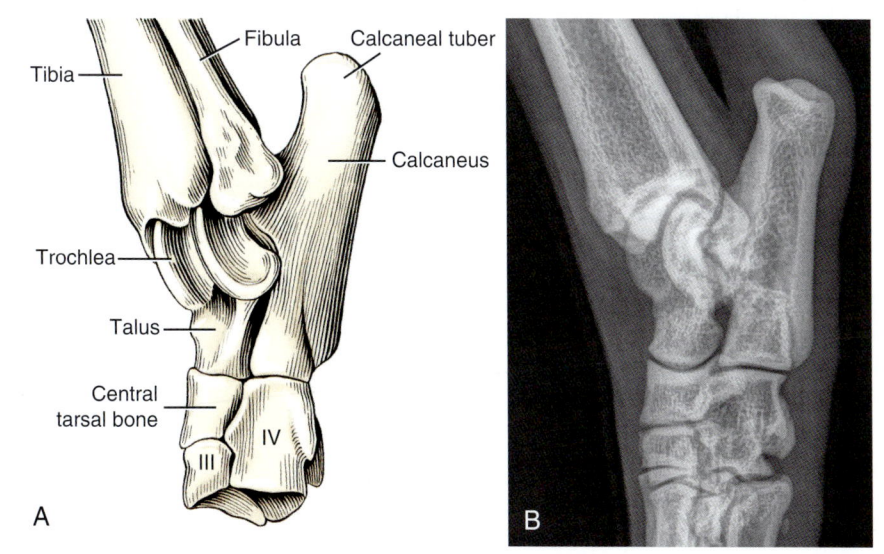

• **Fig. 4.141 A**, Left tarsus, articulated, craniolateral aspect. **B**, Oblique radiograph of left tarsus, articulated.

the talus articulates with the calcaneus by three distinct and separate **calcaneal articular surfaces** (*facies articularis calcanea*). On the plantarolateral surface of the talus is a large, concave articular surface. The lateral part of this articular surface is located on a large, right-angled process that is articular on three sides. It is the **lateral process of the talus** (*processus lateralis tali*). An oval middle articular surface is separated from the lateral part by the deep but narrow *sulcus tali*. The smallest articular surface for the calcaneus is located on the extreme distolateral part of the talus. The **head** (*caput tali*) of the talus is the transversely elongated distal extremity. The distal surface is the **articular surface for the central tarsal** (*facies articularis navicularis*). It is rounded and irregularly oval transversely, and it contacts only the central tarsal. The **neck** (*collum tali*) unites the large, proximally located body with the head. It is smooth and convex medially and lies directly adjacent to the skin.

The **calcaneus**, formerly called the *os calcis* or *fibular tarsal bone*, is the largest and longest bone of the tarsus. The distal half of the bone is wide transversely and possesses three articular surfaces and two processes whereby it is mortised with the talus to form a very stable joint. The *tuber calcanei*, or proximal half of the bone, is a sturdy traction process that serves for the insertion of the common calcanean tendon (*tendo calcaneus communis*). Its slightly bulbous free end contains the medial and lateral processes, which are

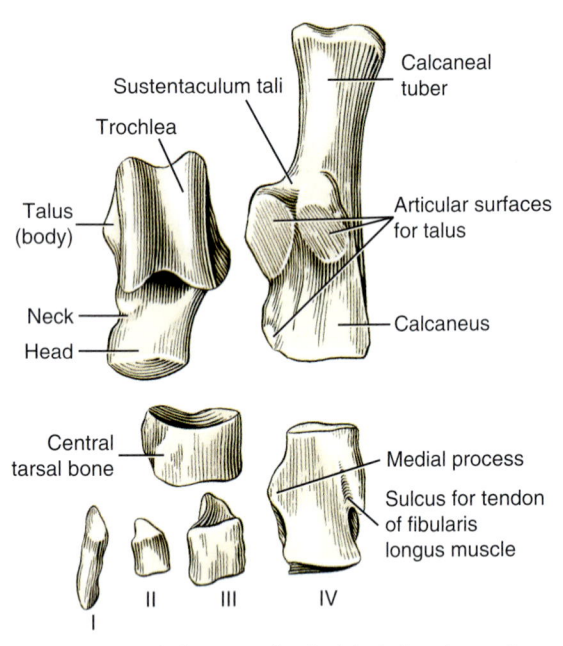

• **Fig. 4.142** Left tarsus, disarticulated, dorsal aspect.

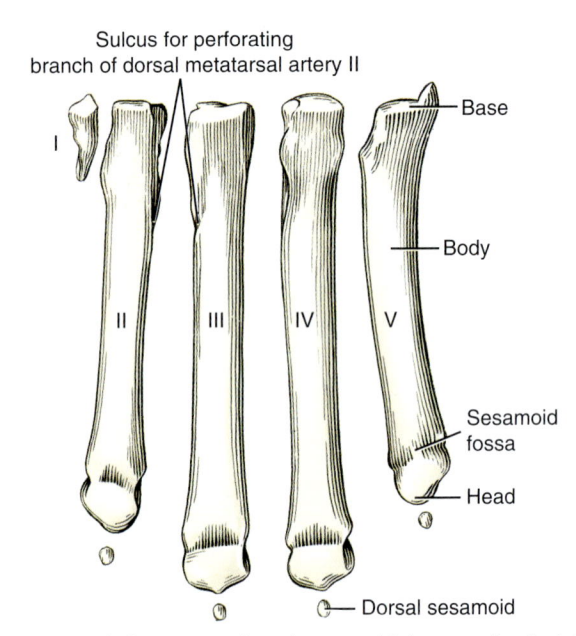

• **Fig. 4.144** Left metatarsal and sesamoid bones, disarticulated, dorsal aspect.

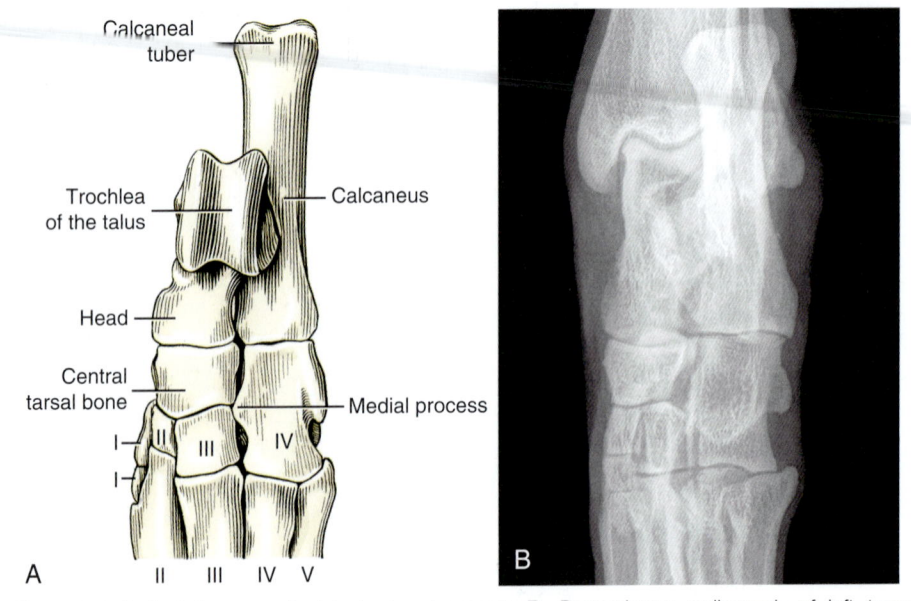

• **Fig. 4.143** **A**, Left tarsus, articulated, dorsal aspect. **B**, Dorsoplantar radiograph of left tarsus, articulated.

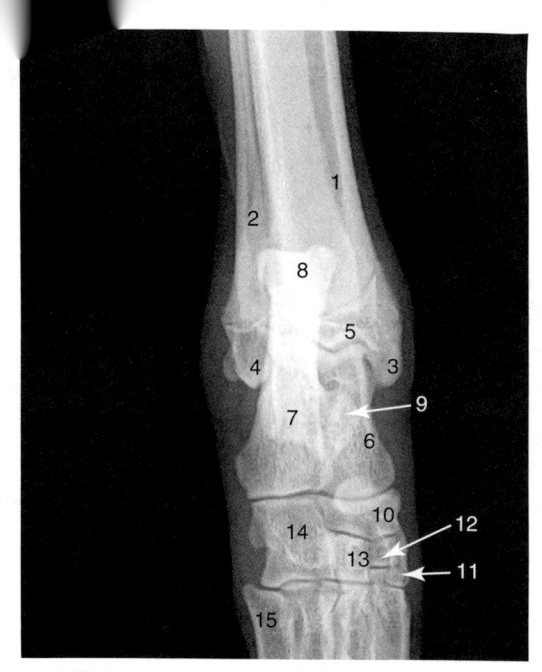

CHAPTER 4 The Skeleton 171

separated by a wide groove. A jutting shelf, the *sustentaculum tali*, leaves the medial side of the bone. On the plantar side of this process is a wide, shallow groove over which the tendon of the m. flexor digitorum lateralis passes. The **articular surfaces** for articulation with the talus (*facies articularis talaris*) consist of a concave oval surface dorsomedially and a convex lateral surface. The most distal and the smallest surface is confluent with a small articular surface for the central tarsal on the distal surface. Between the middle and the distal articular surfaces is the **calcanean sulcus** (*sulcus calcanei*). This sulcus concurs with a similar one of the talus to form the **tarsal sinus** (*sinus tarsi*). On the distal end of the calcaneus is a large flat articular surface (*facies articularis cuboidea*) for articulation mainly with the fourth tarsal and by a small surface with the talus.

The **central tarsal bone** (*os tarsi centrale*) lies in the medial part of the tarsus between the proximal and the distal rows. It articulates with all the other tarsal bones. Proximally it articulates with the talus by a large, concave, roughly oval area. On the proximal surface of the plantar process of the bone, *tuberositas plantaris*, is a small surface for articulation with the calcaneus. The central tarsal articulates distally with the first, second, and third tarsals, and laterally with the proximal half of the fourth tarsal.

The **first tarsal bone** (*os tarsale I*) varies greatly in development. When it does not exist as a separate bone, it is fused with the distally lying first metatarsal bone. It is always compressed transversely. When it is fused with the first metatarsal, it forms a rough, bent plate. The first tarsal bone normally articulates with the central tarsal, the second tarsal, and the first metatarsal. Occasionally the first tarsal bone articulates with the second metatarsal. Other possible variations are described in the discussion of the first digit of the hindpaw, under the section on phalanges.

The **second tarsal bone** (*os tarsale II*) is the smallest of the tarsal bones. It is a wedge of bone that extends toward the plantar side only a short distance. It articulates with the central tarsal proximally, the third tarsal laterally, the first tarsal medially, and the second metatarsal distally. The joint with the second metatarsal is at a higher level than the similar joints lateral to it.

The **third tarsal bone** (*os tarsale III*) is nearly three times larger and two times longer than the second tarsal bone. It articulates proximally with the central tarsal, laterally with the fourth tarsal, distally with the third metatarsal, and medially with the second tarsal and metatarsal. On the plantar side it ends in a rounded plantar tuberosity that is embedded in the joint capsule.

The **fourth tarsal bone** (*os tarsale IV*) is as long as the combined dimensions of the central and third tarsals, with which it articulates medially. The joint between the fourth and the central tarsals slopes proximally and laterally, whereas the joint with the third tarsal slopes distally and medially. Proximally, the fourth tarsal articulates mainly with the calcaneus and slightly with the talus on its dorsomedial edge. Medially, the fourth tarsal articulates with the central and third tarsals and distally with metatarsals

1. Tibia
2. Fibula
3. Medial malleolus
4. Lateral malleolus
5. Tibial cochlea
6. Talus
7. Calcaneus
8. Calcaneal tuber
9. Sustentaculum tali
10. Central tarsal bone
11. First tarsal bone
12. Second tarsal bone
13. Third tarsal bone
14. Fourth tarsal bone
15. Metatarsal V

• **Fig. 4.145** Dorsoplantar radiograph of the tarsus:

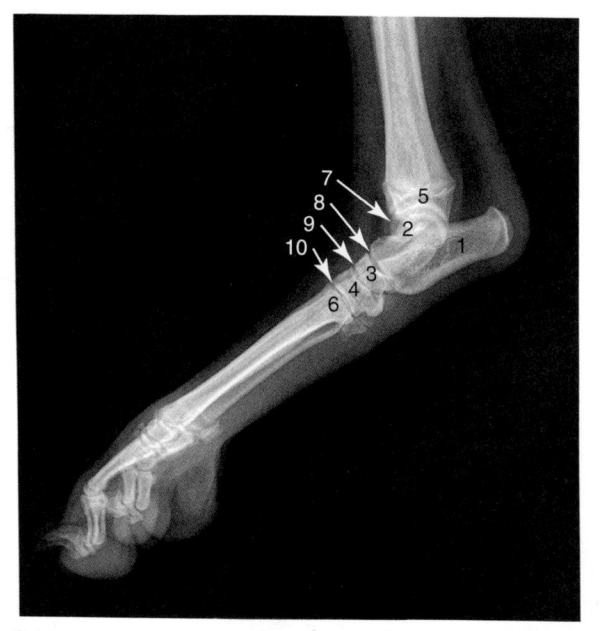

1. Calcaneus
2. Talus
3. Central and fourth tarsal bones
4. First to fourth tarsal bones
5. Tibial cochlea
6. Metatarsal bones (bases)
7. Tarsocrural joint
8. Proximal intertarsal joint
9. Distal intertarsal joint
10. Tarsometatarsal joint

• **Fig. 4.146** Lateral radiograph of the tarsus.

IV and V. The distal half of the lateral surface is widely grooved for the tendon of the m. fibularis longus, forming the *sulcus tendinis m. fibularis longus*. Proximal to the sulcus is the salient tuberosity of the fourth tarsal bone (*tuberositas ossis tarsalis quarti*). Distally there are two indistinct rectangular areas, sometimes partly separated by a synovial fossa, for articulation with metatarsals IV and V. All tarsal bones of the distal row possess prominent plantar processes for the attachment of the heavy plantar portion of the joint capsule.

Metatarsus

The term *metatarsus* refers to the region of the pes, or hindpaw, located between the tarsus and the phalanges (see Figs. 4.140 and 4.144). The **metatarsal bones** (*ossa metatarsalia I–V*) resemble the corresponding metacarpal bones in general form. They are, however, longer. The shortest main metatarsal bone, metatarsal II, is about as long as the longest metacarpal bone. The metatarsus is compressed transversely so that the dimensions of the bases of the individual bones are considerably greater sagittally than they are transversely. Furthermore, as a result of this lateral crowding the areas of contact between adjacent bones are greater and the intermetatarsal spaces are smaller. The whole skeleton of the hindpaw is longer and narrower than that of the forepaw.

The **first metatarsal bone** (*os metatarsale I*) is usually atypical and will be described with the phalanges of the first digit.

Metatarsal bones II, III, IV, and V (*ossa metatarsalia II–V*) are similar. A typical metatarsal bone consists of a proximal base (*basis*), which is transversely compressed and irregular, and a shaft, or **body** (*corpus*), which in general is triangular proximally, quadrangular at midshaft, and oval distally. Each body possesses one large and several small nutrient foramina that enter the proximal halves of the bones from either the contact or the plantar surface. Oblique grooves on the opposed surfaces of the proximal fourths of metatarsals II and III form a space through which passes the proximal perforating branch of the dorsal metatarsal artery II. The distal end of each main metatarsal bone, like each corresponding metacarpal bone, has a ball-shaped **head** (*caput*), which is separated from the body dorsally by a deep transverse **sesamoid fossa** (*fossa sesamoidalis*). On the plantar part of the head the articular surface is divided by a sagittal crest in such a way that the area nearer the axis of the paw is slightly narrower and less oblique transversely than the one on the abaxial side. The four mm. interossei arise from the plantar side of the bases of the main metatarsal bones and intimately cover most of their plantar surfaces. The m. tibialis cranialis inserts on the medial side of the base of metatarsal II and the m. fibularis brevis inserts on the lateral side of the base of metatarsal V.

Phalanges

The phalanges and sesamoid bones of the hindpaw are so similar to those of the forepaw that no separate description is necessary, except for the bones of digit 1.

The term **dewclaw** is applied to the variably first digit of the hindpaw of the dog. Some breeds are recognized by the American Kennel Club (2017) as normally possessing fully developed first digits on their hindpaws. Many individuals of the larger breeds of dogs possess dewclaws in various degrees of development (Kadletz, 1932). In the most rudimentary condition an osseous element bearing a claw is attached only by skin to the medial surface of the tarsus. The proximal phalanx may be absent, and metatarsal I, much reduced in size, may or may not be fused with the first tarsal. Occasionally, two claws of equal size are present on the medial side of the hindpaw. These supernumerary digits probably have no phylogenetic significance. Complete duplication of the phalanges and metatarsal I is sometimes encountered. The first metatarsal may also be divided into a proximal and a distal portion. The distal metatarsal element is never fused to the proximal phalanx. It may be united to its proximal part by fibrous tissue, or a true joint may exist. Although the dewclaw may be lacking, a rudiment of the first metatarsal is occasionally seen as a small, flattened osseous plate that lies in the fibrous tissue on the medial side of the tarsus.

Stockard (1930), in his review of the atavistic reappearance of digits in mammals, noted that in most breeds of domestic and wild dogs there are five digits on the forepaw and four on the hindpaw. (Only the African hunting dog, *Lycaon pictus*, regularly has four digits on each paw.) Stockard crossed St. Bernards having the first digit on the hindpaw (sometimes double), with Great Danes, which always lack it (although they may have a rudimentary hidden first metatarsal). Of 78 hybrid pups from St. Bernard–Great Dane crosses, enough had the first digit present to indicate that it was inherited as a dominant character, even though this feature has almost disappeared in the family Canidae.

Bibliography

Alberch, P. (1985). Developmental constraints: Why St. Bernards often have an extra digit and poodles never do. *Am Nat, 126*, 430–433.

Albrecht, P. (1880). Uber den proatlas, einen zwischen dem occipitale und dem atlas der amnioten wirbelthiere gelegenen wirbel, und den nervus spinalis 1 s. proatlanticus. *Zool Anz, 3*, 450–454, and 472–478.

American Kennel Club (2017). *The new complete dog book* (22nd ed.). Mt. Joy, PA: Fox Chapel Publ.

Badoux, D. M. (1969). Biostatics of the cervical vertebrae in domesticated dogs. *Proc K Ned Akad Wet C, 72*, 478–490.

Badoux, D. M. (1975). General biostatics and biomechanics. In R. Getty (Ed.), *Sisson and Grossman's anatomy of the domestic animals* (5th ed.). Philadelphia: Saunders.

Baum, H., & Zietzschmann, O. (1936). *Handbuch der anatomie des hundes. Band I: Skelette- und muskel-system*. Berlin: Paul Parey.

Bonewald, L. F. (2008). The osteocyte. In *Osteoporosis* (3rd ed.). Amsterdam: Elsevier.

Bourne, G. H. (1972). *The biochemistry and physiology of bone* (2nd ed., Vol. I, II, III). New York: Academic Press.

Bourne, G. H. (1976). *Calcification and physiology* (Vol. IV). New York: Academic Press.

Bressou, C., Pomriaskinsky-Kobozieff, N., & Kobozieff, N. (1957). Étude radiologique de l'ossification du squelette du pied du chien aux divers stade de son évolution, de la naissance à l'âge adulte. *Rec Méd Vet Alfort, 133*, 449–464.

Buckwalter, J. A., Glimcher, M. J., Cooper, R. R., et al. (1995). Bone biology. I. structure, blood supply, cells, matrix, and mineralization, II. Formation, form, modeling, remodeling, and regulation of cell function. *J Bone Joint Surg Am, 77A/8*, 1256–1275, 77A/8, 1276–1289.

Carrig, C. B., & Morgan, J. P. (1975). Asynchronous growth of the canine radius and ulna—early radiographic changes following experimental retardation of longitudinal growth of the ulna. *J Am Vet Radiol Soc, 16*, 121–129.

Casinos, A., Bou, J., Castiella, M. J., et al. (1986). On the allometry of long bones in dogs (*Canis familiaris*). *J Morphol, 190*, 73–79.

Cave, A. J. E. (1975). The morphology of the mammalian cervical pleurapophysis. *J Zool, 177*, 377–393.

Cerny, H., & Čižinauskas, S. (1995). The clavicle of newborn dogs. *Acta Vet Brno, 64*, 139–145.

Chaine, J. (1926). L'os pénien; étude descriptive et comparative. *Actes Soc Linn Bordeaux, 78*, 1–195.

Clutton-Brock, J., Corbet, G. B., & Hills, M. (1976). A review of the family Canidae with a classification by numerical methods. *Bull Br Mus Zool (Nat Hist), 29*(3), 1–99.

Crary, D. D. (1962). Modified benzyl alcohol clearing of alizarine stained specimens without loss of flexibility. *Stain Technol, 37*, 124–125.

Dabanoglu, I., Kara, M. E., Turan, E., et al. (2004). Morphometry of the thoracic spine in German shepherd dog: A computed tomographic study. *Anat Histol Embryol, 33*(1), 53–58.

Debarekeleer, J., Gross, K. L., Zicker, S. C., et al. (2010). Feeding growing puppies. In M. S. Hand, C. D. Thatcher, R. L. Remillard, et al. (Eds.), *Small animal clinical nutrition* (5th ed.). Topeka, KS: Mark Morris Institute.

de Beer, G. R. (1937). *The development of the vertebrate skull*. London: Oxford University Press.

Dingerkus, G., & Uhler, L. D. (1977). Enzyme clearing of alcian blue stained whole small vertebrates for demonstration of cartilage. *Stain Technol, 52*, 229–232.

Dixon, A. D., Sarnat, B. G., & Hoyte, D. A. N. (1991). *Fundamentals of bone growth: Methodology and applications*. Boca Raton, FL: CRC Press.

Dixon, T. F., & Perkins, H. R. (1956). The chemistry of calcification. In G. H. Bourne (Ed.), *The biochemistry and physiology of bone* (pp. 287–317). New York: Academic Press. chapter 10.

Ellenberger, W., & Baum, H. (1943). *Handbuch der vergleichenden anatomie der haustiere* (18th ed.). Berlin: Springer.

Ellis, J. L., Thomason, J., Kebreab, E., et al. (2009). Cranial dimensions and forces of biting in the domestic dog. *J Anat, 214*(3), 362–373.

Erhart, M. B. (1943). Anotacoes craniologicas III: Incidencia do "os preinterparietale" em cranios de "canis familiaris." *Rev Sudam Morfol, 1*, 1–15.

Evans, F. G. (1939). The morphology and functional evolution of the atlas-axis complex from fish to mammals. *Ann N Y Acad Sci, 39*, 29–104.

Evans, H. E. (1948). Clearing and staining small vertebrates, in toto, for demonstrating ossification. *Turtox News, 26*, 42–47.

Evans, H. E. (1958). Prenatal ossification in the dog. *Anat Rec, 130*, 406.

Evans, H. E. (1962). Fetal growth and skeletal development in the dog. *Am Zool, 2*, 521.

Evans, H. E. (1974). *Prenatal development of the dog*. Ithaca, NY: Gaines Symposium.

Fagin, B. D., Aronson, E., & Gutzmer, M. A. (1992). Closure of the iliac crest ossification center in dogs: 750 cases (1980-1987). *J Am Vet Med Assoc, 200*, 1709–1711.

Farnum, C. E., Turgai, J., & Wilsman, N. J. (1990). Visualization of living terminal hypertrophic chondrocytes of growth plate cartilage in situ by differential interference, contrast microscopy and time-lapse cinematography. *J Orthop Res, 8*, 750–763.

Farnum, C. E., & Wilsman, N. J. (1989). Condensation of hypertrophic chondrocytes at the chondro-osseous junction of growth plate cartilage in Yucatan swine: Relationship to long bone growth. *Am J Anat, 186*, 346–358.

Flower, W. H. (1870). *An introduction to the osteology of mammalia*. London: Globe. 3rd ed., Asher, Netherlands, 1966.

Freiberger, R. H., Wilson, P. D., & Nicholas, J. A. (1965). Acquired absence of the odontoid process. A case report. *J Bone Joint Surg, 47A*, 1231–1236.

Gage, E. D., & Smallwood, J. E. (1970). Surgical repair of atlanto-axial subluxation in a dog. *Vet Med Small Anim Clin, 65*, 583–592.

Geary, J. C., Oliver, J. E., & Hoerlein, B. F. (1967). Atlanto-axial subluxation in the canine. *J Small Anim Pract, 8*, 577–582.

Getty, R. (1975). *Sisson and Grossman's anatomy of the domestic animals* (5th ed.). 2 vols. Philadelphia: Saunders Co.

Grässel, S., & Aszódi, A. (2016). *Cartilage. Vol. 1: Physiology and development*. Switzerland: Springer.

Haag, W. G. (1948). *An osteometric analysis of some aboriginal dogs* (Vol. VII, 3, pp. 107–264). Reports in anthropology. Lexington: University of Kentucky.

Haines, R. W. (1942). The evolution of epiphyses and of endochondral bone. *Biol Rev, 17*, 267–292.

Hall, B. K. (1977). Chondrogenesis of the somatic mesoderm. *Adv Anat Embryol Cell Biol, 53*, 1–50.

Hall, B. K. (1978). *Developmental and cellular skeletal biology*. New York: Academic Press.

Hall, B. K. (1988). The embryonic development of bone. *Am Sci, 76*, 174–182.

Hall, B. K. (1989–1992). *Bone: A treatise, The osteoblast and osteocyte, vol. 1, The osteoclast, vol. 2, Bone matrix, vol. 3, Mineralization of bone, vol. 4, Hormones and bone, vol. 5, Bone growth, vol. 6, Fracture repair and regeneration, vol. 7*. New York: Academic Press.

Hall, B. K. (2015). *Bones and cartilage: Developmental and evolutionary skeletal biology* (2nd ed.). Amsterdam: Elsevier.

Hall, B. K., & Newman, S. (1991). *Cartilage: Molecular aspects*. Boca Raton, FL: CRC Press.

Hamon, M. A. *Atlas de la Tete du Chien: Coupes series-radioanatomie-tomographies*. Theses, l'Univ, 1977, Paul Sabatier de Toulouse (Sciences).

Hancox, N. M. (1972). *Biology of bone*. Cambridge: Cambridge University Press.

Hansen, H. (1952). A pathologic-anatomical study on disc degeneration in the dog. *Acta Orthop Scand Suppl, 11*, 1–117.

Hare, W. C. D. (1960). The age at which epiphysial union takes place in the limb bones of the dog. *Wien Tierarztl Monatsschr, 9*(72), 224–245.

Hare, W. C. D. (1961a). Zur ossification und vereinigung der wirbelepiphysen beim hund. *Wien Tierarztl Monatsschr, 9*(72), 210–215.

Hare, W. C. D. (1961b). Radiographic anatomy of the cervical region of the canine vertebral column. *J Am Vet Med Assoc, 139*, 209–220.

Hare, W. C. D. (1961c). The age, at which the centers of ossification appear roentgenographically in the limb bones of the dog. *Am J Vet Res, 22*, 825–835.

Hedhammer, A., Wu, F. M., Krook, L., et al. (1974). Overnutrition and skeletal disease. An experimental study in growing great dane dogs. *Cornell Vet, 64*(2 Suppl. 5), 1–160.

Hildebrand, M. (1954). Comparative morphology of the body skeleton in recent canidae. *Univ Calif Publ Zool, 52*, 399–470.

Hughes, H. V., & Dransfield, J. W. (1953). *Mcfadyean's osteology and arthrology of the domesticated animals*. London: Baillière, Tindall & Cox.

Huja, S., & Beck, F. M. (2007). Bone remodeling in maxilla, mandible, and femur of young dogs. *Anat Rec, 291*, 1–5.

Iwanoff, S. (1935). Variations in the ribs and vertebrae of the dog. *Jb Vet Med Fat Sofia (Bulg), 10*, 461–497.

Jayne, H. (1898). *Mammalian anatomy: Part I. The skeleton of the cat*. Philadelphia: JB Lippincott.

Johnson, K. A. (1981). Retardation of endochondral ossification at the distal ulnar growth plate in dogs. *Aust Vet J, 57*, 474–478.

Jurvelin, J., Lahtinen, T., Kiviranta, I., et al. (1988). Blood flow, histomorphology and elemental composition of the canine femur after physical training or immobilization. *Acta Physiol Scand, 132*(3), 385–389.

Kadletz, M. (1932). *Anatomischer atlas der extremitätengelenke von pferd und hund, Berlin*. Wien: Urban & Schwarzenberg.

Kelly, W. L., & Bryden, M. M. (1983). A modified differential stain for cartilage and bone in whole mount preparations of mammalian fetuses and small vertebrates. *Stain Technol, 58*, 131–134.

Kimmel, D. B., & Jee, W. S. S. (1982). A quantitative histologic study of bone turnover in young adult beagles. *Anat Rec, 203*, 31–45.

Kincaid, S. A., & Van Sickle, D. C. (1983). Bone morphology and postnatal osteogenesis. Potential for disease. *Vet Clin North Am Small Anim Pract, 13*, 3–17.

Koch, D. A., Wiestner, T., Balli, A., et al. (2012). Proposal for a new radiological index to determine skull conformation in the dog. *Schweiz Arch Tierheilk, 154*, 217–220. doi:10.1024/0036-7281/a000331.

König, H. E., & Liebich, H.-G. (2004). *Veterinary anatomy of domestic animals*. Stuttgart: Schattauer.

Kuhn, J. L., Goulendt, R. W., Pappas, M., et al. (1990). Morphometric and anisotropic symmetries of the canine distal femur. *J Orthop Res, 8*, 776–780.

Kumar, M. S. A. (2015). *Clinically oriented anatomy of the dog & cat* (2nd ed.). Ronkonkoma, NY: Linus Learning.

Kuntz, A., & Richins, C. A. (1945). Innervation of the bone marrow. *J Comp Neurol, 83*, 213–222.

Lumer, H. (1940). Evolutionary allometry in the skeleton of the domesticated dog. *Am Nat, 74*, 439–467.

Lindner, D. L., Marretta, S. M., Pijanowski, G. J., et al. (1995). Measurement of bite force in dogs: A pilot study. *J Vet Dent, 12*, 49–52.

Maier, V. (1928). Untersuchungen über die pneumatizität des hundeschädels mit berücksichtigung der rassenunterschiede. *Z Anat Entwicklungsgesch, 85*, 251–286.

Marks, S. C., & Popoff, S. N. (1988). Bone cell biology: The regulation of development, structure, and function in the skeleton. *Am J Anat, 183*, 1–44.

Martin, T. J., & Sims, N. A. (2009). Bone remodeling: Cellular and molecular events. In *Pourquie the skeletal system*. Cold Spring Harbor, NY: Laboratory Press.

McCarthy, P. H., & Wood, A. K. (1988). Anatomic and radiologic observations of the clavicle of adult dogs. *Am J Vet Res, 49*(6), 956–959.

Moore, W. J. (1981). *The mammalian skull*. London: Cambridge University Press.

Nickel, R., Schummer, A., Seiferle, E., et al. (1977). *Lehrbuch der anatomie der haustiere. Band 1: Bewegungsapparat*. Berlin: Paul Parey.

Nap, R. C., & Hazewinkel, H. A. W. (1994). Growth and skeletal development in the dog in relation to nutrition; a review. *Vet Q, 16*, 50–59.

Noden, D. M., & de Lahunta, A. (1985). *The embryology of domestic animals. developmental mechanisms and malformations*. Baltimore, MD: The Williams & Wilkins Co.

Oliver, J. E., & Lewis, R. E. (1973). Lesions of the atlas and axis in dogs. *J Am Anim Hosp Assoc, 9*, 304–313.

Orsini, M. W. (1962). Technique of preparation, study, and photography of benzyle-benzoate cleared material for embryological studies. *J Reprod Fertil, 3*, 283–287.

Owen, R. (1866). *On the anatomy of vertebrates*. London: Longmans and Green.

Pomriaskinsky-Kobozieff, N., & Kobozieff, N. (1954). Étude radiologique de l'aspect du squelette normal de la main du chien aux divers stades de son évolution, de la naissance à l'âge adulte. *Rec Méd Vet Alfort, 130*, 617–646.

Pourquie, O. (2009). *The skeletal system*. Cold Spring Harbor, NY: Cold Spring Harbor Laboratory Press.

Rasmussen, H., & Bordier, P. (1974). *The physiological and cellular basis of metabolic bone disease*. Baltimore, MD: Williams & Wilkins.

Regodon, S., Vivo, J. M., Franco, A., et al. (1993). Craniofacial angle in dolichol-, meso-, and brachycephalic dogs: Radiological determination and application. *Anat Anz, 175*, 361–363.

Richards, M. W., & Watson, A. G. (1991). Development and variation of the lateral vertebral foramen of the atlas in dogs. *Anat Histol Embryol, 20*, 363–368.

Richardson, D. C., Zentek, J., & Hazewinkel, H. A. (2010). Developmental orthopedic disease of dogs. In M. S. Hand, C. D. Thatcher, R. L. Remillard, et al. (Eds.), *Small animal clinical nutrition* (5th ed.). Topeka, KS: Mark Morris Institute.

Roberts, S. (1986). *Veterinary obstetrics and genital diseases* (3rd ed.). Woodstock, VT: S. Roberts.

Romer, A. S., & Parsons, T. (1986). *The vertebrate body* (5th ed.). Philadelphia: Saunders.

Rumph, P. F., & Hathcock, J. T. (1990). A symmetric axis-based method for measuring the projected femoral angle of inclination in dogs. *Vet Surg, 19*(5), 328–333.

Sawin, P. B., Ranlett, M., & Crary, D. D. (1962). Morphogenetic studies of the rabbit. XXIX. Accessory ossification centers at the occipito-vertebral articulation of the dachs (chondrodystrophy) rabbit. *Am J Anat, 111*, 239–257.

Scapino, R. (1965). The third joint of the canine jaw. *J Morphol, 116*, 23–50.

Scapino, R. (1981). Morphological investigation into functions of the jaw symphysis in carnivorans. *J Morphol, 167*, 339–375.

Schaeffer, H. (1934). Die ossifikationsvorgänge im gliedmassenskelett des hundes. *Morph Jahrb, 74*, 472–512.

Schatzker, J., Rorabeck, C. H., & Waddell, J. (1971). Fractures of the dens (odontoid process): An analysis of thirty-seven cases. *J Bone Joint Surg, 53B*, 392–405.

Schebitz, H., & Wilkins, H. (1986). *Atlas of radiographic anatomy of the dog and cat* (4th ed.). Philadelphia: Saunders.

..., J. (1978). First metacarpal bone or proximal phalanx? *J Am Vet Radiol Soc*, *19*, 50–52.

Simoens, P., Poels, P., & Lauers, H. (1994). Morphometric analysis of the foramen magnum in Pekingese dogs. *Am J Vet Res*, *55*(1), 34–39.

Simon, W. T., Bronk, J. T., Pinto, M. R., et al. (1988). Cortical and cancellous bone: Age-related changes in morphologic features, fluid spaces, and calcium homeostasis in dogs. *Mayo Clin Proc*, *63*(2), 154–160.

Singh, B. (2017). *Dyce, Sack and Wensing's textbook of veterinary anatomy* (5th ed.). St Louis, MO: Elsevier.

Slijper, E. J. (1946). Comparative biologic-anatomical investigations on the vertebral column and spinal musculature of mammals. *K Ned Akad Wet Verh (Tweede Sectie)*, *42*(5), 1–128.

Smith, R. N. (1960). Radiological observations of the limbs of young greyhounds. *J Small Anim Pract*, *1*(2), 84–90.

Smith, R. N., & Allcock, J. (1960). Epiphysial fusion in the greyhound. *Vet Rec*, *72*(5), 75–79.

Stockard, C. R. (1930). The presence of a factorial basis for characters lost in evolution: The atavistic reappearance of digits in mammals. *Am J Anat*, *45*, 345–377.

Stockard, C. R. (1941). *The genetic and endocrinic basis for differences in form and behavior. Am. Anat. Memoir 19*. Philadelphia: Wistar Institute of Anatomy and Biology.

Suminski, P. (1975). Investigation and comparison of the skull of the wolf (*Canis lupus* L.) with that of the domestic dog (*Canis familiaris* L.). *Z Jagdwiss*, *21*(2), 129–133.

Taylor, W. R., & VanDyke, G. C. (1985). Revised procedures for staining and clearing small fishes and other vertebrates for bone and cartilage study. *Cybium*, *9*, 107–119.

Trouth, C. O., Winter, S., Gupta, K. C., et al. (1977). Analysis of the sexual dimorphism in the basioccipital portion of the dog's skull. *Acta Anat (Basel)*, *98*, 469–473.

Ueshima, T. (1961). A pathological study on deformation of the vertebral column in the short-spine dog. *Jpn J Vet Res*, *9*, 155–179.

Van Sickle, D. C. (1966). The relationship of ossification to canine elbow dysplasia. *Anim Hosp*, *2*, 24–31.

Wake, M. H. (1979). *Hyman's comparative vertebrate anatomy* (3rd ed.). Chicago: University of Chicago Press.

Watson, A. G. (1981). *The phylogeny and development of the occipitoatlas-axis complex in the dog*, Thesis. Ithaca, NY: Cornell University.

Watson, A. G., & Evans, H. E. (1976). The development of the atlas-axis complex in the dog. *Anat Rec*, *184*, 558.

Watson, A. G., & Stewart, J. S. (1990). Postnatal ossification centers of the atlas and axis in miniature schnauzers. *Am J Vet Res*, *51*, 264–268.

Watson, A. G., de Lahunta, A., & Evans, H. E. (1989). Dorsal notch of foramen magnum due to incomplete ossification of supraoccipital bone in dogs. *J Small Anim Pract*, *30*, 666–673.

Watson, A. G., Evans, H. E., & de Lahunta, A. (1986). Ossification of the atlas-axis complex in the dog. *Anat Histol Embryol*, *15*, 122–138.

Wayne, R. K. (1984). *A comparative study of skeletal growth and morphology in domestic and wild canids*, Thesis, Baltimore, MD: Johns Hopkins University.

Wayne, R. K. (1985). *A comparative study of skeletal growth and morphology in domestic dogs and wild canids*, Thesis, Berkeley: University of California.

Wayne, R. K. (1986). Limb morphology of domestic and wild canids: The influence of development on morphologic change. *J Morphol*, *187*, 301–319.

Williams, E. E. (1959). Gadows arcualia and the development of tetrapod vertebrae. *Q Rev Biol*, *34*, 1–32.

Wollin, D. G. (1963). The os odontoideum: Separate odontoid process. *J Bone Joint Surg*, *45A*, 1459–1471.

Wu, F. (1973). *Overnutrition and skeletal disease, a morphological study in great dane dogs*, Thesis. Ithaca, NY: Cornell University.

Zipkin, I. (1973). *Biological mineralization*. New York: John Wiley & Sons.

5
Arthrology

General

Articulations, or **joints** (*articulationes [juncturae] ossium*), are formed when two or more bones are united by fibrous, elastic, or cartilaginous tissue or by a combination of these tissues. Three main groups are recognized and named according to their most characteristic structural features. Where little movement is required, the union is short, direct, and often transitory. A **fibrous joint** (*junctura fibrosa*), formerly known as a *synarthrosis*, is one of this nature. Such joints include syndesmoses, sutures, and gomphoses. A **cartilaginous joint** (*junctura cartilaginea*), formerly known as an *amphiarthrosis*, permits only limited movement, such as compression or stretching. A **synovial joint** (*junctura synovialis*) formerly known as a diarthrosis or true joint, facilitates mobility. The studies of Kadletz (1932) provide detailed information on the arthrology of the dog, and the well-documented work of Barnett et al. (1961) discusses the structure and mechanics of synovial joints in considerable detail.

The term *syndesmologia* was used in the Basel Nomina Anatomica (BNA) of 1895 for the joints and ligaments. This was changed to *arthrology* in the Birmingham Revision of 1933 and back to the original in Paris in 1955.

At the Tokyo meeting of the International Nomenclature Committee, *arthrologia* was adopted as the most appropriate heading and *articulatio* replaced *junctura*. The sixth edition of *Nomina Anatomica* (the NAV; 1989), retained *arthrologia* and *articulatio*. It should be noted that the discarded original term, *syndesmologia*, for all joints is similar sounding to the term *syndesmosis*, which is used to denote one type of fibrous joint.

Nomina Anatomica Veterinaria (1983) adopted *articulatio* for all joints—fibrous, cartilaginous, and synovial. The term *articulationes synoviales* replaces the former terms *diarthrosis* and *articulus*. This terminology was retained in the revised fifth edition of the *Nomina Anatomica Veterinaria* in 2017.

Fibrous Joints

A **syndesmosis** is a fibrous joint with a considerable amount of intervening connective tissue. The attachment of the hyoid apparatus to the petrous part of the temporal bone is an example of a syndesmosis.

A **suture** (*sutura*) is a fibrous joint of the type that is confined largely to the flat bones of the skull. Depending on the shape of the apposed edges, sutures are further divided into (1) **serrated suture** (*sutura serrata*), one that articulates by means of reciprocally alternating processes and depressions; (2) **squamous suture** (*sutura squamosa*), one that articulates by overlapping of reciprocally beveled edges; (3) **plane suture** (*sutura plana*), one in which the bones meet at an essentially right-angled edge or surface; and (4) **foliate suture** (*sutura foliata*), one in which the edge of one bone fits into a fissure or recess of an adjacent bone. Serrate sutures are found where stable noncompressible joints are needed, such as the parietooccipital and the interparietal unions. Where a slight degree of compressibility is advantageous, such as is required in the fetal cranium at birth, squamous sutures are found. Similarly, the frontonasal and frontomaxillary squamous sutures allow enough movement to absorb the shock of a blow that might otherwise fracture the bones of the face. Examples of plane sutures are those of the ethmoid and those between most of the bones of the face. Where extreme stability is desirable, foliate sutures are formed. The best example of this type is the zygomaticomaxillary suture. The various fibrous sutures of the skull also permit growth to take place at the periphery of the bones. When uneven jagged edges of bones interlock in a fibrous joint, as occurs in several skull bones, it is called a **schindylesis**.

The implantation of a tooth in its alveolus by means of a fibrous union known as a **gomphosis**, or *articulatio dentoalveolaris*. This specialized type of fibrous joint is formed by the periodontal ligament (*periodontium*), which attaches the cementum of the tooth to the alveolar bone of the alveolus and permits slight movement.

Cartilaginous Joints

Many bones are united by cartilaginous joints, which are sometimes referred to as *synchondroses*. Unions of this type may be formed by hyaline cartilage, by fibrocartilage, or by a combination of the two, and they are subject to change with increasing age.

Hyaline cartilage joints, or primary joints, are usually temporary and represent persistent parts of the fetal skeleton or secondary cartilage of growing bones. The epiphysis of an immature long bone is united with the diaphysis by

...physeal plate. When adult stature is reached, ...fusion occurs and a joint no longer exists, although a slight physeal line may mark the union. This osseous union in some anatomic works is called a *synostosis*. Similar transitory hyaline cartilage joints are typical of the spheno-occipital synchondrosis or the union of an apophysis with the extremity (epiphysis) or body (diaphysis) of a long bone such as with the femoral trochanters or the ulnar olecranon tubercle. The humeral tubercles develop from the proximal epiphysis. Some hyaline cartilage joints, such as the costo-chondral junctions, remain throughout life.

Fibrocartilaginous joints, or secondary joints, are sometimes referred to as *amphiarthroses*. The best examples of such joints are those of the pelvic symphysis, the inter-mandibular articulation, sternebrae, and vertebral bodies. The fibrocartilage uniting these bones may have an intervening plate of hyaline cartilage at each end. Occasionally these joints may ossify, as do hyaline cartilage joints.

Synovial Joints

The synovial joints of the extremities permit the greatest degree of movement and are most commonly involved in dislocations. All **synovial joints** (*articulationes synoviales*) are characterized by a **joint cavity** (*cavum articulare*), a **joint capsule** (*capsula articularis*) including an outer fibrous layer and an inner synovial membrane, **synovial fluid** (*synovia*), and **articular cartilage** (*cartilago articularis*). Collateral ligaments are developed in the fibrous layer of the joint capsule. A few of the synovial joints have modifications of their joint capsules peculiar to the functions they perform and may possess intraarticular ligaments, menisci, fat pads, or synovial membrane projections in the form of plicae or villi. These are primarily developments of the fibrous membrane of the joint capsule.

The blood supply of synovial joints is provided by an arterial and venous network from parent trunks in the vicinity of the joint. The vessels supply the capsule and also the epiphyses bordering the joint. Around the articular margins, the blood vessels of the synovial membrane form anastomosing loops, referred to collectively as the *circulus articularis vasculosus*.

Lymphatic vessels are also present in synovial membranes and account for the rapid removal of some substances from the joint cavity.

The nerve supply of synovial joints is derived from cutaneous or muscular branches in the vicinity of the joint. Included in these articular nerves are proprioceptive axons, nociceptor axons, and sympathetic visceral efferent and visceral afferent axons related to vasomotor or vasosensory functions respectively. Some areas of the joint capsule are more richly innervated than others. Four types of joint receptors are present in most animal joints (Polacek, 1966; Zimny, 1988): (1) Ruffini-like receptors in the capsule, (2) Pacinian-like receptors in the capsule, (3) Golgi tendon organs in ligaments, and (4) free nerve endings. If a joint has intraarticular structures, they are usually innervated.

The purpose of the innervation is proprioception and the recognition of angular movement; thus posture is very dependent on these endings. It is likely that the stifle joint with its many ligaments and menisci has the richest innervation of all joints. O'Connor and McConnaughey (1978) and O'Connor (1976, 1984) found both Ruffini endings and Pacinian corpuscles in the menisci of the dog and cat. Sfameni (1902) found single or grouped nerve endings that arose from single axons in the dog and suggested the name *Ruffini endings* because they resembled those described in the skin by Ruffini in 1894. Gardner (1950) reviewed the morphologic and physiologic characteristics of joints in the human, including their innervation, and cites more than 500 references. Ansulayotin (1960) studied the nerves that supply the appendicular joints in the dog.

Structure of Synovial Joints

The **joint capsule** is composed of an inner synovial membrane and an outer fibrous membrane. The **synovial membrane** (*membrana synovialis*) is a vascular connective tissue that lines the inner surface of the capsule and is responsible for the production of synovial fluid. The synovial membrane does not cover the articular cartilage but blends with the periosteum as it reflects onto the bone. Joint capsules may arise postnatally if the need exists, and thus false joints often form following unreduced fractures. Synovial membrane covers all structures within a synovial joint except the articular cartilage and the contact surfaces of fibrocartilaginous plates. Synovial membrane also forms sleeves around intraarticular ligaments and covers muscles, tendons, nerves, and vessels if these cross the joint closely. Adipose tissue often fills the irregularities between articulating bones, and, in some instances, it is aspirated into or squeezed out of the joint as the surfaces of the articulating bones part or come together during movement. Fat in such locations is covered by synovial membrane. A **synovial fold** (*plica synovialis*) is an extension of the synovial membrane; such folds usually contain fat. Around the periphery of some synovial joints the synovial membrane is in the form of numerous processes, or **synovial villi** (*villi synoviales*). These are soft and velvety. The synovial membrane may extend beyond the fibrous layer and act as a bursa deep to a tendon or ligament or may even form a synovial sheath.

The **fibrous membrane** (*membrana fibrosa*) of a joint capsule is composed mainly of white fibrous tissue containing yellow elastic fibers. It is also known as the capsular ligament. In most joints the ligaments are thickenings of the fibrous portion of the joint capsule. In some synovial joints the ligaments appear to be quite separate from the fibrous capsular ligament, such as the patellar ligament of the stifle joint. This may be a reason to consider the patellar ligament to be the tendon of insertion of the quadriceps muscle with a sesamoid (the patella) associated with this insertion. On the other hand, the patellar ligament can be considered to be a development of the fibrous layer of the stifle joint capsule along with the extensive fat pad associated with it.

In those joints where great movement occurs in a single plane the fibrous membrane is usually thin and loose on the flexor and extensor surfaces and thick on the sides of the bone that move the least. Such thickenings of the fibrous layer are known as **collateral ligaments** (*ligg. collateralia*) and are present to a greater or lesser degree in all hinge joints. The fibrous membrane attaches at the margin of the articular cartilage, or at most 3 cm from it, where it blends with the periosteum.

The **synovial fluid** (*synovia*) serves chiefly to lubricate the contact surfaces of synovial joints. In all cases these surfaces are hyaline cartilage or fibrocartilage. Fibrocartilage contains few blood vessels and nerves, and hyaline cartilage has neither. Therefore the synovial fluid serves the additional function of transporting nutrient material to the hyaline cartilage and removing the waste metabolites from it. Synovia also enables the wandering leukocytes to circulate in the joint cavity and phagocytize the products of the wear and tear of the articular cartilage. In many joints there is little, if any, free synovia. The average volume in the stifle joint of adult dogs of various sizes varies from 0.2 mL to 2 mL. The general health and condition of the dog has a marked influence on the amount of synovia present in the joints. Synovia is thought to be a dialysate, although mucin is probably produced by the fibroblasts of the synovial membrane (Davies, 1944). The chemical composition of synovia closely resembles that of tissue fluid. In addition to mucin, it contains salts, albumin, fat droplets, and cellular debris. The quantitative composition of synovia depends largely on the type of tissue underlying the surface fibroblasts and the degree of vascularity of this tissue. Because of its mucin content, the synovia forms a viscous capillary film on the articular cartilage.

The **articular cartilage** (*cartilago articularis*) is usually hyaline cartilage (Freeman, 1979). It covers the articular surfaces of bones where its deepest part may be calcified. It contains no nerves or blood vessels, although it is capable of some regeneration after injury or partial removal (Bennett et al., 1932). It receives its nutrition from the synovia. The articular cartilage varies in thickness in different joints and in different parts of the same joint. It is thickest in young, healthy joints and in joints that bear considerable weight. Its thickness in any particular joint is in direct proportion to the weight borne by the joint, and it may atrophy from disuse. Healthy articular cartilage is translucent, with a bluish sheen. Elasticity and compressibility are necessary physical properties that it possesses. This resiliency guards against fracture of bone by absorbing shock.

A **meniscus** (*meniscus articularis*), or **disc** (*discus articularis*), is a complete or partial fibrocartilaginous plate that divides a joint cavity into two parts. The temporomandibular joint contains a thin, but complete, articular disc, and, because the capsular ligament attaches to the entire periphery of the disc, the joint cavity is completely divided into two parts. Two menisci are found in the stifle joint, and neither is complete, thus allowing all parts of the joint cavity to intercommunicate. Menisci have a small blood and nerve supply and are capable of regeneration. Their principal function, according to MacConaill, is "to bring about the formation of wedge-shaped films of synovia in relation to the weight-transmitting parts of joints in movement." An obvious function is the prevention of injury from concussion. The stifle and temporomandibular joints are the only synovial joints in the dog that possess menisci, or discs.

A **ligament** (*ligamentum*) is a band or a cord of nearly pure collagenous tissue that unites two or more bones. The term has also been used to designate remnants of fetal structures and relatively avascular narrow serous membrane connections. Ligaments, as used in this chapter, unite bone with bone. Tendons unite muscle with bone. Most ligaments are extraarticular but a few are intraarticular, such as in the stifle and hip joints. They always develop initially within the fibrous layer of the joint capsule. The loss of intraarticular components of the joint capsule may result in what appear to be ligaments within a joint unassociated with a joint capsule. They are covered by synovial membrane. They are heaviest on the side of joints where the margins of the bones do not separate but glide on each other. **Hinge** joints with the greatest radii of movement have the longest ligaments. The ligaments often widen at their attached ends, where they blend with the periosteum. Histologically, ligaments are composed largely of long parallel or spiral collagenous fibers, but all possess some yellow elastic fibers also. The integrity of most joints is ensured by the ligaments, but in some (shoulder and hip) the heavy muscles that traverse the joints play a more important part in the function of that joint than do the ligaments. Such muscles and their tendons are sometimes spoken of as active ligaments. In hinge joints ligaments limit lateral mobility, and some (cruciate ligaments of the stifle joint) limit folding, opening, and sliding of the joint as well. In certain ball-and-socket synovial joints the sockets are deepened by ridges of dense fibrocartilage, known as **glenoid lips** (*labia glenoidalia*).

Pathologic Conditions

Articular separations are spoken of as **subluxations** or **luxations** or partial or complete dislocations, respectively. Although most luxations are due to injury or degenerative changes, there are also predisposing genetic factors (often breed-specific) that play an important role.

Classification of Synovial Joints

Synovial joints may be classified according to (1) the number of articulating surfaces involved, (2) the shape or form of the articular surfaces, or (3) the function of the joint (Barnett et al., 1961).

According to the number of articulating surfaces a joint is either **simple** (*articulatio simplex*) or **compound** (*articulatio composita*). A simple joint is formed by two articular surfaces within an articular capsule. When more than two articular surfaces are enclosed within the same capsule, the joint is compound.

synovial joints (*Nomina Anatomica* 2017) is based on the shape or form of the articular surfaces. There are seven basic types:

- A **plane joint** (*articulatio plana*) is one in which the articular surfaces are essentially flat. It permits a slight gliding movement. An example is the costotransverse joint.
- A **ball-and-socket joint** (*articulatio spheroidea*) is formed by a convex hemispherical head that fits into a shallow glenoid cavity (shoulder joint) or into a deep cotyloid cavity (hip joint).
- An **ellipsoidal joint** (*articulatio ellipsoidea*) is similar to a spheroidal joint. It is characterized by an elongation of one surface at a right angle to the other, forming an ellipse. The reciprocal convex (male) and concave (female) elongated surfaces of the antebrachiocarpal articulation form an ellipsoidal joint.
- A **hinge joint** (*ginglymus*) permits flexion and extension with a limited degree of rotation. The most movable surface of a hinge joint is usually concave. An example is the elbow joint.
- A **condylar joint** (*articulatio condylaris*) resembles a hinge joint in its movement but differs in structure. The surfaces of such a joint include rounded prominences, or condyles, that fit into reciprocal depressions or condyles on the adjacent bone, resulting in two articular surfaces usually included in one articular capsule. Examples of condylar joints include the temporomandibular joint and the stifle joint. The stifle joint is best classified as a complex condylar joint because it possesses an intraarticular fibrocartilage that partially subdivides the intraarticular cavity.
- A **trochoid** (*articulatio trochoidea*), or **pivot joint**, is one in which the chief movement is around a longitudinal axis through the bones forming the joint. The median atlantoaxial joint and the proximal radioulnar joint are examples of trochoid joints.
- A **saddle joint** (*articulatio sellaris*) is characterized by opposed surfaces, each of which is convex in one direction and concave in the other, usually at right angles. When opposing joint surfaces are concavo-convex, the main movements are also in planes that meet at right angles. The tarsocrural or interphalangeal joints are examples of this type of articulation.

Movements of Synovial Joints

Joint movements that are brought about by the contraction of muscles that cross the joints are known as *active movements*. Those joint movements caused by gravity or secondarily by the movement of some other joint or by an external force are known as *passive movements*. Synovial joints are capable of diverse movements. **Flexion**, or folding, denotes moving two or more bones so that the angle between them becomes less than 180 degrees. **Extension**, or straightening, denotes movement by which the angle is increased to 180 degrees. It is readily seen that some joints, such as the metacarpophalangeal and metatarsophalangeal joints, are in a resting state of overextension. This is also called *dorsal flexion*. When an animal "humps up," it flexes its vertebral column. Some parts of the vertebral column (the joints between the first few caudal vertebrae) are normally in a state of flexion, whereas others (the joints between the last few cervical vertebrae) are in a state of overextension. Flexion and extension occur in the sagittal plane unless the movement is specifically stated to be otherwise (right or left lateral flexion of the vertebral column). **Adduction** is the term applied to moving an extremity toward the median plane or a digit toward the axis of the limb. **Abduction**, or taking away, is the opposite movement. **Circumduction** occurs when an extremity follows in the curved plane of the surface of a cone. **Rotation** is the movement of a part around its long axis.

Ligaments and Joints of the Skull

Temporomandibular Joint

The **temporomandibular joint** (*articulatio temporomandibularis*) (Figs. 5.1 and 5.2) is a condylar joint that allows considerable sliding movement. The transversely elongated condyle of the mandible does not correspond entirely to the articular surface of the mandibular fossa of the temporal bone. A thin **articular disc** (*discus articularis*) lies between the cartilage-covered articular surface of the condylar process of the mandible and the similarly covered mandibular fossa of the temporal bone.

The loose **joint capsule** extends from the articular cartilage of one bone to that of the other. On the temporal bone

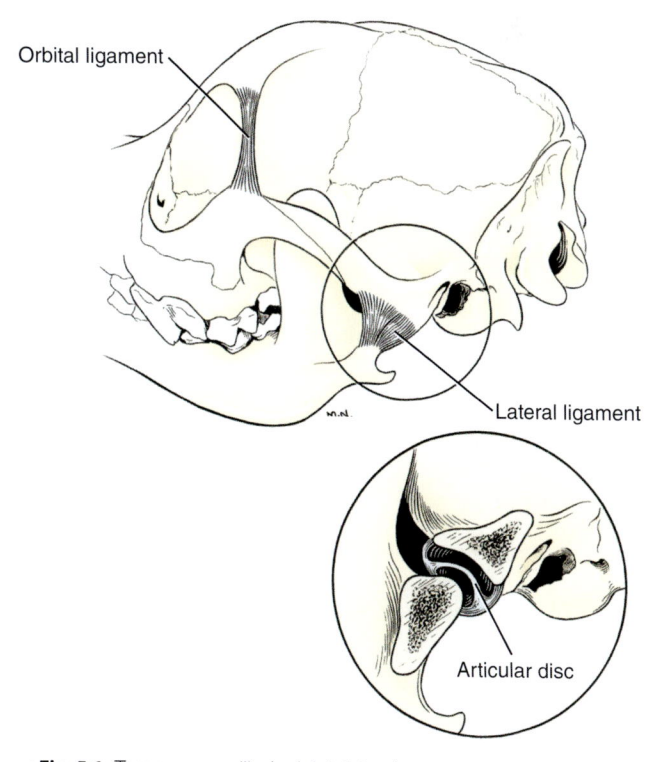

• **Fig. 5.1** Temporomandibular joint, lateral aspect and sagittal section.

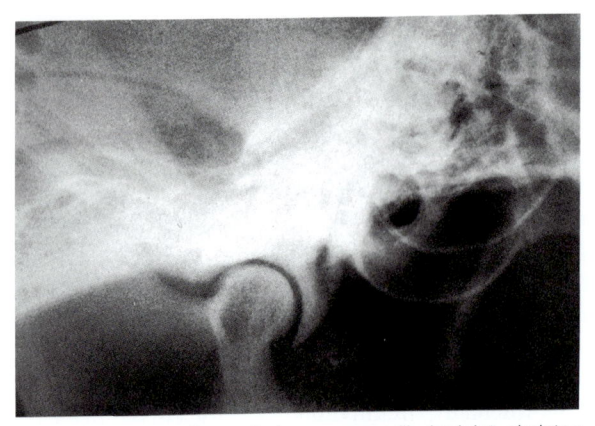

Fig. 5.2 Lateral radiograph, temporomandibular joint, skeleton.

the capsular ligament also attaches to the retroarticular process. It attaches to the entire edge of the disc as it passes between the two bones. The joint cavity is thus completely divided into a *dorsal compartment*, between the disc and temporal bone, and a *ventral compartment*, between the disc and mandible. Laterally the fibrous part of the joint capsule is strengthened by fibrous strands to form the **lateral ligament** (*lig. laterale*). The lateral ligament becomes progressively tighter as the jaws open, and, if one or the other is unduly lax owing to stretching or joint dysplasia, it is possible to dislocate the temporomandibular joint. Robins and Grandage (1977) described open-mouth jaw locking and its surgical correction in two Basset Hounds with temporomandibular joint dysplasia. A subsequent case review details open-mouthed jaw locking in multiple dogs (Gatineau et al., 2008). Differential movement at the joints, when the jaws were opened widely, allowed locking of the coronoid process lateral to the zygomatic arch. A common disorder of dog temporomandibular joint was reported as osteoarthritis localized in the medial aspect of the joint (Arzi et al. 2013).

Vollmerhaus and Roos (1996) described transverse movement of the temporomandibular joint in 20 dogs of various breeds. This movement is important for mastication. Umphlet et al (1988) described the effect of hemimandibulectomy on the joint.

Intermandibular Joint

The **intermandibular articulation** (*articulatio intermandibularis*) includes a small part formed by cartilage. This is the median synchondrosis (*synchondrosis intermandibularis*) uniting right and left mandibular bodies. The larger part of the articulation consists of connective tissue forming a suture (*sutura intermandibularis*). The opposed articular surfaces are interdigitated, and the fibrocartilage of the articulation may persist throughout life.

Scapino (1965, 1981) investigated the morphologic characteristics and function of the intermandibular articulation in the dog and other carnivores. He described four types of articulations, ranging from flexible to synostosed. He considers the dog to have a flexible joint that permits a moderate amount of independent movement of the mandibles and found this to be the most common union in carnivores. When the mandibles of such a joint are separated, the articular surfaces are flat or have low rugosities. A smooth area can be seen rostrodorsally, and the articular space is usually wider caudally than rostrally. The joint is characterized by a single fibrocartilage pad, cruciate ligaments, and a venous plexus. In the wolf and dog the articulation is not stiff, as in the lion and tiger, and is not synostosed, as in the badger and panda.

Joints of Auditory Ossicles

The **joints of the auditory ossicles** (*articulationes ossiculorum auditus*) allow for movement of the malleus, incus, and stapes (see Chapter 20). The head of the malleus articulates with the body of the incus via a synovial **incudomallear joint** (*articulatio incudomallearis*). The lenticular process of the long crus of the incus likewise forms a synovial joint with the head of the stapes, which is called the **incudostapedial joint** (*articulatio incudostapedia*). The footplate, or base, of the stapes attaches to the margin of the vestibular window (*fenestra vestibuli*) by means of a fibrous union (*syndesmosis tympanostapedia*).

The **ligaments of the auditory ossicles** (*ligg. ossiculorum auditus*) function to hold the ossicles in place and to limit their movement. Associated with the malleus (*lig. mallei*) is a short **lateral ligament** between the lateral process of the malleus and the tympanic notch, a **dorsal ligament** joining the head of the malleus to the roof of the epitympanic recess, and a short **rostral ligament** connecting the rostral process of the malleus to the osseous tympanic ring. The body of the incus is attached to the roof of the epitympanic recess by a **dorsal ligament**, and the short crus of the incus is attached to the fossa incudis by a **caudal ligament**. The base of the stapes is attached to the margin of the vestibular window by an annular ligament (*lig. annulare stapedis*).

Joints of Hyoid Apparatus

The tympanohyoid cartilage articulates with the mastoid part of the petrous portion of the temporal bone, forming the *articulatio temporohyoidea*. This articulation is adjacent to the stylomastoid foramen. Except for the temporohyoid joint, there are tightly fitting synovial cavities between all the bones of the hyoid complex, as well as a small synovial cavity between the thyrohyoid bone and the cranial cornu of the thyroid cartilage.

Synchondroses of the Skull

The **synchondroses of the skull** (*synchondroses cranii*) include the following:

Synchondrosis sphenooccipitalis
Synchondrosis petrooccipitalis
Synchondrosis intersphenoidalis

Synchondrosis sphenopetrosa
Synchondrosis intermandibularis
Synchondrosis intraoccipitalis squamolateralis
Synchondrosis intraoccipitalis basolateralis

Sutures of the Skull

The **sutures of the skull** (*suturae capitis*) are described in the discussion of the individual bones of the skull in Chapter 4. The name of each bone in the following list is followed by the names of the sutures in which it participates.

Occipital Bone
    Sutura lambdoidea
    Sutura occipitosquamosa
    Sutura occipitomastoidea
    Sutura occipitointerparietalis
    Sutura occipitotympanica
Parietal Bone
    Sutura parietointerparietalis
    Sutura lambdoidea
    Sutura coronalis
    Sutura squamosa
    Sutura sagittalis
    Sutura sphenoparietalis
Frontal Bone
    Sutura interfrontalis
    Sutura coronalis
    Sutura sphenofrontalis
    Sutura frontonasalis
    Sutura frontomaxillaris
    Sutura frontolacrimalis
    Sutura frontopalatina
    Sutura frontoethmoidalis
    Sutura frontozygomatica
Sphenoid Bone
    Sutura vomerosphenoidalis
    Sutura sphenoethmoidalis
    Sutura sphenopalatina
    Sutura sphenofrontalis
    Sutura sphenosquamosa
    Sutura sphenoparietalis
    Sutura pterygosphenoidalis
Temporal Bone
    Sutura squamosa
    Sutura sphenosquamosa
    Sutura temporozygomatica
Ethmoid Bone
    Sutura sphenoethmoidalis
    Sutura vomeroethmoidalis
    Sutura frontoethmoidalis
    Sutura ethmoidomaxillaris
    Sutura ethmoidonasalis
    Sutura palatoethmoidalis
Incisive Bone
    Sutura maxilloincisiva
    Sutura vomeroincisiva
    Sutura nasoincisiva
    Sutura interincisiva
Nasal Bone
    Sutura internasalis
    Sutura frontonasalis
    Sutura nasomaxillaris
    Sutura nasoincisiva
    Sutura ethmoidonasalis
Maxilla
    Sutura maxilloincisiva
    Sutura nasomaxillaris
    Sutura frontomaxillaris
    Sutura lacrimomaxillaris
    Sutura zygomaticomaxillaris
    Sutura palatomaxillaris
    Sutura palatina mediana
    Sutura ethmoidomaxillaris
    Sutura vomeromaxillaris
Zygomatic Bone
    Sutura zygomaticomaxillaris
    Sutura lacrimozygomatica
    Sutura temporozygomatica
Palatine Bone
    Sutura palatina mediana
    Sutura palatina transversa
    Sutura vomeropalatina
    Sutura palatomaxillaris
    Sutura sphenopalatina
    Sutura pterygopalatina
    Sutura frontopalatina
    Sutura palatoethmoidalis
    Sutura palatolacrimalis
Lacrimal Bone
    Sutura frontolacrimalis
    Sutura lacrimomaxillaris
    Sutura lacrimozygomatica
    Sutura palatolacrimalis
    Sutura palatoethmoidalis
Pterygoid Bone
    Sutura pterygosphenoidalis
    Sutura pterygopalatina
Vomer
    Sutura vomerosphenoidalis
    Sutura vomeroethmoidalis
    Sutura vomeropalatina
    Sutura vomeromaxillaris
    Sutura vomeroincisiva

Ligaments and Joints of the Vertebral Column

Atlantooccipital Articulation

There is a common joint cavity formed by the articulations of the occipital condyles with the atlas, and the atlas with the axis. By means of silicone casts this cavity (Fig. 5.3) has been studied and described as the "composite

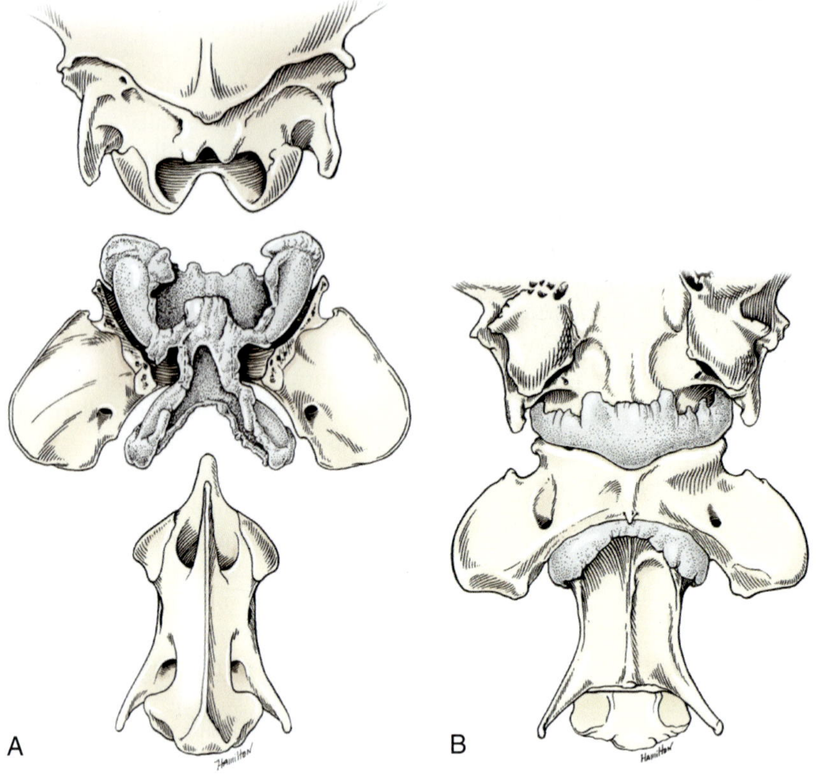

• **Fig. 5.3 A**, An exploded dorsal view of the composite occipito-atlas-axis joint cavity of an adult dog. The dorsal arch of the atlas has been removed to expose the silicone joint cavity cast (*stippled*). **B**, A ventral view of the skull, atlas, and axis, articulated. The ventral portions of the atlantooccipital and atlantoaxial joint cavities (*stippled*) are exposed. (With permission from Watson AG, Evans HE, de Lahunta A: Gross morphology of the composite occipito-atlas-axis joint cavity in the dog, *Zbl Vet Med C Anat Histol Embryol* 15:139–146, 1986.)

occipito-atlas-axis joint cavity" by Watson et al. (1986). A cast of the cavity resembles the shape of an "hourglass" with the ends removed or "popeye" holding up the head. It appears to be a composite of five synovial joints: right and left atlantooccipital joints, a median joint cavity between the ventral articular surface of the dens and the dorsal surface of the ventral arch of the atlas, and right and left atlantoaxial joints. The synovial bursa between the transverse atlantal ligament and the dens does not communicate with the common joint cavity.

The **atlantooccipital joint** (*articulatio atlantooccipitalis*) (see Fig. 5.4) is formed by the dorsolaterally extending occipital condyles and the corresponding concave cranial articular fovea of the atlas. The spacious **joint capsule** (*capsula articularis*) on each side attaches to the margins of the opposed articular surfaces. Ventromedially the two sides are joined so that an undivided U-shaped joint cavity is formed. The atlantooccipital joint cavity communicates with the atlantoaxial joint cavity along the dens. The dorsal and ventral atlantooccipital membranes reinforce the joint capsule at their respective locations.

The **dorsal atlantooccipital membrane** (*membrana atlantooccipitalis dorsalis*) extends between the dorsal edge of the foramen magnum and the cranial border of the dorsal arch of the atlas. Two oblique, straplike thickenings, approximately 8 mm wide, arise on each side of the notch of the squama occipitalis, diverge as they run caudally, and attach to the dorsolateral parts of the atlas. In the triangular space formed by these bands, punctures are made for the removal of cerebrospinal fluid from the cerebellomedullary cistern.

The **ventral atlantooccipital membrane** (*membrana atlantooccipitalis ventralis*) and its synovial layer form the uniformly thin joint capsule located between the ventral edge of the foramen magnum and the ventral arch of the atlas.

The **lateral ligament** (*lig. laterale*) of the atlantooccipital joint (see Fig. 5.5) runs from the lateral part of the dorsal arch of the atlas to the paracondylar process of the occipital bone. Its course is cranioventrolateral, and its caudal attachment is narrower than its cranial one. Another small ligament runs from each side of the inner surface of the lateral part of the ventral arch of the atlas to the lateral part of the foramen magnum. Ventral and medial to these ligaments the unpaired joint cavities between the skull and the atlas and between the atlas and the axis freely communicate.

Atlantoaxial Articulation

The **atlantoaxial joint** (*articulatio atlantoaxialis*) (see Figs. 5.3 to 5.6) is a pivot joint that permits the head and atlas

CHAPTER 5 Arthrology 183

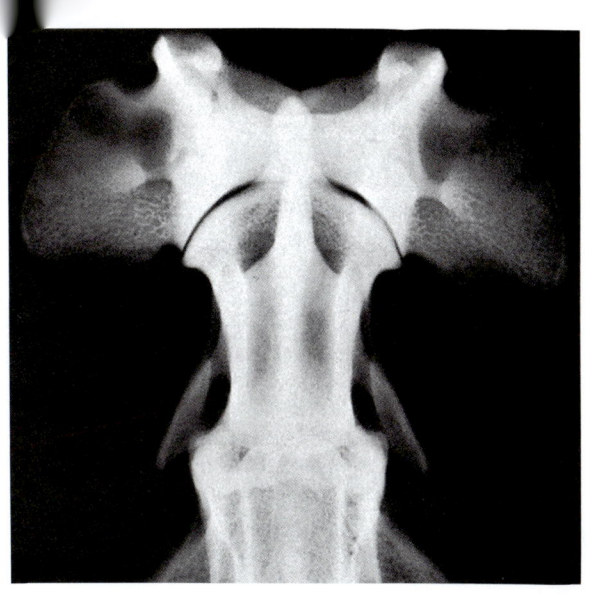

• **Fig. 5.4** Dorsoventral radiograph, atlantoaxial articulation, skeleton.

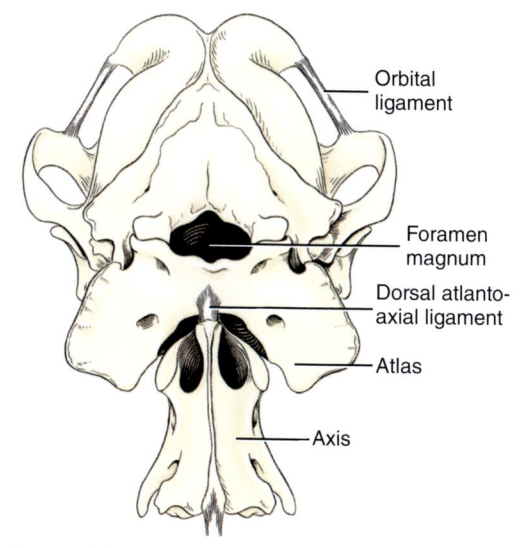

• **Fig. 5.6** Atlantooccipital space, joint flexed, caudal aspect.

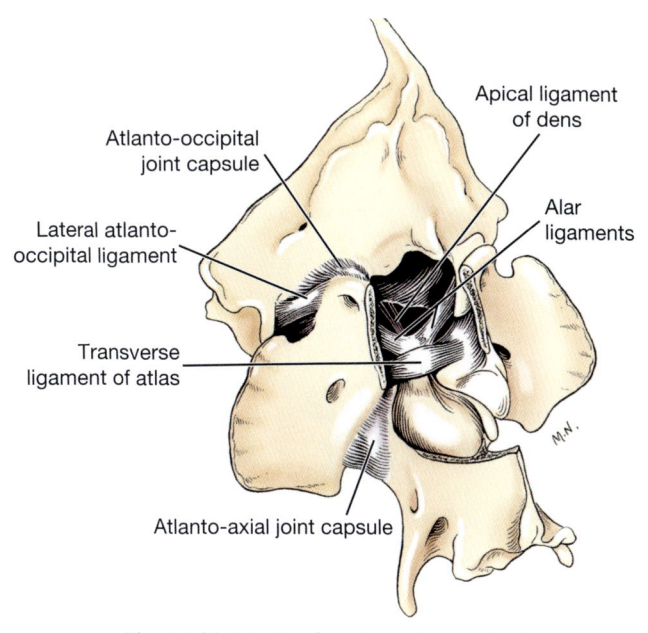

• **Fig. 5.5** Ligaments of occiput, atlas, and axis.

to rotate around a longitudinal axis. The **joint capsule** is loose and uniformly thin as it extends from the dorsal part of the cranial articular surface of one side of the axis to a like place on the opposite side. Cranially it attaches to the caudal margins of the caudal articular foveae and ventral arch of the atlas. The fibrous layer of the joint capsule extends from right to left between the dorsal arch of the atlas and the arch of the axis. This is the **dorsal atlantoaxial membrane**, or *membrana tectoria*.

The **apical ligament of the dens** (*lig. apicis dentis*) (see Fig. 5.5) leaves the apex of the dens and passes straight cranially to the basioccipital bone at the ventral part of the foramen magnum. The apical ligament represents a remnant of the notochord. The two **alar ligaments** (*ligg. alaria*) are wider and heavier than the apical ligament. They attach to the dens on either side of the apical ligament and diverge from each other to attach to the occipital bone medial to the caudal parts of the occipital condyles. The **transverse atlantal ligament** (*lig. transversum atlantis*) is a thick ligament that connects one side of the ventral arch of the atlas to the other. It crosses dorsal to the dens and functions to hold this process against the ventral arch of the atlas. A spacious bursa, not formally named, exists between the ventral surface of the ligament and the dens.

Atlantoaxial subluxation with absence of the dens has been reported frequently, particularly in toy breeds, and has been ascribed to either congenital developmental or degenerative causes. Injury may result in a fracture of the dens. In almost all instances there is a tilting or dorsal displacement of the axis into the vertebral canal, with resultant compression of the spinal cord (Cook & Oliver, 1981; Oliver & Lewis, 1973).

Other Synovial Joints of the Vertebral Column

The synovial joints of the vertebral column caudal to the axis are those that appear in pairs between the articular processes of contiguous vertebrae (*articulations processuum articularum*), also known as *juncturae zygapophyseales*, and the joints between the ribs and the vertebrae (*articulationes costovertebrales*). The articular process joint capsules (*capsular articularis*) are most voluminous in the cervical region and at the base of the tail, where the greatest degrees of movement occur. The articular processes of all vertebrae cranial to the tenth thoracic are in nearly a dorsal plane so that the cranial articular processes face dorsally and the caudal articular processes face ventrally. At the tenth thoracic vertebra the direction of the articular processes changes. From the articulation between the tenth and eleventh thoracic vertebrae and through all the lumbar vertebral articulations there is essentially a sagittal interlocking of the cranial and caudal articular processes. The caudal articular

184 CHAPTER 5 Arthrology

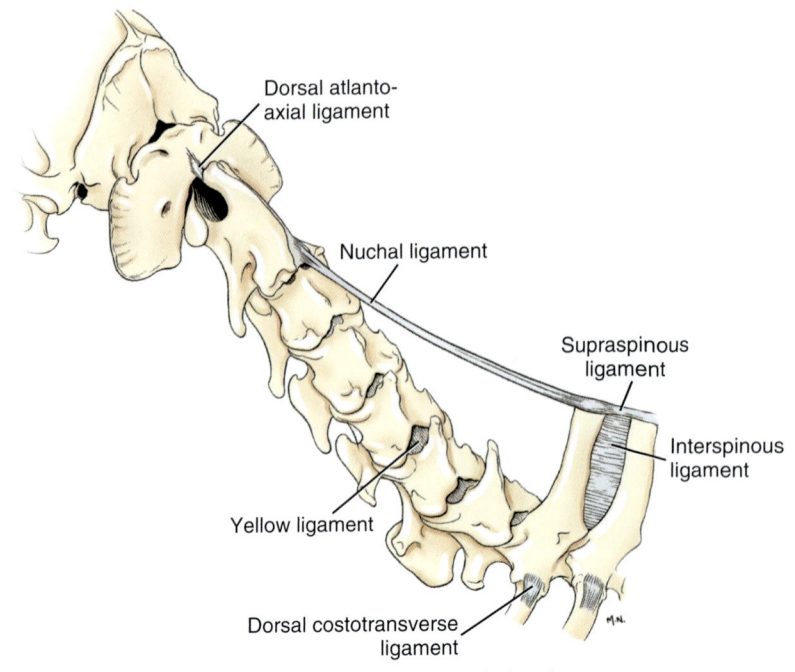

• **Fig. 5.7** Ligaments of the cervical region.

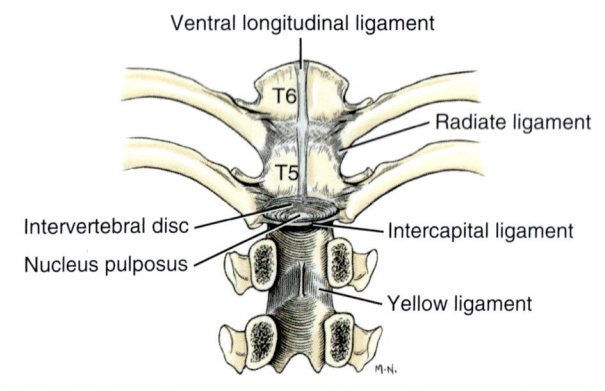

• **Fig. 5.8** Ligaments of thoracic vertebral column and ribs, ventral aspect.

processes of this segment face laterally, and the cranial articular processes face medially.

Long Ligaments of the Vertebral Column

The **nuchal ligament** (*lig. nuchae*) (Fig. 5.7) is composed of longitudinal yellow elastic fibers that attach cranially to the caudal part of the large spinous process of the axis. It extends caudally to the dorsal extremity of the spinous process of the first thoracic vertebra. It is a laterally compressed, paired band that lies between the medial surfaces of the mm. semispinales capiti. The yellow nature of the nuchal ligament continues caudally in the supraspinous ligament to the tenth thoracic spinous process (Baum & Zietzschmann, 1936).

The **supraspinous ligament** (*lig. supraspinale*) (see Figs. 5.7 and 5.12) extends from the spinous process of the first thoracic vertebra caudally to the third caudal vertebra. It is a thick band especially in the thoracic region, where it attaches to the apices of the spines as it passes from one to another. Bilaterally the dense collagenous thoracolumbar fascia imperceptibly blends with it throughout the thoracic and lumbar regions. The thin interspinous ligaments send some strands to its ventral surface, but the supraspinous ligament more than the interspinous ligaments prevents abnormal separation of the spines during flexion of the vertebral column (Heylings, 1980).

The **ventral longitudinal ligament** (*lig. longitudinale ventrale*) (Fig. 5.8) lies on the ventral surfaces of the bodies of the vertebrae. It can be traced from the axis to the sacrum, but it is best developed caudal to the middle of the thorax. The **dorsal longitudinal ligament** (*lig. longitudinale dorsale*) (see Fig. 5.10) lies on the dorsal surfaces of the bodies of the vertebrae. It therefore forms a part of the floor of the vertebral canal. It is narrowest at the middle of the vertebral bodies and widest over the intervertebral fibrocartilages. The dorsal longitudinal ligament attaches to the rough ridges on the dorsum of the vertebral bodies and to the intervertebral fibrocartilages. It extends from the dens of the axis to the end of the vertebral canal in the caudal region. The dorsal longitudinal ligament is thicker than the ventral longitudinal ligament. A narrow longitudinal ligament attaches the dorsal longitudinal ligament of the vertebral column to the overlying dura mater on the ventral midline of the spinal cord. This has been called the *meningovertebral ligament*.

Intervertebral Discs and Short Ligaments of the Vertebral Column

The **intervertebral discs** (*disci intervertebrales*) are interposed in every intervertebral space (except between C1 and C2), uniting the bodies of the adjacent vertebrae (Figs. 5.8 and 5.9). In the sacrum of young specimens, transverse lines indicate the planes of fusion of the discs with the adjoining vertebral bodies. The thickness of the discs is greatest in the cervical and lumbar regions, the thickest ones being between the last few cervical vertebrae. The thinnest discs are in the caudal region. Those between the last few segments being smaller in every way than any of the others. Each intervertebral disc consists of an outer laminated fibrous ring, the **anulus fibrosus** and a central, amorphous, gelatinous center, the nucleus pulposus. The nucleus pulposus of a young dog is proportionally larger than that of an adult and more mucoid than fibroid for 1 to 7 years (King & Smith, 1955). It is a mass of mesodermal cell remnants of the notochord in a homogeneous basophilic intercellular material. Eventually small foci of degeneration and fibrosis occur, which make the disc appear opaque rather than gelatinous and may obscure the boundary with the annulus fibrosus. In chondrodystrophic breeds a chondroid degeneration may occur in young adults that eventually calcifies. There may be ossification within the disc without any adverse effect on surrounding tissues. However, the loss of function of the nucleus pulposus may result in tearing of the anulus fibrosis dorsally with protrusion or extrusion of degenerate nuclear material into the vertebral canal (Smith & King, 1954). This is a common cause of discomfort with or without neurologic deficits caused by spinal cord compression in these chondrodystrophic breeds. A similar but fibroid degeneration may occur in nonchondrodystrophic breeds at an older age.

The **fibrous ring** (*anulus fibrosus*) consists of bands of parallel fibers that run obliquely from one vertebral body to the next. They provide a means for the transmission of stresses and strains that are required by all lateral and dorsoventral movements. These bands of fibers cross each other in a latticelike pattern and are more than eight layers thick ventrally. Near the nucleus pulposus the anulus fibrosus loses its distinctive structure and form and becomes more cartilaginous and less fibrous. The anulus fibrosus is one and a half to three times thicker ventrally than dorsally. Viewed cranially or caudally the disc is oval in outline, with the longest diameter transverse. Willenegger et al. (2005) demonstrated innervation of the periphery of the intervertebral disc in the dog by means of a protein gene marker. They looked at paraffin serial sections of lumbar discs from adult dogs.

The **pulpy nucleus** (*nucleus pulposus*) is a gelatinous remnant of the notochord. Its position and shape are indicated on each end of the vertebral body as a depressed area surrounded by a line displaced dorsally off-center. Its consistency is semifluid, and it is put under pressure by any movements of the vertebral bodies so it bulges when the retaining fibrous ring ruptures or degenerates. Sether et al. (1990) described and illustrated intervertebral disc degeneration in dogs and characterized six types of disc morphology. They found that magnetic resonance imaging was the best available method for the recognition of early disc degeneration. Their study used frozen sections to examine postmortem material. It is said that chondrodystrophic breeds show progressive collagenation and calcification in the nucleus pulposus and inner anulus fibrosus that results in a higher incidence of disc herniation than is seen in nonchondrodystrophic breeds.

Dallman et al. (1991) measured the intervertebral disc space widths of 73 anesthetized dogs. They found that body weight had a significant effect on the craniocaudal length of the disc space, so they used adjusted data for their analysis. Cervical and lumbar spaces tended to be longer than those in the caudal thoracic region. The longest cervical intervertebral spaces were C4–5 and C5–6; the shortest was C2–3. In the lumbar region L2–3 was longest (not L7–S1 as is usually reported), and L4–5 was the shortest. Dachshunds generally had greater mean intervertebral disc space lengths than did other breeds, significantly so between T12–13 and L6–7. Four ligaments are associated with each intervertebral disc. A **dorsal** and a **ventral longitudinal ligament** passes from one vertebral body to another and in so doing fuses with each intervertebral disc.

The **interspinous ligaments** (*ligg. interspinalia*) (see Figs. 5.7 and 5.12) connect adjacent vertebral spines. They consist of laterally compressed bands of tissue interspersed with muscle bundles of the mm. interspinalis. The bands run from the bases and borders of adjacent spinous processes and decussate as they insert on the opposed caudal and cranial borders of adjacent processes near their dorsal ends. The thicker fibers of the interspinous ligaments lie almost vertically. Some of their fibers blend dorsally with the supraspinous ligament. Great variation exists, and there seems to be no correlation with body type.

The **intertransverse ligaments** (*ligg. intertransversaria*) consist of bundles of fibers that unite the craniolaterally directed transverse processes of the lumbar vertebrae. They are not distinct in any of the other regions of the vertebral column.

The **yellow ligaments** (*ligg. flava*) (see Fig. 5.7), formerly *interarcuate ligaments*, are loose, thin elastic sheets between

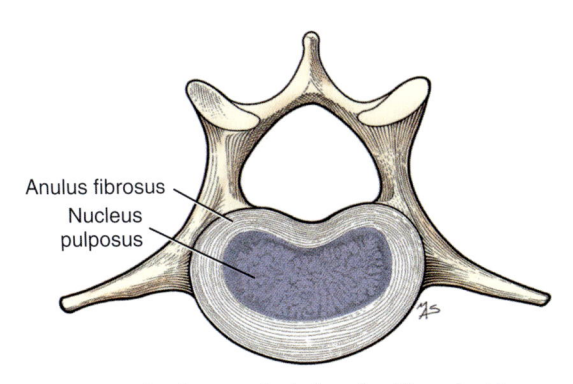

• **Fig. 5.9** Lumbar intervertebral disc of a 10-week-old puppy.

the arches of adjacent vertebrae. Laterally they blend with the articular capsules surrounding the articular processes. Ventral to this ligament is the epidural space, which separates the ligaments and the arches of the vertebrae from the dura covering the spinal cord.

Breit and Kunzel (2004) made a morphometric study of breed-specific features affecting sagittal rotation and lateral bending in the cervical vertebral column (C3–7) of the dog. They found that large breeds have a tendency toward a higher range of motion in sagittal rotation and lateral bending compared with Dachshunds and small breeds. Bergknut et al. (2013) and Smolders et al. (2013a) described the anatomy of normal intervertebral discs as well as features associated with their degeneration in chondrodysplastic dogs. Degeneration of the intervertebral discs appears most commonly in breeds associated with chondrodystrophy (short-limbed breeds, such as the Miniature Dachshund and others: see Smolders et al., 2013a). Gene changes leading to the transformation of notochordal cells to chondrocyte-like cells within the nucleus pulposus may underlie intervertebral disc degeneration (Smolders et al., 2013b).

Ligaments and Joints of the Ribs and Sternum

Each typical rib articulates with the vertebral column by two synovial joints and with the sternum by one. There is usually a slightly enlarged costochondral articulation (synchondrosis) between the rib and its costal cartilage.

The **costovertebral joints** (*articulationes costovertebrales*) (Fig. 5.10) are formed by the articulation of the capitulum of each rib (*articulatio capitis costae*) with the costal fovea on the cranial aspect of the body of the vertebra of the same number as the rib and the articulation of each tuberculum (*articulatio costotransversaria*) with the fovea on the transverse process of the corresponding vertebra. For the first 10 ribs the capitulum also articulates with a fovea on the caudal aspect of the body of the vertebra cranial to the vertebra of the same number as the rib. The articular joints are thin-walled synovial sacs that completely surround each joint and are associated with the four ligaments of the costovertebral articulation. These are two ligaments of the head and the intercapital ligament, for the capitular joint, and the ligament of the neck at the tubercular (costotransverse) joint.

The two **ligaments of the head** are the **radiating head** (*lig. capitis costae radiatum*) (see Fig. 5.12) and the **intraarticular head** (*lig. capitis costae intraarticulare*) ligaments. The radiating head ligament radiates from the ventral surface of the rib head to the bodies of the two adjacent vertebrae. It consists of collagenous bundles that extend from the neck of the rib to the ventral surface of the transverse process and the adjacent lateral surface of the body of the vertebra. The intraarticular head ligament attaches the crest of the rib head to the dorsal surface of the two adjacent vertebrae as well as the intervertebral disc. The last three or four ribs are displaced caudally at their vertebral articulations, and the ligaments also shift caudally and attach to the body of the vertebra and the intervertebral disc of the same number as that rib.

The **intercapital ligament** (*lig. intercapitale*) (Figs. 5.8 and 5.10) is part of the *lig. capitis costae intraarticularis* and runs from the head of one rib over the dorsal part of the intervertebral disc, but ventral to the dorsal longitudinal ligament, to the head of the opposite rib. It grooves the dorsal part of the intervertebral disc. A synovial membrane between the ligament and the intervertebral disc joins the joint capsules of the opposite rib heads. The intercapital ligament is attached both cranially and caudally to the intervertebral disc by a delicate membrane and is attached dorsally to the dorsal longitudinal ligament and dura by areolar tissue. The ligament functions to hold the heads of opposite ribs tightly against their articular surfaces and to prevent excessive cranial and caudal movements of the ribs. The **ligament of the head of the rib** extends the short distance from the rib head to the disc and the two adjacent vertebrae. The intercapital ligament is regularly absent from the first, eleventh, twelfth, and thirteenth ribs, according to King and Smith (1955).

The **costotransverse ligament** (*lig. costotransversarium*) (Fig. 5.11), formerly the *ligament of the tubercle*, is the largest single ligament uniting the rib to the vertebra. It attaches just distal to the articular capsule of the tubercle, crosses the capsule, and blends with the periosteum of the transverse process of the vertebra corresponding to the rib. The costotransverse ligaments of the first five ribs lie cranial to the joints and run obliquely craniomedially from the tubercles to the transverse processes. The ligaments of the next three run almost directly medially to the transverse processes from the dorsal surfaces of the tubercles, and those of the last four incline increasingly caudally as they run from the rib tubercles to the transverse processes of the vertebrae. Great variation in size and position of these ligaments exists in different dogs. The costotransverse ligaments are usually largest on the last four ribs.

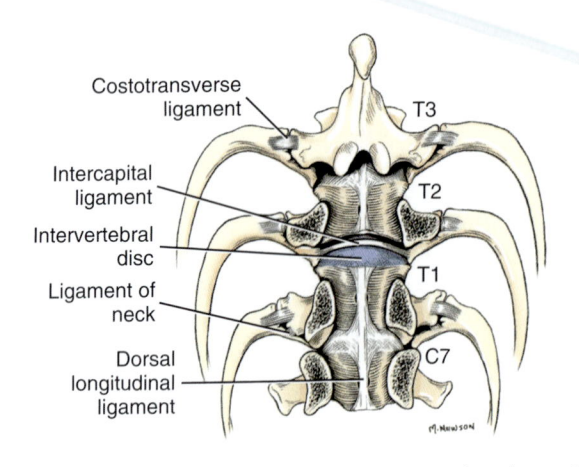

• **Fig. 5.10** Ligaments of vertebral column and ribs, dorsal aspect.

sternocostal joints (*articulationes sternocostales*) (Figs. 5.12 and 5.13) are synovial joints formed by the first eight costal cartilages articulating with the sternum. In the young puppy these sternocostal junctions are usually combinations of synovial joints and synchondroses. Williams (1957) found complete synovial cavities in several joints of 4-month-old puppies along with incomplete and fibrosed joints. The second to seventh pairs of joints are typical, but the first and last pairs present special features. The first sternebra is widened cranially by the formation of lateral shelves of bone that articulate with the transversely compressed costal cartilages of the first ribs. These costal cartilages approach their sternal articulations at a more acute angle than do any of the other costal cartilages. The last sternocostal joints, typically, are formed by the ninth pair of cartilages joining each other and together articulating with the ventral surface of the fibrocartilage between the last two sternebrae, or with the sternebra cranial to the xiphoid process. The ends of the right and left ninth costal cartilages are united by an indistinct collagenous ligament. No synovial joint is found here as the ninth costal cartilages lie closely applied to the eighth costal cartilages. The joint capsule is usually thin, except dorsally and ventrally, where the heavy perichondrium leaving the costal cartilages thickens and spreads out as it goes to the intersternebral fibrocartilages. These are the dorsal and ventral **sternocostal radiate ligaments** (*ligg. sternocostalia radiata*). The dorsal and ventral surfaces of the sternum are covered by white membranous sheets and bands of thickened periosteum, the **sternal membrane** (*membrana sterni*). The dorsal part is divided into two or more strands, whereas the ventral part consists of a single median band. The **costoxiphoid ligaments** (*ligg. costoxiphoidea*) are two flat cords that originate on the eighth costal cartilages. They cross ventral to the ninth costal cartilages and converge and blend as they join the periosteum on the ventral surface of the caudal half of the xiphoid process.

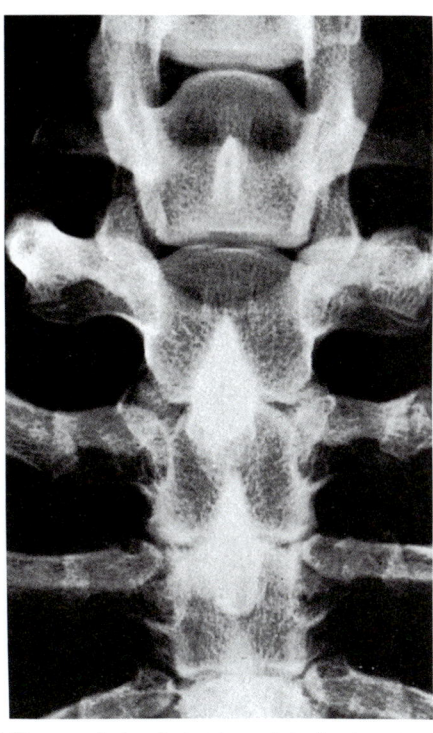

• **Fig. 5.11** Dorsoventral radiograph, vertebral column and ribs, skeleton; C6 through T4 are shown.

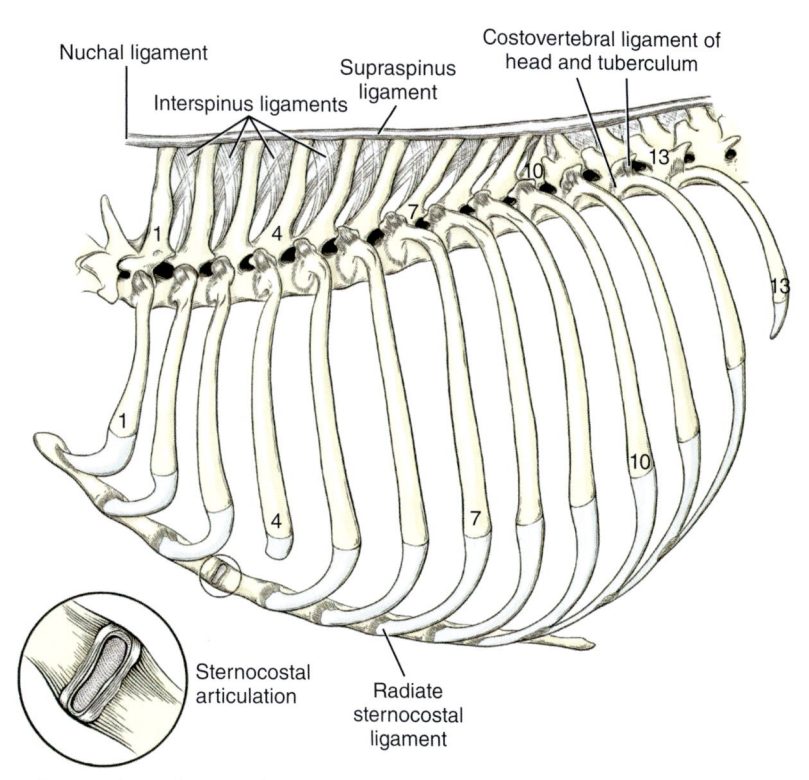

• **Fig. 5.12** Interspinous and supraspinous ligaments of thoracic skeleton, lateral aspect.

188 CHAPTER 5 Arthrology

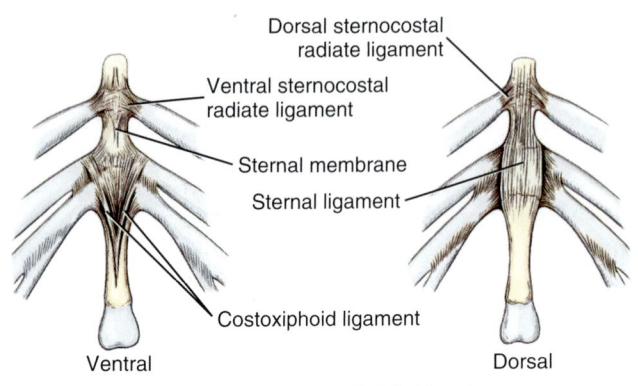

• Fig. 5.13 Ligaments of xiphoid region.

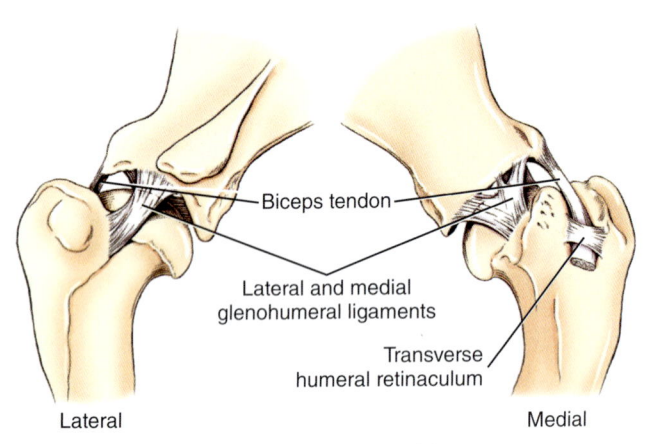

• Fig. 5.14 Left shoulder joint.

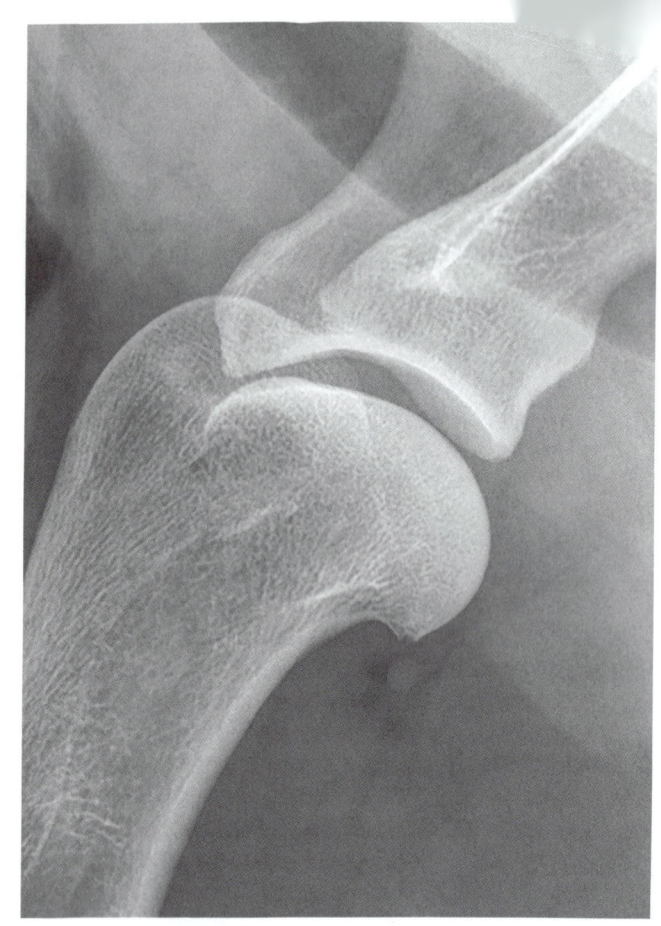

• Fig. 5.15 Lateromedial radiograph, left shoulder joint, skeleton.

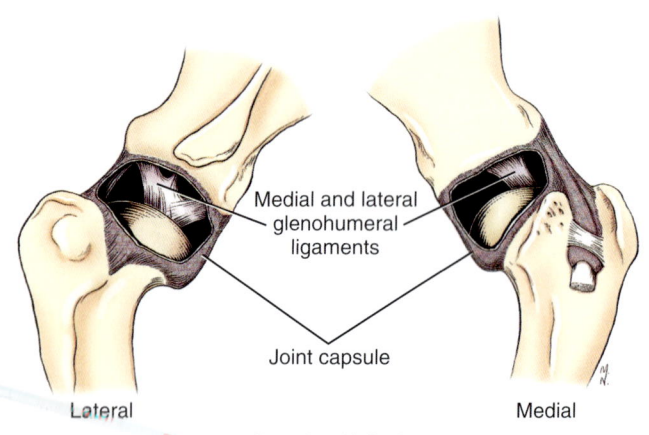

• Fig. 5.16 Capsule of left shoulder joint.

The **costochondral joints** (*articulationes costochondrales*) are the joints between the ribs and the costal cartilages. Apparently, no synovial cavities ever develop here. In puppies these joints are slightly enlarged and appear as a longitudinal line of beads on the ventrolateral surface of the thorax.

Ligaments and Joints of the Thoracic Limb

Shoulder Joint

The **shoulder joint** (*articulatio humeri*) (Figs. 5.14 to 5.17) is the ball-and-socket joint between the glenoid cavity of the scapula and the head of the humerus. It is capable of movement in any direction, but its chief movements are flexion and extension. The shallow, small glenoid cavity of the scapula is increased in size and deepened by the **glenoid lip** (*labrum glenoidale*), which extends 1 or 2 mm beyond the edge of the cavity caudolaterally. The **articular capsule** (*capsula articularis*) forms a loose sleeve that attaches just peripheral to the glenoid lip proximally. In places the capsule attaches several millimeters distal to the articular part of the humeral head, where it blends with the periosteum on the neck of the humerus. A part of the joint capsule surrounds the tendon of origin of the m. biceps brachii and extends distally approximately 2 cm in the intertubercular groove. The tendon with its synovial sheath is held in the groove by the **transverse humeral retinaculum** (*ret. transversum humerale*). The capsule blends with this retinaculum craniomedially and with the tendon of the m. subscapularis medially. Laterally the joint capsule blends with the tendons of the mm. supraspinatus and infraspinatus. Elsewhere, especially caudally, the articular capsule is thin and expansive possessing a number of irregular pouches when it is distended. Medially and laterally the fibrosa of the capsule is irregularly thickened internally to form the **medial** and **lateral glenohumeral ligaments**

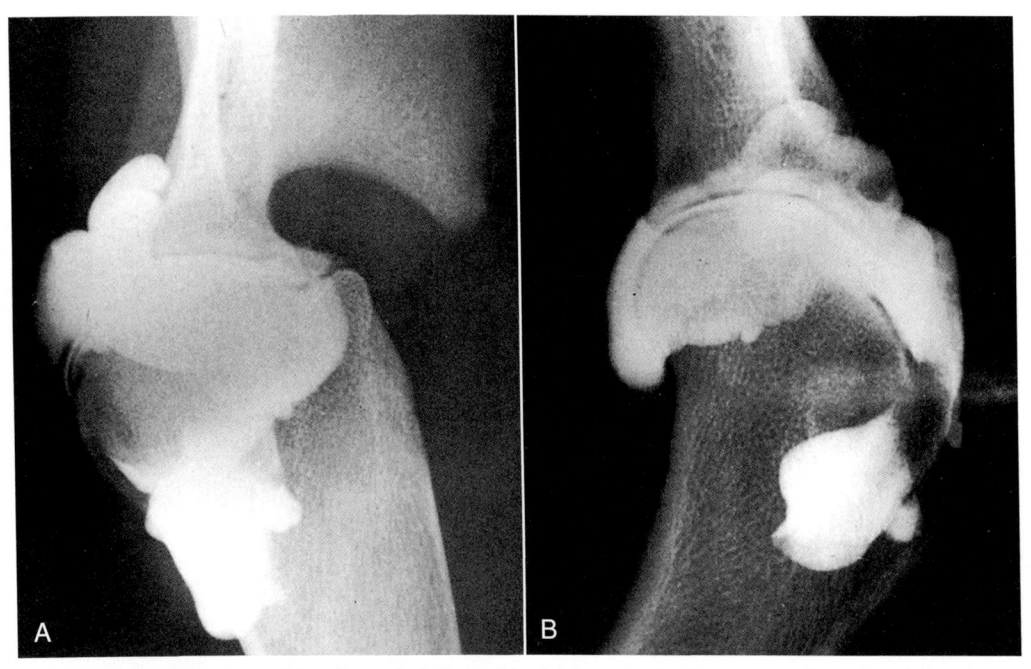

Fig. 5.17 A, Craniocaudal radiograph, left shoulder joint; contrast arthrogram performed to define the synovial space. **B,** Lateromedial radiograph, left shoulder joint; contrast arthrogram performed to define the synovial space. Note the distal extent of the synovial space along the tendon of the biceps brachii.

(*ligg. glenohumeralia medialis et lateralis*). These reinforcing bands protrude appreciably into the joint cavity. The thick tendons that cross the joint function as ligaments. These tendons of the subscapularis, supraspinatus, and infraspinatus provide for this joint's stability and maintain the sagittal plane of movement assisted by the teres minor laterally and the teres major medially.

Hunting dogs that step in a depression and overextend the shoulder often tear the m. infraspinatus at the musculotendinous junction (see de Lahunta et al., 2015), an injury unrelated to nerve damage. When the muscle heals, it has a shortened functional length which creates excessive lateral rotation of the humerus at the shoulder. This is best observed in the non-weight-bearing phase of the gait.

Sidaway et al. (2004) evaluated the effect of transecting the tendon of the biceps brachii, the tendon of the infraspinatus, or the medial glenohumeral ligament on shoulder joint stability in canine cadavers. When the medial glenohumeral ligament was transected complete medial luxation of the humeral heads occurred.

Suter and Carb (1969), using Silastic injections and subsequent maceration, have demonstrated the extent of the shoulder joint capsule. In cranial view a lateral extension of the joint capsule is seen deep to the tendon of the supraspinatus, a large medial synovial sheath extends distally to surround the biceps tendon, and a large medial pouch can be found deep to the broad insertion of the subscapularis.

McCarthy and Wood (1988) have investigated various fascial connections of the clavicle to neighboring structures in 50 dogs of 10 breeds. They noted that a band of connective tissue may connect the clavicle to the caudal border of the scapula, to fascia deep to the latissimus dorsi, to the subscapular fascia, to the clavicular intersection, or to the manubrium of the sternum. Several combinations may exist in the same animal. They speculate on functional implications that may be important.

Elbow Joint

The **elbow joint** (*articulatio cubiti*) (Figs. 5.18 to 5.24) is a composite joint formed by the humeral condyle with the head of the radius, the **humeroradial joint** (*articulatio humeroradialis*), and with the trochlear notch of the ulna, the **humeroulnar joint** (*articulatio humeroulnaris*). The **proximal radioulnar joint** (*articulatio radioulnaris proximalis*) freely communicates with the humeroradial and humeroulnar joints. The humeroradial part of the elbow joint transmits most of the weight supported by the limb (Knox et al., 2003). The humeroulnar part stabilizes and restricts the movement of the joint to a sagittal plane, and the proximal radioulnar joint allows rotation of the antebrachium. Lateral or medial movements of the elbow joint are minimal because of the thick collateral ligaments and the cranial extension of the anconeal process of the ulna into the deep olecranon fossa of the humerus. Enough rotational movement occurs at the radioulnar and carpal joints so that the forepaws can be supinated approximately 90 degrees (De Rycke et al., 2002).

The **joint capsule** is common to all three articular parts. It is taut on the sides but expansive cranially and caudally. On the cranial or flexor surface, it attaches proximal to the supratrochlear foramen and encompasses most of the radial fossa. Caudally, or on the extensor surface, the joint capsule forms a loose, fat-covered synovial pouch that attaches distal

• Fig. 5.18 Left elbow joint, medial aspect.

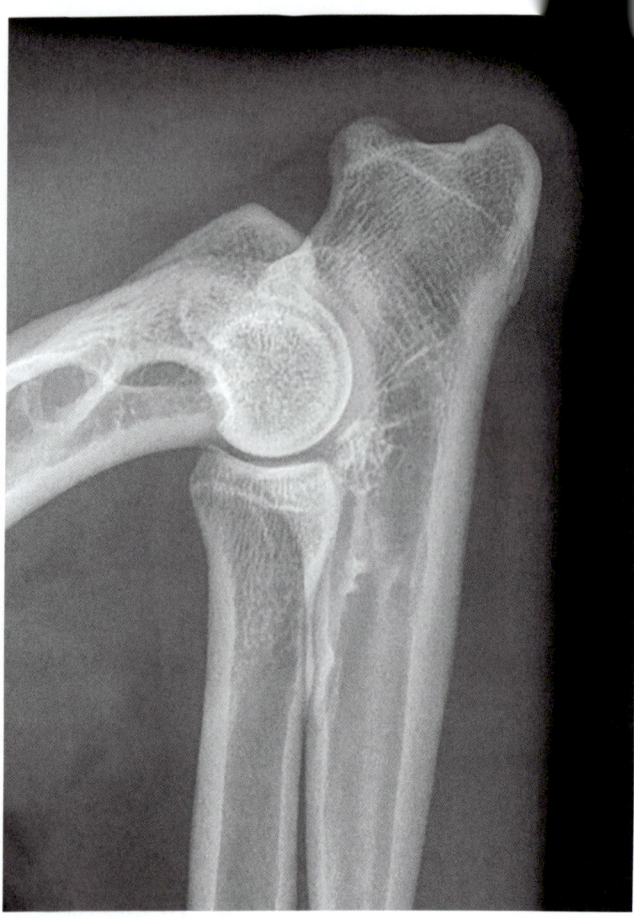

• Fig. 5.19 Lateromedial radiograph, left elbow joint, skeleton.

to the supratrochlear foramen, so that there is no intercommunication between the extensor and flexor pouches through the supratrochlear foramen. The joint capsule extends distally between the radial notch of the ulna and the articular circumference of the radius. Everywhere but cranially the synovial membrane attaches closely to the articular cartilage. Medially it extends a distal pouch deep to the m. biceps brachii, and similar extensions occur laterally deep to the mm. extensor carpi radialis and extensor digitorum communis. On the caudomedial side, extensions of the capsule occur deep to the mm. flexor carpi radialis and m. flexor digitorum profundus, the caput humerale.

The **lateral collateral ligament** (*lig. collaterale cubiti laterale*) attaches proximally to the lateral epicondyle of the humerus. Distally it divides into two crura. The slightly larger cranial crus attaches to a small lateral eminence distal to the neck of the radius. The flatter caudal crus passes to the ulna. At the level of the articular circumference the ligament blends with the annular ligament and, according to Baum and Zietzschmann (1936), often contains a sesamoid bone.

The **medial collateral ligament** (*lig. collaterale cubiti mediale*) is smaller than the lateral collateral ligament, which it resembles. It attaches proximally to the medial epicondyle of the humerus, crosses the annular ligament distally, and divides into two crura. The thinner cranial crus attaches proximal to the radial tuberosity. The thicker caudal crus

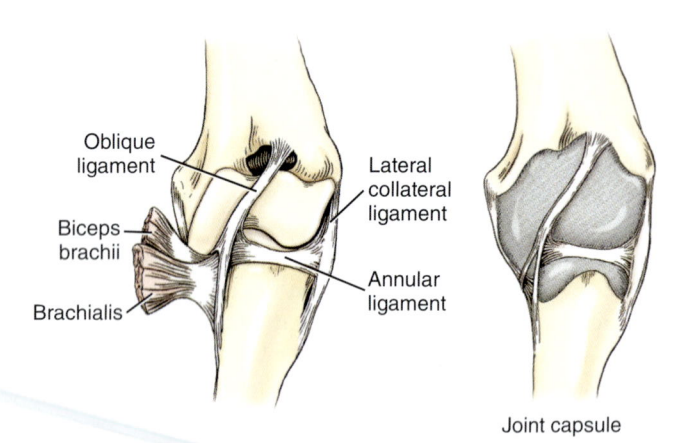

• Fig. 5.20 Left elbow joint, cranial aspect.

passes deeply into the interosseous space, where it attaches mainly on the ulna but also partly on the radius. A morphometric and structural examination of both collateral ligaments was reported by Koch et al. (2005).

The **annular ligament of the radius** (*lig. anulare radii*) is a thin band that runs transversely around the radius. It attaches to the lateral and medial coronoid processes of the ulna that are at either end of the radial notch of the ulna. It lies deep to the collateral ligaments and is slightly blended with the ulnar collateral ligament. In conjunction with the

CHAPTER 5 Arthrology

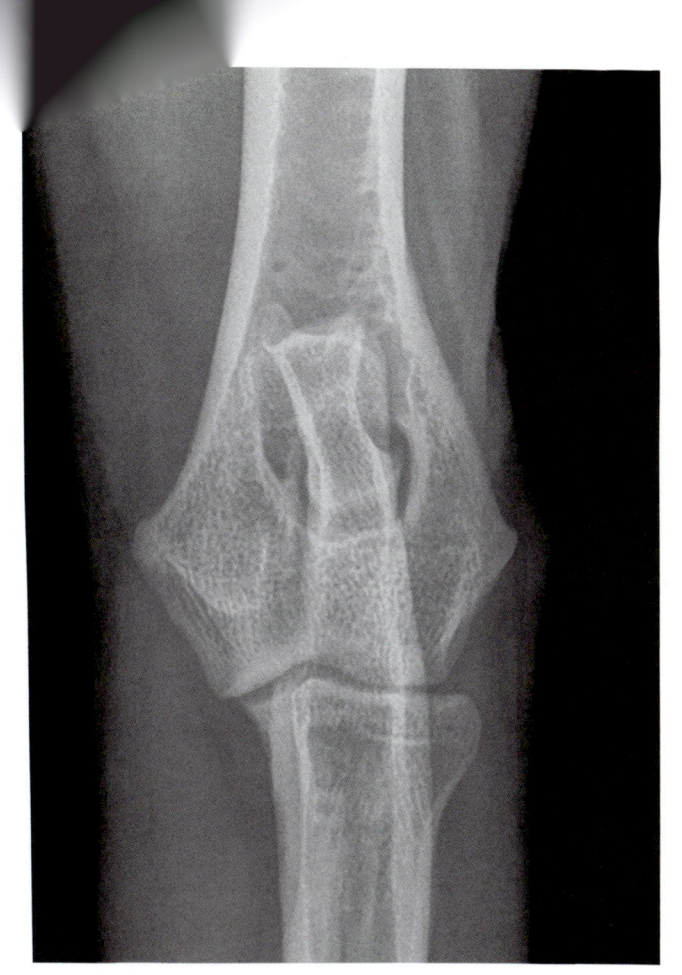

• Fig. 5.21 Craniocaudal radiograph, left elbow joint, skeleton.

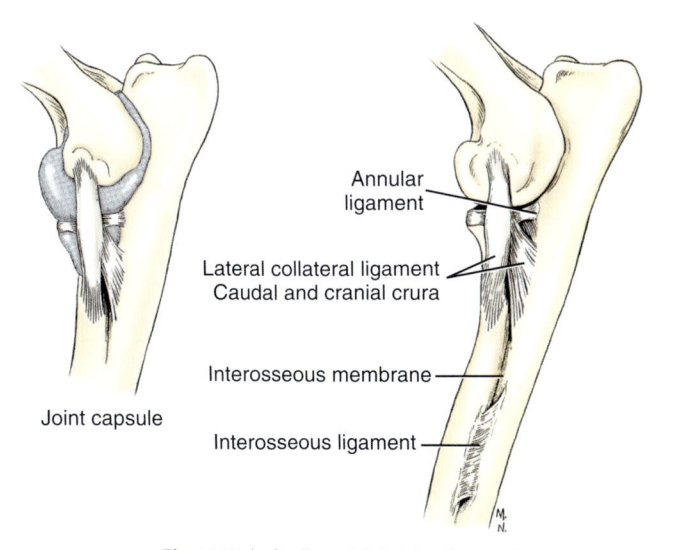

• Fig. 5.22 Left elbow joint, lateral aspect.

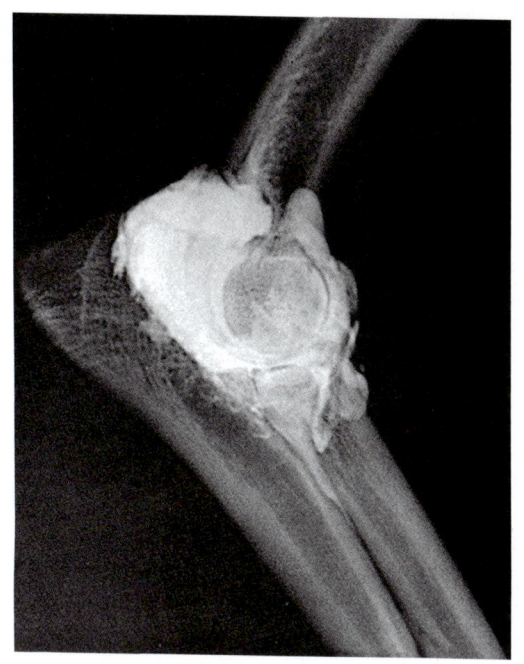

• Fig. 5.23 Lateromedial radiograph, left elbow joint; contrast arthrogram performed to define the synovial space.

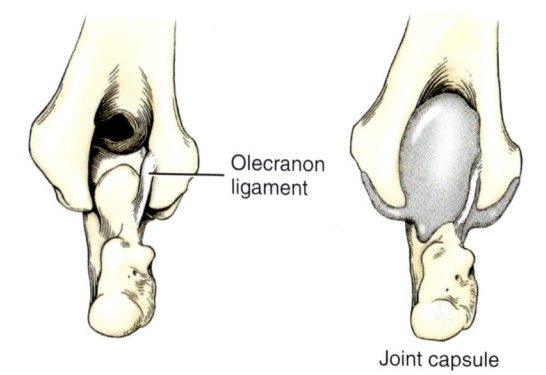

• Fig. 5.24 Left elbow joint, caudal aspect.

ulna, it forms a ring in which the articular circumference of the radius turns when the forearm is rotated.

The **olecranon ligament** (*lig. olecrani*) is an elastic ligament that passes between the craniomedial aspect of the olecranon and the medial border of the olecranon fossa.

The **oblique ligament** is a small but distinct band of fibers in the cranial aspect of the joint capsule that arises on the proximal edge of the supratrochlear foramen and crosses the cranial, flexor, surface of the elbow joint distomedial to the tendons of the mm. biceps brachii and brachialis. At the level of these tendons, directly distal to the annular ligament, it divides into two parts. The shorter part blends with the cranial crus of the medial collateral ligament. The longer branch ends on the medial border of the radius after looping around the tendons of the mm. biceps brachii and brachialis.

Radioulnar Joints

The radius and ulna are united at the proximal and distal radioulnar synovial joints and by the surprisingly thick interosseous ligament and the narrow thin interosseous membrane, which extends both proximally and distally from the interosseous ligament.

The **proximal radioulnar joint** (*articulatio radioulnaris proximalis*), already mentioned as a part of the main elbow joint, extends distally between the articular circumference of the radius and the radial notch of the ulna to a depth of approximately 5 mm. The joint allows rotation of the radius in the radial notch of the ulna. Staszyk and Gasse (1994) discussed the arrangement and attachment of collagen fibers to the bone around the joint capsule in regard to biomechanical forces.

Preston et al. (2000) evaluated the areas of articular contact of the proximal portions of the radius and ulna in normal elbow joints of dogs and the effects of axial load on size and location of these areas. Specific areas of articular contact were identified on the radius, the craniolateral aspect of the *anconeal process*, and the medial coronoid process. They concluded that there are three distinct contact areas in the elbow joint of dogs. Two ulnar contact areas were detected, suggesting that there may be physiologic incongruity of the humeroulnar joint. There was no evidence of surface incongruity between the medial edge of the radial head and the lateral edge of the medial coronoid process. Mason et al. (2005) produced transarticular force maps by placing a tactile array pressure sensor into the elbow joint cavity and loading cadaveric forelimbs in a materials testing system. They found the proximal articular surface of the ulna contributes substantially to load transfer through the canine elbow joint. Breit et al. (2005) examined 234 necropsy dogs ranging in age between 2 days and 17 years to characterize the cross-sectional shape of the humeroantebrachial contact area of the radius and ulna on radioulnar scans of giant, large, mid-sized, small, and chondrodystrophic breeds.

The **interosseous ligament of the antebrachium** (*lig. interossei antebrachii*) (see Fig. 5.22) is a thick but short collagenous ligament that extends across the interosseous space from the apposed rough areas on the radius and ulna. It is approximately 2 cm long, 0.5 cm wide, and 0.2 cm thick. From just distal to the radioulnar joint, it extends distally slightly beyond the middle of the ulna but not quite to the middle of the radius because this bone does not extend as far proximally as the ulna. The long axis of the ligament is slightly oblique so that the distal part is more lateral than the proximal. It is wider distally and is separated from the interosseous membrane by a small fossa, which extends deep to the ligament for approximately half its length. In the fornix of the fossa the interosseous membrane and ligament fuse. The interosseous ligament of the antebrachium is much thicker than the interosseous membrane located both proximal and distal to it. The **interosseous membrane of the antebrachium** (*membrana interossea antebrachii*) (see Fig. 5.22) is a narrow, thin septum that connects the radius and ulna both proximal and distal to the interosseous ligament. It attaches to the apposed interosseous crests of the radius and ulna. The membrane extends from the proximal to the distal radioulnar synovial joints but is perforated proximally for the passage of the common interosseous artery and vein and the interosseous nerve. Distally a smaller perforation in the membrane allows for the passage of the distal dorsal interosseous artery and vein from the caudal side. There are also, throughout the length of the interosseous membrane, small openings for the anastomotic vessels that course between the caudal interosseous and the cranial interosseous vessels.

The **distal radioulnar joint** (*articulatio radioulnaris distalis*), which extends between the distal portions of the radius and the ulna, is a proximal extension of the antebrachiocarpal joint capsule. The distal end of the ulna bears a slight articular convexity, and the adjacent surface of the radius bears a shallow articular cavity. The fibrosa of the joint capsule is continuous with the interosseous membrane and is short and tight cranially forming the **radioulnar ligament** (*lig. radioulnare*). It is the distal pivotal joint for the small amount of rotational movement permitted between the bones of the forearm (Kaiser et al., 2007).

Carpal, Metacarpal, and Phalangeal Joints (*Articulationes Manus*)
Carpal Joints

The **carpal joints** (*articulationes carpi*) (Figs. 5.25 to 5.32) are composite articulations that include proximal, middle, distal, and intercarpal joint surfaces. The **antebrachiocarpal joint** (*articulatio antebrachiocarpea*) is located between the distal part of the radius (the trochlea), and the ulna and the proximal row of carpal bones. The **middle carpal joint** (*articulatio mediocarpea*) is located between the two rows of carpal bones. The **carpometacarpal joints** (*articulationes carpometacarpeae*) are located between the carpus and the metacarpus. Joints between the individual carpal bones of each row constitute the **intercarpal joints** (*articulationes intercarpeae*). The carpal joint as a whole acts as a ginglymus, permitting flexion and extension with some lateral movement. Greatest movement occurs in the antebrachiocarpal and middle carpal joints. Considerably less movement takes place in the intercarpal and carpometacarpal joints.

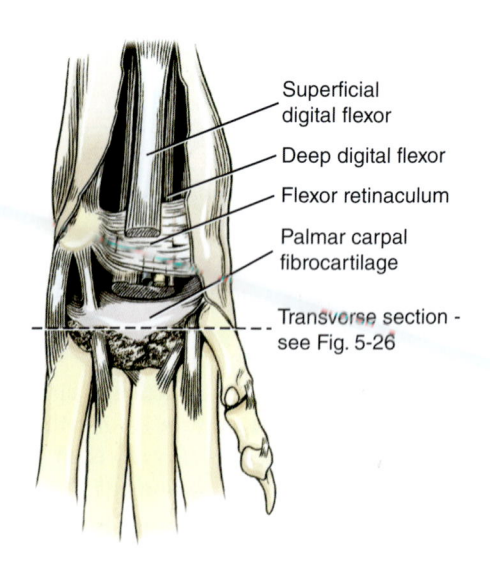

• **Fig. 5.25** Tendons and ligaments of left carpus, palmar aspect.

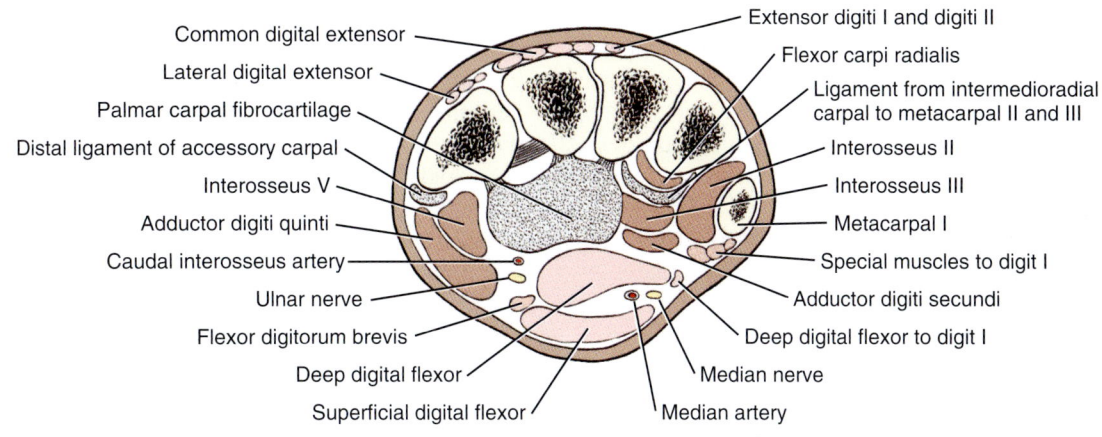

• **Fig. 5.26** Transverse-section through proximal end of left metacarpus.

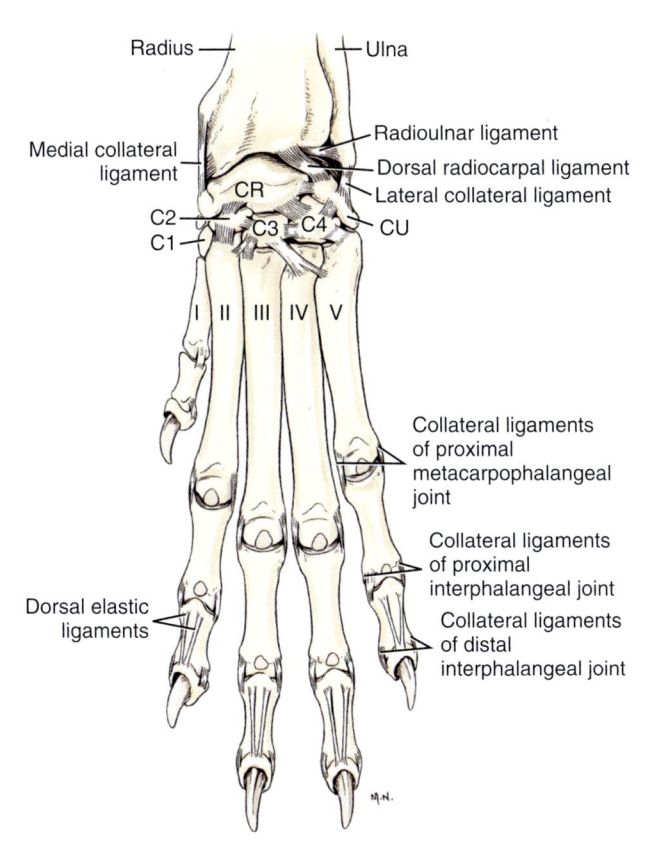

• **Fig. 5.27** Ligaments of left forepaw, dorsal aspect. *C1* to *C4*, First, second, third, fourth carpals; *CR*, intermedioradial carpal; *CU*, ulnar carpal; *I* to *V*, metacarpals.

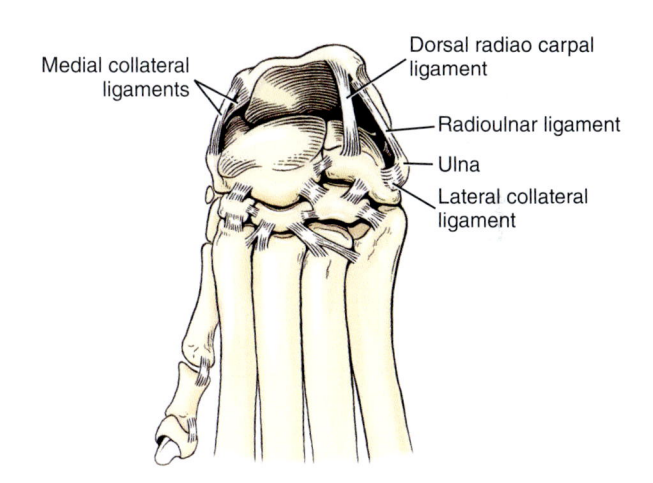

• **Fig. 5.28** Ligaments of flexed carpus, dorsal aspect.

There are no continuous collateral ligaments for the three main joints of the carpus. The dorsal and palmar parts of the joint capsule are much thicker than is usually the case on the extensor and flexor surfaces of hinge joints. Long collateral ligaments are lacking. Two superimposed sleeves of collagenous tissue, with tendons located between them, ensure the integrity of the carpus. The superficial sleeve is a modification of the deep carpal fascia, and the deep sleeve is the fibrous layer of the joint capsule. Laterally and medially, the two sleeves fuse and become specialized in part to form the short collateral ligaments.

The **flexor retinaculum** (*retinaculum flexorum*), formerly called the *transverse palmar carpal ligament* (see Fig. 5.25), is well developed in the dog. It is a modification of the palmar part of the carpal fascia. It attaches laterally to the medial part of the enlarged free palmar end of the accessory carpal bone and widens as it passes medially to attach to the styloid process of the radius and on the palmar projections of the intermedioradial and first carpals. The flexor retinaculum is divided into two parts. One lies superficial and the other lies deeper between the tendons of the superficial and deep digital flexors. The **carpal canal** (*canalis carpi*) on the palmar side of the carpus is formed superficially by the superficial part of the flexor retinaculum and deeply by the palmar carpal fibrocartilage and the palmar part of the joint capsule. The carpal canal is bounded laterally by the accessory carpal bone. It contains the tendons and synovial sheaths of the mm. flexor digitorum superficialis and flexor digitorum profundus and the tendon of the flexor carpi radialis as well as the radial, median, and caudal interosseous arteries and veins and the ulnar and median nerves.

The **palmar carpal fibrocartilage** (*fibrocartilago carpometacarpeum palmare*) (see Figs. 5.25 and 5.26) is not recognized by the NAV but is considered in this text to represent a development of the palmar surface of the fibrous layer of the joint capsule, which includes a plethora of small individual palmar ligaments between adjacent carpal bones. It is quite thick and sharply defined proximally. As it crosses the palmar surfaces of the carpal bones, it attaches to all of their palmar surfaces and has a thick attachment on the dorsomedial border of the accessory carpal bone, just palmar to the articulation of the intermedioradial carpal with the ulnar carpal. The palmar carpal fibrocartilage is thicker distally where it attaches to the palmar surfaces of the distal row of carpal bones and the adjacent surfaces of the proximal parts, the bases, of metacarpals III, IV, and V. The palmar carpal fibrocartilage serves as the origin for most of the special muscles of digits 2 and 5, as well as furnishing part of the origin for the interosseous muscles. It flattens the palmar irregularities at the carpometacarpal joints and

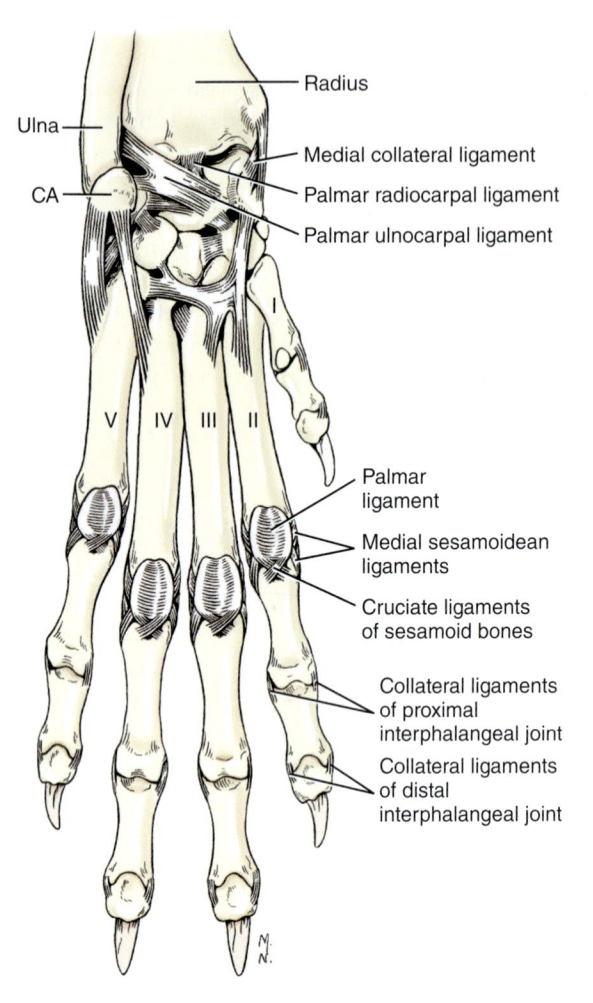

• Fig. 5.29 Deep ligaments of left forepaw, palmar aspect. *CA*, Accessory carpal; *I to V*, metacarpals.

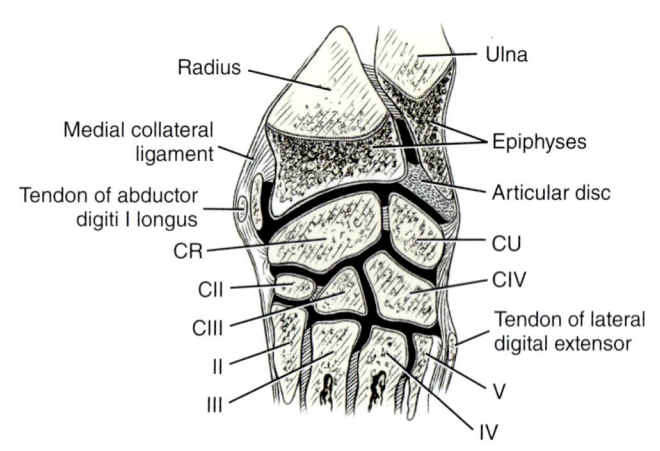

• Fig. 5.30 Schematic section of left carpus, showing articular cavities. *CII, CIII, CIV*, Second, third, fourth carpals; *CR*, intermedioradial carpal; *CU*, ulnar carpal; *II to V*, metacarpals.

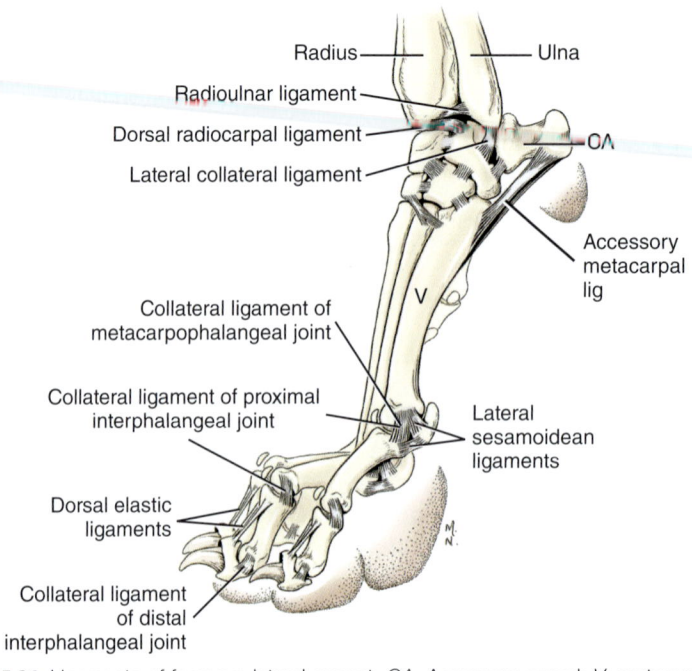

• Fig. 5.31 Ligaments of forepaw, lateral aspect. *CA*, Accessory carpal; *V*, metacarpal V.

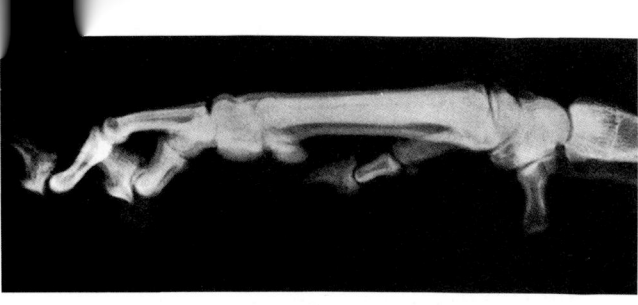

• **Fig. 5.32** Lateromedial radiograph, left forepaw skeleton.

furnishes a smooth, deep surface for the carpal canal. The **special ligaments of the carpus** are treated briefly. Some of the smaller ones are not described, but all are illustrated in Figs. 5.27 to 5.31.

The short **medial collateral ligament** (*lig. collaterale carpi mediale*) consists of a straight and an oblique part. The straight part runs from a tubercle above the radial styloid process to the most medial part of the intermedioradial carpal. The oblique part, after leaving the styloid process, runs obliquely to the palmaromedial surface of the intermedioradial carpal. The tendon of the m. abductor pollicis longus lies between the two parts as it crosses the medial surface of the carpus.

The short **lateral collateral ligament** (*lig. collaterale carpi laterale*) extends from the styloid process of the ulna to the ulnar carpal. In addition to the short collateral ligaments the cranial distal lip of the radius is attached to the dorsal surface of the ulnar carpal by a thick **dorsal radiocarpal ligament** (*lig. radiocarpeum dorsale*). These ligaments diverge as they run distally, thus allowing a free opening on the cranial surface of the antebrachiocarpal joint during flexion. The ulna is securely anchored to the palmar side of the intermedioradial carpal by an obliquely running **palmar ulnocarpal ligament** (*lig. ulnocarpeum palmare*) located just proximal to the accessory carpal bone. From the palmar surface of the radius, near its distal articular cartilage, the **palmar radiocarpal ligament** (*lig. radiocarpeum palmare*) runs to the palmar surface of the intermedioradial carpal. A short leaf of this ligament runs from the midpalmar surface of the radius to the intermedioradial carpal. A flat band nearly 1 cm wide runs from the palmarolateral surface of the radius from within the distal part of the interosseous space to the lateral surface of the intermedioradial carpal adjacent to the ulnar carpal. The accessory carpal bone is secured distally by two **accessory metacarpal ligaments** (*lig. accessoriometacarpeum*) that originate near its enlarged, rounded, free end. Distally one attaches to metacarpal V and the other to metacarpal IV. Many short intercarpal ligaments unite the carpal bones transversely, holding them as units in the two rows.

Metacarpal Joints

The **intermetacarpal joints** (*articulationes intermetacarpeae*) are close-fitting joints between the proximal ends, the bases, of adjacent metacarpal bones. The synovial membrane from the adjacent carpometacarpal joint extends a few millimeters between the metacarpal bones. Distal to the synovial part, the bones are united for variable distances by fibrous tissue, the **interosseous metacarpal ligaments** (*ligg. metacarpea interossea*). Distal to these ligaments are the **interosseous spaces** of the metacarpus (*spatia interossea metacarpi*).

The **metacarpophalangeal joints** (*articulationes metacarpophalangeae*) are the five joints formed by the distal ends, the heads, of the metacarpal bones and the proximal ends, the bases, of the proximal phalanges. To these are added in each of the four main joints the two palmar sesamoid bones. Each joint has a **joint capsule** that runs between the four bones that form the joint with the two **collateral ligaments** that unite the osseous parts. Each pair of palmar sesamoid bones of the four main joints is joined together by a **palmar ligament** (*lig. palmaria*), formerly called the *intersesamoidean ligament*. This short, cartilaginous ligament consists of transverse fibers that unite the paired sesamoid bones and cover their palmar surfaces. The **lateral** and **medial collateral sesamoidean ligaments** (*ligg. sesamoidea collateralia laterale et mediale*) are short, flat bands on each side of the metacarpophalangeal joint. The first part attaches the corresponding lateral and medial surfaces of the sesamoid bones to the distal surfaces of the metacarpal bone palmar to the proximal attachments of the collateral ligaments of the metacarpophalangeal joint. The second part goes to the medial and lateral tubercles of the base of the proximal phalanx. In the dog there are two sets of distal sesamoidean ligaments. From the distal ends of each pair of sesamoid bones, adjacent to the synovial membrane of the joint capsule, there is a thin, flat band that attaches to the palmar side of the proximal phalanx. It is called the **short sesamoidean ligament** (*lig. sesamoideum breve*). On the palmar surface of this short ligament are the **cruciate ligaments of the sesamoid bones** (*ligg. sesamoidea cruciata*) that extend from the bases of the sesamoid bones to the diagonally opposite tubercles on the bases of the proximal phalanx. In the first digit there is usually only one sesamoid bone and therefore only one ligament.

The dorsal sesamoid bones of the metacarpophalangeal joints are secured by delicate fibers from the tendons of the m. extensor digitorum communis and the mm. interossei proximally and by a ligament to the dorsal surface of the middle phalanx distally.

Phalangeal Joints

The **proximal interphalangeal joints** (*articulationes interphalangeae proximales*) are formed by the heads of the proximal phalanges articulating with the articular fovea of the base of the middle phalanges in each of the main digits, II to V. These are saddle-type joints. The **joint capsules** have dorsal walls that are thickened by a bead of cartilage. Here the capsules are intimately united with the extensor tendons so that the sesamoid cartilages appear to be intercalated in the joint capsule. On the palmar side the joint capsules are intimately fused with the flexor tendons. The **collateral ligaments** are stout collagenous bands that do not parallel the axis through the digit but extend in vertical planes as the dog stands. They attach proximally to the depressions on the sides of the heads of the first phalanges and distally to the collateral tubercles on the proximal ends of the middle phalanges. In the first digit, which has only two phalanges, the collateral ligaments attach distally to the proximal end of the distal phalanx.

The **distal interphalangeal joints** (*articulationes interphalangeae distales*) in the second to fifth digits are formed by the heads of the middle phalanges articulating with the saddle-shaped fovea on the bases of the distal phalanges. A single, small, spheroidal, sesamoid cartilage is located on the palmar side of the **joint capsule**. The joint capsule is thickened to form the **collateral ligaments**, which attach proximally to the shallow depressions on each side of the head of the middle phalanx and extend obliquely caudodistally to attach to the sides of the ungual crest of the third, or distal, phalanx. The **dorsal ligaments** are two elastic cords that extend across the dorsal part of the distal interphalangeal joint some distance from its surface. They attach proximally to the dorsal surface of the base of the middle phalanx, where they are approximately 2 mm apart. Distally they attach close together on the dorsal part of the ungual crest. They passively keep the claws retracted, so that the claws do not touch the supporting surface except when their tension is overcome by the m. flexor digitorum profundus or the claws are overgrown.

Metacarpal and Digital Fascia

The palmar annular ligaments are developments of the **palmar fascia** (*fascia palmaris*) in the metacarpophalangeal area. The digital annular ligaments are developments of the **digital fascia** (*fascia digitii*). Superficial to these the fascia of the palmar metacarpophalangeal area thickens to form obliquely oriented fibers that form a continuous superficial, V-shaped ligamentous structure that not only holds the digits together but also acts as a fastening mechanism for the large heart-shaped metacarpal pad. These fibers compose the **deep transverse metacarpal ligament** (*lig. metacarpeum transversum profundum*). These fibers originate bilaterally as small fibrous strands from the abaxial borders of the second and fifth tendons of the m. flexor digitorum superficialis. From their origin proximal to the metacarpophalangeal joints they extend distally to the proximal digital annular ligaments that cross the flexor tendons at these joints of digits II and V. This ligament attaches to the proximal digital annular ligaments of the second and fifth digits and, augmented in size, runs distoaxially to the proximal digital annular ligaments of the third and fourth digits. It attaches to these annular ligaments and again increases in size, reaching a maximum width of 4 mm in large dogs. Continuing distally, it unites in a single broad band located dorsal to the metacarpal pad. The conjoined fibers at the apex of this ligament continue to the integument of the pad and cover the flexor tendons opposite the proximal interphalangeal joints. This is the main supportive structure of the pad, but there are in addition several fibroelastic strands that pass radially into the substance of the pad from the deep transverse metacarpal ligament as it crosses and fused to the annular ligaments. Proximal to this ligament is a feeble collagenous strand that runs from the palmar surface of metacarpal II to a like place on metacarpal V. It is not present in the hindpaw, according to Baum and Zietzschmann (1936).

Ligaments and Joints of the Pelvic Limb

Joints of Pelvic Girdle (*Articulationes Cinguli Membri Pelvinae*)

The right and the left os coxae in young dogs are united midventrally by cartilage to form the **pelvic symphysis** (*symphysis pelvis*). The cranial half is formed by the **pubic symphysis** (*symphysis pubica*), and the caudal half by the **ischial symphysis** (*symphysis ischiadica*). In the adult, the pelvic symphysis ossifies first at the ischial symphysis and later at the pubic symphysis. Occasionally a symphysis is lacking at midpoint. In many, if not most, dogs the pelvic symphysis remains partially unossified until 5 or 6 years of age. The pubic symphysis is subject to periodic resorption as a result of advanced pregnancy in some mammals.

Sacroiliac Joint

The **sacroiliac joint** (*articulatio sacroiliaca*) is a combined synovial and fibrocartilaginous joint. The apposed crescent-shaped auricular surfaces on the wings of the sacrum and ilium are covered by cartilage, and their margins are united by a thin **joint capsule**. The fibrosa of the caudoventral part is so thin that the capsular wall is translucent. Dorsal to the auricular surfaces, the wing of the sacrum and the wing of the ilium are rough and possess irregular projections and depressions that tend to interlock. In life this space is occupied by a plate of fibrocartilage that unites the two wings. When this joint is disarticulated by injury, or by force as in an autopsy procedure, the fibrocartilage usually remains attached to the sacrum. Through the medium of this fibrocartilage, the ilium and sacrum are firmly united, to form the **sacroiliac synchondrosis** (*synchondrosis sacroiliaca*). The sacroiliac synchondrosis is located craniodorsal to the synovial portion of the joint. Gregory et al. (1986) found the sacroiliac joint capable of slight motion.

The **ventral sacroiliac ligament** (*lig. sacroiliacum ventrale*) (Fig. 5.33) consists of many short, fibrous fascicles that are arranged in two groups. Those of the cranial group run medially and caudally from the ilium to the sacrum. Those of the shorter caudal group run medially and cranially. The thin joint capsule appears between them.

The **dorsal sacroiliac ligaments** (*ligg. sacroiliacum dorsale breve et longum*) (Fig. 5.34) are more extensive than the ventral ones. They can be divided into a short and a long part. The short part consists of collagenous bands that extend obliquely caudomedially from the caudal dorsal iliac spine to the cranial two thirds of the lateral border of the sacrum. The long part is dorsocaudal to the short part and is fused to it cranially. It is questionable whether a long

CHAPTER 5 Arthrology 197

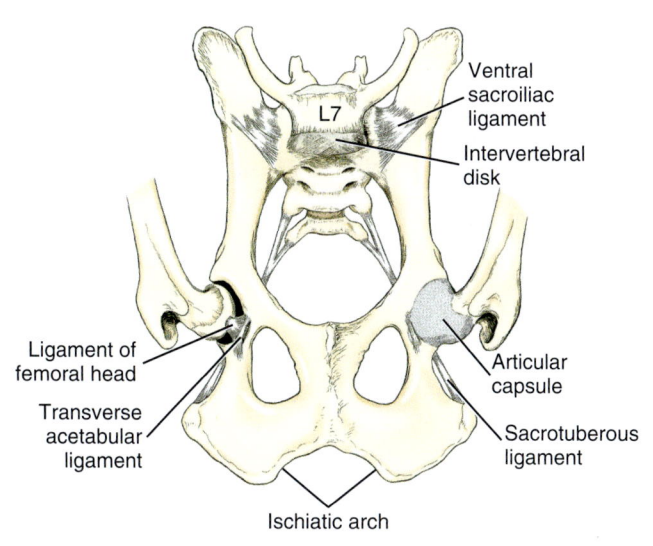

- **Fig. 5.33** Ligaments of pelvis, ventral aspect.

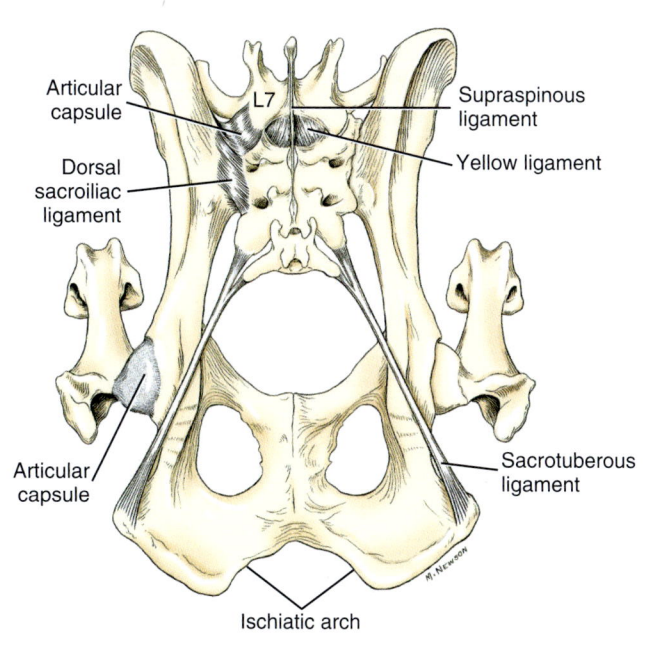

- **Fig. 5.34** Ligaments of pelvis, dorsal aspect.

dorsal sacroiliac ligament should be recognized because it represents largely the attachment of the fasciae of the pelvis and tail. The long part of the ligament extends farther caudally on the sacrum and may even reach the transverse process of the first caudal vertebra.

The **sacrotuberous ligament** (*lig. sacrotuberale*) (see Fig. 5.34) is a fibrous cord that is flattened at both ends. It extends from the caudolateral part of the apex of the sacrum and the transverse process of the first caudal vertebra to the lateral angle of the ischiatic tuberosity. In large dogs the middle part of the ligament may be 3 mm thick, and its flattened ends may be 1 cm wide. The sacrotuberous ligament lies hidden mainly by the m. gluteus superficialis. It forms the caudodorsal boundary of the lesser ischiadic foramen (*foramen ischiadicum minus*). The following muscles arise wholly or in part from it: mm. biceps femoris, gluteus superficialis, piriformis, and abductor cruris caudalis.

Hip Joint

The **hip joint** (*articulatio coxae*) (see Figs. 5.33 and 5.34) is formed by the head of the femur articulating with the acetabulum, the cotyloid cavity of the os coxae (Shively, 1975; Shively & Van Sickle, 1982). Axes through the femur and os coxae meet at the hip joint in a cranially open angle of approximately 95 degrees. Although flexion and extension are the chief movements of the joint, its ball-and-socket construction allows a great range of movement. The action of adjacent muscles restricts this movement similar to that described for the shoulder joint. The deep acetabulum is further deepened in life by a band of fibrocartilage, the **acetabular lip** (*labrum acetabulare*), which is applied to the rim of the acetabulum. It extends across the acetabular notch as a free ligament, the **transverse acetabular ligament** (*lig. transversum acetabuli*). The **joint capsule** is capacious. It attaches, medially, a few millimeters from the edge of the acetabular lip, and, laterally, on the neck of the femur, 1 or 2 cm from the cartilage-covered head. The fibrous coat has various thickenings but no definite ligaments. The most distinct thickening is in the dorsal part of the fibrosa. This causes a nearly horizontal bulging of the synovial membrane, known as the **orbicular zone** (*zona orbicularis*). As it arches from the cranial to the caudal border across the dorsal surface of the neck, it parallels both the dorsal part of the acetabular rim and the dorsal part of the head–neck junction. It presents no definite fiber pattern and appears as a white thickening in the joint capsule, measuring less than 1 mm thick by 2 or 3 mm wide. Other less prominent reinforcements occur cranially as the **iliofemoral ligament** (*lig. iliofemorale*) and caudally as the **ischiofemoral ligament** (*lig. ischiofemorale*).

Maieral et al. (2005) studied the hip joints of 43 dog cadavers of various breeds to describe the biomechanical features as exactly as possible with respect to long-term and momentary loading. Their findings indicate that the articular surfaces of the hip joint are not loaded homogeneously.

The **ligament of the head of the femur** (*lig. capitis femoris*) (see Fig. 5.33), formerly called the *round ligament*, is a short, thick, flattened cord that extends from the fovea in the head of the femur to the acetabular fossa. This ligament is largely intraarticular and not weight-bearing but is still covered by synovial membrane. In large dogs it is approximately 1.5 cm long and 5 mm wide at its femoral attachment. Its acetabular attachment is wide as it blends with the periosteum of the acetabular fossa and the transverse acetabular ligament. The pelvic attachment of the ligament of the femoral head is more than 1 cm wide in large dogs. In and peripheral to the rectangular acetabular fossa there is usually a small quantity of fat.

Hip dysplasia in the dog has a high incidence in some breeds. It is a progressive disparity between muscle mass and bone growth that results in malarticulation and subsequent degenerative joint disease (Riser, 1964, 1973, 1975; King, 2017).

198 CHAPTER 5   Arthrology

- **Fig. 5.35** Ligaments of left stifle joint.

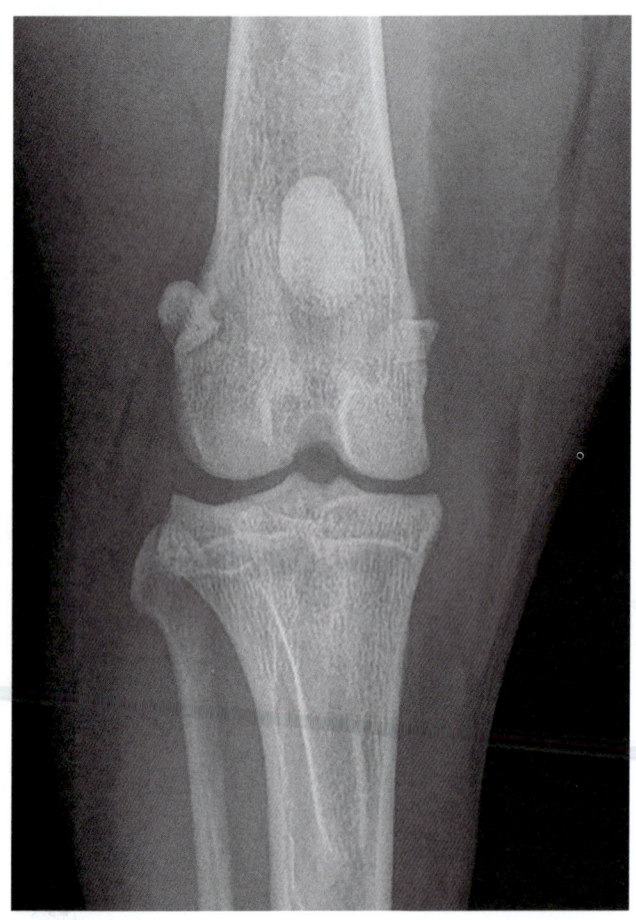

- **Fig. 5.36** Craniocaudal radiograph, left stifle joint, skeleton.

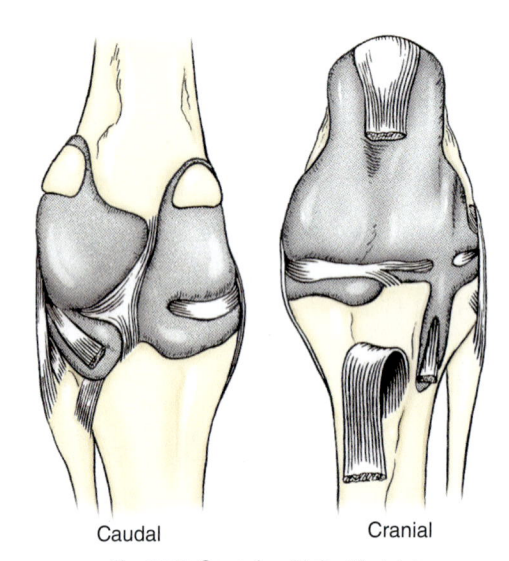

- **Fig. 5.37** Capsule of left stifle joint.

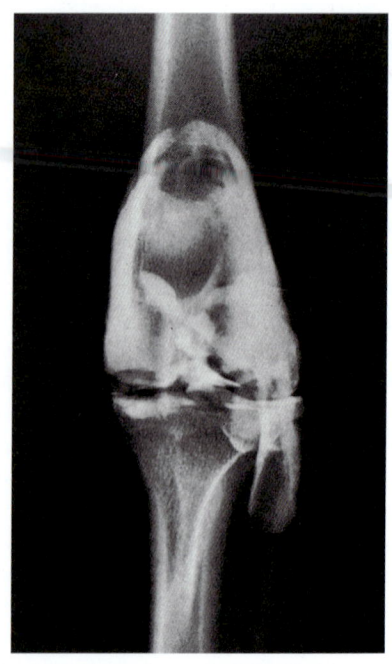

- **Fig. 5.38** Craniocaudal radiograph, left stifle joint; contrast arthrogram performed to define the synovial space.

Stifle Joint

The **stifle joint** (*articulatio genus*) (Figs. 5.35 to 5.45) is a complex condylar synovial joint. The main spheroidal part is formed by the thick, rollerlike condyles of the femur articulating with the flattened condyles of the tibia to form the **femorotibial** or condyloid part of the joint (*articulatio femorotibialis*). Freely connected with this is the **femoropatellar joint** (*articulatio femoropatellaris*), located between the patella and the trochlea of the femur. The two joints are interdependent in that the patella is held to the tibia firmly

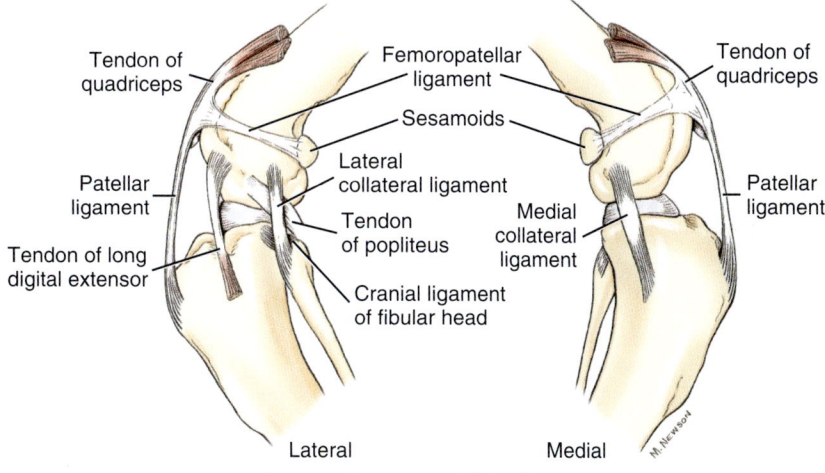

• **Fig. 5.39** Ligaments of left stifle joint.

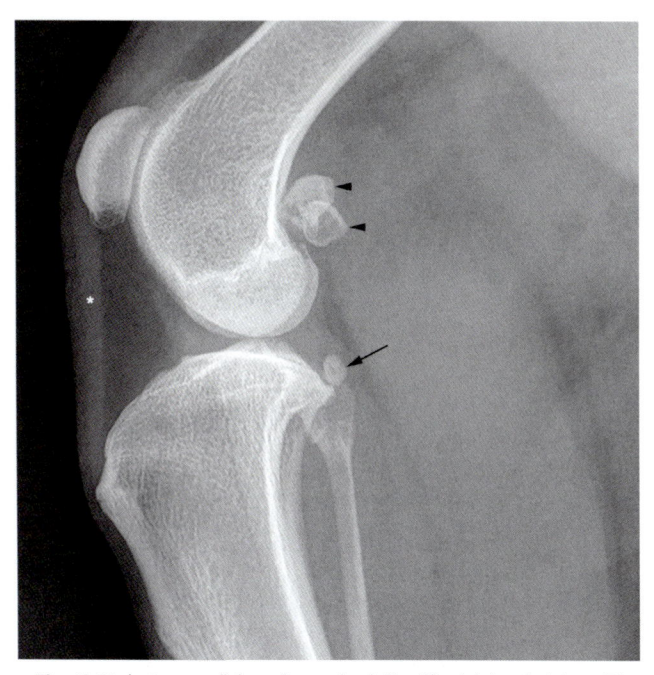

• **Fig. 5.40** Lateromedial radiograph, left stifle joint, skeleton. The patella in the tendon of insertion of the quadriceps is seen on the trochlea of the femur, the superimposed sesamoids (arrowheads) in the heads of the gastrocnemius are located on the proximocaudal surface of the femoral condyles, and the popliteal sesamoid (arrow) rests on the lateral condyle of the tibia.

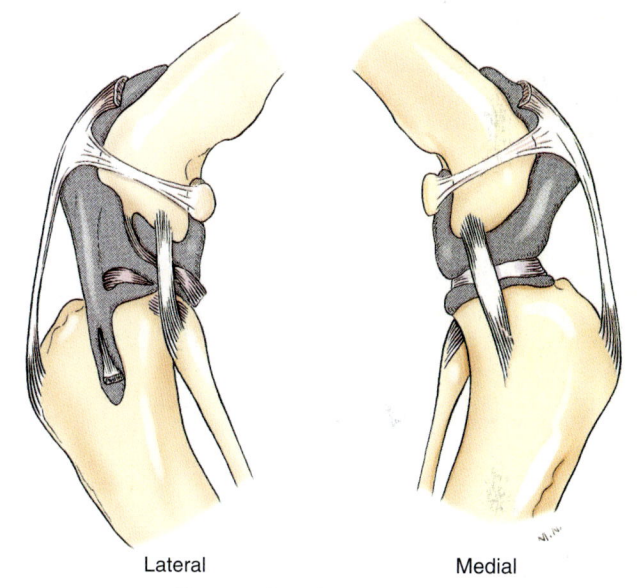

• **Fig. 5.41** Capsule of left stifle joint.

by ligamentous tissue so that any movement between the femur and the tibia also occurs between the patella and the femur. The incongruence that exists between the tibia and the femur is occupied, in life, by two fibrocartilages, or *menisci*, one located between the adjacent medial condyles (*meniscus medialis*) and the other (*meniscus lateralis*) between the adjacent lateral condyles of the femur and tibia. In addition the proximal tibiofibular joint communicates with the stifle joint.

The **joint capsule** of the stifle joint is the largest in the body. It forms three sacs, all of which freely intercommunicate. Two of these are between the femoral and the tibial condyles (*saccus medialis et lateralis*), and the third is beneath the patella. The patellar part of the joint capsule is very capacious. It attaches to the edges of the patella, and, adjacent to the patella, the parapatellar fibrocartilages develop in the fibrosa of this joint capsule. The joint capsule extends beyond these in all directions. Proximally a sac of the femoropatellar joint capsule protrudes 1.5 cm deep to the tendon of the m. quadriceps femoris. Laterally and medially the patellar part of the joint capsule extends approximately 2 cm from the crests of the trochlear ridges toward the femoral epicondyles in large breeds. Distally, the patellar and femorotibial parts join without sharp demarcations. Distal to the patella the fibrous layer of the cranial part of the joint capsule contains a large quantity of fat, the **infrapatellar fat body** (*corpus adiposum infrapatellare*) (see Fig. 5.45), which increases in thickness distally. This fat body develops in the fibrous layer of the joint capsule. The

200 CHAPTER 5 Arthrology

• **Fig. 5.42** Lateromedial radiograph, left stifle joint; contrast arthrogram performed to define the synovial space.

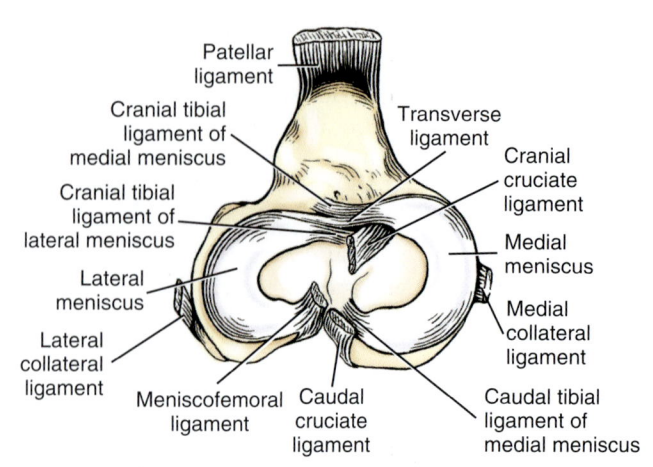

• **Fig. 5.44** Menisci and ligaments of left stifle joint, dorsal aspect.

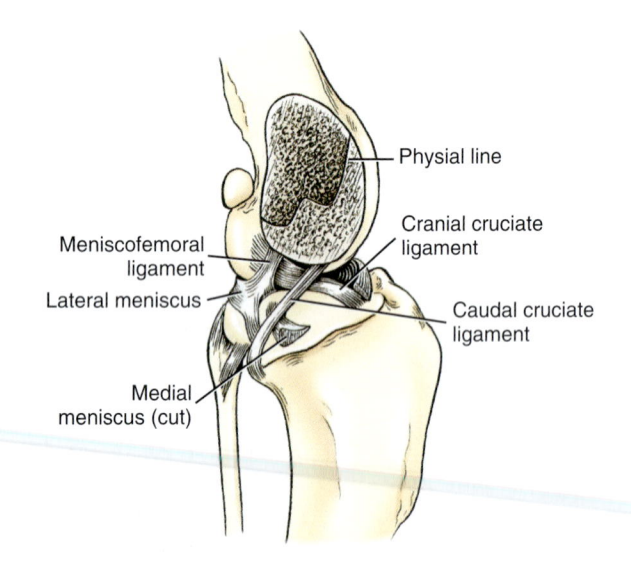

• **Fig. 5.43** Cruciate and meniscal ligaments of left stifle joint, medial aspect. Medial meniscus and part of the medial femoral condyle removed.

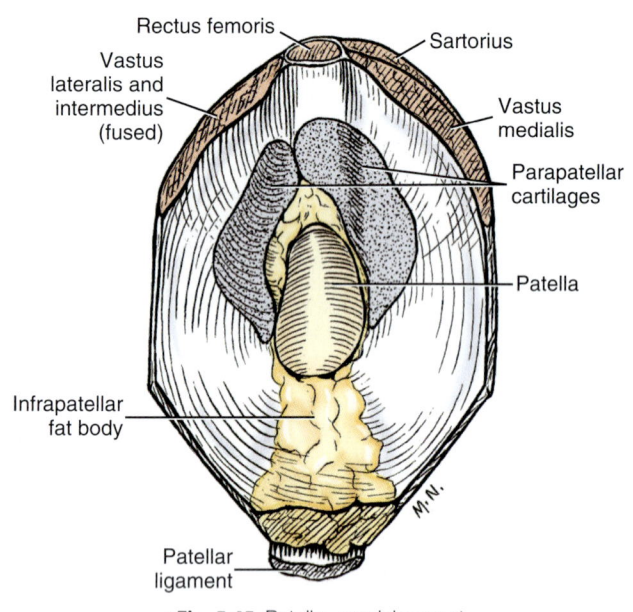

• **Fig. 5.45** Patella, caudal aspect.

femorotibial sacs are considerably smaller than the femoropatellar. Both femorotibial sacs are partly divided by the menisci into femoromeniscal and tibiomeniscal parts. The menisci develop in the fibrous layer of the capsule and the two parts communicate primarily around their concave, sharp-edged axial borders, where the tibial and femoral condyles contact each other. A free transverse communication also exists between the lateral and the medial condyloid parts of the joint. Both the lateral and medial condyloid parts extend between the caudal, proximal parts of the femoral condyles and the fabellae that articulate with them. The lateral femorotibial joint capsule has two other pouches as well as a joint communication in addition to the extension between the lateral fabella and the femur. On the craniolateral aspect of the tibia, lateral to the tibial tuberosity is the sulcus muscularis of the tibia. A pouch extends distally in this sulcus approximately 2 cm forming a sheath for the tendon of the m. extensor digitorum longus. This tendon originates from the extensor fossa of the femur proximal to the sulcus muscularis of the tibia. Its sheath is provided by the synovial membrane of the lateral femorotibial joint capsule. The tendon of origin of the m. popliteus on the lateral condyle of the femur is never completely surrounded by synovial membrane, but it does possess on its deep surface a well-defined synovial pouch of the lateral femorotibial joint capsule that acts as a bursa. At the site of the proximal tibiofibular joint on the caudolateral surface of the lateral tibial condyle, there is a narrow communication between the synovial spaces of the lateral femorotibial and proximal tibiofibular joints. The entire synovial space of the proximal tibiofibular joint is narrow and the joint capsule is tight, accounting for the limited movement of this joint.

The **lateral and medial menisci** (*meniscus lateralis et medialis*) are semilunar, fibrocartilaginous discs with sharp, deeply concave axial, and thick convex abaxial borders. The lateral meniscus is slightly thicker and forms a slightly greater arc than the medial one. In large dogs the peripheral border of the lateral meniscus measures approximately 8 mm. The lateral meniscus does not reach the border of the tibia caudolaterally where the tendon of origin of the m. popliteus passes over the tibial condyle. Similar to ligaments at synovial joints, the menisci are developments of the fibrous layer of the joint capsule and are covered by synovial membrane. The medial meniscus retains its attachment to the joint capsule but this has been lost for the lateral meniscus.

Carpenter and Cooper (2000) reviewed the anatomy of the canine stifle joint and pointed out the highlights of its basic anatomy.

Ligaments of Stifle Joint

The **meniscal ligaments** attach the menisci to the tibia and femur. Four of these, two from each meniscus, go to the tibia. *Nomina Anatomica Veterinaria* 2017 recognizes only two meniscal ligaments: one from the lateral meniscus to the femur and one transverse ligament between menisci. The ligamentous attachments of the menisci to the tibia are described here.

The **cranial tibial ligament of the medial meniscus** goes from the cranial, axial angle of the medial meniscus to the cranial intercondyloid area of the tibia. This attachment is immediately cranial to the transverse ligament, the cranial tibial attachment of the lateral meniscus, and the tibial attachment of the cranial cruciate ligament.

The **caudal tibial ligament of the medial meniscus** goes from the caudal axial angle of the medial meniscus to the caudal intercondyloid area of the tibia. This attachment is just cranial to the tibial attachment of the caudal cruciate ligament.

The **cranial tibial ligament of the lateral meniscus** goes to the cranial intercondyloid area of the tibia, where it attaches caudal to the transverse ligament and the cranial tibial attachment of the medial meniscus.

The **caudal tibial ligament of the lateral meniscus** goes from the caudal axial angle of the lateral meniscus to the popliteal notch of the tibia just caudal to the caudal intercondyloid area of the tibia.

The **femoral ligament of the lateral meniscus** (*lig. meniscofemorale*) is the only femoral attachment of the menisci. It passes from the caudal axial angle of the lateral meniscus dorsally to that part of the medial femoral condyle that faces the intercondyloid fossa.

The **transverse ligament** (*lig. transversum genus*), formerly the *intermeniscal ligament*, is a small transverse fibrous band that leaves the caudal side of the cranial tibial ligament of the medial meniscus and goes to the cranial part of the cranial tibial ligament of the lateral meniscus.

The **femorotibial ligaments** are the collateral and the cruciate ligaments. The **cruciate ligaments of the stifle** (*ligg. cruciata genus*) are located within the stifle joint cavity. The collateral ligaments develop in the fibrous layer of the joint capsule on either side of the stifle. The **medial collateral ligament** (*lig. collaterale mediale*) is a thick ligament that extends between the medial epicondyle of the femur and the medial border of the tibia approximately 2 cm distal to the medial tibial condyle in large breeds. As it passes over the border of this condyle a bursa is interposed between the ligament and the bone. The total length of the ligament is more than 4 cm in medium-sized dogs. It fuses with the medial meniscus.

The **lateral collateral ligament** (*lig. collaterale laterale*) is similar to its fellow in size and length. As it crosses the joint cavity it passes over the tendon of origin of the m. popliteus. It ends distally on the head of the fibula, with a few fibers going to the adjacent lateral condyle of the tibia.

The cruciate ligaments are located centrally in the intercondylar fossa. They limit cranial and caudal sliding (translational) movement of the tibia on the femur. The **cranial cruciate ligament** (*lig. cruciatum craniale*) (see Fig. 5.43) runs from the caudomedial part of the lateral condyle of the femur somewhat diagonally across the intercondyloid fossa to the cranial intercondyloid area of the tibia. Dueland, Sisson, and Evans (1982) described an aberrant origin of the cranial cruciate ligament.

The **caudal cruciate ligament** (*lig. cruciatum caudale*) runs from the lateral surface of the medial femoral condyle caudodistally to the lateral edge of the popliteal notch of the tibia. The caudal cruciate ligament is slightly thicker and definitely longer than the cranial one. As their name implies, the cruciate ligaments decussate, or cross each other. This occurs at their proximal ends in the intercondylar fossa. The caudal cruciate ligament lies medial to the cranial one.

The cruciate ligaments are covered by synovial membrane that, in fact, forms an imperfect sagittal septum in the joint. However, this is incomplete, allowing medial and lateral parts to communicate. Innervation of the cruciate ligaments was described by Newman et al. (1988).

Vasseur and Arnoczky (1981) investigated the anatomic features and functions of the collateral ligaments and made measurements of tension in flexion and extension. They found that the collateral ligaments worked together with the cruciate ligaments to limit medial rotation of the tibia on the femur. In extension the collateral ligaments were the primary check against medial as well as lateral rotation. In flexion, the lateral collateral ligament was less taut and the cruciate ligaments were the primary restraint against medial rotation of the tibia. Lateral rotation was limited only by the collateral ligaments in both flexion and extension.

Excessive cranial movement of the tibia with the joint in extension is positive evidence of a rupture of the cranial cruciate ligament. The cranial cruciate ligament is the one most often torn or severed as a result of trauma or excessive forces applied to the normal joint or normal forces applied to a joint in which there is degeneration of the ligaments. Hyperextension or excessive medial rotation with the stifle flexed are the movements most likely to cause a tear of the cranial cruciate ligament. In extreme instances the collateral ligaments also may be ruptured. Schreiber (1947) has written an anatomical treatise on the canine stifle joint.

Dennler et al. (2006) measured the angles between the patellar ligament and the tibiofemoral contact point throughout the full range of motion of the stifle joint. They studied 16 pelvic limbs of dog cadavers without detectable degenerative joint disease. They concluded that, at approximately 90 degrees of flexion in the stifle joint, the shear force in the sagittal plane exerted on the proximal portion of the tibia shifts the loading from the cranial cruciate ligament to the caudal cruciate ligament.

Although the patella is a large sesamoid bone intercalated in the tendon of insertion of the m. quadriceps femoris, a portion of the tendon from the patella to the tibial tuberosity is spoken of as the **patellar ligament** (*lig. patellae*). The patellar ligament is separated from the synovial membrane of the joint capsule by a large quantity of fat, which is particularly thick distally. Between the distal part of the patellar ligament and the tibial tuberosity, just proximal to its attachment, there is frequently located a small synovial bursa. The patella is held in the trochlea of the femur mainly by the thick lateral femoral fascia, or fascia lata, and the thinner medial femoral fascia. Aiding in this function are the delicate **medial and lateral femoropatellar ligaments** (*ligg. femoropatellare mediale et laterale*). They are narrow bands of loose fibers that partially blend with the overlying femoral fasciae. The lateral band can usually be traced from the lateral side of the patella to the fabella in the lateral head of the m. gastrocnemius. The medial ligament, smaller than the lateral, usually blends with the periosteum of the medial epicondyle of the femur. The sides of the patella are continued into the femoral fascia by the **medial** and **lateral parapatellar fibrocartilages** (*cartilago parapatellaris mediale et lateralis*). These usually meet dorsally. Baum and Zietzschmann (1936) mention a suprapatellar fibrocartilage being present in older dogs in the tendon of the m. rectus femoris. The lateral and medial cartilages ride on the crests of the femoral trochlea and tend to prevent dislocation of the patella. Yahia et al. (1992), using a modified gold-chloride technique, found that the cruciate ligaments of the dog were supplied by abundant mechanoreceptive and proprioreceptive elements. These so-called Ruffini and Pacini receptors were located within the center of the ligaments.

For an illustrated review of the canine stifle joint, see Carpenter and Cooper (2000).

Tibiofibular Joints

The fibula articulates with the tibia at each end by small synovial cavities and, in addition, possesses an extensive tibiofibular syndesmosis. Barnett and Napier (1953) studied the rotatory mobility of the fibula in eutherian mammals and concluded that in the dog no rotation could be demonstrated on passive movements of the pes.

The **proximal tibiofibular joint** (*articulatio tibiofibularis proximalis*) is small and tightly fitting (Figs. 5.35 and 5.39). Its synovial membrane is a distal extension of the membrane for the lateral femorotibial part of the stifle joint capsule. The fibrous layer is not well developed, although a recognizable ligament of short fibers goes from the head of the fibula proximocranially deep to the lateral collateral ligament to the adjacent lateral condyle of the tibia as the **cranial ligament of the fibular head** (*lig. capitis fibulae craniale*). The **caudal ligament of the fibular head** (*lig. capitis fibulae caudale*) is a short band of fibers coursing from the caudal surface of the fibular head to the caudal aspect of the lateral tibial condyle. The **interosseous membrane of the crus** (*membrana interossea cruris*) extends from the proximal to the distal tibiofibular joint. The fibula has many muscles attaching to it, and many of these extend beyond their fibular attachment to the interosseous membrane, which, more than anything else, fastens the fibula to the tibia. The fibers that compose this fibrous sheet decussate, forming a latticelike flat ligament. Proximally an opening exists in the ligament for the passage of the large cranial tibial artery and its small satellite vein.

The **distal tibiofibular joint** (*articulatio tibiofibularis distalis*) receives an extension of the synovial membrane from the lateral side of the talocrural joint. Like the proximal tibiofibular joint, the distal joint is hardly more than a synovial pocket between the lateral malleolus and the distal lateral surface of the tibia. Besides the tight connection to the calcaneus, fourth tarsal, and metatarsal V, by means of the lateral collateral ligament, the lateral malleolus of the fibula has a **cranial tibiofibular ligament** (*lig. tibiofibulare craniale*) that runs a short distance transversely from the cranial edge of the lateral malleolus to the adjacent lateral surface of the tibia. The **caudal tibiofibular ligament** (*lig. tibiofibulare caudale*) passes from the lateral malleolus to the caudolateral surface of the tibia. The lateral collateral ligament has short (deep) and long (superficial) parts (see Fig. 5.49).

Tarsal, Metatarsal, and Phalangeal Joints (Articulationes Pedis)

Tarsal Joints

The **tarsal joints** (*articulationes tarsi*) (Figs. 5.46 to 5.50), like the carpal joints, are composite articulations. The **tarsocrural joint** (*articulatio tarsocruralis*) permits the greatest degree of movement. The trochlea of the talus, formed largely of two articular ridges, fits into reciprocal grooves that form the cochlea of the tibia. The grooves and ridges are not quite in sagittal planes but deviate laterally approximately 25 degrees so that the open angle faces dorsally. This allows the hindpaws to be thrust past the forepaws on their lateral sides when the dog gallops. The **talocalcaneal central joint** (*articulatio talocalcaneocentralis*) is the intertarsal joint between the talus and calcaneus proximally and the central tarsal distally on the medial side (Gorse et al., 1990). The **calcaneoquartal joint** (*articulatio calcaneoquartalis*) is

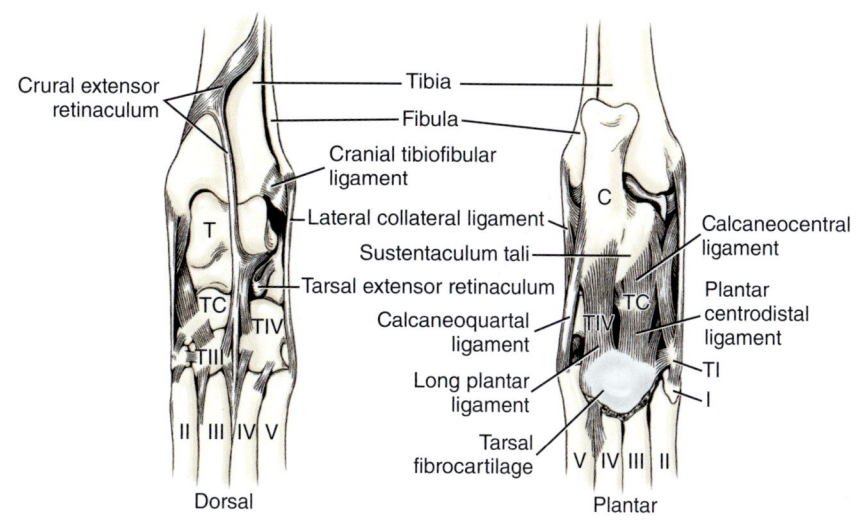

• **Fig. 5.46** Ligaments of left tarsus. *C,* Calcaneus; *I to V,* metatarsals; *T,* talus; *TI, TIII, TIV,* first, third, fourth tarsals; *TC,* central tarsal.

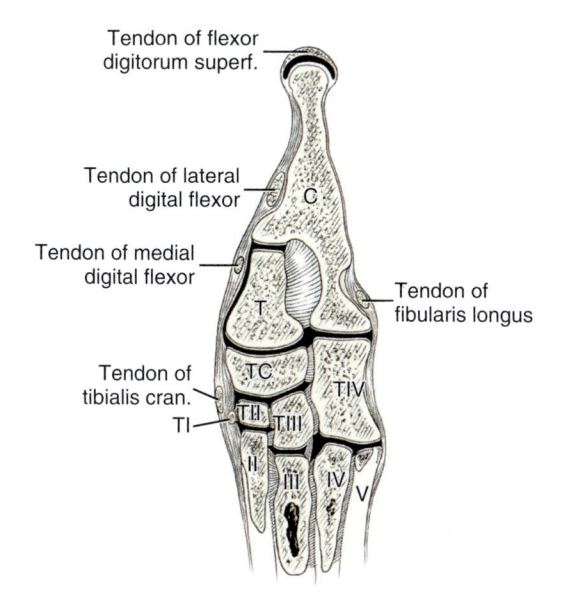

• **Fig. 5.47** Schematic section of left tarsus showing articular cavities, dorsal aspect. *C,* Calcaneus; *II to V,* metatarsals; *T,* talus; *TII, TIII, TIV,* second, third, fourth tarsals; *TC,* central tarsal.

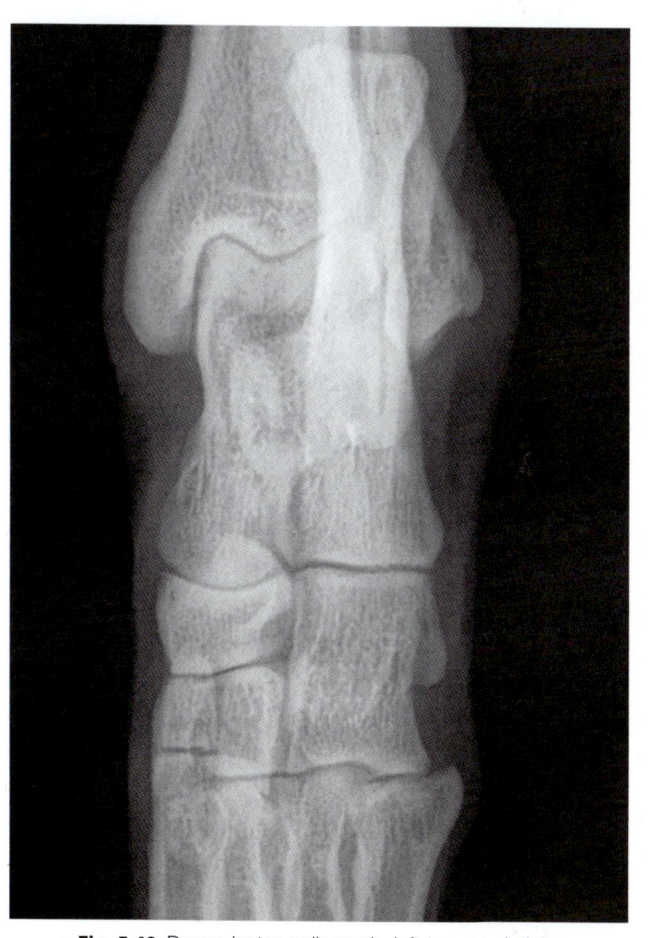

• **Fig. 5.48** Dorsoplantar radiograph, left tarsus, skeleton.

between the calcaneus proximally and the fourth tarsal distally on the lateral side. These joints form one continuous space, the **proximal intertarsal joint**. Some side movement as well as flexion and extension are possible here as the slightly convex distal ends of the talus and calcaneus fit into glenoid cavities of the central and fourth tarsals. The **centrodistal joint** (*articulatio centrodistalis*) is between the central tarsal and tarsals I, II, and III on the medial side. This is also referred to as the **distal intertarsal joint**. The four distal tarsal bones, the first to fourth, articulate with metatarsals I to V, forming the **tarsometatarsal joints** (*articulationes tarsometatarseae*). Vertical **intertarsal joints** occur between the individual bones of the tarsus, all of which are exceedingly rigid.

The fibrous part of the **tarsal joint capsule** extends from the periosteum proximal to the distal articular cartilage of the tibia and fibula to the proximal ends of the metatarsal bones. As the fibrous layer with its contained ligaments covers the individual tarsal bones, it fuses to the free surfaces of the bones. The synovial layer of the joint capsule extends to the edges of the articular cartilages. There are three lateral and four medial joint sacs. Proximally the largest sac lines the most freely movable joint of the tarsus, the tarsocrural

204　CHAPTER 5　Arthrology

- **Fig. 5.49** Ligaments of left tarsus. *C*, calcaneus; *I to V*, metatarsals; *T*, talus; *TII, TIII, TIV*, second, third, fourth tarsals; *TC*, central tarsal.

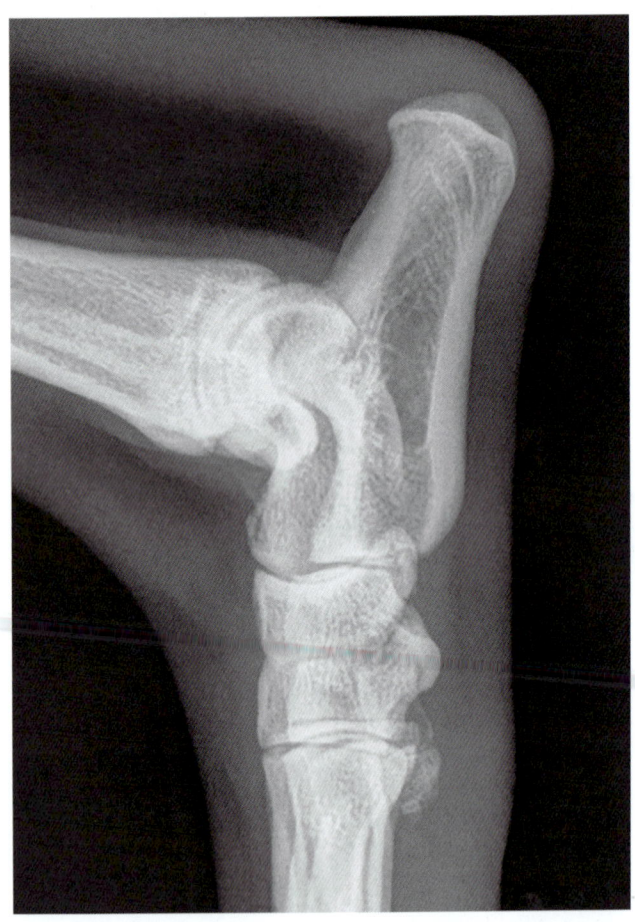

- **Fig. 5.50** Lateromedial radiograph, left tarsus, skeleton.

According to Baum and Zietzschmann (1936), the tarsocrural and the continuous talocalcaneocentral and the calcaneoquartal joint sacs communicate with each other and these communicate with the synovial sheath surrounding the tendon of the m. flexor digitorum lateralis. These authors further state that the centrodistal joint sac communicates with the tarsometatarsal sac, but that the two intercommunicating proximal sacs do not communicate with the two intercommunicating distal sacs.

The **medial collateral ligament** (*lig. collaterale mediale*) (see Fig. 5.49) is divided into a long and a short part. The long, more superficial part is a large band that runs from the medial malleolus to attach firmly to the first tarsal with lesser attachments to metatarsals I and II. As it crosses the tarsus it has a small attachment to the free surface of the talus and larger one to the free surface of the central tarsal. The short part, attaching craniodistal to the long part on the medial malleolus, divides as it passes deep to the proximal attachment of the long part. One part of this division extends on the plantar surface to attach on the talus. The other part is longer and parallels the plantar aspect of the long part of the medial collateral ligament. A few fibers may end distally on the sustentaculum tali of the calcaneus by a fascial connection. However, it attaches primarily to the first tarsal and metatarsal bones.

The **lateral collateral ligament** (*lig. collaterale laterale*), like the medial collateral ligament, is divided into a long and a short part. The long part passes from the lateral malleolus to the base of metatarsal V, attaching along its course to the calcaneus and fourth tarsal. The short part lies deep to the long part proximally. From the lateral malleolus one band extends to the tuber calcanei of the calcaneus. A second band goes to the more dorsally located talus. Both bands run at nearly right angles to the long part of the lateral collateral ligament.

On the dorsal surface of the tarsus there are various short dorsal ligaments. One prominent ligament unites the talus with the third and fourth tarsals. It blends proximally with a distal extension of the **crural extensor retinaculum**,

joint. Distal to this, on the medial side of the tarsus, are the proximal and distal intertarsal sacs of the talocalcaneocentral and centrodistal joints respectively. Laterally, only a single intertarsal sac exists between the calcaneus and the fourth tarsal, the calcaneoquartal joint. Between the tarsus and the metatarsus is the tarsometatarsal joint sac enclosing the joint that extends between the distal row of tarsal bones, the first to fourth, and the bases of metatarsals I to V.

...ons of the extensor digitorum longus, ...gitil longus, and tibialis cranialis to the tibia. A ...all band connects the second and third tarsals. The **dorsal centrodistal ligaments** are oblique bands between the central and second tarsals as well as between the central and third tarsals. The distal row of tarsal bones is joined to the bases of the metatarsal bones by small vertical ligaments on the dorsal surface. The **tarsal extensor retinaculum** is a ligamentous loop that attaches to the calcaneus and surrounds the tendon of the extensor digitorum longus (see Fig. 5.49).

On the plantar surface of the tarsus, the special plantar ligaments are thicker than those on the dorsal side (see Fig. 5.46). Most of these fuse distally with the thickened part of the joint capsule at the tarsometatarsal joints. Several of these ligaments are distinct. The **long plantar ligament** (*lig. plantare longuum*) passes from the body of the calcaneus across the fourth tarsal to which it attaches and continues to the base of the fourth and fifth metatarsals. The **calcaneocentral ligament** (*lig. calcaneocentralis*) leaves the plantar surface of the sustentaculum tali of the calcaneus and attaches to the central tarsal. The **plantar centrodistal ligament** (*lig. centrodistale plantare*) is attached between the central tarsal and the first three tarsal bones and ends in the thickened tarsometatarsal joint capsule. Laterally the **calcaneoquartal ligament** (*lig. calcaneoquartale*) is a conspicuous band that leaves the plantarolateral surface of the calcaneus, blends with the long lateral collateral ligament, and is attached to the fourth tarsal and the base of metatarsal V.

Metatarsal and Phalangeal Joints

The joints and ligaments of the metatarsus and digits are similar to the comparable joints and ligaments of the forepaw.

Bibliography

Ansulayotin, C. (1960). *Nerve supply to the shoulder, elbow, carpal, hip, stifle and tarsal joints of the dog as determined by gross dissection, thesis.* Ithaca, NY: Cornell University.

Arzi, B., Cissell, D. D., Verstraete, F. J., et al. (2013). Computed tomography findings in dogs and cats with temporomandibular joint disorders: 58 cases (2006–2011). *J Am Vet Med Assoc, 242,* 69–75.

Barnett, C. H., & Napier, J. R. (1953). The rotatory mobility of the fibula in eutherian mammals. *J Anat, 87,* 11–21.

Barnett, C. H., Davies, D. V., & MacConaill, M. A. (1961). *Synovial joints: their structure and mechanics.* Springfield, IL: Charles C Thomas.

Baum, H., & Zietzschmann, O. (1936). *Handbuch der Anatomie des Hundes* (2nd ed.). Berlin: Paul Parey.

Bennett, G. A., Bauer, W., & Maddock, S. J. (1932). A study of the repair of articular cartilage and the reaction of normal joints of the adult dogs to surgically created defects of articular cartilage, "joint mice" and patellar displacements. *Am J Pathol, 8,* 499–523.

Bergknut, N., Smolders, L. A., Grinwis, G. C. M., et al. (2013). Intervertebral disc degeneration in the dog. Part 1: Anatomy and physiology of the intervertebral disc and characteristics of inter-vertebral degeneration. *Vet J, 195,* 282–291. doi:10.1016/j.tvjl.2012.10.024.

Breit, S., & Kunzel, W. (2004). A morphometric investigation on breed specific features affecting sagittal rotational and lateral bending mobility in the canine cervical spine (C3-C7). *Anat Histol Embryol, 33*(4), 244–250.

Breit, S., Kunzel, S., & Seiler, S. (2005). Postnatal modeling of the humeroantebrachial contact areas of radius and ulna in dogs. *Anat Histol Embryol, 34*(4), 258–264.

Carpenter, D. H., & Cooper, R. C. (2000). Mini review of canine stifle joint anatomy. *Anat Histol Embryol, 29*(6), 321–329.

Cook, J. R., & Oliver, J. E. (1981). Atlantoaxial luxation in the dog. *Continuing Educ, 3,* 242–252.

Dallman, M. J., Moon, M. L., & Giovannitti-Jensen, A. (1991). Comparison of the width of the intervertebral disc space and radiographic changes before and after intervertebral disc fenestration in dogs. *Am J Vet Res, 52,* 140–145.

Davies, D. V. (1944). Observations on the volume, viscosity, and nitrogen content of synovial fluid, with a note on the histological appearance of the synovial membrane. *J Anat, 78,* 68–78.

de Lahunta, A., Glass, E., & Kent, M. (2015). *Veterinary neuroanatomy and clinical neurology.* Elsevier/Saunders.

Dennler, R., Kipfer, N. M., Tepic, S., et al. (2006). Inclination of the patellar ligament in relation to flexion angle in stifle joints of dogs without degenerative joint disease. *Am J Vet Res, 67*(11), 1849–1854.

DeRycke, L. M., Gielen, I. M., van Bree, H., et al. (2002). Computed tomography of the elbow joint in clinically normal dogs. *Am J Vet Res, 63*(10), 1400–1407.

Dieterich, H. (1931). Die Regeneration des Meniscus. *Deutsch Zeitschrift fur Chirurgie, 230,* 251–260.

Dueland, R., Sisson, D., & Evans, H. E. (1982). Aberrant origin of the cranial cruciate ligament mimicking an osteochondral lesion radiographically: a case history report. *Vet Radiol, 23,* 175–177.

Freeman, M. A. R. (1979). *Adult articular cartilage* (2nd ed.). Tunbridge Wells, England: Pitman Medical Publishing Co.

Gardner, E. (1950). Physiology of movable joints. *Physiol Rev, 30,* 127–176.

Gatineau, M., El-Warrak, A. O., Marretta, S. M., et al. (2008). Locked-jaw syndrome in dogs and cats: 37 cases (1998-2005). *J Vet Dent, 25,* 16–22. doi:10.1177/089875640802500106.

Gorse, M. J., Purinton, P. T., Penwick, R. C., et al. (1990). Talocalcaneal luxation, an anatomic and clinical study. *Vet Surg, 19,* 429–434.

Gregory, C. R., Cullen, J. M., Pool, R., et al. (1986). The canine sacroiliac joint: preliminary study of anatomy, histopathology, and biomechanics. *Spine, 71,* 1044–1048.

Heylings, D. J. A. (1980). Supraspinous and interspinous ligaments in dog, cat, and baboon. *J Anat, 130,* 223–228.

Kadletz, M. (1932). *Anatomischer Atlas der Extremitätengelenke von Pferd und Hund.* Berlin: Wien, Urban & Schwarzenberg.

Kaiser, A., Liebich, H. G., & Maierl, J. (2007). Functional anatomy of the distal radioulnar ligament in dogs. *Anat Histol Embryol, 36,* 466–468.

King, A. S., & Smith, R. M. (1955). A comparison of the anatomy of the intervertebral disc in dog and man: with reference to herniation of the nucleus pulposus. *Br Vet J, 111,* 135–149.

King, M. D. (2017). Etiopathogenesis of canine hip dysplasia, prevalence and genetics. *Vet Clin North Am Small Anim Pract, 47,* 753–767. doi:10.1016/j.cvsm.2017.03.001.

Knox, V. W., Sehgal, C. M., & Wood, A. K. W. (2003). Correlation of ultrasonographic observations with anatomic features and radiography of the elbow joint in dogs. *Am J Vet Res, 64*(6), 721–726.

Koch, R., Hemmes, M. J., Meyer, W., et al. (2005). Morphometric and structural examination of the collateral ligaments of the canine elbow joint. *Anat Histol Embryol, 34*(1), 25–26.

MacConaill, M. (1932). A The function of intra-articular fibrocartilages, with special reference to the knee and inferior radio-ulnar joints. *J Anat, 66,* 210–227.

Maieral, J., Lieser, B., Bottcher, P., et al. (2005). Functional anatomy and biomechanics of the canine hip joint. *Anat Histol Embryol, 34*(1), 32.

Mason, D. R., Schulz, K. S., Fujita, Y., et al. (2005). In vitro force mapping of normal canine humeroradial and humeroulnar joints. *Am J Vet Res, 66*(1), 132–135.

McCarthy, P. H., & Wood, A. K. (1988). Anatomic and radiologic observations of the clavicle of adult dogs. *Am J Vet Res, 49,* 956–959.

Newman, N. H., Carioto, S., Trinh, H., et al. (1988). *Innervation of the cruciate ligaments in the dog.* Can Orthop Res Soc Annual Meeting Ottawa 38.

Nomina Anatomica (1989). *International Anatomical Nomenclature Committee* (6th ed.). London: Churchill Livingstone.

Nomina Anatomica Veterinaria. (1983). *International Committee on Veterinary Gross Anatomical Nomenclature*, ed 2. Ithaca, New York: World Association of Veterinary Anatomists.

Nomina Anatomica Veterinaria. (2017). *International Committee on Gross Veterinary Anatomical Nomenclature*, ed 6. World Association Veterinary Anatomists (with updates as an electronic resource).

O'Connor, B. L. (1976). The histological structure of dog knee menisci with comments on its possible significance. *Am J Anat, 147,* 407–417.

O'Connor, B. L. (1984). The mechanoreceptor innervation of the posterior attachments of the lateral meniscus of the dog knee joint. *J Anat, 138,* 15–26.

O'Connor, B. L., & McConnaughey, J. S. (1978). The structure and innervation of cat knee menisci and their relation to a "sensory hypothesis" of meniscal function. *Am J Anat, 153,* 431–442.

Oliver, J. E., & Lewis, R. E. (1973). Lesions of the atlas and axis in dogs. *J Am Anim Hosp Assoc, 9,* 304–313.

Polacek, P. (1966) *Receptors of the joints: their structure, variability, and classification.* Acta Fact Med Univ Brne 1–107.

Preston, C. A., Schulz, K. K., & Kass, P. H. (2000). In vitro determination of contact areas in the normal elbow joint of dogs. *Am J Vet Res, 61*(10), 1315–1321.

Riser, W. H. (1964). An analysis of the current status of hip dysplasia in the dog. *J Am Vet Med Assoc, 144,* 709–721.

Riser, W. H. (1973). Growth and development of the normal canine pelvis, hip joints, and femurs from birth to maturity: a radiographic study. *J Am Vet Radiol Soc, 14,* 24–34.

Riser, W. H. (1975). The dog as a model for the study of hip dysplasia. *Vet Pathol, 12,* 229–334.

Robins, G., & Grandage, J. (1977). Temporomandibular joint dysplasia and open-mouth jaw locking in the dog. *J Am Vet Med Assoc, 171,* 1072–1076.

Scapino, R. (1965). The third joint of the canine jaw. *J Morphol, 116,* 23–50.

Scapino, R. (1981). Morphological investigation into functions of the jaw symphysis in carnivorans. *J Morphol, 167,* 339–375.

Schreiber, J. (1947). Beiträge zur vergleichenden Anatomie und zur Mechanik des Kniegelenkes. *Wien Tierärztl Monatsschr, 34,* 725–744.

Sether, L. A., Nguyen, C., Yu, S., et al. (19..). ... discs: correlation of anatomy and MR imaging. .. 207–211.

Sfameni, A. (1902). Recherches anatomiques sur l'existence des nerfs et sur leur mode de terminer dans le tissu adipeux dabs le perioste dans le perichondre et dans tissus qui reinforcent les articulations. *Arch Ital Biol, 35,* 49–106.

Shively, M. J. (1975). *Selected morphological parameters of the developing canine coxofemoral joint, Ph.D thesis.* Lafayette, IN: Purdue University.

Shively, M. J., & Van Sickle, D. C. (1982). Developing coxal joint of the dog: gross morphometric and pathologic observations. *Am J Vet Res, 43,* 185–194.

Sidaway, B. K., McLaughlin, R. M., Elder, S. H., et al. (2004). Role of the tendons of the biceps brachii and infraspinatus muscles and the medial glenohumeral ligament in the maintenance of passive shoulder joint stability. *Am J Vet Res, 65*(9), 1216–1222.

Smith, R. N., & King, A. S. (1954). Protrusion of the intervertebral disc in the dog. *Vet Rec, 66,* 1–11.

Smolders, L. A., Bergknut, N., Grinwis, G. C. M., et al. (2013a). Intervertebral disc degeneration in the dog, Part 2: Chondrodystrophic and non-chondrodystrophic dog breeds. *Vet J, 195,* 292–299. doi:10.1016/j.tvjl.2012.10.024.

Smolders, L. A., Meij, B. P., Onis, D., et al. (2013b). Gene expression profiling of early intervertebral disc degeneration reveals a downregulation of canonical Wnt signaling and caveolin-1 expression: implications for development of regenerative strategies. *Arthritis Res Ther, 15,* R23. doi:10.1186/ar4157.

Staszyk, C., & Gasse, H. (1994). The enthesis of the elbow-joint capsule of the dog humerus. *Eur J Morphol, 39*(5), 319–323.

Suter, P. F., & Carb, A. V. (1969). Shoulder arthrography in dogs—radiographic anatomy and clinical application. *J Small Anim Pract, 10,* 407–413.

Umphlet, R. C., Johnson, A. L., Eurell, J. C., et al. (1988). The effect of partial rostral hemimandibulectomy on mandibular mobility and temporomandibular joint morphology in the dog. *Vet Surg, 17,* 186–193.

Vasseur, P. B., & Arnoczky, S. P. (1981). Collateral ligaments of the canine stifle joint: anatomic and functional analysis. *Am J Vet Res, 42,* 1133–1137.

Vollmerhaus, B., & Roos, H. (1996). Die transversale Kieferbewegung (Translationsbewegung) des Hundes, zugleich ein Hinweis auf die Kiefergelenksdysplasie beim Dachshund. *Anat Histol Embryol, 25*(3), 145–149.

Watson, A. G., Evans, H. E., & de Lahunta, A. (1986). Gross morphology of the composite occipito-atlas-axis joint cavity in the dog. *Zbl Vet Med C Anat Histol Embryol, 15,* 139–146.

Willenegger, S., Friess, A. E., Lang, J., et al. (2005). Immunohistochemical demonstration of lumber intervertebral disc innervation in the dog. *Anat Histol Embryol, 34*(2), 123–128.

Williams, M. (1957). Morphology of the sternochondral joints of mammals. *J Morphol, 101,* 275–306.

Yahia, L. H., Newman, N. M., & St. Georges, M. (1992). Innervation of the canine cruciate ligaments. A neuro-histological study. *Anat Histol Embryol, 21,* 1–8.

Zimny, M. L. (1988). Mechanoreceptors in articular tissues. *Am J Anat, 182,* 16–32.

6

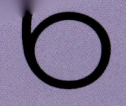

The Muscular System

JOHN W. HERMANSON

Introduction

The muscular system is composed of contractile units of varied morphologic characteristics, activated by voluntary or involuntary nerve impulses or by humoral substances. Muscles provide forces for many functions, including locomotion or posture, respiration, alimentation, and circulation. Both voluntary and involuntary muscles respond to the emotional state of the dog by subtle changes in facial expression or raising the hair, or more overt responses such as wagging the tail and barking. An important feature of muscular action, in addition to providing motive force, is the production of heat for the maintenance of body temperature.

The functional cellular unit is the **muscle fiber**, or **myofiber**. These myofibers are further classified as *smooth* or *striated muscles*. The latter category includes cardiac muscle as well as skeletal muscle.

Smooth muscle fibers are spindle-shaped, with a single central nucleus. Like other muscle cells, they possess myofibrils, but they are homogeneous and not striated. They are found in the walls of hollow organs and in blood vessels as well as in association with glands, and with the spleen, the eyeball, and hair follicles of the skin. Smooth muscle is innervated by the general visceral efferent neurons of the autonomic nervous system and, in many cases, is also under humoral control. Other names that have been used for smooth muscle are *unstriated*, *involuntary*, or *visceral muscle*.

Cardiac muscle fibers form the bulk of the heart. The fibers are arranged in a network of individual multinucleated cellular units with intercalated discs between the cell extremities. They exhibit cross-striations, as do skeletal muscle fibers, and have centrally placed nuclei, which is similar to smooth muscle fibers. Cardiac muscle is capable of rhythmic contractions and is under autonomic control. Specialized cardiac muscle fibers (Purkinje fibers) serve as a conducting system for impulses within the heart.

Skeletal muscle fibers are long, cylindrical, multinucleated cells organized into distinct bundles with connective tissue envelopes. Other names applied to skeletal muscle include *striated*, *voluntary*, or *somatic muscle*. The cells appear striated because the light and dark bands of adjacent myofibrils are in register with each other. Each **muscle fiber** is composed of several hundred or several thousand parallel **myofibrils**, which also exhibit cross-striations. The myofibril is in turn composed of several hundred thick and thin **myofilaments**, which consist of the proteins myosin (thick) and actin (thin). These myofilaments alternate and interdigitate along the length of the myofibril and thus produce the characteristic alternation of the isotropic (I), or light, bands and the anisotropic (A), or dark, bands. The control of skeletal muscles is largely voluntary. Some muscles, such as the retractor penis, have both smooth and skeletal muscle fibers.

Another way of classifying muscles is based on their developmental origin and innervation. Thus, one can speak of somatic muscles with striated fibers and somatic motor innervation versus visceral smooth muscle fibers or cardiac muscle fibers and visceral autonomic motor innervation.

For a consideration of structural detail at the microscopic level, the reader is referred to any of the standard histology texts (Fawcett, 1986; Samuelson, 2007) and for muscle as functional units in regard to mechanics and structure see Basmajian (1974), Lieber (1992), and Biewener (1998). For overviews of biochemistry, physiology, and pharmacology see Bourne (1972, 1973), Peachey (1983), Hoyle (1983), and McMahon (1984). The phylogenetic history of muscles as seen in lower vertebrates offers many insights for explaining observed anomalies, deficiencies, or excesses in mammals (see Peters & Goslow, 1983). For a general review of comparative aspects of the muscular system in vertebrates, see Romer and Parsons (1986), Liem et al. (2000), Hildebrand and Goslow (2001), and Kardong (2008). For domestic animals, see Getty (1975) and Dyce, Sack, and Wensing (2010).

At a gross level, mammalian muscle fibers are classified as red or white muscles, characteristics that are correlated with myoglobin concentration and the aerobic capacity of the muscle. Red muscle fibers (or whole muscles that are distinctly "red" in appearance) are usually specialized for repetitive or postural recruitment, contain many mitochondria, have high specific activity levels for enzymes used in aerobic metabolism such as succinic dehydrogenase (SDH), and are rich in myoglobin. Dog gastrocnemius muscles, for example, are "mixed" muscles containing slow and fast muscle fibers exhibiting high or low oxidative capacity, respectively. The medial head of m. triceps brachii is largely composed of red, aerobic, fatigue-resistant fibers (Armstrong, 1980). Good examples of "red" muscle may be better described in cats and rats in which the m. soleus (a muscle absent in dogs) is predominantly slow-twitch and highly oxidative and contrasts with the adjacent gastrocnemius muscle group. In contrast, white muscle fibers (or whole muscles with a pale "white" appearance) are involved in burst activity that requires short-duration bouts of high-force production and are exemplified by the long head of the m. triceps brachii (Armstrong, 1980). These fast and oxidative fibers are relatively fatigue resistant in dogs and facilitate the long-duration pursuits wild dogs exhibit during the pursuit of prey. These red and white muscle fiber categories have been variously described based on histochemical or immunologic studies. Two predominant systems of classification are based on either a correlation of myosin adenosine triphosphatase (ATPase) staining with metabolic properties (Peter et al., 1972) or an interpretation of myosin ATPase based on stability in acidic or alkaline buffer environments (Brooke & Kaiser, 1970; Snow et al., 1982) and myosin isoform characterization of muscle fibers (Shelton et al., 1985a; Stål et al., 1994). Controversy exists about the exclusive use of either of these systems, and it is useful to be versed in either classification (Table 6.1). Although the summary in Table 6.1 suggests some general agreement between these classifications, the two systems considered interchangeable. For example, it is often that the oxidative potential decreases in the order type I, IIa, and IIb. However, in rat muscles, significant overlap in either glycolytic potential or oxidative potential was found in type IIa and IIb fibers (Nemeth & Pette, 1981; Reichmann & Pette, 1982), or type IIb fibers exhibited more oxidative potential than did type IIa fibers (Reichmann & Pette, 1984). Similarly, type I fibers in rat and guinea pig were found to exhibit less oxidative potential than did type IIa fibers in the same muscle (Reichmann & Pette, 1982). Snow et al. (1982) recognize three predominant fiber types in the locomotory muscles of dogs. First, there are fibers best adapted for slow, low-force postural activity that are classified as type I fibers (Fig. 6.1). These type I fibers of dogs are comparable to type SO in the Peter et al. (1972) classification (an abbreviation referring to the slow-twitch, metabolically oxidative profiles of these fibers). These type I fibers occur in highest density in muscles active in maintaining posture, such as those active during a quiet stance (i.e., medial head of triceps brachii). A second fiber type is called *type IIa* and is characterized by fast-twitch, forceful contractions that are fatigue resistant. It is tempting to correlate these with the type FOG (fast-twitch, with both oxidative and glycolytic attributes that confer fatigue resistance) of other species, such as the cat (Burke, 1981). However, as stated previously, one must be cautious in applying such terminology across species. In dogs, a third

TABLE 6.1 Generalized Descriptors for and Functional Correlates of Histochemical Fiber Type Classifications Based Primarily on Analysis of Cat Triceps Surae Muscles[a,b]

Histochemical	Type I (SO)	Type IIA (FOG)	Type IIB (FG)	Type IIX
Physiologic and Morphologic Characteristics				
Twitch tension	Low	Low	High	Intermediate
Twitch contraction time	Slow	Fast	Fast	Fast
Maximal totanic tension	Low	Intermediate	High	Intermediate
Resistance to fatigue	High	High	Low	Intermediate/high
Mean fiber area	Small	Small to intermediate	Large	Small to intermediate
Capillary supply	Rich	Rich	Sparse	Rich
Histochemical Characteristics				
mATPase stain				
Alkaline preincubation	Low	High	High	High
Acidic preincubation	High	Low	Intermediate	Intermediate/high
Oxidative enzymes	High	High	Low	High
Glycolytic enzymes	Low	High	High	High

FG, Fast glycolytic; *FOG*, fast oxidative glycolytic; *mATPase*, myosin adenosine triphosphatase; *SO*, slow oxidative.
[a]Data for cat medial gastrocnemius modified from Sypert and Munson (1981). Other muscles such as the cat soleus have slightly different values. Similar data summaries are not available for muscles of the dog and must account for the opinion that dogs do not have type IIb fibers in their appendicular muscles (Snow et al., 1982).
[b]This information is provided to allow comparison of the two fiber type nomenclatures commonly used and their measured physiologic properties as generally known.

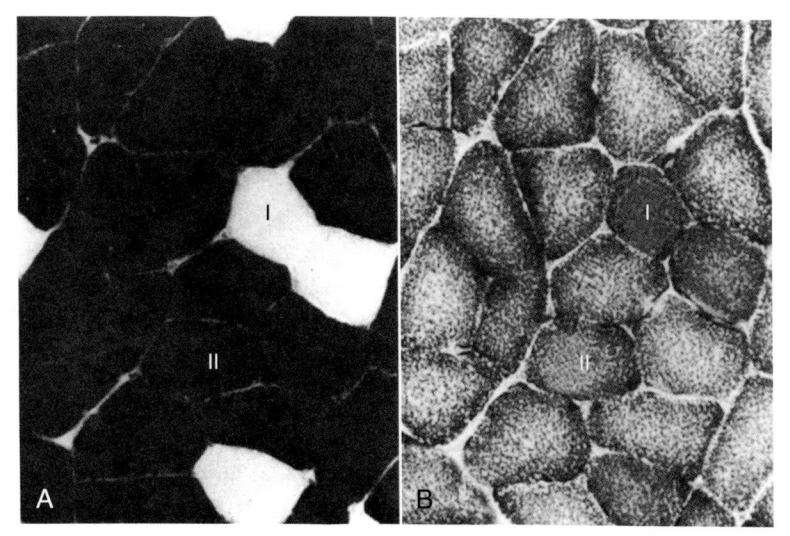

• **Fig. 6.1** Representative serial sections from the m. triceps brachii (caput longus) to illustrate the fiber type classification of appendicular muscles of the dog. Transverse serial sections of the muscle were stained for myofibrillar adenosine triphosphatase (ATPase) following alkaline preincubation (**A**) and for nicotinamide adenine dinucleotide (NADH) tetrazolium reductase (**B**) activities. Dark fibers in the ATPase are classified as type II and are presumed to be fast-twitch. Fibers unstained after ATPase staining are classified as type I (presumed slow-twitch). In dog muscle, most fibers stain intensely for oxidative potential as indicated by the NADH stain. (From Armstrong RB, Saubert CW, Seeherman HJ, Taylor CR: Distribution of fiber types in locomotory muscles of dogs, *Am J Anat* 163:87–98, 1982. Copyright © 1982 Wiley-Liss. Reprinted with permission of the publisher, John Wiley and Sons, Inc.)

fiber type occurs but is immunologically different from the type IIb fibers of cats (Fig. 6.2). Type IIB myosin isoforms have been found in few dog muscles, including some extraocular muscles, laryngeal muscles and sporadically in some fibers of the semimembranosus muscle (Toniolo et al., 2007). Snow et al. (1982) identified these fibers as type II on the basis of antibody reactions and demonstrated that they possessed oxidative and glycolytic properties similar to those of the type IIA fibers. The type IIA fibers could be identified by their histochemical reactions and by positive immunohistochemical staining with a type IIa antibody. The presence of two populations of a "FOG-like" fiber type may represent an adaptation to the natural history of feral dogs, in which it is common to run for long distances. In correlation with muscle-specific function, varying proportions of fiber types are found in various muscles (Fig. 6.3). Studies in other mammals (primarily but not limited to laboratory rats) have demonstrated the presence of a novel myosin heavy chain isoform termed MHC_{2X} (La Framboise et al., 1990; Schiaffino et al., 1989). These "IIX" (or "2X," discussed later in this chapter) fibers are generally found in muscles that undergo repetitive contraction, such as the diaphragm of rats and mice. Based on the difficulty associated with standard histochemical separation of this fiber type population and on the similarity of highly oxidative and glycolytic properties in these unique type II fibers, it is tempting to speculate that dog limb muscles may contain a mixture of type I, IIA, and IIX fibers (see Acevedo & Rivero, 2006). Another myosin heavy chain isoform termed MHC_{2D} was identified by another group and named because of its occurrence in the rat diaphragm (Bär & Pette, 1988).

This 2D form appears to be identical to the 2X form (La Framboise et al., 1990; Termin et al., 1989). One can see that the classification of these various fiber types has become the realm of muscle specialists.

An additional novel fiber type has been reported in selected masticatory muscles of the dog (Mascarello et al., 1982, 1983; Shelton et al., 1985a, b) and in other carnivores (Mascarello et al., 1983; Rowlerson et al., 1981) and referred to as *IIM* or "superfast." This IIM (sometimes called *2M*) has been found to be immunologically differentiated from type II (IIa, IIb, or IIx) fibers of appendicular skeletal muscles of the dog. It is possible that this fiber type has evolved in those muscles associated with the first branchial arch. Reiser et al. (2009) and Toniolo et al. (2008) have shown that this masticatory-related isoform in carnivores and other mammals is, in fact, not fast-twitch, but rather is a high-force–producing muscle isoform based on analysis of isolated single myofibers in vitro. Other muscle-specific fiber types or myosin-based specializations have been reported in the extraocular muscles of mammals; these function extremely rapidly and in the absence of significant external loads (Sartore et al., 1987). For a historical review of this field of fiber types and contractile proteins see Pette and Staron (1990) and Acevedo and Rivero (2006). An additional complication of achieving a straightforward classification of muscle fibers is the observation that some muscles may express multiple "hybrid" fibers that contain one or two myosin heavy chain isoforms (see Wu et al., 2000) and that not all research groups use identical terminology. For example, muscle types may be expressed with a Roman numeral as opposed to a digit (i.e., type IIA as

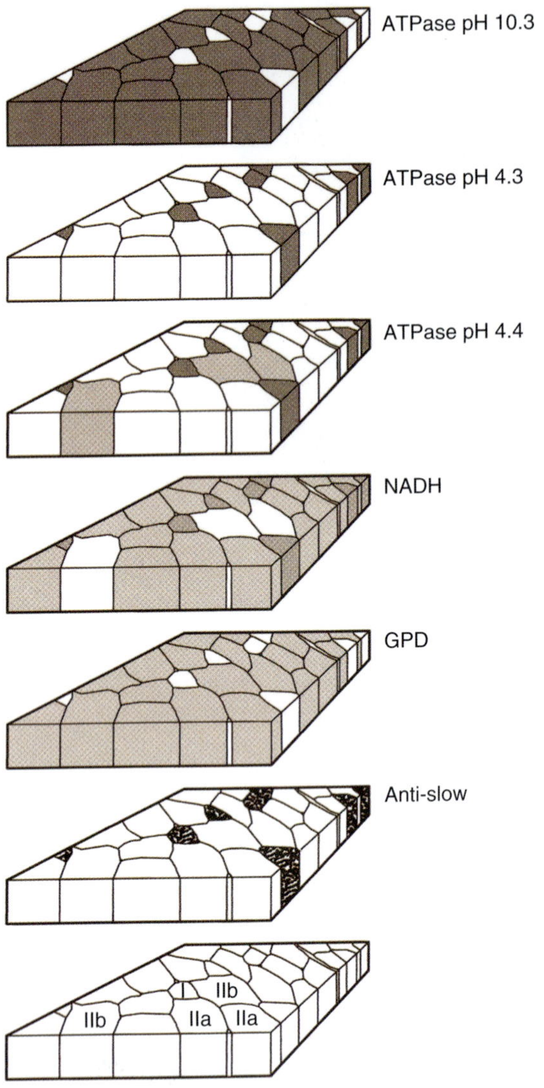

• **Fig. 6.2** Representative serial sections of a mammalian muscle as a histologist might interpret them after staining for myosin adenosine triphosphatase (mATPase) with preincubation at pH 10.3, 4.3, and 4.4. Note the reversal of staining properties after preincubation in acidic and alkaline environments. Oxidative or glycolytic potential is indicated by dark staining after incubation for nicotinamide adenine dinucleotide or glyceraldehyde phosphate dehydrogenase, respectively. Further confirmation of the histochemistry is obtained by staining for myosin heavy chain–specific antibodies, such as an anti-slow antibody. Note the correlation of its reactions with individual fibers staining darkly for mATPase after acidic incubation. Although dogs do not have type IIb fibers, other mammals such as cats have a tripartite fiber division such as is shown here, including type I (presumed slow), type IIa (here a fast and fatigue-resistant fiber), and type IIb (here a fast and fatigable fiber).

compared with type 2A). For present purposes these are interchangeable.

Skeletal Muscles

This chapter is concerned primarily with the axial and appendicular muscles of the body. In mammalian species the skeletal muscles constitute approximately one-third to one-half of the total body weight. According to Gunn (1978b) Greyhounds contain the highest proportion of muscle to live weight at 57%, whereas in other dog breeds (mixed-breed and pure-bred) this proportion is approximately 44%. Skeletal muscles range in size from the minute stapedius muscle of the middle ear to the large gluteus medius muscle of the pelvic region. Each muscle fiber is surrounded by a thin **sarcolemma** and a delicate connective tissue sheath known as the **endomysium**. When several fibers are grouped into a fasciculus they are enclosed by a connective tissue, the **perimysium**. The definitive muscle is composed of several fasciculi wrapped by an **epimysium**, which delimits one muscle from another or occasionally fuses with the intervening fascia. The size of an individual muscle fiber depends on the species and the specific muscle, as well as on the physical condition of the animal, because individual muscle fibers are capable of hypertrophy as well as atrophy.

Lockhart and Brandt (1938) found muscle fibers running the entire length of the sartorius muscle (5 cm) in a human fetus and were able to isolate fibers 34 cm long in a 52-cm sartorius muscle of an adult. Huber (1916) and Van Harreveld (1947), working with rabbit thigh muscles, found that many fibers do not extend from end to end. They concluded that, although the longer fasciculi have longer fibers, many fibers end intrafascicularly. This observation was ignored for many years until Loeb et al. (1987) demonstrated that a majority of fibers do not course the entire length of specific cat muscles. If muscle fibers exceed a certain length they become potentially inefficient because of the different conduction velocities of action potentials along nerves and muscles. Muscle fascicles appear to consist of "in-series" fibers, identified by short transverse bands of neuromuscular endplates. Similar patterns of short, "in-series" fibers have been observed in the diaphragm of dogs and cats, but not in the rabbit and rat in which fibers appear to extend from the central tendon to its costal origin (Gordon et al., 1989). Other examples of long muscles composed of short "in-series" fibers include the m. semitendinosus in the goat (Gans et al., 1989). Trotter (1990) has amplified these findings to demonstrate that tension is transmitted through "in-series" muscle fibers via the endomysium surrounding the individual fibers. Force transmission within a muscle may involve side-to-side transmission from one myofiber to another (Gao et al., 2008).

Muscles take diverse shapes and are usually named according to some structural or functional feature, although other criteria have also been used. The variations encountered in the muscular system within a species are numerous and may constitute a breed-specific feature. Huntington (1903) considered problems of gross myologic research and the significance and classification of muscular variations. The most complete account of the muscles in the dog is by Baum and Zietzschmann (1936). A succinct illustrated summary of dog muscles based on the *Nomina Anatomica Veterinaria* (NAV) is available in Schaller (2007). For an illustrated guide to identify skeletal muscles of the dog, see Evans and de Lahunta (2017).

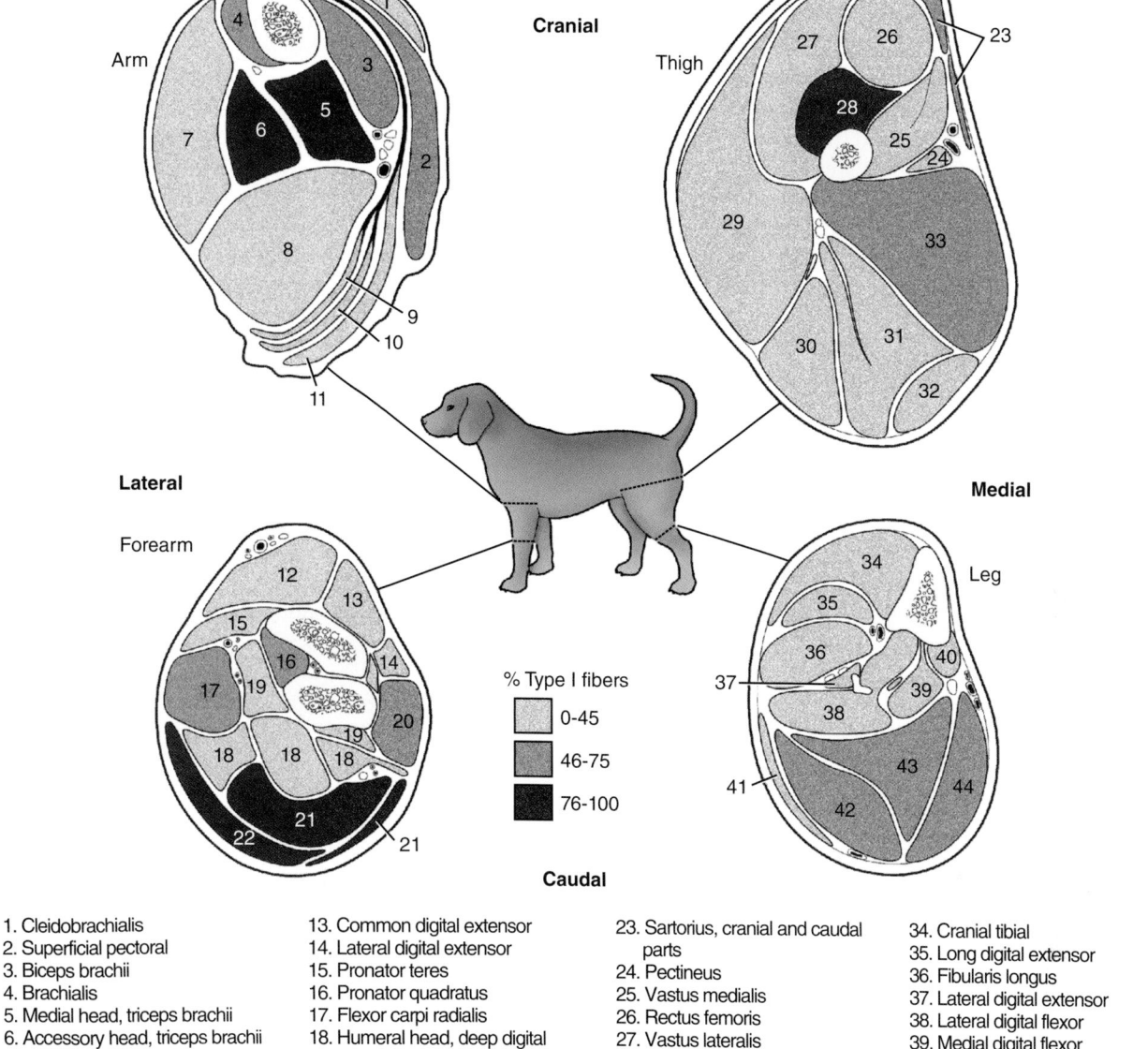

CHAPTER 6 The Muscular System 211

Fig. 6.3 Transverse sections through the arm, forearm, thigh, and crus (leg) of the dog to indicate the distribution of type I histochemical fiber types. (Adapted from Armstrong RB, Saubert CW, Seeherman HJ, Taylor CR: Distribution of fiber types of locomotory muscles of dogs, *Am J Anat* 163:87-98, 1982. Copyright © 1982 Wiley-Liss. Reprinted with permission of John Wiley and Sons, Inc.)

1. Cleidobrachialis
2. Superficial pectoral
3. Biceps brachii
4. Brachialis
5. Medial head, triceps brachii
6. Accessory head, triceps brachii
7. Lateral head, triceps brachii
8. Long head, triceps brachii
9. Tensor fasciae antebrachii
10. Latissimus dorsi
11. Deep pectoral
12. Extensor carpi radialis
13. Common digital extensor
14. Lateral digital extensor
15. Pronator teres
16. Pronator quadratus
17. Flexor carpi radialis
18. Humeral head, deep digital flexor
19. Radial and ulnar heads, deep digital flexor
20. Ulnaris lateralis
21. Flexor carpi ulnaris
22. Superficial digital flexor
23. Sartorius, cranial and caudal parts
24. Pectineus
25. Vastus medialis
26. Rectus femoris
27. Vastus lateralis
28. Vastus intermedius
29. Biceps femoris
30. Semitendinosus
31. Semimembranosus
32. Gracilis
33. Adductor
34. Cranial tibial
35. Long digital extensor
36. Fibularis longus
37. Lateral digital extensor
38. Lateral digital flexor
39. Medial digital flexor
40. Popliteus
41. Biceps femoris
42. Lateral head, gastrocnemius
43. Superficial digital flexor
44. Medial head, gastrocnemius

Origin and Insertion

Most skeletal muscles are attached by connective tissue to a bone or cartilage. Some are attached to an organ (eye, tongue), to another muscle, or to the skin; others lie free beneath the skin and act as sphincters of orifices. The connective tissue attachment may be in the form of a cordlike **tendon** or a flat, sheetlike **aponeurosis**. Some muscles have no demonstrable tendons or aponeuroses but attach directly to the periosteum of bones. Such origins or insertions are spoken of as "fleshy attachments." The more fixed point of muscle attachment is spoken of as the **origin**; the more movable point of attachment is called the **insertion** or **termination**. In the limb the insertion of a muscle is always considered to be distal to its origin, although functionally it may be the most fixed point at some phase of the stride. Certain muscles have equally fixed or mobile attachments, and the naming of an origin and an insertion is rather arbitrary. In such cases the student might choose to refer to "proximal attachment" or "distal attachment" if that provides clarity.

The expanded fleshy portion of a muscle is its belly, the origin is a **head**. Minor divisions of origin or termination are called **slips**. A muscle may have more than one belly (digastric) or more than one head (triceps) and several slips. **Neuromuscular compartments** are regions innervated by a single primary nerve branch and separated from adjacent compartments by connective tissue partitions or epimysium (English & Letbetter, 1982a, b; English & Weeks, 1984; Galvas & Gonyea, 1980). Although functional interpretation of neuromuscular compartments is still controversial, it may provide an anatomic substrate for motor control at a higher hierarchic level than that of the motor unit (see later discussion).

Just as muscles grow and gain mass as well as strength during fetal and postnatal development, muscles show a natural aging process called **sarcopenia**, which includes a loss of mass and strength (Morley et al., 2001). Sarcopenia is well described in humans (Walston, 2012) and in some laboratory rodents, but not as well studied in dogs (Freeman, 2012). Sarcopenia may be responsible for decrements of speed or performance in older dogs and may parallel cachexia associated with disease processes.

Function

Muscles that attach to long bones (the levers) and span one or more joints usually work at a mechanical disadvantage. When a muscle fiber contracts, it does so at its maximal level of activation in an all-or-none fashion. Performance measures such as power or tension generation are complex in that they are influenced by a number of factors, such as muscle fiber length or antagonistic forces being applied against the fiber. The contraction is initiated by a nerve impulse traveling over a motor nerve fiber (axon) to the muscle fibers, or cells. Each motor neuron supplies several muscle fibers by axonal branching. These neuromuscular units are known as **motor units**, and the number of motor units functioning at any time determines the activity of the muscle. In general, a single motor unit corresponds with a single category of muscle fibers, such as slow- or fast-contracting fibers. The orderly recruitment of smaller and sequentially larger motor units thus correlates with the force being generated by a muscle to perform a task. Extensive reviews of motor unit physiology have been written by Burke (1981), Goslow (1985), and Stuart and Enoka (1983). If a muscle has many motor units, each of which includes only a few muscle fibers, then the precision of movement is great (as in the extrinsic muscles of the eyeball). This condition is referred to as a *high innervation ratio*.

It is important to study and experiment with muscles in the living body to appreciate the full significance of precise muscular movement and the value of such movement in a neurologic examination for the determination of intact or defective nerve supply. Electrodiagnostic procedures are an excellent technique for studying living muscles (see Loeb & Gans, 1986).

Of two muscles of equal size and shape, the muscle with the greater physiologic cross-sectional area will produce the most force (Josephson, 1975). Straplike and sheetlike muscles contract to a greater degree than do many muscles of the extremities, in part because their fibers are relatively longer and they can function efficiently over a larger range of excursions (Sacks & Roy, 1982). Examples of straplike muscles include m. gracilis and m. biceps femoris. Muscles possessing tendons throughout their length are known as **pennate muscles**. A muscle with a tendon running along one side is called **unipennate**; if there is a tendon on each side of the muscle, it is **bipennate**; when a muscle has tendons distributed throughout its volume, it is **multipennate**. Pennate muscles can be stronger because they have many short, obliquely arranged fibers and have a relatively greater physiologic cross-sectional area than similarly sized nonpennate muscles (Sacks & Roy, 1982). Examples of pennate architecture in dog muscles include m. biceps brachii and m. flexor digitorum superficialis. Because of their elasticity, tendons can protect muscles from sudden strains. However, all tendons are not constructed similarly. A range of elastic moduli can be observed in tendons obtained from different muscles in one animal.

Muscles that straighten bone alignment, or open a joint, are called **extensors**; those that angulate the bones, or close the joint, are known as **flexors**. Flexion and extension are the primary movements necessary for locomotion. Accompanying movements include **adduction**, or the movement of an extremity toward the median plane; **abduction**, or movement away from the median plane (in the case of the digits the reference point is the axis of the limb); **circumduction**, or moving an extremity in a plane describing the surface of a cone; and **rotation**, or moving a part around its long axis. Opposing rotatory movements around loosely fitting joints like the shoulder or hip are important in maintaining a normal gait. The pattern of movement resulting from muscle contractions, even for apparently simple movements, is brought about by the complex interactions of many muscles.

Ironically, a great deal of work performed by muscles during locomotion occurs while they are electrically active but while the muscles undergo only slight or no intrinsic length changes (Goslow et al., 1981). These *eccentric contractions* (being stretched while electrically active) conserve energy in several ways. First, appendicular muscles that primarily stabilize joints, such as single-joint extensors (supraspinatus, lateral head of triceps brachii), are active while the limb bears weight. By maintaining a rigid limb, the animal literally "pole-vaults" over the limbs and is able to use potential energy accrued from gravity. Second, at the higher speeds of trot and walk, these elastic storage mechanisms might be quite important as the animals store energy by stretching active muscles and subsequently recover this energy as the muscle reaccelerates the limb segment. Valuable discussions of elastic storage mechanisms are provided by Cavagna et al. (1964) and Heglund et al. (1982). The characteristic movement of a joint is produced by a muscle or muscles, called **prime movers**, or **agonists**. The muscles responsible for the opposite action are known as **antagonists**, although they actually aid the prime mover by relaxing in a controlled manner so that the movement will be smooth and precise. For the elbow joint, a prime mover in flexion is the brachialis; the antagonist is the triceps brachii. Conversely, in bringing about extension, the prime mover is the triceps. **Fixation and articular muscles** are those that stabilize joints while the prime movers are acting. **Synergists** are fixation muscles that stabilize intermediate or proximal joints and enable the force of the prime mover to be exerted on a more distal joint.

Accessory Structures

Associated with muscles are accessory structures of great physiologic and clinical importance, such as sesamoid bones, bursae, synovial tendon sheaths, and fascia.

Sesamoid bones are located in certain tendons or joint capsules as small, rounded nodules. Occasionally they develop in response to friction, but usually they form prenatally. The patella is an example of a large sesamoid bone in the tendon of insertion of the quadriceps femoris muscle. Sesamoid bones serve three important functions: (1) they protect tendons that pass over bony prominences, (2) they increase the surface area for attachment of tendons over certain joints, and (3) they serve to redirect the pull of tendons so that greater effective force can be applied to the part being moved.

Bursae are simple connective tissue sacs containing a viscous fluid and serving to reduce friction. They are usually located between a tendon, ligament, or muscle, and a bony prominence. Occasionally they are located between tendons or between a bony prominence and the skin. Inconstant bursae may develop at various sites in response to undue friction, and, conversely, cellular proliferation caused by infection or trauma may eliminate them. **Synovial tendon sheaths** are double-layered, elongated sacs containing synovia that wrap tendons as they pass through osseous or fibrous grooves or cross an osseous surface. The inner layer of the sheath, which is fused to the tendon, attaches to the outer layer of the passageway by its **mesotendon**. The latter is continuous with the outer layer of the sheath. Blood vessels and nerves enter the tendon via the mesotendon. The tendon sheath with its contained synovia serves for reducing friction during movement. An additional anatomic structure to reduce friction during movement is the sleeve formed by the superficial digital flexor tendon around the deep digital flexor tendon at each metapodial joint. This is known as a *manica flexoria*.

Connective Tissue

Fascia is connective tissue that remains after the recognizable mesodermal structures have been differentiated in the fetus. It serves many important functions and has considerable clinical significance. For descriptive purposes it is convenient to distinguish many fascial entities that envelop, separate, or connect muscles, vessels, and nerves. Fascial sheets provide routes for the passage of blood vessels, lymphatics, and nerves, as well as serving for the storage of fat. Intramuscular fascial sheets also may partition neuromuscular compartments. Failure to find primary nerve branches crossing such partitions, in both neonatal and adult muscle, has been used to argue in favor of the significance of such compartments for muscle development and for functional specialization of neuromuscular compartments (Donahue & English, 1989). The superficial fascia beneath the skin is closely associated with the dermis and often includes cutaneous muscle fibers. The deep fascia that covers and passes between the muscles is particularly thick and distinct in the limbs. It functions as a sleeve within which the muscles can operate and often serves as an aponeurosis of origin or insertion. In certain locations fascia blends with the periosteum of bone, forming interosseous membranes or annular bands that confine tendons or redirect their force. Most commonly, distinct fascial septa separate groups of muscles from one another and result in fascial planes along which infection may spread or fluids drain.

The amount of connective tissue present is much greater in some muscles than in others. When the connective tissue content is high, the muscle usually has many pennate fibers and thus has a high tensile strength and tends to be capable of more finely graded movements. Connective tissue elements include collagen fibers, elastic fibers, reticular fibers, fibroblasts, and histiocytes. Increased connective tissue concentrations in a muscle may also be associated with diseases, such as muscular dystrophy (Valentine et al., 1986).

Blood and Nerve Supply

Muscles have a high metabolic rate and are well supplied with blood by branches from neighboring blood vessels. The arteries supplying a muscle enter at rather definite places and often anastomose within the muscle. There is much constancy in arterial supply, although variations do occur. Most dog muscles exhibit a relatively high number of capillaries per fiber compared with other mammals (Kuzon et al., 1989). This rich capillary distribution facilitates oxygen delivery to muscles necessary for endurance running performance. Lymphatics accompany the arteries and, like them, form capillary plexuses around the muscle fibers. Veins also accompany the arteries, and during muscular contraction blood is forced into the larger veins, which, as a rule, are more superficial than the arteries.

Nerves accompany the blood vessels and ramify within the muscle. Approximately half of the axons in nerves are motor and the other half sensory. Efferent neurons form motor endplates, which are neuromuscular junctions on muscle fibers. Sensory receptors of a muscle include neuromuscular and neurotendinous spindles, free nerve endings, and capsulated corpuscles (Golgi tendon organs and paciniform), which discharge proprioceptive impulses in response to relaxation or contraction of the muscle and modify the activities of motor neurons. For a summary of findings related to primary and secondary endings, static and dynamic spindles, feedback loops, and possible mechanisms of muscle spindle operation see reviews by Barker et al. (1974), Matthews (1972), Hunt (1990), and Hulliger (1984). Muscle spindles are not distributed evenly between or within muscles. High densities of muscle spindles have been associated with small or highly oxidative muscles (Buxton & Peck, 1990; Peck et al., 1984; Richmond & Abrahams, 1975a, b; Richmond & Bakker, 1982). Spindles and capsulated corpuscles are apparently not present in some muscles, such as m. digastricus, in which proprioceptive feedback may be replaced by mechanical sensation from the teeth. In extraocular muscles, myotendinous cylinders or palisades are the primary receptor organs (Alvarado-Mallart & Pincon-Raymond, 1979; Richmond et al., 1984).

Regeneration

Mammalian skeletal muscle fibers are capable of regeneration, although the success of the reparative process is variable. Regeneration results from the activation of satellite cells (myosatellitocytus), which are small cells located on the surface of striated muscle fibers. Surgical implants of minced muscle (Carlson, 1972, 1986) regenerate to approximately 25% of their former bulk, whereas transplanted whole muscle regains approximately 80% of its volume and function. The inward progression of regeneration of an implant is correlated with its revascularization. The ability of minced muscle to survive vascular deprivation is one of the striking features of muscle regeneration. The regenerative process may be aborted by conditions that stimulate connective tissue formation, such as circulatory insufficiency, widening of the gap, infection, or presence of foreign bodies. Regulation of skeletal myocyte regeneration has been studied extensively (see reviews by Chargé & Rudnicki, 2004). The process of skeletal muscle regeneration has many applications, such as in clinical repair of injury (Carlson & Faulkner, 1983). Regeneration has been studied to assess myogenic potential during normal development or in adult animals (Ontell, 1986). Adult fiber regeneration does not recapitulate ontogeny: The number and size of myofibers in regenerating muscles are reduced relative to age-matched control subjects. Fiber type–specific deficiencies may result. Manipulation of skeletal muscles can also involve modification and transplantation for cardiac assistance (Acker et al., 1987), surgical rearrangement for orthopedic repairs (Lippincott, 1981), or reconstruction of large wounds (Miller et al., 2007). Such applications need to be performed with knowledge of the basic biologic attributes of muscle cells. The ability of cardiac muscle to regenerate is denied by some authors and supported by others. Field (1960), after reviewing the literature, concluded that, although cardiac muscle has less regenerative capacity than skeletal muscle even under optimal conditions, it does at times exhibit appreciable regeneration. More recent studies have contributed information about stem cell potential to regenerate or salvage damaged heart tissue (Balsam et al., 2004; Grounds et al., 2002; Jackson et al., 2001). Additional work examined developmental stages and inputs during myocyte ontogeny and implications for strategies to regenerate damaged heart muscle (Bu et al., 2009; Zhou et al., 2008). As a whole, the heart is complex because of the interplay of developing endothelial smooth muscle as well as intracardiac cardiomyocytes.

Muscle Description

The following description of individual muscles is organized into eight groups: muscles of the head (*musculi capitis*), muscles of the neck (*musculi colli*), dorsal muscles (*musculi dorsi*), muscles of the thorax (*musculi thoracis*), abdominal muscles (*musculi abdominis*), muscles of the tail (*musculi caudae*), muscles of the thoracic limb (*musculi membri thoracici*), and muscles of the pelvic limb (*musculi membri pelvini*).

Muscles of the Head

The **muscles of the head** are composed of nine groups categorized primarily on the basis of their embryonic origin and their innervation (Box 6.1): (1) the muscles of facial expression innervated by the facial nerves; (2) the masticatory musculature, primarily innervated by the mandibular nerves from the trigeminal nerves; (3) the extrinsic eye musculature, innervated by the oculomotor, trochlear, and abducent nerves; (4) the tongue musculature, supplied by the hypoglossal nerves; (5) the muscles of the pharynx innervated by the glossopharyngeal and vagus nerves; (6) the soft palate muscles innervated by the trigeminal, glossopharyngeal, and vagal nerves; (7) the laryngeal musculature, supplied by the accessory and vagus nerves; (8) the hyoid muscles innervated by the trigeminal, hypoglossal, and cranial cervical nerves; and (9) cervical vertebral muscles that insert on the skull and are innervated by cervical nerves. The cranial muscles of many vertebrates have been described by Edgeworth (1935). The facial musculature of the dog has been described and illustrated by Huber (1922, 1923).

Muscles of Facial Expression
Superficial Muscles

The superficial muscles of the face are derived from three primary layers of the primitive sphincter colli. They include the m. sphincter colli superficialis, platysma, and m. sphincter colli profundus.

The **m. sphincter colli superficialis** (Fig. 6.4) is best developed in the laryngeal region deep to the skin. Its delicate transverse fibers span the ventral borders of the platysma muscles at the junction of the head and neck. Occasionally fibers of the sphincter colli superficialis reach

> **BOX 6.1 The Nine Groups of Head Muscles**

Muscles of facial expression
   Superficial
      Sphincter colli superficialis
      Platysma
      Sphincter colli profundus
   Deep
      Lip and nose
         Orbicularis oris
         Zygomaticus
         Superior and inferior incisivus
         Levator labii superioris
         Caninus
         Buccinator
         Mentalis
         Levator nasolabialis
   Eyelids, forehead, and ears
      Orbicularis oculi
      Retractor anguli oculi lateralis
      Levator anguli oculi medialis
      Levator palpebrae superioris
      Orbitalis
      Occipitalis
      Extrinsic ear muscles
         Rostral
            Superficial scutuloauricularis
            Deep scutuloauricularis
            Frontoscutularis
            Frontalis
            Zygomaticoauricularis
         Dorsal
            Interscutularis
            Parietoscutularis
            Parietoauricularis
         Caudal
            Cervicoscutularis
            Superficial cervicoauricularis
            Middle cervicoauricularis
            Deep cervicoauricularis
            Parotidoauricularis
            Styloauricularis
      Intrinsic ear muscles
         Helicis
         Helicis minor
         Tragicus
         Transversus auriculae
         Oblique auriculae
      Middle ear muscles
         Stapedius
         Tensor tympani
Muscles of mastication
   Masseter
   Temporalis
   Pterygoideus lateralis
   Pterygoideus medialis
   Digastricus
Muscles of bulbus oculi-external
   Dorsal and ventral oblique
   Dorsal, lateral, ventral, and medial rectus
   Retractor bulbi
   Orbicularis
Muscles of the tongue
   Styloglossus
   Hyoglossus
   Genioglossus
   Lingual proper
Muscles of the pharynx
   Hyopharyngeus
   Thyropharyngeus
   Cricopharyngeus
   Stylopharyngeus
   Palatopharyngeus
   Pterygopharyngeus
Muscles of the soft palate
   Tensor veli palatini
   Levator veli palatini
   Palatinus
Muscles of the larynx
   Cricothyroideus
   Cricoarytenoideus dorsalis
   Cricoarytenoideus lateralis
   Thyroarytenoideus
   Vocalis
   Ventricularis
   Arytenoideus transversus
   Hyoepiglotticus
Muscles of the hyoid apparatus
   Sternohyoideus
   Thyrohyoideus
   Mylohyoideus
   Ceratohyoideus
   Geniohyoideus
   Occipitohyoideus
   Stylohyoideus
Muscles of cervical vertebrae
   Rectus capitis ventralis
   Rectus capitis dorsalis major
   Rectus capitis dorsalis minor
   Rectus capitis lateralis
   Obliquus capitis cranialis
   Obliquus capitis caudalis
   Splenius capitis
   Longus capitis

---

the thorax, radiate over the shoulder joint, or blend with the cervical part of the platysma.

The ***platysma*** is a well-developed muscle sheet that takes its origin from the mid-dorsal tendinous raphe of the neck and the skin. The two separate layers of origin fuse near the midline. In its longitudinal course it extends over the parotid and masseter regions to the cheek and commissure of the lips, where it radiates into the m. orbicularis oris. In the lips, the platysma has been designated as the m. cutaneus faciei. The portion in the neck is known as m. cutaneous colli. At the ventral midline these bilateral cutaneous muscles, when they are well developed, approach each other and meet caudal to a transverse plane through the commissures of the lips. The platysma covers large portions of the m. sphincter colli profundus. Its dorsal border, extending from the neck to the commissural portion of

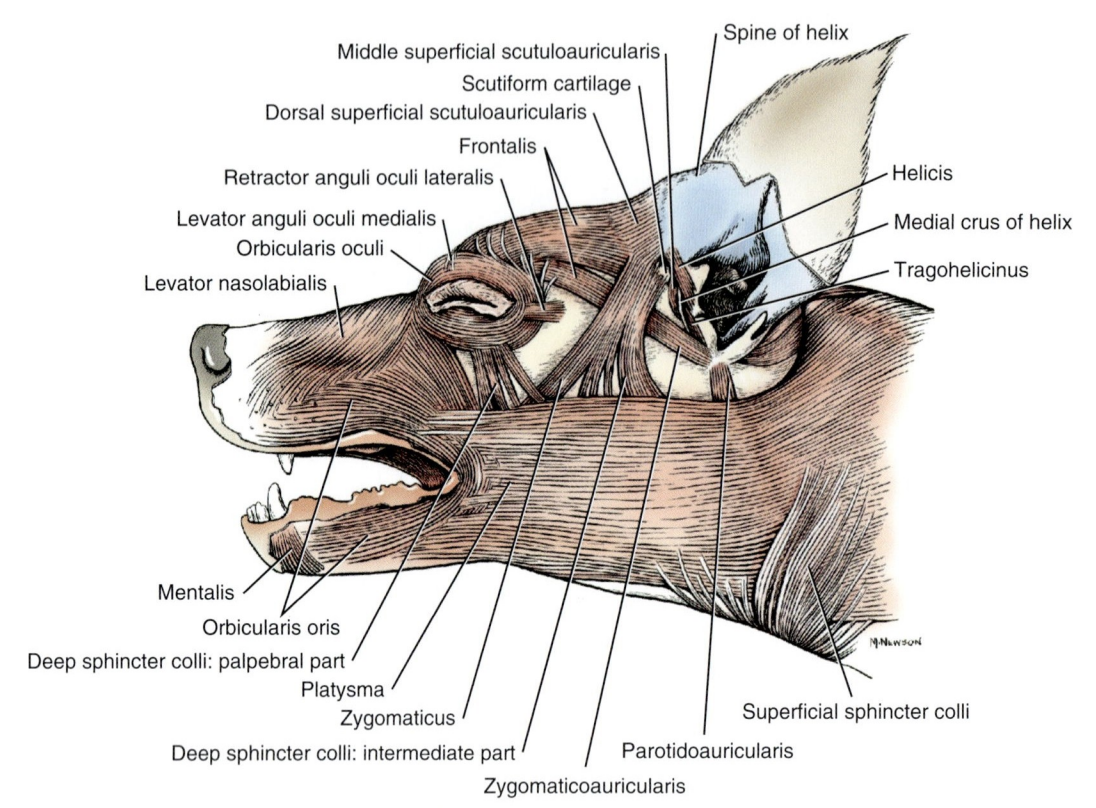

• Fig. 6.4 Superficial muscles of the head, lateral aspect.

the superior lip, is united with the underlying sphincter colli profundus by many fiber bundles. The ventral border has a distinct boundary. Only rarely does the platysma have defects.

Action: To draw the commissure of the lips caudally.
Innervation: Buccal branches and the caudal auricular nerve from the facial nerve (*rami buccales et n. auricularis caudalis, n. facialis*).

The **sphincter coli profundus** consists of a few thin muscle fascicles that extend dorsoventrally from the base of the ear, lateral to the masseter muscle and parotid gland. These fascicles are covered by the platysma and extend across the ventral median plane to fuse with the fascicles of the same muscle on the opposite side. In addition a few fascicles extend dorsoventrally from the orbicularis oculi deep to the platysma.

Deep Muscles of the Lip and Nose

The deep muscles of the lip and nose include the orbicularis oris, zygomaticus, superior and inferior incisivus, levator labii superioris, caninus, buccinator, mentalis, and levator nasolabialis. All are innervated by the facial nerve and almost all by the dorsal or ventral buccal branches of the facial nerve (*rami buccales n. facialis*).

The ***m. orbicularis oris*** (Figs. 6.4 and 6.5), the principal component of the lips, extends from the commissural region into the lips near their free borders. In the rostral median segment of both lips, the muscle is interrupted. It lies between the skin and the mucosa. The other muscles of the lips and the muscles of the cheeks (platysma; mm. buccinator, zygomaticus, and levator nasolabialis) enter the m. orbicularis oris caudally so that here these muscles blend with each other; the m. incisivus is also attached to it rostrally. The portion of the orbicularis oris lying in the superior lip is the thicker component. Separate fibers extend from it to the external naris.

Action: The muscle closes the lips of a closed mouth and is a pressor of the labial glands. Of the bundles extending to the lateral nasal cartilage on either side, the medial ones act to pull the entire nose ventrally (in sniffing), and the lateral bundles act to increase the diameter of the external nares. In strong contractions both the medial and the lateral fiber bundles function to dilate the external nares.

The ***m. zygomaticus*** (Figs. 6.4 to 6.7) arises from the scutiform cartilage. The straplike, long muscle extends from the rostral angle of the scutiform cartilage to the edge of the superior lip and cheek, where it sinks into the orbicularis oris after crossing deep to the rostral fibers of the sphincter colli profundus. Its rostral portion is deep and bears no relationship to the platysma. Proximally it is distinctly separated from the m. frontalis. This portion of the m. zygomaticus is covered by the skin.

Action: To fix the angle of the mouth and draw it caudally, or to fix and draw the scutiform cartilage rostrally.

CHAPTER 6 The Muscular System 217

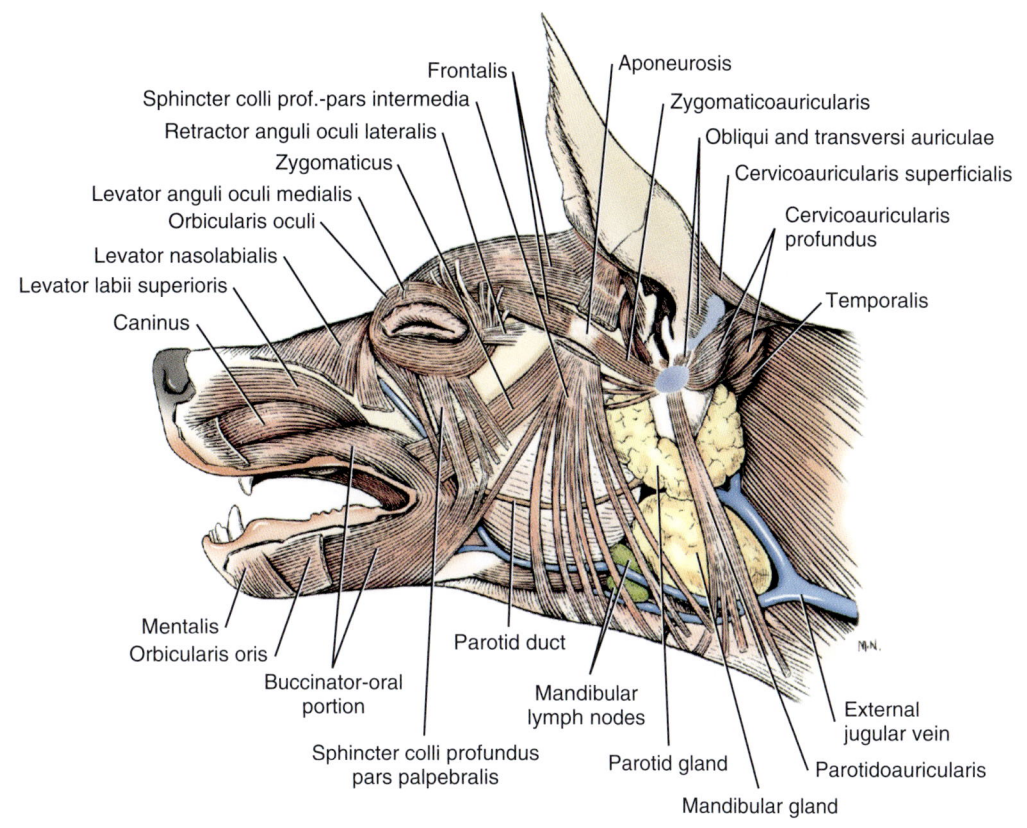

• **Fig. 6.5** Superficial muscles of the head, lateral aspect. (Platysma and sphincter colli superficialis removed.)

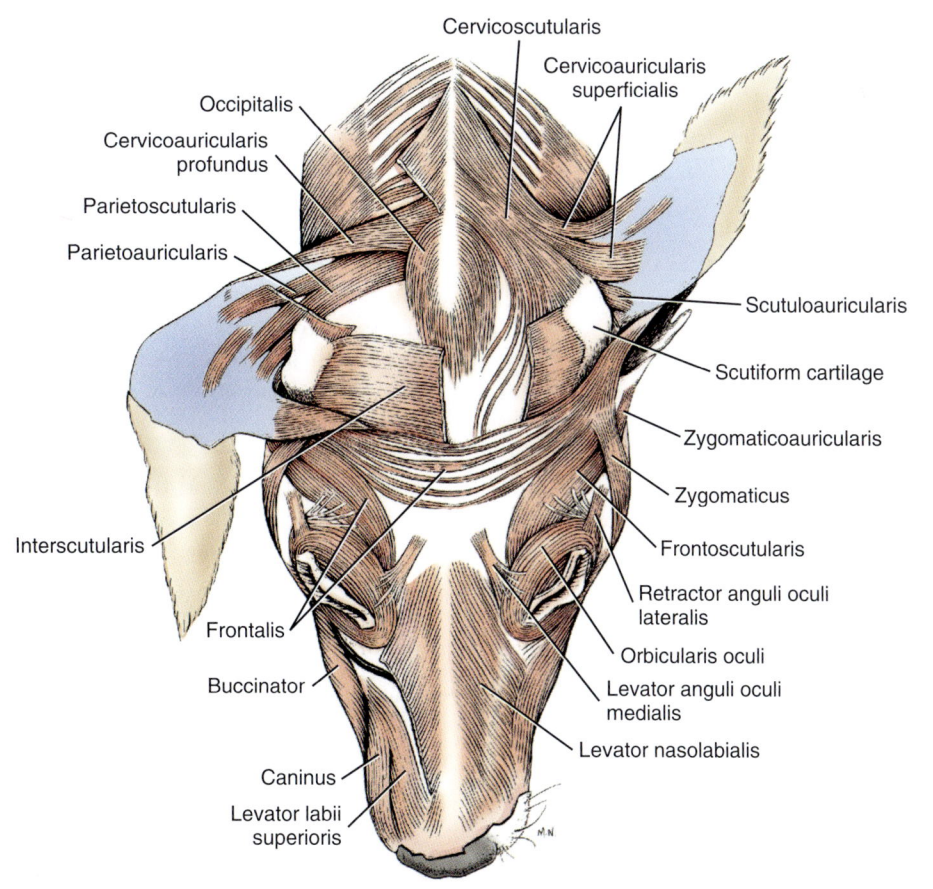

• **Fig. 6.6** Deep muscles of the head and ear, dorsal aspect.

218   CHAPTER 6   The Muscular System

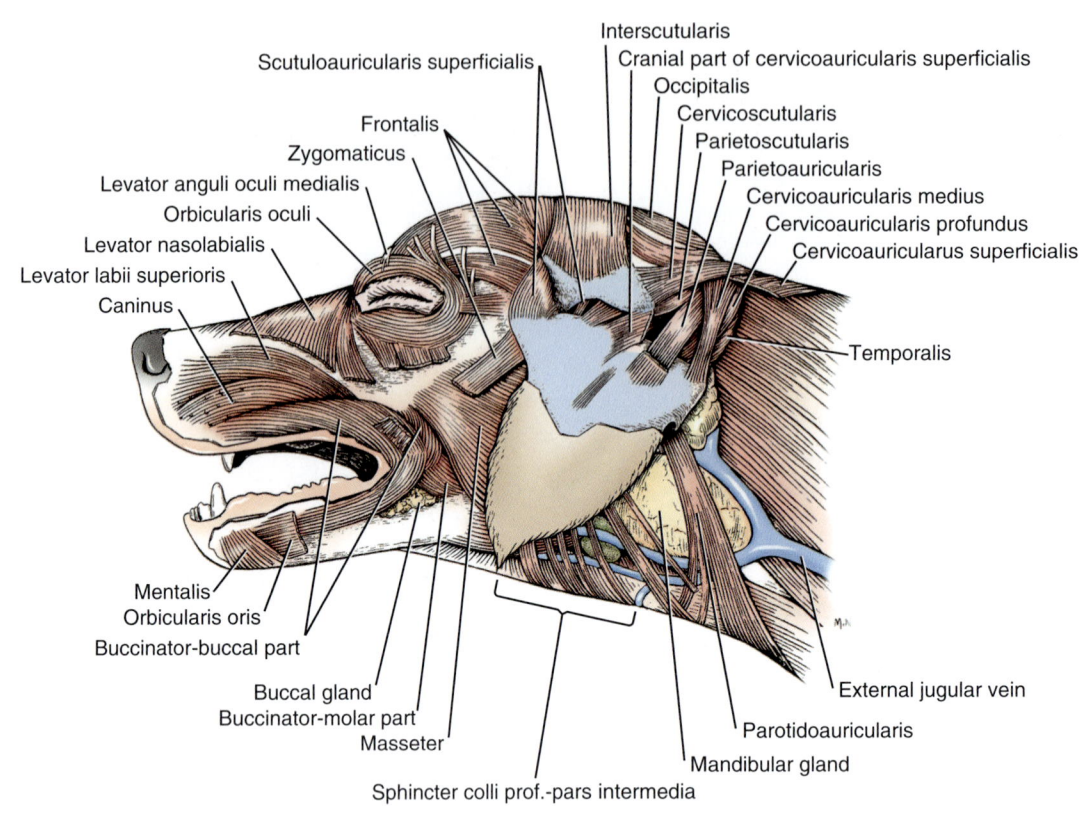

• **Fig. 6.7** Deep muscles of the head and ear, lateral aspect.

The *mm. incisivus superioris et inferioris* lie deep to the orbicularis oris. These are two thin muscles not clearly defined from the orbicularis and buccinator. They arise on the alveolar borders of the incisive bone and mandible as far as the corner incisor teeth and are situated immediately deep to the mucosa of the lips. They extend to the orbicularis oris. According to Huber (1922), the inferior one cannot be isolated as a separate muscle.

Action: The m. incisivus superioris raises the superior lip. The m. incisivus inferioris depresses the inferior lip.

The *m. levator labii superioris* (Figs. 6.5 to 6.7), is a flat muscle that lies deep to the apical end of the levator nasolabialis on the maxilla and incisive bone. It arises from the maxillary bone caudoventral to the infraorbital foramen and courses rostrally along the dorsal border of the caninus muscle. The fibers of insertion spread out as they enter the nasal ala and the superior lip.

The *m. caninus* (Figs. 6.5 to 6.7), is immediately ventral to the levator labii superioris and extends rostrally deep to the labial end of the levator nasolabialis. It terminates rostrally in the superior lip.

Action: To increase the diameter of the external naris and to lift the apical portion of the superior lip.

The *m. buccinator* (Figs. 6.5, 6.6, and 6.7) has developed from the deep part of the orbicularis oris. It is a thick, flat, wide muscle that forms the foundation of the cheek. It is composed of two portions, which extend caudally from the labial commissure. These are the buccalis and molar parts of the buccinator muscle. The **buccal part** (*pars buccalis*), formerly called *pars dorsalis*, is the somewhat larger portion. It arises from the maxilla dorsally and the mandible ventrally deep to the orbicularis oris. It consists primarily of longitudinal fibers where it is located in both lips. Caudally in the cheek the dorsal and ventral portions meet in a raphe that extends caudally from the commissure of the lips. The **molar part** (*pars molaris*) is deep to the buccal part and consists of longitudinal fibers that arise from the ramus of the mandible and course rostrally to fill the cheek and blend with the buccal part as well as with the orbicularis oris. The caudal portion of the molar part is overlapped by the masseter muscle.

Action: To return food from the vestibule to the masticatory surface of the teeth.

The *m. mentalis* (Figs. 6.4, 6.5, and 6.7) arises from the alveolar border and body of the mandible near the third incisor. The fibers unite with those of the opposite side and radiate into the inferior lip, forming a prominent, fat-infiltrated muscle.

Action: To stiffen the inferior lip in the apical region.

The *m. levator nasolabialis* (Figs. 6.4 to 6.7) is a flat, thin, and broad muscle (even in large dogs), lying immediately deep to the skin on the lateral surface of the nasal and

...maxillary bones. It arises in the frontal region between the orbits from the nasofrontal fascia, the medial palpebral ligament, and the maxillary bone. Occasionally a few additional fibers come from the lacrimal bone. Spreading out, it proceeds to the nose and superior lip to insert deep to the orbicularis oris. The caudal portion inserts on the buccinator. The apical, larger portion passes deep to the orbicularis to end near the edge of the lip. The most dorsal and rostral fibers interdigitate with the fibers of the levator labii superioris to attach to the external naris.

Action: To increase the diameter of the naris and lift the apical portion of the superior lip.
Innervation: Auriculopalpebral nerve from the facial nerve (n. auriculopalpebralis, n. facialis).

Deep Muscles of the Eyelids, Forehead, and Ears

The deep muscles of the eyelids, forehead, and ears include the orbicularis oculi, retractor anguli oculi lateralis, levator anguli oculi medialis, levator palpebrae superioris, orbitalis (ocular smooth muscles), occipitalis, and the multiple ear muscles. These are all innervated by the facial nerve except the levator palpebrae superioris (oculomotor nerve) and the orbitalis (sympathetic nerves).

The ***m. orbicularis oculi*** (Figs. 6.4 to 6.7) surrounds the palpebral fissure. Portions of the muscle adjacent to the borders of the lids extend from the medial palpebral ligament dorsal to the superior lid, around the lateral commissure of the lids, and along the inferior lid back to the ligament. Thus, in the dog, this muscle, which originally was divided into dorsal and ventral portions, has become one. Huber (1922) states that the ventral portion comes from the m. zygomaticus, and the dorsal portion comes from the m. frontalis.

Action: To close the palpebral fissure.

The ***m. retractor anguli oculi lateralis*** (Figs. 6.4 to 6.7) arises beside the m. frontalis from the temporal fascia. It extends horizontally to the lateral palpebral angle, and, in so doing, it crosses the orbicularis oculi before it sinks into the fibers of the latter.

Action: To draw the lateral palpebral angle caudally.

The ***m. levator anguli oculi medialis*** (Figs. 6.4 to 6.7) is a small, thick muscle strand that arises from the median line on the frontal bone from the nasofrontal fascia. It extends dorsal to the orbicularis oculi of the medial half of the superior eyelid.

Action: To elevate the superior eyelid, especially its nasal portion, and erect the hairs of the eyebrow.

The ***m. levator palpebrae superioris*** (Fig. 6.13) is the main retractor of the superior eyelid. It arises dorsal to the optic canal between the dorsal rectus and the dorsal oblique muscles. It courses deep to the periorbita and superficial to the extraocular muscles in reaching the superior eyelid. The levator inserts in the superior eyelid by means of a wide, flat tendon that passes between the fascicles of the m. orbicularis oculi.

Action: To lift the superior eyelid.
Innervation: N. oculomotorius.

There are also smooth muscles, ***m. orbitalis***, associated with the eyeball, orbit, and lids. The extraocular components include smooth muscle fascicles in the superior, inferior, and third eyelids as well as the periorbita. Several of these, including the ventral and dorsal palpebral muscles, have been referred to in the past as *muscles of Müller*. Acheson (1938) described and illustrated the inferior and medial smooth muscles of the kitten's eye and showed their relationship to the eyelids and nictitating membrane. In the dog a delicate fan of muscle fibers arises from the trochlear cartilage and inserts in the superior lid. These fibers are nearly continuous at their insertion with the edge of the m. levator palpebrae superioris.

Action: Retract the eyelids and protrude the eyeball.
Innervation: Sympathetic postganglionic axons primarily within the branches of the ophthalmic nerve from V.

The ***m. occipitalis*** (Figs. 6.6 and 6.7) lies superficial to the occipital and parietal bones. From the external sagittal crest, its fibers turn rostrally in bilaterally symmetric arches in such a way that they form an unpaired, oval, thin membranous muscle that can be followed a short distance rostrally deep to the caudal portion of the m. interscutularis. There, on the frontal bone, they spread out into the nasofrontal fascia.

Action: To tense the nasofrontal fascia.

Muscles of the External Ear

The **muscles of the external ear** are organized into five groups. Four of these are groups of extrinsic muscles and one is an intrinsic group. The extrinsic muscle groups are rostral, dorsal, caudal, and ventral. The **intrinsic ear muscles** include the helicis, helicis minor, tragicus, transverse auricular, and oblique auricular. The names of these muscles have been subjected to extensive revisions. Synonyms used in the previous editions of this book are enclosed in parentheses. Other names may be included within the specific descriptions. For external ear cartilages also see Figs. 20.15 and 20.16. For external ear intrinsic muscles see Figs. 20.17 to 20.20.

The ***mm. helicis, helicis minor***, and ***tragicus*** (Fig. 6.4) lie together in one muscle complex that bridges the space between the superimposed conchal cartilage edges at the opening of the conchal cavity. The *concha auriculae* is the funnel-shaped proximal part of the auricle. This muscle aggregate passes from the deep surface of the lateral crus of the helix to the tragus. In certain cases all of these muscles are independent. See Leahy (1949) for further pictorial and descriptive treatment. The m. helicis arises from the external surface of the tragus, the m. helicis minor from the tragus and the conchal canal, and the m. tragicus from the external surface of the concha.

Action: To narrow the entrance to the conchal canal and thus make the concha rigid.

The **rostral extrinsic ear muscles** include the superficial scutuloauricularis, deep scutuloauricularis, frontalis, frontoscutularis, and zygomaticoauricularis.

The *m. scutuloauricularis superficialis* (m. auricularis anterior superior of Huber) (Figs. 6.4 and 6.6 to 6.8) is the dorsal medial rotator of the ear. It consists of two short broad bundles that arise from the lateral border of the scutiform cartilage and attach to the concha and the lateral crus of the helix. It separates dorsocaudally from the m. frontalis, with which it is always partly united. It courses in a fold of skin to the medial border of the concha.

Action: To turn the conchal opening rostrally and medially.

The *m. scutuloauricularis profundus* or large rotator of the concha (see Fig. 6.8), is completely separated from the m. frontalis. It lies deep to the scutiform cartilage and arises on its deep surface to extend to the concha adjacent to the m. temporalis. The muscle has an almost sagittal course.

Action: To turn the conchal fissure caudally.

The *m. frontalis* (Figs. 6.5 to 6.8) is a thin muscle that lies on the temporalis. It arises rostral to the rostral border of the scutiform cartilage, by means of a fascial leaf, and extends to the forehead and toward the superior eyelid. It spans across the midline to unite with the opposite muscle rostral to the m. interscutularis. Rostrally it joins the frontal fascia by which it attaches to the zygomatic process. From the external ear cartilage a considerable number of muscle strands of the m. scutuloauricularis superficialis extend over the scutiform cartilage into the frontalis.

Action: To fix and pull the scutiform cartilage rostrally.

The *m. frontoscutularis* (Fig. 6.6) has formerly been considered part of the frontalis muscle, which is adjacent to its medial border. It arises from the rostral part of the scutiform cartilage and courses rostrally to terminate on the frontal bone and medial palpebral ligament medial to the medial portion of the orbicularis oculi and lateral to the levator anguli oculi medialis.

The *m. zygomaticoauricularis* (Figs. 6.4 to 6.6) is the medial rotator that arises as a rather broad muscle from the tendinous leaf lying rostral to the scutiform cartilage. It is continuous rostrally with the ventral portion of the frontalis and is deep to the sphincter colli profundus. Caudally, it extends ventrally to terminate on the basal portion of the tragus.

Action: To turn the auricular concha rostrally.

The **dorsal extrinsic ear muscles** include the interscutularis, parietoscutularis, and parietoauricularis.

The *m. interscutularis* (Fig. 6.6) is a thin muscle extending from one scutiform cartilage to the other without attaching to the cranial bones. It has developed from the fusion of bilateral portions. The origin is from the entire dorsomedial border of the scutiform cartilage. The caudal portion of the muscle has a distinct border and covers the m. occipitalis and the m. cervicoscutularis, both of which blend with the interscutularis. Rostrally it has no distinct border and encroaches upon the m. frontalis.

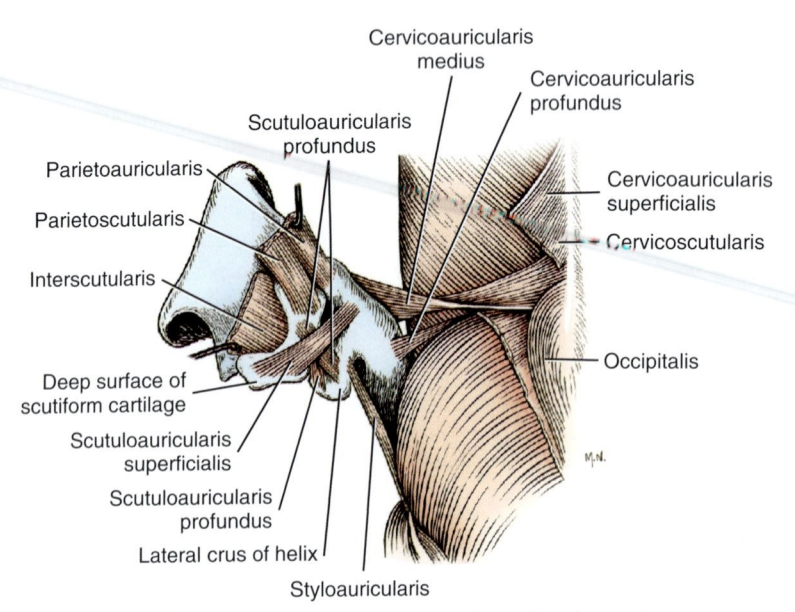

• **Fig. 6.8** Muscles of the right external ear, dorsal aspect.

Action: Fixation of the scutiform cartilage.

The *m. parietoscutularis* (**interparietoscutularis**) (Figs. 6.6 and 6.7) is only exceptionally an independent muscle. It is described by Huber (1923) as the m. cervicoscutularis medius belonging to the middle layer. It arises from the interparietal portion of the external sagittal crest and inserts on the caudal border of the scutiform cartilage, which is completely covered by the superficial layer of this muscle complex.

Action: With other scutular muscles, it aids in fixation of the scutiform cartilage.

The *m. parietoauricularis* (**interparietoauricularis**), or middle levator (cervicoauricularis profundus anterior of Huber) (Figs. 6.6 and 6.7), is only seldom completely isolated. Indeed, it belongs to the deep layer but usually fuses with the m. parietoscutularis, which becomes separate only near the scutiform cartilage. In its entire course it is covered by the superficial layer of the caudal auricular musculature. It arises from the interparietal segment of the external sagittal crest and goes directly to the dorsum of the concha, where it attaches deep to the caudal terminal branch of the m. cervicoauricularis superficialis basal to its insertion.

Action: To raise the concha.

The **caudal extrinsic ear muscles** include the cervicoscutularis, cervicoauricularis superficialis, cervicoauricularis medius, and cervicoauricularis profundus.

The *m. cervicoscutularis* (cervicointerscutularis of Huber) (Figs. 6.6 and 6.7) is a narrow, intermediate portion of the muscle complex that is not clearly defined. It is deep to the interscutularis and passes to the caudal border and the caudomedial angle of the scutiform cartilage. It is united with the deep surface of the interscutularis by means of a few fibers.

Action: To draw the scutiform cartilage ventrally and caudally or fix it when the scutiform cartilage is drawn rostrally at the same time.

The *m. cervicoauricularis superficialis*, or long levator (Figs. 6.6 and 6.7), arises from the cervical midline and the external occipital protuberance. As a broad muscle mass it passes to the concha and ends in two branches on the dorsum of the ear. The rostral branch is made wider by fibers from the lateral border of the scutiform cartilage. These correspond to the m. scutuloauricularis superficialis or short levator of other animals. The caudal branch covers the auricular end of the parietoauricularis.

Action: To raise the concha.

The *m. cervicoauricularis medius* (**cervicoauricularis profundus major**), or long lateral rotator (Figs. 6.7 and 6.8), is a thick, relatively wide muscle that, covered partly by the cervicoauricularis superficialis, arises on the external sagittal crest, the external occipital protuberance, and the neighboring attachment of the nuchal ligament. It extends to the base of the concha and finally ends on the root of the lateral conchal border (antitragus), where it lies next to the insertion of the parotidoauricularis. This muscle covers a portion of the origin of the parietoauricularis, the greater part of the cervicoauricularis profundus, and the m. temporalis of that region.

Action: To turn the conchal fissure laterally and caudally.

The *m. cervicoauricularis profundus* (**cervicoauricularis profundus minor**) or short lateral rotator (Figs. 6.5 to 6.8) is a division of the deep layer of the caudoauricular musculature. At its origin, it is rather variable in that it can be divided into two to five clearly defined muscle bundles. Of these, the caudal one usually comes from the external occipital protuberance, whereas the other portions are more or less shortened and arise by an aponeurosis from the m. temporalis. Covered by the long lateral rotator, the muscle runs to the extended lateral conchal border.

Action: To turn the concha laterally and caudally.

The **ventral extrinsic ear muscles** are composed of the parotidoauricularis muscle and styloauricularis.

The *m. parotidoauricularis* (**parotideoauricularis**) (Figs. 6.4, 6.5, and 6.7), formerly called the *depressor auriculae*, arises caudal to the laryngeal region, on or near the midline, where it blends with the cervical fascia. As a well-defined band, it runs obliquely dorsally toward the concha, crossing the mandibular and parotid glands in its course. The muscle is almost completely covered by the platysma and inserts on the antitragus.

Action: To depress the ear.

The *m. styloauricularis* (**mandibuloauricularis**) (Figs. 6.8 and 6.9) is a muscle of the concha. It is a long, narrow muscle that also bears the name *m. tragicus lateralis* in descriptive nomenclature. It arises tendinously in the niche between the angular and the condyloid processes of the mandible and extends dorsally to the helix covered by the parotid salivary gland. In its course it passes over the root of the zygomatic process of the temporal bone, extends along the rostral side of the concha, and ends opposite the scutuloauricularis profundus. This muscle may undergo great reduction and, in extreme cases, may be represented only by tendinous remains. Often it is connected directly with the m. helicis, whose innervation it shares.

Muscles of the Middle Ear

The *m. stapedius* (see Fig. 20.10) was originally associated with the hyomandibular bone of the primitive mandibular joint. During evolution the hyomandibular became the

The Muscular System

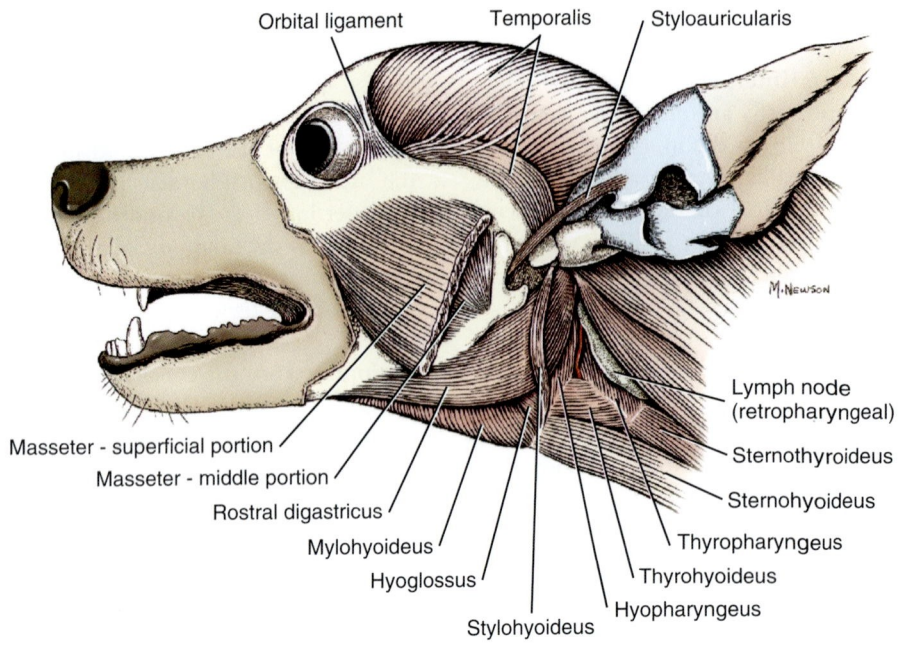

• **Fig. 6.9** Muscles of mastication, lateral aspect.

stapes and, with its associated muscle, was incorporated into the middle ear (for review, see Hildebrand & Goslow, 2001). This muscle, the m. stapedius, innervated by the facial nerve, is described with the ear ossicle muscles in Chapter 20 on the ear.

The **m. tensor tympani**, innervated by the trigeminal nerve, is discussed with muscles of the ear ossicles in Chapter 20 on the ear (see Fig. 20.10). The m. tensor tympani contains a unique myosin, referred to as *2M*, that is not found in the adjacent m. stapedius (Mascarello et al., 1982; Mascarello et al., 1983), supporting an independent origin of these two muscles. The tensor tympani develops from branchial arch 1 with its trigeminal nerve innervation, and the stapedius muscle develops from branchial arch 2 with its facial nerve innervation. The 2M myosin is also found in the trigeminal nerve innervated muscles of mastication derived from branchial arch 1.

Muscles of Mastication

The muscles of mastication include the masseter, temporal, lateral, and medial pterygoid and the digastricus. All are innervated by the mandibular nerve from the trigeminal except for the caudal portion of the digastricus, which is innervated by the facial nerve. See Figs. 6.9 to 6.11 and 6.23.

The **m. masseter** lies on the lateral surface of the ramus of the mandible ventral to the zygomatic arch. It projects somewhat beyond the ventral and caudal borders of the mandible. The muscle is covered by a thick, glistening aponeurosis, and tendinous intermuscular strands are interspersed throughout its depth. The muscle can be divided into three layers (superficial, middle, and deep), using the change of fiber direction as a guide to the separation between the layers.

The superficial layer, the largest part, arises from the ventral border of the rostral half of the zygomatic arch. Its fibers pass caudoventrally and insert, partly, on the ventrolateral surface of the mandible. Some fibers project around the ventral and caudal borders of the mandible and insert on its ventromedial surface, as well as on a tendinous raphe that passes between the masseter and the m. pterygoideus medius. The tendinous raphe continues caudally from the angle of the jaw and attaches on the temporal bone adjacent to the tympanic bulla. In specimens with well-developed masseters, this layer, at its ventral border, projects somewhat over the m. digastricus.

The middle layer, the thinnest part, arises from the zygomatic arch, medial to the origin of the superficial layer and in part caudal to it. Most of its fibers pass ventrally to be inserted on the ventral margin of the masseteric fossa and the narrow area just ventral to the fossa. In some specimens a small bundle of fibers, which belong to this layer, run in a more rostral direction to be inserted on the rostroventral margin of the fossa.

The deep layer is impossible to isolate at its origin because many of its fibers intermingle with those of the temporalis. Some fibers, however, arise from the medial surface of the zygomatic arch. The majority of its fibers are directed caudoventrally and are inserted in the caudal part of the masseteric fossa and on the ridge adjacent to it. A few fibers pass ventrally along the rostral margin of the temporal muscle to be inserted on the rostral ridge of the masseteric fossa. It is tempting to speculate that these three layers may correlate with regional functional properties. The masseter of pigs is a complex muscle exhibiting unique histochemical properties and sarcomeric lengths in different parts of the muscle. These differences correlate with variation in electromyographic (EMG) patterns observed during different

CHAPTER 6 The Muscular System 223

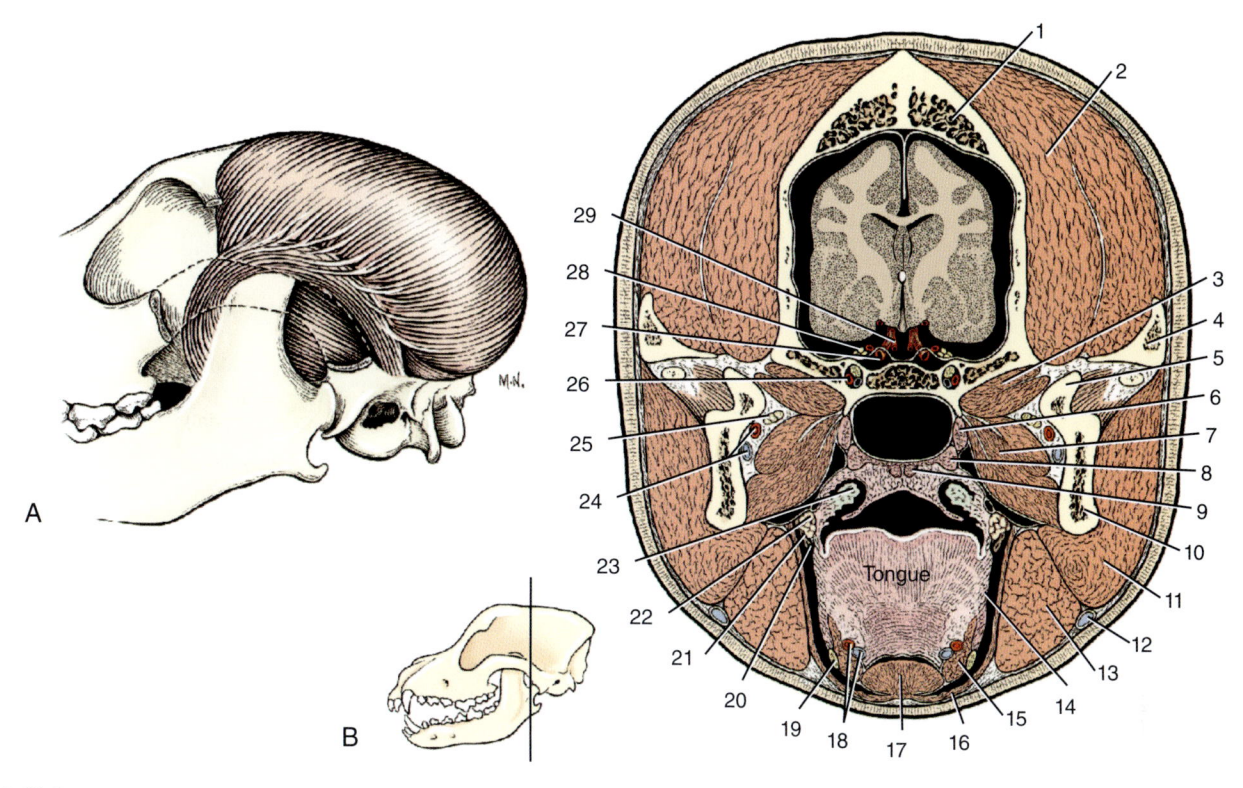

1. Diploe
2. Temporal m.
3. Lateral pterygoid m.
4. Zygomatic process of temporal bone
5. Condylar process
6. Tensor veli palatini
7. Medical pterygoid m.
8. Pterygopharyngeus m.
9. Palatinus m.
0. Mandible
1. Masseter m.
12. Facial vein
13. Digastricus m.
14. Styloglossus m.
15. Hyoglossus m.
16. Mylohyoideus m.
17. Geniohyoideus m.
18. Lingual a. and v.
19. Hypoglossal n.
20. Mandibular duct
21. Major sublingual duct
22. Sublingual salivary gland
23. Palatine tonsil in tonsillar fossa
24. Inferior alveolar a. and v.
25. Mylohyoid, inferior alveolar and lingual nn.
26. Maxillary a., v. and n. in alar canal
27. Internal carotid a. in cavernous sinus
28. Cranial nerves III, IV, and VI and ophthalmic n.
29. Cerebral arterial circle—caudal communicating a.

• **Fig. 6.10** **A,** The m. temporalis, lateral aspect. (Zygomatic arch removed.) **B,** Transection of head through palatine tonsil.

phases of the chewing cycle or with chewing foodstuffs with different hardness properties (Herring et al., 1979). Bubb and Sims (1986) classified the fast fibers in the masseter of dogs as type 2M (superfast), representing approximately 85% of the muscle fibers. Toniolo et al. (2008) reported that nearly all fibers in canine masseter and temporalis muscles contain a unique m-MyHC that produced high force per unit cross-section and moderate shortening speeds. The masticatory myosin heavy chain appears unique to masticatory muscles and is found in other species (Reiser et al., 2009, 2010).

Action: To raise the mandible in closing the mouth.
Innervation: N. massetericus of the n. mandibularis from the n. trigeminus.

The ***m. temporalis*** is the largest muscle of the head. It occupies the temporal fossa, from which it extends ventrally around the coronoid process of the mandible. During the course of its ventral extension, it is related rostrally to the orbit and orbital fat, medially to the mm. pterygoidei, and laterally to the m. masseter. Dorsolaterally it is covered by the caudoauricular muscles, the scutiform cartilage, and the ear. It arises largely from the parietal bone and to a lesser extent from the temporal, frontal, and occipital bones. The margins of the muscle at its origin are the orbital ligament and temporal line rostrally, the zygomatic arch laterally, the dorsal nuchal crest caudally, and the external sagittal crest or temporal line medially. Closely applied to the muscle, within these margins, is a thick, glistening fascia. In dolichocephalic dogs the temporal muscle meets its fellow of the opposite side and forms a mid-dorsal sulcus. In dogs with brachycephalic heads the temporal muscles usually do not meet on the midline, and the area is devoid of muscle, except for the dorsal and caudal auricular muscles. From its large origin, the muscle fibers curve rostrally and ventrally medial to the zygomatic arch to invest and insert on the coronoid process of the mandible, as far ventral as the ventral margin of the massetric fossa. On the lateral side of the coronoid process the fibers are intermingled with fibers of the deep layer of the m. masseter. On the medial side the fibers lie in contact with the mm.

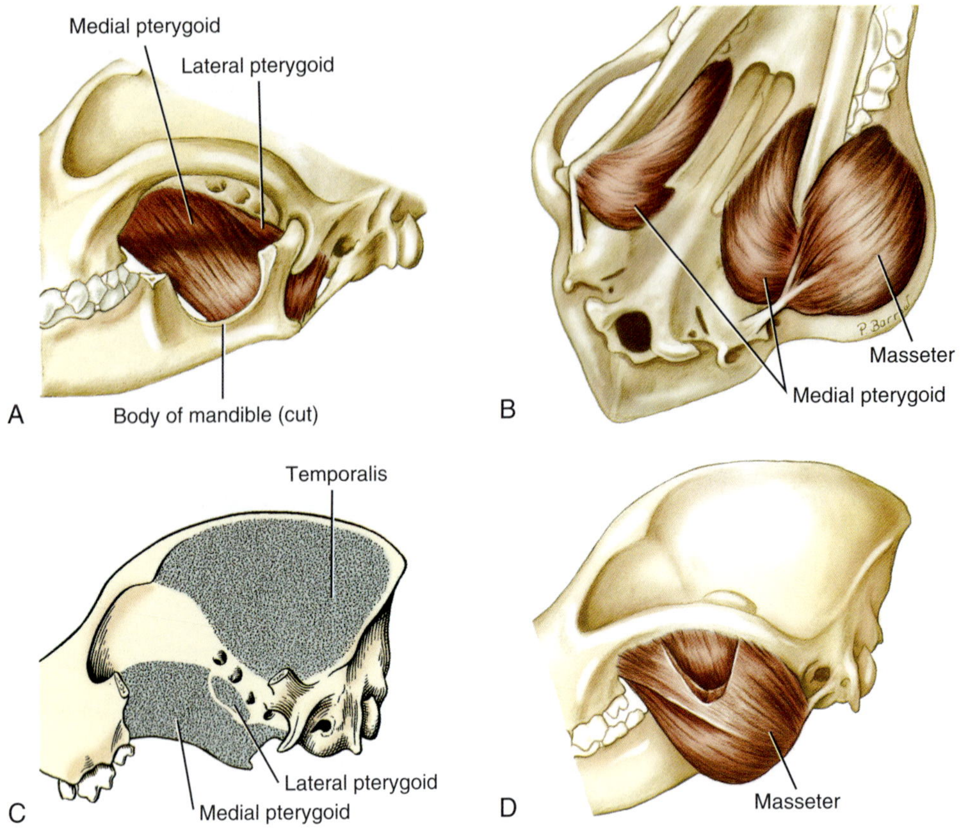

• **Fig. 6.11** Muscles of mastication. **A**, Mm. pterygoideus medialis and pterygoideus lateralis. **B**, Mm. masseter and pterygoideus medialis. **C**, Areas of origin of mm. temporalis, pterygoideus medialis, and pterygoideus lateralis. **D**, M. masseter, cut to show the deep portion.

pterygoidei. A bundle of muscle fibers arise from the nuchal crest, near the base of the zygomatic process of the temporal bone, and sweeps rostrally dorsal and parallel to the zygomatic arch. It blends gradually into the main mass of the muscle.

The dog temporalis muscle contains a unique isoform of myosin common to masticatory muscles of other carnivores (Rowlerson et al., 1981; Shelton et al., 1988). This isoform has been called "superfast myosin" by others (references in Hoh et al., 1988). Although the specific function of this 2M (sometimes called IIM myosin) is not known, it has been demonstrated in dog temporalis and masseter but not in appendicular skeletal muscles (Shelton et al., 1985a). More recent analysis indicates that this unique myosin is, in fact, correlated with high-force and not with superfast-twitch single fiber properties (Reiser et al., 2010; Reiser & Bicer, 2007; Toniolo et al., 2008).

Action: To raise the mandible in closing the mouth.
Innervation: N. temporalis of the n. mandibularis from n. trigeminus.

The *m. pterygoideus lateralis* (Figs. 6.10 and 6.11) is a much smaller and shorter muscle than the m. pterygoideus medialis. It arises from the sphenoid bone in a small fossa, which lies ventral to the alar canal and orbital fissure. The ventral boundary of its origin is a bony ridge also on the sphenoid bone. This short muscle passes ventrolaterally and slightly caudally, to be inserted on the medial surface of the condyle of the mandible just ventral to its articular surface. Tomo et al. (1995) describe a tendinous attachment to the temporomandibular joint articular disc, as well as the main insertion upon the condyle.

Action: To raise the mandible.
Innervation: Nn. pterygoidei of the n. mandibularis from n. trigeminus.

The *m. pterygoideus medialis* arises from the lateral surface of the pterygoid, palatine, and sphenoid bones. It passes caudolaterally to be inserted on the medial and caudal surfaces of the angular process of the mandible and ventral to the insertion of the mm. temporalis and pterygoideus lateralis. Many fibers insert on a fibrous raphe that passes between the insertion of this muscle and the superficial layer of the masseter muscle. When viewed from the pharyngeal side, the medial pterygoid completely covers the lateral one.

The inferior alveolar nerve passes across the lateral face of the m. pterygoideus medialis and the medial surface of the m. pterygoideus lateralis, thus separating the two muscles. The m. pterygoideus medialis extends to the caudal margin of the mandible and is inserted on the caudal margin and slightly on the caudomedial surface.

Action: To raise the mandible.
Innervation: Nn. pterygoidei of the n. mandibularis from n. trigeminus.

The *m. digastricus* (*biventer mandibulae*) runs from the paracondylar process of the occiput to the ventral border of the mandible. Although it appears as a single-bellied muscle in the dog, a tendinous intersection and an innervation by both the n. trigeminus and the n. facialis are evidence of its dual nature. Thus the two parts of the muscle are referred to as the *rostral belly* and the *caudal belly*. Much has been written about this muscle in mammals (Bijvoet, 1908; Chaine, 1914; Rouviere, 1906). Functional study has focused on the m. digastricus of guinea pigs (Byrd, 1981; Lev-Tov & Tal, 1987) and primates (Byrd et al., 1978). EMG patterns in the two bellies (rostral and caudal) in rodents suggest that activity in the caudal belly precedes electrical activity in the rostral belly. This sequential recruitment pattern allows the caudal belly to modulate the length of the rostral belly such that the latter functions at or near an optimal part of its length-tension curve (Lev-Tov & Tal, 1987). In cats, however, EMG activity is synchronous in the two bellies (Gorniak & Gans, 1980). This situation may be most similar to that in the dog because both cats and dogs have a highly reduced myotendinous intersection interposed between the two bellies. Both portions of digastricus were found to contain predominantly type IIa fibers (Bubb & Sims, 1986).

The digastricus lies medial to the parotid and mandibular glands. After crossing the ventrocaudal edge of the insertion of the masseter, it has a fleshy ending on the ventromedial border of the mandible over a distance of approximately 2.5 cm, to the level of the canine tooth. Small muscle bundles extend far rostral toward the chin.

Action: To open the mouth.
Innervation: N. facialis to caudal belly and n. trigeminus to rostral belly.

Muscles of Bulbus Oculi: Extrinsic

There are seven extrinsic muscles of the eyeball: two oblique muscles, four recti muscles, and the retractor bulbi (Figs. 6.12 to 6.13). Closely associated with these, but inserting in the superior eyelid, is the m. levator palpebrae superioris (see Deep Muscles of the Eyes, Forehead, and Ears). All of the extrinsic ocular muscles insert in the fibrous coat of the eyeball near its equator. The level of insertion of the recti muscles is nearer the corneoscleral junction than is that of the four parts of the retractor. In general, the oblique muscles insert in an intermediate zone between the insertions of the recti and retractor groups. All arise from the margin of the optic canal and orbital fissure, except the ventral oblique, which comes from the rostral part of the pterygopalatine fossa. Gilbert (1947) has investigated the origin and development of the extrinsic ocular muscles in the domestic cat. Extraocular muscles are characterized by two layers: a surface region composed of small-diameter fibers and a global region composed of fibers with heterogeneous diameters. Both layers contain myofibers innervated either by single axons or by multiple axons (Harker, 1972; Pachter, 1982, 1983). Myosin heavy chain isoform expression patterns differ between the global and surface layers of dog rectus muscles (Bicer & Reiser, 2009) with more complexity and up to nine isoforms found in the surface layer. There are more myosin heavy chain isoforms in eye muscles than are found in appendicular muscles. (See Chapter 21 for a more complete treatment of the eyeball.)

The *m. obliquus ventralis* arises from the rostrolateral margin of a variably sized opening in the palatine bone adjacent to the suture between the palatine, lacrimal, and maxillary bones. Frequently a groove harbors the origin of the muscle and extends caudally. As the ventral oblique muscle passes ventral to the eyeball, it gradually widens and crosses ventral to the tendon of insertion of the ventral rectus. The ventral oblique divides as it reaches the ventral border of the lateral rectus. Part of its tendon crosses that of the lateral rectus superficially to attach to the sclera lateral to the insertion of the dorsal rectus. The deep part goes medial to the lateral rectus, and ends in the sclera.

Action: To rotate the eyeball around its anterior to posterior axis so that the lateral part is moved laterally and ventrally—extorsion.
Innervation: N. oculomotorius.

The *m. obliquus dorsalis*, or trochlearis, arises from the medial border of the optic canal. It ascends on the dorsomedial face of the periorbita to a cartilaginous pulley located on the medial wall of the orbit near the medial canthus of the eye. The pulley, or *trochlea* is a disc of hyaline cartilage located dorsocaudal to the medial canthus of the lids on the medial wall of the orbit, less than 1 cm from the orbital margin. It is spherical to oval in outline, with its long axis parallel to that of the head. It is approximately 1 cm long by 1.5 mm thick. The trochlea is suspended from the rostral border of the frontal bone and its zygomatic process by three ligamentous thickenings of the periorbita. A long, distinct ligament runs from the rostral end of the trochlea, where the dorsal oblique tendon bends around the cartilage, to the periosteum at the medial canthus. A short but wide thickening of the periorbita anchors the trochlea to the dorsal orbital wall near its margin. The third ligament is a thickening in the periorbita that runs from the caudal pole of the trochlea to the periosteum on the ventral surface of the zygomatic process.

The slender tendon of the dorsal oblique muscle passes through a groove on the medial surface of the ventrorostral end of the trochlear cartilage, where it is held in place by a collagenous ligament. As it passes through this pulley, or trochlea, it bends at an angle of approximately 45 degrees.

The Muscular System

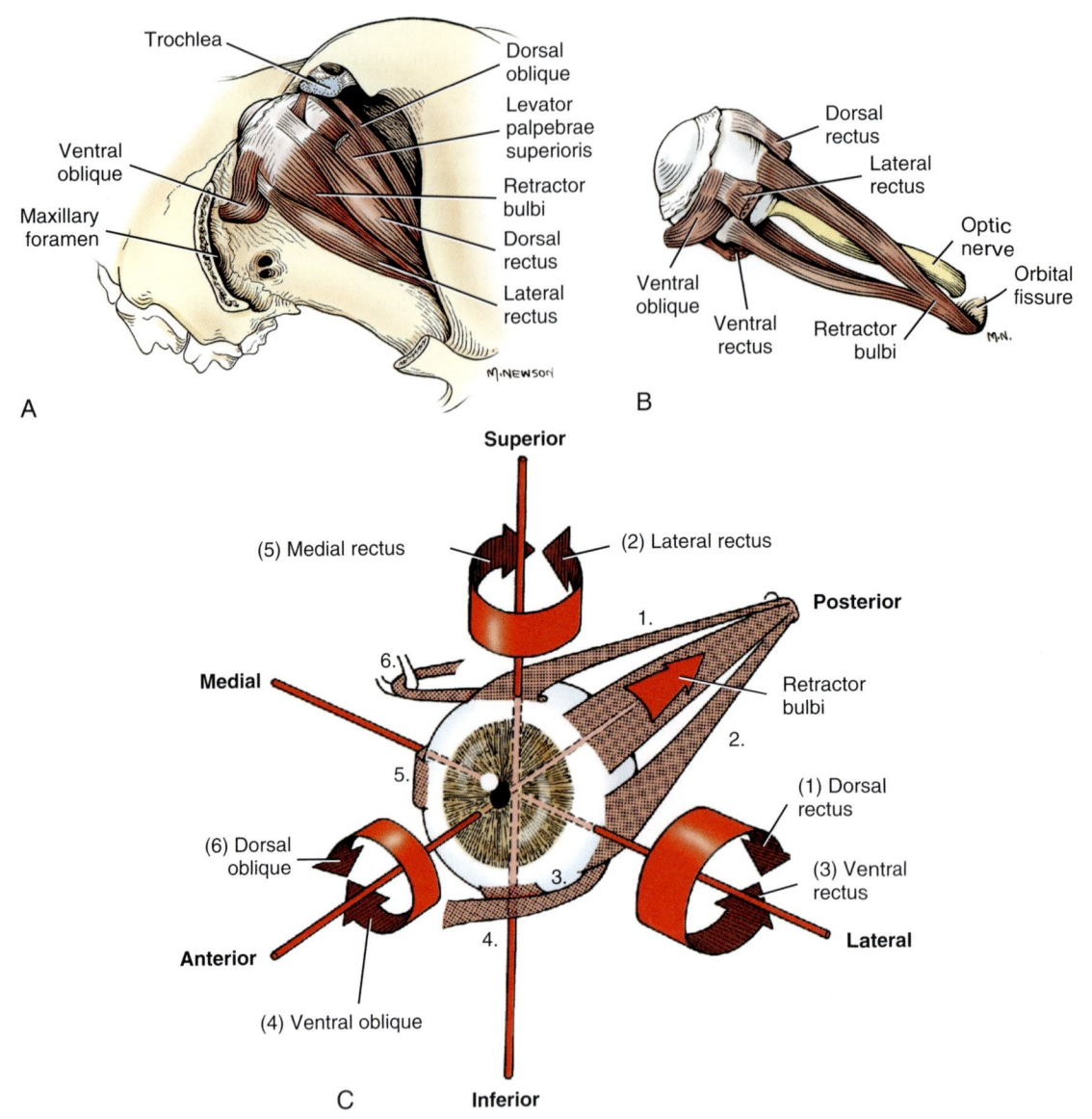

- **Fig. 6.12** Muscles of the eyeball. **A**, Caudolateral aspect. **B**, The m. retractor bulbi, lateral aspect. **C**, Schema of the extrinsic ocular muscles and their action on the eyeball.

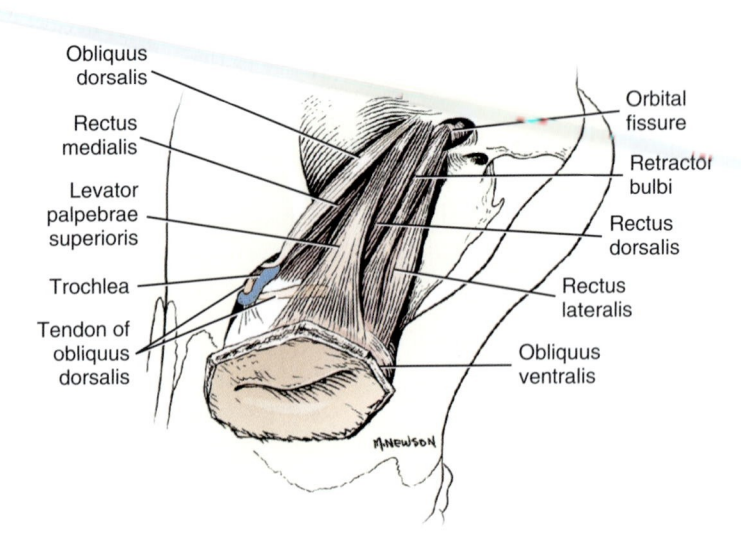

- **Fig. 6.13** A, Extrinsic muscles of the eyeball, dorsolateral aspect.

It passes dorsolaterally and deep to the tendon of the dorsal rectus, at the lateral edge of which it inserts in the sclera. It is the longest and slenderest muscle of the eyeball.

Action: To rotate the eyeball around its anterior–posterior axis so that the dorsal part is pulled medially and ventrally—intorsion.
Innervation: N. trochlearis.

The *mm. recti*, or straight muscles of the eyeball, include the mm. rectus lateralis, rectus medialis, rectus dorsalis, and rectus ventralis. They all arise from a poorly defined fibrous ring that is attached around the optic canal and is continuous with the dural sheath of the optic nerve. The dorsal and medial recti arise farther peripherally from the optic canal than do the others. As the four muscles course rostrally from this small area of origin, they diverge and insert laterally, medially, dorsally, and ventrally on an imaginary line circling the eyeball, approximately 5 mm from the margin of the cornea. The muscles are fusiform, with widened peripheral ends that give rise to delicate aponeuroses. The muscles diverge from each other so that wedgelike spaces are formed between them. In the depths of these spaces the four segments of the m. retractor bulbi lie deep to the fascia and fat. The recti are longer and larger than the parts of the retractor with which they alternate. They therefore insert a greater distance from the caudal pole than do the parts of the retractor. The medial rectus is slightly larger than the others.

Action: The medial and lateral recti rotate the eyeball about a vertical axis through the equator resulting in adduction and abduction; the dorsal and ventral recti rotate the eyeball about a horizontal axis through the equator resulting in elevation and depression.
Innervation: N. oculomotorius to the ventral, medial, and dorsal recti; n. abducens to the lateral rectus.

The *m. retractor bulbi* arises deep to the mm. recti at the apex of the orbit, where they attach to the ventral end of the pterygoid crest and the adjacent orbital fissure. This places the initial part of the muscle lateral to the optic nerve.

The four fasciculi of the m. retractor bulbi diverge as they run to the equator of the eye. The muscle fasciculi can be divided into dorsal and ventral pairs. The optic nerve, as it emerges from the optic canal, passes between the dorsal and the ventral portions. The insertion of the several parts of the retractor on the globe of the eye is approximately 5 mm caudal and deep to the recti.

Action: To retract the eyeball. In addition, because of its essentially alternate attachments with the recti, it aids in bringing about oblique eye movements.
Innervation: N. abducens.

Muscles of the Tongue

The muscles of the tongue include the styloglossus, hyoglossus, genioglossus, and lingual intrinsic muscles. These are all innervated by the n. hypoglossus (Figs. 6.14 to 6.16 and 6.21).

The *m. styloglossus* extends from the stylohyoid bone to the tongue. It is composed of three muscle heads that insert in the tongue at different levels along its long axis.

The short head arises from the distal half of the caudal surface of the stylohyoid bone. It curves ventral and rostral across the lateral surface of the epihyoid bone. Immediately after crossing the epihyoid bone the fibers diverge and insert in the base of the tongue among the inserting fibers of the hyoglossal muscle.

The rostral head arises from the proximal half of the stylohyoid bone. These fibers curve ventrally and rostrally, pass over part of the inserting fibers of the short head, intermingle with fibers of the m. hyoglossus, and insert in the tongue along its ventrolateral surface.

The long head arises just dorsal and lateral to the origin of the fibers of the short head. These fibers immediately cross the stylohyoid bone, then curve ventrally and rostrally along the ventral border of the rostral head. They continue rostrally along the ventral midline of the tongue and across the lateral side of the genioglossus muscle to their insertion on the ventral surface of the rostral half of the tongue, near the median plane.

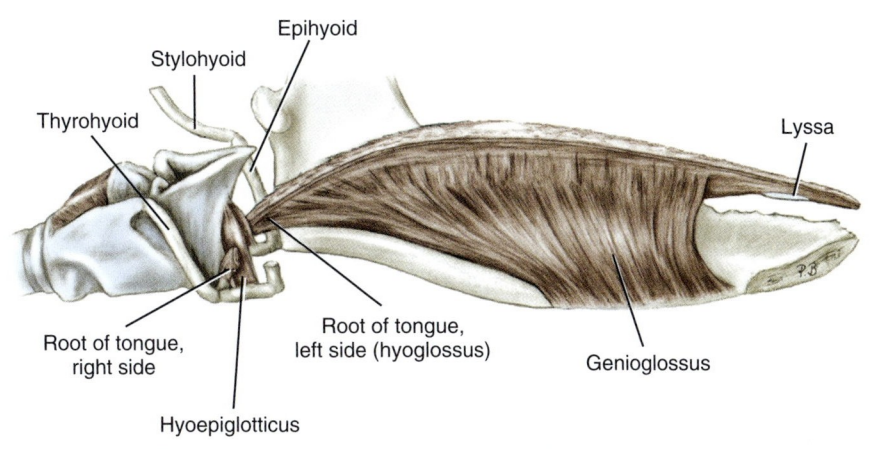

• **Fig. 6.14** The larynx, hyoid apparatus, and left half of the tongue.

The Muscular System

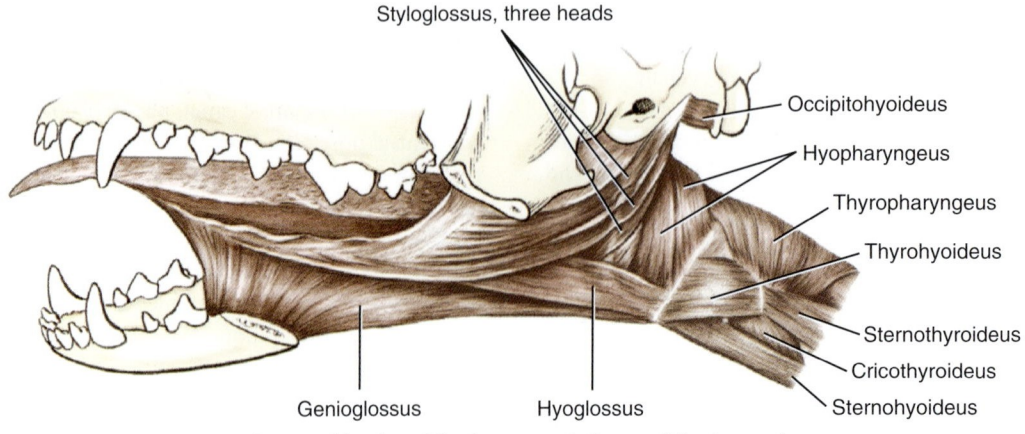

• **Fig. 6.15** Muscles of the tongue and pharynx, lateral aspect.

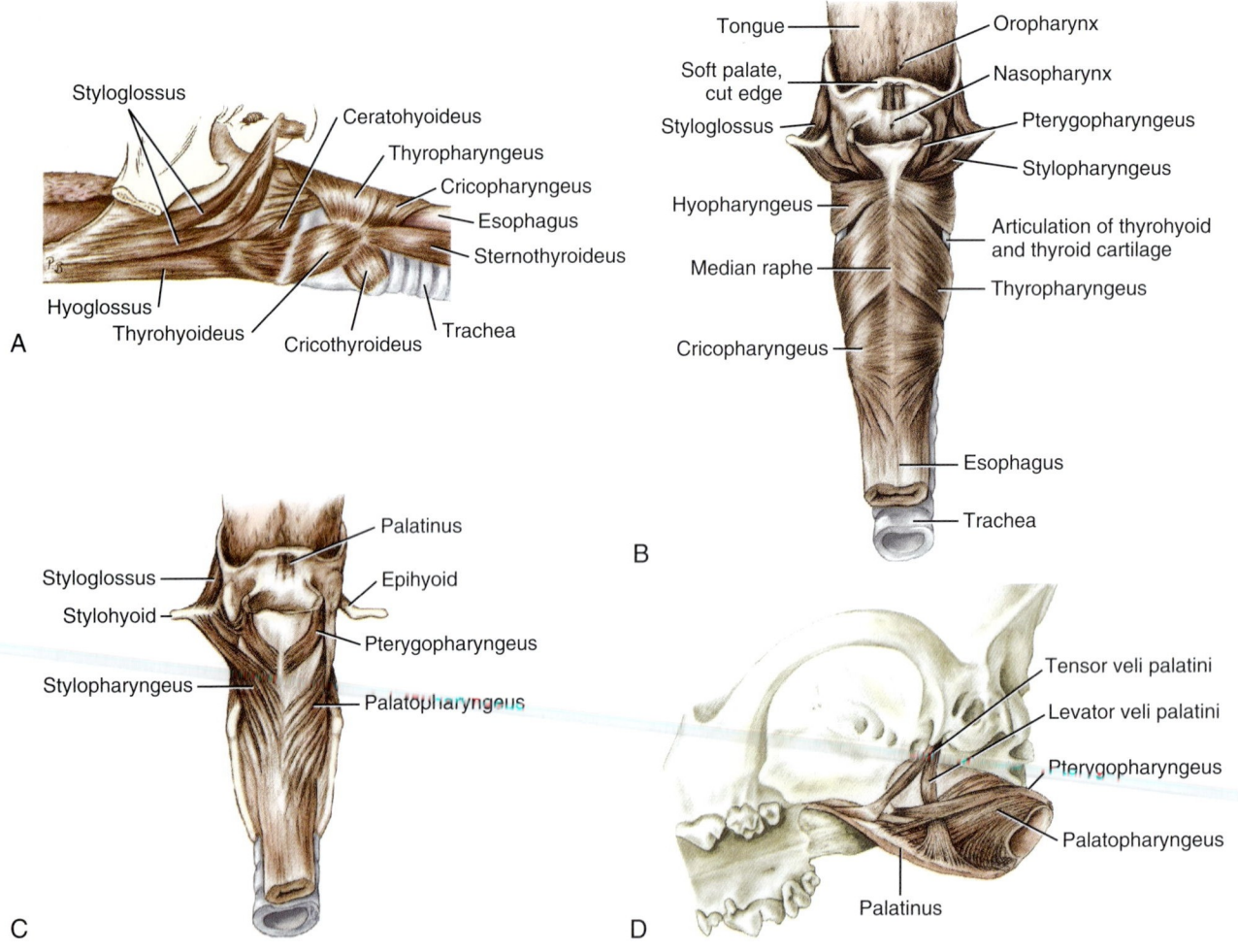

• **Fig. 6.16** **A,** Muscles of the tongue and pharynx, deep dissection, lateral aspect. **B,** Muscles of the pharynx, dorsal aspect. **C,** Muscles of the pharynx, deep dissection, dorsal aspect. **D,** Muscles of the pharynx and palate, deep dissection, ventrolateral aspect.

Action: To draw the tongue caudally when all three heads act together and to elevate the caudal part of the tongue.

The ***m. hyoglossus*** is located in the root of the tongue. It arises from the ventrolateral surface of the basihyoid and the adjoining end of the thyrohyoid bone. It runs rostrally dorsal to the m. mylohyoideus and lateral to the mm. geniohyoideus and genioglossus. At the base of the tongue it crosses the medial side of the m. styloglossus to be inserted in the root and caudal two-thirds of the tongue.

Action: To retract and depress the tongue.

The ***m. genioglossus*** is a thin, triangular muscle that lies in the intermandibular space, in and ventral to the tongue. The apex of this triangular muscle corresponds to its origin on the medial surface of the mandible, just caudal to the origin of the geniohyoideus. The fibers run caudally and dorsally in a sagittal plane. In their course the muscle fibers lie lateral to the m. geniohyoideus and dorsal to the m. mylohyoideus. The most rostral fibers run dorsally and rostrally, to be inserted on the midventral surface of the apex of the tongue. These fibers form the substance of the frenulum. The remaining fibers sweep dorsally and caudally in a fanlike arrangement, to be inserted along the midventral surface of the tongue in close contact with the fibers of the corresponding muscles of the opposite side. A distinct bundle of fibers runs directly caudally, to be inserted on the basihyoid and ceratohyoid bones. This caudal portion is referred to as the *horizontal compartment* and had a slower histochemical profile (84% slow-twitch) than the rostral compartment (Mu & Sanders, 2000).

Action: To depress the tongue. The caudal fibers draw the tongue rostrally; the rostral fibers curl the apex of the tongue ventrally. The caudal portion of the dog m. genioglossus appears to be a dilator of the oropharynx and is thus important to maintain airway patency (Miki et al., 1989). The rostral portion is specialized for fine motor control of the tongue apex. Vertically oriented fibers in the mid-belly of the tongue may depress the midline of the tongue during food manipulation (Mu & Sanders, 2000).

The ***m. propria linguae*** is the intrinsic tongue musculature that consists of many muscular bundles that are located among the fascicles of insertion of the extrinsic muscles of the tongue. They are arranged bilaterally in four poorly delineated fiber groups: (1) fibrae longitudinalis superficialis, (2) fibrae longitudinalis profundi, (3) fibrae transversae, and (4) fibrae perpendiculares. The superficial longitudinal fibers lie directly deep to the dorsal mucosa of the organ and are well developed. The transverse and oblique fibers form a rather wide zone deep to the superficial longitudinal bundles. The perpendicular group are primarily near the median plane of the tongue. A few long muscle strands lie ventral to the previously mentioned zone and compose the deep longitudinal muscle. Thus the muscle bundles run in diverse directions.

Action: To protrude the tongue and bring about complicated intrinsic, local movements; to prevent the tongue from being bitten. The tongue functions in mastication, deglutition, and vocalization as well as serving as the primary organ of taste. Bennett and Hutchinson (1946) have discussed the action of the tongue in the dog.

For the complete structure of the tongue see Chapter 7, The Digestive Apparatus and Abdomen.

Muscles of the Pharynx

The muscles of the pharynx are primarily associated with the laryngopharynx and include the hyopharyngeus, thyropharyngeus, cricopharyngeus, stylopharyngeus, palatopharyngeus, and pterygopharyngeus. These are all innervated by pharyngeal branches of the glossopharyngeal and vagal nerves (*ramus pharyngeus, n. glossopharyngeus et vagus*). The hyopharyngeus, thyropharyngeus, and cricopharyngeus are often referred to as the *constrictors* of the pharynx. See Figs. 6.15 to 6.18 and 6.21.

The ***m. hyopharyngeus*** has two parts based on their separate hyoid bone origin. The larger part arises from the lateral surface of the thyrohyoid bone under cover of the hyoglossal muscle. The smaller part arises from the

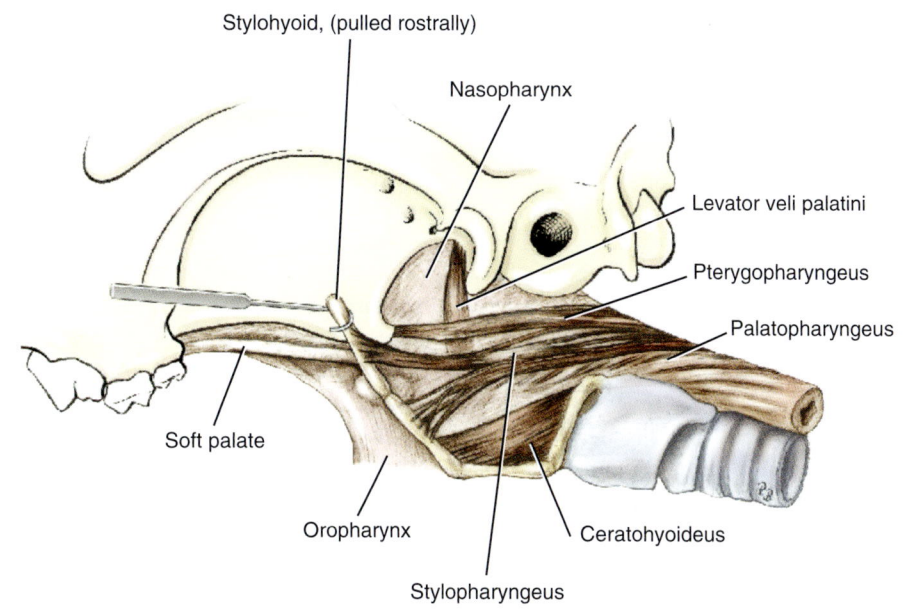

- **Fig. 6.17** Muscles of the pharynx and palate, deep dissection, lateral aspect.

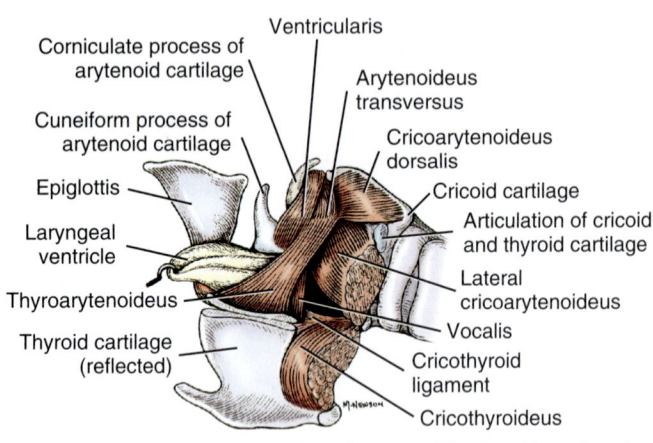

Fig. 6.18 Laryngeal muscles, lateral aspect. (The thyroid cartilage is cut left of midline and reflected.)

ceratohyoid bone. The muscle fibers of both parts form a muscle plate, the fibers of which pass dorsally over the larynx and pharynx to be inserted on the medial dorsal raphe of the pharynx, opposite the insertions of the muscles of the opposite side. Near their insertions the caudal fibers are overlaid by inserting fibers of the m. thyropharyngeus. The m. hyopharyngeus is the most rostral pharyngeal constrictor.

Action: To constrict the rostral part of the pharynx.

The *m. thyropharyngeus* lies on the larynx and pharynx just caudal to the hyopharyngeus muscle. It arises from the oblique line on the lamina of the thyroid cartilage and goes dorsally and rostrally over the dorsal border of the thyroid lamina. The fibers spread out over the dorsal surface of the pharynx and insert on the median dorsal raphe of the pharynx, just caudal to the m. hyopharyngeus. Some of the most rostral fibers of insertion overlie fibers of the m. hyopharyngeus.

Action: To constrict the middle part of the pharynx.

The *m. cricopharyngeus* lies on the larynx and pharynx immediately caudal to the m. thyropharyngeus. It arises from the lateral surface of the cricoid cartilage and passes dorsally to be inserted on the median dorsal raphe. As the muscle fibers pass over the dorsal wall of the pharynx they blend, at their caudal margin, with muscle fibers of the esophagus.

Action: To constrict the caudal part of the pharynx.

The *m. stylopharyngeus* is a small muscle that extends from the stylohyoid bone to the rostrodorsal wall of the pharynx. In most specimens the fibers arise from the caudal border of the proximal end of the stylohyoid bone. On some specimens, however, a few fibers arise on the epihyoid bone. From their origin the fibers run caudally and medially deep to the constrictor muscles on the dorsolateral wall of the pharynx, where they are loosely arranged and intermingle with fibers of the m. palatopharyngeus.

Action: To dilate, elevate, and draw the pharynx rostrally.

The *m. palatopharyngeus* is a poorly developed muscle, medial to the m. tensor veli palatini, whose fibers are loosely associated as they encircle the pharynx. Dyce (1957) divides the muscle into a dorsal and ventral portion. Most of the fibers arise from the soft palate and sweep obliquely dorsal and caudal over the pharynx to the mid-dorsal line. Some fibers of the mm. pterygopharyngeus and stylopharyngeus blend with the m. palatopharyngeus on the dorsal wall of the pharynx. A few fibers run rostrally from their palatine origin and are dispersed in the soft palate, nearly as far rostral as the hamulus of the pterygoid bone.

Action: To constrict the pharynx and draw it rostral and dorsal.

The *m. pterygopharyngeus* arises from the hamulus of the pterygoid bone, passes caudally lateral to the m. levator veli palatini, and continues dorsally over the pharynx to be inserted on the mid-dorsal raphe. Its fibers are intermixed with fibers of the m. palatopharyngeus and the m. stylopharyngeus as they radiate toward their insertions.

Action: To constrict the pharynx and draw it rostrally.

Muscles of the Soft Palate

The muscles of the soft palate are closely associated with the muscles of the pharynx and include the tensor veli palatini, levator veli palatini, and the palatinus. See Figs. 6.16 and 6.17. These muscles are considered essential during swallowing, as well as for pneumatization of the auditory tube and middle ear (Sánchez-Collado et al., 2013).

The *m. tensor veli palatini* is a very small muscle that arises from the muscular process at the rostral margin of the tympanic bulla. From its origin it passes ventrally over the wall of the nasopharynx to the hamulus of the pterygoid bone. At the hamulus the muscular fibers become tendinous and pass over a trochlear ridge on the hamulus. In their distal course these tendinous fibers radiate medially and rostrally and are dispersed in the soft palate.

Action: To stretch the soft palate between the pterygoid bones, to expand the lumen of the nasopharynx.
Innervation: N. mandibularis from n. trigeminus.

The *m. levator veli palatini* is slightly larger than the m. tensor veli palatini. It arises from the muscular process adjacent to the tympanic bulla and passes ventrally and caudally on the wall of the nasopharynx. In its distal course it passes between the m. palatopharyngeus and the m. pterygopharyngeus and radiates to its insertion on the caudal half of the soft palate lateral to the m. palatinus.

Action: To raise the caudal part of the soft palate.
Innervation: Ramus pharyngeus, N. glossopharyngeus et vagus.

The *m. palatinus* (m. uvulae) is a small, straight muscle that runs longitudinally through the soft palate. It arises from the palatine process of the palatine bone and passes with its fellow to the caudal free border of the soft palate. In the dog, the m. palatinus is 98% fast twitch (see Sánchez-Collado et al., 2013).

Action: To shorten the palate and curl the caudal border ventrally, narrowing the intrapharyngeal ostium.
Innervation: Ramus pharyngeus, N. glossopharyngeus et vagus.

Muscles of the Larynx

The larynx, which has evolved from primitive gill arch supports, serves as a protective sphincter mechanism in addition to subserving the function of sound production. The intrinsic muscles of the larynx are innervated by branches of the accessory and vagus nerves. The m. cricothyroideus is innervated by the ramus externus of the n. laryngeus cranialis. All other intrinsic muscles receive their motor supply via the n. laryngeus caudalis, the terminal portion of the n. laryngeus recurrens. The motor axons in the recurrent laryngeal nerve originate from the medulla as branches of the accessory nerve that join the vagus nerve as the latter leaves the cranial cavity (see Chapter 19). Laryngeal muscle innervation in the dog has been investigated by Vogel (1952). Pressman and Kelemen (1955) have reviewed the anatomy and physiology of the larynx in a variety of animals. Piérard (1963) studied the comparative anatomy of the larynx in the dog and other carnivores. Duckworth (1912) considered the plica vocalis and the tendency for subdivision of the thyroarytenoideus muscle mass in the dog and other animals. Hoh (2005) has reviewed the histochemical and biochemical properties of laryngeal muscles. See Figs. 6.18 to 6.20).

The *m. cricothyroideus* (Fig. 6.18) is a thick muscle on the lateral surface of the larynx between the thyroid lamina and the cricoid cartilage. From its attachment on the lateral surface of the cricoid cartilage (ventral to the cricothyroid articulation), it runs dorsally and cranially to attach to the caudal margin and medial surface of the thyroid cartilage. Some cranial fibers may attach ventrally close to the origin of the m. vocalis. Three neuromuscular compartments have been described in the dog's m. cricothyroideus (Zaretsky & Sanders, 1992).

Action: To pivot the cricoid cartilage on its thyroid articulation, thus tensing the vocal cords.

The *m. cricoarytenoideus dorsalis* (Figs. 6.18 and 6.20) arises from the entire length of the dorsolateral surface of the cricoid cartilage. The fibers run craniolaterally and converge at their insertion on the muscular process of the arytenoid cartilage. A few of the most lateral fiber bundles blend with the m. thyroarytenoideus. Three neuromuscular compartments have been identified in the dog's m. cricoarytenoideus dorsalis. The function of the three heads was assessed by Sanders et al. (1993) based on anatomic position and histochemical profiles. The three heads may each contribute mostly to vocal fold abduction during exercise, arytenoid stabilization, or medial to lateral translation of the arytenoid seen during quiet inspiration; however, EMG data were not available.

Action: To open the glottis by abducting the vocal folds.

The *m. cricoarytenoideus lateralis* (Figs. 6.18 and 6.19) arises from the lateral and cranial surface of the cricoid cartilage. Its fibers pass dorsally and slightly cranially to insert on the muscular process of the arytenoid cartilage between the m. cricoarytenoideus dorsalis dorsally and the m. vocalis ventrally.

Action: To pivot the arytenoid cartilage medially and close the rima glottis.

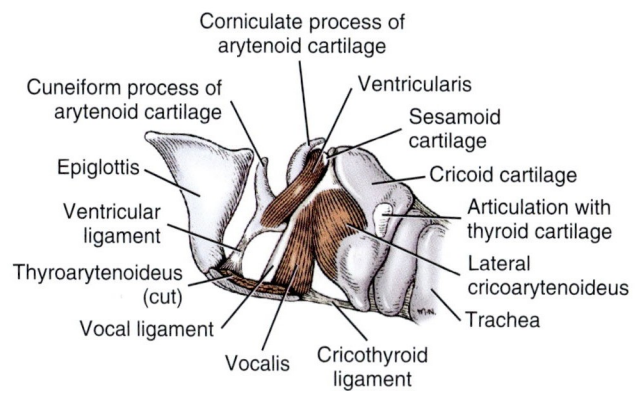

• **Fig. 6.19** Laryngeal muscles, lateral aspect. (The thyroid cartilage is cut left of midline and removed; the mm. thyroarytenoideus, arytenoideus transversus, and cricoarytenoideus dorsalis have also been removed.)

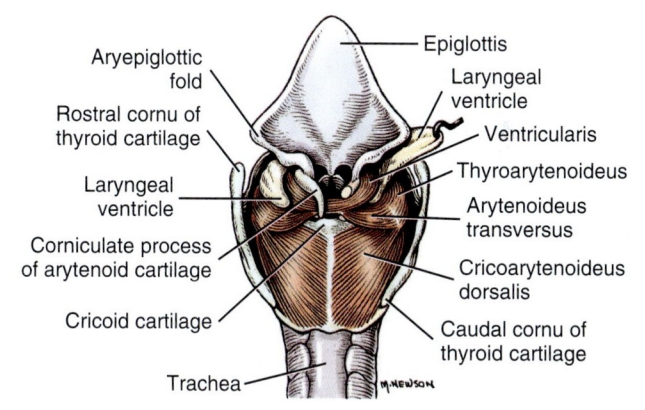

• **Fig. 6.20** Laryngeal muscles, dorsal aspect. (The right corniculate cartilage has been cut, and the right laryngeal ventricle is reflected.)

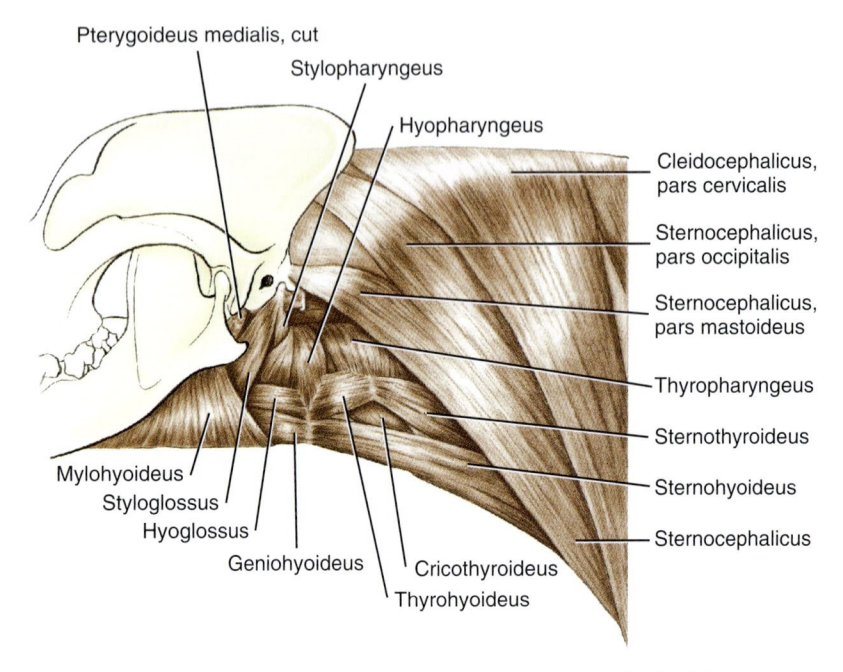

• **Fig. 6.21** The hyoid muscles and muscles of the neck, lateral aspect. (Stylohyoideus and digastricus removed.)

The **m. thyroarytenoideus** (Figs. 6.18 and 6.19) is the parent muscle mass that has given rise to the m. ventricularis and the m. vocalis. It originates along the internal midline of the thyroid cartilage and passes caudodorsally to insert on the arytenoid cartilage at the raphe, which represents the origin of the m. arytenoideus transversus. Dorsally the m. thyroarytenoideus (m. thyroarytenoideus externus of some authors) sends a few fibers to the m. ventricularis rostrally and to the m. cricoarytenoideus dorsalis caudally. The major middle portion of the m. thyroarytenoideus blends with the aponeurosis of the m. arytenoideus transversus superficially and attaches to the muscular process of the arytenoid cartilage deeply. A slower complement of myosin heavy chain isoforms was found in the more medial portions of the muscle (m. vocalis) compared with its lateral or rostral regions (Bergrin et al., 2006; Wu et al., 2000).

Action: To relax the vocal cord and constrict the glottis.

The **m. vocalis** (Figs. 6.18 and 6.19) is a medial division of the original thyroarytenoid muscle mass. It is also known as the m. thyroarytenoideus aboralis (Nickel et al., 1954) or the thyroarytenoideus internus. The m. vocalis originates on the internal midline of the thyroid cartilage medial and partly caudal to the m. thyroarytenoideus. It inserts on the vocal process of the arytenoid cartilage, its greatest bulk being on the lateral side. Attached along the cranial border of the m. vocalis is the vocal ligament, which can be distinguished grossly by its lighter color and finer texture.

Action: To draw the arytenoid cartilage ventrally, thus relaxing the vocal cord.

The **m. ventricularis** (Fig. 6.19) is a cranial division of the thyroarytenoid muscle mass, which has shifted its origin in the dog from the thyroid cartilage to the cuneiform process of the arytenoid cartilage. It is also known as the *thyroarytenoideus oralis* (Nickel et al., 1954). The m. ventricularis lies medial to the laryngeal ventricle and possibly aids in dilating the ventricle. From its ventral origin on the cuneiform process, the ventricularis passes dorsally and slightly caudally to insert on the dorsal surface of the interarytenoid cartilage, where it meets its fellow of the opposite side. Occasionally an unpaired cartilage is present on the dorsal midline, dorsal to the interarytenoid cartilage, onto which the bulk of the fibers may insert. The m. ventricularis receives some connecting fibers from the cranial dorsal surface of the m. thyroarytenoideus.

Action: To constrict the glottis and dilate the laryngeal ventricle.

The **m. arytenoideus transversus** (Fig. 6.20) originates broadly on the muscular process of the arytenoid cartilage at the line of insertion of the thyroarytenoideus. It inserts on the lateral expanded ends and dorsal surface of the interarytenoid cartilage, meets its fellow fibers from the opposite side, and blends with the more dorsally located m. ventricularis, which spans the midline.

Action: To constrict the glottis and adduct the vocal folds.

The **m. hyoepiglotticus**, a small, spindle-shaped muscle, arises from the medial surface of the ceratohyoid bone. It passes medially to the midline, then turns dorsally and passes to the ventral midline of the epiglottis to be inserted. The fibers of fellow muscles blend into a common tendon of insertion, which fades into the ventral surface of the epiglottis.

Action: To draw the epiglottis ventrally.

Muscles of the Hyoid Apparatus

The muscles of the hyoid apparatus include the sternohyoideus, sternothyroideus, thyrohyoideus, mylohyoideus, ceratohyoideus, geniohyoideus, occiptiohyoideus, and stylohyoideus. Collectively they are innervated by the trigeminal, facial, glossopharyngeal, and cervical spinal nerves. See Figs. 6.15, 6.22 to 6.25, and 6.45.

The ***m. sternohyoideus*** is a straplike muscle that arises from the dorsal surface of the manubrium sterni and the cranial edge of the first costal cartilage. It lies in contact with its fellow, and together they extend cranially in the neck, covering the ventral surface of the trachea, to be inserted on the basihyoid bone. At its origin, and throughout its caudal third, the dorsal surface of the m. sternohyoideus is fused to the m. sternothyroideus. The caudal third of the m. sternohyoideus is covered by the m. sternocephalicus, and, in specimens in which there is a decussation of fibers between the sternocephalic muscles, the caudal two-thirds of the muscle will be covered by these cross fasciculi. The cranial portion of the muscle that is not covered by the m. sternocephalicus is the most ventral muscle of that portion of the neck, except for the platysma. A transverse fibrous intersection separates the caudal third from the cranial two-thirds of the muscle.

Occasionally, muscle slips arise from the transverse fibrous intersection of the m. sternohyoideus and pass cranially in the neck to be inserted half in the stylohyoideus muscle, just lateral to the basihyoid bone, and half in the digastricus muscle at the angle of the mandible. The m. digastricus may be considerably smaller than normal and separated by a short intermediate tendon, as is the homologous muscle of man and horse. Leahy (1949) and Evans (1959) have described unilateral and bilateral anomalous slips in the dog.

Action: To pull the basihyoid bone and tongue caudally.
Innervation: Ramus ventralis of nn. cervicales and sometimes hypoglossal nerve (Benson & Fletcher, 1971).

The ***m. sternothyroideus*** lies dorsal to the m. sternohyoideus and has a similar tendinous intersection that divides the muscle into cranial and caudal portions. The m. sternothyroideus arises from the first costal cartilage and passes cranially in the neck covered by the m. sternocephalicus. Although smaller than the m. sternohyoideus, it covers more of the lateral surface of the trachea. It inserts on the lateral surface of the thyroid lamina.

Action: To draw the hyoid apparatus, larynx, and tongue caudally.
Innervation: Ramus ventralis of nn. cervicales.

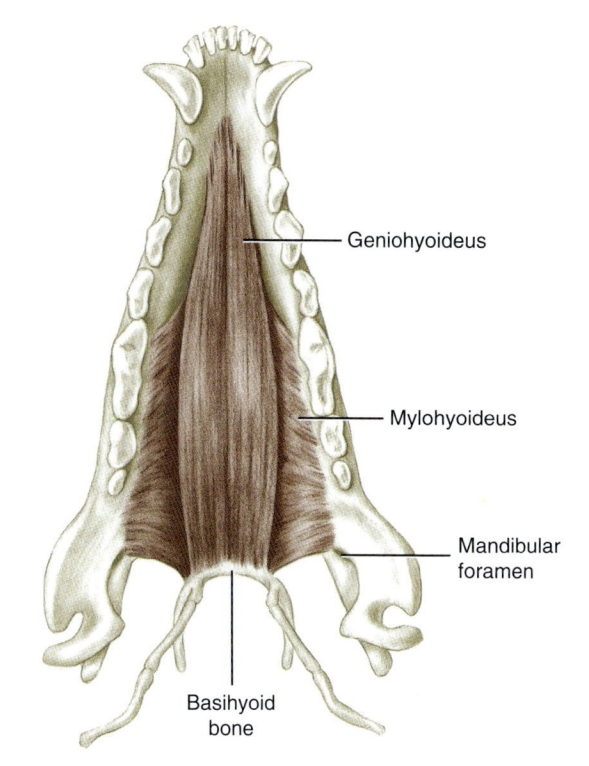

• **Fig. 6.22** Muscles of mandible and basihyoid bone, dorsal aspect.

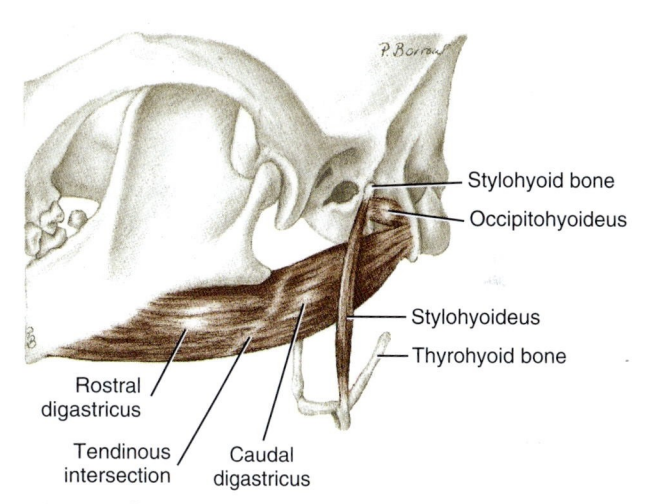

• **Fig. 6.23** Superficial hyoid muscles and the digastricus, lateral aspect.

The ***m. thyrohyoideus*** originates on the lamina of the thyroid cartilage. At the thyroid attachment it is bordered dorsally by the insertion of the m. thyropharyngeus and caudally by the mm. cricothyroideus and sternothyroideus. Its fibers pass obliquely rostrally and ventrally, over the surface of the thyroid lamina, to be inserted along most of the caudal border of the thyrohyoid bone.

Action: To draw the hyoid apparatus caudally and dorsally.
Innervation: Primarily n. hypoglossus and occasionally the first cervical nerve.

The ***m. mylohyoideus*** lies most ventrally in the intermandibular space. Together with the muscle of the opposite

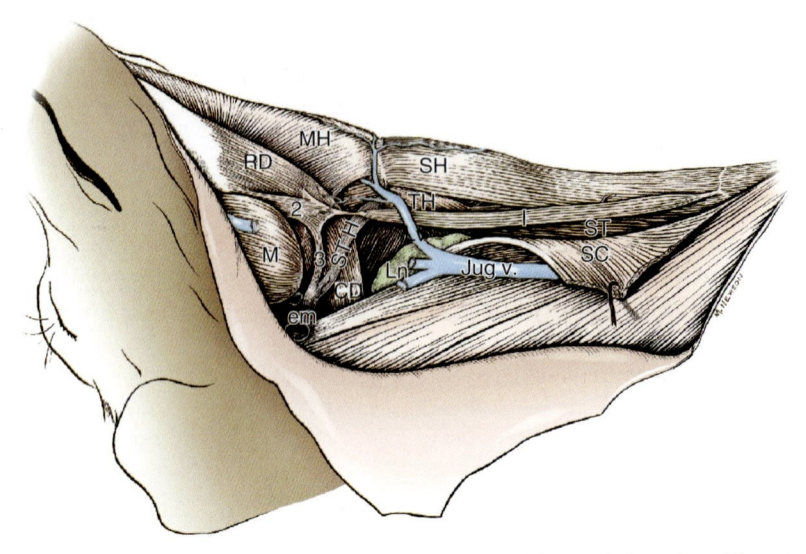

• **Fig. 6.24** Lateral view of anomalous slips of the sternohyoideus *(1)*, rostral digastricus *(2)*, and stylohyoideus *(3)*. (From Evans HE: Hyoid muscle anomalies in the dog, *Canis familiaris*, *Anat Rec* 133:145–162, Wiley-Liss, 1959. *CD*, Caudal digastricus; *em*, external acoustic meatus; *Jug v*, external jugular vein; *Ln*, medial retropharyngeal lymph node; *M*, masseter; *MH*, mylohyoideus; *RD*, rostral digastricus; *SC*, sternocephalicus; *SH*, sternohyoideus; *ST*, sternothyroideus; *STH*, stylohyoideus; *TH*, thyrohyoideus.

side, it forms a sling for the tongue. It has a long origin from the medial side of the mandible. In most specimens the most rostral fibers are opposite the first inferior premolar tooth, and the most caudal fibers are slightly caudal to the last inferior molar tooth. From its origin the muscle fibers extend medially, forming a thin plate that is inserted largely on a median fibrous raphe with its fellow of the opposite side. The most rostral fibers curve and insert on the midline farther rostral than their point of origin. A few of the most caudal fibers curve and pass caudally, to be inserted on the basihyoid bone. The dorsal surface of the muscle is related to the m. geniohyoideus, the tongue, and the oral mucosa.

Action: To raise the floor of the mouth and draw the hyoid apparatus rostrally.
Innervation: N. mandibularis from n. trigeminus.

The ***m. ceratohyoideus*** is a small triangular plate of muscle, one side of which attaches to the rostral border of the thyrohyoid bone. The fibers run rostroventrally from the thyrohyoid bone to the ceratohyoid bone, to be attached along the dorsal border of the bone. In some specimens a few fibers attach to the ventral end of the epihyoid bone. The medial surface of the muscle is related to the root of the tongue and the oral mucosa, and the lateral surface is related to the m. hyopharyngeus.

Action: To decrease the angle formed by the thyrohyoid and ceratohyoid bones.
Innervation: N. glossopharyngeus.

The ***m. geniohyoideus*** is a fusiform muscle that extends from the intermandibular articulation parallel to the midventral line, to the basihyoid bone. It arises by a short tendon from the intermandibular articulation and, muscularly, from the medial surface of the mandible adjacent to the articulation. It passes directly caudad, at first bordered on the lateral side by the m. genioglossus and in its further course by the m. mylohyoideus, which also covers much of its ventral surface. Throughout its length the muscle is in close contact with its fellow of the opposite side. It is inserted on the rostral border of the basihyoid bone.

The m. geniohyoideus appears to act synergistically with other cranial airway muscles to dilate the nasopharynx (Strohl et al., 1987). As such, it performs an important role in breathing as well as during mastication and swallowing (Lakars & Herring, 1987). In cats, the m. geniohyoideus has a fast-twitch contraction profile as assayed by histochemistry and in vitro physiology (Van Lunteren et al., 1990). In awake dogs, m. geniohyoideus showed minimal correlation of EMG activity or of fiber length changes with phasic quiet breathing. However, there was a marked increase of EMG activity and phasic fiber shortening and lengthening during swallowing (Yakoba et al., 2003).

Action: To draw the hyoid apparatus cranially as during swallowing and to maintain a patent airway.
Innervation: N. hypoglossus.

The ***m. stylohyoideus*** is a narrow muscle bundle that proceeds from the tympanohyoid and proximal end of the stylohyoid obliquely across the lateral surface of the m. digastricus to the lateral end of the basihyoid. It inserts by means of a small terminal tendon or aponeurosis that is intimately related to the hyoglossus or mylohyoideus, or both, rostrally and the sternohyoideus caudally. Over much of its course the muscle is hidden from view by the

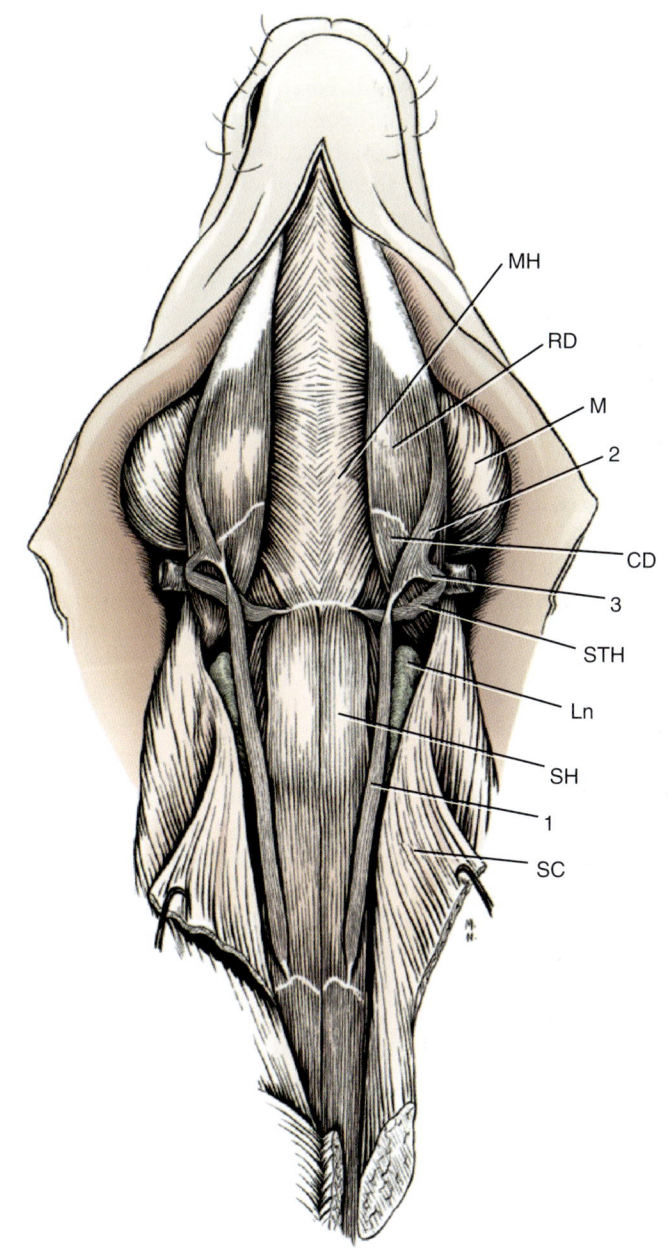

• **Fig. 6.25** Ventral view of anomalous slips of hyoid muscles: sternohyoideus *(1)*, rostral digastricus *(2)*, and stylohyoideus *(3)*. (From Evans HE: Hyoid muscle anomalies in the dog, *Canis familiaris*, *Anat Rec* 133:145–162, 1959. Wiley-Liss.) *CD*, Caudal digastricus; *Ln*, medial retropharyngeal lymph node; *M*, masseter; *MH*, mylohyoideus; *RD*, rostral digastricus; *SC*, sternocephalicus; *SH*, sternohyoideus; *STH*, stylohyoideus.

with the digastricus, mylohyoideus, sternohyoideus, or subhyoidean septum

Action: To raise the basihyoid bone.
Innervation: N. facialis.

The **m. occipitohyoideus** (jugulohyoideus or jugulostyloideus of some authors) is a small rectangular muscle that extends from the paracondylar process of the occiput to the cartilaginous tympanohyoid and proximal end of the stylohyoid. The muscle is partly covered by the cranial end of the mastoid part of the m. sternocephalicus. The m. occipitohyoideus arises on the laterally projecting caudal border, whereas the m. digastricus attaches to the knobby end of the paracondylar process.

Action: To move the stylohyoid bone caudally.
Innervation: N. facialis.

Muscles of the Cervical Vertebrae

At its cranial end the cervical vertebral column serves special functions. There is a corresponding special development of the first two cervical vertebrae, as well as of their joints. The specialized musculature dorsal and ventral to the atlas and axis is adapted to these special functions. The **m. rectus capitis** that runs between regions on the spinous process of the axis, the atlas, and the occipital bone can be compared with the m. interspinalis. There are also two oblique muscles, the mm. obliquus capitis caudalis and cranialis, that can be considered modifications of the m. multifidus or derivatives of the m. intertransversarius. There are six cervical vertebral muscles that insert on the skull and are included with the muscles of the head. These are the rectus capitis ventralis, rectus capitis dorsalis major, rectus capitis dorsalis minor, rectus capitis lateralis, obliquus capitis cranialis, and obliquus capitis caudalis.

The **m. rectus capitis ventralis** (see Fig. 6.28) is a short, thick muscle that lies dorsal to the cranial portion of the m. longus capitis. It extends from the ventral arch of the atlas to the basioccipital bone. As it crosses the atlantooccipital joint, it converges somewhat with its fellow of the opposite side.

Action: Flexion of the atlantooccipital joint.
Innervation: Ramus ventralis of the n. cervicalis 1.

The **m. rectus capitis dorsalis major** (see Fig. 6.31) is a thick, almost triangular muscle. It is covered by the m. semispinalis capitis as it runs between the spinous process of the axis and the squama of the occipital bone. It arises cranial to the attachment of the ligamentum nuchae on the caudal end of the spinous process of the axis, and it ends on the ventrolateral part of the squamous occipital bone. The dorsal portion of the m. obliquus capitis cranialis, which lies on the border of the wing of the atlas, also inserts on the ventrolateral part of the occipital bone.

mandibular gland. Occasionally the muscle divides into two bellies as it crosses the tendinous intersection of the digastricus. Huber (1923) noted the tendency toward reduction of the stylohyoideus and the possible elimination of this muscle in the dog. Evans (1959) described loss and anomaly of the hyoid muscles in mongrels and Beagles that reflected the phylogenetic history of the muscles. The stylohyoideus was frequently absent bilaterally or unilaterally, particularly in Beagles, and also exhibited secondary slips or fusions

The ***m. rectus capitis dorsalis minor*** is a short, flat muscle, lying between the atlas and the occipital bone on the capsule of the atlantooccipital joint immediately next to its fellow of the opposite side. It arises on the cranial edge of the dorsal arch of the atlas and inserts dorsal to the foramen magnum near or on the ventral portion of the occipital crest where it fuses with the m. rectus capitis dorsalis major.

Action: Both rectus dorsalis muscles extend the atlantooccipital joint.
Innervation: Ramus dorsalis of n. cervicalis 1.

The ***m. rectus capitis lateralis*** is a small muscle that lies lateral to the m. rectus capitis ventralis (separated from it by the ventral branch of the first cervical nerve). It originates on the ventral surface of the caudal half of the wing of the atlas (lateral to the m. rectus capitis ventralis); it passes sagittally toward the cranium ventral to the atlantooccipital joint and inserts on the base of the paracondylar process of the occipital bone. This muscle can be considered a special portion of the m. intertransversarius ventralis.

Action: Flexion of the atlantooccipital joint.
Innervation: Ramus ventralis of n. cervicalis 1.

The ***m. obliquus capitis cranialis*** (Fig. 6.31) extends obliquely craniomedially dorsal to the atlantooccipital joint; it lies medial to the m. splenius and can be divided into two portions. The principal part arises on the lateroventral surface and lateral border of the wing of the atlas. Inclined dorsomedially, it passes dorsal to the paracondylar process and inserts on the mastoid part of the temporal bone and from there on the nuchal crest. The accessory portion is a superficial flat belly that takes its origin on the lateral border of the wing of the atlas and, provided with tendinous leaves, inserts between the principal portion and the m. rectus capitis dorsalis major on the nuchal crest.

Action: Extension of the atlantooccipital joint.
Innervation: Ramus dorsalis or n. cervicalis 1.

The ***m. obliquus capitis caudalis*** (see Fig. 6.31) is a thick, flat muscle lying medial to the mm. semispinalis capitis and splenius dorsal to the axis and atlas. It arises along the entire spinous process and the caudal articular process of the axis and runs obliquely craniolaterally dorsal to the capsule of the atlantoaxial joint to insert on the border of the wing of the atlas near the alar notch.

Action: Unilateral: rotation of the atlas and thus the head on the axis; bilateral: fixation of the atlantoaxial joint.
Innervation: Rami dorsales of the nn. cervicales 1 and 2.

Fasciae of the Head

The **superficial fascia of the head** lies directly deep to the skin; for the most part it is easily displaceable, but in the muzzle it fuses with the skin. It contains the cutaneous muscles of the head, portions of the platysma, and the m. sphincter colli profundus. It covers the entire head like a mask and continues on the neck like a cylinder. It is divided into the following regions: buccopharyngeal, masseteric, parotid, and temporal. In many places the special nerves and vessels for the skin pass through the superficial fascia of the head.

The **temporal fascia** (*fascia temporalis*) contains the frontalis muscle and conceals the muscles of the scutular group as well as the scutiform cartilage itself. Medially it goes into the superficial temporal fascia of the other side without attaching to the median system of cranial ridges. Rostrally it continues over the orbital ligament to the eyelids and from there into the nasofrontal region where it contains the levator nasolabialis and spreads to the nose and superior lip. Ventrally it is continuous with the buccopharyngeal, masseteric, and parotid fascia.

The **buccopharyngeal fascia** (*fascia buccopharyngea*) contains the buccal portions of the platysma and the sphincter colli profundus and covers the buccinator and the large facial vessels and nerves. The parotid duct is loosely surrounded by buccopharyngeal fascia as it lies caudal to the labial commissure. The fascia spreads out into the lips. It is continuous dorsally with temporal fascia and caudally with masseteric fascia. Ventromedially it extends into the intermandibular space with the masseteric fascia where it covers the mylohyoideus and the basihyoid bone.

The **masseteric fascia** (*fascia masseterica*) covers the masseter muscle and contains the buccal branches of the facial nerve and the parotid duct. Dorsally this fascia is continuous over the zygomatic arch into the superficial temporal fascia and spreads out on the pinna of the ear. It contains portions of m. sphincter colli profundus and the platysma. It extends ventrally and rostrally with the buccopharyngeal fascia into the intermandibular space.

The **parotid fascia** (*fascia parotidea*) covers the parotid region, which includes the mandibular and parotid glands and the superficial vessels here. It contains the portions of the platysma and sphincter colli profundus that are located there and is continuous rostrally with the masseteric fascia and caudally with the cervical fascia.

Deep fascia is especially well developed where it covers the temporal and masseter muscles. The **deep temporal fascia** (*fascia temporalis profunda*) is thick as it covers the temporal muscle and spreads out and attaches to the temporal line, external sagittal crest, nuchal crest, and the zygomatic arch. If a part of the parietal bone is not covered by the temporal muscle, as frequently occurs in brachycephalic breeds, then this fascia fuses with the periosteum of the bone. Ventrally the deep temporal fascia passes over the zygomatic arch and the masseter as the **deep masseteric fascia** (*fascia masseterica profunda*). It then spreads over the m. buccinator, extends into both lips, and passes over the mandible and larynx, as the **deep buccopharyngeal fascia** (*fascia buccopharyngea*). From the masseter muscle caudally, the **deep parotid fascia** passes around the parotid gland, crosses the digastricus, and passes deep to the mandibular gland and thence into the deep cervical fascia. Everywhere on the head the deep fascia lies deep to the large superficial vessels.

Muscles of the Neck

The muscles of the neck (*musculi colli*) included here are those muscles that are primarily located in the neck with attachments to the head or thoracic limb. These include the brachiocephalicus, omotransversarius, sternocephalicus, splenius, longus capitis, longus colli, scalenus, and serratus ventralis cervicis. Architectural studies of neck muscles of dogs were conducted by Sharir et al. (2006) and document intra- and intermuscular differences in myofiber lengths and physiological cross-sectional areas as related to potential biomechanical modeling.

The **m. brachiocephalicus** (Figs. 6.21, 6.45, 6.48, 6.49) lying on the neck deep to the m. sphincter colli superficialis and platysma as a long, flat muscle, extends between the brachium and the head and neck. Cranial to the shoulder the muscle is traversed by a clavicular remnant, a transverse, often arched, fibrous intersection, plate, or tendon called the **clavicular intersection** (*intersectio clavicularis*). The vestigial clavicle is connected with the medial end of the clavicular intersection and lies deep to the muscle. The three portions of this muscle are named by their relationship to this clavicular intersection. The **m. cleidobrachialis**, 5 to 6 cm broad and 5 to 8 mm thick in large dogs, arises from a narrow part of the distal end of the cranial surface of the humerus. It passes between the m. brachialis, laterally, and m. biceps brachii, medially, and courses dorsocranially covering the cranial aspect of the shoulder joint cranially and somewhat laterally, ends on the clavicular tendon. No muscle fibers cross the clavicular intersection. The **m. cleidocephalicus**, which extends cranially in the neck from the clavicular tendon, is further divided into two portions. In the dog it divides into a thin **cervical part** (*pars cervicalis*), which broadens and gets thinner as it courses dorsocranially and attaches to the dorsal part of the neck (see Fig. 6.21). It serves as a cranial extension of the m. cleidobrachialis from the clavicular tendon to the dorsum of the neck. This cervical part inserts by an aponeurosis on the fibrous raphe of the cranial half of the neck. The **mastoid part** (*pars mastoideus*) is a deep ventromedial portion of the cleidocephalicus that extends from the clavicular intersection to the mastoid part of the temporal bone. It is covered by the cervical part of the cleidocephalicus and the occipital part of the sternocephalicus. It reaches a width of 2.5 to 3 cm and a thickness of 7 to 10 mm and is often split into two round bundles throughout its length. By means of a thick tendon it inserts on the mastoid part of the temporal bone with the mastoid part of the sternocephalicus, which lies ventral to it.

Action: To draw the limb cranially and, acting bilaterally, to fix the neck.

Innervation: M. cleidocephalicus: n. accessorius, rami ventrales of the nn. cervicales; m. cleidobrachialis: rami ventrales of nn. cervicales 6 and 7.

The **m. omotransversarius** (Figs. 6.46 and 6.48) lies lateral to the cervical vertebrae as a flat, narrow muscle. It arises on the distal portion of the scapular spine, as far as the acromion, and from that part of the omobrachial fascia that covers the acromial part of the m. deltoideus. It separates from the m. trapezius cervicis, passes deep to the pars cervicalis of the m. cleidocephalicus, and proceeds lateral to the mm. scalenus and the intertransversarius cervicalis, which cover the transverse processes of the cervical vertebrae dorsally. It terminates at the caudal border of the wing of the atlas. In large dogs it is at first as much as 4 cm wide and 2 to 4 mm thick; cranially it becomes narrower and thicker. Its ventral border is limited by the transverse processes of the cervical vertebrae.

Action: To draw the limb cranially.
Innervation: N. accessorius.

The **m. sternocephalicus** (Figs. 6.21, 6.45, and 6.48) in the dog can be separated into mastoid and occipital parts. In large dogs this flat muscle is 2.5 to 3.5 cm wide at the sternum and 10 to 14 mm thick. It arises as a unit on the manubrium sterni and, covered only by skin, runs to the mastoid part of the temporal bone and to the nuchal crest of the occipital bone. At their origin the muscles of the two sides are intimately joined, but they separate at or caudal to the middle of the neck, and each crosses deep to the external jugular vein of its own side and encroaches closely upon the ventral edge of the ipsilateral m. cleidocephalicus. The **mastoid part** (*pars mastoideus*) is the ventral portion that separates as a large, elliptical bundle that unites with the mastoid part of the cleidocephalicus in a large tendon that inserts on the mastoid part of the temporal bone. The broader, thinner, dorsal **occipital part** (*pars occipitalis*) attaches to the nuchal crest as far as the midline of the neck by means of a thin aponeurosis. Because of the divergence of the two sternocephalic muscles, there is a space ventral to the trachea in which the bilateral mm. sternohyoideus and sternothyroideus appear. Here in the deep cervical fascia, additional fibers for the mastoid part of the sternocephalicus may arise.

Action: To draw the head and neck to one side, lateral flexion.
Innervation: Ventral branches of cervical nerves and branches from accessory nerve (rami ventrales of the nn. cervicales et n. accessorius).

The **m. splenius capitis** (Fig. 6.27) is a flat, fleshy, triangular muscle with the caudal end as the apex and the cranial end as the base of the triangle. It lies on the dorsolateral portion of the neck, extending from the third thoracic vertebra to the skull. Its fibers run in a cranioventral direction and cover the mm. semispinalis capitis, longissimus capitis, and the terminal part of the m. spinalis et semispinalis dorsi. It arises by fleshy fibers from the dorsal end of the first and sometimes of the second thoracic spine, and from approximately 1 cm of the ligamentum nuchae immediately cranial to the first thoracic spine. A third point of origin is from the **median dorsal raphe** of the neck as far cranial as the first cervical vertebra. This tendinous raphe runs from the first thoracic spine, where it fuses with the ligamentum nuchae, cranially to the occipital bone. The final origin of the m. splenius is by an aponeurosis from the cranial border of the thoracolumbar fascia, which extends this muscle's origin caudally to the fifth or sixth thoracic spine. At the cranial border of the atlas the m. splenius is enclosed in a coarse aponeurosis, which inserts on the nuchal crest of the occipital bone and the mastoid part of the temporal bone. The m. splenius may occasionally send a prominent serration to the transverse process of the axis. At the lateral border of the atlas the dorsal surface of the m. longissimus capitis attaches firmly to the m. splenius and, by means of a strong tendon so formed, inserts along with the m. splenius on the mastoid part of the temporal bone.

The m. splenius in cats is composed of predominantly fast-twitch, type II muscle fibers, suggesting an important role in effecting quick responses of head position (Richmond & Abrahams, 1975a). Such observations are in line with the observation that head position is constantly changing during locomotion and that precise control of head and neck position is necessary to facilitate orientation by the vestibular and visual systems.

Action: To extend and raise the head and neck. In unilateral action to draw the head and neck laterally, lateral flexion. It also functions in fixation of the first thoracic vertebra.
Innervation: Nn. cervicales.

The ***m. longus capitis*** (Figs. 6.28 and 6.31) is a long, flat muscle that lies on the lateral and ventral sides of the cervical vertebrae lateral to the m. longus colli. It arises from the caudal branches of the transverse processes of the sixth to the second cervical vertebra and extends cranially to the axis, where it receives a large, tendinous leaf laterally. After crossing the atlantooccipital joint, it inserts (tendinous laterally, muscular medially) on the muscular tubercles of the basioccipital bone, between the tympanic bullae.

Action: To flex the atlantooccipital joint and to draw the neck ventrally.
Innervation: Rami ventrales of the nn. cervicales.

The ***m. longus colli*** (Fig. 6.28) is a long muscle composed of separate bundles; it lies adjacent to its contralateral fellow on the ventral surface of the bodies of the first six thoracic and all of the cervical vertebrae and thus is divided into thoracic and cervical portions. On the neck the bilateral muscle is enclosed by the right and the left m. longus capitis. The thoracic portion consists of three incompletely separated parts that arise on the concave ventral surfaces of the first six thoracic vertebrae. These portions, complicated in their make-up, are provided with tendinous coverings. Diverging cranially from those of the opposite side, the fibers of these three portions become partly tendinous laterally; the medial fibers insert immediately beside this tendon on the ventral border of the transverse processes of the sixth and seventh cervical vertebrae. The continuation of the cervical portion consists of four separate bundles. These bundles arise on the ventral border of the transverse process of the sixth to the third cervical vertebra and end on the ventral spine of the next preceding vertebra. The most cranial segment ends on the ventral tubercle of the atlas.

Action: To flex the neck.
Innervation: Rami ventrales of the nn. cervicales and nn. thoracici I to VI.

The ***m. scalenus*** (Figs. 6.26, 6.29) bridges the space between the first three ribs and the cervical vertebrae. The muscle is divided into two components: a large dorsal part and a medial part. Their origins on the transverse processes of cervical vertebrae are by distinct tendons. The dorsal scalenus arises from the transverse process of cervical vertebrae 4 through 6. It inserts on the lateral surface of the middle of ribs 2 through 8 where it is covered by the m. obliquus abdominis externus. The middle component, ***m. scalenus medius***, arises from the transverse processes of cervical vertebrae 6 and 7 and passes caudally to insert on the dorsal portion of the lateral surface of the first rib. A ventral component, ***m. scalenus ventralis***, which would pass ventral to the nerve roots of the brachial plexus, is not present in the dog. If present it arises from the transverse processes of cervical vertebrae 3 through 6. It consists of longitudinal fibers that pass caudally to insert on the cranial surface of the middle of the first rib.

Action: Inspiratory muscle. It acts by displacing the ribs cranially, which increases the transverse diameter of the thorax (De Troyer & Kelly, 1984). The muscle may act unilaterally to bend the neck laterally or flex the neck ventrally.

The ***m. serratus ventralis cervicis*** (Figs. 6.26 and 6.47) covers the caudal half of the lateral surface of the neck. It is a thick, fan-shaped muscle that arises on the facies serrata of the scapula, its fibers diverging to form an angle of approximately 150 degrees. It ends on the transverse processes of the last five cervical vertebrae as the *m. serratus ventralis cervicis*. This is continuous with a thoracic component, the *m. serratus ventralis thoracis*, that inserts on the first seven or eight ribs, somewhat ventral to their middle. This part of the serratus ventralis is described with the thoracic muscles. In large dogs the muscle is 1.5 to 2 cm thick near the scapula. The terminal serrated edge of the cervical portion is not sharply defined; the individual slips insert between the m. longissimus cervicis and the m. intertransversarius.

CHAPTER 6 The Muscular System   239

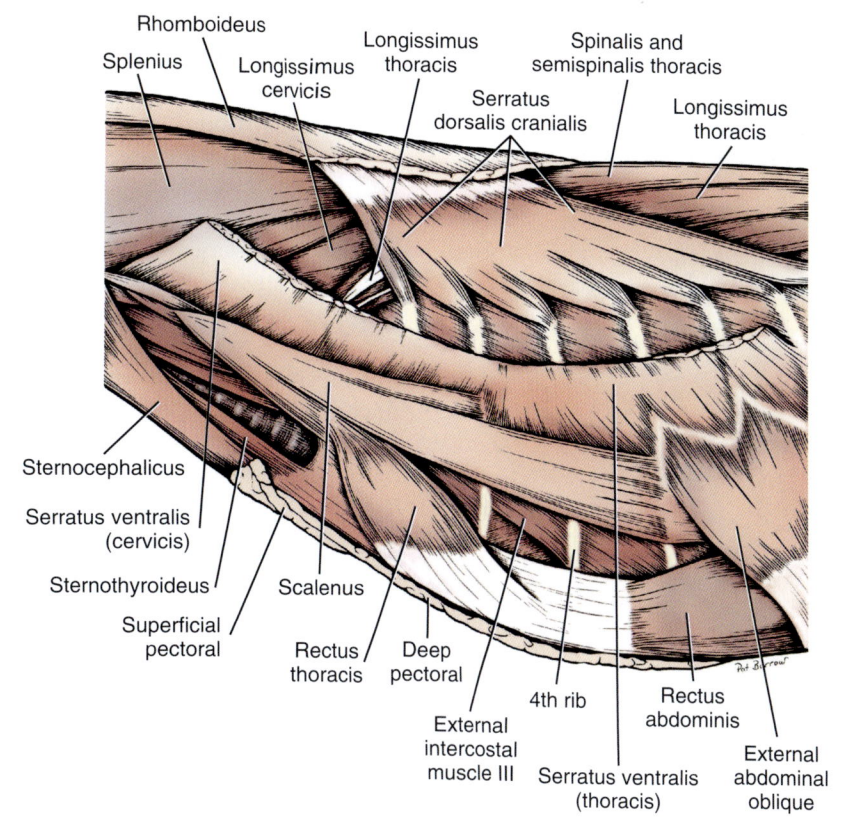

• **Fig. 6.26** Muscles of neck and thorax, lateral aspect.

Labels: Rhomboideus, Splenius, Longissimus cervicis, Longissimus thoracis, Spinalis and semispinalis thoracis, Serratus dorsalis cranialis, Longissimus thoracis, Sternocephalicus, Serratus ventralis (cervicis), Sternothyroideus, Superficial pectoral, Scalenus, Rectus thoracis, Deep pectoral, External intercostal muscle III, 4th rib, Serratus ventralis (thoracis), Rectus abdominis, External abdominal oblique.

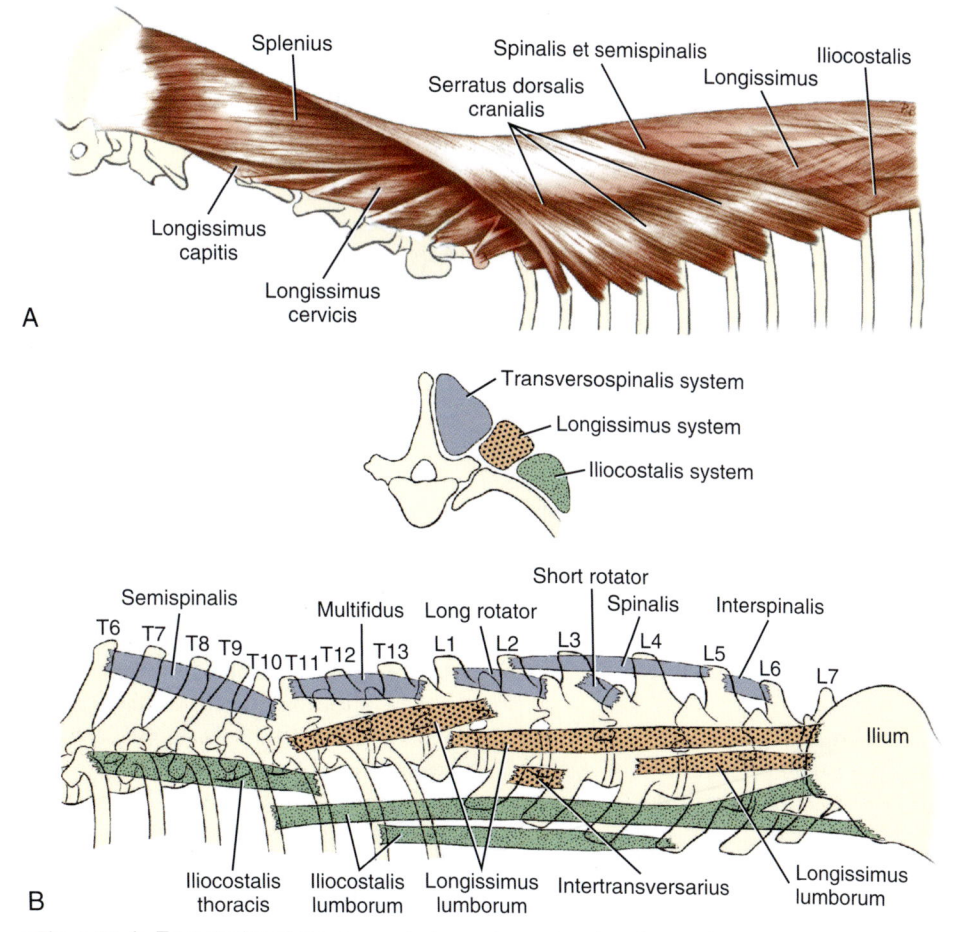

• **Fig. 6.27** A, Topography of the mm. splenius and serratus dorsalis cranialis. B, Schema of epaxial muscles. This is one schema for the organization of epaxial muscles. The text description follows that given in the NAV, which has some minor differences with the schema in this figure.

A labels: Splenius, Spinalis et semispinalis, Serratus dorsalis cranialis, Longissimus, Iliocostalis, Longissimus capitis, Longissimus cervicis.

Cross-section labels: Transversospinalis system, Longissimus system, Iliocostalis system.

B labels: Semispinalis, Multifidus, Long rotator, Short rotator, Spinalis, Interspinalis, T6, T7, T8, T9, T10, T11, T12, T13, L1, L2, L3, L4, L5, L6, L7, Ilium, Iliocostalis thoracis, Iliocostalis lumborum, Longissimus lumborum, Intertransversarius, Longissimus lumborum.

240 CHAPTER 6 The Muscular System

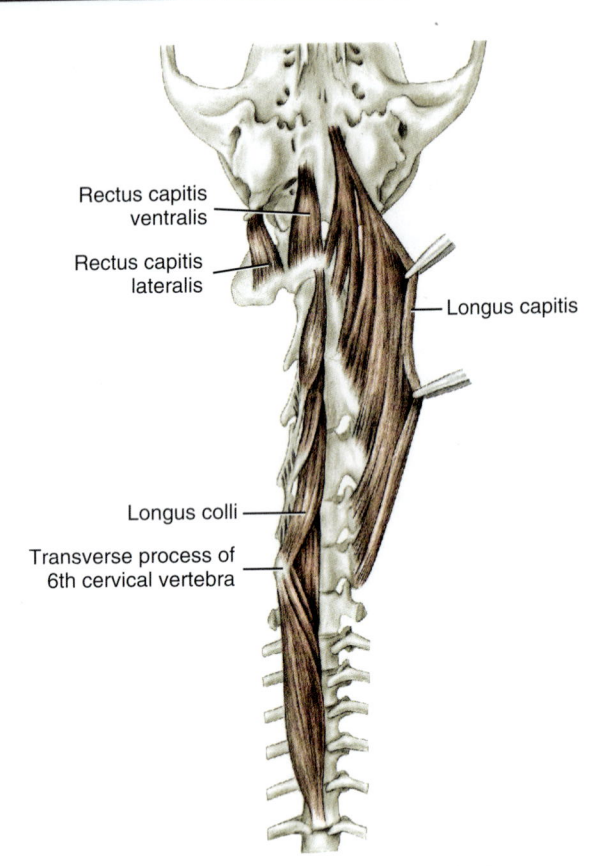

Fig. 6.28 Ventral muscles of the vertebral column.

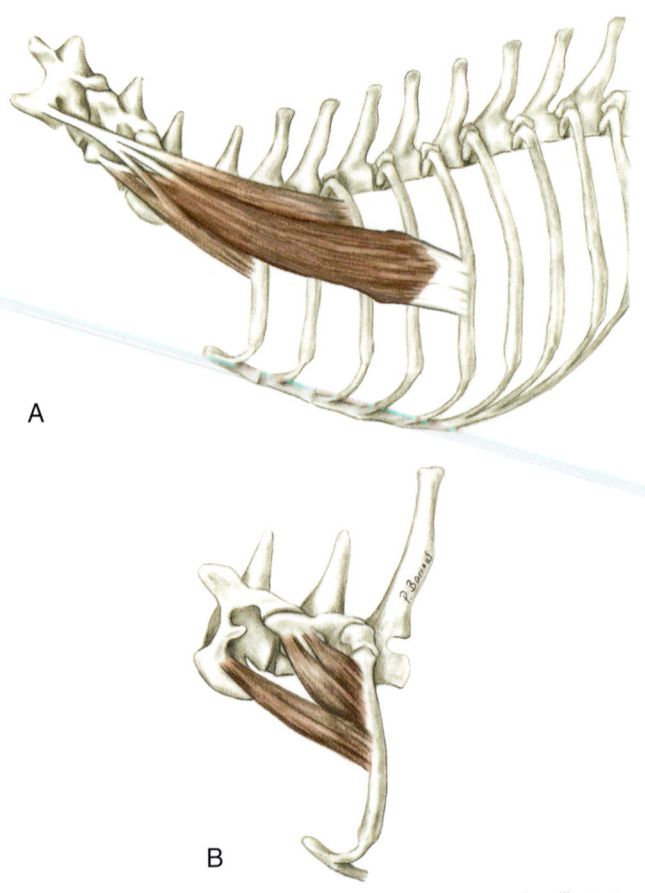

Fig. 6.29 The scalenus muscles. **A,** superficial. **B,** Deep view illustrating attachments along first rib. Part A redrawn by Talia Coppens.

Action: Support of the trunk, to carry the trunk cranially and caudally; inspiration; to carry the shoulder cranial and caudal with respect to the limb. In trotting dogs, the cervical portion of m. serratus ventralis was electrically active during the terminal part of the swing phase and throughout the early and middle portions of the ipsilateral stance phase (Carrier et al., 2006).
Innervation: Rami ventrales of nn. cervicales.

Fasciae of the Neck

The superficial and deep cervical fasciae are the direct continuations of the superficial and deep fasciae of the head. The **superficial fascia** (*lamina superficialis*) of the neck is cylindrical in form as it clothes the whole neck. It is thin, lies directly deep to the skin, and is easily displaced. It originates from the superficial temporal, parotid, and masseteric fasciae, and it continues caudally into the superficial scapular fascia and ventrally into the superficial trunk fascia of the sternal region and axillary fascia. It contains the m. sphincter colli superficialis and the platysma. With these, it covers the mm. trapezius, omotransversarius, cleidocephalicus, and sternocephalicus, and it bridges the external jugular vein that lies in the jugular groove. The bilateral portions of the fascia meet dorsally and ventrally. At the dorsal midline there is no special attachment to the underlying portions (median raphe) so that on the neck, just as on the trunk and pelvic region, this fascia can be lifted in a large fold with the skin. In many places the smaller cutaneous vessels and nerves pass through the superficial fascia.

The **deep fascia** (*lamina profunda*) of the neck is a dense layer that extends deep to the mm. sternocephalicus, cleidocephalicus, and omotransversarius. It covers the mm. sternohyoideus and sternothyroideus superficially and surrounds the trachea, thyroid gland, larynx, and esophagus. It passes over the large cervical vessels and nerves to the superficial surface of the mm. scalenus and longus colli. From these it goes to the superficial surface of the mm. serratus ventralis and rhomboideus, to end in the median raphe of the neck. The layer of deep fascia ventral to the trachea is the **pretracheal fascia** (*lamina pretrachealis*). It is continuous laterally with an extension of the deep fascia that forms the carotid sheath that is a special loose condensation of fascia in which the common carotid artery, internal jugular vein, tracheal duct, and the vagosympathetic trunk are located. Much loose connective tissue is accumulated around both the trachea and esophagus to provide them with a high degree of displaceability. The deep cervical fascia dorsal to the trachea on the ventral surface of the longus colli is the **prevertebral fascia** (*lamina prevertebralis*). Cranially, it is attached to the base of the head. Caudally, it continues with the mm. longi colli on the ventral surface of the first six thoracic vertebrae into the thorax to unite with the **endothoracic fascia** (*fascia endothoracica*).

Cranially, the deep cervical fascia passes deep to the mandibular and parotid glands and ends on the hyoid bone.

Deep to the salivary glands, the deep cervical fascia is united with the deep fascia of the m. masseter. Caudally, the dorsal part of the deep cervical fascia continues over the m. rhomboideus to the superficial surface of the scapula with its muscles and thus runs into the deep fascia of the scapular region. On the surfaces of the cervical parts of the mm. serratus ventralis and scalenus, the deep cervical fascia continues to the thoracic parts of these muscles medial to the scapula and shoulder to become the deep thoracic fascia. Ventral to the m. scalenus it attaches to the first rib and the manubrium sterni. The deep fascia sends various divisions between the layers of muscles of the neck. One of these is a thick leaf that passes medial to the cervical parts of the mm. serratus ventralis, trapezius, and rhomboideus but lateral to the m. splenius.

Muscles of the Dorsum

The muscles of the dorsum, **musculi dorsi**, include extrinsic muscles of the thoracic limb that attach to the thorax and the epaxial muscles that form a continuous column throughout most of the vertebral column. The extrinsic thoracic limb muscles include: trapezius, latissimus dorsi, and rhomboideus. The epaxial muscles are the serratus dorsalis, the erector spinae, transverso spinalis, interspinalis, and intertransversarii.

Extrinsic Thoracic Limb Muscles

The *m. trapezius* is a broad, thin, triangular muscle (Figs. 6.46 to 6.48). It lies deep to the skin and the caudal portion of the platysma in the neck. It arises from the median fibrous raphe of the neck and the supraspinous ligament of the thorax. Its origin extends from the third cervical vertebra to the ninth thoracic vertebra. The insertion is on the spine of the scapula. It is divided into a cervical and a thoracic portion by a tendinous band extending dorsally from the spine of the scapula.

The fibers of the comparatively narrow *pars cervicalis* arise on the mid-dorsal raphe of the neck. They run obliquely caudoventrally to the spine of the scapula, and end on the free edge of the spine. Only a small distal portion of the spine remains free for the attachment of the m. omotransversarius. The latter muscle cannot be separated from the ventral border of the trapezius near the spine.

The *pars thoracica* arises from the supraspinous ligament and the spinous process of the third to the eighth or ninth thoracic vertebra and by an aponeurosis that blends with the thoracolumbar fascia. Its fibers are directed cranioventrally and end on the proximal third of the spine of the scapula.

The fibrous band that divides the m. trapezius varies considerably. Sometimes it is lacking; sometimes it is broad and includes the dorsal border of the middle part of the entire muscle; sometimes it is interrupted. When it is present, it serves as a common attachment for the two parts of the m. trapezius.

Action: To elevate the limb and draw it cranially, to rotate the scapula.
Innervation: Dorsal branch of the n. accessorius.

The *m. latissimus dorsi* (Figs. 6.49B, 6.50A, and 6.52 is a flat, almost triangular muscle that lies caudal to the muscles of the scapula and brachium on the dorsal half of the lateral thoracic wall. It begins as a wide, tendinous leaf from the superficial leaf of the thoracolumbar fascia and thus from the spinous processes of the lumbar vertebrae and the last seven or eight thoracic vertebrae; and it arises muscularly from the last two or three ribs. Its fibers converge toward the shoulder joint. The cranial border of the muscle lies medial to the thoracic part of the trapezius, where it covers the caudal angle of the scapula. The apical end of the muscle is cranioventral where it encroaches on the dorsal edge of the deep pectoral and with it goes medial to the shoulder and arm musculature, ending in an aponeurosis medially on the m. triceps brachii. This aponeurosis partly blends with the tendon of the m. teres major to insert on the teres tubercle and partly joins with the deep pectoral muscle to terminate in the medial fascia of the brachium. Laterally, near the origin of the m. tensor fasciae antebrachii, an extension of the m. cutaneus trunci joins it. Because the ventral border of the m. latissimus dorsi gives off a bundle of fibers that pass laterally over the m. biceps brachii to the m. pectoralis profundus and with it inserts aponeurotically on the crest of the major tubercle, the dog, like the cat, has a "muscular axillary arch" (Heiderich, 1906; Langworthy, 1924).

Action: To draw the trunk cranially and possibly laterally; extend the vertebral column; and support the limb, draw the limb against the trunk, and draw the free limb caudally during flexion of the shoulder joint. To decelerate cranial motion of the limb. Two or three periods of EMG activity occur in this muscle during the step cycles of locomoting dogs (Goslow et al., 1981). A major phase of this activity coincides with the middle to late protraction movement of the limb (swing phase). Another phase is observed as the swing phase ends, prior to paw touchdown. Similar data were reported by Carrier et al. (2008) with EMG activity during the mid to late portions of the swing phase and ending prior to foot touchdown during trotting on level ground, thus braking and reversing the protraction of the thoracic limb. The authors felt that the m. latissimus dorsi did not produce external work during steady-state locomotion such as the trotting in their experiments. However, when these dogs ran uphill on an incline, EMG activity extended midway through the stance phase. Thus m. latissimus dorsi is an important thoracic limb retractor during "vigorous acceleration" and active digging behaviors.
Innervation: Nn. pectorales caudales, and n. thoracodorsalis.

The *m. rhomboideus* (Figs. 6.26, 6.46, and 6.47), covered by the trapezius, fans out on the neck and cranial thorax between the median line of the neck and thorax and the dorsal border of the scapula. It is in part flat and in part thick, and it is divided into three parts.

The cervical part, *m. rhomboideus cervicis*, lies dorsolaterally on the neck from the second or third cervical vertebra to the third thoracic vertebra. It arises on the tendinous median raphe of the neck and the ends of the spinous processes of the first three thoracic vertebrae and inserts on the rough medial surface and on the edge of the dorsal border of the scapula, including the scapular cartilage. Near the scapula in large dogs it becomes as much as 1.5 cm thick. From the cervical part, cranial to the fourth cervical vertebra, the *m. rhomboideus capitis* is given off as a straplike muscle to the occipital bone. The thoracic portion, *m. rhomboideus thoracis*, arises on the spinous processes of the fourth to the sixth or seventh thoracic vertebra and inserts on the medial and partly on the lateral edge of the dorsal border of the scapula. This portion of the m. rhomboideus is covered by the m. latissimus dorsi. The cervical and thoracic portions are never clearly separated from each other and are often intimately bound together.

Action: To elevate the limb, pull the limb and shoulder cranially or caudally; to draw the scapula against the trunk (in common with all the extrinsic muscles).
Innervation: Rami dorsales of nn. cervicales et thoracales.

The *m. serratus dorsalis* (Figs. 6.26, 6.27, and 6.33) is an epaxial muscle that is completely divided into cranial and caudal parts (see the special investigations of Maximenko, 1929, 1930) with different innervation and function. The *m. serratus dorsalis cranialis*, also known as the inspiratory part, lies on the dorsal surface of the cranial thorax, where it is medial to the rhomboideus, serratus ventralis, and latissimus dorsi. The muscle arises by a broad aponeurosis from the superficial leaf of the thoracolumbar fascia and, by means of this, from the tendinous median raphe of the neck as well as from the spinous processes of the first six to eight thoracic vertebrae. This aponeurosis fuses caudally with that of the mm. latissimus dorsi and serratus dorsalis caudalis. The aponeurosis covers the splenius and the fleshy part of the muscle covers the longissimus thoracis and iliocostalis from ribs 2 to 10. The fleshy portion of the muscle begins at approximately the dorsal border of the m. longissimus thoracis and ends immediately lateral to the m. iliocostalis, with distinct serrations on the cranial borders and the lateral surfaces of ribs 2 to 10. The fibers of the muscle, as well as those of its aponeurosis, are directed caudoventrally.

Action: To lift the ribs for inspiration.
Innervation: Adjacent nn. thoracici (branches from the branch to the m. intercostalis externus).

The narrower *m. serratus dorsalis caudalis*, or expiratory part, consists of three rather distinctly isolated portions. These arise by a broad aponeurosis from the lumbar part of the thoracolumbar fascia from which the m. obliquus externus abdominis and m. obliquus internus abdominis also arise. After extending cranioventrally, they end on the caudal border of the eleventh, twelfth, thirteenth, and, occasionally, also the tenth rib.

Action: To draw the last three or four ribs caudally for expiration.
Innervation: Branches from the adjacent nn. thoracici.

Erector Spinae Muscles

The dorsal musculature, associated with the vertebral column and ribs, may be divided into longitudinal muscle masses, each comprising many overlapping fascicles. The muscles act as extensors of the vertebral column and also produce lateral movements of the trunk when acting only on one side. Slijper (1946) described the functional anatomy of the epaxial spinal musculature in a wide variety of mammals. The organization of these epaxial muscles is complex, and considerable variation exists in the literature. Fig. 6.27B is one schematic version. The following description complies with the organization described in the NAV fifth edition.

The **erector spinae muscles** (*m. erector spinae*) are the dorsal muscles that include the epaxial muscles located on the dorsal surface of the vertebral column and ribs. These are represented by the various divisions of the iliocostalis, longissimus, and spinalis muscles.

Iliocostalis muscles (*m. iliocostalis*) (Fig. 6.30) consist of a series of fascicles lateral to the other epaxial muscles that form a narrow longitudinal muscle mass that runs cranioventrally over many segments. The caudal members of the series arise on the ilium and constitute a lumbar portion, whereas the cranial fascicles extend to the first thoracic vertebra and constitute the thoracic portion. The last fascicle inserts on the seventh cervical vertebra and constitutes the cervical portion.

The *m. iliocostalis lumborum* is a thick muscle mass that arises from the pelvic surface of the wing of the ilium, the iliac crest, and from an intermuscular septum located between the m. iliocostalis and m. longissimus. This septum is attached to the ilium and the deep surface of the thoracolumbar fascia. As the fibers of the muscle run cranioventral, large lateral fascicles from the ends of all the lumbar transverse processes join them. The cranial end of the lumbar portion runs toward the ribs and is distinctly separated from the m. longissimus. With increasingly smaller fleshy serrations, the m. iliocostalis lumborum attaches to the thirteenth, twelfth, eleventh, and tenth ribs, and occasionally, by a long delicate tendon, to the ninth rib also.

The *m. iliocostalis thoracis* is a long, narrow muscle mass extending cranially from the ribs, except the first and last. Its origin lies medially deep to the cranial segments of the m. iliocostalis lumborum. It lies lateral to the m. longissimus and reaches its greatest size between the fifth and third ribs. It is composed of individual portions that originate on

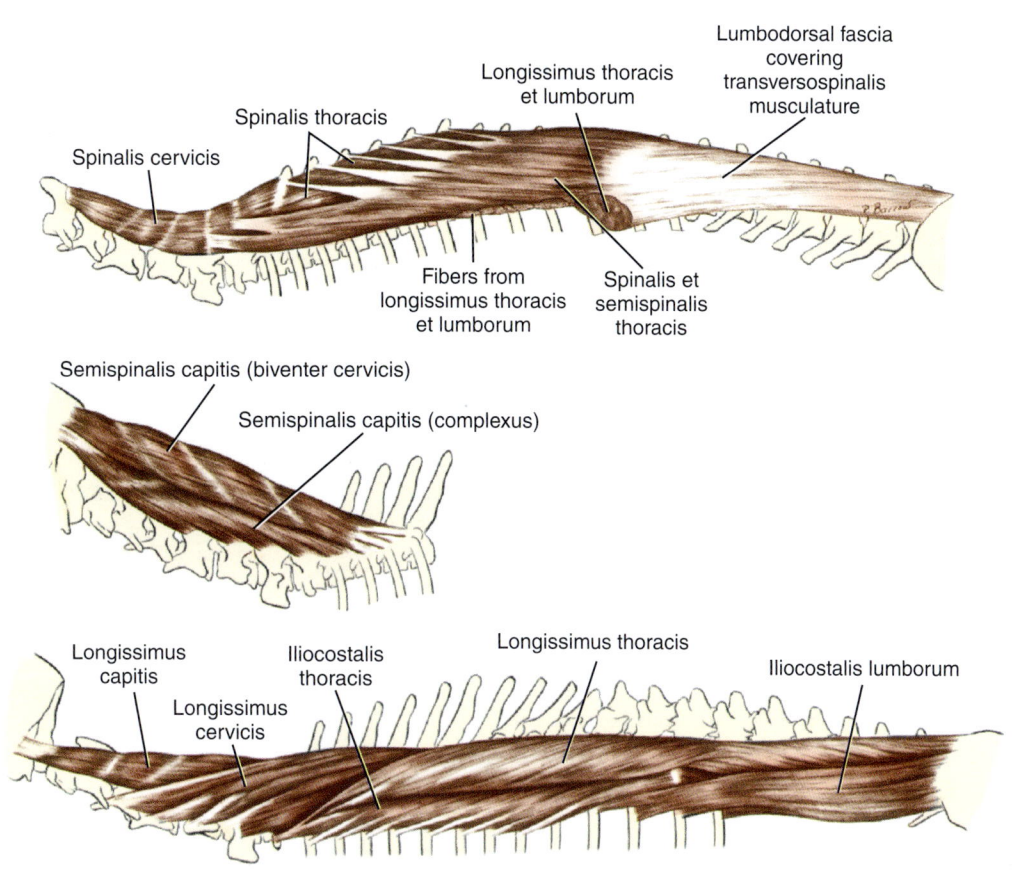

• Fig. 6.30 The superficial epaxial muscles.

the cranial borders of the vertebral end of the ribs; they extend craniolaterally and, after passing over one rib, form a common muscle belly. From this belly, terminal serrations arise that, by means of long tendons, are larger cranially and on the costal angles of the ribs. The most cranial termination is on the transverse process of the seventh cervical vertebra and is referred to as *m. iliocostalis cervicis*.

Action: Fixation of the vertebral column or lateral movement when only one side contracts; aids in expiration by pulling the ribs caudally.
Innervation: Dorsal branches of the nn. thoracici and lumbales.

The **longissimus muscle** (*m. longissimus*) (Figs. 6.26, 6.30, 6.31, 6.40A) is the erector spinae muscle that lies medial to the m. iliocostalis. It comprises the major portion of the epaxial muscle mass and consists of overlapping fascicles that extend from the ilium to the head. The m. longissimus consists of lumbar, thoracic, cervical, atlantal, and capital regional divisions. The m. sacrocaudalis dorsalis lateralis can be regarded as the caudal continuation of the m. longissimus on the tail; this muscle is discussed with the tail muscles.

The thoracolumbar part of the longissimus muscle mass is the largest muscle of the trunk (see Webster et al., 2014). Lateral to the spinous processes of the lumbar and thoracic vertebrae (which are covered by deeper muscles), and dorsal to the lumbar transverse processes and the ribs, it runs from the iliac crest to the last cervical vertebra. In the lumbar region, it is intimately fused with the m. iliocostalis lumborum. The thoracolumbar division reaches its greatest development in the cranial part of the lumbar region; in the thoracic region it gradually narrows, whereas the m. iliocostalis gets larger. The **m. longissimus lumborum** (Eisler, 1912) is covered by an exceptionally dense aponeurosis that is separated from the thoracolumbar fascia by fat. It arises caudally from the iliac crest and medial surface of the ilium and medially from the spinous processes and supraspinous ligament. Its fibers run craniolaterally. The aponeurosis is divided into many large tendinous strands between which narrower intermediate portions extend. Cranially, it is dissipated at the fifth rib. In the lumbar region the m. longissimus lumborum sends off seven medially directed fascicles from the ilium and the intermuscular septum. These fascicles cover the roots of the lumbar transverse processes and end on the accessory processes of the sixth to first lumbar vertebra. The smallest, most caudal portion runs to a fleshy insertion on the arch of the seventh lumbar vertebrae and to the intervertebral disc of the lumbosacral joint. There are also independent, more dorsally placed medial tendons going to the cranial articular processes of the seventh, sixth, and fifth lumbar vertebrae.

244 CHAPTER 6 The Muscular System

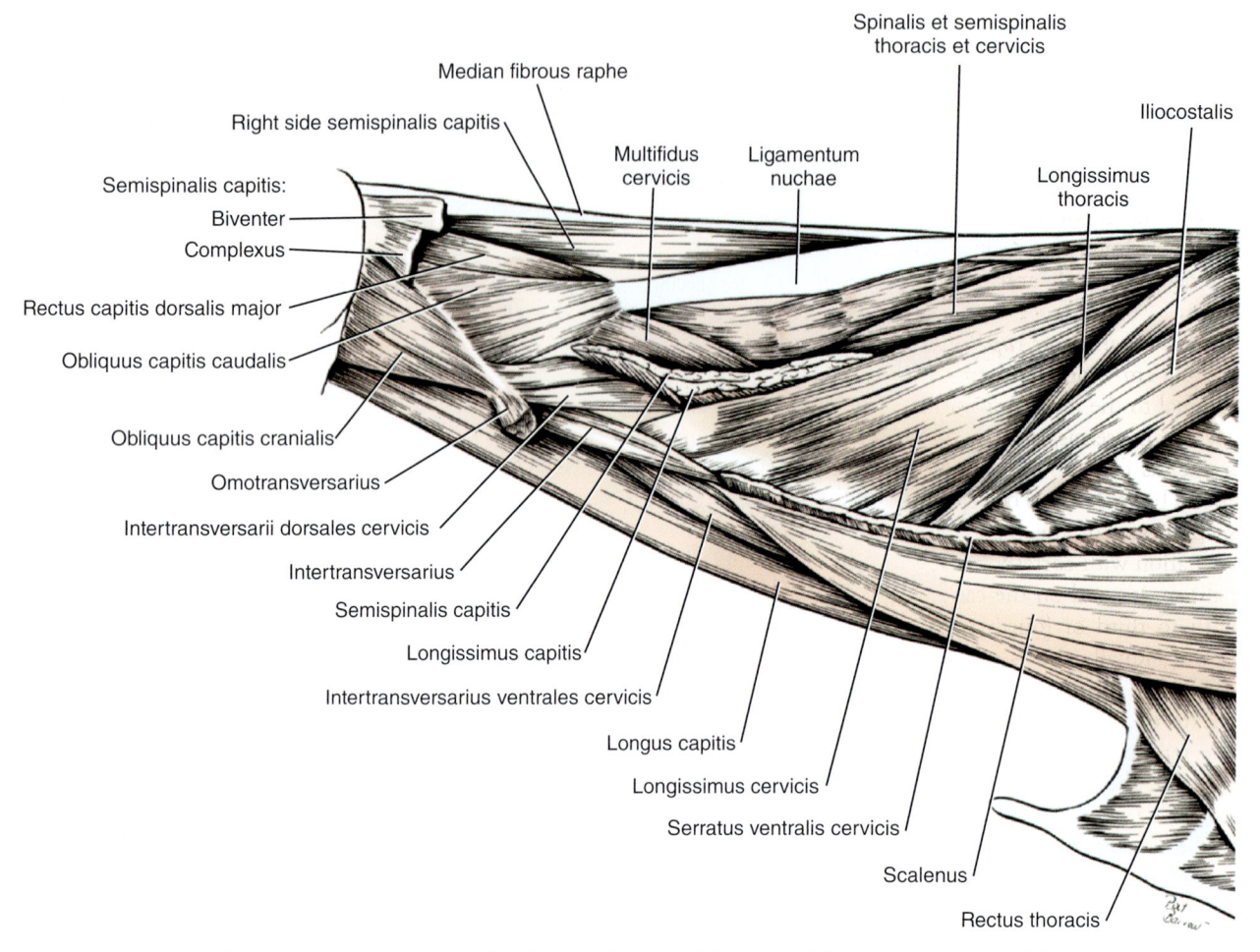

• **Fig. 6.31** Muscles of neck and head, deep dissection, lateral aspect. Serratus ventralis cervicis.

The ***m. longissimus thoracis*** has serrations that run to the caudal borders of the ribs by means of broad tendinous leaves. Each tendinous leaf separates into a medial and a lateral terminal tendon with thick edges. Between these tendons pass the dorsal branches of the thoracic nerves. The medial tendons of these ventral serrations end on the accessory processes of the thirteenth to sixth thoracic vertebrae. Because accessory processes are lacking from the fifth to first thoracic vertebrae, the medial tendons insert on the caudal ends of the transverse processes. The lateral tendons of the m. longissimus thoracis insert on the thirteenth to sixth ribs, where they attach medial to the attachment of the m. iliocostalis on the edge of a flat groove adjacent to the costal tubercle. Cranial to the sixth rib the muscle becomes so narrow that its tendons appear undivided. The terminal tendons end on the costal tubercles of the fifth to first ribs immediately lateral to the costotransverse joint. Occasionally, further divisions of the terminal tendon insert on the transverse processes of the sixth and fifth cervical vertebrae, where they fuse with serrations of the m. longissimus cervicis.

Action: For the thoracolumbar portion of the longissimus muscles, extension of the vertebral column. During trotting, EMG activity is biphasic, with major activity during the ipsilateral stance phase and a period of lesser activity during the ipsilateral swing phase (Schilling & Carrier, 2009). The thoracolumbar part of the longissimus muscle must stabilize the trunk against rotational moments imposed on the pelvis by hindlimb muscles (Ritter et al., 2001). In conjunction with other muscles, it permits fixation of the vertebral column, deflection of the trunk by fixation of the cervicothoracic junction, and sudden raising of the caudal portion of the body, which is initiated by means of the pelvic limbs.

Innervation: Dorsal branches of the thoracic and lumbar nerves (*nn. thoracici et lumbales*).

The m. longissimus in the lumbar and thoracic regions gives rise to serrations from its deep medial part. These follow the fiber direction of the m. longissimus, but, in contrast to it, they pass over only a small number of vertebrae. These are described under the system of the mm. intertransversarii.

The ***m. longissimus cervicis*** (Figs. 6.26, 6.27, 6.30, and 6.31) is a continuation of the m. longissimus thoracis, lying in the angle between the cervical and thoracic vertebrae. It is triangular in form and in large dogs is 1 to 1.5 cm thick. The muscle complex is composed of four serrations that are incompletely separable; each consists of a long lateral bundle and several short medial bundles. They are so arranged that a caudal serration partly covers its cranial neighbor. These serrations turn ventrally and insert on the transverse processes of the sixth to third cervical vertebrae.

Innervation: Dorsal branches of cervical and thoracic nerves (nn. cervicales and thoracici).
Action: To extend the neck; in unilateral action to extend the neck obliquely and turn it to one side.

The *m. longissimus capitis* (Fig. 6.30) is a large muscle 3.5 to 4.5 cm wide and 5 to 7 mm thick in large dogs; it lies medial to the mm. longissimus cervicis and splenius. It covers the m. semispinalis capitis along its ventral border and extends from the first three thoracic vertebrae to the temporal bone. It arises by separate bundles from the transverse processes of the third to first thoracic vertebrae in combination with corresponding serrations of the m. semispinalis capitis and on the caudal articular processes of the seventh to third or fourth cervical vertebrae. The muscle narrows gradually and is divided by one or two tendinous intersections. It runs over the dorsal surface of the atlas and, by means of a large tendon, inserts on the mastoid process of the temporal bone. At the level of the atlas, it unites firmly with the m. splenius. In many dogs there is a deep portion, the *m. longissimus atlantis*, whose fibers come from the articular processes of the seventh to fourth cervical vertebrae and end on the border of the wing of the atlas (Bogorodsky, 1930).

Action: Extension of the atlantooccipital joint. The atlantal portion in unilateral action rotates the atlantoaxial joint, whereas in bilateral action it fixes the atlantoaxial joint.
Innervation: Dorsal branches of the cervical nerves (nn. cervicales).

The **m. spinalis** (Figs. 6.30 and 6.31) is the most medial of the erector spinae group of muscles that consists of thoracic and cervical parts. These muscle fibers attach to spinous processes of the thoracic and cervical vertebrae. They are medial to the longissimus and semispinalis muscles and lateral to the multifidus group. The fibers of the spinalis muscles are closely related to and often difficult to separate from the semispinalis muscles. As a large, partly unsegmented, longitudinal muscle that consists primarily of incompletely isolated segments, the *m. spinalis thoracis* lies lateral to the spinous processes of the thoracic vertebrae and dorsomedial to the m. longissimus thoracis. It is continuous cranially with the cervical spinalis muscles. The *m. spinalis cervicis* (Fig. 6.30) is the medial, flat muscular strand bearing four tendinous inscriptions. It arises from the cranial border of the first thoracic spinous process, but it also receives a few bundles from the spinous process of the seventh cervical vertebra. Separated from the muscle of the opposite side only by the median ligamentous septum, it runs cranially ventral to the ligamentum nuchae. It inserts on the spinous processes of the fifth to second cervical vertebrae.

Action: To fix the thoracic vertebral column and to extend the neck.
Innervation: Medial branch of the dorsal branches of the cervical and thoracic nerves (*nn. cervicales et thoracici*).

Transversospinalis Muscle

The **transversospinalis muscle** is a medial epaxial muscle mass composed of a number of different systems of fascicles that join one or more vertebrae (Fig. 6.27). The nomenclature employed by various authors varies considerably (Plattner, 1922; Slijper, 1946; Winckler, 1939). The following adheres to the NAV description. The transversospinalis muscle is a collective term for those epaxial muscles that are primarily medial to the iliocostalis and longissimus muscles and lateral to the spinalis, interspinalis, and intertransversarius groups. The three muscle groups that compose the transversospinalis muscle are the semispinalis, multifidus, and rotators.

The *semispinalis thoracis* lies lateral to the spinous processes of the thoracic vertebrae and dorsomedial to the m. longissimus thoracis. It is closely associated with the spinalis thoracis muscle but lateral to it. It arises from the mamillary processes of thoracic vertebrae and courses over the lateral surface of the spinalis thoracis to the dorsal aspect of the spinous processes.

The *m. semispinalis cervicis* is continuous with the semispinalis thoracis and fused medially with the spinalis cervicis.

Action: To fix the thoracic vertebral column and to extend the neck.
Innervation: Medial branch of the dorsal branches of the cervical and thoracic nerves.

The *m. semispinalis capitis* (Figs. 6.30 and 6.31) is the large continuation to the head of the spinalis and semispinalis thoracic and cervical muscles. The capital portion of the semispinalis strand is lateral to and covers the cranial end of the spinalis and semispinalis cervical muscles. Its broad origin is covered by the mm. longissimus and splenius. The muscle lies rather deep as it extends from the first five thoracic vertebrae and the last cervical vertebra to the occipital bone. It surrounds each half of the ligamentum nuchae laterally and dorsally, meeting its fellow of the opposite side. The left and right muscles are separated only by the nuchal ligament and the median fibrous raphe. The semispinalis capitis is divided into two distinct parts, the dorsally located m. biventer cervicis and the ventrally placed m. complexus. These two muscles can be separated as far as their insertions, despite the intimate connections between them.

The *m. biventer cervicis* (Fig. 6.30) is dorsal and medial to the m. complexus. It arises by three strong serrations medial to the m. longissimus cervicis and capitis, from the transverse processes of the fourth, third, and second thoracic vertebrae. Fascial strands also come from the lateral surfaces of the spinous processes deep to the m. semispinalis thoracis. Other fibers are added to the dorsal border from the thoracolumbar fascia at the level of the cranial thorax. The m. biventer cervicis is firmly connected with the median fibrous raphe of the neck. It appears to be divided by four (rarely five) very oblique tendinous inscriptions into separate portions having longitudinal fibers. It inserts on a distinct, oval, rough area ventrolateral to the external occipital protuberance on the caudal surface of the skull. In cats, the m. biventer cervicis is divided by tendinous inscriptions into five in-series compartments. Each compartment has a distinct architecture with deeply lying fiber bundles containing predominantly type I fibers and more superficial regions containing predominantly fast-twitch, type II fibers (Richmond & Armstrong, 1988). The m. biventer cervicis of cats contains a high concentration of muscle spindles, as do other deep neck muscles, suggesting a role in providing fine control of neck and head movements during locomotion (Richmond & Abrahams, 1975b). Another kind of muscle proprioceptive receptor, the neurotendinous spindle (Golgi tendon organ), is commonly found at the musculotendinous interfaces provided by these intramuscular septa (Richmond & Bakker, 1982). These neurotendinous spindles often appear to be arranged alongside or in a dyad arrangement with the muscle spindles of adjacent muscle tissue. If the similar pattern of multiple connective tissue septa in dogs is an indication, the anatomy and function of the neck muscles is critical to coordination of the head and neck for orientation and for efficient locomotion.

The **m. complexus** (Fig. 6.30) is lateral and ventral to the biventer cervicis muscle. It arises from the caudal articular processes of the first thoracic to the third cervical vertebra in common with the m. longissimus capitis (laterally) and the m. multifidus (medially). The caudal segments are more fleshy. The one arising on the first thoracic vertebra has a tendinous covering medially, which is also related to one of the portions of the m. multifidus. Fibers also arise in the fascia of the m. obliquus capitis caudalis somewhat cranial to the caudal border of the atlas. The fibers run craniomedially to end laterally on the nuchal crest by means of a tendon coming from a thick superficial fibrous covering. According to Richmond and Armstrong (1988), the m. complexus of cats contains the highest density of muscle spindles of any of the epaxial neck muscles.

Action: To extend the head and neck; in unilateral action to flex the head and neck laterally.
Innervation: Dorsal branches of the nn. cervicales.

The **m. multifidus** (Figs. 6.27, 6.31, 6.32, and 6.40A) is a muscle composed of numerous individual portions that overlap in segments and extend from the sacrum to the second cervical vertebra. It consists of a continuous deep series of muscle bundles that course dorsocranially from mamillary, transverse, or articular processes of caudally lying vertebrae to spinous processes of cranially lying ones. As a rule, two vertebrae are passed over by each bundle. The m. multifidus is continuous in the tail with the sacrocaudalis dorsalis medialis muscle.

The lumbar portion of this muscle is a large, seemingly homogeneous muscle that runs from the sacrum to the spinous process of the eighth or ninth thoracic vertebra. It is divided into 11 individual, flat portions that are united with each other. They originate from the three articular

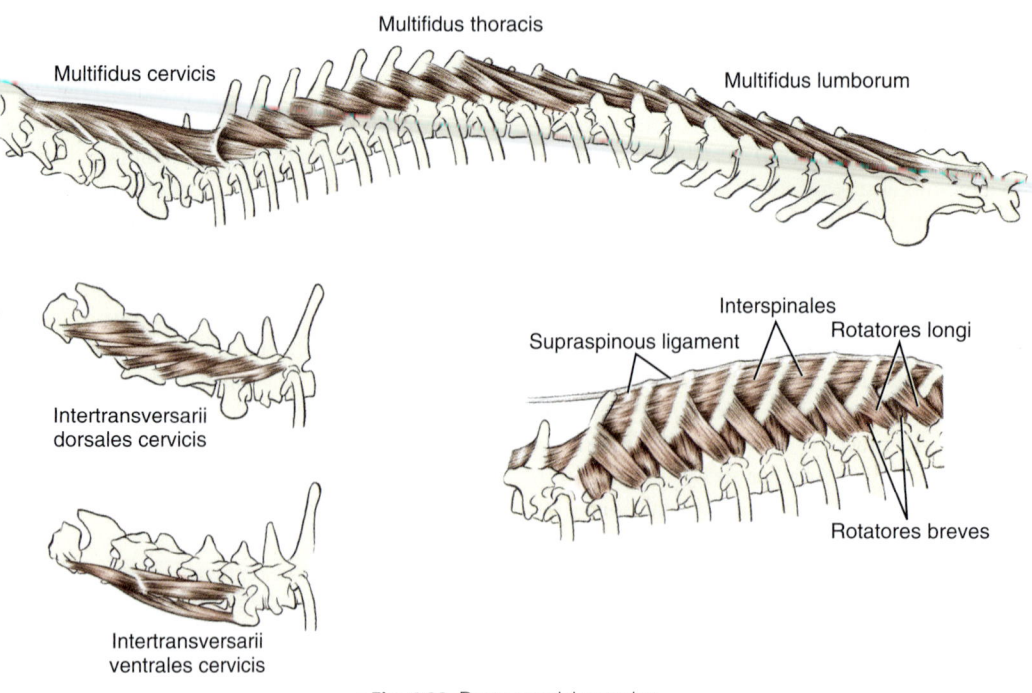

• **Fig. 6.32** Deep epaxial muscles.

processes of the sacrum and the mamillary process of the first caudal vertebra and the seventh lumbar to the twelfth thoracic vertebra. After the several parts pass over two segments, they end laterally on the ends of the spinous processes of the sixth lumbar to the ninth (occasionally eighth) thoracic vertebra immediately ventral to the supraspinous ligament. The thoracic portion of the multifidus lies more ventrally on the vertebral column, and its segments are more vertical than those of the lumbar part. It arises by nine distinctly isolated portions on the mamillary and transverse processes of the eleventh to the third thoracic vertebra and inserts on the spinous processes of the eighth thoracic to the seventh cervical vertebra. The cervical part is covered by the m. semispinalis capitis. It appears deep to the ventrolateral border of the m. spinalis, m. semispinalis thoracis, and m. semispinalis cervicis, where it extends from the articular process of the second thoracic vertebra to the spinous process of the axis. It consists of six incompletely separable individual portions that themselves are again partially divided into lateral principal, medial accessory, and deep accessory parts, according to Stimpel (1934). Collectively they arise essentially from the articular processes.

Action: As a whole, the m. multifidus, along with the other epaxial muscles, fixes the vertebral column, especially in bilateral action.
Innervation: Medial branches of the rami dorsales in the lumbar, thoracic, and cervical regions (rami mediales nn. lumbales, thoracici, cervicales).

From the medial surface of the m. multifidus certain deep muscles have become extensively differentiated. These are the mm. rotatores longi and breves. In addition, throughout the vertebral column there are the mm. interspinales between the spinous processes and the mm. intertransversarii, which in general run between the transverse processes.

The ***mm. rotatores*** (Figs. 6.27B, 6.32) are developed as eight long and nine short rotators; in the dog they are confined strictly to the cranial thoracic region, where the pairs of articular processes are tangentially placed, thus allowing rotary movements. The long rotator muscles extend between the transverse and spinous processes of two alternate vertebrae. The most caudal extends from the transverse process of the tenth thoracic vertebra to the spinous process of the eighth thoracic vertebra ventral to the insertion of the corresponding segment of the multifidus. The most cranial long rotator extends between corresponding points of the third and the first thoracic vertebrae. These segments are more vertical than those of the m. multifidus, along the caudal border of which they appear. The short rotators are situated more deeply than are the long rotators. The most caudal belly runs between the transverse process of the tenth and the spinous process of the ninth thoracic vertebra. The most cranial belly passes between similar points on the second and the first thoracic vertebrae. Often this portion is surrounded extensively by tendinous tissue (Krüger, 1929).

Action: Rotation of the cranial portion of the thoracic vertebral column about the longitudinal axis in unilateral action; otherwise, fixation.
Innervation: Medial branches of the rami dorsales of the thoracic nerves (rami medialis, rami dorsales nn. thoracici).

Interspinal Muscles

The ***mm. interspinales*** (Fig. 6.32) are distinctly separable into lumbar, thoracic, and cervical portions; the lumbar portion is covered by the m. multifidus. In the thoracic region, after removal of the mm. semispinalis and longissimus, the mm. interspinales are visible at the ends of the spinous processes. They run between contiguous edges of spinous processes and overlap these edges somewhat. They also extend between the spinous processes of the first thoracic to the fifth cervical vertebra.

Action: Fixation of the vertebral column.
Innervation: Medial branches of the dorsal branches of the spinal nerves (rami medialis, rami dorsales nn. spinalis).

Intertransverse Muscles

The ***mm. intertransversarii*** (Fig. 6.32) are deep segments split off from the longissimus system. They are separable into caudal, lumbar, thoracic, and cervical parts, and, as delicate muscle bundles, they pass over one or two, or, at most, three vertebrae. They pass between transverse processes, between articular and transverse processes, or between mamillary and transverse processes. These are small muscles in the lumbar (***mm. intertransversarii lumborum***) and thoracic (***mm. intertransversarii thoracis***) regions where they overlap. These separate parts run between the mamillary processes of the seventh lumbar to the thirteenth or twelfth thoracic and the accessory processes of the fifth lumbar to the ninth thoracic vertebrae and between the transverse processes of the twelfth to the eighth and those of the eighth to the fourth thoracic vertebrae. The ***mm. intertransversarii dorsales cervicis*** lie between the lines of insertion of the mm. longissimus cervicis, longissimus capitis, and semispinalis capitis. As a segmental muscle strand it extends from the eminence on the cranial articular process of the first thoracic vertebra to the wing of the atlas. Its individual bundles run craniolaterally in the form of five indistinctly separated bellies from the first thoracic and the seventh to fourth cervical vertebrae to the transverse processes of the sixth to second cervical vertebrae. The cranial portion of the muscle extends from the eminence of the third and second cervical vertebrae to the caudal border of the wing of the atlas. The ***mm. intertransversarii medii cervicis*** form a strand that is composed of five or six distinctly separable, thin parts that extend only between transverse processes. They lie ventral to the insertion of the m. serratus ventralis cervicis and dorsal to the m. scalenus and are partly covered by these two muscles. The segments course between the terminal tubercles of the ends of the transverse processes from the

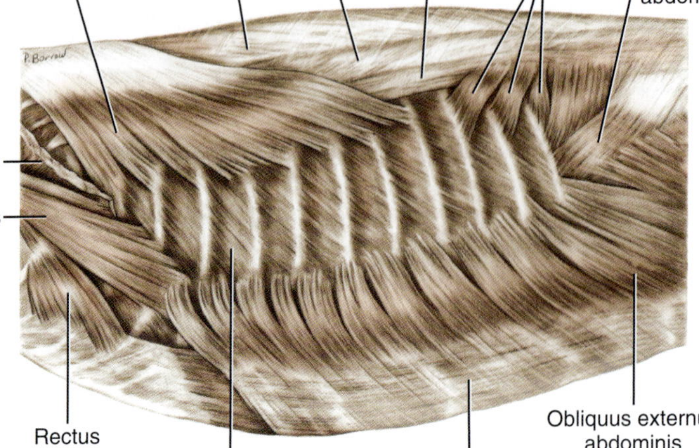

• **Fig. 6.33** Superficial muscles of thoracic cage, lateral aspect. (M. serratus ventralis [thoracis] has been removed.)

first thoracic to the second cervical vertebra. On the sixth cervical vertebra it is on the transverse process proper, and, from the fifth cervical vertebra cranially it is on the caudal branch of the transverse process and the border of the wing of the atlas. The most cranial portion runs deep to the dorsal m. intertransversarius of the axis. The deep fibers pass from segment to segment; the superficial ones pass over one segment. The **mm. intertransversarii ventrales cervicis** run cranially from the m. scalenus and form a homogeneous longitudinal strand. This is found ventral to the m. scalenus and dorsal to the m. longus colli; it extends from the ventral border of the winglike transverse process of the sixth cervical vertebra to insert by three separate terminal segments on the caudal branch of the transverse process of the fourth, third, and second cervical vertebrae. This strand is covered by the m. scalenus caudally and by the intermediate portion of the mm. intertransversarii cranially.

Muscles of the Thoracic Wall (Musculi Thoracis)

The spaces between the ribs are filled by the mm. intercostales, which appear in a double layer, internal and external, and cross each other. Each m. intercostalis externus is adjacent to m. levator costarum dorsally. The fibers that make up the almost spindle-shaped belly of the m. levator costarum do not come from the following rib, but come rather from the transverse process of the corresponding thoracic vertebra. Cranially, on the thorax, the m. rectus thoracis covers the superficial ventral ends of the first ribs; the m. transversus thoracis crosses the internal surface of the cartilages of the sternal ribs and the sternum. The mm. retractor costae and subcostalis are special muscles of the last rib.

The **mm. intercostales externi** (Figs. 6.33, 6.34, and 6.38) form the thicker external layer in the intercostal spaces. They are 4 or 5 mm thick in large dogs but become thinner in the region of the floating ribs. They extend ventrally from the mm. levatores costarum, which are indistinctly set apart, to the costochondral junctions; they may also extend into the spaces between the costal cartilages. The fibers of the external intercostal muscle arise on the caudal border of each rib and run caudoventrally to the cranial border of the next rib. This muscle is lacking in the first two or three interchondral spaces because the external intercostals end proximal to or at the costochondral junctions. Distal to the ends of the external intercostals, the internal intercostals make their appearance. With each successive segment, the external intercostal muscles extend farther distally, so that the ninth and the tenth interchondral spaces are completely filled, although occasional defects in the muscle are found. Although the external intercostals are rather well developed in the false or asternal interchondral spaces, the muscle is completely absent in the twelfth interchondral space.

Action: Inspiration; draws the ribs together so as to enlarge the thoracic cavity. For a discussion of function in these muscles see De Troyer et al. (1985). Carrier (1996) reported correlation of EMG activity with inspiration during quiet breathing but noted some correlation with locomotor cycles during active locomotion (trotting).

Innervation: Muscular branches of the nn. intercostales 1 to 12.

The **mm. levatores costarum** (Fig. 6.34) are present as 12 special formations of the external intercostal muscles.

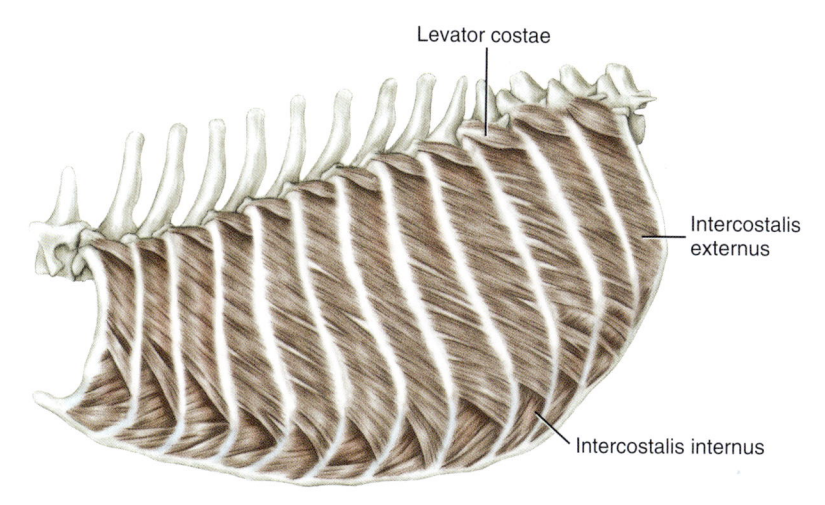

• Fig. 6.34 Deep muscles of thorax, lateral aspect.

They are flat, spindle-shaped muscles covered by the mm. longissimus thoracis and iliocostalis thoracis. They are fleshy at their origins on the transverse processes of the first to twelfth thoracic vertebrae. After running caudoventrally to the angle of the rib next caudad, they end on the cranial borders of the second to thirteenth ribs. They overlap the proximal ends of the external intercostal muscles.

Action: Inspiration; the fixed point is the transverse process of the vertebra.
Innervation: Small branches of the nn. intercostales 1 to 12.

The **mm. intercostales interni** (Figs. 6.34, 6.36, and 6.38) form the thinner internal layer of the intercostal musculature. This layer is 2 or 3 mm thick in large dogs. The internal intercostals extend from the vertebral column, where they leave free only a small triangular space adjacent to the vertebrae, to the distal ends of the ribs including the cartilaginous portion. The fibers course cranioventrally from the cranial border of one rib to the caudal border of the rib next cranial to it. In this cranioventral course, the fibers attain angles of inclination which from the vertebral column to the sternum decrease from 78 to 71 degrees to 68 to 54 degrees. Thus, they are steeper than the mm. intercostales externi, which they cross. The internal intercostals fill the interchondral spaces where they are 4 to 5 mm thick and covered laterally by the rectus abdominis. The different fiber directions observed in the mm. intercostales externi et interni may provide resistance to twisting movements imposed on the thorax during locomotion (De Troyer et al., 1985).

Action: Expiration, to draw the ribs together so as to narrow the thoracic cavity. EMG activity showed strong correlation with expiration (Carrier, 1996).
Innervation: Nn. intercostales.

The **mm. subcostales** are located medial to the internal intercostal muscles at the vertebral ends of the caudal ribs, especially ribs 9 to 11. The fibers are directed cranioventrally across several ribs.

The **m. rectus thoracis** (Figs. 6.26, 6.31, and 6.33), formerly known as the *m. transversus costarum*, is a flat, almost rectangular muscle that runs caudoventrally from its origin on the first rib, opposite the most ventral portion of the m. scalenus to its insertion over the ventral ends of ribs 2, 3, and 4. Its aponeurosis of insertion obliquely crosses the lateral surface of the cranial portion of the aponeurosis of the m. rectus abdominis and blends with the deep fascia of the trunk.

Action: Inspiration.
Innervation: Lateral branch of the nn. intercostales.

The **m. retractor costae** (Fig. 6.35) is a thin muscle lying deep to the tendon of origin of the m. transversus abdominis. It bridges the space between the transverse processes of the first three or four lumbar vertebrae and the last rib (Iwakin, 1928). At these transverse processes it is attached to the thoracolumbar fascia. Seen from the interior, this thin muscle lies directly adjacent to the peritoneum and transversalis fascia. Its fibers cross those of the m. transversus abdominis. The arcus lumbocostalis of the diaphragm crosses over the ventral surface of its cranial border. Farther distally the caudal fiber bundles extend on the last rib and partly encroach on the peritoneal surface of the pars costalis of the diaphragm. The m. retractor costae belongs to the system of the m. intercostalis internus and is innervated by the last thoracic nerve (Kolesnikow, 1928).

The **m. transversus thoracis** (sometimes referred to as the *triangularis sterni* or the *sternocostalis internus* (Reighard & Jennings, 1938) (Fig. 6.36) is a flat, fleshy muscle lying on the dorsal surfaces of the sternum and adjacent costal cartilages. It forms a continuous triangular leaf that covers the second to eighth costal cartilages. A delicate, special bundle may be given off to the first costal cartilage. Its fibers arise by a narrow aponeurosis, on the dorsolateral surface of the sternum, from the second sternebra to the caudal end

Fig. 6.35 Diaphragm, abdominal surface. *a*, Medial; *b*, intermediate; *c*, lateral portions of pars lumbalis. Label: lumbocostal arch.

of the xiphoid process. They end with indistinct segmentations on the second to seventh costal cartilages, somewhat ventral to the costochondral articulation.

Action: The m. transversus thoracis contributes to expiration (De Troyer & Ninane, 1986).

Diaphragm

The **diaphragm** (*diaphragma*) (Figs. 6.35 and 6.36) is a musculotendinous plate between the thoracic and the abdominal cavities. It projects cranially into the thoracic cavity like a dome. On the thoracic side, it is separated from the parietal pleura by the endothoracic fascia; on the abdominal side, it is separated from the parietal peritoneum by the transversalis fascia. Peripherally, this wall that separates the body cavities attaches to the ventral surfaces of the lumbar vertebrae, the medial surfaces of the ribs, and the dorsal surface of the sternum. The fibers of the diaphragm arise on these skeletal parts and radiate toward the tendinous center. The diaphragm has been described as two function-based muscles by De Troyer et al. (1981).

The **central tendon** (*centrum tendineum*) of the diaphragm, in the dog, occupies approximately 21% of the surface area of the diaphragm (Gordon et al., 1989). It consists of a triangular central area with dorsal extensions on each side. From the cranial aspect this tendinous area appears to be displaced somewhat ventrally. The two-layered disposition of the tendon fibers is easily followed. To the right, at the base of the body of the tendon, there is a concentric arrangement of thick fibers about the foramen venae cavae that courses slightly cranioventrally. On the columns of the central tendon, fibers run in an arch from the crural

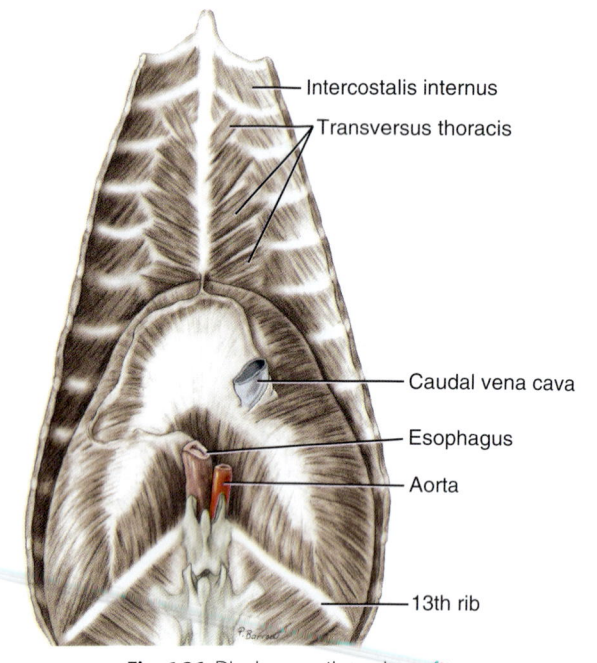

Fig. 6.36 Diaphragm, thoracic surface.

musculature directly to those of the costal parts. Special thick reinforcements extend lengthwise along the borders. Fibers from the muscle surrounding the esophagus radiate on the body of the tendon to the sternal and ventral parts of the costal diaphragmatic musculature. Transverse fibers course from one side to the other as a reinforcing apparatus. Peculiar whorls are formed near the bases of both columns. Muscle fibers from the costal portion often radiate into the dorsal border of the foramen venae cavae (Pancrazi, 1928).

The muscular part of the diaphragm surrounds the central tendon on all sides, and its fibers stream into the latter in a radial direction. It is divided into the pars lumbalis and a pars costalis on each side, and the pars sternalis.

The **lumbar part** (*pars lumbalis*) of the diaphragmatic musculature is formed by the right and left diaphragmatic crura. At the aortic hiatus (*hiatus aorticus*) they enclose the aorta, the azygos and hemiazygos veins, and origin of the thoracic duct from the cisterna chyli. Although at first glance they appear to be symmetric, they are not symmetric in their construction or in the thickness of their fibers. The right crus is considerably larger than the left. Each crus arises by a long bifurcate tendon, one part of which is longer and larger and comes from the cranial edge of the body of the fourth lumbar vertebra. The shorter and somewhat smaller part of the tendon comes from the body of the third lumbar vertebra. Both portions of the tendon of each side unite to form an almost sagittal tendon that appears medial to the m. psoas minor. The right crural tendon is considerably larger than the left crural tendon. The bilateral tendons are closely adjacent to the aorta, and, from their lateral surfaces in particular, they give rise to more and more muscle fibers. This results in a flat, fan-shaped muscle that bears a medial tendon of origin. The muscle parallels the dorsal thoracic wall. Immediately cranial to the celiac artery, a tendinous strand descends on each side of the aorta to form the aortic hiatus. Seen from the abdominal cavity, each crus of the diaphragm is a triangular muscle plate with borders that give rise to the tendinous portions. As a whole, this plate of muscle radiates cranially toward the concavity of the diaphragmatic tendon. The muscle fiber arrangement is somewhat different in the two crura.

The lateral portion of the lumbar right crus originates mainly from the tendon of origin coming from the third lumbar vertebra. It extends ventral to the psoas muscles in an almost transverse **lumbocostal arch** (*arcus lumbocostalis*). The pleura and peritoneum encroach directly on one another dorsal to the arch. After crossing the lumbar musculature, the fiber bundles of the lateral crus run toward those of the pars costalis, with which they coalesce into a narrow tendinous band. This band is the extension of the end of the column of the tendinous center. In the wedge between these portions is a triangular area that is free of muscle with only fascial coverings of the diaphragmatic musculature radiating into it. This portion of the peripheral diaphragmatic attachment crosses the ventral aspect of the m. retractor costae and the last rib. On each side the splanchnic nerves and the sympathetic trunk cross dorsally to the lumbocostal arch. The lateral portion of the left lumbar crus arises in a similar way from its corresponding tendon. However, it has another special lateral division that radiates into the lumbocostal arch from the ventral border of the psoas muscles. Thus on the left side this triangular area is muscular. The course of the fibers into the tendinous center is the same as on the right side.

The intermediate portion of the right lumbar crus derives its fibers from the principal part of the tendon of origin and from the right column of the tendinous aortic hiatus. On the left side, the fibers of this part come from the left column of the hiatus along its entire length. These fibers on both sides radiate into the medial borders of the bilateral columns of the central tendon.

The musculature of the medial portion of the right lumbar crus is the thickest (5 or 6 mm) and originates from the terminal portion of the right column of the aortic hiatus. It extends ventrally, surrounds the esophageal hiatus, and blends ventrally with the dorsal border of the body of the central tendon. The muscular border of this hiatus is thick. The **esophageal hiatus** (*hiatus esophageus*) transmits the esophagus with its vessels and the two vagal nerve trunks.

The generally homogeneous **costal part** (*pars costalis*) on each side consists of bundles of muscle fibers radiating from the costal wall to the tendinous center. Each bundle consists of a number of muscle fibers arranged in-series such that four to six fibers, each being 1 to 6 cm, may be interposed between attachments on the ribs and the central tendon (Gordon et al., 1989). This muscle arises by indistinct serrations from the medial proximal part of the thirteenth rib, distal part of the twelfth rib, and costochondral articulation of the eleventh rib, as well as the whole length of the tenth and ninth, and at the bend on the eighth costal cartilage. In the caudal part of the line of origin the serrations encroach distally on those of the m. transversus abdominis. In the region of the tenth, ninth, and eighth costal cartilages (often only the eighth alone) openings may be found that allow the passage of the first three cranial serrations of the m. transversus abdominis. The serrations of the diaphragm reach beyond those of the m. transversus abdominis and insert cranial and caudal to them on the corresponding costal cartilages. Interspersed with many radial, fatty strands, the bundles of the costal part run centrally into the lateral borders of the columns and body of the central tendon.

The **sternal part** (*pars sternalis*) of the diaphragm may not exist in the dog. It is an unpaired medial part unseparated from the bilateral costal portions. Its fibers arise on the base of the xiphoid cartilage, the adjacent transversalis fascia, and the eight costal cartilages. They extend dorsally to the apex of the body of the central tendon.

Regional differences in histochemical fiber type composition exist in the diaphragm of dogs. Reid et al. (1987) reported that no IIb fibers were present and that costal diaphragm contained approximately 46% type I fibers, whereas the fibers of the right crus located on the left side of the esophageal hiatus contained 64% type I fibers. Such differences appear to correlate with regional specializations of function. For example, Decramer et al. (1984) demonstrated asynchronous EMG activity in costal and crural parts of the diaphragm in controlled, resting respiration.

The diaphragm projects far into the thoracic cavity, and its costal part lies on the internal surface of the last few ribs. A capillary space is formed between the layers of pleura lining the diaphragm and the ribs. This is the **costodiaphragmatic recess** (*recessus costodiaphragmaticus*). This decreases on inspiration but increases in size on expiration. During active flattening of the summit of the diaphragm, the inflated lung pushes into the opened space, and, on cessation of the diaphragmatic action, it is again pushed out of the space. Even during the most extreme inspiration the space is not entirely filled by the lung. Similar relationships exist in the region dorsal to the diaphragmatic crura and ventral to the vertebra covered by the psoas muscles. This bilateral **lumbodiaphragmatic recess** (*recessus lumbodiaphragmaticus*) extends caudally to the middle of the lumbar vertebrae. In the midplane the diaphragm forms an arch bulging into the thoracic cavity. This arch extends freely ventrally from the first few lumbar vertebrae, passing cranioventrally over more than half of the height of the thoracic cavity. Near the sternum it turns in a caudoventral direction. The summit or most cranial portion of this arch of the diaphragm is the **cupula** (*cupula diaphragmatis*) of the diaphragm. This cupula lies at the junction of the middle and ventral thirds of the muscle. On expiration the diaphragm undergoes an excursion of at least one and half thoracic segments at each respiration. The cupula has also been shown to move cranially and caudally in a coordinated fashion during locomotion (for review, see Bramble, 1989). As a dog trots or runs, deceleration of cranial movement occurs briefly when the two forelimbs strike the ground. At this time, abdominal viscera move cranially and push the diaphragm cranially into the thoracic cavity. This model, sometimes termed the *visceral piston hypothesis*, suggests that cranial movement of the abdominal viscera may assist in expiration. Caudal movement of the abdominal viscera occurs during the cranial acceleration of the body as the forelimbs move through the stance or propulsion phase of locomotion (Bramble & Jenkins, 1993). This latter movement can assist in pulling the diaphragm caudally, contributing to inspiration. Challenges to the visceral piston model (Ainsworth et al., 1996, 1997) showed diaphragm activity was driven by "respiratory neuromuscular events." In particular, these studies showed a correlation between phasic diaphragm activity and changes in esophageal pressure and less correlation with gait or foot placement than had been advocated by Bramble and Jenkins.

The muscle of the diaphragm is covered on the convex thoracic side by the fascia endothoracica and the pleura. On the concave abdominal side it is covered by a continuation of the fascia transversalis and the peritoneum. Both the fascia and serosa are so thin in the dog that over the tendinous portion they can only be seen microscopically.

The convex thoracic side of the diaphragm lies against the surface of the lungs, from which it is separated by a potential space. At about the midplane of the thorax where the mediastinum descends from the thoracic vertebrae, the two pleural leaves on either side of the mediastinum separate on the diaphragm to become its pleural covering. The attachment of the mediastinum is median only from the dorsal portion of the diaphragm to the esophagus. Ventral to the esophagus the mediastinum makes a strong deflection to the left, to return to the midplane just dorsal to the sternum. Here the mediastinal pleura connecting to the caudal vena cava branches off in a convex arch to form the plica vena cava.

In the dorsal part of the mediastinum the aorta, the azygos and hemiazygos veins, and the thoracic duct extend to the hiatus aorticus. The esophagus passes to the hiatus esophageus with the dorsal and ventral vagal nerve trunks. On the right side the esophagus is covered by pleura, which comes from the mediastinum. In the ventral part of the mediastinum the left phrenic nerve lies in its own mediastinal fold, and the phrenicopericardial ligament runs to the diaphragm near the midline. The caudal vena cava and the right phrenic nerve reach the diaphragm in the plica vena cava. The stomach and liver attach by ligaments to the concave peritoneal surface of the diaphragm.

Action: Retraction of the diaphragmatic cupula and thus inspiration (Ainsworth et al., 1989); maintaining the position of abdominal viscera during locomotion. Inhibition of activity in the crural diaphragm is important to allow passage of swallowed food through the esophageal hiatus (Monges et al., 1978). During emesis there is a differential function with the diaphragm with the costal region exhibiting EMG activity and myofiber shortening and the crural regions having decreased EMG activity and myofiber lengthening (Abe et al., 1993; Sprung et al., 1989).

Innervation: Nn. phrenici (from the ventral branches of the fifth, sixth, and seventh cervical nerves).

Endothoracic fascia (*fascia endothoracica*) lines the inner surface of the thoracic wall where it is located between the musculoskeletal wall including the diaphragm and the parietal pleura.

Muscles of the Abdominal Wall (*Musculi Abdominis*)

From external to internal the abdominal muscles are the rectus abdominis, the obliquus externus abdominis, the obliquus internus abdominis, the transversus abdominis, and quadratus lumborum. The m. rectus abdominis extends longitudinally in the ventral abdominal wall on each side of the linea alba from the external surface of the thorax to the pecten ossis pubis. The mm. obliqui and the transversus are in the lateral abdominal wall. In general these muscles arise from the lateral surface of the ribs, the lumbar region, or the tuber coxae to pass in the lateral wall to the ventral abdominal wall or to the pelvis. The quadratus lumborum is in the dorsal wall of the abdomen and consists of longitudinal fibers ventral to the bodies of last thoracic vertebrae and the lumbar transverse processes (Fig. 6.35). In the ventral wall the aponeuroses of the two oblique muscles cross the rectus muscle superficially, whereas the aponeurosis of the transverse muscle crosses deeply. In this way the "sheath of the rectus" (see Fig. 6.39) is formed. The

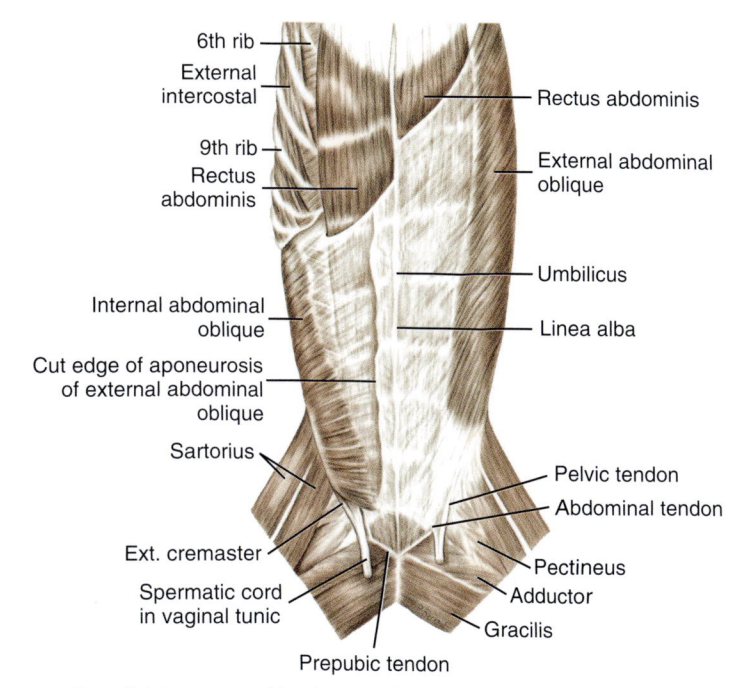

Fig. 6.37 Superficial muscles of trunk, ventral aspect. (M. pectoralis profundus removed.)

abdominal muscles are covered superficially by the extensive cutaneous muscle of the trunk (m. cutaneous trunci).

The oblique muscles, the fibers of which cross each other at about right angles, form the oblique girdle of the abdomen. The straight and transverse muscles, which also cross each other at right angles, form the straight girdle of the abdomen.

The **m. obliquus externus abdominis** (Figs. 6.33, 6.37, and 6.39) is an expansive sheet covering the ventral half of the lateral thoracic wall and the lateral and ventral parts of the abdominal wall. According to its origin, the muscle can be considered to have two parts, costal and lumbar. The costal part arises by indistinct serrations in a caudally rising line from the middle parts of the fourth or fifth to the twelfth rib and the adjacent deep trunk fascia, which covers the external intercostal muscles. It is partly covered by the ventral edge of the m. latissimus dorsi at its origin. The unserrated lumbar part arises from the last rib and, in common with the costal part of the obliquus internus abdominis, from the principal lamina of the thoracolumbar fascia.

The cranial serrations of the muscle extend between the serrations of origin of the m. serratus ventralis thoracis and cover the terminal tendon of the longest part of the m. scalenus, the scalenus dorsalis. The caudal serrations are more dorsal on the costal wall than the cranial ones; thus the line of origin of the lumbar portion meets the lateral border of the m. iliocostalis.

The fibers of the external abdominal oblique muscle run caudoventrally, the caudal part being more horizontal than the cranial. In the ventral abdominal wall, 6 to 8 cm from the midline in large dogs, it forms a wide aponeurosis. In the caudal abdomen, a slit or oval opening occurs in this aponeurosis that is the **superficial inguinal ring** (*anulus inguinalis superficialis*). This is at the level of the femoral triangle just cranial to the iliopubic eminence. The craniomedial border of this ring is the **medial crus** (*crus mediale*), and the caudolateral border is the **lateral crus** (*crus laterale*). The medial crus has been referred to as the *abdominal tendon* and the lateral crus as the *pelvic tendon* (Fig. 6.37).

The aponeurosis of the external abdominal oblique extends craniocaudally nearly the entire length of the abdominal wall and nearly half of its width, starting from the linea alba. This broad aponeurosis serves as the insertion for both the costal and lumbar parts of this muscle. This flat tendon extends across the ventral surface of the m. rectus abdominis to the linea alba, where it unites with that of the opposite side. Caudally it attaches to the pecten ossis pubis. The deep trunk fascia closely adheres to the aponeurosis, obscuring the direction of its fibers. Near the lateral border of the rectus abdominis, this aponeurosis fuses deeply with the aponeurosis of the m. obliquus internus abdominis and with it forms the **external lamina** (*lamina externa*) of the **sheath of the rectus abdominis** (*vagina m. rectus abdominis*). It lies closely upon the superficial surface of the m. rectus abdominis, where it is intimately connected with the tendinous inscriptions of the rectus. Cranial to the iliopubic eminence, the superficial inguinal ring develops as a slit in this aponeurosis. At the cranial end of this ring fibrous strands, *fibrae intercrurales*, extend across between the medial and lateral crura to reinforce this angle of the ring. Embedded in the caudal end of this ring is a small palpable iliopubic cartilage, sometimes bone (Baumeier, 1908). This is in the tendon of origin of the pectineus. In the dog, the thickened caudal border of the aponeurosis of the external abdominal oblique is poorly associated with the inguinal ligament (*arcus inguinalis*), which is a fascial band that extends from the ilium and iliac fascia to the prepubic tendon at the iliopubic eminence. This is described next.

The **prepubic tendon** (*tendo prepubicus*) is a strong, collagenous mass composed primarily of the tendons of the paired rectus abdominis muscles and the tendons of origin of the paired pectineus muscles. It is firmly attached to the median ventral pubic tubercle situated on the external surface of the symphysis caudal to the free edge and the adjacent cranial rami of the pubic bones. The prepubic tendon develops as the attachments of fetal and neonatal muscles become tendinous. It extends from the iliopubic eminence and tendon of origin of the m. pectineus of one side to the same structures of the opposite side. The iliopubic cartilages are included at the lateral extent of the prepubic tendon. Included in the prepubic tendon are the aponeurotic attachments of the abdominal oblique muscles. To achieve homology with large domestic animal structure, the concept of the prepubic tendon of the dog, according to Habel (1990), should include the pectineus tendons, rectus abdominis tendons, abdominal oblique attachments, and the transversus abdominis terminations. The iliopubic cartilages (which sometimes ossify) would be included. The relationship of the lateral crus (pelvic tendon) of the superficial inguinal ring to the iliopubic cartilage and the prepubic tendon is well illustrated by Habel and Budras (1992). The prepubic tendon extends from the ventral pubic tubercle of the pubis to the tubercle of the psoas minor on the ilium. The prepubic tendon is a confluence of muscle attachments and incorporates the iliopubic cartilages on each side to which the pectineus tendon and external abdominal oblique attach.

Action: Along with other abdominal muscles, compression of the abdominal viscera. This action, known as *abdominal press*, aids in such vital functions as expiration, urination, defecation, and parturition. Flexion of the vertebral column when fellow muscles contract. Lateral bending (lateral flexion) of the vertebral column.

Innervation: Lateral branches of the last eight or nine nn. intercostales and the lateral branches of the nn. costoabdominalis, iliohypogastricus, and ilioinguinalis.

The **m. obliquus internus abdominis** (Figs. 6.33, 6.37 to 6.39) is a flat muscle lying medial to the m. obliquus externus abdominis in the lateral and ventral abdominal wall, where it is almost completely covered by the external oblique. Its fibers arise from the principal lamina of the thoracolumbar fascia caudal to the last rib, in common with the lumbar portion of the m. obliquus externus abdominis. This fascia provides attachment to the transverse and spinous processes of the lumbar vertebrae. Caudal to this it originates from the tuber coxae. Some fibers arise also from the fascia covering the m. iliopsoas and the dorsal portion of the inguinal ligament. Its fibers in general run cranioventrally and thereby cross those of the external oblique muscle at approximately a right angle. The thick cranial or costal part is often separated from the middle part by a distinct

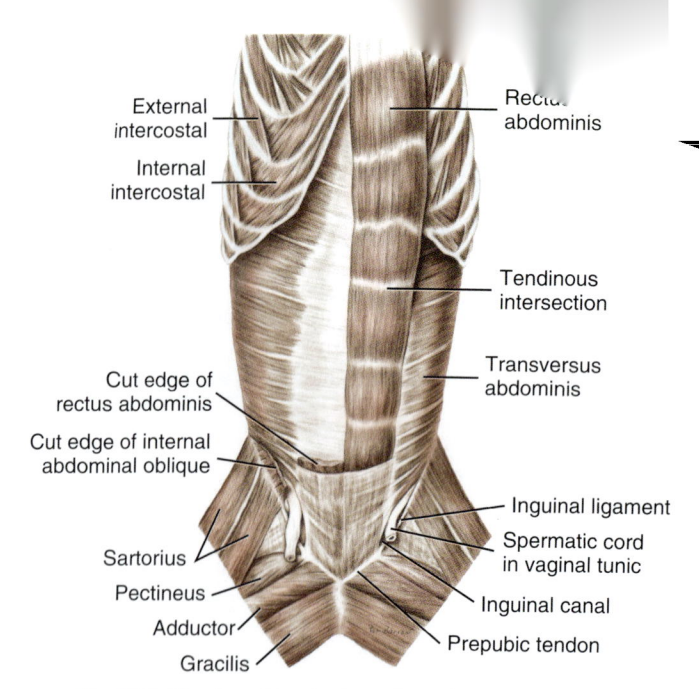

• **Fig. 6.38** Muscles of trunk, deep dissection, ventral aspect.

fissure that contains vessels of the abdominal wall. Its fleshy ending is on the thirteenth rib and on the cartilage of the twelfth rib. The middle abdominal portion gives rise to a broad aponeurosis at the lateral border of the m. rectus abdominis. This line of transition from muscle to aponeurosis (tendon) is often irregular. It extends from the bend of the twelfth costal cartilage to the iliopubic eminence. This long abdominal aponeurosis joins that of the external abdominal oblique and extends over the external surface of the rectus abdominis as part of the superficial leaf of the rectus sheath. It ends on the linea alba. A narrow cranial lamina of the aponeurosis is split off from the principal portion and runs over the internal surface of the rectus abdominis to aid in forming the **internal lamina** (*lamina interna*) or deep leaf of the rectus sheath.

According to Kassianenko (1928), this muscle becomes amplified at its cranial border (in 30% of dogs) by one to three slender muscle bundles that arise from the medial surface of the thirteenth, twelfth, and eleventh costal angles. Their tendons are related to that portion of the tendon of the internal abdominal oblique muscle that helps make up the deep leaf of the rectus sheath.

The caudal portion of the m. obliquus internus abdominis is rather distinctly separated from the middle portion by a fissure containing vessels of the abdominal wall. This part of the muscle comes from the tuber coxae, by means of a short aponeurosis, and from the inguinal ligament. Ventrally it forms the cranial border of the deep inguinal ring. This portion of the internal abdominal oblique extends caudal to the caudal border of the external abdominal oblique. Ventral to the inguinal canal, its most distal muscle fibers join the aponeurosis of the more cranial part and extend with the lateral lamina of the sheath to attach to the linea alba. Arising from the caudal free border of the

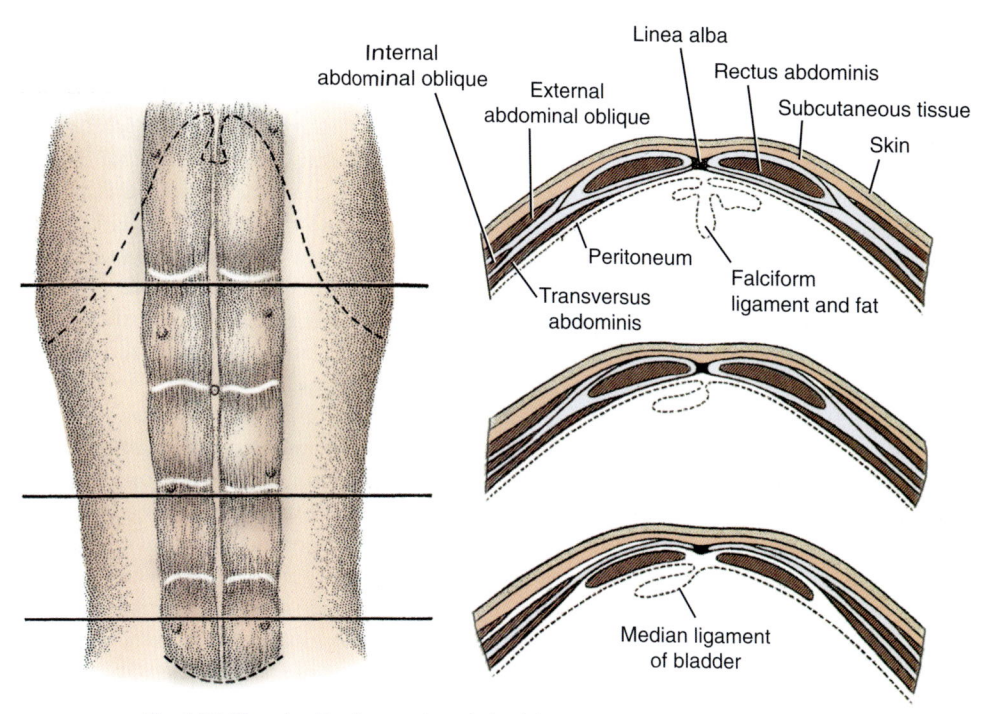

• Fig. 6.39 The sheath of m. rectus abdominis with cross-sections at three levels.

internal oblique muscle are fibers which form the cremaster muscle in the male (Figs. 9.10 and 9.14). These fibers pass through the inguinal canal in the fascia of the vaginal tunic.

Action: Compression and support of the abdominal viscera.
Innervation: Medial branches of the last few nn. intercostales and the nn. costoabdominalis, iliohypogastricus, and ilioinguinalis.

The *m. transversus abdominis* (Figs. 6.35, 6.38, and 6.39) is the deepest abdominal muscle and, like the oblique muscles, it is developed into an extensive leaf that reaches a thickness of 2 to 4 mm in large dogs. It lies in the lateral and ventral abdominal wall where its muscle fibers course transversely on the internal surface of the m. obliquus internus abdominis and adjacent costal cartilage. It arises medially from a line extending from the eighth costal cartilage to the last lumbar transverse process and thence caudally to the tuber coxae.

The lumbar part arises by broad, short tendons from the transverse processes of all the lumbar vertebrae via the deepest division of the thoracolumbar fascia. This fascia completely surrounds the longissimus lumborum and iliocostalis lumborum muscles. Its superficial layer provides the origin for the internal and external abdominal oblique muscles that extend within the abdominal wall superficial to the transversus abdominis. At the last rib the lumbar part is continuous with the costal part with no clear separation. Here the transversus abdominis muscle arises on the medial sides of the thirteenth and twelfth ribs and the eleventh to eighth costal cartilages in such a way that its line of origin crosses that of the diaphragm. From one to three serrations have parietal pleural coverings. The entire costal part of this muscle extends ventrally and slightly caudally from the internal surface of the last 4 or 5 ribs, 3 or 4 cm cranial to the origin of the m. obliquus internus abdominis. The medial branches of the ventral divisions of the last few thoracic and the first few lumbar nerves run over the superficial surface of the m. transversus abdominis. The muscle is marked by these into several (usually six) "segments" that occur in the part caudal to the last rib, the remainder appearing medial to the costal arch. The muscle extends to the linea alba on the internal surface of the m. rectus abdominis by a long aponeurosis that begins on this internal surface near the lateral border to the m. rectus abdominis. From cranial to caudal this aponeurosis forms a laterally convex line, the summit of which lies at the region of the umbilicus, 5 cm from the midline. Toward the xiphoid cartilage it lies only 1.5 cm from the midline. This aponeurosis forms most of the internal layer (*lamina interna*) of the sheath of the rectus abdominis. It unites inseparably at the linea alba with the external leaf. Cranially this aponeurosis of the transversus abdominis is joined by an internal extension of the aponeurosis of the internal abdominal oblique to complete the internal lamina at that level.

The cranial part of the muscle, by the development of incomplete fissures, encroaches directly upon the m. transversus thoracis, and the aponeurosis covers the outer surface of the free end of the xiphoid cartilage. The caudal part of this aponeurosis does not cross the internal surface of the rectus abdominis muscle. Instead it traverses the external surface to join the aponeuroses of the two oblique muscles in the formation of the external lamina of the rectus sheath. Toward the pelvis, it fuses with a tendinous strand of the rectus. On the internal surface of the pelvic end of the rectus abdominis, there is no aponeurotic covering. There is only a thin continuation of the transversalis fascia and parietal peritoneum.

Action and Innervation: Same as for the internal abdominal oblique.

The **transversalis fascia** (*fascia transversalis*) covers the inner surfaces of the mm. transversi abdominis. It runs between the iliac fascia on the ventral, lateral border of the mm. psoas major and minor and the ventral midline of the abdomen. During its course, it covers the pelvic part of the m. rectus abdominis, which is free of the aponeurosis of the transversus abdominis. Farther cranially, it fuses with the internal lamina of the rectus abdominis sheath. In the lateral abdominal wall, it runs cranially to the diaphragm and continues on the abdominal surface of the latter, which it completely covers. The fascia transversalis may contain much fat. The fascia contains dense reinforcements of coarse elastic fibers that run in anastomosing strands from caudal to cranial, thus crossing the course of the fibers of the m. transversus abdominis. These fibers come from the entire length of the m. iliopsoas and are especially dense ventrally. Deep to the point of separation of the m. cremaster from the caudal border of the m. obliquus internus abdominis, the elastic masses are the thickest. Toward the ribs they become correspondingly thinner. At the inguinal canal the peritoneum everts as the vaginal process in the female and the vaginal tunic in the male. The transversalis fascia covers this eversion and encloses the m. cremaster in the male on the lateral and caudal sides of the vaginal tunic.

The **inguinal ligament** (*arcus inguinalis* [*lig. inguinale*]) (Fig. 6.38) is closely related to the fascia transversalis and, like it, contains much elastic tissue. In comparison with other domestic animals, in the dog this inguinal ligament is a relatively incomplete structure and independent of the external abdominal oblique. It is a distinct band extending in the iliac fascia from the tuber coxae obliquely over the m. iliopsoas, marking the caudal border of origin of the fascia transversalis. Together with this fascia it extends ventrolaterally along the m. iliopsoas. The main part of the inguinal ligament continues distally between the deep inguinal and femoral rings to attach to the lateral border of the prepubic tendon. By taking this course it forms the caudal border of the deep inguinal ring. Fibers from this ligament are continuous with the transversalis fascia that extends through the inguinal canal with the vaginal process, forming its internal spermatic fascia. At its ilial end, this ligament gives origin to part of the m. obliquus internus abdominis. The fusion of this ligament with the iliac, pelvic, and transversalis fasciae acts as a binder in closing the potential space that might exist between the pelvic and abdominal walls.

Budras and Wünsche (1972) substitute a concept of an inguinal arch for the inguinal ligament. Their inguinal arch is composed of lateral, middle, and medial parts, of which the lateral and middle parts often form an inconstant inguinal tract that joins the caudal border of the aponeurosis of the external abdominal oblique and continues on the tendon of origin of the pectineus at the prepubic tendon.

The ***m. rectus abdominis*** (Figs. 6.33, 6.37 to 6.39) is a long, flat, relatively narrow (compared with the other abdominal muscles) muscle that extends from the first costal cartilage to the pecten ossis pubis. The two muscles are adjacent to the ventral median plane of the thorax and abdomen. In the abdomen, the muscles are separated by the linea alba and contained between the internal and external laminae that compose the sheath of the rectus abdominis. Cranially, in large dogs, this muscle is 7 to 8 cm broad. Caudally, it gradually narrows to 3.5 to 4 cm. Its thickness is 5 to 7 mm, decreasing toward the lateral border. The fibers of the muscle course longitudinally. It arises by a broad, flat aponeurosis (tendon) from the cranial sternum and the first costal cartilage and rib, where it is covered by the terminal tendon of the m. rectus thoracis. It also has a fleshy origin by means of a special serration from the sternal portion of the ninth costal cartilage. As it passes over the ventral abdominal wall, it lies in a nearly horizontal position, with the medial border facing the linea alba. Occasionally the terminal portion of the muscle is wide enough to help in the formation of the medial wall of the inguinal canal and to appear at the level of the superficial inguinal ring. United by the linea alba and covered externally by a thick tendinous covering, the two recti end on the pecten ossis pubis, from one iliopubic eminence to the other. At its insertion at the pubis each muscle unites with the tendon of origin of the m. pectineus and, along with contributions from the aponeuroses of the other abdominal muscles, forms the prepubic tendon. A conical, paired segment of superficial fibers continues farther and ends on the tubercle on the ventral surface of the pelvic symphysis. This crosses the thickened border of the external leaf of the rectus sheath. This long muscle is divided into segments by three to six (usually five) transverse, zigzag, tendinous intersections (*intersectiones tendineae*). Their distinctness varies. Their number does not correspond with the number of entering nerves. Intimately attached to the tendinous intersections are fibers of the external lamina of the rectus sheath. The fibers of the internal lamina of the sheath are not as firmly attached. The first intersection is at the level of the seventh costal cartilage; the last segment is usually the longest; all other relations vary (Strauss, 1927).

Action: All functions that depend on abdominal press, such as expiration, urination, defecation, and parturition; support of the abdominal viscera; to bring the pelvis cranial; flexion of the trunk.

Innervation: Medial branches of the branches of the nn. intercostales and medial branches of the nn. costoabdominalis, iliohypogastricus, and ilioinguinalis.

The **sheath of the rectus abdominis** (*vagina m. recti abdominis*) (Figs. 6.37 to 6.39) covers both surfaces of the rectus abdominis muscle. It is formed primarily by the aponeuroses of the other abdominal muscles. The **external** *lamina externa*) of the rectus sheath consists of the wide and long aponeuroses of the m. obliquus externus abdominis, most of the aponeurosis of the m. obliquus internus abdominis, and, near its caudal end, a portion of the aponeurosis of the m. transversus abdominis. The **internal lamina** (*lamina interna*) of the rectus sheath is formed by the end aponeurosis of the m. transversus abdominis, the fascia transversalis, and cranially by an internal leaf of the aponeurosis of the m. obliquus internus abdominis. At its pelvic end, the m. rectus abdominis lacks an internal aponeurotic covering, being covered here by only a thin continuation of the transversalis fascia and parietal peritoneum.

The **inguinal canal** (*canalis inguinalis*) (Figs. 6.38 and 9.12) in both sexes is a connective tissue-filled fissure between the abdominal muscles and their aponeuroses in the caudoventral abdominal wall. In the male the inguinal canal serves as the passageway for the fetal vaginal process and the descent of the testis. After this descent, the canal contains spermatic fascia, the vaginal tunic and its spermatic cord, the cremaster muscle, external pudendal vessels, and the genitofemoral nerve. In the female it contains fascia, the vaginal process and its round ligament, much fat, the external pudendal vessels, and the genitofemoral nerve. It is relatively short. It begins at the deep inguinal ring, which is formed by (1) the ventral end of the inguinal ligament, (2) the fleshy caudal border of the internal abdominal oblique muscle, and (3) the lateral border of the rectus abdominis muscle. The inguinal canal is covered externally by the aponeurosis of the m. obliquus externus abdominis. The path of the canal is determined by the processus vaginalis. Because the latter pushes over the caudal border of the m. obliquus internus abdominis for a short distance, the medial wall of the inguinal canal is formed by the superficial surface of this muscle. The superficial surfaces of the aponeuroses of the mm. transversus abdominis and rectus abdominis also aid in forming the medial wall. The lateral wall is formed solely by the aponeurosis of the external oblique. The canal is open to the outside because a narrow, oval slit forms in the aponeurosis of the external abdominal oblique. This is the superficial inguinal ring (anulus inguinalis superficialis). This ring has medial and lateral borders, crura, formed by this aponeurosis. Where the borders meet, the cranial and caudal angles, or commissures, are formed. The caudal commissure contains the iliopubic cartilage, which is located in the tendon of origin of the pectineus. The cranial commissure is much thinner as the parallel strands of collagenous tissue that form the two crura in the aponeurosis of the external oblique are held together mainly by the transversalis fascia.

The **linea alba** (Figs. 6.37 and 6.39) is a midventral strip of collagenous tissue that extends from the xiphoid process to the symphysis pelvis. It serves for the main insertion of the abdominal transverse and external and internal oblique muscles. The medial borders of the right and left rectus muscles lie closely against its lateral borders. At the level of a transverse plane through the last ribs, the linea alba contains a scar, the **umbilicus** (*anulus umbilicalis*), a remnant of the umbilical ring and cord. The linea alba is a little more than 1 cm wide and less than 1 mm thick just caudal to the xiphoid process. It gradually narrows and thickens caudally. Caudal to the umbilicus it appears as a line, being less than 1 mm wide but considerably thicker. It blends with the prepubic tendon and attaches to the cranial edge of the pelvic symphysis.

The quadratus lumborum is listed as an abdominal muscle in the NAV, but in this text it is described with the lumbar hypaxial muscles.

The ***m. cutaneus trunci*** (Fig. 6.48), according to Langworthy (1924), is a derivative of the m. pectoralis profundus. As a thin leaf it covers almost the entire dorsal, lateral, and ventral walls of the thorax and abdomen. It begins caudally in the gluteal region and, running cranially and ventrally, covers the dorsal and lateral surfaces of the abdomen and thorax. It ends in the axilla and on the caudal border of the deep pectoral. It lies in the superficial trunk fascia and is not attached to the vertebral spinous processes. It is principally a longitudinal muscle with its origin in the superficial gluteal fascia. The dorsal borders of the muscle on each side run parallel along the spinous processes of the lumbar and thoracic vertebrae. Only in the region caudal to the scapula, where the muscle begins to extend ventrally on the thorax, do the fibers arise from the dorsal midline and meet those of the opposite side. Because this part of the muscle is also not attached to the spinous processes of the vertebrae, it is free over the vertebral column to be included in raised folds of the skin. Its ventral border crosses in the fold of the flank to the lateral and ventral abdominal wall. The course of the fibers is predominantly ventrocranial. Its craniodorsal border covers the m. trapezius, a portion of the m. infraspinatus, and the m. latissimus dorsi, and ends by means of the muscular axillary arch in the medial brachial fascia. The principal part of the muscle, however, with its loose fiber bundles, passes to the superficial surface of the m. pectoralis profundus adjacent to its free edge, where it ends in the superficial thoracic fascia. The fibers of the ventral border coming from the flank reach each other in the midventral line caudal to the sternum.

The ***m. preputialis cranialis*** consists of longitudinal muscle strands filling the space between the opposite abdominal portions of the two cutaneous trunci muscles in the region of the xiphoid cartilage in the male. Toward the umbilicus a pair of muscular strands arises from the m. preputialis. They radiate into the prepuce in such a way that they come together archlike in the prepuce ventral to the glans. In so doing they are firmly united with each other and with the prepuce. Dogs do not have a m. preputialis caudalis.

The ***m. supramammaricus*** of the bitch is homologous with the m. preputialis of the male. In contrast to the muscle in the male, this muscle is more delicate and narrower and is paired from its beginning. From the region caudal to the xiphoid cartilage, the muscle fibers extend caudally in loose bundles, dorsal to the mammary gland complex, to the pubic region. Cranial to the paired inguinal mammary glands, each blends with the ipsilateral m. cutaneous trunci.

Action: The m. cutaneus trunci shakes the skin to remove foreign bodies and increase heat production. It also tenses the skin when required. The preputial muscle draws the prepuce over the glans after erection. The supramammary muscle aids in support of the mammary glands and perhaps in milk ejection.

Innervation: Efferent supply, lateral thoracic nerve (Langworthy, 1924); afferent supply, lateral thoracic and lateral branches of the intercostal nerves and the nn. costoabdominalis, iliohypogastricus, ilioinguinalis, and genitofemoralis. Note that the lateral thoracic nerve has muscle afferents but no cutaneous afferents.

Muscles of the Tail (*Musculi Caudae*)

The caudal vertebrae are largely enclosed in muscles. The mm. sacrocaudalis dorsalis lateralis and medialis, dorsal in location, are extensors or levators of the tail. The mm. sacrocaudalis ventralis lateralis and medialis, ventral in location, are flexors or depressors of the tail. The mm. coccygeus, levator ani, and the intertransversarii caudae, lateral in location, are the lateral flexors of the tail. The dorsal muscles are direct continuations of the epaxial musculature of the trunk. The caudal muscles lie on the lumbar vertebrae, sacrum, and caudal vertebrae, and insert on the caudal vertebrae, exclusively. They have fleshy endings as well as tendinous ones of variable length. The most caudal tendons go to the last caudal vertebrae. Cranially the muscles, as well as the vertebral bodies, are larger. The caudal muscles of the dog resemble those of the cat (Schumacher, 1910).

The **m. sacrocaudalis dorsalis lateralis**, or long levator of the tail (Fig. 6.40), is a flat, segmental muscle strand that becomes larger toward its dorsal border. It may be regarded as a continuation of the m. longissimus on the tail. In the caudal part of the lumbar region it lies between the m. longissimus, laterally, and the mm. multifidus lumborum and sacrocaudalis dorsalis medialis, medially. It has a fleshy origin from the aponeurosis of the m. longissimus and a tendinous origin from the mamillary processes of the first to sixth lumbar vertebrae, the articular processes of the sacrum, and the mamillary processes of at least the first eight caudal vertebrae. It is indistinctly divided into long individual parts that partly cover one another. From this muscular belly, which extends from the second sacral to the fourteenth caudal vertebra (when 20 caudal segments are present), there appear 16 thin, long tendons. These are arranged into a flat bundle by the accumulation of successive tendons. They lie embedded in the thick, deep caudal fascia. The first tendon ends on the mamillary process of the fifth caudal vertebra, the next ends on the sixth, and so on, to the last one. Cranial to their terminations a few take on a little tendon of the underlying segment of the m. sacrocaudalis dorsalis medialis.

Action: Extension or lifting of the tail, possibly also it to one side.

Innervation: Branches of the plexus caudalis dorsalis.

The **m. sacrocaudalis dorsalis medialis**, or short levator of the tail (Fig. 6.40), is the direct continuation on the tail of the m. multifidus and, like the latter, it is composed of relatively short, individual segments. It lies next to the median plane on the sacrum and caudal vertebrae and extends from the seventh lumbar to the last caudal vertebra. The individual segments can be isolated at the root of the tail. They are composed of deep, short muscle masses and a larger, superficial, long part that possesses a small tendon that spans four or five vertebrae. These individual muscles run between the spinous processes of cranial vertebrae and the dorsolaterally located tubercles, as well as on the mamillary processes on the cranial ends of more caudal vertebrae. Toward the tip of the tail the muscle segments become shorter, smaller, and more homogeneous. They arise from the small processes that are dorsolateral to the caudal edge of the rodlike caudal vertebrae. They pass over only one segment and end on dorsolateral humps that correspond to the mamillary processes of the lumbar vertebrae. The superficial tendons end in common with the long tendons of the m. sacrocaudalis dorsalis lateralis. Muscle fibers also accompany the tendons.

Action: Extension of the tail, possibly also lateral flexion.
Innervation: Branches of the plexus caudalis dorsalis.

The **m. sacrocaudalis ventralis lateralis**, or long depressor of the tail (Fig. 6.41), is large in large dogs. It consists of numerous long, individual parts that are arranged like those of the long levator and that end by means of long tendons from the sixth to the last segment. The first segment comes from the ventral surface of the body of the last lumbar vertebra and from the sacrum. The remaining segments arise from the ventral surfaces and the roots of the transverse processes of the caudal vertebrae. From the segmented bellies of the third and successive segments caudally, the individual long tendons arise and are embedded in the thick, deep caudal fascia. The first of these is attached to the ventrolateral tubercle (*processus hemalis*) of the proximal end of the sixth caudal vertebra, the second on the corresponding elevation of the seventh, and so on to the last caudal vertebra. Before inserting, each of these tendons acquires the small tendon of the segment of the short depressor, which has been crossed by the segment of the long depressor.

Action: Flexion of the tail and, occasionally, lateral movement.

Innervation: Branches of the plexus caudalis ventralis.

The **m. sacrocaudalis ventralis medialis**, or short depressor of the tail (Fig. 6.41), consists of segmental, short individual parts extending from the last sacral vertebra

CHAPTER 6 The Muscular System   259

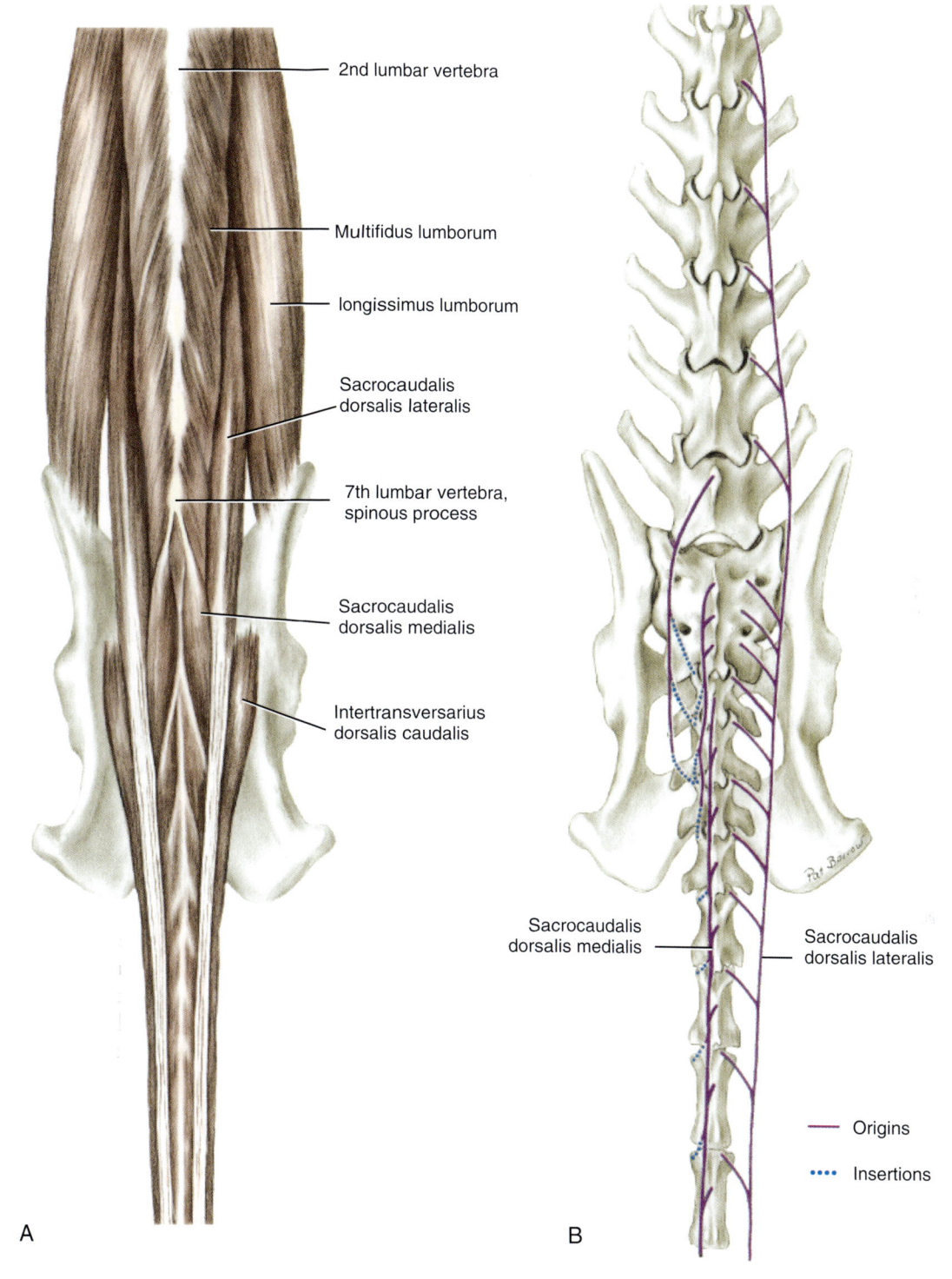

- **Fig. 6.40** Muscles of lumbocaudal region. **A**, Epaxial muscles, dorsal aspect. **B**, Diagram of sacrocaudal muscles, dorsal aspect.

throughout the length of the tail. It lies against the ventral surface of the vertebrae and, with the muscle of the opposite side, forms a deep furrow (for the a. caudalis). At the pelvic outlet the bundles are very large and the segmentation is indistinct. However, more distally, independent segments are separated out. The fibers of each of these segments arise essentially from the ventral surface of one vertebra. Superficially, a small, flat tendon is then formed. This unites with the tendon of the sacrocaudalis ventralis lateralis, which lies immediately lateral to it, and this common tendon then passes over the following segment to end on the hemal process of the next following vertebra.

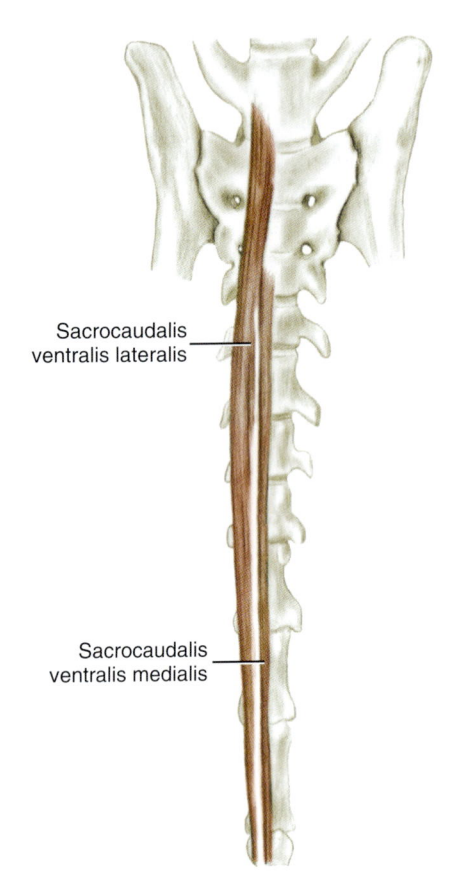

• Fig. 6.41 Sacrocaudal muscles, ventral aspect.

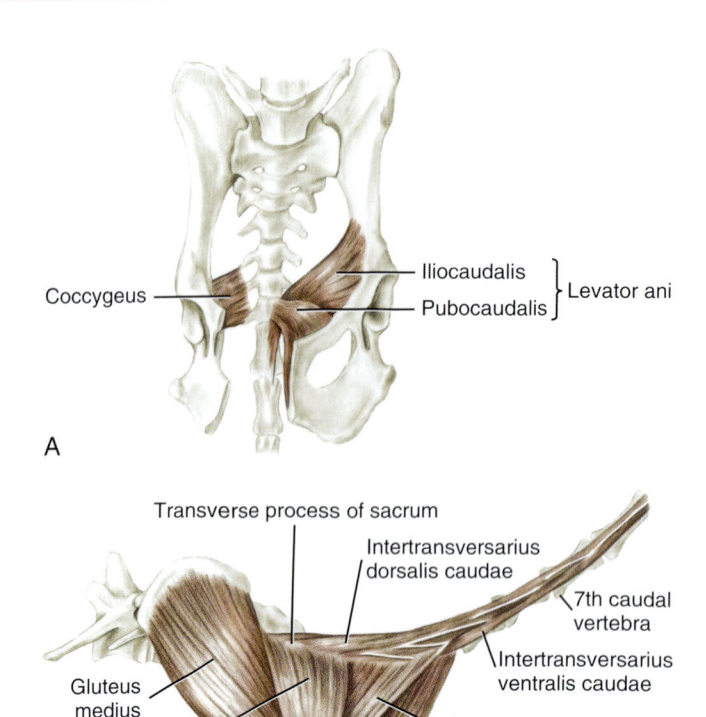

• Fig. 6.42 Muscles of the pelvis. A, Mm. levator ani and coccygeus, ventral aspect. B, Caudal and gluteal muscles, lateral aspect.

Action and Innervation: Same as for the m. sacrocaudalis ventralis lateralis.

The **m. intertransversarius dorsales caudae** (Figs. 6.40A and 6.42B) lies between the sacrum and the middle of the tail. In general, it consists of short individual parts, of which only the first is well developed. This portion arises on the long, dorsal sacroiliac ligament, on the lateral part of the third sacral vertebra, and forms a large, round muscle belly that ends on the transverse process of the fifth or sixth caudal vertebra by means of a long tendon. In its course it receives supplementary fibers from the transverse processes of the first few caudal vertebrae. These deep elements gradually become independent muscles that extend from one transverse process to that of the following vertebra. They lie on the dorsal surfaces of the transverse processes or their rudiments, where they are partly covered by the long tendons of the levators. These muscle segments become so small in the caudal half of the tail that they are difficult to isolate. Superficial parts of the first large segment give rise to two or three long, flat tendons that extend to the thick caudal fascia and to the rudiment of the transverse process of the sixth or seventh or even the eighth caudal vertebra.

Action: With the m. intertransversarius ventralis caudalis, lateral flexion of the tail.
Innervation: Branches of the plexus caudalis ventralis.

The **m. intertransversarius ventrales caudae** (Fig. 6.42B) situated ventral to the transverse processes, begins at the third caudal vertebra. It forms a round belly, composed of segments, and, at the base of the tail, is smaller than the dorsal muscle. However, it has a more constant size and is well segmented, and thus is easily traced to the end of the tail. Ventrally the muscle is covered by the long tendons of the long depressor of the tail. From the third to the fifth caudal vertebra, the ventral and dorsal mm. intertransversarii are separated by the m. coccygeus; otherwise they are separated by a strong intermuscular septum of the caudal fascia.

Action and Innervation: Same as for the m. intertransversarius dorsalis caudalis.

The **pelvic diaphragm** (*diaphragma pelvis*) in quadrupedal mammals is the vertical closure of the pelvic cavity through which the rectum passes. The two muscles of the pelvic diaphragm are the m. coccygeus and the m. levator ani.

The **m. coccygeus**, formerly called the *m. coccygeus lateralis* (Figs. 6.42, 6.43, 6.70, and 6.82), is a thick muscle arising by means of a narrow tendon on the ischiatic spine cranial to the internal obturator muscle. It crosses the medial aspect of the sacrotuberous ligament and, spreading like a fan, extends to the lateral surface of the tail. There it

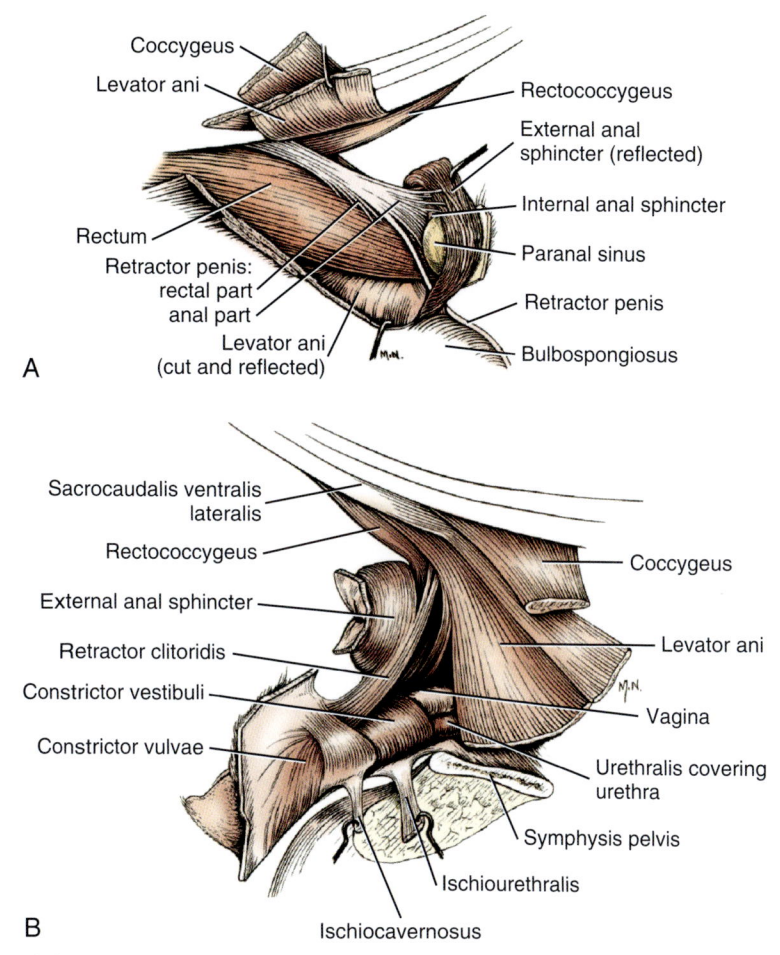

• **Fig. 6.43** **A**, Muscles of the male anal region, lateral aspect. **B**, Constrictor muscles of female genitalia, lateral aspect.

ends, ventral to the m. intertransversarii dorsales caudae, on the transverse processes of the second to fifth caudal vertebrae. It is partially covered by the caudal portion of the m. gluteus superficialis.

Action: Bilateral: to press the tail against the anus and genital parts and, in conjunction with the depressors, to draw the tail between the pelvic limbs. Unilateral: lateral flexion.
Innervation: Ventral branches of the third sacral nerve.

The **m. levator ani**, formerly known as the *m. coccygeus medialis* or the *m. ilio-, ischio-,* or *pubococcygeus* (Figs. 6.42, 6.43, and 6.70), lies cranial and medial to the coccygeus. It is a broad triangular muscle originating on the medial edge of the shaft of the ilium, on the dorsal surface of the ramus of the pubis, and on the entire pelvic symphysis. Bilaterally, the muscles spread out and radiate dorsocaudally toward the root of the tail. In so doing, they surround a large median, fatty mass, as well as the genitalia and the rectum. Caudally, each encroaches upon the dorsal surface of the m. obturator internus. After decreasing in size, the muscle then appears at the caudal edge of the m. coccygeus, passes into the caudal fascia, and ends on the hemal process of the seventh caudal vertebra by means of a prominent tendon immediately next to the tendon of its fellow of the opposite side. This muscle can be divided into a **m. iliocaudalis** and a **m. pubocaudalis**, based on their origins. The n. obturatorius passes between them. The fibers of both parts enter the tendon at an angle. The deep surface of the muscle is firmly covered by the pelvic fascia, which is also connected with the m. sphincter ani externus. Pettit (1962) has summarized many cases of perineal hernia in the dog and described their surgical repair with regard to the muscles of the pelvic diaphragm.

Action: Bilateral: to press the tail against the anus and genital parts; unilateral: to bring the tail cranially and laterally. The mm. levatores ani, in combination with the levators of the tail, cause the sharp angulation between the sixth and seventh caudal vertebrae, which is characteristic for defecation; compression of the rectum.
Innervation: Ventral branches of the third (last) sacral and the first caudal nerve.

The **m. rectococcygeus** (Fig. 6.43) is a paired smooth muscle composed of fibers from the external longitudinal musculature of the rectum. The fibers sweep caudodorsally from the sides of the rectum and pass through the fascial arch formed by the attachment of the external anal sphincter to the fascia of the tail. Right and left portions of the muscle fuse beneath the third caudal vertebra. The median muscle thus formed lies between the ventral sacrocaudal muscles and passes caudally to insert on the fifth and sixth caudal vertebrae. The attachment of the rectococcygeus muscle on the tail serves to anchor the rectum and provide for caudal traction in defecation. Extension of the tail during defecation aids in evacuating the rectum because of the attachments of the mm. rectococcygeus, coccygeus, and levator ani. The mm. coccygeus and levator ani cross the rectum laterally and tend to compress it. The m. rectococcygeus, by shortening the rectum, aids in evacuation of the fecal column.

Action: To aid in defecation.
Innervation: Autonomic fibers from pelvic plexus.

The **m. sphincter ani internus** (Fig. 6.43) is the caudal, thickened portion of the circular coat of the anal canal. It is composed of smooth muscle fibers and is smaller than the striated external anal sphincter. Between the two sphincter muscles on either side lies the paranal sinus (*sinus paranalis*). The duct from the paranal sinus crosses the caudal border of the internal sphincter muscle.

The **m. ani externus** (Fig. 6.43), composed of striated muscle fibers, surrounds the anus, covers the internal sphincter except caudally, and is largely subcutaneous. The cranial border of the external sphincter is united by fascia to the caudal border of the levator ani. Dorsally the external sphincter attaches mainly to the caudal fascia at the level of the third caudal vertebra. This attachment is such that a cranially directed concave fascial arch is formed, through which the rectococcygeus muscle passes. Approximately half of the fibers of the external sphincter encircle the anus ventrally. The remaining superficial ventral fibers end on the urethral muscle and the bulbocavernosus muscle of the male. In the female, comparable fibers blend with the constrictor vulvae.

The **m. retractor penis, clitoridis** (Fig. 6.43) is a band of muscle that arises ventrally on each side of the sacrum or first two caudal vertebrae. It was called the caudoanal or caudocavernosus muscle in the cat by Straus-Durckheim (1845) and in the dog by Langley and Anderson (1895). It was illustrated as the coccygeoanalis muscle in the dog by Miller et al. (1964). This muscle is now referred to as the *m. retractor penis* or *clitoridis* with a *pars analis* and a *pars rectalis*. At its origin on the vertebrae there is a considerable decussation of fibers ventral to the rectococcygeus muscle. Each band passes ventrocaudally across the lateral surface of the rectum, to which it contributes some fibers. It becomes wider distally as it passes caudal to the paranal sinus and into the sphincters. The bulk of its fibers appear to end near the duct of the paranal sinus, although some fibers insert in the external sphincter. Occasionally, a rudiment of a ventral anal loop may be present. In the male, a ventral portion of the muscle band, in combination with some fibers from the external sphincter, continues distally as the retractor penis muscle. In the female this is the retractor clitoridis. Superficially these retractor muscles are covered by the levator ani, with which there may be some fiber interchange.

Fasciae of the Trunk and Tail

On the trunk, as on other parts of the body, there is a superficial and a deep fascia, known collectively as the *external fascia of the trunk*. It covers the muscles and bones of the thorax and abdomen. In addition, there is an internal fascia of the trunk, which serves a special function in the formation of the body cavities.

The **internal fascia of the trunk** lies on the deep surfaces of the muscles of the body wall and on the superficial surfaces of the serous coverings of the cavities. In the thoracic cavity, it is the *fascia endothoracica*; in the abdominal cavity, the *fascia transversalis*. The latter covers the m. transversus abdominis on its deep surface and fuses ventrally with its aponeurosis. Cranially the fascia transversalis covers the diaphragm as a thin membrane. The internal trunk fascia is reinforced by yellow elastic tissue wherever it covers a movable or expansible structure, such as the diaphragm. The *fascia iliaca* covers the lumbar hypaxial muscles and is connected with the last few lumbar vertebral bodies and with the ilium. The *fascia pelvis* clothes the pelvic cavity; it lies deeply on the bones and gluteal muscles concerned, and it continues on the pelvic surface of the muscles of the pelvic diaphragm. In obese dogs it contains much fat.

The **superficial external fascia of the trunk** (*fascia trunci superficialis*) is relatively thick; it covers the thorax and abdomen in a manner similar to that on other parts of the body. It extends cranially, dorsally, and laterally to the scapular region and neighboring parts of the brachium. The ventral part uses the axillary and sternal region to gain the neck and also sends connections to the superficial fascia of the medial surface of the thoracic limb. Caudally direct continuations are found in the superficial gluteal fascia and, by means of the thigh, on the cranial crural portions to the lateral and medial crural fasciae, and, finally, in the pubic region, to correspondingly superficial fascial parts. There are no attachments with the dorsal ends of the thoracic and lumbar vertebrae. Thus, as on the neck, the fascia can be picked up with folds in the skin. There are ventral fascial leaves to the prepuce and to the mammary glands. The superficial trunk fascia covers the mm. trapezius and latissimus dorsi, as well as parts of the pectoral muscles, omotransversarius, deltoideus, and triceps brachii. In relation to the underlying structures, all parts of the superficial fascia are extremely displaceable. Only on the scapula is this mobility limited. Wherever there is great mobility in well-nourished animals large quantities of subfascial fat are deposited.

The **deep external fascia of the trunk** (*fascia thoracolumbalis*) is a dense, thick, shining, tendinous membrane.

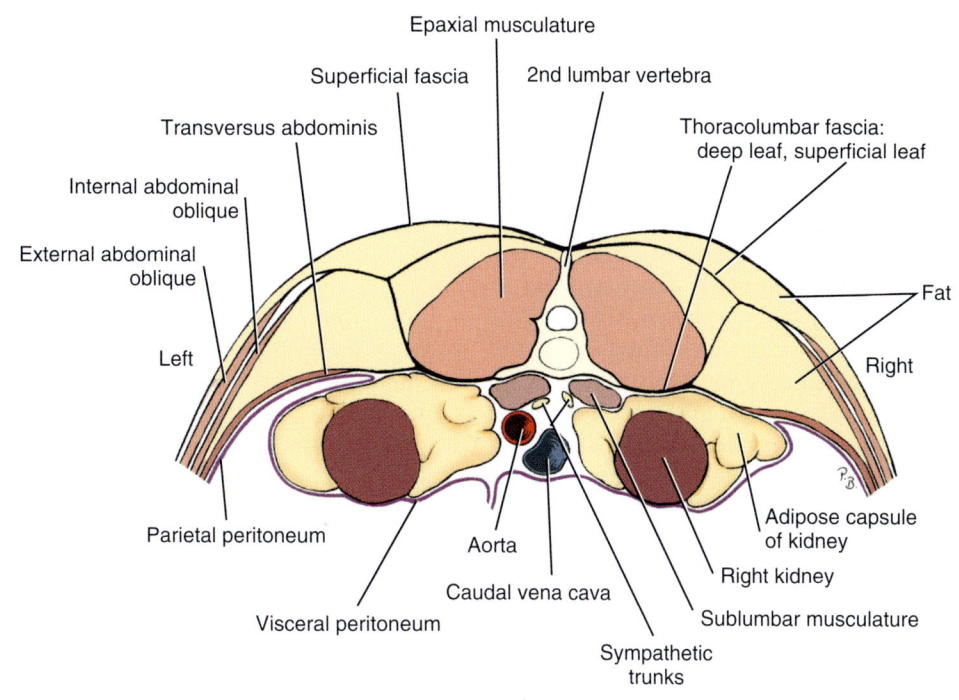

• **Fig. 6.44** Schematic transverse section through lumbar region, showing the fascial layers.

It begins on the ends of the spinous processes of the thoracic and lumbar vertebrae, from the supraspinous ligament. It passes over the epaxial musculature to the lateral thoracic and abdominal wall, to fuse with the fascia of the opposite side at the linea alba. In the sternal region it passes deep to the pectoral musculature on the sternum and costal cartilages. Caudally it is attached to the ilium.

The thoracolumbar fascia covers the epaxial, erector spinae muscles and has two leaves (Fig. 6.44). The superficial leaf gives rise to the latissimus dorsi cranially and the two oblique abdominal muscles and the serratus dorsalis caudalis caudally. The deep leaf gives rise to the splenius and the serratus dorsalis cranialis cranially and the transversus abdominis caudally. Medial to the scapula, the deep leaf is medial to the rhomboideus and lateral to the erector spinae muscles. Laterally it attaches to the scapula. In the caudal thoracic and abdominal region, the fused layers of the thoracolumbar fascia provide an aponeurosis for the longissimus and iliocostalis muscles. A deep extension forms an intermuscular septum between these muscles. Laterally it attaches to the lumbar vertebral transverse processes where its deep leaf provides origin for the transversus abdominis muscle.

As the relatively thin thoracolumbar fascia passes to the lateral wall of the abdomen and thorax, it continues on the superficial surface of the m. obliquus externus abdominis and on the thoracic serrations of the m. serratus ventralis, with which it is firmly fused. Over the m. serratus ventralis thoracis and deep to the scapula, the deep thoracic fascia is connected with the deep cervical fascia. These two fasciae meet on the superficial surface of the mm. serratus ventralis cervicis and scalenus. In the abdominal region and in the caudal thoracic region the deep fascia of the trunk descends over the external surface of the external sheath of the rectus abdominis. Caudally it is more or less firmly united with the crura of the superficial inguinal ring. At the commissures of the crura it unites the diverging collagenous strands especially at the cranial commissure, which is thought to prevent enlargement of the ring during herniation. At the caudal commissure it blends with the tendon of origin of the m. pectineus. From the crura, especially the medial one, the deep fascia extends on the vaginal process or tunic and its contents. In the male this is known as the *external spermatic fascia*. Caudal to the lumbar region, the deep fascia of the trunk becomes the deep gluteal fascia, and from the lateral abdominal wall it becomes the crural fascia.

The **superficial** and **deep fasciae of the tail** (*fasciae caudae*) arise from the corresponding leaves of the gluteal fascia. The superficial fascia is insignificant. The thick, deep leaf provides thick connective tissue masses for special ensheathment of the long tendons of the mm. sacrocaudalis dorsalis lateralis and sacrocaudalis ventralis lateralis.

Muscles of the Thoracic Limb

Extrinsic Muscles

The extrinsic muscles of the thoracic limb originate on the neck and thorax and extend to the scapula or humerus as far distally as the elbow joint. They include a superficial layer of muscles lying directly on the fascia of the scapula and brachium, and a second, deeper layer, being in part medial and in part lateral to the scapula and brachium. According to the points of attachment, the extrinsic muscles can be divided into those from the trunk to the scapula and those from the trunk to the humerus. Included in these extrinsic muscles are the brachiocephalicus, omotransversarius, trapezius, latissimus dorsi, rhomboideus, and serratus ventralis cervicis, which have already been described with the neck or thoracic muscles. A description of the superficial and deep pectorals follows.

The **mm. pectorales superficiales** consist of a small **descending pectoral muscle** (*m. pectoralis descendens*) and a large **transverse pectoral muscle** (*m. pectoralis transversus*) (Figs. 6.45, 6.48, and 6.49). They lie deep to the skin on the cranioventral part of the thorax between the cranial end of the sternum and the humerus. Both arise paramedially on the cranial end of the sternum, run laterally and distally, and cover the m. biceps brachii. Then, with the m. cleidobrachialis, they pass between the mm. biceps brachii and brachialis and end, except for a small distal part, on the entire crest of the major tubercle of the humerus. Three divisions of the muscle are discernible because there are two slips of the more cranial descending pectoral.

Action: To support the limb, draw the limb medially (adduction), draw the limb cranially or caudally according to its position, and draw the trunk laterally.
Innervation: Nn. pectorales craniales and also branches from nn. cervicales 7 and 8 (Langworthy, 1924).

The **m. pectoralis profundus**, or ascending pectoral (*m. pectoralis asendens*) (Figs. 6.45 and 6.49B) is a broad muscle lying ventrally on the thorax; it can be divided into a major portion and a minor superficial, lateral portion. It extends between the sternum and the humerus. It arises from the first to the last sternebra and, with a superficial marginal portion as the pars abdominalis, from the deep fascia of the trunk in the region of the xiphoid cartilage. Its fibers run cranially and laterally toward the brachium. It covers the

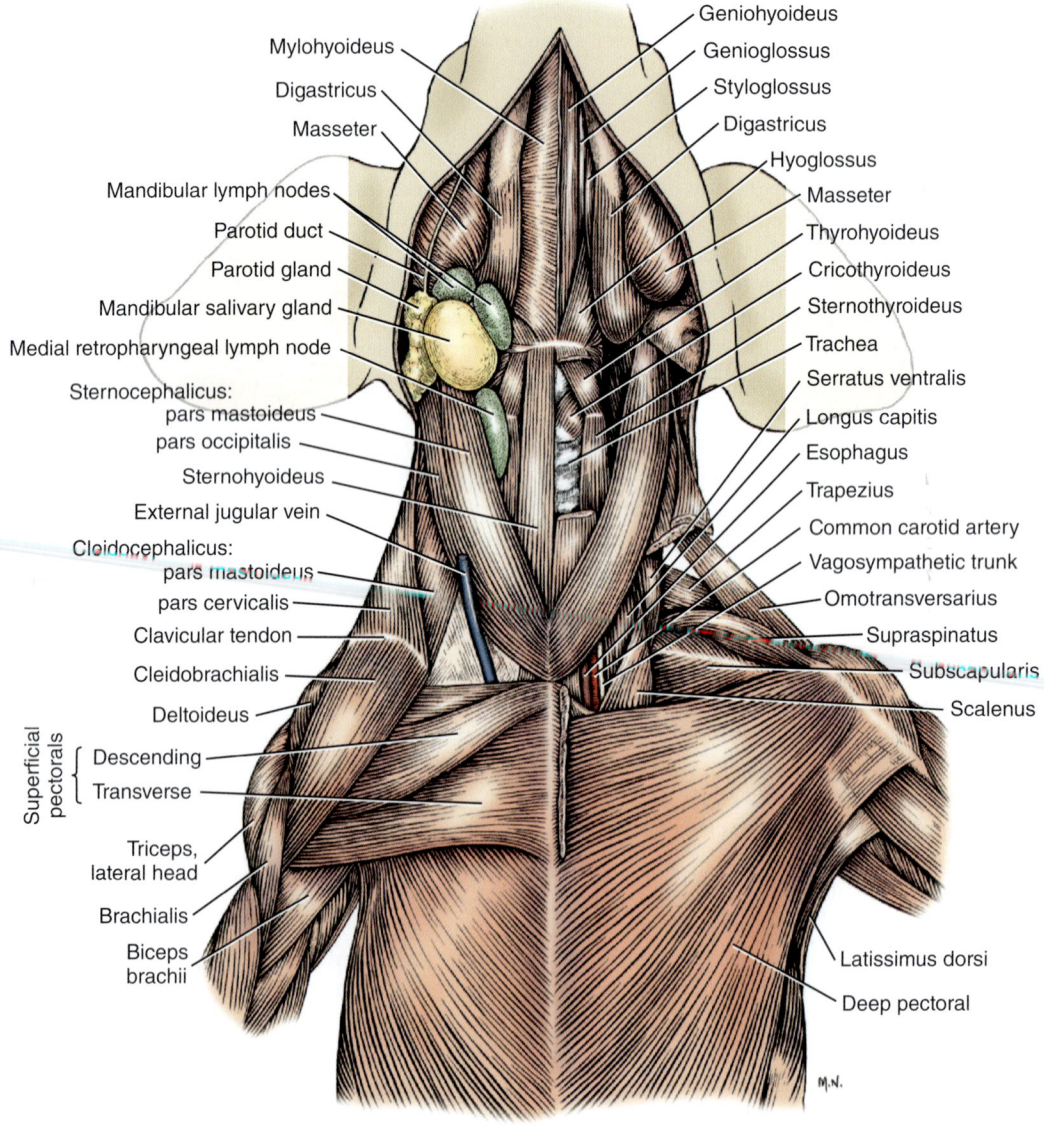

- Fig. 6.45 Superficial muscles of neck and thorax, ventral aspect.

sternum and the cartilages of the sternal ribs from which it is separated by the aponeurosis of the mm. rectus abdominis and rectus thoracis. After passing deep to the superficial pectoral, the major part of the muscle largely inserts, partly muscularly and partly tendinously, on the lesser tubercle of the humerus. An aponeurosis passes over the m. biceps brachii to the major tubercle. The superficial part, which originates from the abdominal fascia, and which is crossed laterally by the terminal fibers of the m. cutaneus trunci, goes to the middle of the humerus. There the m. latissimus dorsi and the m. cutaneus trunci attach to it. It then radiates into the medial fascia of the brachium.

The muscle in large dogs is 2 to 2.5 cm thick in its cranial part; caudally it is thinner. The m. pectoralis superficialis covers it cranially.

Action: During locomotion, to move the trunk cranially over the advanced limb; extend the shoulder joint; draw the limb caudally. According to Slijper (1946), the m. pectoralis profundus, along with the m. serratus ventralis, plays an important role in supporting the trunk because its humeral insertion is considerably dorsal to its sternal origin. EMG activity was pronounced during the late swing phase of the ipsilateral limb during steady speed trotting, during similar time frames as the adjacent m. latissimus dorsi (Carrier et al., 2008). The period of EMG activity lengthened into the stance phase while trotting uphill on an incline; this suggests that positive work is performed by the muscle during active acceleration or digging motions. Trunk support may be more important in the transverse portions of the m. pectoralis superficialis than in the more caudally placed m. pectoralis profundus.

Innervation: Nn. pectorales caudales and also branches from nn. cervicalis 8 and thoracicus 1.

The *m. serratus ventralis thoracis* (Figs. 6.26 and 6.47) covers the cranial half of the lateral thoracic wall; it is a very thick, fan-shaped muscle. This muscle is related to the *m. serratus ventralis cervicalis*, which has been described with *muscles of the neck*. It attaches on the *facies serrata* of the scapula, its fibers diverging to form a broad angle. It ends on the first seven or eight ribs, somewhat ventral to their middle, as the m. serratus ventralis thoracis. Cranially it is related to the m. serratus ventralis cervicalis. In large dogs, the muscle is 1.5 to 2 cm thick near the scapula. The thoracic portion of serratus ventralis has well-defined serrations that are covered in part by the m. scalenus. Its three or four caudal serrations interdigitate with those of the m. obliquus externus abdominis.

Action: Support of the trunk, to carry the trunk cranially and caudally; inspiration; to carry the shoulder cranially and caudally with respect to the limb. EMG activity occurs during the early to middle period of ipsilateral limb support, emphasizing the crucial role of this muscle in weight support (Carrier et al., 2006).

Innervation: N. thoracalis longus.

Intrinsic Muscles

The intrinsic muscles of the thoracic limb have their origins and insertions on the bones of the thoracic limb and no direct association with the neck or trunk. For descriptive purposes these are grouped by the regions where they are located.

Lateral Scapular Muscles

The lateral scapular muscles, mm. supraspinatus and infraspinatus, occupy the scapular fossae. Superficially, the m. deltoideus and the m. teres minor traverse the flexor angle of the shoulder joint laterally.

The ***m. supraspinatus*** (Figs. 6.46, 6.49, and 6.50) is covered by the L2 mm. trapezius cervicis and omotransversarius. It fills the supraspinous fossa and curves over the lateral edge of the neck of the scapula. It arises from the entire surface of the supraspinous fossa, including the spine of the scapula, and from the edge of the neck of the scapula by numerous tendons from which the subscapularis also partly originates. Distally the strong muscular belly curves

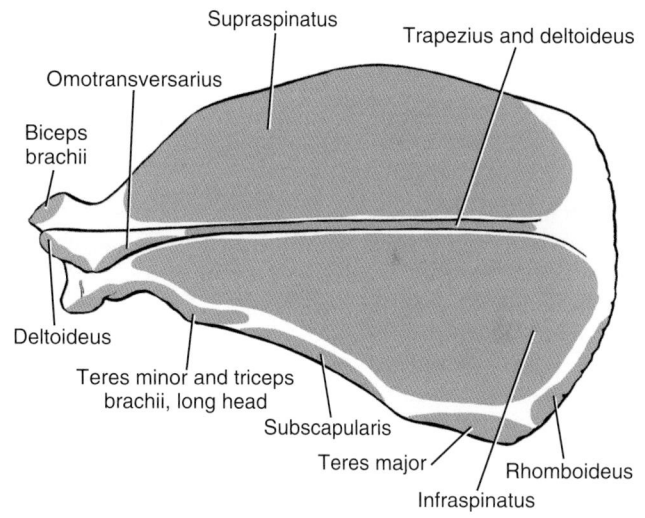

• **Fig. 6.46** Left scapula, showing areas of muscle attachment, lateral aspect.

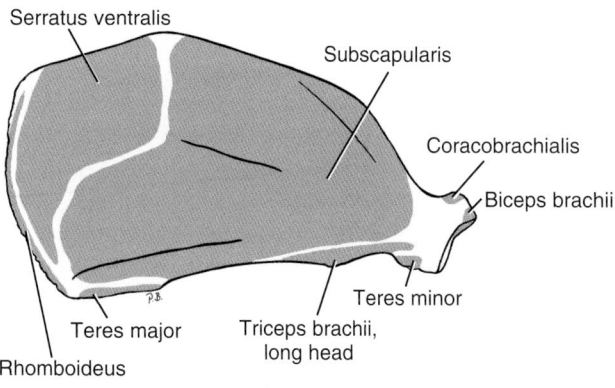

• **Fig. 6.47** Left scapula, showing areas of muscle attachment, medial aspect.

far around the neck of the scapula so that it also appears on the medial surface of the shoulder joint. The entire muscle attaches with a short, extremely thick tendon on the free edge of the greater tubercle of the humerus. In the distal third of the muscle, a thick tendinous fold develops that extends into the terminal tendon and the distal end of the muscle is pennate. The caudal half of the muscle is covered by a glistening tendinous sheet from the spine of the scapula.

Action: Extension of the shoulder joint and advancement of the limb. On the basis of EMG, the muscle is important to stabilize and prevent collapse of the shoulder joint (Goslow et al., 1981). It is active during 65% to 80% of the stance phase, including a period during which the muscle is being stretched.
Innervation: N. suprascapularis.

The *m. infraspinatus* (Figs. 6.46, 6.48B, 6.49A, 6.50B, and 6.51A) is covered largely by the scapular part of the m. deltoideus. It lies in the infraspinous fossa and extends caudally somewhat beyond the fossa. It arises from the fossa, the scapular spine, the caudal border of the scapula, and from the tendinous sheet that covers it. The latter is the scapular aponeurosis of origin of the scapular part of the m. deltoideus. At the shoulder joint the fleshy muscle becomes a thick tendon that crosses the caudal part of the greater tubercle. The **infraspinous bursa** (*B. subtendinea m. infraspinati*) is found here. The muscle ends on a smooth round face, *facies m. infraspinati*, distal to the tubercle. This tendon originates from the middle of the muscle so that it is pennate in form. Proximal to the infraspinous bursa, which is approximately 1 cm in diameter in large dogs, there is constantly found a second, smaller one.

Action: The muscle is the lateral rotator and abductor of the humerus and a flexor or extensor of the shoulder joint, depending on the position of the joint when the muscle contracts. Its tendon functions as a lateral collateral ligament of the shoulder joint. EMG activity is quite similar to that observed in m. supraspinatus: the muscle is electrically active throughout much of the stance phase of locomotion (Tokuriki, 1973a, b). Such activity is consistent with stabilization of the shoulder joint during locomotion. This muscle actively prevents medial rotation of the humerus.
Innervation: N. suprascapularis.

The *m. teres minor* (Figs. 6.46, 6.47, 6.49A, and 6.51) lies distocaudally on the scapula on the flexor side of the shoulder joint, where it is covered by the m. deltoideus and the m. infraspinatus. It arises by an aponeurosis that lies on the long head of the m. triceps brachii, from the distal third of the caudal edge of the scapula and primarily from the infraglenoid tubercle. It inserts by a short, stout tendon on a special eminence of the crest of the major tubercle proximal to the deltoid tuberosity. It is covered on both sides by a tendinous sheet.

Action: Flexion of the shoulder joint.
Innervation: N. axillaris.

The *m. deltoideus* (Figs. 6.46, 6.48, 6.49A, and 6.50B) is composed of two portions lying side by side, the scapular and acromial parts. The **scapular part** of the deltoideus (*m. deltoideus pars scapularis*) is superficial directly deep to the scapular fascia between the scapular spine and the proximal half of the humerus and is covered by an opalescent aponeurosis, from

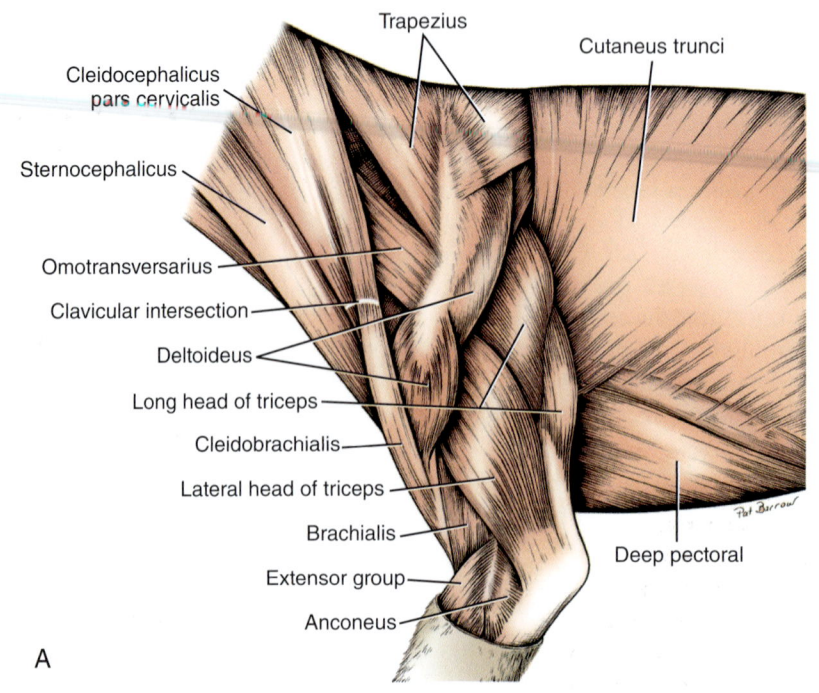

• **Fig. 6.48** Muscles of scapula, shoulder joint and arm, lateral aspect. **A,** Superficial muscles.

CHAPTER 6 The Muscular System 267

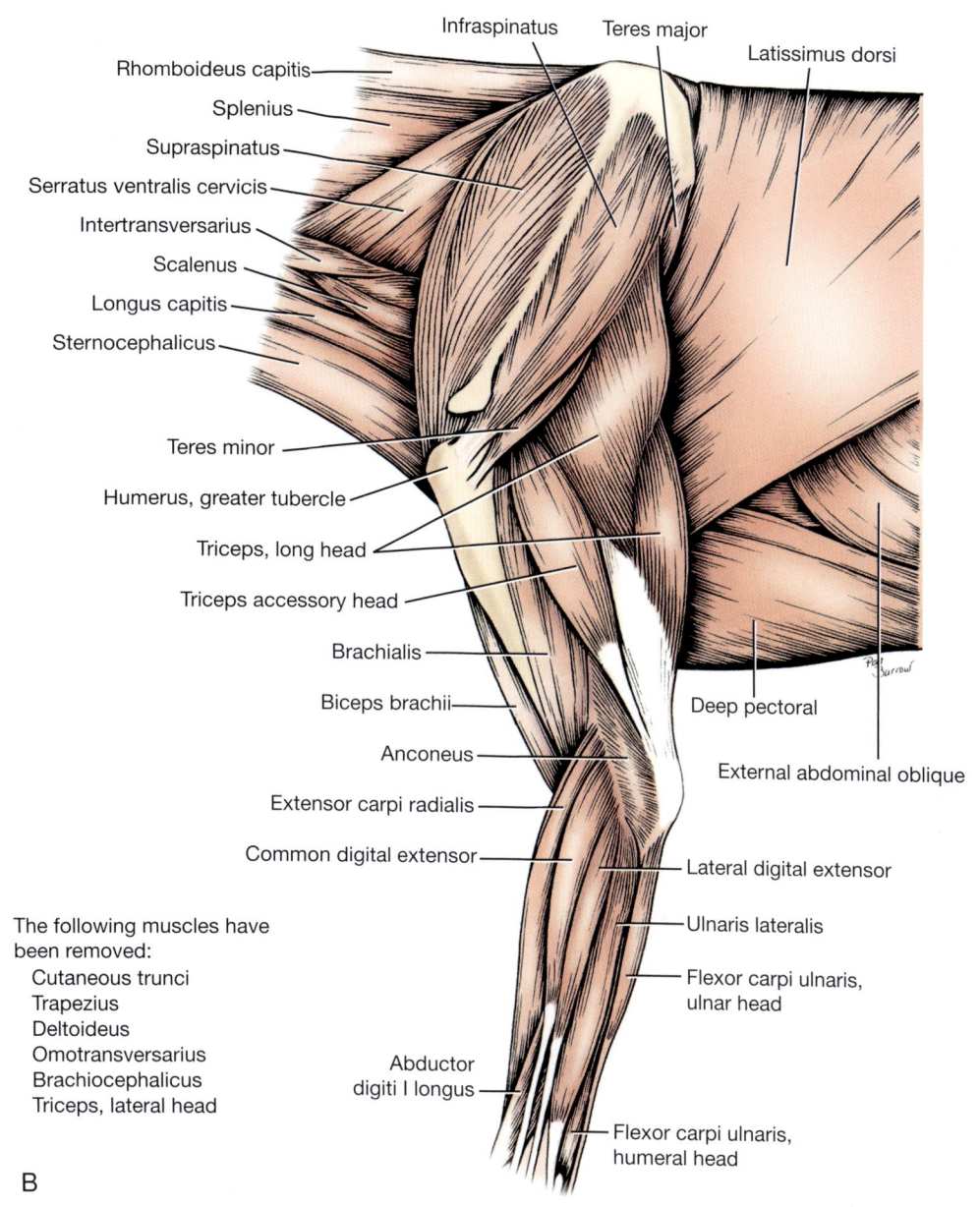

Infraspinatus
Teres major
Latissimus dorsi
Rhomboideus capitis
Splenius
Supraspinatus
Serratus ventralis cervicis
Intertransversarius
Scalenus
Longus capitis
Sternocephalicus
Teres minor
Humerus, greater tubercle
Triceps, long head
Triceps accessory head
Brachialis
Biceps brachii
Deep pectoral
Anconeus
External abdominal oblique
Extensor carpi radialis
Common digital extensor
Lateral digital extensor
Ulnaris lateralis
Flexor carpi ulnaris, ulnar head

The following muscles have been removed:
  Cutaneous trunci
  Trapezius
  Deltoideus
  Omotransversarius
  Brachiocephalicus
  Triceps, lateral head

Abductor digiti I longus
Flexor carpi ulnaris, humeral head

B

• **Fig. 6.48, cont'd** B, Deeper muscles.

which myofibers arise. This aponeurosis blends with the m. infraspinatus and comes from the scapular spine. Distal to the shoulder joint it becomes a tendinous sheet that passes medially deep to the acromial part. The **acromial part** (*m. deltoideus pars acromialis*) arises at the acromion. Its oval, flat belly, which in large dogs is 1.25 to 1.5 cm thick, crosses the lateral side of the shoulder joint, unites with the tendinous sheet of the scapular part, and ends partly in tendon and partly in muscle on the deltoid tuberosity. More than half of the acromial part is covered by an aponeurotic sheet composed of radiating fibers from which two distinct tendinous processes penetrate into the body of the muscle. The medial surface of both portions has an aponeurosis, which is thin distally as it attaches to the deltoid tuberosity. Between the acromial part and the tendon of the m. infraspinatus there is occasionally found a synovial bursa.

Action: Flexion of the shoulder joint, abduction of the humerus. Involvement in flexing the shoulder joint is shown by EMG activity at several speeds of locomotion (Tokuriki, 1973a, 1973b, 1974).
Innervation: N. axillaris.

Medial Scapular Muscles

The medial scapular muscles fill the subscapular fossa—m. subscapularis, or cross the flexor angle of the shoulder joint medially—the m. teres major.

The broad, flat ***m. subscapularis*** (Figs. 6.46, 6.47, 6.49B, and 6.50A) lies in the subscapular fossa and overhangs the caudal edge of the scapula. It is covered by a shiny, tendinous sheet that sends four to six tendinous bands that divide the muscle into broad pennate portions. Three or

268 CHAPTER 6 The Muscular System

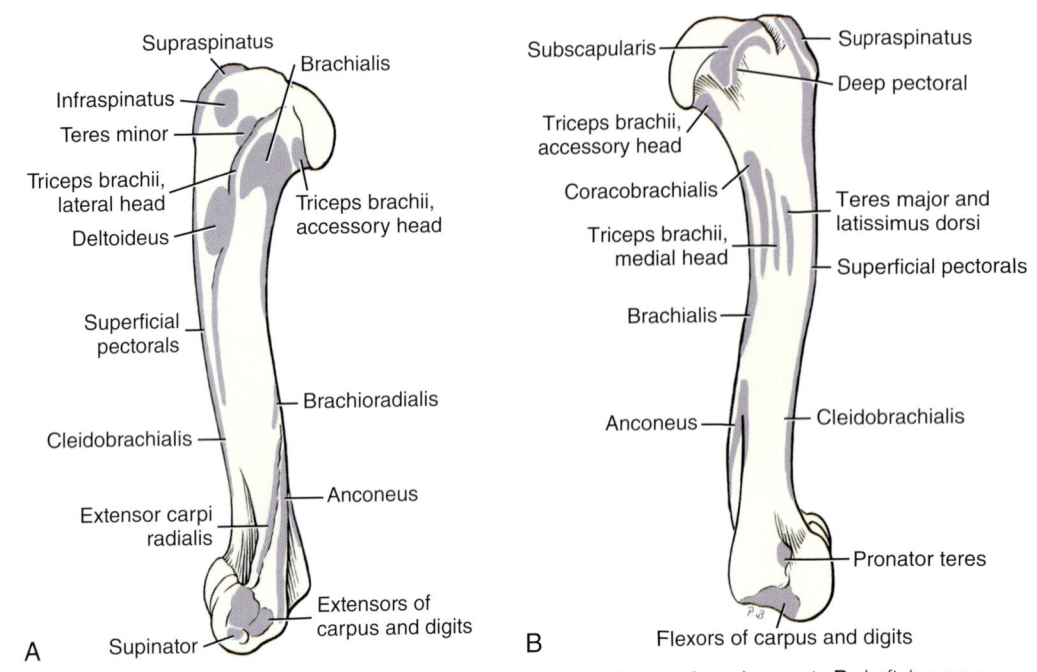

- **Fig. 6.49** **A**, Left humerus, showing areas of muscle attachment, lateral aspect. **B**, Left humerus, showing areas of muscle attachment, medial aspect.

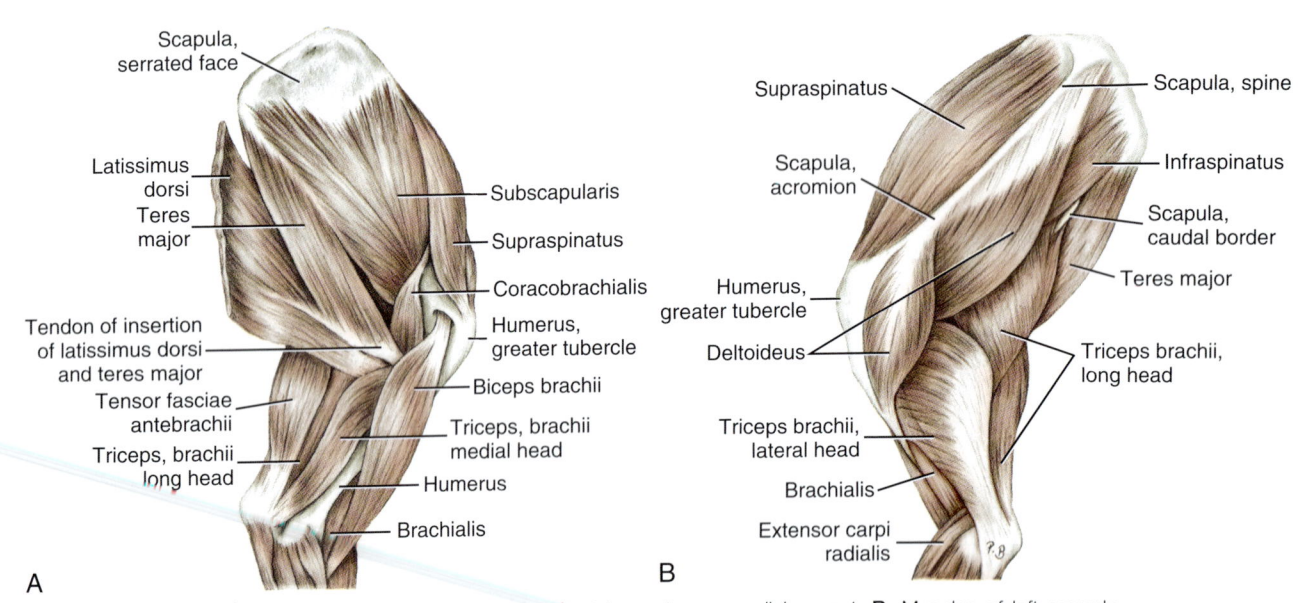

- **Fig. 6.50** **A**, Muscles of left scapula, shoulder and arm, medial aspect. **B**, Muscles of left scapula, shoulder and arm, lateral aspect.

four of these portions have separate tendinous coverings on their free medial side. In the interior of the muscle there are tendinous bands that parallel the surface of the muscle. Correspondingly, the muscle has an exceedingly complicated system of fasciculi that run in many different directions. The m. subscapularis arises in the subscapular fossa, especially from the muscular lines on the caudal edge of the scapula and on the curved boundary line between the facies serrata and subscapular fossa. The muscle becomes narrower and is partly tendinous as it passes over the shoulder joint medially. It inserts by means of a short, very thick tendon on the lesser tubercle of the humerus. The tendon unites intimately with the joint capsule.

Action: Primarily to adduct and extend the shoulder joint and to draw the humerus cranially during flexion of the joint. It aids in maintaining flexion. It rotates the humerus medially and thus prevents lateral rotation of the humerus. Its tendon functions as a medial collateral ligament.

Innervation: Nn. subscapularis and axillaris.

The *m. teres major* (Figs. 6.46, 6.47, 6.49B, and 6.50) is a fleshy, slender muscle lying caudal to the m. subscapularis. It, as well as the m. subscapularis, arises at the caudal angle and the adjacent caudal border of the scapula. Distally it crosses the mm. triceps brachii and coracobrachialis as it diverges from the m. subscapularis. It inserts on the teres

CHAPTER 6 The Muscular System 269

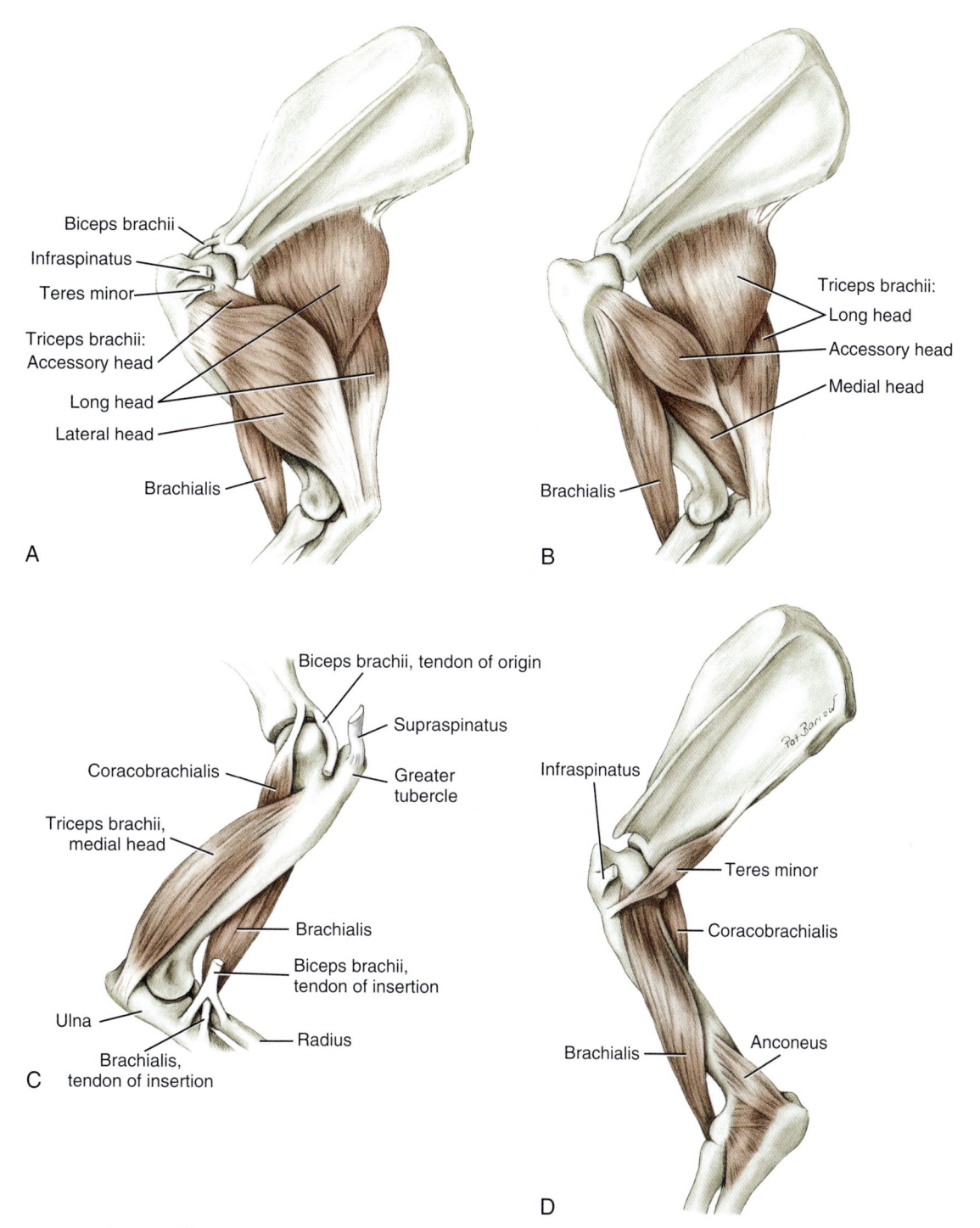

- **Fig. 6.51** Deep muscles of the brachium. **A,** Lateral aspect. **B,** Lateral aspect. (Lateral head of triceps removed.) **C,** Medial aspect. (Biceps brachii muscle removed.) **D,** Caudolateral aspect. (Triceps brachii removed.)

major tuberosity by a short, flat tendon, which blends with that of the m. latissimus dorsi. The lateral surface of the muscle bears a tendinous sheet which is thick distally. A similar tendinous sheet from the m. latissimus dorsi blends into it.

Action: Flexion of the shoulder joint, to draw the humerus caudally. Medial rotation of the shoulder joint and thus prevents lateral rotation. Electrical activity in the muscle occurs throughout the stance phase and continues into the earliest part of the swing phase of locomotion (Tokuriki, 1973a, 1973b, 1974).

Innervation: Branch of the n. axillaris.

Brachial Muscles

The muscles of the brachium completely surround the humerus except for a small portion, mediodistally, which is

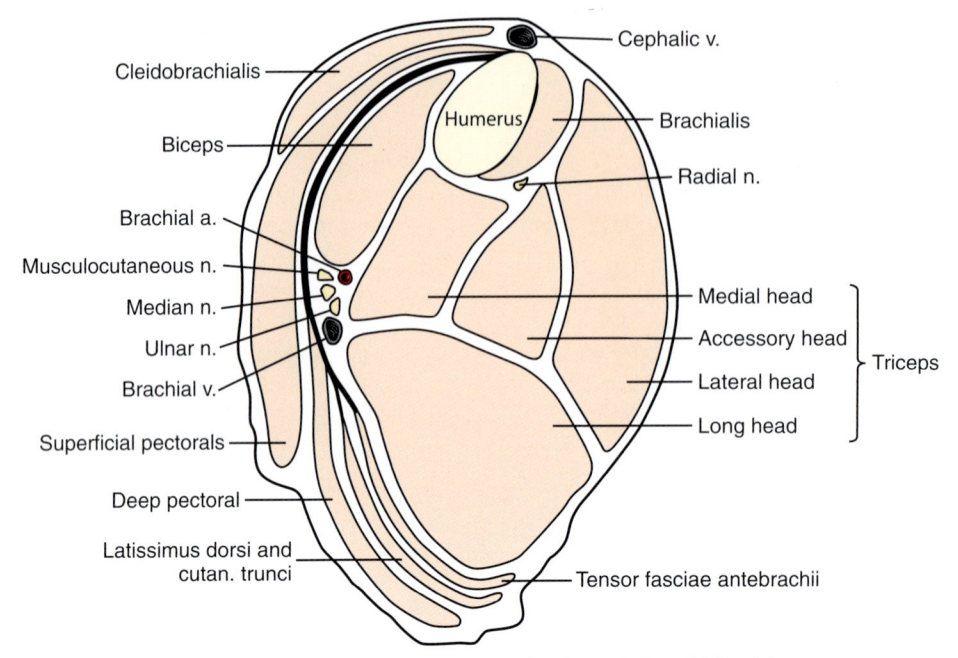

• Fig. 6.52 Schematic plan of transverse section through the middle of the arm.

left bare. Cranially are the extensors of the shoulder joint or flexors of the elbow joint—the mm. biceps brachii, coracobrachialis, brachialis. Caudally are the extensors of the elbow—the mm. triceps brachii, anconeus, and tensor fasciae antebrachii. The scapula is so attached to the lateral thoracic wall that the wall is covered caudally as far as the third intercostal space. Accessibility of the heart for clinical examination would be diminished if the limb could not be drawn cranially.

Cranial Brachial Muscles

The cranial brachial muscles include the m. biceps brachii, m. brachialis, and m. coracobrachialis.

The **m. biceps brachii** (Figs. 6.46, 6.47, 6.50A, 6.51 to 6.53, 6.58, and 6.59) is attached proximally at the supraglenoid tubercle by means of a long tendon of origin that crosses the shoulder joint in a sharp curve to gain the cranial surface of the humerus through the intertubercular groove. Cranially it invaginates the joint capsule deeply and is held in place by a transverse band (*retinaculum transversum*) between the greater and lesser tubercles. The joint capsule reflects around the tendon as its synovial sheath. Distal to the intertubercular sulcus the tendon becomes a wide, spindle-shaped muscle, which in large dogs is 3 to 4 cm thick in the middle and which extends from the medial to the cranial surface of the humerus. In the region of the elbow joint the tendon of insertion splits into two parts. The larger of the two inserts on the ulnar tuberosity and the smaller one inserts on the radial tuberosity. The terminal tendon of the m. brachialis inserts between the two parts of the tendon of insertion of the m. biceps brachii. Beginning at the tendon of origin, the muscle is covered by two extensive fibrous sheets that cover three-fourths to four-fifths of its length. The narrower one is applied to the side of the

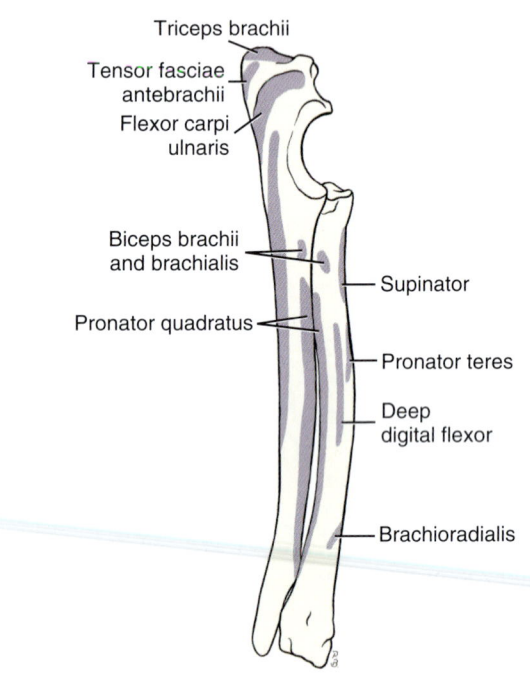

• Fig. 6.53 Left radius and ulna, showing areas of muscle attachment, medial aspect.

muscle next to the bone; the other is broader and covers the cranial and medial surfaces. Pushed into the interior of the muscle is a strong tendinous fold that, externally, is manifested by a groove. The fold does not reach the proximal tendon of origin. It makes the m. biceps brachii in the dog double pennate. The fibers of the m. biceps brachii run obliquely from both fibrous coverings to the interior fibrous fold, so that their length is less than one-fifth that of the entire muscle. The m. biceps brachii in the dog shows the first step toward the acquisition of a passive tendinous apparatus (Krüger, 1929), which in the quadrupeds is necessary for the fixation of the shoulder joint when standing. Sidaway et al. (2004) demonstrated the role of the proximal tendon of the m. biceps brachii in stabilizing the shoulder joint based on ablation studies in cadaver limbs. Transection of the biceps brachii tendon resulted in shoulder joint instability, including cranial, lateral, and medial translation of the humerus relative to the glenoid axis. Distally from the interior fold, there extends a tendinous strand in the groove between the m. extensor carpi radialis and the m. pronator teres; it crosses these muscles and spreads out in the antebrachial fascia. It corresponds to the lacertus fibrosus in the horse. This mechanical arrangement is strengthened by a high percentage of type I (presumed slow-twitch) muscle fibers that are fatigue resistant and well suited for postural maintenance (Armstrong et al., 1982). The overall contribution of passive extension of the shoulder and of active flexion of the elbow was investigated by Williams et al. (2008). These authors examined muscle moment arms, myofiber lengths, and tendon lengths and concluded that the m. biceps brachii was most important in elbow flexion, perhaps at the extreme of elbow extension during the stance phase. They concluded that passive elastic energy storage was not significant in this muscle, nor in most other thoracic limb muscles of dogs.

Action: Flexion of the elbow joint and extension and stabilization of the shoulder joint during quiet standing or during the stance phase of locomotion (Goslow et al., 1981).
Innervation: N. musculocutaneus.

The **m. brachialis** (Figs. 6.48, 6.49A, 6.50 to 6.52, 6.58, and 6.59) arises muscularly from the proximal part of the caudal surface of the humerus or proximal part of the spiral brachial groove for the brachialis muscle (*sulcus m. brachialis*). It extends laterally as far as the humeral crest, and medially as far as the medial surface. The muscle winds from the caudolateral to the cranial surface of the humerus in its course distally in this groove. At the distal third of the humerus it becomes narrower, goes over the flexor surface of the elbow joint to the medial side of the joint, lateral to the m. biceps brachii, and ends partly fleshy on that part of the tendon of the m. biceps brachii that goes to the radial tuberosity. The remainder becomes the tendon of insertion, which goes to the ulnar tuberosity between the two tendons of the m. biceps brachii. The muscle is mostly covered by the m. triceps brachii. Medially it is covered by a closely adherent fascial leaf that extends distally to the m. extensor carpi radialis. Similar to the m. biceps brachii, the m. brachialis contains a high proportion (approximately 47%) of type I (presumed slow-twitch) fibers. One difference, however, is that m. brachialis is electrically active during the swing phase while the limb is being held off the ground (Goslow et al., 1981).

Action: Flexion of the elbow joint.
Innervation: N. musculocutaneus.

The **m. coracobrachialis** (Figs. 6.47, 6.49B, 6.50A, and 6.51), short and rather thick, arises on the coracoid process of the scapula by a long, narrow tendon that is surrounded by a synovial sheath (*vagina synovialis m. coracobrachialis*). The tendon extends obliquely caudodistally over the medial side of the shoulder joint and thus lies in a groove close to the tendon of insertion of the m. subscapularis. The muscle runs between the medial and the accessory heads of the m. triceps brachii, ending on the crest of the minor tubercle, as well as caudal to the crest between the medial head of the m. triceps brachii and the m. brachialis. From its insertion a delicate tendinous leaf extends proximally over almost the entire muscle belly.

Action: Extension and adduction of the shoulder joint.
Innervation: N. musculocutaneus.

Caudal Brachial Muscles

The muscles that fill in the triangular space between the scapula, humerus, and olecranon are important antigravity muscles. They are primarily the extensors of the elbow joint. The principal part of this musculature is formed by the m. triceps brachii. The other extensors of the elbow joint in the dog are the m. anconeus and the m. tensor fasciae antebrachii.

The **m. triceps brachii** (Figs. 6.46 to 6.54) consists of four heads: *caput longum, caput laterale, caput mediale,* and *caput accessorium,* with a common insertional tendon to the olecranon tuber. Where this tendon crosses the grooves and prominences of the olecranon tuber, a synovial bursa (*B. subtendineae m. tricipitis brachii*) is interposed.

The **long head** (*caput longum m. triceps brachii*) forms a triangular muscle belly with a base that lies on the caudal edge of the scapula and the apex on the olecranon. The muscle

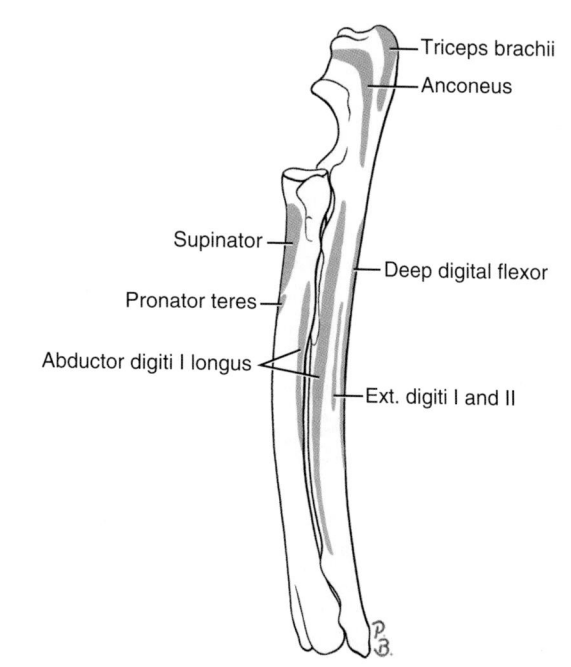

• **Fig. 6.54** Left radius and ulna, showing areas of muscle attachment, lateral aspect.

arises partly fleshy and partly tendinously on the distolateral two-thirds of the caudal border of the scapula and chiefly by tendon on the infraglenoid tuberosity. Its fibers, which are covered laterally by a rather thin and somewhat extensive fascia, converge toward the olecranon tuber and end in a short, thick, round tendon. This tendon is attached to the caudal part of the olecranon tuber, but deep to the lateral head, it is supplemented by a fascial sheet that is thick distally and that radiates between the long head and the lateral head in a proximal direction. This fascia also embraces the cranial edge of the muscle. The interior of the muscle reveals a thin, tendinous strand that is parallel to the surface. Between the terminal tendon and the cranial, grooved portion of the olecranon tuber, there is a synovial bursa, which may be more than 1 cm wide. There is abundant fat located at this insertion. The muscle is interspersed with several tendinous bands and manifests distinct subdivisions. Near the scapula, the mm. deltoideus and teres minor are found laterally and the m. teres major lies medially. EMG recordings showed electrical activity throughout 47% to 70% of the stance phase of several gaits. During all periods of EMG activity, the muscle shortened, suggesting that it does not store elastic energy during locomotion (Goslow et al., 1981). Because this muscle spans two joints, it has a role in shoulder flexion and elbow extension. This muscle contains only approximately 30% to 35% type I (slow-twitch) fibers (Armstrong et al., 1982; Reid et al., 1987). Because the muscle has a combination of large size (compared with adjacent elbow extensors) and relatively short muscle fascicles, Williams et al. (2008) conclude that the long head is capable of producing large forces during locomotion, important in stiffening the shoulder and elbow during accelerative movements.

The **lateral head** (*caput laterale m. triceps brachii*) is a large, almost rectangular muscle lying between the long head and the humerus. This muscle, which blends with the accessory head and which lies on the m. brachialis, arises by an aponeurosis on the tricipital line between the tuberosity for the teres minor and the deltoid tuberosity. This aponeurosis in small dogs is approximately 1 cm wide. After emerging from the caudal border of the m. deltoideus, its fibers run toward the olecranon tuber and terminate in a broad, short tendon that blends partially with the tendon of the long head and partially with the deep leaf of the antebrachial fascia. EMG analysis shows this muscle to be quiescent during walking but active through 64% to 70% of the stance phase during the trot or gallop (Goslow et al., 1981). Because elbow flexion was observed during the early part of the EMG bursts of the lateral head, this muscle underwent a cycle of eccentric activity (lengthening) followed by active shortening during each stance phase. Thus the muscle probably stores elastic energy during locomotion. The lateral head contains approximately 75% type II (fast) fibers, suggesting a dynamic role in locomotion (Armstrong et al., 1982).

The **medial head** (*caput mediale m. triceps brachii*) is a spindle-shaped muscle that arises tendinously on the crest of the minor tubercle between the point of insertion of the teres major and that of the m. coracobrachialis. A thick, tendinous fascia extends over the proximal two-thirds of the muscle. It attaches medially and independently on the olecranon tuber. In addition, the tendon blends with that of the long head and continues into the antebrachial fascia. The bursa associated with this muscle insertion is deep to the tendon of the medial head.

The **accessory head** (*caput accessorium m. triceps brachii*), which is irregularly rectangular in cross-section, lies on the caudal side of the humerus between the other heads of the m. triceps brachii and the m. brachialis. It arises from the proximal caudal part of the neck of the humerus and becomes tendinous at the distal third of the humerus. The tendon is elliptical in cross-section and blends with that of the long and lateral heads and thus inserts on the olecranon tuber. The common tendon lies caudal to the subtendinous bursa. A significant postural role for the accessory head is suggested by a high percentage of type I (slow) muscle fibers in the muscle (Armstrong et al., 1982).

Action: Extend the elbow joint.
Innervation: N. radialis.

The *m. anconeus* (see Figs. 6.48, 6.49, 6.51, and 6.54) lies on the caudal side of the distal half of the humerus between the epicondyles. It arises on the lateral epicondylar crest, the lateral epicondyle, and, because it almost completely fills the olecranon fossa, part of the medial epicondyle also. It ends on the lateral surface of the proximal end of the ulna and is mostly covered by the m. triceps brachii. It covers the proximal surface of the elbow joint capsule and one of its out-pocketings. The m. anconeus is composed entirely of type I (slow) muscle fibers, all with a relatively high aerobic potential (Armstrong et al., 1982). This composition suggests an important role in resisting elbow flexion during quiet standing. This muscle also contains a high density of muscle spindles compared with the adjacent parts of the m. triceps brachii (Buxton & Peck, 1990) and thus may provide important proprioceptive information about the elbow joint to the central nervous system.

Action: The m. anconeus, with the m. triceps brachii, extends the elbow joint, and helps tense the antebrachial fascia.
Innervation: N. radialis.

The *m. tensor fasciae antebrachii* (Figs. 6.50A, 6.52, and 6.53) is a flat, broad, straplike muscle that, in large dogs, is only 2 mm thick; it lies on the caudal half of the medial surface and on the caudal edge of the long head of the m. triceps brachii. It arises above the "axillary arch" from the thickened epimysium of the lateral surface of the m. latissimus dorsi. It ends, in common with the m. triceps brachii, in a tendon on the olecranon tuber, and independently in the antebrachial fascia. Occasionally one finds a synovial bursa between the muscle and the medial surface of the olecranon tuber.

Action: Supports the action of the m. triceps brachii and is the chief tensor of the antebrachial fascia.
Innervation: N. radialis.

Antebrachial Muscles

The muscles of the forearm embrace the bones in such a way that the distal two-thirds of the medial side of the antebrachial skeleton (especially the radius) is uncovered. The extensors of the carpus and digits lie cranially and laterally. The carpal and digital joints of the thoracic limb have equivalent angles; that is, their extensor surfaces are directed dorsally. On the palmar side are the flexors of the joints. The mm. pronator teres and supinator serve to turn the forepaw about the long axis; these are found in the flexor angle of the elbow joint. Because most of the muscles appear on the palmar side, the antebrachium of the dog appears to be compressed laterally. Because the muscle bellies are located proximally and the slender tendons distally, the extremity tapers toward the paw.

Craniolateral Antebrachial Muscles

The craniolateral group of antebrachial muscles are represented chiefly by the extensors of the carpal and digital joints. These are the mm. extensor carpi radialis, extensor digitorum communis, extensor digitorum lateralis, ulnaris lateralis (extensor carpi ulnaris), extensor digiti I et II, and abductor digiti I longus. To these are added the mm. brachioradialis and the supinator in the flexor angle of the elbow joint. The majority of these muscles arise directly or indirectly from the lateral (extensor) epicondyle of the humerus.

The *m. brachioradialis* (Figs. 6.53, 6.55A, and 6.56), much reduced and occasionally lacking, is a long, narrow muscle in the flexor angle of the elbow joint. This muscle has also been called the *m. supinator longus*. Wakuri and Kano (1966) found the muscle present in 35 of 90 dogs examined. It is cranial in position between the superficial and the deep antebrachial fascia and is intimately bound to

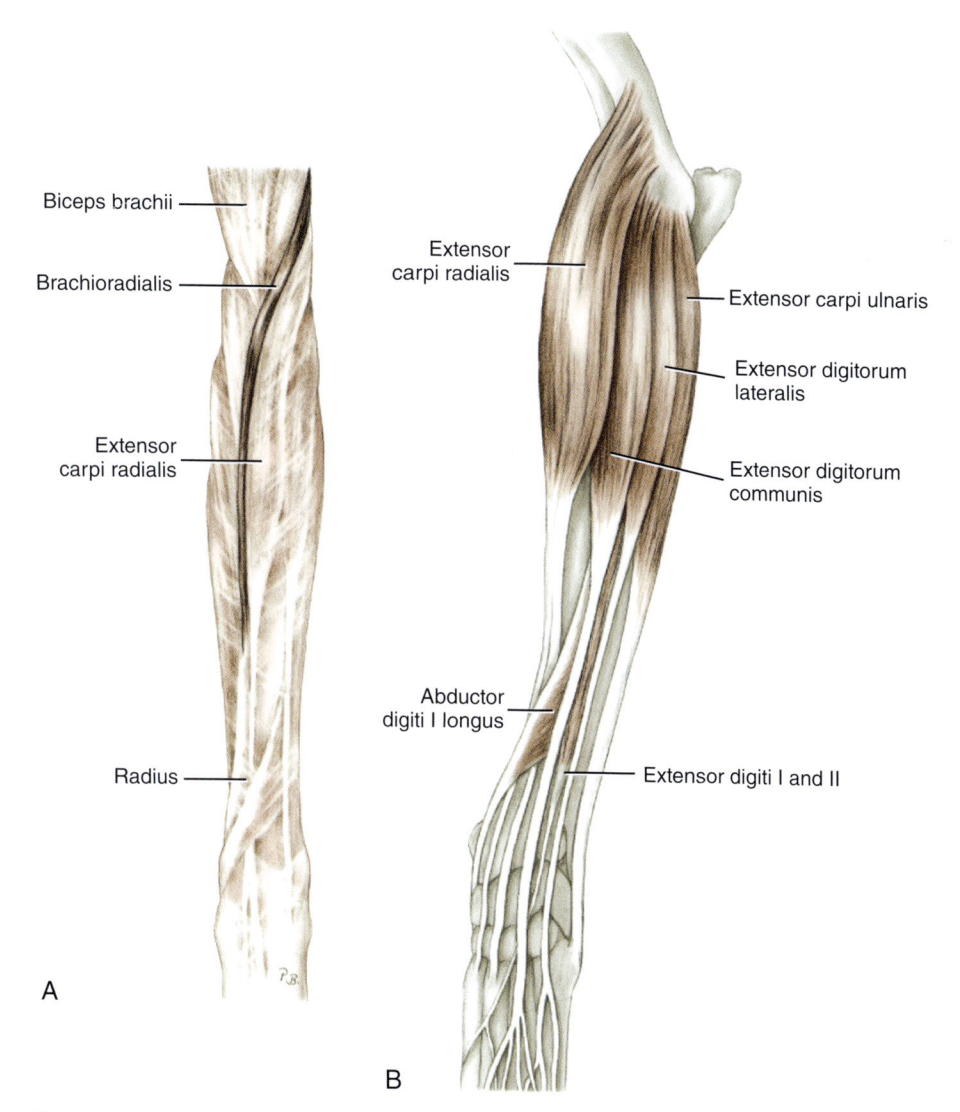

• **Fig. 6.55** A, Forearm with antebrachial fascia, cranial aspect. B, Superficial antebrachial muscles, craniolateral aspect.

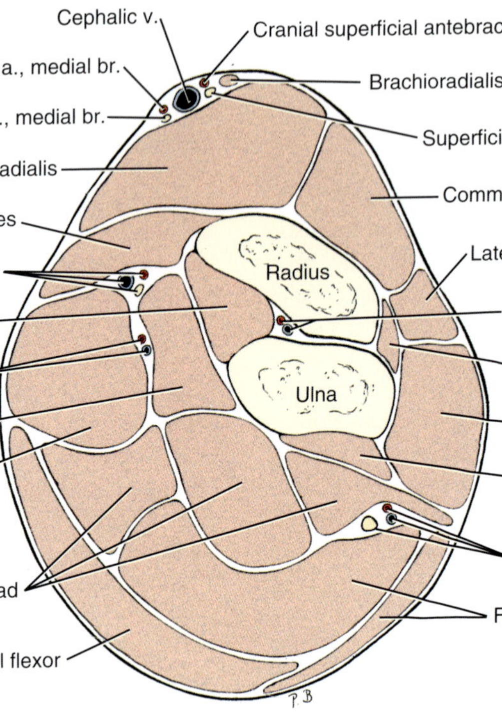

• **Fig. 6.56** Schematic plan of transverse section of the forearm between the proximal and middle thirds.

the superficial leaf of the latter fascia. It arises on the proximal end of the lateral epicondylar crest of the humerus directly proximal to the m. extensor carpi radialis. It extends cranially at first beside the m. extensor carpi radialis, then turns more medially and extends distally in the groove between the m. extensor carpi radialis and the radius. Between the third and the distal fourth of the bone it ends on the periosteum of the radius by a thin aponeurosis.

Action: Rotation of the radius craniolaterally, supination.
Innervation: N. radialis.

The **m. extensor carpi radialis** (Figs. 6.49A, 6.50B, 6.55 to 6.58A, 6.65A, and 6.66) is a long, thick, fleshy muscle lying on the cranial surface of the radius medial to the m. extensor digitorum communis. It is the first muscle encountered after the free surface of the radius, when one palpates from the medial to the cranial surface. The m. extensor carpi radialis arises on the lateral epicondylar crest of the humerus, united with the m. extensor digitorum communis for a short distance by an intermuscular septum. It forms a muscle belly that fades distally and splits into two flat tendons at the distal third of the radius. Both tendons are closely approximated as they extend distally along the radius. By way of the middle sulcus of the radius, they gain the dorsal, extensor, surface of the carpus, where they lie in a groove covered by the extensor retinaculum. They are often surrounded by a synovial sheath. The tendons separate; one inserts on a small tuberosity on metacarpal II (*m. extensor carpi radialis longus*) and the other on metacarpal III (*m. extensor carpi radialis brevis*). The muscle bellies for these two tendons are partially fused in the dog. From the aponeurosis covering the medial surface of the m. brachialis arises a fascial leaf that extends over the proximal medial surface of the belly of the m. extensor carpi radialis, as does a fascial leaf from the m. biceps brachii. The most proximal part of the muscle lies on the joint capsule, which forms a bursalike pocket at this point. In approximately half of all specimens the tendons are completely or almost completely surrounded by a common tendon sheath (*vag. tendinis m. extensor carpi radialis*), which extends from the beginning of the tendon to the proximal end of the metacarpus. A synovial bursa may exist at the proximal row of carpal bones deep to both tendons or only deep to the lateral tendon. A second bursa is occasionally found deep to the lateral tendon at the distal row of carpal bones. In other specimens, in place of the synovial sheath, one finds loosely meshed tissue. EMG studies in dogs show a long burst of electrical activity in m. extensor carpi radialis during the swing phase of walking (Tokuriki, 1973a). Such activity is consistent with a role in elbow flexion. During trot and gallop, the muscle is quiet during the midswing phase, and there is a distinct early- and late-swing phase burst (Tokuriki, 1973b, 1974). The late burst precedes paw placement by 15 to 20 msec and is consistent with carpal extension that occurs immediately prior to paw touchdown.

Action: Extension of the carpal joint and flexion of the elbow joint.
Innervation: N. radialis, deep ramus.

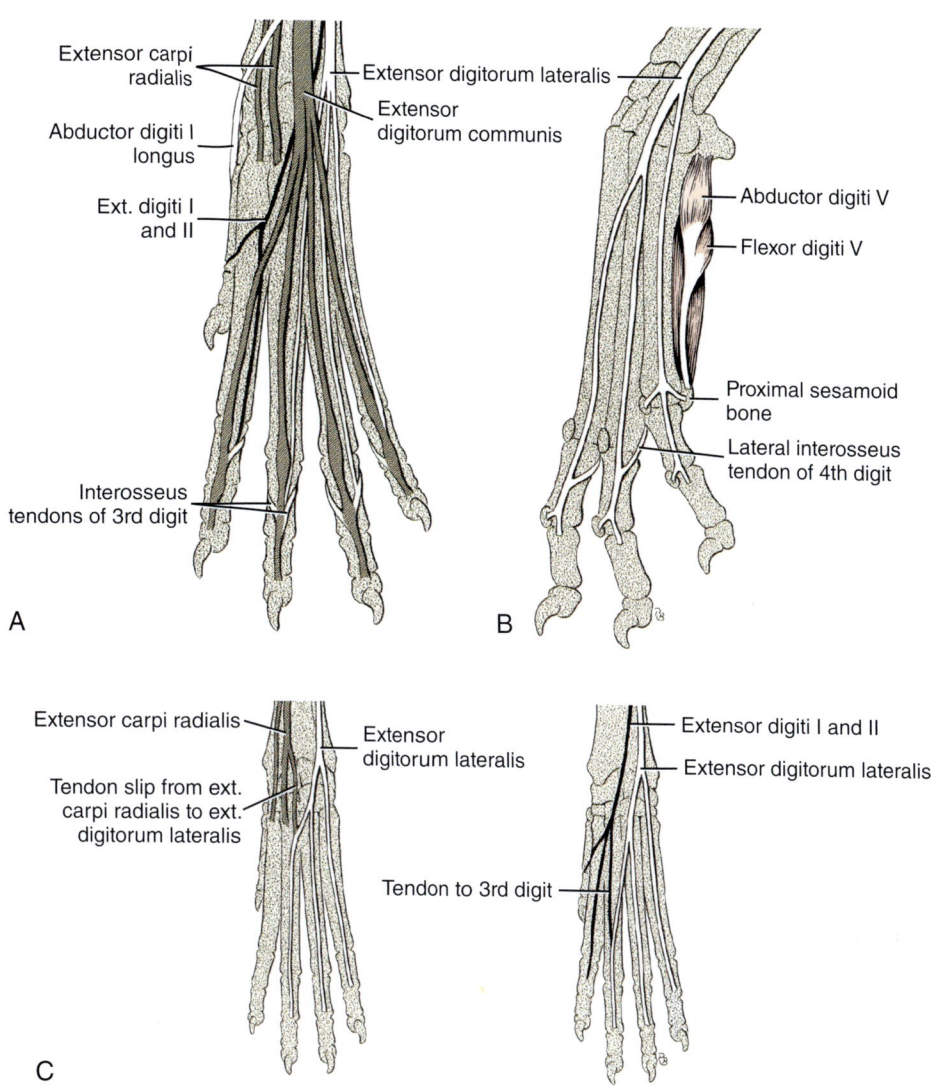

• **Fig. 6.57** Tendons on the dorsum of the left forepaw. **A,** Insertion of the common digital extensor. **B,** Lateral aspect, tendons of the common digital extensor removed. **C,** Two common variations.

The ***m. extensor digitorum communis*** (Figs. 6.49A, 6.55 to 6.57, 6.64, 6.65A, and 6.66) lies on the craniolateral surface of the radius between the m. extensor carpi radialis and the m. extensor digitorum lateralis. It arises on the lateral epicondyle somewhat cranial and proximal to the attachment of the lateral collateral ligament of the elbow joint and with a smaller portion from the antebrachial fascia. At its origin it is fused deeply with the m. extensor carpi radialis by a common aponeurosis that separates into two parts distally, one for each muscle. After the appearance of a corresponding number of superficial tendinous bands, the slender belly divides into four bellies and tendons distally; at first these lie so close together that the whole tendon appears to be undivided. At the same time the deep muscle fibers extend over to the medial tendon. The compound tendon, enclosed in a common synovial sheath (*vag. tendinis extensoris digit communis*), extends distally on the m. abductor digiti I longus and passes through the lateral distal sulcus of the radius, where it is covered by a thick, indistinct extensor retinaculum (*retinaculum extensorum*). After the tendon crosses the dorsal, extensor, surface of the carpal joint, the individual tendons separate from each other and pass on the dorsal surface of the corresponding metacarpal bones and phalanges to the distal phalanges of digits II to V, inclusive. Here each tendon broadens into a caplike structure and ends on the dorsal portion of the ungual crest of the distal phalanx, covered by the crura of the dorsal ligaments (*ligg. dorsalis*). The m. extensor digitorum communis is composed of digital extensors II, III, IV, and V. Each tendon, at the distal end of the proximal phalanx, receives bilaterally a thin extension of the tendons of insertion of the interosseous muscles that cross obliquely from the palmar surface. The tendons of the lateral digital extensor unite with the tendons of the common digital extensor on digits III, IV, and V. Thus all extensor tendons are deeply embedded in the dorsal fibrous tissue of the digits.

Deep to the origin of the m. extensor digitorum communis there extends an outpouching of the elbow joint capsule. The separation of the terminal portion of the muscle is usually described as distinct, although an undivided muscle

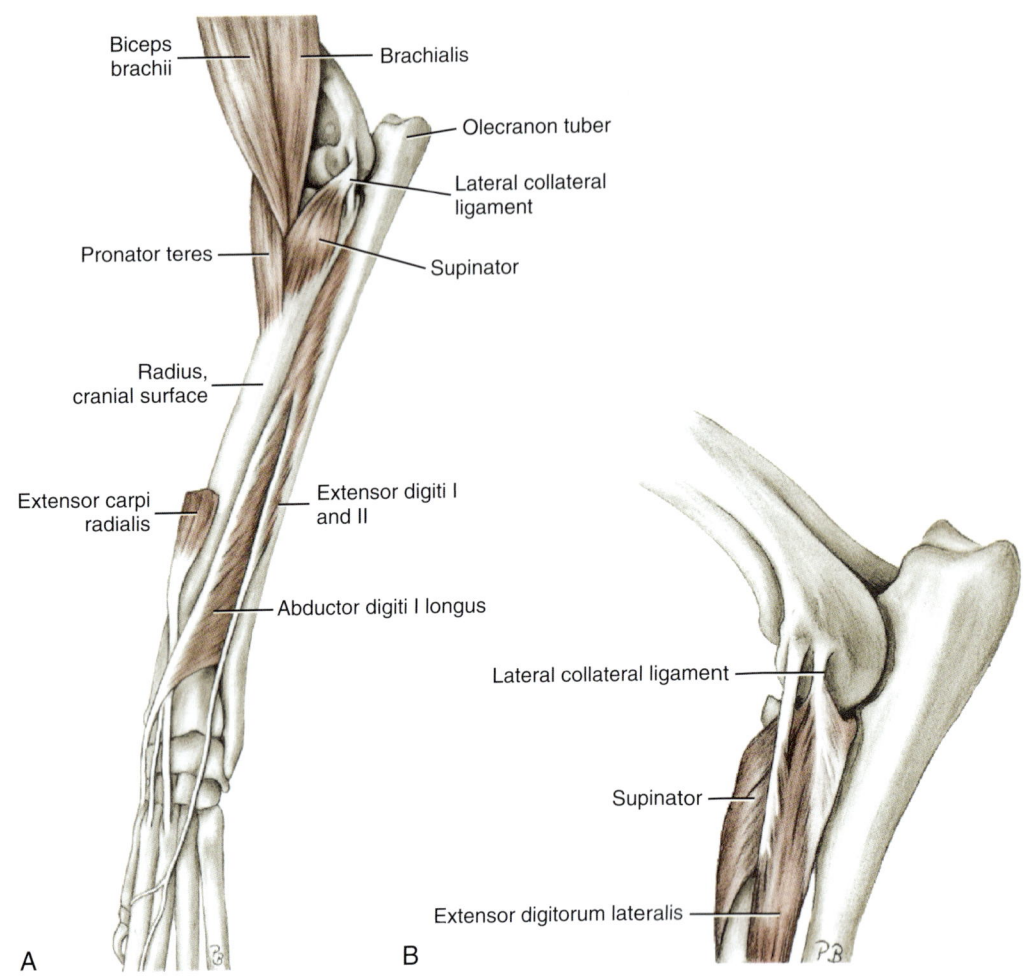

Fig. 6.58 Antebrachial muscles. **A,** Deep antebrachial muscles, craniolateral aspect. **B,** Origins of supinator and extensor digitorum lateralis.

is simulated. On the other hand, the tendons may fuse in part with one another; this is especially true for the tendons of digits IV and V. The muscle branch for digit II is the longest and becomes tendinous at the middle of the antebrachium. The three remaining muscle branches reach only to the middle third of the antebrachium. The synovial sheath that surrounds the tendon bundle of this muscle and that of the m. extensor digiti I longus et digiti II begins shortly distal to where the muscle has become tendinous (in large dogs 3 to 4 cm proximal to the carpus). It reaches at least to the middle of the carpus, often to the proximal end of the metacarpus. Its fibrosa fuses with the periosteum of the radius and with the joint capsule of the carpus. Its mesotendon, which appears at its medial border, first covers the tendon of the m. extensor digiti I longus et digiti II and then the four tendons of the m. extensor digitorum communis. At the metacarpophalangeal joint the tendon glides on the sesamoid element, which is embedded in the joint capsule; this sesamoid has an ossified nucleus, whereas those at the proximal interphalangeal joints remain cartilaginous.

Action: Extension of the joints of the four principal digits.
Innervation: N. radialis, deep ramus.

The *m. extensor digitorum lateralis* (Figs. 6.49A, 6.55 to 6.57, 6.58B, 6.65A, and 6.66) lies in the antebrachium laterally on the radius between the m. extensor digitorum communis and the m. ulnaris lateralis. It covers the m. abductor digiti I longus. The muscle has two bellies. It arises on the cranial edge of the lateral collateral ligament of the elbow joint, and on the lateral epicondyle of the humerus. In the distal half of the forearm, the two muscle bellies are continued by distinct tendons. The tendon adjacent to the common digital extensor is the smaller one and comes from a slender, distal fascial sheet. The other tendon arises from a considerably larger, distal fascial leaf that lies next to the m. ulnaris lateralis. The tendons lie close together and usually are enclosed in a common synovial sheath. They pass through the groove between the distal ends of the radius and ulna, over the dorsolateral border of the carpus to the metacarpus, and then diverge from each other. The tendon of the larger caudal belly extends from metacarpal V to the proximal phalanx of digit V, unites with the corresponding tendon of the m. extensor digitorum communis and ends with it on the distal phalanx as well as on the dorsal surface of the proximal ends of the proximal and middle phalanges. The tendon of the smaller belly divides at the carpus into two branches that extend obliquely deep to the tendons of the m. extensor digitorum communis medially to the third and fourth metacarpophalangeal joints. On the proximal phalanx of digits III and IV they unite with the corresponding tendons of the common digital extensor; often they also unite with one or both of the distal ligaments that come from the m. interossei. The tendons end principally on the distal phalanges of digits III and IV. The tendons of the lateral digital extensor are only approximately one-third the width of those of the common digital extensor. This muscle has a relatively long tendon and short muscle fibers (fascicle length of <90 mm), suggesting some potential for elastic energy storage during locomotion. However, its lateral location on the limb may make it more critical for stabilizing or as a "damper" to attenuate vibrations within the limb during high speed locomotion (Williams et al., 2008).

In approximately one-half of all specimens, both tendons of m. extensor digitorum lateralis are enclosed in a common synovial sheath (*vag. tendinis extensoris lateralis manus*), which in large dogs begins 2.5 to 3 cm proximal to the carpus and often reaches the metacarpus. In other specimens there is no distinct synovial sheath, but rather there is a space under both tendons bounded by the fascia. In exceptional specimens the tendon for digit III is independent and arises from the fascia distal to the carpus (Ziegler, 1929).

Action: Extension of the joints of digits III, IV, and V.
Innervation: N. radialis.

The large **m. extensor carpi ulnaris** (*m. extensor carpi ulnaris* and formerly called ulnaris lateralis) (Figs. 6.55, 6.56, 6.61, 6.65, and 6.66) lies on the caudolateral side of the ulna, and is directly deep to the fascia. It arises on the lateral epicondyle of the humerus caudal to the lateral collateral ligament of the elbow joint by a long, relatively large tendon. At the middle of the antebrachium the large distal tendinous band of the lateral surface, which eventually goes into the large terminal tendon, takes on the delicate distal tendinous leaf of the medial surface. On the medial surface of the terminal tendon, fibers of the deeper muscle mass radiate into the broad tendon as far as the carpus; the tendon passes laterally over the carpus, being held in place by connective tissue without a sulcus in which to glide. It ends laterally on the base of metacarpal V. From the accessory carpal bone, two fiber bundles arise from the antebrachial fascia and cross each other to blend with the tendon of the m. extensor carpi ulnaris at the carpus. A tendinous fold, which parallels the surface, is concealed in the interior of the muscle. Deep to the tendon of origin of the muscle in older dogs, there is constantly a synovial bursa (*b. subtendinea m. ulnaris carpi ulnaris*), 1 to 2 cm in diameter. A second bursa is found occasionally, between the tendon and the distal end of the ulna. The m. extensor carpi ulnaris is generally a flexor of the carpus and a lateral rotator, supinator, of the forearm. However, the anatomic insertion close to the axis of joint rotation in the carpus leads to several interpretations. The m. extensor carpi ulnaris is active

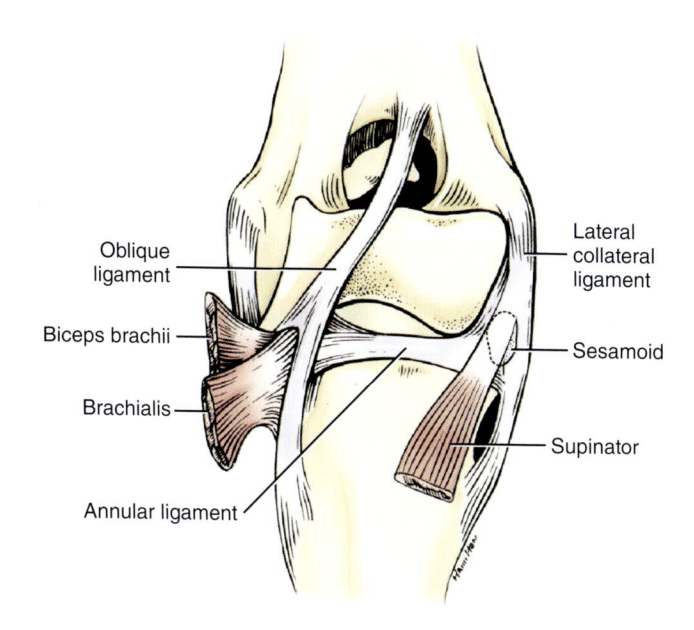

• **Fig. 6.59** Cranial view of left elbow joint.

during the last part of the swing phase and through the first one-third to one-half of the subsequent stance phase during all gaits (Tokuriki, 1973a, 1973b, 1974). It is essentially coactive with the adjacent m. flexor carpi ulnaris.

Action: Abduction and lateral rotation of the carpal joint; support of the carpus when extended to bear weight.
Innervation: N. radialis.

The **m. supinator** (Figs. 6.49A, 6.53, 6.54, 6.58, and 6.59) is broad and flat and is almost completely covered by a delicate fascia. It lies laterally on the flexor surface of the elbow, covered by the m. extensor carpi radialis and the digital extensors. It lies directly on the joint capsule and radius. It arises by a short, thick tendon on the lateral collateral ligament of the elbow joint, and on the lateral epicondyle. There is usually a sesamoid bone in the tendon of origin of the supinator muscle (Fig. 6.59) that articulates with the lateral aspect of the head of the radius. It extends obliquely distomedially covering the proximal fourth of the radius and ends on its cranial surface as far as the medial border. The muscle extends a short distance deep to the border of the m. pronator teres.

Action: Supination of the paw so that the palmar surface faces medially.
Innervation: N. radialis.

The **m. extensor digiti I et II**, formerly called *m. extensor pollicis longus et indicis proprius* (Figs. 6.54, 6.55, 6.57, 6.58, 6.60, and 6.65A), is a combination of two muscles that is an exceedingly small, slender, flat muscle on the lateral side of the antebrachium, where it is covered by the m. extensor carpi ulnaris, and the lateral and common digital extensors.

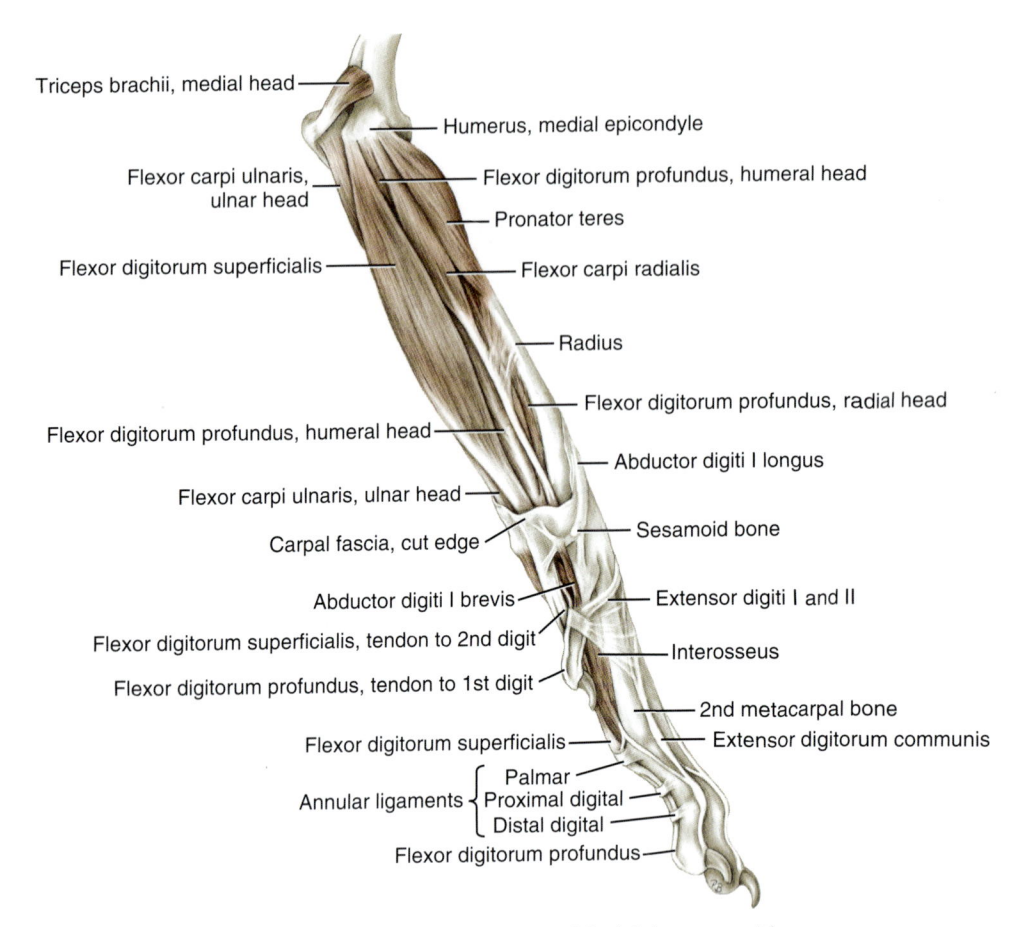

Fig. 6.60 Muscles on the medial surface of the left forearm and forepaw.

After arising from approximately the middle third of the dorsolateral border of the ulna, adjacent to the m. abductor digiti I longus, it runs distally, parallel to the ulna. Its fibers run obliquely distomedially. The muscle gradually crosses deep to the extensors, so that its extremely delicate tendon appears medial to the common extensor tendons at the carpal joint, where the two tendons are surrounded by a common synovial sheath. On the dorsal surface of metacarpal III the tendon divides into two parts. The medial portion expands over metacarpal II to the head of metacarpal I, where it is buried in the fascia. The lateral portion, after passing deep to the tendon of the m. extensor digitorum communis to digit II, unites with it at the metacarpophalangeal joint. Rarely another small tendon goes to digit III, and occasionally the muscle splits into two bellies.

Action: Extension of digits I and II and adduction of digit I.
Innervation: N. radialis.

The *m. abductor digiti I (pollicis) longus* (Figs. 6.54, 6.55 to 6.58, 6.60, and 6.65B), almost completely covered by the digital extensors, lies in the lateral groove between the radius and the ulna. It arises on the lateral surface of the radius and ulna and the interosseous membrane. Its fibers, which are directed obliquely medially and distally, blend into a narrow tendinous band that proceeds along the craniomedial border of the muscle and which becomes the terminal tendon toward the carpus, after it has bridged the gap between the tendons of the m. extensor digitorum communis and the m. extensor carpi radialis. In the distal forearm its tendon crosses the tendon of the m. extensor carpi radialis, passes into the medial sulcus of the radius, and crosses the medial border of the carpus deep to the short collateral ligament. Finally, the tendon inserts medially on the base of metacarpal I, where a sesamoid bone is embedded in it.

Where the tendon goes over that of the m. extensor carpi radialis, there is usually a bursa or a short synovial sheath.

Action: Abduction and extension of the first digit; medial deviation of the forepaw.
Innervation: N. radialis.

Caudal Antebrachial Muscles

The caudal group of antebrachial muscles consists of the flexors of the carpus and digits: mm. flexor carpi radialis, flexor carpi ulnaris, flexor digitorum superficialis, and flexor digitorum profundus. To these are added the small mm. pronator teres and pronator quadratus, which do not extend beyond the antebrachium. Most of these muscles come from the medial or flexor epicondyle. They form the caudal and medial part of the antebrachium.

CHAPTER 6 The Muscular System 279

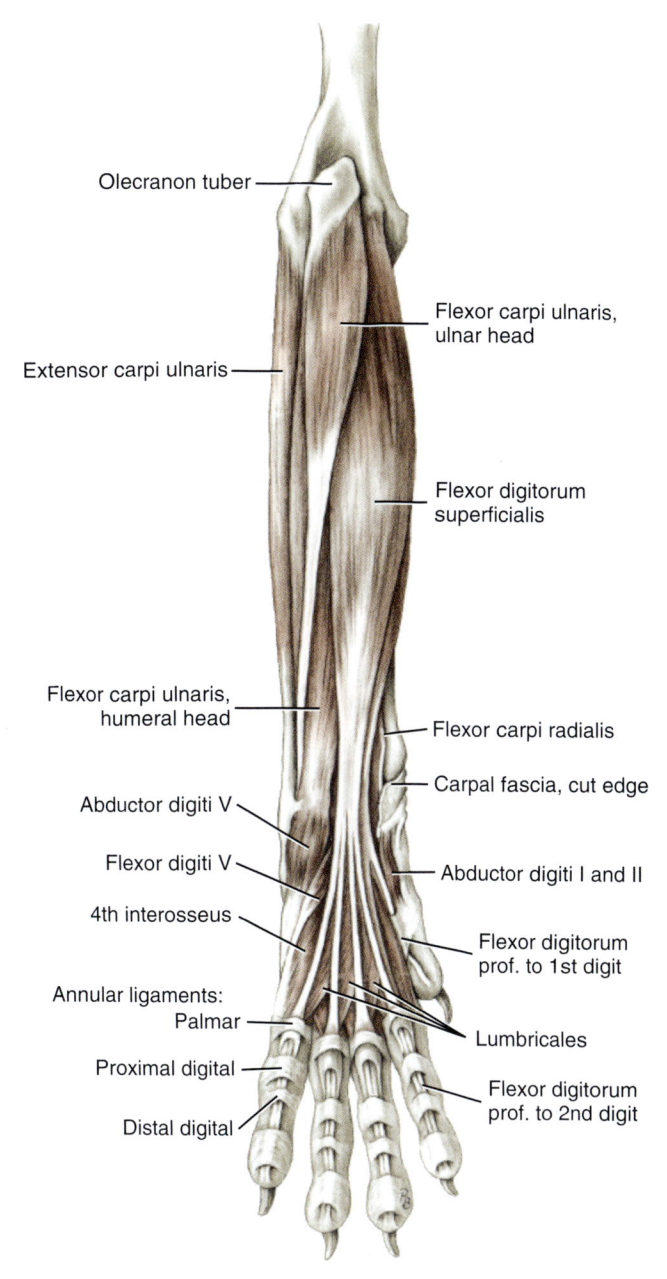

• Fig. 6.61 Antebrachial muscles, caudal aspect.

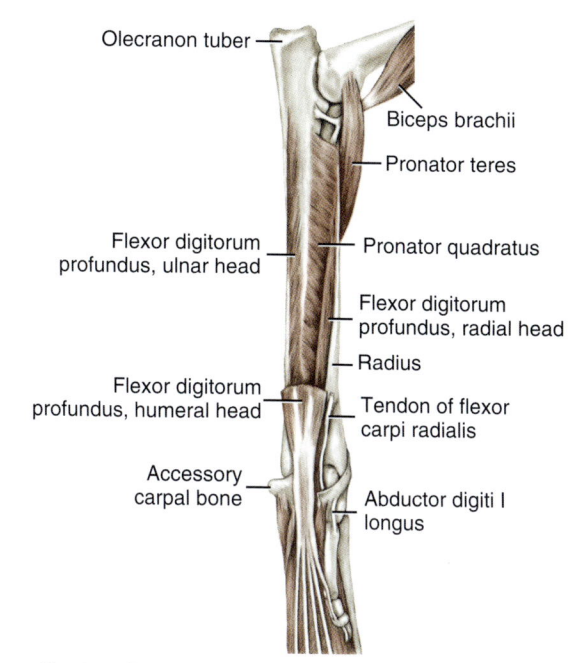

• Fig. 6.62 Deep antebrachial muscles. Caudomedial aspect.

When viewed medially, the muscles appear in the following order, beginning cranially: mm. pronator teres (only the proximal third of the forearm), flexor carpi radialis, flexor digitorum profundus (only the proximal third of the forearm), flexor digitorum profundus (only the distal half of the forearm), flexor digitorum superficialis, and caput ulnare of the m. flexor carpi ulnaris (only in a very insignificant and proximal segment of the antebrachium). Seen from the caudal aspect, the caput ulnare of the m. flexor carpi ulnaris is lateral to the m. flexor digitorum superficialis. However, at the distal half of the antebrachium, the caput humerale of the m. flexor carpi ulnaris appears between these two. The m. extensor carpi ulnaris is adjacent to the m. flexor carpi ulnaris on the lateral surface of the forearm.

The *m. pronator teres* (Figs. 6.49B, 6.53, 6.54, 6.56, 6.58, 6.60, and 6.62), round in transverse section, crosses the medial surface of the elbow joint. It lies deep to the skin and fascia largely on the proximal third of the radius. It arises from the medial epicondyle cranial to the m. flexor carpi radialis. The body of the muscle extends obliquely craniodistally and, upon forming a thick tendinous band, ends distal to the m. supinator on the medial border of the radius as far as its middle. Its internal surface is provided with a strong, proximal tendinous band.

Action: It rotates the forearm so that the dorsal surface of the manus tends to become medial, which is pronation. It may function only as a flexor of the elbow joint (Zimmermann, 1928).
Innervation: N. medianus.

The *m. flexor carpi radialis* (Figs. 6.56, 6.60 to 6.63B, 6.65B, and 6.66) lies in the medial part of the antebrachium directly deep to the skin and antebrachial fascia, where it covers the m. flexor digitorum profundus. It arises on the medial epicondyle caudal to the medial collateral ligament of the elbow joint between the m. pronator teres and the caput humerale of the m. flexor digitorum profundus. It extends distally between the m. pronator teres and the m. flexor digitorum superficialis and, forming a short, thick fusiform belly, merges into a flat tendon near the middle of the radius. It receives a delicate supporting fascia from the radius throughout its entire length. At the flexor surface of the carpus it runs through the carpal canal deep to the flexor retinaculum, where it is enclosed in a synovial sheath (*vag. tendinis m. flexoris carpi radialis*). At the metacarpus, it splits into two distinct tendons that end on the palmar side of

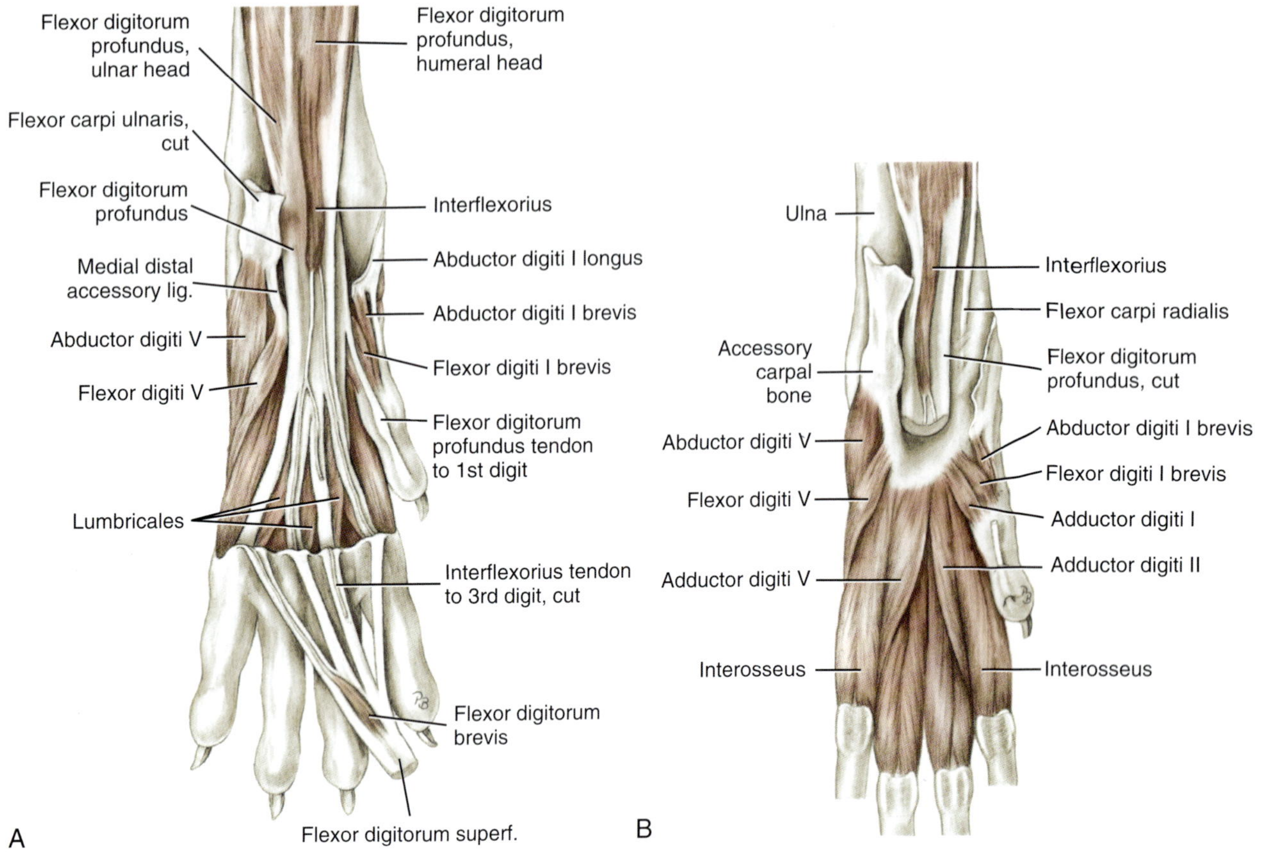

• **Fig. 6.63** Muscles of left forepaw. **A**, Superficial muscles, palmar aspect. **B**, Deep muscles, palmar aspect.

the base of metacarpals II and III, very close to the proximal articular surface. A projection from the elbow joint capsule extends deep to the muscle at its origin. The m. flexor carpi radialis was described by McConathy et al. (1983) as "compartmentalized" and as being histochemically composed of relatively more slow fibers than is the same muscle of cats (62% vs. 37% slow muscle fibers). The implications of this finding seem to reinforce the notion that dog muscle contains many fatigue-resistant muscle fibers to permit long duration bouts of locomotion. Intramuscular specialization was suggested by LaTorre et al. (1993) who described many large type I (slow) fibers in the medial compartment that differed from the lateral compartment (these are proximal subdivisions of the main muscle belly arising from the epicondyle), which contained fewer and smaller type I fibers. These authors suggested that the humeral compartment, containing a more robust fast-fiber population of muscle fibers may be more important in carpal flexion during locomotion.

Action: Flexion of the carpal joint. EMG activity was recorded throughout the late swing phase and first half of the stance phase during walking in dogs (Tokuriki, 1973a). Such activity during the stance phase (a period when the carpus is extended) could either stabilize the carpus during the stance (m. flexor carpi radialis acting antagonistically to the carpal extensors) or provide a component of cranial thrust during the middle to late part of the stance phase.

Innervation: N. medianus.

The strong, flat ***m. flexor digitorum superficialis*** (Figs. 6.56, 6.60, 6.61, 6.63A to 6.65B, and 6.66) in dogs, in contrast with that in other animals, lies directly deep to the skin and antebrachial fascia in the caudomedial part of the antebrachium. It covers the m. flexor digitorum profundus and the humeral head of the m. flexor carpi ulnaris. It arises by a short but thick tendon on the medial or flexor epicondyle cranial to the humeral head of the m. flexor carpi ulnaris and somewhat proximal to the flexor digitorum profundus. The fleshy muscle belly reaches far distally and becomes tendinous only a short distance proximal to the carpus. Its tendon is large, elliptical in cross-section, approximately 1 cm wide and 0.5 cm thick. This tendon runs over the flexor surface of the carpus medial to the accessory carpal bone enclosed in a superficial layer of the flexor retinaculum (*retinaculum flexorum*). It is separated from the deep flexor tendon by a thick deep layer of the flexor retinaculum. In the proximal third of the metacarpus the tendon of the superficial digital flexor splits into four parts, which diverge to the second to fifth metacarpophalangeal joints. Lying in a palmar relationship to the corresponding

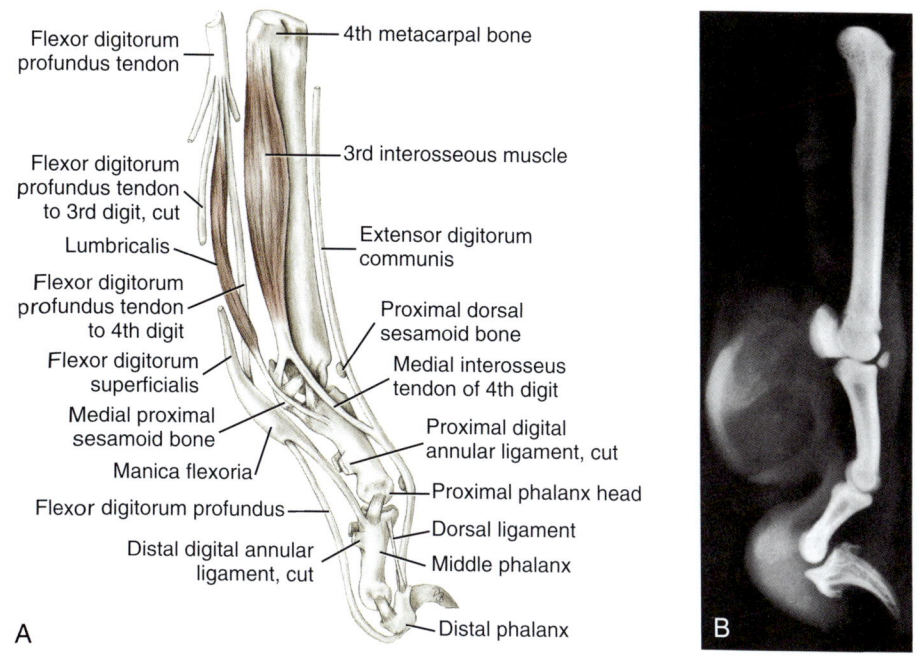

Fig. 6.64 **A**, The fourth digit, medial aspect. (Palmar annular ligament removed.) **B**, Lateral radiograph of a digit.

terminal tendons of the deep flexor tendon, each continues over the respective proximal phalanx and ends on the palmar surface of the base of the middle phalanx after being "perforated" by one of the deep flexor tendons passing to a distal phalanx. Each branch of the superficial tendon, at the metacarpophalangeal joint, forms a tubelike enclosure around the deep flexor tendon called a *manica flexoria*. The proximal edge of this sleeve projects a short distance proximally beyond the articular surfaces of the sesamoid bones. Distal to the sesamoids at the metacarpophalangeal joints, the tube is so split for the passage of the deep digital flexor tendon that the superficial tendon appears to be in two branches when it is viewed from the palmar side. The deep part of the sleeve, however, is undivided and accompanies the enclosed tendon farther and attaches to the palmar surface of the base of the middle phalanx throughout its breadth. The four terminal tendons of the muscle are as a rule of equal size (in large dogs, approximately 5 mm wide and 0.5 mm thick). The branch to digit V is much smaller. At the metacarpophalangeal joint and both proximal and distal to the proximal interphalangeal joint, the branches of the superficial and deep digital flexor tendons are bridged by the three well-defined annular ligaments: the palmar annular ligament at the metacarpophalangeal joint, and the proximal and distal digital annular ligaments on the palmar surface of the proximal phalanx, respectively.

Deep to the origin of the superficial digital flexor there is a synovial bursa 2 to 2.5 cm long in large dogs. This communicates with a second bursa beneath the origin of the caput humerale of the m. flexor carpi ulnaris. Each of the four terminal tendons has a long digital synovial sheath. This sheath is described more fully later in this chapter, in the discussion of the m. flexor digitorum profundus.

Action: Flexion of the metacarpophalangeal and proximal interphalangeal joints of the four principal digits and thereby of the whole forepaw.
Innervation: N. medianus.

The ***m. flexor carpi ulnaris*** (Figs. 6.53, 6.56, 6.60, 6.61, 6.63, and 6.65B) consists of two bellies, which converge into a single tendon ending on the accessory carpal bone. The muscle lies caudolaterally on the antebrachium, with its smaller ulnar head most superficial and lateral to and partly covering the m. flexor digitorum superficialis. The much larger humeral head is in the second layer of the palmar musculature deep to the m. flexor digitorum superficialis and superficial to the m. flexor digitorum profundus.

The rather flat **ulnar head** (*caput ulnare*), which is straplike in small dogs, arises medially on the palmar border of the proximal end of the ulna and is covered at its origin by the terminal tendon of the medial head of the m. triceps brachii. Proximal to the middle of the antebrachium, the ulnar head becomes a flat tendon that extends distally, lateral and caudal to the m. flexor digitorum superficialis covering the humeral head. Toward the accessory carpal bone the tendon of the ulnar head gradually courses deep to the terminal tendon of the humeral head and ends independently on the accessory carpal bone. The strong antebrachial fascia fuses with it throughout its length.

The much larger **humeral head** (*caput humerale*) arises on the medial epicondyle of the humerus by a short, thick

282 CHAPTER 6 The Muscular System

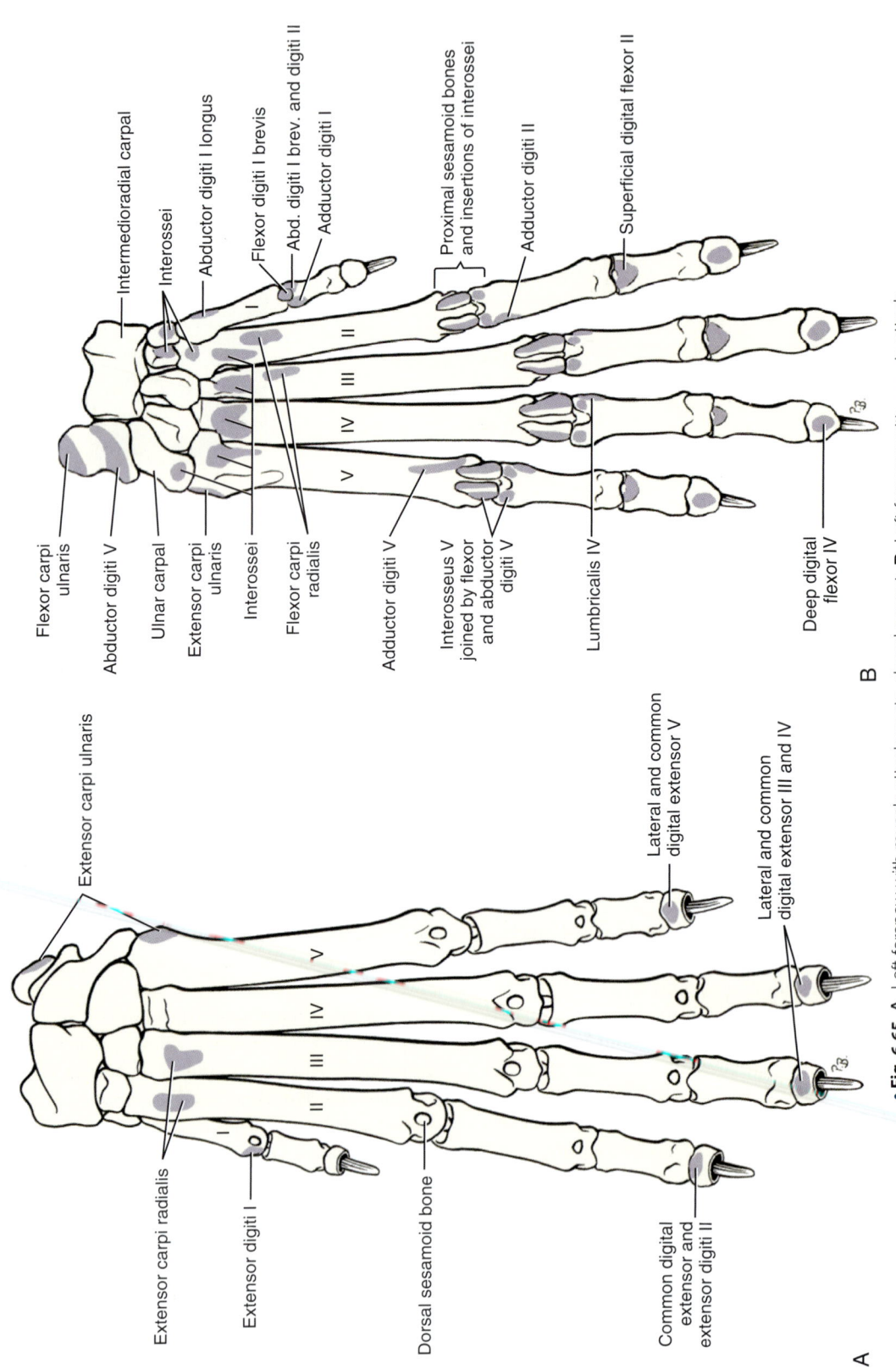

- **Fig. 6.65** **A,** Left forepaw with muscle attachments, dorsal aspect. **B,** Left forepaw with muscle attachments, palmar aspect.

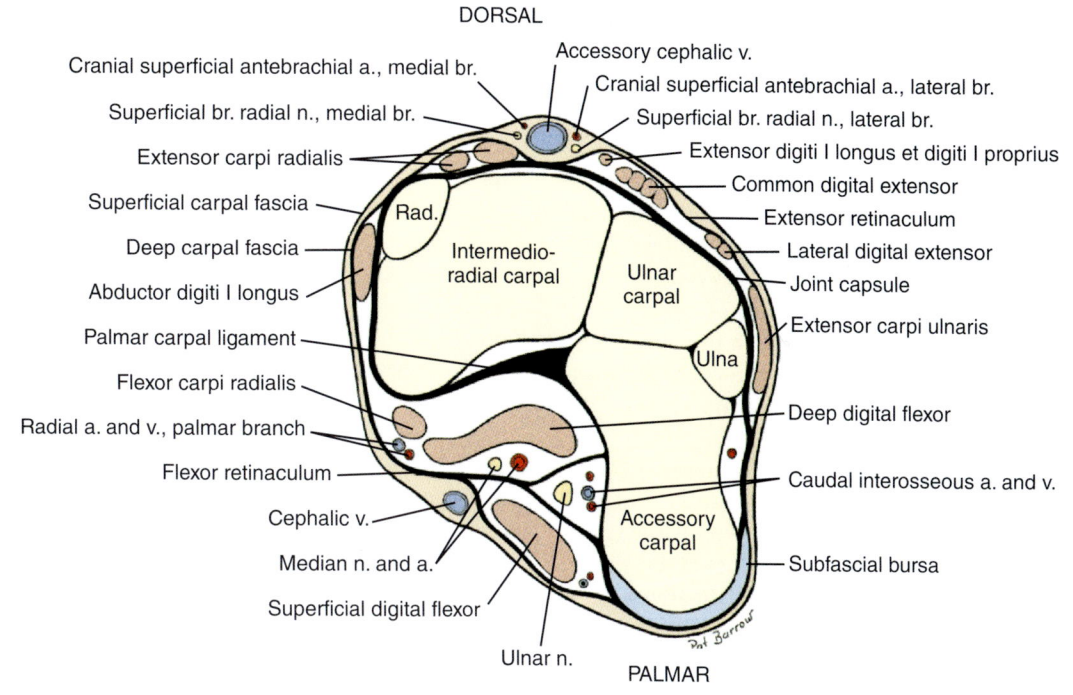

• Fig. 6.66 Schematic transverse section of forepaw through accessory carpal bone.

tendon that is adjacent to that of the m. flexor digitorum superficialis. It ends by an equally short, thick tendon on the accessory carpal bone. This thick, flat muscle, as much as 3 cm wide and 1 cm thick, in the dog, in contrast with that in other mammals, is almost completely covered by the m. flexor digitorum superficialis. Only the lateral edge of its distal half and its terminal tendon encroach on the antebrachial fascia. Both surfaces of its body are covered by a tendinous sheet. The caudal sheet is almost entirely a distal one; the cranial tendinous sheet is equally extensive proximally and distally and is provided with a narrow tendinous sulcus that, near the middle, appears to be displaced somewhat medially. Thus the muscle has a complicated fiber structure.

Both heads of m. flexor carpi ulnaris in mongrel dogs were reported to contain more than 50% type I fibers, whereas the overall mean was 77% type I fibers for both heads (Armstrong et al., 1982). Similar studies showed that the same muscle in cats contained approximately 50% slow oxidative (SO), or type I, fibers for the caput humerale and 36% type SO fibers in the caput ulnare. Gonyea et al. (1981) suggested that the m. flexor carpi ulnaris of cats and, in particular, the caput humerale contained significantly more slow, postural muscle fibers than did any of the other forearm muscles. Support for the histochemical data was provided by Glenn and Whitney (1987), who measured contraction times that were slow in the m. flexor carpi ulnaris of cats relative to contraction times of other carpal flexors. Glenn and Whitney concluded that the caput humerale was probably important in performing an antigravity role during stance and locomotion, based on a significantly slower contraction time and a higher fatigue index than was observed in the caput ulnare. These data suggest the possibility of differing roles for the two heads of m. flexor carpi ulnaris in cats and suggest that similar situations might be present in the dog.

Deep to the origin of this muscle is found a synovial bursa that communicates with the one deep to the origin of the m. flexor digitorum superficialis. A second bursa, deep to the terminal tendon, in large dogs extends proximally 1 to 1.5 cm from the accessory carpal bone.

Action: Flexion of the forepaw with abduction.
Innervation: N. ulnaris.

The *m. flexor digitorum profundus* (see Figs. 6.53, 6.54, 6.56, 6.60 to 6.64, and 6.65B) consists of three heads and, generally speaking, forms the deepest layer of the caudal musculature of the forearm. It is covered by the mm. flexor carpi radialis, flexor digitorum superficialis, and flexor carpi ulnaris. Its bellies, along with the m. pronator quadratus, lie directly on the caudal surface of the radius and ulna. It consists of humeral, radial, and ulnar heads, which represent completely separate muscles whose tendons fuse to form the thick deep digital flexor tendon. The homologization of these three muscles is still in dispute (Kajava, 1922).

The **humeral head** (*caput humerale*) of the m. flexor digitorum profundus, as the largest division of the entire muscle, consists of three bellies that are difficult to isolate. It is provided with tendinous sheets and bands and thus has a very complex fiber arrangement. The three bellies arise by a common short, thick tendon on the medial epicondyle of the humerus, immediately caudal to the tendon of origin of the m. flexor carpi radialis and covered by that of the m. flexor digitorum superficialis, and the humeral head of the m. flexor carpi ulnaris. The complexly constructed body of the muscle lies on the caudomedial side of the antebrachium in such a way that it appears partly enclosed between the radial head medially and deeply and the ulnar head laterally. Near the carpus, or at the border between the carpus and the antebrachium, the tendons of the humeral head fuse into a flat, but thick, main tendon that is grooved on its palmar surface. Just proximal to the groove the smaller tendons of the radial and ulnar heads converge to form the deep flexor tendon.

The **radial head** (*caput radiale*) of the m. flexor digitorum profundus lies on the caudomedial surface of the radius, along the mm. pronator quadratus, pronator teres, flexor carpi radialis, and the humeral head of the flexor digitorum profundus. It arises, as the smallest division of the entire muscle, from the medial border and for a small distance also on the caudal surface of the proximal three fifths of the radius. Near the carpus it forms a thin, flat tendon that runs from a slender tendinous sheet on the proximal, caudal border of the muscle. This joins the large tendon of the humeral head at the proximal border of the carpus. After being united for a short distance with the principal tendon, it again splits away to insert on digit I. Exceptionally, the branch of the deep tendon going to the first digit is independent in the dog (Ziegler, 1931).

The **ulnar head** (*caput ulnare*) of the m. flexor digitorum profundus is larger than the radial head. It is a flat muscle at the caudal side of the ulna, located among the m. extensor carpi ulnaris, flexor carpi ulnaris, and the humeral head of the m. flexor digitorum profundus. It is covered superficially by both the m. flexor carpi ulnaris and extensor carpi ulnaris. It arises on the caudal border of the ulna from the distal portion of the medial ridge of the olecranon to the distal fourth of the ulna. Its fibers run obliquely distally and caudally to a large, broad tendinous sheet that accompanies the palmar edge of the muscle almost from the level of the elbow joint. At the distal fourth of the antebrachium the muscle ends in a tendon, which after a short course is united with the common tendon of the m. flexor digitorum profundus.

The deep flexor tendon crosses the flexor surface of the carpus in a groove that is converted into the carpal canal by the flexor retinaculum. The tendon is very wide and, because of great thickening of its edges, forms a palmar groove. In the proximal portion of the metacarpus, from its medial border, the deep flexor tendon gives off the round, small tendon to digit I. Shortly thereafter the principal tendon divides into four branches for digits II to V, which run distally, covered by the corresponding grooved branches of the m. flexor digitorum superficialis. At the level of the sesamoids of the metacarpophalangeal joints of digits II to V the deep digital flexor tendons pass through the tubular sheaths (*manica flexoria*) formed by the branches of the superficial digital flexor tendons. They emerge from the palmar sheaths, extend over the flexor surface of the distal interphalangeal joints, and end on the tuberosities of the distal phalanges of digits II to V.

The two digital flexor tendons on each of the four main digits are held in place by three annular ligaments. The proximal one, lig. metacarpeum transversum superficiale (*lig. anulare palmare*), or palmar annular ligament, lies at the metacarpophalangeal joint and runs between the collateral borders of the sesamoid bones. The middle one, proximal digital annular ligament, lies on the proximal phalanx, at approximately its middle, and the distal one, distal digital annular ligament, lies immediately distal to the proximal interphalangeal joint. The distal one is lacking in digit I.

Deep to the origin of the humeral head of the m. flexor digitorum profundus is a synovial bursa. The terminal tendon of the muscle, as it passes through the carpal canal, is partly or wholly surrounded by a synovial sheath (see Fig. 6.66). This extends from the distal end of the radius to the metacarpus. It may be replaced by a sac with rough, thin walls, without synovia. In the digits the digital synovial sheaths are formed around the individual branches of the deep flexor tendon. The branch going to the first digit has its own sheath, which extends from the middle of metacarpal I to the tuberosity of the distal phalanx. The principal tendons going to digits II to V, however, bear synovial sheaths, which are also common for the superficial flexor tendons. These extend from the ends of the metacarpal bones to the tuberosities of the distal phalanges. These common synovial sheaths begin in large dogs 1 to 1.5 cm proximal to the metacarpophalangeal articulations immediately proximal to the sesamoid bones in the region of the proximal ends of the sheathes formed by the superficial flexor tendons. At their origin the sheaths enclose only the deep flexor tendons. Somewhat farther distally, they also enclose the superficial flexor tendons. Here their fibrosa fuses with the proximal transverse or palmar annular ligaments. To each collateral border of the deeply situated and flattened superficial flexor tendons, there extends a mesotendon. Distally the synovial sheaths also enclose the proximal digital annular ligaments of the flexors so that they receive mesotendons extending to their proximal edges. Farther distally the deep branches alone are surrounded by synovial sheaths. The distal digital annular ligaments, however, do not push into the synovial spaces, but fuse with the palmar and lateral walls of the synovial sheaths. The transverse palmar and digital annular ligaments are developments of the fibrous portion of the synovial sheaths. Mesotendons connect the synovial sheaths with the flexor tendons.

Action: The m. flexor digitorum profundus is the flexor of the forepaw (carpus and digital joints).

Innervation: The radial head as well as the deep and medial portions of the humeral head: n. medianus; the lateral portion of the humeral head and the ulnar head: n. medianus and n. ulnaris (Agduhr, 1915).

The *m. pronator quadratus* (Figs. 6.53, 6.56, and 6.62) fills in the space between the radius and the ulna medially. It is rhomboidal in outline, and covers the interosseous membrane, a portion of the medial surface of the ulna, and the caudal surface of the radius, except for the proximal and distal ends. It is covered by the m. flexor digitorum profundus. Its fibers run from the ulna obliquely, distally and medially, to insert on the radius.

Action: Turn the forepaw medially, which is pronation.
Innervation: N. medianus.

Muscles of the Forepaw

In the forepaw are the tendons of the antebrachial muscles, which insert on the metacarpal bones and phalanges, as well as the special muscles that are confined to the palmar surface of the forepaw. The four metacarpals and digits I to V are thus covered by many palmar muscles. A portion of these special muscles lies between the large flexor tendons; another portion lies between these and the skeleton, either lying directly on the four large metacarpal bones or occurring as special muscles of digits I, II, and V.

Muscles Associated with the Flexor Tendons

These muscles include the m. interflexorius, m. flexor digitorum brevis, and the mm. lumbricales.

The small *m. interflexorius* (Fig. 6.63) is the longest of the group. It arises at the level of the distal fourth of the antebrachium from the palmar tendinous sheet of the lateral superficial belly of the humeral head of the m. flexor digitorum profundus. As a slender, rounded muscle belly, it runs to the carpal joint lying between the digital flexors. It crosses deep to the flexor retinaculum on the palmar surface of the deep flexor tendon, and its thin tendon splits into two (or three) branches at the middle of the metacarpus. These accompany the branches of the m. flexor digitorum superficialis for digits III and IV, and occasionally digit II, and fuse with them.

Ellenberger and Baum (1943) designate it as the m. palmaris longus accessorius. The name *m. interflexorius* is derived from Agduhr (1915) and Pitzorno (1905). According to Kajava (1923), the muscle could be designated *m. interflexorius profundosublimis*.

Action: Flexion of the forepaw.
Innervation: N. medianus.

The *m. flexor digitorum brevis* (Fig. 6.63), the smallest of this group, is a delicate, only slightly fleshy muscle, which arises distal to the carpus from the palmarolateral surface of the superficial flexor tendon branch for digit V. It goes into a flat tendon, which occasionally takes the place of the whole muscle. It ends on the palmar annular ligament at the metacarpophalangeal joint.

According to Kajava (1923), however, one would have to regard this as a muscle mass in the carpal pad. Ellenberger and Baum (1943) describe this muscle as the *m. palmaris brevis accessorius*.

The *mm. lumbricales* (Figs. 6.61, 6.63, and 6.64) are three small muscles that are associated with the tendons of the flexor digitorum profundus. The first muscle arises from the contiguous sides of the flexor digitorum profundus tendons to the second and third digits, the second from the tendons to the third and fourth digits, and the third from the tendons to the fourth and fifth digits. They pass obliquely distally and laterally and end in thin tendons that are inserted on the medial surface of the base of the first phalanges of the third, fourth, and fifth digits. The tendon of the first muscle inserts on the third digit, the second on the fourth, and the third on the fifth (Leahy, 1949).

Action: Flexion of the metacarpophalangeal joints.
Innervation: Deep branch of the n. ulnaris.

Muscles Associated with the Palmar Side of the Metacarpal Bones

These include the interosseous muscles.

The fleshy **mm. interossei** (Figs. 6.60, 6.63, to 6.65B) are four in number. They lie on the palmar side of the four large metacarpal bones deep to the tendon branches of the flexor digitorum profundus. They are relatively large and border on one another. They arise from the proximal ends (the bases) of metacarpals II, III, IV, and V, and from the carpometacarpal joint capsule, and cover the entire palmar surfaces of these metacarpal bones. After coursing a short distance, each muscle divides into two branches that attach by tendons to the base of the first phalanx. A sesamoid is embedded in each tendon. A portion of each tendon extends over the collateral borders of the joint and runs distally on the dorsal surface of the proximal phalanx to unite with the common extensor tendon. These are referred to as "check ligaments."

Morphologically each of these muscles results from the fusion of two muscles. According to Kajava (1923), they represent the mm. flexores breves profundi, which are placed dorsal to the ramus palmaris profundus of the n. ulnaris and are innervated by it. Each of the four muscles is collaterally covered by a considerable tendinous fascia that extends far distally. According to Forster (1916), each muscle is invaginated by a tendinous sheet that comes from the diverging portions and that extends proximally, causing the duplicity of each muscle to be much more marked.

Action: Flexion of the metacarpophalangeal joints.
Innervation: Deep branch of the n. ulnaris.

Special Muscles of Digit I

The rudimentary first, or medial, digit has three special muscles: an abductor, a flexor, and an adductor.

The *m. abductor digiti I (pollicis) brevis* (Figs. 6.60, 6.61, and 6.65B) arises from the flexor retinaculum and passes to the tendon of the m. abductor digiti I longus located on the medial side of the carpus. It ends in the ligamentous tissue at the metacarpophalangeal joint of digit I. According to Kajava (1923), the muscle represents the radial head of the m. pollicis brevis profundus.

Action: Abduction and flexion of digit I.
Innervation: Deep branch of the n. ulnaris.

The **m. flexor digiti I (pollicis) brevis** (Figs. 6.63 and 6.65B) is larger than the special abductor just described and lies between it and the m. adductor digiti I. It arises on the radiate carpal ligament (part of what was formerly called the palmar carpal ligament, a connective tissue on the palmar surface of the carpal bone region), runs obliquely to digit I, and ends on the sesamoid bone or on the proximal phalanx.

Action: Flexion of digit I.
Innervation: Deep branch of the n. ulnaris.

The **m. adductor digiti I (pollicis)** (Figs. 6.63 and 6.65B) is the largest muscle of digit I. It arises as a small, fleshy muscle body between the special flexor and the m. interosseus of digit II on the flexor retinaculum and ends on the lateral surface of the proximal phalanx of digit I.

Action: Adduction and flexion of digit 1.
Innervation: Deep branch of n. ulnaris.

Special Muscles of Digit V

The fifth digit, like the first, also has three special muscles: an adductor, a flexor, and an abductor.

The **m. adductor digit V** (Figs. 6.63 and 6.65B) arises from the radiate carpal ligament (part of what was formerly called the *palmar carpal ligament*) and extends as a slender belly obliquely in a lateral direction to end on the medial surface of metacarpal V and the proximal phalanx of digit V. Its proximal portion lies on the mm. interossei III and IV, and its distal portion lies between mm. interossei IV and V.

Action: Adduction of digit V.
Innervation: Deep branch of the n. ulnaris.

The **m. flexor digiti V** (Figs. 6.63 and 6.65B) arises on the ligament from the accessory carpal bone to metacarpal IV, runs obliquely over the m. interosseus of the fifth digit laterally, and, by a thin tendon, joins that of the m. abductor digiti V.

Action: Flexion of the digit V.
Innervation: Deep branch of the n. ulnaris.

The **m. abductor digiti V** (Figs. 6.63 and 6.65B) is larger than the flexor muscle and arises on the accessory carpal bone. It ends by means of a tendon that unites with the m. flexor digiti V on the lateral sesamoid and frequently by a thin tendon on the proximal phalanx of the fifth digit. It lies directly deep to the skin on the flexor retinaculum. On its deep surface the fusiform body bears a delicate, proximal tendinous leaf.

Action: Abduction of digit V.
Innervation: Deep branch of the n. ulnaris.

Special Muscles of Digit II

The second digit has only one special muscle, an adductor.

The **m. adductor digiti II** (Figs. 6.63B and 6.65B) arises on the radiate carpal ligament between the m. interosseus 2 and the m. adductor digiti V, runs distally between the mm. interossei 2 and 3, and ends by means of a tendon on the base of the proximal phalanx of digit II.

Action: Adduction of digit II.
Innervation: Deep branch of the n. ulnaris.

Forster (1916) includes the adductors of the first, second, and fifth digits under the name mm. contrahentes digitorum, which in the dog are represented separately but which, when better developed, constitute a "contrahentes leaf." They lie palmarly on the ramus profundus of the n. ulnaris and are innervated by it.

Fasciae of the Thoracic Limb

The superficial and deep fasciae of the neck and thorax extend laterally over the scapula and there form the superficial and deep fasciae of the scapula, which continues distally in the thoracic limb. The whole limb is covered by this double system of connective tissue, the parts of which take their name from the portion of the limb that they cover.

The **superficial fascia** on the scapula and brachium covers these portions of the extremity as a bridge laterally from the superficial neck and superficial trunk fasciae. In the distal brachial region, however, it is completely closed into a cylinder because that portion of the superficial fascia in the region of the sternum extends to the medial brachial surface. Cranially and laterally this covers the mm. brachiocephalicus, deltoideus, and triceps brachii, on which it unites firmly with the deep leaf of the brachial fascia. It covers the m. pectoralis superficialis medially. The v. cephalica is covered laterally by the superficial fascia and, as it crosses the flexor surface of the elbow joint, it lifts the fascia into a fold. Distal to the elbow joint the closely applied superficial fascia is extremely delicate and less easily movable with respect to the deep tissue. The superficial fascia of the forearm, carpus, metacarpus, and digits, contain the cutaneous vessels and cutaneous nerves that extend over long distances before they actually enter the skin.

The **deep fascia** of the thoracic limb includes the axillary, brachial, and antebrachial fascia. The **axillary fascia** (*fascia axillaris*) covers the medial muscles at the level of the shoulder joint. Dorsally this is continuous with the deep cervical and thoracolumbar fascia. The deep fascia of the neck covers the m. rhomboideus and is continuous with the superficial leaf of the thoracolumbar fascia, which covers the mm. latissimus dorsi and trapezius. The latter deep fascia is firmly attached to the spine of the scapula after it has covered the mm. infraspinatus, supraspinatus, deltoideus, and triceps brachii, or as much of these muscles as make their appearance laterally. The deep fascia of the scapular region is continuous distally with the brachial fascia, *fascia brachii*, which attaches to the crest of the major tubercle of the humerus between the mm. deltoideus and brachialis on one side and the m. cleidobrachialis on the other. Distally, where the m. brachialis is free in the triangle between the mm. triceps brachii and cleidobrachialis, the fascia is especially thick. Here it extends deep to the cephalic vein and surrounds the muscle loosely with intermuscular septa that extend deep to the m. cleidobrachialis. Farther medially it covers the m. biceps brachii. The deep fascia is thinner and more firmly attached to the long and lateral heads of the m. triceps brachii than it is elsewhere. Axillary fascia arises from the inner surface of the mm. subscapularis and teres major and passes distally as brachial fascia over the m. triceps brachii and the medial surface of the humerus to merge into the deep antebrachial fascia at the elbow joint. This medial brachial fascia forms a thick fold, which is readily palpated. The *fascia antebrachii* covers the muscles of the forearm as a closely applied tube that is thickest medially. Between the extensor and the flexor muscles it sends septa to the periosteum of the radius and ulna; these septa enclose the individual muscles, as well as small groups of muscles. The fascia is intimately united with the extensors, more loosely covers the flexors, and is firmly fused to all free portions of the bones of the antebrachium. In the distal antebrachial region it is intimately joined with the connective tissue found between the tendons. In the groove between the tendons of the mm. extensor carpi ulnaris and flexor carpi ulnaris proximal to the accessory carpal bone, the fascia invaginates more deeply. At the carpus it becomes the **fascia of the forepaw** (*fascia manus*), which, as the dorsal and palmar deep fascia, ensheathes all tendons and superficial muscles of the forepaw distally and attaches to all projecting parts of bones. Even the cushions of all of the pads are closely united with the deep fascia. From the cushion of the carpal pad an especially thick band of the fascia extends directly laterally and slightly proximally toward the distal end of the ulna. On the medial side another such band, the *flexor retinaculum* (Fig. 6.66), goes to the medial border of the carpus, bridging over the digital flexor tendons. On the dorsal surface of the carpus are found transverse supporting fibers, the extensor retinaculum. On the dorsal surface of the metacarpus, there is formed a triangular, fibrous leaf that extends from metacarpal I obliquely laterally and distally to the branches of the common digital extensor tendon for digits II, III, and IV. Palmarly, on the metacarpophalangeal joints, thickened portions of the deep fascia form palmar annular ligaments that attach primarily to the sesamoid bones.

Muscles of the Pelvic Limb

Muscles of the Pelvis and Thigh

The pelvis and thigh are covered on all sides by muscles that are, for the most part, common to both of these body regions, so that the two groups cannot be sharply differentiated. The so-called hip muscles belong to the pelvic group and act mostly on the hip joint, but a few act also on the sacroiliac joint. The muscles of the thigh act primarily on the stifle, the femorotibial joint. The pelvic muscles are divided into three groups. The **lumbar hypaxial** muscles lie on the ventral surfaces of the lumbar vertebrae and ilium and include mm. psoas minor, psoas major, and quadratus lumborum. The **lateral pelvic** muscles lie on the lateral side of the pelvis and include mm. gluteus superficialis, medius, and profundus, piriformis, and tensor fasciae latae. The **medial pelvic** muscles are deep and partly inside the pelvis: mm. obturator internus, gemelli, external obturator, and quadratus femoris. The muscles of the **thigh** are designated as to their cranial, caudal, and medial positions. To the caudal group belong the mm. biceps femoris, semitendinosus, and semimembranosus (sometimes called the *hamstring muscles*). They form a large, fleshy mass on the caudal side of the femur. The m. biceps femoris is lateral; the m. semimembranosus medial and the m. semitendinosus is caudal and between the other two muscles. To the cranial group belongs the m. quadriceps femoris, which forms the fleshy foundation of the cranial half of the thigh. A small m. capsularis and the m. sartorius cranialis are associated with it. The medial group includes the mm. gracilis, pectineus, adductores, and sartorius caudalis.

Lumbar Hypaxial Muscles

The lumbar hypaxial muscles arise on the ventral surfaces of the caudal thoracic and lumbar vertebrae and insert on the os coxae and femur. They lie on one another in several layers.

The ***m. psoas minor*** (Figs. 6.67 to 6.70) runs toward the pelvis ventromedially as it lies between the iliac fascia and the peritoneum and transversalis fascia ventrally and the mm. psoas major and quadratus lumborum dorsally. Its muscular belly is smaller than that of the m. psoas major. It arises from the tendinous fascia of the m. quadratus lumborum at the level of the last thoracic vertebrae and on the ventral surface of the last thoracic vertebra and the first four or five lumbar vertebrae; it is separated from its fellow of the opposite side by an interval gradually increasing caudally so that the bodies of the lumbar vertebrae become visible. The large flat tendon fused with the iliac fascia comes out of a shining, tendinous leaf at the fifth lumbar vertebra. It runs to the arcuate line and inserts on this line as far as the iliopubic eminence.

Action: To steepen the pelvis by flexion of the lumbosacral joint or to flex the lumbar part of the vertebral column.

288 CHAPTER 6 The Muscular System

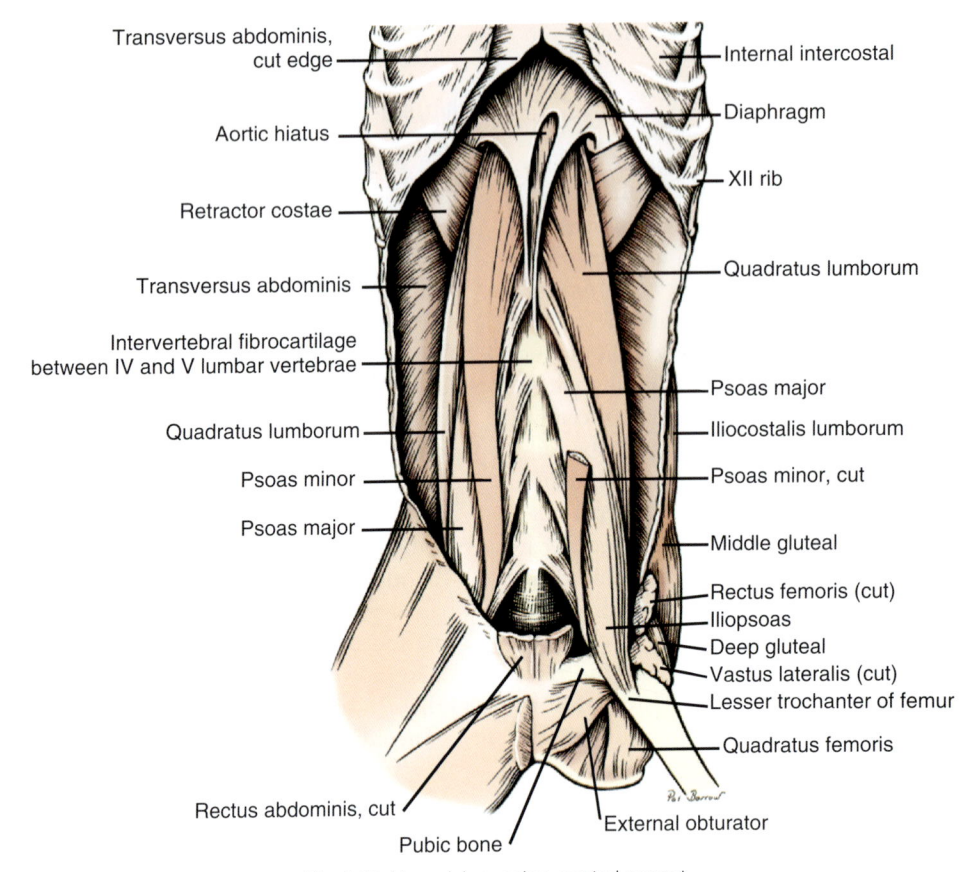

- Fig. 6.67 Hypaxial muscles, ventral aspect.

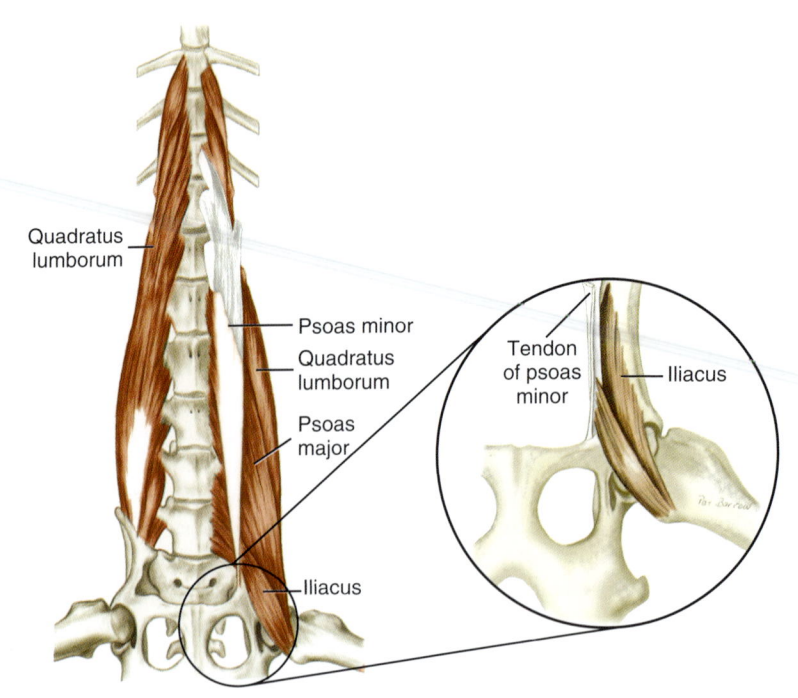

- Fig. 6.68 Hypaxial muscles, deep dissection, ventral aspect.

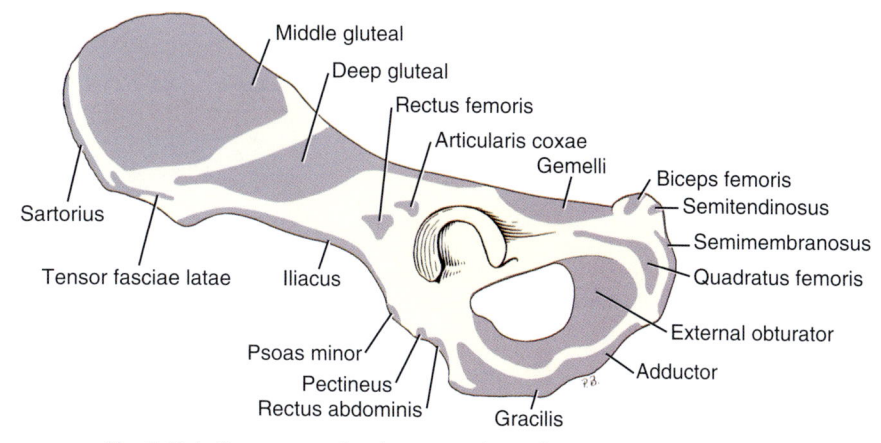

Fig. 6.69 Left os coxae, showing areas of muscle attachment, lateral aspect.

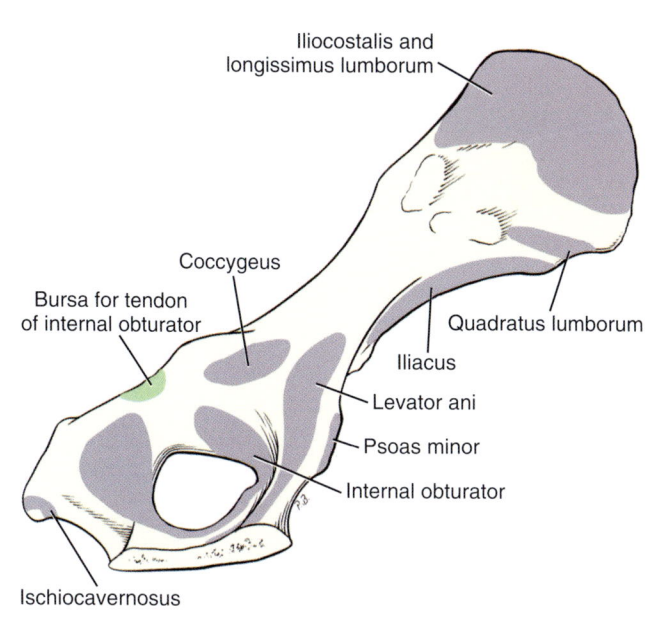

Fig. 6.70 Left os coxae, showing areas of muscle attachment, medial aspect.

Innervation: Lateral branches of the rami ventrales of lumbar nerves 1 to 4 or 5.

The ***m. psoas major*** (Figs. 6.67, 6.68, and 6.72) lies ventral to the m. quadratus lumborum and dorsal to the m. psoas minor. It is narrow and tendinous at its origin on the transverse processes of lumbar vertebrae 2 and 3, where it lies medial to the m. quadratus lumborum. It also attaches by means of the ventral aponeurosis of this muscle on lumbar vertebrae 3 and 4, and, finally, on the ventral and lateral surfaces of lumbar vertebrae 4 to 7. As this caudal portion of the m. psoas major passes along the cranioventral border of the ilium it receives the ***m. iliacus*** from the smooth ventral surface of the ilium between the arcuate line and the lateral border of the ilium. The two muscle masses (m. psoas major and m. iliacus) compose the ***m. iliopsoas***, which can be easily isolated. The m. iliopsoas attaches to the trochanter minor of the femur.

Action: To draw the pelvic limb cranial by flexion of the hip joint. When the femur is fixed in position, flexion and fixation of the vertebral column. When the limb is extended caudally, it draws the trunk caudally. May cause some lateral rotation of the femur.

Innervation: Branches of the rami ventrales of the lumbar nerves.

The ***m. quadratus lumborum*** (Figs. 6.67, 6.68, and 6.70) is the most dorsal of the lumbar hypaxial muscles. It lies directly ventral to the bodies of the last three thoracic and all the lumbar vertebrae as well as ventral to the proximal portions of the last two ribs and the transverse processes of the lumbar vertebrae. Caudal to the first lumbar vertebra it is covered ventrally by the psoas minor and caudal to the fourth lumbar vertebra by the psoas major. It has a thoracic and a lumbar portion. The thoracic portion of this muscle, which is rather large in the dog, consists of incompletely isolated bundles that become tendinous. These bundles extend more or less distinctly caudolaterally from the bodies of the last three thoracic vertebrae to the transverse processes of the lumbar vertebrae as far caudally as the seventh. It is covered by tendinous leaves dorsally and ventrally. It ends on the medial surface of the wing of the ilium between the articular surface and the cranial ventral iliac spine. The lateral portion of the muscle overhangs the transverse processes of the lumbar vertebrae, so that it also comes to lie on the ventral surface of the tendon of origin of the m. transversus abdominis.

Action: Flexion and fixation of the lumbar vertebral column.
Innervation: Rami of the ventral branches of nn. lumbales.

Pelvic Muscles

The pelvic muscles extend between the pelvis and the thigh and include a lateral and medial group.

The **lateral pelvic muscles** are arranged in several layers and include the tensor fascia lata, three gluteal muscles, and the piriformis.

The ***m. tensor fasciae latae*** (Figs. 6.69 and 6.71) is a triangular muscle that attaches proximally to the ilium

290 CHAPTER 6 The Muscular System

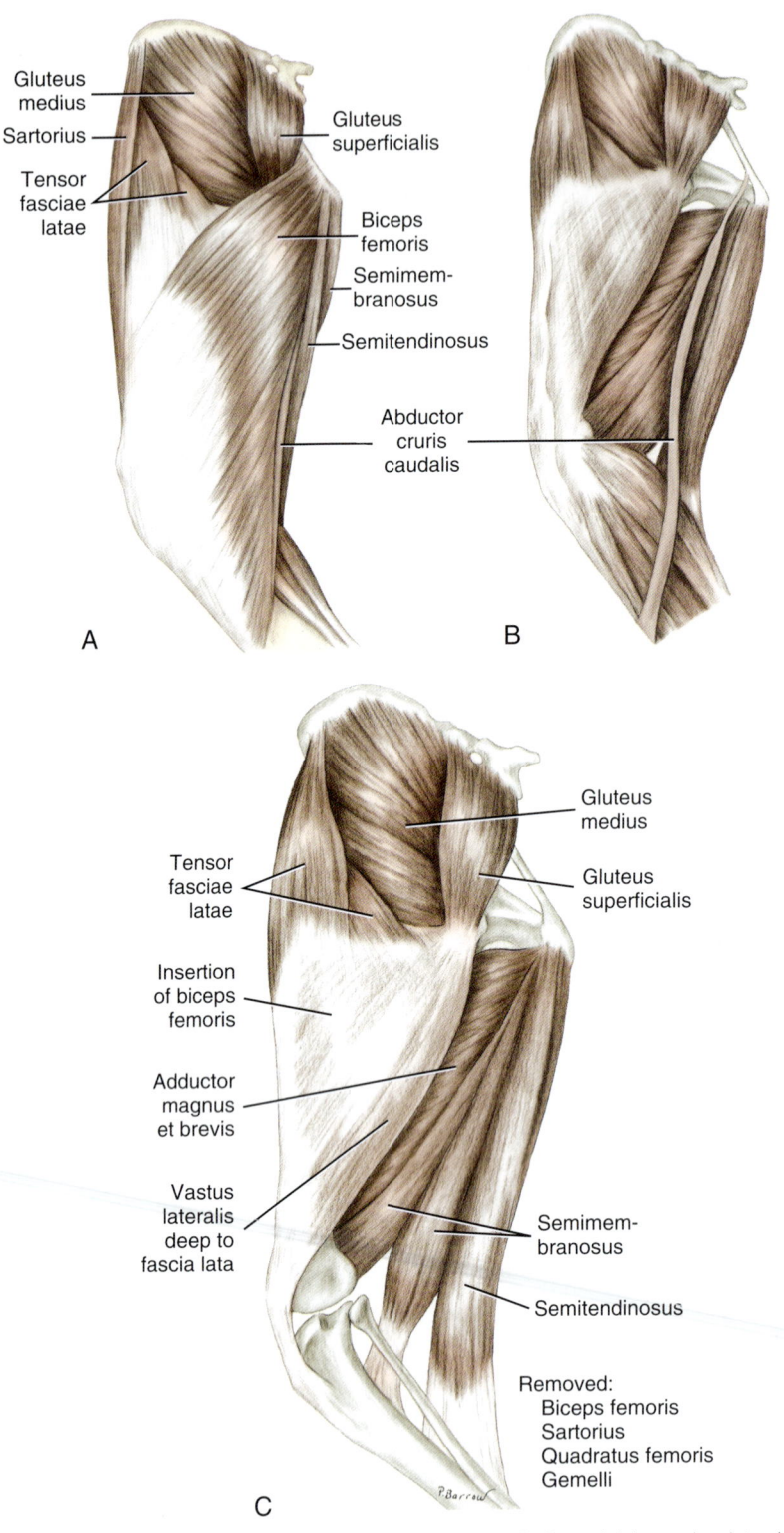

- **Fig. 6.71** Muscles of thigh. **A,** Superficial muscles, lateral aspect. **B,** Superficial muscles, lateral aspect. (Biceps femoris removed.) **C,** Deep muscles, lateral aspect. (Internal obturator removed.)

from the tuber coxae to the alar spine. It lies between the sartorius cranially, the middle gluteal caudodorsally and the quadriceps femoris distomedially. Part of its caudodorsal surface is attached to the middle gluteal near its origin. The muscle can be divided into two portions. The cranial more superficial portion is inserted on the lateral femoral fascia, which radiates over the quadriceps and blends with the fascial insertion of the biceps femoris. The deeper caudal portion is inserted on a layer of lateral femoral fascia that runs deep to the biceps femoris toward the stifle on the lateral surface of the vastus lateralis.

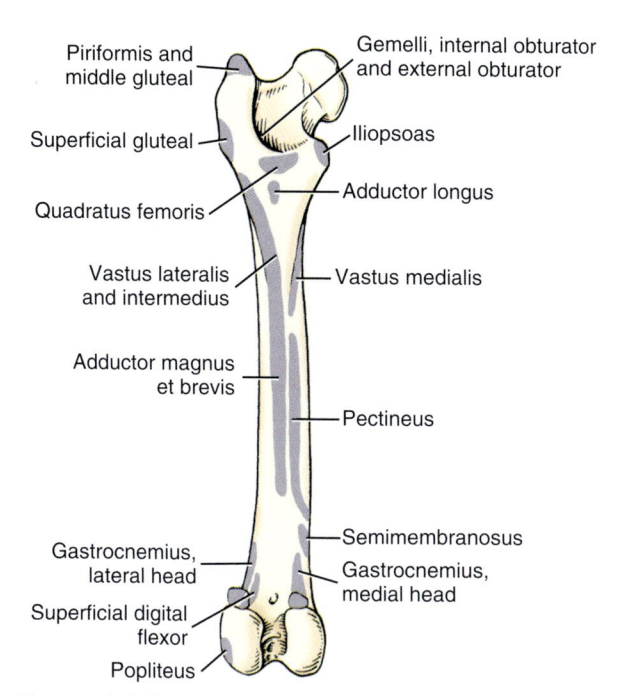

• **Fig. 6.72** Left femur, showing areas of muscle attachment, caudal aspect.

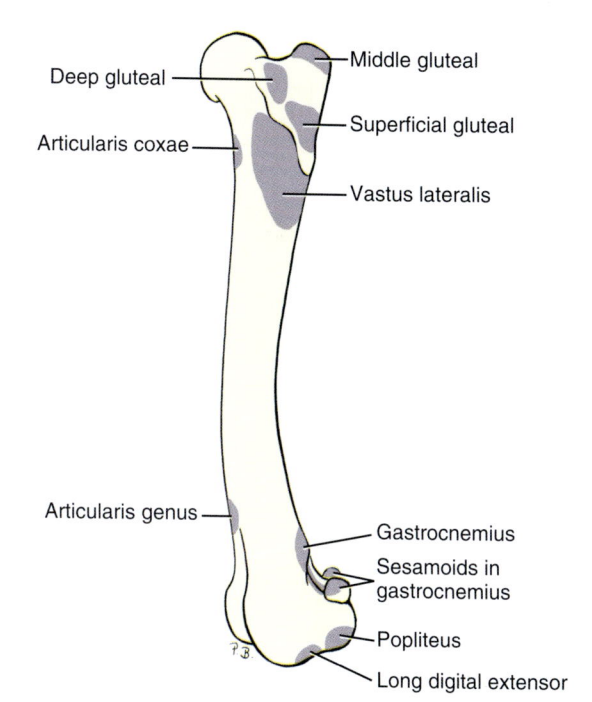

• **Fig. 6.73** Left femur, showing areas of muscle attachment, lateral aspect.

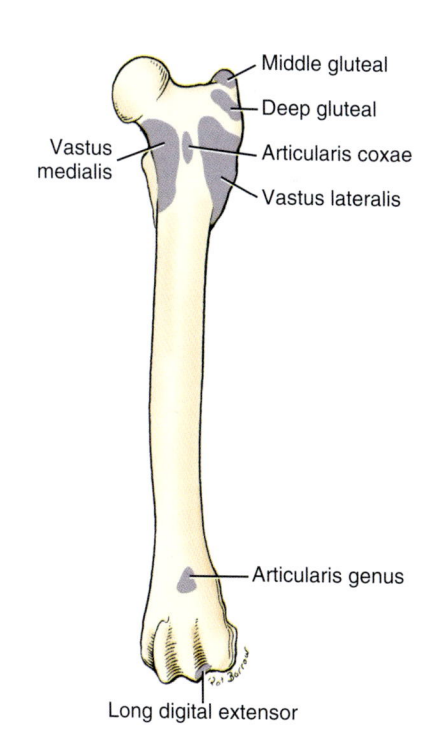

• **Fig. 6.74** Left femur, showing areas of muscle attachment, cranial aspect.

Action: To flex the hip, abduct the limb and extend the stifle joint.
Innervation: N. gluteus cranialis.

The *m. gluteus superficialis* (Figs. 6.71 to 6.73), the most superficial of the gluteal muscles, is a rather small, flat, almost rectangular muscle. It extends between the sacrum and the first caudal vertebra proximally and the trochanter tertius distally. The gluteal fascia covers this muscle loosely. It fuses with the muscle more intimately only at the proximal two-thirds of its cranial portion. The muscle arises from the gluteal fascia, a deep fascia, and thereby from the tuber sacrale of the ilium. Neighboring portions come from the caudal fascia. The thick caudal portions come from the lateral part of the sacrum, from the first caudal vertebra, and from more than half of the proximal part of the sacrotuberous ligament. Its fibers converge laterally and become tendinous. The tendon runs over the trochanter major and inserts on the small trochanter tertius. This tendon fuses with the aponeurosis of the m. tensor fasciae latae. The m. gluteus superficialis covers portions of the mm. gluteus medius and piriformis, and also the sacrotuberous ligament. In large dogs it is 5 to 7 cm wide and more than 1 cm thick caudally. A thin, deep portion was seen by Ziegler (1934), lying deep to the caudal border of the muscle and having a special origin on the sacrotuberous ligament. Deep to its terminal tendon on the trochanter tertius in approximately one-third of the specimens, there is a synovial bursa approximately 1 cm wide.

Action: Extension of the hip joint.
Innervation: N. gluteus caudalis.

The large *m. gluteus medius* (Figs. 6.69, 6.71 to 6.76) lies on the gluteal surface of the ilium, from which it takes its principal origin. It also arises from the iliac crest and most of the tuber sacrale. Some fibers also come from the dorsal portion of the sacroiliac ligament and from the deep surface of the gluteal fascia, a deep fascia that is fused with the muscle caudal to the iliac crest. A large part of the muscle lies deep to the gluteal fascia and skin, and only

292 CHAPTER 6 The Muscular System

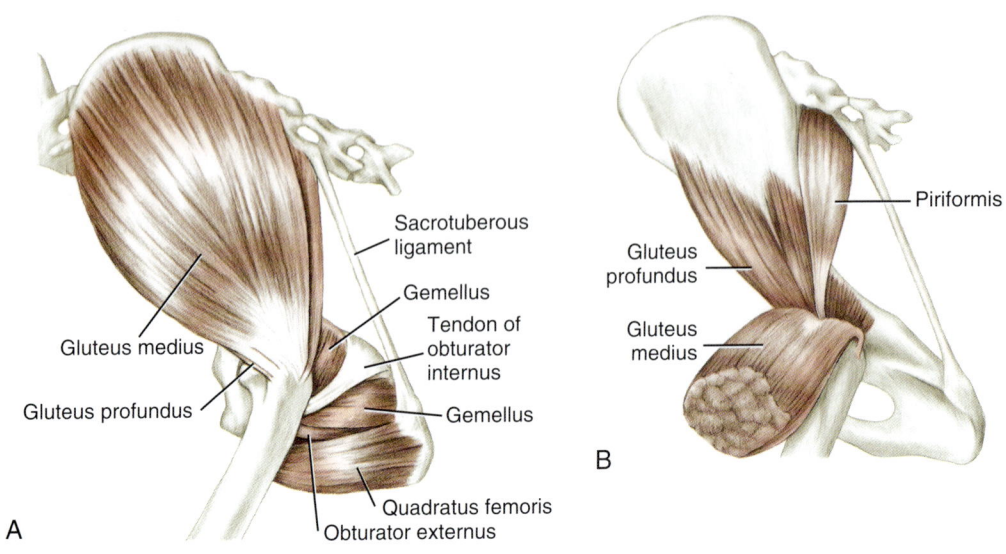

• **Fig. 6.75** Muscles of the gluteal region. **A**, Superficial muscles. **B**, Deep dissection.

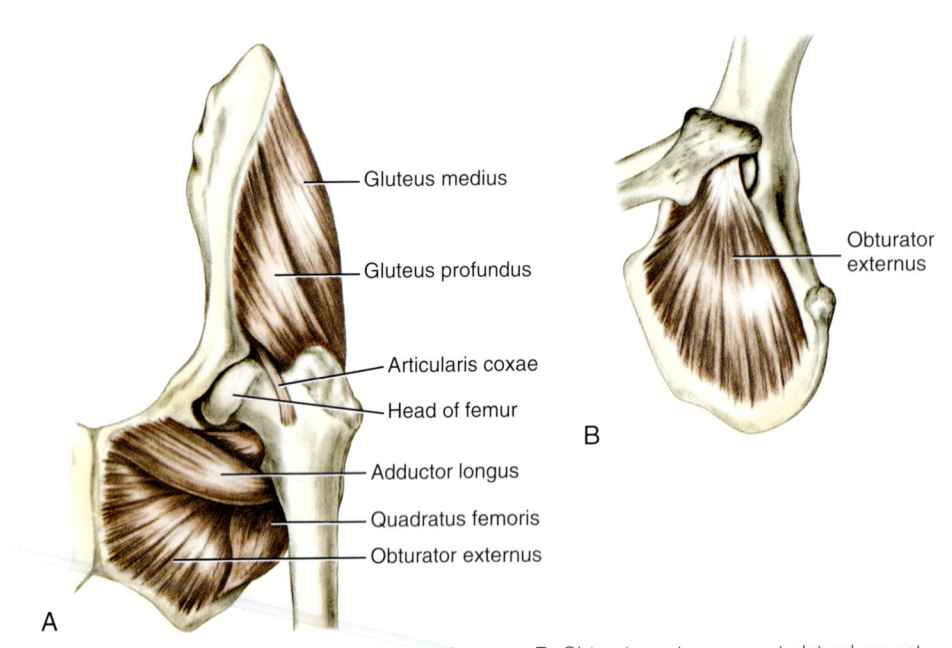

• **Fig. 6.76** Muscles of the hip joint. **A**, Ventral aspect. **B**, Obturator externus, ventrolateral aspect.

caudally is it covered by the superficial gluteal muscle. In a caudodistal direction it extends over the m. gluteus profundus and ends by a short, thick tendon on the free end of the trochanter major. The muscle is 2.5 to 3.5 cm thick and 7 to 9 cm wide. From the caudal border of the m. gluteus medius, a narrow but thick, deep belly can be defined that does not correspond to the m. gluteus accessorius of other animals. This deep portion arises on the transverse processes of the last sacral and first caudal vertebrae and on the sacrotuberous ligament and ends on the trochanter major by a narrow tendon that sinks into the principal tendon.

Action: Extension of the hip joint. Medial rotation of the hip and prevention of lateral rotation during weight bearing.
Innervation: N. gluteus cranialis.

The **m. piriformis** (Figs. 6.72, 6.75, and 6.82) lies caudal and medial to the m. gluteus medius and is completely covered by the m. gluteus superficialis. The m. piriformis arises on the lateral surface of the third sacral and first caudal vertebrae. Its tendon of insertion joins that of the m. gluteus medius on the major trochanter. Designation of a m. piriformis in dogs is questionable. Some authors consider this muscle to be the caudal portion of the m. gluteus profundus. For an illustrated consideration of this muscle and the gluteal region, see Henning (1965).

Action: Extension of the hip joint.
Innervation: N. gluteus caudalis.

The broad, fan-shaped **m. gluteus profundus** (Figs. 6.69, 6.73 to 6.77, and 6.82) is the deepest of the gluteal muscles.

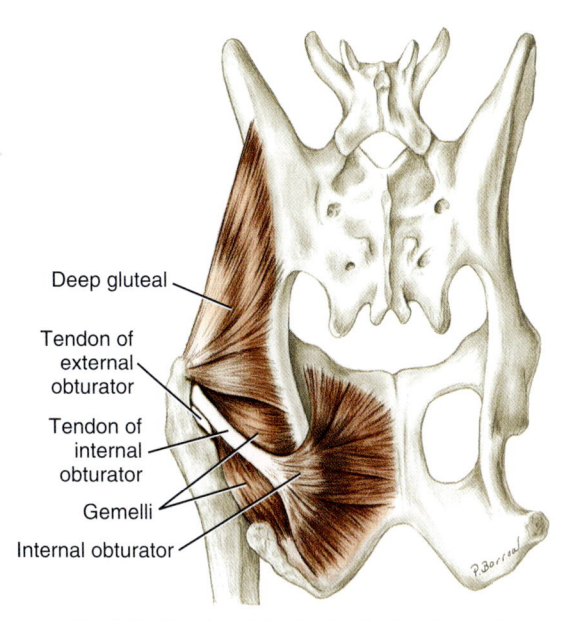

Fig. 6.77 Muscles of the hip joint, dorsal aspect.

It is completely covered by the mm. gluteus medius and piriformis. At the same time it extends, for a considerable distance, caudal to the deep portion of the gluteus medius. It takes its origin from the lateral surface of the body of the ilium near the ischiatic spine. Its fibers converge over the hip joint distolaterally and form a short, thick tendon that ends cranially on the trochanter major distal to the insertion of the m. gluteus medius. Deep to the tendon of insertion, there is often a small synovial bursa.

Action: Extension of the hip joint, with some abduction of the pelvic limb. Medial rotation of the hip and prevention of lateral rotation on weight bearing.
Innervation: N. gluteus cranialis.

The **medial pelvic muscles** are also called the "small pelvic association muscles" and include a group of short muscles that lie caudal to the m. gluteus profundus and the hip joint. They extend from the inner and outer surfaces of the ischium to the femur. These are the mm. obturator internus, the gemelli, the obturator externus, and the quadratus femoris.

The ***m. obturator internus*** (Figs. 6.70, 6.72, 6.75, and 6.77) is a large, fan-shaped muscle that covers the obturator foramen internally. It arises medial to the foramen on the pelvic surfaces of the rami of the pubis and ischium, the ischiatic table and from the ischiatic arch. Its fibers converge laterally and pass over the smooth surface of the lesser ischiatic notch directly caudal to the ischiatic spine and ventral to the sacrotuberous ligament. As the muscle passes over this notch, a prominent tendon forms and turns ventrolaterally almost at right angles and continues distolaterally where it is embedded deeply between the edges of the broader mm. gemelli that lie deep to it. The overhanging portions of the mm. gemelli, bearing a shining distal tendinous sheet, run from the edge of the lesser ischiatic notch into the internal obturator tendon, so that the triple tendinous apparatus ends undivided in the trochanteric fossa. Caudally the tendon of the m. obturator externus accompanies it. Where the muscle glides over the lesser ischiatic notch, there is a very thin-walled synovial bursa (*B. ischiadica m. obturatorii interni*), 1.5 to 2 cm wide, that surrounds the edges of the tendon and may extend out on the underlying mm. gemelli. A second bursa (*B. subtendinea m. obturatorii interni*), 2 to 3 mm wide, lies deep to the mm. obturator internus and gemelli tendons in the trochanteric fossa between the trochanter major and the joint capsule.

Action: Lateral rotation of the hip joint and prevention of medial rotation on weight bearing.
Innervation: N. ischiadicus.

The ***mm. gemelli*** (Figs. 6.69, 6.72, 6.75, and 6.77) represent a muscle that has been formed by the fusion of two parts and that lies between the terminal portions of the mm. obturator internus and obturator externus caudal to the m. gluteus profundus and the hip joint. It overhangs the tendon of the m. obturator internus cranially and caudally. The mm. gemelli arise together on the lateral surface of the body of the ischium in the arch ventral to the lesser ischiatic notch and are covered superficially by a shining fascia that forms the floor of the groove for the internal obturator tendon. Altogether this tendon apparatus ends undivided in the trochanteric fossa.

Action: Lateral rotation of the hip joint and prevention of medial rotation on weight bearing.
Innervation: N. ischiadicus.

The ***m. obturator externus*** (Figs. 6.69, 6.72, 6.75 to 6.77) is fan-shaped and arises on the ventral surface of the pubis and ischium adjacent to the pelvic symphysis. It is separated from the ischial symphysis by the mm. adductores. It covers the obturator foramen externally. Its caudal border is covered by the quadratus femoris, whereas the cranial border is hidden by the adductor muscle. On some of its pennate parts, the muscle body bears delicate tendinous strands from the origin of the muscle. The fibers converging toward the trochanteric fossa appear deep to the lateral aspect of the ischium and form a thick tendon that passes between the terminations of the gemelli and internal obturator dorsally and the quadratus femoris ventrally. This tendon joins that of the internal obturator and the gemelli to insert in the trochanteric fossa.

Action: Lateral rotation of the hip joint and prevention of medial rotation on weight bearing.
Innervation: N. obturatorius.

The short, fleshy ***m. quadratus femoris*** (Figs. 6.69, 6.72, 6.75, and 6.76) arises on the ventral surface of the ischium medial to the lateral angle of the ischial tuberosity. It is surrounded by the origins of the mm. adductor magnus et brevis, semimembranosus, semitendinosus, biceps femoris, and obturator externus. Medial to the m. biceps femoris, it extends in an almost sagittal direction cranially. It bends slightly laterally and runs distally to reach the distal portion of the trochanteric fossa between the mm. obturator externus and adductor magnus et brevis. It ends on the intertrochanteric crest just proximal to the level of the trochanter tertius.

Action: Extension and lateral rotation of the hip joint and prevention of medial rotation on weight bearing.
Innervation: N. ischiadicus.

Caudal Muscles of the Thigh

The caudal thigh muscles are grouped about the ischial tuberosity, and some of them run to the lateral side of the stifle—the mm. biceps femoris and abductor cruris caudalis; others run to the medial side of the stifle—the mm. semitendinosus and semimembranosus. These are collectively referred to as the "hamstring muscles."

The **m. biceps femoris** (see Figs. 6.69, 6.71, 6.81A, 6.81B, 6.83, 6.84, 6.86D, and 6.90A) is a large, long muscle lying in the lateral part of the thigh and extending from the region of the ischial tuberosity to the calcaneus. It arises by two unequal heads, a cranial, superficial one, and a caudal, much smaller, deep head. The principal superficial head arises from the ventrocaudal end of the sacrotuberous ligament and partly from the lateral angle of the ischial tuberosity, where it is firmly united with the m. semitendinosus in an intermuscular leaf. The fibers of this muscle run nearly parallel. New fiber bundles, which arise from a thick, tendinous leaf on the deep surface of the muscle, are added distally. A portion of these laterally located fibers can be differentiated from the main mass of the cranial head as the middle branch of the m. biceps femoris. The caudal deep head arises from the ventral side of the lateral angle of the ischiatic tuberosity by a long tendon. This is deep to the medial tendinous origin of the superficial head where it covers the deep head. There appear to be three components of the biceps femoris based on the broad termination of its tendinous fibers. In the region of the femorotibial joint the entire m. biceps femoris, with slightly diverging fibers, runs on the lateral surface of the vastus lateralis and the gastrocnemius group, and, as an aponeurosis, radiates into the fascia lata and the fascia cruris. By means of this aponeurosis the cranial head, by fusing with the covering of the m. quadriceps femoris, attaches to the patella and the patellar ligament and by this to the tibial tuberosity. The middle and caudal portions radiate into the fascia lata and crural fascia as these enclose all of the cranial and lateral muscles of the thigh and crus to insert on the cranial border of the tibia (formerly the "tibial crest"). The deep surface of the muscle is covered by a distinct perimysium, which continues distally as a distinct tendon. Where the muscle passes over the deep surface of the m. abductor cruris caudalis (which accompanies the caudal border of the m. biceps femoris), the tendon reaches a width of 5 mm. It lies deep to the abductor and, by means of the crural fascia, runs distally along the m. gastrocnemius. It curves cranial to the main part of the common calcanean tendon to end on the dorsal surface of the tuber calcanei after it has united with a thick, tendinous strand coming from the mm. semitendinosus and gracilis. The **common calcanean tendon** (*tendo calcaneus communis*), also known as the *Achilles tendon*, consists of all those structures attaching to the tuber calcanei of the calcaneus. The tendons of the mm. flexor digitorum superficialis and gastrocnemius are its main components, although the mm. biceps femoris, semitendinosus, and gracilis also contribute to its formation. From the proximal end of the strand of the biceps femoris, which aids in forming the calcanean tendon, fibers pass to the medial lip of the caudal surface of the femur. Dense connective tissue fibers of the interfascicular septa of the m. biceps femoris enter the tendon and, without the aid of muscle fiber attachment, fasten it intimately so that a single functional unit results.

Armstrong et al. (1982) reported a mean of 32% type I (presumed SO or "slow oxidative") fibers in the biceps femoris muscles of three dogs. The remaining fibers were described as type II (presumed fast twitch), and all exhibited high oxidative capacity as measured by nicotinamide adenine dinucleotide activity (assayed histochemically) or by SDH activity (succinic dehydrogenase activity, assayed in vitro). In contrast, Chanaud et al. (1991) detected a predominance of fast (type II) fibers of the m. biceps femoris of cats, with type I fibers constituting only 3% to 6% of the muscle fibers sampled. Neurophysiologic studies of cat m. biceps femoris showed an anatomic partitioning of the muscle into "cranial," "middle," and "caudal" parts (English & Weeks, 1987). These seemed to correlate with hip extensor, hip extensor and stifle flexor, or stifle flexor motor functions, respectively. Analysis of EMG activity during stance or locomotion demonstrates discrete recruitment patterns among the three defined regions of the biceps femoris. For example, the "cranial" head of the cat biceps femoris was active during the stance phase, seeming to function as a hip extensor (Chanaud et al., 1991; English & Weeks, 1987; Goslow et al., 1981; Rasmussen et al., 1978). "Caudal" portions of biceps femoris of the cat were most active during faster gaits and then predominantly during the swing phase of the gait, when it functioned as a stifle flexor. The Ia sensory nerves supplying these muscle regions had a cranial to caudal topographic distribution in the biceps femoris motor nucleus of the spinal cord, supporting the idea of neuromuscular compartmentalization within the m. biceps femoris (Botterman et al., 1983). Thus although the grossly visible divisions in the m. biceps femoris may seem trivial, they appear to have important functional correlates. None of the studies of the cat reported an innervation of the cranial part of the m. biceps femoris by the caudal gluteal nerve.

Action: There appear to be region-specific functions effected by the cranial, middle, and caudal regions of this muscle.

Wentink (1976) recorded EMG activity of cranial and caudal regions of the m. biceps femoris and found them to differ. The cranial part exhibited a single burst of EMG activity associated with paw placement and the stance phase of locomotion. Thus the cranial part seems to perform an antigravity role as a hip extensor and perhaps to a lesser degree as a stifle extensor. The caudal part of the muscle exhibited two EMG bursts: a short burst somewhat coactive with the cranial part, and a second short burst associated with stifle flexion at the start of the swing phase of locomotion. By virtue of the insertion of the caudal part on the crural fascia, tarsal joint extension is also an important role.

Innervation: N. ischiadicus. Cranial part: ramus distalis of the n. gluteus caudalis. Middle and caudal parts: ramus muscularis proximalis of the n. tibialis (Nickel et al., 1954; Skoda, 1908; Ziegler, 1934). This double innervation supports the hypothesis that the m. biceps femoris of the dog is a m. gluteobiceps. Its cranial belly is to be regarded as split off from the m. gluteus superficialis.

The straplike **m. abductor cruris caudalis** (Figs. 6.71, 6.82, 6.83 and 6.84), 10 mm wide and 1 mm thick, lies deep to the caudal edge of the m. biceps femoris. This muscle has been called *m. tenuissimus* in cats. It arises by a long, flat tendon, which lies on the aponeurosis of the deep surface of the m. biceps femoris on the ventrocaudal edge of the sacrotuberous ligament near the ischial tuberosity. It extends deep to the m. biceps femoris on the lateral surface of the mm. quadratus femoris, adductor, and semimembranosus. At the level of the popliteal space, it appears superficially between the mm. biceps femoris and semitendinosus and, keeping close to the edge of the m. biceps femoris, crosses the crus in an arc and goes into the crural fascia, where it often extends beyond the end of the m. biceps femoris to the digital extensors. Because of its innervation, receiving a separate nerve coursing from the N. ischiadicus, this muscle has not been looked on as a division of the m. biceps femoris.

Action: With the caudal branch of the m. biceps femoris, it abducts the limb and flexes the stifle.
Innervation: N. ischiadicus.

The **m. semitendinosus** (Figs. 6.69, 6.71, 6.78, 6.81 to 6.83) is 2.5 to 3.5 cm thick, and has four edges in cross-section. The m. semitendinosus arises on the caudal and ventrolateral parts of the lateral angle of the ischiatic tuberosity between the mm. biceps femoris and semimembranosus. It lies in the caudal part of the thigh between the cranial and the lateral parts of the m. biceps femoris and the medial and cranial parts of the m. semimembranosus. It extends in an arc between the ischial tuberosity and the proximal segment of the crus, where it forms a large part of the caudal contour of the thigh. It extends distally at the caudal edge of the m. biceps femoris and diverges from it at the popliteal space to the medial side of the gastrocnemius where it follows the m. semimembranosus. By means of a prominent, flat tendon it passes deep to the aponeurosis of the m. gracilis. Both of these aponeuroses represent portions of the crural fascia and, as such, attach to the medial surface of the tibia cranial to the flexor muscles. Separate strands of both tendons, however, extend in the fascia in an arc cranially and proximally toward the rough surface on the distal end of the cranial border of the tibia. From the caudal edge of the tendon of the m. semitendinosus (close to its origin) a tendon is separated that unites with a distinct strand from the tendon of the m. gracilis. The conjoined tendons extend

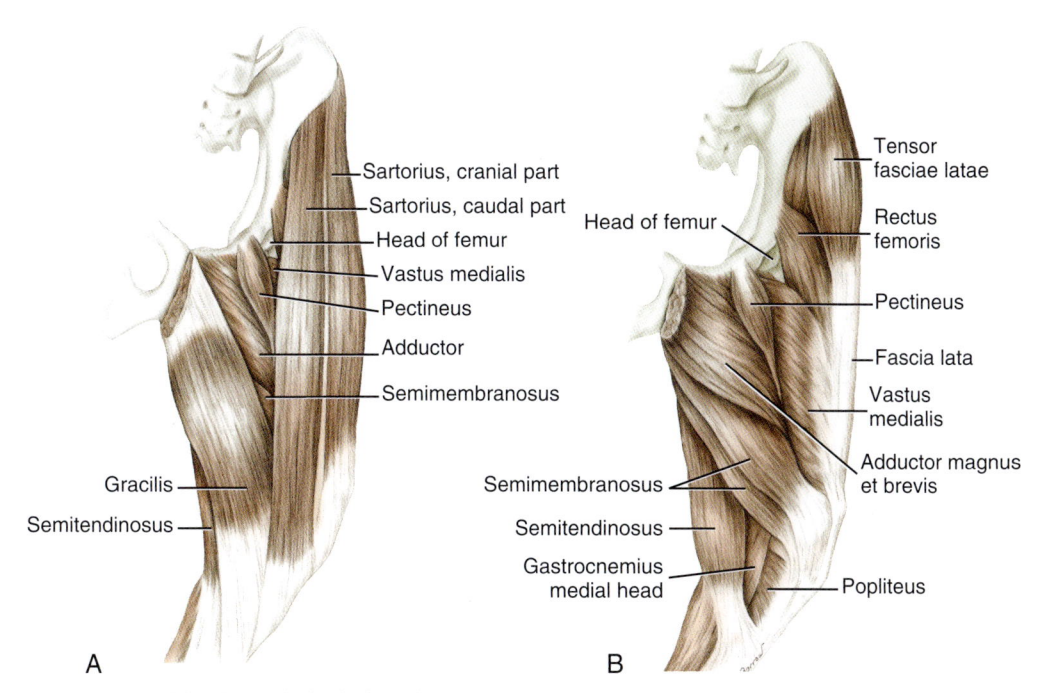

• **Fig. 6.78** Muscles of thigh. **A**, Superficial muscles, medial aspect. **B**, Deep muscles, medial aspect.

on the medial surface of the m. gastrocnemius medialis to the common calcanean tendon and thus to the tuber calcanei. It joins the corresponding tendon of the m. biceps femoris proximal to the calcaneus and cranial to the gastrocnemius tendon by a fascial bridge, which distally becomes progressively thicker.

Between the proximal and the middle third of the semitendinosus, and visible on the free surface, there is a delicate, but complete, tendinous inscription. This intercalation is probably the remains of the tendon of the m. caudofemoralis, which in lower mammals divides the semitendinosus transversely. This muscle has disappeared, but its tendon remains as the inscription. The proximal portion of the muscle is to be regarded as a division of the m. gluteus superficialis. The two portions of the m. semitendinosus are provided with individual nerves.

The division of m. semitendinosus into proximal and distal parts appears to be a common feature among mammals, being documented in goats (Gans et al., 1989), cats (Chanaud et al., 1991; English & Weeks, 1987), rabbits, and rodents (Roy et al., 1984). The in-series arrangement of fibers in the proximal and distal heads, and their innervation by separate primary motor nerves, suggests an interesting biomechanical problem in terms of efficient motor control. If a lesson can be taken from cat anatomy, the m. semitendinosus has a primary role as a flexor of the stifle. However, its underlying anatomy is complex. Proximal and distal regions of cat m. semitendinosus exhibit divergent histochemical fiber type compositions (Chanaud et al., 1991). Armstrong et al. (1982) reported that approximately 27% of the muscle fibers of the dog m. semitendinosus were type I, but did not specify sample sites. Gunn (1978a) demonstrated significant variation in fiber type composition of canine m. semitendinosus within a single transverse section. In non–Greyhound dogs, the deep and medial parts contained significantly more fibers with slow ATPase activity, similar to type I fibers, than did the superficial portions. This complexity may underlie the observation by Wentink (1976) of two bursts of EMG activity during walking in dogs. A first period was observed at the initiation of the swing phase; a second period was observed at the beginning of the stance phase, and it continued through approximately one-third of the stance.

Action: Extension of the hip and tarsal joints; flexion of the stifle joint in the free non–weight-bearing limb.
Innervation: Ramus muscularis proximalis of the n. tibialis (special branches for the part found proximal to and the part found distal to the tendinous inscription).

The **m. semimembranosus** (Figs. 6.69, 6.71, 6.72, 6.78, 6.79, and 6.81 to 6.83) is entirely fleshy, has parallel fibers, and is oval to triangular in cross-section. It crosses the m. semitendinosus medially and lies between the mm. biceps femoris and semitendinosus laterally, and the mm. adductor and gracilis medially. It arises caudal and medial to the m. semitendinosus on the ventral surface of the rough portion of the tuber ischiadicum. After a short distance it splits into two equally large bellies that extend in a slight arch to the medial side of the stifle joint. The cranial belly, which is 3 to 3.5 cm thick, joins the m. adductor magnus et brevis and ends in a short, flat tendon that attaches to the distal end of the medial lip of the femur, which runs distally on the shaft as a rough line to the medial condyle. Part of this insertion distally is on the aponeurosis of origin of the m. gastrocnemius. The caudal belly partly covers the cranial belly from the lateral side. It goes into a somewhat longer, narrower tendon, which extends over the m. gastrocnemius

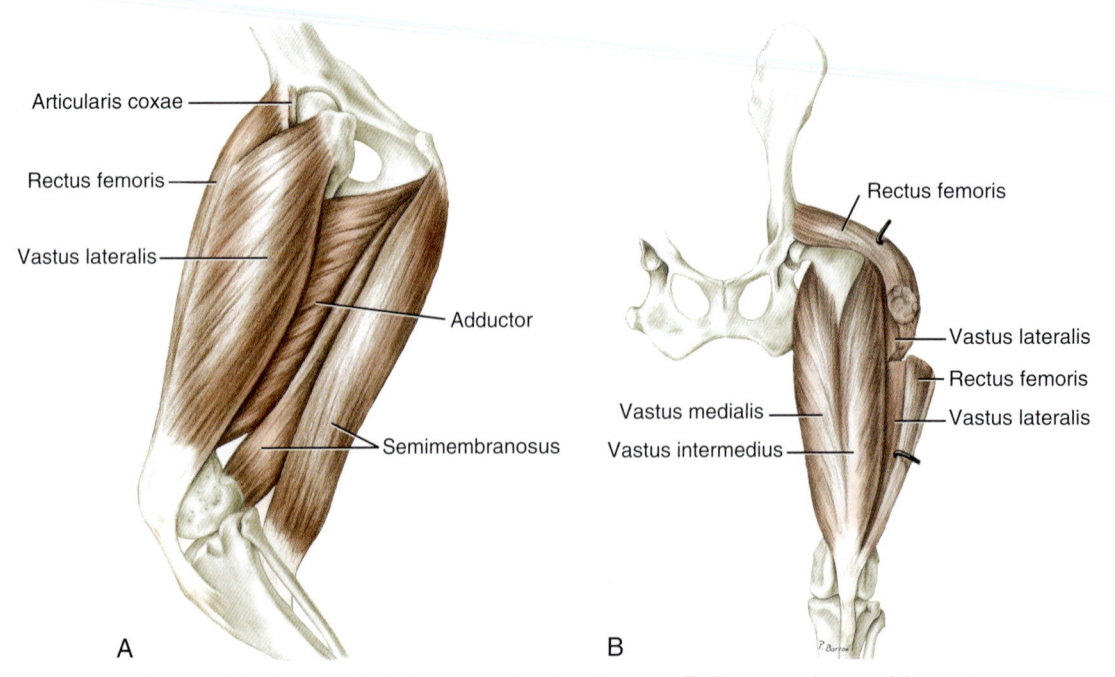

• **Fig. 6.79** Muscles of thigh. **A**, Deep muscles, lateral aspect. **B**, Deep muscles, cranial aspect.

medialis to end deep to the medial collateral ligament of the femorotibial joint on the margin of the medial condyle of the tibia.

The two heads of m. semimembranosus exhibit different EMG patterns during the walk (Wentink, 1976). In the caudal head, there was a period associated with the early swing phase of locomotion and a second period associated with the stance phase. In contrast, the cranial head exhibited a single period of EMG activity associated with the early stance phase (coactive with the caudal head of m. semimembranosus). Although Armstrong et al. (1982) reported the m. semimembranosus to be approximately 27% type I fibers, similar to the adjacent m. semitendinosus, there are no comparative analyses for the cranial versus the caudal head of m. semimembranosus. Physiologic analyses of the m. semimembranosus in cats demonstrated significant differences in the cranial and caudal heads (Peters & Rick, 1976). In cats, the cranial head of m. semimembranosus produces maximal tension over a large range of excursion. The caudal head produced its maximal tension within a narrow range of muscle excursion, suggesting a functional division of labor within the m. semimembranosus. Clearly, the one-joint and two-joint morphology of the two heads of m. semimembranosus in dogs relates to differing abilities for hip extension or stifle flexion.

Action: The m. semimembranosus extends the hip when the paw is placed on a solid substrate. The cranial head extends the hip and is active during the stance phase of locomotion. The caudal head is a two-joint muscle and can flex the stifle and contribute to hip extension.

Innervation: Ramus muscularis proximalis of the n. tibialis.

Cranial Muscles of the Thigh

The cranial thigh muscles extend between the pelvis and the femur proximally and the patella and tibial tuberosity distally. The four subdivisions of the m. quadriceps femoris form the bulk of the group. To this is added the insignificant muscle of the joint capsule of the hip, the m. capsularis, and the m. articularis genus proximal to the stifle joint.

The large ***m. quadriceps femoris*** (Figs. 6.69, 6.71 to 6.73, 6.78, 6.79, 6.81 to 6.83) covers the femur cranially, laterally, and medially. Distally it forms a tendon that includes the patella and ends on the tibial tuberosity as the ligament of the patella. It fuses with the fascia lata and thereby with the aponeurosis of the mm. biceps femoris and sartorius. The quadriceps muscle consists of the rectus femoris (cranial), vastus lateralis (lateral), vastus medialis (medial), and sometimes a fourth belly, the vastus intermedius, directly deep to the rectus femoris and covering the cranial surface of the femur.

The ***m. rectus femoris***, 2 to 3 cm thick in large dogs, is round in cross-section proximally and is laterally compressed distally. It is enclosed between the vasti in such a way that it overhangs them somewhat cranially. It arises by a short, thick tendon from the lateral and medial areas for the m. rectus femoris on the body of the ilium just cranial to the acetabulum and appears between the m. sartorius and the m. tensor fasciae latae. Covered cranially and laterally by the cranial belly of the m. tensor fasciae latae, it extends between the vastus lateralis and the vastus medialis to the patella, which is included in its large tendon as a sesamoid bone. This tendon continues distally as the ligament of the patella, over the cranial surface of the stifle joint, to insert on the tibial tuberosity. Proximal to and at the sides of the patella, islands of cartilage are found buried in the tendon. (For details, see the description of the stifle joint in Chapter 5.) The tendons of the vastus lateralis, vastus medialis, and the m. tensor fasciae latae fuse intimately with the patellar portion of the rectus tendon. Each collateral surface of the rectus bears a prominent tendinous leaf. The lateral surface takes on tendinous strands from the vastus lateralis. The rectus femoris flexes the hip and contributes to stifle extension.

The ***m. vastus medialis***, 4 to 5 cm wide and up to 2.5 cm thick, arises in the proximal fifth of the femur craniomedially on the line for the vastus medialis and, somewhat farther distally, on the proximal portion of the medial lip. It is laterally compressed and covers the distal portion of the rectus medially. Laterally and cranially it bears large distal tendinous leaves; medially it bears a large proximal one. Between these two tendinous systems the muscle fibers extend rather obliquely. Only proximal to the patella do its tendinous elements fuse with those of the rectus femoris. The muscle ends on the patella, covered by the cranial bellies of the m. sartorius and m. tensor fasciae latae and its principal portions encroach upon the mm. sartorius and pectineus. The vastus intermedius sends many fibers into the tendinous leaf.

The larger ***m. vastus lateralis*** (Fig. 6.79) arises on the craniolateral part of the proximal fifth of the femur on the transverse line and on the line of the vastus lateralis to the lateral lip. It covers the rectus femoris laterally to some extent. Laterally, at the origin, it bears a large tendinous leaf from which the majority of the muscle fibers extend obliquely medially and cranially. The proximal fibers go to the rectus femoris and radiate into its lateral aponeurotic covering as far as the terminal tendon. The vastus lateralis is inseparably united with the rectus femoris and its terminal tendon except proximally. The caudal fibers of the muscle are more longitudinal in direction; they extend from the lateral lip rather directly to the stifle joint, where their tendinous portion unites intimately with the joint capsule. There are firm connections with the fascia lata and with a prominent aponeurotic leaf between the vastus lateralis and the m. biceps femoris which attaches to the bone (see Fig. 6.74). The vastus lateralis shows EMG activity consistent with stifle extension during the stance phase (Goslow et al., 1981).

The ***m. vastus intermedius*** (Fig. 6.79) is the smallest portion of the quadriceps. It arises with the vastus lateralis, which covers it, and also from the lateral part of the

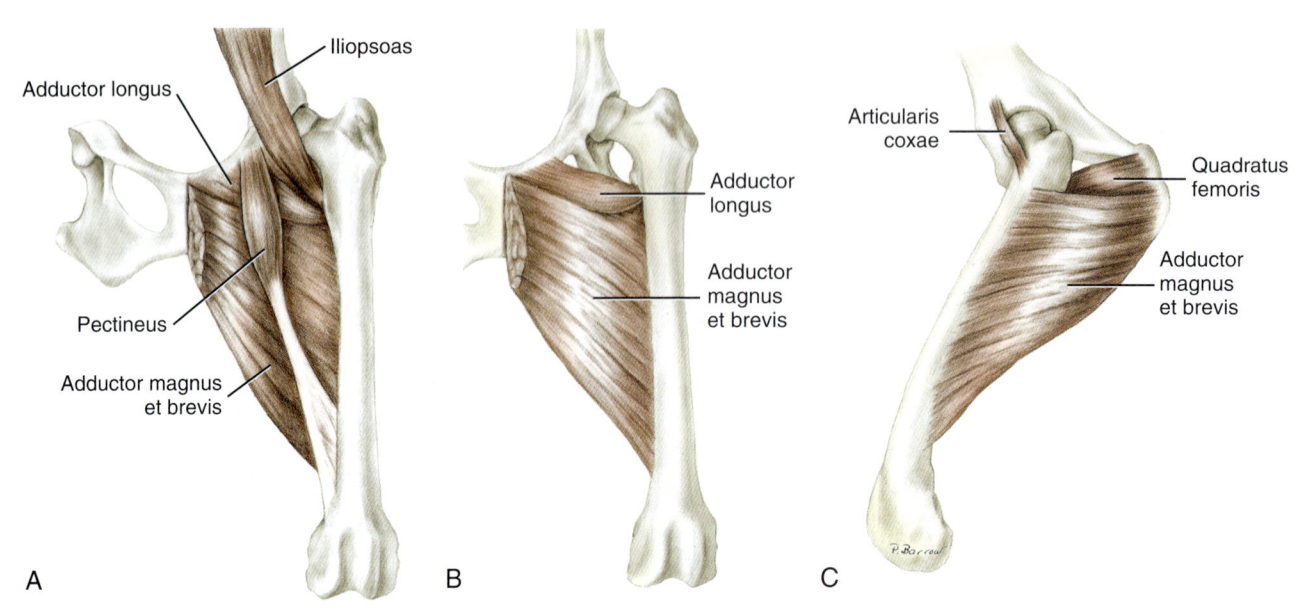

Fig. 6.80 Muscles of thigh. **A**, Mm. adductor magnus et brevis, adductor longus, pectineus, and iliopsoas, cranial aspect. **B**, Mm. adductor magnus et brevis and adductor longus, cranial aspect. **C**, Mm. adductor magnus et brevis, quadratus femoris, and articularis coxae, lateral aspect.

proximal fourth of the femur. Lying deep to the rectus, directly on the femur, its terminal tendinous leaf radiates into the m. vastus medialis.

Bursae

Deep to the tendon of origin of the m. rectus femoris, a small, synovial bursa is occasionally found. There is almost constantly a bursa (0.5 to 1.5 cm in diameter) between the distal third of the muscle and the femur. A small (0.5 cm) bursa is usually present deep to the terminal tendons of the vastus medialis and the vastus lateralis. In addition, the patellar joint capsule has a considerable proximal out-pocketing deep to the tendon of the quadriceps.

The mm. rectus femoris, vastus lateralis, and vastus medialis contained approximately 40% type I fibers, in contrast with the deeply situated m. vastus intermedius, which contained 88% type I fibers (Armstrong et al., 1982).

EMG studies of the m. vastus lateralis of dogs demonstrated a clear correlation of electrical activity with the stance phase of locomotion during the walk (Goslow et al., 1981; Wentink, 1976) as well as trot and gallop (Goslow et al., 1981). Such activity is consistent with an antigravity action at the stifle joint. However, at the trot and the gallop, the muscle is stretched on foot touchdown and then shortened to effect stifle extension (Goslow et al., 1981). This activity pattern allows alternate storage and release of energy during locomotion. The biarticular m. rectus femoris, spanning from ilium to tibia, exhibits two periods of activity during walking in dogs (Wentink, 1976). A burst of activity during the swing phase suggests that the m. rectus femoris contributes to hip flexion and pelvic limb protraction. The second burst of EMG activity during stance suggests a synergistic function with the other heads of the quadriceps femoris.

Action of the m. quadriceps: Extension of the stifle joint, tension of the fascia cruris, flexion of the hip.
Innervation: N. femoralis.

The **m. articularis coxae** (Figs. 6.69, 6.74, 6.76, and 6.80C) is a small, spindle-shaped muscle 2 to 4 cm long in the region of the hip joint. It is placed laterally and caudally from the ilium adjacent to the attachment of the rectus femoris and passes cranially and laterally over the capsule of the hip joint to the neck of the femur, where it attaches to the common ridge between the origins of the lateral and the medial vastus muscles.

Action: Flexion of the hip joint. A very small muscle, so its contribution to hip flexion is minimal. It may also adjust position of the hip joint capsule.
Innervation: N. femoralis.

The **m. articularis genus** (Figs. 6.73, 6.74) is a small, 2 mm wide, short muscle that arises from the cranial surface of the femur several centimeters proximal to the trochlea for the patella. It inserts on the deep surface of the femoropatellar joint capsule, in parallel with the distal attachment of the m. vastus intermedius. It is separated from the main portion of the m. quadriceps femoris by a delicate intermuscular septum. It is closely related on its deep surface to the proximal pouch of the stifle joint capsule as the muscle courses distally.

Action: Extension of the stifle joint and possibly tension of the proximal pouch of the stifle joint capsule. Kincaid et al. (1996) suggest the muscle may be a proprioceptor monitoring stifle joint motion.
Innervation: N. femoralis.

Medial Muscles of the Thigh

The adductors are a large group of muscles on the medial side of the thigh. Proximally, the long belly of the m. tensor fasciae latae lies on the medial side; distally, the m. semitendinosus takes part in the caudal border of the medial surface of the thigh. The adductors are arranged in superficial and deep layers. The superficial group includes the mm. sartorius and gracilis; the deep group is represented by the mm. pectineus and adductor. Between the m. sartorius and the m. gracilis a broad gap exists proximally at the site of the femoral triangle. In its depth the mm. adductor and pectineus can be seen caudally; the rectus femoris and vastus medialis cranially. Superficially, this gap is closed by the medial femoral fascia.

The **m. sartorius** (Figs. 6.69, 6.71A, 6.78A, 6.81, 6.82, and 6.83) is a long, flat muscle that extends in two straplike strands, each 3 to 4 cm wide on the cranial contour of the thigh from the region of the tuber coxae to the medial surface of the stifle joint.

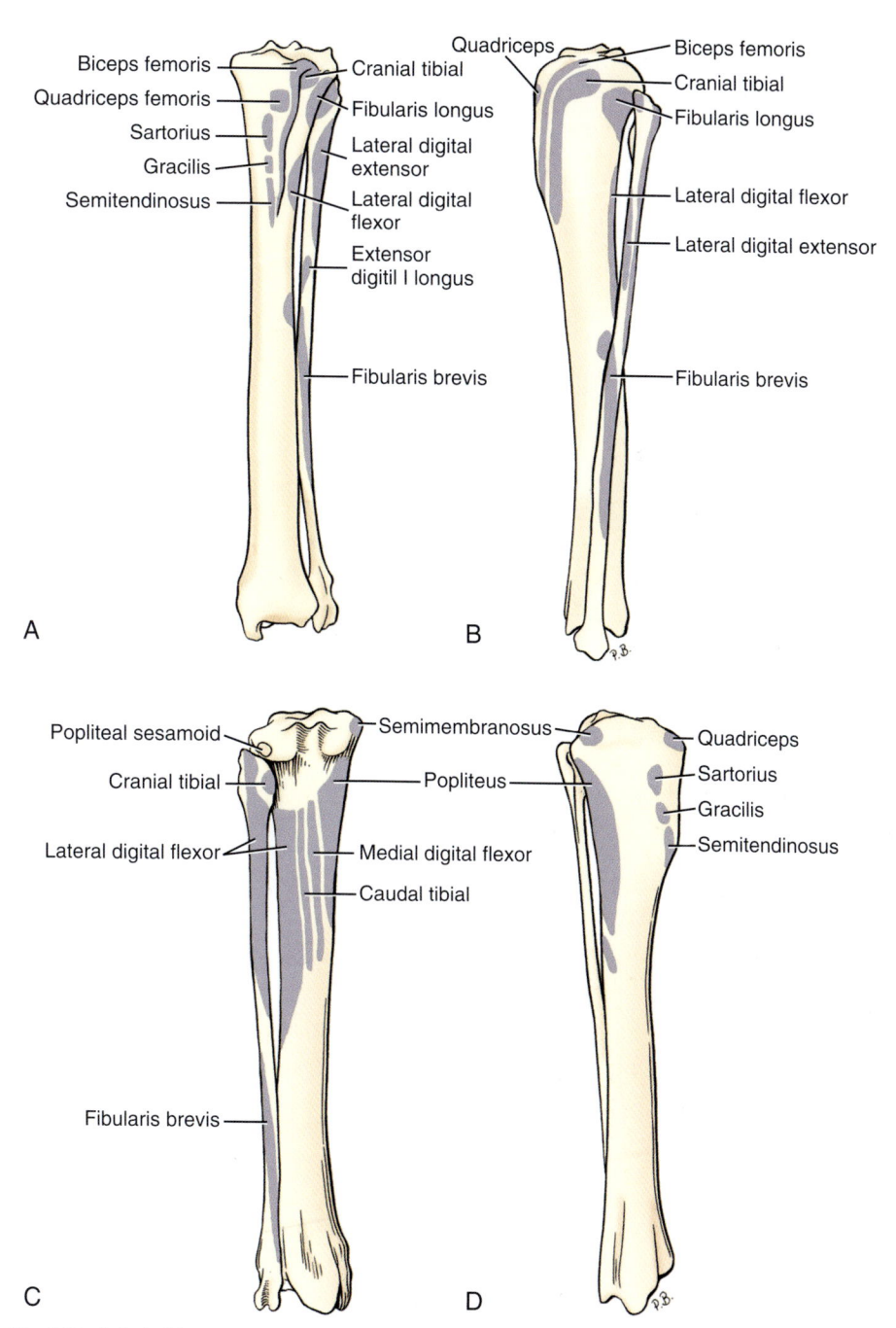

• Fig. 6.81 **A**, Left tibia and fibula, showing areas of muscle attachment, cranial aspect. **B**, Left tibia and fibula, showing areas of muscle attachment, lateral aspect. **C**, Left tibia and fibula, showing areas of muscle attachment, caudal aspect. **D**, Left tibia and fibula, showing areas of muscle attachment, medial aspect.

300 CHAPTER 6 The Muscular System

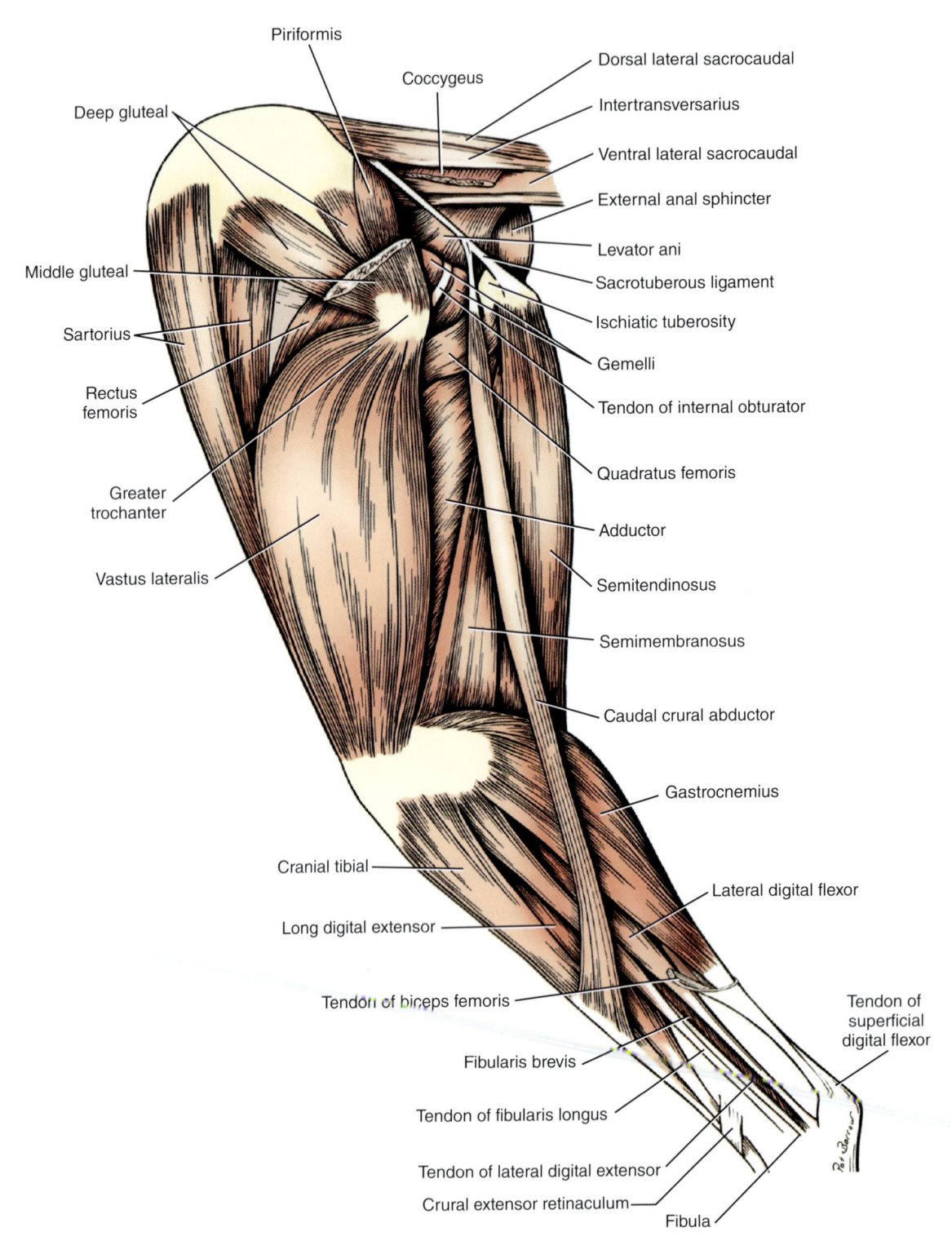

• **Fig. 6.82** Deep muscles of pelvic limb, lateral aspect.

The **cranial part** arises on the iliac crest and the cranial ventral iliac spine, as well as from the thoracolumbar fascia. Along with the caudal belly it bounds the m. quadriceps femoris cranially and medially, and with the m. tensor fasciae latae it also bounds the muscle laterally. The cranial belly of the m. sartorius is visible proximally on the lateral aspect of the thigh cranial to the m. tensor fasciae latae. From the cranial border it passes to the medial surface of the thigh, to pass into the medial femoral fascia just proximal to the patella. There is a firm union with the tendon of the rectus femoris and the vastus medialis.

The **caudal part** lies adjacent to the cranial part, entirely on the medial surface of the thigh. It arises on the tuber coxae of the ilium. Here it is between the m. iliopsoas and

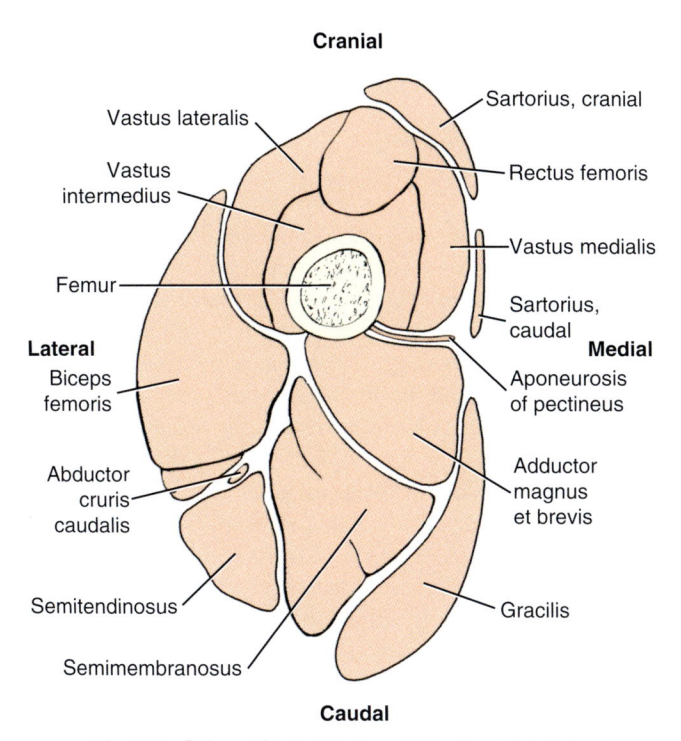

Fig. 6.83 Schematic transverse section through left thigh

the lumbar portion of the m. iliocostalis on the one side, and the mm. tensor fasciae latae and gluteus medius on the other. It passes over the medial surfaces of the vastus medialis and stifle joint and forms an aponeurosis, which blends with that of the m. gracilis. Radiating into the crural fascia, it ends on the cranial border of the tibia.

The m. sartorius has been studied intensively in the cat because it exhibits a longitudinal separation of the muscle into two parts, usually described as the "anterior" (cranial) and "medial" (caudal) parts (Hoffer et al., 1987). Although there is no complete anatomic separation of these two parts except for their distributed insertion from the patella to the medial surface of the tibia in the cat, the cranial part consistently exhibits two bursts of electrical activity during locomotion, whereas the caudal part exhibits a single phase of activity during the swing phase of locomotion. The caudal part, by virtue of its insertion on the tibia and its single EMG burst during swing phase, was interpreted to be a flexor of the hip and stifle as the limb was lifted from the ground and protracted. The cranial part had a burst of EMG activity associated with the swing phase but also exhibited a major burst of electrical activity during the stance or propulsive phase of locomotion. Thus some contribution to hip and stifle flexion as well as some degree of stifle extension (transmitted via its attachments to the patella) could be predicted. Based on these data and on recent analysis of reflex partitioning within the muscle, Pratt and Loeb (1991) concluded that the cranial and caudal parts of m. sartorius represent the smallest functional units into which the muscle can be partitioned. Loeb et al. (1987) described this muscle as composed of many interdigitated short fibers arranged in-series along the length of the muscle.

Fibers within either the cranial or caudal parts exhibited synchronous activation patterns.

Similar analyses of the m. sartorius are not available for dogs. EMG data presented by Goslow et al. (1981) for the cranial part of the m. sartorius demonstrated a single burst of activity during walk, trot, or gallop, similar to data for the caudal part of the m. sartorius of the cat. Wentink (1976) and Tokuriki (1973a, 1973b, 1974) presented similar uniphasic EMG data for m. sartorius of locomoting dogs but did not specify whether recordings were made from the caudal or cranial parts of the muscle. Histochemical data provided by Armstrong et al. (1982) suggested a partitioning of the m. sartorius of dogs. The pars cranialis contained approximately 51% type I fibers, whereas the pars caudalis contained a mean of 69%; however, the statistical significance of this difference was not stated.

Action: To flex the hip and stifle while the limb is being protracted and to contribute to stifle extension during stance. The actions of the cranial and caudal parts of this muscle should be interpreted separately.
Innervation: N. saphenous (*pars muscularis*) for both parts.

The ***m. gracilis*** (see Figs. 6.69, 6.78A, 6.81, and 6.83) in the dog forms an extensive, broad muscular sheet that is found in the superficial layer of the caudal portion of the medial surface of the thigh. Caudally the muscle thickens where it can be seen to a small extent from the lateral aspect. Its aponeurosis covers the medial surface of the m. adductor magnus et brevis. The muscle arises from the pelvic symphysis via a **symphysial tendon** (*tendo symphysialis*) that also serves as the origin for the m. adductor. The line of origin for the m. gracilis presents a distally convex arc that passes from the pecten ossis pubis to the ischial arch. Tendinous fibers extend from one side of this median, unpaired tendinous plate to the other. The m. gracilis passes over the medial surface of the m. adductor magnus et brevis as well as both bellies of the m. semimembranosus. At approximately the edge of this latter muscle it becomes a flat tendon that passes deep to the m. sartorius, continues over the popliteal space with the m. gastrocnemius medialis and the distal end of the m. semitendinosus, to insert along the entire length of the cranial border of the tibia. This terminal aponeurosis also spreads out into the crural fascia, and from its caudal border it sends a well-developed reinforcing band to the common calcanean tendon of the semitendinosus. According to Frandson and Davis (1955), the caudal part of the gracilis, the part that attaches to the tuber calcanei after joining the calcanean tendon of the semitendinosus, may rupture in racing dogs. Their findings suggest that the caudal part of the gracilis is an important extensor of the tarsus in the racing greyhound. EMG data for m. gracilis suggest a primary activity related to the early portion of the stance phase (Tokuriki, 1973a, 1973b, 1974; Wentink, 1976) while the limb is being extended and retracted. Armstrong et al. (1982) reported a high percentage of fast-twitch fibers in this muscle.

Action: Adduction of the limb, extension of the hip joint, flexion of the stifle, and extension of the tarsus.
Innervation: N. obturatorius.

The ***m. pectineus*** (Figs. 6.69, 6.72, 6.78, 6.80, and 6.83) belongs to the deeper group of adductors. It is cranial to the m. gracilis, covered by medial fascia of the thigh, closely applied to the m. adductor magnus et brevis caudally, but is separated from the cranially lying m. sartorius by the femoral fascia and vessels in the femoral canal. Its spindle-shaped body is circular in cross-section and may reach a thickness of 2 or 3 cm. It has a fleshy origin on the iliopubic eminence and cartilage and a tendinous origin on the prepubic tendon and from the abdominal muscles that join this tendon. Distally the muscle becomes flatter after it has passed deep to the caudal part of the m. sartorius. It fills the narrow space between the vastus medialis and the adductor in such a way that its wide and long tendon coming from tendinous sheets on two surfaces of the muscle passes over to the caudal surface of the femur after turning obliquely. The elongate thick tendon inserts along the distal end of the medial lip of the caudal rough surface of the femur medial to the insertion of the adductor magnus et brevis. Its distal insertion on this lip is in common with the insertion of the cranial belly of the m. semimembranosus.

Although appearing to be a small and relatively insignificant muscle, the m. pectineus has been studied intensively to assess its possible role in the onset of canine hip dysplasia. A number of studies recognized that the muscle is hypotrophic in dogs predisposed toward clinically defined hip dysplasia (Cardinet et al., 1972; Ihemelandu et al., 1983; Lust et al., 1972). However, it remains debatable whether an abnormal development or biomechanical performance by the m. pectineus causes hip dysplasia or whether the abnormalities seen in the muscle are a secondary consequence of the articular disturbance. According to Ihemelandu et al. (1983), there is a significant decrease in myofiber size and an increase in the ratio of connective tissue to myofiber volume within the m. pectineus of dysplastic dogs. Despite the interest in m. pectineus, few functional data are available. Wentink (1976) reports two periods of EMG activity during each step cycle in walking dogs: there is a brief burst of activity at the onset of the stance phase and a longer period of activity associated with the swing phase. The muscle is anatomically positioned to effect adduction of the pelvic limb.

Action: Adduction of the thigh.
Innervation: N. obturatorius.

The ***mm. adductores*** (see Figs. 6.69, 6.71C, 6.72, 6.76A, 6.78 to 6.80, 6.82, and 6.83) form the caudal part of the deep group of muscles next to the m. pectineus. In the dog they are represented by two separable muscles: the small fusiform m. adductor longus and the much larger m. adductor magnus et brevis. Both extend distally and laterally from the pelvic symphysis to the femur. See Budras (1972) for an illustrated review of the homology of the mm. adductores and the m. pectineus in domestic mammals, including the dog.

The ***m. adductor longus*** is partly covered medially by the proximal fleshy part of the m. pectineus as well as the large part of the adductor. From its origin on the pubic tubercle, it extends laterally cranial to the m. obturator externus and inserts on the proximal part of the lateral lip of the rough surface of the femur near the third trochanter. Its tendon covers the insertion of the m. quadratus femoris.

The ***m. adductor magnus et brevis*** arises along the entire pelvic symphysis and on the neighboring parts of the ischiatic arch, but primarily from the symphysial tendon of the pelvic symphysis. The large muscle belly of this part of the adductor extends obliquely lateral and deep to the m. gracilis and m. pectineus. Lateral and deep to the m. sartorius, the pectineus and its narrow tendon are compressed between the large adductor and the vastus medialis. Here the m. adductor magnus et brevis exhibits a glistening tendinous leaf that unites firmly with the tendon of the m. pectineus. The large adductor muscle inserts over the whole length of the lateral lip of the rough surface of the femur, from the trochanter tertius to a place near the origin of the m. gastrocnemius laterale from the lateral supracondylar tuberosity. Its tendon, with that of the m. pectineus, blends with the periosteum of the popliteal surface of the femur. Laterally the muscle is covered by the m. biceps femoris. It extends between the m. quadratus femoris and the m. semimembranosus to the caudal surface of the femur. From the broad muscle body of the adductor magnus et brevis a less distinct portion can regularly be separated.

According to Tokuriki (1973a, 1973b, 1974) and Wentink (1976), the adductor muscles are active briefly during the earliest parts of the stance phase of locomotion at all speeds. The exact sampling location within the muscles is not specified. There are different histochemical fiber populations in the m. adductor magnus et brevis compared with the m. adductor longus, the latter containing significantly more type I fibers (Armstrong et al., 1982).

Action: Adduction and extension of the hip joint.
Innervation: N. obturatorius.

The Femoral Triangle and Associated Structures

The opening caudal to the abdominal wall for the passage of the iliopsoas muscle and its contained femoral nerve is known as the **muscular lacuna** (*lacuna musculorum*). It is bounded laterally and caudally by the ilium, medially by the rectus abdominis, and cranially by the inguinal ligament and iliac and transversalis fascia. The iliac fascia also separates the muscular lacuna from the vascular lacuna (see Fig. 6.38).

The **vascular lacuna** (*lacuna vasorum*) lies craniomedial to the muscular lacuna, separated from it by the iliac fascia. It is bounded cranially by the caudal muscular border of the internal abdominal oblique and the inguinal ligament and medially by the rectus abdominis. It is separated from the superficial inguinal ring, which lies only a few millimeters craniolateral to it, by the inguinal ligament. It contains the femoral artery and vein and the saphenous nerve. The transversalis fascia that surrounds the femoral vessels as they pass through the vascular lacuna is continuous with the medial femoral fascia in the femoral canal. Whereas the vascular lacuna is the space between the inguinal ligament and the os coxae for passage of the femoral vessels, the **femoral ring** (*anulus femoralis*) is the entrance from the abdominal cavity into the femoral canal at the inguinal ligament. The **femoral canal** (*canalis femoralis*) is the space occupied by the femoral vessels and the saphenous nerve on the medial side of the proximal thigh. The **femoral triangle** (*trigonum femorale*) forms the borders of this canal consisting of the caudal part of the sartorius cranially and the pectineus caudally. The lateral border of the femoral canal is formed proximally for a short distance by the m. iliopsoas. The m. pectineus and m. vastus medialis complete this boundary. Superficially, the femoral artery and vein and the lymphatics are covered by the medial femoral fascia and skin. Because of the superficial position of the artery in the femoral triangle it is a favorable site for taking the pulse of the dog.

Muscles of the Crus

Other terms used for the crus are the true leg, gaskin, or shank. On the crus, the muscles lie on the cranial, lateral, and caudal surfaces of the tibia or fibula, whereas the medial surface of the tibia is essentially left free. Flexor and extensor groups are not separated on the crus as they are on the antebrachium. Cranially and laterally are found extensors of the digital joints and flexors of the tarsus. Caudally lie flexors of the digital joints and extensors of the tarsus. These functional muscle groups are mixed on the crus because the tarsal joint is set at an angle opposite to that of the digital joints. The tarsal joint has its flexor surface dorsally, whereas each of the digital joints has its extensor surface dorsally. Therefore the muscles lying over the dorsal surface must be flexors of the tarsus and extensors of the digital joints.

Craniolateral Muscles of the Crus

The flexors of the tarsal joint that lie on the craniolateral side of the crus are the mm. tibialis cranialis, fibularis (peroneus) longus, extensor digitorum longus, extensor digitorum lateralis, and extensor digiti I longus.

The *m. tibialis cranialis* (Figs. 6.81, 6.82, 6.84, 6.85, 6.88A, and 6.90) is a superficial, somewhat flattened muscle lying on the cranial surface of the tibia. It arises lateral to the sulcus extensorius on the cranial portion of the articular margin of the lateral tibial condyle and on the laterally arched edge of the cranial border of the tibia. From its origin the muscle, which is approximately 3 cm wide, passes over the craniomedial surface of the crus and, near its distal third, becomes a thin, flat tendon. This tendon extends obliquely over the tarsus to the medial side where it turns

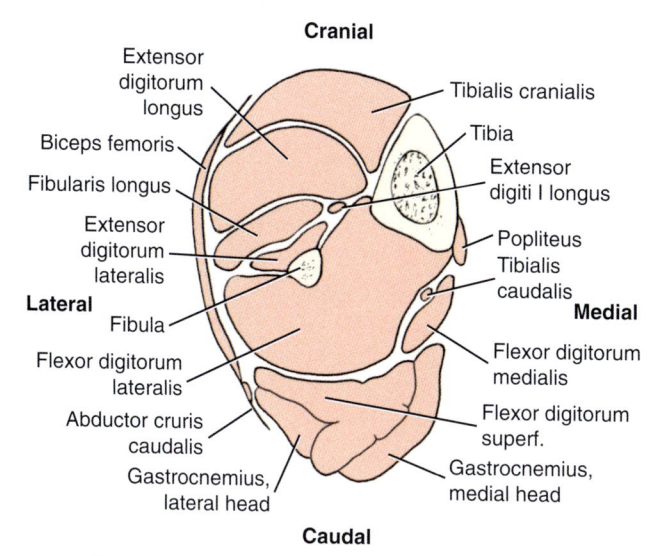

• **Fig. 6.84** Schematic transverse section through left crus.

around the medial border to the plantar side. Here it attaches to the plantar surface of the rudiment of metatarsal I, which is very often fused with the first tarsal bone and to the proximal end, the base, of metatarsal II.

The threadlike tendon of the *m. extensor digiti I longus* encroaches closely on the lateral edge of this tendon throughout its extent as far as the metatarsus, both turning toward the medial edge of the tarsus. The tendon of insertion of the cranial tibial becomes increasingly removed from the long digital extensor, as the latter passes to the metatarsus lateral to the axis of the pes. On the distal part of the tibia all three tendons are bridged over by the broad crural extensor retinaculum (see Fig. 6.85), which extends obliquely from proximolateral to distomedial. The long digital extensor tendon passes deep to the tarsal extensor retinaculum as it crosses the tarsus. This is a collagenous loop coming from the calcaneus. The end of the tendon of the cranial tibial muscle often shows variations that frequently are associated with variations in the m. extensor digiti I longus (Grau, 1932). The fascia is thickened into a strand on the medial side of the cranial tibial muscle that reaches from the cranial border of the tibia to the crural extensor retinaculum, and farther, a strand continues to the proximal end of metatarsal III. In its entirety, this strand may, perhaps, be comparable to the m. fibularis tertius of the horse. The terminal tendons of the mm. tibialis cranialis and extensor digiti I longus are, according to Walter (1908), surrounded by a synovial sheath between the crural extensor retinaculum and the middle of the tarsus.

The m. tibialis cranialis is composed of predominantly type II presumed fast-twitch muscle fibers (Armstrong et al., 1982; Newsholme et al., 1988; Rodríguez-Barbudo et al., 1984), although Newsholme et al. cautioned that muscle biopsy studies should be carefully designed both because of significant individual variation and because of higher variation of fiber type composition in superficial

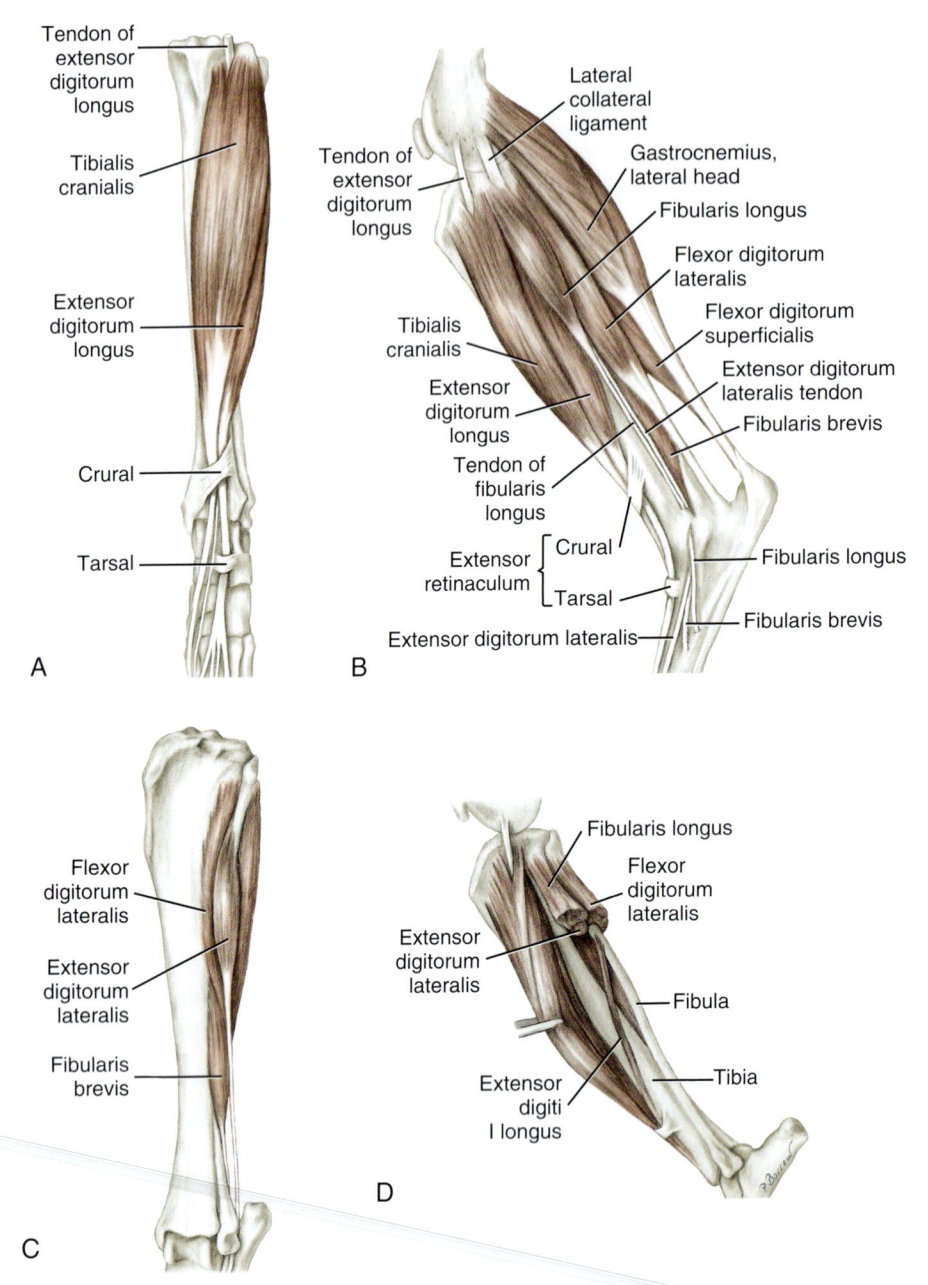

Fig. 6.85 Muscles of left crus. **A**, Superficial muscles, cranial aspect. **B**, Superficial muscles, lateral aspect. **C**, Deep muscles, cranial lateral aspect. **D**, Deep muscles, lateral aspect.

portions of the muscle than in deep portions. EMG activity was confined to the swing phase during walking or trotting in dogs (Tokuriki, 1973a, b; Wentink, 1976). This recruitment pattern supports a hypothesized primary role of tarsal flexion.

Action: To flex the tarsus and rotate the paw laterally: supination.
Innervation: N. fibularis.

The **m. extensor digitorum longus** (Figs. 6.73, 6.74, 6.82, 6.84, 6.85, and 6.88), spindle-shaped and at most 2 to 2.5 cm thick, lies in the group of digital extensors on the tibia between the m. tibialis cranialis and the m. fibularis longus. Proximally it is covered by the m. tibialis cranialis. Distally it lies free lateral and caudal to the m. tibialis cranialis. It arises in the extensor fossa on the lateral aspect of the articular surface of the lateral condyle of the femur and passes through the sulcus extensorius of the tibia. The muscle belly bears a large distal, cranial, tendinous leaf toward which all fibers converge. Near the tarsus it goes into its terminal tendon, which consists of four branches. This tendon runs along the tendon of the m. tibialis cranialis and that of the m. extensor digiti I longus, both of which are medial to it. At the distal fourth of the crus these tendons are held in place by the crural extensor retinaculum. Toward the tarsus the long digital extensor tendon diverges from the other tendons and on the flexor surface of the tarsus it is it may be 2 cm thick. It arises on the lateral condyle of the tibia, the lateral collateral ligament of the femorotibial joint, and the head of the fibula. Near the middle of the tibia it becomes an elliptical tendon that is enclosed in a thick fascial mass with the tendons of the mm. extensor digitorum lateralis and fibularis brevis. From the lateral surface of the tarsus, the tendon of fibularis longus runs through the sulcus of the lateral malleolus. Running distally, cranial to the distal tibiofibular ligament, it crosses superficially from medial to lateral, the tendon of the m. extensor digitorum lateralis and the m. fibularis brevis and passes through the groove on the lateral side of the fourth tarsal. From here it continues in a sharp curve deep to the tendinous m. abductor digiti V to the plantar surface of the metatarsus, which it crosses transversely. It inserts on the fourth tarsal and the plantar surfaces of the base of all of the metatarsals. The synovial sheath of the m. fibularis longus (*vag. tendinus m. fibularis longi*) begins 3 to 4 cm proximal to the lateral malleolus and is provided with a mesotendon on its deep surface. It reaches approximately the end of the tarsus and may be divided. Deep to the plantar end of the tendon there is a synovial bursa, which communicates with the joint capsule between the third and fourth tarsals.

The m. fibularis longus contains approximately 40% type I, presumed slow-twitch muscle fibers (Armstrong et al., 1982). According to Wentink (1976), this muscle is active during the swing phase of walking in dogs. Such a pattern is consistent with the muscle contributing to tarsal flexion during locomotion.

Action: Rotation of hindpaw medially so that the plantar surface faces laterally, pronation; flexion of the tarsus.
Innervation: N. fibularis.

The ***m. extensor digitorum lateralis*** (Figs. 6.81, 6.82, and 6.84 to 6.88) is a small muscle (1 cm wide; 2 to 3 cm thick) that lies between the m. fibularis longus and the m. flexor digitorum lateralis (lateral deep digital flexor) on the m. fibularis brevis and fibula. It arises on the proximal third of the fibula. Superficially it has a distal tendinous covering that becomes a thin tendon at the middle of the crus. This tendon lies between the cranially located tendon of the m. fibularis longus and the caudally located tendon of the m. fibularis brevis as these traverse the sulcus on the lateral malleolus of the fibula. At the level of the proximal lateral surface of the tarsus, the tendon of the lateral digital extensor usually lies medial to that of the m. fibularis brevis. It unites with the long digital extensor and the m. interosseus of the proximal phalanx of the fifth digit. The tendon of the lateral digital extensor is enclosed in a synovial sheath (*vag. tendinis m. extensoris digit. lat. pedis*), having a medial mesotendon in common with that of the m. fibularis brevis. In large dogs this begins 1.5 to 2.5 cm proximal to the lateral malleolus, reaches almost to the middle of the tarsus, and almost always communicates with the capsule of the talocrural joint.

Action: Extension and abduction of digit V.
Innervation: N. fibularis.

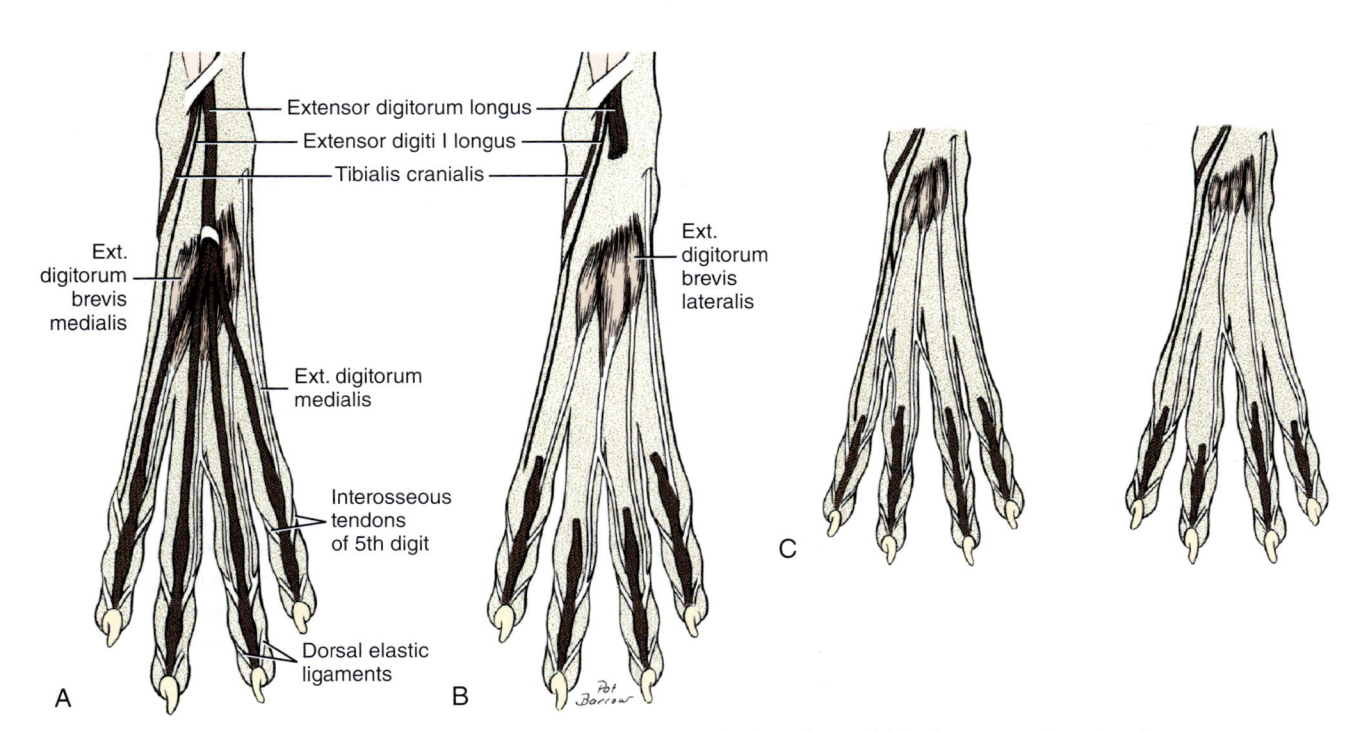

• **Fig. 6.88** Extensor muscles of left hindpaw. **A,** Schematic plan of superficial extensor muscles, dorsal aspect. **B,** Schematic plan of deep extensor muscles, dorsal aspect. **C,** Two variations of the extensor digitorum brevis.

The ***m. fibularis (peroneus) brevis*** (Figs. 6.81, 6.82, 6.85, 6.87C, and 6.90) is a deep crural muscle that first appears distally deep to the lateral digital extensor between the m. fibularis longus and the m. flexor digitorum lateralis (lateral deep digital flexor). It arises from the lateral surface of the distal two-thirds of the fibula and tibia, almost as far distal as the lateral malleolus. Here the muscle becomes completely tendinous after beginning far proximal as a narrow leaf. After crossing the long lateral collateral ligament of the tarsus and the tendon of the m. fibularis longus, it runs farther between the tendons of the m. fibularis longus and the lateral digital extensor, to attach to the base of metatarsal V. The tendon of the fibularis brevis is included in a common synovial sheath with the tendon of the m. extensor digitorum lateralis. An insignificant bursa lies under the tendon at its insertion.

Action: Flexion of the tarsal joint.
Innervation: N. fibularis profundus.

Caudal Muscles of the Crus

On the caudal side of the crus lie the extensors of the tarsal joint and the flexors of the digital joints. These include the gastrocnemius and superficial and deep digital flexors. In addition the caudal tibial and popliteus muscles are in the caudal crus.

The ***m. gastrocnemius*** (Figs. 6.72, 6.73, 6.82, 6.84 to 6.87, and 6.90) is the largest muscle in the caudal crus and is divided into a lateral and a medial head covered by strong tendinous leaves and infiltrated by tendinous strands. The **lateral head** (*caput laterale*) arises by a large tendon on the lateral supracondylar tuberosity of the femur. The **medial head** (*caput mediale*) arises on the medial supracondylar tuberosity. Each tendon of origin has a prominent sesamoid bone, the lateral and the medial sesamoids (formerly called *fabellae*). These are covered by articular cartilage on the distal surface that faces the femur. They articulate with the corresponding femoral condyle on a small, flat area. The femorotibial joint capsule attaches to the border of the articular surface of each sesamoid. The two heads of the m. gastrocnemius almost completely enclose the m. flexor digitorum superficialis, which arises in common with the lateral head. The two gastrocnemius heads fuse with each other distally, forming a flat (in large dogs 5 to 6 cm wide) muscle, the duplicity of which is accentuated distally by a middle tendinous plate. After crossing the superficial flexor tendon laterally, the tendon of the m. gastrocnemius attains its deep surface and inserts on the dorsoproximal surface of the tuber calcanei. Proximally the muscle is covered laterally by the m. biceps femoris and medially by the mm. semitendinosus, semimembranosus, and gracilis. Distally it lies deep to the fascia and skin. Deep to the m. gastrocnemius, directly on the tibia and fibula, are located the m. popliteus, the m. tibialis caudalis, and the two heads of the m. flexor digitorum profundus.

The **common calcanean tendon** (*tendo calcaneus communis*) is the aggregate of those structures that attach to the tuber calcanei. The tendon of the m. gastrocnemius, the main component, is crossed medially by that of the superficial digital flexor, which first lies cranial to the tendon of the gastrocnemius but attains its caudal surface at the tuber calcanei. Joining these two tendons are those of the mm. biceps femoris laterally and the semitendinosus and gracilis medially. Histologically, the common calcanean tendon transitions from having parallel-arranged collagen fibers in its proximal and middle region, to having fibrocartilage elements in its distal region, particularly over the calcanean tuber (Jopp & Reese, 2009). Elements of the common calcanean tendon never fully fuse together from their origins in the gastrocnemius, superficial digital flexor muscles, and from the accessory ischial muscles (i.e., biceps femoris) but are contained within a unifying connective tissue sheath.

Wentink (1976) found insignificant differences in the time of activity of the medial and lateral heads of m. gastrocnemius, with both being active essentially throughout the stance phase. Detailed analysis of EMG activity and joint angle changes during locomotion demonstrated that the medial head of m. gastrocnemius was active during much of the stance phase during walk, trot, or gallop (Goslow et al., 1981). In all gaits the medial head was active through approximately 80% to 85% of the stance phase, and, at higher speeds such as during the gallop, the early period of EMG activity was correlated with flexion at the stifle and tarsal joints. This yield of the latter joints when the limb first contacts the ground surface would passively stretch the active muscle in a mode known as eccentric contraction (stretch during electrical activity: Cavagna et al., 1977) and would result in storage of elastic energy for release during later parts of the propulsive stance phase. This mechanism permits the conservation of kinetic energy generated by the vertical oscillations of the body during locomotion such that some of the energy can be redirected to produce propulsion. Even at slow speeds (walk), the medial head was active. Armstrong et al. (1982) reported that approximately 50% of the muscle fibers in the medial and lateral heads were type I, presumed slow-twitch. Many of these slow fibers were probably active both during quiet standing and during all speeds of locomotion (Armstrong et al., 1982; Walmsley et al., 1978). Comparable recruitment patterns have been described for the medial and lateral gastrocnemii of cats (Rasmussen et al., 1978). Taken together, these studies support a hypothesis that the m. gastrocnemius is the primary muscle extending the tarsal joint during stance (resisting gravity) or locomotion (producing propulsive forces). This role is somewhat synergistic with the adjacent m. flexor digitorum superficialis. According to Bonneau et al. (1983), complete avulsion of the gastrocnemius portion of the tendo calcaneus communis results in slight flexion at the tarsal joint because of the similar course of the superficial flexor tendon over the calcaneal tuber. In these animals the tension on the superficial digital flexor causes digital flexion.

Action: Primarily extends the tarsal joint; slight flexion of the stifle joint.
Innervation: N. tibialis.

The ***m. flexor digitorum superficialis*** (Figs. 6.72, 6.82, 6.84 to 6.87, and 6.90), infiltrated by tendinous strands, lies on the mm. flexor digitorum profundus, tibialis caudalis, and popliteus. It is enclosed to a great extent by the heads of the m. gastrocnemius and is compressed to an angular body that flattens distally and becomes broader. A small portion of the proximal segment and a narrow portion of the distal border appear beyond the m. gastrocnemius and thus encroach on the fascia. The muscle is multipennate because of the numerous tendinous folds that course through it. Proximally, it is firmly united with the lateral head of the m. gastrocnemius. It arises with the lateral head on the femur and along with the lateral head of the gastrocnemius contains the lateral sesamoid that articulates with the caudodorsal aspect of the lateral femoral condyle. At the middle of the tibia the tendon of the m. flexor digitorum superficialis winds medially around the tendon of the m. gastrocnemius to gain its caudal surface. On the tuber calcanei it broadens like a cap and inserts collaterally on the tuber calcanei, united with the crural fascia. The tendon continues distally on the plantar surface of the tuber calcanei where it covers the long plantar ligament and divides twice, at the distal row of tarsal bones, forming four branches. These extend distally over metatarsals II, III, IV, and V. At the metatarsophalangeal joints, the branches are enclosed, in common with the corresponding branches of the deep flexor tendon, by a plantar annular ligament. Here the superficial digital flexor tendons form the sheaths (*manica flexoria*), as on the thoracic limb, for the passage of the tendons of the deep digital flexor. The synovial apparatus and the annular ligaments correspond with those of the thoracic limb. Deep to the tendon on the tuber calcanei and extending proximally along the gastrocnemius tendon and distally from the tuber, there is an extensive synovial bursa, the *bursa calcanea m. flexoris digit. superficialis*. Its proximal portion lies between the superficial digital flexor tendon and the tendon of the m. gastrocnemius; its distal portion lies between the superficial flexor tendon and the long plantar ligament.

Wentink (1976) reported that the superficial digital flexor muscle is active throughout much of the stance phase of walking locomotion in the dog. The muscle is composed of approximately 55% type I fibers, compared with the adjacent m. flexor digitorum profundus, which contains only approximately 29% type I fibers (Armstrong et al., 1982). Thus, despite the similar topographic positions, the two digital flexor muscles may be specialized for particular roles.

Action: Flexion of the digits; extension and fixation of the tarsus, flexion of the stifle joint.
Innervation: N. tibialis.

The ***mm. flexor digitorum profundi*** lies on the caudal surface of the tibia, covered by the m. gastrocnemius and the superficial digital flexor. It consists of the large, laterally located lateral digital flexor (flexor digitorum lateralis), formerly m. flexor hallucis longus, and the smaller medially located medial digital flexor (flexor digitorum medialis), formerly m. flexor digitorum longus. The latter muscle, short and spindle-shaped, lies on the caudal surface of the tibia, between the m. popliteus and the m. tibialis caudalis. In hoofed animals the m. tibialis caudalis, whose tendon joins that of the m. flexor digitorum lateralis, constitutes a third head of the deep digital flexor muscle. The caudal tibial muscle is independent of the two heads of the deep digital flexor in carnivores.

The ***m. flexor digitorum lateralis*** (Figs. 6.81, 6.82, 6.84 to 6.87, and 6.89) arises from the caudal surface of the proximal three fifths of the fibula and the proximal caudolateral border of the tibia. It also arises from the interosseous membrane. It has many tendinous strands, resulting in formation of the multipennate muscle. Caudally it is covered by a prominent tendinous leaf from which the principal tendon arises and runs distally. It passes over the sustentaculum tali on the medial side of the calcaneus. At the level of the middle row of tarsal bones it fuses with the smaller tendon of the m. flexor digitorum medialis to form the deep digital flexor tendon. Becoming wider and flatter, it divides into four branches at the middle of the metatarsus; these behave as do the tendons of the m. flexor digitorum profundus of the thoracic limb. In the region of the sustentaculum tali and proximal and distal to it, a synovial sheath (*vag. tendinis m. flexoris digit lateralis*) is formed, which communicates with the capsule of the talocrural joint. Its mesotendon passes to the plantar surface of the tendon. The tendon of the lateral head of the deep digital flexor is bound in the groove over the sustentaculum tali of the calcaneus by the flexor retinaculum.

The small ***m. flexor digitorum medialis*** (Figs. 6.81*C*, 6.84, 6.86, 6.87A, and 6.89), the medial head of the deep digital flexor, is a short, flat muscle lying medial to the m. flexor digitorum lateralis and m. tibialis caudalis and lateral to the m. popliteus. At its origin, it is narrow and arises on the head of the fibula, the popliteal line, and the fascial leaf separating it from the m. flexor digitorum lateralis. Proximal to the middle of the tibia it becomes a fine tendon that runs along the caudomedial border of the tibia with the even finer tendon of the m. tibialis caudalis. Both tendons pass through the groove of the medial malleolus, with the tendon of the tibialis caudalis lying cranial to that of the m. flexor digitorum medialis. In this position they accompany the medial collateral ligament of the tarsus to the level of the talus, where the tendon of the m. flexor digitorum medialis unites with the tendon of the m. flexor digitorum lateralis to form the deep digital flexor tendon. The synovial sheath of the muscle (*vag. tendinis m. flexoris digit. medialis*) begins 1 to 1.5 cm proximal to the medial malleolus and extends distally on the tendon to its union with the lateral tendon. A variable mesotendon passes to the tendon laterally. Distal to the fusion of these two tendons, the common tendon divides into four separate deep digital

310 CHAPTER 6 The Muscular System

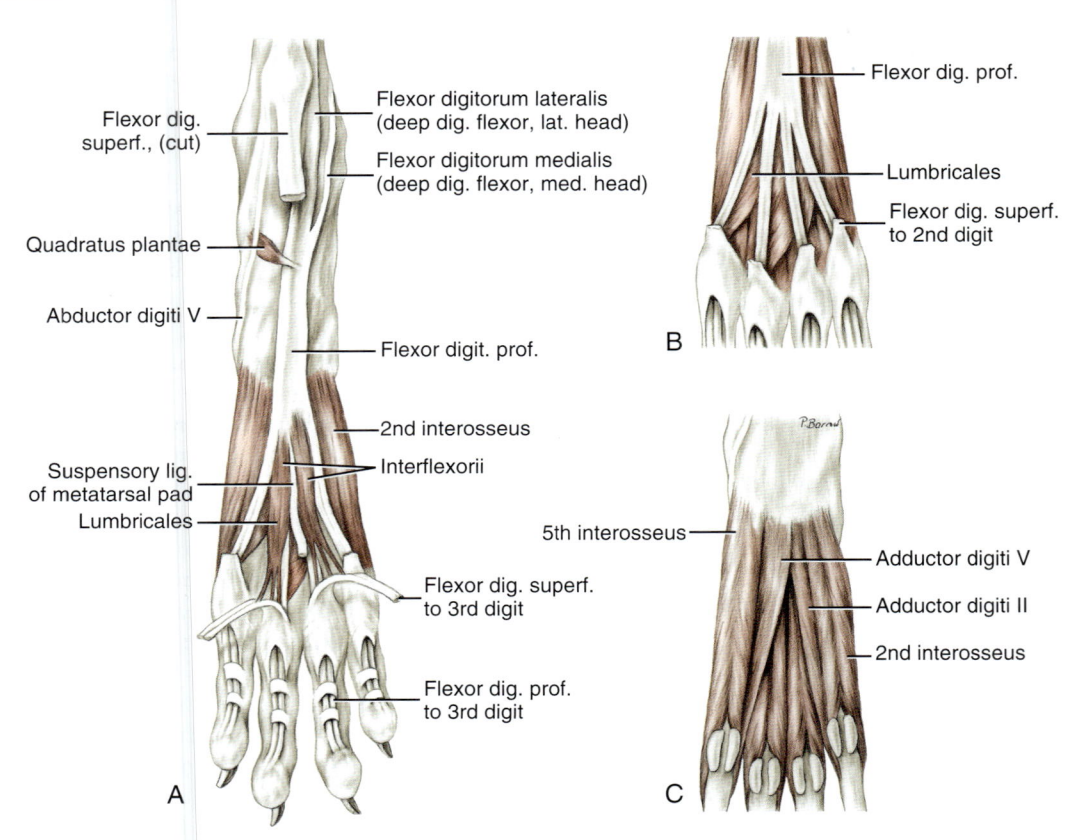

- **Fig. 6.89** Muscles of left hindpaw. **A**, Superficial muscles, plantar aspect. **B**, Deep muscles, plantar aspect. **C**, Deep muscles, plantar aspect. (Flexor digitorum profundus and lumbricales removed.)

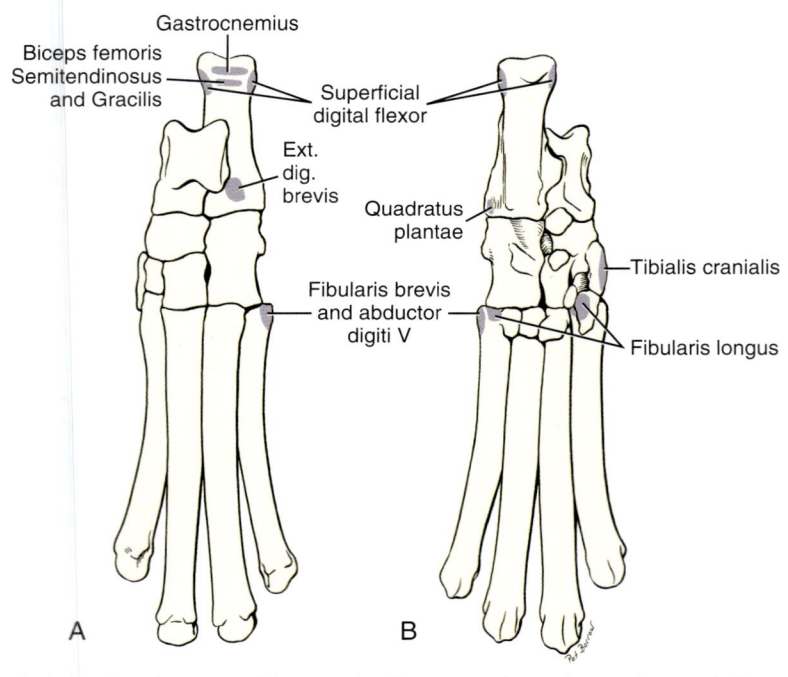

- **Fig. 6.90** Left tarsal and metatarsal bones, showing areas of muscle attachment. **A**, Dorsal aspect. **B**, Plantar aspect.

flexor tendons at the level of the proximal metatarsus. Each tendon passes distally through the manica flexoria at the metatarsophalangeal joints, similar to the condition seen in the thoracic limbs, to insert on the flexor tubercles of the distal phalanges.

EMG studies of the m. flexor digitorum profundus demonstrate that the muscle is largely active during the first three-quarters of the stance phase at walking, trotting, and galloping speeds (Tokuriki, 1973a, 1973b, 1974). Wentink (1976) specified the same EMG pattern for the m. flexor digitorum lateralis. The muscle appears to be composed primarily of type II (presumed fast-twitch) muscle fibers (Armstrong et al., 1982).

Action: Flexion of the digits.
Innervation: N. tibialis.

The *m. tibialis caudalis* (see Figs. 6.81C, 6.84, and 6.86), deep and medially placed, is completely separated in the dog from the two heads of the flexor digitorum profundus, in contrast with the condition in the hoofed animals. As an insignificant spindle-shaped muscle, it lies between the two heads of the m. flexor digitorum profundus. It is covered by the m. flexor digitorum medialis and lies directly on the caudal surface of the tibia. It arises on the medial part of the proximal end of the fibula and after a short course forms a very delicate tendon that extends distally cranial to the somewhat larger tendon of the m. flexor digitorum medialis. The tendon of m. tibialis caudalis ends on the medial ligamentous tissue of the tarsus.

Exceptionally, the muscle may be lacking.

Action: Extension of the tarsus; lateral rotation of the pes: supination.
Innervation: N. tibialis.

The *m. popliteus* (Figs. 6.72, 6.73, 6.81, 6.84, and 6.86) is a relatively short, triangular muscle lying in the space on the proximocaudal surface of the tibia just distal to the popliteal notch and proximal to the popliteal line. It covers the caudal aspect of the stifle joint capsule and the medial half of the proximal third of the tibia. It is covered caudally by the mm. gastrocnemius and flexor digitorum superficialis. It encroaches medially on the m. semitendinosus and fascia. The popliteus arises on the caudal aspect of the articular surface of the lateral condyle of the femur by a long tendon that contains a sesamoid bone. This sesamoid bone articulates with the caudolateral surface of the lateral tibial condyle. McCarthy and Wood (1989) reported the incidence of ossification of the sesamoids in the tendon of origin of the popliteus muscle to be 84%, using anatomic and radiographic techniques in 50 randomly selected Australian dogs. This tendon invaginates the femorotibial joint capsule, which serves as a sheath for the tendon as it crosses deep to the lateral collateral ligament of the femorotibial joint. The triangular muscle extends obliquely medially over the popliteal space to the medial border of the tibia and ends on its proximal third. The m. popliteus contains a significantly higher density of muscle spindles compared with adjacent muscles of the hindlimb (Buxton & Peck, 1990). Such an observation suggests an important role in providing proprioceptive information about stifle position to the central nervous system. The potential as a joint motion sensor is also of significance to a hypothesis that the m. popliteus functions as a stifle extensor, as proposed by Fuss (1989). In this argument, mechanical and computer-based models demonstrate an increase in the length of m. popliteus during joint flexion, countering the traditional view that the muscle is a flexor of the stifle. Fuss suggests that the activity of m. popliteus effects medial rotation of the tibia relative to the femur during the flexion or swing phase of locomotion and that the muscle is largely inactive and ineffective as a flexor during stifle flexion.

Action: Traditionally considered a flexor of the stifle joint, but this is not tenable based on the previous discussion. Also, the muscle effects medial rotation of the crus relative to the femur.
Innervation: N. tibialis.

Muscles of the Pes
Muscles of the Dorsal Surface of the Pes

Only one muscle, the m. extensor digitorum brevis, is found on the dorsal surface of the pes.

The small *m. extensor digitorum brevis* (Figs. 6.88 and 6.90) is a flat muscle, 2.5 to 3 cm wide, on the dorsum of the pes. It lies on the distal row of tarsal bones and on the metatarsal bones. It is covered by the tendons of the m. extensor digitorum longus, the fascia, and skin. It consists of three heads, of which the middle is the longest. The heads arise from the distal part of the calcaneus and on the ligamentous tissue on the flexor surface of the tarsus. Of the three terminal tendons, the lateral one goes to digit IV, the intermediate one to digits III and IV, and the medial one to digits II and III. Three other variations have been described in the distribution of insertional tendons to digits II to V (Wakuri et al., 1988). Only the branch going to digit II radiates directly into the corresponding branch of the long digital extensor. All others unite on the proximal phalanx with the tendinous branches of the mm. interossei. The latter go to the dorsum of the digits and thereby unite secondarily with the digital extensor tendons.

Action: Extension of the digits.
Innervation: N. fibularis.

Muscles of the Plantar Surface of the Pes

The muscles of the plantar surface of the pes include the *mm. interossei*, adductor digiti II, adductor digiti V, and lumbricales. These all behave as do the corresponding ones in the thoracic limb. The mm. abductor digiti V and interflexorii, which are united with the suspensory ligament of the metatarsal pad, are modified. When the first digit (dewclaw) is lacking, its muscles are also lacking, and there is no special flexor of the fifth digit as there is in the manus of the dog.

These muscles belong to the region of innervation of the n. tibialis and n. cutaneus surae caudalis distalis.

The *mm. lumbricales* (Fig. 6.89) lie between the four branches of the deep flexor tendon and are covered on their plantar surfaces by the mm. interflexorii and the suspensory ligament of the metatarsal pad. They are similar to those of the thoracic limb.

The *mm. interflexorii* (Fig. 6.89) are two flat, relatively large muscles that are shorter than the corresponding unpaired muscle of the thoracic limb. They are located between the deep and the superficial flexor tendons. They arise, with the suspensory ligament of the metatarsal pad, from the plantar surface of the tendon of the m. flexor digitorum profundus proximal to the middle of the tarsus. They end approximately 2 cm proximal to the metatarsophalangeal joints on the tendons of the m. flexor digitorum profundus of digits III and IV, which partly cover them. The flat ligament for the metatarsal pad appears between the mm. interflexorii.

The *mm. adductores digiti II et V* (Fig. 6.89) lie on the plantar surfaces of the mm. interossei.

The *m. quadratus plantae* (Figs. 6.87, 6.89, and 6.90) is insignificant. It is the tarsal head of the m. flexor digitorum profundus. It arises on the lateral tuberosity of the calcaneus and the lateral collateral ligament of the tarsus. Directed mediodistally as a delicate muscle, it passes dorsal to the superficial flexor tendon to unite with the deep digital flexor tendon. This is near the point where the tendon of the m. flexor digitorum medialis joins the main tendon.

The *m. abductor digiti V* (Figs. 6.87 and 6.89) is a very small, mostly tendinous muscle. It arises from the lateral aspect of the tuber calcanei, deep to the tendon of the m. flexor digitorum superficialis. It courses distally superficial to the m. fibularis longus to insert with the m. fibularis brevis on the base of the fifth metatarsal bone.

Special Muscles of Digit I

The first digit of the dog is usually absent. When it is developed, it is known as the *dewclaw.*

If the first digit is completely developed on the pes of the dog, it receives special branches from an extensor and a flexor. Its own muscles include m. abductor digiti I, m. flexor digiti I brevis, and adductor digiti I. The fleshy *m. flexor digiti I brevis* extends from the first tarsal bone and from the proximal end of metatarsal I by a short tendon to the base of the proximal phalanx or to the sesamoid apparatus found there.

Fasciae of the Pelvic Limb

The fasciae of the pelvic limb are classified as superficial and deep. These can be further divided in certain places, but the layers cannot always be separated from each other. In general, the deep one is the thicker.

The superficial fascia of the trunk continues dorsally on the lumbosacral region as the **superficial gluteal fascia** and passes over to the tail as the **superficial caudal fascia**. In obese specimens it is mainly separated from the deep fascia by a thick layer of fat. This is found primarily between the base of the tail and the ischial tuberosity. Blood vessels and nerves pass through it on their way to the skin. From the lateral abdominal wall the superficial trunk fascia continues on the lateral surface of the thigh. Here, as the **superficial lateral fascia of the thigh**, as well as in the gluteal region, it conceals the origins of the m. cutaneus trunci. The superficial fascia passes over to the thigh almost as far as the patella. In the entire region of the m. biceps femoris there is an intimate union with the deep fascia. Otherwise the superficial fascia encloses the distal portion of the femur like a cylinder. A leaf of the superficial fascia covers the m. sartorius and the femoral canal, as well as the m. gracilis, to unite firmly with the deep leaf of the superficial fascia. The superficial fascia also envelops the crus, tarsus, metatarsus, and digits, as it does on the thoracic limb. Cutaneous vessels and nerves can be seen through the fascia over long distances before they themselves pass to the skin. The v. saphena medialis (*magna*) on the medial side, and the v. saphena lateralis (*parva*) on the lateral side, are located in the superficial fascia.

The **deep fascia of the pelvic limb** surrounds all portions of the extremity, with its bones, muscles, and tendons, like a tube. In the gluteal region is the **gluteal fascia**. This comes from the thoracolumbar fascia over the crest of the ilium; it continues as the deep caudal fascia on the tail. It is rather thick and covers the m. gluteus medius, which partly takes its origin from it. It is less firmly attached to the m. gluteus superficialis. Over these muscles and the m. tensor fasciae latae it radiates into the thick **fascia lata**, lateral femoral fascia, on the lateral surface of the thigh. Because the terminal aponeurosis of the m. tensor fasciae latae dips into its deep surface, it is two-leaved over a considerable distance. The m. biceps femoris is covered firmly, but parts of the mm. semitendinosus and semimembranosus are covered more loosely. The fascia passes over both the caudal and cranial contours of the thigh, to its medial surface. The fascia lata and the **medial femoral fascia** thus join to form a cylinder on the thigh. The fascia lata passes from the m. biceps femoris cranially and covers the individual portions of the m. quadriceps femoris toward the medial surface as far as the vastus medialis. The medial fascia of the thigh reaches the medial surfaces of the mm. adductor and semimembranosus after going deep to the branches of the m. sartorius and after bridging the femoral canal. Into this fascia the m. gracilis sinks proximally. However, this muscle, like the caudal belly of the m. sartorius in particular, is also covered superficially by a thin leaf of the deep medial femoral fascia, which unites with the deeper lamella over its caudal edge. Distally, on the medial surface of the thigh, the a. and v. saphena and the n. saphenus are included between the two leaves. The fascia lata is attached to the lateral lip of the femur by an intermuscular septum between the m. biceps femoris and the vastus lateralis. The medial fascia is attached to the medial lip of the femur by a septum caudal to the vastus medialis. Toward the stifle both portions of the fascia (lateral and medial) attach to the patella and to the corresponding condyles of the femur. The **fascia of the stifle joint** (*fascia genus*) is demarcated by its thickness and appears to be intimately united with the straight patellar ligament. Distally, it becomes the **crural fascia** (*fascia cruris*). The fascia of the crus is two-leaved. The superficial leaf of the crural fascia is essentially the continuation of the lateral and medial femoral fasciae. It partially fuses with the superficial and deep fascia of the crus. The superficial leaf of the crural fascia is completely lost on the metatarsus after passing over the tarsus. The deep leaf covers the muscles of the crus and the free-lying surfaces of the crural skeleton. Laterally the fibers of the caudal branch of the m. biceps femoris and the m. abductor cruris caudalis radiate into it. Where the two leaves are united with each other, rigid fibrous strands are present, especially in the region of the calcanean tendon of the mm. biceps femoris and semitendinosus. Two other distinct strands exist on the medial side of the crus. One extends from the distal terminal tendon of the m. semimembranosus over the m. popliteus to the cranial border of the tibia, and the other extends along the caudal border of the m. tibialis cranialis to its terminal tendon. The deep leaf forms special sheaths about the mm. tibialis cranialis, extensor digitorum longus, fibularis longus, extensor digitorum lateralis, flexor digitorum profundus, and popliteus, and, with the superficial flexor tendon, about the gastrocnemius group. On the individual portions of the pes, the relationships of the **fascia dorsalis pedis** and **fascia plantaris** are essentially the same as those of the fascia of the manus. There are, however, special relationships to the calcaneal tuber, the tendons, the malleoli, and the collateral ligaments of the tarsal joints.

Bibliography

Abe, T., Kusuhara, N., Katagiri, H., et al. (1993). Differential function of costal and crural diaphragm during emesis in canines. *Respir Physiol, 91*, 183–193.

Acevedo, L. M., & Rivero, J.-L. (2006). New insights into skeletal muscle fibre types in the dog with particular focus towards hybrid myosin phenotypes. *Cell Tiss Res, 323*, 283–303.

Acheson, G. H. (1938). The topographical anatomy of the smooth muscle of the cat's nictitating membrane. *Anat Rec, 72*, 297–311.

Acker, M. A., Mannion, J. D., Brown, W. E., et al. (1987). Canine diaphragm muscle after 1 yr of continuous electrical stimulation: its potential as a myocardial substitute. *J Appl Physiol, 62*, 1264–1270.

Agduhr, E. (1915). Anatomische, statische und experimentelle untersuchungen über N. medianus und N. ulnaris, bes. deren motorisches innervationsgebiet im vorderarm von haustieren, nebst einigen bemerkungen über die muskulatur desselben gebietes und über N. musculocutaneus. *Anat Hefte, 52*, 497–647.

Ainsworth, D. M., Smith, C. A., Eicker, S. W., et al. (1997). Pulmonary-locomotory interactions in exercising dogs and horses. *Resp Physiol, 110*, 287–294.

Ainsworth, D. M., Smith, C. A., Eicker, S. W., et al. (1989). The effects of locomotion on respiratory muscle activity in the awake dog. *Respir Physiol, 78*, 145–162.

Ainsworth, D. M., Smith, C. A., Henderson, K. S., et al. (1996). Breathing during exercise in dogs: passive or active? *J Appl Physiol, 81*, 586–595.

Alvarado-Mallart, R. M., & Pincon-Raymond, M. (1979). The palisade endings of cat extraocular muscles: a light and electron microscope study. *Tissue Cell, 11*, 567–584.

Armstrong, R. B. (1980). Properties and distribution of the fiber types in the locomotory muscles of mammals. In K. Schmidt-Nielson, L. Bolis, & C. R. Taylor (Eds.), *Comparative physiology: primitive mammals*. Cambridge: Cambridge University Press.

Armstrong, R. B., Saubert, C. W., IV, Seeherman, H. J., et al. (1982). Distribution of fiber types in locomotory muscles of dogs. *Am J Anat, 163*, 87–98.

Balsam, L. B., Wagers, A. J., Christensen, J. L., et al. (2004). Haematopoietic stem cells adopt mature haematopoietic fates in ischaemic myocardium. *Nature, 428*, 668–673.

Bär, A., & Pette, D. (1988). Three fast myosin heavy chains in adult rat skeletal muscle. *FEBS Lett, 235*, 153–155.

Barker, D., Hunt, C. C., & McIntyre, A. K. (1974). Muscle receptors. In *Handbook of sensory physiology* (Vol. III/2). Berlin: Springer Verlag.

Basmajian, J. V. (1974). *Muscles alive: their functions revealed by electromyography* (ed. 3). Baltimore, MD: Williams & Wilkins.

Baum, H., & Zietzschmann, O. (1936). *Handbuch der anatomie des hundes. Band I: skelett und muskel-system*. Berlin: Paul Parey.

Baumeier, M. (1908). *Zur vergleichenden anatomie und morphologie des musculus obliquus abdominis ext. und der fascia flava*. Dissertation of University of Bern.

Bennett, G. A., & Hutchinson, R. C. (1946). Experimental studies on the movements of the mammalian tongue; protrusion mechanism of the tongue (dog). *Anat Rec, 94*, 57–83.

Benson, R. O., & Fletcher, T. F. (1971). Variability of the ansa cervicalis in dogs. *Am J Vet Res, 32*, 1163–1168.

Bergrin, M., Bicer, S., Lucas, C. A., et al. (2006). Three-dimensional compartmentalization of myosin heavy chain and myosin light chain isoforms in dog thyroarytenoid muscle. *Am J Physiol, 290*, C1446–C1458.

Bicer, S., & Reiser, P. J. (2009). Myosin isoform expression in dog rectus muscles: patterns in global and orbital layers and among single fibers. *Invest Ophthalmol Vis Sci, 50*, 157–167.

Biewener, A. A. (1998). Muscle properties and organismal function: shifting paradigms—muscle function *in vivo*: a comparison of muscles used for elastic energy savings versus muscles used to generate mechanical power. *Amer Zool, 38*, 703–717.

Bijvoet, W. F. (1908). Zur vergleichenden morphologie des musculus digastricus mandibulae bei den säugetieren. *Ztschr Morph u Anthropol, 11*, 249–316.

Bogorodsky, B. W. (1930). Der laterale strang der dorsalmuskulatur bein den fleischcarnivoren tieren. *Anat Anz, 69*, 82–121.

Bonneau, N. H., Oliveri, M., & Breton, L. (1983). Avulsion of the gastrocnemius tendon in the dog causing flexion of the hock and digits. *J Am Anim Hosp Assoc, 19*, 717–722.

Botterman, B. R., Hamm, T. M., Reinking, R. M., et al. (1983). Localization of monosynaptic ia excitatory post-synaptic potentials in the motor nucleus of the cat biceps femoris muscle. *J Physiol, 338*, 355–377.

Bourne, G. H. *The structure and function of muscle*, Vol. I, *Structure, part I* (1972); Vol. II, *Structure, part 2* (1973); Vol. III, *Physiology and biochemistry* (1973); Vol. IV, *Pharmacology and disease* (1973). (ed. 2, pp. 1972–1973). New York: Academic Press.

Bramble, D. M. (1989). Axial-appendicular dynamics and the integration of breathing and gait in mammals. *Am Zool, 29,* 171–186.

Bramble, D. M., & Jenkins, F. A., Jr. (1993). Mammalian locomotor-respiratory integration: implications for diaphragmatic and pulmonary design. *Science, 262,* 235–240.

Brooke, M. H., & Kaiser, K. K. (1970). Muscle fibre types: how many and what kind? *Arch Neurol, 23,* 361–379.

Bu, L., Jiang, Z., Martin-Puig, S., et al. (2009). Human ISL1 heart progenitors generate diverse multipotent cardiovascular cell lineages. *Nature, 460,* 113–117.

Bubb, W. J., & Sims, M. H. (1986). Fiber type composition of rostral and caudal portions of the digastric muscle in the dog. *Am J Vet Res, 47,* 1834–1842.

Budras, K. D. (1972). Zur homologisierung der mm. adductores und des M. pectineus der haussäugetiere. *Zbl Vet Med C, 1,* 73–91.

Budras, K. D., & Wünsche. (1972). Arcus inguinalis und fibrae reflexae des hundes. *Morph Jb, 117,* 408–419.

Burke, R. E. (1981). Motor units: anatomy, physiology and functional organizations. In V. B. Brooks (Ed.), *Handbook of physiology, sec. I. the nervous system.* Bethesda, MD: American Physiological Society.

Buxton, D. F., & Peck, D. (1990). Density of muscle spindle profiles in the intrinsic forelimb muscles of the dog. *J Morphol, 203,* 345–359.

Byrd, K. E. (1981). Mandibular movement and muscle activity during mastication in the Guinea pig. *J Morphol, 170,* 147–169.

Byrd, K. E., Milberg, D. J., & Lusehei, E. S. (1978). Human and macaque mastication: a quantitative study. *J Dent Res, 57,* 834–843.

Cardinet, G. H., III, Fedde, M. R., & Tunell, G. L. (1972). Correlates of histochemical and physiologic properties in normal and hypotrophic pectineus muscles of the dog. *Lab Invest, 27,* 32–38.

Carlson, B. M. (1972). *The regeneration of minced muscles.* Basel, Switzerland: Karger.

Carlson, B. M. (1986). Regeneration of entire skeletal muscles. *Fed Proc, 45,* 1456–1460.

Carlson, B. M., & Faulkner, J. A. (1983). The regeneration of skeletal muscle fibers following injury: a review. *Med Sci Sports Exer, 15,* 187–198.

Carrier, D. R. (1996). Function of the intercostal muscles in trotting dogs: ventilation or locomotion. *J Exp Biol, 199,* 1455–1465.

Carrier, D. R., Deban, S. M., & Fischbein, T. (2006). Locomotor function of the pectoral girdle "muscular sling" in trotting dogs. *J Exp Biol, 209,* 2224–2237.

Carrier, D. R., Deban, S. M., & Fischbein, T. (2008). Locomotor function of forelimb protractor and retractor muscles of dogs: evidence of strut-like behavior at the shoulder. *J Exp Biol, 211,* 150–162.

Cavagna, G. A., Heglund, N. C., & Taylor, C. R. (1977). Walking, running and galloping: mechanical similarities between different animals. In J. T. Pedley (Ed.), *Scale effects in animal locomotion.* London: Academic Press.

Cavagna, G. A., Saibene, F. P., & Margaria, R. (1964). Mechanical work in running. *J Appl Physiol, 19,* 249–252.

Chaine, J. (1914). Le digastique abaisseur de la mandibule des mammifères. *J Anat, 50,* 248–319, 393–417, 529–703.

Chanaud, C. M., Pratt, C. A., & Loeb, G. E. (1991). Functionally complex muscles of the cat hindlimb. V. the roles of histochemical fiber-type regionalization and mechanical heterogeneity in differential muscle activation. *Exp Brain Res, 85,* 300–313.

Chargé, B. P., & Rudnicki, M. A. (2004). Cellular and molecular regulation of muscle regeneration. *Physiol Rev, 84,* 209–238.

Decramer, M., De Troyer, A., Kelly, S., et al. (1984). Mechanical arrangement of costal and crural diaphragms in dogs. *J Appl Physiol, 56,* 1484–1490.

De Troyer, A., & Kelly, S. (1984). Action of neck accessory muscles on rib cage of dogs. *J Appl Physiol, 56,* 326–332.

De Troyer, A., & Ninane, V. (1986). Triangularis sterni: a primary muscle of breathing in the dog. *J Appl Physiol, 60,* 14–21.

De Troyer, A., Sampson, M., Sigrist, M., et al. (1981). The diaphragm: two muscles. *Science, 213,* 237–238.

De Troyer, A., Kelly, S., Macklem, P. T., et al. (1985). Mechanics of intercostal space and actions of external and internal intercostal muscles. *J Clin Invest, 75,* 850–857.

Donahue, S. P., & English, A. W. (1989). Selective elimination of cross-compartmental innervation in rat lateral gastrocnemius muscle. *J Neurophysiol, 9,* 1621–1627.

Duckworth, W. L. H. (1912). On some points in the anatomy of the plica vocalis. *J Anat, 47,* 80–115.

Dyce, K. M. (1957). The muscles of the pharynx and palate of the dog. *Anat Rec, 127,* 497–508.

Dyce, K. M., Sack, W. O., & Wensing, C. J. G. (2010). *Textbook of veterinary anatomy* (4th ed.). St Louis, MO: Saunders.

Edgeworth, F. H. (1935). *The cranial muscles of vertebrates.* Cambridge: Cambridge University Press.

Eisler, P. (1912). *Die muskeln des stammes.* Jena: G Fischer.

Ellenberger, W., & Baum, H. (1943). *Handbuch der vergleichenden anatomie der haustiere* (18th ed.). Berlin: Springer.

English, A. W., & Letbetter, W. D. (1982a). Anatomy and innervation patterns of cat lateral gastrocnemius and plantaris muscles. *Am J Anat, 164,* 67–77.

English, A. W., & Letbetter, W. D. (1982b). A histochemical analysis of identified compartments in cat lateral gastrocnemius muscle. *Anat Rec, 204,* 123–130.

English, A. W., & Weeks, O. I. (1984). Compartmentalization of single motor units in cat lateral gastrocnemius. *Exp Brain Res, 56,* 361–368.

English, A. W., & Weeks, O. I. (1987). An anatomical and functional analysis of cat biceps femoris and semitendinosus muscles. *J Morphol, 191,* 161–175.

Evans, H. E. (1959). Hyoid muscle anomalies in the dog (*Canis familiaris*). *Anat Rec, 133,* 145–162.

Evans, H. E., & de Lahunta, A. (2017). *Guide to the dissection of the dog* (8th ed.). St. Louis, MO: Elsevier.

Fawcett, D. W. (1986). *A textbook of histology.* Philadelphia: Saunders.

Field, E. J. (1960). Muscle regeneration and repair. In G. H. Bourne (Ed.), *Structure and function of muscle* (Vol. III). New York: Academic Press.

Forster, A. (1916). Die mm. contrahentes und interossei manus in der säugetierreihe und beim menschen. *Arch Anat Phys,* 101–378.

Frandson, R. D., & Davis, R. W. (1955). "Dropped muscle" in the racing greyhound. *J Am Vet Med Assoc, 126,* 468–469.

Freeman, L. M. (2012). Cachexia and sarcopenia: emerging syndromes of importance in dogs and cats. *J Vet Intern Med, 26,* 3–17. doi:10.1111/j.1939-1676.2011.00838.x.

Fuss, F. K. (1989). An analysis of the popliteus muscle in man, dog, and pig with a reconsideration of the general problems of muscle function. *Anat Rec, 225,* 251–256.

Galvas, P. E., & Gonyea, W. J. (1980). Motor-end-plate and nerve distribution in a histochemically compartmentalized pennate muscle in the cat. *Am J Anat, 159,* 147–156.

Gans, C., Loeb, G. E., & deVree, F. (1989). Architecture and consequent physiological properties of the semitendinosus muscle in domestic goats. *J Morphol, 199*, 287–297.

Gao, Y., Waas, A. M., Faulkner, J. A., et al. (2008). Micromechanical modeling of the epimysium of the skeletal muscles. *J Biomech, 41*, 1–10.

Getty, R. (1975). *Sisson and Grossman's anatomy of the domestic animal* (5th ed.). Philadelphia: Saunders.

Gilbert, P. W. (1947). The origin and development of the extrinsic ocular muscles in the domestic cat. *J Morphol, 81*, 151–194.

Glenn, L. L., & Whitney, J. F. (1987). Contraction properties and motor nucleus morphology of the two heads of the cat flexor carpi ulnaris muscle. *J Morphol, 191*, 17–23.

Gonyea, W. J., Marushia, S. A., & Dixon, J. A. (1981). Morphological organization and contractile properties of the wrist flexor muscles in the cat. *Anat Rec, 1099*, 321–339.

Gordon, D. C., Hammond, C. G., Fisher, J. T., et al. (1989). Muscle-fiber architecture, innervation, and histochemistry in the diaphragm of the cat. *J Morphol, 201*, 131–143.

Gorniak, G. C., & Gans, C. (1980). Quantitative assay of electromyograms during mastication in domestic cats (*Felis catus*). *J Morphol, 163*, 253–281.

Goslow, G. E., Jr. (1985). Neural control of locomotion. In M. Hildebrand, D. M. Bramble, K. F. Liem, & D. B. Wake (Eds.), *Functional vertebrate morphology*. Cambridge, MA: Harvard University Press.

Goslow, G. E., Jr., Seeherman, H. J., Taylor, C. R., et al. (1981). Electrical activity and relative length changes of dog limb muscles as a function of speed and gait. *J Exp Biol, 94*, 15–42.

Grau, H. (1932). Über einige muskelvarietäten bei haustieren besonders über varietäten des M. extensor hallucis longus und des M. tibialis anterior beim hunde. *Anat Anz, 74*, 218–227.

Grounds, M. D., White, J. D., Rosenthal, N., et al. (2002). The role of stem cells in skeletal and cardiac muscle repair. *J Histochem Cytochem, 50*, 589–610.

Gunn, H. M. (1978a). Differences in the histochemical properties of skeletal muscles of different breeds of horses and dogs. *J Anat, 127*, 615–634.

Gunn, H. M. (1978b). The proportions of muscle, bone and fat in two different types of dog. *Res Vet Sci, 24*, 277–282.

Habel, R. E. (1990). The prepubic tendon continued: does it exist in the dog? *Anat Histol Embryol, 19*, 84.

Habel, R. E., & Budras, K. D. (1992). Anatomy of the prepubic tendon in the horse, cow, sheep, goat, and dog. *Am J Vet Res, 53*, 2183–2195.

Harker, D. W. (1972). The structure and innervation of sheep superior rectus and levator palpebrae extraocular muscles. I. extrafusal muscle fibers. *Invest Ophthal, 11*, 956–969.

Heglund, N. C., Fedak, M. A., Taylor, C. R., et al. (1982). Energetics and mechanics of terrestrial locomotion. IV. Total mechanical energy changes as a function of speed and body size in birds and mammals. *J Exp Biol, 97*, 57–66.

Heiderich, F. (1906). Die faszien und aponeurosen der achselhöhle. *Anat Hefte, 30*, 517–557.

Henning, P. (1965). Der M. piriformis und die nn. clunium medii des hundes. *Zbl Vet Med, 12*, 263–275.

Herring, S. W., Grimm, A. F., & Grimm, B. R. (1979). Functional heterogeneity in a multipinnate muscle. *Am J Anat, 154*, 563–576.

Hildebrand, M., & Goslow, G. (2001). *Analysis of vertebrate structure* (5th ed.). New York: Wiley.

Hoffer, J. A., Loeb, G. E., Sugano, N., et al. (1987). Cat hindlimb motoneurons during locomotion. III. Functional segregation in sartorius. *J Neurophysiol, 57*, 554–562.

Hoh, J. F. Y. (2005). Laryngeal muscle fibre types. *Acta Physiol Scand, 183*, 133–149.

Hoh, J. F. Y., Hughes, S., Hale, P. T., et al. (1988). Immunocytochemical and electrophoretic analyses of changes in myosin gene expression in cat posterior temporalis muscle during postnatal development. *J Musc Res Cell Motil, 9*, 48–58.

Hoyle, G. (1983). *Muscles and their neural control*. New York: Wiley.

Huber, E. (1922–1923). Über das muskelgebiet des N. facialis beim hund, nebst allgemeinen betrachtungen über die fascialismuskulatur. *Morph Jahrb, 52*, 1–110, 354–414.

Huber, G. C. (1916). On the form and arrangement of fasciculi of striated voluntary muscle fibers. *Anat Rec, 11*, 149–168.

Hulliger, M. (1984). The mammalian muscle spindle and its central control. *Rev Physiol Biochem Pharmacol, 101*, 1–110.

Hunt, C. C. (1990). Mammalian muscle spindle: peripheral mechanisms. *Physiol Rev, 70*, 643–663.

Huntington, G. S. (1903). Present problems of myological research and the significance and classification of muscular variations. *Am J Anat, 2*, 157–175.

Ihemelandu, E. C., Cardinet, G. H., III, Gufly, M. M., et al. (1983). Canine hip dysplasia: differences in pectineal muscles of healthy and dysplastic German shepherd dogs when two months old. *Am J Vet Res, 44*, 411–416.

Iwakin, A. A. (1928). Zur frage über die homologie der ventralen lumbaimuskulatur: I. über den M. retractor costae ultimae. *Morph Jahrb, 59*, 179–195.

Jackson, K. A., Majka, S. M., Wang, H., et al. (2001). Regeneration of ischemic cardiac muscle and vascular endothelium by adult stem cells. *J Clin Invest, 107*, 1395–1402.

Jopp, I., & Reese, S. (2009). Morphological and biomechanical studies of the common calcaneal tendon in dogs. *Vet Comp Orthop Traumatol, 22*, 119–124.

Josephson, R. K. (1975). Extensive and intensive factors determining the performance of striated muscle. *J Exp Zool, 194*, 135–154.

Kajava, Y. (1922). Über homologisierung einiger muskeln der hand unserer haussäugetiere. *Verhdlg Anat Ges, 55*, 136–153.

Kajava, Y. (1923). Die volare handmuskulatur. *Act Soc Med Fennic Duodecim, 4*, 1–184.

Kardong, K. V. (2008). *Vertebrates: comparative anatomy, function, evolution* (5th ed.). New York: McGraw Hill.

Kassianenko, W. (1928). Zur vergleichenden anatomie der mm. intercartilaginei bei den säugetieren. *Ztschr Anat u Entw, 85*, 166–177.

Kincaid, S. A., Rumph, P. F., Garrett, P. D., et al. (1996). Morphology of the musculus articularis genus in dog with description of ectopic muscle spindles. *Anat Histo Embryol, 25*, 113–116.

Kolesnikow, W. (1928). Zur morphologie des M. iliocostalis. *Ztschr Anat u Entw, 88*, 397–404.

Krüger, W. (1929). *Über den bau des M. biceps brachii in seinen beziehungen zur funktion beim menschen und bei einigen haussäugetieren*. Hannover, Germany: Baum Festschrift.

Kuzon, W. M., Jr., Rosenblatt, D., Pynn, B. R., et al. (1989). A comparative histochemical and morphometric study of canine skeletal muscle. *Can J Vet Res, 53*, 125–132.

La Framboise, W. A., Daood, M. J., Guthrie, R. D., et al. (1990). Electrophoretic separation and immunological identification of type 2x myosin heavy chain in rat skeletal muscle. *Biochim Biophys Acta, 1035*, 109–112.

Lakars, T. C., & Herring, S. W. (1987). Polymorphous geniohyoid muscles of mice, rats and hamsters. *Arch Oral Biol, 32*, 421–427.

Langley, J. N., & Anderson, H. K. (1895). The innervation of the pelvic and adjoining viscera: III. The external generative organs. *J Physiol, 19,* 85–121.

Langworthy, O. R. (1924). The panniculus carnosus in cat and dog and its genetic relation to the pectoral musculature. *J Mammal, 5,* 49–63.

La Torre, R., Gil, F., Vazquez, J. M., et al. (1993). Morphological and histochemical characteristics of muscle fiber types in the flexor carpi radialis of the dog. *J Anat, 182,* 313–320.

Leahy, J. R. (1949). *Muscles of the head, neck, shoulder and forelimb of the dog,* Thesis. Ithaca, NY: Cornell University.

Lev-Tov, A., & Tal, M. (1987). The organization and activity patterns of the anterior and posterior heads of the Guinea pig digastric muscle. *J Neurophysiol, 58,* 496–509.

Lieber, R. L. (1992). *Skeletal muscle structure and function.* Baltimore, MD: Williams and Wilkins.

Liem, K. F., Bemis, W., Walker, W. F., et al. (2000). *Functional anatomy of the vertebrates: an evolutionary perspective* (3rd ed.). Florence, KY: Brooks Cole.

Lippincott, C. L. (1981). Improvement of excision arthroplasty of the femoral head and neck utilizing a biceps femoris muscle sling. *J Am Anim Hosp Assoc, 17,* 668–672.

Lockhart, R. D., & Brandt, W. (1938). Length of striated muscle fibers. *J Anat, 72,* 470.

Loeb, G. E., & Gans, C. (1986). *Electromyography for experimentalists.* Chicago: University of Chicago Press.

Loeb, G. E., Pratt, C. A., Chanaud, C. M., et al. (1987). Distribution and innervation of short, interdigitated muscle fibers in parallel-fibered muscles of the cat hindlimb. *J Morphol, 191,* 1–15.

Lust, G., Craig, P. H., Ross, G. E., Jr., et al. (1972). Studies on pectineus muscles in canine hip dysplasia. *Cornell Veterinarian, 62,* 628–645.

Mascarello, F., Carpene, E., Veggetti, A., et al. (1982). The tensor tympani muscle of cat and dog contains IIM and slow-tonic fibres: an unusual combination of fibre types. *J Muscle Res Cell Motil, 3,* 363–374.

Mascarello, F., Veggetti, A., Carpene, E., et al. (1983). An immuno-histochemical study of the middle ear muscles of some carnivores and primates, with special reference to the IIM and slow-tonic fibre types. *J Anat, 137,* 95–108.

Matthews, P. B. C. (1972). *Mammalian muscle receptors and their central actions.* Baltimore, MO: Williams & Wilkins.

Maximenko, A. (1929). Material zum studium der mm. serrati dorsales der säugetiere. *Ztschr Anat u Entw, 89,* 156–170. (1930). 92:151–177.

McCarthy, P. H., & Wood, A. K. W. (1989). Anatomical and radiological observations of the sesamoid bone of the popliteus muscle in the adult dog and cat. *Anat Histol Embryol, 18,* 58–65.

McConathy, D., Giddings, C. J., & Gonyea, W. J. (1983). Structure-function relationships of the flexor carpi radialis muscle compared among four species of mammals. *J Morphol, 175,* 279–292.

McMahon, T. A. (1984). *Muscles, reflexes, and locomotion.* Princeton, NJ: Princeton University Press.

Miki, H., Hida, W., Shindoh, C., et al. (1989). Effects of electrical stimulation of the genioglossus on upper airway resistance in anesthetized dogs. *Am Rev Respir Dis, 140,* 1279–1284.

Miller, J. M., Lanz, O. I., & Degner, D. A. (2007). Rectus abdominis free muscle flap for reconstruction in nine dogs. *Vet Surg, 36,* 259–265.

Miller, M. E., Christensen, G. C., & Evans, H. E. (1964). *Anatomy of the dog.* Philadelphia: Saunders.

Monges, H., Salducci, J., & Naudy, B. (1978). Dissociation between the electrical activity of the diaphragmatic dome and crura muscular fibers during esophageal distension, vomiting, and eructation: an electromyographic study. *J Physiol, 74,* 541–554.

Morley, J. E., Baumgartner, R. N., Roubenoff, R., et al. (2001). Sarcopenia. *J Lab Clin Med, 137,* 231–243.

Mu, L., & Sanders, I. (2000). Neuromuscular specializations of the pharyngeal dilator muscles: II. Compartmentalization of the canine genioglossus muscle. *Anat Rec, 260,* 308–325.

Nemeth, P. M., & Pette, D. (1981). Succinic dehydrogenase activity in fibres classified by myosin ATPase in three hind limb muscles of rat. *J Physiol, 320,* 73–80.

Newsholme, S. J., Lexell, J., & Downham, D. Y. (1988). Distribution of fibre types and fibre sizes in the tibialis cranialis muscle of beagle dogs. *J Anat, 160,* 1–8.

Nickel, R., Schummer, A., & Seiferle, E. (1954). *Lehrbuch der anatomie der haustiere. Band 1: bewegungsapparat.* Berlin: Paul Parey.

Ontell, M. (1986). Morphological aspects of muscle fiber regeneration. *Fed Proc, 45,* 1461–1465.

Pachter, B. R. (1982). Fiber composition of the superior rectus extraocular muscle of the rhesus macaque. *J Morphol, 174,* 237–250.

Pachter, B. R. (1983). Rat extraocular muscle. 1. Three dimensional cytoarchitecture, component fibre populations and innervation. *J Anat, 137,* 143–159.

Pancrazi, G. (1928). Intorno al "foramen venae cavae" del diaframma dei mammiferi. *Atti Soc Nat Modena, 7,* 191–192.

Peachey, L. D. (1983). Skeletal muscle. In *Handbook of physiology.* Bethesda, MD: American Physiological Society.

Peck, D., Buxton, D. F., & Nitz, A. (1984). A comparison of spindle concentrations in large and small muscles acting in parallel muscle combinations. *J Morphol, 180,* 243–252.

Peter, J. B., Barnard, R. J., Edgerton, V. R., et al. (1972). Metabolic profiles of three fibre types of skeletal muscle in Guinea pigs and rabbits. *Biochemistry, 11,* 2627–2633.

Peters, S. E., & Goslow, G. E., Jr. (1983). From salamanders to mammals: continuity in musculoskeletal function during locomotion. *Brain Behav Evol, 22,* 191–197.

Peters, S. E., & Rick, C. (1976). The actions of three hamstring muscles of the cat: a mechanical analysis. *J Morphol, 152,* 315–327.

Pette, D., & Staron, R. S. (1990). Cellular and molecular diversities of mammalian skeletal muscle fibers. *Rev Physiol Biochem Pharmacol, 116,* 1–76.

Pettit, G. D. (1962). Perineal hernia in the dog. *Cornell Veterinarian, 52,* 261–279.

Piérard, J. (1963). *Comparative anatomy of the carnivore larynx,* Thesis. Ithaca, NY: Cornell University.

Pitzorno, M. (1905). Musculi accessorii ad flexorum perforatum. Studi sassarei anno 4. *Schwalbes Jahresbericht, 3,* 207.

Plattner, F. (1922). Über die ventral innerviete und die genuine rückenmuskulatur bei drei anthropomorphen. *Morphol Jahrb, 52,* 241.

Pratt, C. A., & Loeb, G. E. (1991). Functionally complex muscles of the cat hindlimb. I. patterns of activation across sartorius. *Exp Brain Res, 85,* 243–256.

Pressman, J. J., & Kelemen, G. (1955). Physiology of the larynx. *Physiol Rev, 35,* 506–554.

Rasmussen, S., Chan, A. K., & Goslow, G. E., Jr. (1978). The cat step cycle: electromyographic patterns for hindlimb muscles during posture and unrestrained locomotion. *J Morphol, 155,* 253–269.

Reichmann, H., & Pette, D. (1982). A comparative microphotometric study of succinate dehydrogenase activity levels in type I, IIA and IIB fibres of mammalian and human muscles. *Histochemistry, 74,* 27–41.

Reichmann, H., & Pette, D. (1984). Glycerolphosphate oxidase and succinate dehydrogenase activities in IIA and IIB fibres of mouse and rabbit tibialis anterior muscles. *Histochemistry, 80*, 429–433.

Reid, M. B., Ericson, G. C., Feldman, H. A., et al. (1987). Fiber types and fiber diameters in canine respiratory muscles. *J Appl Physiol, 62*, 1705–1712.

Reighard, J., & Jennings, H. S. (1938). *Anatomy of the cat* (3rd ed.). New York: Henry Holt and Company. (Edited by R. Elliott).

Reiser, P. J., & Bicer, S. (2007). High force generation and moderate shortening velocity in jaw-closing muscle fibers expressing masticatory ('superfast') myosin. *Biophys J, Suppl S*, 191A.

Reiser, P. J., Bicer, S., Chen, Q., et al. (2009). Masticatory ('superfast') myosin heavy chain and embryonic/atrial myosin light chain 1 in rodent jaw-closing muscles. *J Exp Biol, 212*, 2511–2519.

Reiser, P. J., Bicer, S., Patel, R., et al. (2010). The myosin light chain 1 isoform associated with masticatory myosin heavy chain in mammals and reptiles is embryonic/atrial MLC1. *J Exp Biol, 213*, 1633–1642.

Richmond, F. J. R., & Abrahams, V. C. (1975a). Morphology and enzyme histochemistry of dorsal muscles of the cat neck. *J Neurophysiol, 38*, 1312–1321.

Richmond, F. J. R., & Abrahams, V. C. (1975b). Morphology and distribution of muscle spindles in dorsal muscles of the cat neck. *J Neurophysiol, 38*, 1322–1339.

Richmond, F. J. R., & Armstrong, J. B. (1988). Fiber architecture and histochemistry in the cat neck muscle, biventer cervicis. *J Neurophysiol, 60*, 46–59.

Richmond, F. J. R., & Bakker, D. A. (1982). Anatomical organization and sensory receptor content of soft tissues surrounding upper cervical vertebrae in the cat. *J Neurophysiol, 48*, 49–61.

Richmond, F. J. R., Johnston, W. S. W., Baker, R. S., et al. (1984). Palisade endings in human extraocular muscles. *Invest Ophthal Vis Sci, 25*, 471–476.

Ritter, D. A., Nassar, P. N., Fife, M. M., et al. (2001). Epaxial muscle function in trotting dogs. *J Exp Biol, 204*, 3053–3064.

Rodríguez-Barbudo, V., Vaamonde, R., Agüera, E., et al. (1984). Estudios histoquimico y morfometrico del musculo tibial craneal en perros de diferentes aptitudes dinamicas (galgo, pastor aleman y fox terrier). *Anat Histol Embryol, 13*, 300–312.

Romer, A. S., & Parsons, T. S. (1986). *The vertebrate body*. Philadelphia: Saunders.

Rouviere, H. (1906). Étude sur le development phylogenetique de certain muscles sushyoidiens. *J Anat, 42*, 487–540.

Rowlerson, A., Pope, B., Murray, J., et al. (1981). A novel myosin present in cat jaw-closing muscles. *J Muscle Res Cell Motil, 2*, 415–438.

Roy, R. R., Powell, P. L., Kanim, P., et al. (1984). Architectural and histochemical analysis of the semitendinosus muscle in mice, rats, Guinea pigs, and rabbits. *J Morphol, 181*, 155–160.

Sacks, R. D., & Roy, R. R. (1982). Architecture of the hind limb muscles of cats: functional significance. *J Morphol, 173*, 185–195.

Samuelson, D. A. (2007). *A textbook of veterinary histology*. St Louis, MO: Saunders.

Sanders, I., Jacobs, I., Wu, M. D., et al. (1993). The three bellies of the canine posterior cricoarytenoid muscle: implications for understanding laryngeal function. *Laryngoscope, 103*, 171–177.

Sánchez-Collado, C., Vazquez, J. M., Rivero, M. A., et al. (2013). Distribution pattern of muscle fibre types in soft palate of the dog (canis familiaris, L.). *Anat Histol Emb, 43*, 56–63. doi:10.1111/ahe.12048.

Sartore, S., Mascarello, F., Rowlerson, A., et al. (1987). Fibre types in extraocular muscles: a new myosin isoform in the fast fibres. *J Muscle Res Cell Motil, 8*, 161–172.

Schaller, O. (Ed.), (2007). *Illustrated veterinary anatomical nomenclature* (2nd ed.). Stuttgart, Germany: Enke Verlag.

Schiaffino, S., Gorza, L., Sartore, S., et al. (1989). Three myosin heavy chain isoforms in type 2 skeletal muscle fibres. *J Muscle Res Cell Motil, 10*, 197–205.

Schilling, N., & Carrier, D. R. (2009). Function of the epaxial muscles during trotting. *J Exp Biol, 212*, 1053–1063.

von Schumacher, S. (1910). Die segmentale innervation des säugetierschwanzes als beispiel fúr das vokommen einer "kollateralen" innervation. *Anat Hefte, 120*(Bd. 40), 47–94.

Sharir, A., Milgram, J., & Shahar, R. (2006). Structural and functional anatomy of the neck musculature of the dog (Canis familiaris). *J Anat, 208*, 331–351.

Shelton, G. D., Bandman, E., & Cardinet, G. H., III. (1985a). Electrophoretic comparison of myosins from masticatory muscles and selected limb muscles in the dog. *Am J Vet Res, 46*, 493–498.

Shelton, G. D., Cardinet, G. H., III, & Bandman, E. (1985b). Fiber type specific autoantibodies in a dog with eosinophilic myositis. *Muscle Nerve, 8*, 783–790.

Shelton, G. D., Cardinet, G. H., & Bandman, E. (1988). Expression of fiber type specific proteins during ontogeny of canine temporalis muscle. *Muscle Nerve, 11*, 124–132.

Sidaway, B. K., McLaughlin, R. M., Elder, S. H., et al. (2004). Role of the tendons of the biceps brachii and infraspinatus muscles and the medial glenohumeral ligament in the maintenance of passive shoulder joint stability in dogs. *Am J Vet Res, 65*, 1216–1222.

Skoda, C. (1908). Eine beim pferde vorkommende scheinbare homologie des M. abductor cruris posterior der carnivoren. *Anat Anz, 32*, 216–221.

Slijper, E. J. (1946). Comparative biologic-anatomical investigations of the vertebral column and spinal musculature of mammals. *Kon Ned Akad Wet Verh (Tweede Sectie), 42*(5), 1–128.

Snow, D. H., Billeter, R., Mascarello, F., et al. (1982). No classical type IIB fibres in dog skeletal muscle. *Histochemistry, 75*, 53–65.

Sprung, J., Deschamps, C., Hubmary, R. D., et al. (1989). In vivo regional diaphragm function in dogs. *J Appl Physiol, 67*, 655–662.

Stål, P., Eriksson, P. O., Schiaffino, S., et al. (1994). Differences in myosin composition between human oro-facial, masticatory and limb muscles: enzyme-, immunohisto-, and biochemical studies. *J Mus Res Cell Motil, 15*, 517–534.

Stimpel, J. (1934). Die morphologie des medialen muskelstranges der stammzone bei den haustieren. *Morph Jahrb, 74*, 337–363.

Straus-Durckheim, H. (1845). *Anatomie descriptive et comparative du chat, type des mammifères en général det des carnivores en particulier* (Vol. II). Paris: Syndesmologie et Ia Myologie.

Strauss, L. H. (1927). Der rectus abdominis. *Bruns Beiträge z klin Chir, 141*, 684–698.

Strohl, K. P., Wolin, A. D., Van Lunteren, D., et al. (1987). Assessment of muscle action on upper airway stability in anesthetized dogs. *J Lab Clin Med, 110*, 221–230.

Stuart, D. G., & Enoka, R. M. (1983). Motoneurons, motor units, and the size principle. In R. G. Grossman & W. D. Willis (Eds.), *The clinical neurosciences, section V, neurobiology*. New York: Churchill Livingstone.

Sypert, G. W., & Munson, J. B. (1981). Basis of segmental motor control: motoneuron size or motor unit type? *Neurosurgery, 8*, 608–621.

Termin, A., Staron, R. S., & Pette, D. (1989). Myosin heavy chain isoforms in histochemically defined fiber types of rat muscle. *Histochemistry, 92*, 453–457.

Tokuriki, N. (1973a). Electromyographic and joint-mechanical studies in quadrupedal locomotion. I. walk. *Jpn J Vet Sci, 35*, 433–448.

Tokuriki, N. (1973b). Electromyographic and joint-mechanical studies in quadrupedal locomotion. II. Trot. *Jpn J Vet Sci, 35*, 525–535.

Tokuriki, N. (1974). Electromyographic and joint-mechanical studies in quadrupedal locomotion, III, Gallop. *Jpn J Vet Sci, 36*, 121–132.

Tomo, S., Nakajima, K., Tomo, I., et al. (1995). The morphology and innervation of the lateral pterygoid muscle of the dog. *J Anat, 186*, 435–439.

Toniolo, L., Maccatrozzo, L., & Patruno, M. (2007). Fiber types in canine muscles: myosin isoform expression and functional characterization. *Am J Physiol Cell, 292*, C1915–C1926. doi:10.1152/ajpcell.00601.2006.

Toniolo, L., Cancellara, P., Maccatrozzo, L., et al. (2008). Masticatory myosin unveiled: first determination of contractile parameters of muscle fibers from carnivore jaw muscles. *Am J Cell Physiol, 295*, C1535–C1542.

Trotter, J. A. (1990). Interfiber tension transmission in series-fibered muscles of the cat hindlimb. *J Morphol, 206*, 351–361.

Updike, S. J. (1985). A redescription of the gross anatomy of the canine extensor digitorum longus muscle. *Zbl Vet Med C Anat Histol Embryol, 14*, 342–347.

Valentine, B. A., Cooper, B. J., Cummings, J. F., et al. (1986). Progressive muscular dystrophy in a golden retriever dog: light microscope and ultrastructural features at 4 and 8 months. *Acta Neuropathol, 71*, 301–310.

Van Harreveld, A. (1947). On the force and size of motor units in the rabbit's sartorius muscle. *Am J Physiol, 151*, 96–106.

Van Lunteren, E., Salomone, R. J., Manubay, P., et al. (1990). Contractile and endurance properties of geniohyoid and diaphragm muscles. *J Appl Physiol, 69*, 1992–1997.

Vogel, P. (1952). The innervation of the larynx of man and the dog. *Am J Anat, 90*, 427–440.

Wakuri, H., & Kano, Y. (1966). Anatomical studies on the brachioradial muscle in dogs. *Acta Anat Nipponica, 41*, 222–231.

Wakuri, H., Mutoh, K., & Ikeda, F. (1988). Variations of the extensor digitorum brevis muscle in the dog. *Anat Histol Embryol, 17*, 164–168.

Walmsley, B., Hodgson, J. A., & Burke, R. E. (1978). Forces produced by medial gastrocnemius and soleus muscles during locomotion in freely moving cats. *J Neurophysiol, 41*, 1203–1216.

Walter, C. (1908). *Die sehnenscheiden und schleimbeutel der gliedmassen des hundes*. Dissertation. Dresden-Leipzig.

Walston, J. D. (2012). Sarcopenia in older adults. *Curr Opin Rheumatol, 24*, 623–627. doi:10.1097/BOR.0b013e328358d59b.

Webster, E. L., Hudson, P. E., & Channon, S. B. (2014). Comparative functional anatomy of the epaxial musculature of dogs (*Canis familiaris*) bred for sprinting vs. fighting. *J Anat, 2014*, 317–327. doi:10.1111/joa.12208.

Wentink, G. H. (1976). The action of the hindlimb musculature of the dog in walking. *Acta Anat, 96*, 70–80.

Williams, S. B., Wilson, A. M., Daynes, J., et al. (2008). Functional anatomy and muscle moment arms of the thoracic limb of an elite sprinting athlete: the racing greyhound (*Canis familiaris*). *J Anat, 213*, 373–382.

Winckler, G. (1939). Contribution à l'étude de la morphogénèse du muscle spinalis dorsi. *Arch Anat Hist Embr, 27*, 99.

Wu, Y. Z., Crumley, R. L., & Caiozzo, V. J. (2000). Are hybrid fibers a common motif of canine laryngeal muscles? *Arch Otol Head Neck Surg, 126*, 865–873.

Yakoba, M., Hawes, H. G., & Easton, P. A. (2003). Geniohyoid muscle function in awake canines. *J Appl Physiol, 95*, 810–817.

Zaretsky, L. S., & Sanders, I. (1992). The three bellies of the canine cricothyroid muscle. *Ann Otol Rhinol Laryngol, 101*(Suppl. 156), 3–16.

Zhou, B., Ma, Q., Rajagopal, S., et al. (2008). Epicardial progenitors contribute to the cardiomyocyte lineage in the developing heart. *Nature, 454*, 109–113.

Ziegler, H. (1929). Muskelvarietäten bei haustieren. *Ztschr Anat u Entw, 91*, 442–451.

Ziegler, H. (1931). Die innervationsverhältnisse der beckenmuskeln bei haustieren im vergleich mit denjenigen beim menschen. *Morph Jahrb, 68*, 1–45.

Ziegler, H. (1934). Weitere untersuchungen, über den M. glutaeobiceps von hund (*Canis familiaris*) and katze (*Felis catus dom.*). *Morph Jahrb, 73*, 385–391.

Zimmermann, A. (1928). Zur vergleichenden anatomie des M. pronator teres. *Verhdlg Anat Ges, 66*, 281–282.

7

The Digestive Apparatus and Abdomen

The **digestive system** (*apparatus digestorius*) consists of the oral cavity, pharynx, alimentary canal, and accessory organs. The accessory organs include the teeth, tongue, salivary glands, liver, gallbladder, pancreas, and paranal sinus.

The wall of the digestive tube is richly supplied with secretory epithelium and intrinsic glands. It is lined throughout by a mucous membrane that is continuous with the surface integument at the mouth and anus.

Oral Cavity

The **mouth** (*os. oris*) in anatomic terms includes only the opening between the lips (*rima oris*) into the vestibule of the oral cavity. The **oral cavity** (*cavum oris*) is divided into the **vestibule** and the **oral cavity proper** and contains salivary glands, teeth, and the tongue.

Vestibule

The **vestibule of the oral cavity** (*vestibulum oris*) is the space external to the teeth and gums and internal to the lips and cheeks. It opens to the outside rostrally by means of the U-shaped slit, the mouth or **oral fissure** (*rima oris*), between the lips. This opening is in a dorsal plane. When the mouth is closed, the vestibule communicates with the oral cavity proper by means of the interdental spaces, which vary greatly in size. A space on either side, caudal to the last cheek tooth and nearly 1 cm long in large dogs, also establishes free communication between the two parts of the oral cavity.

The parotid and zygomatic salivary ducts open into the dorsocaudal part of the vestibule. The parotid duct opens through the cheek on the small **parotid papilla** (*papilla parotidea*), located opposite the caudal part of the superior fourth premolar tooth, approximately 5 mm from the fornix of the vestibule, which is formed by a reflection of the mucosa from the cheek to the gum. The main duct of the zygomatic gland opens lateral to the caudal part of the superior first molar tooth on a small papilla near the vestibular fornix (Fig. 7.1). A small mucosal ridge connects the main zygomatic and parotid duct openings. Usually one to four small accessory ducts from the zygomatic gland open caudal to the main duct. The submucosal labial and ventral buccal glands are few and are confined to the inferior lip and the adjacent part of the cheek. The secretion of these glands is discharged through approximately 10 openings located opposite the four inferior premolar teeth near the fornix of the vestibule.

Lips

The **lips** (*labia oris*) form the rostral and most of the lateral external boundaries of the vestibule. Superior and inferior lips (*labium superius et labium inferius*), formerly upper and lower lips, meet at the angles of the mouth (*angulus oris*). The lips bound the oral fissure, the external opening (the mouth) into the vestibule. Their margins are narrow and devoid of hair except the rostral two-thirds of the superior lip on either side. Toward the angle on either side, the caudal third progressively increases in width to form a rounded border measuring as much as 1 cm. The margin of the inferior lip as far caudally as a level through the canine teeth is devoid of hair over a zone approximately 5 mm wide. Caudal to the canine teeth this smooth zone increases to 1 cm in width, and the narrow border becomes serrated by the formation of approximately 15 conical papillae several millimeters high.

No definite frenulum, or median mucosal fold, attaches the inferior lip to the gum, and the median mucosal fold of the superior lip is poorly developed, being thick but narrow. The mucosa of the inferior lip is firmly attached to the gum on either side in the space between the canine and the first premolar tooth (interdental space). A deep, straight, narrow cleft, the *philtrum*, marks the union of the two halves of the superior lip rostrally. The hair of both lips slopes caudoventrally. It is thinner and shorter rostrally, longer and thicker caudally. A few of these are **tactile hairs** (*pili tactiles*). On the superior lip and adjacent dorsal part of the muzzle the tactile hairs are imperfectly arranged in four rows. The wide orbicularis oris muscle and the insertions of several other facial muscles form the media of the lips.

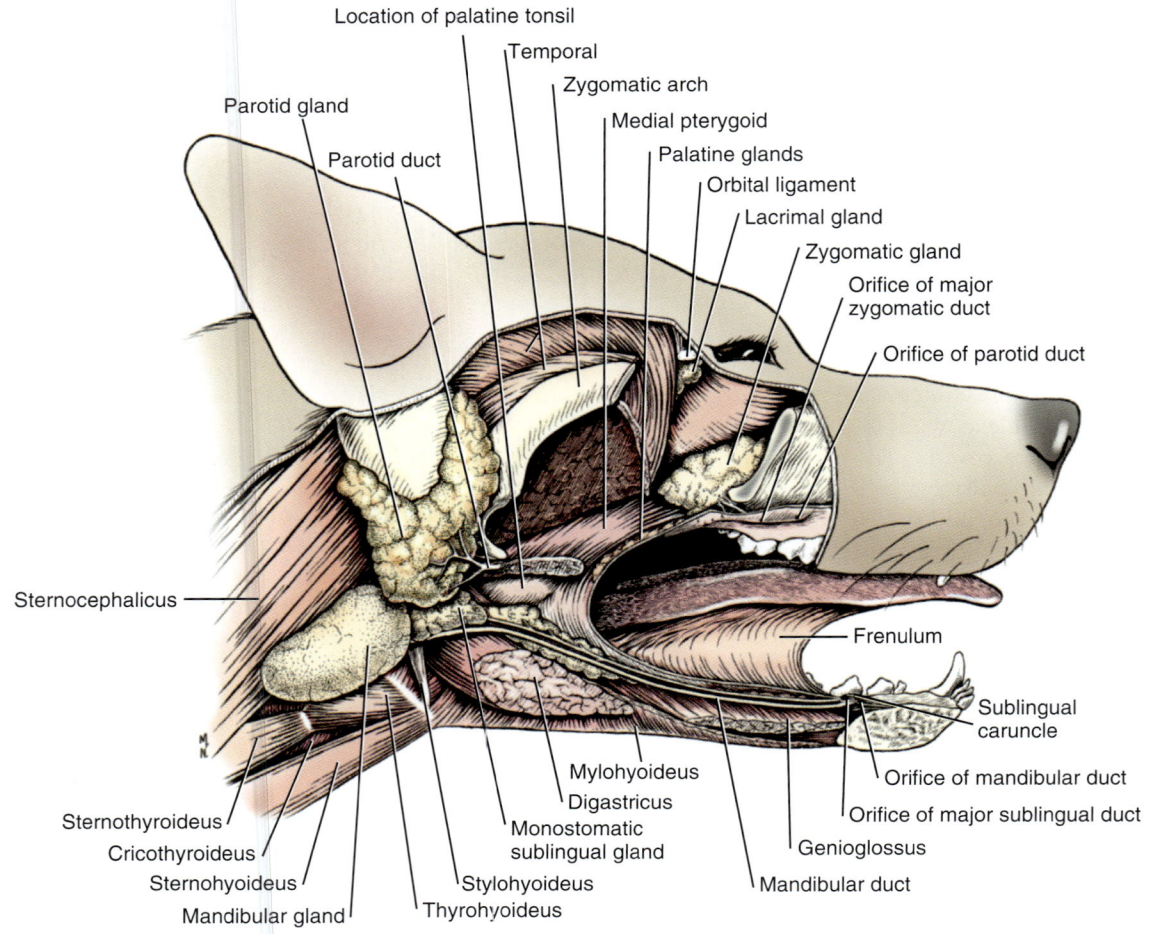

Fig. 7.1 Salivary glands. (The right half of the mandible is removed.)

Cheeks

The **cheeks** (*buccae*) form the caudal portion of the lateral walls of the vestibular cavity. The cheeks are small in the dog because of the large mouth opening. The cavity of the cheeks runs medial to the masseter muscles and extends as far caudally as the attachment of the buccinator muscles on the mandible and maxilla at their alveolar borders opposite the last two cheek teeth of the maxilla and mandible and the intervening rostral border of the basal half of the coronoid process. In rodents and most herbivores the cheeks are large and serve as storage space, especially during mastication and transportation. This function is of minor importance to the dog.

The morphologic characteristics of the cheeks are closely related to that of the lips, with which they are continuous. The lips and the cheeks consist of three basic layers. The external layer is the hairy integument, the middle layer consists of muscle and fibroelastic tissue, and the inner layer consists of the mucosa. Projecting caudolaterally from the caudal part of the skin of the cheek are usually two coarse tactile hairs, 3 to 5 cm long. The middle layer of the cheek consists primarily of the buccinator muscle, although lateral to this are the m. zygomaticus and some fasciculi of the cutaneous fascia. The dorsal buccal glands in carnivores are consolidated to form the **zygomatic gland** (*Glandula zygomatica*), a large mixed salivary gland located in the rostroventral part of the orbit. The ventral buccal glands consist of a few small, solitary glands located in the submucosa, rostral to the masseter muscle and medial to the fibers of the ventral part of the buccinator. The mucosa of the lips and cheeks is thinly cornified, stratified squamous epithelium that, in some breeds, is partly or wholly pigmented. Although the lips are not used as prehensile organs, the various muscles in them provide for movement and expression of emotions, such as anger or fear.

Oral Cavity Proper

The **oral cavity proper** (*cavum oris proprium*) is bounded dorsally by the hard palate and a small part of the adjacent soft palate. Laterally and rostrally the dental arches and teeth form its boundary. The tongue and the reflected mucosa ventral and lateral to it form the floor of this cavity. When the mouth is closed the tongue nearly fills the oral cavity proper. The monostomatic sublingual and mandibular gland ducts open rostrally ventral to the body of the tongue, on the inconspicuous **sublingual caruncle** (*caruncula sublingualis*).

Extending caudally from the caruncle, lateral to the frenulum, to about a transverse plane through the inferior shearing or carnassial teeth is a low ridge of mucosa approximately 2 mm wide and 1 mm high. This is the **sublingual fold** (*plica sublingualis*). It lies close to the body of the mandible and is formed by the underlying mandibular and major sublingual ducts and a variable number of lobules of the polystomatic portion of the sublingual gland.

Just caudal to the superior central incisor teeth is the **incisive papilla** (*papilla incisiva*), a rounded eminence that extends caudally to blend with the first transverse ridge formed of the mucosa covering the hard palate. On each side of this papilla an **incisive duct** (*ductus incisivus*) opens. This duct, formerly the nasopalatine duct, leaves the oral cavity by a slitlike opening and extends caudodorsally for 1 or 2 cm through the palatine fissure to open into the floor of the nasal cavity. Before opening into the nasal cavity, the duct communicates with the vomeronasal duct and organ.

The oral cavity is continuous caudally with the **isthmus of the fauces** (*Isthmus faucium*), the orifice between the oral cavity and the oral pharynx.

Palate

The **palate** (*palatum*) (Fig. 7.2) is a partly bony, partly membranous partition separating the respiratory and digestive passages of the head. The nasal cavities and nasal pharynx lie above it; the oral cavity and oral pharynx lie below it. The bony hard palate is rostral, and the soft palate caudal. The **hard palate** (*palatum durum*) is formed by processes of the palatine, maxillary, and incisive bones on each side. The mucosa on the nasal side consists of pseudostratified ciliated columnar epithelium; that on the oral side consists of stratified squamous epithelium that is cornified. The hard palate is nearly flat. Laterally and rostrally it inclines slightly ventrally, and it is continuous with the portions of the incisive and maxillary bones that contain the alveoli of the superior teeth. Six to ten ridges (*rugae palatinae*) and depressions cross it transversely on the oral side. Not all of these ridges are complete. In extremely brachycephalic heads they become nearly straight. Close inspection of the ridges reveals small blunt eminences.

The **soft palate** (*palatum molle* or formerly called *velum palatinum*) continues caudally from the hard palate at an irregularly transverse level, passing just caudal to the last superior molar teeth in mesaticephalic heads. In extremely brachycephalic heads the junction of the hard and soft palates is more than 1 cm caudal to this transverse level. The soft palate is particularly long in the dog. In preserved heads the epiglottis is usually seen to lie above the thick caudal border of the soft palate. Occasionally it may lie ventral to the palate or even be recessed in the caudal margin of the soft palate. In brachycephalic breeds the soft palate may be so long as to interfere with the passage of air into the larynx. In the average dog's head the soft palate is 6 cm long, 3 cm wide, and 5 mm thick where it is continuous

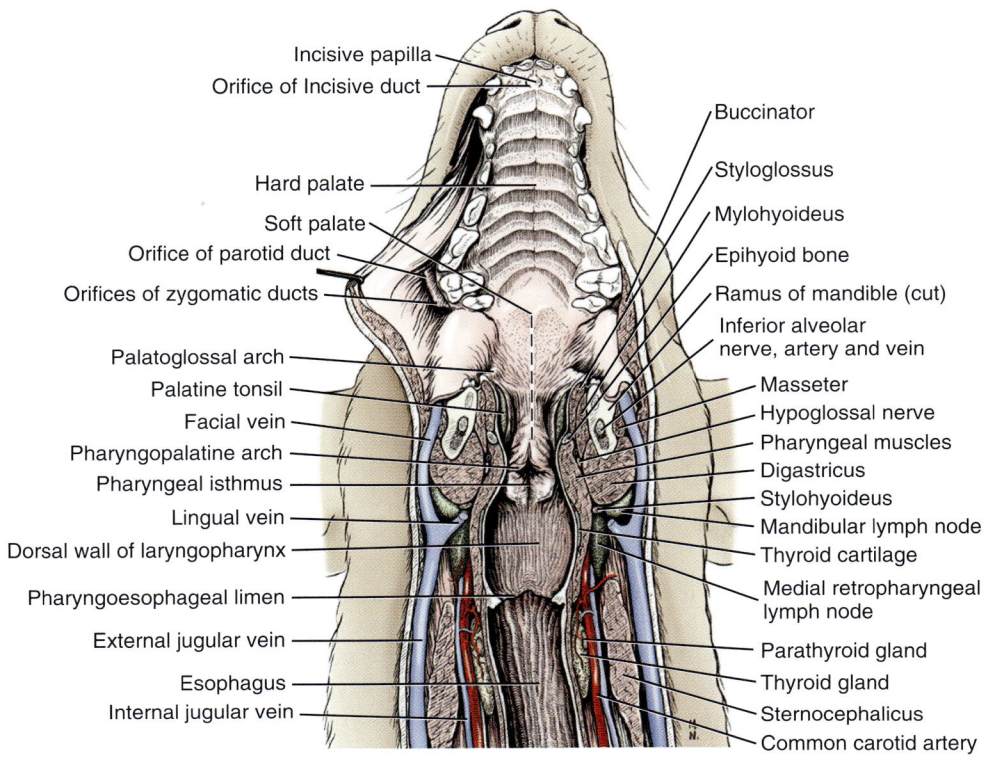

• **Fig. 7.2** Dorsal plane section of head and neck through the digestive tube, ventral aspect.

with the hard palate. The soft palate gradually thickens, so that at the junction of its middle and caudal thirds it is approximately 1 cm thick, after which it becomes slightly thinner and ends caudally in a concave border when viewed dorsoventrally. From its ventrolateral part a thin elliptical fold extends laterally to form the medial and ventral wall of the tonsillar sinus.

Each side the caudal border of the soft palate is continued to the dorsolateral wall by the **palatopharyngeal arch** (*arcus palatopharyngeus*), or caudal pillar of the soft palate. This serves a part of the boundary between the nasal pharynx and the laryngopharynx. The **palatopharyngeal muscle** (*m. palatopharyngeus*) and the mucosa that covers it form this pillar. When the tongue is forcibly withdrawn from the mouth and moved to one side, a **palatoglossal arch** (*arcus palatoglossus*) is developed on the opposite side, running from the body of the tongue to the initial part of the soft palate. This serves as part of the boundary between the oral cavity and the oral pharynx. That portion of the soft palate caudal to a transverse plane through the caudal borders of the pterygoid bones is known as the **palatine veil** (*velum palatinum*). No uvula, a conical projection at the caudal end of the human soft palate, is present on the caudal border of the soft palate.

Structure of the Soft Palate

The soft palate, from the ventral to the dorsal surface, consists of the following layered structures.

Soft Palate Epithelium. Stratified squamous epithelium, a continuation of that of the hard palate, covers the ventral surface of the soft palate. Unless stretched, it is thrown into many fine longitudinal folds and a few larger transverse ones. The mucosal folds are evidence of the mobility and slight elasticity of the soft palate. The stratified squamous epithelium does not end at the caudal border but curves around the border and runs rostrally a few millimeters on the dorsal, respiratory surface. The remainder of the dorsal surface is covered by a pseudostratified ciliated columnar epithelium.

Palatine Glands. The **palatine glands** (*glandulae palatinae*) form the thickest stratum of the organ. They are mixed glands opening on the oral surface of the soft palate by approximately 200 openings per square centimeter rostrally. Caudally the number decreases, but the openings increase in size. Near the caudal margin there are only approximately 10 openings per square centimeter. The region of the palatine glands in the rostral half of the soft palate is approximately 4 mm thick, the glandular layer gradually becoming thicker and then thinner before it ends in the concave caudal border. The stratum formed by the palatine glands is bounded on each side by the large medial pterygoid and the styloglossal muscles.

Palatine Muscles. The muscles of the soft palate consist of the paired **palatine muscles** (*mm. palatini*) and the end ramifications of the paired **tensor** and **levator veli palatini muscles** (Fig. 7.3), which are nearly equal in size. These muscles are described with the muscles of the head. The right and left intrinsic palatine muscles lie close together on each side of the median plane, ventral to the palatine aponeurosis. The end ramifications of the paired extrinsic muscles, the levator and tensor veli palatini, blend with the palatine aponeurosis. The right and left **pterygopharyngeal muscles** pass lateral to the caudal part of the soft palate from origins on the pterygoid bones. Right and left **palatopharyngeal muscles** arise near the median plane from the palatine aponeurosis. They sweep laterally and dorsocaudally in the pharynx, forming the bases for the palatopharyngeal arches.

Palatine Vessels. The right and left **major palatine arteries** (*aa. palatinae majores*) are the main arteries to the hard palate. The main arteries to the soft palate are the **minor palatine arteries** (*aa. palatinae minores*), aided by the **ascending pharyngeal** (*a. pharyngea ascendens*) and the major palatine. They are dwarfed by the **palatine plexus** of veins of the soft palate, which lies mainly lateral to the two slender palatine muscles. The main part of the palatine plexus is located in the deep part of the glandular mantle of the soft palate. It arises from the smaller, less developed venous plexus of the hard palate, which is located in the submucosa covering the bony palate. The lymphatics go to the **medial retropharyngeal lymph nodes**.

Palatine Nerves. The predominant source of sensory innervation to the palate is from branches of the **maxillary nerve** (*n. maxillaris*) from the **trigeminal nerve** (*n. trigeminus*). The major palatine nerve courses through the major palatine canal and supplies sensory fibers to the oral side of the hard palate. The nasal side is supplied by the caudal nasal nerve. The minor palatine nerve supplies the soft palate, which follows the minor palatine artery to enter the rostral end of the soft palate. Branches from the **glossopharyngeal nerve** (*n. glossopharyngeus*) and the **vagus nerve** (*n. vagus*) also enter the soft palate and supply motor innervation to the palatinus, pterygopharyngeal, and palatopharyngeal muscles. The vagus nerves contributes most of the nerve supply to these muscles. The glossopharyngeal nerves supply sensory branches to the lateral walls of the oral pharynx and, to a lesser extent, the soft palate. They are sensory also to the caudal part of the tongue.

Palatine Aponeurosis. The **palatine aponeurosis** (*raphe palati*) consists essentially of the thin, fanned-out terminal tendons of the right and left tensor veli palatini muscles. It is located between the ventral margins of the right and left perpendicular parts of the palatine bones and the pterygoid bones, and attaches rostrally to the caudal margin of the hard palate.

Lying directly dorsal to the palatine aponeurosis are the small mixed dorsal **palatine glands**. The epithelium that covers them, and on which their numerous ducts open, is of the pseudostratified ciliated columnar type. It is continued rostrally on the dorsum of the hard palate to line the nasal pharynx. Caudally before reaching the caudal border of the soft palate, it is continued by stratified squamous epithelium, which is the epithelium of the entire ventral surface of the palate.

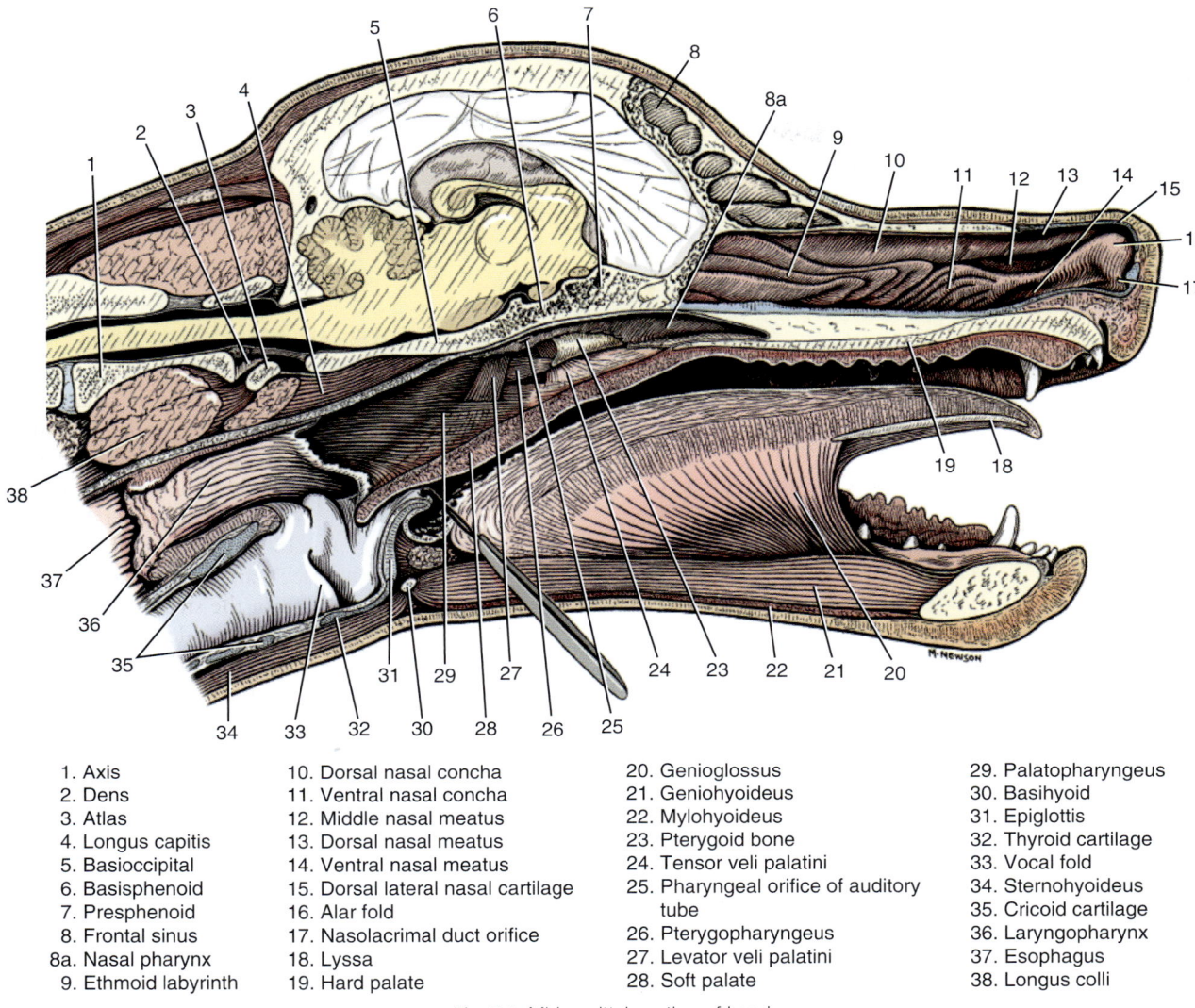

CHAPTER 7 The Digestive Apparatus and Abdomen   323

- Fig. 7.3 Mid-sagittal section of head.

1. Axis
2. Dens
3. Atlas
4. Longus capitis
5. Basioccipital
6. Basisphenoid
7. Presphenoid
8. Frontal sinus
8a. Nasal pharynx
9. Ethmoid labyrinth
10. Dorsal nasal concha
11. Ventral nasal concha
12. Middle nasal meatus
13. Dorsal nasal meatus
14. Ventral nasal meatus
15. Dorsal lateral nasal cartilage
16. Alar fold
17. Nasolacrimal duct orifice
18. Lyssa
19. Hard palate
20. Genioglossus
21. Geniohyoideus
22. Mylohyoideus
23. Pterygoid bone
24. Tensor veli palatini
25. Pharyngeal orifice of auditory tube
26. Pterygopharyngeus
27. Levator veli palatini
28. Soft palate
29. Palatopharyngeus
30. Basihyoid
31. Epiglottis
32. Thyroid cartilage
33. Vocal fold
34. Sternohyoideus
35. Cricoid cartilage
36. Laryngopharynx
37. Esophagus
38. Longus colli

Teeth

The **teeth** (*dentes*) (Fig. 7.4) are highly specialized structures that serve for the procuring, cutting, and crushing of food as well as for social interaction. Each tooth is divided into three parts. The **crown** (*corona dentis*) is the exposed portion of tooth that extends beyond the **gingiva** or "gums" (*gingiva*) and is covered by a thin layer of enamel. This has been defined by the American Veterinary Dental College (https://www.avdc.org/Nomenclature/Nomen-Dental_Anatomy.html) to include an anatomical crown as the part of the tooth that is coronal to the cementoenamel junction, and a clinical crown that is the part of the tooth coronal to the gingival margin. With the exception of the canine teeth, all crowns in the dog end in **cusps** (*apex cuspidis*). The **neck** or cervical region (*cervix dentis*) of the tooth lies at the cementoenamel junction, the interface between the crown and the root. The neck includes the most coronal region of the root and the level of the epithelial attachment of the gingiva. The term,

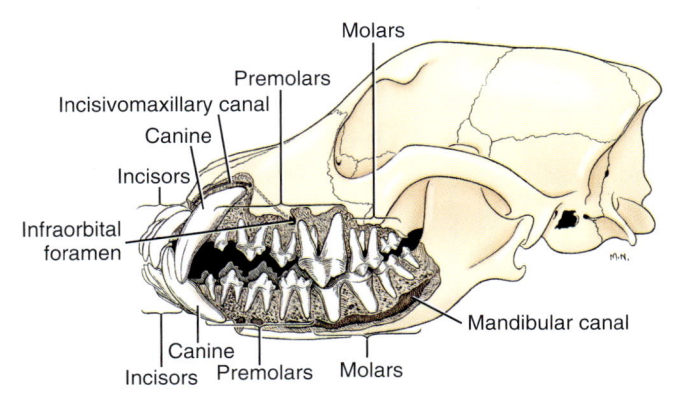

- Fig. 7.4 Jaws and teeth of an adult dog. Lateral view of jaws, sculpted to show tooth roots.

CHAPTER 7 The Digestive Apparatus and Abdomen

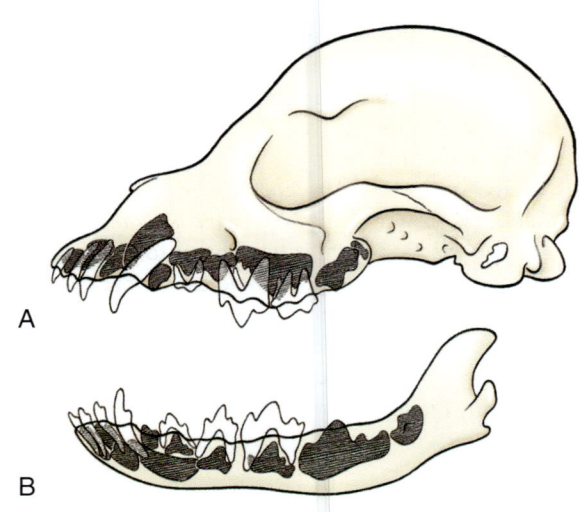

• **Fig. 7.5** The dentition of a Beagle pup at 3 months, 10 days. The seven superior (A) and seven inferior (B) deciduous teeth have erupted. The permanent teeth, none of which have erupted through the gum, are shown cross-hatched. Note there is not a grossly visible tooth germ for the lower third molar.

"enamel bulge" (Fig. 7.7), is a lay term referring to the widening of the tooth at the base of the crown. The **root** (*radix dentis*) is the portion of the tooth located beyond the level of the attached gingiva, embedded in alveolar bone. The root tip is termed the **apex of the root** (*apex radicis dentis*). Many teeth have more than one root. A dog's dentition is diphyodont, meaning there are two sets of teeth that develop sequentially. Once teeth are fully erupted in the dog they achieve adult stature but may continue to undergo developmental changes. For example, secondary dentin deposition continues to occur throughout lifetime. The first set is fully erupted and functional early in the second month after birth (Fig. 7.5). These teeth, known as **deciduous teeth** (*dentis decidui*), serve the animal during its most active puppyhood. Lawson et al. (1967) described the development and eruption of teeth and illustrated several stages by a series of radiographs. They found that eruption of deciduous teeth begins on approximately the twentieth day and is completed by the thirty-fifth day.

Esaka (1982) studied the development of premolar tooth germs and their rotation by means of radiographs, dissections, serial sections, and reconstructions. He found that the direction of rotation of the teeth varied along the dental arch. His accompanying table showed the rotation and contact relationship of permanent tooth germs with deciduous teeth from birth to 6 months. Upon approaching maturity at 6 months of age, when the bones that contain the teeth have become larger, the small deciduous teeth are no longer adequate; they are shed (exfoliated) and replaced by the **permanent teeth** (*dentes permanentes*) (Fig. 7.6), which last throughout adult life. Permanent teeth are larger and stronger than deciduous teeth. As the maxilla and mandible continue to grow over the next two to three months permanent molar teeth erupt caudal to the premolar teeth. There are two molar teeth in each maxilla and three in each mandible. In an experimental study of diet and teeth, Mellanby (1929) began with a detailed review of dental structure in dogs that included the development of the teeth.

Observations on the development of the deciduous teeth in the fetal dog have been reported by Satrapa-Binder (1959), Williams (1961), and Williams and Evans (1978). Postnatal calcification and eruption of the deciduous and permanent teeth have been studied by Meyer (1942),

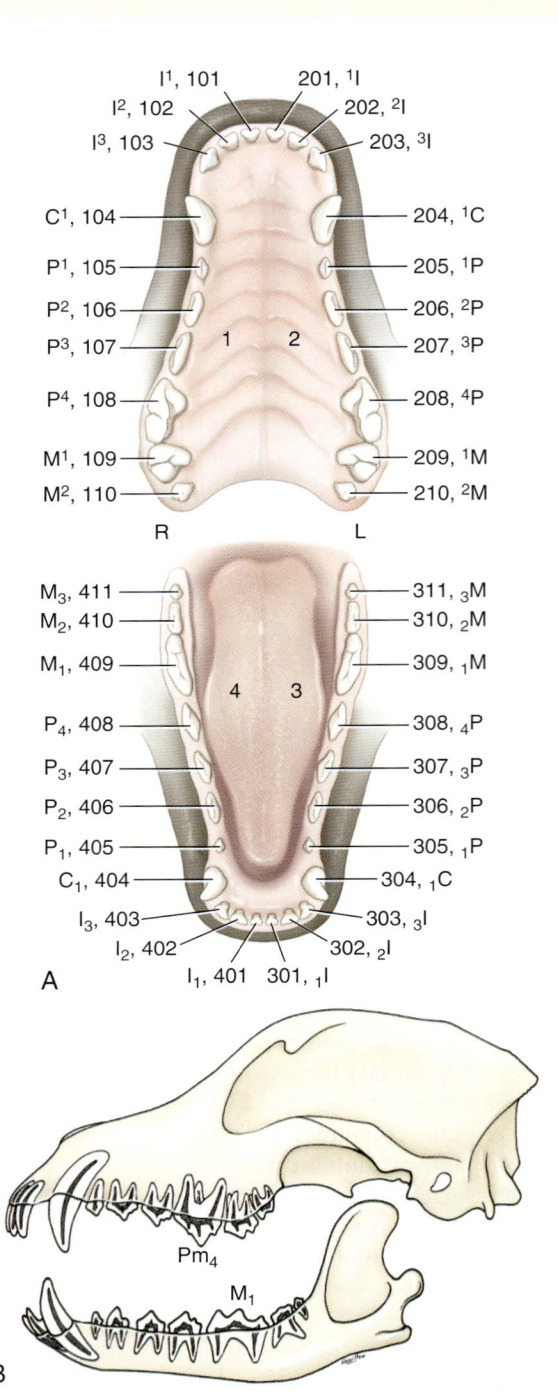

• **Fig. 7.6** A, An open-mouth view of the dog with teeth identified by the anatomic and Modified Triadan System of nomenclature. B, The dentition of an adult Beagle. The teeth were decalcified and sectioned to show the pulp cavity.

Höppner (1956), Arnall (1961), and Kremenak (1967). Cahill and Marks (1982) studied exfoliation of the third deciduous mandibular premolar in mongrels and purebred beagles from the thirteenth to the twenty-seventh postnatal week. They used radiographs and histologic sections to correlate bone, tooth, and soft-tissue events. The timing and sequence were the same in Beagles and mongrels. Eruption of the permanent third premolars began during the sixteenth postnatal week and was completed in 7 weeks.

The central and intermediate deciduous incisors (deciduous i1 and i2) and the canine teeth of both superior and inferior arches have usually erupted by the end of the first month. The corner incisors (i3) erupt during the fifth or sixth week: the deciduous premolars between the fourth and eighth weeks. Most permanent teeth, with the exception of the superior canine teeth, erupt lingual to their deciduous counterparts while the permanent superior fourth premolar erupts buccal to the deciduous fourth premolar. The permanent superior canine teeth erupt mesially relative to their deciduous counterpart. Teeth erupt earliest in the large breeds. Table 7.1 gives the normal range of time for the eruption of each of the permanent teeth, which erupt at approximately the same time in each arch.

Eruption of permanent teeth requires a coordinated resorption and formation of alveolar bone on opposite sides of the developing and erupting tooth. During eruption a pathway is formed by resorption of the overlying bone and deciduous tooth roots. As root formation of the permanent tooth begins there is considerable bone deposition. Although it is known that the presence of a dental follicle is necessary to trigger eruption, the full sequence of dental eruption has yet to be completely understood. Overall, eruption of permanent teeth can vary by a few weeks to a couple of months depending on the breed, nutrition, and systemic health.

Tetracycline antibiotics concentrate in growing bones and teeth and can inhibit bone growth or interfere with enamel formation. Because they fluoresce yellow or orange under ultraviolet light, they have been used to study incremental growth of bones and teeth. Owen (1963) studied the effects of tetracycline ingestion on the teeth of dogs and noted that dentine, cementum, and enamel can all incorporate the fluorescent component. Therefore the use of tetracycline or its derivatives is discouraged in animals younger than 6 months of age.

The teeth are arranged as **superior** (maxillary) and **inferior** (mandibular) **dental arches** (*arcus dentalis superior et inferior*). The inferior arch is anisognathic, narrower and shorter than the superior arch; therefore, superior incisors are located slightly rostral to the inferior incisors. Incisors function mainly to nibble or nip during mastication, grooming, and social interactions. From the superior corner (3rd) incisor to the superior fourth premolar, superior and inferior teeth alternate in position along the dental arch resulting in a scissor-like bite. Canine teeth are used for puncturing and grasping. Stockard (1941) referred to the area between the canine and carnassial teeth as the "premolar carrying space," in reference to hunting breeds. Overlap of the carnassial teeth, the superior fourth premolars, and the inferior first molars allows for optimal shearing of food. Direct occlusal contact of the superior and inferior molars provides for grinding of food (Fig. 7.7A). In dogs, food is mostly swallowed without mastication and complete occlusal contact is not necessary. Wood and Wood (1933) commented on the genetic and phylogenetic significance of a third superior molar in the modern dog.

Tooth Structure

The dense, outer layer of the crown is **enamel** (*enamelum*). It is the hardest substance in the body, being 96% inorganic, composed of millions of crystals of hydroxyapatite. It cannot regenerate when damaged. Enamel is relatively translucent. It is thickest on the occlusal surfaces of the teeth, and its hardness gradually increases in the first year of life. Skobe et al. (1985) studied the ultrastructure of dog enamel and found three layers to be present: a rodless (aprismatic) surface layer, a middle layer of parallel rods that was not constant at all sites, and an inner layer with prominent Hunter-Schreger bands. Enamel rods of the dog tooth, as seen after acid etching of the surface, appear to be primarily hexagonal, although semicircular and spiral shapes are also present. The enamel rod is a column of mineral that extends from the dentinoenamel junction to the coronal surface of the tooth. They are perpendicular to the surface and each rod has two parts: a core of hydroxyapatite and a sheath of organic fibrous substance. A study of dental enamel in dogs was made by Glock et al. (1942).

Dentin (*dentinum*), which is similar to bone in chemical composition, forms the bulk of the tooth and encloses the pulp cavity. It is capable of some regeneration. Odontoblasts of the dentin layer may permit some change throughout the life of a tooth. Dentin consists of horizontal mineralized tubules that are stacked vertically. There are three forms of dentin: all of the dentin present when a tooth erupts is primary dentin, secondary dentin is laid down as the tooth ages, and tertiary or reparative dentin is created in response to wear or damage to the tooth. This latter form of dentin

TABLE 7.1 Eruption of Permanent Teeth

Group	Tooth	Eruption Period
Incisors	Central	2 to 5 months
	Intermediate	2 to 5 months
	Corner	Most breeds 4 or 5 months
Canine		5 or 6 months
Premolars	First	4 or 5 months
	Second	6 months
	Third	6 months
	Fourth	4 or 5 months
Molars	First	5 or 6 months
	Second	6 or 7 months
	Third	6 or 7 months

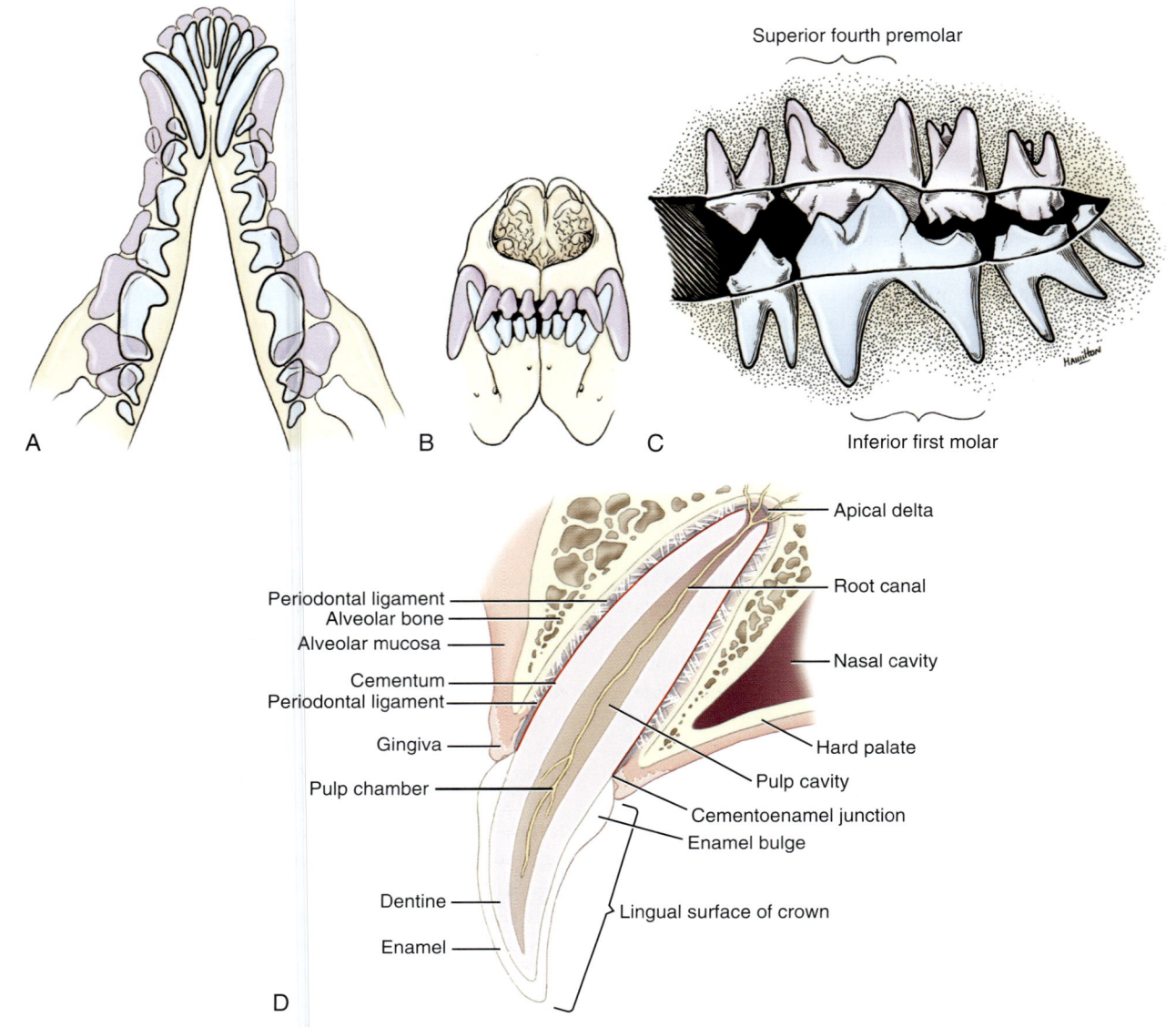

Fig. 7.7 A, Superimposition of superior and inferior dental arches. (Superior teeth in light pink bite lateral to the inferior teeth.) **B,** Bite of the incisor and canine teeth; note that the inferior canine tooth bites rostral to the superior canine. **C,** Bite of the shearing teeth. Medial view, right dentition. **D,** Diagrammatic section through a superior canine of an adult dog. The epithelial attachment is the site where the alveolar mucosa meets the tooth.

is relatively disorganized, and it stains faster than surrounding primary or secondary dentin. Gradual loss of enamel and dentin by wear that may occur in the aged is not accompanied by nociception, as the conducting axons recede or calcify in advance of the wearing surface.

The **cementum** in the dog is a thin covering found only on the roots. Cementum is a calcified tissue that is relatively less durable than either enamel or dentin. It is produced throughout life and its collagen fibers are interwoven with the connective tissue of the surrounding periodontal ligament. Grossly, the cementum cannot be differentiated from the dentin it covers. Cementum is largely void of cells, having an acellular region and a cellular region. The cementoblast cells (the resident stem cells within the cellular part of cementum) lie within lacunae, similar to the positioning of osteoblasts within bony lacunae (Kumar, 2015). The cementum provides anchorage for the periodontal ligament on the root.

The **pulp** (*pulpa dentis*), is soft tissue contained in a tooth (see Fig. 7.7). It is composed of sensory nerves, arteries, veins, lymphatic capillaries, and a connective tissue that holds those structures together. The pulp is contained in the **pulp cavity** (*cavum dentis*) The portion of the pulp cavity that is within the crown is the **pulp chamber** (*cavum coronale dentis*). That portion of the pulp chamber that is within the tooth root is the **root canal**. An **apical delta** (*foramen apices dentis*) at the apex of each root consists of multiple small channels, thus the name "delta," that allow free passage of the vessels and nerves in and out of the **root canal** (*canalis radicis dentis*).

Tooth Surfaces

The surface of the tooth that faces the lip or cheek is the **vestibular surface** (*facies vestibularis*), formerly called *labial* or *buccal surface*, and the surface that faces the tongue is the **lingual surface** (*facies lingualis*). The surface adjacent to the next tooth in the dental arch is the **contact surface** (*facies contactus*). For all teeth the contact surfaces are mesial and distal. The **mesial surface** is the contact surface adjacent to the next rostral or medial tooth, and the **distal surface** is the contact surface adjacent to the next caudal or lateral tooth. The surface that faces the ipsilateral opposite superior or inferior dental arch is the **occlusal surface** (*facies occlusalis*). In addition, direction along a tooth is indicated by the terms **coronal**, toward the crown, and **apical**, toward the apex of the root.

Tooth Groupings

The superior teeth are attached in the alveoli of the incisive and maxillary bones. Those with roots embedded in the incisive bones are the **incisor teeth** (*dentes incisivi*). The incisor tooth nearest the midplane on each side in each incisive bone is incisor 1, the central incisor. The second is incisor 2, the intermediate incisor, and the third is incisor 3, the corner incisor. They are long slender teeth, arched slightly rostral and laterally compressed. Superior incisors increase in size from the central to the corner incisor. The crowns of the superior corner incisors are largest and slightly hooked caudally with its conformation more anatomically similar to a small canine tooth. The superior central and intermediate incisors have three cusps each. Of the three incisal cusps, the central one is largest and extends farthest coronally; the small mesial and distal cusps have been called *mamelons* (a term more commonly used in newly erupted human incisors), and a V-shaped ridge of crown with its apex nearest the gingiva, connects the side cusps on the lingual surface. The lingual crown enlargement at the most apical aspect of the superior central and middle crowns is termed the **cingulum**, and when the mouth is closed the inferior incisor occlusal surfaces rest on the cingulum. Inferior incisors are similar in size and shape to the superior central and intermediate incisors. Depending on the occlusion and chewing habits of the dog, the cusps and crown (particularly the incisive margins (*Margo incisalis*) may slowly wear throughout life. The **canine teeth** (*dentes canini*) are separated from the corner superior incisors by an interdental space matching the width of the inferior canine tooth (approximately 4 to 10 mm) and from the corner inferior incisors by a space of roughly 1 to 3 mm. The canine teeth are by far the longest teeth in the dog having large roots that are nearly two times as long as their crowns. All four canine teeth are similar in length and width. They are transversely compressed with an oval cross-section. When the mouth is closed, the crown of the inferior canine tooth occupies the interdental space between the superior corner incisor and the superior canine tooth (Fig. 7.7B). The superior roots produce an arciform alveolar juga and all four canine roots are located adjacent to the root apices of the first and second premolar teeth. Canine tooth roots are slightly wider in the midalveolar region and taper down to a rounded apex. Whereas the superior canine tooth root runs parallel to the maxillary bone, the inferior canine tooth root crosses the width of the rostral mandible making extraction challenging. The size, shape, and course of canine tooth roots necessitate a surgical approach for extraction unless significant alveolar bone loss has occurred. Lorber et al. (1979) found differences between male and female canine teeth in the dog. In the male, crowns were 23% longer, and roots were 40% longer than in females. Likewise, in the male, the width of the crown of the canine tooth was 26% wider, and the width of the root was 50% wider. The smaller crown-to-root ratio in males, together with greater root width, indicated to the authors a difference in the tooth anchorage mechanism. All teeth caudal to the canines are often referred to as the *cheek teeth* (St. Clair & Jones, 1957). They are divided into premolars and molars. In the permanent dentition, there are four **premolar teeth** (*dentes premolares*) in each of the four dental quadrants. There are no deciduous first premolar or molar teeth. The first premolar erupts between the fourth and fifth postnatal month and usually remains throughout life. The placement of the premolar teeth may be altered by changing the shape of the head through selective breeding, but regardless of head shape the teeth remain relatively constant in form and size (Stockard, 1941). This leads to tooth crowding in smaller breeds, which predisposes them to periodontal disease. The first premolar is the smallest, and has a single root. The fourth premolar is the largest. In the superior dental arch, it has three roots—mesiobuccal (also called *mesiovestibular*), mesiolingual, and distal—and in the inferior arch only two roots—mesial and distal. The second and the third premolar teeth are similar in all quadrants. Each premolar has two roots, mesial and distal. The crowns of the first three premolar teeth are similar in all quadrants. All three have a singular pyramidal shape. The first premolar tooth has one cusp. The second and third premolars have similar crowns with an additional small cusp on the distal aspect. The enamel bulge at the neck of the tooth is more prominent on the lingual surface (Fig. 7.7). On each tooth the mesial border slopes slightly distal. The distal border of the largest cusp is steep. Adjacent to the base of the main cusp on this border is a second smaller cusp 1 or 2 mm high. The most distal surface of the crowns of the second and third premolars can be irregular with additional small cusps located in this region.

The superior fourth premolars and the inferior first molars are the largest shearing teeth in the mouth. They are the **carnassial** or **sectorial teeth** (*dens sectorius*) (Fig. 7.7C). The superior fourth premolar teeth have three stout diverging roots. The mesiobuccal and mesiolingual roots are more slender than the wide distal root. The space between all roots is referred to as the **furcation**, which is normally filled with interradicular bone. The mesiobuccal and distal roots form prominent alveolar juga that end just ventral to the ventral border of the infraorbital canals. The distal root of each superior fourth premolar tooth is triangular and somewhat transversely flattened, becoming wide at the neck. The mesiolingual root is flattened in an oblique plane; a small cusp extends lingually off the mesial developmental ridge of the crown indicating the position of this root. A developmental groove separates the largest mesial cusp from a more prominent distal cusp.

The **molar teeth** (*dentes molares*) have no deciduous predecessors. There are two in each superior quadrant and three in each inferior quadrant. In each quadrant the first are the largest and the last are the smallest. The masticatory surfaces of the superior molars have multiple cusps at two levels. The buccal (vestibular) cusps are higher than the low lingual cusp. The occlusal surfaces of the superior molar teeth are irregularly flattened and make occlusal contact with the last two inferior molars and the distal third of the first inferior molar. The inferior molars are also have multiple cusps.

Each superior molar tooth has three slightly diverging roots. The lingual root of each of these teeth is more massive than either of the two vestibular roots, although it is shorter. It is slightly compressed rostrocaudally and is so shaped that the greatest compression force is transmitted through it to the compact bone that lies adjacent to the neck of the tooth.

The inferior first molar tooth is greater than twice the size of the second and third molar teeth. The distal third of the first molar inferior teeth is adapted for crushing and grinding; the mesial portion is sharp and pointed, and is well-suited for shearing. The shearing portion of each inferior first molar possesses the largest cusp of any inferior cheek teeth and it is roughly quadrilateral in form. A small indentation formed in the hard palate mucosa slightly lingual to the midportion of the superior fourth premolar tooth receives the coronal tip of this large cusp when the mouth is closed. For a discussion of the terminology used for tooth cusps and crests, see Szalay (1969) and Every (1972, 1974). Szalay uses a modified Cope-Osborn terminology for mammalian tritubercular cusps and crests, whereas Every proposes a new term for each. We have used the word "cusp" instead of tubercle in our description of teeth, following Constantinescu and Schaller (2012) and the Nomina Anatomica Veterinaria (2017). The terms "tubercle" is used in description of some bovid incisors and is likely a relict of "tritubercular nomenclature" initially proposed for the evolution of mammalian teeth (for an early review, see Gregory, 1934).

Dental Formulae

Because teeth are grouped according to position and form, it is possible to express their arrangement as a dental formula. The abbreviation representing the particular teeth (incisor [I], canine [C], premolar [PM], molar [M]) is followed by the number of such teeth on one side of the superior and inferior arches.

The formula for the **deciduous dentition** of the dog (see Fig. 7.5) is:

$$I3/3 C1/1 PM3/3 \times 2 = 28$$

The key to understanding deciduous teeth is twofold. First, as mentioned previously, there are no deciduous first premolar and any molar teeth. Second, the deciduous premolar teeth take on the crown shape of the distally adjacent permanent tooth. The deciduous fourth premolar crown mimics the shape of the permanent first molar, and the deciduous third premolar crown mimics the shape of the permanent fourth premolar.

The formula for the **permanent dentition** of the dog (see Fig. 7.6) is:

$$I3/3 C1/1 PM4/4 M2/3 \times 2 = 42$$

A formula for remembering the number of roots of the cheek teeth (premolars and molars) is useful for dental applications.

Superior cheek teeth   1,2,2,3,3,3
Inferior cheek teeth   1,2,2,2,2,2,1

Dental Nomenclature

Veterinary dentists require a user-friendly numbering system to identify teeth to facilitate clinical diagnosis, monitoring of therapy, computer record keeping, and transmittal of information for referrals or publication. A human system uses two digits to identify the dentition, dental arch, quadrant, and tooth. A similar system for domestic animals requires three digits because of their increased number of teeth.

The first digit identifies the kind of dentition (deciduous or permanent) and the quadrant of the dental arch where the tooth is located (superior or inferior). The American Veterinary Dental College uses the terms "maxillary" or "mandibular" for superior and inferior, respectively (American Veterinary Dental College web site: https://www.avdc.org/Nomenclature/Nomen-Dental_Anatomy.html). Other references will use "upper" and "lower" to good effect (Singh, 2017).

Numbers 1 to 4 indicate permanent teeth, with 1 referring to the superior right quadrant, 2 for the superior left quadrant, 3 for the inferior left quadrant, and 4 for the inferior right quadrant.

In a similar fashion 5 to 8 are used for the deciduous teeth.

The second and third digits identify the specific tooth. Numbering is consecutive and starts with the most mesial tooth (incisor 1) and progresses distally to the last cheek tooth. Where a tooth did not develop, that number is deleted. In domestic animals the pig has more teeth (relative to dogs) and thus uses all of the designated numbers. This system is referred to as the *Modified Triadan System*. For example, in the dog, the permanent superior right canine is tooth 104, the permanent superior left second molar is tooth 210, the inferior left first premolar is 305, and the inferior right third molar is 411 (see Fig. 7.6A).

De Forge and Colmery (2008) in *An Atlas of Veterinary Dental Radiology* provide an extensive glossary of dental and anatomic terms borrowed from the human literature. In the appendix, there is a description and rationalization for a Modified Triadan System of Dental Nomenclature proposed by Professor Triadan in 1972 for human teeth. Included is a reprinted article from the *Journal of Veterinary Dentistry* by Michael Floyd, who explains how this system has been modified for use with domestic animals (1991).

Dental Anomalies

Deviations from the normal number or placement of the teeth are the most common dental anomalies reported in all dogs and are most frequent in brachycephalic breeds. As the muzzle is shortened, deviation in placement and number of the teeth results. The size of the teeth does not decrease proportionately with a reduction in the length or width of the bones containing them (Stockard, 1941). The result is crowded large teeth in small mouths predisposing toy breeds and breeds smaller than 20 pounds to a higher incidence of periodontal disease.

Supernumerary teeth are occasionally found in all breeds. Dole and Spurgeon (1998) reported supernumerary teeth in 20 of 55 Greyhounds. Extra incisors and premolars are most common. Supernumerary first premolars are foremost among the premolars, and supernumerary incisors can be located within the dental arch or lingual/vestibular to the arch. Supernumerary teeth are usually unilateral and occur in the superior arcade more frequently than in the inferior arch.

The third superior premolar is most prone to development of a supernumerary root, and it is the first tooth to rotate as the muzzle is shortened by selective breeding. Later, all superior premolars may be rotated. The second and third premolars may rotate either clockwise or counterclockwise, although rotation that brings their rostral roots nearer the median plane is more common. Little additional room is gained by rotation of the first premolar because its width nearly equals its length. The molar teeth seem to be little affected by rotation. All anomalous placements of teeth are more common in the superior than in the inferior dental arch.

Partially erupted or deformed teeth are seen occasionally in all animals. Schamberger et al. (2010) described a young dog with a partially erupted, malformed superior canine tooth having clinical, radiographic, and histologic features of odontodysplasia. These teeth are often reduced in size, discolored, and rough. Surgical extraction may be indicated although resorption along the alveolar margin is a likely consequence. For terms used in dental studies, see Heasman and McCracken (2007) "Dental Dictionary." For a retrospective review of developmental dental defects, see Boy et al. (2016).

Periodontium

The **periodontium** (Fig. 7.7D) is a term used to designate the supporting tissues of the teeth. These include the **cementum** on the root, the **alveolar bone** of the socket, and the **periodontal ligament** or **periodontal membrane** (*Periodontium*), which connects the two across the periodontal space. The periodontal ligament is composed of collagenous and elastic connective tissue and contains blood vessels, lymphatics and nerves. Thus, the tooth is anchored by a cushion of tissues, which allows for limited movement of teeth during mastication.

Gingiva

The **gingiva,** also called the *gums* (*gingivae*), surround the teeth and are composed of dense fibrous tissue covered by smooth, richly vascularized mucosae. They bleed readily and heal quickly. Gingiva are thick around the necks of the teeth and extend down into the alveoli to be continuous with the alveolar periosteum. The labial surface of the alveolar mucosa is continuous with the mucosa of the vestibule. The gingiva and the alveolar mucosa are separated by the mucogingival junction, which is a clinically discernible line. The mucogingival junction is clinically relevant because it is often where draining tracts of odontogenic origin are found. Internally the gingivae blend with the floor of the oral cavity proper and the hard palate. In those breeds with pigmented mucosae the gingivae are likewise pigmented.

Comprehensive accounts concerning the anatomy, pathologic characteristics, and surgery of oral structures and teeth can be found in the older literature by Staple (1964–1966) and Miles (1967). More recent veterinary literature includes books by Holmstrom et al. (1992), Emily and Penman (1994), Wiggs and Lobprise (1997), Kessel (2000), Holmstrom et al. (2004), Gorrel and Derbyshire (2005), Gorrel (2004, 2008), DuPont and DeBowes (2008), and Verstraete and Lommer (2012). Special mention should be made of the well-illustrated manual of the British Small Animal Veterinary Association entitled *Canine and Feline Dentistry*, by Tutt, Deeprose, and Crossley (2007).

Tongue

The **tongue** (*lingua*), composed primarily of skeletal muscle, appears embryologically as a mesodermal swelling on the floor of the stomodeum and rostral foregut, overlying the first, second, and third branchial arches. There are two **lateral swellings** (*tuberculum linguale laterale*), one **median tongue bud** (*tuberculum lingulae medium*), and one **median proximal swelling** (*tuberculum linguale proximale [copula]*) immediately caudal to the median tongue bud (Fig. 7.8). These muscular swellings arise partly as a result of cellular migration from three occipital myotomes. Migrating cells form a condensation in the vicinity of the developing root fibers of the hypoglossal nerve, which innervates the glossal musculature. This glossal muscle mass contributes most of the intrinsic and extrinsic lingual musculature by a ventrorostral migration into the floor of the foregut.

The tongue is an organ of prehension, important for moving food boluses within the mouth and for moving water or other liquids from an external source through the oral cavity and to the esophagus. This can be a physical challenge given that a standing dog propels liquids vertically

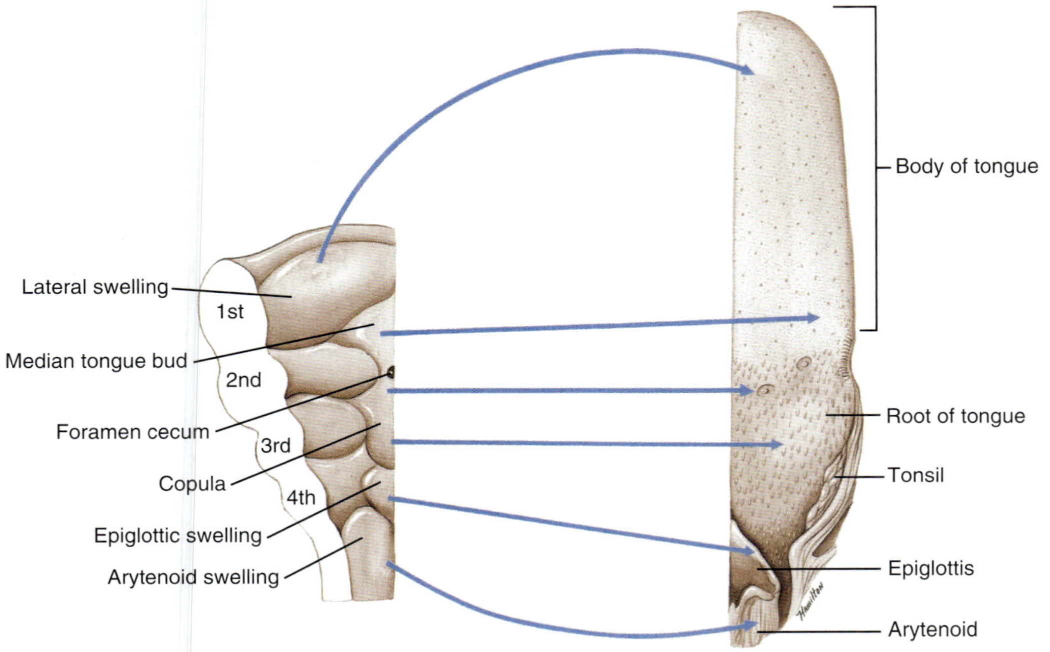

• Fig. 7.8 Parts of the tongue and their origin from structures on the floor of the pharynx.

within the oral cavity. A number of studies have elucidated tongue function during intraoral transport in adult as well as in suckling neonates (for pigs: Thexton et al., 1998; for dogs: Crompton & Musinsky, 2011; Gart et al., 2015).

Part of the lingual musculature seems to develop in situ from the mesodermal swelling on the floor of the stomodeum. This view is supported by experimental results in the dog tongue that indicate that some facial motor neurons assist in the innervation of lingual musculature. Although the number of facial motor neurons involved is minimal when compared with the overwhelming contribution from the hypoglossal nerve, the finding supports a dual origin of the lingual musculature: in situ and occipital myotomic origins. The dual origin of lingual musculature has for a long time been a subject of much debate (Bates, 1948; Kingsbury, 1926; Langman, 1975). Doran (1975) has reviewed the evolution and phylogeny of the mammalian tongue and Baggett et al. (1971) considered the structure and functional classification of mammalian tongues. Bennett and Ramsay (1941) studied movements of the split tongue in the dog.

The tongue has a **body** (*corpus linguae*) and a **root** (*radix linguae*) separated by a row of **vallate papillae** (*papillae vallatae*) arranged in the form of a V. The rostral two-thirds of the tongue (body) is covered by the mucous membrane derived from ectodermal epithelium of the stomodeum. This portion of lingual epithelium receives sensory innervation from the lingual nerve branch of the mandibular nerve from the trigeminal nerve (V) for nociception, temperature, and touch sensations, and from the chorda tympani, a branch of the facial nerve (VII), for taste (Chibuzo et al., 1980). There is no visible foramen cecum or sulcus terminalis, the site of origin of the thyroid gland. The mucous membrane, covering the root of the tongue, is derived from the endoderm of the foregut and receives its sensory innervations from the glossopharyngeal nerve (IX) for all sensations, including taste. Developmentally, these cranial nerves are associated with structures on sequential branchial arches: hence the trigeminal nerve (V) is the nerve of the first (mandibular) arch, the facial (VII) is the nerve of the second (hyoid) arch, the glossopharyngeal (IX) is the nerve of the third arch, and the pharyngeal branch of the vagus nerve (X) is the nerve of the fourth arch. The hypoglossal nerve (XII) to the musculature of tongue was developmentally associated with occipital myotomes. Because these cranial nerves also supply different parts of the tongue, they reflect the embryologic origin of the tongue and other lingual structures that they innervate.

The tongue of an adult dog (Fig. 7.9) is an elongated, mobile, muscular organ covered by cornified stratified squamous epithelium. It extends from its attachment on the basihyoid bone to its free tip, the **apex** (*apex linguae*) at the intermandibular articulation. The dorsal surface of the tongue (*dorsum linguae*), unlike the ventral surface (*facies ventralis linguae*), is very rough owing to the presence of five types of cornified lingual papillae: filiform, fungiform, vallate, foliate, and conical papillae. The dorsum linguae is divided into two lateral halves by a **median groove** (*sulcus medianus linguae*) that extends from the apex of the tongue to the level of the caudal pair of the vallate papillae.

The **margin of the tongue** (*margo linguae*) separates the dorsal and ventral surfaces. The two margins meet rostrally in the formation of the **apex**, the thinnest and narrowest end of this muscular organ. Caudal to the apex, the tongue widens and gradually increases in thickness as more intrinsic and extrinsic lingual muscles are incorporated into the body of the tongue. The body is long and slender and lies between the apex and the root of the tongue. The root is the caudal one-third that bears conical, vallate, and foliate papillae (Figs. 7.9 through 7.13).

Filiform and fungiform papillae are located together on the ectodermally derived mucous membrane of the oral portion or body of the tongue, whereas the foliate, vallate, and conical papillae are located on the endodermally derived mucous membrane of the caudal one-third, or pharyngeal part, the root, of the tongue. These two zones are demarcated in the fetus by the terminal sulcus. In the fetus it forms the rostral border of the V-shaped arrangement of the vallate papillae.

The **lingual mucosa** (*tunica mucosa linguae*) is thick and heavily cornified on the dorsal surface of the tongue but thin and less cornified on the ventral surface. It is composed of stratified squamous epithelium and a dermis of connective tissue. This mucosa forms papillae on the dorsum of the tongue. On the ventral surface of the tongue it forms an unpaired, median mucosal fold, the **lingual frenulum** (*frenulum linguae*), which primarily connects the body of the tongue to the floor of the mouth.

Filiform Papillae

The **filiform papillae** (*papillae filiformes*) are the smallest in size and the most numerous of all lingual papillae. Like the **fungiform papillae**, they are located on the dorsum of the rostral two-thirds (the body) of the tongue. Rarely do

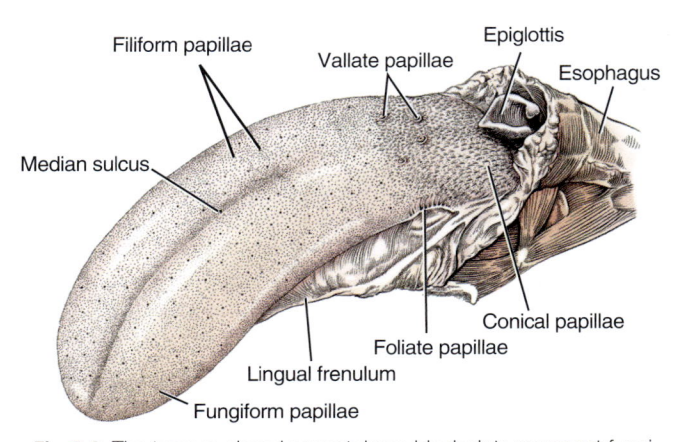

• **Fig. 7.9** The tongue, dorsal aspect: large black dots represent fungiform papillae; finer dots represent filiform papillae.

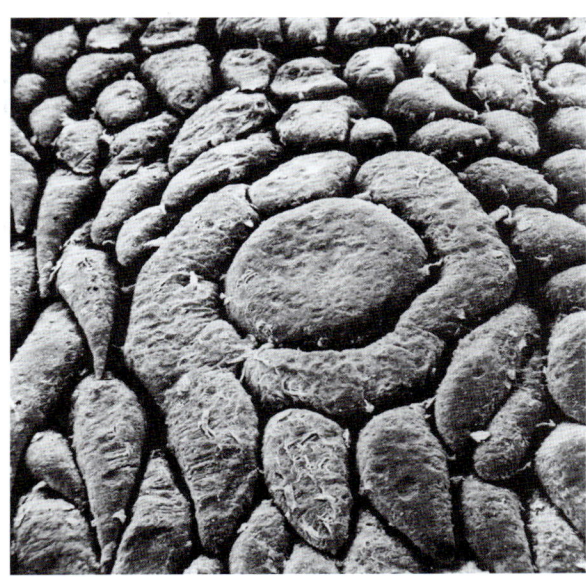

• **Fig. 7.11** Vallate papilla of a puppy. (Reproduced from Beidler LM: In Pfaffmann C, editors, *Olfaction and taste III*, New York, 1969, Rockefeller University Press. By copyright permission of the Rockefeller University Press.)

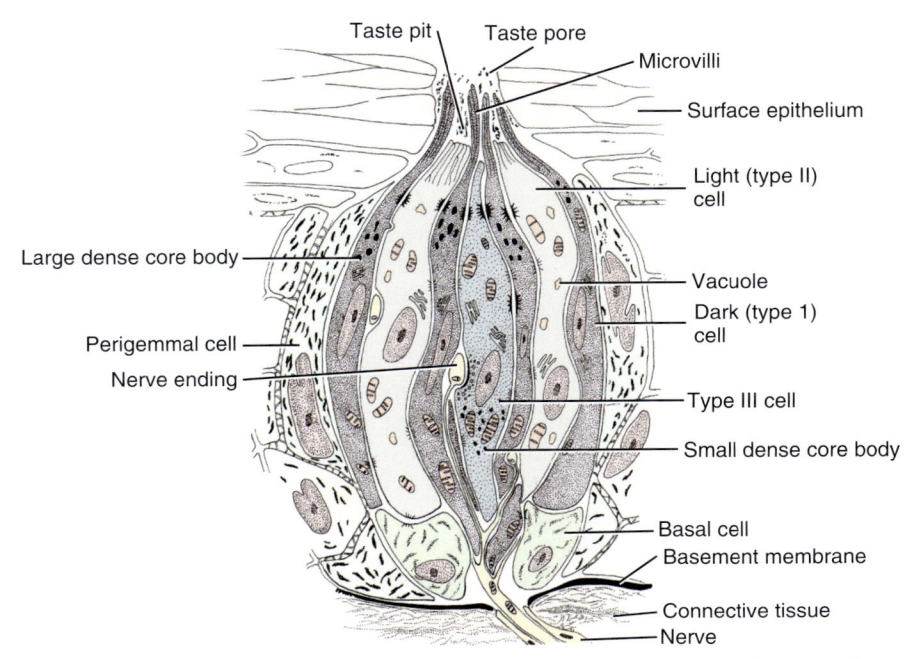

• **Fig. 7.10** Schematic longitudinal section of a taste bud. Electron microscopic composite.

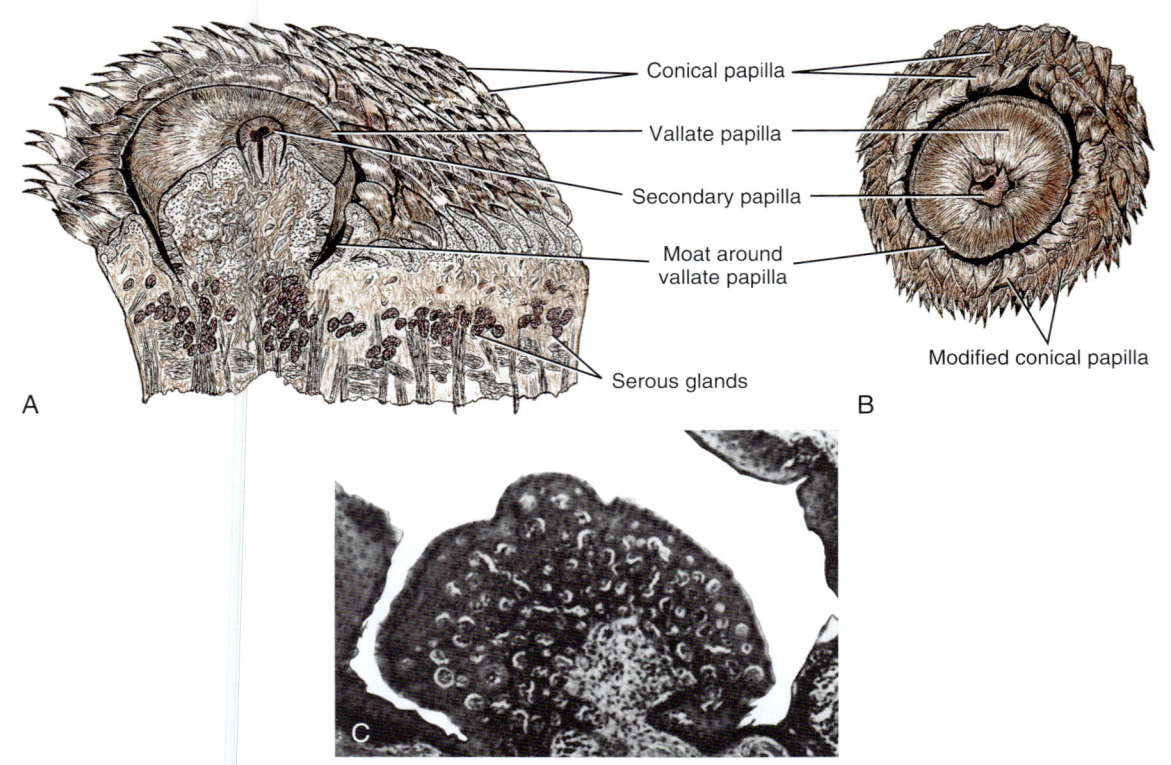

• **Fig. 7.12** Vallate papilla. **A**, Longitudinal section. **B**, Dorsal view. **C**, Tangential section.

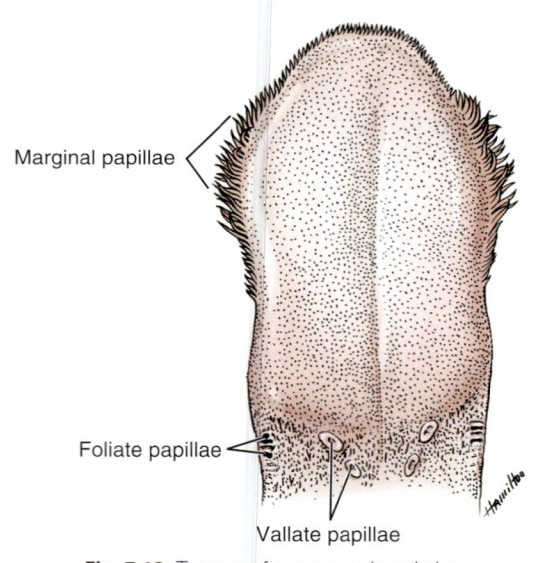

• **Fig. 7.13** Tongue of a puppy, dorsal view.

they extend caudal to the level of the vallate papillae. Filiform papillae are not threadlike, as the name implies, but rather each papilla is a complex of primary, secondary, and tertiary serrations. Each complex has a broad base with a dermal core. The dermal core forms the axis of the centrally placed single primary filiform papilla. Each secondary filiform papilla of each complex arises from the basal end of the primary and, like the latter, has a dermal core branching directly off the base of the primary basal core. There are generally four to six secondary filiform papillae around the base of the centrally placed primary filiform papilla. Generally, tertiary filiform papillae arise from the secondary. They are smaller than the secondary papillae and lack dermal cores. They are, therefore, totally made up of epithelial tissue.

These filiform papillae are inclined so that their tips point caudally. The surfaces of these papillae are well cornified to aid in licking and to protect deeper structures from injury. The cornification is greatest at the apex of the primary and secondary filiform serrations and least at their bases, which are bathed in a film of saliva and less exposed to wear. The tertiary filiform serrations, on the other hand, are completely cornified.

It is through the dermal cores (which are absent in the tertiary serrations) that the blood vessels and nerves reach these papillae. Only the lingual nerve, a branch of the mandibular nerve from the trigeminal nerve, innervates the filiform papillae, unlike the fungiform papillae, which receive a dual innervation from both the lingual nerve and the chorda tympani, a branch of the facial nerve (Cheal & Oakley, 1977; Miller, 1974).

Generally, 8 to 10 filiform papilla complexes are spaced around a single fungiform papilla. This arrangement creates a depression containing a fungiform papilla central to a circular arrangement of 8 to 10 taller filiform papilla complexes. The significance of this arrangement is explained later.

Fungiform Papillae

The **fungiform papillae** (*papillae fungiformes*) are mushroom-shaped papillae on the rostral two-thirds of the tongue, among the rougher, more numerous filiform papillae. Occasionally, some are found caudal to the vallate papillae. They are the second most numerous lingual papillae and are most concentrated at the apex and sides of the tongue. The fungiform papillae in these locations are smaller in size than those elsewhere on the tongue. The median sulcus is devoid of fungiform papillae.

Fungiform papillae are shorter, broader, and less numerous than filiform papillae. Though their surfaces are covered by cornified, stratified squamous epithelium, the cornification is much thinner than that in the filiform papillae. Each fungiform papilla has a proximal narrow base and an expanded distal end. The base may bear spinous cornified projections on only one side. Because the fungiform papillae are very thinly cornified but very well vascularized, the blood they contain gives them a dark pink appearance in the living state, making them prominent among the taller filiform papillae.

A scanning electron microscopic study of fungiform papillae shows that some of them contain taste pores (*porus gustatorius*) on their expanded surfaces. These are openings in the epithelium at the tip of **taste buds** (*caliculus gustatorius*) (Fig. 7.10). As many as eight taste pores have been seen on some papillae, but some contain no taste pores. These taste pores open in the form of a rounded crater fringed by a thin shelf of cornified epithelium. The rim of each fungiform taste pore is often slightly elevated above the surrounding surface of the papilla. At the center of this rim is a depression that contains numerous microvilli on the apices of gustatory cells that stand out distinctly at high magnifications. It is through these pores that oral fluids reach the taste buds. The depression created by the tall filiform papillae surrounding each short fungiform papilla tends to provide an environment for an adherent pool of oral fluid around the fungiform papillae and the associated taste pores.

A sagittal section of a fungiform papilla reveals a centrally located primary dermal core. Secondary dermal cores branch out from the primary core. Some of these secondary dermal cores border the taste buds that are located on the dorsal surface of the tongue and contact the oral cavity through the microvilli projecting into the taste pores. Each taste bud passes through the total thickness of epithelium and rests on a secondary dermal papilla. Except where taste pores exist, tight junctions prevent penetration of fluids through the lingual epithelium (Holland et al., 1989). It is through the secondary dermal cores that nerves reach the taste buds and the adjacent epithelium. Some fungiform papillae do not contain any taste buds. The fungiform papillae receive innervation from two sources: the chorda tympani to the taste buds and the lingual nerve to the epithelium of the papillae (Ferrell, 1984; Miller, 1974). The terminal ends of taste nerves are nonmyelinated. The dermal cores also offer passage for the blood vessels. The chorda tympani also supplies mechanoreceptors and thermal receptors to the rostral two-thirds of the tongue.

Vallate Papillae

In the dog, the **vallate papillae** (*papillae vallatae*) (Fig. 7.9) are located on the caudal third of the dorsum of the tongue. They mark the boundary between the filiform papillae of the oral part and the conical papillae of the pharyngeal part of the tongue. Like the foliate papillae, they are endodermal in origin. Usually there are three to six vallate papillae in the dog, most commonly four. Whenever an even number (four or six) are present, they are arranged in the form of a V evenly located on both sides of the sulcus medianus linguae. The point of the V is always directed caudally. When there is an odd number (three or five), they are asymmetrically arranged. When asymmetrical, the V arrangement is absent because the dog, unlike humans, does not have a median vallate papilla.

Each papilla may be simple or complex. The simple types are more prevalent in the even-numbered arrangement, whereas the complex types are seen more often in the odd-numbered arrangement. On the average, the diameter of vallate papillae is 1.5 to 2.5 mm. A simple vallate papilla (Fig. 7.11) has a deep moat around it. This moat, in the dog, is deficient on one side, and hence the old term *circumvallate* is not applicable. The dorsal surface of each papilla contains a central depression through which projects a secondary papilla (Fig. 7.12A and B), the significance of which is not known. This arrangement creates a complete central moat around the secondary papilla. In scanning micrographs the exposed surface of some of the secondary papilla flares, displaying a rim around a central convexity. Although this central elevation does not show a pit, it obviously is very uneven, being peppered with numerous tiny projections. A simple vallate papilla, therefore, has two moats. The central moat within the papilla itself is complete and surrounds the secondary papilla. The outer moat, which is external to the papilla, is incomplete as it surrounds the vallate papilla. The wall of the outer moat is formed by modified conical papillae arranged side by side in a closely packed manner around the vallate papilla.

Although the vallate papillae and, occasionally, the walls of their moats contain taste buds, the secondary papillae contain none. The connective tissue core (the dermal papilla) forms secondary dermal papillae only on the dorsal half of the vallate papilla. Most taste buds are located ventral to the level of the secondary dermal papillae on the epithelium of the basal half of the papillae. A tangential section that cuts only the epithelium of the vallate papilla contains 6 to 12 vertical rows of taste buds (Fig. 7.12C). Each row circles the papilla with taste buds. The number of taste buds per vallate papilla varies greatly. It is through the dermal papillae that blood vessels and nerves, which are terminal branches of the glossopharyngeal nerve, reach the taste buds.

Complex vallate papillae occur occasionally, and, when present, are generally on the side of the tongue with the least number of vallate papillae. Like the simple one, a complex vallate papilla has an outer moat. However, there are two to four individual simple vallate papillae inside this common outer moat. Each papilla of this complex resembles the simple type in every manner, including taste bud distribution. A central moat surrounds the secondary taste bud–free papilla of each member of the component vallate papilla.

Serous gustatory glands (*glandulae gustatoriae*), or von Ebner's glands, exist at the base of the vallate papillae. They empty their secretions into the bottom of the moat. Associated with the ducts of these glands are lymphatic aggregates.

Foliate Papillae

There are two groups of **foliate papillae** (*papillae foliatae*) in the dog. They are covered by cornified, stratified squamous epithelium. Each group is located on the dorsolateral aspect of the caudal third of the tongue immediately rostral to the palatoglossal arch. Such a group contains 8 to 13 papillae, alternating with 9 to 14 crypts that parallel the papillae and separate them from one another in a leaflike arrangement. The long axes of these papillae (except the most central one) run obliquely from the side of the tongue toward the dorsum of the tongue in a radiating manner. The papillae, rostral and caudal to the central ones, spread out dorsally. The narrower ventrolateral end of this arrangement converges in an epithelial elevation. The oral fluids that drain out of the crypts are temporarily retarded by this elevation. The crypts are deepest and longest in the center of a group of foliate papillae and shallowest and shortest at the margins. The central crypts extend medially as diverticula deep to the surface epithelium. Their walls contain several taste buds with pores that empty into the diverticula. Similarly, the papillae at the center of a foliate group are broader and longer than those located closer to the margins. Each group of foliate papillae is bordered dorsally, rostrally, and caudally by conical papillae. The lateral boundary is devoid of conical papillae. The epithelium in this area is very thinly cornified and contains the elevation cited previously. The papillae at the caudal and rostral parts of a group are small in size and very irregular in shape. They may resemble the adjacent conical papillae except that they are larger and lie between crypts.

An individual foliate papilla has a central primary dermal core. The secondary dermal papillae arise from the primary. The taste buds are located on the secondary dermal papillae and extend the total thickness of the epithelium. The majority of the taste buds are found on the sides of the central papillae. They occupy the dorsal half of the lateral walls of these papillae and are not found on the ventral half. The taste pores open into the crypts. Unlike the vallate papillae, foliate papillae may contain taste pores that open on their dorsal surfaces. Irrespective of location in the diverticula, in the crypts, or on the dorsum of a papilla, foliate taste pores are in the form of circular craters with an almost uniform diameter. Scanning electron microscopy of these pores reveals a large number of gustatory cell microvilli.

The ducts of subepithelial serous gustatory salivary glands (glands of von Ebner), are located at the bases of the papillae and open into the gustatory crypts. Also associated with the bases of some of the papillae are aggregates of lymphatic tissue. The foliate papillae are innervated by the glossopharyngeal nerve.

Conical Papillae

The **conical papillae** (*papillae conicae*) are found on the dorsum of the caudal one-third of the tongue. Each stands on a wide circular base and narrows to a thin, firm point at its apex. The caudally directed apex is more heavily cornified than the base. The area immediately rostral to the rostral pair of vallate papillae is a transitional zone containing a mixture of filiform and conical papillae. The conical papillae in the transitional zone are smaller in size than those caudal to it. The largest conical papillae are found caudal to the palatoglossal arch, but they are less crowded here. Scanning electron micrographs reveal that the unevenness of their surfaces is due to flakes of surface cornification about to fall out. Some conical papillae are modified to form the wall of the outer moat of the vallate papillae. In scanning electron micrographs it is common to see small conical papillae arising between the bases of full-sized conical papillae. The dermal core of the conical papillae contains secondary dermal papillae. Conical papillae, like filiform papillae, are mechanical and tactile rather than gustatory in function. They are innervated by the glossopharyngeal nerve.

Marginal Papillae

The **marginal papillae** (*papillae marginales*) function in suckling and are present in newborn dogs. They disappear as the pups change from liquid to solid diets. They help in preventing milk from spilling over the tongue and aid in sealing the lips around the nipple for suction. These papillae (Fig. 7.13) are distributed along the margins of the rostral half of the pup's tongue (Habermehl, 1952). They are least developed at the margin of the apex of the tongue, best developed at the margins of the tongue in the premolar carrying space, and absent at the margins of the caudal half of the tongue. The premolar carrying space is the area of lack of occlusal contact which extends from the canine teeth to the third premolars. Loss of liquid diet (milk) through this space is prevented by the dorsomedial folding of both the margins of the rostral half of the tongue and the associated marginal papillae during suckling. The marginal papillae adjacent to this space are each from 2 to 4 mm long and are arranged in a single compact row so as to obliterate spaces between successive papillae. These papillae are threadlike and narrower at their apices. Those located at the margin of the apex of the tongue are very small, and some may be less than 0.75 mm long. The marginal papillae are mechanical and tactile rather than gustatory in function. In addition to the transient marginal papillae, all the permanent lingual papillae described previously are present in newborn dogs (Kobayashi et al., 1987).

Tongue Muscles

The complex but precise movements of the dog's tongue are important for lapping water, food prehension, mastication, swallowing, and prevention of accidental biting of the tongue. These movements depend on the coordinated actions of the **extrinsic** and **intrinsic muscles** of the tongue (*musculi linguae*) (Brand & Isselhard, 1994). The extrinsic

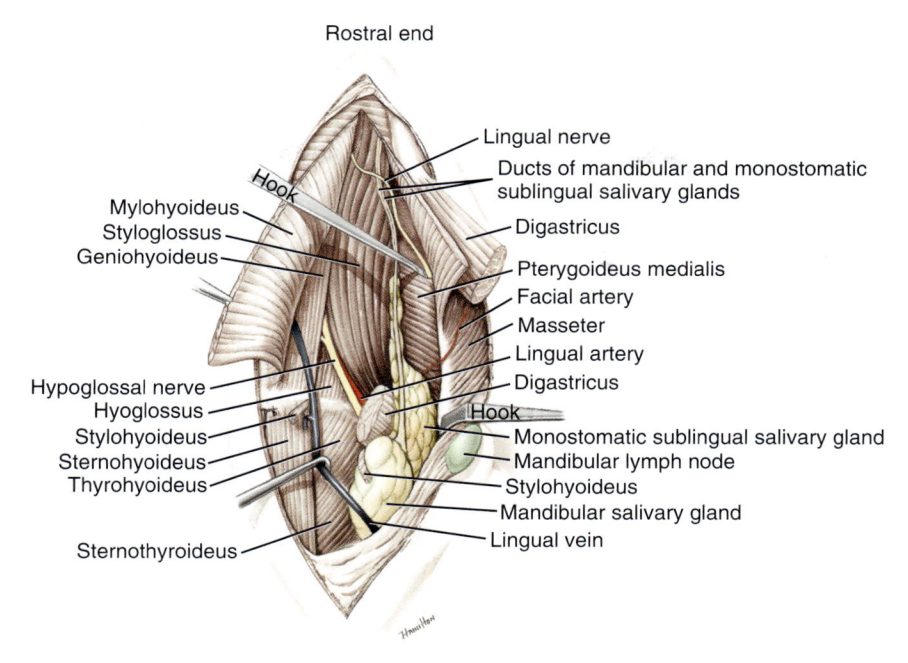

• **Fig. 7.14** Ventral view of the left half of the intermandibular space and hyoid region. Monostomatic sublingual gland.

muscles are the m. styloglossus, the m. hyoglossus, and the m. genioglossus. The intrinsic muscle of the tongue (m. lingualis proprius) contains superficial longitudinal (fibrae longitudinales superficiales), deep longitudinal (f. long, profundae), perpendicular (f. perpendiculares), and transverse (f. transversae) muscle fibers.

The **styloglossus muscle** (*m. styloglossus*) is the most lateral of the extrinsic lingual muscles seen at the caudal third of the tongue. The medial border of the middle part of this muscle (Fig. 7.14) parallels the part of the hypoglossal nerve seen at this level. It is narrow proximally but wide and thin rostrally. Its fibers curve ventrally and rostrally to insert in the tongue (Fig. 7.15). The styloglossus muscle has three heads that insert at different levels along the axis of the tongue. In a caudorostral sequence these are the short, the long, and the rostral heads of the m. styloglossus. The short head arises from the distal half of the caudal surface of the stylohyoid bone and curves ventrally and rostrally over the epihyoid bone. Rostral to the epihyoid bone, its fibers spread out to insert on the proximal part of the tongue with the inserting fibers of the m. hyoglossus. The long head also curves ventrally and rostrally. It arises from the stylohyoid bone immediately dorsolateral to the origin of the short head. Rostrally, its fibers are lateral to those of the rostral head. These fibers curve ventrally and rostrally along the ventral surface of the tongue and cross the lateral surface of the genioglossus muscle to insert on the ventral surface of the rostral half of the tongue adjacent to its midline.

The rostral head of the m. styloglossus arises from the rostrodorsal surface of the proximal half of the stylohyoid bone. Its fibers pass dorsal to the insertion of the short head to insert along the lateral surface of the caudal part of the tongue. The fibers of insertion of the rostral head of the styloglossus mingle with those of the m. hyoglossus.

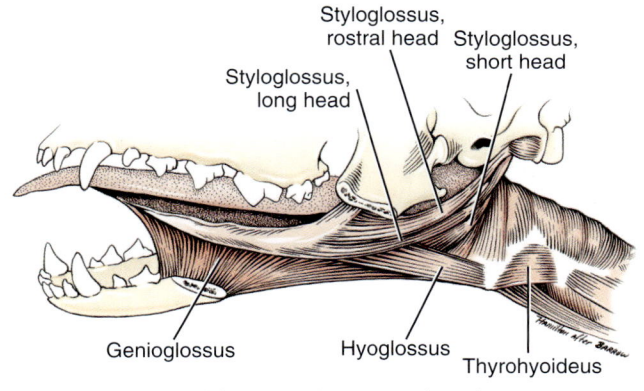

• **Fig. 7.15** Muscles of the tongue, lateral aspect.

Action: Acting as a unit, the three muscle heads draw the tongue caudally and elevate the root of the tongue.
Innervation: N. hypoglossus.

The **hyoglossus muscle** (*m. hyoglossus*) is located in the root of the tongue (Fig. 7.15). It arises from the ventrolateral surface of the basihyoid and the adjacent end of the thyrohyoid bone. Rostrally, it is dorsal to the m. mylohyoideus but lateral to mm. geniohyoideus and genioglossus. At the base of the tongue, it crosses the medial side of the m. styloglossus and then inserts in the root and caudal two-thirds of the tongue.

Action: Retracts and depresses the tongue.
Innervation: N. hypoglossus.

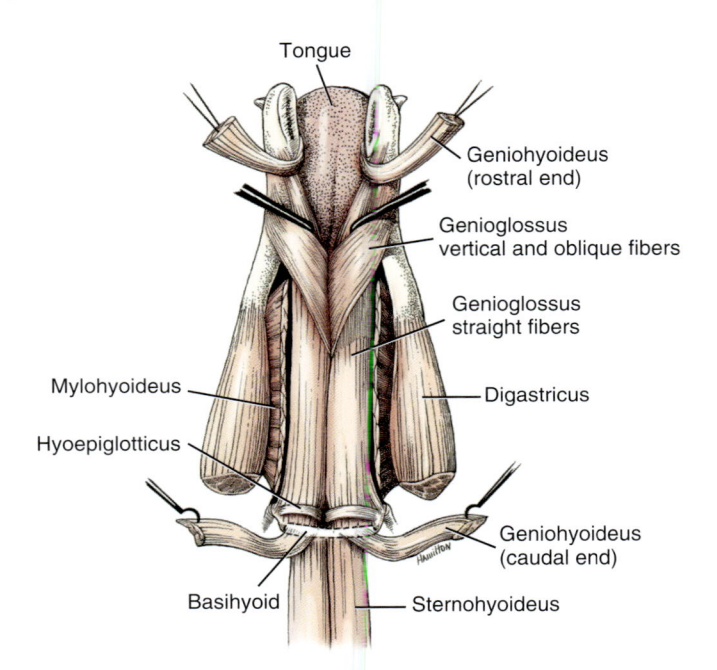

• **Fig. 7.16** Muscles of the intermandibular space, ventral aspect.

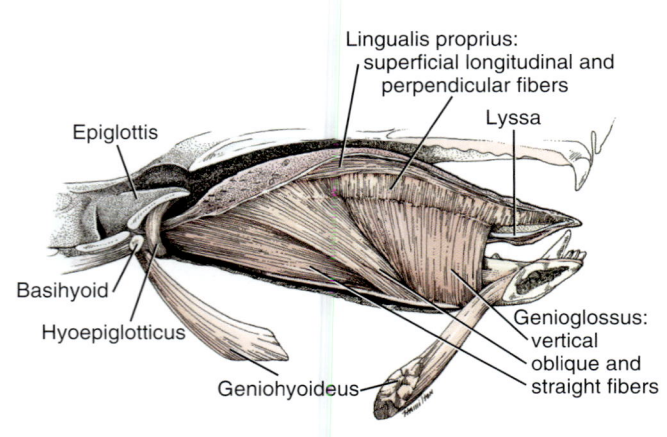

• **Fig. 7.17** Median section through the tongue.

The **genioglossus muscle** (*m. genioglossus*) (Figs. 7.15 to 7.17) is a fan-shaped muscle lying dorsal to the geniohyoideus. Its narrow end originates from the medial surface of the mandible adjacent to the intermandibular articulation just caudal to the origin of the m. geniohyoideus. Easy surgical access and isolation of the genioglossus muscle at its origin has made it very useful for physiologic studies (Gordon & Herring, 1987; Issa et al., 1988; Miki et al., 1987). It is composed of three muscle bundles best seen on its medial surface. Each bundle has a distinct mandibular origin near the intermandibular articulation. The bundles of the m. genioglossus are composed of the vertical, the oblique, and the straight fibers (Fig. 7.17).

The **vertical bundle** is located at the rostral part of m. genioglossus and inserts on the rostral half of the tongue just caudal to the lyssa. None of these fibers curves rostrally to the apex of the tongue. The vertical bundle arises from the ventromedial surface of the rostral end of the mandible caudal to the intermandibular articulation. It depresses the rostral half of the tongue just caudal to the lyssa.

The **oblique bundle** lies caudal to the vertical bundle. Some of its rostral fibers intermingle with the caudal fibers of the vertical bundle. It is narrower, longer, and more oblique than the vertical bundle. The fibers run ventrodorsal from its small ventral site of origin on the ventromedial aspect of the mandible, adjacent but caudal to the origin of the vertical bundle. It inserts on the caudal half of the tongue and, by its oblique orientation, helps to protrude the tongue.

The **straight bundle of the m. genioglossus** lies lateral to both the vertical and the oblique bundles. Its orientation parallels the body of the mandible. It originates with the m. geniohyoideus from the caudal border of the intermandibular articulation. However, its fibers of origin are medial to those of the geniohyoideus. It has three insertion sites: the caudal one-third of the tongue, the basihyoid bone, and the ceratohyoid bone. Its principal action is to protrude the tongue. Caudally one straight bundle is separated from its contralateral fellow by the m. hyoepiglotticus (see Fig. 7.17), which is located on the ventromedial surface of the basihyoid insertion of the straight bundle of genioglossus. Each m. hyoepiglotticus continues ventrally from the rostral side of the epiglottis to form a loop around the ventral surface of the insertion of the ipsilateral m. genioglossus on the basihyoid bone.

Action: As a unit, the genioglossus depresses and protrudes the tongue.
Innervation: N. hypoglossus.

The **proper lingual muscles** (*m. lingualis proprius*) are the intrinsic muscles of the tongue. These muscles form the core of the tongue and are arranged bilaterally in four groups: superficial longitudinal, deep longitudinal, transverse, and perpendicular.

The **superficial longitudinal fibers** (*fibrae longitudinales superficiales*) are located immediately deep to the dorsal lingual mucosa. They are best developed in the caudal half of the tongue (Fig. 7.18), where the fibers are organized into a compact mass on either side of the dorsal part of the septum of the tongue. The latter is a thin fibrous sheet between the two halves of the tongue deep to the median sulcus. More rostrally (Fig. 7.19), the superficial longitudinal fibers are well spaced in distinct small groups arranged symmetrically so that the largest bundles are next to the septum of the tongue, while the smallest bundles are situated next to the edge of the tongue.

The **deep longitudinal fibers** (*fibrae longitudinales profundae*) are located in the ventral half of the tongue. They are less numerous and less organized than the superficial longitudinal fibers. They often intermingle with the inserting fibers of the extrinsic lingual muscles and the transverse and perpendicular fibers of the intrinsic muscles. Rostrally,

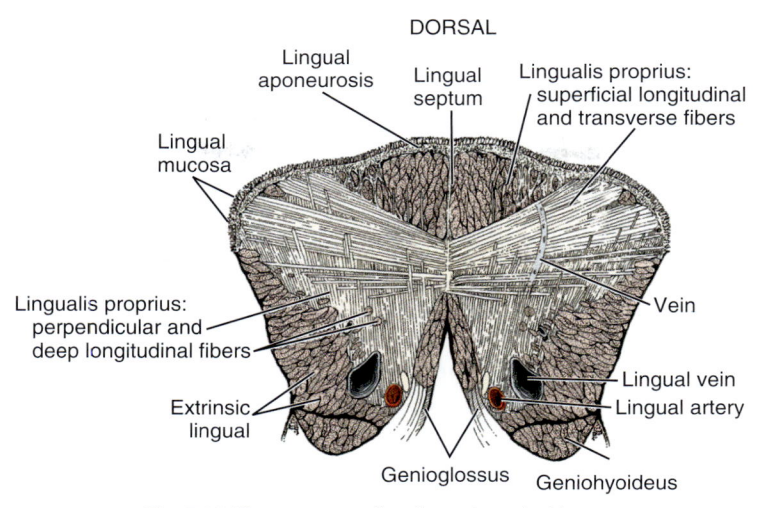

Fig. 7.18 Transverse section through root of tongue.

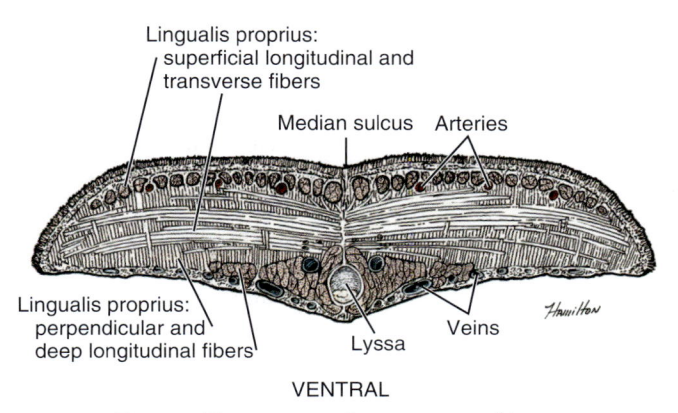

Fig. 7.19 Transverse section near apex of tongue.

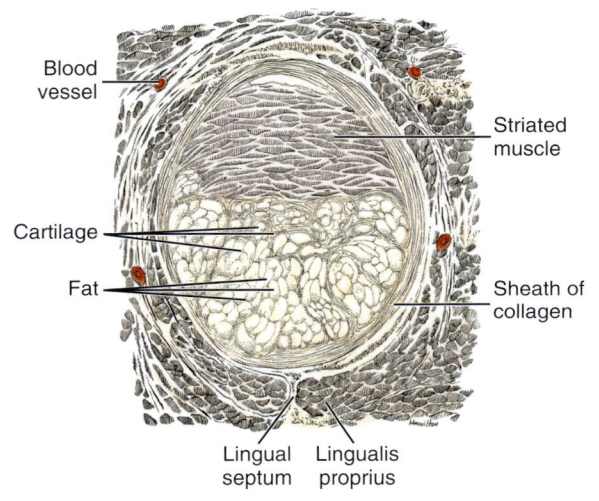

Fig. 7.20 Transverse section of the lyssa.

however, the deep longitudinal fibers organize into a compact mass. Here they also surround the lyssa (see Figs. 7.17 and 7.19).

The **transverse** (*fibrae transversae*) and the **perpendicular** (*fibrae perpendiculares*) fibers form an intricate network between the superficial and the deep longitudinal muscle fibers. They occupy a wide area in the center of the tongue.

Action: As a unit, the intrinsic muscles protrude the tongue, bring about complicated intricate local movements, and prevent the tongue from being bitten.
Innervation: N. hypoglossus.

According to Abdel-Malek (1938), the superficial longitudinal portion of the m. lingualis proprius is the only contralateral deviator of the tongue. The deep longitudinal portion of the m. lingualis proprius, the styloglossus muscle, and the rostral fibers of hyoglossus and genioglossus besides being homolateral deviators, are ventroflexors of the apex of the tongue (Abdel-Malek, 1938, 1955; Bennett & Hutchinson, 1946). The tongue takes part in all stages of mastication. During the "preparation" stage, the tongue becomes troughlike. During the "throwing" stage, it moves the food between the teeth. During the "guarding" stage, the tongue action prevents the food from falling back from the teeth. During the "sorting out" stage, the well-ground food particles are selected for molding into boluses, which are formed during the "bolus formation" stage prior to swallowing.

Lyssa

The **lyssa** (Figs. 7.17, 7.19, and 7.20), also known as the *lytta* in older literature, is a rodlike, flexible body, approximately 4 cm long in a medium-sized dog, which lies on the ventral median plane in the free end of the tongue. It extends from almost the apex of the tongue to the level of the rostral part of the vertical fibers of the genioglossus muscle (Figs. 7.17 and 7.19). Its rostral end is superficial deep to the ventral mucosa, whereas its caudal end is buried among striated muscle fibers. It is encapsulated by a dense sheath of connective tissue. Adipose tissue, striated muscle, and, occasionally, islands of cartilage fill the capsule (Dellmann & Brown, 1976; Trautmann & Fiebiger, 1957). Whereas adipose tissue predominates in its ventral half, striated muscle occupies most of its dorsal half, especially in the middle part of the lyssa. It receives blood vessels and branches of the hypoglossal nerve. Bennett (1944) demonstrated that the lyssa was elongated when the tongue muscles were stimulated via the hypoglossal nerve and suggested that the lyssa may act as a stretch receptor.

Tongue Glands
The tongue is rich in **salivary glands** (*glandulae linguales*) of both serous and mucous types (Gómez, 1961; Rakhawy, 1975). Glands that are associated with the base of vallate or foliate papillae are exclusively serous. They are the **gustatory glands** (*glandulae gustatoriae*) attributed to Von Ebner, with ducts that open into the gustatory furrow or moat. Exclusively serous glands are also present among the bundles of the intrinsic muscles of the tongue, especially in the caudal one-third of the tongue (Chibuzo & Cummings, 1986). Mucoserous glands are abundantly distributed in the lingual submucosa at the caudal one-third of the tongue. The lateral margins of the tongue also contain seromucous glands in the submucosa. Small ganglionic neuronal cell bodies in groups or in isolation are present near the acini and among the acinar cells (Gómez, 1961; Rakhawy, 1972). These are parasympathetic cell bodies of postganglionic axons that are innervated by preganglionic axons whose cell bodies are located in the parasympathetic nuclei of the facial and glossopharyngeal nerves (Chibuzo et al., 1979a). These axons reach the glands of the tongue through the chorda tympani and glossopharyngeal nerves, which are considered to be secretory motor nerves (Chibuzo et al., 1979a, b).

Tongue Blood Vessels
The arterial supply to the tongue is primarily through the paired lingual arteries (Fig. 7.18) that enter the tongue deep to the hypoglossal nerve (Fig. 7.14). The **lingual artery** (*arteria lingualis*) crosses the medial surface of the m. hyoglossus at the root of the tongue and gives off muscular branches to the intrinsic and extrinsic muscles of the tongue as it runs to the apex of the tongue. Daigo et al. (1961) illustrated the distribution and anastomoses of arteries in the dog's tongue. They found that the right and left lingual arteries anastomosed in the apex, body, and root of the tongue. The mm. genioglossus and geniohyoideus also receive some collateral arterial blood supply through the **sublingual artery** (*a. sublingualis*). According to Nikolov and Schumacher (1973), primary arteries or muscular arterial branches of the lingual artery break up into secondary arteries, which form a capillary rete in the muscles. All lingual tributary veins (Fig. 7.19) are valveless (Nikolov & Schumacher, 1973) and do not have parietal musculature except at their openings into the **lingual vein**. Brown (1937) and Pritchard and Daniel (1953) demonstrated the presence of many arteriovenous anastomoses in the dog's tongue. They are innervated by a sympathetic nerve plexus (Iijima et al., 1987). Their superficial location in the tunica propria covering the dorsal surface of the tongue is indicative of their thermoregulatory function (Brown, 1937). According to Kishi et al. (1988), arteriovenous anastomoses are most numerous at the apex of the tongue, followed by the body, and less numerous at the root of the tongue. They identified 2292 arteriovenous anastomoses in the lamina propria covering half of the dorsal surface of the dog's tongue.

Tongue Nerve Supply
The tongue is innervated by the lingual (V), chorda tympani (VII), glossopharyngeal (IX), and hypoglossal (XII) nerves (Figs. 7.14 and 7.21).

The **lingual nerve** (*n. lingualis*), a branch of the mandibular nerve from the trigeminal nerve (V), contains the general somatic afferent fibers that convey exteroceptive (tactile, noxious, and thermal) impulses from the rostral two-thirds of the lingual mucosa. Their cell bodies of origin are situated in the trigeminal ganglion, from which their axons enter the brain stem at the pons and terminate in the pontine sensory trigeminal nucleus or course caudally in the spinal tract of the trigeminal nerve to terminate in the nucleus of the spinal tract of the trigeminal nerve.

The *chorda tympani*, a branch of the facial nerve, carries mechanoreceptor and thermoreceptor afferent fibers as well as taste fibers. The gustatory fibers innervate the fungiform taste buds distributed to the mucosa of the rostral two-thirds of the tongue. The cell bodies of origin of these neurons are located in the geniculate ganglion and their axons enter the solitary tract in the medulla and terminate on neurons in the nucleus of the solitary tract. Parasympathetic general visceral efferent postganglionic axons innervate the glands of the tongue. Their cell bodies are within or close to these glands in the tongue substance (Gómez, 1961; Mikhail et al., 1980; Rakhawy, 1972). Their preganglionic cell bodies are located in the parasympathetic nucleus of the facial nerve in the medulla (Chibuzo et al., 1979a,

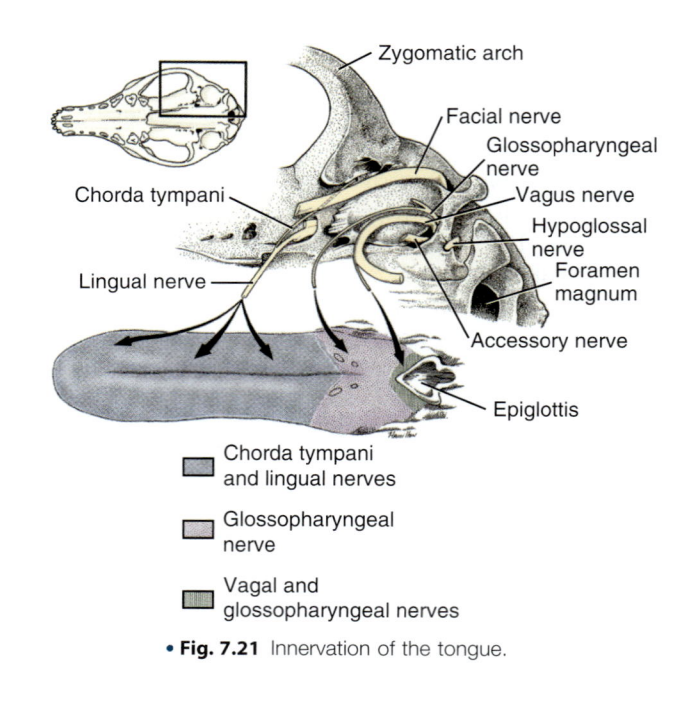

• Fig. 7.21 Innervation of the tongue.

1981). These general visceral efferent fibers are secretory and are vasodilators to the glands of the tongue.

The lingual branch of the **glossopharyngeal nerve** (*n. glossopharyngeus*) carries special visceral afferent, general visceral afferent, and general visceral efferent fibers to the caudal one-third of the tongue. The special visceral afferent fibers innervate the vallate and foliate taste buds and therefore carry gustatory impulses from the caudal one-third of the tongue. The cell bodies of origin of these fibers are located in the distal or proximal ganglion of the glossopharyngeal nerve. These ganglia are joined together in the dog. The distal ganglion was formerly called the *petrosal ganglion*. Their axons enter the solitary tract in the medulla. The general visceral afferent fibers carry exteroceptive (tactile, noxious, and thermal) impulses from the mucosa of the caudal one-third of the tongue. The cell bodies of origin of this component are also situated in the proximal or distal ganglion of the glossopharyngeal nerve, from which their axons enter the solitary tract in the medulla. The general visceral efferent component of the glossopharyngeal nerve sends secretory and vasodilator fibers to the lingual glands located in the caudal part of the tongue. Their parasympathetic cell bodies of the postganglionic axons are located in the tongue substance close to or among these glands. The preganglionic cell bodies are in the parasympathetic nucleus of the glossopharyngeal nerve (Chibuzo et al., 1979a).

The **hypoglossal nerve** (*n. hypoglossus*) (Fig. 7.14) contains the general somatic efferent axons that innervate the mm. genioglossus, hyoglossus, styloglossus, and lingualis proprius. The cell bodies of these motor neurons are located in the long hypoglossal nucleus in the medulla. These muscles have been shown to be somatotopically represented in the hypoglossal nucleus (Chibuzo & Cummings, 1982; Uemura-Sumi et al., 1988). It has also been demonstrated that this nerve in the dog (Sobusiak et al., 1967) contains ganglionic cell bodies throughout its peripheral course. It has been suggested that these neuronal cell bodies are sensory for deep sensation and are probably lingual proprioceptive afferent neurons (Adatia & Gehring, 1971; Pearson, 1945). It has also been demonstrated that some sensory neurons from the cranial cervical spinal ganglia reach the muscles of the tongue via the hypoglossal nerve. These neurons are also considered to be for lingual proprioception (Chibuzo, 1979; Chibuzo & Cummings, 1981; Kubota et al., 1988).

Anomalies. Hutt and de Lahunta (1971, 1972) described a lethal hereditary defect of the tongue in two pups called to their attention by a breeder. The curled, overly narrow tongue (Fig. 7.22), which they called *bird tongue*, presumably prevented pups from suckling and resulted in their death from starvation. The pups showed no interest in suckling and could not be coaxed to nurse or swallow. Normal reflex sucking and swallowing is a function of glossopharyngeal, vagal, and hypoglossal nerves, which in these pups appeared normal. During a period of 7 years at this kennel there were 12 litters that included one or more such pups (54 normal pups, 22 with abnormal tongues). The

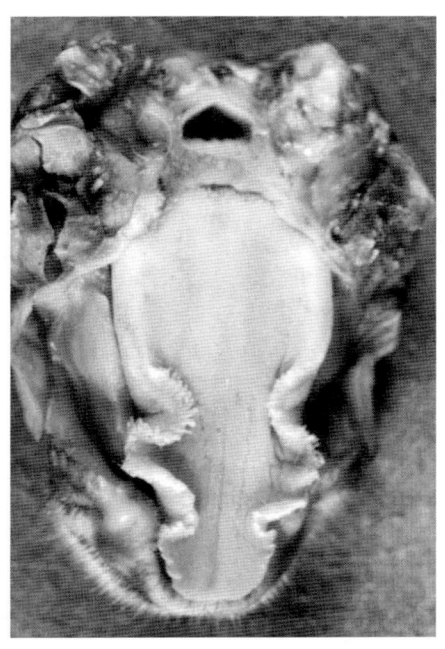

• **Fig. 7.22** One of two pups described as "bird tongue" by Hutt and de Lahunta (1971). They showed no interest in suckling. (With permission *J Hered* 62:291–293, 1971.)

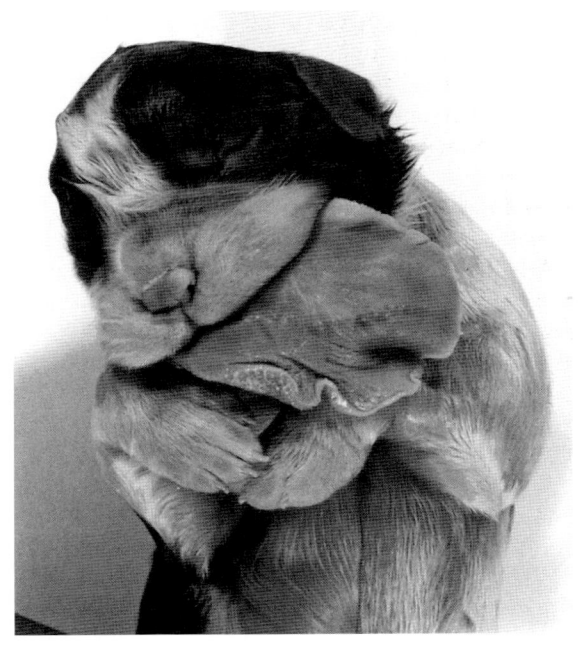

• **Fig. 7.23** A newborn Springer Spaniel with an oversized tongue that prevented suckling. This rare condition in humans is called *primary macroglossia*. (Specimen courtesy RG Wiswall; photograph, Evans [1994]).

breeder traced this defect to a foundation sire, and the authors ascribed this abnormality to a simple recessive autosomal gene in the homozygous state.

The opposite condition of an oversized tongue that protruded from the mouth and prevented suckling (Fig. 7.23) was sent to Howard Evans by a practitioner who had received it alive from a breeder of Springer Spaniels. The other four pups in this litter were normal. This anomaly, reported several times as "macroglossia" in the human, has not been reported in dogs and did not recur at this kennel.

Salivary Glands

The salivary glands that compose the glands of the oral cavity or **oral glands** (*glandulae oris*), broadly speaking, are all of those glands that pour their secretions into the oral cavity. These include both **minor** and **major salivary glands** (*gll. glandulae salivariae minores et majores*). The major salivary glands include the parotid, mandibular, monostomatic and polystomatic sublingual, and zygomatic glands. The minor salivary glands include labial, buccal, molar, lingual, and palatine. Radiographic examination of the contrast injected duct system of the major salivary glands (sialography) is a practical means of discovering and treating salivary sialocele (Glen, 1972; Harvey, 1970).

Parotid Gland

The **parotid gland** (*glandula parotis*) (Fig. 7.24) lies at the junction of the head and neck overlying the basal portion of the auricular cartilage. Its outline is V-shaped as viewed from the surface with the apex directed ventrally. The parotid gland is bounded caudally by the mastoid part of the sternocephalicus and cervical part of the cleidocephalicus muscles and rostrally by the masseter muscle and the temporomandibular joint. The gland weighs approximately 7 g and has an overall length of approximately 6 cm. It is thickest ventrally, measuring approximately 1.5 cm. The gland is a dark flesh color, with coarse lobulations visible through its thin capsule. It is divided into superficial and deep portions.

The **superficial portion** (*pars superficialis*) of the parotid gland consists of the two limbs of the V and the dorsally concave, thin-edged portion that connects the two limbs.

The **deep portion** (*pars profunda*) of the parotid gland is wedge-shaped and lies ventral to the cartilaginous external acoustic meatus. It is dorsal to the rostral pole of the mandibular gland and extends medially toward the tympanic bulla and wall of the nasal pharynx.

Of the **three angles** of the parotid gland, one points dorsorostrally, one dorsocaudally, and the third ventrally. The **borders** are dorsal, rostral, and caudal. The **superficial surface** is nearly flat transversely and only slightly convex longitudinally. It is crossed vertically by the strap-like m. parotidoauricularis (formerly m. depressor auriculae), which, in turn, is covered ventrally by fascicles of the platysma. Near the ventral angle the gland is usually tunneled by the maxillary vein. From deep to its rostral border emerge the palpebral, auriculotemporal, and the dorsal and ventral buccal branches of the facial nerve. The parotid lymph node usually lies for the most part deep to the rostral border of the rostral limb of the superficial part of the gland. The rostral auricular artery and vein and the transverse facial artery run deep to or along the rostral border. The caudal border is circled by branches of the intermediate auricular

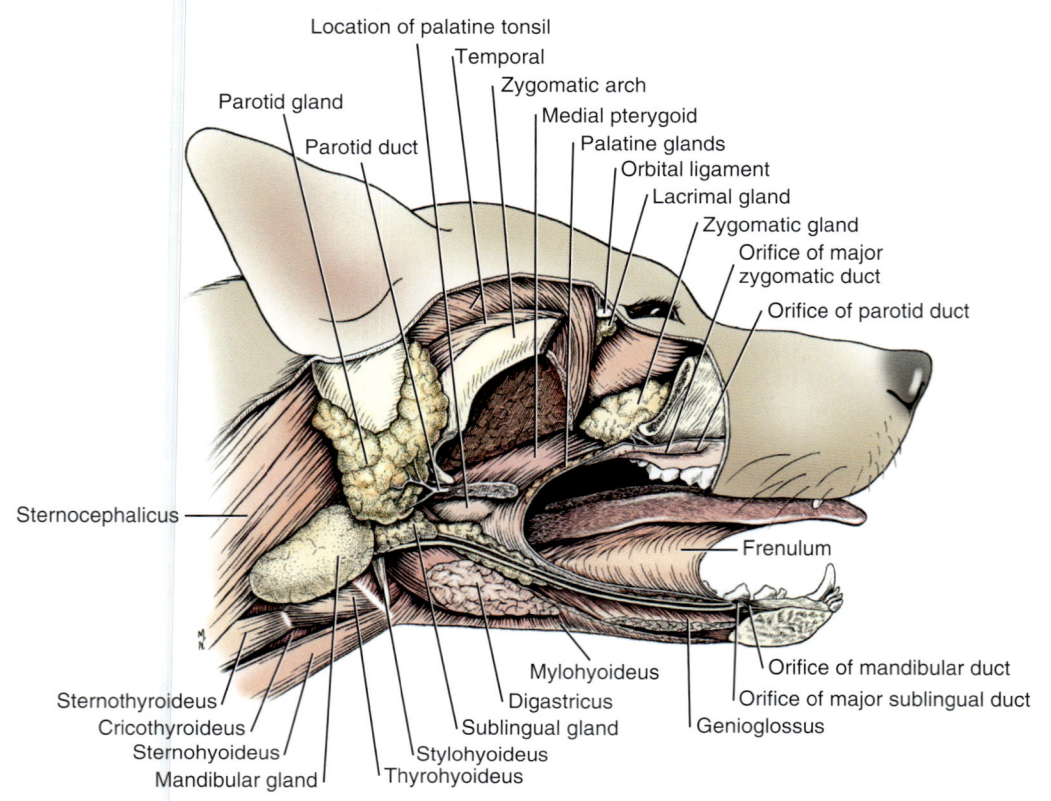

• Fig. 7.24 Salivary glands. (The right half of the mandible was removed.)

blood vessels. Some of these structures may run through the gland.

The dorsal border is not related to any large nerves or vessels, but its position is important because of its close proximity to the cartilaginous part of the external acoustic meatus. Surgical procedures that treat chronic otitis externa by removing the lateral wall of the cartilaginous external acoustic meatus require ventral displacement of the superficial part of the parotid gland to avoid its injury. The caudal deep part of the parotid gland is related to the facial nerve and its terminal branches as they emerge from the stylomastoid foramen caudal to the osseous external acoustic meatus. The rostral deep portion of the gland is also related to the maxillary and superficial temporal arteries. The maxillary vein is related to the parotid gland at a more ventral and superficial level than are the nerves and arteries.

The **parotid duct** (*ductus parotideus*) (Figs. 7.24 and 7.25, *radiographs 1 and 2*) is approximately 1.5 mm in diameter and 6 cm long and can be palpated where it crosses the masseter muscle (McCarthy, 1978). It is formed by two or three converging radicles, which leave the ventral third of the rostral border of the gland and unite with each other on the masseter muscle several millimeters from the gland. The duct is rather closely united to the lateral surface of the masseter muscle by superficial fascia as it runs straight rostrally to the cheek, parallel, or nearly parallel, to the fibers of the masseter. Testoni et al. (1977) described the terminal part of the parotid duct as having two right-angle curves, one medially and the other ventrally, before passing through the buccal mucosa. It opens into the buccal cavity at the rostral end of a blunt ridge of mucosa by a small papilla. This is located opposite the caudal margin of

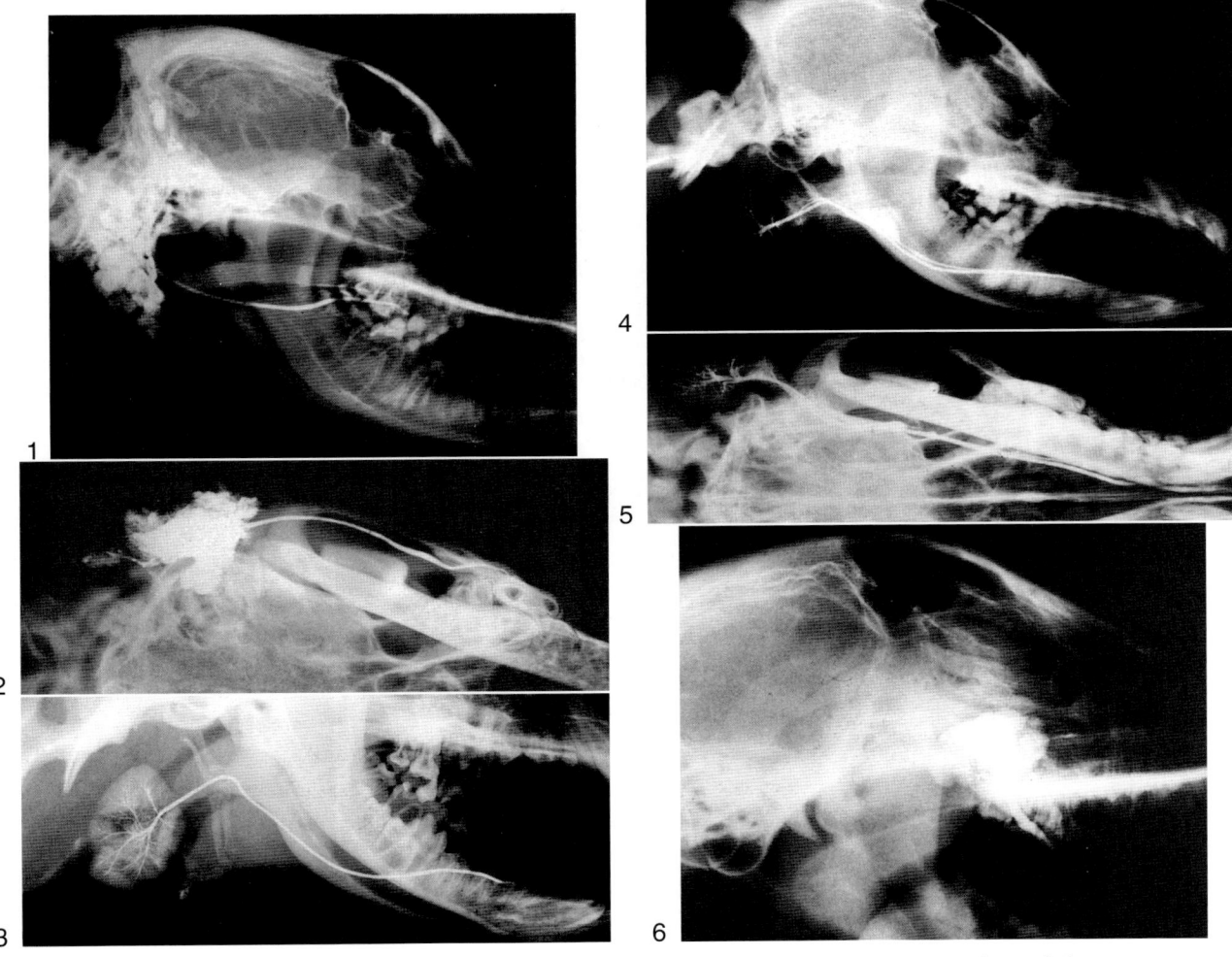

• **Fig. 7.25 Radiograph 1**, Lateral contrast radiograph of the parotid gland and its duct. **Radiograph 2**, Dorsoventral contrast radiograph of the parotid gland and its duct. **Radiograph 3**, Lateral contrast radiograph of the mandibular gland and its duct. **Radiograph 4**, Lateral contrast radiograph of the mandibular and monostomatic sublingual glands and their ducts. The monostomatic sublingual gland lies rostral to and in contact with the mandibular gland. **Radiograph 5**, Dorsoventral radiograph of the mandibular and monostomatic sublingual glands and their ducts. The monostomatic sublingual gland lies rostral to and in contact with the mandibular gland. **Radiograph 6**, Lateral radiograph of the zygomatic gland and its ducts.

the superior fourth premolar, or shearing tooth. The ridge of mucosa, on the rostral end of which the duct opens, runs caudally to the end of the dental arch lying in or near the fornix formed by the attachment of the cheek to the maxilla.

Accessory parotid glands (*glandulae parotis accessoria*) are usually present on one or both sides. They range in size from single lobules to small oval glandular masses more than 1 cm long. They usually lie dorsal to the parotid duct and may be placed at any level along it. Their small ducts empty into the main parotid duct.

The fascia covering the parotid gland is thin and of the areolar type. At the borders of the gland it blends with the superficial fascia of the head, ear, and neck. Similar fascia lines the space in which the gland lies. The fascia separating the lobules is abundant and loose.

The **parotid artery**, a branch of the external carotid, is wholly distributed to the parotid gland and usually is its main blood supply. The caudal auricular, transverse facial, and rostral auricular arteries all send branches to the parotid gland. The veins that drain the parotid are radicles of the **superficial temporal** and **caudal auricular veins**. The lymphatics from the parotid gland drain into the **parotid** and **medial retropharyngeal lymph nodes**. The parotid gland receives parasympathetic nerve fibers through the **auriculotemporal nerve**, a branch of the mandibular nerve from the trigeminal nerve (V). Preganglionic cell bodies are in the parasympathetic nucleus of the glossopharyngeal nerve in the medulla. The axons course in the glossopharyngeal nerve and enter the tympanic cavity in the tympanic nerve to form a tympanic plexus. The preganglionic axons leave the plexus in the minor petrosal nerve and just caudal to the oval foramen; these axons enter the otic ganglion to synapse on cell bodies of postganglionic axons. These postganglionic axons enter the auriculotemporal nerve, a branch of the mandibular nerve, to be distributed to the parotid gland. Sympathetic postganglionic axons from the cranial cervical ganglion follow the arteries that supply the parotid gland.

Histologically, the parotid salivary gland is a seromucous type gland containing dense secretory granules, according to Nagato and Tandler (1986). The intercalated ducts are short, and each drains several acini. According to the latter authors, the parotid gland of the dog resembles those of other carnivores on histochemical grounds, but at the ultrastructural level major differences are apparent in the secretory granules and striated ducts.

Mandibular Gland

The **mandibular gland** (*glandula mandibularis*) (Fig. 7.24, radiograph 3) is an ovoid body lying largely between the linguofacial and maxillary veins just caudal to the angle of the mandible. It weighs approximately 8 g, being slightly heavier than the parotid gland. Its lobules, which are of approximately the same dimensions as the parotid lobules, are fitted together much more compactly, with less connective tissue separating them. The whole organ is a light buff color and is not sharply separated from the smaller monostomatic portion of the sublingual gland. This portion of the sublingual gland lies adjacent to the ventral part of the rostral pole of the mandibular gland, on which it leaves a nearly flat, oblique impression.

From a superficial gross appearance this portion of the sublingual gland constitutes the pointed rostral pole of the salivary mass in this location because both of the glands are contained within the same heavy fibrous capsule. The common capsule is a specialization of the buccopharyngeal fascia and does not send trabeculae into the glands. It is derived primarily from the deep cervical fascia. The mandibular gland has rostral and caudal poles and superficial and deep surfaces. Its rostral pole is truncate and is related to the caudal portion of the monostomatic sublingual gland. The caudal pole forms an even arc vertically as it unites the superficial and deep surfaces at an acute angle. The superficial surface is slightly rounded in all planes and is grooved dorsally for the maxillary vein. Its rostrodorsal part is variably overlapped by the parotid gland. Ventrally it is related to the mandibular lymph node, or nodes, lying dorsal to the linguofacial vein. The deep surface is further divided into subsurfaces by the following structures on which it lies: the muscle and terminal tendon of the mastoid part of the sternocephalicus, dorsocaudally; the medial retropharyngeal lymph node and larynx, medially; and the digastricus and ribbonlike stylohyoid muscles, rostrally.

The mandibular gland is a mixed gland. Stormont (1928) gives a brief review of the literature concerning the histology of the salivary glands of carnivores.

The **mandibular duct** (*ductus mandibularis*) leaves the medial surface of the gland near the ventromedial part of the impression formed by the sublingual gland. As the initial part of the duct runs rostromedially, it lies in relation to the medial surface of the monostomatic sublingual gland adjacent to the major sublingual duct. In their course into the oral cavity the mandibular duct and monostomatic sublingual gland lie between the masseter muscle and mandible laterally, and the digastricus medially. In this location the gland and duct run obliquely rostromedially. On reaching the lateral part of the pharyngeal mucosa, the mandibular duct arches rostrally and, with lobules of the rostral part of the monostomatic sublingual gland, runs in the intermuscular septum between the medially located m. styloglossus and the laterally located m. mylohyoideus. Throughout the remaining part of its course the mandibular duct is closely related to the major sublingual duct and is described with it following the description of the monostomatic sublingual gland.

The largest artery supplying the mandibular gland, the glandular branch of the **facial artery**, enters the gland where the mandibular duct leaves it. Entering the dorsal part of the deep surface of the gland are one or two small branches from the **caudal auricular artery**. The chief vein draining the gland leaves its deep surface and terminates usually in the **lingual vein** as this vessel joins the facial vein. A second vein leaves the caudal part of the gland and terminates in the **facial, maxillary,** or **lingual vein.** The parasympathetic secretory visceral efferent innervation consists of preganglionic neuronal cell bodies in the parasympathetic nucleus of the facial nerve. The preganglionic axons course through the facial nerve to the level of the tympanic cavity where they enter the chorda tympani and traverse the tympanic cavity. At the oval foramen where the mandibular nerve from the trigeminal nerve (V) emerges from the cranial cavity, the preganglionic axons join the lingual nerve as it branches from the mandibular nerve. As the lingual nerve crosses the major sublingual and mandibular ducts these preganglionic axons terminate in the **mandibular ganglion** where they synapse on the neuronal cell bodies of postganglionic axons that course caudally to innervate the mandibular gland. Sympathetic postganglionic axons from the cranial cervical ganglion follow the arterial blood supply to the mandibular gland. The lymphatics drain into the medial retropharyngeal lymph node.

Sublingual Glands

There are two sublingual glands: the monostomatic and the polystomatic (*glandula sublinguali monostomatica et polystomatica*) (Figs. 7.24 and 7.25). These are the smallest of the four pairs of major salivary glands. The **monostomatic sublingual salivary gland** has all of its secretion enter the oral cavity through one opening on the sublingual caruncle adjacent to the rostral portion of the frenulum of the tongue. This sublingual gland weighs approximately 1 g and consists of an aggregation of two or more lobulated masses. The nearly flat, truncated base, or caudal surface, of the largest division of the gland is closely related to the blunt rostral end of the mandibular gland. Both glands are enclosed in the same fibrous capsule, the monostomatic sublingual gland being distinguishable by its rostral position and its slightly darker color. The tapered extremity of the gland extends rostromedially between the caudomedial border of the masseter muscle laterally and the digastricus medially. It curves rostrally on reaching the lateral surface of the styloglossus, so that it lies medial to the body of the mandible.

Usually separated from the rostral end of this portion of the gland is an ovoid cluster of lobules, which may reach a length of 3 cm and a width of 1 cm. These lobules lie directly deep to the mucosa, which reflects from the mandible to the tongue. Their secretion is poured into the major sublingual duct through four to six short excretory ducts. The major sublingual duct lies ventral to the gland. The **polystomatic sublingual gland** consists of that portion of the sublingual gland that discharges its secretion directly into the oral cavity without its passing through the major sublingual duct. The gland consists of 6 to 12 small, usually isolated lobules of salivary tissue, which lie deep to the mucosa on each side of the body of the tongue rostral to the lingual nerve. They are so small that no definite sublingual fold is formed by them. They open into the oral cavity adjacent to the tongue by several ducts.

The **major sublingual duct** (*ductus sublingualis major*) is closely related to the dorsal aspect of the mandibular duct throughout its course in the intermandibular space. On reaching the caudal margin of the mylohyoid muscle which is located in a transverse plane less than 1 cm rostral to the angle of the mandible, the two ducts pass medial and dorsal to this muscle. Rostral to the lingual branch of the trigeminal nerve, which crosses the lateral surfaces of the ducts at a transverse level just caudal to the orbital openings, the ducts lie between the genioglossal and mylohyoid muscles. The ducts open on a small **sublingual caruncle** (*caruncula sublingualis*), which is located lateral to the rostral end of the frenulum at its attachment caudal to the intermandibular articulation. When the openings are separate, which is usually the case, the mandibular opening lies rostral to the sublingual.

The glandular branch of the **facial artery** supplies the monostomatic sublingual gland and the **sublingual artery**, a branch of the lingual, supplies the small polystomatic gland. These arteries are accompanied by satellite veins that drain the **gland**. Parasympathetic innervation is similar to that of the mandibular gland except the preganglionic axons synapse in the small **sublingual ganglion** located near where the lingual nerve crosses the major sublingual duct. Lymphatic drainage is into the **medial retropharyngeal lymph node**.

Zygomatic Gland

The **zygomatic gland** (*glandula zygomatica*) (Fig. 7.24), formerly known as the *orbital gland*, weighs approximately 3 g and is located ventromedial to the zygomatic arch. Found only in the dog and cat, among the domestic mammals it represents a caudal condensation of the largely unilobulated dorsal buccal glands of other mammals. It is globular to pyramidal in shape, with its base directed dorsally and caudally and lying against the ventral part of the periorbita. It is surrounded by soft fat outside a poorly developed capsule. Because of the soft tissue adjacent to it, its lobules are much more distinct than are those of the mandibular gland, which it resembles in color. From its blunt apex, which lies lateral to that part of the maxilla containing the roots of the last superior molar tooth, it sends one major duct and two to four minor ducts to the caudodorsal part of the vestibule. The major duct opens approximately 1 cm caudal to the parotid papilla on the ridge of mucosa that extends to a plane through the caudal surface of the last superior cheek tooth. The smaller, minor ducts open on this ridge, caudal to the opening of the major duct.

Usually, the first branch of the **infraorbital artery**, as it enters the infraorbital canal, supplies the zygomatic gland. The main vein that leaves it enters the **deep facial vein**, which grooves its lateral surface. Parasympathetic preganglionic axons in the glossopharyngeal nerve continue in the tympanic nerve into the tympanic plexus in the tympanic cavity. They leave the cavity in the minor petrosal nerve to synapse in the otic ganglion. Postganglionic axons travel in

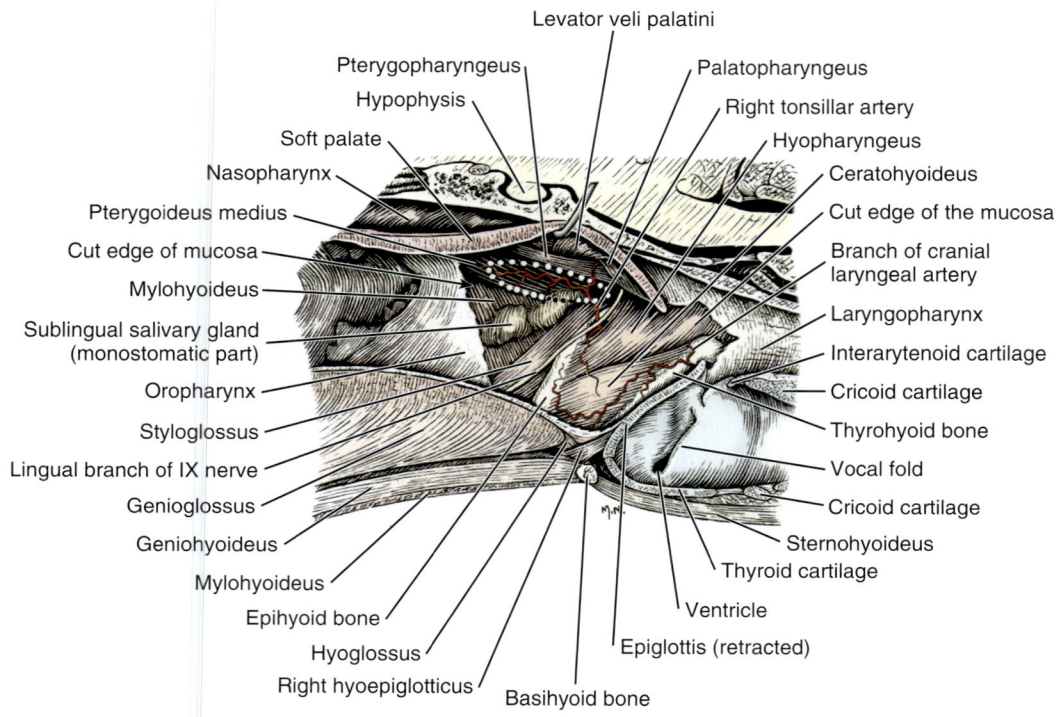

Fig. 7.26 Median section through the pharynx. The location of the right palatine tonsil is indicated by a dotted circle. The buccopharyngeal fascia deep to the tonsil was removed and the soft palate elevated.

the buccal nerve, a branch of the mandibular nerve, to innervate the zygomatic salivary gland.

Pharynx

The **pharynx** (*cavum pharyngis*) (Fig. 7.26) is a passage that is, in part, common to both the respiratory and the digestive systems. It is a musculomembranous junction of the respiratory and digestive tubes between the oral and nasal cavities rostrally and the esophagus and larynx caudally. It extends approximately from a transverse plane through the head at the level of the orbital openings to a similar plane through the second cervical vertebra. The pharynx of the dog consists of nasal, oral, and laryngeal parts (Fig. 7.27).

Nasal Pharynx

The **nasal pharynx** (*pars nasalis pharyngis*) (Fig. 7.28) is the respiratory portion dorsal to the soft palate and extends from the choanae of the nasal cavity to the intrapharyngeal opening of the pharynx. In the dorsolateral wall at about the level of the middle of the soft palate is a slit approximately 5 mm long, which is the **pharyngeal opening of the auditory tube** (*ostium pharyngeum tubae auditivae*). The caudal end of this tube opens into the tympanic cavity. Pharyngeal and tubal tonsils associated with the wall of the nasal pharynx are usually not grossly visible.

The **intrapharyngeal opening** (*ostium intrapharyngeum*), formerly called the *pharyngeal isthmus* or *pharyngeal chiasma*, is the opening of the nasal pharynx into the laryngopharynx. It is formed by the free caudal border of the soft

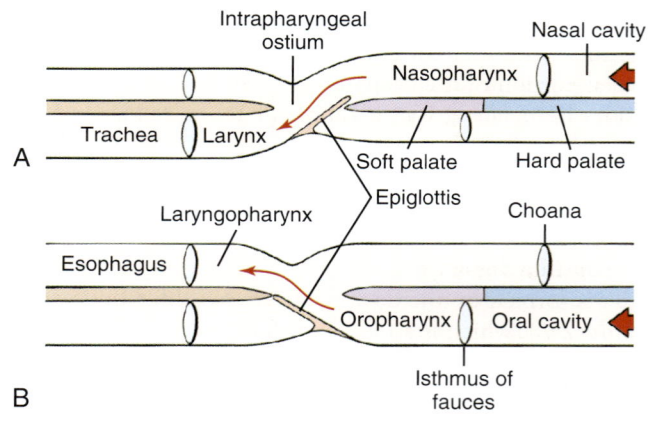

Fig. 7.27 Diagram of the pharynx and the intrapharyngeal opening (*ostium intrapharyngeus*). **A,** During respiration. **B,** During deglutition.

palate and the right and left palatopharyngeal arches. During nasal respiration this opening faces the epiglottis ventrally. Caudal to the intrapharyngeal opening the digestive tube is continued dorsal to the larynx as the laryngeal part of the pharynx, and the respiratory tube is continued ventrally as the larynx, which in turn is continuous with the trachea.

Oral Pharynx

The **isthmus of the fauces** (*isthmus faucium*) (Fig. 7.27) is the orifice between the oral cavity and the oral part of the pharynx. It is bounded on each side by the palatoglossal arch (*arcus palatoglossus*), ventrally by the tongue, and

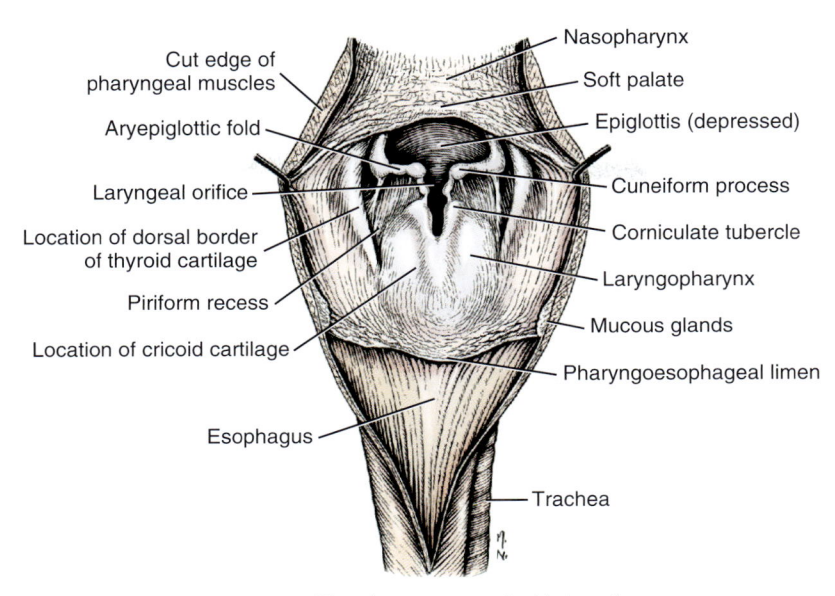

Fig. 7.28 The pharynx opened mid-dorsally.

dorsally by the soft palate. Lateral to the palatoglossal arch is the **pterygomandibular fold** (*plica pterygomandibularis*) which is a fold of mucosa between the soft palate and the mandible caudal to the last molar. The **oropharynx** (*pars oralis pharyngis*) extends from the isthmus of the fauces to the base of the epiglottis. It is bounded dorsally by the soft palate, ventrally by the root of the tongue, and laterally by the tonsillar fossa, with its contained palatine tonsil. The rostral portion of the oropharynx where the palatine tonsil resides in its lateral wall is called the **fauces**. The **palatine tonsil** (*tonsilla palatina*) is a long, relatively thin lymphoid organ, located in the lateral wall of the oral part of the pharynx (fauces), just caudal to the palatoglossal arch. It is hidden from casual observation because of its position in the **tonsillar fossa** (*fossa tonsillaris*). The medial wall of the fossa is formed by the thin, falciform **tonsillar fold** (*plica semilunaris*), which is a fold from the ventral surface of the lateral portion of the soft palate.

The palatine tonsil is divided into a protruding fusiform portion that composes the major portion of the organ, and a usually smaller, deeper, minor portion that lies deep to the mucosa, forming the rostral part of the lateral wall of the tonsillar fossa. The deep portion of the gland may be formed as a result of tonsillitis because it is usually absent in young, healthy specimens. It develops in the submucosa directly in the thick buccopharyngeal fascia. Lateral to this fascia lies the lingual branch of the glossopharyngeal nerve and the styloglossal and medial pterygoid muscles.

The palatine tonsil has a long, narrow hilus that may be thickened in its middle so that rostral and caudal fossae are formed that separate the main portion of the tonsil from the lateral wall of the tonsillar fossa. When the major portion of the organ is forcibly pulled out of the tonsillar fossa, the deeper, minor portion is also drawn ventrally in a fold of mucosa formed by the traction, so that complete extirpation of the organ is made possible. The average dimensions of the major portion are a length of 2.5 cm, a width of 0.5 cm, and a thickness of 0.4 cm. The pointed ends of the fusiform organ are not free but are firmly attached to the dorsolateral parts of the wall of the fossa. The palatine tonsil has no afferent lymphatics. Its efferent vessels drain into the **medial retropharyngeal lymph node**. It receives its nutrition mainly from the **tonsillar artery**, which is derived from the lingual. The tonsillar artery enters the middle or widest portion of the tonsil by approximately three branches. The caudal pole of the tonsil may receive branches from the hyoid branches of the lingual. The small veins from the tonsil enter the **palatine plexus of veins**. In addition to the palatine tonsils, other lymphoid tissue lies in the base of the tongue and in the nasal part of the pharynx. These are referred to as the *lingual* and *pharyngeal tonsils*. The **lingual tonsil** (*tonsilla lingualis*) is so diffuse it cannot be seen on gross examination.

Laryngeal Pharynx

The **laryngeal pharynx** (*pars laryngea pharyngis*) or **laryngopharynx** (Fig. 7.28) is that portion of the pharynx that lies dorsal to the larynx. It extends from the intrapharyngeal ostium and the nasal part of the pharynx rostrally to the beginning of the esophagus caudally. Its caudal limit, therefore, reaches to a transverse plane that passes through the caudal border of the cricoid cartilage and the middle of the axis. The pharyngoesophageal junction in the dog is distinctly marked by an annular ridge of tissue known as the *limen pharyngoesophageum*, formerly called the *annular fold*.

Although the function of the laryngeal part of the pharynx is both respiratory and alimentary, its chief importance is in deglutition. The bolus of food ingested is conveyed to it by the plungerlike movement of the base of the tongue. Six pairs of extrinsic muscles control the shape and size of the nasal and laryngeal parts of the pharynx. Three pairs of these muscles are constrictors, two pairs are shorteners, and the muscles of one pair act as a dilator. Dyce (1957) uses the name *laryngopharyngeus* to designate the combined cricopharyngeal and thyropharyngeal muscles, which are the two caudal pairs of constrictors. These two muscles are largely fused to each other, and they are also blended caudally with the spiral muscular coat of the esophagus. The muscles of the pharynx are described in Chapter 6.

The laryngopharynx receives its nutrition through the paired **pharyngeal branches of the cranial thyroid** and the **ascending pharyngeal arteries**. The soft palate, the dorsal wall of the oral part of the pharynx, receives most of its nutrition from the paired **minor palatine arteries**. Innervation is from the pharyngeal branches of the glossopharyngeal and vagus nerves.

The Alimentary Canal

Esophagus

The esophagus (Fig. 7.29), the first part of the alimentary canal, is the connecting tube between the laryngeal part of the pharynx and the stomach. In medium-sized dogs it is approximately 30 cm long and 2 cm in diameter when it is collapsed. Because this passage traverses most of the neck and all of the thorax, and ends on entering the abdomen, it is divided into cervical, thoracic, and abdominal portions. It begins opposite the middle of the axis dorsally, and the caudal border of the cricoid cartilage ventrally. A plicated ridge of mucosa, the *limen pharyngoesophageum*, most prominent ventrally, is the internal demarcation between the pharynx and the esophagus. The esophagus ends at the cardia of the stomach. The dorsal part of the esophagus, as it terminates, lies ventral to the last thoracic vertebra, and the ventral part lies slightly cranial to this level. The site of termination of the esophagus may vary a vertebral segment cranially or caudally.

The **cervical portion** (*pars cervicalis*) of the esophagus is related mainly to the left longus colli and longus capitis muscles dorsally, and to the trachea ventrally and to the right. At its origin it starts to incline to the left, so that at the thoracic inlet it usually lies left lateral to the trachea. Its position here varies; in some specimens it is left dorsal and in others it is left ventral to the trachea. On the left side, the left common carotid artery, vagosympathetic nerve trunk, internal jugular vein, and tracheal duct run in the angle between the esophagus and the longus capitis muscle. The corresponding structures on the right side are located lateral to the trachea.

The **thoracic portion** (*pars thoracica*) of the esophagus extends from the thoracic inlet to the esophageal hiatus of the diaphragm Figs. 8.23, 8.30, 8.31, 8.34, 11.34, and 11.35). At first, it usually lies to the left of the trachea between the widely separated leaves of the dorsal part of the cranial mediastinum. It obliquely crosses the left face of the trachea to gain its dorsal surface as the trachea bifurcates into the principal bronchi ventral to the fifth and sixth thoracic vertebrae. In reaching this level it crosses the right face of the aortic arch and lies ventral to the right and left longus colli muscles. It is separated from these muscles here,

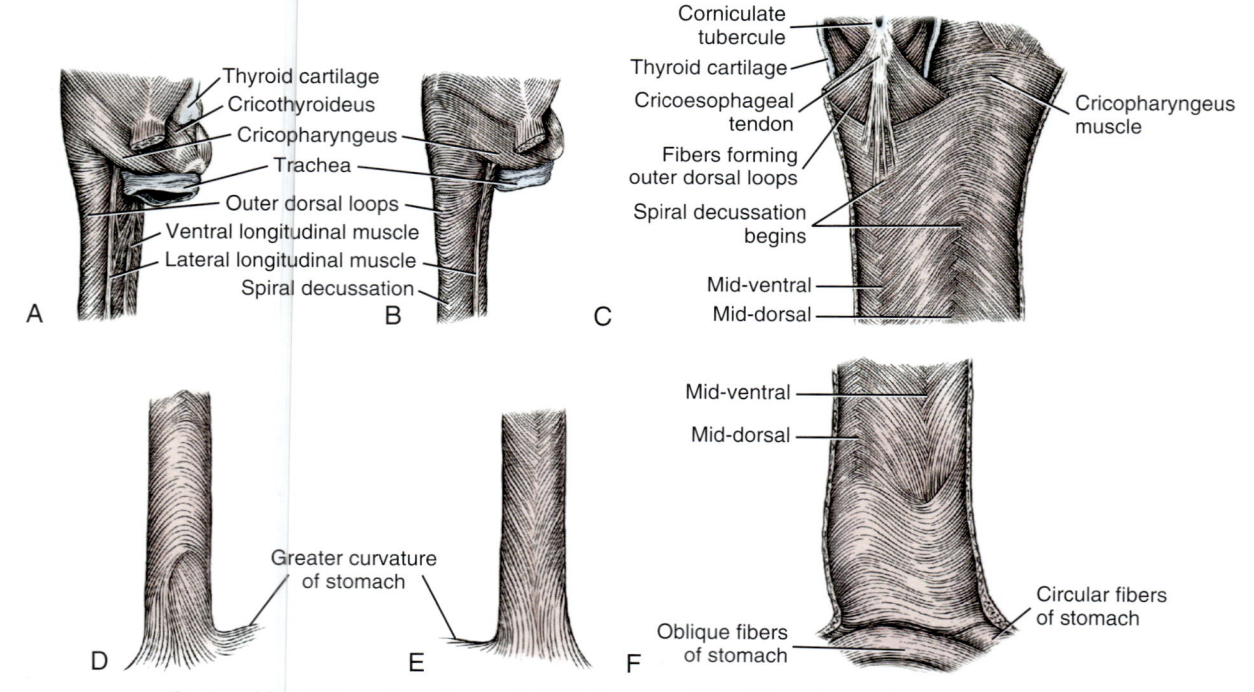

• **Fig. 7.29** Musculature of esophagus. A, Outer layer, cranial end, lateral ventral aspect. B, Outer layer, cranial end, lateral dorsal aspect. C, Inner layer, cranial end. (Esophagus opened on left side.) D, Outer layer, caudal end, ventral aspect. E, Outer layer, caudal end, dorsal aspect. F, Inner layer, caudal end. (Esophagus opened on right side.)

as well as in the neck, by the prevertebral fascia. Caudal to a transverse plane through the termination of the trachea the esophagus lies nearly in the median plane as it passes in the mediastinum between the two pleural sacs.

The aorta obliquely crosses the left side of the esophagus between the fifth and ninth thoracic vertebrae and thereafter diverges from it in a progressive manner caudally so that at the diaphragm the two structures are separated by approximately 3 cm. The dorsal branches of both right and left vagal nerves run dorsocaudally across the sides of the esophagus and unite with each other on the dorsum of the esophagus, 2 to 4 cm cranial to the dorsal part of the esophageal hiatus. The dorsal vagal trunk, so formed, continues to and passes through the dorsal part of the esophageal hiatus. The right and left ventral branches of the vagi unite immediately caudal to the root of the lungs to form the ventral vagal trunk. This trunk at first lies in contact with the esophagus and then arches ventrally in the caudal mediastinum before it passes through the esophageal hiatus with the esophagus.

The **abdominal portion** (*pars abdominalis*) of the esophagus is its wedge-shaped terminal part. Dorsally, the esophagus immediately joins the stomach. Ventrally it notches the thin, dorsal border of the caudate lobe of the liver.

The esophagus is not uniform in either the thickness of its wall or the diameter of its lumen. In the cervical portion its wall averages approximately 4 mm in thickness and in the thoracic portion, 2.5 mm; the wall is thickest in the abdominal portion, measuring approximately 6 mm where it joins the stomach. As determined by the size of the approximately 10 primary longitudinal folds of its mucosa, the whole tube is capable of great dilatation. The least distensible parts occur at both its beginning and its end and as it passes through the thoracic inlet.

Coats of the Esophagus

The esophagus has four coats: fibrous, muscular, submucous, and mucous. In the cervical region, the **fibrous coat**, or **adventitia** (*tunica adventitia*), blends with the deep cervical fascia dorsally and on the left, and with the fascia that forms the carotid sheath on the left. The adventitia of the thoracic and abdominal portions of the esophagus blends with the endothoracic and the transversalis fascia, respectively. It is largely covered by pleura in the thorax and with peritoneum in the abdomen. Where the esophagus is not covered by serosa, its adventitia blends with that proper fascia of the organs with which it comes in contact.

The **muscular coat** (*tunica muscularis*) (see Fig. 7.29) consists essentially of two oblique layers of striated muscle fibers. The external muscular coat arises on the ventral side of the esophagus from the medial dorsal crest of the cricoid and the corniculate portions of the arytenoid cartilages by means of the **cricoesophageal tendon** (*tendo cricoesophageus*). This tendon is a distinct thin band of collagenous tissue approximately 0.5 cm wide and 1 cm long. It tapers to a point caudally as muscle fibers leave each side of it. It, more than any other structure, serves as the fixed point of cranial attachment of the esophagus (Sauer, 1951).

The first few muscle fibers to arise arch sharply lateral and dorsal on each side and meet dorsally as transverse fibers. They are not distinct from the caudal fibers of the cranially lying cricopharyngeal muscles. Helm (1907) appropriately called this initial portion of the external esophageal muscle coat the *cricoesophageal muscle*. The fibers from each side do not decussate mid-dorsally but blend with each other without demarcation. Although the first few fibers are nearly transverse in direction, the subsequent fibers become increasingly more oblique so that in fusing with their fellows they form progressively narrower loops or ellipses caudally.

The main musculature of the esophagus caudal to the cricoesophageal fibers is in the form of spiral fibers. These start approximately 5 cm from the beginning of the esophagus and continue to within 5 to 10 cm of the cardia of the stomach. The superficial fibers on one side become the deep ones on the other side. These apparently continuous oblique bundles spiral around the esophagus in such a way that they cross each other at nearly right angles in making up the two main muscular coats of the organ. The lines of decussations are dorsal and ventral in position. The line of ventral decussation seems to stop approximately 10 cm from the cardia, whereas the dorsal decussations end approximately 5 cm from it. The decussations do not end abruptly as there is a gradual shifting of the direction of the fibers of the inner and outer muscle coats.

The fibers of the inner coat become more transverse in direction, whereas those of the outer coat become more longitudinal, especially dorsally as they approach the cardia. Approximately 3 cm from the cardia, ventrally, many of the oblique fibers of the inner coat, instead of becoming more transverse, become nearly longitudinal and pass to the outside. They continue on the visceral wall of the stomach as its outer longitudinal layer. The longitudinal fibers of the dorsal surface of the esophagus (*m. esophageus longitudinalis dorsalis*) continue on the dorsal wall of the stomach. The nearly transverse, inner muscular fibers of the esophagus partly blend with the circular and oblique fibers of the stomach. The division between the striated musculature of the esophagus and the smooth musculature of the stomach cannot be determined by gross examination.

The cervical portion of the esophagus possesses, in addition to the two oblique coats, several poorly developed groups of longitudinal fibers. The right and left lateral longitudinal bands (*m. esophageus longitudinalis lateralis*) are best developed. They arise deep to the cricopharyngeal muscles from the fascia adjacent to the lateral borders of the dorsal cricoarytenoid muscles. Some fibers contributing to these bands come from the cricoesophageal tendon. The muscles are 1 to 2 mm wide. They usually fade away on the caudal portion of the cervical part of the esophagus, but they may extend to the midthoracic part. Inner and outer ventral longitudinal esophageal muscle fibers (*m. esophageus longitudinalis ventralis*) can usually also be recognized. The inner ones arise from the cricoesophageal tendon and, after running approximately 2 cm, become dispersed on the main inner muscular coat. They lie on the dorsal surface of the ventral decussations that they partly cover. The outer longitudinal muscle fibers lie ventral to the ventral decussations. They are so feeble that they cannot always be dissected in gross with certainty. In some specimens extremely delicate longitudinal muscle bundles have been seen lying between the inner and outer muscular coats in the cranial part of the cervical portion of the esophagus.

The **submucous coat** (*tela submucosa*) loosely connects the mucous and the muscular coats. It allows the relatively inelastic mucous coat to be thrown into heavy longitudinal folds when the esophagus is contracted. It contains blood vessels, nerves, and mucous glands. Trautmann and Fiebiger (1957) state that the **esophageal glands** (*gl. esophageae*) form a continuous stratum that extends to the vicinity of the stomach. The **muscular layer of the mucosa** (*lamina muscularis mucosae*), according to these authors, is present only in the caudal half of the esophagus and forms a continuous layer of smooth muscle only near the stomach.

The **mucous coat** (*tunica mucosa*) is composed of a superficially cornified, stratified squamous epithelium that contains the openings, at approximately 1 mm intervals, of the ducts of the esophageal glands. In the collapsed esophagus it forms large and numerous longitudinal rugae or folds. Cardiac glands exist in the distal part of the esophagus.

Vessels of the Esophagus

The arteries to the cervical portion of the esophagus are primarily branches from the cranial and caudal **thyroid arteries**. The glandular mantle underlying the limen pharyngoesophageum is richly supplied by branches from the cranial thyroid artery. In the region of the thoracic inlet on the left side, a long but small descending branch from the left caudal thyroid artery anastomoses with an ascending branch from the bronchoesophageal. From this small anastomotic trunk, branches go to the esophagus. The esophageal portion of the **bronchoesophageal artery** is the main source of blood to the cranial two-thirds of the thoracic portion of the esophagus (Figs. 7.30 and 11.34). The remaining part is supplied by esophageal branches of the aorta or **dorsal intercostal arteries**, and the terminal portion is supplied by the esophageal branch of the **left gastric artery**.

The veins that drain the esophagus are essentially satellites of the arteries that supply it. Those veins from the thoracic portion empty largely into the **azygos vein**, with the vein that accompanies the esophageal branch of the left gastric artery being a tributary of the portal system. Adjacent veins, like the arteries, anastomose with each other on the esophagus. According to Baum (1918), lymph vessels from the esophagus drain into the **medial retropharyngeal, deep cervical, bronchial, portal, splenic, gastric,** and **jejunal lymph nodes**.

Nerves of the Esophagus

The cricopharyngeal muscle and the cervical portion of the esophagus are supplied with motor fibers from the **pharyngeal plexus** that receives pharyngeal branches from the **glossopharyngeal** and **vagal** nerves. These pharyngeal branches arise close to the distal ganglia of these two cranial nerves (Hwang et al., 1948). These investigators also found that a variable portion of the cervical part of the esophagus contracted when the peripheral ends of the vagus or the recurrent laryngeal nerves were stimulated at the base of the neck. Most nerve branches to the esophagus are too small to be seen in gross. There is probably an overlapping in the amount of the cervical part supplied by the pharyngeal plexus and recurrent laryngeal nerves. It is further evident from physiologic experiments that these two nerves are reciprocal in the amount of the cervical portion of the esophagus that they supply.

Hwang et al. (1948) found that a small branch from the pharyngeal branch of the vagus passed deep to the pharyngeal muscles to reach the esophagus. Stimulation of this branch produced contraction of the cranial half of the cervical portion. It is probable that the recurrent laryngeal nerves carry afferent (Chauveau, 1886) and efferent fibers to the cervical portion of the esophagus as well as providing both the motor and sensory nerve supply to the thoracic part as far caudally as the heart. The dorsal and ventral branches of the vagi and the vagal trunks they form supply the esophagus caudal to the heart.

Watson (1974) described three major regions of the esophagus in the dog as characterized by their innervation (Fig. 7.31): a cervical region supplied by paired pharyngoesophageal and paired pararecurrent laryngeal nerves, a cranial thoracic region supplied mainly by the left pararecurrent laryngeal nerve, and a caudal thoracic and abdominal region supplied by the vagal trunks. For most of its course in the neck the recurrent laryngeal nerve was paralleled by a slightly smaller nerve lying more dorsally and giving branches to both the trachea and the esophagus. This latter nerve was called the *pararecurrent laryngeal nerve* by Lemere (1932), and, as Watson pointed out, it is always present. (Lemere claimed that the pararecurrent nerves are motor, secretomotor, and sensory to the caudal two-thirds of the cervical esophagus.)

Khurana and Petras (1991) studied the sensory innervation of the dog esophagus, stomach, and duodenum using the horseradish peroxidase technique. Their data showed that the area of innervation for each viscus overlapped its neighbor significantly, although there is a field of peak innervation. Craniocaudal innervation of the esophagus spanned as many as 23 paired spinal ganglia (C1 to L2). There were two peak innervation fields for the cervical (C2 to C6 and T2 to T4) and the thoracic (T2 to T4 and T8 to T12) sectors of the esophagus. The sensory innervation of the stomach extended over as many as 25 paired spinal ganglia (C2 to L5). The peak innervation levels for the stomach spanned an area from T2 to T10. The duodenum was innervated by as many as 15 paired thoracolumbar spinal ganglia (T2 to L3), with a peak innervation in the middle and caudal thoracic spinal ganglia and cranial lumbar (T6 to L1). Vagal afferent innervation of the esophagus, stomach, and duodenum was bilateral and originated primarily but not entirely from the distal ganglia. Neurons from the proximal ganglia were more frequent in the esophagus than they were in the stomach or duodenum.

Holland, Satchell, and Farrow (1996) studied vagal esophagomotor nerve function and esophageal motor performance in 16 control dogs and 4 with congenital idiopathic megaesophagus. Their conclusions were that, in dogs with congenital idiopathic megaesophagus, the vagal efferent innervation to the esophagus is likely to be normal. A primary esophageal myopathy is unlikely to be present, and the observed reduction in esophageal motor performance may arise as a secondary consequence of altered biomechanical properties rather than from a primary neuromuscular abnormality.

Abdomen

Regions of the Abdomen

The abdomen is between the thorax and the pelvic cavity, and includes viscera that are coexistent within these regions (Fig. 7.32). For convenience of description the abdomen is divided into several primary regions by three transverse

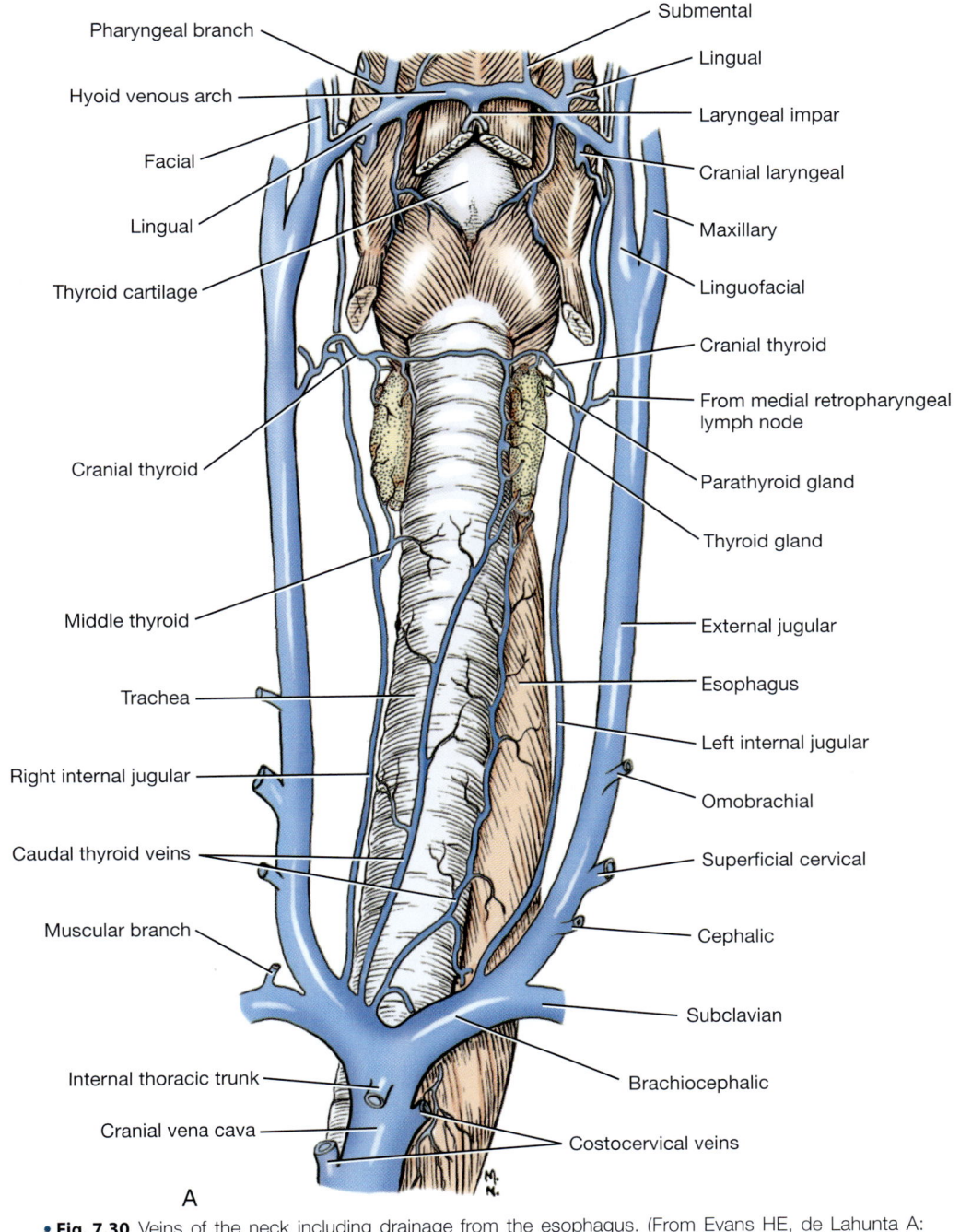

• **Fig. 7.30** Veins of the neck including drainage from the esophagus. (From Evans HE, de Lahunta A: *Guide to the Dissection of the Dog*, 8th ed., St. Louis, 2017, Elsevier.) *Continued*

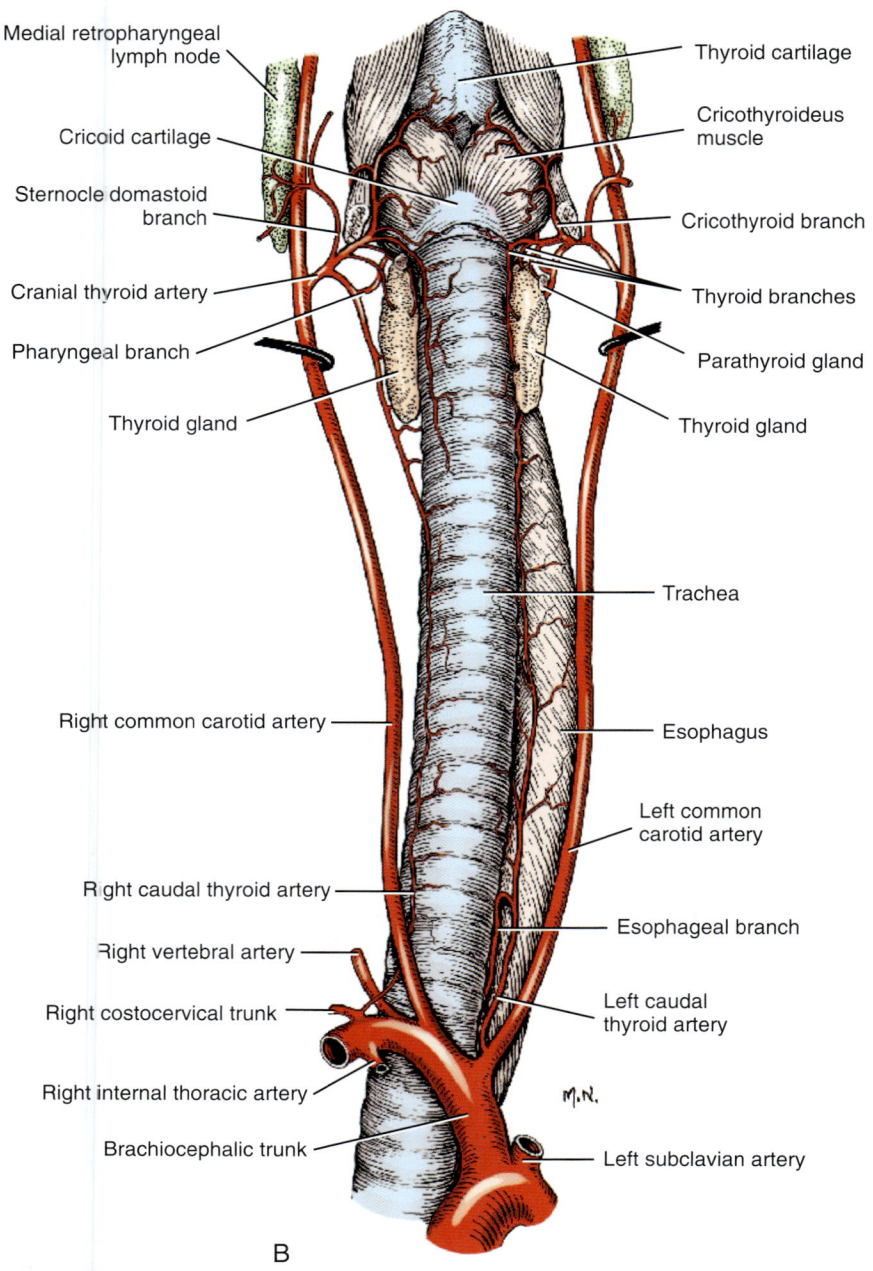

• **Fig. 7.30, cont'd** The relation of the common carotid arteries to the larynx, trachea, esophagus, and related structures, ventral aspect.

planes. Each of the regions has three subdivisions defined by these sagittal planes (see Fig. 7.33).

The middle of the three transverse planes passes through the most caudal border of the costal arch. This plane therefore passes through the caudal portion of the second lumbar vertebra. The more caudal of the three transverse planes crosses the body at a level through the ventral cranial iliac spines, or the most cranial parts of the wings of the ilia. This plane bisects the caudal part of the sixth lumbar vertebra. By means of these three planes the abdomen is divided into three segments, which are named the *cranial, middle,* and *caudal abdominal regions.* Of these three segments, the cranial abdominal region is by far the largest as it extends far cranial between the ribs of each side, where it is limited cranially by the diaphragm. The caudal abdominal region is smallest as it ends caudally at the pelvic inlet. An atlas for the cranial abdomen by means of computed tomography was made by Rivero et al. (2009). A similar study including the thorax was made by Smallwood and George (1993).

The two imaginary sagittal planes, which further divide the abdomen into smaller regions, pass on each side midway between the ventral cranial iliac spine and the median sagittal plane. The three parts of the cranial abdominal region are the **right** and **left hypochondriac regions** (*regio*

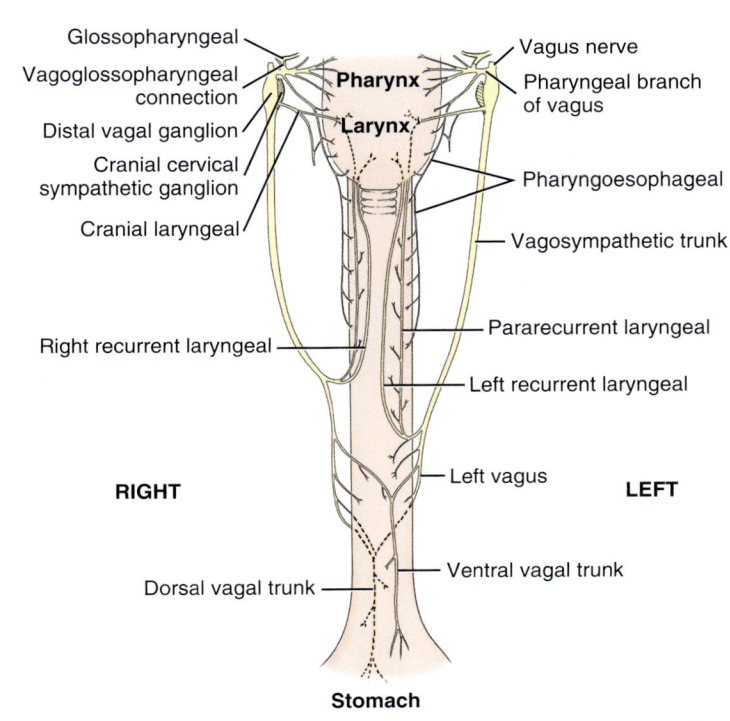

Fig. 7.31 Innervation of the esophagus. (After Watson AG: *Some aspects of the vagal innervation of the canine esophagus: an anatomical study,* Master's thesis, New Zealand, 1974, Massey University.)

hypochondriaca dextra et sinistra) and the median **xiphoid region** (*regio xiphoidea*). The middle abdominal region includes the unpaired, median ventral area of the abdomen, known as the **umbilical region** (*regio umbilicalis*), and the **right** and **left lateral regions** (*regio lateralis dextra et sinistra*). The lateral regions include the **fold of the flank** (*regio plicae lateris*), and each contains an expansive **paralumbar fossa** (*fossa paralumbalis*), which forms a ventral arc and a dorsal, straight base located ventrolateral to the transverse processes of the lumbar vertebrae and the iliocostalis muscle. The three parts of the caudal abdominal segment are the **right and left inguinal regions** (*regio inguinalis dextra et sinistra*) and the median unpaired **pubic region** (*regio pubica*). In addition to the abdominal regions already named, there are preputial and mammary regions.

The **abdomen** (abdominal region or *regiones abdominis*) (Figs. 7.32 to 7.34) is that part of the trunk that extends from the diaphragm to the pelvis. It contains the largest cavity in the body, the **abdominal cavity** (*cavum abdominis*). Caudally the abdominal cavity is continuous with the pelvic cavity, the division between the two being a plane through the pelvic inlet, or brim of the pelvis. The abdominal cavity is a muscle and bone bounded cavity. It is lined internally by the transversalis fascia, which in turn is covered in most places by the peritoneum.

The peritoneum forms the lining wall of the **peritoneal cavity** (*cavum peritonei*), which is contained largely, but not exclusively, within the abdominal cavity. In both sexes the pelvic cavity contains the pelvic portion of the peritoneal cavity. The vaginal tunica, always well developed in the male and the vaginal process, usually present in the female, also exist as extraabdominal extensions of the peritoneal cavity. The abdominal cavity is truncate and cone-shaped, with a domed cranial end or base. It contains the abdominal viscera, which include primarily the flexuous alimentary canal and its two associated glands, the liver and the pancreas. Also included are the spleen, female reproductive tract, deferent ducts in the male, many nerve plexuses, vessels, lymph nodes, kidneys, ureters, bladder, and proximal urethra. It is bounded cranially by the diaphragm; dorsally by the lumbar vertebrae and lumbar hypaxial muscles and the crura of the diaphragm, the two oblique and transverse abdominal muscles, and a small portion of the shaft of the ilium on each side. Ventrally the right and left rectus abdominis muscles and their sheaths form the abdominal wall.

There are three unpaired apertures in the diaphragm: the **esophageal hiatus**, for passage of the esophagus, vagal nerve trunks, and esophageal vessels; the **caval foramen**, for passage of the caudal vena cava; and the **aortic hiatus**, for passage of the aorta, thoracic duct, and the azygos and hemiazygos veins. Paired slitlike openings existing dorsal to the diaphragm are formed ventrally by the dorsal edge of the diaphragm, the lumbocostal arch, and dorsally by the psoas muscles. At these sites the pleura and peritoneum are separated only by the fused endothoracic and transversalis fasciae. The sympathetic trunk and splanchnic nerves pass dorsal to the lumbocostal arch on each side.

Caudally the abdominal cavity communicates freely with the pelvic cavity at the pelvic inlet. In the fetus, there is a relatively large opening, the umbilical aperture, located midventrally, which serves for the passage of the umbilical blood vessels, the small vitelline duct, and the stalk of the

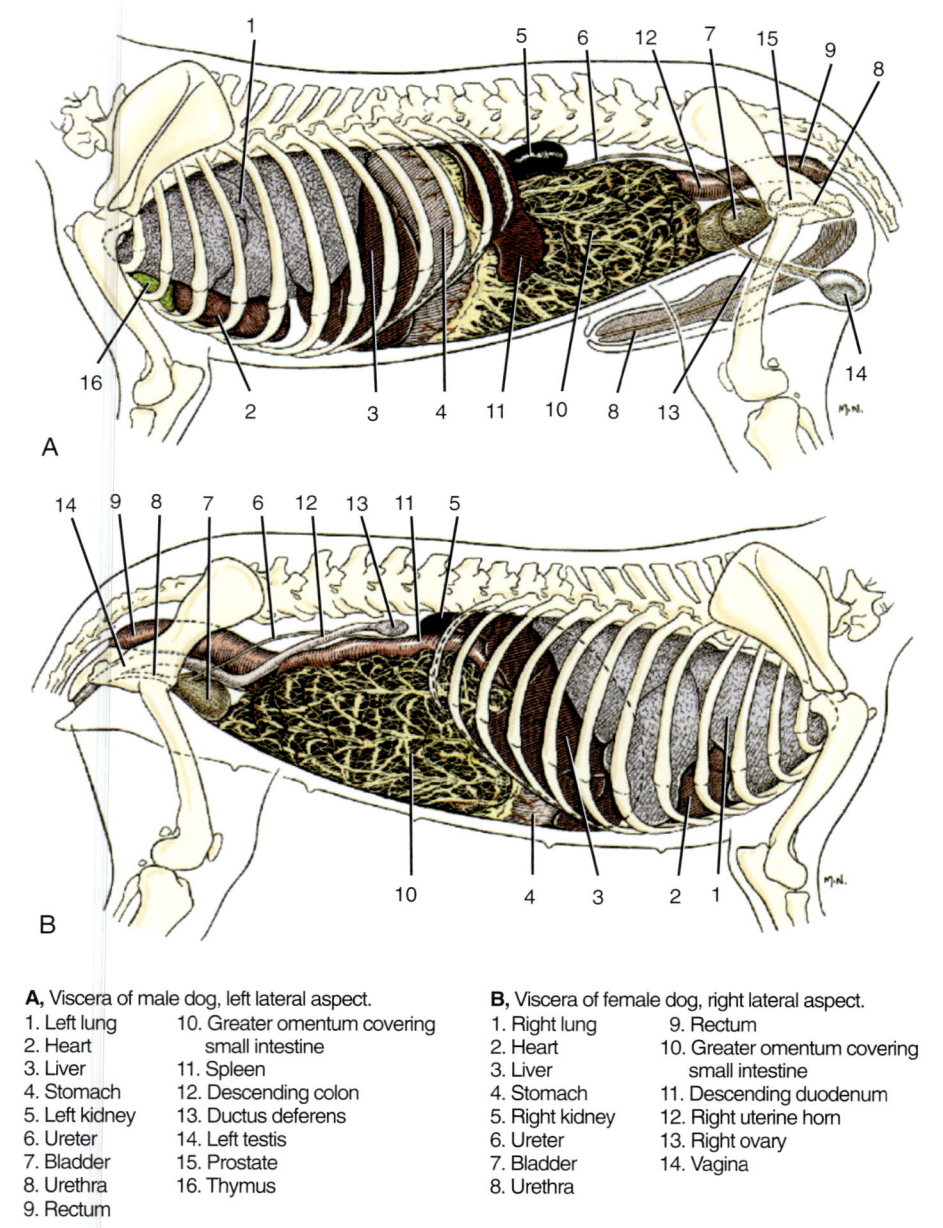

352   CHAPTER 7   The Digestive Apparatus and Abdomen

A, Viscera of male dog, left lateral aspect.

1. Left lung
2. Heart
3. Liver
4. Stomach
5. Left kidney
6. Ureter
7. Bladder
8. Urethra
9. Rectum
10. Greater omentum covering small intestine
11. Spleen
12. Descending colon
13. Ductus deferens
14. Left testis
15. Prostate
16. Thymus

B, Viscera of female dog, right lateral aspect.

1. Right lung
2. Heart
3. Liver
4. Stomach
5. Right kidney
6. Ureter
7. Bladder
8. Urethra
9. Rectum
10. Greater omentum covering small intestine
11. Descending duodenum
12. Right uterine horn
13. Right ovary
14. Vagina

• **Fig. 7.32** Viscera of the dog. (The location of the diaphragm is indicated by a dotted circle.)

allantois. After these structures are disrupted at birth, this opening rapidly closes, forming a faint scar, the umbilicus, on the midventral line. There is a passage on each side in the caudoventral part of the abdominal wall, called the *inguinal canal*, for the passage of the vaginal tunic and the spermatic cord in the male and the vaginal process and round ligament of the uterus in the female. In both sexes the external pudendal vessels and the genitofemoral nerve pass through the caudal part of the inguinal canal. Another pair of abdominal openings in the caudal part of the abdominal wall are the right and left vascular lacunae. The femoral artery, vein, lymphatics, and saphenous nerve, surrounded by transversalis fascia, pass through each vascular lacuna.

The **pelvic cavity** (*cavum pelvis*) can be considered as a caudal continuation of the abdominal cavity and, in a broad sense, is regarded as a division of it. It begins at the **cranial pelvic aperture** (*apertura pelvis cranialis*) also known as the pelvic inlet. This aperture is bordered by the **terminal line** (*linea terminalis*), which is a circular line from the sacral promontory across the sacroiliac articulation, along the arcuate line of the ilium to the pectin of the pubis. The pelvic cavity extends caudally to the **caudal pelvic aperture** (*apertura pelvis caudalis*), also known as the *pelvic outlet*, which is bounded dorsally by the first caudal vertebra, laterally by the sacrotuberous ligament, and ventrally by the ischial arch. The lateral walls of the pelvic cavity include the ilium, middle gluteal, levator ani, and coccygeus muscles.

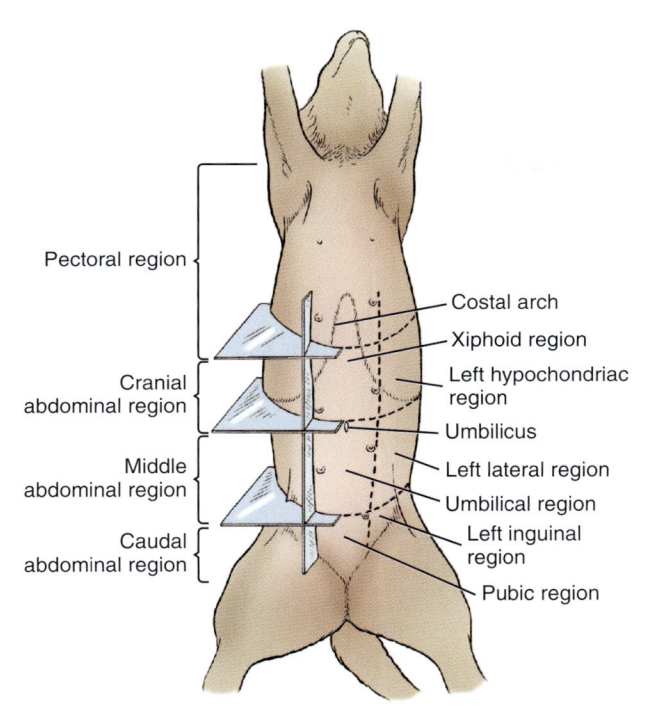

• **Fig. 7.33** Regions of the abdomen as determined by sagittal and transverse planes.

The pelvic cavity contains the rectum and the urethra in both sexes, the vagina and part of the vestibule in the female, and a part or all of the prostate in the male.

The abdominal and pelvic cavities are lined by fascia throughout. In most places this fascia attaches to muscles or bones peripherally and is adhered to the parietal layer of the peritoneum centrally. The fascia was previously named according to the region or parts it covered, so that parts of it were known by such names as *diaphragmatic, transversalis, iliac, internal spermatic,* and *pelvic fascia*. The term **transversalis fascia** (*fascia transversalis*) is used to include all of these fascial divisions. In obese specimens the large fat deposits around the kidneys, in the falciform ligament, in the pelvis, and around the vaginal rings are located in a layer of the transversalis fascia.

Relations of Abdominal Organs

The greater omentum, or epiploon (Fig. 7.34), is a fat-streaked, lacy, double reflection of peritoneum that covers most of the abdominal contents ventrally and on the sides. It lies principally between the parietal peritoneum and the intestinal mass. The greatest caudal extension of the liver occupies the right hypochondriac region.

The stomach, when empty, does not contact the abdominal wall, but when moderately filled it lies against the xiphoid and left hypochondriac portions of this wall caudal to the liver. The completely filled stomach, especially in pups, lies largely in contact with the xiphoid and umbilical regions, ventrally, and the right and left lateral portions of the abdominal wall, and reaches caudally to a transverse plane just caudal to the umbilicus.

The left kidney contacts the dorsal part of the left lateral abdominal wall. The spleen, separated from the greater curvature of the stomach by the gastrosplenic ligament, contacts an oblique zone of the abdominal wall from the left kidney to the midventral line or even beyond this. A small portion of the right kidney immediately caudal to the last rib and a large portion of the descending part of the duodenum lie directly in contact with the dorsal part of the right lateral abdominal region. The urinary bladder, adjacent to the greater omentum but not covered ventrally by it, is the only visceral organ which lies in contact with the abdominal wall in the pubic region.

All abdominal organs vary normally in size and position. The stomach, uterus, urinary bladder, and spleen vary more than the other organs because of their ability to undergo marked changes in size and shape. The gravid uterus alters the position of all the other movable abdominal organs more markedly than do any of the others. It always occupies the most ventral position in the abdomen because it contains no gas and is therefore the heaviest freely movable abdominal organ. In advanced pregnancy it nearly completely fills the ventral half of the abdominal cavity. It is impossible to assign a constant position for any one of the abdominal organs, especially those attached by elongate peritoneal folds. Imaging (magnetic resonance imaging [MRI], computed tomography [CT], ultrasound) and hardened anatomic preparations clearly reveal the normal variations that exist from time to time and in different specimens.

Peritoneum

The peritoneum is a **serous membrane** (*tunica serosa*) that, like other serous membranes, is made up of a surface mesothelium composed of squamous epithelial cells and a connective tissue ground work, or stroma. The connective tissue stroma is composed of yellow elastic and white fibrous tissue. A serous membrane is histologically largely connective tissue, whether it is found in the thoracic, pericardial, or abdominal cavity. The transversalis fascia serves to attach the peritoneum to the underlying muscle and bone.

The lining of the abdominal cavity and its coextensive pelvic and scrotal cavities, as well as the covering of and the reflections from the organs of the abdomen, is peritoneum. It is distributed as though in the embryo all the organs developed in the walls of the abdominal, pelvic, or scrotal cavities and, as they grew, pushed the peritoneum before them as elastic veils. Some structures, such as the liver, kidneys, and gonads, do develop in this way. The abdominal part of the alimentary canal arises very early in the embryo between the two layers of peritoneum, which form a midsagittal partition separating the abdominal part of the celom into right and left parts. Most of the ventral part of this fold becomes obliterated shortly after it forms. The parts that are left go to the liver, the stomach, and the beginning of the duodenum cranially and the bladder caudally. Because most of the primitive ventral mesentery (that ventral to the digestive tube before it has rotated) becomes obliterated, the definitive appearance of the tube suggests that it migrated ventrally from the dorsal abdominal wall; actually it develops between the two peritoneal layers.

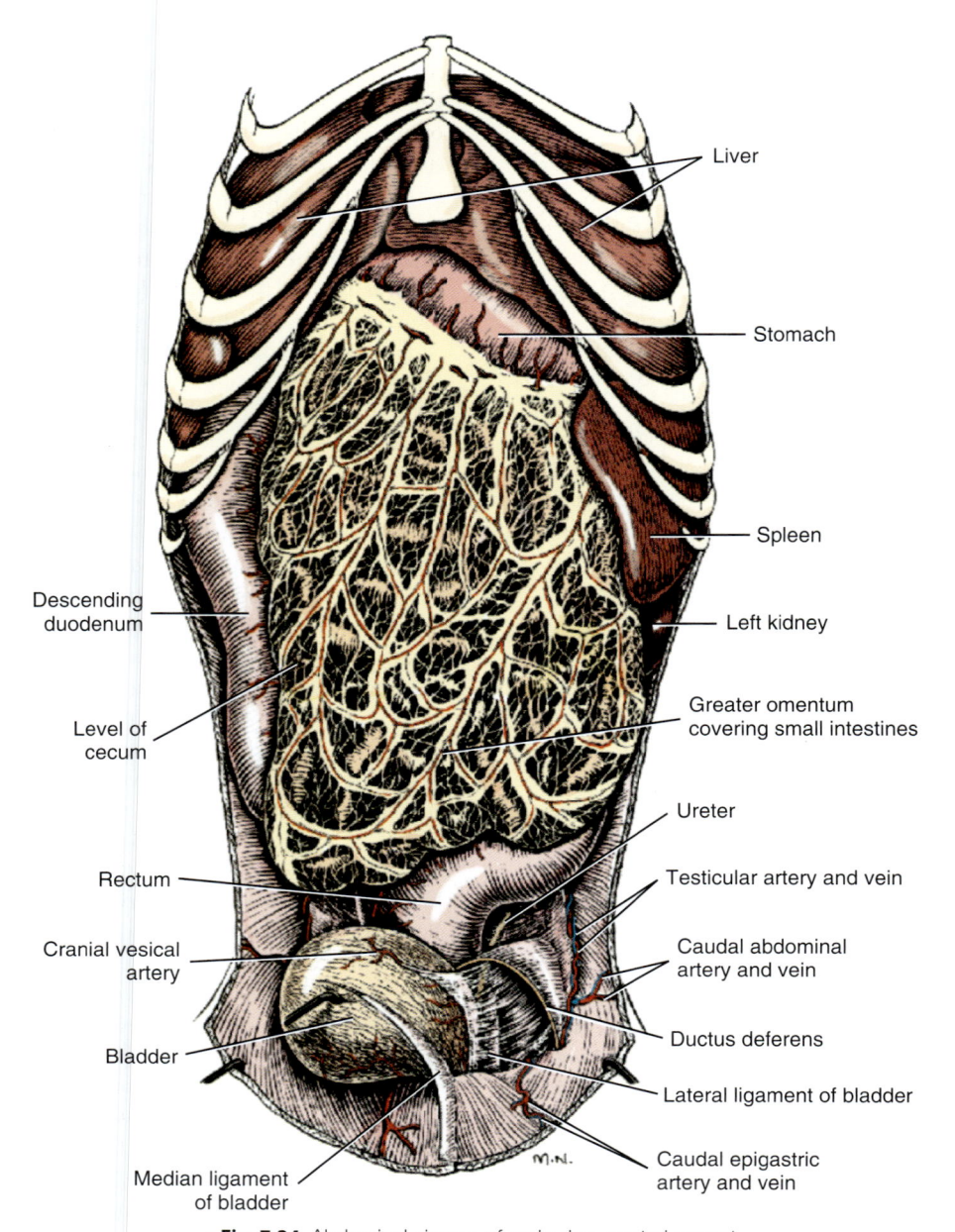

Fig. 7.34 Abdominal viscera of male dog, ventral aspect.

The peritoneum serves to reduce friction between parts. A small amount of viscous fluid is produced for this purpose. Whenever two peritoneal surfaces in contact fail to move for an appreciable time, the mesothelium of the apposed surfaces is absorbed and the connective tissue reinforcement, the stroma, ceases to be differentiated from that of adjacent parts; thus peritoneal sheets become obliterated, and viscera adhere to neighboring structures. From a relatively simple disposition in the embryo, the arrangement of the peritoneum in an adult becomes a complicated maze of mesenteries and ligaments.

The peritoneum may be divided into:

The **parietal peritoneum** (*peritoneum parietale*) covers in large part the inner surface of the walls of the abdominal, pelvic, and scrotal cavities.

The **visceral peritoneum** (*peritoneum viscerale*) covers the organs of the abdominal, pelvic, and scrotal cavities, wholly or in part.

The **connecting peritoneum** consists of double sheets of peritoneum extending between organs or connecting them to the parietal peritoneum. These peritoneal folds are referred to as *mesenteries*, *omenta*, or *ligaments*. A **mesentery** (*mesenterium*), in a restricted sense, passes from the abdominal wall to the jejunum and ileum. It is long and contains many vessels and nerves. In a broader sense, a mesentery is any long, serous fold that attaches organs to a wall and serves as a route by which the nerves and vessels reach the organs. A **ligament** passes from a wall to an organ, or from an organ to an organ, and is usually narrow and contains few vessels.

The cavities enclosed by serous membrane are closed cavities, except for the peritoneal cavity in most female animals. In the bitch there is an opening at the abdominal end of each uterine tube and thus, through the genital tract, to the outside. No organs or tissues are located in the peritoneal cavity (except at the time of ovulation, when an oocyte emerges from the ovary and passes to the opening into the uterine tube). In life this is an almost nonexistent cavity containing only enough lubricating fluid to moisten the apposed peritoneal surfaces, both between different organs and between the organs and the parietal peritoneum.

Organs that lie against the walls of the abdominal or pelvic cavities and that are covered only on one surface by peritoneum are said to be retroperitoneal. Most of these organs are small and are embedded in fat. Organs that project freely into the abdominal, pelvic, and scrotal cavities and receive a nearly complete covering of peritoneum are termed intraperitoneal.

At an early stage in development the alimentary canal is relatively straight, thus allowing the primitive dorsal mesentery (*mesenterium dorsale primitivum*) to exist as a simple median partition. When the parts of the digestive tube differentiate, those parts of the primitive dorsal mesentery going to the several organs receive specific names, as follows: to the stomach, *mesogastrium*; to the duodenum, *mesoduodenum*; to the jejunoileum, *mesojejunoileum* or *mesentery*; to the colon, *mesocolon*; and the rectum, *mesorectum*. In fat dogs, the apposed surfaces of the two layers of the connecting peritoneum are separated by fat that is deposited along the arteries, and, because of this, neither the abdominal aorta nor the caudal part of the caudal vena cava is visible. This continuous connecting peritoneum is the peritoneal fold that leaves the dorsal abdominal wall and reflects, directly or indirectly, around most of the freely movable organs of the abdominal cavity. It can be demonstrated by grasping the abdominal part of the digestive tube along with the pancreas and spleen and moving them ventrally. In thin dogs it can be seen to leave the aorta, providing a route by which the celiac, cranial, and caudal mesenteric arteries; autonomic nerves; lymphatics; and radicles of the portal vein pass to or from the intestine and other organs. It is the retained part of the serous partition that divided the celom dorsal to the alimentary canal into right and left halves.

The primitive ventral mesentery disappears between the stomach cranially and the rectum and bladder caudally. Remnants of this cranially are the lesser omentum, liver serosa and hepatic ligaments, and the falciform ligament. Caudally the only remnant is the median ligament of the bladder.

A transverse section of the caudal abdomen reveals the disposition of the peritoneum in its simplest form. Follow the peritoneum starting from where it covers the inner surface of the left rectus abdominis. Here it is closely united with the internal sheath of the rectus abdominis by transversalis fascia. Progressing to the right the peritoneum forms a fold at the linea alba that continues from the umbilicus cranially to the bladder caudally. This is the median ligament of the bladder. In the fetus this contains the stalk of the allantois (the urachus) and the two umbilical arteries but in the adult there are no remnants of these fetal structures. On the right side of this ligament the peritoneum covers the internal sheath of the right rectus abdominis. Further dorsally on the lateral abdominal wall in the male, the peritoneum sends a thin narrow plica ventromedially that surrounds the testicular vessels and nerves. In the female this plica surrounds the uterine horn and contains the branches of the uterine blood vessels and nerves. This plica of connecting peritoneum is called the *broad ligament* (*lig. latum uteri*). At this level a lateral fold of this broad ligament surrounds the round ligament of the uterus that is running between the cranial end of the uterine horn and the vaginal ring.

In the ventral lumbar region, the peritoneum loosely covers the ureter as the latter crosses the external iliac vessels. Near the median plane it covers the right sympathetic trunk and opposite the lumbar vertebral column it turns ventrally to extend to and surround the descending colon from which it continues back dorsally to the lumbar vertebral column. This connecting peritoneal fold is called the *descending mesocolon* (*mesocolon descendens*).

Pelvic Peritoneal Excavations

The peritoneum in the pelvic cavity can be traced by following it in a sagittal section just lateral to the median plane. By starting ventrally at a transverse plane passing through the tuber coxae and advancing caudally, one finds the peritoneum runs on the sheath of the rectus abdominis and passes over the ventral part of the pelvic inlet into the pelvic cavity. Within the first 2 cm after entering the pelvic cavity the peritoneum reflects dorsally on the neck of the bladder of the female or on the prostate gland of the male, forming the shallow **pubovesical pouch** (*excavatio pubovesicalis*). After reflecting cranially around the cranial surface of the bladder, the peritoneum leaves the dorsal surface of its neck in the female and forms the **vesicogenital pouch** (*excavatio vesicogenitalis*) as it reflects cranially on the ventral surface of the vagina and uterus. In the male this pouch is formed between the prostate ventrally and the genital fold dorsally with the deferent ducts. The reflection of peritoneum between the genital organs ventrally and the rectum dorsally is the **rectogenital pouch** (*excavatio rectogenitalis*). The caudal extension of the rectogenital pouch is not as great in the female as in the male. The caudal angles of the reflections of the peritoneum from one pelvic organ to the next dorsal to it are located progressively farther caudally in the male when they are traced in parasagittal planes from the pubis to the tail. A line drawn from a point approximately 1 cm caudal to the cranial border of the pubis to the transverse process of the third caudal vertebra indicates their most caudal extensions in the male. In the female, the rectogenital pouch extends farther caudally than the vesicogenital, but neither extends as far caudally as does the rectogenital pouch in the male.

Cranial Abdominal Connecting Peritoneum

To understand the definitive positions of the connecting peritoneum to the cranial abdominal alimentary tract and the liver, it is helpful to recall the primary rotations the tube makes and the differential growth that certain parts undergo. Early in development, the dorsal part of the stomach grows faster than the ventral part forming the greater curvature of the stomach. This causes it to rotate on its longitudinal axis to the left (counterclockwise as seen from caudal to cranial). Simultaneously with this rotation the stomach rotates on its vertical axis (counterclockwise as seen from dorsal to ventral) so that it lies in nearly a transverse position with the outlet located on the right while the inlet remains to the left in nearly the median plane. Distal to the stomach the anlagen of the liver and pancreas appear as diverticula of the mucosa of the duodenum. The liver grows ventrally between the peritoneal layers that form the primitive ventral mesentery. The ventral pancreas initially grows from the proximal duodenum on into the primitive ventral mesentery with the liver anlagen. With development, it rotates so that it grows into mesoduodenum on the right side. The dorsal pancreas grows from the proximal duodenum into the mesogastrium and with growth of the latter remains in the deep leaf of the greater omentum.

The intestinal part of the alimentary canal grows many times the length of the abdominal cavity. Therefore the parts with long mesenteries, mainly the jejunum and to a lesser extent the ileum, become greatly folded and occupy no constant location in the abdominal cavity. During development a part of the tube, in the form of an elongate U-shaped loop, is accommodated in a normal umbilical hernia caused by space restrictions in the fetal abdominal cavity. This hernia lasts but a short time. The cranial mesenteric artery lies in the mesentery, which connects the two limbs of the loop. As the loop is withdrawn into the abdomen, it rotates about three-fourths of a circle in a counterclockwise direction, as viewed from ventral to dorsal, around the axis of the artery. Because of this rotation, the proximal part of the small intestine, the duodenum, passes caudally on the right side of the cranial mesenteric artery and forms a hook shape, the caudal duodenal flexure, as it passes caudal to the artery and then cranially on its left side. At the same time the proximal part of the colon passes cranial to the artery and forms a hook shape, the transverse colon, as it passes to the right side and caudally to form the ascending colon. The descending duodenum on the right and the descending colon on the left side remained in the abdomen and were not part of the herniated intestine.

The following describes the various derivatives of the primitive dorsal mesentery and ventral mesentery as they run between the abdominal wall and the various parts of the alimentary canal.

The peritoneal folds, which in the adult leave approximately the greater and lesser curvatures of the stomach, are known as the greater and lesser omentum, respectively. The greater omentum, the most specialized serous fold in the body, is derived from the dorsal mesogastrium. The lesser omentum, small and relatively simple, is that portion of the ventral mesogastrium that extends between the liver and the lesser curvature of the stomach and the initial part of the duodenum.

Greater Omentum

The **greater omentum** (*omentum majus*), or epiploon (Figs. 7.34 to 7.36) is the dorsal mesogastrium that has been elongated into a large fold between the stomach and the dorsal body wall. By folding, the greater omentum has a superficial wall (*paries superficialis*) attached to the greater curvature of the stomach and facing the ventral abdominal wall and a deep wall (*paries profundus*) that faces the jejunoileum and attaches to the dorsal body wall cranial to the cranial mesenteric artery. The peritoneal space enclosed by these two walls is the large caudal recess of the omental bursa (*recessus caudalis omentalis*). This greater omental fold extends from the stomach caudally to the bladder where it turns cranially to near the stomach and continues to the dorsal body wall. This fold covers the coils of the jejunoileum ventrally and on the sides but remains medial to the descending duodenum and descending colon. Its deep wall passes ventral to the kidneys and lumbar hypaxial muscles. Thus the jejunoileum is covered by two layers of the greater omentum. Each wall of the greater omentum is composed of a double peritoneal sheet in which there are streaks of fat located around the arteries that run through it. The omentum forms one of the major fat storehouses in obese specimens. Between the streaks of fat the peritoneum is transparent because of its thinness. During surgery and in the postmortem specimen, the omentum appears as a fenestrated membrane that can be manually separated into its superficial and deep walls.

The more superficial, ventral wall (layer or leaf) (*paries superficialis*) was formerly called the *parietal part*, and the deeper, dorsal wall (layer or leaf) (*paries profundus*) was known as the *visceral part*. Between these two layers is a potential cavity, a portion of the peritoneal cavity, called the *lesser peritoneal cavity*, or the caudal recess of the omental bursa. Except for the constant opening, the epiploic foramen, the omental bursa is a closed sac. The entire **omental bursa** (*bursa omentalis*) is the potential peritoneal space enclosed by the greater and the lesser omenta, the stomach and liver. Another portion of the omental bursa, the mediastinal serous cavity (*cavum mediastini serosum*), extends cranially through the diaphragm and adjacent to the esophagus as a potential space within the dorsal part of the caudal mediastinum (Gendron et al., 2017). The largest portion of the omental bursa is the caudal recess between the two walls of the greater omentum. The **epiploic foramen** (*foramen omentale-epiploicum*) connects the greater and lesser peritoneal cavities. It is bounded ventrally by the peritoneum covering the portal vein in the hepatoduodenal ligament, dorsally by that covering the caudal vena cava, caudally by the hepatic artery covered by mesoduodenum, and cranially by the liver. It faces the

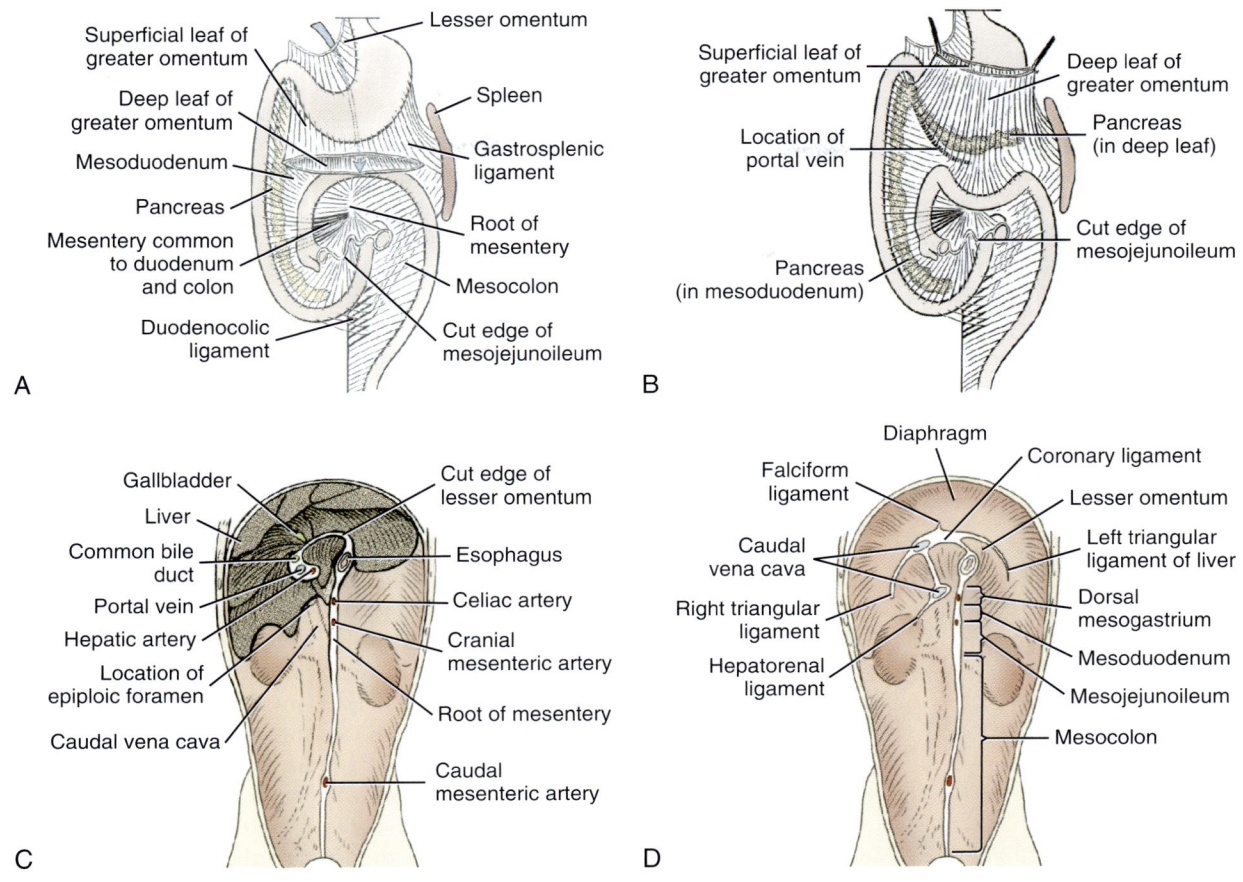

• **Fig. 7.35** Peritoneum. **A**, Plan of visceral and connecting peritoneum, ventral aspect. The greater omentum is transected caudal to the stomach. Red arrow in epiploic foramen. **B**, Plan of peritoneum with greater omentum reflected cranially. The transverse colon is displaced caudally. **C**, Plan of the dorsal reflections of the connecting and parietal peritoneum. The stomach and intestines removed. **D**, Plan of the dorsal reflections of the connecting and parietal peritoneum. All abdominal viscera removed.

right side. During surgery, placing a finger in this foramen and compressing its ventral border will deprive the liver of its blood supply coursing through the portal vein and hepatic artery.

Four portions of the greater omentum form three ligaments and a veil. The most extensive ligament is the **gastrosplenic ligament** (*lig. gastrolienale*). This portion extends from the hilus of the spleen to the greater curvature of the fundus and body of the stomach. The spleen itself develops within the dorsal mesogastrium where it bulges laterally to be enclosed by the superficial layer of peritoneal mesothelium of the part of the greater omentum where the latter folds from the superficial wall to the deep wall on the left side. This ligament is represented at the spleen by the peritoneal attachment along the entire length of the hilus of the spleen. When taut the gastrosplenic ligament is approximately 5 cm wide ventrally. The large splenic vessels that approach the spleen near the middle of the hilus give origin to the short gastric and left gastroepiploic vessels that course through this ligament to the greater curvature and fundus of the stomach.

The attachment from the gastrosplenic ligament to the left crus of the diaphragm is the **phrenicosplenic ligament** (*lig. phrenicolienale*). The portion of the greater omentum that attaches the left crus of the diaphragm to the fundus of the stomach is the **gastrophrenic ligament** (*lig. gastrophrenicum*). The gastrosplenic ligament is the most well developed of these three ligaments in the dog.

The **omental veil** (*velum omentale*) is a sagittal membrane connecting the deep wall of the greater omentum with the left side of the descending colon. It has a free caudal border and is not involved with the formation of the omental bursa. It contains between its peritoneal leaves, cranially, the left extremity and caudal margin of the left lobe of the pancreas. Its borders form approximately a rectangle, each lateral margin measuring approximately 20 cm in length. The cranial margin is approximately 10 cm long and the caudal one 7 cm. The right, or mesocolic, margin blends with the left peritoneal layer of the left mesocolon opposite the attachment of the duodenocolic ligament that blends with the right peritoneal layer of the left mesocolon. Its left margin is free and usually contains a fine but strong

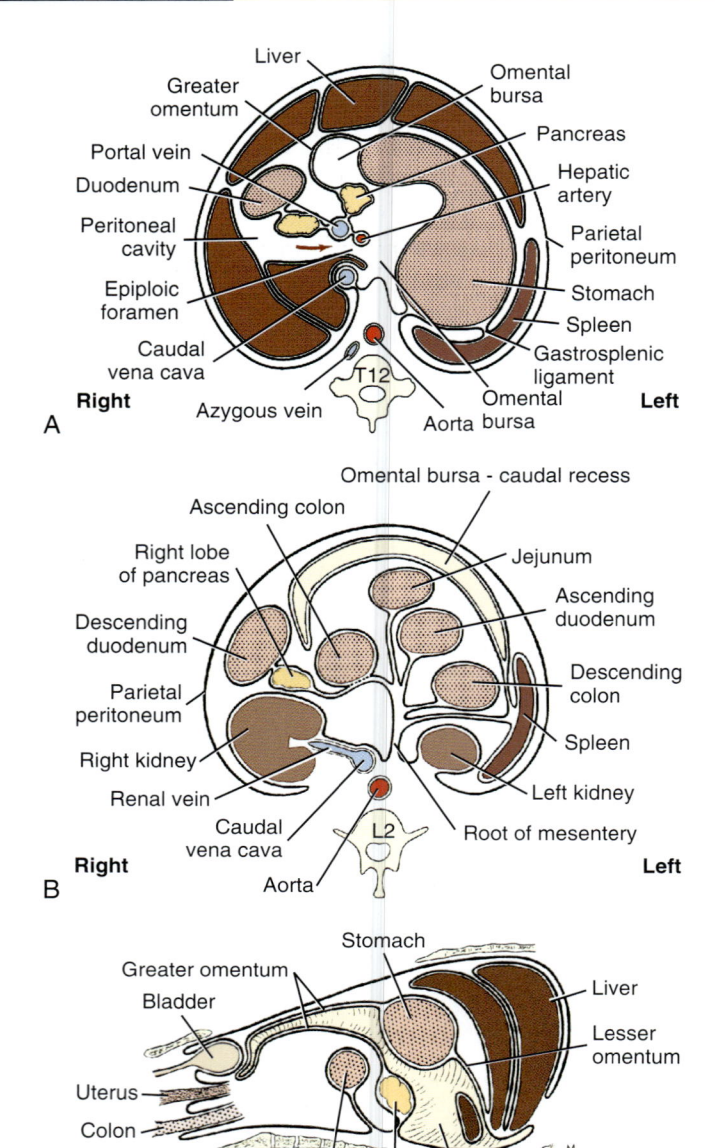

• Fig. 7.36 Peritoneal schema as viewed with the dog in a supine position. **A**, Transverse section through the epiploic foramen (*red arrow*). **B**, Transverse section through the root of the mesentery. **C**, Sagittal section.

filament. Its cranial margin blends with the dorsal peritoneal layer of the deep wall of the greater omentum. A relatively fat-free side plica leaves the left lateral peritoneal layer of the main portion of the omental veil. Cranially this side fold attaches to the visceral surface of the spleen, usually at the beginning of the distal fourth, where it extends at a right angle to the hilus and runs toward the caudal border of the organ.

The greater omentum has many functions, yet when it is largely removed, it does not regenerate. Webb and Simer (1940) removed the greater omentum in three dogs and found that the health of the dogs was not impaired in any way. The greater omentum is used frequently by the surgeon because of the important part it plays aiding in the revascularization of tissues that have had their normal blood supply impaired. The mobility of the omentum is facilitated by peristalsis. Higgins and Bain (1930) found that there are two systems of lymphatic drainage from the abdomen, one associated with the gastrointestinal tract that passes through the mesenteries to the cisterna and the other associated with the omentum and the diaphragm that passes through the ventral portion of the mediastinum to the cervical lymph ducts. The omental lymphatics function more to hold and isolate foreign material in the peritoneal cavity than they do to transport such material to larger channels.

Lesser Omentum

The **lesser omentum** (*omentum minus*) is the largest derivative of the ventral mesogastrium but it is not nearly as voluminous or as complex as is the greater omentum, which it resembles in structure, although it contains less fat. It loosely spans the distance from the lesser curvature of the stomach and the initial part of the duodenum to the porta of the liver. Between the liver and the cardia of the stomach it attaches to the margin of the esophageal hiatus of the diaphragm. It becomes continuous with the mesoduodenum on the right. The papillary process of the caudate lobe of the liver is loosely enveloped by the lesser omentum as it projects into the vestibule of the omental bursa. The greater portion of the lesser omentum that passes from the liver to the stomach is the **hepatogastric ligament** (*lig. hepatogastricum*). The right border of the lesser omentum that goes to the duodenum from the liver is known as the **hepatoduodenal ligament** (*lig. hepatoduodenale*). This is the ventral border of the epiploic foramen and contains the portal vein, hepatic artery, and the bile duct.

Omental Bursa

The **omental bursa** (*bursa omentalis*) (see Fig. 7.36), or lesser peritoneal cavity, is collapsed in life. The organs bounding it cranially are the visceral wall of the stomach, the caudate lobe of the liver, and the left lobe of the pancreas, which is located largely in the deep wall of the greater omentum. The omental bursa has but one large, constantly present opening into the greater peritoneal cavity, which is called the **epiploic foramen** (*foramen epiploicum*). It is a narrow passage, approximately 3 cm long, which lies to the right of the median plane, medial to the caudate process of the liver. It is bounded dorsally by the caudal vena cava, caudally by the hepatic artery, ventrally by the portal vein in the hepatoduodenal ligament, and cranially by the liver. The foramen leads into the **vestibule** (*vestibulum bursae omentalis*) or antechamber of the omental bursa, from which three recesses radiate.

The **dorsal recess** (*recessus dorsalis omentalis*) is that portion of the omental bursa into which projects the papillary process of the liver. It is bounded ventrally by the lesser omentum, dorsally and cranially by the liver, and caudally partly by the lesser curvature of the stomach. It freely communicates with the caudal recess over the dorsal wall of the stomach.

The **caudal recess** (*recessus caudalis omentalis*) is the main cavity of the omental bursa. It is enclosed by the bursal portion of the greater omentum and extends caudally and laterally from the stomach to the urinary bladder. The two parts, superficial and deep, of the greater omentum do not fuse with each other caudally but are apposed to each other, which reduces the size of the omental bursa.

The omental bursa is closed caudally from the superficial wall reflecting on itself to form the deep wall. Cranially the closure of the omental bursa is more involved. The dorsal wall of the stomach and the liver largely fill the "mouth" of the bursa. At the cardia, the inner peritoneal layer of the greater omentum becomes continuous with the similar layer of the lesser omentum as the two layers are connected by the visceral peritoneum covering the dorsum of the cardia. On the right side the inner peritoneal layers of the two omenta converge on the medial surface of the cranial part of the duodenum, thus closing the bursa at this site. At other places around its periphery the inner peritoneal layers of the deep and superficial walls become continuous. The other peritoneal layers of the two walls are also continuous except on the left, where the veil portion of the greater omentum is formed.

The **splenic recess** (*recessus lienalis*) is largely nonexistent unless the abdominal cavity is opened and the spleen displaced. In such instances, it is a recess of the left extremity of the omental bursa opposite the hilus of the spleen enclosed by the gastrophrenic, gastrosplenic, and phrenicosplenic ligaments.

Three folds invaginate the inner peritoneal sheet of the omental bursa or the whole bursa wall. These are formed by the three branches of the celiac artery and the nerve plexuses that surround them. The **hepatopancreatic fold** (*plica hepatopancreatica*) is a low peritoneal fold that contains the hepatic artery. It extends obliquely across the medial face of the portal vein just within the vestibule from the epiploic foramen as part of the hepatoduodenal ligament. The **gastropancreatic fold** (*plica gastropancreatica*) is formed by the left gastric artery and nerve plexus. It is short and extends from the celiac artery to the left extremity of the lesser curvature of the stomach. Surrounded by fat, it continues on the dorsal wall of the body of the stomach just caudal to the attachment of the lesser omentum. A large fold is also formed by a dorsal displacement of the bursal wall produced by the splenic artery and nerves and their continuation opposite the hilus of the spleen as the left gastroepiploic artery and nerve plexus.

The various peritoneal folds that attach the liver and digestive tube to the abdominal wall or to other viscera are treated in the descriptions of the several organs.

Stomach

The **stomach** (*ventriculus*, *gaster*) (Figs. 7.37 to 7.43), the largest dilation of the alimentary canal, is a musculoglandular organ interposed between the esophagus and the small intestine. It varies greatly in size. It stores and partly mixes the food, and its intrinsic glands intermittently add enzymes, mucus, and hydrochloric acid. During embryonic development of the caudal foregut, the region

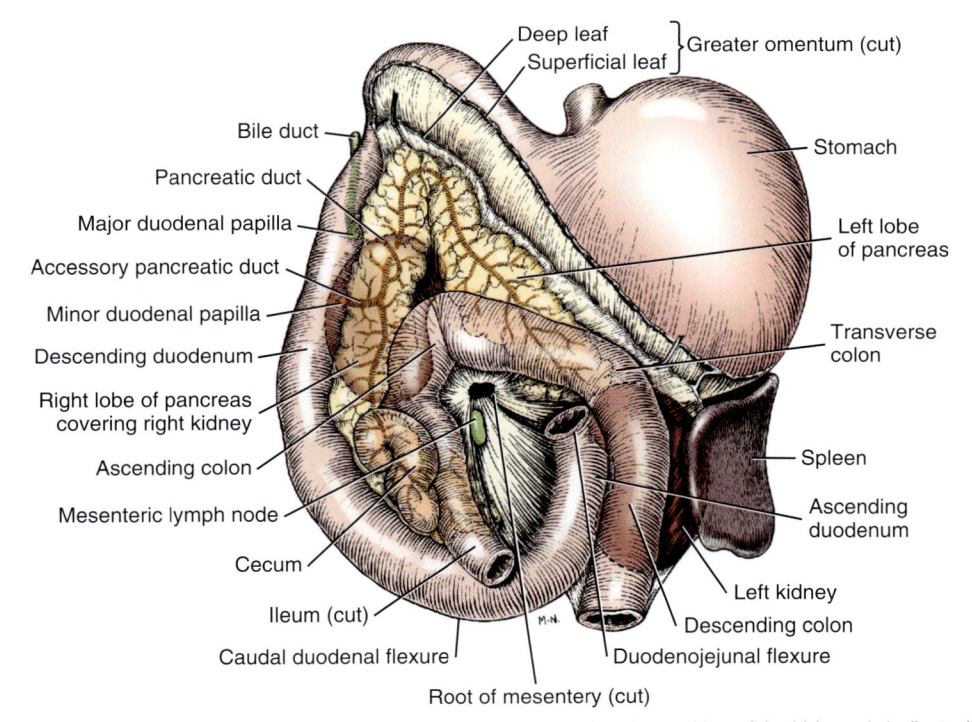

• **Fig. 7.37** Abdominal viscera, ventral aspect. The pancreas in situ; the position of the kidneys is indicated by a dotted line.

360 CHAPTER 7   The Digestive Apparatus and Abdomen

destined to form the stomach first appears as a short swelling that grows more rapidly on its dorsal surface forming the embryonic greater curvature. As the stomach grows, it undergoes two simultaneous rotations. One is approximately 90 degrees counterclockwise around its longitudinal axis when viewed from caudal to cranial and the other approximately 90 degrees counterclockwise around a dorsoventral axis when viewed from dorsal to ventral. This results in a C-shaped structure with the cranial end, the cardia, on the left about on the median plane and the caudal end, the

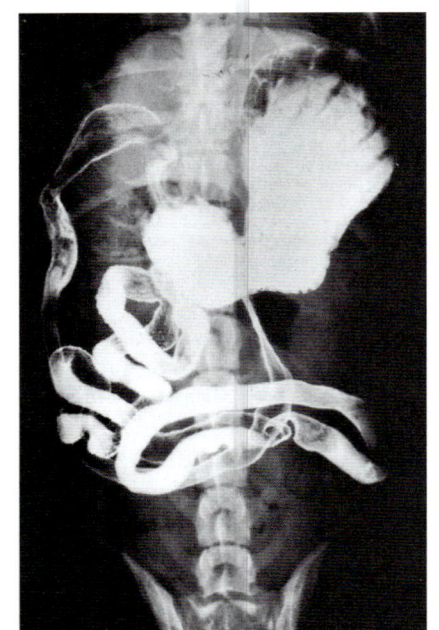

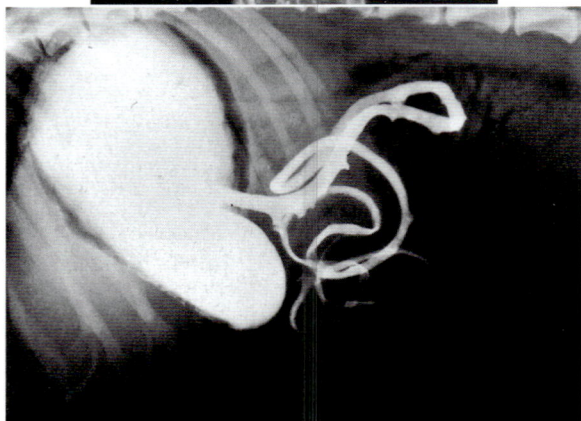

- **Fig. 7.38 Radiograph 1** (*top*), Dorsoventral contrast radiograph of the stomach and small intestine 8 minutes after the administration of contrast medium. Dog's left side is on the right side of the radiograph. **Radiograph 2** (*bottom*), Lateral contrast radiograph of the stomach and duodenum.

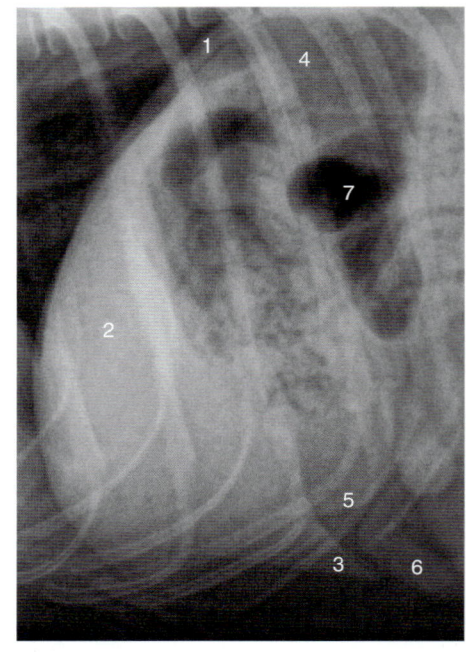

1. Left crus of diaphragm
2. Liver
3. Left lateral lobe of liver
4. Fundus of stomach
5. Greater curvature of stomach
6. Small intestine
7. Transverse colon

where the body becomes the pyloric part

- **Fig. 7.40** Lateral radiograph of the cranial abdomen.

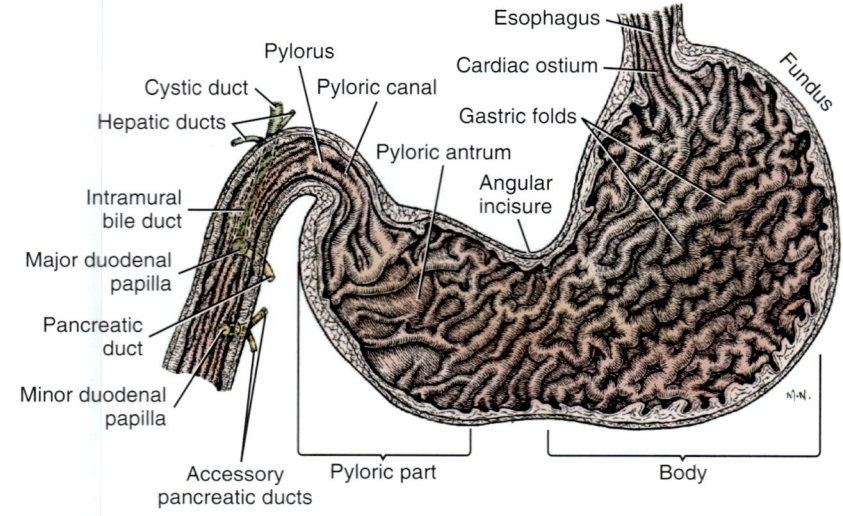

- **Fig. 7.39** Longitudinal section of stomach and proximal portion of duodenum.

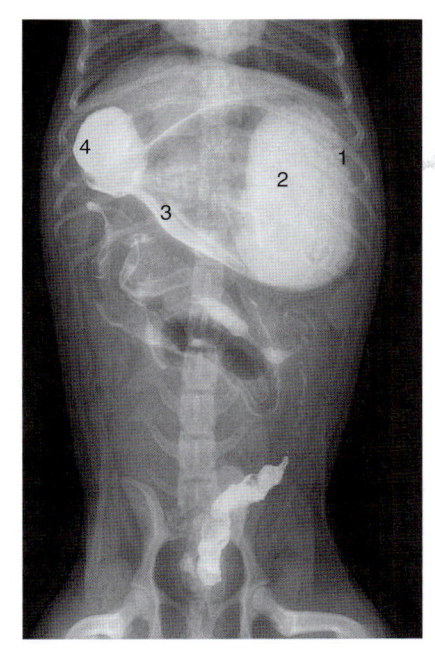

CHAPTER 7 The Digestive Apparatus and Abdomen   361

1. Fundus of stomach
2. Body of stomach
3. Pyloric part of stomach
4. Pylorus

• **Fig. 7.41** Ventrodorsal radiograph of the abdomen with barium.

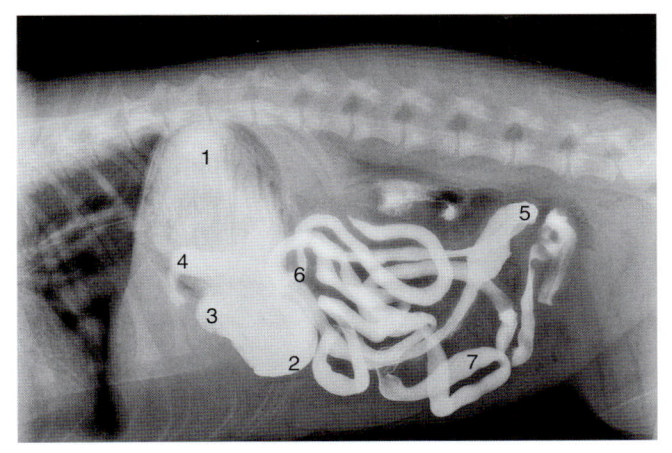

1. Fundus of stomach
2. Body of stomach
3. Pylorus of stomach
4. Cranial duodenum
5. Caudal duodenal flexure
6. Duodenojejunal flexure
7. Jejunum

• **Fig. 7.42** Lateral radiograph of the abdomen with barium.

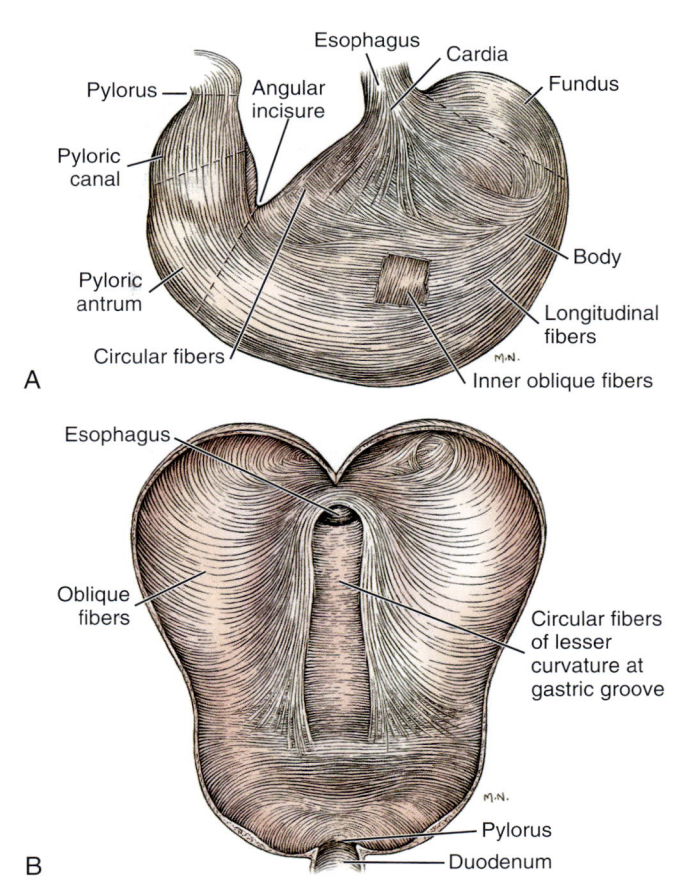

• **Fig. 7.43** Musculature of stomach. **A**, Outer layer, ventral aspect. Window cut to show inner oblique fibers. **B**, Inner layer, the stomach opened along the greater curvature.

The **visceral surface** (*facies visceralis*) presents a convex outer surface that faces mainly dorsally, but also caudodextrally. It lies in contact with the left lobe of the pancreas in the deep wall of the greater omentum and is separated from the intestinal mass and left kidney by the deep wall of the greater omentum. The **parietal surface** (*facies parietalis*) faces to the left and cranially as well as ventrally. In the contracted state this surface of the stomach lies in contact with the liver, in which it produces an extensive gastric impression. The dilated stomach extends beyond the liver chiefly to the left and ventrally and in contact with the abdominal wall.

Curvatures of the Stomach

The **greater curvature** (*curvatura ventriculi major*) forms the convex border of the stomach, which extends from the cardia to the pylorus. It is approximately 30 cm long in a stomach moderately filled. The superficial wall of the greater omentum attaches to the greater curvature except on the left, where its line of attachment runs obliquely across the dorsal wall of the stomach to form, with the lesser omentum at the cardia, a closure of the omental bursa at this site.

The **lesser curvature** (*curvatura ventriculi minor*) forms the concave border of the stomach, which also runs from the cardia to the pylorus and is the shortest distance between

pylorus, slightly on the right of the median plane and the greater curvature facing caudoventral and to the left. The fully developed stomach lies largely in a transverse position, more to the left of the median plane than to the right of it. It lies in an extensive concavity on the caudal surface of the liver, and, when it is empty, it is located completely cranial to the costal arches. The inlet of the stomach is called the **cardia** and the outlet the **pylorus**. The major divisions of the stomach are the cardiac portion, fundus, body, and pyloric portion. It possesses visceral and parietal surfaces and greater and lesser curvatures.

these two parts. It does not form an even concavity but is in the form of a 50- to 70-degree angle, the **angular incisure** (*incisura angularis*). Lying within this angle is the papillary process of the liver. The pyloric part of the stomach lies to the right of the angular incisure, and the body of the stomach lies to the left of it. The caudal edge of the lesser omentum attaches to the lesser curvature and covers the papillary process.

Regions of the Stomach

The **cardiac part** (*pars cardiaca*) of the stomach is the portion that blends with the esophagus. The four coats of both organs blend with each other. The greatest differences occur in the muscular and mucous layers as these are traced from the esophagus to the stomach. The opening into the stomach is the *ostium cardiacum*.

The **fundus of the stomach** (*fundus ventriculi*) is the rather large blind outpocketing located to the left and dorsal to the cardia. The esophagus joins the stomach in such a way that, on the right, its surface continues with that of the lesser curvature of the stomach without definite demarcation. On the left, the **cardiac incisure** (*incisura cardiaca*) is formed between the cardia and the bulging fundic part. The **body of the stomach** (*corpus ventriculi*) is the large middle portion of the organ. It extends from the fundus on the left to the pyloric part on the right. If two transverse planes are projected through the stomach at right angles to its curved long axis, one through the caudal face of the cardia dorsally and the other through the angular incisure ventrally, these planes will limit the beginning and end of the body of the stomach. The shortest path that ingesta can take in passing from the cardia to the pyloric part of the stomach is known as the **gastric groove** (*sulcus ventriculi*). This path follows the lesser curvature of the stomach.

The **pyloric part** (*pars pylorica*) (Figs. 7.39 and 7.43) is approximately the distal third of the stomach as measured along the lesser curvature from the angular incisure to the duodenum. It is always somewhat sacculated as it unites the body of the organ to the duodenum. The pyloric part is irregularly funnel-shaped toward the pylorus, which is directed cranially. The initial two-thirds is thin-walled and expanded to form the **pyloric antrum** (*antrum pyloricum*). The distal third is contracted and bent so that the greater curvature (caudal side) is three or four times longer than the cranial side. The **pylorus** (*pylorus*) is largely surrounded by a thick, double muscular sphincter at the entrance to the duodenum. This forms the narrowest part of the cavity of the stomach. The lumen of the pylorus is the *ostium pyloricum*. The **pyloric canal** (*canalis pyloricus*) is the short narrow segment between the pyloric antrum and the pylorus.

Shape, Position, and Capacity

The empty, contracted stomach is not only contained within the cranial abdomen medial to the ribs but is also nestled within the caudal concavity of the liver, being completely separated from the abdominal wall. When the stomach increases in size as the result of filling, the fundus enlarges first and pushes caudodorsally on the left. It tends to displace the liver ventrally as the stomach comes in contact with the left lateral abdominal wall and diaphragm. The body of the stomach is the second part to fill and expand. It is the largest division of the organ, as well as the part capable of the greatest dilation. During filling, it migrates caudoventrally and makes extensive contact with the abdominal wall. It is particularly distensible in puppies, and, when maximally expanded, it may extend from a transverse plane through the eighth thoracic vertebra to a plane caudal to the umbilicus. This necessitates an expansion of the abdomen and a crowding of the intestinal mass and spleen caudally and slightly dorsally. According to Grey (1918) the normal stomach possesses a striking capacity to adjust its size to the volume of its contents with only minimal changes in intragastric pressure.

Secord (1941) states that food remains in the dog's stomach from 10 to 16 hours. Zietzschmann (1938) states that the pylorus varies least in position as the stomach fills. It is always more cranial and ventral than the cardia. The pyloric part is the last part to expand, the antrum expanding more than the canal. The pyloric part functions chiefly as an ejection mechanism by which the partly digested stomach contents, the *chyme*, is forced through the pyloric canal and pylorus and squirted into the duodenum. The empty or the partly filled stomach is shaped like a C, with its convex surface facing caudoventrally and to the left.

The capacity of the stomach varies from 0.5 to 8 liters. Greater ranges in relative size are present in puppies than in adult dogs. Ellenberger and Baum (1943) cite Neumayer, who gives the capacity as 100 to 250 cc per kilogram of body weight. The average empty stomach of a 15-kg dog weighs approximately 100 g.

Coats of the Stomach

The **serous coat** (*tunica serosa*) covers the stomach and is continuous with the greater and lesser omenta. The serous coat covers the organ completely except for an extremely narrow line, not covered directly by peritoneum on the proximal half of the greater curvature, that continues obliquely across the dorsal surface of the stomach to the cardia. A second similar line on the stomach that is not covered by peritoneum extends from the cardia along the lesser curvature to the duodenum. These lines lie along the attachment of the two omenta on the stomach. The smooth peritoneal sheets of serous membrane that intimately cover the dorsal and ventral walls of the stomach fuse just distal to these lines to form the greater and lesser omenta. In obese specimens a small irregular strip of fat and the nerves and vessels serving the organ widen the line along which the omenta arise. The two peritoneal layers that form these folds separate at the cardia to extend cranially on the abdominal portion of the esophagus. The peritoneal leaves of the lesser omentum become continuous with those of the mesoduodenum over the bile duct. The serosa of the stomach is extremely thin and elastic. It adheres closely to the stomach musculature by a scanty amount of subserous connective tissue, the *tela subserosa*.

The **muscular coat** (*tunica muscularis*) of the stomach (see Fig. 7.43) consists essentially of an outer longitudinal and an inner circular layer of smooth muscle fibers. To these layers are added oblique fibers over the body of the stomach.

The outer **longitudinal layer** (*stratum longitudinale*) is continuous with the essentially outer longitudinal layers of both the duodenum and the esophagus. The longitudinal fibers on and adjacent to the lesser curvature, as traced from the esophagus, spray out and end before reaching the angular incisure. Those fibers on the dorsal and ventral walls of the body of the stomach end before reaching the middle of the body, whereas the longitudinal fibers on the greater curvature continue uninterruptedly from the esophagus to the duodenum. On both the dorsal and ventral walls of the stomach at approximately the junction of the fundus and body there is a kind of muscular whorl formed by the bundles of fibers and the longitudinal layer changing position and direction. At and adjacent to the angular incisure there are no longitudinal fibers, so that the circular fibers of the inner coat become superficial. As the longitudinal fibers cover the pyloric portion they are particularly thick on the sides between the curvatures, but no definite pyloric ligaments are formed.

The inner **circular layer** (*stratum circulare*) of the stomach is more complete and specialized than is the longitudinal layer. At the cardia the circular layer is thickened to form the small **cardiac sphincter** (*m. sphincter cardiae*). This sphincter is augmented on the greater curvature by the acquisition of a condensation of the transversely running inner oblique fibers. At the approximate junction of the fundus and the body on both the dorsal and ventral walls, the circular coat enters into the formation of a muscular fiber interchange with the longitudinal coat. The circular coat is not covered by the longitudinal coat in and adjacent to the angular incisure so that in this region it receives a peritoneal covering, superficially. Deeply, throughout the length of the lesser curvature from the cardia to the pyloric antrum, there is a muscular trough, approximately 2 cm wide, which is formed on the sides by the parallel longitudinal parts of the oblique fibers and deeply by the circular fibers. This corresponds to the gastric groove.

Surrounding the pyloric canal, the inner circular layer is well developed, as Torgersen (1942) has pointed out. The musculature is thickest as it crosses the greater curvature. The pylorus, which opens into the duodenum, is also surrounded by a circular muscle termed the **pyloric sphincter** (*m. sphincter pylori*).

The **oblique fibers** (*fibrae obliquae*) are adjacent to the submucosa. They appear to arise from a heavy transverse stratum that is arched across the dorsal (greater curvature) boundary of the cardiac orifice. These fibers run distally and outward toward the pylorus and the greater curvature in each wall. The oblique fibers thus are spread like a fan; in a moderately distended, medium-sized stomach, those bundles nearest the lesser curvature are essentially parallel.

The fibers next peripheral to the parallel ones fan out and end on the inner surface of the circular fibers of the distal part of the body of the stomach. The most proximal oblique fibers become almost transverse proximally and blend with those of the circular layer in augmenting the size of the dorsal part of the small cardiac sphincter.

The **submucous coat** (*tela submucosa*) consists of a dense but thin elastic layer of areolar tissue that more firmly attaches to the mucosa than to the muscularis. It contains the finer branches of the gastric vessels and nerves. In the contracted organ it is thrown into folds that occupy the centers of the relatively inelastic plicae of the mucous coat.

The **mucous coat** (*tunica mucosa*) in carnivores is entirely glandular. It consists of a columnar surface epithelium, a glandular lamina propria, and a lamina muscularis mucosae consisting of muscular fibers which may be irregularly interwoven or stratified (Trautmann & Fiebiger, 1957). In the contracted empty or even a moderately distended organ, the mucosa and much of the underlying submucosa are thrown into folds, the *plicae gastricae*. These folds are largely longitudinal in direction and very tortuous except adjacent to the lesser curvature, where the folds are less crowded and are relatively straight. In a strongly contracted stomach the mucosal folds, which may be 1 cm high, lie closely adjacent to each other. The normal color of the mucosa in the body and fundus of a fresh stomach is pink to grayish red. In the pyloric region it is lighter in color. The color varies with the amount of contained blood, as well as the freshness of the material.

Under magnification the mucosa is seen to possess approximately 40 raised areas for every square centimeter. These are the *areae gastricae*. In the pyloric region these areas are elongated in a longitudinal direction, but elsewhere they are polygonal and rendered distinct by small surrounding furrows. Each of the small gastric areas on their surfaces and sides is stippled with numerous minute openings, the *foveolae gastricae*. The foveolae are longest, approximately 0.68 mm in the pyloric region. They gradually shorten toward the cardia and disappear, so that none exist in the cardiac gland region which is adjacent to the esophagus (Mall, 1896). According to Mall, there are 1,000,000 foveolae in the stomach of the dog, and each of these has about 16 gastric glands opening into it. There may be folds, *plicae villosae*, between the gland openings.

Glands of the Stomach

The glands of the stomach are known as the **gastric glands** (*glandulae gastricae*). They are branched tubular glands with necks and bodies that reach nearly to the lamina muscularis mucosae. According to Trautmann and Fiebiger (1957), in older carnivores a double-layered lamina subglandularis intervenes between the lamina muscularis mucosae and the blind ends of the glands. According to these authors, the lamina propria contains the gastric glands, and, in certain areas exclusive of the cardiac gland zone, the glands are divided into groups by heavier strands of supporting tissue that contain muscle fibers from the lamina muscularis mucosae. Three types of gastric glands are recognized in the dog. These are the cardiac glands, the gastric glands proper, and the pyloric glands.

The **cardiac glands** (*glandulae cardiacae*), according to Haane (1905), are found in a narrow zone around the cardia. Cardiac glands are also scattered along the lesser curvature, according to Ellenberger (1911).

The **gastric glands proper** (*glandulae gastricae [propriae]*), or fundic glands, occupy approximately two-thirds of the gastric mucosa. This includes the left extremity, or fundus, and the body of the stomach. It is exclusive of the pyloric part and the cardiac gland region.

The **pyloric glands** (*glandulae pyloricae*) are found in the pyloric part of the stomach. Between the pyloric and gastric glands proper, according to Bloom and Fawcett (1994), there exists in the dog a zone of intermediate glands which reaches a width of 1 to 1.8 cm. Harvey (1906) states that when the stomach is flattened out the intermediate zone is 2 to 3 cm wide. The difference between the various gland zones is in the type of cells they contain, and therefore in the nature of the secretion they produce. The mucosal regions of the stomach are not coextensive with the gross divisions of the organ with the same or comparable names. There is considerable intermixing of the glands of each gland area with those of adjacent areas. The intermediate gland zone is formed in this manner. The cardiac glands of the stomach are similar to the cardiac glands in the caudal portion of the esophagus. The pyloric glands imperceptibly blend with those of the duodenum, and, as they do, they come to lie in the submucosa. Both the type of cells in the gastric glands and their morphologic characteristics and location have influenced the naming of the mucosal areas of the stomach.

According to Bloom and Fawcett (1994), four types of glandular cells are found in the stomach mucosa. These are (1) chief, or zymogenic, cells, which contain granules that are believed to contain pepsinogen, the precursor of the chief gastric enzyme, pepsin; (2) parietal cells, which are spherical or pyramidal cells lying next to the basement membrane and are considered the source, probably indirectly, of the hydrochloric acid of the gastric juice; (3) mucous neck cells, which are located in the necks of the gastric glands, filling the spaces between the parietal cells, and producing mucus; and (4) argentaffin cells, which are moderately abundant in the proper gastric glands, less frequent in the pyloric glands, and numerous in the first part of the small intestine. The glands of the cardiac, intermediate, and pyloric regions function mainly to produce mucus; the proper gastric glands produce hydrochloric acid indirectly and the enzyme pepsin. As in most other areas of the alimentary canal, lymph nodules are scattered throughout the mucosa of the stomach. Some of these extend through the lamina muscularis mucosae into the submucosa (Bensley, 1902).

Vessels of the Stomach

The main arteries to the stomach are the **left** and **right gastric arteries**, which run along the lesser curvature, and the **left** and **right gastroepiploic arteries**, which run along the greater curvature. The larger left gastric artery anastomoses with the right gastric at the beginning of the pyloric antrum. The epiploic vessels anastomose with each other on the greater curvature of the body of the stomach. In addition to these arteries, two or more long branches leave the terminal part of the splenic artery and supply a portion of the fundus of the stomach by **short gastric arteries**. The arterial branches that actually enter the musculature of the organ along the greater curvature run greater distances under the serosa and are more nearly vertical to the parent trunks than the comparable branches along the lesser curvature. The veins from the stomach are satellites of the arteries supplying the organ. The **left gastric** and **left gastroepiploic veins** are tributaries of the splenic vein. The **right gastric** and **right gastroepiploic veins** are tributaries of the gastroduodenal vein. The blood from the stomach enters the liver through the portal vein. The lymphatics from the stomach all eventually drain into the **hepatic lymph nodes**. Baum (1918) stated that most of these vessels drain into the left hepatic node after first having passed through the splenic and gastric nodes. A few lymphatics from the stomach drain into the right hepatic node after first having passed through the duodenal node.

Nerves of the Stomach

The stomach is supplied by parasympathetic fibers from the **vagi** and by sympathetic fibers from the **celiac plexus**. The ventral vagal trunk, after passing through the esophageal hiatus, immediately sends two to four small branches to the pylorus and liver. Other branches go to the lesser curvature of the stomach. The dorsal vagal trunk also sends branches to the lesser curvature and to the ventral wall of the stomach and continues across the celiac plexus to reach and follow branches of the celiac and cranial mesenteric arteries. The sympathetic fibers to the stomach reach it by traveling on the numerous gastric branches of the celiac artery. They come from the **celiacomesenteric plexus**. Khurana and Petras (1991) studied the sensory innervation of the dog's stomach using the horseradish peroxidase technique. Their data showed that the sensory innervation of the stomach came from the distal ganglia of the vagus nerve and extended over as many as 25 paired spinal ganglia (C2 to L5). The peak innervation levels for the stomach spanned an area from T2 to T10. There is consensus that vagal afferents monitor stomach volume or distension but not nutritive status (Powley & Phillips, 2004; Williams et al., 2016).

Small Intestine

The **small intestine** (*intestinum tenue*) extends from the pylorus of the stomach to the ileocolic orifice leading into the large intestine. It is the longest portion of the alimentary canal, having an average length, in the living animal, of 3.5 times the length of the body. After death and the cessation of peristaltic contractions, the intestine increases in length owing to the loss of muscular tonus. Williams (1935),

Alvarez (1948), and Nickel et al. (1973) cite intestinal measurements in the dog. The small intestine consists of three main parts, the relatively fixed and short proximal loop, or **duodenum**; the freely movable, long, middle and distal portions, the **jejunum**; and the very short terminal part, the **ileum**.

Duodenum

The duodenum (see Fig. 7.37) is the first and most fixed part of the small intestine. It is approximately 25 cm, or 10 inches, long. It begins in the dorsal half of the right hypochondriac region opposite the ninth intercostal space. It runs mainly caudally to a transverse level through the tuber coxae, makes a U-shaped turn, and runs obliquely craniosinistrally to be continued by the jejunum to the left of the root of the mesentery. Both the pancreatic ducts and the bile duct open into the duodenum (see Fig. 7.39). The acid chyme that enters it from the stomach is mixed with the alkaline secretions from the liver, pancreas, and small intestinal glands. Because of the high nutritive content of the material ingested, most free-living intestinal parasites are found in the duodenum. For descriptive purposes the duodenum is divided into four portions and two flexures. These are the cranial, cranial duodenal flexure, descending, caudal duodenal flexure, transverse (caudal), and ascending portions.

The **cranial portion** (*pars cranialis*) of the duodenum is short between the pylorus and cranial duodenal flexure. It arises from the pylorus and almost immediately turns acutely to the right and caudally as the **cranial duodenal flexure** (*flexura duodeni cranialis*). The pyloric part of the stomach runs cranially, whereas the cranial duodenal flexure runs essentially caudally. The cranial portion of the duodenum is also known as the *duodenal cap* or *bulb*. This region lies opposite the ninth and tenth ribs and the intervening intercostal space. Ventrally it is separated from the stomach by the greater omentum. Dorsally and laterally it lies in contact with the liver, and medially it is in contact with the pancreas (see Fig. 7.37).

The **descending portion** (*pars descendens*) of the duodenum, approximately 15 cm long, runs caudally from the cranial portion nearly to the pelvic inlet. Its lateral surface lies in contact with the right lateral and right medial lobes of the liver, cranially and with the parietal peritoneum of the dorsolateral abdominal wall caudally. Dorsally the right lobe of the pancreas lies in contact with it. Medially it is related primarily to the cecum caudally and the ascending colon cranially, but it is separated from these by the infolded greater omentum.

The **caudal duodenal flexure** (*flexura duodeni caudalis*) is between the descending and transverse parts of the duodenum.

The **transverse portion** (*pars transversa [pars caudalis]*) of the duodenum connects the descending and ascending portions from right to left and is approximately 5 cm long. It lies in a dorsal (horizontal) plane, starting at the caudal duodenal flexure. The transverse portion usually lies ventral to the body and right transverse process of the sixth lumbar vertebra. A full bladder and colon would force it cranially. The initial segment of this portion, at the right, lies in contact with the parietal peritoneum of the sublumbar region and the uterine horn ventral to the deep circumflex iliac vessels. It is continued by a rounded angle which is somewhat less than a U-turn as the ascending portion of the duodenum diverges slightly from the descending portion. The transverse portion of the duodenum is related to the terminal portion of the ileum and to the jejunum ventrally.

As the **ascending portion** (*pars ascendens*) of the duodenum runs obliquely cranially and to the left from the transverse part, it crosses obliquely the dorsally lying ureters, sympathetic trunks, caudal vena cava, aorta, and lumbar lymphatic trunks. Ventrally the ascending portion is related to the coils of the jejunum. On the left it approaches the descending colon, and makes a sweeping curve ventrally to form the **duodenojejunal flexure** (*flexura duodenojejunalis*). At this flexure the jejunum continues the duodenum ventrally, caudally, and to the left, and enters into the formation of numerous coils and kinks (festoons), which constitute most of the intestinal mass.

Attachments and Peritoneal Relations

The first two parts of the duodenum on the right are located in the free border of the *mesoduodenum*. On leaving the right portions of the duodenum, the two peritoneal leaves that form the mesoduodenum as traced to the left extend directly to the right lobe of the pancreas or merge for a short distance before covering this portion of the gland. The peritoneal leaves merge again on leaving the left side of the right pancreatic lobe and pass to and cover the ascending part of the duodenum. On leaving the ascending duodenum, the mesoduodenum becomes continuous with the right peritoneal leaf of the descending mesocolon. Caudally the two peritoneal layers of the mesoduodenum form a triangular fold with a free caudal border that runs from the mesocolon in the region of the pelvic inlet obliquely craniodextrally to the caudal duodenal flexure. This triangular attachment of the initial part of the ascending duodenum is called the **duodenocolic fold** (*plica duodenocolica*).

The **caudal duodenal recess** (*recessus duodenali caudalis*) (Fig. 7.44A), formerly called the *duodenal fossa*, may be absent, or, when present, it may admit the end of the little finger. It varies in length up to 4 cm. Its opening faces cranially and is usually situated approximately 2 cm caudal to the duodenojejunal flexure. The fossa runs caudally along the attached border of the ascending duodenum. When maximally developed, it reaches a transverse level through the most cranial extension of the duodenocolic fold.

Jejunum and Ileum

The jejunum and ileum compose the remainder and the majority of the small intestine with the jejunum being the longest portion. The jejunum begins at the left of or caudal to the root of the mesentery at the duodenojejunal flexure, and the ileum ends by opening into the initial portion of

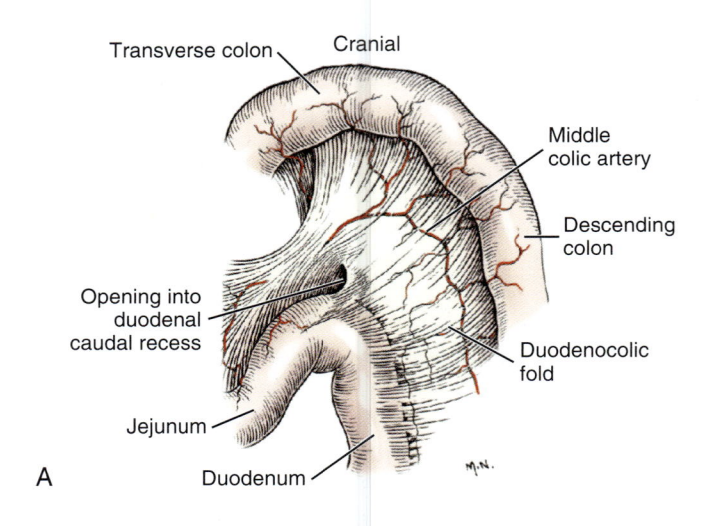

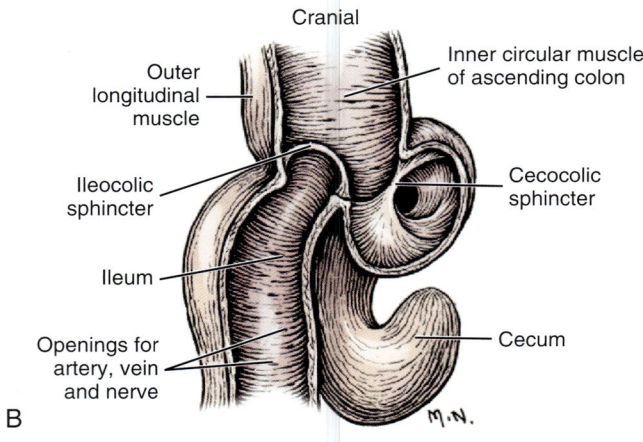

Fig. 7.44 A, Duodenal recess, ventral aspect. B, Dissection of inner circular and outer longitudinal muscle layers of ileum, cecum, and colon, dorsal aspect.

the ascending colon as the **ileal papilla** (*papilla ilealis*) with an **ileal orifice** (*ostium ileale*) and an associated circular **sphincteric muscle** (*m. sphincter ilex*). The orifice lies at a level usually between the descending and ascending portions of the duodenum. In contrast to the relatively fixed duodenum, the jejunoileum is the most mobile and free part of the entire alimentary canal. It is suspended by the long mesentery (consisting of mesojejunum and mesoileum) from the cranial part of the sublumbar region and is therefore also known as the mesenteric portion of the small intestine (*pars intestinum tenue mesenteriale*). No definite gross, microscopic, or developmental manifestations mark the division between jejunum and ileum. This division was made by early investigators from the gross appearance of this portion of the bowel. According to Field and Harrison (1947), Galen applied the term *jejunum* to the middle portion of the small intestine because it is usually empty or appears emptier than the rest. The term *ileum* is applied to the relatively short, contracted terminal portion of the small intestine in domestic animals. Although there are distinctive differences, particularly in the mucosa, between a typical portion of the jejunum and that of the ileum, there are no sufficiently marked gross differences in the character of the walls to differentiate the jejunum from the ileum. The ileum of the dog is approximately the last 15 cm of the small intestine.

Position of the Small Intestine

The *jejunum* is located ventrocaudal to the empty stomach. It is separated from the ventral and lateral abdominal wall only by the deep and superficial walls of the greater omentum. It is related dorsally to the large intestine, duodenum, pancreas, kidneys, ovaries and nongravid uterus, caudal vena cava, aorta, sympathetic nerve trunks, and lumbar lymphatics. The jejunum rarely extends into the pelvic cavity caudally because the urinary bladder and the rectum largely fill the pelvic inlet. The spleen, through the greater omentum, is related to the craniosinistral part of the jejunum. The ileum is the terminal part of the small intestine. Most veterinary anatomists regard only the short, terminal, usually contracted part of the small intestine as ileum. In the dog the ileum contains fewer aggregated lymph nodules than the more proximal part of the small intestine, including the duodenum (Titkemeyer & Calhoun, 1955). The ileum is readily identified by the ileocecal fold and its contained antimesenteric ileal vessels.

Mesentery of the Small Intestine

The **ileocecal fold** (*plica ileocecalis*) is a narrow but usually long, variably developed plica of peritoneum that continues proximally on the antimesenteric surface of the ileum from the area of adhesion of the cecum to the ileum. It is rarely more than 1 cm wide at its origin, and when it is double at this site it is considerably narrower. It varies in length from 2 to 30 cm. A streak of fat located in its ileal attachment surrounds the antimesenteric ileal vessels. Its distal end is reduced to a low ridge of peritoneum formed by the underlying vessels and fat. Frequently the vessels can be traced proximally on the ileum beyond the ending of the fold.

The **mesentery** (*mesenterium*) (Fig. 7.35) is also known as the great or proper mesentery, or the mesojejunoileum, to differentiate it from the various other portions that are derived from the primitive dorsal mesentery. In the adult it is continuous cranially with the mesoduodenum and caudally with the descending mesocolon. Embryonically, the mesentery is continuous with the mesoduodenum cranially and with the ascending mesocolon caudally. Through rotation, torsion, and differential growth of the various portions of the alimentary canal the definitive continuations of the mesentery have been altered. The mesentery is in the form of a large fan hanging from the cranial part of the sublumbar region. In its free distal border is located the convoluted jejunum and ileum. It is approximately 20 cm wide and 5 mm thick. Its length or greatest dimension varies greatly, depending on where the measurement is taken. It is only approximately 1.5 cm long at its parietal attachment to the aorta and diaphragmatic crura opposite the second lumbar vertebra. This portion of the mesentery is known as the **root of the mesentery** (*radix mesenterii*). It is the thickest portion because it includes the cranial mesenteric artery, intestinal lymphatics, and the extensive mesenteric plexus of nerves that surround the artery. The free, or intestinal, border of the mesentery is its longest part. It extends from the duodenojejunal flexure, proximally, to the ileocolic junction, distally. It is as long as the jejunoileum, or approximately 250 cm in life. It is greatly folded or ruffled as it follows the turns of the intestine. The peripheral part of the mesentery is much thinner than the root. Even in obese specimens the mesentery does not contain a great amount of fat, and it is deposited most abundantly only along the larger vessels, so that large translucent areas are present between the vascular branches and arcades.

Coats of the Small Intestine

The small intestine, like the other parts of the alimentary tract, is composed of mucous, submucous, muscular, and serous tunics.

The **mucous coat** (*tunica mucosa*), throughout the small intestine of the dog, presents a free surface that is velvety owing to the presence of innumerable **intestinal villi** (*villi intestinales*). The single-layered epithelial surface cells are of two types. One type consists of the columnar cells, which function in absorption, and the other type consists of the goblet, mucus-producing cells. The deeper part of the mucosa is occupied largely by the **intestinal glands** (*glandulae intestinales*) and diffuse lymphoid tissue and single nodules. In approximately 22 areas throughout the small intestine of the dog the lymphoid nodules are grouped together to form the **aggregated lymph nodules** (*noduli lymphatici aggregati*). Titkemeyer and Calhoun (1955) found the aggregated nodules to be circumscribed elevations measuring approximately 2 by 1.5 cm. They are more numerous in the proximal portion of the small intestine than in the ileum, many being found in the duodenum. In the distended bowel they are visible through the serosa and are more numerous in the side walls of the intestines than in that part of the wall opposite the mesentery. Titkemeyer and Calhoun also described a special connective tissue layer approximately 30 μm thick between the intestinal glands and the lamina muscularis mucosae. This layer, found only in the dog, is apparently similar to the layer in a comparable location in the stomach. The *lamina muscularis mucosae*, according to the previously mentioned investigators, was found to be three times thicker in the dog than it was on average in the other domestic animals studied. It is definitely divided into inner circular and outer longitudinal layers. In the dog, the **duodenal glands** (*glandulae duodenales*) differ from the intestinal glands in that they closely resemble the pyloric glands of the stomach. They are located only around a narrow zone of the duodenum adjacent to the pylorus. The main portion of each gland is located in the submucosa, and a portion may extend into the lamina propria of the mucosa. Warren (1939) estimates that the ratio of mucosal area to serosal area for the whole small intestine of the dog is 8.5 to 1. The villi account for most of this large surface area because the dog has no circular mucous folds.

The **submucous coat** (*tela submucosa*) resembles that of the stomach and large intestine. It loosely binds together the mucous and muscular layers. The smaller blood vessels, lymphatics, and the submucous nerve plexus are located in it. Trautmann and Fiebiger (1957) state that the aggregated nodules are located mainly in the submucosa, with only a small portion in the lamina propria of the mucosa.

The **muscular coat** (*tunica muscularis*) consists of a relatively thin outer longitudinal layer (*stratum longitudinale*) and a thicker inner circular layer (*stratum circulare*).

The **serous coat** (*tunica serosa*) of the small intestine is composed of the peritoneum, which completely covers the duodenum except along the lines where it is attached, including the duodenocolic fold and a small elongated area where it leaves the pancreas to reflect around the duodenum. The jejunum and ileum are also truly intraperitoneal organs. The only parts not covered by peritoneum are along the lines of the mesenteric attachment and on the antimesenteric side of the terminal portion of the ileum where the cecum is loosely fused to the ileum and where this attachment is continued by the ileocecal fold.

Vessels of the Small Intestine

The large middle portion of the small intestine, the jejunum, is supplied by 12 to 15 **jejunal arteries**, which are branches of the cranial mesenteric. The duodenal branches from both the **cranial** and **caudal pancreaticoduodenal arteries** supply the duodenum, the most proximal jejunal artery anastomosing with the most distal duodenal branch of the caudal pancreaticoduodenal artery. The ileum is supplied on its mesenteric side by ileal branches from the **ileocolic artery** and on its antimesenteric side it is supplied by the antimesenteric ileal branches of the **cecal artery**. The main antimesenteric ileal branch runs in the areolar tissue, connecting the cecum to the ileum. Upon leaving the adhered area between the two viscera, it continues in the ileocecal fold along the whole ileum as the *ramu ilei antimesenterialis* and anastomoses with the most distal jejunal artery in the musculature of the small intestine. From the terminal arcades that lie closely adjacent to the intestine the short, irregular *vasa recti*, upon reaching the intestine, run variable distances on the mesenteric half of the musculature before perforating it to supply the submucosa and the mucosa (Noer, 1943; Sommerova, 1980). According to Morton (1929), the duodenum has a much richer blood supply than does the ileum, and it produces 5 to 10 times more fluid.

The lymph vessels from the jejunum and ileum drain primarily into the **jejunal lymph nodes**. Some lymph from the duodenum is carried to the **hepatic lymph nodes** and to the **pancreaticoduodenal lymph node**, when it is present. Lymphatics from the ileum also drain into the **colic lymph nodes**.

Nerves of the Small Intestine

The nerve fibers to the mesenteric portion of the small intestine come to it from the **vagus** and **splanchnic nerves** by way of the **celiac** and **cranial mesenteric plexuses**. The sensory innervation of the duodenum was studied with horseradish peroxidase by Khurana and Petras (1991), who found that it was innervated by as many as 15 paired thoracolumbar spinal ganglia (T2 to L3), with a peak innervation in the middle and caudal thoracic spinal ganglia and cranial lumbar spinal ganglia (T6 to L1). Vagal afferent innervation of the duodenum originated primarily but not entirely from their distal ganglia. Recent research in mice demonstrated strong evidence for combined vagal afferent responses, thus detailing both the filling (volumetric) and nutritive (chemosensory) information that underlie hormonal responses of the small intestine after feeding (Williams et al., 2016).

Large Intestine

The **large intestine** (*intestinum crassum*) is short and unspecialized. The large intestine of the dog and cat is much simpler than that of the other domestic animals. Neither haustra nor tenia exists; nor are flexures or spirals present. In general, it is a simple tube, only slightly larger in diameter than the small intestine. Its most important function is the dehydration of its fecal contents. The large intestine is divided into cecum, colon, rectum, and anal canal. It begins at the ileal papilla and ends at the anus.

Cecum

The **cecum** (Figs. 7.44 through 7.47) is usually described as the first part of the large intestine, but this is not true in the dog because the ileum, the terminal part of the small intestine, communicates only with the colon, and the cecum exists as a diverticulum of the proximal portion of the colon, the ascending colon. The openings of the ileum and cecum into the ascending colon are closely associated. The cecum is extremely variable in size and form. In the live animal it is approximately 5 cm long and 2 cm in diameter at its colic end. It irregularly tapers to the rather blunt **apex** (*apex ceci*), which is less than 1 cm in diameter and usually points caudoventrally or is located transversely. The large middle portion of the organ may be referred to as the **body** (*corpus ceci*). When it is detached and straightened, the length of the cecum is more than twice what it is when the cecum is attached. The only communication of the cecum is with the beginning of the ascending colon by means of the **cecocolic orifice** (*ostium cecocolicum*). This opening lies approximately 1 cm from the ileocolic orifice. The **cecal sphincter** (*m. sphincter ceci*) is a specialization of the inner circular muscular coat that guards the cecocolic orifice. It is approximately 0.5 cm in diameter when partly constricted. The cecum is attached to the terminal portion of the ileum by fascia and peritoneum throughout most of its length. At the apical end of the body beyond its attachment to the ileum extends the single or double **ileocecal fold** (*plica ileocecalis*). When single, this fold is triangular, with its free caudal border measuring 0.5 to 1 cm in width and only slightly more in length. It does not leave the apex of the cecum but

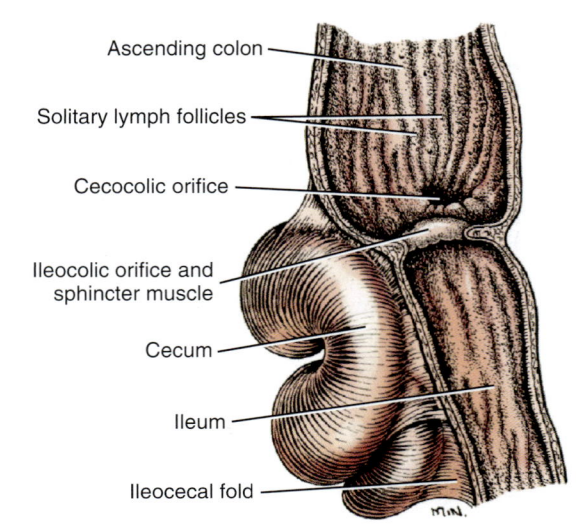

• **Fig. 7.45** Longitudinal section through ileocolic orifice, ventral aspect.

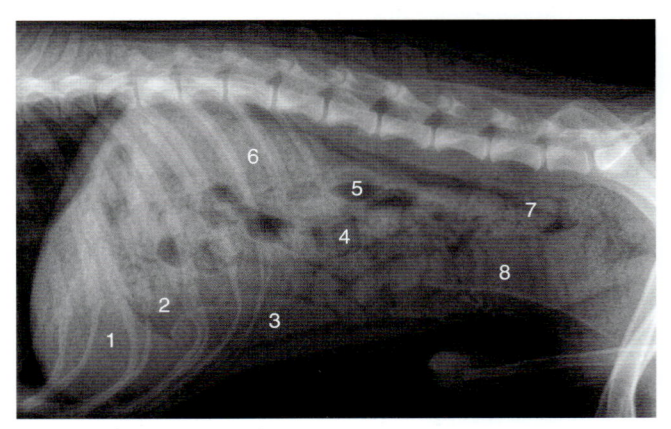

1. Liver
2. Greater curvature of stomach where the body becomes the pyloric part
3. Spleen
4. Small intestine
5. Cecum
6. Transverse colon
7. Descending colon
8. Bladder

• **Fig. 7.46** Lateral radiograph of the abdomen.

the concavity of the terminal flexure. A low peritoneal ridge containing fat and the antimesenteric ileal vessels continues beyond the fold as far as 30 cm. Kadletz (1929) described a smaller fold extending from the proximal body of the cecum to the ascending colon and named it the accessory cecocolic fold. It may also be double, enclosing a small peritoneal fossa. The peritoneal folds affect the definitive form of the cecum. The twisting of the cecum is less marked in puppies than in adults (Mitchell, 1905). Bradley and Grahame (1948) imply that the variations of its flexures are formed by its not having a wide mesentery. As the cecum grows out from the colon, it is apparently restrained from growing in a straight line by its attachment to the ileum. The flexures develop quite irregularly. In its simplest form the cecum is sigmoid in shape, but more often it is in the form of an irregular corkscrew with a large U-shaped kink extending to the left from its ileal attachment. The cecum

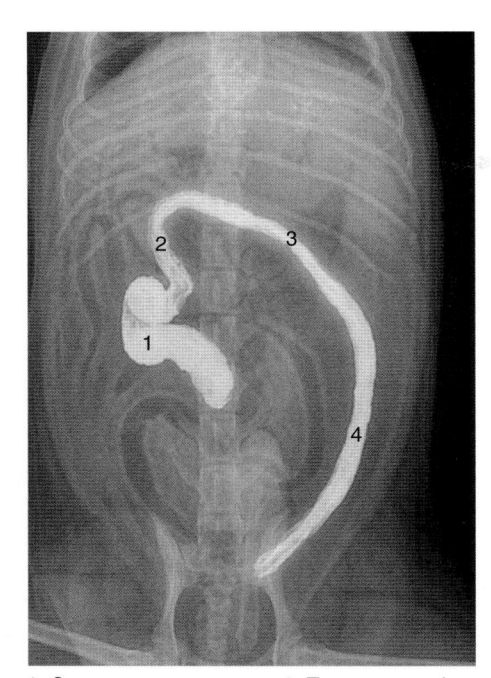

1. Cecum
2. Ascending colon
3. Transverse colon
4. Descending colon

• **Fig. 7.47** Ventrodorsal radiograph of the abdomen with barium. The dog's left side is viewed on the right side of this radiograph.

is located to the right of the median plane, usually within the duodenal loop. It lies dorsal to and occasionally partly surrounded by the coils of the jejunum, ventral to the right transverse processes of the second to fourth lumbar vertebrae. In rare instances it contacts the right lateral abdominal wall.

Colon

The **colon** (see Fig. 7.37) is divided into ascending, transverse, and descending portions and their connecting flexures. The colon lies in the dorsal part of the abdominal cavity and is shaped like a shepherd's crook or question mark. The proximal hooked part of the colon lies cranial and to the right of the root of the mesentery. The cranial part of the crook is the transverse colon; the short right portion is the ascending colon. The flexure that unites these two parts is known as the **right colic flexure** (*flexura coli dextra*). The transverse colon is continued by the descending colon at the flexure located to the left of the root of the mesentery. This bend is called the **left colic flexure** (*flexura coli sinistra*). The colon measures approximately 2 cm in diameter throughout its length and is approximately 25 cm long in a Beagle-type preserved specimen. Because of its shorter mesentery, the colon does not vary as much in position or in length as does the small intestine.

The **ascending colon** (*colon ascendens*) begins at the ileal ostium, runs cranially, and ends at the right-angled right colic flexure. It usually is approximately 5 cm long but this varies greatly. In rare instances the ascending colon is lacking, or it may lie cranial or even to the left of the mesenteric root. In these specimens apparently the whole gut failed to rotate around the cranial mesenteric artery as it usually does. Typically, the ascending colon is related to the mesoduodenum and the right lobe of the pancreas dorsally, where it lies ventral to the right kidney. The descending part of the duodenum bounds it on the right. The small intestinal mass lies adjacent to the ascending colon ventrally and on the left. Cranially the ascending colon lies in contact with the stomach unless this viscus is greatly distended, in which case the stomach displaces the small intestinal mass caudally and lies ventral to the relatively fixed ascending colon. The cecum enters the ascending colon at the cecocolic ostium just cranial to the ileal ostium.

The **transverse colon** (*colon transversum*) forms an arc that runs from right to left cranial to the cranial mesenteric artery and the dorsal part of the mesojejunoileum or root of the mesentery. Like the ascending colon, with which it is continuous at the right colic flexure, it may fail to form or be placed to the left of the mesenteric root owing to the failure of the gut to rotate sufficiently. It is related cranioventrally to the stomach and craniodorsally to the left lobe of the pancreas. Ventrally and caudally it lies in contact with the coils of the small intestine. It is approximately 7 cm long.

The **descending colon** (*colon descendens*) is the longest segment of the colon. It extends from the left colic flexure to a transverse plane passing through the pelvic inlet, where it is continued by the rectum without demarcation. It is approximately 12 cm long and usually quite straight. It follows the curvature of the left lateral abdominal wall from the dorsal part of the left costal arch to a point ventral to the promontory of the sacrum. It lies closely applied dorsally to the psoas major muscle, but at its beginning it lies in contact with the left lateral or occasionally with the ventral surface of the left kidney. The left ureter lies dorsal to its medial border initially, but farther caudally this tube obliquely crosses the dorsal surface of the colon and curves around the caudal part of its lateral border before emptying into the bladder.

Usually the ascending portion of the duodenum lies adjacent to its medial or mesenteric border and the spleen crosses it laterally. The intestinal mass covered by greater omentum is ventromedial to it. The uterus and the bladder lie ventral to its terminal part. The body of the uterus always lies in contact with it, and the bladder, if it is distended sufficiently to extend cranial to the uterine body, lies in contact with it at a more cranial level. In the male an enlarged prostate gland replaces the uterus as a ventral boundary.

Mesentery of the Colon

The **mesocolon** (Fig. 7.35) is divided into the same parts as the colon that it suspends. No part of the colon of the dog is retroperitoneal, nor does any part of the greater omentum attach to it. As the proximal part of the colon hooks around the cranial side of the root of the mesentery, the mesocolon of this part attaches to it. The two peritoneal sheets that largely compose the mesocolon do not uninterruptedly at all places to their central attachments. Therefore the various parts will be described separately. The **ascending mesocolon** (*mesocolon ascendens*) is the mesentery of the ascending colon. It is shortest at its origin, where the ileum, colon, and cecum come together. In some specimens these parts are directly attached by areolar tissue to the left jejunal lymph node, but usually a short mesentery exists. Cranially this mesentery is the beginning of the ascending mesocolon; caudally, it is the end of the mesentery or the mesoileum. The medial peritoneal sheet of the ascending mesocolon attains a width of 2 to 3 cm at the right colic flexure. Its length varies with the length of the ascending colon. It is continuous centrally with the mesojejunoileum, which covers the right jejunal lymph node, cranial mesenteric vessels, and nerves. A small colic fossa is usually formed by a thin, circular plica of peritoneum that bridges between the ascending and transverse colon at the right colic flexure.

The **transverse mesocolon** (*mesocolon transversum*) runs directly to the mesenteric root. It is approximately 3 cm long at the right colic flexure, but as it crosses the median plane, it increases in length to approximately 5 cm at the left colic flexure. The length of the transverse mesocolon, determined by the length of the transverse colon, is usually approximately 7 cm. It is continuous at the right colic flexure with the ascending mesocolon and at the left colic flexure with the descending mesocolon. The **descending mesocolon** (*mesocolon descendens*) is continuous without demarcation from the mesorectum at the pelvic inlet. The dorsal part of the descending mesocolon represents the primitive dorsal mesentery and attaches to the aorta approximately in the median plane. Both its right and left peritoneal leaves are interrupted in a dorsal plane approximately 1 cm from their aortic attachments. The secondary fold that blends with the right peritoneal sheet is the duodenocolic fold. It extends as far caudally as the pelvic inlet before it is effaced. On the left side, a loose, fat-streaked plica, a fold from the deep leaf of the greater omentum and spleen, the omental velum, blends with the peritoneal (left) sheet of the descending mesocolon. It attaches at the same dorsoventral level as does the duodenocolic fold on the right side and fades completely a few centimeters cranial to the pelvic inlet. In addition to carrying the caudal mesenteric artery and the large cranially coursing caudal mesenteric vein and fat, one to several left colic lymph nodes are located around the terminal branches of the caudal mesenteric artery in the descending mesocolon.

The ascending colon, transverse colon, and left colic flexure are supplied by vagal general visceral afferents and vagal parasympathetic preganglionic axons. Sympathetic postganglionic axons reach these parts via the cranial mesenteric plexus.

The descending colon and rectum receive sympathetic innervation from the caudal mesenteric ganglion and plexus. The parasympathetic supply is via the pelvic nerve and pelvic plexus.

Rectum

The **rectum** (Fig. 7.48) begins at the pelvic inlet, where it is continuous cranially with the descending colon; it ends ventral to the second or third caudal vertebra, at the beginning of the anal canal. It is straight, approximately 5 cm long, and 3 cm in diameter. Dorsally the rectum is attached to the ventral surface of the sacrum by the thin *mesorectum*. Caudally the mesorectum becomes shorter and ends at a point usually opposite the second caudal vertebra. The peritoneal sheets of the mesorectum are continued dorsally on the sides of the pelvis as the parietal peritoneum. Caudally the visceral peritoneum from the rectal surface reflects cranially at an acute angle in a dorsal plane to become coextensive with the parietal peritoneum, which is derived from the lateral portion of the mesorectum. In this manner, a **pararectal fossa** (*fossa pararectalis*) is formed on each side, right and left of the terminal portion of the rectum (Fig. 7.49). Ventrally the peritoneum blends with that of the rectogenital excavation. The rectum is bounded dorsally by the right and left ventral sacrocaudal muscles. Laterally it is bounded primarily by the levator ani muscle. Many vessels and nerves cross the rectum but at least initially within the connective tissue of the parietal peritoneum of the pararectal fossa. The internal pudendal artery obliquely crosses the lateral side of the initial portion of the rectum. The first branch, prostatic (male) or vaginal (female) artery, continues the direction of the parent vessel, and the internal pudendal runs parallel to the rectum for approximately 2 cm before passing lateral to the coccygeus and levator ani muscles. In a craniocaudal sequence the rectum is crossed laterally first by the obturator, then by the ischiatic, pelvic, and pudendal nerves. The pelvic plexus lies lateral to the middle portion of the rectum. The hypogastric nerve enters it from cranially, and the pelvic nerve or nerves enter it from dorsally. Ventrally the rectum is bounded by the vagina in the female, and by the urethra in the male. When the prostate gland is small, it lies within the pelvis or at the pelvic

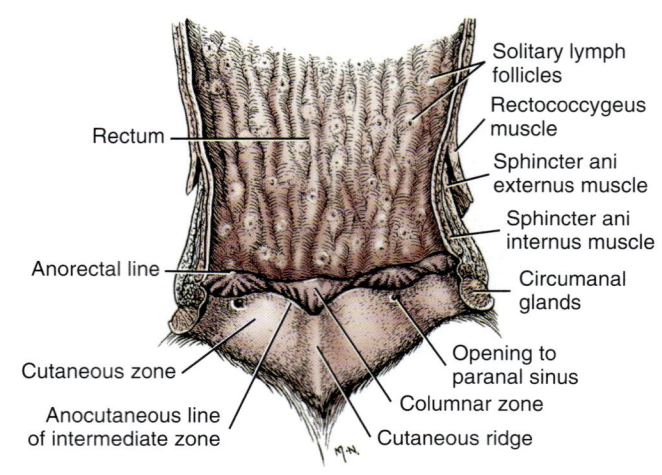

• **Fig. 7.48** The rectum and anal canal, opened to the left of the mid-dorsal line.

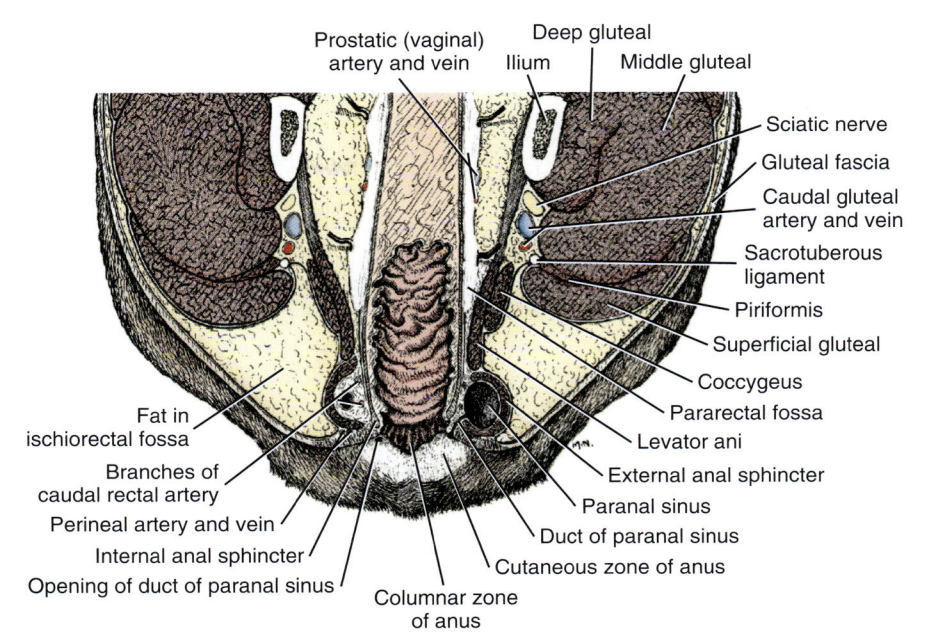

• **Fig. 7.49** Section through the anus in a dorsal plane. (Note that the right side is cut at a lower level, through the duct of the paranal sinus.)

brim, and bounds the rectum at that place. When it is large, the prostate lies largely cranial to the pelvic inlet. The most prominent feature of the rectal mucosa is the presence of approximately 100 **solitary lymph nodules** (*lymphonoduli solitarii*). These nodules are each approximately 3 mm in diameter and 1 mm high. The free surface of each is umbilicated, forming a crater, or rectal pit.

Anal Canal

The **anal canal** (*canalis analis*) (Figs. 7.48 and 7.49) is the terminal, specialized portion of the alimentary canal lined by stratified squamous epithelium. It is approximately 1 cm long and extends from the termination of the rectum to the anus. The anal canal lies ventral to the fourth caudal vertebra and is surrounded by both the smooth and the striated anal sphincter muscle. The mucosa of the anal canal is divided into cutaneous, intermediate, and columnar zones.

The **cutaneous zone** (*zona cutanea*), the most caudal of the three zones of the anal canal, is divided into external and internal portions. The **anus**, the terminal opening of the alimentary canal, may be located in a plane separating the two portions of the cutaneous zone. Thus the external cutaneous zone is not properly a zone of the anal canal because it lies outside the canal. It is feasible, however, to describe the two zones together as the division between them varies with the movement of the tail and the degree of fullness of the rectum. Except during defecation, the anus is closed. In an animal's normal position, with the tail hanging, the anus is indicated by a transverse groove; however, if the tail is slightly raised, the boundaries of the anus form an irregular isosceles triangle. The dorsal or longer border is not straight in old male dogs but is ventrally arched owing to the large mass of gland tissue located deep

to it. The shorter ventrolateral borders converge in forming a V with the apex pointing ventrally. A low ridge, approximately 2 mm wide and 8 mm long, continues from the apex of the V toward the perineum. The internal, cranial, portion of the cutaneous zone is approximately 4 mm wide, and, in life, its surface is moist. The duct from the paranal sinus opens on this zone, approximately 2 mm from its cranial limit and in the depths of the lateral angle of the anus. The external, caudal part of the cutaneous zone may be defined as the relatively hairless zone peripheral to the anus. It varies greatly in width, particularly in adult male dogs, owing to the varied development of the deeply lying circumanal glands. Because these glands probably grow throughout life in the male (Parks, 1950) and their full development tends to result in a loss of hair, the external cutaneous zone may attain a width of 4 cm in large, old male dogs. The cutaneous zone of the dog is studded by small elevations that relate to the circumanal glands deep to them.

The **anocutaneous line** (*linea anocutanea*) is the boundary between the mucous membrane and the skin and cannot be differentiated from the intermediate zone. It completely encircles the anal canal. Its mucosa, like the surface of the cutaneous zone, is also stratified squamous epithelium.

The **intermediate zone** (*zona intermedia*) is between the anocutaneous line and the columnar zone. It is usually less than 1 mm wide and is in the form of an irregular, sharp-edged scalloped fold, which is divided into four arcs. It is lined by stratified squamous noncornified epithelium.

The **columnar zone** (*zona columnaris*) (Fig. 7.48) is so named because it contains longitudinal or oblique ridges, or **anal columns** (*columnae anales*), which run cranially from the intermediate zone for approximately 7 mm. The line that represents the cranial extent of these columns is the **anorectal line** (*linea rectalis*) where the simple columnar epithelium of the rectum meets the stratified squamous epithelium of the anal canal. Caudally the adjacent anal columns are united by the fold that forms the intermediate zone. In this way, a large number of pockets are formed, called **anal sinuses** (*sinus anales*). The anal sinuses are contained within the four arches of the intermediate zone thus producing its scalloped appearance. The smaller of the four arches are dorsal and ventral; the larger ones are located laterally. The columns are not uniform in either length or direction. Some disappear after running only a few millimeters cranially; most end in the anorectal line that encircles the anal canal.

The **paranal sinuses** (*sinus paranalis*) (Fig. 7.49), usually referred to as *anal sacs*, consist of two sinuses with one on each side of the anal canal. They are approximately spherical sinuses that are located between the inner smooth and the outer striated sphincter muscle of the anus. These sinuses vary in size from a pea to a marble, the average diameter being a little less than 1 cm. The excretory duct of each sinus is approximately 5 mm long and 2 mm in diameter and opens near the cranial end of the furrow between the dorsal and lateral parts of the inner cutaneous zone of the anus adjacent to the anocutaneous line and intermediate zone. In about 10% of dogs the opening of the paranal sinus is located in the broad depression formed by the lateral arch of the anocutaneous line on each side. The paranal sinuses are of considerable clinical importance. They frequently become enlarged owing to accumulated secretion from the **paranal sinus glands** (*gll. sinus paranalis*) that lie in the wall of the sinus, or they may become abscessed and painful, causing constipation. Infrequently they rupture to the outside, lateral to the anus, producing anal fistulas (Budsberg et al., 1985). For a discussion of the paranal sinuses and its secretions, see Grau (1935), Ewer (1973), and Doty and Dunbar (1974). The paranal sinus functions for territorial scent marking as in wolves (Asa et al., 1985).

Glands of the Anus

Three gland areas are located in relation to the anus. These are the circumanal glands, the anal glands, and the glands of the paranal sinuses.

The **circumanal glands** (*glandulae circumanales*) are located around the anus in a subcutaneous zone that may reach a radius of 4 cm and a thickness of 8 mm. Circumanal gland elements are also found in the walls of the paranal sinus ducts (Parks, 1950) and may extend peripherally a short distance deep to the skin, which contains abundant hair. Parks found that the circumanal gland is a bipartite structure consisting of a superficial sebaceous portion and a deep nonsebaceous part. Because the nonsebaceous cell is capable of transforming and in certain cases does transform into a sebaceous cell, Parks concluded that the circumanal gland is potentially a sebaceous gland. Isitor and Weinman (1979) and Isitor (1983) studied the origin, early development, and mode of secretion of the circumanal

glands that they considered as hepatoid cells derived from the external hair follicle. Konig et al. (1985) investigated both the circumanal glands and the tail glands of dogs and found similar cells. They denote only the deeper hepatoid lobules as circumanal glands, contrary to other authors. They never observed bursting of "retention" cysts or emptying of contents, thus these nonvacuolated hepatoid glands are not exocrine. Vacuolated hepatoid cells were found only in the circumanal glands of newborn and young puppies, and they do not have ducts.

Scattered among the circumanal glands are apocrine glands, and sweat glands are located in a zone 2 to 4 mm wide directly peripheral to the anal orifice. Probably because the circumanal glands continue to grow throughout life in the unaltered male, adenomas of this region are common in old male dogs.

Atoji et al. (1998) concluded that, although the circumanal glands have many characteristics of epidermis, they should not be classified as glandular tissue. They considered the controversy as to whether they should be classified as exocrine or endocrine or something else altogether. In addition they investigated cell degeneration in lobules of the circumanal glands in relation to apocrine glands. The cysts in lobules can be interpreted as closed hair canals.

The **anal glands** (*glandulae anales*), according to Trautmann and Fiebiger (1957), are tubuloalveolar glands that open to the outside in the intermediate zone. Their secretion is fatty in the dog. Bradley and Grahame (1948) state that the microscopic anal glands are laterally located, cranial to the circumanal glands. Ellenberger and Baum (1943) describe these as a band of grape-shaped glands, 5 mm wide. Budsberg and Spurgeon (1983) found anal glands to be present in the zona columnaris and zona intermedia of the anal canal. Sebaceous, circumanal, and apocrine sweat glands were restricted to the zona cutanea.

The **paranal sinus glands** (*gll. sinus paranalis*) lie in the wall of the sinus and open into it. They are composed of large, coiled, apocrine, sudoriparous tubules. Similar tubules lie in the wall of the duct, which also contains sebaceous acini. The paranal sinus, therefore, is a reservoir for the secretion of the glands of its wall, the secretion being a foul-smelling, serous to pasty liquid. According to Montagna and Parks (1948), both the paranal sinus and its duct are lined by cornified, stratified squamous epithelium, subjacent to which lies a thick mantle of glandular tissue embedded in a connective tissue stroma rich in diffuse lymphatic tissue.

Special Muscles of the Rectum and the Anal Canal

The **internal anal sphincter** (*m. sphincter ani internus*) (Figs. 6.43A and 7.48) is the caudal thickened part of the circular coat of the anal canal. It is composed of smooth, and therefore involuntary, muscle. It is lined by submucosa on its inner surface, and is separated from the external anal sphincter by a small amount of fascia. On its lateral external surface on each side lies the paranal sinus, which is interposed largely between the two sphincter muscles. The duct from the sinus crosses the caudal border of the internal sphincter, which extends slightly farther caudally than does the external anal sphincter. The internal anal sphincter receives its postganglionic sympathetic axons solely via the hypogastric nerves and pelvic plexus. The **external anal sphincter** (*m. sphincter ani externus*) (see Figs. 7.48 and 7.49) averages approximately 1.5 cm in width and 0.5 to 1.5 mm in thickness. It is more than 2 cm wide (craniocaudal distance) dorsally and usually approximately 1 cm wide ventrally. On the sides, because of the underlying paranal sinuses, it forms variably developed bulges. It is largely a circular band of striated and therefore voluntary muscle and is the chief guardian of the lumen of the anal canal. It lies largely subcutaneously on the side. Ventrally its fibers decussate somewhat and may spread out and end on the urethral muscle and the origin of the bulbospongiosus muscle of the male. In the female, the comparable fibers blend with the constrictor vulvae. Approximately half of the deeper fibers of this sphincter from each side continue across to the other side, ventrally. In both sexes the fibers of the superficial half blend with the muscles of the external genitalia. On the sides, the cranial border of the external anal sphincter is united by fascia to the caudal borders of the levator ani muscles. Dorsally the muscle becomes wider and attaches mainly to the fascia of the tail opposite the third caudal vertebra. This attachment is made in such a way that a cranially facing, concave fascial arch is formed through which the paired rectococcygeal muscles pass.

The retractor muscles of the penis and clitoris have anal and rectal components proximally. A band of smooth muscle fibers approximately 3 mm wide and less than 1 mm thick arises on each side from the ventral surface of the sacrum or first caudal vertebra and sweeps caudoventrally. As it obliquely crosses the rectum, it contributes some fibers to it and then fans out between the paranal sinus and the internal anal sphincter. This band of muscle fibers composes the **pars analis of the retractor penis muscle** (*pars analis m. retractor penis*) or retractor clitoridis muscle (pars analis m. retractor clitoridis). The major portion of this muscle appears to end near the duct of the paranal sinus, with some fibers inserting in the external anal sphincter *pars rectalis*. The minor ventrolateral portion of the pars analis, in combination with fibers from the external anal sphincter, continues distally as the mixed (smooth and striated) pars pennia of the **retractor penis muscle** of the male. The anatomy of this muscle is the same in the female except that it is the **retractor clitoridis muscle** (*m. retractor clitoridis*) and the distal part is *pars clitoridae*.

The **rectococcygeal muscle** (*m. rectococcygeus*) (Figs. 6.43 and 9.42) is a paired, smooth muscle at its origin, composed of a condensation of many of the outer longitudinal fibers from each side of the rectum. These fibers sweep caudodorsally from the sides of the rectum and pass dorsally through the fascial arch formed by the attachment of the external anal sphincter to the fascia of the tail. Right and left portions lie closely together at this site, ventral to the third caudal vertebrae, and fuse. Caudally the muscle lies on the bodies of successive caudal vertebrae, in the groove formed by the apposed ventral sacrocaudal muscles, and runs caudally to attach on the bodies of the fifth and sixth caudal vertebrae. The attachment of the rectococcygeus on the tail serves as an anchorage whereby the muscle can stabilize the anal canal and rectum and prevent their being pulled cranially by a peristaltic wave, or, by its contraction, it can move the anal canal and rectum caudally during defecation. The movement of the tail during the act of defecation has a direct influence on evacuating the rectum not only through the action of the rectococcygeus but also by the action of the coccygeus and levator ani muscles. The coccygeus muscles cross the rectum laterally and tend to compress the tube while the rectococcygeus, by shortening, aids the circular muscle coat in moving the fecal column to the outside.

Vessels and Nerves of the Anal Canal

The mucosa of the anal canal and the sphincter muscles that surround it receive their blood mainly from the **right** and **left caudal rectal arteries, branches of the internal pudendals,** that anastomose in the anal sphincters. The long **cranial rectal artery from the caudal mesenteric** may extend far enough caudally to furnish some blood to the anal canal. Thus the blood from the anal canal returns to the heart both by the portal system, through the **cranial rectal, caudal mesenteric, portal,** and **hepatic veins** and by the **caudal vena cava** of the systemic system, through the **caudal rectal** and **perineal veins**, which are usually tributaries of the internal pudendal vein. The internal pudendal and caudal gluteal veins unite to form the internal iliac vein. The internal and external iliac veins unite to form the common iliacs, which in turn unite to form the caudal vena cava. The venous blood is returned from the anal canal through the veins that are the satellites of the arteries of supply. The skin of the perineum and the underlying circumanal glands are served largely by the perineal vessels, usually from both the internal pudendal and the caudal gluteal arteries. The lymph vessels from the anal canal drain into the **sacral lymph nodes**, if present, and the **medial iliac lymph nodes**. The external anal sphincter muscle, being striated and voluntary, is supplied by the caudal rectal nerve, a branch of the **pudendal nerve**. The involuntary, smooth internal anal sphincter and rectococcygeus are supplied by autonomic axons from the **pelvic plexuses**. The parasympathetic portion comes to it through the **pelvic nerves**, branches from usually the first, second, and third sacral nerves, and the sympathetic portion is derived from the **hypogastric nerves**, which arise from the caudal mesenteric ganglion.

Coats of the Large Intestine

Except for the terminal part, all of the large intestine has the usual four coats as found in the small intestine. These are the mucous, submucous, muscular, and serous tunics, or coats.

The **mucous coat** (*tunica mucosa*) of the large intestine differs from that of the small intestine in that there are no aggregated lymph nodules or intestinal villi. Solitary lymph nodules, however, are numerous and can be counted from the outside in the dilated gut. Although present throughout the large intestine, they are most numerous in the rectum. The mucosa of the large intestine, except in the anal canal, contains many folds that are similar to those of the contracted stomach. However, these large intestinal folds cannot be effaced by distention. Depending on the type of contraction, these plicae are either longitudinal or circular.

The **intestinal glands** (*glandulae intestinales*) of the large intestine are longer, straighter, and richer in goblet cells than are those of the small intestine (Trautmann & Fiebiger, 1957). They are lined by a columnar epithelium that is continuous with the columnar epithelium of the mucosal surface of the lumen of the gut. The *lamina muscularis mucosae* consists of muscle fibers that are poorly arranged in two strata.

The **submucous coat** (*tela submucosa*) does not differ appreciably from that of the small intestine. Many of the solitary lymph nodules are located partly within it. This tunic contains the submucous nerve plexuses and many vessels in the meshes of loose connective tissue.

The **muscular coat** (*tunica muscularis*) is uniform in thickness. The *stratum longitudinale* is not concentrated in muscular bands (taenia), as it is in the horse and pig, and no haustra are present. The fibers forming the longitudinal stratum sweep dorsocaudally from the sides of the rectum and, opposite the first or second caudal vertebra, leave the dorsum of the rectum to form the smooth *m. rectococcygeus*, which passes dorsal to the external anal sphincter and attaches to the bodies of the fifth and sixth caudal vertebra. The *stratum circulare* of the large intestine resembles that of the small intestine, except that it is thicker. Its caudal portion forms the **internal anal sphincter muscle**.

The **serous coat** (*tunica serosa*) resembles that of the small intestine. It covers the colon, cecum, and much of the rectum as the visceral peritoneum. The anal canal and the caudal portion of the rectum are retroperitoneal. See the description of the pararectal and rectogenital excavations in the previous discussion of the peritoneum.

Perineum

The perineum is the region of the pelvic outlet. It includes the anal and urogenital regions. On the surface of the body of the dog it is limited by the tail dorsally, by the scrotum or ventral commissure of the vulva ventrally, and by the skin that covers the paired superficial gluteal and internal obturator muscles and the tubera ischiadicum laterally. Deeply, the perineum is bounded by the third caudal vertebra dorsally, the sacrotuberous ligaments laterally, and by the arch of the ischium ventrally. The digestive system terminates in the anus. The bones, muscles, blood vessels, nerves, and glands of the pelvic outlet are described in the appropriate chapters. Here only the ischiorectal fossa, and the perineal and, to a lesser extent, the pelvic fasciae are described. The perineal region holds much interest for the surgeon because of the frequency of occurrence of adenomas and perineal hernias in old male dogs.

The **ischiorectal fossa** (*fossa ischiorectalis*) is the deep, wedge-shaped depression located lateral to the terminal pelvic portions of the digestive and urogenital tubes and pelvic diaphragm. The medial boundary of the fossa is the levator ani and coccygeus muscles that obliquely cross the lateral surface of these tubes as the muscles pass essentially sagittally from the os coxae to the caudal vertebrae. The most caudal part of the medial boundary is the external anal sphincter dorsally and the constrictor vulvae of the female and the retractor penis of the male ventrally. The ventrolateral and ventral boundary is formed by the internal obturator muscle, the lateral boundary by the sacrotuberous ligament, the dorsal and dorsolateral boundary by the superficial gluteal muscle. Cranially and ventrally the fossa forms a narrow fornix where the medially located coccygeus muscles arise adjacent to the origin of the laterally located internal obturator muscle. This angle is located opposite the bodies of the ilium and ischium and along the entire pelvic symphysis. The ischiorectal fossa in well-nourished dogs is filled with fat, which is bounded peripherally by the skin.

The **perineal fascia** (*fascia perinei*) is a term used by veterinary anatomists to include those parts of the adjacent fasciae from the tail, pelvic region, and thigh that converge at the anus, enclosing the pelvic outlet. It is divided into superficial and deep strata.

The **superficial perineal fascia** (*fascia perinei superficialis*) forms the feeble matrix in which the fat of the ischiorectal fossa is elaborated. It is a single-layered, loose fascia, but it is abundantly developed. The numerous small perineal vessels and nerves that stream caudally over the ventral part of the pelvic outlet lie in the superficial perineal fascia. It is continuous with the superficial fascia of the pelvis, thigh, and tail.

The **deep perineal fascia** (*fascia perinei profunda*) covers the dorsomedial surface of the internal obturator muscle. It firmly attaches to the dorsal subcutaneous portion of the tuber ischii ventrally, and the adjacent portion of the obliquely running sacrotuberous ligament caudolaterally. Craniolaterally it becomes continuous with the deep gluteal fascia of the superficial gluteal muscle. The combination of this pelvic fascia and the paired coccygeus and levator ani muscles is referred to as the **pelvic diaphragm** (*diaphragma pelvis*).

In the male the deep perineal fascia is tightly applied to the dorsal surfaces of the right and left ischiourethralis and ischiocavernosus muscles and to the unpaired bulbospongiosus muscle that lies between them. In both sexes the deep perineal fascia, but no muscle fibers, extends cranially between the digestive and urogenital tubes at the pelvic outlet. Developed in the caudal part of this dorsal plane of fascia is the retractor penis muscle of the male and the constrictor vulvae muscle of the female. Just cranial to the muscles that pass from the external anal sphincter to the pudenda in both sexes, collagenous fibers directly unite the complex musculature between the anal canal and the vagina or the bulb of the penis. This median fascial union, if sufficiently large or differentiated as a fibromuscular node, is the **perineal body** (*centrum tendineum perinei*).

Liver

The **liver** (*hepar*) (Figs. 7.50 and 7.51) is the largest gland in the body. It is both exocrine and endocrine in function. The bile, which is its exocrine product, is stored largely in the gallbladder before being poured into the descending portion of the duodenum. Its endocrine substances released into the bloodstream function in the intermediary metabolism of fats, sugars, and some nitrogenous products.

Physical Characteristics

The average weight of the liver in 91 dogs was 450 g. The average weight of these dogs was 13.3 kg. In this sampling of adult mongrel dogs of both sexes the weight of the liver averaged 3.38% of the body weight. Thus the liver weighed approximately a pound in those dogs whose average weight was approximately 27 pounds. The liver is relatively much heavier in the puppy than in the aged dog. The fresh liver is a deep red color, firm in consistency, but friable. In a 30-pound, hound-type dog, its dorsoventral dimension is 14 cm, its width 12 cm, and its thickness 6 cm.

Surfaces, Borders, and Relations

The **diaphragmatic surface** (*facies diaphragmatica*), or parietal surface, of the liver is strongly convex in all directions as it lies mainly in contact with the diaphragm. It is so strongly convex that more of this surface faces bilaterally and dorsally than faces cranially and ventrally. In general terms, the right part is largest as it extends from the cranial extent of the liver at the level of the sixth intercostal space to the last, or twelfth, intercostal space. On the left side the caudal border usually lies opposite the tenth intercostal space. The cranial part may exhibit a shallow, broad, indistinct cardiac impression that is located largely to the left of the median plane. The dorsal part is deeply notched, approximately in the median plane, by the caudal vena cava (*sulcus venae cavae*) and the esophagus (*impressio esophagea*). The caudal vena cava lies to the right of the esophagus as they groove the liver.

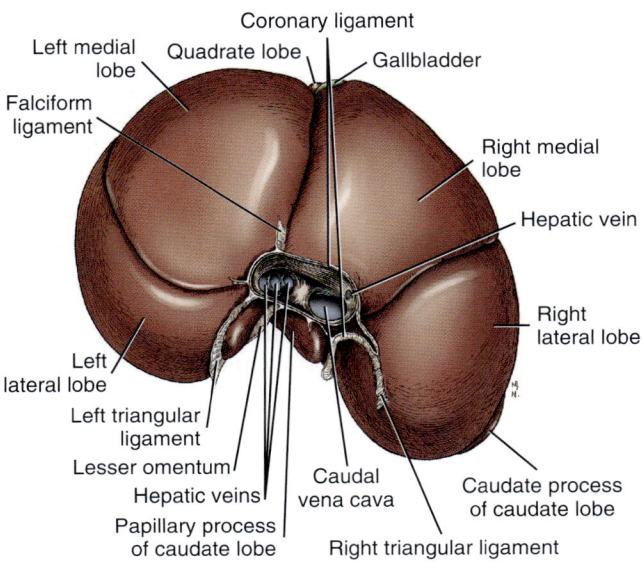

• **Fig. 7.50** Liver, diaphragmatic aspect.

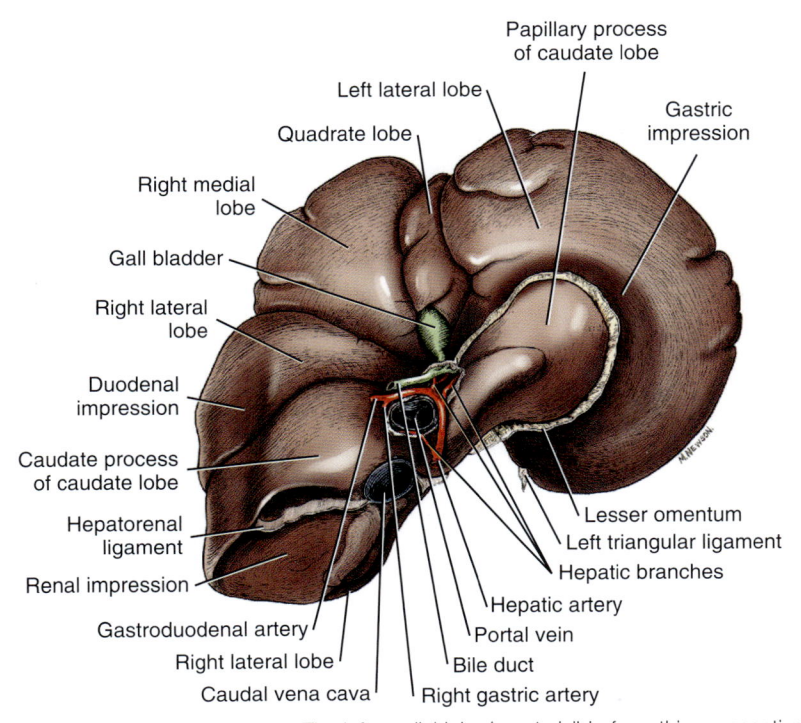

• **Fig. 7.51** Liver, visceral aspect. The left medial lobe is not visible from this perspective.

The **visceral surface** (*facies visceralis*) of the liver is irregularly concave and faces mainly caudoventrally and to the left. It lies in contact with the stomach, duodenum, pancreas, and right kidney. All but the pancreas produce impressions on the organ. The liver is completely invested with peritoneum except at the hilus and where the gallbladder is fused to it. The centrally located **papillary process** (*processus papillaris*) of the caudate lobe, which protrudes caudally from its dorsal part, a prominent feature of the visceral surface.

The **gastric impression** (*impressio gastrica*) occupies the whole left half of the visceral surface. When the stomach is moderately full it resides in this impression. The pyloric part, owing to its relatively fixed position, produces an oblique impression across the middle portion of the gland, where it lies in contact with the caudal face of the gallbladder. When the stomach is empty, the coils of small intestine contact the visceral surface of the liver through the greater omentum but leave no impressions on it.

The **duodenal impression** (*impressio duodenalis*) begins at the junction of the right and quadrate lobes as the most cranial indentation of the visceral surface. This impression at first runs to the right, then it makes a sweeping arch caudoventrally and finally runs caudodorsally, essentially paralleling and lying dorsal to the right ventral border of the organ. The right lobe of the pancreas lies dorsomedial to the cranial and descending portions of the duodenum in contact with the liver, but leaves no impression on it.

The **renal impression** (*impressio renalis*) is a deep, nearly hemispheric fossa formed by the cranial pole of the right kidney projecting into the most caudodorsal portion of the liver, the caudate process of the caudate lobe. Ventrally the liver covers more than half of the kidney. Because of the close proximity of the caudal vena cava to the right adrenal gland, this gland does not leave an impression on the liver.

The **porta of the liver** (*porta hepatis*) is the hilus of the organ. The hepatic vessels and nerves and the hepatic ducts communicate with the gland through the porta. The nerves and arteries enter the porta dorsally, the hepatic ducts leave ventrally, and the portal vein enters between the two (Fig. 7.50). It is located on the dorsal third of the visceral surface, ventrodextral to the attachment of the papillary process. From the porta, the deep fissures that subdivide the organ diverge toward the lateral and ventral surfaces, so that the liver, opposite and dorsal to the porta, is especially thick.

Dorsal, **ventral**, **right**, and **left borders** (*margo dorsalis, ventralis, dexter, et sinister*) are recognized. They are sharp-edged and continuous around the periphery of the organ except dorsally, where this circumferential margin is effaced by the deep, broad notch that contains in its depths the caudal vena cava and esophagus. In addition to the main clefts that subdivide the liver into lobes, there are a few short fissures that cut into the borders of the organ. In the dog, the **fissure for the round ligament** (*fissura lig. teretis*) is the caudoventral portion of the interlobar fissure between the quadrate lobe on the right and the left medial lobe on the left. In the puppy, the round ligament (umbilical vein of the fetus) runs from the umbilicus to the porta of the liver in or just caudal to this cleft.

Lobes and Processes

The liver is divided into four lobes and four sublobes, as well as two processes, by deeply running fissures.

The **left hepatic lobe** (*lobus hepatis sinister*) is that portion of the liver that lies entirely, or almost entirely, to the left of the median plane. This lobe forms from a third to nearly a half of the total liver mass. Its parenchyma is usually completely divided into two sublobes, as follows: The **left lateral hepatic lobe** (*lobus hepatis sinister lateralis*) begins dorsally deep to the left crus of the diaphragm, where it is approximately 3 cm wide. Traced ventrally, it crosses ventral to the left portion of the tendinous center and then ventral to the left portion of the muscular periphery of the diaphragm. Its diaphragmatic surface gradually becomes wider, until it reaches a width of 4.5 to 5 cm in its middle, after which it gradually becomes narrower and ends in a point dorsal to the last sternebra. The lateral border may protrude as much as 2 cm caudal to the ventral portion of the costal arch, but in some specimens it is completely contained within the rib wall. The dorsal portion partially caps the body of the stomach. The visceral surface of the left lateral lobe is concave peripherally as it lies on the fundus and body of the stomach. Centrally it is partly covered by the papillary process of the caudate lobe. This central portion of the left lateral lobe is slightly convex, forming the **omental tuber** (*tuber omentale*). It lies adjacent to the lesser omentum covering the papillary process and is formed by the moldable hepatic tissue protruding toward the lesser curvature of the stomach.

The **left medial hepatic lobe** (*lobus hepatis sinister medialis*) varies from being nearly triangular to oval in outline as seen from the diaphragmatic surface. The fissure that separates it from the left lateral lobe begins from 1.5 to 3 cm from the most caudoventral portion of the organ. It exists as a deep, curved cleft, which usually completely separates the left medial and left lateral lobes of the liver. It extends to the porta. Dorsally in some specimens, the left medial and left lateral lobes are joined by a narrow but deep bridge of liver tissue. Otherwise, the two lobes are joined together only by the intrahepatic vessels and nerves. The left medial lobe is separated from the quadrate and right medial lobe by a deep fissure, nearly midsagittal in location, which extends to the porta and nearly to the esophageal notch. This fissure contains the round ligament of the liver in the free edge of the falciform ligament.

The **quadrate lobe** (*lobus quadratus*) is a deep wedge of liver tissue that lies essentially in the median plane, where it is interposed in the fissure that separates the right medial and the left hepatic lobe, being fused to a certain extent to the former. Its diaphragmatic surface is fusiform, and it extends neither to the ventral border nor to the notch for the esophagus and caudal vena cava. The middle of its right surface is smoothly excavated by the left half of the **fossa** for the gallbladder (*fossa vesicae felleae*). In nearly half of the specimens examined, the quadrate lobe did not reach the visceral surface of the liver.

The **right hepatic lobe** (*lobus hepatis dexter*) is smaller than the left hepatic lobe and lies completely to the right of the median plane. It lies between transverse planes passed through the dorsal portions of the sixth and the tenth intercostal spaces. Like the left hepatic lobe, it is divided into medial and lateral sublobes.

The **right medial hepatic lobe** (*lobus hepatis dexter medialis*) is fused to the medially lying quadrate lobe. The degree of fusion varies; in some specimens only the dorsal portions of these always closely adjacent lobes are fused; in others the fusion extends nearly to the fossa for the gallbladder, leaving only a short fissure extending dorsally from the fossa to separate the two lobes. The right medial lobe is always longer than the right lateral lobe and is the portion that extends caudally beyond the ventral portion of the costal arch if any portion of the right hepatic lobe protrudes beyond it. Its diaphragmatic surface is in the form of a curved triangle. It is also triangular in cross-section as it is wedge-shaped, possessing a concave, slightly fissured medial border that extends to the visceral surface of the organ. The right half of the **fossa for the gallbladder** is located on its medial face opposite the comparable excavation on the quadrate lobe.

The **right lateral hepatic lobe** (*lobus hepatis dexter lateralis*) is shaped roughly like a laterally compressed hemisphere with a slightly concave base. Cranially it is overlapped by the right medial lobe; caudally it overlaps the caudate process of the caudate lobe and is usually fused to it, lateral to the caudal vena cava. Its most ventral extension lies opposite the distal portion of the middle third of the caudal border of the right medial lobe.

The **caudate lobe** (*lobus caudatus*) is composed of the caudate and papillary processes and the isthmus of liver tissue that connects them. This isthmus is compressed between the caudal vena cava dorsally and the portal vein ventrally. It is a bridge of hepatic tissue that is approximately 1.5 cm long, 1 cm wide, and 0.5 cm thick.

The **papillary process** (*processus papillaris*) is pyramidal to tongue-shaped and is usually partly subdivided by one or two fissures. The more constant fissure separates the frenular part from the body of the process. This process is loosely enveloped by the lesser omentum and lies in the lesser curvature of the stomach. It projects by an acute angle to the left and cranially from its attachment to the caudate lobe.

The **caudate process** (*processus caudatus*) forms the most caudal portion of the liver as it extends to a plane through the twelfth intercostal space or last rib on the right side. Its caudolateral portion is deeply recessed by the cranial half of the right kidney. The outline of its diaphragmatic surface forms nearly an equilateral triangle as it lies mainly ventral to the right kidney. The parenchyma of the caudate lobe is usually partly fused to the right lateral lobe, but occasionally the two portions are completely separated or other variations may exist.

Peritoneal Attachments and Fixation

The liver is almost completely enveloped by peritoneum, which forms its **serous coat** (*tunica serosa*). The serous coat is fused to the underlying *tela subserosa* and **fibrous capsule** (*tunica fibrosa*), a thin but dense layer, composed mainly of collagenous tissue, that closely invests the surfaces of the liver and sends interlobular trabeculae into the gland substance. At the porta the fibrous coat becomes thicker and is continued into the interior of the liver in association with the vascular and nervous structures that serve the gland. These extensions from the fibrous capsule along the hepatic ducts and the branches of the hepatic artery and portal vein within the liver are referred to as *capsula fibrosa perivascularis* (formerly *Glisson's capsule*). The only parietal attachment of the liver is to the diaphragm by means of continuations of its serous and fibrous coats in the form of the coronary ligament and several small folds that radiate from it. These folds form the right triangular, the left triangular, and the falciform ligaments. The hepatorenal ligament and the lesser omentum also attach to the liver. The serous coat and these ligaments are remnants of the primitive ventral mesentery of the stomach, the ventral mesogastrium. The dorsal remnant is the lesser omentum.

The **coronary ligament of the liver** (*lig. coronarium hepatis*) (Fig. 7.50) is not a true peritoneal ligament because the two sheets of peritoneum that form it are not in the form of a fold but are irregularly separated. The term refers to the line of peritoneum that reflects around a triangular "bare area" (*area nuda*) of the liver, approximately 2 cm long on each side, and is continued on the dorsal surface of the caudal vena cava and the tributaries that enter it from the diaphragm. The coronary ligament is irregular in outline. It reflects the close embryonic relationship between the diaphragm and the liver. Its stellate border gives rise to the triangular ligaments and is coextensive with the dorsal part of the falciform ligament.

The **right triangular ligament** (*lig. triangulare dextrum*) (Fig. 7.50) is a plica of peritoneum that extends between the diaphragm and the dorsal part of the right lateral lobe. Its free lateral border is 1 to 5 cm wide. As it passes medially, it becomes progressively narrower until its two formative peritoneal layers become continuous with the right peritoneal leaf of the coronary ligament as this bounds the bare area of the liver on the right. It is usually longer than it is wide. The right triangular ligament includes a fold from the diaphragm to the diaphragmatic surface of the right medial lobe. Other smaller but similar plicae are present.

The **left triangular ligament** (*lig. triangulare sinitrum*), like the comparable right ligament, may have multiple components. The cranial component runs from the left lateral lobe to the diaphragm. If there are two components, the caudal member is larger than the cranial and contains the **fibrous appendix of the liver** (*appendix fibrosa hepatis*) when this is present. This fibrous appendix is a narrow, thin tapering band of atrophic hepatic tissue located in or near the free border of the ligament. It is present in only a small number of adult specimens.

The **falciform ligament of the liver** (*lig. falciforme hepatis*) (Fig. 7.50) is a remnant of the primitive ventral mesentery that extends between the liver and the diaphragm and ventral body wall caudally to the umbilicus. The middle portion of the falciform ligament in the dog usually becomes wholly or partly obliterated before birth so that the umbilical vein, which in early fetal life is located in its free border, usually has no peritoneal attachment immediately before birth. The portion of the falciform ligament that extends from the umbilicus to the diaphragm remains as a fat-filled irregular fold that may weigh several pounds in obese specimens. Cranially the falciform ligament may disappear completely at the liver, but usually it remains as a thin, avascular fold that extends from the dorsal end of the fissure between the right and the left medial lobes to the coronary ligament. When present, the left peritoneal sheet of the falciform ligament becomes coextensive with the left portion of the coronary ligament, and the right peritoneal sheet becomes coextensive with the ventral portion of the coronary ligament. Ventrally the falciform ligament is between the quadrate and left medial lobes.

The **hepatorenal ligament** (*lig. hepatorenale*) (Fig. 7.51) is a delicate peritoneal fold that extends from the medial portion of the renal fossa to the ventral surface of the right kidney lateral to the fat that fills its hilus. It is not constant. The **lesser omentum** (*omentum minus*) is a thin, lacy, fat-streaked, loose peritoneal fold that is that remnant of the primitive ventral mesentery (*ventral mesogastrium*) that extends from the liver to the lesser curvature of the stomach and cranial part of the duodenum.

Structure

The free surface of the liver is firmly covered by the thin peritoneum superficially (tunica serosa) and the equally thin fibrous capsule (tunica fibrosa) that sends septa into the gland. On close observation the surface of the liver presents a finely mottled appearance. The delicate dappling is due to the contrast in color between the dark, small, polygonal units of liver parenchyma and the lighter connective tissue surrounding them. These units, called **hepatic lobules** (*lobuli hepatis*), are the smallest grossly visible functional divisions of the organ. Each lobule is approximately 1 mm in diameter and is composed of curved sheets of cells that enclose numerous, blood-filled cavities known as the liver sinusoids. According to Elias (1949), the sinusoids of the dog are intermediate in form between the saccular and the tubular types that are found in some other mammals. The sheets or plates of cells that form the sinusoidal walls are one cell thick and contain openings that allow free passage of the intersinusoidal blood.

Blood and Lymph Vessels

In the centers of the lobules there are typically the single **central veins** (*venae centrales*). These constitute the beginning of the efferent, or outgoing, venous system of the liver. Adjacent central veins fuse to form the **interlobular veins** (*venae interlobulares*). The interlobular veins unite with each other to form finally the **hepatic veins** (*vv. hepaticae*), which empty into the caudal vena cava. Arey (1941) and others have shown that, in the dog but not in the cat, there are spiral and circular muscle fibers in the walls of the central and interlobular veins. The sphincter action produced by these muscle fibers restricts venous drainage, producing precisely the effects of experimental shock. The hepatic veins convey to the caudal vena cava all the blood that the liver receives through the portal vein and hepatic arteries. These hepatic veins enter the caudal vena cava progressing from the right lobes to the left lobes in a caudal to cranial direction as the caudal vena cava crosses the liver.

The **portal vein** (*v. portae*) (Fig. 7.51) brings the functional blood to the liver from the stomach, intestines, pancreas, and spleen. Approximately four-fifths of the blood entering the liver reaches it by the portal vein (Markowitz et al., 1949). The **hepatic arteries** (*aa. hepaticae*) furnish the liver with the blood that nourishes its cells—the oxygenated nutritional supply. The parenchymal cells are bathed by mixed blood from the portal vein and hepatic arteries so that they receive nutrition from both. The hepatic arteries supply primarily the liver framework, including its capsules and the walls of the blood vessels, the intrahepatic biliary duct system, and the nerves (see Oishi et al., 2015).

Although only approximately one-fifth of the blood coming to the liver reaches it through the hepatic arteries, their occlusion usually results in death if such occlusion is not accompanied by massive doses of penicillin. Markowitz et al. (1949) found that, without antibiotic treatment following ligation of the arteries at the portal fissure, gangrene results. In research on the arterial blood supply to the liver, it should not be overlooked that there are never fewer than two, and, in some specimens, there are as many as five visible branches that leave the hepatic artery at the hilus of the liver, and most of these arteries branch before they enter the lobes of the liver. See the treatise of Payer et al. (1956) on the surgical anatomy of the arteries to the liver of the dog.

In the fetal pup there is a shunt from the umbilical vein to the hepatic venous system, known as the *ductus venosus*. The ductus venosus develops within the liver between the left intrahepatic branch of the portal vein where the umbilical vein joins it and the caudal vena cava where the last (most cranial) hepatic vein enters the caudal vena cava from the left hepatic lobe. The ductus venosus becomes fibrotic after birth and is known as the *ligamentum venosum*. In the stillborn pup it is several millimeters long and approximately 2 mm wide. It extends obliquely from left to right in the liver parenchyma, where it lies ventral to the attachment of the papillary process.

Lohse and Suter (1977) found that closure of the ductus venosus began within 48 hours after birth. Olivera et al. (1979), in a larger series of pups, confirmed that the ductus venosus began to close at approximately 2 days of age and, by 6 days postpartum, was closed in all pups. The lymph vessels from the liver freely anastomose with those of the gallbladder (McCarrell et al., 1941). They drain into the **hepatic** and **splenic lymph nodes**.

Nerves

The liver is supplied by both afferent and efferent axons through the vagi and by sympathetic axons from the **celiac plexus**. The vagal axons reach the abdomen by passing through the diaphragm with the esophagus as the dorsal and ventral vagal nerve trunks. Chiu (1943) has shown that, in a representative dog, two branches leave the ventral vagal trunk and one leaves the dorsal at the level of the cardia. They pass obliquely to the right in the lesser omentum toward the porta and supply the liver parenchyma and biliary system. McCrea (1924) describes the abdominal distribution of the vagi in the rabbit, cat, and dog. Possibly the liver also receives vagal axons through the portion of the dorsal vagal trunk that joins the celiac plexus. Chiu (1943) also mentions the possibility of a coronary nerve reaching the liver in the dog. The sympathetic axons reach the liver through the **splanchnic nerves**, **celiac ganglia**, and **celiac plexus** and continue on the hepatic arteries and their lobar branches as the plexuses of these arteries. Alexander (1940) states that in some specimens the biliary system receives afferent axons from the phrenic nerves. He also confirmed that the hepatic artery receives only sympathetic axons.

Bile Passages and Gallbladder

The bile, produced by the sheets of liver cells surrounded by the blood sinuses, is discharged into the minute bile canaliculi (*canliculus bilifer*) that lie between these cells. The canaliculi unite to form the **biliary ductules** (*ductuli biliferi*), which continue into plexiform **interlobular ductules** (*ductuli interlobularis bilifer*), which lie in the interstitial tissue between the lobules. These interlobular ducts are found in the portal triads with branches of the hepatic artery and portal vein. Larger interlobular bile ducts form by the anastomosis of interlobular ductules. Finally the interlobular ducts of various sizes unite to form the lobar intrahepatic ducts, which are variable in number and termination and from which the extrahepatic ducts arise. The extrahepatic bile passages consist of the **hepatic ducts** (*ductuli hepaticae*) (Fig. 7.52) from the liver. These are variable in number. The **cystic duct** (*ductus cystica*) joins the gall bladder with two or more hepatic ducts to form the **bile duct** (*ductus choledochus*) that enters the duodenum on the major duodenal papilla. One of the many possible patterns of hepatic duct termination is illustrated by Fig. 7.52.

The **gallbladder** (*vesica fellea*) (see Fig. 7.52) stores and concentrates the bile. The function of its mucoid secretion, like that of mucus generally, is for lubrication and protection (Ivy, 1934). The gallbladder epithelium is able to absorb lipid-soluble compounds, including cholesterol. Bile is secreted into the duodenum as a suspension of fatty compounds that can be absorbed in the small intestine. Although the vagal nerve axons are motor to its musculature, Winkelstein and Aschner (1924) state that the gallbladder displays variations in tonicity but seems to possess little contractile power. Nawar and Kamel (1975) investigated the intrinsic innervation of the gallbladder in dogs. Intraabdominal pressure chiefly caused by the inspiratory phase of respiration effects a large variation in pressure within the gallbladder. The gallbladder is a pear-shaped vesicle that lies between the quadrate lobe of the liver medially and the right medial lobe laterally. When distended, it extends through the thickness of the liver to its diaphragmatic surface and contacts the diaphragm. Its capacity in a Beagle-sized dog is 15 mL (Mann et al., 1920). It is approximately 5 cm long and 1.5 cm in its greatest width in such specimens. The blind, rounded, cranial end of the gallbladder is known as the **fundus** (*fundus vesicae felleae*); the large middle portion, as the **body** (*corpus vesicae felleae*); and its slender, tapering caudodorsally directed extremity, as the **neck** (*collum vesicae felleae*).

The **cystic duct** (*ductus cysticus*) (Fig. 7.53) in a topographic sense may be regarded as the beginning of the biliary duct system. It extends from the neck of the gallbladder to the site of its junction with the first tributary from the liver. The cystic duct was at least 5 mm long in 80% of the dogs studied by Imagawa et al. (2009). The **bile duct** (*ductus choledochus*) in dogs is formed after the last hepatic duct joins the excretory duct system. Higgins (1926) has recorded double cystic and bile ducts in dogs. In dogs, the lobar ducts do not unite to form a single hepatic duct, but all converge to enter the main trunk of the excretory tree that constitutes the beginning of the cystic duct (see Fig. 7.53). Imagawa et al. (2009) reported that the hepatic duct was formed by four major tributaries in 70% of dogs studied and by three tributaries in the remaining dogs ($N = 50$). These authors also noted that the lobar branches from the right medial and quadrate lobes often enter the hepatic duct system "proximal to the gallbladder," or presumably proximal relative to the position of the cystic duct's merger with the hepatic duct. This information can be useful during

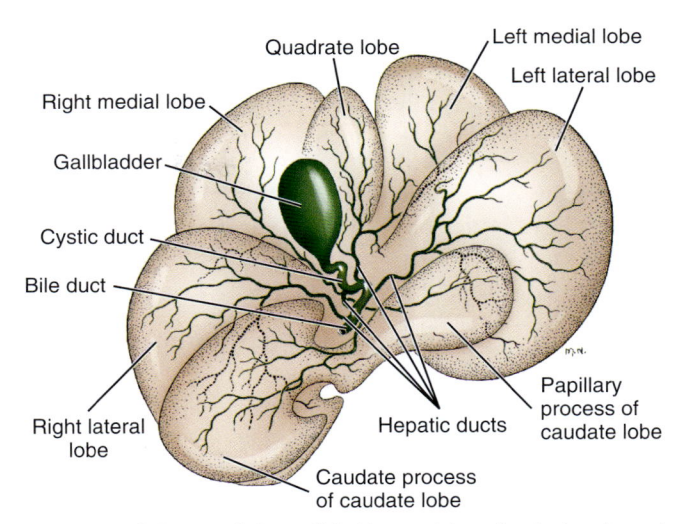

• **Fig. 7.52** Schema of the gallbladder and hepatic ducts, visceral aspect.

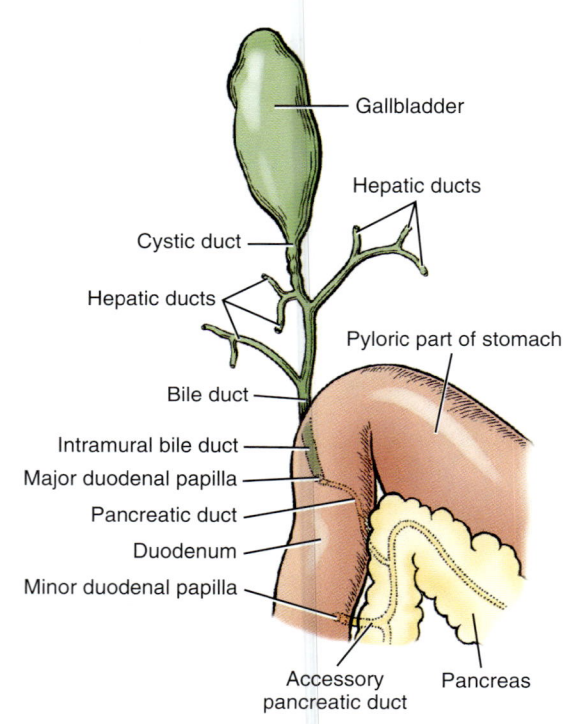

• Fig. 7.53 Bile, hepatic, and pancreatic ducts.

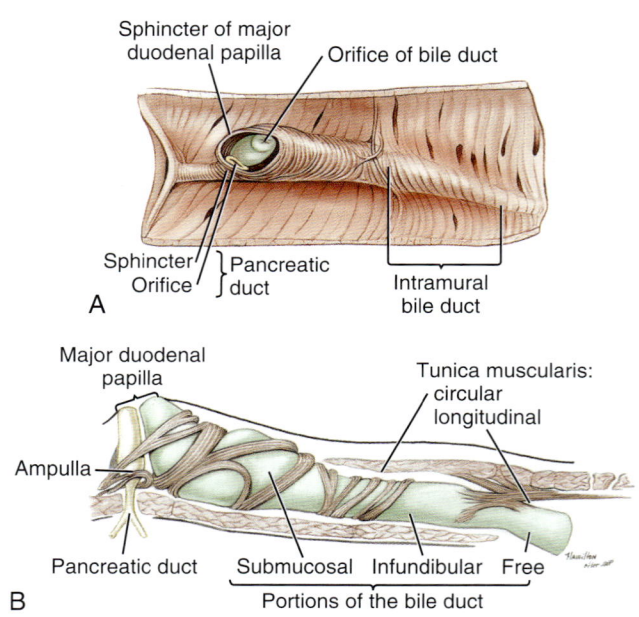

• Fig. 7.54 Reconstruction of the intramural course of the bile duct and the termination of the pancreatic duct at the major duodenal papilla in the dog. (After Eichhorn EP Jr, Boyden EA: The choledochoduodenal junction in the dog—a restudy of Oddi's sphincter, *Am J Anat* 97:431–451, 1955. Copyright © 1955 Wiley-Liss. Reprinted by permission of Wiley-Liss, a Division of John Wiley and Sons, Inc.) **A**, Interior of the duodenum with the mucosa removed. Note that the pancreatic duct opens separately from the bile duct. **B**, Sagittal reconstruction of the intramural course of the bile duct and pancreatic duct in a young dog. The encircling musculature of the bile duct constitutes a choledochal sphincter, the m. sphincter ductus choledochi. The smooth muscle bundles around the ampullae of the bile and pancreatic ducts, at the major duodenal papilla, can be considered as the m. sphincter ampullae hepatopancreaticae.

surgical resection of the gall bladder. Imagawa's report agreed, in general, with an earlier study (Sleight & Thomford, 1970) regarding numbers of hepatic or lobar branches contributing to the hepatic duct. The distal or caudal portion of the bile duct enters the dorsal or mesenteric wall of the duodenum. This portion of the bile duct is known as the *free portion*, in contrast with the intramural portion, which extends obliquely through the duodenal wall. The free portion is approximately 5 cm long and 2.5 mm in diameter as it courses through the hepatoduodenal ligament, the right border of the lesser omentum. The intramural portion of the duct and its mode of emptying into the lumen of the duodenum have been studied by many investigators.

Eichhorn and Boyden (1955) have analyzed the structure of the choledochoduodenal junction in the dog. They illustrate and describe from wax reconstructions and maceration specimens the intramural portion of the bile duct and its musculature in both the fetus and the adult (Fig. 7.54). In their review of the literature they call attention to the early work by Oddi (1887), which included studies on the dog. The bile duct has an intramural length of 1.5 to 2 cm. It terminates on a small hillock located at the end of a low longitudinal ridge representing its intramural course. The bile duct opens in the center of a small rosette on the hillock, and to one side is the slitlike opening of the pancreatic duct. The site of this combined opening of the bile duct and the pancreatic duct is the **major duodenal papilla** (*papilla duodeni major*). Approximately 3 cm distal to this opening lies a second low hillock, on which the accessory pancreatic duct from the dorsal pancreas opens, the **minor duodenal papilla** (*papilla duodeni minor*).

Eichhorn and Boyden (1955) have verified the existence of a double layer of smooth muscle around the intramural portion of the bile duct. The outer layer is formed by the *tunica muscularis* of the duodenum. The inner layer, formed by the musculus proprius of the bile duct, begins in the infundibular portion of the bile duct and extends in the submucosa to the termination of the duct as the sole investing muscle. As such, the musculus proprius forms a variable ring of muscle that surrounds the terminations of the bile and pancreatic ducts to form the *m. sphincter ampullae hepatopancreaticae*. Ensheathing the remaining intramural portion of the bile duct the musculus proprius constitutes the *m. sphincter ductus choledochi*. Eichhorn and Boyden point out that, in the dog, the downgrowth of a septum of the tunica muscularis on the mucosal side of the duct creates a muscular funnel through which the bile duct must pass. This feature makes the discharge of bile dependent to a large degree on the activity of the duodenum (see Fig. 7.54).

Apparently, great variation exists in the amount of musculature that is present at the termination of the bile duct. In fact, there are conflicting interpretations of the presence or absence of a sphincter function along the length of the cystic or bile ducts. Halpert (1932) found proper muscle present in only 1 of 25 dogs he examined. Casas (1958) states that in the dog the bile duct sphincter previously described as the sphincter of Oddi consists of three layers of muscle. MacPherson et al. (1984) studied the muscle layers within the gall bladder and cystic duct and reported the muscular layer to be thickest in the gall bladder and progressively thinner moving along the cystic and bile ducts. They emphasized that the muscular organization was relatively "loose," with separate bundles of smooth muscles interspersed among patches of connective tissue (see Fig. 7.54B) and that no anatomic sphincter (no coalescence of muscle bundles at one location) was present. However, Doyle and Farrar (1969) measured intraluminal pressures and demonstrated the development of pressure gradients between regions of the duct system, suggesting the existence of a sphincter mechanism along the length of the cystic duct.

Pancreas

The pancreas (Figs. 7.37 and 7.53) is yellowish gray when preserved and pinkish gray in life. It is a rather coarsely lobulated, elongate gland. The lobules, as Revell (1902) has pointed out, produce a nodular surface with irregularly crenated margins. The pancreas is located in the dorsal part of both the cranial and right lateral abdominal regions, caudal to the liver. Like the liver, the pancreas has both an exocrine and an endocrine function. Its exocrine secretion, the pancreatic juice, the most important of the digestive secretions, is conveyed to the descending portion of the duodenum by one or several ducts, usually two. It is a clear alkaline secretion containing three principal enzymes, one of which reduces proteins, one fats, and the third carbohydrates. Insulin, a protein hormone, is a major endocrine secretion produced by the islet cells. This hormone keeps the sugar content of the blood at a constant level, and, in its absence, a fatal metabolic disorder, diabetes mellitus, occurs. Tsuchitani et al. (2016) reported that the proportion of endocrine (relative to exocrine) cells increased along an axis from the right to the left pancreatic lobes, suggesting the existence of functional specialization within lobes of the pancreas.

The weight of the pancreas averaged 31.3 g in 76 dogs, with an average weight of 13.8 kg. The pancreas weighs approximately 1 ounce in a dog whose weight is approximately 30 pounds. These data compare favorably with Mintzlaff's (1909) findings in 30 dogs, although his specimens were, on average, larger. The average total length of the pancreas in a 30-pound dog is approximately 25 cm, or 10 inches.

The pancreas, when hardened in situ, is in the form of a V that lies in a dorsal plane with the apex pointing cranially and to the right. The gland is basically divided into a thin, slender right lobe and a shorter, thicker, and wider left lobe. The two lobes are united at the body, formerly called the *pancreatic angle*, which lies caudomedial to the pylorus.

Lobes and Relations

The **right lobe** of the pancreas (*lobus pancreatis dexter*) lies in the mesoduodenum near or in contact with the dorsal portion of the right abdominal wall, the paralumbar fossa. It extends from a transverse plane through the middle of the ninth intercostal spaces to one through the fourth lumbar vertebra. The right lobe varies in width from 1 to 3 cm and in thickness up to 1 cm. Its length is approximately 15 cm, or 6 inches, in a Beagle-type dog. The right lobe is positioned in the mesoduodenum in such a way that its round, flat, caudal extremity lies in the concavity of the duodenal loop. By traction the gland can be separated for a distance of approximately 3 cm from the various parts of the duodenum that form the loop because the mesoduodenum at this site is loose.

As the right lobe runs obliquely cranially toward the pylorus it becomes narrow and flattened dorsoventrally, so that dorsal and ventral surfaces are formed. On contacting the initial part of the descending duodenum, it becomes molded to this organ. The caudal part of the right lobe of the pancreas is related to the sublumbar fat containing the ureter and to the ventral surfaces of the right kidney and the caudate process of the liver. The right lobe of the pancreas is related ventrally to the ileum and cecum caudally, and to the ascending colon cranially. Loops of the jejunum contact those portions of its ventral surface that are not already in contact with more fixed viscera. In some specimens the right lobe of the pancreas and the adjacent descending part of the duodenum have gravitated lateral and even ventral to the jejunal coils.

The **body** of the pancreas (*corpus pancreatis*) unites the two lobes of the pancreas in an angle of approximately 45 degrees, which is open sinistrocaudally. Cranially it lies closely applied to the caudosinistral portion of the pyloric region, which forms a large concave impression on the cranial portion of the body. Caudal to this impression, the pancreas is approximately 1 cm thick and 3 cm wide. The portal vein crosses the dorsal portion of the body. As the pancreaticoduodenal artery and gastroduodenal vein disappear into the pancreas at this place, they are crossed on their right side by the bile duct, which lies adjacent to the duodenum.

The **left lobe** of the pancreas (*lobus pancreatis sinister*) lies in the deep wall of the greater omentum. It begins at the body and runs caudosinistrally. It is approximately two-thirds as long and half again as wide as the right lobe, measuring 10 cm, or 4 inches, in length, and 4 cm, or 1.6 inches, in width. Its **dorsal surface** (*facies dorsalis*), on the right, is related to the caudate process of the liver and then, in succession on the left, to the portal vein, caudal vena cava, and aorta. It ends in the left part of the sublumbar region in close relation to the cranial pole of the left kidney and the middle portion of the spleen. A full stomach alters these relations. The **ventral surface** (*facies ventralis*) of the left lobe of the pancreas is related ventrocaudally to the transverse colon and ventrocranially to the dorsal wall of the stomach.

An **accessory pancreas** (*pancreas accessorium*) is occasionally found in the dog. Baldyreff (1929) cites cases in which the aberrant gland was located in the wall of the gallbladder and in the caudal part of the mesentery.

Pancreatic bladders have been described by various authors as occurring in the cat, but none has been recorded in the dog (Boyden, 1925).

Ducts of the Pancreas

The pancreas nearly always has two excretory ducts (see Figs. 7.37 and 7.39), in conformity with the dual origin of the gland, one anlage arising dorsally from the duodenum and the other ventrally at the termination of the bile duct (Revell, 1902). Within the pancreas, these two ducts usually intercommunicate, or they may cross within the gland because the parenchyma of the whole gland is elaborated around them. In the adult, the two portions of the gland are fused without any demarcation to indicate their dual origin. Revell, however, points out that, when the two ducts do not communicate within the gland, the **pancreatic duct** drains the right lobe, or embryonic ventral pancreas, and the **accessory pancreatic duct** drains the left lobe, or embryonic dorsal pancreas. Although this is the basic pattern by which the pancreatic ducts form in the domesticated mammals, great variations exist among the different species and within the same species.

The largest excretory duct of the pancreas in the dog is the **accessory pancreatic duct** (*ductus pancreaticus accessorius*), which opens into the duodenum on the minor duodenal papilla. The **pancreatic duct** (*ductus pancreaticus*) is the smaller duct in the dog and may occasionally be absent. The latter is associated with the opening of the bile duct and usually enters the duodenum on the major duodenal papilla alongside the bile duct (Fig. 7.54). From its formation at the union of the ducts from the two lobes in the dog to the site where it perforates the intestinal wall, the accessory pancreatic duct is approximately 3 to 4 mm long and 2 mm wide. The union of the two lobar ducts to form the main duct (accessory pancreatic duct) may occur at any level up to the intestinal wall, or rarely, the two lobar ducts may open separately (Revell, 1902). According to Bottin (1934), the pancreatic and the accessory pancreatic duct open separately into the duodenum in approximately 75% of dog specimens, and they always communicate with each other in the gland.

In the 50 dogs of all ages and breeds and of both sexes that Nielsen and Bishop (1954) studied by the use of radiopaque medium, the duct system of the canine pancreas could be divided into five main types. In type 1 (46%), a single main duct is formed by a tributary from each lobe uniting in a Y junction that entered the duodenum at the minor duodenal papilla. In this group there was also an additional duct, arising from the left lobar duct, that frequently followed a most indirect and tortuous route and entered the duodenum at or near the major duodenal papilla. Type 2 (22%) was similar to type 1, except that the small pancreatic duct arose from the right lobar duct instead of the left and crossed over the duct of the left lobe before entering the duodenum. In type 3 (16%), each lobe had its own excretory duct. The ducts crossed, the one from the right lobe emptying into the major duodenal papilla with the bile duct and that from the left lobe emptying on the minor duodenal papilla. A fine and often tortuous shunt connected the two ducts. In type 4 (8%), the ducts from the two lobes anastomosed in a Y formation. In two of the four specimens there was a small anastomosis within the pancreas between the ducts of the two lobes. In type 5 (8%), there were three orifices into the duodenum from the ducts from the pancreas, and in one specimen there were two additional small ducts, one emerging on either side of the minor duodenal papilla.

Other variations of the ducts of the canine pancreas exist, as Revell (1902) and Mintzlaff (1909) have shown. The main duct from each lobe occupies the approximate center of the lobe and is joined at right angles by tributaries from the adjacent parenchyma. Because the gland is ribbonlike, the small ducts from the adjacent parenchyma enter largely on opposite sides, the openings being spaced at 0.5 to 1.5 cm intervals.

The opening of the pancreatic duct is closely associated with that of the bile duct (see Fig. 7.54). In two out of three specimens Eichhorn and Boyden (1955) found the slitlike orifice of the pancreatic duct located distal to that of the bile duct; others have described this opening as proximal to that of the bile duct. The accessory pancreatic duct usually opens into the duodenum 28 mm from the opening of the bile duct into the duodenum, or approximately 8 cm from the pyloric sphincter (Nielsen & Bishop, 1954). Its entry into the duodenum resembles that of the bile duct in that a ridge of mucosa is formed with a slight elevation at its distal end on which the opening is located.

The accessory pancreatic duct, like the pancreatic duct but, unlike the bile duct, runs through the duodenal wall rather directly. The opening through the mesenteric wall of the proximal portion of the descending duodenum is frequently located to the left of the cranial pancreaticoduodenal vessels, whereas the bile and pancreatic ducts open to the right of these vessels.

Eichhorn and Boyden (1955) described and illustrated the musculature of the pancreatic and bile ducts of the dog (sphincter of Oddi). Kyösola and Rechardt (1974) described its innervation.

Blood and Lymph Vessels

The main vessels to the right lobe of the pancreas are the pancreatic branches of the **cranial** and **caudal pancreaticoduodenal arteries** that anastomose in the gland. The left extremity of the left lobe of the pancreas is supplied primarily by the pancreatic branch of the **splenic artery**. It also receives small branches from the **hepatic artery** as this vessel may groove the dorsal surface of the organ, and the left lobe regularly receives, near the pancreatic body, one or two branches from the **gastroduodenal artery**. Small pancreatic branches directly from the **celiac artery** may supply a small portion of the left lobe of the pancreas near its free end.

The **caudal pancreaticoduodenal vein**, a satellite of the artery of the same name, is the principal vein from the right pancreatic lobe. It is the last tributary to enter the cranial mesenteric vein, and, unlike the intestinal veins that empty into it, it enters the larger vessel from the cranial side. The left lobe of the pancreas is drained primarily by two veins that terminate in the last 2 cm of the splenic vein. The venous satellite of the small branch of the cranial pancreaticoduodenal artery that supplies the left lobe near the pancreatic body drains this part of the gland.

The lymphatics from the pancreas drain into the **duodenal lymph node**, if present, and into the **hepatic**, **splenic**, and **jejunal lymph nodes**.

Nerves

Most sympathetic axons come from the **celiac plexus** and reach the organ by following the pancreatic branches of the cranial pancreaticoduodenal and celiac arteries. It is probable that the caudal part of the right lobe receives sympathetic axons from the **cranial mesenteric plexus** that follow the caudal pancreaticoduodenal artery and its pancreatic branches. McCrea (1924) states that, in the dog, vagal (parasympathetic) axons reach the pancreas as fine branches that run with the splenic branch of the celiac artery and with the cranial mesenteric artery, presumably along the caudal pancreaticoduodenal branch.

Bibliography

Abdel-Malek, S. (1938). A contribution to the study of the movements of the tongue in animals with special reference to the cat. *J Anat, 73*, 15–30.

Abdel-Malek, S. (1955). The part played by the tongue in mastication and deglutition. *J Anat, 89*, 250–255.

Adatia, A. K., & Gehring, E. N. (1971). Proprioceptive innervation of the tongue. *J Anat, 110*, 215–220.

Alexander, W. F. (1940). The innervation of the biliary system. *J Comp Neurol, 72*, 357–370.

Alvarez, W. C. (1948). *An introduction to gastro-enterology* (3rd ed.). New York: Paul B. Hoeber.

American Veterinary Dental College (2017). Retrieved from: https://www.avdc.org/Nomenclature/Nomen-Dental_Anatomy.html.

Arey, L. B. (1941). Throttling veins in the livers of certain animals. *Anat Rec, 81*, 21–33.

Arnall, L. (1961). Some aspects of dental development in the dog: Calcification of crown and root of the deciduous dentitions. *J Small Anim Pract, 1*, 169–173.

Asa, C. S., et al. (1985). Deposition of anal-sac secretions by captive wolves (canis lupus). *J Mammal, 66*, 89–93.

Atoji, Y., Yamamoto, Y., Komatsu, T., et al. (1998). Circumanal glands of the dog: A new classification and cell degeneration. *Anat Rec, 250*, 251–267.

Baggett, H., et al. (1971). A structural and functional classification of mammalian tongues. *J Mammal, 52*, 427–429.

Baldyreff, E. B. (1929). Report of an accessory pancreas on the ileum of a dog. *Anat Rec, 43*, 47–51.

Bates, M. N. (1948). The early development of hypoglossal musculature in the cat. *Am J Anat, 83*, 329–355.

Baum, H. (1918). *Das lymphgefässystem des hundes*. Berlin: Hirschwald.

Bennett, G. A. (1944). The lyssa of the dog (Abstr). *Anat Rec, 88*, 422.

Bennett, G. A., & Hutchinson, R. C. (1946). Experimental studies on the movements of the mammalian tongue: The protrusion mechanism of the tongue (dog). *Anat Rec, 94*, 57–83.

Bennett, G. A., & Ramsay, A. J. (1941). Experimental studies on the movements of the mammalian tongue: Movements of the split tongue (dog). *Anat Rec, 79*, 39–51.

Bensley, R. R. (1902). The cardiac glands of mammals. *Am J Anat, 2*, 105–156.

Bloom, W., & Fawcett, D. W. (1994). *A textbook of histology* (12th ed.). Philadelphia: Saunders.

Bottin, J. (1934). Contribution à l'étude de l'anatomie des canaux excréteurs du pancréas chez le chien. *C R Soc Biol (Paris), 117*, 825–827.

Boy, S., Crossley, D., & Steenkamp, G. (2016). Developmental structural tooth defects in dogs- experience from veterinary dental referral practice and review of the literature. *Front Vet Sci, 3*, 9. doi:10.3389/fvets.2016.00009.

Boyden, E. A. (1925). The problem of the pancreatic bladder. *Am J Anat, 36*, 151–183.

Bradley, O. C., & Grahame, T. (1948). *Topographical anatomy of the dog* (5th ed.). London: Oliver & Boyd.

Brand, R. W., & Isselhard, D. E. (1994). *Anatomy of orofacial structures* (4th ed.). St Louis: Mosby.

Brown, M. E. (1937). The occurrence of arteriovenous anastomoses in the tongue of the dog. *Anat Rec, 69*, 287–292.

Budsberg, S. C., & Spurgeon, T. L. (1983). Microscopic anatomy and enzyme histochemistry of the canine anal canal. *Anat Histol Embryol, 12*, 295–316.

Budsberg, S. C., Spurgeon, T. L., & Liggitt, H. D. (1985). Anatomic predisposition to perianal fistulae formation in the German shepherd dog. *Am J Vet Res, 46*, 1468–1472.

Cahill, D. R., & Marks, S. C., Jr. (1982). Chronology and histology of exfoliation and eruption of mandibular premolars in dogs. *J Morphol, 171*, 213–218.

Casas, A. P. (1958). Contribution à l'étude du sphincter d'Oddi chez canis familiaris. *Acta Anat (Basel), 34*, 130–153.

Chauveau, A. (1886). *The comparative anatomy of the domestic animals*. New York: D. Appleton & Company.

Cheal, M., & Oakley, B. (1977). Regeneration of fungiform taste buds: Temporal and special characteristics. *J Comp Neurol, 172*, 609–626.

Chibuzo, G. A. (1979). *Locations of primary motor and sensory cell bodies that innervate the dog's tongue*. Ph.D. Thesis. Ithaca, NY: Cornell University.

Chibuzo, G. A., & Cummings, J. F. (1981). The origins of afferent fibers to the lingual muscles of the dog, a retrograde labelling study with horseradish peroxidase. *Anat Rec, 200*, 95–101.

Chibuzo, G. A., & Cummings, J. F. (1982). An enzyme tracer study of the organization of the somatic motor center for the innervation of different muscles of the tongue: Evidence for two sources. *J Comp Neurol, 205*, 273–281.

Chibuzo, G. A., & Cummings, J. F. (1986). The zonal distribution of lingual glands and ganglia in the dog: The chorda tympani and glossopharyngeal contribution. *Zarya Vet, 1*, 56–64.

Chibuzo, G. A., Cummings, J. F., & Evans, H. E. (1979a). Experimental investigation of the salivatory centers in the dog; evidence for trigeminal innervation. *Anat Rec, 193*, 162.

Chibuzo, G. A., Cummings, J. F., & Evans, H. E. (1979b). Surgical procedures for exposure of the chorda tympani in dogs: A ventral approach. *Cornell Vet, 69*, 295–301.

Chibuzo, G. A., Cummings, J. F., & Evans, H. E. (1980). Autonomic innervation of the tongue: A horseradish peroxidase study in the dog. *J Auton Nerv Syst*, 2, 117–129.

Chibuzo, G. A., Cummings, J. F., & Evans, H. E. (1981). The distribution and central projection of the lingual ganglia: An enzyme tracer study. *Anat Histol Embryol*, 10, 89.

Chiu, S. L. (1943). The superficial hepatic branches of the vagi and their distribution to the extrahepatic biliary tract in certain mammals. *Anat Rec*, 86, 149–155.

Constantinescu, G. M., & Schaller, O. (2012). *Illustrated veterinary anatomical nomenclature* (3rd ed.). Stuttgart: Enke Verlag.

Crompton, A. W., & Musinsky, C. (2011). How dogs lap: Ingestion and intraoral transport in *Canis familiaris*. *Biol Lett*, 7, 882–884. doi:10.1098/rsbl.2011.0336.

Daigo, M., Morita, S., & Ogami, E. (1961). Stereoroentgenographic studies on the arteries of the tongue and vicinity. 1. Arteries of the tongue of the dog. *Bull Nippon Vet Zootech Coll*, 10, 18–22.

De Forge, D. H., & Colmery, B. H. (2008). *An atlas of veterinary dental radiology* (2nd ed.). Ames: Iowa State University Press.

Dellmann, H. D., & Brown, E. M. (1976). *Textbook of veterinary histology*. Philadelphia: Lea & Febiger.

Dole, R. S., & Spurgeon, T. L. (1998). Frequency of supernumerary teeth in a dolichocephalic canine breed, the greyhound. *Am J Vet Res*, 59(1), 16–17.

Doran, G. (1975). Review of the evolution and phylogeny of the mammalian tongue. *Acta Anat (Basel)*, 91, 118–129.

Doty, R. L., & Dunbar, I. (1974). Color, odor, consistency and secretion rate of anal sac secretions from male, female, and early-androgenized female beagles. *Am J Vet Res*, 35, 729–731.

Doyle, S., & Farrar, J. T. (1969). A sphincteric mechanism in the cystic duct of dogs. *Ir J Med Sci*, 2, 109–117.

DuPont, G. A., & De Bowes, L. J. (2008). *Atlas of dental radiography in dogs and cats*. St Louis: Saunders.

Dyce, K. M. (1957). The muscles of the pharynx and palate of the dog. *Anat Rec*, 127, 497–508.

Eichhorn, E. P., Jr., & Boyden, E. A. (1955). The choledochoduodenal junction in the dog—a restudy of Oddi's sphincter. *Am J Anat*, 97, 431–451.

Elias, H. (1949). A re-examination of the structure of the mammalian liver: Parenchymal architecture. *Am J Anat*, 84, 311–333.

Ellenberger, W. (1911). *Handbuch der vergleichenden mikroskopischen anatomie der haustiere* (Vol. 3). Berlin: Paul Parey.

Ellenberger, W., & Baum, H. (1943). *Handbuch der vergleichenden anatomie der haustiere* (18th ed.). Berlin: Springer.

Emily, P., & Penman, S. (1994). *Handbook of small animal dentistry* (2nd ed.). London: Pergamon Press.

Esaka, S. (1982). Development of rotation of mandibular premolar tooth germs in the dog. *Acta Anat (Basel)*, 114, 211–227.

Evans, H. E. (1994). Macroglossia in a new-born dog: Program summary. In *AAVA* (p. 12). University of California–Davis.

Every, R. G. (1972). *A new terminology for mammalian teeth founded on the phenomenon of theogosis*. Christchurch, NZ: Pegasus Press.

Every, R. G. (1974). Thegosis in prosimians. In R. D. Martin, G. A. Doyle, & A. C. Walkers (Eds.), *Prosimian biology*. London: Duckworth.

Ewer, R. (1973). *The carnivores*. Ithaca, NY: Cornell University Press.

Ferrell, F. (1984). Gustatory nerve response to sugars in neonatal puppies. *Neurosci Biobehav Rev*, 8, 185–190.

Field, E. J., & Harrison, R. J. (1947). *Anatomical terms: Their origin and derivation*. Cambridge: Heffer.

Floyd, M. (1991). The Triaden system of dental nomenclature. *J Vet Dent*, 8(4).

Gart, S., Socha, J. J., Vlachos, P. P., & Jung, S. (2015). Dogs lap using acceleration-driven open pumping. *Proc Natl Acad Sci USA*, 112, 15798–15802. doi:10.1073/pnas.1514842112.

Gendron, K., McDonough, S. P., Flanders, J. A., et al. (2017). The pathogenesis of paraesophageal empyema in dogs and constancy of radiographic and computed tomography signs are linked to involvement of the mediastinal serous cavity. *Vet Radiol Ultrasound*, 1–11. doi:10.1111/vru.12582.

Glen, J. B. (1972). Canine salivary mucoceles: The results of sialographic examination and surgical treatment of fifty cases. *J Small Anim Pract*, 13, 515–526.

Glock, G. E., Mellanby, H., Mellanby, M., et al. (1942). A study of the development of dental enamel in dogs. *J Dent Res*, 21, 183–199.

Gómez, H. (1961). The innervation of lingual salivary glands. *Anat Rec*, 139, 69–76.

Gorrel, C. (2004). *Veterinary dentistry for the general practitioner*. St Louis: Saunders.

Gorrel, C. (2008). *Saunders solutions in veterinary practice: Small animal dentistry*. St Louis: Elsevier.

Gorrel, C., & Derbyshire, S. (2005). *Veterinary dentistry for the nurse and technician*. St Louis: Butterworth-Heinemann.

Gordon, K. R., & Herring, S. W. (1987). Activity patterns within the genioglossus during suckling in domestic dogs and pigs: Interspecific and intraspecific plasticity. *Brain Behav Evol*, 30, 249–262.

Grau, H. (1935). Der after von hund und katze unter biologischen und praktischen gesichtspunkten. *Tierarztl Rundsch*, 41, 351–354.

Gregory, W. K. (1934). A half century of trituberculy: The Cope-Osborn theory of dental evolution, with summary of molar evolution from fish to man. *Proc Am Philos Soc*, 73, 169–317.

Grey, E. G. (1918). Observations on the postural activity of the stomach. *Am J Physiol*, 45, 272–285.

Haane, G. (1905). Über die cardiadrüsen und die cardiadrüsenzone des magens der haussäugetiere. *Arch Anat Physiol*, 11–32.

Habermehl, K. H. (1952). Uber besondere randpapillen an der zunge neilgeborener saugetiere. *Z Anat Entwicklungsgesch*, 116, 355–372.

Halpert, B. (1932). The choledocho-duodenal junction—a morphological study in the dog. *Anat Rec*, 53, 83–102.

Harvey, B. C. H. (1906). A study of the gastric glands of the dog and of the changes they undergo after gastroenterostomy and occlusion of the pylorus. *Am J Anat*, 6, 207–239.

Harvey, C. E. (1970). Sialography in the dog. *J Am Vet Radiol Soc*, 10, 18–27.

Heasman, P., & McCracken, G. (2007). *Harty's dental dictionary* (3rd ed.). London: Churchill Livingstone.

Helm, R. (1907). *Vergleichende anatomische und histologische Untersuchungen über den Oesophagus der Haussäugetiere*. Inaugural Dissertation. Zürich.

Higgins, G. M. (1926). An anomalous cystic duct in the dog. *Anat Rec*, 33, 35–41.

Higgins, G. M., & Bain, C. G. (1930). The absorption and transference of particulate material by the greater omentum. *Surg Gynecol Obstet*, 50, 851–860.

Holland, C. T., Satchell, P. M., & Farrow, B. R. (1996). Vagal esophagomotor nerve function and esophageal motor performance in dogs with congenital idiopathic megaesophagus. *Am J Vet Res*, 57(6), 906–913.

Holmstrom, S. E., Frost, P., & Gammon, R. L. (1992). *Veterinary dental techniques for the small animal practitioner*. Philadelphia: Saunders.

Holmstrom, S. E., Fitch, P. F., & Eisner, E. R. (2004). *Veterinary dental techniques for the small animal practitioner* (3rd ed.). St Louis: Saunders.

Holland, V. F., Zampighi, G. A., & Simon, S. A. (1989). Morphology of fungiform papillae in canine lingual epithelium: Location of intercellular junctions in the epithelium. *J Comp Neurol, 279,* 13–27.

Höppner, N. (1956). *Röntgenologische Untersuchungen über Gebiss und Zahnentwicklung beim Hunde von Geburt bis zum Ende des Zahnwechsels.* Vet Dissertation. Berlin: Free University.

Hutt, F. B., & de Lahunta, A. (1971). A lethal glossopharyngeal defect in the dog. *J Hered, 62*(5), 291–293.

Hutt, F. B., & de Lahunta, A. (1972). "Bird tongue" puppies. In *Gaines dog research progress.* Fall.

Hwang, K., Grossman, M. I., & Ivy, A. C. (1948). Nervous control of the cervical portion of the esophagus. *Am J Physiol, 154,* 343–357.

Iijima, T., Kondo, T., & Hasegawa, K. (1987). Autonomic innervation of the arteriovenous anastomoses in the dog tongue: A histological, chemical and ultrastructural study. *Cell Tissue Res, 247,* 167–177.

Issa, F. G., Edwards, P., Szeto, E., et al. (1988). Genioglossus and breathing responses to airway occlusion: Effect of sleep and route of occlusion. *J Appl Physiol, 64,* 543–549.

Isitor, G. N. (1983). The nature and mode of secretion of canine hepatoid circumanal glands (Abst). *Anat Histol Embryol, 12,* 92.

Isitor, G. N., & Weinman, D. E. (1979). Origin and early development of canine circumanal glands. *Am J Vet Res, 40,* 487–492.

Ivy, A. C. (1934). The physiology of the gall bladder. *Physiol Rev, 14,* 1–102.

Kadletz, M. (1929). Über eine blinddarmvarietät beim hund, nebst bemerkungen über die lage, Gestalt und entwicklungsgeschichte des hundeblinddarmes. *Morph Jb, 60,* 469–479.

Imagawa, T., Ueno, T., Tsuka, T., et al. (2009). Anatomical variations of the extrahepatic ducts in dogs: Knowledge for surgical procedures. *J Vet Med Sci, 72,* 339–341.

Kessel, M. L. (2000). *Veterinary dentistry for the small animal practitioner.* Amers: Iowa State Press.

Khurana, R. K., & Petras, J. M. (1991). Sensory innervation of the canine esophagus, stomach, and duodenum. *Am J Anat, 192,* 293–306.

Kingsbury, B. F. (1926). Branchiomerism and the theory of head segmentation. *J Morphol, 42,* 83–109.

Kishi, Y., So, S., Harada, Y., et al. (1988). Three-dimensional SEM study of arteriovenous anastomoses in the dog's tongue using corrosive resin casts. *Acta Anat (Basel), 132,* 17–27.

Kobayashi, K., Miyata, K., & Iino, T. (1987). Three-dimensional structures of the connective tissue papillae of the tongue in newborn dogs. *Arch Histol Jpn, 50,* 347–357.

Konig, M., Mosimann, W., & Devaux, R. E. (1985). Micromorphology of the circumanal glands and the tail gland area of dogs. *Vlaams Diergeneeskd Tijdschr, 54,* 278–286.

Kremenak, C. R., Jr. (1967). Dental exfoliation and eruption chronology in Beagles. *J Dent Res, 46,* 686–693.

Kubota, K., Narita, N., Takada, L., et al. (1988). Origin of lingual proprioceptive afferents in Japanese monkey, M. fuscata fuscata. Studied by HRP-labelling technique. *Anat Anz, 166,* 141–148.

Kumar, M. S. A. (2015). *Clinically oriented anatomy of the dog and cat* (2nd ed.). Ronkonkoma, New York: Linus Learning.

Kyösola, K., & Rechardt, L. (1974). The anatomy and innervation of the sphincter of Oddi in the dog and cat. *Am J Anat, 140,* 497–533.

Langman, J. (1975). *Medical embryology.* Baltimore: Williams & Wilkins.

Lawson, D. D., Nixon, G. S., Noble, N. W., et al. (1967). Development and eruption of the canine dentition. *Br Vet J, 123,* 26–30.

Lemere, F. (1932). Innervation of the larynx. I. innervation of laryngeal muscles. *Am J Anat, 51,* 417–437.

Lohse, C. L., & Suter, P. F. (1977). Functional closure of the ductus venosus during early postnatal life in the dog. *Am J Vet Res, 38,* 839–844.

Lorber, M., Alvo, G., & Zontine, W. J. (1979). Sexual dimorphism of canine teeth in dogs. *Arch Oral Biol, 24,* 585–590.

MacPherson, B. R., Scott, G. W., Chansouria, J. P. N., & Fisher, A. W. F. (1984). The muscle layer of the canine gallbladder and cystic duct. *Acta Anat (Basel), 120,* 117–122.

Mall, F. (1896). The vessels and walls of the dog's stomach. *Johns Hopkins Hosp Rep, 1,* 1–36.

Mann, F. C., Brimhall, S. D., & Foster, J. P. (1920). The extrahepatic biliary tract in common domestic and laboratory animals. *Anat Rec, 18,* 47–66.

Markowitz, J., Rappaport, A., & Scott, A. C. (1949). The function of the hepatic artery in the dog. *Am J Dig Dis, 16,* 344–348.

McCarrell, J. D., Thayer, S., & Drinker, C. K. (1941). The lymph drainage of the gallbladder together with the composition of liver lymph. *Am J Physiol, 133,* 79–81.

McCarthy, P. H. (1978). The anatomy of the parotid duct (ductus parotideus) of the Greyhound as appreciated by the sense of touch. *Anat Histol Embryol, 7,* 311–319.

McCrea, E. D. (1924). The abdominal distribution of the vagus. *J Anat, 59,* 18–40.

Mellanby, M. (1929). *Diet and teeth: An experimental study. Part I. Dental structure in dogs. The normal structure and development of dog teeth* (pp. 15–26). Special report series 140. London: Medical Research Council. Chap. II.

Meyer, L. (1942). *Das Gebiss des deutschen Schäferhundes mit besonderer Berücksichtigung der Zahnalterbestimmung und der Zahnanomalie.* Vet Dissertation. Zürich.

Mikhail, Y., El-Raham, S. A., & Morris, L. (1980). Observations on the structure of the subepithelial nerve plexus in the tongue. *Acta Anat (Basel), 107,* 311–317.

Miki, H., Hida, W., Shindoh, C., et al. (1987). Effect of electrical stimulation of genioglossus muscle on upper airway resistance in anesthetized dogs. *Tohoku J Exp Med, 153,* 397–398.

Miles, A. E. W. (1967). *Structural and chemical organization of teeth.* New York: Academic Press.

Miller, I. J. (1974). Branched chorda tympani neurons and interactions among taste receptors. *J Comp Neurol, 158,* 155–166.

Mintzlaff, M. (1909). *Leber, Milz, Magen, Pankreas des Hundes.* Dissertation. Leipzig.

Mitchell, P. C. (1905). Intestinal tract of mammals. *Trans Zool Soc Lond, 17,* 437–536.

Montagna, W., & Parks, H. F. (1948). A histochemical study of the glands of the anal sac of the dog. *Anat Rec, 100,* 297–318.

Morton, J. (1929). The differences between high and low intestinal obstruction in the dog: An anatomic and physiologic explanation. *Arch Surg, 18,* 1119–1139.

Nagato, T., & Tandler, B. (1986). Ultrastructure of dog parotid gland. *J Submicrosc Cytol, 18,* 67–74.

Nawar, N. N. Y., & Kamel, I. (1975). Intrinsic innervation of the gall bladder in the dog. *Acta Anat (Basel), 92,* 411–416.

Nickel, R., Schummer, A., Seiferle, E., et al. (1973). *The viscera of the domestic animals.* Translated and revised by W. O. Sack. (2nd ed.). New York: Springer-Verlag.

Nielsen, S. W., & Bishop, E. J. (1954). The duct system of the canine pancreas. *Am J Vet Res, 15*, 266–271.

Nikolov Von Sp, D., & Schumacher, G. H. (1973). Zur frage der blutgefassversorgung der zunge; mikrovaskularisation der zungenmuskeln des hundes. *Dtsch Stomatol, 23*, 337–343.

Noer, R. (1943). The blood vessels of the jejunum and ileum: A comparative study of man and certain laboratory animals. *Am J Anat, 73*, 293–334.

Nomina Anatomica Veterinaria. (2017). *International Committee on Veterinary Gross Anatomical Nomenclature (6th ed.).* Hanover, World Assoc Veterinary Anatomists.

Oddi, R. (1887). D'une disposition a sphincter speciale de l'ouverture du canal choledoque. *Arch Ital Biol, 8*, 317–332.

Oishi, Y., Tani, K., Nakazawa, H., et al. (2015). Anatomical evaluation of hepatic vascular system in healthy beagles using X-ray contrast computed tomography. *J Vet Med Sci, 77*, 925–929.

Olivera, M. C., Pinto, P., Silver, E., et al. (1979). Anatomical observations about the closure of the ductus venosus in the dog (canis familiaris). *Anat Anz, 145*, 353–358.

Owen, L. N. (1963). The effects of administering tetracyclines to young dogs with particular reference to localization of the drugs in the teeth. *Arch Oral Biol, 8*, 715–727.

Parks, H. F. (1950). *Morphological and cytochemical observations on the circumanal glands of dogs.* Thesis. Ithaca, NY: Cornell University.

Payer, V. J., Riedel, J., Minar, J., et al. (1956). Der extrahepatale abschnitt der leberarterie des hundes vom gesichtspunkt der chirurgischen anatomie. *Anat Anz, 103*, 246–257.

Pearson, A. A. (1945). Further observations on the intramedullary sensory type neurons along the hypoglossal nerve. *J Comp Neurol, 82*, 93–100.

Powley, T. L., & Phillips, R. J. (2004). Gastric satiation is volumetric, intestinal satiation is nutritive. *Physiol Behav, 82*, 69–74.

Pritchard, M. M. L., & Daniel, P. M. (1953). Arteriovenous anastomosis in the tongue of the dog. *J Anat, 87*, 66–74.

Rakhawy, M. T. (1972). Phosphatases in the nervous tissue: The nature of the ganglionic nerve cells in the tongue. *Acta Anat (Basel), 83*, 356–366.

Rakhawy, M. T. (1975). Phosphatases in the lingual glands of man and dog. *Acta Anat (Basel), 92*, 607–614.

Revell, D. G. (1902). The pancreatic ducts of the dog. *Am J Anat, 1*, 443–457.

Rivero, M. A., Vazquez, J. M., Gil, F., et al. (2009). CT-soft tissue window of the cranial abdomen in clinically normal dogs: An anatomical description using macroscopic cross-sections with vascular injection. *Anat Histol Embryol, 38*, 18–22.

Satrapa-Binder, N. (1959). *Ein Beitrag zur Zahnentwicklung im Unterkiefer von Hundefeten.* Vet Dissertation. Wien.

Sauer, M. E. (1951). The cricoesophageal tendon. *Anat Rec, 109*, 691–699.

Schamberger, G., Marretta, S. A., Dubielzig, R., et al. (2010). Regional odontodysplasia in a juvenile dog. *J Vet Dent, 27*, 98–103.

Secord, A. C. (1941). Small animal dentistry. *J Am Vet Med Assoc, 98*, 470–476.

Singh, B. (2017). *Dyce, Sack, and Wensing's textbook of veterinary anatomy* (5th ed.). St. Louis: Elsevier.

Skobe, Z., Prostak, K. S., & Trombly, P. L. (1985). Scanning electron microscope study of cat and dog enamel structure. *J Morphol, 184*, 195–203.

Sleight, D. R., & Thomford, N. R. (1970). Gross anatomy of the blood supply and biliary drainage of the canine liver. *Anat Rec, 166*, 153–160.

Smallwood, J. E., & George, T. F. (1993). Anatomic atlas for computed tomography in the mesaticephalic dog: Thorax and cranial abdomen. *Vet Radiol Ultrasound, 34*, 65–83.

Sobusiak, T., Zimny, R., Obrebosski, A., et al. (1967). Ganglionic cells of the hypoglossal nerve in the dog. *Folia Morphol, 26*, 298–306.

Sommerova, J. (1980). Contribution to the comparative anatomy of jejunoileal arcades in mammals. *Folia Morphol (Praha), 28*, 282–285.

Staple, P. H. (1964). *Advances in oral biology* (Vol. I and II). New York: Academic Press.

St Clair, L. E., & Jones, N. D. (1957). Observations on the cheek teeth of the dog. *J Am Vet Med Assoc, 130*, 275–279.

Stockard, C. R. (1941). *The genetic and endocrinic basis for differences in form and behavior* Amer Anat Memoirs 19. Philadelphia: The Wistar Institute of Anatomy and Biology.

Stormont, D. L. (1928). The salivary glands. In E. V. Cowdry (Ed.), *Special cytology.* New York: Paul B. Hoeber.

Szalay, F. S. (1969). Mixodectidae, microsyopidae, and the insectivoreprimate transition. *Bull Am Mus Nat Hist, 140*, 193–330.

Testoni, F. J., Lohse, C. L., & Hyde, R. J. (1977). Anatomy and cannulation of the parotid duct in the dog. *J Am Vet Med Assoc, 170*, 831–834.

Thexton, A. J., Crompton, A. W., & German, R. Z. (1998). Transition from suckling to drinking at weaning: A kinematic and electromyographic study in miniature pigs. *J Exp Zool, 280*, 327–343.

Titkemeyer, C. W., & Calhoun, M. L. (1955). A comparative study of the structure of the small intestines of domestic animals. *Am J Vet Res, 16*, 152–157.

Torgersen, J. (1942). The muscular build and movements of the stomach and duodenal bulb. *Acta Radiol Suppl, 45*, 1–191.

Trautmann, A., & Fiebiger, J. (1957). *Fundamentals of the histology of domestic animals.* Ithaca, NY: Comstock Publishing Assoc. Translated and revised from the 8th and 9th German editions, 1949, by R. E. Habel and E. L. Biberstein.

Triadan, H. (1972). Tierzahnheilkunde: Zahnerhaltung (fullungstherapie mit "comsite materials" und endodontie) bei affen und raubtieren. *Schweiz Arch Tierheilkd, 114*, 292.

Tsuchitani, M., Sato, J., & Kokoshima, H. (2016). A comparison of the anatomical structure of the pancreas in experimental animals. *J Toxicol Pathol, 29*, 147–154. doi:10.1293/tox.2016-0016.

Tutt, C., Deeprose, J., & Crossley, D. (2007). *Manual of canine and feline dentistry* (3rd ed.). Quedgeley, UK: British Small Animal Veterinary Association.

Uemura-Sumi, M., Itoh, M., & Mizuno, N. (1988). The distribution of hypoglossal motoneurons in the dog, rabbit and rat. *Anat Embryol, 177*, 389–394.

Verstraete, F., & Lommer, M. (2012). *Oral and maxillofacial surgery in dogs and cats* (1st ed.). St. Louis: Saunders.

Warren, R. (1939). Serosal and mucosal dimensions at different levels of the dog's small intestine. *Anat Rec, 75*, 427–437.

Watson, A. G. (1974). *Some aspects of the vagal innervation of the canine esophagus, an anatomical study.* Master's Thesis. New Zealand: Massey University.

Webb, R. L., & Simer, P. H. (1940). Regeneration of the greater omentum. *Anat Rec, 76*, 449–454.

Wiggs, R. B., & Lobprise, H. B. (1997). *Veterinary dentistry principles and practice.* Philadelphia: Lippincott-Raven.

Williams, E. K., Chang, R. B., Strochlic, D. E., et al. (2016). Sensory neurons that detect stretch and nutrients in the digestive system. *Cell, 166*, 209–221. doi:10.1016/j.cell.2016.05.011.

Williams, R. C. (1961). *Observations on the chronology of deciduous dental development in the dog*. Thesis. Ithaca, NY: Cornell University.

Williams, R. C., & Evans, H. E. (1978). Prenatal dental development in the dog, Canis familiaris: Chronology of tooth germ formation and calcification of deciduous teeth. *Anat Histol Embryol, 7*, 152–163.

Williams, T. (1935). The anatomy of the digestive system of the dog. *Vet Med, 30*, 442–444.

Winkelstein, A., & Aschner, P. W. (1924). The pressure factors in the biliary duct system of the dog. *Am J Med Sci, 168*, 812–819.

Wood, A. E., & Wood, H. E. (1933). The genetic and phylogenetic significance of the presence of a third upper molar in the modern dog. *Am Midl Nat, 14*, 36–48.

Zietzschmann, O. (1938). Lage und form des hundemagens. *Berl Munch Tierarztl Wochenschr, 10*, 138–141, and *Vet Rec, 50*, 984–985.

8

The Respiratory System

LINDA A. MIZER

The **respiratory system** (*apparatus respiratorius*) uses the nose, nasal cavity, pharynx, larynx, trachea, bronchi, and smaller passageways to bring air to alveoli, the sites of gaseous exchange within the lungs. Various structures associated with these passageways modify or regulate the flow of air, serve as olfactory receptors, facilitate water and heat exchange, and make phonation possible.

The mucosa lining the **nasal cavity** and the **conchae** (also called *turbinates*) warms and moistens the air and removes foreign material. The **pharynx** serves as a passageway for both the respiratory and the digestive systems. The **larynx** guards the entrance to the **trachea**, functions in vocalization, and regulates both the flow of air during inspiration and the expiration. The trachea is a cartilage-reinforced tube lined by pseudostratified ciliated epithelium. It terminates at the **carina** as two **principal bronchi** that continue into the two lungs and sequentially branch to form **lobar bronchi**, **segmental bronchi**, **bronchioles**, **alveolar ducts**, **alveolar sacs**, and **alveoli**. The elastic, well-vascularized lungs, passively expand and collapse in response to changes in intrathoracic pressure, created by the action of the muscles of the diaphragm and thoracic wall.

The **nose** (*nasus*), in a broad sense, refers to the **external nose** (*nasus externus*) and its associated **nasal cartilages** (*cartilagines nasi*) surrounding the **external nares**, as well as to the internal nose, or **nasal cavity** (*cavum nasi*) containing scrolls of mucous membrane-covered conchae. The facial portion of the respiratory system and the rostral portion of the digestive system collectively constitute what is called the **muzzle**. In dolichocephalic breeds (e.g., Greyhound) the muzzle is long and may account for half of the total length of the skull. In brachycephalic breeds (e.g., Bulldog), the shortened muzzle often is the cause of respiratory difficulties because of the crowded conchae that restrict the passage of air between within the **meatuses** of the nasal cavity.

When referring to nasal structures or diseases the root **rhin-**, from the Greek *rhinos,* for nose, is frequently employed.

External Nose

The external nose is the part of the face rostral to the frontal bone and dorsal to the infraorbital, buccal, and oral regions. It consists of a fixed bony case and a cartilaginous framework. The cartilaginous portion is movable by virtue of several skeletal muscles associated with the external nose (Chapter 6). The short hair on the skin of the nose is directed caudally on the mid-dorsal surface and gradually slopes in a caudoventral direction laterally, where it is continued to the lips. The apical portion of the nose (*apex nasi*) is flattened and devoid of hair. It is called the **nasal plane** (*planum nasale*) and includes the **nostrils** (*external nares*), which are separated from each other by a groove, or *philtrum* (Fig. 8.1). The integument of the nasal plane is hairless and nonglandular, being moistened from nasal gland secretions and tear drainage. It presents epithelial elevations (areae) or papillary ridges that result in patterns characteristic for each individual. For this reason nose prints may be used as a means of identification in the dog, similar to the way fingerprints are used in human beings (Horning et al., 1926; Coldea, 1994; Meadows, 2005; Wee et al., 2014).

The lateral walls of the bony portion of the nose are formed by the incisive bones rostrally and maxillae laterally, whereas the roof is formed dorsally by the paired nasal bones. The concave rostral ends of the nasal bones, dorsally, and the incisive bones, laterally and ventrally, bound the largest opening into the skull. This opening, called the **bony nasal aperture** (*apertura nasi ossea*), is wider ventrally than dorsally and lies in an oblique plane. In life this opening is bounded rostrally by the nasal cartilages. The aggregate of these cartilages, with their ligaments and covering skin, composes the **movable portion of the nose** (*pars mobilis nasi*). The movable part of the nose ends in a truncated **apex** (*apex nasi*).

Cartilages of the Nose

The mobile part of the external nose has a framework composed entirely of the nasal hyaline cartilages (see Fig. 8.1). These include the unpaired septal cartilage, the paired dorsal lateral and ventral lateral nasal cartilages, and the paired lateral accessory cartilages. Related to the ventral part of the septal cartilage is the vomeronasal cartilage, enclosing the vomeronasal organ.

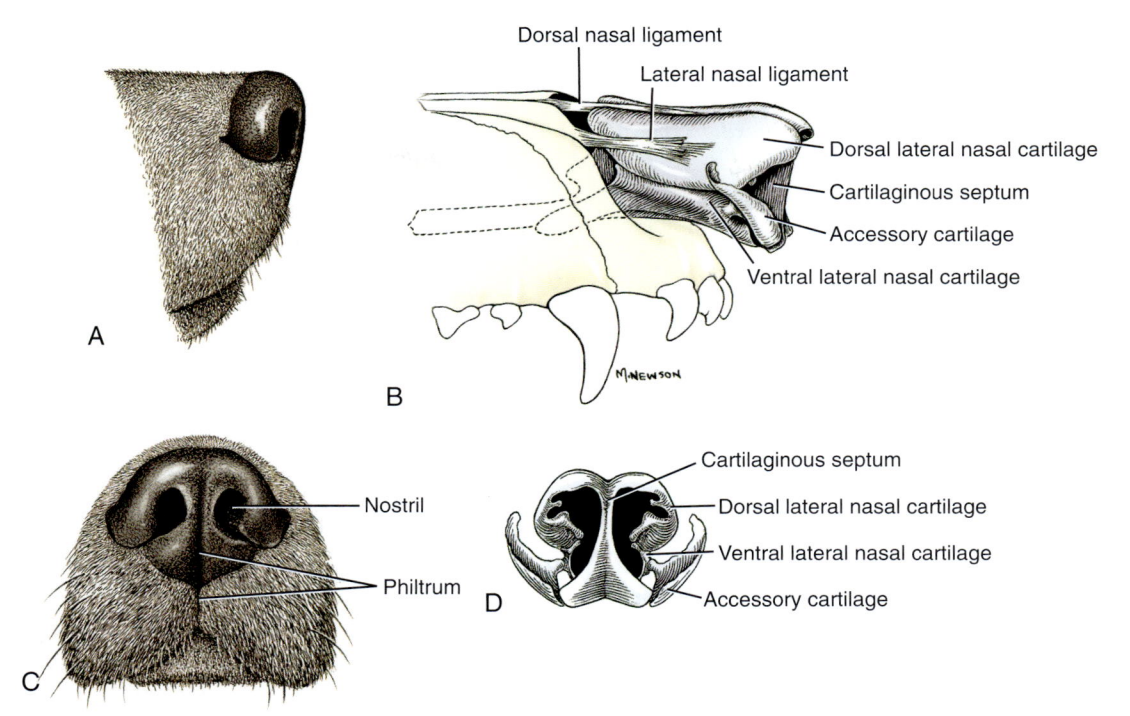

• **Fig. 8.1** External nose and nasal cartilages. **A**, Nose, lateral aspect. **B**, Nasal cartilages, viewed as in A. **C**, Nose, rostral aspect of planum nasale. **D**, Nasal cartilages, as viewed in C.

The **septal cartilage of the nose** (*cartilago septi nasi*) is a perpendicular median plate that separates most of the nasal airway into right and left nasal cavities. It is a rostral continuation of the perpendicular plate of the ethmoid bone that does not ossify. In the region of the aperture of the osseous skull, the septum is lacking in cartilage over a distance of approximately 1 cm so that the nasal septum in this region is formed by the **membranous nasal septum** (*pars membranacea septi nasi*), which connects the cartilaginous immovable caudal part with the mobile rostral part.

The caudal part of the cartilaginous nasal septum is thicker ventrally, where it lies in the septal groove of the vomer, than it is dorsally, where it blends with the thin, conjoined ventral processes of the nasal bones. It presents a prominent caudal process on the median plane that occupies the space between the osseous perpendicular lamina of the ethmoid dorsally and the groove in the vomer ventrally.

The rostral part of the cartilaginous nasal septum continues a median course rostrally from the membranous portion of the nasal septum (Fig. 8.2). It lies between the right and the left **nasal vestibule**. The rostral border of this portion of the septum is divided into right and left laminae. The cleft between the two laminae is deeper and much wider ventrally than it is dorsally. It forms a depressed triangular area ventrally. The dorsal portion of each lamina is rolled laterally to form the dorsolateral nasal cartilage. Arising from the ventral portion of the rostral part of the septal cartilage is the small ventrolateral nasal cartilage, which turns dorsally and medially toward the dorsolateral nasal cartilage (Fig. 8.1D). The accessory cartilage is united by collagenous tissue to the ventrolateral nasal cartilage.

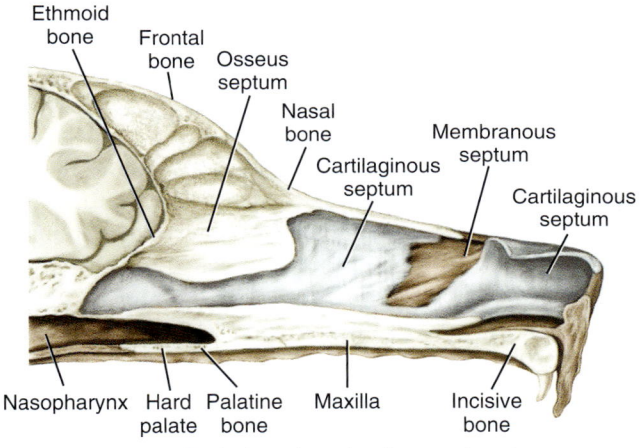

• **Fig. 8.2** Sagittal section, showing nasal septum.

The **dorsolateral nasal cartilage** (*cartilago nasi lateralis dorsalis*) is the most expansive of the cartilages in the mobile part of the external nose. On each side it is a continuation of half of the dorsal portion of the septal cartilage. From this dorsal origin it is rolled into a tube by curving laterally, ventrally, and medially. Its widest portion is its rostral half. Caudally it joins the dorsal part of the bony aperture, to which it is attached by fibrous tissue along the concave border of the nasal bone. The free rolled-in border of the dorsolateral nasal cartilage is greatly thickened rostrally and contains a plexus of blood vessels that form a meshwork in the collagenous tissue directly caudal to the nostril. It becomes much thinner caudally. At a transverse plane through the bony aperture it blends with the rostral extremity of the ventral nasal concha (formerly *maxilloturbinate*). The free medial border of the dorsolateral cartilage curves ventral to the thicker free lateral border of the ventrolateral cartilage to a transverse plane through the caudal angle of the midlateral slit of the nostril.

The **ventrolateral nasal cartilage** (*cartilago nasi lateralis ventralis*) (Fig. 8.1B, D) is a continuation of the rostral portion of the lateral half of the septal cartilage. Caudally its origin moves obliquely dorsad on the lateral surface of the ventral part of the septal cartilage. It is slightly shorter and approximately one-fourth as wide as the dorsolateral cartilage. As it rolls dorsally, it is neither of uniform thickness nor of uniform curvature. Rostrally, it runs into the apex of the nose. It ends caudal to the lateral leaf of the septal cartilage adjacent to the articulation of this cartilage with the accessory cartilage. Caudally it assumes a sigmoid shape in cross-section, being bent in such a way that its free border is added to the free border of the dorsolateral cartilage in forming the cartilaginous basis of the **alar fold** (*plica alaris*) that continues the ventral nasal concha to the vestibule.

The **accessory cartilage** (*cartilago accessoria*) (see Fig. 8.1B, D) is a laterally convex leaf that articulates with the ventrolateral angle of the wide ventrally divided portion of the septal cartilage and extends dorsocaudally to the lateral surface of the expanded portion of the dorsolateral nasal cartilage. For a considerable portion of its length, it lies directly deep to the integument that covers the ventral surface of the midlateral slit in the nostril.

A second small accessory cartilage is occasionally located directly dorsal to the septal cartilage in the groove formed by the origins of the right and left dorsolateral cartilages. Its position is only a few millimeters rostral to the internasal suture.

When sniffing for olfactory purposes the mobile part of the nose is moved and the shape of the nostrils is altered. This is accomplished by the action of intrinsic muscles and of the nasal part of the levator labii superioris and of the levator nasolabialis muscles, which are inserted on these cartilages.

Vomeronasal Organ

The paired **vomeronasal organ** (*organum vomeronasale*) (Figs. 8.3, 8.6, and 8.7), long known as *Jacobson's organ,* is located in the rostral base of the nasal septum as a tubular pocket of olfactory epithelium partially enclosed by a scroll of cartilage (*cartilago vomeronasalis*).

Each vomeronasal organ opens rostrally into an incisive duct that connects the nasal and oral cavities (see Fig. 8.3). Adams and Wiekamp (1984) investigated the surface and transsectional anatomy of the vomeronasal organ in the dog and described its epithelium in detail. They observed both receptor and nonreceptor areas. The receptors in the vomeronasal organ of the dog were unusual in that the cilia did not appear to be of the motile type (no dynein arms or radial spokes) and did not resemble the cilia of the cat or rabbit. Dog receptor cells did have basal bodies and apical mitochondria. The lateral wall of the vomeronasal organ has an extensive venous plexus. The neural pathways used to transmit stimuli from the vomeronasal mucosa to the brain are distinct from those of normal olfactory mucosa (Adams, 1992; Scalia & Winans, 1976).

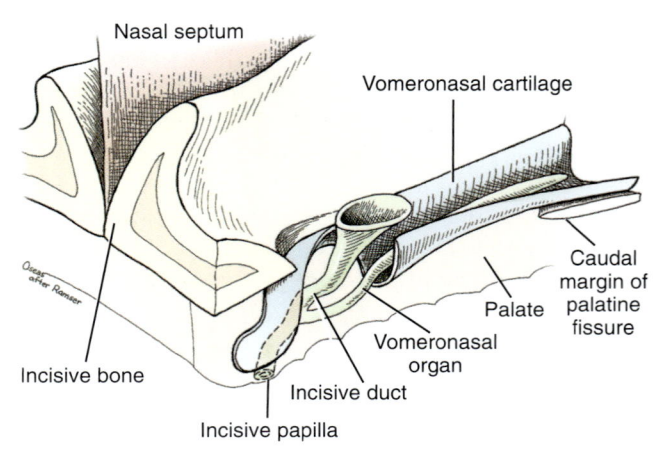

• Fig. 8.3 Schematic view of the incisive duct and the vomeronasal organ. (From Ramser R: *Zur Anatomie des Jakobsonschen Organs beim Hunde,* Dissertation, Berlin, 1935, Friedrich Wilhelms University.)

The olfactory nature of this organ in mammals was long suspected, and now we know that it plays a role in sexual behavior and kin recognition via pheromones, some of which have been identified chemically. The vomeronasal organ and its innervation was investigated by Read (1908) and Ramser (1935) in the cat and dog, McCotter (1912) in the opossum and other mammals, Mann (1961) in the bat, Kratzing (1971) in the sheep, Estes (1972) in several ungulates, and Salazar et al. (1984) in the dog. The role of olfaction in social communication in mammals was been reviewed by Eisenberg and Kleiman (1972). The effects of olfaction on the reproduction of mammals were considered by several authors in Doty (1976).

Associated with the sexual role of the vomeronasal organ is the behavioral "olfactory reflex" or "lip-curl" seen in many mammals and described by Schneider (1930) as *flehmen.* This curling of the superior lip, which exposes the gums and teeth and allows air to be drawn in, clears the passageway to the vomeronasal organ and helps aspirate pheromones so they may contact the mucus in the vicinity of the incisive duct and be drawn into the organ to reach receptor sites. Goodwin et al. (1979) made extracts from the vaginal fluid of dogs in estrus and reported that the major component of the sexual attractant was methyl *p*-hydroxybenzoate. Some recent reports dispute this and suggest methyl paraben (methyl *p*-hydroxybenzoate) was not detectable in urine sampled from bitches during different reproductive phases (Dzięcioł et al., 2014).

The **incisive duct** (*ductus incisivus*), formerly called the *nasopalatine duct* or *Stensen canal* (Figs. 8.3 and 8.7), passes through the palatine fissure and connects the nasal and oral cavities. The oral orifice of each duct lies lateral to the incisive papilla, caudal to the superior central incisor teeth. Dogs have been observed to make rapid licking movements with the apex of the tongue, across the incisive papilla, while holding their lips slightly curled (*flehmen*) and their incisor teeth slightly apart. The paired incisive ducts pass dorsocaudally to open into each nasal cavity, and the vomeronasal organ exits from it before it reaches the cavity. The incisive duct is not enclosed in a bony canal, nor does it contact the margin of the palatine fissure through which it passes.

Ligaments of the Nose

Three ligaments, composed of one pair and one unpaired, attach the mobile part of the nose to the dorsal portion of the osseous nose (Fig. 8.1B). The **dorsal nasal ligament** (*lig. nasale dorsale*) is a single band of collagenous tissue that runs from the caudodorsal end of dorsolateral nasal cartilage to the dorsum of the nasal bones. The **lateral nasal ligament** (*lig. nasale laterale*), one on either side, is a collagenous band that runs from the midlateral surface of the caudal aspect of the dorsolateral nasal cartilage to the border of the bony nasal aperture directly dorsal to the end of the nasomaxillary suture. The ligaments of the nose are best developed in old dogs of the working breeds.

Nasal Cavity

The **nasal cavities** (*cava nasi*) are the facial portion of the respiratory passageway. They extend from the **nostrils** (*nares*) to the choanae, being separated by the nasal septum. The **septum** (Fig. 8.2) consists of a bony portion (*septum nasi osseum*), a cartilaginous portion (*cartilago septi nasi*), and a membranous portion. Each nasal cavity has a respiratory and an olfactory region.

Each nasal cavity begins at the nostril with the nasal vestibule and ends with the nasopharyngeal meatus and choana. Each nasal cavity is divided into four principal air channels and several smaller ones (Figs. 8.5 and 8.6). During development the growth of laminae from the lateral and dorsal walls of the nasal cavity results in the formation of conchae that largely fill the cavity and restrict the flow of air. The air passages thus created between the conchae are called the *nasal meatuses*.

The **nostril** (*naris*), the opening into the nasal vestibule, is a curved opening that is much wider dorsomedially than it is ventrolaterally. It possesses more than usual importance because, in some brachycephalic dogs, the opening is too restricted and interferes with respiration. Leonard (1956) devised an operation whereby the transverse diameter of the nostril may be increased.

The **alar fold** (*plica alaris*) (Figs. 8.4 and 8.5), which is an extension of the ventral nasal concha, terminates within the vestibule by a bulbous enlargement that fuses to the wing of the nostril. The **wing of the nostril** (*ala nasi*) is the thickened dorsolateral portion of the nostril. The wing of the nostril contains much of the dorsolateral and accessory nasal cartilages. It is the most mobile portion of the nostril

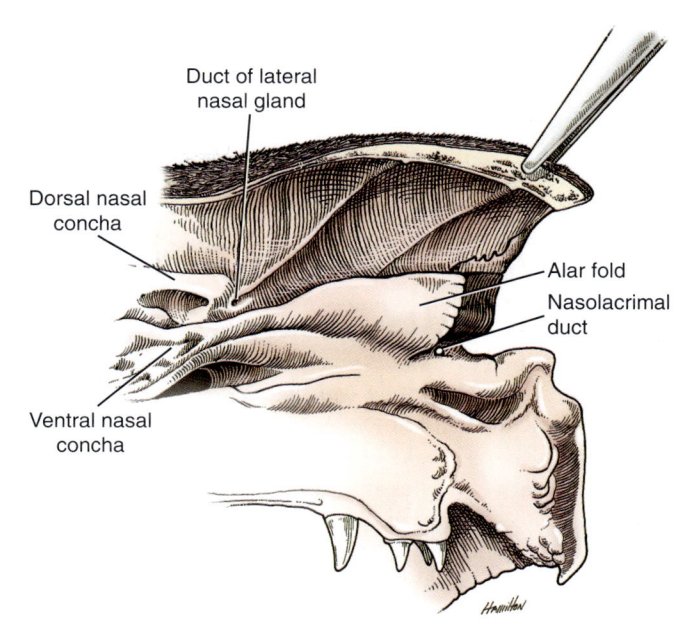

• **Fig. 8.4** The nasal vestibule opened to show the entrance of the duct of the lateral nasal gland and the nasolacrimal duct.

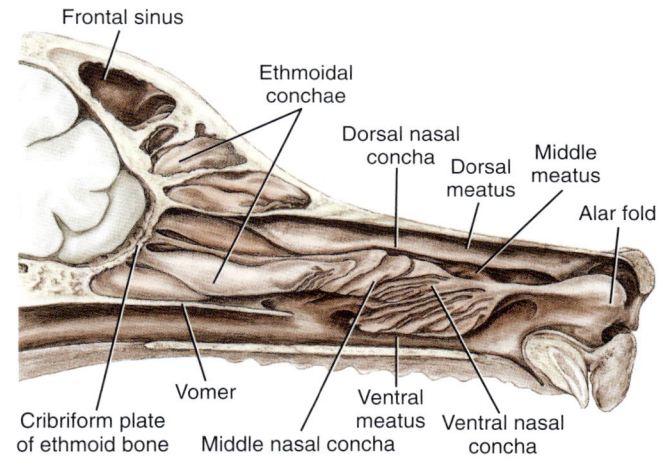

• **Fig. 8.5** Sagittal section, showing the conchae.

because it receives the terminal fibers of the nasal portions of the mm. levator labii superioris and levator nasolabialis.

The **nasal vestibule** (*vestibulum nasi*) is not an empty antechamber but rather it is largely obliterated by the large bulbous end of the alar fold that extends into it. Because the end of the alar fold is fused to the medial surface of the wing of the nostril, it acts to divert the incoming air. On entering the vestibule through a nostril, air is diverted medially and ventrally into the largest meatus of the nasal cavity, the ventral nasal meatus. The **nasolacrimal duct** (*ductus nasolacrimalis*), which conducts the lacrimal secretion from the eye, opens into the vestibule by an orifice located at the rostral end of the attached margin of the alar fold. The small duct of the **lateral nasal gland** opens on the oblique fold into the dorsal vestibule where it is continuous with the atrium of the dorsal nasal meatus. This is dorsocaudal to the opening of the nasolacrimal duct (Fig. 8.4).

Nasal Conchae

The **nasal conchae** (*conchae nasales*) are cartilaginous or ossified scrolls covered with nasal mucosa that occupy the major portion of each nasal cavity. They include the dorsal, ventral, and ethmoidal conchae, which were formerly called the *dorsal nasoturbinate*, the *maxilloturbinate*, and the *ethmoturbinate*, respectively. The individual ethmoidal conchae are still identified as *ethmoturbinates*.

The **dorsal nasal concha** (*concha nasalis dorsalis*) (Figs. 8.4 and 8.5) consists of an elongated, slightly curled scroll of the first endoturbinate that is attached to the **ethmoid crest** (*crista ethmoidalis*) of the ethmoid and nasal bones. A mucosal fold continues the concha into the vestibule of the nose.

The **ventral nasal concha** (*concha nasalis ventralis*) (Figs. 8.5 and 8.6) is a tightly folded series of scrolls that occupies the rostral part of the nasal cavity and is attached to the **conchal crest** (*crista conchalis*) on the medial surface of the maxilla. It extends from the level of the first to the third premolar teeth. The alar fold is an extension of this ventral concha into the vestibule.

The **middle nasal concha** (*concha nasalis media*) is formed by a rostral extension of the second endoturbinate of the ethmoidal labyrinth. It fills the short space between

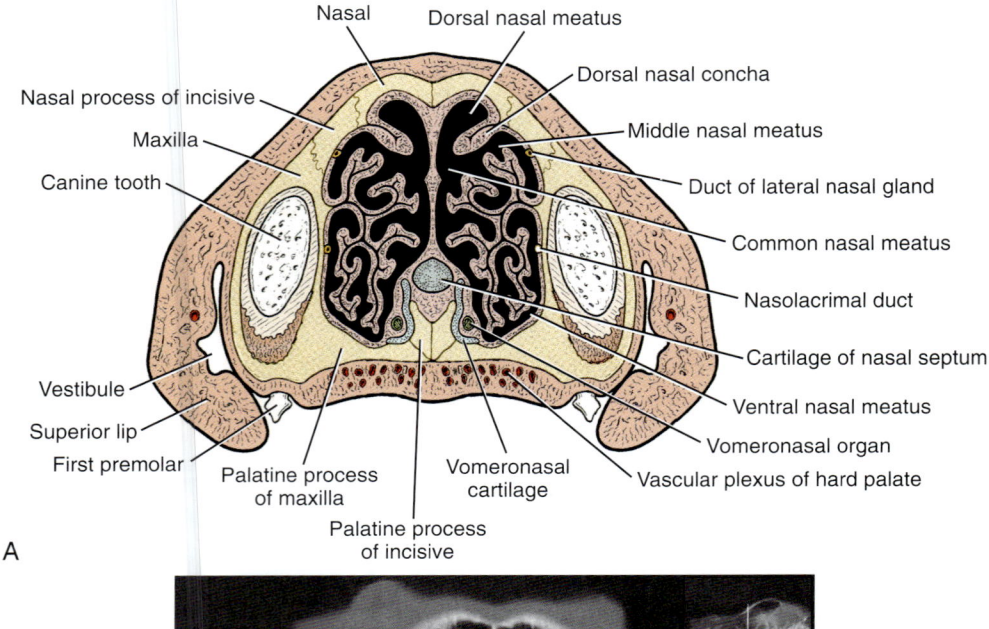

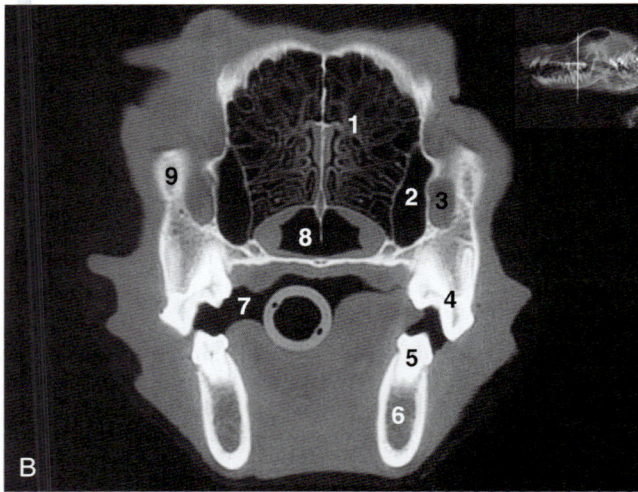

1. Ethmoidal labyrinth
2. Maxillary recess
3. Maxillary foramen
4. Superior molar 1
5. Inferior molar 1
6. Body of the mandible
7. Oral cavity
8. Rostral nasopharynx just caudal to the choanae
9. Zygomatic bone

• **Fig. 8.6** A, Transverse section of the nasal cavities at the level of the first premolar teeth. B, Transverse CT image of the caudal nasal cavities and nasopharynx. (From Evans HE, de Lahunta A: *Guide to the Dissection of the Dog,* 8th ed., St Louis, 2017, Elsevier.)

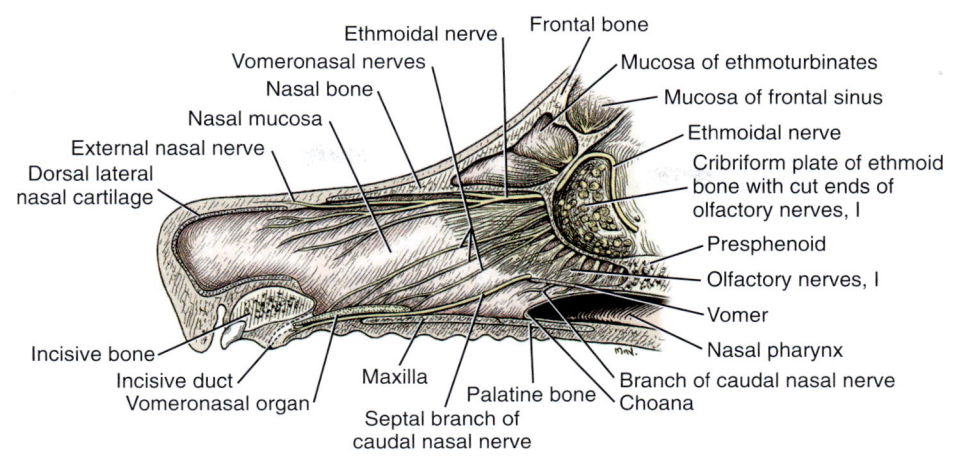

• **Fig. 8.7** Sagittal section, showing distribution of nerves on the septal mucosa. Note vomeronasal organ.

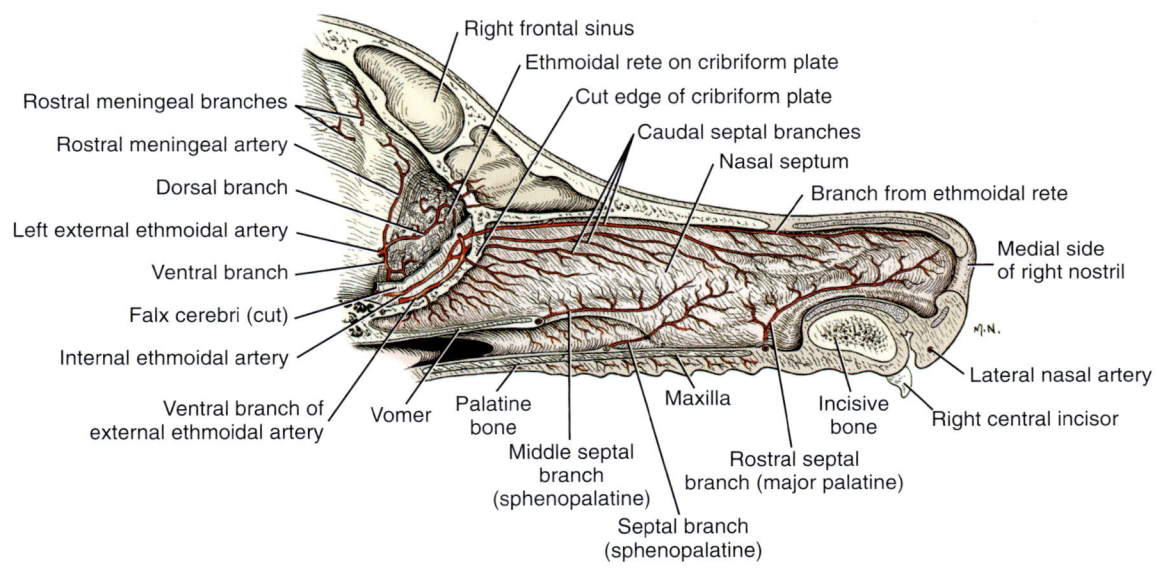

• **Fig. 8.8** Sagittal section, showing arteries of the nasal septum.

the scrolls of the ventral nasal concha and the ethmoid labyrinth.

The **ethmoidal conchae** (*conchae ethmoidales*) (Figs. 4.24 and 4.25, 8.5) form the ethmoidal labyrinth (*labyrinthus ethmoidalis*) that fills the caudal part of the nasal cavity. Developmentally, they are outgrowths of the ethmoid bone covered with nasal mucosa. The numerous delicate, bony scrolls are known as *ethmoturbinates* and are further subdivided into ectoturbinates and endoturbinates. All are attached to the orbital lamina and cribriform plate of the ethmoid. The six ectoturbinates are small and lie on the dorsal aspect of the labyrinth, whereas the four endoturbinates lie ventrally and fill the caudal portion of the nasal cavity. The first endoturbinate extends rostrally and forms the bony scroll for the concha nasalis dorsalis, and the second endoturbinate forms the middle nasal concha (Graeger, 1958). One or more scrolls of the ectoturbinates usually extend into the frontal sinus.

Olfactory nerves ramify in the mucosa of the ectoturbinate scroll(s) that extends into the frontal sinus. The epithelium on the olfactory part of the sinus has a brown color. The mucosa of the nasal cavity is richly supplied with nerves and blood vessels (Figs. 8.7 and 8.8). Olfactory nerves supply approximately half of the ethmoturbinates, the caudal half of the nasal septum, and a significant portion of the roof and lateral walls of the nasal cavity.

After the inhaled air leaves the nasal vestibule, it traverses the longitudinal **nasal meatuses** to reach the nasal part of the pharynx.

Nasal Meatuses

The **dorsal nasal meatus** (*meatus nasi dorsalis*) (Figs. 8.5 and 8.6) is a passage through the dorsal part of each nasal cavity. It lies between the dorsal nasal concha and the ventral surface of the nasal bone. Laterally it is limited by the ethmoidal crest, from which the concha arises. Medially the dorsal nasal meatus becomes confluent with the common nasal meatus.

The **middle nasal meatus** (*meatus nasi medius*) lies between the dorsal nasal concha dorsally and the dorsal part of the numerous scrolls composing the ventral nasal concha, ventrally. Throughout the long middle portion of the middle nasal meatus its width is approximately 1 mm. At its rostral end it presents a dilatation, and caudally its lateral portion is divided into several parts.

The **atrium of the middle nasal meatus** (*atrium meatus nasi medius*) is an ellipsoidal dilation that connects the nasal vestibule with the middle nasal meatus. The atrium is formed ventrally by the narrow handle of the club-shaped mucosal alar fold that runs rostral and dorsal from the ventral nasal concha. Dorsally it is bounded by the relatively straight rostral portion of the dorsal nasal concha. In large mesaticephalic heads it is approximately 5 mm deep, 5 mm wide, and 2 cm long. Rostrally the orifice of the duct from the lateral nasal gland opens into this atrium.

Laterally the caudal part of the middle nasal meatus is divided by the scrolls of the middle nasal concha, which is an extension of the second endoturbinate from the ethmoid bone into several air passages that lie between these scrolls.

The **ventral nasal meatus** (*meatus nasi ventralis*) is located between the ventral nasal concha and the dorsal surface of the hard palate. It is narrow rostrally as it leaves the nasal vestibule. It gradually widens caudally and attains a width of 1 cm at the large nasomaxillary opening into the maxillary recess, where it continues ventral to the basal lamina of the ethmoid bone as the nasopharyngeal meatus. This wide portion of each nasal cavity is located in a transverse plane through the caudal portions of the fourth superior premolar teeth, where the middle, ventral, and common nasal meatuses converge.

The **common nasal meatus** (*meatus nasi communis*) (Fig. 8.6) is a longitudinal narrow space on either side of the nasal septum. Laterally, it is bounded by the dorsal nasal concha and ventral nasal concha. Dorsal, ventral, and between these bones it is coextensive with the dorsal, ventral, and middle nasal meatuses, respectively.

The **nasopharyngeal meatus** (*meatus nasopharyngeus*) extends on either side from the caudal dilated portion of the ventral nasal meatus to the choana. It is a short passage with a much longer lateral than medial wall. It is bounded laterally by the maxillary and palatine bones, dorsally by the basal lamina of the ethmoid bone, ventrally by the palatine bone, and medially by the vomer. It represents where all four nasal meatuses of each nasal cavity converge and continue as the nasopharyngeal meatus to the choanae where the nasal pharynx begins. The *choanae* are the openings, where the caudal portion of the vomer attaches to the hard palate, of the two nasopharyngeal meatuses into the nasal portion of the pharynx. The choanae are located where the caudal portion of the vomer attaches to the hard palate (Fig. 8.6). They are oval in shape and oblique in position.

Paranasal Sinuses

The paranasal sinuses, which are also connected with the respiratory passageways, are described with the skeletal system. They include a maxillary recess, a frontal sinus, and a sphenoidal sinus. The maxillary recess is not called a sinus because it is not enclosed in the maxilla. However, the opening to the recess, in life, is narrowed considerably by the mucosa-covered orbital lamina of the ethmoid bone and the lateral nasal gland located there. The frontal sinus is divided into rostral, medial, and lateral compartments. The sphenoidal sinus of the dog is in the presphenoid bone. It is only a potential cavity because it is filled by an endoturbinate scroll. Negus (1958) discusses the comparative anatomy of the nose and paranasal sinuses in various mammals.

De Rycke et al. (2003) used computed tomography (CT) and magnetic resonance imaging (MRI) to provide a detailed description of the nasal cavities and paranasal sinuses in clinically normal mesaticephalic dogs. MRI scans are superior to CT scans for determining soft tissue structures.

Nasal Mucosa

The various types of epithelia that line the nasal cavity and coat its associated structures are spoken of collectively as the *nasal mucosa*. The transition from the more peripheral respiratory type of epithelium to the deeper lying olfactory epithelium is not abrupt. The receptors for the sense of smell are located primarily on the ethmoturbinates, which lie in the caudomedial and caudodorsal parts of the nasal cavity. The olfactory epithelium and sensory nerves, so beautifully demonstrated by various techniques in several mammals by Bojsen-Møller (1964, 1967, 1975), are developed from the olfactory placode and include olfactory nerves, vomeronasal nerves, and the nervus terminalis. A richly vascularized and innervated mucosa (see Figs. 8.7 and 8.8) is present in the nasal cavity, vomeronasal organ, and in some mammals on a small area of the septum called the *septal olfactory organ*. Allison (1953) reviewed the olfactory system of vertebrates. Recent reviews of vertebrate olfactory system structure and function may be found in Eisthen (1997) and Taniguchi and Taniguchi (2014).

Under normal conditions of inspiration, the respiratory and olfactory currents of air are associated. When a dog deliberately wants to sample the environment, the nostrils are dilated, and, with a forced inspiration, the dog sniffs the air. This act provides a greater volume of inspired air, which takes a more dorsal course around the ethmoturbinates, where the olfactory receptors are most numerous. Craven et al. (2007) claim that, functionally, the dorsal meatus is a bypass for odorant-bearing inspired air around the complicated ventral nasal concha during sniffing for olfaction. They show that within both the ventral nasal concha and ethmoturbinate air flow must be laminar.

Pearsall and Verbruggen (1982) wrote a practical guide for training dogs to track scents. They include many useful

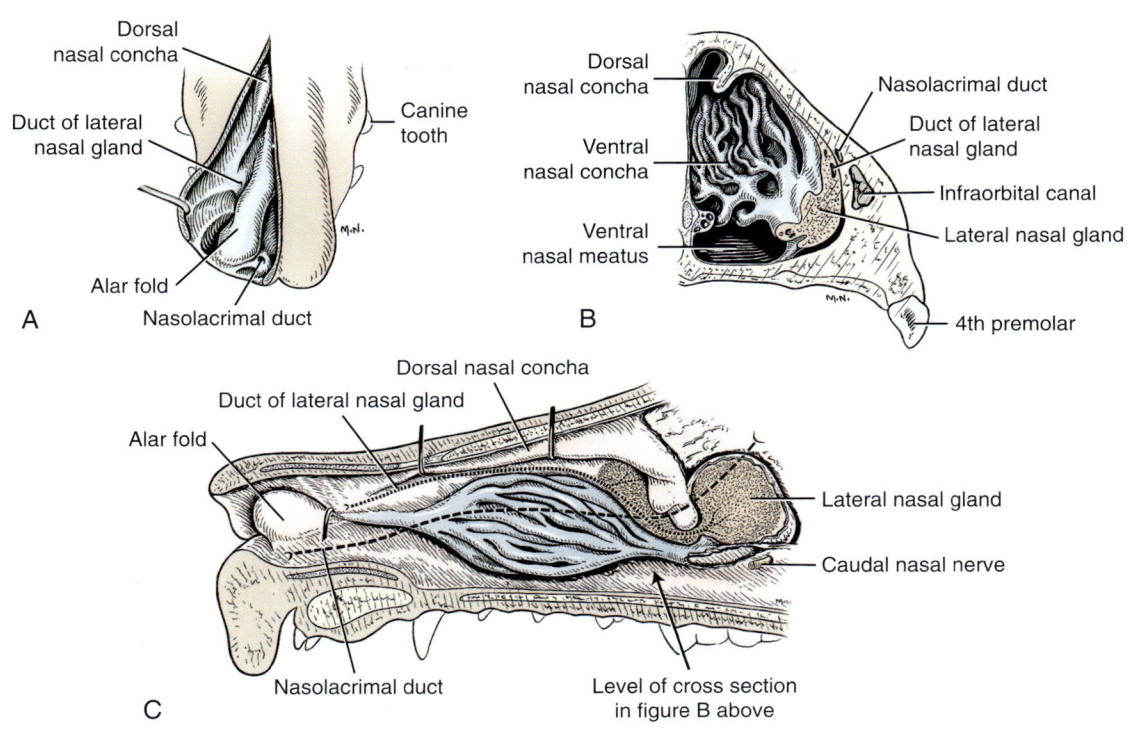

• **Fig. 8.9** Topography of the nasal cavity and the lateral nasal gland with its duct. **A**, Dorsal view of the entrance to the right nasal cavity opened parasagittally. (Note that the duct of the lateral nasal gland opens midway between the dorsal nasal concha and the alar fold.) **B**, Transverse section of the left nasal cavity to show the position of the lateral nasal gland in the maxillary recess. **C**, Medial view of the right nasal cavity. The ethmoidal labyrinth has been removed to expose the lateral nasal gland.

behavioral observations that help delimit olfactory perception. Zanoni et al. (1998) discussed the significance of both dog and handler training in the use of dogs as forensic search dogs. Dorriety (2007) analyzed prior studies of the use of "cadaver dogs" as a forensic tool, and dogs have been trained in water searches to locate submerged bodies, Osterkamp (2011).

Glands of the Nose

The **lateral nasal gland** (*glandula nasalis lateralis*) (Fig. 8.9) is a serous gland that is located in the mucosa of the maxillary recess near the opening of this recess into the nasal cavity (Evans, 1977). The lateral nasal gland was first described in the dog by Steno in 1662 and in other mammals by Bojsen-Møller (1964). The functional significance of the lateral nasal gland as part of the thermoregulatory system in the dog was postulated by Schmidt-Nielsen et al. (1970), based on airflow studies. This was confirmed by Blatt et al. (1972), who measured the amount of secretion correlated with heat-load and panting. Adams et al. (1981) described the structure of the lateral nasal gland in the dog and analyzed its secretions.

The lateral nasal gland is thickest at the level of the fourth superior premolar, where its ducts unite and pass rostrally to form one major duct that opens on the lateral wall of the vestibule (Fig. 8.9). The opening of the nasolacrimal duct into the ventral vestibule is visible externally, whereas the opening of the duct of the lateral nasal gland into the dorsal vestibule is hidden from view by the alar fold (Figs. 8.4 and 8.9). The lateral nasal gland duct can be entered by a cannula with a diameter of 0.038 to 0.048 mm after surgical reflection of the dorsal wall of the vestibule. The opening lies dorsal and caudal to that of the nasolacrimal duct, where air flow is most rapid because of the narrowness of the passageway.

The lamina propria of the mucosa of the respiratory part also contains serous, mucous, and mixed tubuloalveolar glands. These glands are also present in the mucosa of the nasal vestibule. Goblet cells are present throughout the respiratory region, and olfactory glands that contain yellow pigment granules are located in the olfactory epithelium. Adams and Hotchkiss (1983) described the nasal mucosa of the dog.

The **nasolacrimal duct** (*ductus nasolacrimalis*) carries the serous secretion from the conjunctival sac to the nasal vestibule (Fig. 8.4). A characteristic of a healthy dog is a moist nose, which is maintained in part by the combined secretions of the lacrimal and lateral nasal glands.

Functional Considerations

The rostral end of the nose in the dog is stiffened by cartilages and moved by the levator nasolabialis and levator labii superioris muscles (Figs. 6.4 to 6.7). Dilation of the nostril alters the conformation of the nasal vestibule and changes the flow pattern of inspired air. This is most noticeable when the dog is presented with a stimulating scent, which, for analysis, must reach the deeper ethmoturbinates. There may also be a relationship between changes in air-flow pattern and the functioning of the vomeronasal organ.

Much evaporative cooling in the dog is accomplished by heat exchange from the lungs and respiratory passageways. Schmidt-Nielsen et al. (1970) suggested that the lateral nasal gland supplies the water necessary for heat dissipation during panting. This function of the lateral nasal gland is in a sense analogous to that of the sweat glands of humans. Hyperventilation to get rid of excess heat can result in drying and hypertrophy of the respiratory mucosa unless moisture is provided. The nasal glands of mammals provide the necessary fluid. Blatt et al. (1972) cannulated the duct of the lateral nasal gland, subjected the dogs to various heat-loads, and collected the secretions. It was found that a rise from 25° to 40°C results in an increased flow approximately 40 times.

The nasal vestibule of the dog is restricted to a residual cavity encircling the bulbous end of the alar fold, which extends into it. The alar fold is an extension of the ventral nasal concha that attaches to the wing of the nostril. Air entering the nostril is diverted dorsally, medially, and ventrally around the obstructing alar fold, with a resultant increase in velocity and evaporative effect. Perhaps the alar fold or ridges in the vestibule act as a swell body to produce cyclic alternating changes in the air passageway to protect the nasal mucosa from constant desiccation. In humans there is a cyclic distention of the cavernous tissues in the conchae and septum that results in an alternating air flow through right and left nasal chambers. Bojsen-Møller and Fahrenkrug (1971) found a similar nasal cycle in rabbits and rats.

Nasal Portion of the Pharynx

The **nasal portion of the pharynx** (*pars nasalis pharyngis*), also called the **nasopharynx**, extends from the choanae to the intrapharyngeal ostium. The **intrapharyngeal ostium** (*ostium intrapharyngeum*), formerly called the *pharyngeal isthmus*, is formed rostral to the larynx by the crossing of the digestive passageway (oropharynx) and the respiratory passageway (nasopharynx) (Fig. 8.10). The rostral part of the nasopharynx is bounded by the hard palate ventrally, the vomer dorsally, and the palatine bones bilaterally. Although the middle and caudal portions of the nasopharynx are bounded dorsally by the base of the skull and the muscles that attach to it, its ventral boundary is the mobile, long soft palate (Fig. 8.11). At each act of swallowing, the cavity of the caudal part of the nasopharynx is obliterated by the pressure of the material swallowed and the root of the tongue forcing the soft palate dorsally.

On each lateral wall of the nasopharynx, dorsal to the middle of the soft palate, is an oblique slit-like opening, approximately 5 mm long, that is the **pharyngeal opening of the auditory tube** (*ostium pharyngeum tubae auditivae*).

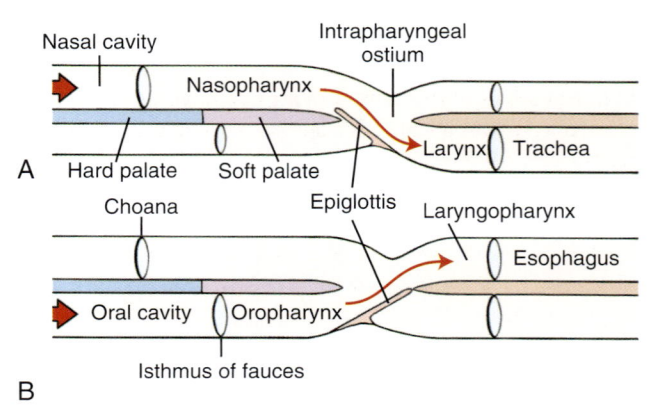

• **Fig. 8.10** Diagram showing relation of portions of pharynx to esophagus and trachea. **A**, During normal respiration. **B**, During swallowing.

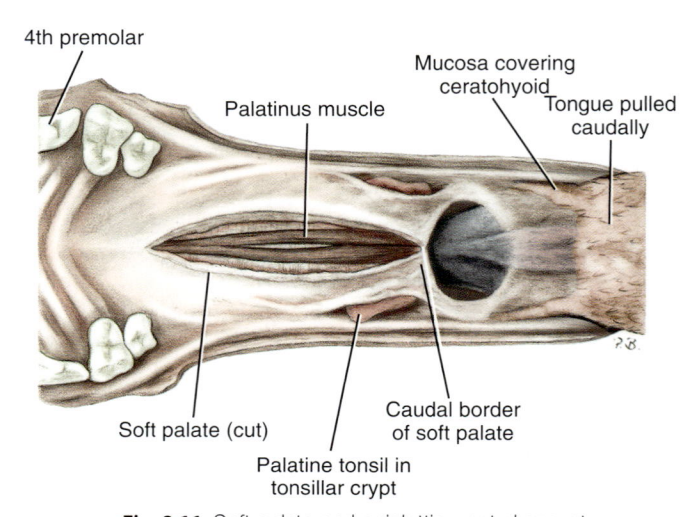

• **Fig. 8.11** Soft palate and epiglottis, ventral aspect.

The opening is located directly caudal to the caudal border of the pterygoid bone and faces rostroventrally. Schreider and Raabe (1981) discuss the anatomy of the nasopharyngeal airway of experimental animals.

The **auditory tube** (*tuba auditiva*), formerly Eustachian tube, extends between the cavity of the middle ear and the cavity of the nasopharynx. It serves to equalize the atmospheric pressure on the two sides of the tympanic membrane and to allow drainage of epithelial glandular secretions.

Larynx

The larynx (Figs. 8.12 to 8.22) is a musculocartilaginous organ guarding the entrance to the trachea, which serves as an air passageway, aids vocalization, and prevents the inspiration of foreign material. The valvular function of the larynx, by means of the epiglottis, is vital because it is across its inlet that all substances swallowed must pass in their course from the oropharynx through the laryngopharynx to the esophagus. Negus (1949) has described and illustrated the comparative anatomy of the larynx from fish through mammals, and Piérard (1965) studied the dog and other carnivores. The larynx is located directly caudal to the root of the tongue, oropharynx, and the soft palate, ventral to the atlas. It is approximately 6 cm long in a medium-sized dog, nearly half of this length being occupied by the epiglottic cartilage, which lies at the laryngeal opening. The intrinsic muscles of the larynx control the size of the laryngeal inlet, the size and shape of the glottis, and the positions of the laryngeal cartilages. Sound production with the aid of the larynx serves an important social function in canids (Tembrock, 1976). Vasquez et al. (1990) studied the normal dog larynx by MRI.

Cartilages of the Larynx

The **laryngeal cartilages** (*cartilagines laryngis*) (see Figs. 8.12 and 8.13) are the epiglottic, thyroid, cricoid, arytenoid, sesamoid, and interarytenoid cartilages. Only the arytenoid cartilage is paired.

The **epiglottic cartilage** (*cartilago epiglottica*) (Figs. 8.12 to 8.22) forms the basis of the epiglottis. In outline,

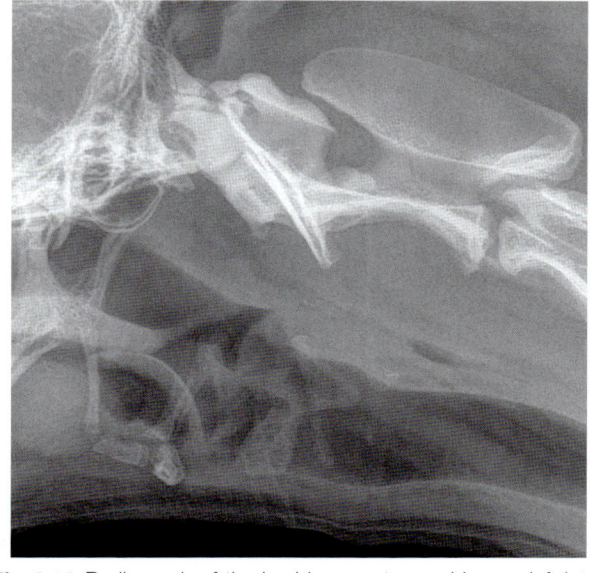

• **Fig. 8.14** Radiograph of the hyoid apparatus and larynx, left lateral view.

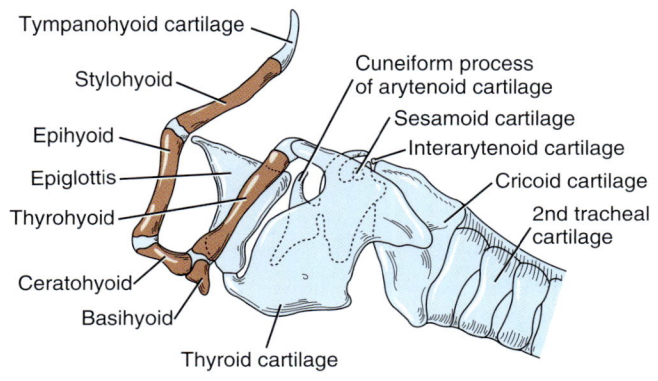

• **Fig. 8.12** Hyoid apparatus, larynx, and trachea, left lateral view. The rostral cornu of the thyroid cartilage of the larynx articulates with the thyrohyoid bone of the hyoid apparatus. The hyoid apparatus is suspended from the mastoid process of the skull by the tympanohyoid cartilage on each side.

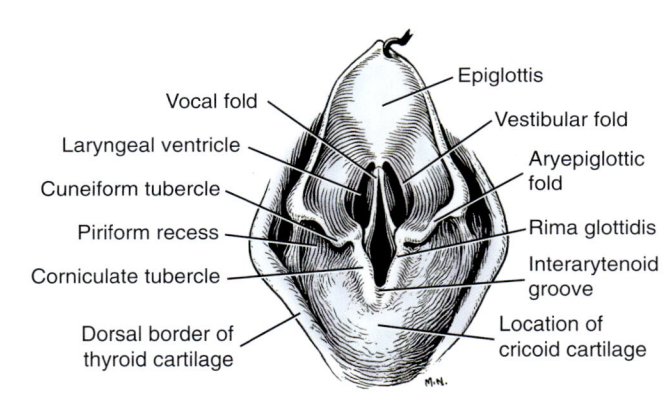

• **Fig. 8.15** Dorsal aspect of larynx, showing vocal and vestibular folds.

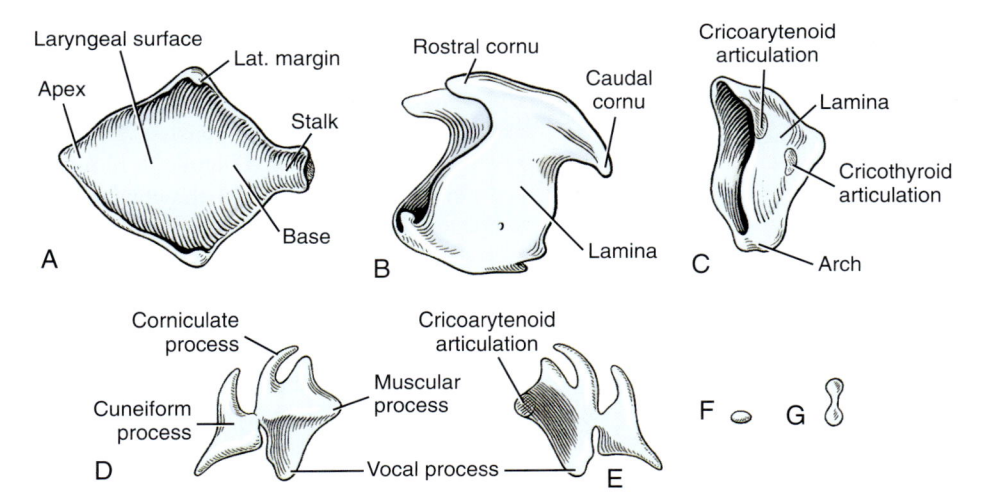

• **Fig. 8.13** Laryngeal cartilages disarticulated. **A**, Epiglottis, dorsal aspect. **B**, Thyroid cartilage, lateral aspect. **C**, Cricoid cartilage, lateral aspect. **D**, Left arytenoid cartilage, lateral aspect. **E**, Left arytenoid cartilage, medial aspect. **F**, Interarytenoid cartilage. **G**, Sesamoid cartilage, dorsal aspect.

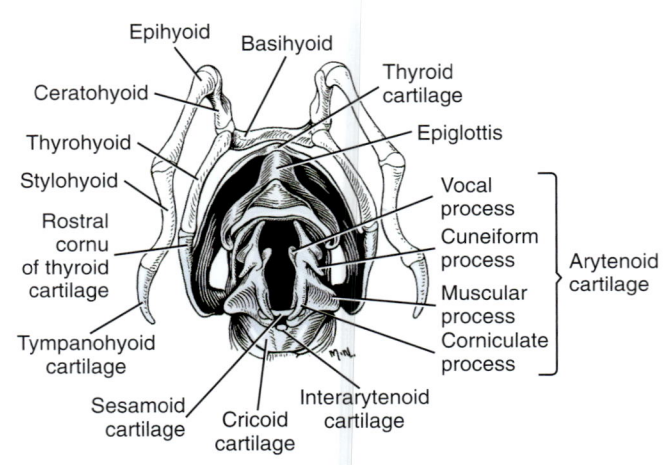

• **Fig. 8.16** Laryngeal cartilages and hyoid apparatus, dorsal aspect.

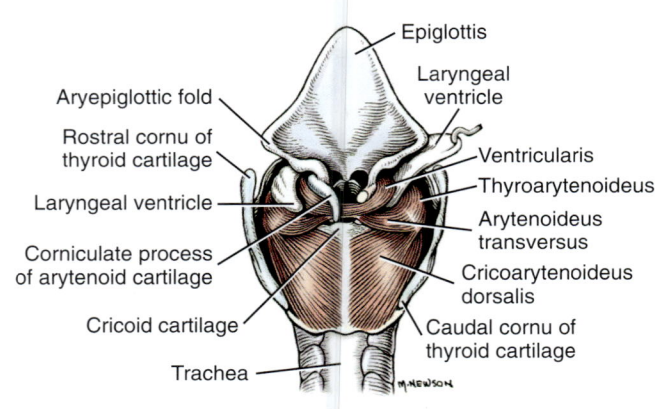

• **Fig. 8.17** Laryngeal muscles, dorsal aspect. (The right corniculate cartilage has been cut, and the right laryngeal ventricle reflected.)

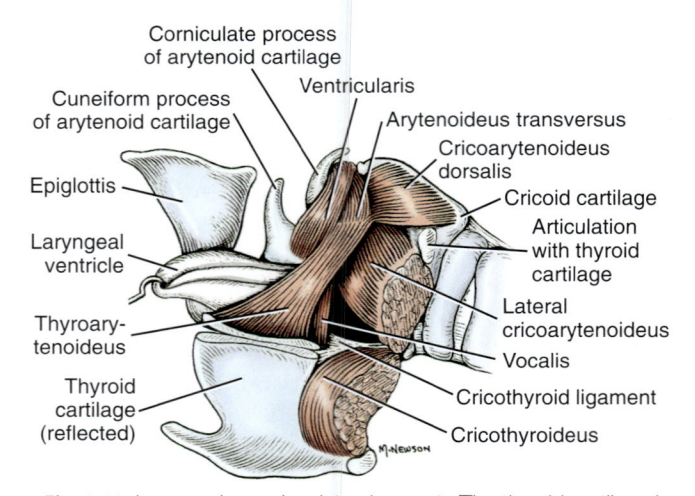

• **Fig. 8.18** Laryngeal muscles, lateral aspect. (The thyroid cartilage is cut to the left of the midline and reflected as is the attached cricothyroideus muscle.)

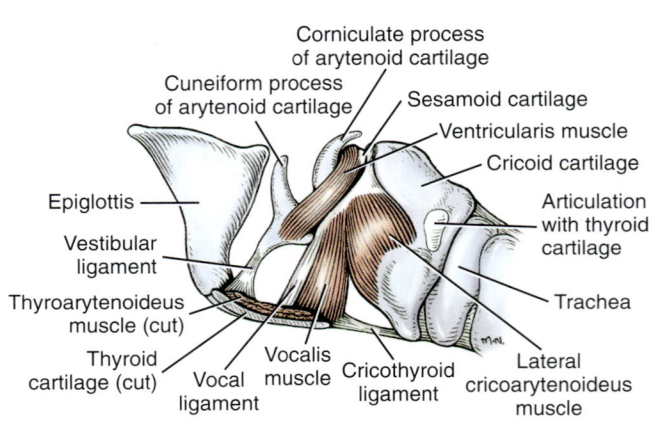

• **Fig. 8.19** Laryngeal muscles, lateral aspect. (The thyroid cartilage is cut to the left of the midline and removed. The mm. thyroarytenoideus, arytenoideus transversus, and cricoarytenoideus dorsalis have been removed.)

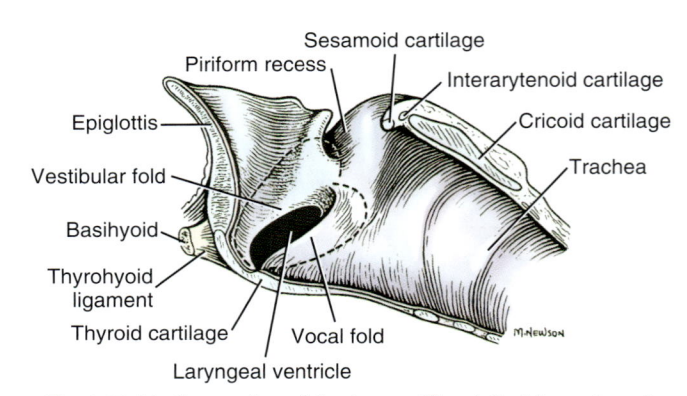

• **Fig. 8.20** Median section of the larynx. (The dotted lines show the extent of the laryngeal ventricle.)

the rostral margin of the cartilage forms a thin, dorsally concave triangle with its **apex** pointing rostrally. The **epiglottis** resembles a sharp-pointed spade. Its **laryngeal surface** (*facies laryngea*) formerly aboral surface, is concave and faces dorsocaudally. The opposite **lingual surface** (*facies lingualis*), formerly the *oral surface,* is convex and faces the oropharynx. The lingual surface is attached to the middle of the body of the basihyoid bone by the short, stout hyoepiglottic muscle. On either side of the median mucosal fold that covers the muscle is a deep pocket of mucosa, called the **vallecula** (*vallecula epiglottica*), which may attain a depth of 1.5 cm. Each vallecula is limited laterally by a small fold of stratified squamous epithelium running from the lingual surface of the epiglottis near its caudolateral angle to the lateral wall of the laryngeal part of the pharynx. The **stalk** of the epiglottis (*petiolus epiglottidis*) is in the form of a thickened handle of fibrous tissue that unites the mid-caudal portion of the epiglottis and the dorsal rostral surface of the thyroid cartilage. The normal position of the epiglottis allows the apex to rest dorsal to the soft palate.

The **thyroid cartilage** (*cartilago thyroidea*) (Figs. 8.13 to 8.22) is the largest cartilage of the larynx. It forms the middle portion of the laryngeal skeleton and is open dorsally. It consists of **right** and **left laminae** (*lamina dextra et sinistra*), which are united ventrally to form a short but deep trough. An inconspicuous **oblique line** (*linea obliqua*) on the lateral surface serves primarily for the attachment of the sternothyroid muscle. Each lamina is expanded dorsally to form transversely thin processes, the **rostral** and **caudal cornua** (*cornu rostralis et caudalis*).

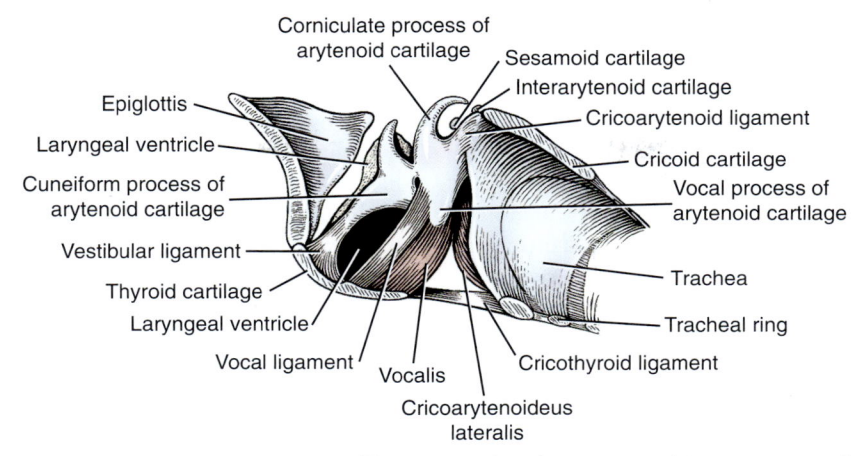

- **Fig. 8.21** Median section of the larynx. (The mucosa has been removed to expose muscles and ligaments.)

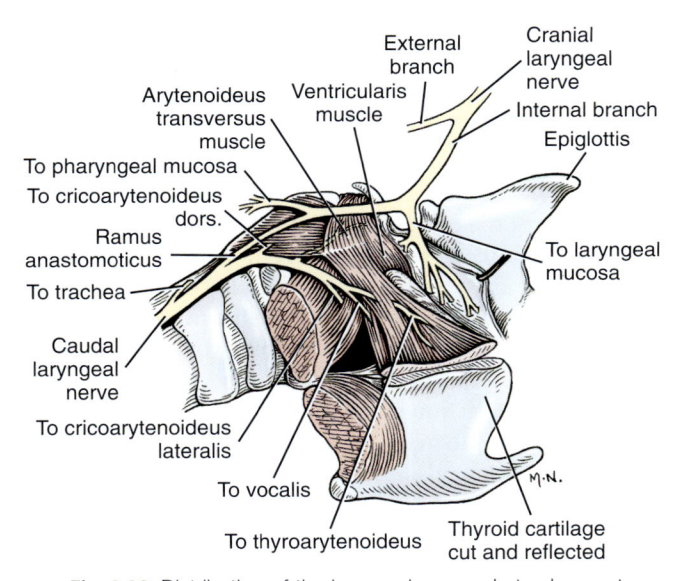

- **Fig. 8.22** Distribution of the laryngeal nerves. Lateral aspect.

The rostral cornu has a **hyoid articular surface** (*facies articularis hyoidea*) on its medial side for articulation with the thyrohyoid bone. Similarly, on the medial side of the caudal cornu is a **cricoid articular surface** (*facies articularis cricoidea*) for articulation with the caudolateral aspect of the lamina of the cricoid cartilage. Separating the rostral cornu from the thyroid lamina is the **thyroid fissure** (*fissura thyroidea*). The cranial laryngeal nerve and the cranial laryngeal artery pass through this fissure. Where the two laminae fuse ventrally, a slight ventral **laryngeal prominence** (*prominentia laryngea*) is formed. The laryngeal prominence, known as the *Adam's apple* in humans, is not visible externally in the dog, but it can be palpated.

The ventral caudal border of the thyroid cartilage possesses the median deep **caudal thyroid notch** (*incisura thyroidea caudalis*), whereas the rostral border is slightly convex from side to side. The caudal border of the thyroid cartilage is united to the ventral arch of the cricoid cartilage by the **cricothyroid ligament** (*ligamentum cricothyroideum*). The cranial border is joined to the basihyoid and thyrohyoid bones by the **thyrohyoid membrane** (*membrana thyrohyoidea*).

The **cricoid cartilage** (*cartilago cricoidea*) (Figs. 8.13 to 8.22) is the only cartilage of the larynx that forms a complete ring. The dorsal portion is approximately five times wider than the ventral portion. The expanded dorsal part is the **lamina of the cricoid cartilage** (*lamina cartilaginis cricoideae*). It possesses a **median crest** (*crista mediana*) for muscle attachment. Occasionally a pair of vascular foramina is located in the lamina, one on each side of the cranial portion of the crest. The **arch of the cricoid cartilage** (*arcus cartilaginis cricoideae*) extends ventrally from the lamina and completes the enclosure of the caudal part of the cavity of the larynx. It is bilaterally concave in a transverse direction. The cricoid cartilage possesses two pairs of articular surfaces. An indistinct pair of thyroid articular surfaces (*facies articularis thyroidea*) for articulation with the apices of the caudal cornua of the thyroid cartilage are located at the junction of the lamina and the arch about 1 mm from the caudal border. A more prominent pair of arytenoid articular surfaces (*facies articularis arytenoidea*), for articulating with the arytenoid cartilages, are located on the rostral border of the lamina lateral to the median crest. Both pairs of articular surfaces are enclosed in articular capsules and form synovial joints with the cartilages with which they articulate. The sides of the ventral arch of the cricoid cartilage are gradually reduced in width ventrally. Mid-ventrally in a medium-sized dog, the narrowest part of the arch is only 5 mm long; in such a dog the mid-dorsal lamina would be approximately 2 cm long.

The **arytenoid cartilage** (*cartilago arytenoidea*) (Figs. 8.11 and 8.12 and 8.16 to 8.19) is an irregular cartilage, one on either side, that articulates with the rostrodorsal border of the cricoid cartilage. When the laryngeal cartilages are viewed laterally, the arytenoid is largely hidden from view by the thyroid lamina.

The morphologic characteristics of the arytenoid cartilage vary greatly in different species of mammals, so that what may appear as a process of the arytenoid in one species may be a separate cartilage in another. In the dog, the arytenoid cartilage embodies the corniculate cartilage and the cuneiform cartilage of other mammals. As a result, this compound cartilage may be described as possessing a corniculate process, a muscular process, a vocal process, and a cuneiform process.

The **articular surface** (*facies articularis*) is a slightly oval, concave surface on the caudal border of the arytenoid, which faces caudomedially and joins the arytenoid articular surface of the cricoid cartilage to form the cricoarytenoid articulation (*articulatio cricoarytenoidea*). The **muscular process** (*process muscularis*) is a relatively thick, rounded process that is located directly lateral to the articular surface. The m. cricoarytenoideus dorsalis attaches to this process. The **corniculate process** (*processus corniculatus*) is the longer and more caudal of the two dorsal processes that form the dorsal margin of the laryngeal inlet. The **vocal process** (*processus vocalis*) is a caudal ventral projection of the arytenoid cartilage. It is approximately 3 mm thick and 5 mm long at its base. The vocal ligament and the m. vocalis, from the thyroid cartilage, attach to the vocal process (Fig. 8.21).

The **cuneiform process** (*processus cuneiformis*) is the most rostral portion of the arytenoid cartilage. It is connected by a narrow neck (Figs. 8.12 and 8.13) to the main portion of the arytenoid cartilage and is considered by some authors to be a separate cartilage. In the dog, the cuneiform process is roughly triangular in shape. The ventral portion lies in the vestibular fold, and the dorsal portion serves as the medial attachment of the aryepiglottic fold and aids in forming the laryngeal inlet. Attached to the cuneiform process are the ventricular ligament and the m. ventricularis (Fig. 8.19). Duckworth (1912) suggested that the cuneiform cartilage arose in mammals from the lateral margin of the epiglottis.

The **sesamoid cartilage** (*cartilago sesamoidea*) (Figs. 8.19 to 8.21) is an oval or dumbbell-shaped nodule located cranial to the cricoid lamina and between the arytenoid cartilages. It is occasionally paired, in which case an intersesamoid ligament or fibrous union joins the two. Primarily, the sesamoid cartilage appears to be intercalated in the transverse arytenoid muscle. There is frequently a small contact surface with the dorsal portion of each arytenoid cartilage.

The **interarytenoid cartilage** (*cartilago interarytenoidea*) (Figs. 8.16 & 8.20) is small, flat, and easily overlooked. It lies cranial to the cricoid lamina and caudodorsal to the transverse arytenoid muscle and sesamoid cartilage. In this superficial position the interarytenoid cartilage is embedded in connective tissue that attaches the arytenoid cartilages and the cricoesophageal tendon to the cricoid lamina.

Muscles of the Larynx

See Chapter 6.

Cavity of Larynx and Laryngeal Mucosa

The **cavity of the larynx** (*cavum laryngis*) is divided into five transverse segments: the aditus laryngis, vestibule, vestibular cleft, cleft of the glottis and the infraglottic cavity.

The **laryngeal inlet** (*aditus laryngis*) (Fig. 8.15) lies directly caudal to the intrapharyngeal ostium bounded by the epiglottis. Air entering or leaving the larynx can travel either by way of the nasal part or by way of the oral part of the pharynx. In lolling (rapid breathing with the tongue hanging out), most of the air passes through the mouth and oropharynx; in slow, shallow breathing it passes through the nasal cavity and nasopharynx. The margin of the laryngeal opening forms an imperfect triangle, with the base located caudally. The margin of the epiglottis forms its lateral boundaries and apex. The caudal boundary is formed by the right and left aryepiglottic folds.

Each **aryepiglottic fold** (*plica aryepiglottica*) (Fig. 8.15) runs from the dorsal portion of the arytenoid cartilage and the closely associated corniculate cartilage to the caudolateral angle of the epiglottic cartilage. Two prominent tubercles that are separated by a deep notch are present in the fold. The more dorsocaudal tubercle, formed by the underlying corniculate process, is called the **corniculate tubercle** (*tuberculum corniculatum*). It is a rounded process approximately 1 cm long and 0.5 cm wide. It and the opposite tubercle form the most dorsal and the least expandable part of the laryngeal opening. Ventral to these tubercles the dorsal parts of the two arytenoid cartilages lie close together to form the **interarytenoid groove** (*incisura interarytenoidea*). This groove communicates dorsally with the middle of the rostral portion of the laryngopharynx and ventrally with the rima vestibuli and rima glottidis. The **cuneiform tubercle** (*tuberculum cuneiforme*) forms a relatively large cone-shaped projection that is united in a sagittal plane with the corniculate tubercle; it is also united in a transverse plane to each lateral angle of the epiglottic cartilage by means of a loose plica of mucosa. The channel lying external to each aryepiglottic fold is called the **piriform recess** (*recessus piriformis*). When food or fluid is forced past the closed laryngeal opening in deglutition, it largely occupies these recesses, which constitute the ventrolateral portions of the laryngeal pharynx.

The **laryngeal vestibule** (*vestibulum laryngis*) extends from the laryngeal aditus to the vestibular folds. It is a funnel-shaped cavity that opens freely dorsocranially. It is bounded ventrally by the mucosa covering the caudal part of the large, dorsally concave epiglottis. The rostral part of the wall on either side is also composed of the epiglottis. Rostrodorsal to the vestibular folds the flattened cuneiform processes form its wall. The vestibule opens caudally into the rima vestibuli.

The **vestibular cleft** (*rima vestibuli*) is the portion of the laryngeal cavity bounded bilaterally by the vestibular folds and the mucosa covering the cuneiform processes. The ventral boundary is formed by the mucosa covering the thyroid cartilage directly caudal to the thyroepiglottic ligament. The **vestibular fold** (*plica vestibularis*) (Fig. 8.20) is a short, wide plica of mucosa, containing a few elastic fibers, that runs from the expanded ventral margin of the cuneiform cartilage to the rostrodorsal surface of the thyroid cartilage. It is less than one-half the dorsoventral diameter of the larynx, and its width approximates that of the vocal fold that lies caudal to it.

The **rima glottidis** (*rima glottidis*) or **cleft of the glottis** is the portion of the laryngeal cavity between the vocal folds and arytenoid cartilages. The **glottis** consists of the vocal folds, arytenoid cartilages, and the rima glottidis. The portion of the rima glottidis between the vocal folds is the **intermembranous part** (*pars intermembranacea*); that between the medial surfaces of the arytenoid cartilages is the **intercartilaginous part** (*pars intercartilaginea*). The rima glottidis is the most important part of the larynx from the standpoint of veterinary medicine because it is the narrowest part of the laryngeal passageway, and it contains the vocal folds that are important for vocalization—barking, baying, whining, and growling—and for optimal ventilation in racing breeds. Flanders and Thompson (2009) discussed surgical correction in two cases of dyspnea in dogs caused by retroversion of the epiglottis and occlusion of the rima glottidis.

The **vocal fold** (*plica vocalis*) (Figs. 8.15 and 8.19 to 8.21), on either side, extends from the vocal process of the arytenoid cartilage to the dorsocaudal part of the trough of the thyroid cartilage. It is approximately 13 mm long and 6 mm wide in a medium-sized dog. It is separated from the vestibular fold by the slitlike opening of the laryngeal ventricle. The **vocal ligament** (*lig. vocale*) is a strap of elastic fibers that is enclosed in the vocal fold. It forms the supporting framework for the cranial border of the vocal fold and is covered by mucous membrane. It measures 1 to 2 mm in maximum thickness and has a thin cranial border. Caudally it is continuous with the vocalis muscle, which is a portion of the thyroarytenoideus muscle mass.

The **laryngeal ventricle** (*ventriculus laryngis*) (Figs. 8.15, 8.20, and 8.21) is a small mucosal sac between the vestibular and vocal folds medially and the thyroid lamina laterally. Its border is attached to these two folds where its lumen opens into the laryngeal cavity at the junction of the rima vestibuli and the rima glottidis. This opening maintains a constant width of approximately 1.5 mm and a length equal to that of the rostral border of the vocal fold that forms the caudal border of the opening. In the production of sound the vocal and vestibular folds can vibrate into the cavity of the glottis.

The **infraglottic cavity** (*cavum infraglotticum*) of the larynx extends from the rima glottidis to the cavity of the trachea. It constitutes the fifth subdivision of the laryngeal cavity. The infraglottic cavity is wide dorsally, corresponding to the lamina of the cricoid cartilage, and narrow ventrally. Because of this disparity in the lengths of the dorsal and the ventral wall of the infraglottic cavity, the cavity of the larynx is in nearly a dorsal plane, whereas that of the trachea is in an oblique caudoventral plane.

Pressman and Kelemen (1955), in their review of laryngeal physiology, consider the comparative functional anatomy responsible for the sphincter action of the larynx. Closure or constriction of the larynx may be accomplished at three levels: at the inlet (aryepiglottic folds) by muscular action during deglutition, at the vestibular folds by passive action for creating intrathoracic or intraabdominal pressure, and at the vocal folds by muscular action during phonation. All three levels may be involved in normal closure, or only one level may be. Subsequent reviews of laryngeal function may be found in Bartlett (1986), Widdicombe (1986), and Strohl et al. (2012).

Innervation of the Larynx

The muscles of the larynx were described in Chapter 6. The nerves are described here and also with the cranial nerves in Chapter 19. The nerves of the larynx in the dog (Fig. 8.22) have been reported on by Franzmann (1907), Lemere (1932a, 1932b, 1933), Vogel (1952), and Bowden and Scheuer (1961).

The **cranial laryngeal nerve** leaves the vagus at the level of the distal vagal ganglion. At the larynx, it divides into an external branch, which supplies the cricothyroideus muscle, and an internal branch, which receives axons from the mucosa of the larynx rostral to the vocal folds. The internal branch usually anastomoses (*ramus anastomoticus*) with the caudal laryngeal nerve. A nerve from the pharyngeal plexus (pharyngeal rami of the glossopharyngeal and vagus nerves) may also supply the cricothyroideus muscle. The cranial laryngeal nerve probably innervates taste buds on the epiglottis and the luminal mucosa of the larynx. It is these receptors that initiate reflex closing of the glottis cleft during swallowing.

The **caudal laryngeal nerve** (Fig. 8.22) is the motor supply to all of the intrinsic muscles of the larynx except the cricothyroideus muscle. It is the terminal segment of the recurrent laryngeal nerve, which in turn originates in the thorax by leaving the vagus. The somatic efferent axons have their neuronal cell bodies in part of the nucleus ambiguus in the medulla. They leave the medulla in the cranial roots of the accessory nerve that form its internal branch. This branch joins the vagus nerve as these two cranial nerves exit the skull. They follow the vagus nerve into the thorax and return to the larynx in the recurrent laryngeal nerve. The somatic efferent axons that innervate the cricothyroideus muscle leave the medulla in the roots of the vagus nerve. Réthi (1951) reports that cutting the intracranial portion of the accessory nerve results in degeneration of the vast majority of the axons in the recurrent laryngeal nerve. Cutting the intracranial portion of the vagus prior to its receiving the components of the cranial roots of the accessory nerve leaves the motor axons of the recurrent laryngeal nerve intact, whereas the motor component of the cranial laryngeal nerve shows complete degeneration. When the recurrent laryngeal nerve is cut on its course along the trachea, there are bundles of afferent axons in the distal component that do not degenerate. These are baroreceptor and chemoreceptor primary afferents, which have their cell bodies in the distal ganglion of the vagus. These afferents reach the larynx via the cranial laryngeal nerve and continue in the ramus anastomoticus to join the caudal laryngeal nerve on their way to the aortic arch (Andrew, 1954; Vogel, 1952). Several investigators—Lemere (1932a), Piérard (1963), and Watson (1974)—describe an inconstant extravagal pararecurrent nerve that leaves the recurrent near its origin in the thoracic cavity, parallels the recurrent nerve along the trachea, and has variable anastomoses along its course. It is continuous cranially with the ramus anastomoticus of the cranial laryngeal nerve.

Trachea

The trachea (Fig. 8.23) runs from a transverse plane through the middle of the body of the axis to a similar plane through the fibrocartilaginous disc between the fourth and fifth thoracic vertebrae. It is a relatively noncollapsible tube that extends from the cricoid cartilage of the larynx to its **bifurcation** (*bifurcatio tracheae*) dorsal to the cranial part of the base of the heart. Done (1978) has reported on collapse of the trachea in dogs. The crest of the partition at the site where the trachea divides into the two principal bronchi is called the **tracheal carina** (*carina tracheae*). Approximately 35 C-shaped hyaline **tracheal cartilages** (*cartilagines tracheales*) form the skeleton of the trachea. The diameter and thickness of the tracheal rings is smallest at the level of the thoracic inlet (Dabanoglu et al., 2001). The space left by failure of these cartilages to meet dorsally is bridged by fibers of the smooth, transversely running **tracheal muscle** (*musculus trachealis*) and connective tissue. The rings so formed are united in a longitudinal direction by bands of fibroelastic tissue, called the **annular ligaments of the trachea** (*ligg. anularia [trachealia]*). They are approximately 1 mm wide, compared with the 4-mm width of each tracheal cartilage. The annular ligaments allow considerable intrinsic movement of the trachea without breakage or collapse of the tube. Macklin (1922) reconsidered the network of longitudinal elastic fibers in the tunica propria of the trachea and bronchial tree. This elastic membrane deep to the epithelium is thick in the trachea and larger bronchi, but thin in the terminal respiratory passageways. It provides a recoil mechanism for the lung.

Bronchi

The bronchial tree (*arbor bronchialis*) (Figs. 8.23 to 8.26) begins at the bifurcation of the trachea by the formation of a right and a left **principal bronchus** (*bronchus principals [dexter et sinister]*). Each principal bronchus divides into **lobar bronchi** (*bronchi lobares*), formerly *secondary bronchi*, which is the basis for the identification of the lung lobes. These supply the various lobes of the lung and are named according to the lobe supplied. Within the lobe of the lung the lobar bronchus divides into **segmental bronchi** (*bronchi segmentales*), which are sometimes referred to as *tertiary bronchi*. The segmental bronchi and the lung tissue that they ventilate are known as **bronchopulmonary segments** (*segmenta bronchopulmonalia*). Ishaq (1980) studied 37 pairs of dog lungs and suggested a system for designating the bronchi. Schlesinger and McFadden (1981) discuss the morphometry of the proximal bronchial tree in six mammalian species. Adjacent bronchopulmonary segments normally communicate with each other in the dog. Various injection and reconstruction techniques have been employed to delineate these segments in the dog (Angulo et al., 1958; Boyden & Tompsett, 1961; Kilpper & Stidd, 1973; Tucker & Krementz, 1957a,b) (Fig. 8.26). For bronchoscopic purposes Amis and McKiernan (1986) described a system of letters and numbers to identify lobar, segmental, and

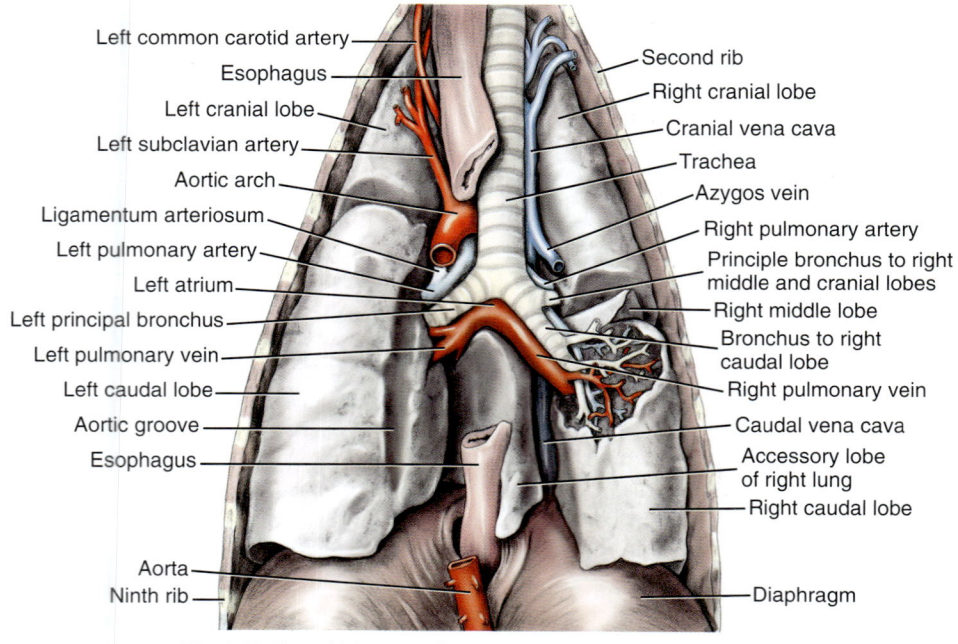

• **Fig. 8.23** Bronchial tree and associated structures, dorsal aspect.

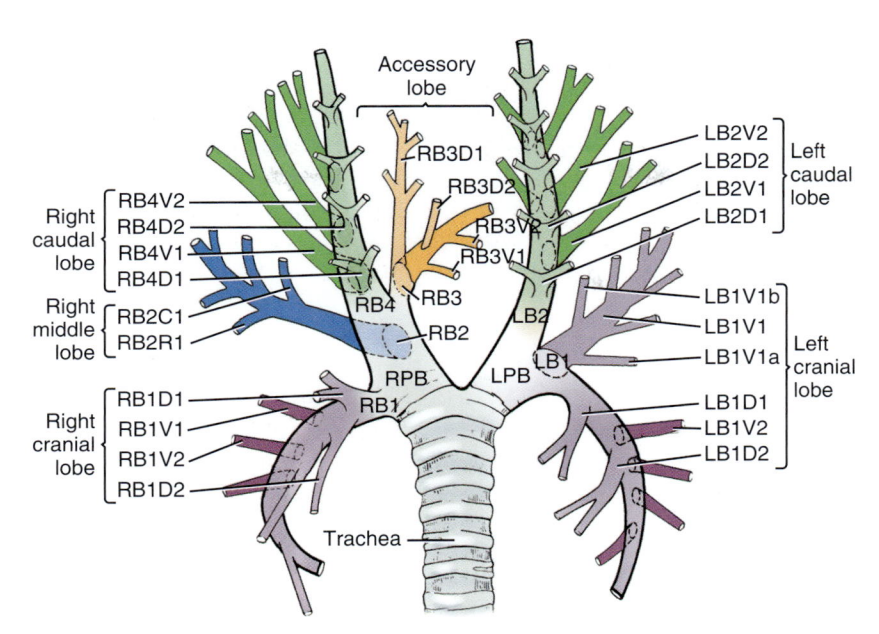

• **Fig. 8.24** Schematic bronchial tree of the dog in dorsal view. Letters and numbers identify the principal, lobar and segmental bronchi by their bronchoscopic order of origin and their anatomical orientation. Lower case *a* and *b* represent subsegmental bronchi. (Modified from Amis TC, McKieran BC: Systematic identification of endobronchial anatomy during bronchoscopy in the dog, *Am J Vet Res* 47:2649–2657, 1986.)

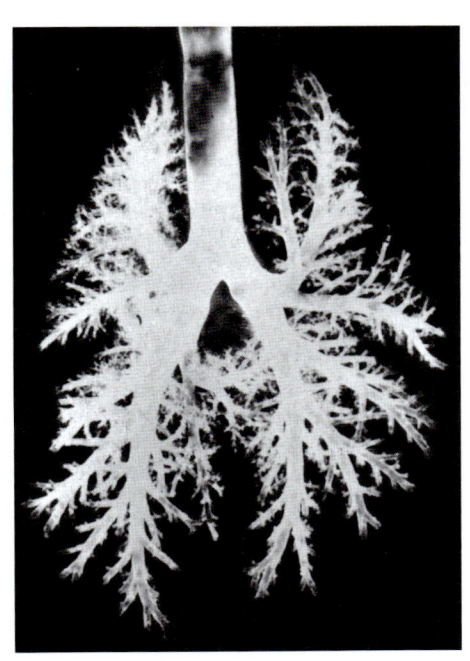

• **Fig. 8.25** Contrast radiograph. The bronchial tree, anatomical specimen.

subsegmental bronchi on the basis of their origination and anatomic orientation. The segmental bronchi arise from the dorsal and ventral surfaces of the lobar bronchi of all the lung lobes except the right middle lobe where they arise from the cranial and caudal surfaces (Fig. 8.24).

DeLorenzi et al. (2009) endoscopically studied abnormalities of the bronchial pathways in 40 brachycephalic dogs with stertorous breathing and clinical signs of respiratory distress. Included were 20 Pugs, 13 English Bulldogs, and 7 French Bulldogs. Bronchial collapse was a common finding associated with laryngeal collapse. The left cranial bronchus was the most commonly affected.

The segmental bronchi usually branch dichotomously (Miller, 1937) into small bronchi. This process of branching continues until the respiratory bronchioles are formed. The bronchi are cylindrical tubes that are kept by flattened, overlapping, curved cartilages. The cartilaginous elements end when the diameter of the conducting system is reduced to 1 mm or less. In addition, the bronchioles have spiral bands of smooth muscle in their walls that continue peripherally on the respiratory (alveolar) bronchioles.

The **respiratory bronchioles** (*bronchioli respiratorii*) give rise to **alveolar ducts** (*ductuli alveolares*), **alveolar sacs** (*sacculi alveolares*), and **pulmonary alveoli** (*alveoli pulmonis*). The respiratory portion of the bronchial tree in the dog, including the arteries, veins, and lymphatics, was modeled and described by Miller (1900, 1937). Boyden and Tompsett (1961), in their excellent paper on the postnatal growth of the lung in the dog, point out the substantial reduction postnatally in the number of nonrespiratory branches of both the axial bronchus and the peripheral bronchioles. At birth, many nonrespiratory peripheral bronchioles lined by cuboidal epithelium are converted into respiratory units. Concomitantly, new alveoli and alveolar sacs arise along the terminal bronchioles. Boyden and Tompsett conclude that the number of nonrespiratory branches on the axial stem (dorsocaudal bronchus of the accessory lobe) is reduced from 38 rami before birth to 32 at maturity.

- **Fig. 8.26 A,** Silicone cast of the bronchial tree of a Beagle pruned through the terminal bronchioles. **B,** Silicone cast of the bronchial tree, differentially pruned. (Reprinted with permission from Kilpper RW, Stidd PJ: A wet-lung technique for obtaining Silastic rubber casts of the respiratory airways, *Anat Rec* 176: 279–287, 1973. Copyright © 1973, Wiley-Liss, a Division of John Wiley and Sons, Inc.)

Loosli (1937) studied the microscopic structure of adult alveoli in several species of mammals, including the dog. He described and illustrated interalveolar communications, formerly called the pores of Köhn, in both normal and pathologic lungs and pointed out the significance of these pores in the normal mechanism of respiration and in the spread of infection.

Thoracic Cavity and Pleurae

To obtain a clear understanding of the lungs and how they function passively in the mechanical act of breathing, it is necessary first to understand the morphologic characteristics of the thoracic cavity and its lining membrane, the pleurae.

Thoracic Cavity

The **thoracic cavity** (*cavum thoracis*) (Figs. 8.27, 8.28, and 8.33), in a narrow sense, is bounded by the subserous endothoracic fascia. In a wider sense, its walls are formed by the ribs, thoracic vertebrae, sternum, and associated muscles, including the diaphragm. It is cone-shaped with the apex between the first pair of ribs and the base at the diaphragm.

Rivero et al. (2005) provided a new reference for interpretation of the normal anatomy of the canine thorax imaged by CT. A similar study by Cardoso et al. (2007) used a helical scanner and intravenous contrast media to visualize the lung.

The **endothoracic fascia** (*fascia endothoracica*) is the loose connective tissue that attaches the costal and diaphragmatic pleurae to the underlying muscles, ligaments, and bones. The endothoracic fascia is scanty where it closely attaches the costal pleura to the ribs. Dorsally and ventrally it extends into the mediastinal space and becomes the connective tissue that invests the organs and other structures that lie in the mediastinum. Cranially it passes through the thoracic inlet and is continued into the neck where it blends with the deep cervical fascia, particularly with the prevertebral portion of this fascia. Caudally it blends with the transversalis fascia at the hiatuses of the diaphragm and at the lumbosacral arches.

The thoracic wall is formed bilaterally by the ribs and the intercostal muscles, and dorsally by the bodies of the thoracic

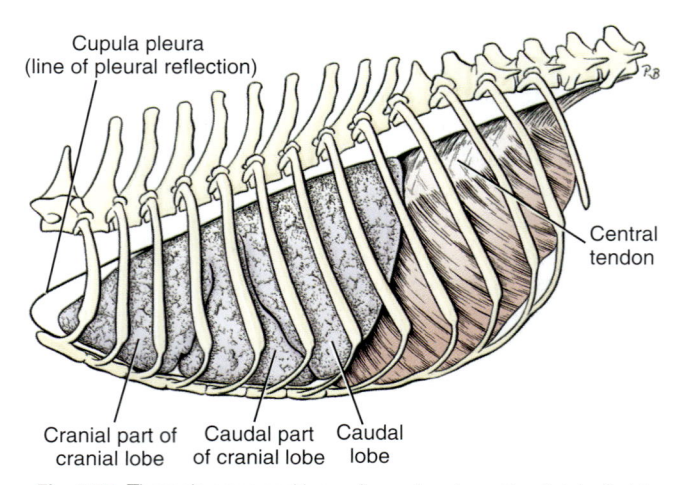

- **Fig. 8.27** Thoracic cage and lungs (lungs hardened in situ). Left side.

- Fig. 8.28 Lateral radiograph of the thorax.

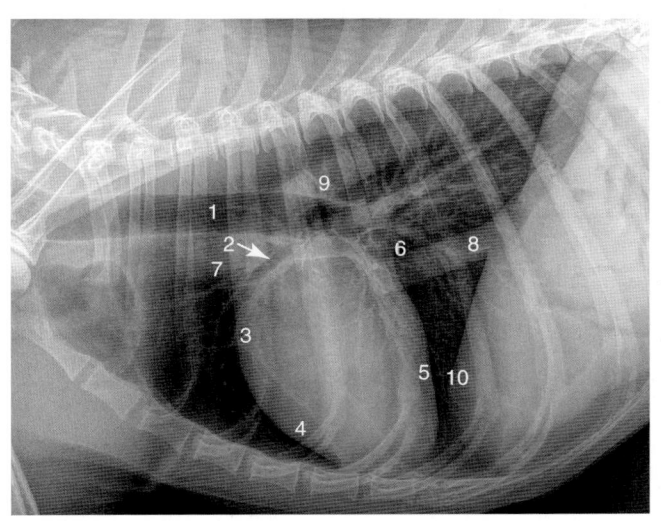

1. Trachea
2. Bronchus to right cranial lung lobe
3. Right auricle
4. Right ventricle
5. Left ventricle
6. Left atrium
7. Cranial vena cava
8. Caudal vena cava
9. Aorta
10. Cupula of diaphragm

vertebrae and the intervening fibrocartilages. Cranial to the sixth thoracic vertebra the right and left longus colli muscles cover the thoracic vertebral bodies and lie directly deep to the pleura and endothoracic fascia. Ventrally the narrow sternum and the paired flat transversus thoracis muscles contribute to the thoracic wall. Caudally the base of the thoracic cavity is formed by the dome-shaped, obliquely placed, musculotendinous diaphragm.

The shape of the thoracic cavity of the dog (Figs. 8.27 and 8.30) varies between breeds of dogs. Its walls are laterally compressed, with the result that in dogs of usual proportions, its average dorsoventral dimension is greater than either the average lateral or craniocaudal measurement. Cranially the thoracic cavity opens to the cervical region at the thoracic inlet. The external contour of the thorax differs from the internal limits of the thoracic cavity. In cross-section the thorax is roughly oval in shape, wider dorsally than ventrally, and long dorsoventrally. A transverse section of the thoracic cavity cranial to the diaphragm is heart-shaped, with the apex located ventrally (Fig. 8.31). The base of the transverse section of the thorax, located dorsally, is widened to accommodate the epaxial muscles, thoracic vertebral bodies, aorta, and smaller associated structures. The thorax is a laterally compressed cone with a base (diaphragm) that is convex cranially. The greatest cranial encroachment of the diaphragm is to a transverse plane through the sixth intercostal spaces and approximately 5 cm dorsal to the sternum. In addition to being convex, the diaphragm is oblique in position. The most cranial dorsal attachment is approximately eight vertebral segments caudal to its most cranial ventral attachment. From attachments on the medial surfaces of the ribs, including the costal cartilages and the lumbar vertebrae, the diaphragm bilaterally extends almost directly cranially, forming a slitlike space or recess at its attachments. The recess is formed by the diaphragm centrally, and the ribs and intercostal structures and lumbar vertebrae peripherally. In normal respiration the diaphragm undergoes a craniocaudal excursion of approximately one and a half vertebral segments, yet, even in forced inspiration, the margin of the lungs never completely invades the recesses so created. In a Beagle-type dog the diaphragm protrudes cranially from its costal attachment for a maximum distance of 6 cm. For the details of the intrinsic structure of the diaphragm, see Figs. 6.35 and 6.36. The thoracic cavity contains the trachea, lungs, heart, thymus gland, esophagus, lymph nodes, vessels, and nerves. The structures that partly or completely traverse the thoracic cavity are the aorta, cranial vena cava and caudal vena cava, azygos and hemiazygos veins, thoracic duct and smaller lymph vessels, esophagus, and the vagal, phrenic, and sympathetic nerves.

The **thoracic inlet** (*apertura thoracis cranialis*) is the roughly oval opening into the cranial part of the thoracic cavity. It is bounded bilaterally by the first pair of ribs with their cranially extending costal cartilages. In a Beagle-type dog its dorsoventral dimension is approximately 4 cm. Its greatest width is approximately one-fourth less than its dorsoventral dimension. The aperture is wider dorsally than ventrally. The first thoracic vertebra and the paired longus colli muscles bound the thoracic inlet dorsally; the manubrium of the sternum bounds it ventrally. Traversing the aperture are the trachea, esophagus, vagosympathetic nerve trunks, recurrent laryngeal nerves, phrenic nerves, first two thoracic nerves, and several vessels. The apices of the pleural cavities lie in the thoracic inlet, as the *cupula pleurae*.

Mediastinum

The mediastinum is the space and the mediastinal pleurae that enclose this space between the right and left pleural cavities. It is divided by the heart into three transverse divisions. The middle division is further divided by the heart into two more divisions dorsal and ventral to it.

The **cranial mediastinum** (*mediastinum craniale*) (Figs. 8.29 and 8.30) is the portion of the mediastinum lying cranial to the heart that contains the trachea, esophagus, thymus, sternal and cranial mediastinal lymph nodes, and many vessels and nerves. Dorsally it attaches to the longus colli muscles and ventrally it attaches to the sternum. Ventrally it reflects over the internal thoracic vessels as they course toward the sternum to pass deep to the transverse "thoracis muscles".

The **ventral mediastinum** (*mediastinum ventrale*) is that portion ventral to the heart that contains the thymus cranially and the **phrenicopericardial ligament** (*lig. phrenicopericardiacum*), a band of connective tissue between the fibrous pericardium and the diaphragm, caudally.

The **middle mediastinum** (*mediastinum medium*) (Fig. 8.31) is the portion containing the heart. Here the mediastinal pleura are fused with the fibrous pericardium. A single layer of tissue separates the pleural cavity from the pericardial cavity. From the pleural cavity to the pericardial cavity, this layer consists of the mediastinal pleura, the fibrous pericardium and the parietal layer of the serous pericardium. On each side the phrenic nerves course across the heart through the fibrous pericardium where they are covered by middle mediastinal pleura. At the base of the heart the vagal nerves cross the heart deep to the middle mediastinal pleura.

The **dorsal mediastinum** (*mediastinum dorsale*) is that part dorsal to the heart containing the major pulmonary vessels, the aorta and its initial branches, thoracic duct, tracheal bifurcation, esophagus, and lymph nodes. At the tracheal bifurcation the dorsal mediastinal pleura reflects on to the lungs as the pulmonary pleura.

The **caudal mediastinum** (*mediastinum caudale*) is that part of the mediastinum lying caudal to the heart. It is reflected to the left by the accessory lung lobe of the right lung and contains the aorta and thoracic duct dorsally and the esophagus with vagal branches and trunks more centrally.

1. Trachea
2. Esophagus
3. Aorta
4. Brachiocephalic trunk
5. Left subclavian artery
6. Sternal lymph nodes
7. Right cranial lung lobe
8. Cranial part of left cranial lung lobe

• **Fig. 8.29** Transverse computed tomographic image of the cranial thorax.

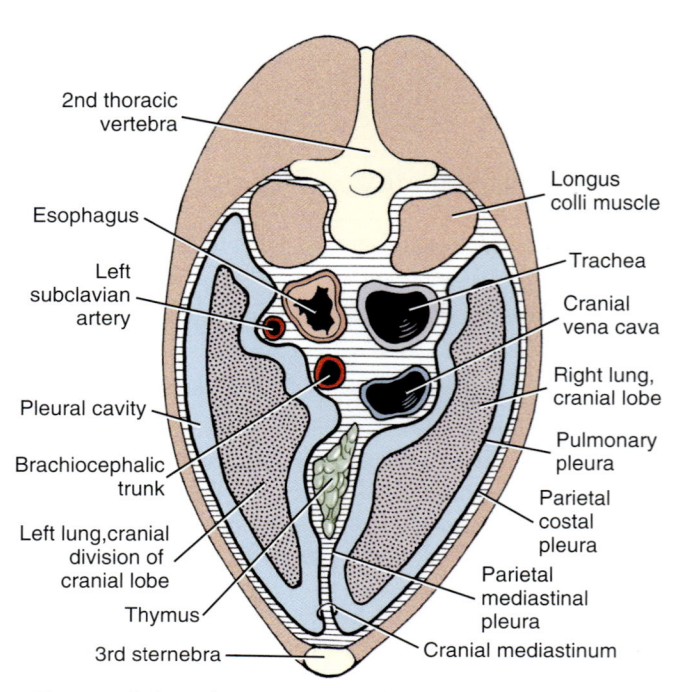

• **Fig. 8.30** Schematic transverse section of thorax through cranial mediastinum and lungs. Caudal aspect. Orientation differs from that of Fig. 8.29.

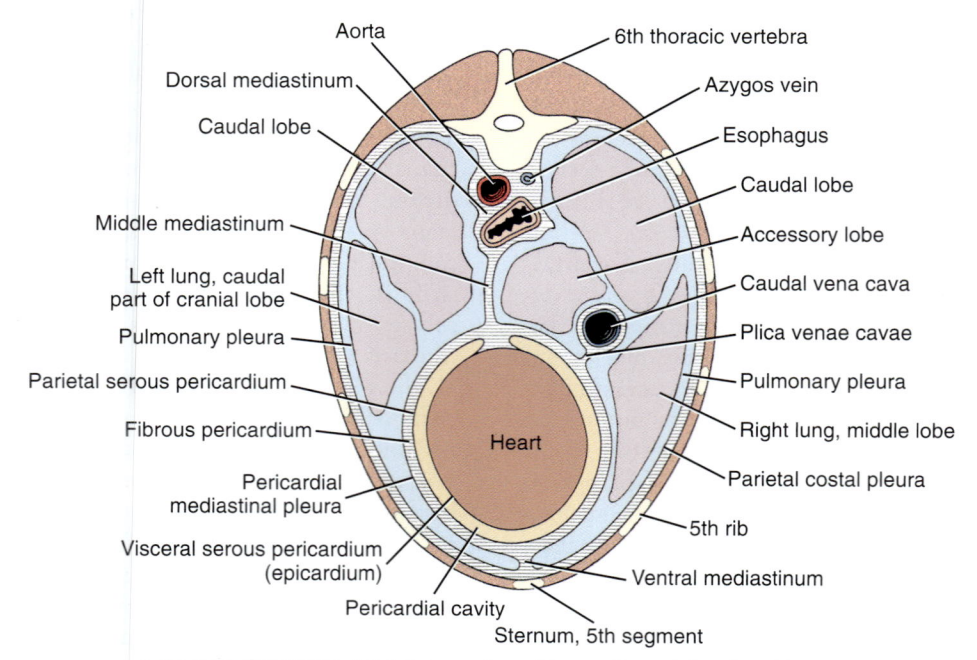

• **Fig. 8.31** Schematic transverse section of thorax through heart and lungs.

A separate fold of the right caudal mediastinal pleura projects dorsally from the level of the sternum to surround the caudal vena cava and right phrenic nerve approximately one-third of the distance between the sternum and the vertebral column. This fold is the **plica vena cava** (*plica venae cavae*). The pleural cavity space created between this plica and the caudal mediastinum is the **mediastinal recess** (*recessus mediastini*) that contains the accessory lobe of the right lung. In the dog the tissue in the mediastinum is extremely scanty, but the pleura that covers it is not fenestrated. Therefore, one lung can be collapsed independently of the other.

The **mediastinal serous cavity** (*cavum mediastini serosum*) is a potential space that represents a cranial extension of the peritoneal serous membranes (greater omentum) within the caudal mediastinum (Gendron et al., 2018). This cavity lies to the right of the esophagus and is lined with mesothelial cells. The serous nature of this space may allow for cranial "sliding" motion of the esophagus and the gastroesophageal junction (Kunath, 1977). The mediastinal serous cavity may be related to congenital or primary type paraesophageal hernia and may be related to sliding hiatal hernia in humans (Karpelowsky et al., 2006). In dogs, empyema and mesothelioma have occurred in this space (Gendron et al., 2018). For illustration of the mediastinal serous cavity, the reader is referred to Gendron et al. (2018) for CT and anatomic images.

Pleurae

The pleurae are the serous membranes that cover the lungs, line the walls of the thoracic cavity, and cover the structures in the mediastinal space. The pleurae form two complete sacs, one on either side, which are known as the *pleural cavities* (Figs. 8.30 and 8.31).

Each **pleural cavity** (*cavum pleurae*) in life is essentially only a potential cavity because it contains only a capillary film of serous fluid that moistens the simple squamous layer of mesothelial cells paving its surface. Except for this capillary fluid, the visceral pleura of the lungs, or pulmonary pleura, lies in contact with the parietal pleura. Only when gas (air) or fluid collects between the pulmonary and parietal pleurae and prevents a lung from expanding does it exist as a real cavity. The right pleural cavity is larger than the left because of displacement of the caudal mediastinal wall to the left side. The pleural cavities do not communicate with each other, although their medial walls and the tissue between them are extremely thin.

For purposes of description, the pleura is designated as the parietal and the pulmonary pleura. The **parietal pleura** (*pleura parietalis*) forms the walls of the pleural cavities. It is further designated as **costal**, **mediastinal**, and **diaphragmatic**.

The **costal pleura** (*pleura costalis*) is the portion of the parietal pleura that attaches to the medial surfaces of the lateral walls of the thoracic cavity. The costal pleura firmly adheres to the medial surfaces of the ribs and is thin. The costal pleura, which covers the medial surfaces of the intercostal muscles and related structures, is thicker and less firmly attached to them. The pleura and the underlying endothoracic fascia possess considerable elasticity.

The **mediastinal pleura** (*pleura mediastinalis*) (Figs. 8.30 and 8.31) forms the wall of the mediastinal space and may be divided into the five parts described previously: cranial, dorsal, middle, ventral, and caudal. The pleural reflection from the mediastinal pleura to the costal pleura both dorsally and ventrally forms a **costomediastinal recess** (*recessus costomediastinalis*) where the lung borders reside.

The **diaphragmatic pleura** (*pleura diaphragmatica*) is the pleural covering of the diaphragm. It is thicker at the muscular periphery of this dome-shaped partition and more loosely attached than it is on the tendinous center. Where the diaphragm is attached to the medial aspect of the lateral thoracic wall the diaphragmatic pleura reflects acutely cranially to form the costal pleura. In life a capillary space is present on each side between the diaphragm and the caudal lateral wall of the thorax. These spaces are called the **right** and **left costodiaphragmatic recesses** (*recessus costodiaphragmatici*). After death the diaphragm and its pleura lie in contact with the costal pleura throughout a circular zone that is approximately 4 cm in width. The right and left costodiaphragmatic recesses extend cranioventrally on each side of the mediastinal pleura as the right and left **costomediastinal recesses** (*recessus costomediastinales*). These pleural spaces are formed between the ventral aspect of the mediastinum and the lateral thoracic walls. Although in cross-section they form acute angles, they are large enough to receive the ventral borders of the lobes of the lungs during inspiration.

The apical portion of each pleural sac extends through the thoracic inlet into the base of the neck, forming a pleural pocket at the line of pleural reflection (Figs. 8.27 and 8.33) known as the **pleural cupula** (*cupula pleurae*). The left cupula is the larger and extends further cranial to the first rib than does the right. The right pleural cupula is wide dorsoventrally but extends only approximately half as far cranial as does the left.

The **pulmonary pleura** (*pleura pulmonalis*), or visceral pleura, tightly adheres to the surfaces of the lungs and follows all of their irregularities. Its greatest intrapulmonary extensions correspond to the adjacent free surfaces of the lobes of the lungs. In all interlobar fissures, except that between the cranial and caudal parts of the cranial lobe of the left lung, the pleura extends to the lobar bronchus of the lung. Between the two parts of the left cranial lobe of the lung, the fissure does not extend to the bronchus, and therefore the pleura does not extend as deeply in this fissure as it does in others. In some specimens the borders of the lungs are notched or fissured by clefts of varying depth. These clefts occur more often on the cranial lobes.

The **pulmonary ligament** (*lig. pulmonale*) (Figs. 8.34 and 8.35) is a triangular fold of pleura that leaves the respective caudal lung lobe on each side, caudal to the hilus. It is continuous with the pleura covering the root or hilus of the lung and contains no visible structures. On the left side, it extends approximately 3 cm caudodorsally from the large pulmonary vein leaving the caudal lobe of the left lung, and ends in a falciform border that stretches from the medial surface of the lung to the left sheet of mediastinal pleura directly ventral to the aorta. The right pulmonary ligament is approximately the same size and shape as the left. It leaves the acute dorsal border of the right caudal lobe, extends along the right portion of the accessory lobe, and becomes continuous with the right sheet of mediastinal pleura that covers the esophagus and aorta. It ends in a falciform border approximately 1 cm cranial to the diaphragm. The pulmonary ligaments are relatively avascular. The pleurae that form them are continuous with the caudal portions of the dorsal mediastinal pleurae that reflect on the roots of the lungs. Small connecting pleural plicae occasionally extend between adjacent lobes of a lung at its hilus.

The *plica venae cavae* is a thin, loose fold of pleura that surrounds the caudal vena cava. The plica occupies the triangular space bounded by the caudal vena cava dorsally, the pericardium cranially, and the diaphragm caudally. Because of its delicate nature the right portion of the accessory lobe of the right lung is visible through it. The space is known as the **mediastinal recess** (*recessus mediastini*). The plica venae cavae leaves the ventral third of the diaphragm approximately 1 cm peripheral to its tendinous center. Ventrally it blends with the sagittal portion of the caudal mediastinal pleura. The plica venae cavae on the right and the oblique portion of the caudal mediastinal pleura on the left form a pocket between the heart and the diaphragm. This is the mediastinal recess in which is located the accessory lobe of the right lung. The right phrenic nerve runs from the base of the heart to the diaphragm in a separate plica, only a few millimeters wide, that leaves the right pleural leaf of the main plica immediately ventral to the caudal vena cava.

Histologically, the pleura is more delicate in the dog than it is in other domestic animals. It contains smooth muscle fibers and, deep to the epithelium, is a dense network of elastic fibers that separate the true serosa (mesothelium) from the collagenous subserosa. The subserosa also contains elastic fibers, mainly on its deep surface, where they communicate with those of the lobules of the lung. The surface of the pleura is covered by a simple squamous layer of mesothelial cells. In life the pleura is covered by a capillary film of fluid so that the friction between the pulmonary pleura and the parietal pleura or between adjacent layers of the pulmonary pleura is minimized. Elastic fibers are also present in the parietal pleura, so that both pulmonary and parietal pleura are capable of stretching. The pulmonary pleura is more tightly adherent to the lung parenchyma than is the parietal pleura to the thoracic wall.

Lungs

The **lung** (*pulmo*) (Figs. 8.27 to 8.36) is the organ in which oxygen from the atmosphere and carbon dioxide from the blood are exchanged. The lungs serve a passive function in the mechanical act of respiration. The diaphragm, when it contracts, enlarges the pleural cavity by moving caudally.

When the intercostal muscles contract and draw the ribs cranially, the size of the thoracic cavity is also increased, and thus air is drawn into the lungs because of the negative pressure that is produced. Aiding in expulsion of the air from the lungs are the abdominal muscles, which contract and force the abdominal viscera against the caudal surface of the diaphragm. The effects of age on lung function and structure were reviewed by Mauderly and Hahn (1982). In general, there is considerable fibrosis and loss of function in the lungs of old dogs. Robinson (1982) summarized some functional consequences of species differences in lung anatomy. There is no explanation for the great variation seen in lung lobation of domestic and wild mammals.

The two lungs (*pulmo sinister et dexter*) possess many features in common. Each has a slightly concave **base** (*basis pulmonis*), which lies adjacent to the diaphragm, and an **apex** (*apex pulmonis*), which lies in the thoracic inlet. The apex of the left lung is more pointed and extends farther cranially than the apex of the right lung (Bourdelle & Bressou, 1927). The curved lateral surface of each lung is called the **costal surface** (*facies costalis*), and the flattened surface, which faces the mediastinum, is called the **medial surface** (*facies medialis*). Because the vertebral bodies protrude ventrally from the dorsal wall of the thorax and intervene between the two lungs, this dorsal portion of the medial surface of each lung is known as the **vertebral part** (*pars vertebralis*). The remaining ventral portion of each medial surface faces the mediastinum and is known as the **mediastinal part** (*pars mediastinalis*). The medial surface of each lung is deeply indented by the heart over an area between the third and the sixth ribs. This is called the **cardiac impression** (*impressio cardiaca*). On each side, the mediastinal pleura covering the pericardial sac are displaced sufficiently by the underlying heart so that its ventral portion lies in contact with the costal pleura. The **cardiac notch of the right lung** (*incisura cardiaca pulmonis dextri*) (Fig. 8.33) is V-shaped, with the apex located dorsally. The right cardiac notch is formed by the ventrally diverging borders of the cranial and middle lobes. Its dorsal apex lies opposite the beginning of the distal fourth of the fourth rib. On the left side usually no obvious cardiac notch is formed.

Each lung has a **diaphragmatic surface** (Figs. 8.34 and 8.35) (*facies diaphragmatica*) that is concave because it lies against the convex surface of the diaphragm. The diaphragmatic surface of the right lung is approximately one-third larger than that of the left lung, this larger area being caused by the accessory lobe of the right lung extending ventrally and to the left, ending in a process at the apex of the heart.

The margin along the vertebral part of the lung is the **dorsal margin** (*margo dorsalis [obtusus]*) (Fig. 8.35) and extends from the apex to the base of the lung. The costal surface of each lung is continuous with the medial surface at an acute angle ventrally, lying in the costomediastinal recess. This margin, extending from the apex to the base of the lung, is called the **ventral margin of the lung** (*margo ventralis*). Caudally the ventral margin of the lung is continuous with the peripheral margin of the base of the lung,

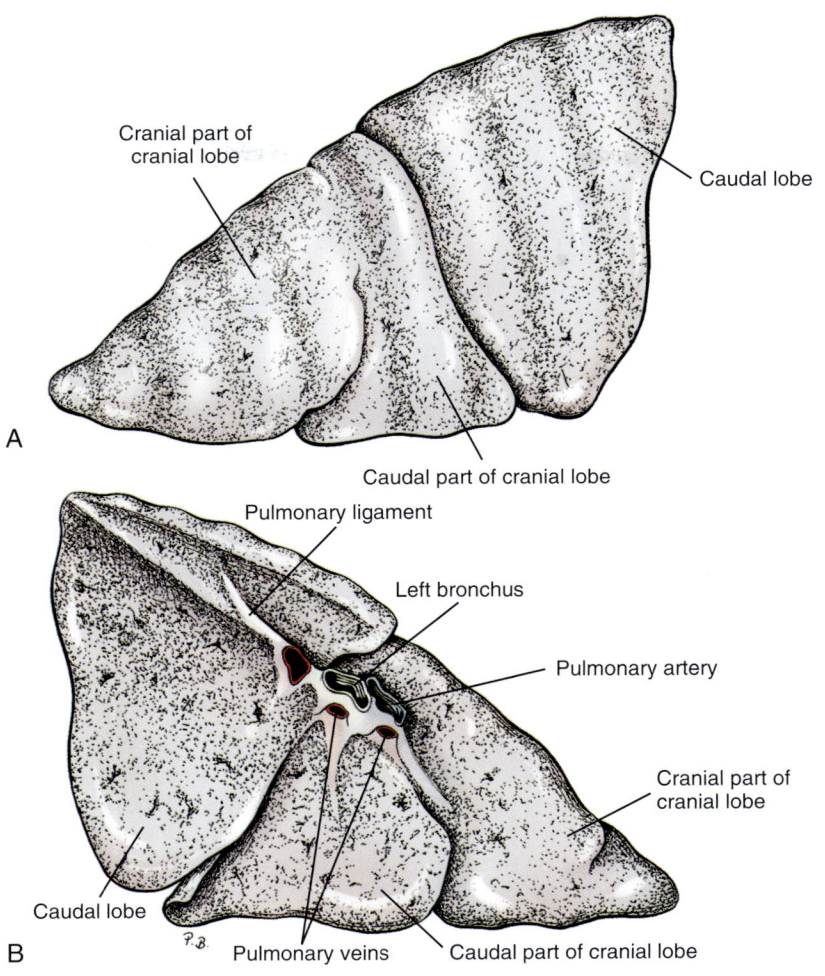

Fig. 8.32 Left lung. **A,** Lateral aspect. **B,** Medial aspect.

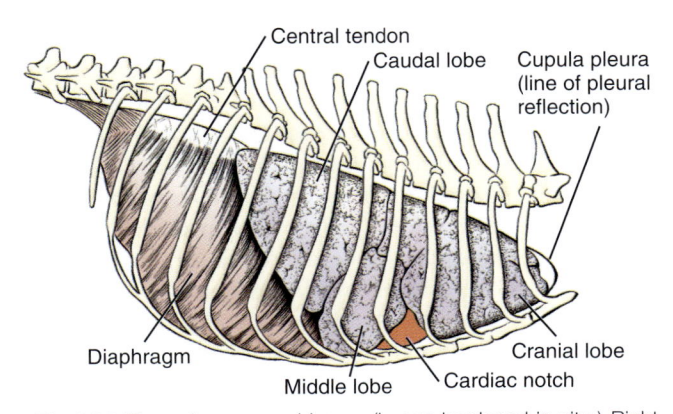

Fig. 8.33 Thoracic cage and lungs. (Lungs hardened in situ.) Right side.

or the **basal margin** (*margo basalis*). The basal margin is where the costal and diaphragmatic surfaces meet. This margin extends into the costodiaphragmatic recess. The combined ventral and basal margins constitute the **acute margin** (*margo acutus*).

The area of each lung that receives the principal bronchi and furnishes passages for the pulmonary and bronchial vessels and nerves is known as the **hilus of the lung** (*hilus pulmonis*).

The **root of the lung** (*radix pulmonis*) consists of the aggregate of those structures that enter or leave the organ at the hilus. Lung lobes are determined by the pattern of branching of the principal bronchi. Interlobar fissures are the external indications of these divisions. The **caudal interlobar fissure** (*fissura interlobalis caudalis*) is between the middle and caudal lobes of the right lung and the cranial and caudal lobes of the left lung. The **cranial interlobar fissure** (*fissura interlobaris cranialis*) is between the cranial and middle lobes of the right lung. The surfaces of adjacent lobes that lie in contact with each other are called the **interlobar surfaces** (*facies interlobares*).

Shape of Lobes and Position of Interlobar Fissures

Lung lobes are named for the branching of principal bronchi into lobar bronchi. The left principal bronchus has two lobar bronchi, cranial and caudal. The cranial lobar bronchus immediately divides into two segmental bronchi that serve the cranial and caudal parts of the cranial lobe. The

410 CHAPTER 8 The Respiratory System

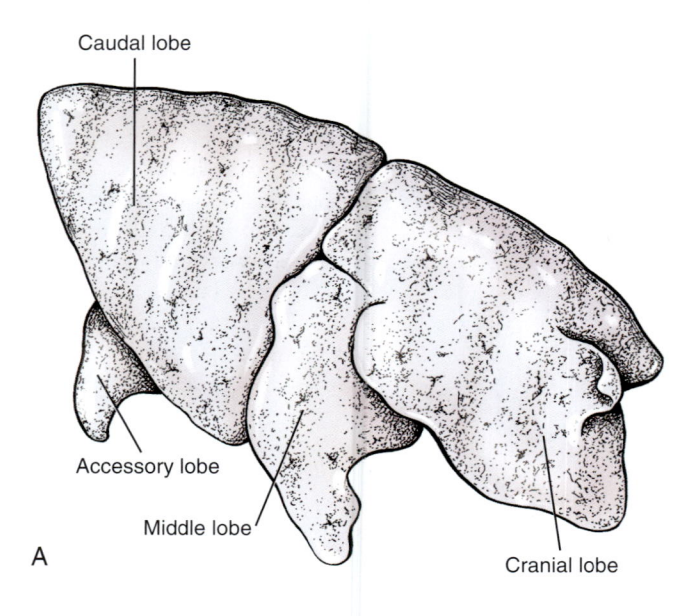

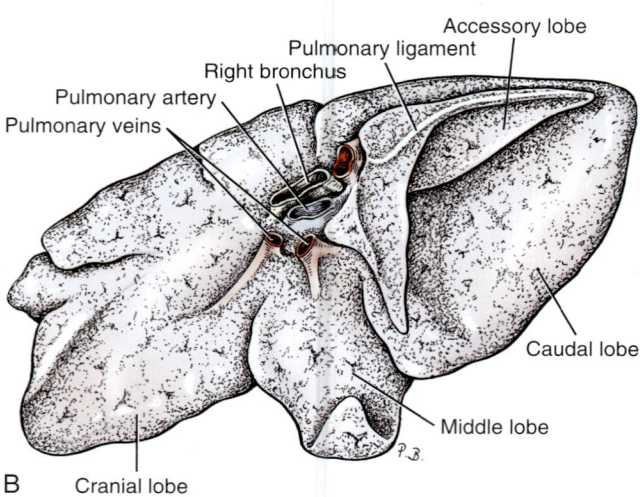

Fig. 8.34 Right lung. **A,** Lateral aspect. **B,** Medial aspect.

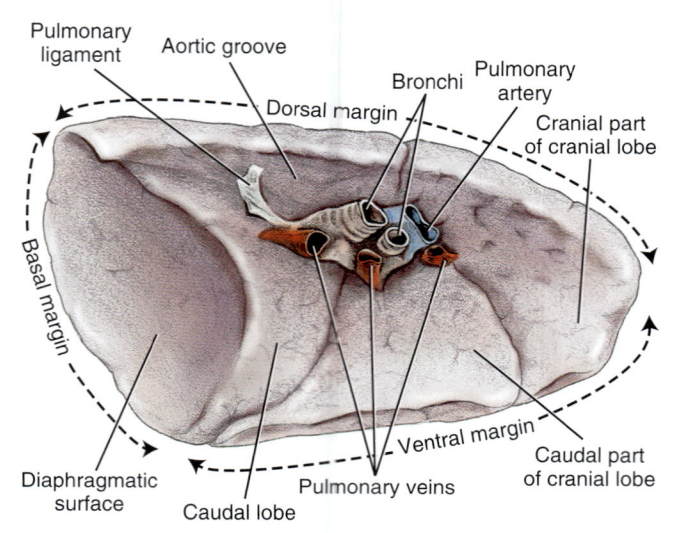

Fig. 8.35 Margins and surfaces of the left lung, medial view.

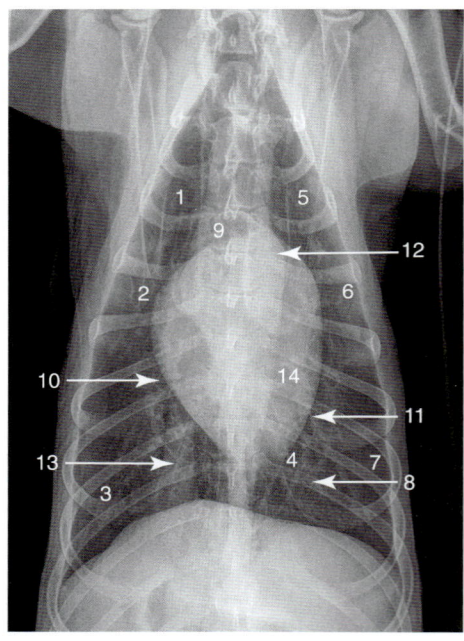

1. Right cranial lung lobe
2. Right middle lung lobe
3. Right caudal lung lobe
4. Accessory lung lobe
5. Cranial part of left cranial lung lobe
6. Caudal part of left cranial lung lobe
7. Left caudal lung lobe
8. Caudal mediastinum
9. Trachea
10. Right ventricle
11. Left ventricle
12. Aorta
13. Caudal vena cava
14. Heart

Fig. 8.36 Dorsoventral radiograph of the thorax.

right principal bronchus has four lobar bronchi, one to each of its four lobes.

Left Lung

The **cranial part of the cranial lobe of the left lung** (*pulmo sinistra, lobus cranialis, pars cranialis*), formerly the *apical lobe* (Fig. 8.32), is transversely compressed between the heart and the lateral thoracic wall. In a 22-pound dog it is 10 cm long, 3 cm wide. It extends from the dorsal part of the fifth rib to and through the thoracic inlet, where its apex lies not only cranial to a transverse plane through the first ribs but also largely to the right of the median plane. The parenchyma of the cranial and caudal parts of the left cranial lobe are fused over a transverse distance of 2.5 cm from the vertebral border to the fissure between the lobe parts.

The **caudal part of the cranial lobe of the left lung** (Fig. 8.32) (*pulmo sinister, lobus cranialis, pars caudalis*) was formerly called the *cardiac lobe*. It presents a thin dorsocranially convex border that overlies the caudal thickened portion of the cranial part of the cranial lobe, or these features and positions of the adjacent lobes are reversed. The ventral margin of the caudal part of the cranial lobe of the left lung lies nearly in a dorsal plane 1 cm from the midventral line. The left lung does not possess a cardiac notch.

The **caudal lobe of the left lung** (*pulmo sinister, lobus caudalis*), formerly *diaphragmatic lobe*, is pyramidal in shape and is completely separated from the cranially lying caudal part of the cranial lobe by the caudal interlobar fissure, which extends from the costal surface to the root of the lung. When the lungs are moderately distended, the fissure begins at the vertebral end of the sixth rib and ends near the costochondral junction of the seventh rib.

Right Lung

The right lung (Fig. 8.34) is divided into cranial, middle, accessory, and caudal lobes. The cranial interlobar fissure separates the cranial and middle lobes of the right lung. The caudal interlobar fissure separates the right middle and caudal lobes.

The **cranial lobe of the right lung** (*pulmo dexter, lobus cranialis*), formerly the *apical lobe*, extends from the dorsal part of the cranial interlobar fissure cranially and ventrally to the right of the median plane. It does not end in a definite apex, as does the left lung, but rather its most cranial and ventral part has a gentle curved convex border that goes from an acute, cranial, and dorsal margin to a slightly convex surface cranial to the heart. This portion of the cranial lobe extends across the median plane to the left side, whereas its most cranioventral portion lies adjacent to the caudal portion of the apex of the left lung that extends across the midline to the right side separated from each other by the cranial mediastinum. The caudoventral margin of the cranial lobe of the right lung is separated from the craniodorsal portion of the middle lobe by the curved **cranial interlobar fissure** (*fissura interlobalis cranialis*).

The **middle lobe of the right lung** (*pulmo dexter, lobus medius*) begins at the cranial interlobar fissure, where its costal surface is broad and tapers to a narrow, pyramid-shaped ventral extremity that lies caudal or caudosinistral to the apex of the heart. Its medial surface is deeply excavated by the heart, resulting in the cardiac impression. The cranioventral one-fourth of its border diverges sharply from the rounded transversely located caudal portion of the cranial lobe, thus exposing a portion of the atrial surface of the heart to the thoracic wall. This notch in the right lung is the **cardiac notch** (*incisura cardiaca pulmonis dextri*).

The **accessory lobe of the right lung** (*pulmo dexter, lobus accessorius*) (Fig. 8.34), formerly *intermediate lobe*, is the most irregular of all of the lobes of the lungs. Caudally it is molded against the diaphragm. Cranially it lies in contact with the apex of the heart and the adjacent portion of the right caudal lobe. The caudal mediastinum separates it from the left caudal lobe. The accessory lobe possesses a thickened middle portion and three processes—a dorsal, a ventral, and a right lateral. The dorsal process is a sharp-pointed pyramid-shaped eminence that extends caudally in contact with the caudoventral face of the dorsomedial portion of the caudal lobe of the right lung. Its free caudal apex does not reach as far caudally as do the caudal lobes. The ventral process of the accessory lobe runs almost directly ventrally to the dorsal surface of the sixth sternebra. It is wedged in the mediastinal recess, the space between the diaphragm and the apex of the heart. Separating the dorsal and the right lateral processes is the notch through which the caudal vena cava and the right phrenic nerve pass.

The **caudal lobe of the right lung** (*pulmo dexter, lobus caudalis*) is similar in shape and comparable in location to the left lobe, except that it lies to the right of the median plane. It is smaller than the left caudal lobe, and does not extend as far ventrally as does the left caudal lobe. Furthermore, its diaphragmatic surface is irregularly excavated in its central part by the accessory lobe. Around its periphery it is concave in all directions, in conformity with the convex surface of the diaphragm against which it lies.

Relationship of Lungs to Other Organs

The heart (Fig. 8.36) produces large impressions on the medial surface of each lung. The **cardiac impression of the right lung** (*impressio cardiaca pulmonis dextri*) is a deep excavation of the medial or mediastinal surfaces of the right cranial lobe cranially, the middle lobe laterally, and the accessory lobe caudally. Ventrally and on the right the cranial and middle lobes fail to cover the heart, so that the pericardial mediastinal pleura lies in contact with the costal pleura over an area that is V-shaped, with the apex located dorsally. This notch in the right lung is called the **cardiac notch of the right lung** (*incisura cardiaca pulmonis dextri*). The cardiac notch exposes approximately 5 square cm of the atrial surface of the heart to the thoracic wall. The ventral margin of the left cranial lobe is arciform. It is located, approximately in a sagittal plane, approximately 1 cm from the median plane, ventrally. The **notch for the caudal vena cava** (*sulcus venae cavae caudalis*) (see Fig. 11.2) is located between the dorsal and the right lateral processes of the accessory lobe. Passing through this notch in close association with the caudal vena cava is the right phrenic nerve as it runs to the diaphragm. Both structures are surrounded by the plica venae cavae, which attaches to the diaphragm. The medial surfaces of the cranial lobes of the lungs lie in contact with the mediastinum covering the thoracic portion of the thymus gland when the thymus is present. At its fullest development, the thymus gland ends caudally opposite the left fifth costal cartilage. It therefore enters into the formation of the cardiac impression of the caudal part of the left cranial lobe.

Pulmonary Vessels

The pulmonary arteries carry non-oxygenated blood from the right ventricle of the heart to the lungs for gaseous exchange. The pulmonary veins return aerated blood from the lungs to the left atrium of the heart. McLaughlin et al. (1961) have shown that the spatial and functional arrangements of the pulmonary vessels differ greatly among various species. In the dog, the pulmonary artery, in addition to supplying the distal portion of the respiratory bronchiole, alveolar duct, and alveoli, continues on to supply the thin pleura.

The **pulmonary trunk** (*truncus pulmonalis*) is the stem artery arising from the fibrous pulmonary ring, the connective tissue of which extends into the tunica media of the pulmonary trunk. It serves for the attachment of muscle fibers from the conus arteriosus. The pulmonary trunk bifurcates into the left and right pulmonary arteries, which ramify in the left and right lungs. The **left pulmonary artery** (*a. pulmonalis sinistra*) (Fig. 8.35) curves dorsally cranial to the vein from the cranial part of the cranial lobe that crosses the lobar bronchus to that lobe. Just prior to this crossing, a large branch of the left pulmonary artery arises and bifurcates. The larger terminal branch runs cranially as the main vessel to the cranial part of the left cranial lobe. The branch to the caudal part of the left cranial lobe lies cranial to the bronchus and caudal to the large vein. The veins from all of the lobes compose the most ventral part of the root of the lung (Fig. 8.35).

The **right pulmonary artery** (*a. pulmonalis dextra*) is shorter than the left. It runs caudolaterally across the heart base from left to right. It passes ventral to the left lobar bronchi and dorsal to the large left lobar veins. The artery divides unequally into a small branch that runs to the right cranial lobe and a large branch that courses caudally into the right caudal lobe. Near the origin of the large artery to the caudal lobe the relatively small right middle lobar artery runs laterally and enters the dorsal third of the lobe. It is related to the dorsal surface of its satellite vein and lies dorsocranial to the right middle lobar bronchus. It may arise from the right cranial lobar artery. The pulmonary lobar artery to the accessory lobe of the right lung enters the thickened middle portion of the lobe and trifurcates into a branch supplying each of the three processes of the lobe. This lobar artery lies ventral to the bronchus to this lobe and dorsal to its satellite vein.

The **pulmonary veins** (*vv. pulmonales*) (Figs. 8.34 and 8.35) are variable in number. All of the blood distributed to the bronchial tree is returned by the pulmonary veins except for a limited area around the hilus drained by bronchial veins. There is one pulmonary vein from each lobe, although there may be two veins that drain the right cranial lobe. The latter veins anastomose to form a larger vein that immediately receives the vein from the right middle lobe so that blood from all of these areas is returned to the right lateral part of the left atrium by a single large vein 1 cm in diameter. The blood from the right caudal and accessory lobes is drained by a single vessel that lies to the right of a similar vessel from the left caudal lobe. The pulmonary lobar veins from the left lung usually open individually into the dorsum of the left atrium. At the hilus of the lung the pulmonary veins lie most ventrally. The pulmonary arteries are dorsal to the veins, and the lobar bronchi are insinuated between the arteries and the veins. Holt et al. (2005) provided a revised anatomic description of the pulmonary veins of the right caudal and accessory lobes of the dog's lung. They described similar conditions in the nine dogs they dissected. The pulmonary vein from the right caudal lung lobe initially paralleled the right caudal lung lobe bronchus, running cranially, medially, and ventrally. It diverged from the bronchus at the level of the pulmonary artery and bronchus of the accessory lung lobe. At this point the pulmonary vein from the right caudal lobe coursed dorsal to the pulmonary artery and bronchus of the accessory lobe. Medial to the bronchus of the accessory lobe, it received the pulmonary vein from the accessory lobe on its ventral surface. Within the pericardium this common venous trunk merged with the caudal aspect of the left atrium either with, or immediately adjacent to, the left caudal pulmonary vein.

Barone (1957), Ishaq (1980), Phalen and Oldham (1983), Amis and McKiernan (1986), and Shishkin et al. (1989) consider various aspects of the bronchial tree and lung in the dog. Holt et al. (2005) revised the anatomic description and embryologic implications of the right caudal and accessory lobe pulmonary veins.

Bronchial Vessels

The small **bronchial arteries** are variable in origin, although in the majority of dogs the parent trunk is the bronchoesophageal artery (Figs. 11.34 and 11.35) that arises from the right fifth intercostal artery close to its origin from the aorta. The bronchoesophageal artery crosses the left face of the esophagus and contributes an esophageal branch before entering the root of each lung as the bronchial artery. In its course, the bronchial artery supplies the tracheobronchial lymph nodes, peribronchial connective tissue, and the bronchial mucous membrane. At the level of the respiratory bronchiole the bronchial artery terminates in a capillary bed that is continuous with that of the pulmonary artery. Miller (1937), McLaughlin et al. (1961), and, more recently, Laitinen et al. (1989) were unable to demonstrate normally occurring bronchial artery-pulmonary artery anastomoses in the dog. Laitinen et al. (1989) have described the structure of tracheal and bronchial blood vessels in the Greyhound using vascular corrosion casts as well as electron micrographs. They found two networks of vessels of different types and sizes in the mucosa. One, a rich capillary network close to the epithelial basement membrane, converged to form venules that then extended to a deeper mucosal plexus formed by larger venules and arterioles.

Notkovitch (1957) found single bronchial arteries on each side in 75% of his specimens, and double bronchial arteries on each side in 10%. In all cases they arose from the first to the fourth right intercostal artery. Berry et al. (1931) found that the right and left bronchial arteries arose from the right sixth intercostal artery by a common trunk, which also supplied branches to the esophagus. They also described small bronchial vessels that supplied the hilus of the lung and that arose from the pericardiacophrenic or internal thoracic arteries. Michel (1982) demonstrated qualitative and quantitative morphologic differences between small pulmonary arteries and veins. Pulmonary arteries of the dog gradually taper and change from elastic to transitional, to muscular, partially muscular, and, finally, nonmuscular arteries.

True **bronchial veins** are found only at the hilus of the lung. They empty into the azygos vein or intercostal vein at the level of the seventh thoracic vertebra.

Pulmonary Lymphatics

The afferent lymph vessels from the lobes of each lung run to the **tracheobronchial lymph nodes** of the respective side and to the middle tracheobronchial lymph node. From these locations lymph is drained via a chain of cranial mediastinal lymph nodes (Correll & Langston, 1958). Refer to Chapter 13 and to Fig. 13.16 for further information on the pulmonary lymphatics.

Bibliography

Adams, D. R. (1992). Fine structure of the vomeronasal and septal olfactory epithelia and of glandular structures. *Microsc Res Tech*, 23, 86–97.

Adams, D. R., & Hotchkiss, K. K. (1983). The canine nasal mucosa. *Anat Histol Embryol*, 12, 109–125.

Adams, D. R., & Wiekamp, M. D. (1984). The canine vomeronasal organ. *J Anat*, 138, 771–788.

Adams, D. R., Deyoung, D. W., & Griffith, R. (1981). The lateral nasal gland of dog: its structure and secretory content. *J Anat*, 132, 29–38.

Allison, A. C. (1953). The morphology of the olfactory system in the vertebrates. *Biol Rev*, 28, 195–244.

Amis, T. C., & McKiernan, B. C. (1986). Systematic identification of endobronchial anatomy during bronchoscopy in the dog. *Am J Vet Res*, 47, 2649–2657.

Andrew, B. L. (1954). A laryngeal pathway for aortic baroreceptor impulses. *J Physiol (Lond)*, 125, 352–360.

Angulo, A. W., Kownacki, V. P., & Hessert, E. C., Jr. (1958). Additional evidence of collateral ventilation between adjacent bronchopulmonary segments. *Anat Rec*, 130, 207–211.

Barone, R. (1957). Arbre bronchique et vaisseaux pulmonaires chez le chien. *Compt Ren Assoc Anat*, 44, 132–144.

Bartlett, D. (1986). Upper airway motor systems. In N. S. Cherniack & J. G. Widdicombe (Eds.), *Handbook of physiology* (Vol. 2). Control of breathing. Bethesda, MD: Amer Physiol Soc.

Berry, J. L., Brailsford, J. F., & Daly, I. B. (1931). The bronchial vascular system in the dog. *Proc R Soc Lond B*, 109, 214–228.

Blatt, C. M., Taylor, C. R., & Habal, M. B. (1972). Thermal panting in dogs: the lateral nasal gland, a source of water for evaporative cooling. *Science*, 177, 804–805.

Bojsen-Møller, F. (1964). Topography of the nasal glands in rats and some other mammals. *Anat Rec*, 150, 11–24.

Bojsen-Møller, F. (1967). Topography and development of anterior nasal glands in pigs. *J Anat*, 101, 321–331.

Bojsen-Møller, F. (1975). Demonstration of terminalis, olfactory, trigeminal, and perivascular nerves in the rat nasal septum. *J Comp Neurol*, 159, 245–256.

Bojsen-Møller, F., & Fahrenkrug, J. (1971). Nasal swell bodies and cyclic changes in the air passage of the rat and rabbit nose. *J Anat*, 110, 25–37.

Bourdelle, E., & Bressou, C. (1927). Le cul de sac anterieur de la caveté pleurale chez les carnivores en particulier chez le chien et chez le chat. *Rec Méd Vét*, 103, 457–466.

Bowden, R. E. M., & Scheuer, J. L. (1961). Comparative studies of the nerve supply of the larynx in eutherian mammals. *Proc Zool Soc London*, 136, 325–330.

Boyden, E. A., & Tompsett, D. H. (1961). The postnatal growth of the lung in the dog. *Acta Anat (Basel)*, 47, 185–215.

Cardoso, L., Gil, F., Ramirez, G., et al. (2007). Computed tomography (CT) of the lungs of the dog using a helical CT scanner, iodine contrast medium, and different CT windows. *Anat Histol Embryol*, 36(5), 328–331.

Coldea, N. (1994). Nose prints as a method of identification in dogs. *Vet Q*, 16(sup1), 60. doi:10.1080/01652176.1994.9694497.

Correll, N. O., Jr., & Langston, H. T. (1958). Pulmonary lymphatic drainage in the dog. *Surg Gynecol Obstet*, 107, 284–286.

Craven, B. A., Newberger, T., Paterson, E. G., et al. (2007). Reconstruction and morphometric analysis of the nasal airway of the dog (*Canis familiaris*) and implications regarding olfactory airflow. *Anat Rec*, 290(11), 1325–1340.

Dabanoglu, I., Ocal, M. K., & Kora, M. E. (2001). A quantitative study on the trachea of the dog. *Anat Histol Embryol*, 30(1), 57–59.

De Rycke, L. M., Saunders, J. H., Gielen, I. M., et al. (2003). Magnetic resonance imaging, computed tomography, and cross-sectional views of the anatomy of normal nasal cavities and paranasal sinuses in mesaticephalic dogs. *Am J Vet Res*, 64(9), 1093–1098.

DeLorenzi, D. D., Bertoncello, D., & Drigo, M. (2009). Bronchial abnormalities found in a consecutive series of 40 brachycephalic dogs. *J Am Vet Med Assoc*, 235, 835–840.

Done, S. H. (1978). Canine tracheal collapse: aetiology, pathology, diagnosis, and treatment. *Vet Ann*, 18, 255–260.

Dorriety, J. K. (2007). Cadaver dogs as a forensic tool: an analysis of prior studies. *J Forensic Ident*, 57(5), 717–725.

Doty, R. L. (1976). *Mammalian olfaction, reproductive processes and behavior*. New York: Academic Press.

Duckworth, W. L. H. (1912). On some points in the anatomy of the plica vocalis. *J Anat Physiol*, 47, 80–115.

Dzieciol, M., Politowicz, J., Szumny, A., & Niżański, W. (2014). Methyl paraben as a sex pheromone in canine uring- is the question still open? *Pol J Vet Sci*, 17, 601–605. doi:10.2478/pjvs-2014-0090.

Eisenberg, J. F., & Kleiman, D. G. (1972). Olfactory communication in mammals. *Annu Rev Ecol Systemat*, 3, 1–32.

Eisthen, H. L. (1997). Evolution of vertebrate olfactory systems. *Brain Behav Evol*, 50, 222–233.

Estes, R. (1972). The role of the vomeronasal organ in mammalian reproduction. *Mammalia*, 36, 315–341.

Evans, H. E. (1977). The lateral nasal gland and its duct in the dog. *Anat Rec*, 187, 574–575.

Flanders, J. A., & Thompson, M. S. (2009). Dyspnea caused by epiglottic retroversion in two dogs. *J Am Vet Med Assoc*, 235, 1330–1335.

Franzmann, A. F. (1907). *Beiträge zur vergleichenden anatomie und histologie des kehlkopfes der Säugetiere mit besonderer Berücksichtigung der Haussaügetiere*. Bonn: C. Georgi.

Gendron, K., McDonough, S. P., Flanders, J. A., et al. (2018). The pathogenesis of paraesophageal empyema in dogs and constancy of radiographic and computed tomography signs are linked to involvement of the mediastinal serous cavity. *Vet Radio Ultrasound*, 2, 1–11. doi:10.1111/vru.12582.

Goodwin, M., Gooding, K. M., & Regnier, F. (1979). Sex pheromone in the dog. *Science*, 203, 559–561.

Graeger, K. (1958). Die Nasenhöhle und die Nasennebenhöhlen beim hund unter Besonderer berucksichtigung der Siebbeinmuscheln. *Dtsch Tierärztl Wschr, 65,* 425–429, 468–472.

Holt, D. E., Cole, S. G., Anderson, R. B., et al. (2005). The canine right caudal and accessory lobe pulmonary veins: revised anatomical description, clinical relevance, and embryological implications. *Anat Histol Embryol, 34*(4), 273–275.

Horning, J. G., McKee, A. J., Keller, H. E., et al. (1926). Nose printing your cat and dog patients. *Vet Med, 21,* 432–453.

Ishaq, M. (1980). A morphological study of the lungs and bronchial tree of the dog: with a suggested system of nomenclature for bronchi. *J Anat, 131,* 589–610.

Karpelowsky, J. S., Wieselthaler, N., & Rode, H. (2006). Primary paraesophageal hernia in children. *J Pediatr Surg, 41,* 1588–1593.

Kilpper, R. W., & Stidd, P. J. (1973). A wet-lung technique for obtaining silastic rubber casts of the respiratory airways. *Anat Rec, 176,* 279–287.

Kratzing, J. (1971). The structure of the vomeronasal organ in the sheep. *J Anat, 108,* 247–260.

Kunath, U. (1977). Die bedeutung der Bursa infracardiaca für die Pathogenese der Hiatusgleithernie. *Langenbecks Arch Surg, 343,* 161–172.

Laitinen, A., Laitinen, L. A., Moss, R., et al. (1989). Organization and structure of the tracheal and bronchial blood vessels in the dog. *J Anat, 165,* 133–140.

Lemere, F. (1932a). Innervation of the larynx. I. innervation of laryngeal muscles. *Am J Anat, 51,* 417–437.

Lemere, F. (1932b). Innervation of the larynx. II. Ramus anastomoticus and ganglion cells of the superior laryngeal nerve. *Anat Rec, 54,* 389–407.

Lemere, F. (1933). Innervation of the larynx. III. Experimental paralysis of the laryngeal nerves. *Arch Otolaryngol, 18,* 413–424.

Leonard, H. C. (1956). Surgical relief for stenotic nares in a dog. *J Am Vet Med Assoc, 128,* 530.

Loosli, C. G. (1937). Interalveolar communications in normal and in pathologic mammalian lungs. *Arch Pathol, 24,* 743–776.

Macklin, C. C. (1922). A note on the elastic membrane of the bronchial tree of mammals with an interpretation of its functional significance. *Anat Rec, 24,* 119–135.

Mann, G. (1961). Bulbus olfactorius accessorius in chiroptera. *J Comp Neurol, 116,* 135–144.

Mauderly, J. L., & Hahn, F. F. (1982). The effects of age on lung function and structure of adult animals. *Adv Vet Sci Comp Med, 26,* 35–77.

McCotter, R. E. (1912). The connection of the vomeronasal nerves with the accessory olfactory bulb in the opossum and other animals. *Anat Rec, 6,* 299–317.

McLaughlin, R. F., Tyler, W. S., & Canada, R. O. (1961). A study of the subgross pulmonary anatomy in various mammals. *Am J Anat, 108,* 149–165.

Meadows, L. B. (2005). *Pet identification system and method,* US Patent No.: US6,845,382 B2.

Michel, R. P. (1982). Arteries and veins of the normal dog lung: qualitative and quantitative structural differences. *Am J Anat, 164,* 227–241.

Miller, W. S. (1900). Das Lungenläppchen, seine Blutund Lymphgefässe, *Arch Anat Physiol Anat Abtheilung* 197–228.

Miller, W. S. (1937). *The lung.* Springfield, IL: Charles C Thomas.

Negus, V. E. (1949). *The comparative anatomy and physiology of the larynx.* London: W. Heinemann Ltd.

Negus, V. E. (1958). *The comparative anatomy and physiology of the nose and paranasal sinuses.* Edinburgh: Livingstone.

Notkovitch, H. (1957). Anatomy of the bronchial arteries of the dog. *J Thorac Surg, 33,* 242–253.

Osterkamp, T. (2011). K9 water searches: scent and scent transportation considerations. *J Forensic Sci, 56*(4), 907–912.

Pearsall, M. D., & Verbruggen, H. (1982). *Scent: training to track, search, and rescue.* Loveland, CO: Alpine Pub.

Phalen, R. F., & Oldham, M. J. (1983). Tracheobronchial airway structure as revealed by casting techniques. *Am Rev Respir Dis, 128,* 1–4.

Piérard, J. (1963). *Comparative anatomy of the carnivore larynx, Thesis.* Ithaca, NY: Cornell University.

Piérard, J. (1965). Anatomie comparée du larynx du chien et d'autres carnivores. *Can Vet J, 6,* 11–15.

Pressman, J. L., & Kelemen, G. (1955). Physiology of the larynx. *Physiol Rev, 35,* 506–554.

Ramser, R. (1935). *Zur anatomie des jakobsonschen organs beim hunde, Dissertation.* Berlin: Friedrich Wilhelms University.

Read, E. A. (1908). A contribution to the knowledge of the olfactory apparatus in dog, cat, and man. *Am J Anat, 8,* 17–47.

Réthi, A. (1951). Histological analysis of the experimentally degenerated vagus nerve. *Acta Morph Acad Sci Hung Tome I Fasc, 2,* 221–230.

Rivero, M. A., Ramirez, J. A., Vazquez, J. M., et al. (2005). Normal anatomical imaging of the thorax in three dogs: computed tomography and macroscopic cross-sections with vascular injection. *Anat Histol Embryol, 34,* 215–219.

Robinson, N. E. (1982). Some functional consequences of species differences in lung anatomy. *Adv Vet Sci Comp Med, 26,* 1–33.

Salazar, I., Rueda, A., & Cifuentes, J. M. (1984). Anatomy of the vomeronasal organ in the dog. *Folia Morphol (Praha), 32,* 331–341.

Scalia, F., & Winans, S. S. (1976). New perspectives on the morphology of the olfactory system: olfactory and vomeronasal pathways in mammals. In R. L. Doty (Ed.), *Mammalian olfaction, reproductive processes, and behavior.* New York: Academic Press.

Schlesinger, R. B., & McFadden, L. A. (1981). Comparative morphometry of the upper bronchial tree in six mammalian species. *Anat Rec, 199,* 99–108.

Schmidt-Nielsen, K., Bretz, W. L., & Taylor, C. R. (1970). Panting in dogs: unidirectional air flow over evaporative surfaces. *Science, 169,* 1102–1104.

Schneider, K. M. (1930). Das flehmen. *Zeit f Gesamte Tiergartnerei Leipzig, 3,* 183–198.

Schreider, J. P., & Raabe, O. G. (1981). Anatomy of the nasal-pharyngeal airway of experimental animals. *Anat Rec, 200,* 195–205.

Shishkin, G. S., Valitskaia, R. I., & Voevoda, T. V. (1989). Quantitative analysis of the bronchial tree structure in dogs and polar foxes. *Arkh Anat Gistol Embriol, 97,* 47–49.

Strohl, K. P., Butler, J. P., & Malhotra, A. (2012). Mechanical properties of the upper airway. *Compr Physiol, 2,* 1853–1872. doi:10.1002/cphy.c110053.

Taniguchi, K., & Taniguchi, K. (2014). Phylogentic studies on the olfactory system in vertebrates. *J Vet Med Sci, 76,* 781–786.

Tembrock, G. (1976). Canid vocalizations. *Behav Process, 1,* 57–75.

Tucker, J. L., Jr., & Krementz, E. T. (1957a). Anatomical corrosion specimens. I. heart-lung models prepared from dogs. *Anat Rec, 127,* 655–665, 667–676.

Tucker, J. L., Jr., & Krementz, E. T. (1957b). Anatomical corrosion specimens. II. Bronchopulmonary anatomy in the dog. *Anat Rec, 127,* 667–676.

Vasquez, J. M., Arencibia, A., Gil, F., et al. (1990). Magnetic resonance imaging of the normal canine larynx. *Anat Histol Embryol, 27*(4), 263–270.

Vogel, P. H. (1952). The innervation of the larynx of man and the dog. *Am J Anat, 90*, 427–447.

Watson, A. G. (1974). *Some aspects of the vagal innervation of the canine esophagus: an anatomical study,* Masters thesis. New Zealand: Massey University.

Wee, N. S., Choi, S. J., & Kim, H. M. (2014). *Device and method for recognizing animal's identity by using animal nose prints,* US 20160259970 A1.

Widdicombe, J. G. (1986). Reflexes from the upper respiratory tract. In N. S. Cherniack & J. G. Widdicombe (Eds.), *Handbook of physiology* (Vol. 2). Bethesda, MD: Amer Physiol Soc.

Zanoni, M. M., Morris, A., Messer, M., & Martinez, R. (1998). Forensic evidence canines: status, training and utilization. Paper presented at the annual meeting of the American Academy of Forensic Sciences, San Francisco, CA.

9
The Urogenital System

Urinary Organs

The **urogenital system** (*apparatus urogenitalis*) is so named because of similar embryologic origins of several component parts and some of the same functional structures in the adults of both sexes. Urinary organs are the first to develop, and several of the early kidney ducts are appropriated by the male reproductive system. There are remnant structures in each sex that are functional components of the other. Because of this commonality in development and the fact that genetic anomalies or hormonal influences in early development can alter the morphologic characteristics of the system, there are frequent instances of malformation. Hollow remnants in either sex are prone to forming fluid-filled cysts.

Intersexes and disorders of sexual development in the dog are common (Hare, 1976; Meyers-Wallen & Patterson, 1986). A dog may be a genetic female with a bicornuate uterus and have abdominal testes (Bodner, 1987 in a Doberman; Stewart et al., 1972 in a Pug). For a comprehensive review of intersexes and freemartins and a well-referenced general treatment of the reproductive system in vertebrates see van Tienhoven (1983) and Lamming (1990). A perceptive book by Willis (1962) provides a background for an understanding of pathologic problems resulting from the duality in development of the urogenital system, as does the embryology text by Noden and de Lahunta (1985) and McGeady et al. (2009). Pathologic conditions of the reproductive system have been discussed by McEntee (1990) and congenital malformations by Szabo (1989).

Urinary organs (*organa urinaria*) include the **kidneys** (*renes*), **ureters**, **bladder** (*vesica urinaria*), and **urethra** (*urethra masculina, urethra feminina*).

Kidneys

The **kidney** (*ren*), *nephros* in Greek (Figs. 9.1 to 9.5), is a reddish-brown, paired structure lying against the lumbar hypaxial muscles on either side of the vertebral column. Each kidney has a cranial and a caudal pole, a medial and a lateral border, and a dorsal and a ventral surface. The cranial and caudal extremities are joined by a convex lateral border. The medial border has an indentation, the **hilus**, that defines a space, the **renal sinus**. The sinus contains the ureter, renal artery and vein, lymph vessels, and nerves. Of these structures, the renal artery is the most dorsal and the renal vein the most ventral. Commonly the renal vein is paired on one or both sides, and sometimes the renal artery may also be paired. The nerves and lymphatics lie in close relationship to the renal vein (Bulger et al., 1979).

Both kidneys are retroperitoneal. The dorsal surface is in contact with lumbar hypaxial muscles and often surrounded by fat; the ventral surface is covered by transparent parietal peritoneum. Each lies lateral to the aorta and caudal vena cava. The dorsal surface of each kidney is less convex than the ventral surface. The cranial pole of each kidney is covered with peritoneum on both the dorsal and the ventral surfaces, whereas only the ventral surface of the caudal pole is covered.

The kidneys lie in an oblique position, tilted cranioventrally. The right kidney is more firmly attached to the dorsal wall than is the left and has a correspondingly larger retroperitoneal area. Both kidneys are invested with a fibrous capsule surrounded by adipose tissue and are held in position by transversalis fascia. They are not rigidly fixed and may move during respiration or may be displaced by a full stomach. In some lean animals it is possible to palpate the kidneys, especially the left kidney. The right kidney lies more cranially than the left (see Fig. 9.1) and is in contact with the liver. Grandage (1975) has considered some effects of posture on the radiographic appearance of the kidney.

The kidney of an average-sized dog measures 6 to 9 cm in length, 4 to 5 cm in width, and 3 to 4 cm in thickness. The weight of the freshly excised kidney averages 25 to 35 g. Finco et al. (1971) made kidney measurements on radiographs of 27 normal male dogs prior to direct measurement at necropsy to establish a basis for estimating kidney size radiographically. Kidney weight and volume were highly correlated; kidney length was best correlated with kidney weight. Several tables of normal values and variations were presented.

Fixation

A thin **fibrous capsule** (*capsula fibrosa*) covers the surface of the kidney. The capsule follows the hilus to line the walls of the sinus and to form the adventitia of the renal pelvis. It also invests the renal vessels and nerves before they pass into the sinus. The fibrous capsule of normal kidneys is easily removable, except in the renal sinus, where it is adherent to blood vessels and to the **renal pelvis** (*pelvis renalis*). Fat of

CHAPTER 9 The Urogenital System 417

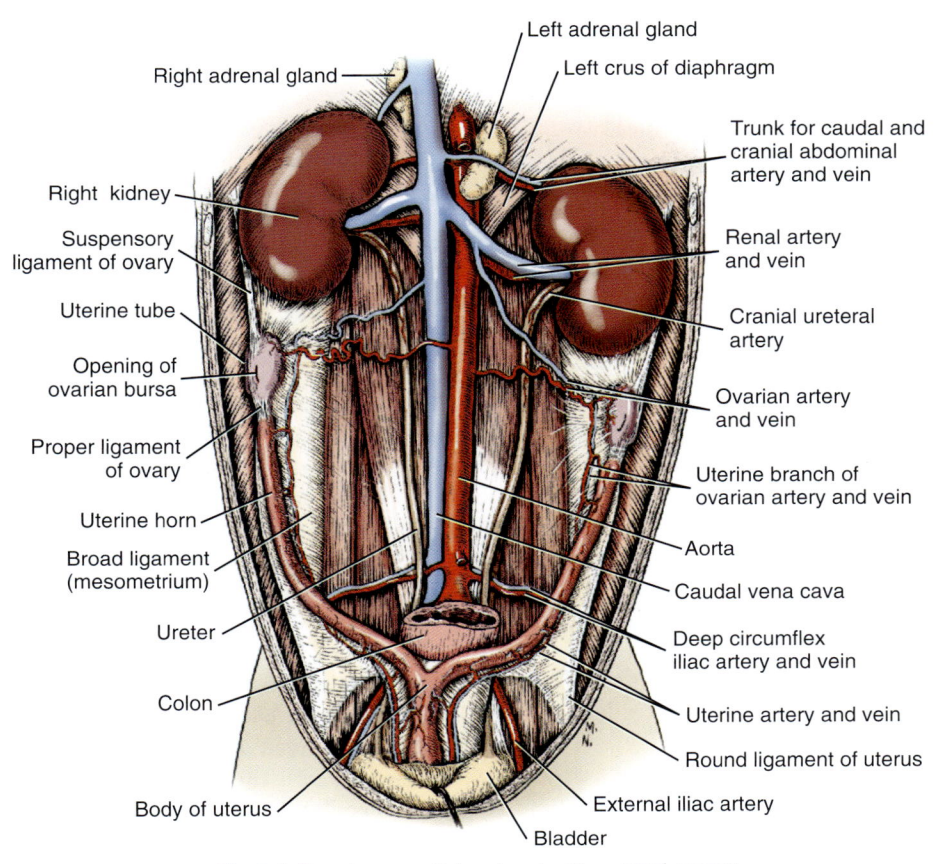

• **Fig. 9.1** Female urogenital system in situ, ventral aspect.

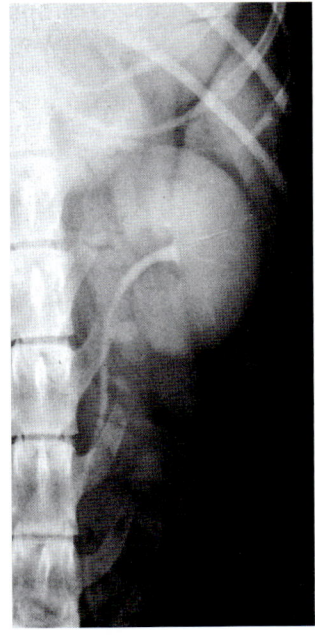

• **Fig. 9.2** Dorsoventral contrast radiograph of the left kidney and ureter.

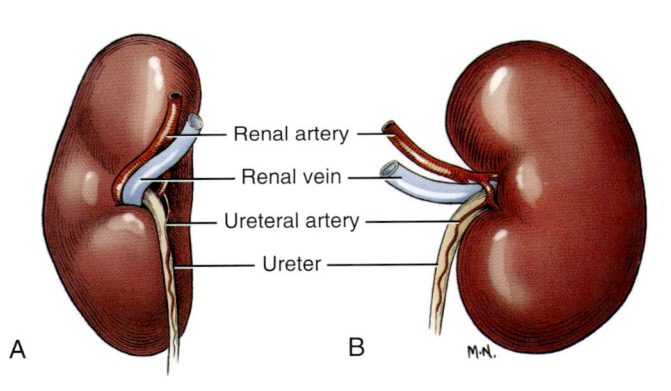

• **Fig. 9.3** Right kidney, and vessels of hilus. A, Medial aspect. B, Dorsal aspect.

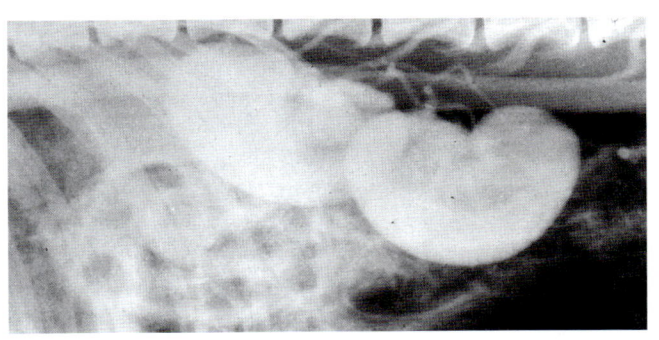

• **Fig. 9.4** Left to right lateral contrast abdominal radiograph of the kidneys. The right kidney is more firmly attached to the dorsal wall and is cranial to the left.

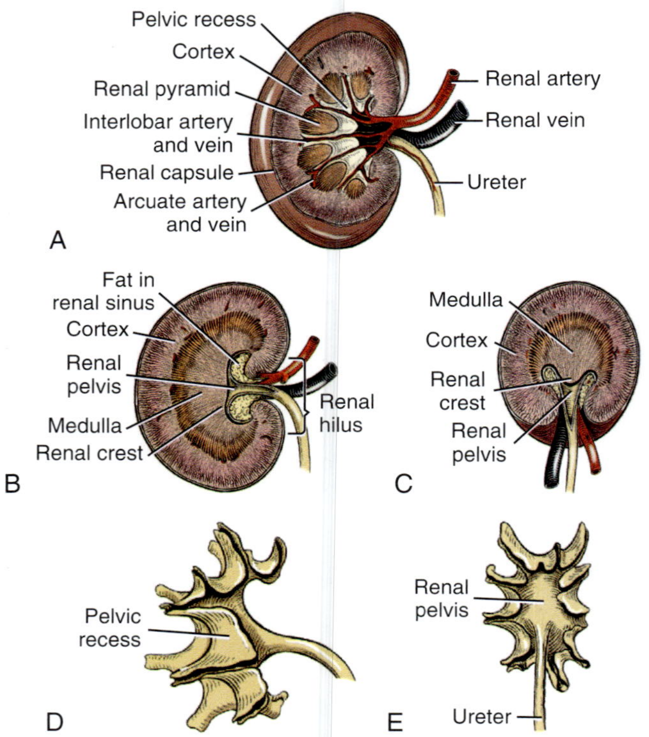

Fig. 9.5 Details of structure of left kidney. **A**, Dorsal aspect, dissected in dorsal plane. **B**, Dorsal aspect, internal surface mid-dorsal plane. **C**, Cross-section. **D**, Cast of renal pelvis, dorsal aspect. **E**, Cast of renal pelvis, medial aspect.

the **adipose capsule** (*capsula adiposa*), in which the kidney is partially embedded is external to the fibrous capsule and extends through the hilus into the sinus.

Position and Relations

The craniolateral surface of the left kidney is in contact with the dorsal end of the medial surface of the spleen, the greater omentum, and the greater curvature of the stomach. Cranially it is in contact with the left lobe of the pancreas and left adrenal gland. Dorsally the kidney, with its adipose capsule, is related to the quadratus lumborum, transversus abdominis, and psoas muscles, as well as to the deep layer of the thoracolumbar fascia underlying the retroperitoneal or pararenal fat. Caudally the left kidney of the female is in contact with the descending colon and the mesovarium. The peritoneum on the ventral surface of the kidney blends with the peritoneum suspending the ovary. In the male, the renal peritoneum is reflected onto the dorsal body wall as parietal peritoneum. Medially the left kidney of the male is related to the left adrenal gland descending colon, mesocolon, and ascending duodenum. The descending colon is also related to the ventral surface of the kidney. The medial edge of the left kidney is located approximately 1 cm from the mid-dorsal line in an average-sized dog; the cranial pole lies approximately 5 cm caudal to the dorsal third of the last rib.

The right kidney has its cranial pole embedded in the fossa of the caudate process of the caudate lobe of the liver. This extremity is located at the level of the thirteenth rib. It may be a few centimeters craniad or caudad, depending on the degree of gastric or, in the female, uterine distention. It may be in contact with the diaphragm and retractor costae muscle. The right adrenal gland is also related to the cranial pole of the right kidney. Medially the right kidney is in close proximity to the caudal vena cava, and, ventrally, it is in contact with the right lobe of the pancreas and the ascending colon.

The kidney has an indentation or cavity on its medial border referred to as the **renal hilus** (*hilus renalis*). The space defined by the walls of the hilus is the **renal sinus** (*sinus renalis*) (see Figs. 9.3 and 9.5). The sinus contains the renal pelvis, a variable amount of adipose tissue, and branches of the renal artery, vein, lymphatics, and nerves. After they pass through the sinus, the vessels and nerves enter the parenchyma of the kidney.

The **renal pelvis** (*pelvis renalis*) (see Fig. 9.5) is a funnel-shaped structure that receives urine from the papillary ducts of the kidney and passes it into the ureter. The pelvis of the kidney is elongated in a craniocaudal direction and is curved to conform with the lateral border of the kidney. It extends into the renal parenchyma both dorsally and ventrally by means of curved diverticula, the recesses of the renal pelvis (*recessus pelvis*). There are generally five or six recesses curving peripherally from each border of the pelvis.

Structure

The parenchyma of the kidney is made up of an internal **medulla** (*medulla renis*) and an external **cortex** (*cortex renis*) (see Fig. 9.5). When cut transversely (see Fig. 9.5C) the peripheral portion of the renal parenchyma or cortex appears granular, owing to the presence of numerous renal corpuscles and convoluted tubules (nephrons). When the kidney is cut in a dorsal plane, numerous cut ends of arcuate arteries and veins are apparent at the corticomedullary junction. The thickness of the renal cortex is approximately the same as the transverse diameter of the renal medulla. The peripheral surface of the cortex is covered by the fibrous capsule.

A median plane longitudinal section of the kidney shows the medulla as a continuous striated structure with its free edge facing the renal pelvis. This is the **renal crest** (*crista renalis*). Similar dorsal plane longitudinal sections on either side of the renal crest show the medulla separated into cone-shaped **renal papillae** (*papilla renalis*) with interlobar vessels between them. These renal papillae are the apices of the **renal pyramids** (*pyramides renales*), the base of which is at the level of the renal cortex. These pyramids extend from the cortex on the dorsal and ventral surfaces of the kidney into the center where they fuse into the renal crest. A variable number **papillary foraminae** (*foramina papillaria*) open on the border of the renal crest that faces the renal pelvis. These are the openings of the **papillary ducts** (*ductus papillares*) that pass urine into the renal pelvis, which leads to the ureter. These foraminae compose the **area cribrosa** of the renal crest. The renal papillae of the pyramids are surrounded by extensions of the renal pelvis called **pelvic**

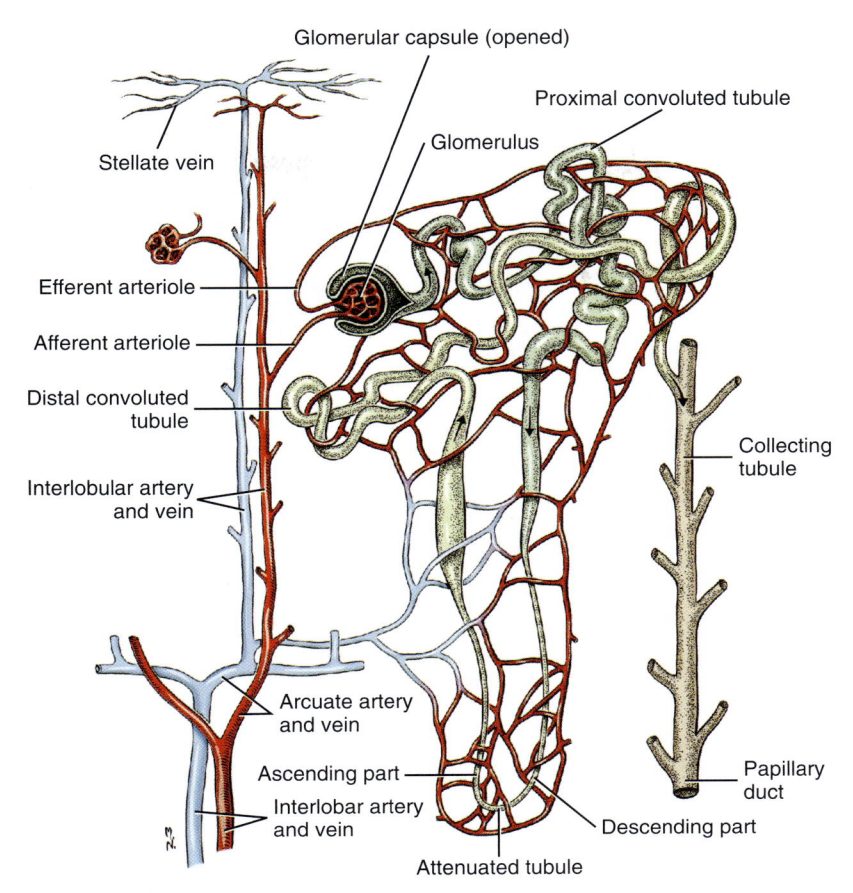

Fig. 9.6 Schema of vessels around the nephron or renal tubule.

recesses (*recessus pelvis*) but there are no papillary foraminae on these papillae.

The Nephron

The **nephron** (*nephronum*) (Fig. 9.6) is a continuous contorted tube that serves for urine production and for the regulation of the volume and composition of the extracellular fluid (Reese, 1991). There are approximately 500,000 nephrons in the dog kidney. Each nephron begins at the double-layered **glomerular capsule** (*capsula glomeruli*), which is invaginated by a spherical rete of blood capillaries, the **glomerulus**. Vimtrup (1928) commented on the number, shape, and structure of glomeruli in several mammals. The glomerulus and capsule together form the **renal corpuscle** (*corpusculum renale*) (see Fig. 9.6). Renal corpuscles are present in the renal cortex, but not in the medulla. The following components compose the tubular nephron in order from the glomerular capsule to the collecting tubules and papillary ducts in the renal medulla: proximal convoluted tubule, proximal straight tubule, attenuated (thin) tubule that forms a loop, distal straight tubule, and distal convoluted tubule.

Eisenbrandt and Phemister (1979) investigated normal postnatal development of the dog kidney in puppies between 2 and 200 days of age. They found a subcapsular nephrogenic zone was present until approximately 8 days of age. This zone produced new nephrons and interstitial tissues. Deep to the nephrogenic zone there were renal corpuscles of increasing maturity at successively deeper levels. They estimated the total number of nephrons to be 445,000 per kidney, and this did not vary significantly during subsequent growth. The corpuscular volume per nephron increased 249% between day 14 and day 200, whereas the increase in the tubular volume per nephron was 303%.

Books on renal morphology and function include Smith (1951); *The Kidney*, in four volumes, by Rouiller and Muller (1969–1971); and *The Kidney*, in two volumes, by Brenner and Rector (1991).

Vessels and Nerves

The kidney is a highly vascular organ, as would be expected (Fuller & Heulke, 1973; Morison, 1926). Briefly, blood enters the renal artery from the aorta, goes through end arteries, interlobar vessels, arcuate vessels, interlobular arteries, and finally to glomeruli via afferent arterioles. Efferent arterioles leave the glomeruli and course directly into the outer layer of the medulla, giving rise to long capillary nets that extend to the apical end of the pyramid, or they branch directly into intertubular capillary networks. The intrarenal vascular system of the puppy kidney was described by Evan et al. (1979).

The **renal artery** (*arteria renis*) bifurcates into dorsal and ventral branches. The site of bifurcation is extremely variable (Christensen, 1952). Variations in the renal artery are common, ranging from a single vessel to one with numerous branches or to completely doubled renal arteries. The two primary branches of the renal artery, end branches, divide into two to four **interlobar arteries** (*aa. interlobares renis*). These branch into arcuate arteries at the corticomedullary junction. The **arcuate arteries** (*aa. arcuatae*) radiate toward the periphery of the cortex, where they redivide into numerous **interlobular arteries** (*aa. interlobulares*). **Afferent arterioles** (*arteriola glomerularis afferens*) leave these to supply the glomeruli and thence the **efferent arterioles** (*arteriola glomerularis efferens*). The mean glomerular diameter in a 35-pound dog is 170 μm. According to Rytand (1938), there are 408,100 glomeruli in one canine kidney, with a total glomerular volume of 1247 mm^3. Finco and Duncan (1972) found a correlation between kidney and nephron size and the body size of the dog.

Venous drainage of the kidney stems from the numerous **stellate veins** (*venulae stellatae*) in the fibrous capsule. These connect with veins of the adipose capsule and empty into **interlobular** (*vv. interlobulares*), **arcuate** (*vv. arcuatae*), and **interlobar veins** (*vv. interlobares*) before entering the main trunk of the **renal vein** (*vena renis*), which joins the caudal vena cava. Venous arcuate vessels, unlike their arterial counterparts, unite to form elaborate arches. Arcuate veins span the medulla to join the dorsal and ventral parts of the kidney. Evan et al. (1979) investigated the vascular system of the puppy kidney between 1 and 21 days after birth. They found the vascular system of the puppy kidney to be strikingly different from that of the adult. The most obvious difference was the lack of peritubular capillaries throughout the cortex. In their place were large sinusoidal vessels directly continuous with the venous system. The vascular arrangement of the efferent arterioles and the sinusoidal vessels appeared to function as a postglomerular shunt.

Bentley et al. (1988) examined the architecture and vasculature of the dog kidney using a dynamic spatial reconstructor. This device is a high-speed, volume-scanning, computed, radiotomographic imaging system, which, when used in conjunction with radiopaque methacrylate injections, allowed them to compare casts with the reconstructed images. Interlobar arteries and occasionally arcuate arteries could be clearly detected. Analysis of artery-to-vein transit times showed some to be as short as 3 seconds.

Capsular and parenchymal lymphatics are connected to interlobular plexuses that pass into trunks that leave the kidney at the hilus. They terminate in the lumbar lymph nodes. According to Peirce (1944) lymphatics in the kidney accompany the interlobular, arcuate, and interlobar vessels, surrounding them in an irregular network. The periarterial rete is thicker than the perivenous network. Cortical and perirenal lymphatics anastomose (O'Morchoe & Albertine, 1980).

A **renal plexus** (*plexus renalis*) surrounds the renal arteries where they enter the renal sinus. This plexus consists of postganglionic sympathetic axons with their cell bodies in **aorticorenal ganglia** (*ganglia aorticorenalia*). The plexus also contains preganglionic parasympathetic axons from the vagus nerve. Innervation is provided to the nephrons, blood vessels, and muscle in the renal pelvis.

Anomalies

Malformations of the kidney are fairly common. Congenital renal cysts and polycystic kidneys occur, although isolated renal cysts are more commonly found. Other congenital anomalies include hypoplasia and aplasia (Hofliger, 1971; Pearson & Gibbs, 1971). Fetal lobation of the kidney may persist in the adult dog.

Ureters

The **ureters** (Figs. 9.1, 9.2, 9.7, and 9.8) carry urine from the kidneys to the bladder. The diameter of a single ureter measures 0.6 to 0.9 cm when it is distended. The length of

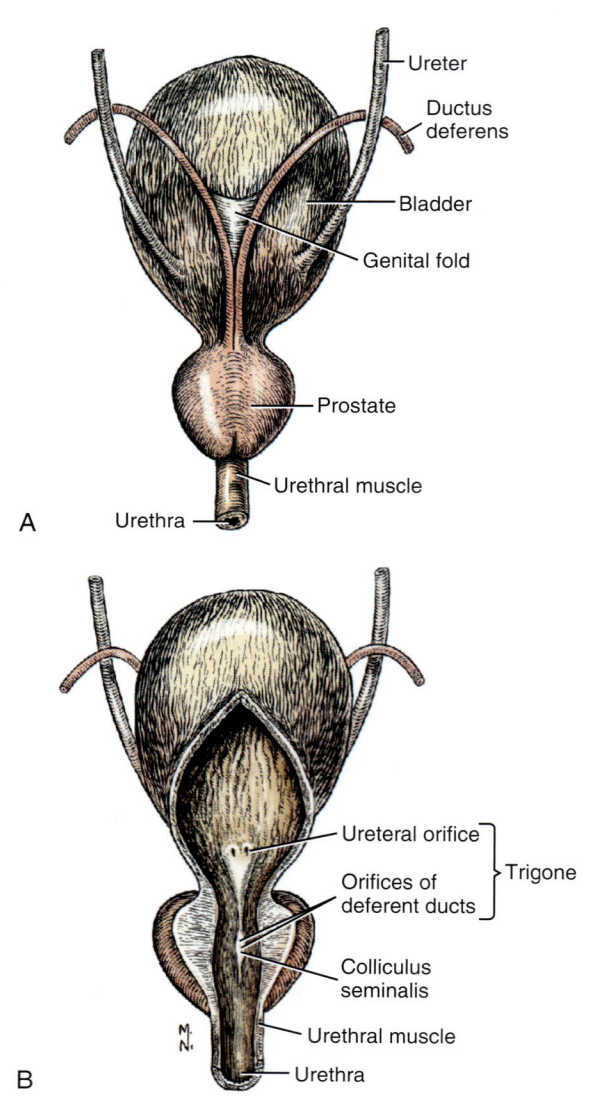

• **Fig. 9.7** Bladder and prostate. **A**, Dorsal aspect. **B**, Ventral aspect, partially opened on midline.

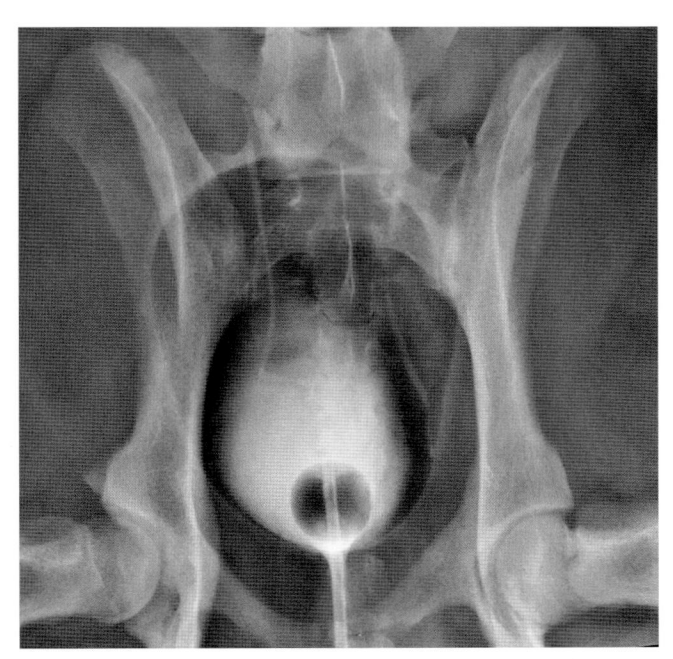

Fig. 9.8 Dorsolateral ventral radiograph of the bladder and ureters.

the ureter depends on the size of the animal, averaging between 12 and 16 cm in a 35-pound dog. The right ureter is slightly longer than the left because of the more cranial position of the right kidney.

The abdominal part of the ureter begins at the renal pelvis, which receives urine from the renal crest. Running caudoventrally and mesially toward the urinary bladder, it is retroperitoneal being bound dorsally by the psoas muscles and ventrally by the peritoneum (see Fig. 9.1). The ureters lie dorsal to the testicular vessels in the male and to the ovarian artery and vein in the female. The right ureter lies in close association with the caudal vena cava and is 1 to 2 cm lateral to the aorta. The ureters pass ventral to the deep circumflex iliac and external iliac arteries and veins. In the male, the ureter crosses dorsal to the ductus deferens, 2 cm from the junction of the ductus deferens with the pelvic urethra. The pelvic part of the ureter enters between the two layers of peritoneum forming the lateral ligament of the bladder and reaches the dorsolateral surface of the bladder just cranial to its neck. In the female, it reaches the lateral ligament of the bladder after being associated with the broad ligament of the uterus. The ureters enter the bladder obliquely and after a short intramural course open by means of two slitlike orifices.

Woodburne and Lapides (1972) studied the size and shape of the dog ureter during peristaltic enlargement. They found it to enlarge 17 times during diuresis by thinning of the muscle coats. The collapsed ureter has a stellate lumen with the epithelial surfaces in contact.

Structure

The muscular wall of the ureter is divided into three thin layers: an outer longitudinal, a middle circular, and an inner longitudinal. Only longitudinal fibers are present at the junction of the ureter with the bladder. The **ureteral mucosa** (*tunica mucosa*) is made up of transitional epithelium.

Vessels and Nerves

The cranial ureteral artery to the ureter is derived from the **renal artery**, whereas the caudal ureteral artery comes from the **prostatic** or **vaginal artery**. Cranial and caudal ureteral arteries anastomose on the ureter. The ureteral arteries have venous counterparts. The autonomic nerves to the ureter come from the celiac and pelvic plexuses.

Anomalies

Congenital anomalies include duplication, ectopic openings into the vagina, ureteral atresia, or dilation of the renal pelvis. The latter condition may result from an obstructed ureter. Obstruction may be caused by calculi, tumors, scars, ligatures, or developmental anomalies.

Urinary Bladder

The **urinary bladder** (*vesica urinaria*) (see Fig. 9.7) is a hollow, musculomembranous organ that varies in form, size, and position, depending on the amount of urine it contains. The bladder in a 25-pound dog is capable of holding 100 to 120 mL of urine without being overly distended. When relaxed, the bladder in a 25-pound dog measures 17.5 cm in diameter and 18 cm in length. When contracted, it measures 2 cm in diameter and 3.2 cm in length. The bladder may arbitrarily be divided into a **neck** (*cervix vesicae*) connecting with the urethra, a **body** (*corpus vesicae*), and a blind cranial part, the **apex** (*apex vesicae*). The visceral peritoneum of the ventral surface of the bladder is separated from the parietal peritoneum of the abdominal wall, just cranial to the pubis. The greater omentum frequently occupies the space between these peritoneal layers. The median ligament of the bladder is the peritoneal fold that attaches the ventral surface of the bladder to the linea alba and symphysis pubis. Dorsally the bladder is in contact with the small intestine (jejunum and frequently ileum) and with the descending colon cranial to the divergence of the uterine horns from the body of the uterus. In the male the deferent ducts and their genital fold lie dorsal to the neck of the bladder, whereas in the female the cervix and body of the uterus are in contact with the dorsal surface of the bladder. When empty, the bladder lies entirely, or almost entirely, within the pelvic cavity. The space on each side of the bladder is occupied by the small intestine.

Structure

There are three layers of muscle in the wall of the urinary bladder, similar to the arrangement of muscle fibers in the ureter: outer and inner longitudinal layers, and a relatively thick middle circular layer. The muscle fibers all take on an oblique appearance at the urethral-bladder junction. This bladder muscle is often referred to as the *detrusor muscle*.

The tunica mucosa of the urinary bladder, like that of the ureter and renal pelvis, is made up of transitional epithelium. It is irregularly folded when the bladder is empty but the mucosal folds disappear during distention. A loose tela submucosa lies between the mucosa and the muscular layer. Internally, a triangular area near the neck of the bladder is termed the **trigone of the bladder** (*trigonum vesicae*). The apex of the trigone is at the urethral orifice, and the base is indicated by a line connecting the ureteral openings. This area is free from the characteristic mucosal folds, but poorly developed ridges, converging toward the urethral crest, denote the boundaries of the trigone.

Fixation

The reflection of the peritoneum from the lateral and ventral surfaces of the urinary bladder to the lateral walls of the pelvis and to the ventral abdominal wall are known as ligaments of the bladder. These are made up of double layers of peritoneum separated by intercalated blood vessels, nerves, lymphatics, and adipose tissue, as well as by the ureters, deferent ducts, and vestiges of embryonic structures. The largest peritoneal fold, the **median ligament of the bladder** (*lig. vesicae medianum*) is reflected from the ventral surface of the bladder to the symphysis pelvis and the linea alba of the abdominal wall as far cranially as the umbilicus. It is median in position and triangular in shape. In the fetus the median ligament contains the urachus (stalk of the embryonic allantois) and the umbilical arteries. These normally disappear shortly after birth, leaving only the peritoneal fold. A vestigial fibrous urachus may sometimes be found in the free edge of the ligament. In an average-sized dog this median ligament has its greatest height caudally (6 cm) and narrows cranially to form an acute angle with the abdominal wall at the umbilicus. Caudally the ligament ends approximately at the level of the vaginovestibular junction in the female and at the level of a transverse plane through the middle of the prostate gland in the male.

The **lateral ligaments of the bladder** (*lig. vesicae laterales*) (Fig. 9.9) connect the lateral surfaces of the bladder to the lateral pelvic walls. They are also triangular in shape. The lateral ligaments of the bladder contain the round ligament of the bladder and the ureter. In the fetus each lateral ligament contains a large umbilical artery that extends cranially along the rudimentary bladder and courses in the median ligament of the bladder with the urachus to the umbilicus. The urachus is the stalk of the allantois, which connects from the apex of the rudimentary bladder to the allantoic portion of the fetal membranes. Before birth, the bilateral umbilical arteries (branches of the internal iliac arteries) carry blood from the fetus to the placenta and are components of the umbilical cord. When the umbilical cord is severed at birth, the arteries retract and become fibrous cords between the bladder and the umbilicus that disappear in the young dog and are rarely visible in adult dogs. The narrowed lumen of each umbilical artery remains patent between the internal iliac artery and the bladder, where the relatively minute cranial vesical artery leaves the umbilical artery to vascularize the apex and body of the bladder. The remnants of these arteries in the lateral ligaments of the bladder are referred to as the **round ligaments of the bladder** (*lig. teres vesicae*). The ureter and round ligament of the bladder cross at nearly right angles to each other at the junction of the broad and lateral ligaments. The ureter is the more mesial of the two structures. The lateral ligaments of the bladder, in the female, blend laterally with the **broad ligament of the uterus** (*mesometrium*) as well as with the lateral pelvic wall. In the male, the ureter and ductus deferens cross each other a few centimeters from the entrance of the ureters into the bladder (see Fig. 9.7). The ductus deferens is suspended by the mesoductus deferens, a fold of peritoneum, which at the vaginal ring separates from the mesorchium, which is the peritoneal fold containing the testicular vessels and nerves. The ductus deferens and its mesoductus deferens course dorsocaudally, dorsal to the ureters in the lateral ligaments of the bladder to terminate in the prostatic urethra. Dorsal to the bladder a short fold of peritoneum connects between each ductus deferens. This is the **genital fold** (*plica genitalis*). In the female this genital fold connects between the two uterine horns. The peritoneal

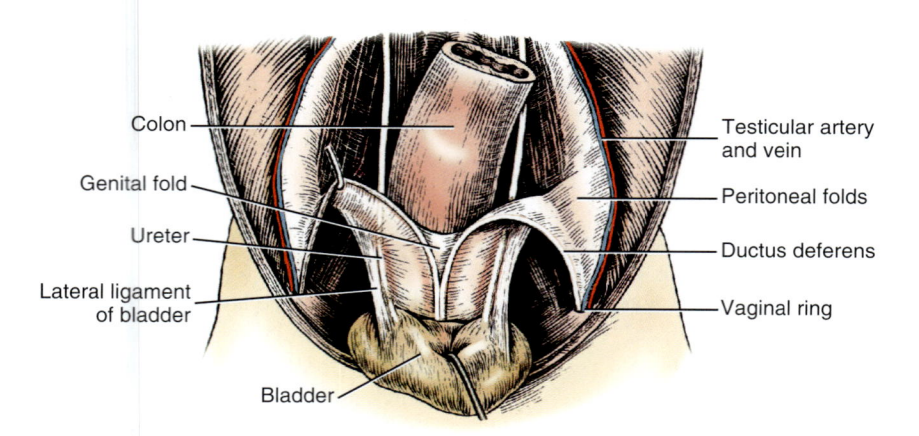

• **Fig. 9.9** Urogenital ligaments of the male, ventral aspect.

pocket between the rectum and the genital fold and the two ductus deferens or the initial part of the two uterine horns, the uterus and cranial vagina is the **rectogenital pouch** (*excavatio rectogenitalis*). A small **pubovesical pouch** (*excavatio pubovesicalis*) is present between the bladder and its lateral ligaments and the pubis

Vessels and Nerves

The urinary bladder receives its major blood supply through the **caudal vesical arteries**. These are branches of the vaginal or prostatic arteries that are branches of the internal pudendals from the internal iliac arteries. The small **cranial vesical artery** from the umbilical supplies the bladder apex. The venous plexus on the urinary bladder drains primarily into the internal pudendal veins. The lymphatics of the bladder drain into the **hypogastric** and **lumbar lymph nodes** (Baum, 1918).

Bladder innervation is complex from an anatomic as well as a physiologic understanding. The bladder receives autonomic innervation from both the sympathetic and parasympathetic general visceral efferent neurons (Drake, 2007). The sympathetic innervation primarily functions in urine storage, and the parasympathetic innervation primarily functions in evacuation of urine. Sympathetic preganglionic cell bodies are located in the lateral horn of the first four lumbar spinal cord segments. Preganglionic axons enter the abdomen through the lumbar sympathetic trunk and splanchnic nerves to synapse on cell bodies of postganglionic axons in the **caudal mesenteric ganglion** or in the bladder wall. For the former, postganglionic axons leave the caudal mesenteric ganglion in the **hypogastric nerves** and course to the **pelvic plexus**, which is associated with the vaginal or prostatic artery. These axons follow the branches of the artery to the bladder to innervate the detrusor muscle with inhibitory synapses and the bladder neck sphincter muscle with excitatory synapses. The sympathetic preganglionic axons that did not synapse in the caudal mesenteric ganglion course to the bladder wall through the hypogastric nerves, the pelvic plexus, and its branches that follow the arteries to the bladder. Synapse occurs on cell bodies of short postganglionic axons within the wall of the bladder. Parasympathetic cell bodies of preganglionic axons are located in the lateral intermediate substance (substantia inermedia lateralis) of the sacral spinal cord segments. The preganglionic axons course into the **pelvic nerve** through the ventral branches of the sacral spinal nerves. The pelvic nerve courses to the pelvic plexus and synapses on cell bodies of postganglionic axons in **pelvic plexus ganglia** or on cell bodies in the bladder wall. These axons of postganglionic cell bodies are excitatory to the detrusor muscle causing contraction and bladder evacuation. The striated **urethralis muscle** which functions to store urine is innervated by general somatic efferent neurons with their cell bodies in the ventral horn of sacral spinal cord segments. Their axons are distributed to this muscle through the sacral plexus and the branches of the **pudendal nerve**. The axons of visceral afferent neurons that innervate the bladder and urethra reverse the pathway of the efferent neurons. Their cell bodies are in cranial lumbar and sacral spinal ganglia. This complex reflex pathway of innervation is under voluntary control by cranially projecting sensory spinal cord pathways, centers in the caudal brainstem, and caudally projecting upper motor neuronal pathways.

Petras and Cummings (1978) describe the location of the cells of origin for the sympathetic and parasympathetic innervation of the urinary bladder and urethra in the dog. Their study, using horseradish peroxidase injected into the bladder and urethra and counterstained with cresyl violet, demonstrates the presence of both sympathetic and parasympathetic intramural ganglia and axons. Thus there is a direct preganglionic sympathetic pathway to the urinary bladder and urethra in addition to the postganglionic sympathetic innervation.

Anomalies

Anomalies of the urinary bladder include diverticula, strictures of the neck of the bladder, urachal cysts, and patent urachus. An enlarged prostate may be the indirect cause of dilation of the bladder.

Reproductive Organs

The reproductive system in vertebrates is a most varied assemblage of primary and accessory organs and parts, which begin developmentally in a similar fashion but result in strikingly different forms in the adult. In recent years the study of reproduction in animals (theriogenology) has made great strides, and, as a result of our new understanding, we are now able to manipulate the system in many ways such as to facilitate artificial insemination, egg or embryo transfer, freezing and storage of eggs and embryos, and cloning of various species. For explanations of developmental processes in domestic animals see Noden and de Lahunta (1985). For an overall view of the reproductive system from fish to humans, there is nothing better than *Marshall's Physiology of Reproduction*. The most recent revision of *Marshall's* by Lamming (1990–1992) devotes one volume to a consideration of reproductive cycles and female anatomy, a second to reproductive structures and functions of the male, and a third to pregnancy and lactation. Other books on the reproductive system include Austin and Short (1982), Segal et al. (1973), and Cupps (1991). For information on the reproductive habits, cycles, and gestations of mammals of the world, including canids, reference should be made to *Asdell's Patterns of Mammalian Reproduction: A Compendium of Species-Specific Data* by Hayssen and van Tienhoven (1993).

Male Genital Organs

The canine male genital organs (*organa genitalia masculina*) (Figs. 9.10 to 9.34) consist of the **scrotum**, the **testes**, the **epididymides**, the **deferent ducts**, the **spermatic cord, the prostate** gland, the **penis**, and the **urethra**.

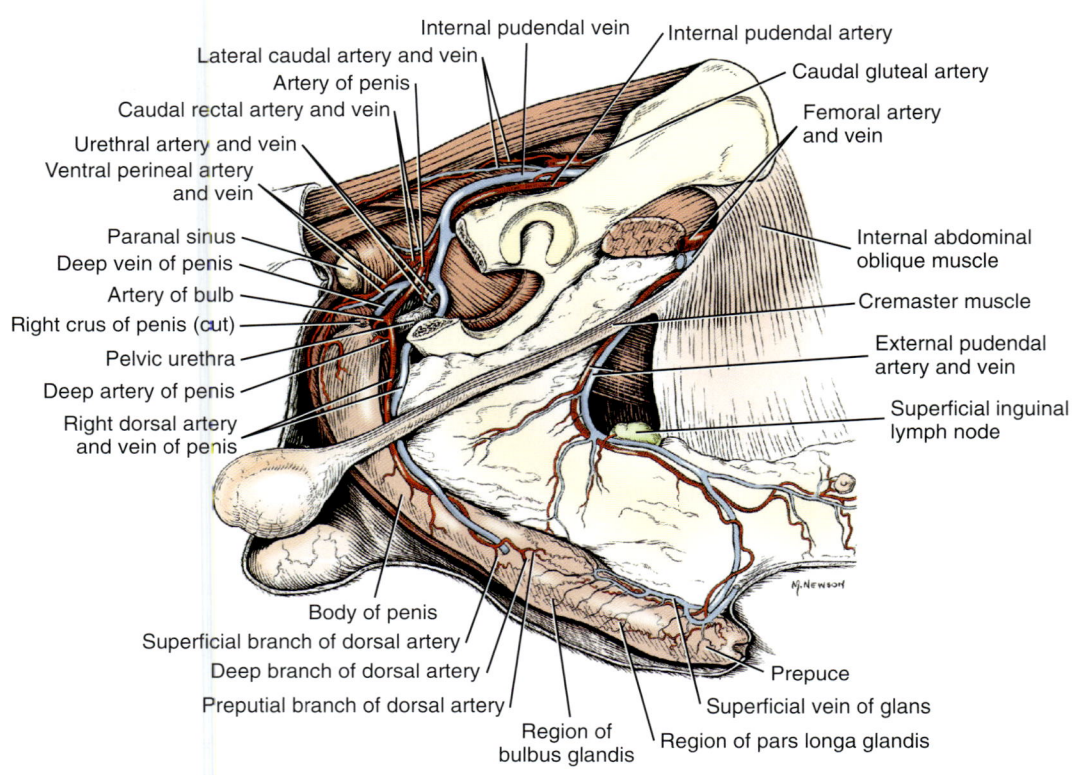

Fig. 9.10 Topographic relations of the penis and other pelvic structures. (The right ischium is removed.) (From Christensen GC: *Angioarchitecture of the canine penis and its role in the process of erection*, Ph.D. Thesis, Ithaca, NY, 1953, Cornell University.)

Scrotum

The **scrotum** (see Figs. 9.14 to 9.16) is a pouch of skin divided by a median septum into two components, each of which is occupied by a testis, an epididymis, and the first part of the spermatic cord. The **scrotal septum** (*septum scroti*) is a median partition that is made up of all the layers of the scrotum except the skin. In the dog, the scrotum is located approximately two-thirds of the distance from the preputial opening to the anus. It lies between the caudal aspect of the thighs and has a spherical shape, indented in an oblique craniocaudal direction by an indistinct raphe scroti. The left testis is usually farther caudad than the right, allowing the surfaces of the testes to glide on each other more easily and with less pressure.

The scrotal integument is pigmented and covered with fine scattered hairs. Sebaceous and tubular (sudoriparous) glands are well developed. Deep to the outer integument of the scrotum is a poorly developed layer of smooth muscle mixed with collagenous and elastic fibers that is sometimes spoken of as the ***tunica dartos***. Dorsally the tissue forming the septum blends with the abdominal fascia. Contraction of the dartos causes the integument of the scrotum to retract and draw the testes close to the body.

Extending into each scrotal sac is an evaginated pouch of peritoneum, the **vaginal tunic** (*tunica vaginalis*) (see Figs. 9.12 and 9.14), covered by spermatic fascia of the abdominal wall. The vaginal tunic and fascia wrap the descended testis and spermatic cord in such a way as to result in a double-walled extension of abdominal peritoneum. This was a vaginal process before the descent of the testis with its duct system, vessels, and nerves (see Figs. 9.12 and 9.15) Zietzsehmann (1928). The outer wall, or parietal layer of the vaginal tunic, is separated by a space, the vaginal canal (*canalis vaginalis*) or vaginal cavity (*cavum vaginale*), from the visceral layer of the vaginal tunic. The vaginal canal surrounds the spermatic cord and the vaginal cavity surrounds the testis. The vaginal canal is continuous with the peritoneal cavity at the vaginal ring.

The development of the vaginal tunic in the male and the vaginal process in the female is similar. As the evaginating peritoneum passes through the deep inguinal ring, it is invested by the **transversalis fascia;** as it emerges from the superficial inguinal ring it is joined by the superficial and deep abdominal fascia. The combined fascias form the **spermatic fascia**, which covers the parietal layer of the vaginal tunic (see Fig. 9.12).

The **cremaster muscle** (see Fig. 9.14) arises from the caudal free border of the internal abdominal oblique (or occasionally from the transversus abdominis) and inserts on the spermatic fascia and parietal layer of the vaginal tunic. The action of the muscle is protective in that it reflexly pulls the testis closer to the body in response to cold.

The scrotum, because of its thin, hairless skin, its lack of subcutaneous fat, and its ability to contract toward the body, functions as a temperature regulator for the tail of

CHAPTER 9 The Urogenital System   425

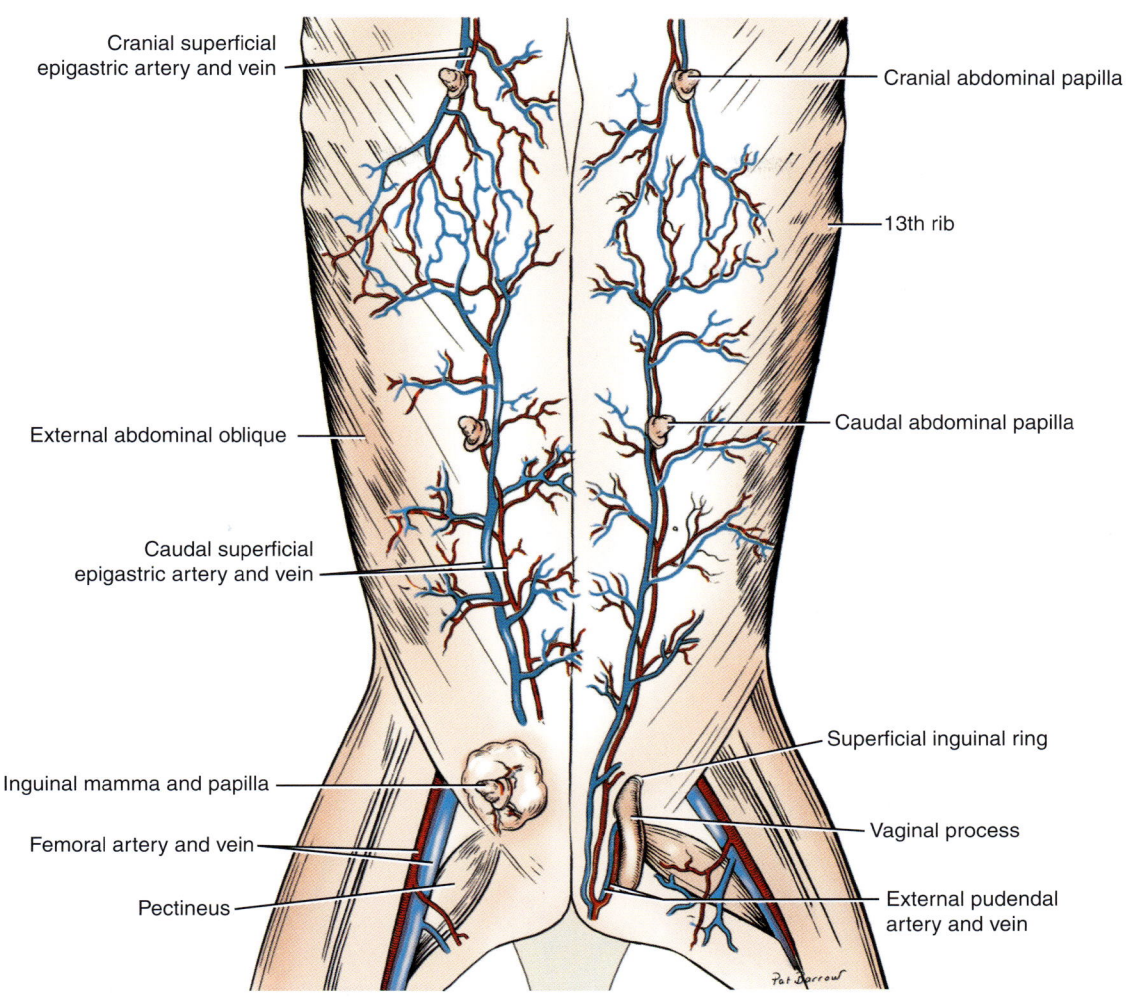

- **Fig. 9.11** Ventral view of the abdomen. The left inguinal mammary gland has been removed to expose the superficial inguinal ring with the vaginal process of the female extending through it. (Fig. 9.13 is a transection of the process to show that it is collapsed and wrapped around fat and the round ligament of the uterus.)

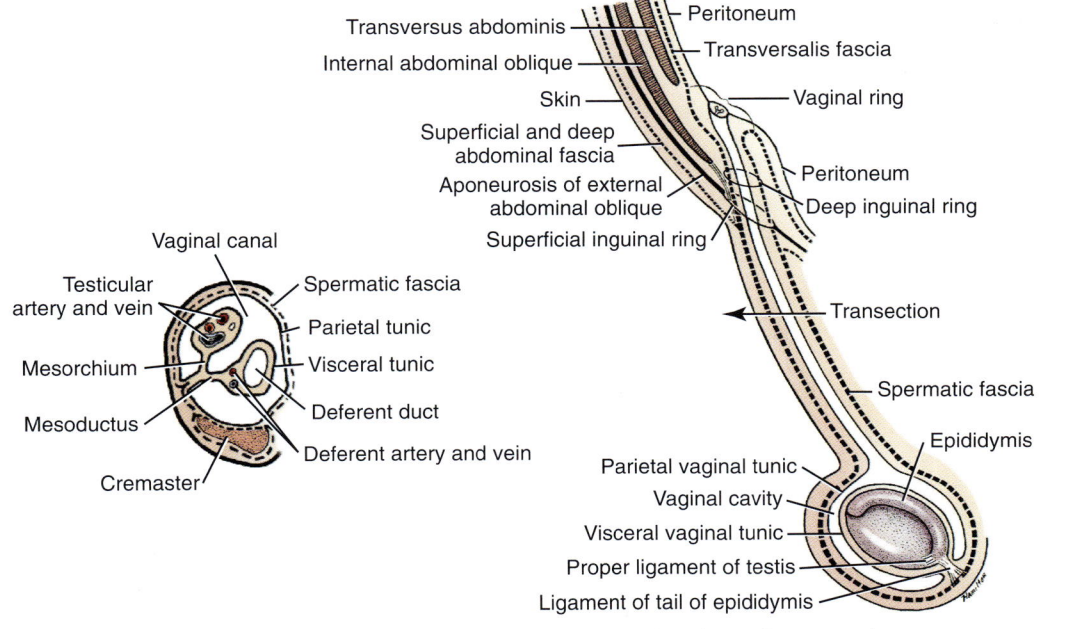

- **Fig. 9.12** Schema of the vaginal tunic in the male with an inset of a transection.

426 CHAPTER 9 The Urogenital System

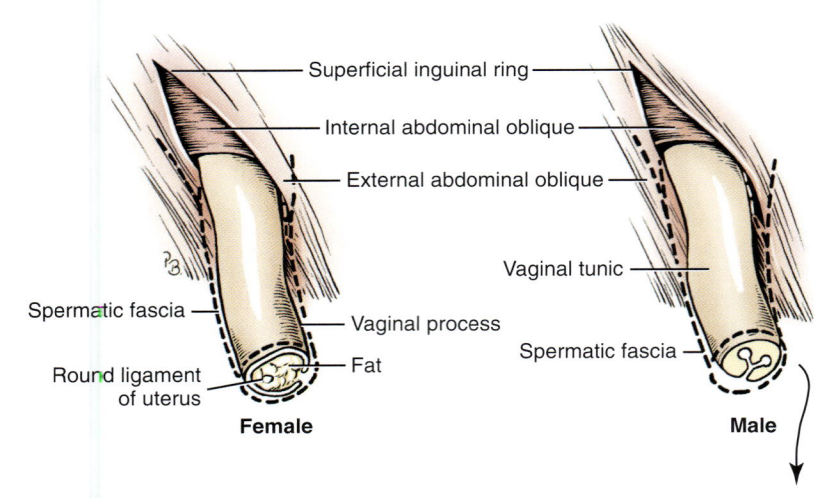

- **Fig. 9.13** Diagram of transected vaginal process in male and female. (*Dotted lines* indicate spermatic fascia. In the male the contents of the vaginal tunic are not shown. See Fig. 9.12.)

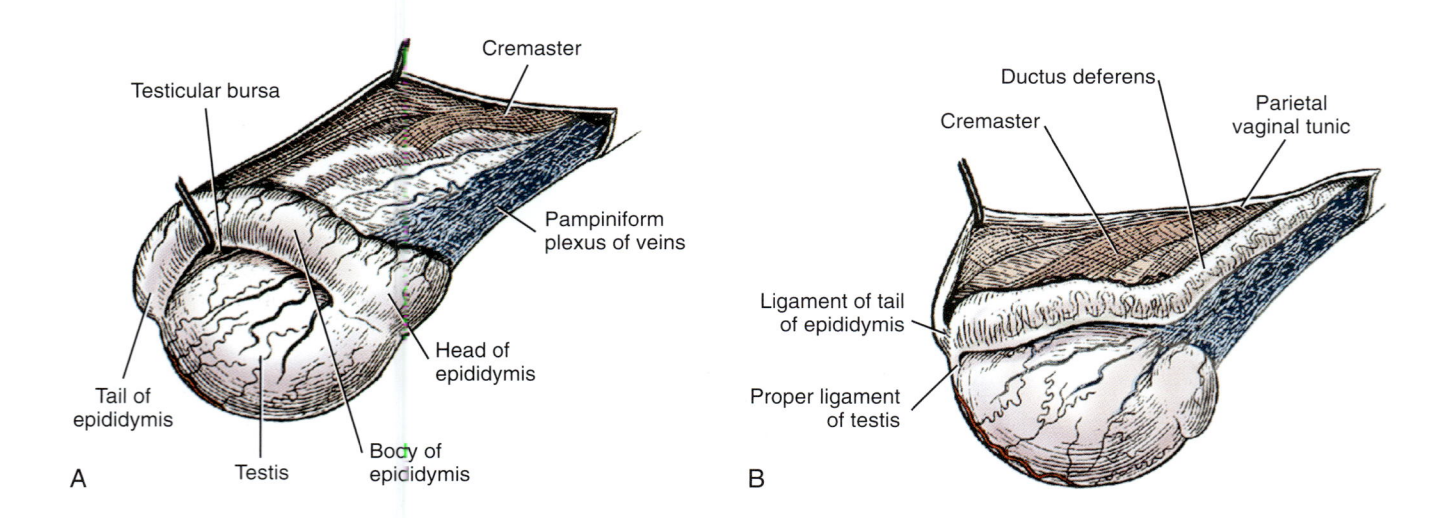

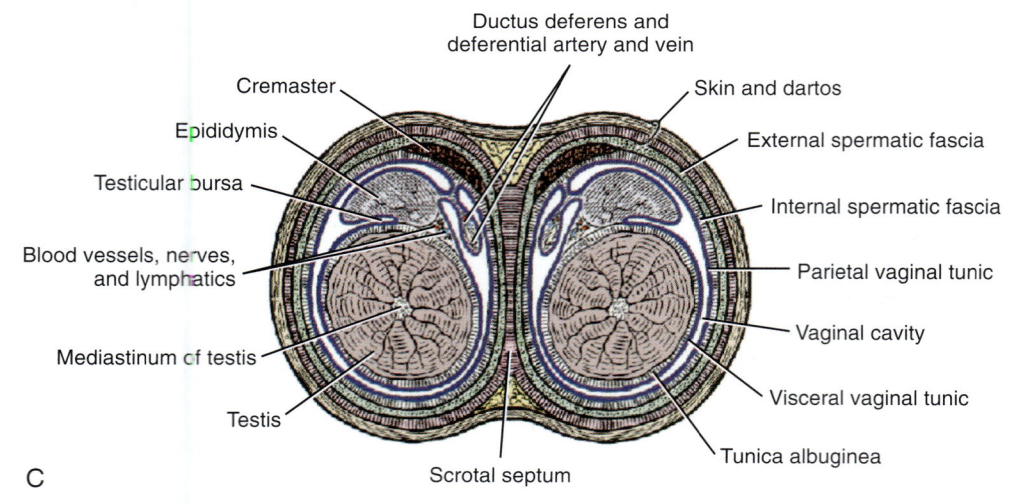

- **Fig. 9.14** Structures of testes and scrotum. **A,** Right testis, lateral aspect. **B,** Left testis, medial aspect. **C,** Schematic cross-section through scrotum and testes.

the epididymis. Evidence indicates that the epididymis, as the site of sperm storage, is the most heat-sensitive region of the male reproductive tract (Bedford, 1978). When the question is raised as to why a scrotum exists in some animals and not in others (there are approximately 1500 ascrotal species), we still do not have a satisfactory answer. Freeman (1990) has reviewed the question and came to the conclusion that the scrotum evolved to provide a cool environment for sperm storage, and testicular descent evolved because it improves sperm quality so that fewer are needed. He provides tables that show the proportional size of the testes in many species of animals. There are six mammalian orders that have species with internal testes as well as species with external testes.

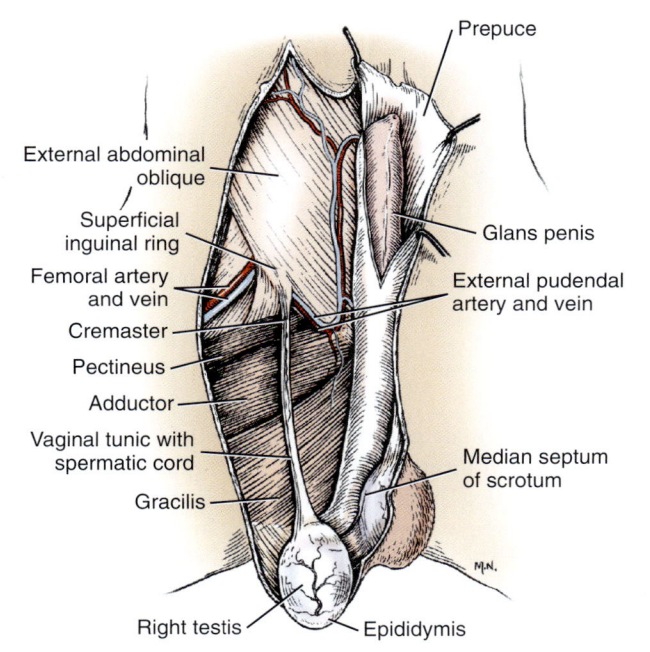

- Fig. 9.15 Male genitalia, ventral view. As the vaginal tunic with spermatic cord leaves the superficial inguinal ring, it is joined by muscle fibers of the internal abdominal oblique that form the cremaster muscle.

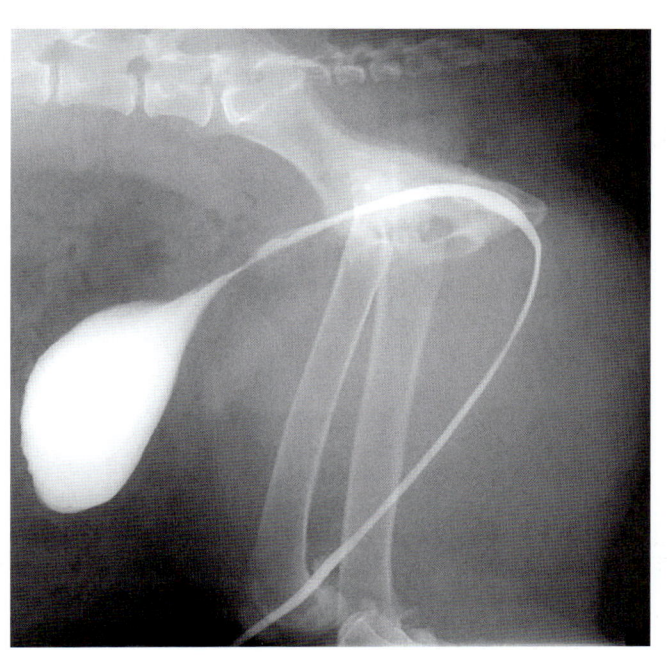

- Fig. 9.17 Lateral contrast radiograph (contrast urethrogram) of the bladder and urethra in the male.

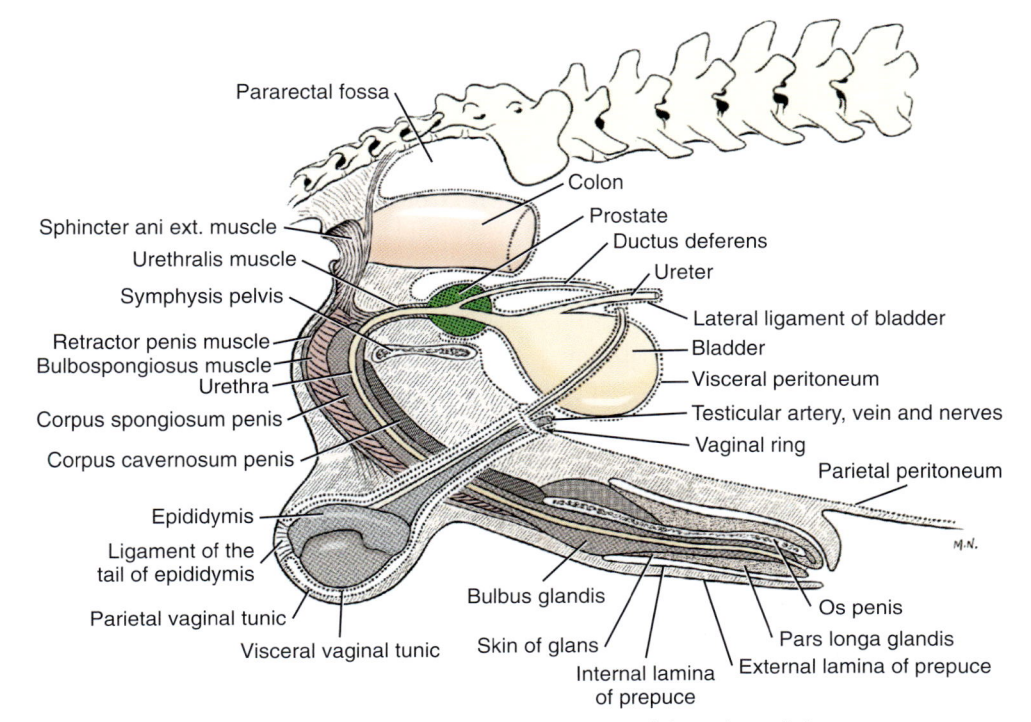

- Fig. 9.16 Diagram of peritoneal reflections and the male genitalia.

• **Fig. 9.18** Male perineum. **A,** Superficial muscles, caudal aspect. **B,** Dorsal section through pelvic cavity. The bilobed bulb of the penis is transected, and the proximal portion removed.

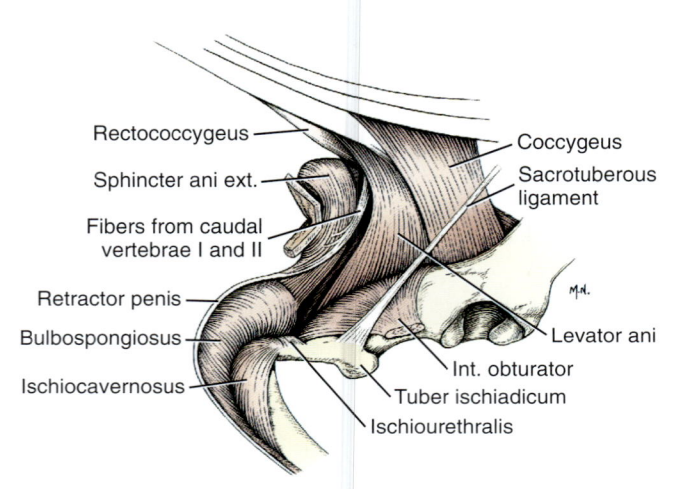

• **Fig. 9.19** Anal region and root of the penis with superficial muscles, right lateral aspect.

Vessels and Nerves

The principal blood vessel to the scrotum is the **ventral scrotal branch** of the **external pudendal artery**. The **cremasteric artery** arises from the deep femoral artery. The **scrotal arteries** run along the cranioventral surface of the testis, superficial to the parietal layer of the vaginal tunic. The perineal branches of the internal pudendal artery supply dorsal scrotal arteries. The draining veins follow the same course in reverse.

The **genital rami**, branches of the genitofemoral nerve from the ventral branches of the third and fourth lumbar nerves, innervate the skin of the prepuce. The **superficial perineal nerve**, a branch of the pudendal from sacral nerves 1, 2, and 3, supplies all of the scrotum, according to Spurgeon and Kitchell (1982). Postganglionic sympathetic axons supplying the tunica dartos enter via the sacral plexus and the pudendal and superficial perineal nerves.

Testes

The **testis**, or male gonad (see Fig. 9.14), is oval in shape and located within the scrotum. The length of the testis in a 25-pound dog averages 3 cm and the width 2 cm. The fresh organ weighs approximately 8 g. In normal position, the testis of the dog is situated obliquely, with the long axis running dorsocaudally. The epididymis is adherent to the dorsolateral surface of the organ, with its head located at the cranial end and its tail at the caudal extremity of the testis.

The surface of the testis is invested by the **tunica albuginea**, a dense, white fibrous capsule. Covering the testis most immediately is the **visceral vaginal tunic**, a serous membrane continuous with the peritoneum of the spermatic cord and the abdominal cavity. The tunica albuginea joins the centrally located mediastinum testis by means of interlobular connective tissue lamellae (*septula testis*), which converge centrally. The **mediastinum testis** is a cord of connective tissue running lengthwise through the middle of the testis. The *lobuli testes* (wedge-shaped portions of testicular parenchyma) are bounded by the septula. The lobuli contain the **convoluted seminiferous tubules** (*tubuli seminiferi contorti*), a large collection of twisted canals. Spermatozoa are formed within the epithelial lining of the tubules, which contains spermatogenic cells and sustentacular (Sertoli) cells. The organization, motility, and structure of sperm cells have been reviewed by André (1982). The longevity of spermatozoa in the reproductive tract of the bitch can be several days (Doak et al., 1967) and at least 6 days as shown by Concannon, et al. (1983).

Straight seminiferous tubules (*tubuli seminiferi recti*) are formed by the union of the convoluted seminiferous tubules of a lobule. The mediastinum testis contains a network of confluent spaces and ducts called the **rete testis**. These connect the straight tubules with the **efferent ductules** (*ductuli efferentes testis*). Testicular blood vessels and

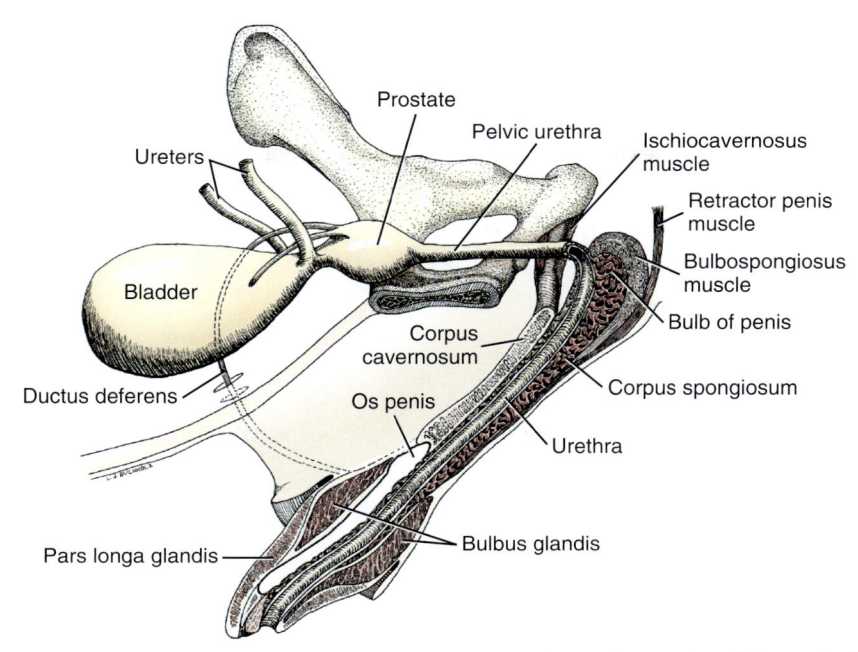

• **Fig. 9.20** Schematic left lateral aspect of pelvic structures and a median section of the penis. (Drawn by L. Buchholz, DVM Class of 1994.)

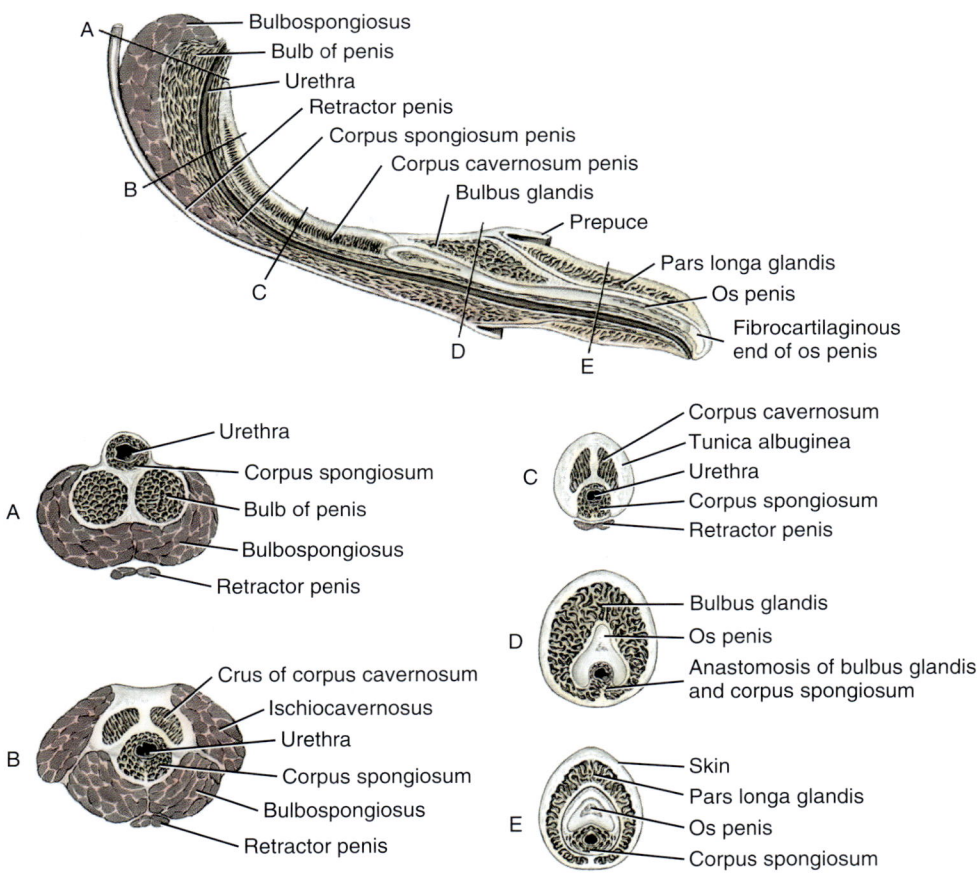

• **Fig. 9.21** Internal morphologic characteristics of the penis. Upper drawing, a sagittal section. A to E, Cross-sections at five levels indicated by letters on upper drawing. (From Christensen GC: *Angioarchitecture of the canine penis and its role in the process of erection*, Ph.D. Thesis, Ithaca, NY, 1953, Cornell University.)

Fig. 9.22 Corrosion preparation of proximal half of the penis. (From Christensen GC: *Angioarchitecture of the canine penis and its role in the process of erection*, Ph.D. Thesis, Ithaca, NY, 1953, Cornell University.)

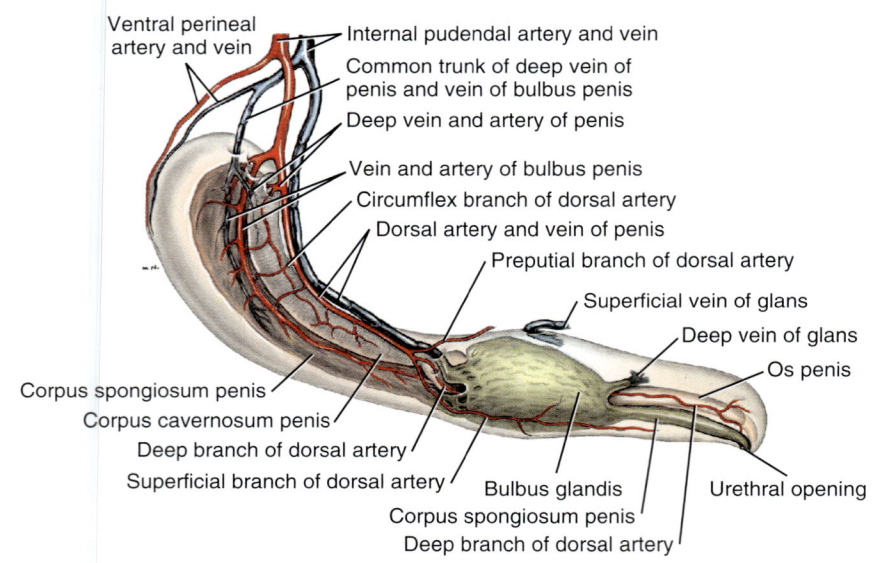

Fig. 9.23 Semidiagrammatic view of penis. The pars longa glandis and the muscles of the root are illustrated as if transparent. The vessels of only one side are shown. (From Christensen GC: *Angioarchitecture of the canine penis and its role in the process of erection*, Ph.D. Thesis, Ithaca, NY, 1953, Cornell University.)

lymphatics enter and leave through the mediastinum. The lobuli testis also contains interstitial cells (of Leydig) between tubular elements. Johnson et al. (1970) and Setchell (1978) consider the anatomy, physiology, biochemistry, and other parameters of the testis.

Attachments

The short **proper ligament of the testis** (*lig. testis proprium*) attaches the testis to the tail of the epididymis. This is continued by the short **ligament of the tail of the epididymis** (*lig. caudae epididymidis*) that attaches the tail of the epididymis to the reflections of the layers of the vaginal tunic at its most distal extent as well as to the spermatic fascia. These two ligaments are remnants of the two divisions of the embryonic gubernaculums testis. The **scrotal ligament** (*lig. scroti*) is a thin layer of connective tissue between the tunica dartos and the tail of the epididymis. These latter two ligaments are difficult to distinguish from each other. These ligaments, as well as the spermatic cord, provide stability to the testis.

Vessels and Nerves

The **testicular artery** and the **artery of the ductus deferens** supply the testis and epididymis. The testicular artery (homologue of the ovarian artery of the female) arises from the ventral surface of the aorta at the level of a transverse

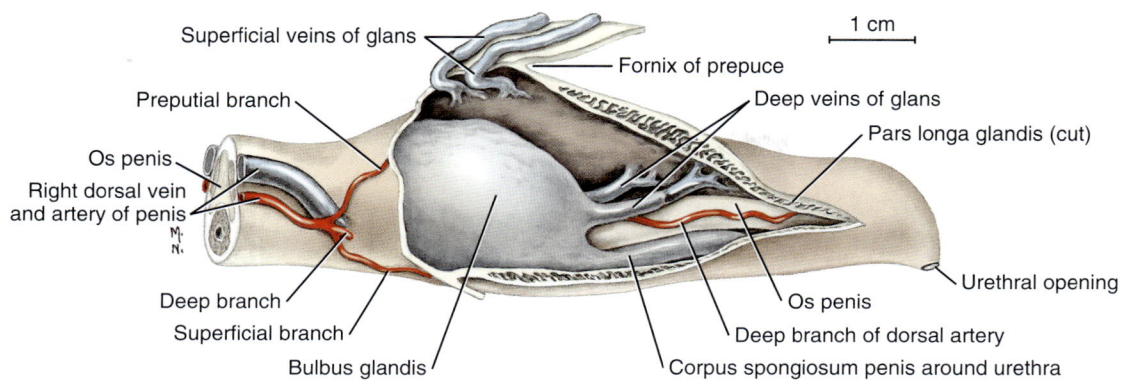

• **Fig. 9.24** Internal morphologic characteristics of the glans penis. (The pars longa glandis has been slit and partially reflected.) (From Christensen GC: *Angioarchitecture of the canine penis and its role in the process of erection*, Ph.D. Thesis, Ithaca, NY, 1953, Cornell University.)

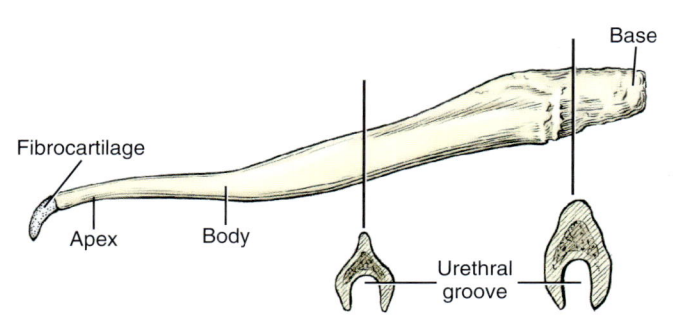

• **Fig. 9.25** Os penis, lateral aspect with two transections.

plane through the fourth lumbar vertebra. The right artery originates cranial to the left, corresponding to the embryonic positions of the testes. The artery of the ductus deferens, a branch of the prostatic artery from the internal pudendal, follows the ductus deferens into the spermatic cord to the level of the epididymis. It sends branches to the epididymis and anastomoses with the testicular artery. The **testicular vein** follows the arterial pattern but forms an extensive **pampiniform plexus** (*plexus pampiniformis*) in the spermatic cord, surrounding the testicular artery lymphatics, and nerves. The right testicular vein empties into the caudal vena cava at the level of the origin of its arterial counterpart. The left drains into the left renal vein. Harrison (1949) made a detailed comparative study of the vascularization of the mammalian testis.

The testicular and epididymal lymphatics anastomose into a variable number of trunks that drain into the lumbar lymph nodes (see Chapter 13).

The nerve supply to the testis is derived from the sympathetic division of the general visceral efferent component of the autonomic nervous system. The nerves of the **testicular plexus** accompany the testicular arteries distally and enter the testis with either the blood vessels or the efferent ducts. Indirectly they are derived from the fourth, fifth, and sixth lumbar sympathetic trunk ganglia. The testicular plexus is derived from the abdominal aortic plexus at the level of the origin of the testicular arteries. These testicular vessels, lymphatics, and nerves are suspended in the spermatic cord by the ***mesorchium***, which is a fold of the visceral layer of the vaginal tunic. This is continued in the abdomen as a fold of the parietal layer of the peritoneum. The blood vessels and smooth muscle fibers in the testis receive a sympathetic nerve supply, but the seminal epithelium and the interstitial secretory tissue do not. Elimination of the sympathetic nerve supply to the testis is followed by degeneration of the seminal epithelium and hypertrophy of the interstitial secretory tissue (Kuntz, 1919b). The degenerative changes are considered to be the result of paralysis of the blood vessels in the spermatic cord and testis.

Anomalies

Cryptorchidism, or failure of the testis to descend, is the most important congenital anomaly of the testis. This condition is comparatively frequent and is believed to be hereditary in some instances. Cox et al. (1978) investigated 12 cases of cryptorchidism in Miniature Schnauzers. Five were unilateral and seven were bilateral. All of the unilateral cases had retained testes on the right side. When retained testes were bilateral the right testis was always smaller. Their observations suggested a multigene defect. In a cryptorchid animal one or both testes are retained either in the abdominal cavity (in the region of the inguinal canal) or between the superficial inguinal ring and the scrotum. Sterile, cryptorchid dogs usually possess normal sexual desire. For a discussion of cryptorchidism see Wensing and van Straten (1980). Hayes et al. (1985) studied 1.8 million documented medical records and identified 2912 dogs (in 104 different breeds) that had cryptorchid testes. There were 14 breeds with significantly high risk.

According to Runnells (1954) testicular tumors of dogs have been reported to cause anatomic alterations, such as atrophy of the opposite testis and enlargement of the prepuce and prostate gland. Hayes et al. (1985) reported that testicular tumors were found in 5.7% of the 2912

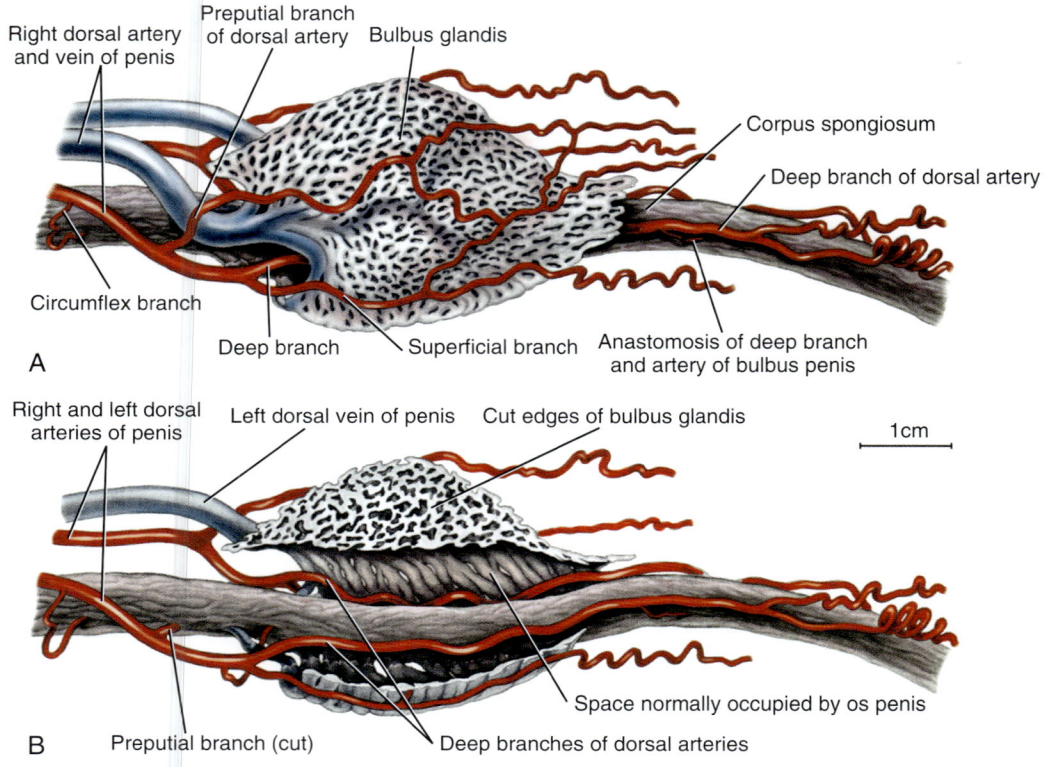

Fig. 9.26 Drawings of corrosion specimen of bulbus glandis and part of corpus spongiosum. (The os penis has been removed.) **A**, Superficial view showing distribution of branches of dorsal artery of the penis. **B**, The near half of the bulbus glandis is cut away, showing the route of the deep branches of the dorsal arteries. (From Christensen GC: *Angioarchitecture of the canine penis and its role in the process of erection*, Ph.D. Thesis, Ithaca, NY, 1953, Cornell University.)

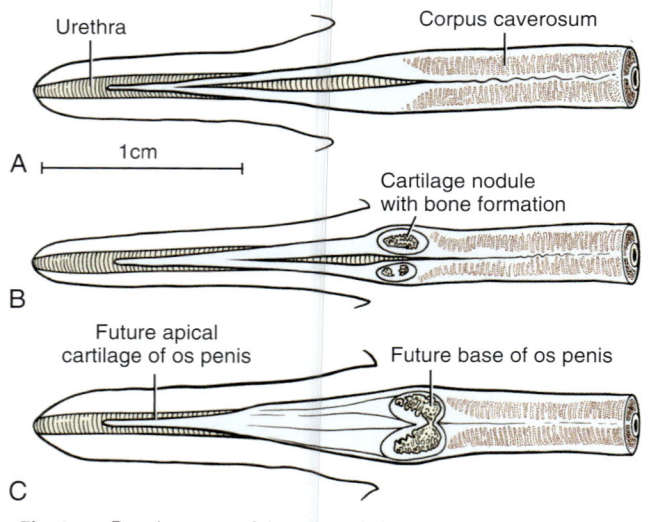

Fig. 9.27 Development of the os penis in littermate Beagles 35 days after birth. The first stages of ossification as seen after clearing in glycerine and staining with alizarine red. Dorsal view. **A**, There is no indication of cartilage or bone in the penis of this pup. Note that the proximal part of each corpus cavernosum consists of fibrous trabeculae with cavernous spaces. The distal right and left fibrocartilaginous portions of the corpora cavernosa fuse dorsal to the urethra. **B** and **C**, Paired cartilaginous nodules with ossification plaques form in the noncavernous portion of each corpus cavernosum in the region of the future base of the os penis. The entire distal portion of the corpora cavernosa will eventually fuse completely and ossify except for the distal tip, which remains cartilaginous. (Figs. 9.27 to 9.30 drawn by M. Simmons from preparations of H. Evans.)

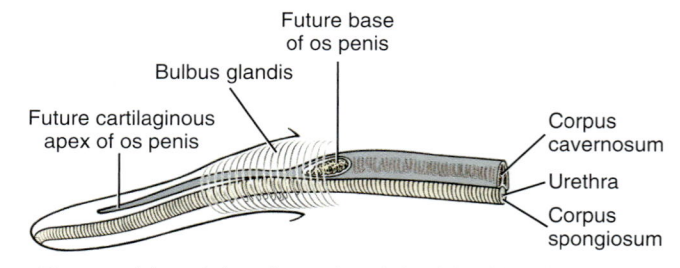

Fig. 9.28 A lateral view shows the relationship of the developing os to the urethra.

cryptorchid dogs whose records they reviewed. Half had Sertoli cell tumors, and one-third had seminomas. Liao et al. (2009) reported that nearly 17% of dogs studied had testicular tumors and that cryptorchidism was associated with development of mixed germ cell–stromal tumors, Sertoli cell tumors, and seminomas. Grieco et al. (2008) reported 27% of male dogs in a separate population had some form of testicular tumor.

Male pseudohermaphroditism and true hermaphroditism have been reported in the dog by Lee and Allam (1952), Brodey et al. (1954), and Bodner (1987). Female pseudohermaphroditism, considered rare (Meyers-Wallen & Patterson, 1986), was reported by Olson et al. (1989) in three sibling Greyhounds.

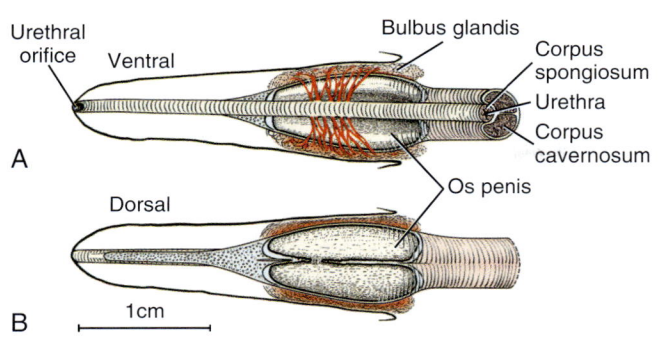

• **Fig. 9.29** Right and left bony plaques, surrounded by a cartilaginous capsule, are beginning to fuse on the mid-dorsal line. The distal fibrocartilage is destined to ossify except for the terminal end, which will remain cartilaginous in the adult (see Fig. 9.33). The vascular connections to the bulbus glandis, seen leaving the corpus spongiosum surrounding the urethra, are shown coursing over the ventrolateral margin of each bony plaque. **A**, Ventral view. **B**, Dorsal view.

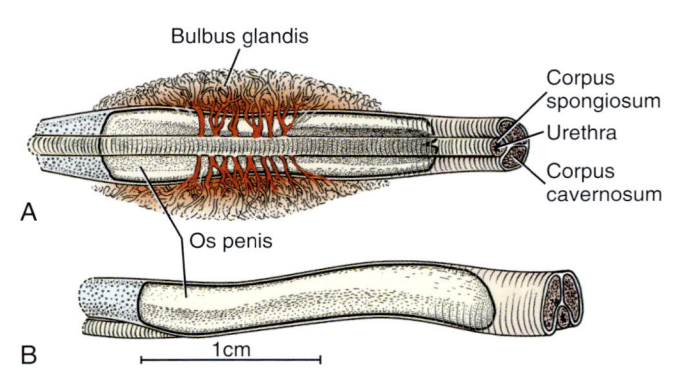

• **Fig. 9.30** The middle portion of the developing penis in a Beagle pup 65 days after birth. **A**, Ventral view. By this stage the right and left ossifications in the corpora cavernosa have elongated and fused completely except for a slight notch at the proximal end. Vascular connections from the corpus spongiosum surrounding the urethra are shown forming the bulbus glandis. **B**, Lateral view of the os penis to show that the urethra is hidden within the urethral groove.

Descent of the Testes

In the majority of mammalian species the testes migrate from their developmental position within the abdomen near the kidneys to a location outside of the body wall, usually in a scrotum (see Fig. 9.15). For these species, including the dog, if neither testis descends (bilateral cryptorchid) spermatogenesis is eliminated and the animal is infertile. If only one testis descends (monorchid or unilateral cryptorchid) fertility is lessened. (Many rodents have testes that descend periodically coincident with breeding. In such species the testes can be gently squeezed back into the body cavity at any time because of the large inguinal canal.)

Much important research on testicular descent in domestic animals has been conducted at the Institute of Veterinary Anatomy of the State University at Utrecht, the Netherlands, by Wensing and co-workers: Wensing (1968, 1973a, 1973b, 1980); Baumans et al. (1981, 1982, 1983); Baumans (1982); Wensing and Colenbrander (1986).

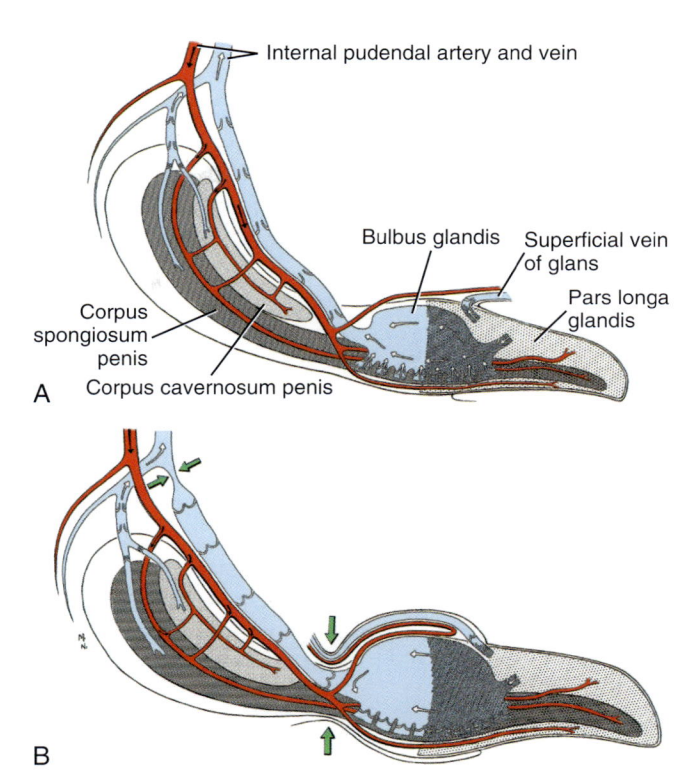

• **Fig. 9.31** Diagrams of circulatory pathways of the penis. **A**, In nonerection. **B**, In erection. The upper arrows on each side of the dorsal vein of the penis represent the effect of contraction of the ischiourethral muscles. The lower arrows, caudal to the bulbus glandis, represent the effect applied externally by the constrictor vestibulae muscles of the female during intromission. (From Christensen GC: *Angioarchitecture of the canine penis and its role in the process of erection*, Ph.D. Thesis, Ithaca, NY, 1953, Cornell University.)

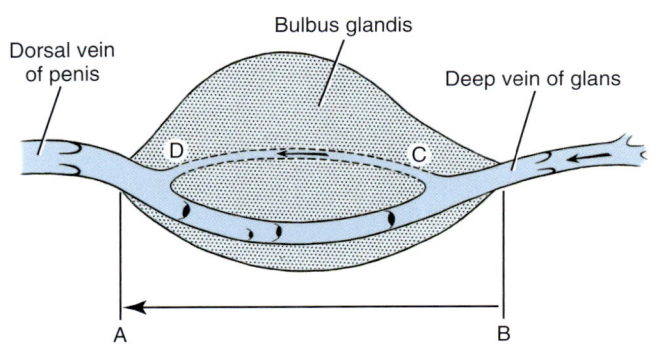

• **Fig. 9.32** Diagram of venous pathways in the bulbus glandis connecting the deep vein of the glans and the dorsal vein of the penis. The ventral shunt (*B to A*) is the principal route when the penis is relaxed; the dorsal shunt (*C to D*) is used during erection. (From Christensen GC: *Angioarchitecture of the canine penis and its role in the process of erection*, Ph.D. Thesis, Ithaca, NY, 1953, Cornell University.)

Whereas in most mammals testicular descent occurs in fetal life, in the dog it occurs at approximately the time of birth, and this makes the dog a good subject for the study of the mechanics and hormonal control of descent. A descriptive and illustrated experimental study of normal development and the factors responsible for the descent of

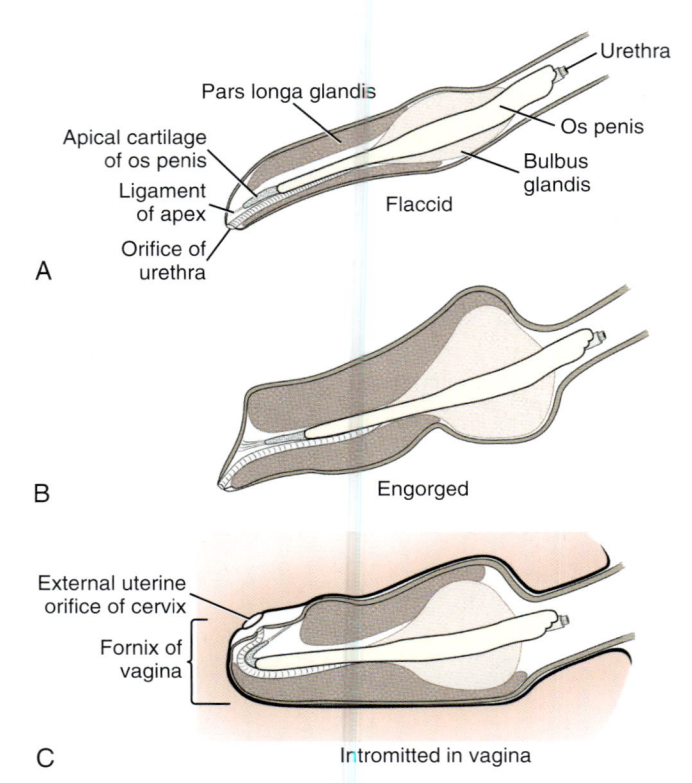

Fig. 9.33 A schematic interpretation of changes in shape of the glans penis during erection and copulation. **A,** Resting state. **B,** Erection as blood fills the cavernous spaces of the bulbus glandis and pars longa glandis. **C,** Intromission and engorgement during copulation when contraction of the ischiourethral muscle in the male and the constrictor vestibulae of the female results in venous occlusion of the veins draining the penis. When the penis is in the fornix of the vagina, the ligament of the cartilage of the os deforms the distal end of the glans to form a corona glandis. When this shape is attained, the opening of the urethra faces dorsally in close proximity to the cervix.

the testes in the dog was published as a thesis in the Netherlands by Baumans (1982). (Included in the thesis are six papers with co-workers, each with a bibliography.) Baumans found that the major factors essential for the descent were first an outgrowth and then a regression of the gubernaculum testis. The gubernaculum is a mesenchymal mass enclosed in a fold of peritoneum that extends from the testis across the mesonephros (kidney ridge) to the inguinal area. It is attached to the caudal pole of the testis and epididymal part of the mesonephric duct. Its distal end continues through the abdominal wall where the inguinal canal forms around it. Here, the gubernaculum is invaded by an outgrowth of parietal peritoneum, the vaginal process. During fetal growth the testis moves caudally to the level of the inguinal canal as the trunk elongates. There are two phases of the migration of the testis through the inguinal canal and into the scrotum. In the first phase the extraabdominal part of the gubernaculum increases enormously in length and volume expanding beyond the inguinal canal and dilating it. When this expansion exceeds the size of the testis and passive resistance is reduced, the testis passes through the canal adjacent to the vaginal process. Here it rests in a mass of swollen gubernaculum, which is still covered by vaginal process peritoneum. An important feature of this testicular migration is that the testis brings with it the visceral peritoneum that formed around it at its site of development in the dorsal abdominal wall. Completion of this first phase of testicular descent initiates the second phase in which the gubernaculum is transformed by tissue degeneration from an expanded mucoid mass into a small fibrous structure in the scrotal sac, thus making room for the testis. This converts the gubernaculum into the proper ligament of the testis, which attaches the tail of the epididymis to the testis,

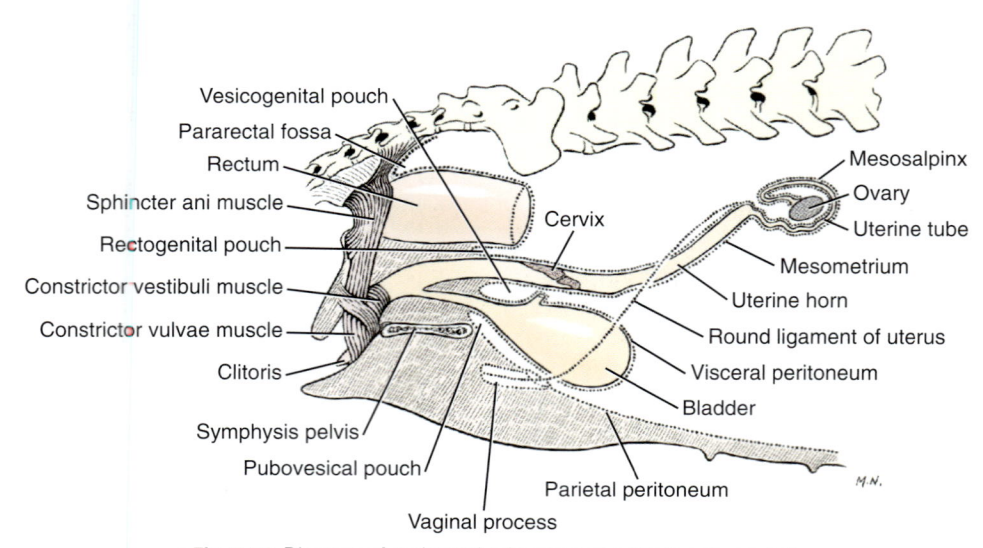

Fig. 9.34 Diagram of peritoneal reflections and the female genitalia.

and the ligament of the tail of the epididymis, which attaches the tail to the distal portion of the vaginal tunic and spermatic fascia. The latter is derived from the remnants of the gubernaculum that surrounds the vaginal tunic. The degeneration of the gubernaculum results in the testis being located at the distal extent of the vaginal tunic.

Baumans found that on the day of birth the testis was located halfway between the kidney and the deep inguinal ring. The gubernaculum had reached its maximum development and was beginning to show signs of regression histologically and histochemically. By day 3 or 4 after birth the testis passes through the inguinal canal and the gubernaculum regresses. By 35 to 40 days after birth the testis reaches its definitive position in the scrotum.

To test the factors responsible for gubernacular growth and regression, Baumans removed the testes in fetal dogs and found that gubernacular outgrowth ceased and there was no epididymal descent. Removal of the testis at birth resulted in retarded gubernacular regression and a delayed epididymal descent. After further investigation it was concluded that the testis induces gubernacular outgrowth and regression and thereby regulates its own descent. It was found that testicular hormones, particularly testosterone, are synthesized in the testis. In the first phase of descent an unidentified testicular factor stimulated gubernacular proliferation and swelling. Sustentacular cells are thought to be the source of this factor. In the second phase of descent testosterone induced gubernacular regression. In regard to the mechanical role of the gubernaculum, it was found that a connection between the testis and the gubernaculum was essential for normal testicular descent. By the end of the second phase of descent the testis plays a mechanical role in distending the scrotum.

Wensing and Colenbrander (1986), in discussing normal and abnormal descent of the testis, make a distinction between the morphologic characteristics of testicular descent in mammals with a striplike cremaster muscle (ungulates, dog, and humans) and those with a saclike cremaster muscle (rodent, lagomorph). They believe that the bilaminar saclike cremaster muscle of rodents and lagomorphs continues to grow and increase in size even after the regression of the gubernaculum and thus plays a role in descent of the testis. Regardless of the morphologic characteristics of the cremaster muscle, they stress the importance of a normal gubernacular outgrowth and regression for affecting testicular descent. Their experimental results showed that the first phase in the descent process (gubernacular outgrowth) does not depend on the presence of active interstitial cells, testosterone, testosterone receptors, or gonadotropins, although the presence of the testis is essential.

Epididymis

The **epididymis** (see Fig. 9.14) is where spermatozoa are stored before ejaculation. It is comparatively large in the dog and consists of an elongated convoluted tube, the coils of which are held together by collagenous connective tissue. The epididymis lies along the dorsolateral border of the testis. The **head** (*caput*) begins on the cranial medial surface of the testis but immediately twists around the cranial extremity to attain the lateral side. It is slightly larger than the remainder of the epididymis. It continues as the **body** (*corpus*), which runs along the dorsolateral surface of the testis, and then as the **tail** (*cauda epididymidis*), which is attached to the caudal extremity of the testis by the proper ligament of the testis. Beyond the tail this duct is continued craniodorsally as the ductus deferens which becomes part of the spermatic cord along with the testicular vessels and nerves. The epididymis has its concave surface in juxtaposition with the testis. Its medial edge is attached to the testis by visceral vaginal tunic, the **distal mesorchium** (*mesorchium distale*). The latter extends medially between the lateral edge of the body of the epididymis and the testis, forming a potential space, the **testicular bursa** (*bursa testicularis*). The bursa is limited cranially and caudally by the epididymal head and tail, which adhere tightly to the testis.

Structure

The epididymis, especially the caudal portion, has a lower temperature than the rest of the body because of its position in the scrotum and is a favorable storage place for spermatozoa before their passage into the ductus deferens (Bedford, 1978). Circular smooth muscle fibers aid seminiferous tubule secretion in moving the germ cells. The length of the epididymis and the slowness of spermatozoa movement are important in allowing the spermatozoa to complete their maturation process, called *capacitation* (Mason & Shaver, 1952).

Ductus Deferens

The **deferent duct** (*ductus deferens*) (see Figs. 9.7, 9.9, 9.14, and 9.16) is the continuation of the duct of the epididymis. Beginning at the tail of the epididymis, it passes cranially along the dorsomedial border of the testis, continues dorsally in the spermatic cord, and enters the abdominal cavity through the inguinal canal. Running in a fold of peritoneum, the mesoductus deferens, it crosses ventral to the ureter at the lateral ligament of the bladder and penetrates the prostate to open into the pelvic urethra, lateral to the colliculus seminalis (Fig. 9.7).

In a 25-pound dog, the ductus deferens averages 17 to 18 cm in length and 1.6 to 3 mm in diameter. The epididymal end of the duct is slightly tortuous, but it straightens out in its course along the medial surface of the testis. It is attached to the testis, along with the artery and vein of the ductus deferens, by a special fold of the visceral vaginal tunic called the ***mesoductus deferens***. At the cranial extremity of the testis the mesoductus deferens blends with the peritoneal fold containing the testicular vessels, nerves, and lymphatics, the **proximal mesorchium** (*mesorchium proximale*) (see Fig. 9.12). In the abdominal cavity at the vaginal ring the deferential fold of peritoneum leaves the vaginal ring, to which it is attached at one edge, and courses caudodorsally to reach the dorsal surface of the bladder. The ductus deferens lies 3.4 cm from the body wall when the deferential fold of peritoneum is stretched out. Dorsal to the bladder, the right and left deferent ducts come into close apposition approximately 2 cm before they penetrate the prostate gland. For approximately 1.5 cm before they contact each other, the ducts are joined by a fold of peritoneum, the **genital fold** (*plica genitalis*). Peritoneum covering the pelvic portion of the ductus is reflected ventrally onto the prostate, bladder, and ureters. Dorsally it is reflected over the prostate and then onto the ventral surface of the rectum at the rectogenital fossa.

Structure

The layers of the ductus deferens are the *tunica adventitia, t. muscularis*, and *t. mucosa*. Three layers of smooth muscle are generally recognized: an outer and an inner longitudinal and a middle circular. The mucosa is made up of simple or pseudostratified columnar epithelium. The terminal portion of the ductus deferens and the adjacent area of the urethra contain branched tubular glands. A distinct ampulla of the deferent duct is not obvious in the dog.

Vessels and Nerves

The **artery of the ductus deferens** is a branch of the prostatic artery, which, in turn, arises from the internal pudendal. It accompanies the ductus deferens to the epididymis, which it also supplies with blood. The artery of the ductus deferens anastomoses with the testicular artery in the spermatic cord. The **vein of the ductus deferens** runs in the spermatic cord with the deferent duct, and empties into the internal iliac vein. The lymphatics drain into the **hypogastric** and **medial iliac lymph nodes**. Nerves to the ductus deferens are autonomic, arising from the pelvic plexus. The **hypogastric nerves** (sympathetic), via the pelvic plexuses, supply the pelvic part of the ductus deferens. Parasympathetic axons are thought to be distributed via the pelvic plexus only to the epididymis and musculature of the ductus deferens.

Spermatic Cord

Each **spermatic cord** (*funiculus spermaticus*) (see Figs. 9.12 and 9.16) is composed of the ductus deferens and its vessels, and the testicular vessels and nerves, along with their serous membrane coverings, the *mesoductus deferens* and the *mesorchium*. These structures pass through the inguinal canal during the descent of the testis. The spermatic cord begins at the vaginal ring, the point at which its component parts converge to leave the abdominal cavity via the inguinal canal. The ductus deferens, which arises from the tail of the epididymis, leaves the vaginal ring, runs caudomedially in the deferential fold of peritoneum, and enters the prostate gland before opening into the prostatic part of the pelvic urethra. The ductus deferens is accompanied by the small artery of the ductus deferens, which arises from the prostatic artery and the vein of the ductus deferens, which drains into the internal iliac vein. The testicular artery originates from the ventral surface of the aorta. The testicular arteries arise cranial to the origin of the caudal mesenteric artery.

The testicular artery runs laterally and caudally, crossing the ventral surface of the ureter, at which point it is joined by the testicular vein and nerve. The left testicular vein empties into the left renal vein and the right into the caudal vena cava. The peritoneal fold, the proximal mesorchium, enclosing the testicular vessels is attached to the abdominal wall in a line slightly lateral to the junction of the transversus abdominis and psoas muscles. The plexus of the testicular nerves arises from the area of the sympathetic trunk between the third and the sixth lumbar sympathetic trunk ganglia. The testicular lymph vessels pass to the lumbar lymph nodes.

The components of the spermatic cord are joined together by loose connective tissue and are surrounded by the visceral layer of the **vaginal tunic**. The peritoneal ring formed by the vaginal tunic passing through the deep inguinal ring is termed the **vaginal ring** (see Fig. 9.12). There is usually an irregular mass of fat at the vaginal ring, covered by peritoneum. It overlaps the cranial border of the ring and probably acts as a valve to decrease the possibility of intestinal or omental herniation. The fat mass may be in two separate parts.

The ductus deferens, with its vessels, is enveloped by one fold of peritoneum at the vaginal ring, the mesoductus deferens; and the testicular vessels and nerves are covered by another, the mesorchium. The double layer of peritoneum uniting these two folds to each other and to the edge of the vaginal ring is termed the **mesofuniculus** (Fig. 9.12). It may be compared to the mesentery, which attaches the intestines to the abdominal wall.

Along the path of the spermatic cord from the deep inguinal ring to the testis, the relationship of the vaginal tunic and the enclosed structures remains constant. The tunic also reflects over the testis as its visceral peritoneum which joins the distal mesorchium along the dorsomedial border of the organ. A small, circumscribed area on the tail of the epididymis is free of tunic, allowing the **ligament of the tail of the epididymis** (embryonic *gubernaculum testis*) to attach the epididymis to the spermatic fascia.

The **inguinal canal** (see Fig. 9.12) is a fissure through the abdominal muscles that connects the **deep** and the **superficial inguinal ring** (Ashdown, 1963; McCarthy, 1976). It is located approximately 1 cm craniomedial to the femoral ring. The femoral ring affords passage for the femoral vessels. The inguinal canal is bounded medially by the rectus abdominis muscle, cranially by the internal oblique muscle, and both laterally and caudally by the aponeurosis of the external abdominal oblique muscle. The **superficial ring**, located 2 to 4 cm lateral to the linea alba, is merely a slit in the aponeurosis of the external abdominal oblique muscle. It represents where the abdominal wall formed around the gubernaculum in the fetus. The cranial wall of the inguinal canal is made up of the transversus abdominis and internal abdominal oblique muscles, as well as the aponeurosis of the external abdominal oblique muscle. Only the latter forms the caudal wall of the canal.

As the spermatic cord and testis pass through the inguinal canal surrounded by the peritoneum of the vaginal tunic, transversalis fascia (underlying parietal peritoneum) is reflected onto them and is here known as **internal spermatic fascia**. The combined superficial and deep abdominal fascia, from the external surface of the external abdominal oblique muscle, is reflected onto the vaginal tunic as it emerges from the inguinal canal. It then lies superficial to the internal spermatic fascia and is known as the **external spermatic fascia**. The cremaster muscle, a caudal fasciculus of the internal abdominal oblique muscle, lies adjacent to the vaginal tunic between the internal and the external spermatic fascia.

Both scrotal and inguinal hernias may occur in male dogs. In both of these hernias abdominal organs (greater omentum or a loop of jejunum) enter the canal of the vaginal tunic. Inguinal hernias remain in the inguinal canal. The hernia may be bilateral or unilateral. For a description of surface palpation of the superficial inguinal ring, see McCarthy (1976). Inguinal hernia (intestines or omentum pushing into the inguinal canal within the vaginal canal) is recognizable as a soft, fluctuating enlargement to one side of the penis.

Prostate Gland

The **prostate gland** (*prostata*) (see Figs. 9.7, 9.16, 9.18, and 9.20) completely envelops the proximal portion of the male pelvic urethra at the neck of the bladder. It is the only accessory sex gland present in the male dog. The prostate develops from a series of symmetric buds of the pelvic urethra that appear at approximately the sixth week of gestation (Price, 1963). The size and weight of the prostate varies, depending on the age, breed, and body weight of the dog (Berg, 1958a; O'Shea, 1962). In most dogs, progressive enlargement occurs with age (Schlotthauer & Bollman, 1936). The latter authors found that in all dogs in which there was more than 0.7 g of prostate per kg of body weight, the prostate was abnormal on histologic examination. They suggested 0.7 g prostate per kg of body weight as the upper limit of normality for the dog. O'Shea (1962) divided prostatic growth into three phases: normal growth in the young adult, hyperplasia during the middle of adult life, and senile involution.

The prostate is bounded dorsally by the rectum and ventrally by the symphysis pubis and ventral abdominal wall. Its craniocaudal position is age-dependent, as discussed by Gordon (1961). The prostate lies entirely within the abdominal cavity until the urachal remnant breaks down at approximately 2 months of age. From that time until sexual maturity the gland is confined to the pelvic cavity. With sexual maturity it increases in size and extends cranially. By 4 years of age more than half of the gland is abdominal, and by 10 years of age the entire gland is in the abdomen. The degree of bladder distention was not found to alter these relationships to any significant degree. The prostate is androgen-dependent, and castration at any age results in a marked reduction in size (Hansel & McEntee, 1977).

The dorsal surface of the prostate is separated from the ventral surface of the genital fold and the two ductus deferentia by the two layers of the fold of peritoneum that bounds the vesicogenital space. The ventral surface of the prostate is retroperitoneal; the ventral sheet of the lateral ligament of the bladder is not continued onto the prostate. A layer of fat usually covers the ventral surface. In mature dogs, the caudal third of the dorsal surface of the prostate is attached to the rectum by a fibrous band (Gordon, 1960).

The prostate is semioval in transverse section; the dorsal surface is flattened. A mid-dorsal sulcus is usually palpable per rectum. The prostatic part of the pelvic urethra passes through the gland somewhat dorsal to its center. A prominent median septum divides the gland into right and left lobes. Each lobe is further divided into lobules by capsular trabeculae. The lobules consist of numerous compound tubuloalveolar glands lined by columnar epithelium. Ducts from these glands enter the urethra throughout its circumference. The **capsule of the prostate** (*capsula prostatae*) is comparatively thick. Smooth muscle fibers are found throughout the capsule, and muscle fibers from the wall of the urinary bladder extend onto the dorsal surface of the capsule.

The two deferent ducts enter the craniodorsal surface of the prostate. They lie adjacent to each other, one on either side of the median plane. They run caudoventrally through the dorsal part of the gland to open into the urethra by two slits on each side of the **seminal colliculus** (*colliculus seminalis*) (see Fig. 9.7). The latter is a small round eminence in the center of the **urethral crest** (*crista urethralis*), which is a short longitudinal fold on the dorsal wall of the prostatic part of the pelvic urethra. The distal portion of the ductus deferens that enters the urethra is referred to as the **ampulla** (*ampulla ductus deferentis*) because of its enlargement resulting from the presence of mucosal glands. In the dog this ampulla is very small and difficult to recognize.

The function of the prostate is not entirely understood. Prostatic secretion contains citrate, lactate, cholesterol, and a number of enzymes. It is believed to be essential to provide an optimum environment for sperm survival and motility. Dog semen is unique in its absence of reducing sugars supplied by the accessory glands in other species; the source of readily metabolizable energy for the spermatozoa is unknown (Hansel & McEntee, 1977).

Vessels and Nerves

The blood and nerve supply of the prostate have been studied by Gordon (1960) and Hodson (1968). The **prostatic artery** (*a. prostatica*) arises from the internal pudendal at the level of the second or third sacral vertebrae, although it may arise from the umbilical (Hodson, 1968) near its origin. The prostatic artery gives rise to the **artery of the ductus deferens** (*a. ductus deferentis*), which is homologous with the uterine artery in the female. The artery of the ductus deferens gives rise to the **caudal vesicle artery** (*a. vesicalis caudalis*). The caudal vesicle artery gives branches to the ureter (*ramus uretericus*) and urethra (*ramus urethralis*) and then ramifies on the surface of the bladder, anastomosing with the contralateral caudal vesicle and cranial vesicle arteries. When the cranial vesicle artery is not present, the caudal vesicle supplies the entire bladder.

The prostatic artery continues caudoventrally and gives rise to the small **middle rectal artery** (*a. rectalis media*) before ramifying on the surface of the prostate. These branches penetrate the capsule on the dorsolateral surface of the gland to become subcapsular arteries (Hodson, 1968). Radial tributaries pass along the capsular septae toward the urethra to supply the glandular tissue. Cavernous tissue, continuous with the corpus spongiosum, surrounds the pelvic urethra. It is supplied by the artery of the bulb of the penis.

Anastomoses occur between the prostatic vessels and the urethral artery (internal pudendal), the cranial rectal artery (caudal mesenteric) and the caudal rectal artery (internal pudendal). These anastomoses complicate prostatectomy. The venous network of the gland drains by way of the **prostatic** and **urethral veins** into the internal iliac vein. The prostatic lymph vessels empty into the **iliac lymph nodes**. The nerve supply to the prostate is closely allied to the vasculature. The **hypogastric nerve**, which supplies sympathetic innervation to the prostate, follows the prostatic artery from the pelvic plexus. The **pelvic nerve**, which may be single or double (Gordon, 1960), accompanies the prostatic artery as far as the lateral surface of the rectum. Here it forms the **pelvic plexus**, together with branches of the hypogastric nerve. The middle portion of the pelvic plexus forms the **prostatic plexus**, which innervates the gland. Parasympathetic stimulation increases the rate of glandular secretion.

Pathologic Conditions

Prostatic hypertrophy, a feature shared by men and dogs (Berg, 1958b), is common in older male dogs, and excessive enlargement leads to urinary obstruction and interference with defecation. Perineal hernia often accompanies prostatic hypertrophy (Greiner & Betts, 1975).

Carcinoma of the prostate occurs much more commonly in the dog than in any other domestic animal (Berg, 1958b; Leav & Ling, 1968). Cysts of the prostate are common in dogs 3 years of age and older. Occasionally these cysts reach enormous proportions and require surgical drainage. Prostatic abscesses and, less frequently, prostatic calculi are also encountered.

Extrinsic Muscles of the Penis

There are four paired extrinsic penile muscles in the dog (see Figs. 9.18 to 9.20). The **retractor penis muscles**, composed principally of smooth muscle fibers (Fisher, 1917), arise indirectly from the first and second caudal vertebrae and blend with the anal sphincters and levator ani muscles. Each runs ventrally along the peripheral border of the anal sphincter to the urethral surface of the penis, and inserts in the penis at the fornix of the prepuce. Bands of muscle fibers leave the retractor penis at the level of the caudal edge of the scrotum and disperse in the septum scroti. The short, broad, paired **ischiocavernosus muscles** cover the crura of the penis. Each originates from the ischial tuberosity and has a broad insertion upon the proximal corpus cavernosum. The **bulbospongiosus muscles**, consisting mainly of transverse fibers, cover the superficial surface of the bulb of the penis. These fibers arise from the tunica albuginea lateral to the corpus spongiosum. Some ventral fibers of the external anal sphincter may be continuous with this muscle, and some fusion occurs with the retractor penis muscle at the proximal third of the body of the penis. The **ischiourethralis muscle** (Fig. 9.18) consists of skeletal muscle fibers that course from each side of the ischial arch, arising from the dorsal surface of the ischial tuberosities. These muscles pass medially where on the midline they end in a common fibrous band, the transverse perineal ligament (*lig. transversum perinei*). This ligament forms a ring around the common trunk of the dorsal veins of the penis. When the muscle contracts, this tenses the ligament and reduces or blocks blood flow exiting the penis from the dorsal veins of the penis. A strong short ligament attaches the fibrous ring to the concave surface of the penis at the level of the ischial arch. The muscle plays an active role in penile erection by slowing the flow of blood out of the cavernous tissues. Innervation is from the pudendal nerve. Innervation and function of this muscle has been studied by Fournier et al. (1987) in dogs and by Dail and Sachs (1991) in rats.

Penis

Topographically the **penis** is composed of three principal divisions: the **root** (*radix penis*), the **body** (*corpus penis*), and the **glans** (*glans penis*). The root of the penis is composed of the two crura and the bulb of the penis. The body is primarily comprised of the two adjacent corpora cavernosa. The glans is subdivided into a bulbus glandis and a pars longa glandis. In the nonerect state the glans penis is entirely withdrawn into the prepuce. The prepuce is attached to the ventral abdominal wall except for its distal open end, which is free. The penis has two primary surfaces, a **dorsal** (*dorsum penis*) and a **ventral** or **urethral surface** (*facies urethralis*). Measurements of the nonerect penis in more than 150 mature dogs of assorted breeds show that its length ranges from 6.5 to 24 cm, with an average of 17.9 cm.

The **crus of the penis** (*crus penis*) is the proximal end of the corpus cavernosum penis that is attached to the lateral aspect of the ischial arch and is covered by the ischiocavernosus muscle (see Figs. 9.10 and 9.19). The thick tunica albuginea that covers the corpus cavernosum penis provides for this attachment. Within each crus is the blood-filled corpus cavernosum penis that extends distally into the body of the penis. The caudal external surface of each root is covered by an **ischiocavernosus muscle** (see Figs. 9.18 and 9.19), which arises from the medial end of the ischial tuberosity.

The **bulb of the penis** (*bulbus penis*) (see Figs. 9.20 and 9.21), formerly urethral bulb, is a partially bilobed, spongy, blood-filled sac that lies between the crura close to the ischial arch (see Fig. 9.20). The bulb is continuous with the corpus spongiosum (see Fig. 9.20) surrounding the caudal part of the pelvic urethra and all of the penile urethra. The external surface of the bulb is covered by the median **bulbospongiosus muscle** (see Figs. 9.18 and 9.20).

The **corpus penis**, or body, begins where the two crura join distal to the bulb. The cavernous bodies of each crus remain distinct as they join to form the body because each is enveloped by a thick covering of collagenous and elastic fibers, the **tunica albuginea**. On transection (see Fig. 9.21) the paired corpora cavernosa appear somewhat triangular and are separated by a median fibrous septum. Ventrally they form a groove for the ventrally lying penile urethra with its surrounding corpus spongiosum. The latter is not wrapped by the tunica albuginea. The body of the penis at midlevel is compressed in such a manner that its cross-sectional diameter is greatest dorsoventrally. This allows for lateral bending without twisting it upside down as the male dismounts to face in the opposite direction. This was described by Grandage (1972) as "flexible rigidity." At the level of the glans the paired corpora have very thick fibrous wrappings and are fused with each other on the midline. They end by attaching to the base of the os penis. (In reality the os penis develops within the terminations of the corpora cavernosa and thus they are attached by virtue of their manner of formation [see Figs. 9.27 and 9.28], as shown by Evans [1986].)

The **corpus spongiosum**, a continuation of the bulbus penis (see Fig. 9.22), has its origin surrounding the urethra at the level of the prostate gland and extends caudally around the pelvic urethra and entire penile urethra. At the ischial arch it expands dorsocaudally into the bulb of the penis. It continues through the penile body and glans to the termination of the penile urethra. Thus the corpus spongiosum lies within the urethral groove of the os penis. Within the proximal glans there are numerous shunts from the corpus spongiosum that pass ventral to the margins of the urethral groove to supply the surrounding bulbus glandis with blood. The **bulbus glandis** is the most distensible portion of the penis in the dog. From one to four valves are located in each of the venous connections between the bulbus glandis and the corpus spongiosum, preventing blood from leaving the bulbus glandis by this route. At the distal quarter of the glans the urethra and its corpus spongiosum lie beneath the cartilaginous termination of the os penis before turning ventrally to terminate at the urethral orifice.

Glans

The glans of the dog is a compound structure, consisting of a proximal ringlike **bulbus glandis** and a distal elongated **pars longa glandis**, which forms the apex of the penis.

The **bulbus glandis** (see Figs. 9.20, 9.23, 9.24, and 9.26) is a barrel-shaped cavernous expansion of the corpus spongiosum, which surrounds the proximal third of the os penis. In the nonerect state it is not distinct from the rest of the glans, but when engorged with blood it expands greatly and is well delineated. It functions to provide the "tie" or "lock" during copulation. The bulbus glandis contains large venous sinuses and numerous trabeculae rich in elastic tissue. The pars longa glandis and bulbus glandis are separated from each other by a connective tissue septum. There is no connection between the corpus spongiosum and the pars longus glandis. A short, large vein on each side drains the pars longa glandis into the cavernous bulbus glandis. The latter drains into the dorsal vein of the penis on each side.

The **pars longa glandis** changes its shape drastically during intromission when its distal end deforms into a flattened **corona glandis** within the fornix of the vagina (see Fig. 9.33). This deformation is possible because of the ligamentous attachment that passes from the distal cartilage of the os penis to the connective tissue of the glans dorsal to the urethra. This connection restricts the cranial movement of the central area of the pars longa glandis, which then flattens to form a corona with a central urethral process (Hart & Kitchell, 1965). Thus the opening of the urethra is shifted from the ventral to the dorsal surface of the glans, and the resulting position of the distal end of the glans aids in directing the ejaculate to the cervical os. The apparent function of the os, aside from adding rigidity for intromission, is to deform the apex of the penis into a corona glandis (see Fig. 9.33).

Os Penis

The **os penis** (see Figs. 9.21 and 9.25), or baculum, is a feature of most mammals (Ruth 1934). It is always present in the male dog. It forms from a paired ossification center in the corpora cavernosa at 35 days of age (see Fig. 9.27). In large dogs it is approximately 10 cm long, 1.3 cm wide, and 1 cm thick. The bone forms a rigid axis of the glans penis, through which it passes. The caudal part, or base of the os penis, is truncate and attached to the termination of the corpora cavernosa within which it formed (see Fig. 9.27). The cranial part, or **apex**, tapers gradually and ends in a cartilaginous tip, which is attached by a fibrous strand to the deep surface of the corona of the glans. The body of the os penis is straight and long having as its most distinctive feature a **urethral groove** (*sulcus urethrae*), which runs ventrally along the base and body of the bone. The urethral groove is of clinical importance because the narrow entrance to the groove at its base may obstruct the passage of urinary calculi through the urethra and require surgical intervention. The groove is approximately 7 mm deep and 4 mm wide near the base and gradually becomes narrower and shallower distally until a groove no longer exists, although the urethra still lies ventral to the bone. The urethra, along its entire course in the penis, is surrounded by the corpus spongiosum, which at approximately midpoint along the bone sends vascular channels out of the urethral groove on both sides (see Figs. 9.26 and 9.30) that enter the bulbus glandis. The os penis usually has indentations on the margins of the groove caused by the passage of these vessels.

The term **os genitale** has been used to include the **os penis** of male mammals (*os priapi* in Greek) and the less frequent **os clitoridis** of the female. The presence of a bone or baculum in the penis is a characteristic feature of males in most mammalian orders, and its morphologic characteristics have been used by mammalogists as a diagnostic feature for genera of Bats, Rodents, Insectivores, and Carnivores (Chaine, 1926; Didier, 1946; Hildebrand, 1954; Pohl, 1911). The bone may be bipartite or trifurcate in rodents and have synovial joints (Arata et al., 1965). An os penis is not present in monotremes, marsupials, ungulates, elephants, or man. The homologous os clitoridis of the female is less frequently present in mammals and only occasionally reported in the dog (Figs. 9.40 and 9.41).

The first indication of external sexual differentiation in the dog fetus is seen approximately halfway through gestation (see Chapter 2). By 35 days of gestation (35 mm) the penis and clitoris are similar in shape and structure but differ in position relative to the anus (closer together in the female). During fetal life there is a condensation of tissue at approximately 34 days and a chondrification at 46 days to form distinctive corpora cavernosa. By the end of gestation external genital features are well differentiated, but it is not until 35 days postpartum that the formation of an os penis can be distinguished by alizarine staining (Evans, 1986). Urgel and Lacalle (1970) observed ossification histologically in a 30-day-old puppy.

Development of the Os Penis

In the month-old Beagle puppy, each corpus cavernosum at midlevel of the penis appears as a slightly compressed column, which dips ventrally as it passes through the bulbus glandis. The internal fibrous trabeculae of the corpus cavernosum appear as transverse striations in cleared specimens (Fig. 9.27). At the level of the bulbus glandis the striated trabecular columns become homogeneous fibrocartilages, without trabecular spaces, which fuse on the midline dorsal to the urethra and reach almost to the tip of the glans.

The first ossifications to form in the penis of the dog appear on the surface of cartilaginous nodules that form within the corpora cavernosa at 35 days after birth (Evans 1985, 1986). The rate of ossification may not be the same in all littermates, as shown in Fig. 9.27. In four littermate Beagles stained with alizarine and cleared in potassium hydroxide and glycerine (Fig. 9.28), one had no ossification, whereas the other three had bilateral single or double ossifications within cartilaginous nodules. The fact that the pup without any ossification did not have a cartilaginous nodule indicates that the bone and the cartilage develop almost simultaneously. One pup already had trabeculae joining right and left ossifications (Figs. 9.27A and 9.28). By 55 days postpartum (Fig. 9.29) the right and left ossifications in each fibrous column of the corpus cavernosum have elongated, flattened, and begun to fuse on the midline dorsal to the urethra. This results in the formation of a prominent urethral groove. As lengthening of the bone progresses, the base widens and the groove deepens.

In the adult male the base of the os is firmly attached to the tunica albuginea surrounding the corpora cavernosa because it developed within this sheath. The widest region of the os is at the level of the bulbus glandis, which surrounds it. The ventral margins of the os are roughened by the passage of vascular channels over the surface that connects the corpus spongiosum to the bulbus glandis. These channels can be seen developing in the 55- and 65-day pup (Figs. 9.29 and 9.30).

Thus the sequence of bone formation for the os penis in the dog is progressive fibroplasia of the terminal portions of the corpora cavernosa, followed by cartilage formation, perichondral bone formation, endochondral ossification, fusion of right and left ossifications, and subsequent bone growth by secondary cartilage ossification at the ends and deposition by an osteoblastic periosteum.

The apex of the os remains cartilaginous (Fig. 9.25) throughout life and has a fibrous continuation to the surface of the glans dorsal to the urethral orifice. It is this fibrous connection that during intromission deforms the glans within the fornix of the vagina and causes it to flatten dorsally as a "corona glandis" (Fig. 9.33).

Vessels and Nerves

Christensen (1954) investigated the normal blood flow through the penis of the dog and the mechanical factors involved in initiating and maintaining erection. Special attention was given to the morphologic characteristics and function of the arteries and veins of the glans penis. More recent studies by Ninomiya et al. (1989) confirm most of these findings.

The latter authors add observations based on corrosion casts and histologic sections to explain the hemodynamics. They found many cushions of epithelioid cells in the arterioles of the erectile bodies, which throttle blood flow into the cavernous spaces when the penis is flaccid, but yield to the pressure of increased flow during erection. Pressure changes in the cavernous spaces appear to be the result of relaxation of smooth muscle of the penis (allowing distension of the corpus cavernosum; see, e.g., Giuliano & Rampin, 2004), contractions of the ischiourethralis muscle which compresses the dorsal vein of the penis, contractions of the bulbospongiosus muscle, which compresses the bulb against the pelvic symphysis, and contractions of the external anal sphincter across the surface of the bulb. Aiding tumescence is the slowed egress of blood from the engorged cavernous spaces caused in part by compression of the internal pudendal vein by the contraction of the levator ani, coccygeus, and the internal obturator muscles.

The principal source of blood to the penis is the **internal pudendal artery** (Fig. 9.22), a ramification of the internal iliac. This is augmented by the **external pudendal artery**, which anastomoses with the preputial branch of the dorsal artery of the penis. After giving off the prostatic and urethral arteries, the internal pudendal gives rise to the ventral **perineal artery**, which supplies the superficial part of the penile root and the perineum. The internal pudendal artery terminates as the **artery of the penis,** which supplies the penis via three principal arteries: the artery of the bulb, the deep artery of the penis, and the dorsal artery of the penis. Typically, the artery of the bulb arises from the artery of the penis proximal to the deep artery of the penis. At this point, the artery of the penis is continued by the dorsal artery (Fig. 9.23).

The paired **arteries of the bulb** diverge into two or three branches, which divide again before entering the corpus spongiosum of the bulbus penis. These supply the spaces and tissue of the corpus spongiosum, the penile urethra, and the pars bulbus glandis (Christensen, 1954). The principal trunk is partially coiled in the nonerect state. Its branches anastomose with the end branches of the dorsal artery of the penis as well as with branches of the deep artery.

The **deep artery of the penis** gives off two to five branches and passes through the tunica albuginea to enter the corpus cavernosum. In this cavernous body, the artery again divides into clumps of spiral or looped vessels, the **helicine arteries**, which open directly into the cavernous spaces. According to Vaerst (1938) and Kiss (1921), helicine arteries retain their spiral shape in the nonerect penis, owing to contracted myoepithelium.

The **dorsal artery of the penis** runs diagonally distally to the bulbus glandis, anastomosing with the deep artery and artery of the bulb. Proximal to the glans penis, the dorsal artery trifurcates into a preputial branch, a deep branch, and a superficial branch (Fig. 9.24). The preputial branch runs dorsodistally over the bulbus glandis, supplying the dorsal surface of the pars longa glandis as well as anastomosing with the external pudendal artery in the parietal wall of the prepuce (Ninomiya & Nakamura, 1981a). The superficial branch runs ventrodistally deep to the epithelium of the skin of the glans, extending almost to the cranial end of the glans. The deep branch of the dorsal artery enters the terminal tunica albuginea and distally reaches the dorsolateral surface of the os penis, deep to the bulbus glandis (Figs. 9.24, 9.26). It passes into the pars longa glandis, terminating near the penile tip. Distal to the bulbus glandis, a large anastomotic branch is given off to the corpus spongiosum. The three branches of the dorsal artery of the penis and the external pudendal artery supply blood to the pars longa glandis.

The **internal** and **external pudendal veins** drain blood from the penis. The internal pudendal joins the internal iliac vein, and the external pudendal drains into the external iliac. The iliac veins on each side unite to form the common iliac vein, and the two common iliac veins then converge into the caudal vena cava. The intrinsic penile veins partially parallel the arteries at the root of the penis (Fig. 9.22). The dorsal veins of the penis are united at the ischial arch for a short distance before they diverge into the right and left internal pudendal veins. Unlike the corresponding arteries, the deep vein of the penis and the vein of the bulb unite in a common vein, the vein of the penis, which enters the internal pudendal vein. The ventral perineal vein also empties into this vein of the penis.

The dorsal veins of the penis arise from either side of the bulbus glandis and run along the dorsolateral surface of the penile body as far as the ischial arch. The superficial vein of the glans runs from the dorsal surface of the pars longa glandis to the external pudendal vein (Fig. 9.24).

The **dorsal vein of the penis** (Deysach, 1939), in its course between the bulbus glandis and the ischial arch where it unites with the opposite dorsal vein of the penis, has distinct semilunar valves regularly spaced along its entire length (Fig. 9.31). The **vein of the bulb** drains the cavernous spaces of the proximal half of the corpus spongiosum, arising at the junction of its proximal and middle thirds. Typically, two valves are located in the vein of the bulb between its emergence from the cavernous body and its junction with the deep vein of the penis. One to five valves are present between the origin of the vein of the penis and where it is joined by the ventral perineal vein.

The **superficial vein of the glans** arises from the deep surface of the pars longa glandis, which it helps to drain, and runs dorsocaudally to the fornix of the prepuce, where it bends acutely cranially and drains into the external pudendal vein by two or more connections (Fig. 9.23). One or more valves are present in each branch of the vein.

The **deep vein of the glans** (Fig. 9.24) drains blood from the pars longa glandis into the bulbus glandis. It arises on each side of the midline from the middle of the deep surface of the pars longa glandis and runs proximally along the dorsolateral surface of the os penis to enter the bulbus glandis. A semilunar valve prevents blood in the bulbus glandis from going to the pars longa glandis.

There is a double connection on each side of the os penis, between the deep vein of the glans and the dorsal vein of the penis (Fig. 9.32). A ventral shunt, through irregularly located openings, receives blood from the venous spaces of the bulbus glandis and the corpus spongiosum. The openings are directed proximally and are bordered distally by a lip of endothelium that diverts blood toward the dorsal vein of the penis. There is also a dorsal shunt through the bulbus glandis, which is narrower in diameter and less clearly defined than the ventral shunt. Numerous branches go from the dorsal shunt into the spaces of the bulbus. Blood going through the dorsal shunt disseminates into cavernous spaces of the bulbus, whereas blood in the ventral shunt is directed into the dorsal vein of the penis without detouring through the venous sinuses of the bulbar erectile tissue.

Nerves leaving the pelvic and sacral plexuses supply the penis. These are the paired **pelvic nerve** and the paired **pudendal nerve,** respectively. The **pelvic plexus** lies on the pelvic wall dorsal to the prostate gland, lateral to the rectum. It receives sympathetic postganglionic axons through the hypogastric nerve, which runs caudally from the caudal mesenteric plexus and ganglion. Sympathetic postganglionic axons may also arise from the sacral sympathetic trunk, enter the sacral plexus, and continue into the pudendal nerve to innervate the penis. The pelvic plexus receives parasympathetic preganglionic axons through the pelvic nerve from ventral branches of the first, second, and sometimes the third sacral nerves. Infrequently, only axons from the second sacral nerve go to the plexus. Axons leave the pelvic plexus and go to the bladder, prostate, pelvic urethra, rectum, and the penis. Sensory (afferent) fibers are present in the pelvic nerve, as well as efferent parasympathetic fibers, according to Gruber (1933). The **hypogastric nerves** (sympathetic) are responsible for ejaculation and prostatic secretion.

The pudendal nerve (mixed) arises from the sacral plexus, which is formed from all three sacral spinal nerve ventral branches. The pudendal nerve gives off superficial and deep perineal nerves and a caudal rectal nerve before continuing as the **dorsal nerve of the penis**. Superficial perineal nerves supply the skin around the anus and the scrotum (Spurgeon & Kitchell, 1982). The caudal rectal nerve supplies the external anal sphincter. Deep perineal nerve branches supply the ischiocavernosus, bulbospongiosus, ischiourethralis, and the retractor penis muscles. The smooth muscle fibers of the retractor penis also receive sympathetic and parasympathetic impulses. The retractor penis muscles receive postganglionic sympathetic axons via the deep perineal nerves (which cause contraction) and postganglionic parasympathetic axons via the pelvic plexus (which cause relaxation). The dorsal nerves of the penis pass cranially, on the dorsolateral surface of the body to the glans penis as sensory nerves of the glans. They give off numerous preputial branches before entering the glans. These branches supply the skin around the preputial orifice (Spurgeon & Kitchell, 1982).

Lymph vessels from the penis drain into the **superficial inguinal lymph nodes**.

Mechanism of Erection

Erection in the dog results from the filling of the spaces of the cavernous bodies with blood. The phenomenon of delayed erection in the dog is due to slow engorgement of the bulbus glandis and the pars longa glandis. There are two phases in the process of filling the erectile tissue of the penis with blood. One phase occurs prior to intromission and one post intromission. For intromission to occur the penis must be stiffened. This primarily involves the corpus cavernosum penis in the body of the penis. Presumably olfactory stimuli initiate activity in the brain that in turn activates sacral spinal cord segments. Pelvic nerve stimulation increases penile blood pressure, partial inhibition of venous drainage (see Figs. 9.31 and 9.33) and dilation of arteries in the penis (Christensen, 1954; Hanyu, 1988). Activation of sacral parasympathetic neurons inhibits the smooth muscle in the helicine branches of the deep arteries and the arteries of the bulb of the penis, allowing them to relax, which results in increased blood flow to the cavernous bodies. Activation of sacral somatic efferent neurons results in rhythmic contractions of the ischiocavernous muscles to help force blood into the corpus cavernosum penis.

Arterial blood pressure in the penis rises, but venous outlets are still sufficient to accommodate the increased inflow of blood. The corpus spongiosum receives the greater share of the blood through the artery of the bulb of the penis. Venous blood continues to flow into the bulbus glandis and into the vein of the bulb. Arterial blood is shunted from the artery of the bulb into the corpus cavernosum via anastomotic branches. The deep vein of the penis is not of sufficient diameter to drain the increased amount of arterial blood emptying into the cavernous spaces from the helicine arteries. Internal pressure against the tunica albuginea causes a stiffening of the corpus cavernosum. The intrinsic veins tend to be compressed. Intromission occurs prior to engorgement of the bulb of the glans.

In the second phase of penile erection that follows intromission, the process of intromission stimulates sacral somatic afferent dendritic zones in the skin of the penis (Hart & Kitchell, 1966). This results in reflex activation of sacral somatic efferent neurons that innervate penile muscles. A rhythmic contraction of the bulbospongiosus muscles occurs and is visible in the copulating male. This forces the blood in the expanding bulb of the penis distally in the corpus spongiosum. At the level of the caudal portion of the os penis the vascular spaces in the corpus spongiosum surrounding the urethra are continuous around the os penis into the bulb of the glans. This permits the expanding blood volume in the corpus spongiosum to expand into the bulb of the glans. A tonic contraction of the two ischiourethralis muscles contributes to maintaining stasis in the erectile tissue by restricting outflow of blood in the dorsal vein of the penis where they form a common trunk.

When the paired ischiourethral muscles contract, the fibrous ring (encircling the common venous trunk) (Figs. 9.18B and 9.31B) is pulled caudally and laterally, narrowing the lumen of the ring and partially squeezing the vein. The fibrous ring is anchored to the symphysis pelvis by a short, thick ligament. Muscular contraction does not affect the arteries, which lie outside the encircling fibrous ring. The ischiocavernosus and bulbospongiosus muscles, upon contracting, slow down egress of blood through the deep vein, the vein of the bulb of the penis, and their union as the vein of the penis. Before intromission, the superficial veins of the glans, as well as the dorsal veins of the penis, allow free flow of venous blood away from the glans. With constriction of the veins leaving the two cavernous bodies, venous blood is further directed into the bulbus glandis via shunts from the corpus spongiosum. More arterial blood enters the capillaries of the pars longa glandis through the branches of the dorsal artery of the penis and the artery of the bulb.

Intromission also stimulates sacral somatic afferent neuronal dendritic zones in the skin and mucosa of the vulva and vestibule of the female, resulting in a reflex tonic contraction of the constrictor vulvae and vestibuli muscles. This contraction is on the body of the penis caudal to the engorged bulb of the glans restricting outflow of blood in the dorsal veins of the penis (Fig. 9.31). This contraction of the female's constrictor vestibuli muscle also prevents blood from leaving the pars longa glandis through the superficial vein of the glans. Because of their relatively thick muscular walls and greater intrinsic pressure, the arteries of the penis are not occluded by extrinsic muscular contraction.

Because the superficial veins of the glans no longer permit outflow of blood, all blood in the pars longa is directed toward the deep veins of the glans. The spaces of the bulbus glandis receive venous blood from two sources: deep veins of the glans and the corpus spongiosum. When the dorsal veins of the penis permit free exit of blood from the bulbus, the blood traverses the ventral shunt in the bulbus without expanding the erectile tissue. With the dorsal veins partially occluded, and the inflow of blood greatly increased, blood entering the bulbus through the deep vein of the glans is forced into the dorsal bulbar shunt (Fig. 9.32). Because of the abundance of openings in the dorsal shunt, excess venous blood is permitted to enter and engorge the spaces of the bulbus glandis. The caliber of the dorsal veins of the penis is not sufficient for them to accommodate this increased amount of blood. Valves in the deep veins of the glans and in the venous connections with the corpus spongiosum prevent blood from leaving the bulbus by any route except through the now inefficient dorsal penile veins.

The engorgement of the bulbus glandis and pars longa glandis is facilitated by relaxation of the smooth muscles of the intersinusoidal trabeculae and by stretching of the elastic fibers in the trabeculae.

The branches of the dorsal artery of the penis lose their helicine-like appearance as the pars longa glandis is distended. The deep branch of the dorsal artery uncoils and straightens out during the height of erection. As the glans penis becomes engorged and firm, less arterial blood can be accommodated, and it is shunted from the dorsal artery to the corpus cavernosum, increasing its stiffness. After ejaculation, the extrinsic penile muscles relax and arterial blood pressure drops to normal. Venous pressure declines as the erectile bodies shrink. The bulbus glandis decreases in diameter sooner than the pars longa glandis, owing to its greater venous drainage. Elastic recoil of the intersinusoidal trabeculae helps force blood out of the glans.

For a historical discussion of the mechanism of erection, refer to Eckhard (1863), Francois-Franck (1895), and Langley (1896). For more recent interpretations see Christensen (1954), Hart and Kitchell (1965), Nitschke (1966), Dorr and Brody (1967), Grandage (1972), Ninomiya (1980), and Ninomiya et al. (1989). Hart (1972) recorded tonic contractions of the ischiourethralis muscle, which inhibits venous return in the dorsal vein, and rhythmical contractions of the bulbospongiosus, which forces blood distally. Purohit and Beckett (1976) found high arterial pressures in the corpora cavernosa that were correlated with contractions of the ischiocavernosus muscles. This indicates a more active role for the corpora cavernosa than was previously believed, although their small blood volume and inexpansible tunica albuginea would not indicate it.

Grandage (1972) divides coitus into a first stage (mounted) and a second stage of longer duration, when the male dismounts with the engorged penis still within the vestibule and vagina and faces in the opposite direction during the "tie" or "lock." During the second stage there is a 180-degree bend in the middle of the body of the penis, which occludes the emissary veins and prevents detumescence. Using radiographic techniques, Grandage was able to determine that the penis displaced the cervix to the level of the sacral promontory. The glans and approximately 3 cm of the body enter the vagina. During this paradox of flexible rigidity, the dorsal surface of the penis remains dorsal because it is a bend of the corpus penis and not a twist. Although the sperm-rich fraction of the ejaculate is passed within 80 seconds of first-stage coitus (following intromission), another 30 mL of seminal fluid is produced during second-stage coitus, which probably aids passage into the uterus and possibly stimulates peristaltic contractions of the uterine tubes.

The "tie," or "lock," depends on the reflex contraction of the ischiourethral muscle by stimulation of deep receptors caudal to the bulbus glandis and by the contraction of the constrictor vestibuli muscle of the female during copulation. Anesthesia of the receptors caudal to the bulbus glandis will result in a partial erection followed by copulation and ejaculation but no locking. Section of the ischiourethral muscle prevented enlargement of the bulbus glandis and locking but did not interfere with copulation or ejaculation (Hart, 1972).

The flaccid penis varies greatly in length and diameter, depending on individual variations as well as on breed and size of the animal. Physiologic changes caused by temperature, urination, and sexual excitement also contribute to marked variations of size.

Male Urethra

The male **urethra** (*urethra masculina*) carries urine, semen, and seminal secretions to the distal end of the penis. In a 25-pound mature dog, the urethra averages 25 cm in length. It is divisible into a pelvic part (*pars pelvina*) and a penile part (*pars penina*). The pars pelvina includes a preprostatic portion and a prostatic portion. In the dog the preprostatic part is essentially absent.

The **prostatic portion** (*pars prostatica*) of the urethra passes through the prostate gland (Fig. 9.16). The walls of the prostatic urethra are made up of a variable number of longitudinal mucosal folds. When distended, all the folds, except the dorsally located **urethral crest** (*crista urethralis*), are obliterated. The **seminal hillock** (*colliculus seminalis*) is an oval enlargement, located at the center of the urethral crest, which protrudes into the lumen of the urethra. The ampullae of the deferent ducts open on each side of the colliculus seminalis. The opening of each duct is usually not visible macroscopically unless fluid is forced from the ducts and ampullae into the urethra. Numerous prostatic ducts also open into the urethra adjacent to and surrounding the urethral crest. Instead of being round or oval, a cross-section through the middle of the prostatic urethra appears U-shaped. The center of the colliculus seminalis contains a minute opening into a tiny tube, the *uterus masculinus*, which runs craniodorsally into the prostate. The uterus masculinus, also known as the *prostatic utricle* and *utriculus prostaticus*, is a homologue of the caudal portion of the paramesonephric ducts in the female. Caudal to the prostate, the pelvic urethra contains a thin layer of vascular tissue, the stratum spongiosum. This cavernous tissue is continued into the penile part of the urethra as the corpus spongiosum, which includes its expansion at the ischial arch as the bulb of the penis.

The **penile part of the urethra** is a continuation of the pelvic part located in the pelvis. The penile part begins at the ischial arch. It is surrounded by corpus spongiosum for its entire length. At the ischial arch, the bulb of the penis is an expansion of this spongy tissue.

The **stratum spongiosum** of the urethra is composed of vascular erectile tissue that is continuous in the penis with the corpus spongiosum. Peripheral to the vascular layer of the pelvic urethra is the **urethral gland** layer (*glds. urethrales*) consisting of isolated small branched glands. The **muscular layer** (*tunica muscularis*) consists of smooth muscle, primarily longitudinal, which extends from the prostate, which it overlaps slightly, to the point where the stratum spongiosum ends at the bulb of the penis. Within the pelvis, peripheral to the smooth muscle layer, is the thick striated **m. urethralis**, which consists of transversely running fibers that are separated dorsally by a thin, longitudinal fibrous raphe.

Vessels and Nerves
The prostatic part of the pelvic urethra is supplied with blood through the **prostatic artery**. The stratum spongiosum is supplied by small **urethral arteries** that branch off the internal pudendal, urethral, or prostatic arteries. The penile part is supplied through the **artery of the bulb of the penis**. The **urethral veins** are satellites of the arteries, draining into the internal pudendal vein. The smooth muscles of the urethra are innervated by the autonomic nerves derived from the **pelvic plexus**. The striated urethralis muscle is innervated by somatic efferent axons in the pudendal nerve.

Anomalies and Variations
The length and diameter of the urethra vary within wide limits. When the penis is flaccid, the urethral mucosa is folded longitudinally and the lumen is obliterated. During urination or ejaculation, the urethral walls are distended. Only that part of the cavernous urethra that passes in the ventral groove of the os penis is limited in its expansion. Fracture of the os (Stead, 1972) can obstruct the urethra. The urethra may infrequently open on the ventral surface of the penis (hypospadias) or on the dorsal surface (epispadias). Hypospadias (Ader & Hobson, 1978) is considered to result from failure of the urethral groove to close normally, whereas epispadias is caused by an embryonic displacement of cells forming the cloacal membrane, resulting in a reversal of the cloacal membrane location.

Prepuce
The **prepuce** (*preputium*) (Fig. 9.16) is a fold of skin covering the glans of the penis in the retracted state. It consists of an **external lamina** (*lamina externa*) and an **internal lamina** (*lamina interna*), which are continuous at the **preputial orifice** (*ostium preputiale*). The internal lamina terminates at the fornix, where it becomes continuous with the skin of the glans, in a transverse plane through the bulbus glandis. The external lamina is the haired skin of the outer surface. In erection the internal lamina is reflected from the preputial orifice onto the bulbus glandis and body of the penis, thus eliminating the **preputial cavity** and **fornix**.

The **preputial muscle** (*protractor preputii*) is a small divergent strip of cutaneous trunci muscle that extends from the area of the xiphoid cartilage to the dorsal wall of the prepuce. Two functions are attributed to the preputial muscles: to prevent the cranial free end of the prepuce from hanging loosely in nonerection and to pull the prepuce back over the glans penis after retraction. During erection, the preputial muscles are relaxed.

Vessels and Nerves
The internal lamina of the prepuce is supplied by an intricate, anastomosing network of arteries. The arteries are branches of the external pudendal artery and the preputial branch of the dorsal artery of the penis (Fig. 9.10). The skin of the glans that covers the glans penis is supplied by the three anastomosing branches of the **dorsal artery** of the penis, the **external pudendal artery**, and, to a lesser degree, by the **artery of the bulb** of the penis.

Ninomiya (1980) studied the cavernous system of the erect and nonerect penis in the dog by injecting acrylic resin. His findings agree with Christensen (1954) and Nitschke (1966) and he illustrates them with figures of entire and transected casts. Ninomiya and Nakamura (1981b) studied the capillary loops in the dermal papillae of the penile skin and noted differences in their configuration at various sites. In the corona glandis there were hairpin loops, in the prepuce near the apex there were simple loops, and near the fornix of the prepuce there were more complicated capillary networks in each dermal papilla. They suggest that the arteriovenous anastomoses seen in the subpapillary area over the collum and bulbus glandis play an active role in passing blood directly to the subpapillary venous plexus, which in turn sends venules into the cavernous spaces.

The veins from the internal lamina drain into the **external pudendal vein**. The skin of the glans is drained by the **superficial vein of the glans** into the external pudendal vein and, deeply, by the **dorsal vein of the penis** via the deep vein of the glans and the bulbus glandis. Preputial lymph vessels enter the **superficial inguinal lymph nodes**.

Sensory (afferent) innervation of the surface of the glans is through preputial branches of the **dorsal nerve of the** penis. These same branches supply the preputial orifice. The remainder of the prepuce is innervated by lateral cutaneous branches of the genitofemoral nerve (Spurgeon & Kitchell, 1982).

Anomalies and Variations

The two most common anomalies of the prepuce are phimosis and paraphimosis. Phimosis is the existence of an abnormally small preputial opening, which prevents protrusion of the penis. Paraphimosis is the inversion of the preputial opening, forming a constrictive ring after penile protrusion, which prevents the return of the glans penis into the preputial cavity. Persistence of the preputial frenulum may also result in the inability to protrude the penis.

Female Genital Organs

The female genital organs (*organa genitalia feminina*) consist of **ovaries**, **uterine tubes**, **uterus**, **vagina**, **vestibule**, **pudendum femininum** (vulva), and **clitoris**. The ovaries contain the **oocytes** (called *ovocytes* per the 2005 NAV, but *oocytes* in Noden & de Lahunta, 1985; Konig & Liebich, 2004; Kumar, 2015), which are periodically ovulated, engulfed by the infundibulum, fertilized or not in the uterine tube, and transported to the uterus. If fertilization takes place the blastocysts develop in the uterine tube and are passed into the uterine horns to be distributed and implanted in either uterine horn (Fig. 9.34). Also see Abe et al. (2010) for position of embryos within the uterus and uterine horn subsequent to artificial insemination.

It is often the case that one ovary ovulates more oocytes than the other, but it is usual to have an even distribution of blastocysts in the uterine horns. The change from one side to the other takes place by transuterine migration through the body of the uterus. Evans (1974) documented transuterine migrations in 13 Beagles (see Table 2.1).

Broad Ligaments

The ovaries, uterine tube, and uterus are attached to the dorsolateral walls of the abdominal cavity and to the lateral walls of the pelvic cavity by paired double folds of peritoneum called the right and left **broad ligament** (*ligamentum latum uteri*). Each broad ligament contains an ovary, uterine tube, and uterine horn. It also contains vessels and nerves to the genitalia and fingerlike streaks of fat. It does not support or suspend the genitalia in the body cavities, but rather unites its components.

The broad ligament is attached dorsally along or near the junction of the psoas and transversus abdominis muscles. Cranially it is attached by means of the suspensory ligament of the ovary to the junction of the middle and distal thirds of the last rib. The ligament is reflected off the vagina onto the rectum dorsally, ventrally onto the urethra and bladder, and in a curved line laterally onto the wall of the pelvic cavity as far as the deep inguinal ring. The ligament is broadest at the level of the ovary, tapering from there to its cranial and caudal extremities. In a 25-pound dog, the distance spanned by the broad ligament at the ovarian level varies from 6 to 9 cm. A peritoneal fold arises from the lateral surface of the broad ligament and extends from the ovary to or through the inguinal canal. It contains the round ligament of the uterus in its free border (Figs. 9.1 and 9.35A, B). The peritoneal pouch that extends through the inguinal canal into the subcutaneous region of the vulva is known as the **vaginal process** (see Figs. 9.11 and 9.13). A similar peritoneal pouch in the male, which extends into the scrotum, forms the vaginal tunic that surrounds the structures in the spermatic cord and testis. The vaginal process and round ligament of the female may be obscured by fat. Both may extend into the subcutaneous tissue of the labia. The round ligament of the uterus and the ovarian ligaments contained in the broad ligament are described more fully in the discussions of the uterus and ovaries.

Morphologically, the broad ligament is divided into three regions: **mesovarium**, **mesosalpinx**, and **mesometrium**. The *mesovarium* (Fig. 9.35) is that part of the broad ligament that attaches the ovary to the dorsolateral region of the abdominal wall. The cranial boundary of the broad ligament, where the suspensory ligament of the ovary attaches to or near to the thirteenth rib, marks its beginning, and it ends at a transverse plane just caudal to the ovary. It contains the ovarian vessels.

The *mesosalpinx* (Fig. 9.35A), another double fold of peritoneum, extends laterally from the dorsal peritoneal layer of the mesovarium. It curves around the dorsal and ventrolateral borders of the ovary to attach to the medial surface of the broad ligament just dorsal to the ovary. It encloses the ovary within a small pouch of the peritoneal cavity, the ovarian bursa. The **ovarian bursa** (*bursa ovarica*) (Fig. 9.35) is variable in size, depending on the age and size of the animal. It averages 2 cm in length in a 25-pound dog. The amount of fat between the peritoneal layers of the mesosalpinx depends on the condition of the animal. The bursa is open to the peritoneal cavity by a narrow slit on its medial surface (Fig. 9.35). In a 25-pound dog, the opening averages 0.8 cm in length. Close to the opening of the bursa lies the proper ligament of the ovary and the suspensory ligament of the ovary. Within the opening of the bursa and protruding from it are the numerous fimbriae of the infundibulum. At the time of ovulation these fimbriae are tumescent and plug the opening of the bursa, which prevents the escape of oocytes into the peritoneal cavity. The entire uterine tube, ascending and descending, lies within the peritoneal layers of the mesosalpinx.

The *mesometrium* begins at the cranial edge of the uterine horn, where it is continuous with the mesovarium, and extends caudally to a point where the peritoneum of the broad ligament reflects onto the bladder and the colon. It leaves the uterine horn, the body of the uterus, the cervix, and the cranial part of the vagina to attach along the abdominal and pelvic walls. The uterine artery and vein and the uterine branch of the ovarian artery and vein run between the peritoneal layers of the mesometrium.

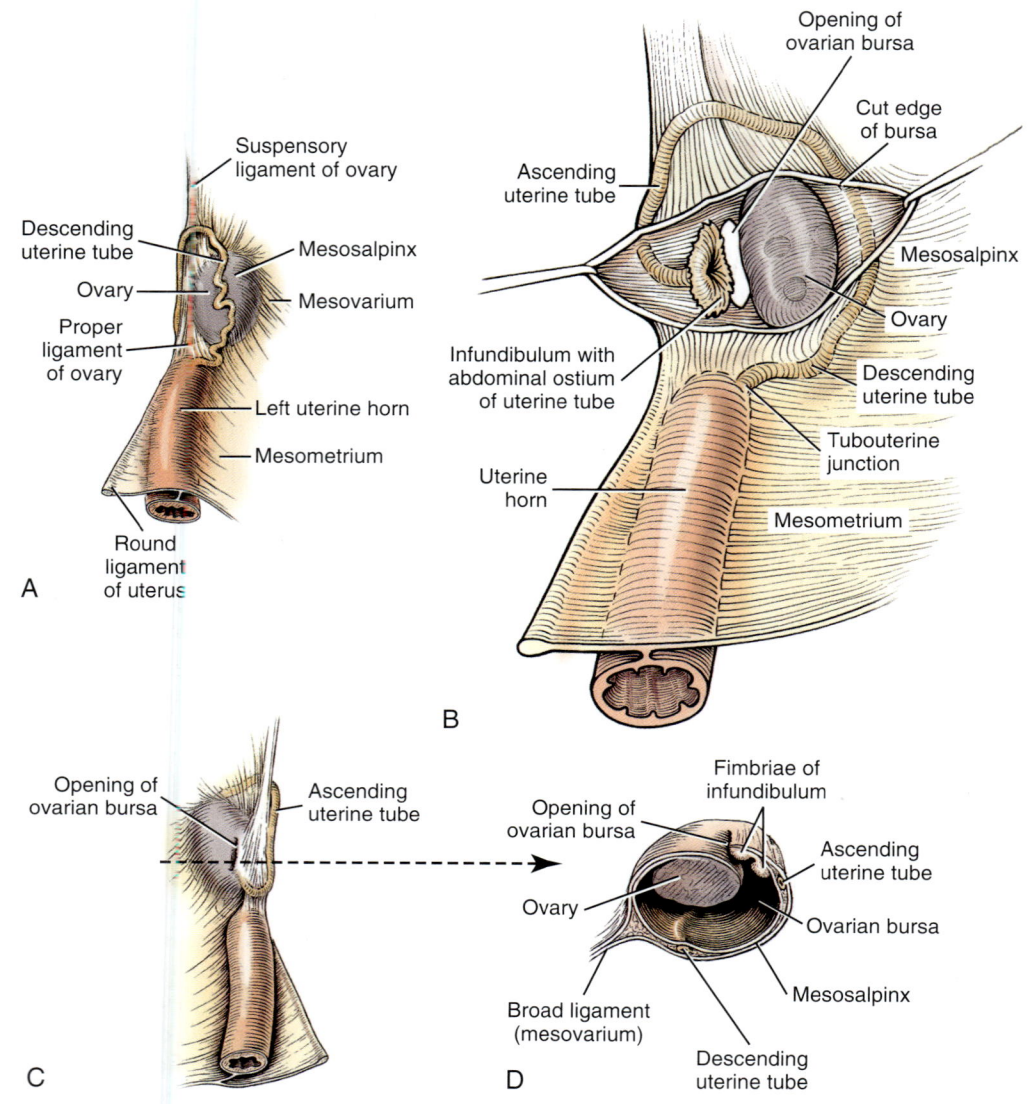

• **Fig. 9.35** Relations of left ovary and ovarian bursa. **A,** Dorsolateral aspect. **B,** Dorsolateral aspect, ovarian bursa opened. **C,** Ventromedial aspect. **D,** Section through ovary and ovarian bursa.

Ovaries

The **ovary**, or female gonad, is a paired oval organ, attached by a mesovarium to the body wall and by the mesosalpinx. The mesovarium proximale extends from the body wall to the origin of the mesosalpinx, and the mesovarium distale extends from the origin of the mesosalpinx to the ovary and forms part of the wall of the ovarian bursa. The ovary lies caudal to the kidney (see Figs. 9.1) and contains all of the oocytes that the female will ovulate in her lifetime (Mossman & Duke, 1973). It is also the source of several hormones. In a 25-pound dog, an ovary averages 1.5 cm in length, 0.7 cm in width, 0.5 cm in thickness, and 0.3 g in weight. In its normal position, an ovary may be described as having tubal and uterine extremities, a free border, and medial and lateral surfaces. The tubal end is nearest the infundibulum. The uterine end is the end attached to the uterus by the proper ligament of the ovary. The ovary is smooth in appearance before estrus, which occurs for the first time between 6 and 9 months of age. In multiparous bitches (several litters) the surface may be rough and nodular. At times the ovaries are dissimilar in size, in which case the left ovary is usually larger.

A laparoscopic study of the ovary of a cycling bitch was made by Wildt et al. (1977). In a sexually mature, 25-pound dog, the left ovary is located approximately 12 cm caudal to the middle of the thirteenth rib and 1 to 3 cm caudal to the corresponding kidney. Typically, it lies between the abdominal wall and the descending colon. The right ovary is located approximately 10 cm caudal to the last rib of the right side. The ventral border and medial surface of the ovary are in contact with the mesovarium. In a young animal it lies ventral to the adipose capsule of the right kidney and dorsal to the descending duodenum. In animals that have undergone numerous pregnancies, both right and left ovaries shift caudally and ventrally. Frequently fat is deposited within the mesosalpinx partially obscuring the ovary.

Ligaments

In addition to the mesovarium, the ovary has two other ligamentous attachments. The **suspensory ligament of the ovary** (*lig. suspensorium ovarii*) is attached cranially to the middle and ventral thirds of the last one or two ribs. Caudally it attaches to the ventral aspect of the ovary and mesosalpinx, lying between the opening of the ovarian bursa and the ascending uterine tube (Fig. 9.35). The suspensory ligament lies between the two layers of peritoneum in the free border of the mesovarium, which is the cranial portion of the broad ligament. It is continued caudally by the **proper ligament of the ovary** (*lig. ovarii proprium*). This in turn attaches the uterine end of the ovary to the cranial end of the uterine horn. There it is continuous with the round ligament of the uterus, which extends caudally toward the inguinal canal and passes through it to be wrapped by the vaginal process before it ends near the vulva. Both the proper and the suspensory ovarian ligament are composed of connective tissue mixed with smooth muscle fibers.

Structure

The ovary has a medulla and a cortex. The **medulla** (*medulla ovarii [zona vasculosa]*) contains blood vessels, nerves, lymphatics, smooth muscle fibers, and connective tissue fibers. The **cortex** (*cortex ovarii [zona parenchymentosa]*) consists of a connective tissue stroma that contains a large number of follicles. For a review of ovarian structures in several mammals, including the dog, see Mossman and Duke (1973). The most comprehensive work is that of Zuckerman (1971).

The connective tissue condenses to form the tunica albuginea around the ovary. The tunica albuginea is covered by visceral peritoneum referred to as the **superficial epithelium of the ovary**. (The latter term replaces the unsuitable but much used name *germinal epithelium*.) Follicles are present deep to the tunica albuginea. A **primordial follicle** consists of an oocyte and its surrounding granulosa cells enclosed in a basement membrane that separates the follicle from the ovarian stroma.

With each estrus a number of follicles mature. The granulosa cells at first form a single cuboidal layer around the oocyte, which constitutes a **primary follicle** (*folliculus ovaricus primarius*). With further maturation, several layers of granulosa cells are formed around the oocyte. Eventually, a cavity filled with follicular fluid forms within the granulosa cell mass. Such a follicle is designated as a **tertiary** or **vesicular follicle** (*folliculus ovaricus tertiarius [vesiculosus]*), formerly termed a Graafian follicle. At one end of the cavity there is a hillock, the cumulus oophorus, which contains the maturing oocyte. In intimate contact with the oocyte is a clear membrane, the zona pellucida. This is surrounded by a layer of radially arranged granulosa cells, the corona radiata. As the **follicular fluid** (*liquor follicularis*) increases,

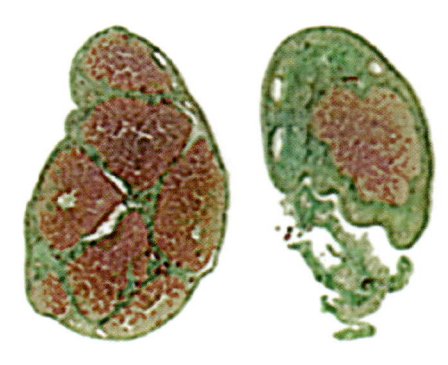

• **Fig. 9.36** Longitudinal section of left and right ovaries of a Beagle, early in gestation. There are seven corpora lutea in the left ovary and one in the right. The uterus contained four embryos in the left horn and three in the right, indicating that at least two blastocysts migrated from the left uterine horn to the right. (From Evans HE: *Gaines symposium*, Ithaca, NY, 1974.)

the follicle migrates to the periphery of the ovary. When the follicle ruptures, the oocyte is released into the **ovarian bursa** and is swept by ciliary action into the infundibulum of the uterine tube (Fig. 9.35). Not all follicles that begin to mature proceed to ovulation. The vast majority of follicles degenerate at different stages of development throughout life, as they do in all mammals (Perry, 1972; Zuckerman, 1971).

After ovulation, relatively slight hemorrhage occurs in the ovary. The follicular cavity tinged by blood is called a **corpus hemorrhagicum** and as this is resorbed, a **corpus luteum** (Fig. 9.36) is formed from the granulosa and theca interna cells. If fertilization does not take place, the corpus luteum gradually degenerates into a connective tissue scar, the **corpus albicans**. If the oocyte is fertilized, the corpus luteum remains fully developed throughout pregnancy and produces progesterone. After parturition, it regresses. Involution of the corpus luteum again allows vesicular follicles to mature.

An ovulated oocyte is visible to the naked eye when held in fluid against a dark background. Recent birth control studies using the oocytes of several animals have resulted in a patent being issued in 1991 to Bonnie Dunbar of Baylor College of Texas for a genetically engineered vaccine based on proteins from the zona pellucida, which surrounds the oocyte. When the protein is injected, the animal produces antibodies that bind to the zona pellucida and prevent sperm from entering the oocyte. Clinical trials of dogs have been authorized by the U.S. Food and Drug Administration.

Estrous Cycle

Estrus in the bitch usually occurs twice a year, in the spring and again in the fall, although it may occur in any month of the year and may vary in occurrence from year to year. Sokolowski et al. (1977) report that Basset Hounds and Cocker Spaniels have mean interestrous intervals of approximately 5 months, whereas the German Shepherd Dog has the shortest interestrous interval, 149 ± 28.5 days. The mean occurrence of estrus for the German Shepherd Dog is 2.4 times per year and for other breeds it is 1.5 times per year. Neither natural nor artificial light has any effect on estrus. Periods of sexual receptivity in the bitch can be recognized by behavioral patterns: lordosis, presenting to the stud, excitement of the stud, cytologic changes in the vaginal epithelium (blood cells and cornification as seen in a smear), visual changes of the vaginal epithelium as seen with an endoscope (Lindsay, 1983), and, more recently, by hormone levels, particularly luteinizing hormone (LH) in the circulating blood (Concannon, 1991).

The changes through which the nonpregnant uterus passes were designated by Heape (1900) as **proestrum**, **estrum**, **metestrum**, and **anestrum**. These terms were used by Evans and Cole (1931), Griffiths and Amoroso (1939), and other early investigators of the dog's estrous cycle. Later workers suggested that the phase of estrus during which the reproductive organs are mainly under the influence of progesterone should be designated as *diestrus*, leaving the term *metestrus* for the short transition stage between estrus and diestrus when the corpora lutea are becoming functional. Investigations by Holst and Phemister (1971, 1974), Concannon et al. (1975), and Concannon (1991) have facilitated a redefinition of the estrous cycle.

Proestrus is a period of increasing levels of estrogen, the discharge of serosanguineous fluid, vaginal cornification, and swelling of the vulva. Pheromones attractive to the male are secreted toward the end of the period, which may be as brief as 3 days or as long as 3 weeks, with a mean of approximately 9 days. During most of this period the bitch will not allow the stud to mount. She may turn and growl, sit down, or lie on her side.

Estrus is a period of heightened sexual activity in response to a decline in estrogen facilitated by a rise in progesterone. Estrous behavior includes standing firmly for the male to mount, deviation of the tail, and lordosis. Concannon (1991) has shown (Fig. 9.37) that the onset of estrus most often occurs within a day or two of the preovulatory LH surge. However, it may occur 4 days before or 6 days after the LH surge. Estrus may be as brief as 3 days or last for several weeks, although the average length is 9 days.

Some breeders prefer to mate their dogs toward the end of the estrous period to ensure that a maximum number of

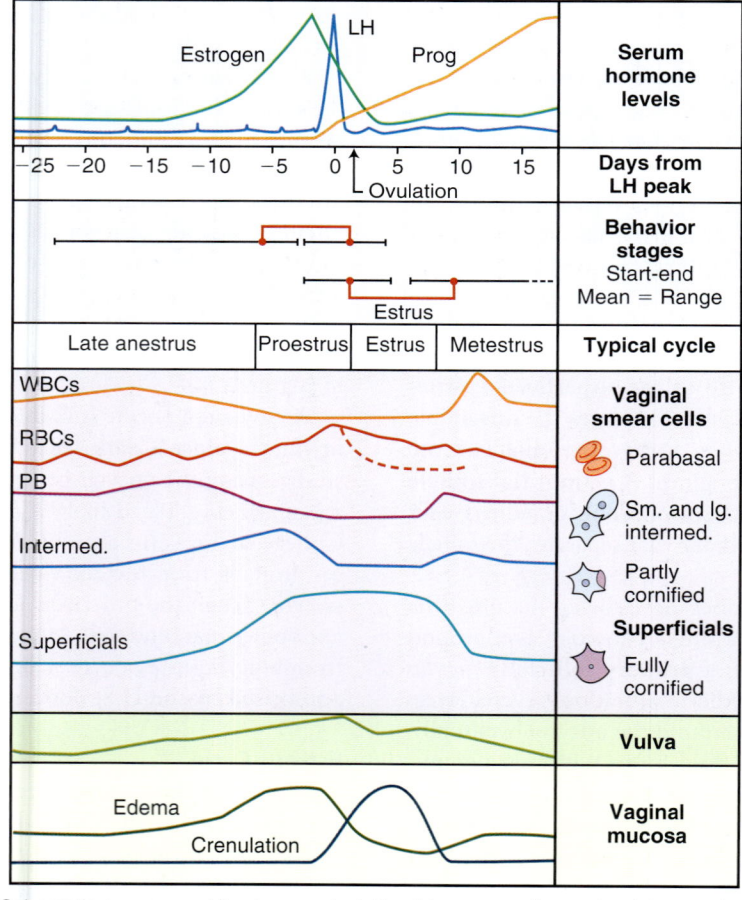

• **Fig. 9.37** Schematic summary of the temporal relationships among the periovulatory endocrine events, behavioral and vulval changes, and changes in the vaginal smear during proestrus, estrus, and early metestrus in the bitch. (From Concannon P, Lein DH: Hormonal and clinical correlates of ovarian cycles, ovulation, pseudopregnancy, and pregnancy in dogs, In Kirk RW, editor: *Current veterinary therapy X*, Philadelphia, 1989, Saunders.)

ova will have been ovulated, but this does not appear to be necessary. The embryos and fetuses used for description in Chapter 2 of this text were collected by Evans from more than 40 Beagle bitches bred to one stud 24 hours after they would first stand firmly and accept the stud. The conception rate for these matings early in estrus resulted in litters that averaged 6.7 pups per litter, which indicates that most ovulations had already occurred or sperm remained viable until the oocytes were ovulated. It is known that dog sperm can live for several days in the female reproductive tract (average 2 or 3 days) and that a mature oocyte can also live for several days (average 3 or 4 days). The average time of ovulation according to Concannon and Lein (1989) is 2 days after the LH surge. They found the peak period of fertility for natural matings ranged from 1 day before the preovulatory LH surge (= day 0) until day 5 or 6 after the LH surge. Based on their studies it can be said that breeding twice, between days 0 and 4, is probably best to ensure conception. This is probably what the normal bitch does if permitted. The length of gestation in the dog as timed by Concannon, using the day of the LH surge as day 0, results in gestation lengths of 64, 65, or 66 days, although the interval from mating to parturition may vary from 56 to 69 days. Evans (1974) considered day 0 to be 24 hours after first acceptance by the bitch, which resulted in an average gestation length of 60 to 63 days in his Beagles.

Metestrus is now synonymous with **diestrus**. It is a period without sharp boundaries when the corporea lutea are becoming functional and progesterone dominant. As this period begins the bitch may or may not accept the stud and there is an increase in the number of noncornified cells from the deeper layers of the vaginal epithelium. Vulval tumescence decreases but mammary development increases. Holst and Phemister (1971, 1974) described the onset of diestrus with regard to the characteristics of the vaginal epithelium and backdated from these signs to show correlations with the early stages of development. Diestrus minus 1 day was the stage of a two-cell cleavage; D minus 3 = fertilization; D minus 4 = formation of a secondary oocyte; D minus 5 = beginning of meiosis; D minus 6 = ovulation. They found that if the day of fertilization (diestrus minus 3 days) is counted as day 1 then the Beagle had a gestation period of 60 days and whelping took place on day 57 of diestrus.

Anestrus is a period of quiescence of the reproductive system with a fall in circulating hormone levels and an absence of sexual behavior. It lasts 2 to 10 months, with an average of 4 months. Some bitches are consistent in interval; others are not. Changes in sexual behavior correlated with hormone levels have been reported by Concannon et al. (1977), but now that it is practical to measure the level of LH in the bitch it is possible to use the LH peak as the most fixed point in the ovulatory cycle. Ovulation usually occurs 2 days after the LH peak and birth will take place about 65 days after the LH peak.

Concannon et al. (1983) in their early studies of gestation length in the dog, reported that in 290 dogs in which apparent gestation length was estimated as the interval from the day of first mating to the day of parturition ranged from 57 to 72 days and averaged 65.3 days. The interval from the day of the peak in LH to parturition was less variable and ranged from 64 to 66 days and averaged 65 days. Fertile single matings 3 days before the LH peak provided evidence that the potential postcoital fertile longevity of canine sperm is at least 6 days and this contributed, along with variability in the onset of estrus, to the observed variation in apparent gestation length in the dog. The limited range in the interval from the day of the preovulatory LH peak to the day of parturition (64, 65, or 66 days) demonstrates considerable regularity in the sequential events of gestation in the dog.

Raps (1948) made a study of the developmental changes in the dog ovary, from 2 days after birth to the sixth postnatal month. His data show that primordial oocytes (ovogonia) surrounded by follicular epithelial cells are present at 4 days of age, that at 15 days true primary follicle formation with granulosa cell development occurs, and that antrum formation is not observable until 6 months of age. Ultrasonographic studies by Yeager and Concannon (1990) and by Yeager et al. (1992) have correlated the LH peak with the echographic appearance of the conceptus (see Chapter 2).

Vessels and Nerves

The ovary is supplied with blood through the **ovarian artery** (Fig. 9.1). Homologous to the testicular artery of the male, the ovarian artery arises from the aorta approximately one-third to one-half the distance from the renal arteries to the deep circumflex iliac arteries. Usually the right ovarian artery arises slightly cranial to the left. The degree of uterine development determines the tortuosity and size as well as the position of the artery. In a nulliparous animal the artery extends laterally almost at right angles from the aorta, whereas in late pregnancy it is drawn cranioventrally, along with the ovary, by the enlarged, heavy uterus. In addition to supplying the ovary, the ovarian artery supplies branches to the adipose and fibrous capsules of the kidney. In addition, small tortuous branches supply the uterine tube and uterus. Caudally the uterine branch of the ovarian artery anastomoses with the **uterine artery**, a branch of the vaginal artery (formerly urogenital artery) (Fig. 11.73). Through this anastomotic connection, the uterine artery may be considered as a supplementary source of arterial blood to the ovary. The arteries to the ovary supply the parenchyma of the medulla and cortex as well as the thecae of the follicles. Capillary loops become extensive during follicular enlargement but recede or disappear during corpus luteum regression.

The right and left **ovarian veins** have different terminations (See Chapter 12). The right vein drains into the caudal vena cava, whereas the left enters the left renal vein. Similar to the corresponding arteries, the **uterine vein** and ovarian vein anastomose between the peritoneal layers of the broad ligament. The ovarian vein receives a tributary that comes from the medial edge of the suspensory ligament of the ovary and the lateral surface of the kidney. In some instances, the vein will also anastomose with the deep circumflex iliac vein. The arteries and veins of the ovaries in the dog have been studied by Del Campo and Ginther (1974). The lymphatics drain into the **lumbar lymph nodes**. Polano (1903) has demonstrated the ovarian lymphatics of the dog.

The nerve supply to the ovaries is from the sympathetic division of the autonomic nervous system. The nerves reach the ovaries by way of the **renal and aortic plexuses**, which receive axons from the fourth, fifth, and sixth lumbar sympathetic trunk ganglia. They accompany the ovarian artery to the ovary. The ovarian blood vessels receive an abundant sympathetic nerve supply, but, according to Kuntz (1919a), the ovarian follicles and interstitial secretory tissue are devoid of sympathetic innervation. Chien et al. (1991) investigated the origins of the sympathetic nerves innervating the ovary of the dog using the horseradish-peroxidase technique. Their findings indicated that the ovary receives sensory nerve fibers from the spinal ganglia of thoracic 10 to lumbar 4 segments. The highest concentrations of labeled neurons were at the thoracolumbar junction, T13 to L3. It has been suggested that nerves reaching the ovary play a role in follicle maturation and ovulation.

Anomalies and Variations

The ovaries may be hypoplastic, displaced, or completely missing. Rarely, an ovary may descend through the inguinal canal, in the manner of a testis, to rest in the vulvar region. Follicular cysts rarely occur. According to McEntee and Zepp (1953), ovarian tumors are relatively infrequent in the dog. Wenzel and Odend'hal (1985) reviewed the literature on the development and presence of the rete ovarii, the homologue of the rete testis. The rete ovarii of the adult dog appears as a mass of tubules in the hilus of the ovary, and the authors conclude that the rete ovarii is important in the control of meiosis and contributes cells to the ovarian follicle. As is true of most hollow remnant structures, cysts may develop from rete remnants.

Uterine Tube

The **uterine tube** (*tuba uterina*) (Fig. 9.35), still called *oviduct* in most zoology texts, transports the oocytes to the uterus. Each uterine tube is located between the peritoneal layers of the mesosalpinx and connects the peritoneal cavity with the uterine cavity. The uterine tube averages 4 to 7 cm in length and 1 to 3 mm in diameter. The ovarian extremity of the tube, the **infundibulum** (*infundibulum tubae uterinae*), is located near the edge of the opening into the **ovarian bursa** (*bursa ovarica*). The infundibulum has a small opening, the **abdominal ostium** (*ostium abdominale tubae uterinae*). The edges of the infundibulum are fringed by numerous diverging, fingerlike processes, the fimbriae. **Fimbriae** are usually visible projecting out of the opening of the ovarian bursa. They mark the junction of peritoneum (mesosalpinx) with the mucous membrane lining the uterine tube. The fimbriae are most visible from within the ovarian bursa. They are very vascular. From the time of ovulation until envelopment by the fimbriae, oocytes are actually in the peritoneal cavity. At the time of ovulation, the fimbriae are swollen and capable of movement so as to engulf an ovulated oocyte and block the entrance to the ovarian bursa. Follicular fluid and tubal mucus also play a role in drawing the oocyte into the uterine tube. In the dog all oocytes ovulated reach the uterine horns.

From the abdominal ostium, the uterine tube at first runs craniolaterally between the ventral layers of the mesosalpinx. Approximately halfway between the uterine end of the ovary and the cranial tip of the uterine horn, the uterine tube bends sharply cranially and runs along the free edge of the suspensory ligament of the ovary. Approximately 0.5 cm cranial to the gonad, it swings onto the dorsal aspect of the suspensory ligament and, still between peritoneal layers of the mesosalpinx, runs in a tortuous manner caudomesially toward the ovary. At the middle of the ovary the uterine tube curves caudolaterally toward the cranial end of the uterine horn, where the uterine tube terminates. The opening of the uterine tube into the horn of the uterus is called the **uterine ostium** (*ostium uterinum tubae*) and is the site of tubouterine junction, an important physiologic regulating sphincter for the passage of sperm cranially in the tube as well as the passage of blastocysts caudally in the tube (Anderson, 1927; Boyd et al., 1944; Hook & Hafez, 1968). Oocytes, zygotes, and blastulae are moved caudally in the uterine tube toward the uterus principally by peristaltic movements as well as by action of cilia. Fertilization, the union of oocyte and sperm, normally takes place close to or in the infundibulum. (An ovum never exists in the dog because first-stage meiosis occurs at ovulation, and second-stage meiosis does not occur until it is penetrated by a sperm cell to form a zygote.)

Structure

The uterine tube is covered by a **tunica serosa**, which is composed of peritoneum that forms the mesosalpinx. The muscular layer of the uterine tube is composed primarily of circular bundles of fibers, but a variable number of longitudinal and oblique fibers are also present. The muscular layer reaches its greatest development near its union with the circular muscles of the uterine horn, where it forms the tubouterine junction. The innermost layer (*tunica mucosa*) is made up of partially ciliated simple columnar epithelium. Sawyer et al. (1984) investigated the effects of progesterone on the uterine tubal epithelium in estrogen-primed prepubertal dogs and found that low cuboidal cells of the uterine tubal epithelium gave rise to columnar ciliated and secretory cells within 12 days after injection.

Vessels and Nerves

The uterine tube is supplied by the **ovarian and uterine arteries**. The two vessels anastomose near the cranial extremity of the uterine horn. The veins are satellites of the arteries. The lymphatics follow the ovarian lymph ducts to the **lumbar lymph nodes**. Sampson (1937) and Ramsey (1946) have worked out the detailed anatomy of the lymphatics of the uterine tube in various species of mammals. For the most part, the numerous lymphatic channels in the mucosal folds of the infundibulum and fimbriae, as well as those of the tube, drain into the lymph vessels of the mesosalpinx.

Nerves to the uterine tube are derived primarily from the thoracolumbar sympathetic trunk and pass through the **aortic and renal plexuses**. Parasympathetic axons from the **pelvic plexus** also innervate the uterine tube (Mitchell, 1938).

Anomalies and Variations

The **epoophoron** are a complex of vestigial tubules that occasionally give rise to cysts in the mesovarium or mesosalpinx. These are remnants of the embryonic mesonephric duct. The **paroophoron** are cystic structures that occur in the mesosalpinx near the uterine extremity of the ovary and are remnants of mesonephric tubules.

Congenital stenosis of the oviduct has been observed.

Uterus

The uterus serves for the conduction of sperm to the uterine tube for the fertilization of the oocyte, and for the conduction, implantation, and nourishment of the developing young. Hypertrophy of the tunica mucosa (endometrium) forms with the fetal membranes a placenta to serve as a source of embryonic and fetal nourishment (Anderson, 1969; Barrau et al., 1975).

The **uterus** consists of a **neck** (*cervix uteri*), a short **body** (*corpus uteri*), and two **horns** (*cornua uteri dextrum et sinistrum*). It is Y-shaped and communicates with the uterine tubes cranially and the vagina caudally (Figs. 9.1 and 9.38). Its size varies considerably, depending on age, previous pregnancies, stage of the estrous cycle, and whether the animal is currently pregnant. In females that have never had young (nulliparous) the uterine horns of a 25-pound dog average 10 to 14 cm in length and 0.5 to 1 cm in diameter. They diverge from the body of the uterus at a point 4 to 5 cm cranial to the symphysis pelvis. The uterine body is 1.4 to 3 cm long and 0.8 to 1 cm in diameter. The cervix averages 1.5 to 2 cm long. A small caudal portion of the cervix may protrude into the vagina. The diameter of this intravaginal cervix is approximately 0.8 cm. The gravid uterus in the latter third of pregnancy may occupy any portion of the abdominal cavity, and the uterine horns frequently change position in relation to one another, although they are somewhat limited by the suspensory and round ligaments. During uterine distention, the horns bend upon themselves and may rest entirely upon the ventral wall the abdomen.

The **uterine horns** are usually of the same size and unite at an acute angle with the body of the uterus. The cranial

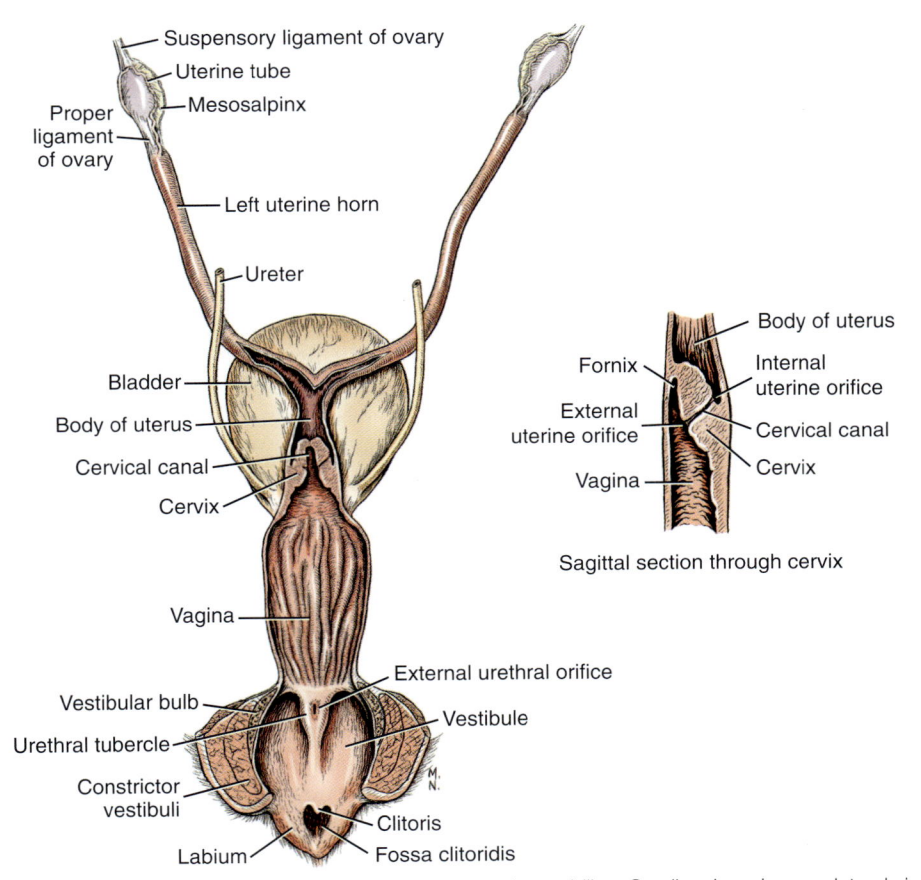

• **Fig. 9.38** Dorsal view of female genitalia, partially opened on midline. Smaller view shows a lateral view of a sagittal section through cervix; the fornix is ventral.

end of each uterine horn is connected to the ovary by the proper ligament of the ovary. The uterine tube opens via the tubouterine junction into the cranial end of the uterine horn.

The **body** of the uterus is usually located in both the pelvic and the abdominal cavities. Generally, the largest portion is in the abdomen, and, in multiparous bitches, the entire uterine body may be located cranial to the brim of the pelvis. The body extends from the point of convergence of the uterine horns to the cervix (Fig. 9.38). An internal partition, the **uterine velum** (*velum uteri*) projects approximately 1 cm into the body of the uterus, separating the horns, and it has been claimed that this feature causes an alternation of births from right and left horns. The partition is not discernible externally. The ventral border of the **cervix** attaches to the uterine wall cranial to its dorsal attachment and the canal of the cervix is directed caudoventrally from uterus to vagina. Therefore the cervix lies diagonally across the uterovaginal junction. Consequently, the **internal orifice** of the cervical canal (*ostium uteri internum*) faces almost directly dorsally, whereas the **external orifice** (*ostium uteri externum*) is directed ventrally toward the vaginal ventral wall. The external uterine orifice opens on a hillock projecting into the vagina on a dorsal median fold (Pineda et al., 1973). The cervical canal averages 0.5 to 1 cm in length and is closed during pregnancy by a mucus plug.

Spaces and Folds

The **rectogenital pouch**, an extension of the peritoneal cavity between the rectum and the uterus, is continuous with the pararectal fossa. The **vesicogenital pouch** extends between the urinary bladder and the uterus with its attached broad ligament.

The **broad ligaments**, containing some fat and unstriped muscle, attach the uterus and ovaries to the body wall. The *mesometrium* is that part of the broad ligament that attaches the uterus to the dorsolateral body wall. The *mesovarium* and *mesosalpinx* have been discussed in the descriptions of the ovary and of the uterine tube. The mesometrium begins on a transverse plane through the cranial end of the uterine horn and extends caudally as far as the cranial end of the vagina. It is attached peripherally to the lateral pelvic wall. The medial surfaces of the uterine horns are connected to each other for approximately 1 cm by a triangular-shaped double layer of peritoneum, the **genital fold** (*plica genitalia*) (Fig. 9.1). The mesometrium and the lateral ligament of the bladder fuse at their attachments to the pelvic wall.

The **round ligament of the uterus** (*ligamentum teres uteri*) is attached to the cranial tip of the ipsilateral uterine horn and is a caudal continuation from the proper ligament of the ovary. These two ligaments are remnants of the embryonic gubernaculum testis in the male. These ligaments consist largely of smooth muscle, allowing for stretching during pregnancy. The round ligament runs in the free edge of the peritoneal fold given off from the lateral surface of the mesometrium. It extends caudally, ventrally, and mesially, toward the deep inguinal ring. In most bitches the round ligament, with its investment of peritoneum, the vaginal process, passes through the inguinal canal and terminates subcutaneously in or near the vulva. The vaginal process is accompanied in its course through the inguinal canal by the genitofemoral nerve, the external pudendal artery and vein, and fat. The fascial layers enveloping the vaginal process are the same as those described with the vaginal tunic of the male.

Structure

The *tunica muscularis* (*myometrium*) consists of a thin, longitudinal outer layer and a thick, circular inner layer of involuntary muscle. Within the circular layer, close to its junction with the longitudinal layer, is a vascular layer containing blood vessels, nerves, and circular and oblique muscle fibers. The circular layer is especially thick in the region of the cervix. In describing the process of labor in the bitch, Rudolph and Ivy (1930) discuss the action of uterine musculature in detail. Briefly, the fetus is advanced by a strong circular contraction that progresses like a cylindrical band and by a longitudinal shortening. The "retreat" of the fetus is prevented by a persistent longitudinal contraction. In the body of the uterus, transverse circular contraction, with some longitudinal shortening, moves the fetus into the vagina. Contraction of the abdominal muscles, as well as of the vaginal musculature, causes the final expulsion of the fetus. Reynolds (1937) describes uterine motility, during estrus, as being a series of simple myometrial contraction waves because intermediation of an intrinsic innervation is not essential to it. Verma and Chibuzo (1974) found that sectioning the hypogastric and pelvic nerves did not alter the frequency or the amplitude of uterine contractions.

For an account of birth in the dog see Naaktgeboren and Slijper (1970); for endocrine parameters of pregnancy and parturition see Concannon (1991). For an account of fetal development and associated hypertrophy of the uterus see Chapter 2.

Evans (1961), reporting on successive cesarean operations of Beagles at various stages of gestation, found that within 10 minutes of the removal of the conceptus (fetus and its fetal membranes) there was considerable contraction of the uterus. Within 5 days after the operation, involution and healing of the uterus was well advanced, and, by the next pregnancy, there was little or no evidence of the uterine incision when chromic gut was used for closure. In those instances where evidence of previous uterine incisions was visible, it was clear that subsequent implantations were not located at the same sites. Serial removals of embryos did not appear to interfere with subsequent reproductive activity. One Beagle bitch that had four fetuses removed from the right uterine horn at 37 days postinsemination gave birth at 63 days to four normal pups. This dog later whelped two litters, one of five pups and another of eight.

The *tunica mucosa* (*endometrium*) is the thickest of the three uterine tunics. Facing the lumen of the uterus is a layer of low columnar epithelium with cells that are periodically ciliated. Simple branched tubular glands are present in the lamina propria. Opening into the uterine cavity, these glands are generally very long and are separated by shorter, inconstant glands or crypts. The long glands in the bitch show relatively little branching or coiling, in contrast with those of the mare or cow. They generally traverse the entire thickness of the endometrium. Grossly, the mucosal surface of the uterus is reddish in color and may be smooth or contain low longitudinal ridges that obliterate the uterine cavity in the nonpregnant state. The cervical canal does not contain the relatively high mucosal folds observed in other domestic animals, but is closed in pregnancy by a collagenous plug.

Vessels and Nerves
The uterus is supplied with arterial blood via the **ovarian** and **uterine arteries**. See Del Campo and Ginther (1974) for the details of vascularization as seen in cleared tissues. The origin of the ovarian arteries from the aorta has been discussed with the description of the ovaries and of the uterine tubes. The uterine branch of the ovarian artery anastomoses with the uterine artery, one of the principal branches of the vaginal artery. The artery enters the mesometrium at the level of the cervix (see Fig. 9.1). On entering the broad ligament, the artery lies relatively close to the body of the uterus. It diverges from the uterine horn until it approaches the cranial extremity of the horn, where it anastomoses with the uterine branch of the ovarian artery. The uterine artery ramifies in the wall of the uterus and in the mesometrium. Branches supply both sides of the uterine horn.

The **uterine** and **ovarian veins** follow a course similar to that of the arteries, except at their terminations. The right ovarian vein empties into the caudal vena cava at the level of the right ovary, whereas the left enters the left renal vein (Fig. 9.1). Both ovarian veins are very tortuous in their course between the peritoneal layers of the broad ligament.

Studying the physiologic aspects of uterine circulation during pregnancy, Reynolds (1949) found two distinct phases in the adjustment of the uterine vessels to the shape and size of the conceptus. First, there is progressive stretching of the blood vessels, and, second, the blood vessels during the latter part of gestation separate from one another without increase of length. Burwell and his coworkers (1938) found that blood pressure in the femoral and uterine veins was elevated during pregnancy in the dog. However, pressure in the uterine vein is higher than in the femoral vein. The uterine veins drain into the caudal vena cava. Two of the principal functions served by rhythmic uterine contractions during estrus, according to Fagin and Reynolds (1936), may be production of an increased volume flow of blood through enlarged, hyperemic vessels and removal of any edematous fluid. The lymphatics from the uterus pass to the **hypogastric** and **lumbar lymph nodes**. The vagina possesses a dense plexus of lymphatics in its tunica propria.

The uterus receives sympathetic and parasympathetic innervation via the pelvic plexus. Sympathetics reach the pelvic plexus as right and left hypogastric nerves. The parasympathetics reach the pelvic plexus via the pelvic nerves. Visceral afferent fibers reach the uterus via the pelvic nerves and the pelvic plexus.

Vagina
The **vagina** is a dilatable canal, extending from the uterus to the vestibule. Cranially the vagina is limited by the fornix, which extends ventral to the cervix (Fig. 9.38). The cervix may protrude 0.5 to 1 cm into the vagina, and is 0.8 cm in diameter. The fornix is the deepest part of the vagina and lies ventral and cranial to the cervix. The length of the dorsal vaginal wall is less than that of the ventral wall because of the oblique position of the cervix. The vagina ends caudally just cranial to the urethral opening. It is demarcated from the vestibule by a transverse mucosal ridge that extends 1 cm dorsally on each side of the midventral line. No definite hymen is present at this point in the bitch, although its vestige may sometimes be found at the vaginovestibular junction. In a 25-pound dog, the vagina averages 12 cm long and 1.5 cm in diameter. Both the length and diameter of the vagina increase considerably during pregnancy and during parturition. The longitudinal folds (*rugae*) of the vaginal mucosa are high, allowing for great expansion in diameter (Fig. 9.38). Smaller transverse folds connecting the longitudinal folds permit craniocaudal stretching of the vagina.

Relations
The cranial portion of the vagina within the pelvic cavity is covered dorsally by peritoneum that reflects onto the colon, forming the **rectogenital pouch** (Fig. 9.34). Ventrally this portion of the vagina has a peritoneal covering that reflects onto the bladder, forming the **vesicogenital pouch**. Laterally the dorsal and ventral peritoneal coverings of the vagina fuse and become part of the broad ligaments. The caudal half of the vagina is retroperitoneal, being connected dorsally to the rectum and ventrally to the urethra by means of loose connective tissue. Laterally the caudal part of the vagina is related to the vaginal blood vessels and nerves and to the ureters. The right and left ureters, with their peritoneal coverings, cross the lateral surface of the uterovaginal junction (Fig. 9.38). The portion of the vagina that is located retroperitoneally depends to a large extent on the fullness of the bladder and rectum.

Structure
The vaginal walls are made up of an inner mucosal layer, a middle smooth muscle layer, and an external coat of connective tissue and peritoneum (cranially). The tunica mucosa is nonglandular, stratified squamous epithelium. The epithelium changes in appearance during the various stages of the estrous cycle as can be seen with a laparoscope and confirmed with vaginal smears (Roszel, 1975). The *tunica muscularis* is composed of a very thin inner layer of longitudinal muscle, a thick circular layer, and a thin outer longitudinal layer. The inner longitudinal and circular layers

encircle the external uterine orifice. The outer longitudinal layer blends with the muscular layer of the body of the uterus. The submucous tissue contains a rich plexus of blood vessels. On the caudoventral wall of the vagina, vestigial ductus deferens (ducts of Gartner), vestigial remains of the caudal portion of the embryonic mesonephric duct, are usually absent.

Vessels and Nerves

Arterial blood is supplied to the vagina via the vaginal artery (formerly urogenital), a branch of the internal pudendal (Fig. 11.73). In addition to its vaginal distribution, the artery also supplies branches to the bladder, urethra and vestibule. Its urethral branches anastomose with the caudal vesical artery. The vaginal veins are satellites of the arteries and drain into the internal pudendal veins. The lymphatics drain into the medial iliac lymph nodes. The vagina is innervated by sympathetic and parasympathetic nerves from the pelvic plexus and by sensory afferent fibers via the pudendal nerve.

Vestibule

The **vestibule** (*vestibulum vaginae*) is the space connecting the vagina with the external genital opening, the vulva (Figs. 9.38 and 9.39). It develops from the embryonic urogenital sinus, the common opening for genital and urinary tracts. The space is variable in size, depending on the size of the animal and whether or not she is pregnant. In a nonpregnant, mature 25-pound dog, the external vulvar opening, the rima pudendi, is approximately 3 cm long. The distance from the ventral commissure of the vulva to the urethral opening is 5 cm, and the diameter of the vaginovestibular junction is 1.5 to 2 cm. The **urethral tubercle** is a ridgelike projection on the cranioventral wall of the vestibule, near the vaginovestibular junction. It contains the **external urethral orifice** (*ostium urethrae externum*). The tubercle, widest cranially, narrows caudally to an apex located at a point approximately half the distance from the urethral opening to the clitoris. A shallow fossa or depression is present on each side of the tubercle. The mucosa of the

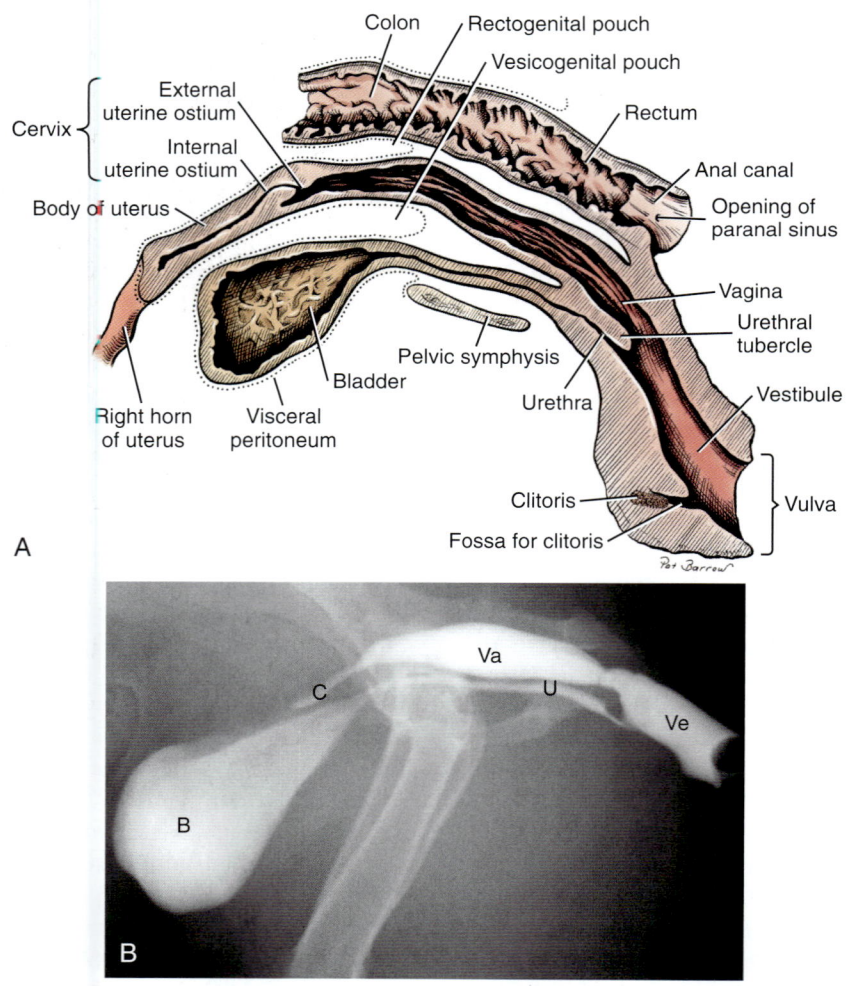

• **Fig. 9.39** A, Female pelvic viscera, median section, left lateral view. B, Lateral contrast radiograph of female pelvic viscera, showing contrast distributed to the vaginal and cervix, dorsally, and to the urethra and bladder ventrally. *B*, bladder; *C*, cervix; *Va*, vagina; *U*, urethra.

vestibule is not covered with distinct ridges, as is the mucosa of the vagina, but is relatively smooth and red.

External Genitalia

The external genitalia of the female dog include the pudendum femininum (vulva), clitoris, and urethra feminina (Fig. 9.39).

Pudendum Femininum

The ***pudendum femininum*** (***vulva***) lies caudal to the vestibule and consists of two lips, **labii** (*labium pudendi* [*vulvae*]) joined dorsally and ventrally by **commissures** (*commissura labiorum dorsalis et ventralis*) and separated by a narrow cleft, the **rima pudendi**. The *labia* form the external boundary of the vulva and in part are homologous with the scrotum of the male. The labia are soft and pliable, being composed of fibrous and elastic connective tissue, striated muscle fibers (*m. constrictor vulvae*), and an abundance of fat. The vaginal processes, containing the round ligaments of the uterus, often end in the subcutaneous connective tissue of the labia. The distance between the dorsal commissure of the labia and the anus is 8 to 9 cm. The dorsal commissure lies at or slightly ventral to the dorsal plane passing through the symphysis pelvis. The ventral portions of the labia, with their uniting commissure, form a pointed projection extending ventrally and caudally from the body, usually with a tuft of hair.

Clitoris

The **clitoris** (Figs. 9.39 to 9.41), the homologue of the male penis, is composed of paired **roots** (*crura clitoridis*), a **body** (*corpus clitoridis*), and a **glans** (*glans clitoridis*). The roots and body are homologues of the male corpora cavernosa penis, and the glans clitoridis is homologous with the glans penis, although it is not bipartite in structure. The body of the clitoris in the dog has both fatty and erectile tissue. It is covered by a tunica albuginea. The clitoris of the dog does not normally contain a bone but an **os clitoridis** can be present (Figs. 9.40B and 9.41). In the normal bitch, there are elongate masses of erectile tissue lying deep to the vestibular mucosa and united to each other dorsally by an isthmus. These are the **vestibular bulbs** (*bulbus vestibuli*) that correspond to the bulb of the penis in the male (Fig. 9.38). The bulbs are each supplied by a terminal branch of the internal pudendal artery, homologous to the artery of the bulb in the male. The glans clitoridis, erectile in structure, is very small and projects into the **fossa clitoridis** (Fig. 9.38). The wall of the fossa is partially folded over the glans clitoridis dorsally. This fold corresponds to the male prepuce (*preputium clitoridis*). The free part of the clitoris (glans) is approximately 0.6 cm long and 0.2 cm in diameter in an average-sized dog; the distance from the ventral commissure of the vulva to the glans clitoridis is 2 to 3 cm and that from the ventral commissure to the fundus of the fossa of the clitoris is 3 to 4 cm. The opening of the fossa is approximately 1 cm in diameter. Nitschke (1970) has described the structure of the clitoris and vagina in the dog. Lindsay

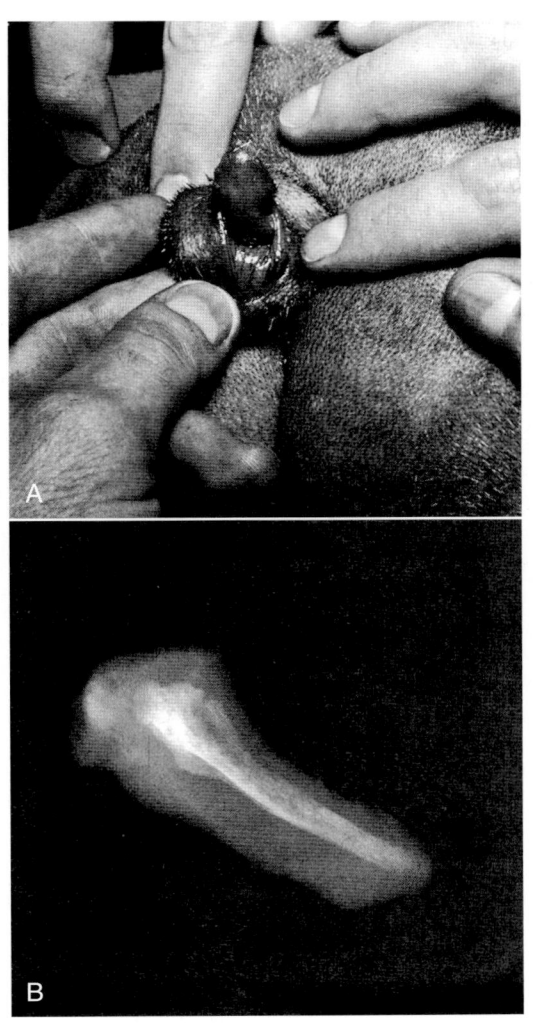

• **Fig. 9.40** A, An enlarged clitoris containing an os clitoridis in a 1-year-old female German Shorthair Pointer. The owner noticed protrusion of the clitoris at 7 months of age in the first heat period. B, Radiograph of the os clitoridis (5 cm actual length). (Case data and photograph A courtesy Dr. R. Kirk.)

(1983) has described and illustrated the endoscopic appearance of the vestibule, vulva, and vagina in the cyclic, noncyclic, and spayed bitch. Her endoscopic photographs, in color, show clearly that the changes in mucosal appearance at different phases of the estrous cycle can be recognized grossly.

An **os clitoridis** can develop in response to an altered hormone balance and may be more than 2.5 cm long. Grandage and Robertson (1971) reported an os clitoridis in a normal Welsh Corgi bitch that subsequently mated and whelped. The bone was seen radiographically to be 13 mm long, laterally compressed, and pointed at its apex.

Although it is said that the dog usually lacks an os clitoridis, it may only be that it is rarely looked for and rarely reported. In four cases that came to Evans's attention, one was less than a centimeter long and three were large. The small one was presented because of a urinary problem,

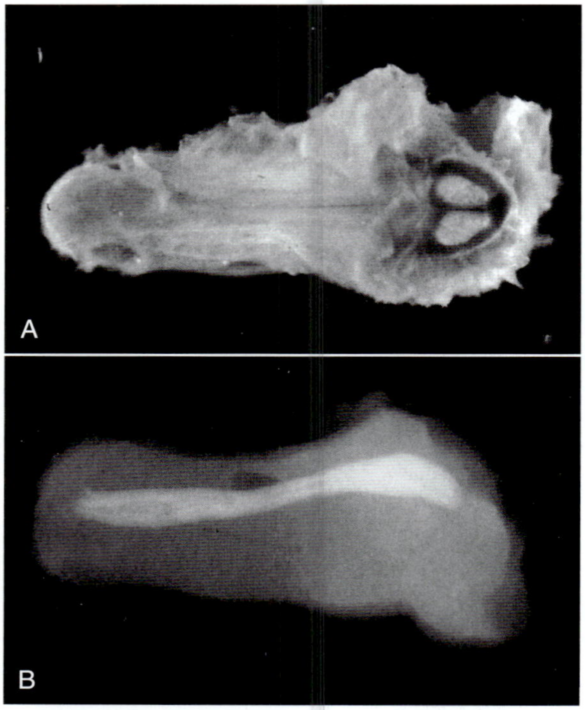

Fig. 9.41 The clitoris of a female Kerry Blue Terrier at 2 years, 9 months. The owner noticed that the clitoris was prominent and inflamed due to mechanical irritation. There was a large fossa of the clitoris and a very small entrance to the vagina. **A,** Cleared clitoris, dorsal surface. Note the transected corpora cavernosa. There is no urethra present and therefore no corpus spongiosum (4 cm long). **B,** Radiograph to show the os clitoridis, which is 3.5 cm long (lateral view). (Specimen courtesy Dr. A. Latschar.)

which was solved by the removal of the clitoris. Two of the large ones (a Kerry Blue Terrier with a 4-cm clitoris and 3.5-cm os (Fig. 9.41) and a Shorthair German Pointer with a 6-cm clitoris and 5-cm os (Fig. 9.40) were brought in by practitioners after surgical removal because of an inflamed clitoris. The fourth os was found in a dissection specimen. When an os clitoridis is present it may be associated with a natural endocrine disturbance or more probably is the result of androgen or progestin therapy. Shane et al. (1969) fed methyltestosterone (150 μg per kg body weight per day) to female Beagles starting on the day of first mating and continuing through pregnancy, parturition, and lactation, and for 9 months thereafter. A total of 87 pups were born to 14 females. Of these pups 42 were intersexes, and 45 were normal males. All of the intersex pups tested (nine) were genetic females. The intersex pups had a phallus that was partially hypospadiac in some. Urine was voided through the phallus and the position assumed for urination was that of a female dog. No scrotum or vulva was present, but a bone was sometimes present in the phallus. On the basis of karyotype studies, the intersex pups were classified as female pseudohermaphrodites, and thus the phallus can be considered a hypertrophied clitoris, which in some cases has an os clitoridis. The development of the ovary and uterine tubes appeared to be normal in all female pups.

When adult, some of these female pseudohermaphrodites ovulated, formed corpora lutea, and accumulated fluid in the uterus. The latter finding is consistent with progesterone secretion.

Structure

Recognition of the location of the external urethral orifice is important for the purpose of catheterization. It is common for the fossa clitoridis to be mistaken for the urethral opening, and the catheterization attempt is unsuccessful. The urethra opens on a tubercle 4 to 5 cm cranial to the ventral commissure of the vulva at the level of the ischial arch.

The mucosal surface of the vulva is covered by stratified squamous epithelium. A variable number of lymph nodules may cause prominences to appear on the mucosa. Small minor vestibular glands, lobular in structure, open ventrally on each side of the median ridge connected to the urethral tubercle. These mucosal glands are located deep to the vestibular smooth muscles and the striated constrictor vestibuli muscles. The body of the clitoris consists of fat, elastic connective tissue, and a peripheral tunica albuginea. The glans clitoridis, made up of erectile tissue, contains numerous sensory nerve endings. The vestibular bulbs are also composed of cavernous tissue. The labia, covered with stratified squamous epithelium, are rich in sebaceous and tubular glands and also contain fat, elastic tissue, and smooth and striated muscle fibers.

Muscles

In addition to the usual unstriped muscle fibers, similar to those of the vagina, the vestibule and vulva each possesses a striated circular muscle (Figs. 9.42 and 9.43). The most cranial of the two is the larger **vestibular constrictor muscle** (*m. constrictor vestibuli*). It is incomplete on the dorsal surface of the vestibule, but fuses along its dorsocaudal border to the external sphincter of the anus. Its fibers run diagonally in a cranioventral direction, encircling the urethra, vestibule, and caudal portion of the vagina before it joins its fellow of the opposite side. It constricts the vestibule.

Immediately caudal to the m. constrictor vestibuli is the relatively thin **constrictor vulvae muscle** (*m. constrictor vulvae*), which is the muscle of the labia. This muscle is continuous dorsally with the external anal sphincter, arising from the caudal fascia ventral to the first and second caudal vertebrae and encircling the vulva and vestibule approximately 1 cm caudal to the point where the urethra enters the genital tract. The constrictor vulvae muscle blends with the vestibular constrictor to a slight degree. The vulvar constrictors fuse together below the vulva, cranial to the ventral commissure. They lift the labia dorsally prior to intromission of the penis, allowing it to enter the vagina more easily. The vestibular and vulvar constrictors together are homologous with the bulbospongiosus muscles of the male. They lie superficial to the vestibular bulbs. Their counterparts in the male are peripheral to the bulb of the penis. The **ischiourethralis muscles** (Figs. 9.42 and 9.43)

CHAPTER 9 The Urogenital System

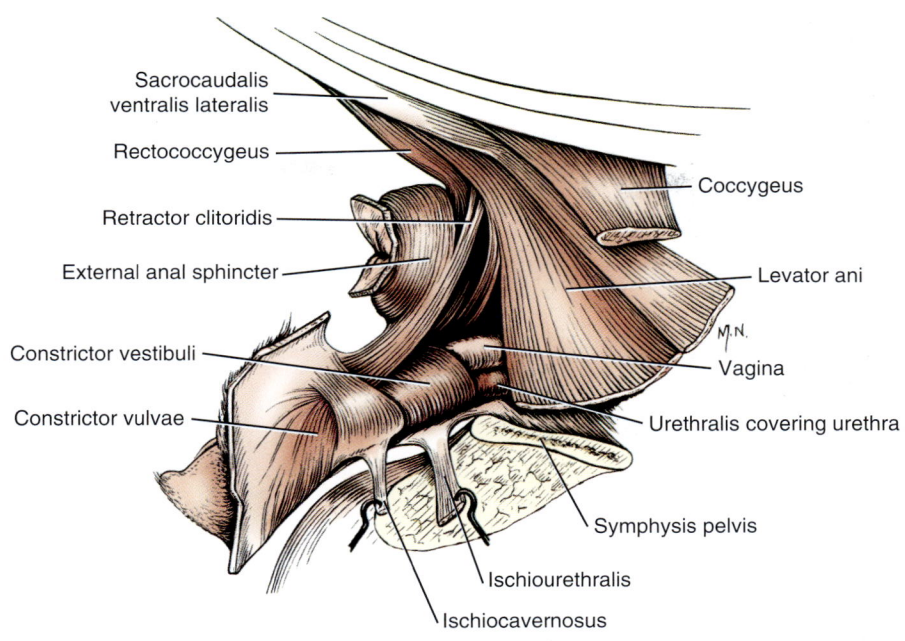

Fig. 9.42 Constrictor muscles of female anus and genitalia, lateral aspect.

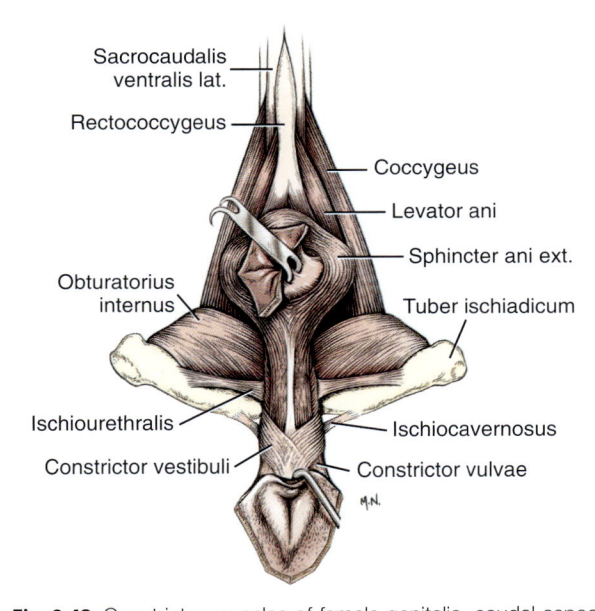

Fig. 9.43 Constrictor muscles of female genitalia, caudal aspect.

arise from the caudomedial surface of the tuber ischii, on each side, and insert upon the poorly developed central tendon of the perineum.

The **ischiocavernosus muscles** (Figs. 9.42 and 9.43) are small in the female. They arise bilaterally from the caudal edge of the ischium and attach to the crura clitoridis. This is similar to the manner in which they insert upon the corpora cavernosa in the male.

Female Urethra

The urethra of the bitch (*urethra feminina*) (Figs. 9.38 and 9.39) corresponds to the preprostatic part of the pelvic urethra in the male. It is approximately 0.5 cm in diameter and 7 to 10 cm long. It originates from the urinary bladder at or near the cranial edge of the symphysis pelvis. It extends caudodorsally to enter the genital tract caudal to the vaginovestibular junction on the urethral tubercle (Fig. 9.44). Its dorsal wall is in close apposition to the ventral wall of the vagina. Structurally, the female urethra resembles that of the male. It is lined by folded mucous membrane, allowing the urethral lumen to expand considerably when under pressure. The mucosa is nonglandular, and the submucosa is highly vascular. Lymph nodules are also present. The musculature of the female urethra consists of outer and inner longitudinal and middle circular layers of unstriped muscle. The smooth muscles become less conspicuous near the entrance of the urethra into the vestibule. At the external urethral orifice, voluntary striated muscle (*m. urethralis*) encircles all but the dorsal surface of the urethra, which is in close contact with the vestibule. These circular fibers form a prominent sphincter at the external orifice.

Vessels and Nerves

The external genitalia and urethra of the female are supplied with blood through the **vaginal** and the **external** and **internal pudendal arteries**. In the inguinal region the external pudendal artery sends branches to the labia (cranial labial artery), corresponding to the scrotal branches in the male. The vaginal artery supplies the vulva by means of the cranial and caudal vestibular branches. The ventral perineal artery supplies branches to the labia dorsally. The clitoris is supplied by branches of the internal pudendal artery, corresponding to the dorsal and deep penile arteries. The vestibular bulb is also supplied by the internal pudendal artery (homologous to the artery of the bulb in the male).

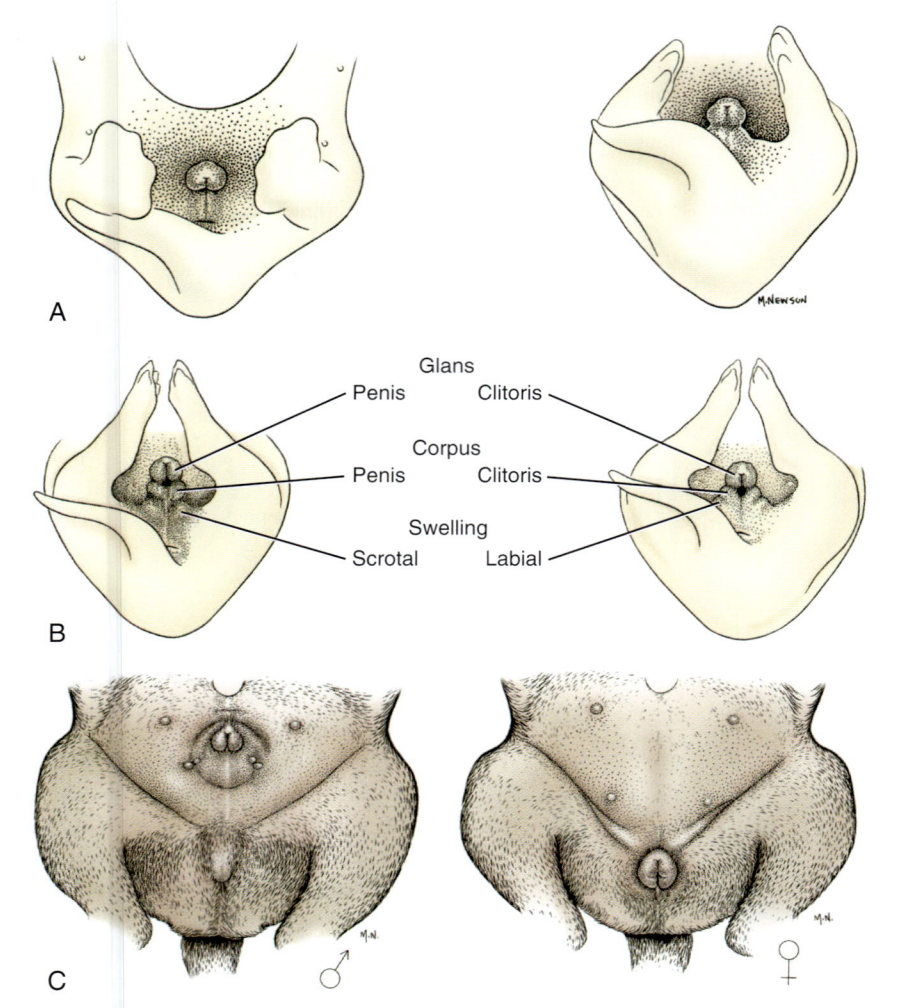

• Fig. 9.44 A, Undifferentiated genital tubercule of a 30 day Beagle embryo. B, Differentiated male and female external genitalia at 35 days of gestation in the Beagle. C, The external genitalia of male and female newborn Beagles (60 days).

The bilateral **dorsal veins** from the clitoris join each other at the ischial arch and then separate again (after a distance of 1 or 2 cm) into **internal pudendal veins**, which drain into the internal iliac veins. The vestibular bulb is drained by a separate tributary of the internal pudendal. Valves are apparent in most of the veins, including the common trunk of the dorsal veins of the clitoris. The dorsal arteries and veins of the clitoris are not actually dorsal to the clitoris, in the manner of the comparable penile vessels. They curve ventrally around the ischial arch and run caudoventrally along the ventral surface of the clitoris that corresponds to the dorsum of the penis. Lymphatic drainage compares with that of the external genitalia of the male.

The sensory afferent nerves to the external genitalia are derived from the pudendal nerves (Spurgeon & Reddy, 1986). According to these authors the genital branches of the genitofemoral nerve do not reach the external genitalia.

The glans clitoridis receives its sensory nerves from the pudendal (**dorsal nerve of the clitoris**). Motor impulses to the urethral muscle and to the vestibular and vulvar constrictors also pass through the pudendal nerve. Autonomic innervation to the external genitalia and urethra in the female is through the **hypogastric** and **pelvic nerves**. It includes principally sympathetic fibers that innervate the musculature of the blood vessels.

Mammae

The presence of **mammary glands** (*glandula mammaria*) and the process of lactation are unique to mammals. Although we know a great deal about the composition of the gland secretion, milk, we still seek to explain the evolutionary origin of nursing our young and the physiologic basis for the great differences between species in the composition of milk (Larson, 1974; Neville & Daniel, 1987; Pond, 1984). The production of milk for the feeding of the newborn (or newly hatched in the case of the echidna and platypus) allows mammals some freedom from daily foraging by allowing them to accumulate fat reserves over time and provide a reliable source of sustained nutrients for the young regardless of temporary environmental constraints.

The basic developmental feature that is responsible for the presence and location of normal or supernumerary mammae is the prenatal development of the **mammary ridge** (Figs. 9.45 and 9.46), which extends in an arc from the axilla to the inguinal region. In the dog the mammary ridge is well developed by 14 mm crown-rump length (25 days), and, shortly thereafter, by 19 mm (30 days). Paired individual **nipples** (*papilla mammae*) can be seen along the former mammary ridges. The formation of mammae is not always symmetric, and uneven numbers of functional mammae are common. Wakuri (1966a, b) reported several instances of seven and nine mammae and noted the occasional loss of the most cranial thoracic mammae. In the male fetus the development of the prepuce results in early involution and loss of the inguinal mammae (Fig. 9.46).

Each *mamma* consists of the glandular complex associated with a single papilla (nipple) covered by skin. The mammary gland is an accessory gland of the skin and resembles a sweat gland in its mode of development. In the male the **mammae masculina** remain rudimentary throughout life, but in the female they are subject to conspicuous changes during pregnancy and during and after lactation.

The mammary glands are typically arranged in two bilaterally symmetric rows extending from the ventral thoracic to the inguinal region (Figs. 9.47 to 9.49). The nipples indicate the position of the glands in the male or in the nonlactating female. The number of glands varies from 8 to 12. Most commonly, there are a total of 10 glands, and 8 are more frequently seen than 12. When 10 glands are present, the relatively small cranial 4 are the thoracic

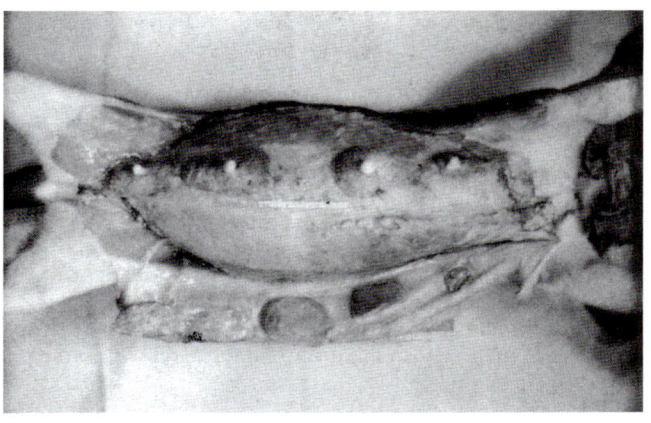

• **Fig. 9.47** The mammary glands of a young, embalmed Beagle, 32 days into gestation. On the left side the mammary glands have been reflected with the skin, whereas on the right the skin has been removed from the glands.

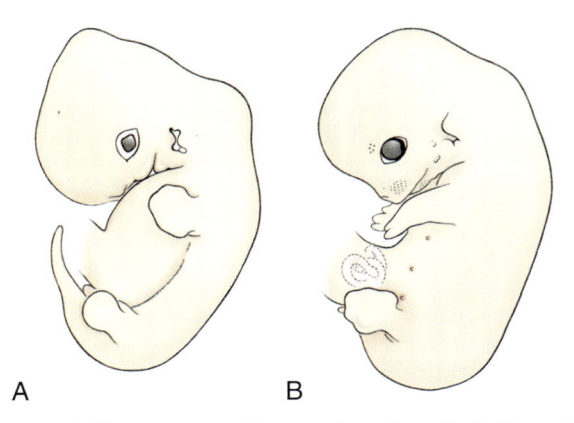

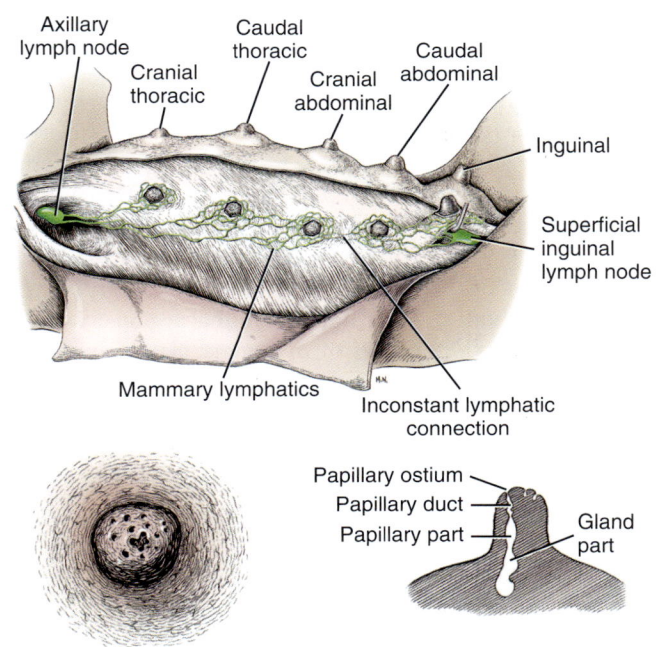

• **Fig. 9.45 A**, The mammary ridge runs from the axilla to the groin in a 14-mm Beagle, approximately 25 days of gestation. **B**, By 19 mm, or 30 days of gestation, distinct papillae have appeared along the former mammary ridge. The intestine lies partly in the umbilical cord. (Evans and Sack, 1973).

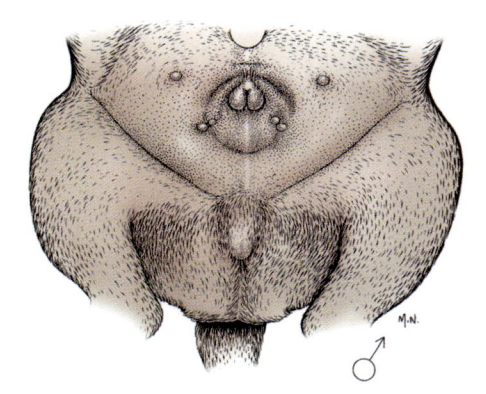

• **Fig. 9.46** Involution of the inguinal mammae owing to prepuce formation in a male Beagle, 1 week prior to birth.

• **Fig. 9.48** Mammary glands, topography, and structure.

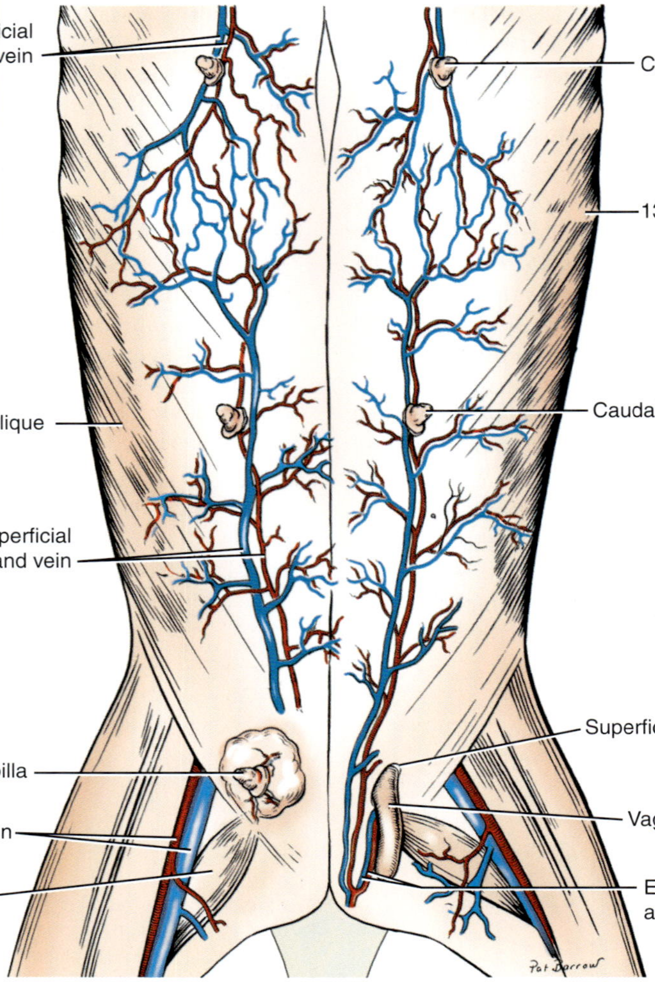

• **Fig. 9.49** Superficial blood vessels of the abdomen showing the epigastric arteries and veins that supply and drain the mammae. The cranial and caudal thoracic papillae and the left inguinal are not shown.

mammae, the following 4 are the abdominal mammae (median in size), and the relatively large caudal 2 are the inguinal mammae. In some instances, especially during involution of the glands following lactation, the relative sizes of the glands may digress from the typical pattern. Under these circumstances, the caudal abdominal mammae may rarely be slightly larger than the inguinal glands. Turner and Gomez (1934) examined 20 dogs and found 10 glands in each of 16 dogs, 9 in 3, and 8 in 1. Supernumerary glands are found in both thoracic and abdominal regions. Wakuri (1966a) found the number of mammary gland nipples in mongrel dogs (29 fetuses, 9 newborn, and 40 adults) to vary between 6 and 10, with a mean of 9.4 in fetuses, 8.8 in newborns, and 8.1 in adults. There appears to be a loss of mammae as the dog matures, particularly in the cranial thoracic region. Study of the mammary glands of the dog has been comparatively neglected.

Structure

The **mammary gland** (*glandula mammaria*) consists of epithelial glandular tissue (*lobuli glandulae mammariae*) and connective tissue.

The secretory tissue is present to a significant degree only during pregnancy, pseudopregnancy, the period of lactation when pups are nursing, and for 40 to 50 days following weaning. After this postpartum period, the alveoli and lobules are reduced to a shrunken system of ducts with relatively few remnants of lobules. For a general discussion of lactation structures, see Larson (1974), Falconer (1971), and Cowie and Tindal (1971).

The number of ducts opening on a nipple varies. In a study of the nipple openings of nine mature dogs of different breeds, as few as 7 and as many as 16 ducts were observed on a teat. The duct openings are located on the blunt end of the nipple in an irregular, sievelike pattern. The peripheral ducts tend to form a circle, whereas the centrally placed ones form an irregular design. Turner (1939) described 8 to 14 ducts in one case and 12 to 22 in another.

Each **papillary duct** (*ductus papillares*) occupies approximately one-third of the length of the nipple. It is lined by stratified squamous epithelium. The epithelium usually lies in folds near the margin of the papillary sinus.

The **lactiferous sinus** (*sinus lactifer*) (Fig. 9.49) has a **glandular part** (*pars glandularis*) and a **papillary part** (*pars* *papillaris*). The sinus extends from the papillary duct into the parenchyma of the gland. In large dogs, the sinus system may be seen upon gross examination of the sectioned gland. The epithelium of the papillary duct changes gradually in the lactiferous sinus, from stratified squamous to columnar.

In the middle portion of the nipple there is an intermingling of diversely running smooth muscle fibers and connective tissue elements. The circular musculature radiates from the axis of the central zone of the nipple into the area among the papillary ducts. The musculature encircles the ducts and joins or condenses into the **sphincters of the ducts** (*m. sphincter papillae*). Elastic fibers radiate among the papillary ducts, forming an extensive network. Essentially, the tunica propria of the nipple is composed of bands of loose connective tissue, blood vessels, and smooth muscle and elastic fibers.

According to Turner (1939), the lactiferous sinus unfolds when filled with milk and shows no constrictions or circular folds between the two divisions of the sinuses. Each **gland sinus** is separated from surrounding sinuses by connective tissue septa and has a distinct glandular area composed largely of minute alveoli.

The skin is very thin over the distal tip of the nipple. It increases in thickness near the base. The corium contains elastic elements, smooth muscle fibers, and blood vessels. The epidermis may be pigmented, in which case the pigment is present in the germinal layer. Although the distal blunt end of the nipple is bare, the rest of it is covered by very fine hairs, which are accompanied by sebaceous glands. Turner (1939) found sweat glands at the base of the teat.

Vessels and Nerves

The mammary glands are highly vascular. Veins are more extensive than arteries. The thoracic mammae receive their arterial blood supply from the perforating cranial branches of the internal thoracic arteries. These penetrate the thoracic wall through the intercostal spaces. Intercostal and lateral thoracic arteries may also contribute blood to the thoracic glands. Abdominal and inguinal mammae are supplied by mammary branches of the superficial epigastric arteries. The cranial superficial epigastric artery arises from the cranial epigastric artery, a branch of the internal thoracic. It penetrates the rectus abdominis muscle approximately 2 to 4 cm from the midventral line, mesial to the costal arch. It sends mammary branches to the cranial abdominal gland and anastomoses with the caudal superficial epigastric artery (Fig. 9.50). The latter artery, a branch of the external pudendal, runs cranially on the surface of the rectus abdominis, deep to the inguinal mamma, which it supplies. The artery continues cranially to supply the abdominal mammae and terminates in numerous superficial branches that anastomose with the end branches of the cranial superficial epigastric artery.

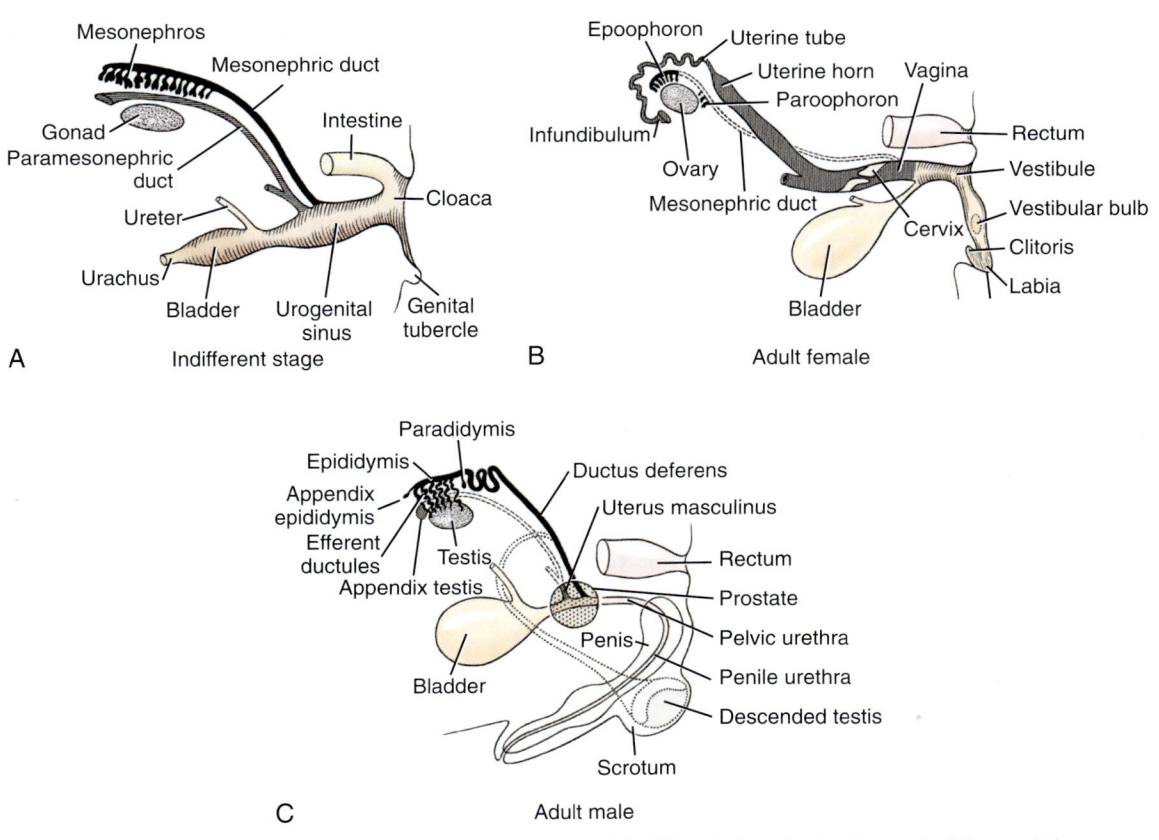

• **Fig. 9.50** Schematic representations of the embryonic indifferent stage in development of the genital system compared to the adult.

The veins of the mammae in the dog parallel the course of the arteries to a large degree. The cranial and caudal superficial epigastric veins are the major veins of the glands. The abdominal and inguinal glands drain into the caudal superficial epigastric veins. The thoracic mammae drain into the cranial superficial epigastric veins, as well as directly into the internal thoracic veins as far cranially as the fifth intercostal space.

Lymphatic drainage of the mammary glands on each side sometimes interconnect, but there are no connections across the midline. Studies by Baum (1918), Stalker and Schlotthauer (1936), and Patsikas and Dessiris (1992) using injections of Berlin Blue, India ink, and Lipiodol followed by dissection or radiographic examination have provided us with a general understanding of the lymphatic flow, but many variations are found. Each gland has its own plexus of lymphatic channels that anastomose and encircle the base of the nipple (see Figs. 9.48 and 13.10B). Lymphatic plexuses are found in the parenchyma, subcutis, and nipple. Usually one to three main channels leave each glandular plexus and pass superficially to the nearest lymph node. The thoracic mammae drain directly, by separate lymphatics, to the axillary node. Typically, the caudal abdominal gland drains into the lymphatic meshwork of the inguinal mammary gland and also directly to the superficial inguinal lymph node. The inguinal mammary gland has an extensive interlocking lymphatic plexus that drains into the adjoining superficial inguinal lymph node. The drainage of the cranial abdominal mamma is inconsistent. Although draining toward the axillary lymph node in most instances, its lymphatics may join those of the caudal abdominal gland and drain toward the superficial inguinal lymph node. Ruberte et al. (1990) found that only the cranial abdominal mammary gland had direct drainage to both the axillary and the superficial inguinal lymph nodes. Schlotthauer (1952) postulates that there may be direct connections between the lymphatics of the mammae and the vascular system, accounting for the direct internal metastasis of tumors. Turner (1939) was able to trace lymphatic ducts from the cranial abdominal gland into the thoracic cavity and directly into the sternal lymph nodes. This has not been verified by other investigators.

Patsikas and Dessiris (1992, 1996) studied the lymph drainage of the mammary glands of 129 lactating bitches using a contrast medium to delineate the possible routes of tumor metastases. (For a full account of procedures and findings see the Ph.D. thesis by M. N. Patsikas, 1992, Aristotelian University, Thessaloniki, Greece.) They found that lymph from the cranial thoracic gland usually drained to the axillary lymph node, but in some instances it passed to both the axillary and the superficial cervical nodes. Lymph from the caudal thoracic gland drained only to the axillary node. The cranial abdominal (third gland) usually sent its lymph to both the axillary and the superficial inguinal lymph nodes. However, in some cases, lymph was drained only to the axillary node or, more rarely, only caudally to the superficial inguinal nodes. The caudal abdominal mamma (fourth gland) usually drained to the superficial inguinal node or, more rarely, into the medial iliac lymph node as well. Lymph from the inguinal mamma (fifth gland) drained into the superficial inguinal lymph nodes. Although there are no direct lymphatics between the right and the left mammae, Patsikas and Dessiris (1992) found connections between the right and the left superficial inguinal nodes and right and left axillary nodes.

The axillary lymph nodes are drained by the sternal nodes within the thoracic cavity. The superficial inguinal lymph nodes drain into the iliac nodes through the lymphatics of the inguinal canal.

The cranial thoracic mammary gland is innervated by lateral cutaneous branches of the fourth, fifth, and sixth thoracic nerve ventral branches (intercostal). The caudal thoracic gland receives its nerve supply from the lateral cutaneous branches of the sixth and seventh thoracic nerve ventral branches (intercostal). The abdominal and inguinal mammae are innervated by the genitofemoral nerve and the ventral cutaneous branches of the first three lumbar nerves: cranial iliohypogastric, caudal iliohypogastric, and ilioinguinal. Sympathetic fibers accompany the blood vessels to the mammae. Nerves are distributed to the parenchyma of the gland, to the blood vessels, to the smooth muscle of the nipple, and to the skin. In addition to being subject to nervous control, secretion of the mammary glands is influenced by hormones from the hypophysis and other organs, brought to them by the blood.

Embryologic Characteristics of the Urogenital System

The development of the mammalian urogenital system is briefly summarized here. For specific details see the textbooks of embryology by Noden and de Lahunta (1985), Latshaw (1987), and McGeady et al. (2009). The homologic characteristics of the structures in the male and female are shown in Box 9.1.

In the classical evolutionary approach to the development of the urinary system there is the formation of three kidneys, the pronephros, mesonephros, and metanephros, that develop in sequence from cranial to caudal along the urogenital ridge of intermediate mesoderm.

The **pronephros** is rudimentary and nonfunctional in mammals. It consists of seven to eight pairs of pronephric tubules that form briefly adjacent to somites 7 to 14. Simultaneously a duct forms from the mesothelium of the adjacent somatopleura and grows caudally on the edge of the intermediate mesoderm to enter the metenteron (hindgut-cloaca). At this stage this duct is called the **pronephric duct**. The pronephric tubules do not usually join this duct in the dog. Following this, adjacent to somites 9 to 26, 70 to 80 pairs of **mesonephric tubules** develop that are more extensive and on one end form a renal corpuscle with a glomerulus that develops from branches of the aorta. Venous drainage is provided by branches of the various cardinal

> **BOX 9.1 Homologies of Genital Organs in Male and Female Mammals**

Male	Female
Testis	Ovary
Mesorchium	Mesovarium
Appendix testis	Abdominal ostium of uterine tube
Proper ligament of testis, lig. of tail of epididymis	Proper ligament of ovary, round ligament of uterus
Pelvic urethra	Urethra
Penile urethra	Vestibule
Penis	Clitoris
Os penis	Os clitoridis (inconstant)
Glans penis	Glans clitoridis
Corpus spongiosum	Vestibular bulb
Corpus cavernosum	Corpus cavernosum
Scrotum	Labia
Scrotal raphe	Dorsal commissure of labia
Prepuce	Fold of fossa clitoridis

veins. The other end of these embryonic nephrons attaches to the pronephric duct, which changes its name to the **mesonephric duct.** As these mesonephric nephrons develop, the pronephric tubules and the adjacent pronephric duct degenerate. Compared with other domestic animals, the size of the canine mesonephros is relatively small. The functional period of the mesonephros is brief, and degeneration from cranial to caudal commences as formation of the metanephric kidney is initiated.

Development of the **metanephros** begins with an outgrowth from the mesonephric duct close to its entrance into the urogenital sinus. This follows the partitioning of the hindgut by the urorectal septum into the rectum and urogenital sinus. This evagination is the **ureteric bud** and this occurs adjacent to somites 26 through 28. The ureteric bud grows dorsally into the intermediate mesoderm where it expands to form the structure that will be the **renal pelvis.** Further branching forms **papillary ducts** and **collecting tubules.** Each of the collecting tubules induces the adjacent intermediate mesodermal cells to form a cluster of cells that will develop into a **nephron.** Each nephron is associated with a glomerulus developed from branches of the aorta that supply the metanephric intermediate mesoderm. The metanephric duct that originated as the ureteric bud becomes the **ureter,** which enters the portion of the urogenital sinus that gives rise to the bladder. A modified mesonephros is the functional kidney of anamniotes (fish and amphibians). The metanephros is the functional kidney of adult amniotes (reptiles, birds, and mammals). Gersh (1937) investigated the correlation of structure and function in the developing mesonephros and metanephros.

The genital system develops simultaneously with this development of the urinary system. The first indication is the proliferation of intermediate mesoderm on the medial side of the middle of the developing mesonephros. This is the **genital ridge.** The proliferating "gonadal" mesodermal cells here are invaded by migrating **primary germ cells.** Further development of the gonad depends on the presence or absence of the Y chromosome and its sex-determining SRY gene in these intermediate mesodermal cells. A testis develops if these cells have a Y chromosome with this gene. An ovary develops if there are only X chromosomes in these genital ridge cells.

Prior to this gonadal sex determination, two duct systems are present: the mesonephric duct that developed with the embryonic urinary system and an adjacent duct that formed on the border of the intermediate mesoderm and grew caudally to enter the urogenital sinus. This is the **paramesonephric duct**, which is not joined by any mesonephric tubules (Fig. 9.50). The caudal ends of the two paramesonephric ducts fuse medially before entering the urogenital sinus. Further development of these duct systems depends on the gonadal sex and the production of endocrine substances in the male gonad.

In the male these endocrine substances induce the caudal mesonephric tubules to form **efferent ductules** in the testis and the caudal mesonephric duct to form the **epididymis** and **ductus deferens.** An additional testicular endocrine inhibits the development of the entire paramesonephric duct, which degenerates. In the female the absence of this paramesonephric duct inhibitory substance permits the paramesonephric ducts to form the **uterine tubules**, the **uterus** and the **cranial vagina**. The mesonephric duct degenerates in the female. Remnants of these degenerating duct systems include in the female, adjacent to the ovary, the **paroophoron (mesonephric tubules)** and the **epoophoron** (mesonephric tubules and duct). In the floor of the caudal vagina is the **vestigial ductus deferens** (Gartner's ducts; caudal mesonephric ducts). In the male, adjacent to the testis, the remnant of the mesonephric duct is the appendix epididymis, and the remnant of the mesonephric tubules is the paradidymis. Remnants of the paramesonephric ducts in the male include the **appendix testis** and the **uterus masculinus (prostatic utricle)** in the seminal colliculus.

The development of external genitalia also depends on the presence or absence of endocrine secretions from the male gonad. In the female, the **urogenital sinus** gives rise to the bladder, urethra, caudal vagina, vestibule, and vulva. In the male, in addition to the bladder and pelvic urethra, the testicular endocrine substances induce the formation of the penis and penile urethra from the **genital tubercle** and the prostate from the pelvic urethra. The genital tubercle in the female forms the clitoris.

Although prenatal mammary development has been studied in carnivora as well as in many other species of mammals, the developing mammae of the fetal dog have not been investigated extensively. The mammary ridge is present at 25 days of gestation and by the thirtieth day has differentiated into five pairs of nipples (Fig. 2.12). Involution of the mammae in the male fetus is illustrated in Chapter 2 (Figs. 2.20 to 2.25). Turner and Gomez (1934) have studied the development of the gland during the estrous cycle, pregnancy, and pseudopregnancy. A few workers have studied mammary growth in dogs as influenced by estrogen and progesterone (Trentin et al., 1952).

Male mammae, and female mammae from birth until the approach of the first estrus, consist of small primary ducts extending a short distance below the base of the nipple. During estrus, the duct system of the gland grows rapidly and the alveolar system develops. Marshall and Halnan (1917) reported that, within a week after estrus, slow growth of the tissues of the gland (a few ducts surrounding the nipple) changes to a period of rapid development in the pregnant animal. The growth phase appears to be completed between day 30 and 40 after initiation of estrus. There is then a gradual increase in the size of the gland, owing to secretory activity of the alveolar epithelial cells.

Turner and Gomez (1934) made a detailed study of the gross and microscopic glandular changes during pregnancy. Ten days after conception the growth of the gland is grossly perceptible. At 20 days, the peripheral borders of adjoining glands in each row begin to unite and to extend toward the midventral line. The glandular systems on each side of the midline always remain intrinsically separate, however. On microscopic examination, the connective tissue stroma is reduced, adipose cells are present, and the growth of the duct system is very marked. At 30 days, a typical duct and lobule system is present, as well as anlagen of alveoli. Individual alveoli with lumina are seen at 40 days, and, for the next 20 days, there is a gradual enlargement of the gland owing to initiation of secretion by the alveolar epithelial cells. Within 1 day after parturition, the alveoli become greatly reduced, compared with the total amount of parenchyma. Changes in the mammary gland during pseudopregnancy are essentially identical to those of pregnancy, except that secretory activity at 60 days is less well developed.

Approximately 10 days after parturition, the size of the mammae is greatly reduced, the lobule-alveolar structures being affected sooner than the duct system. By 40 days the lobule-alveolar system is largely degenerated, and the ducts are shrunken. After cessation of lactation, the mammary gland in the dog regresses to a simple duct system.

Bibliography

Abe, Y., Suwa, Y., Asano, T., et al. (2010). Cryopreservation of canine embryos. *Biol Reprod, 84*, 363–368. doi:10.1095/biolreprod.110.087312.

Ader, P. L., & Hobson, H. P. (1978). Hypospadias: a review of the veterinary literature and a report of three cases in the dog. *J Am Anim Hosp Assoc, 14*, 721–727.

Anderson, D. (1927). The rate of passage of the mammalian ovum through various portions of the fallopian tube. *Am J Physiol, 82*, 557–569.

Anderson, J. W. (1969). Ultrastructure of the placenta and fetal membranes of the dog. 1. The placental labyrinth. *Anat Rec, 165*, 15–36.

André, I. (1982). *The sperm cell. fertilizing power, surface properties, motility, nucleus, and acrosome evolutionary aspects.* Dordrecht: Martinus Nijhoff Publishers.

Arata, A. A., Negus, N. C., & Downs, M. S. (1965). Histology, development, and individual variation of complex muroid bacula. *Tulane Stud Zool, 12*, 51–64.

Ashdown, R. R. (1963). The anatomy of the inguinal canal in the domesticated mammals. *Vet Rec, 75*, 1345–1351.

Austin, C. R., & Short, R. V. (1982). *Reproduction in mammals, books 1 to 5* (2nd ed.). Cambridge: Cambridge University Press.

Barrau, M. D., Abel, J. H., Torbit, C. A., & Tietz, W. J. (1975). Development of the implantation chamber in the pregnant bitch. *Am J Anat, 143*, 115–130.

Baum, H. (1918). *Das lymphgefassystem des hundes.* Berlin: Hirshwald.

Baumans, U. (1982). *Regulation of testicular descent in the dog, Thesis, Utrecht.* The Netherlands: Rijksuniv.

Baumans, U., Dijkstra, G., & Wensing, C. J. G. (1981). Testicular descent in the dog. *Zbl Vet Met C Anat Histol Embryol, 10*, 97–110.

Baumans, U., Dijkstra, G., & Wensing, C. J. G. (1982). The effect of orchidectomy on gubernacular outgrowth and regression in the dog. *Int J Androl, 5*, 387–400.

Baumans, U., Dijkstra, G., & Wensing, C. J. G. (1983). The role of nonandrogenic testicular factor in the process of testicular descent in the dog. *Int J Androl, 6*, 541–552.

Bedford, J. M. (1978). Anatomical evidence for the epididymis as the prime mover in the evolution of the scrotum. *Am J Anat, 152*, 483–508.

Bentley, M. D., Hoffman, E. A., Fiksen-Olsen, M. J., et al. (1988). Three-dimensional canine renovascular structure and circulation visualized in situ with the dynamic spatial reconstructor. *Am J Anat, 181*, 77–88.

Berg, O. S. (1958a). The normal prostate gland of the dog. *Acta Endocrinol, 27*, 129–139.

Berg, O. S. (1958b). Parenchymatous hypertrophy of the canine prostate gland. *Acta Endrocrinol, 27*, 140–154.

Bodner, E. (Oct 14 1987). *Male pseudohermaphroditism in a doberman pinscher,* Senior seminar, College of veterinary medicine. Ithaca, NY: Cornell University.

Boyd, J. D., Hamilton, W. J., & Hammond, J. (1944). Transuterine (internal) migration of the ovum in sheep and other mammals. *J Anat, 78*, 5–14.

Brenner, B. M., & Rector, F. C., Jr. (1991). *The kidney* (4th ed.). Philadelphia: Saunders.

Brodey, R. S., Martin, J. E., & Lee, D. G. (1954). Male pseudohermaphroditism in a toy terrier. *J Am Vet Med Assoc, 125*, 368–370.

Bulger, R. E., Cronin, R. E., & Dobyan, D. C. (1979). Survey of the morphology of the dog kidney. *Anat Rec, 194*, 41–66.

Burwell, C. S., Strayhorn, W. D., Flickinger, D., et al. (1938). Circulation during pregnancy. *Arch Intern Med, 62*, 979–1003.

Chaine, J. (1926). L'os penien: etude descriptive et comparative. *Actes Soc Linne Bordeaux, 78*, 1–195.

Chien, C. H., Li, S. H., & Shen, C. L. (1991). The ovarian innervation in the dog: a preliminary study for the base for electroacupuncture. *J Auton Nerv Syst, 35*, 185–192.

Christensen, G. C. (1952). Circulation of blood through the canine kidney. *Am J Vet Res, 13*, 236–245.

Christensen, G. C.: *Angioarchitecture of the canine penis: its role in the process of erection,* Ph.D. thesis, Ithaca, NY, 1953, Cornell University.

Christensen, G. C. (1954). Angioarchitecture of the canine penis and the process of erection. *Am J Anat, 95*, 227–262.

Concannon, P. W. (1991). Reproduction in the dog and cat. In H. Cole & P. T. Cupps (Eds.), *Reproduction in domestic animals* (3rd ed.). Orlando, FL: Academic Press.

Concannon, P., & Lein, D. H. (1989). Hormonal and clinical correlates of ovarian cycles, ovulation, pseudopregnancy, and pregnancy in dogs. In R. W. Kirk (Ed.), *Current veterinary therapy X*. Philadelphia: Saunders.

Concannon, P., Hansel, W., & Visek, W. J. (1975). The ovarian cycle of the bitch: plasma estrogen, LH, and progesterone. *Biol Reprod, 13*, 112–121.

Concannon, P. W., Whaley, S., Lein, D., & Wissler, R. (1983). Canine gestation length: variation related to time of mating and fertile life of sperm. *Am J Vet Res, 44*, 1819–1821.

Concannon, P., Hansel, W., & McEntee, K. (1977). Changes in LH, progesterone and sexual behavior associated with preovulatory luteinization in the bitch. *Biol Reprod, 17*, 604–613.

Cowie, A. T., & Tindal, J. S. (1971). *The physiology of lactation*. London: Arnold.

Cox, V. S., Wallace, L. J., & Jessen, C. R. (1978). An anatomic and genetic study of canine cryptorchidism. *Teratology, 18*, 233–240.

Cupps, P. T. (1991). *Reproduction in domestic animals* (4th ed.). Orlando, FL: Academic Press.

Dail, W. G., & Sachs, B. D. (1991). The ischiourethralis muscle of the rat: anatomy, innervation, and function. *Anat Rec, 229*, 203–208.

Del Campo, C. H., & Ginther, O. J. (1974). Arteries and veins of uterus and ovaries in dogs and cats. *Am J Vet Res, 35*, 409–415.

Deysach, L. T. (1939). The comparative morphology of the erectile tissue of the penis with especial emphasis on the probable mechanism of erection. *Am J Anat, 64*, 111–131.

Didier, R. (1946). Etude systematique de l'os penien des mammiferes. *Mammalia, 10*, 78–91.

Doak, R. L., Hall, A., & Dale, H. E. (1967). Longevity of spermatozoa in the reproductive tract of the bitch. *J Reprod Fert, 13*, 51–58.

Dorr, L. D., & Brody, M. J. (1967). Hemodynamic mechanisms of erection in the canine penis. *Am J Physiol, 213*, 1526–1531.

Drake, M. J. (2007). The integrative physiology of the bladder. *Ann Roy Coll Vet Surg England, 89*, 580–585. doi:10.1308/003588407X205585.

Eckhard, C. (1863). Untersuchungen uber die erektion des penis beim hunde. *Beitr Anat Physiol, 3*, 123–166.

Eisenbrandt, D. L., & Phemister, R. D. (1979). Postnatal development of the canine kidney: quantitative and qualitative morphology. *Am J Anat, 154*, 179–193.

Evan, A. P., Stoeckel, J. A., Loemker, V., & Baker, J. T. (1979). Development of the intrarenal vascular system of the puppy kidney. *Anat Rec, 194*, 187–200.

Evans, H. E. (1961). Prenatal growth and development of the dog. *Rep NY State Veterinary College, 7960-61*, 23–24.

Evans, H. E.: *Prenatal development of the dog: twenty-fourth Gaines Veterinary Symposium*, Ithaca, NY, 1974.

Evans, H. E. (1985). Development of the os penis in the dog. *Proc Amer Assoc Vet Anat Davis, CA*.

Evans, H. E. (1986). Development of the os penis in the dog. *Zbl Vet Med C Anat Histol Embryol, 15*, 170, (abstr).

Evans, H. E., & Sack, W. O. (1973). Prenatal development of domestic and laboratory animals. *Zbl Vet Med C Anat Histol Embryol, 2*, 11–45.

Evans, H. M., & Cole, H. H. (1931). An introduction to the study of the oestrus cycle in the dog. *Mem Univ Calif, 9*, 65–103.

Fagin, J., & Reynolds, S. R. M. (1936). The endometrial vascular bed in relation to rhythmic uterine contractility, with a consideration of the functions of the intermittent contractions of oestrus. *Am J Physiol, 117*, 86–91.

Falconer, I. R. (1971). *Lactation*. London: Butterworths.

Finco, D. R., & Duncan, J. R. (1972). Relationship of glomerular number and diameter of body size of the dog. *Am J Vet Res, 33*, 2447–2450.

Finco, D. R., Kneller, S. K., & Barrett, R. B. (1971). Radiologic estimation of kidney size of the dog. *J Am Vet Med Assoc, 159*, 995–1002.

Fisher, H. G. (1917). Histological structure of the retractor penis muscle of the dog. *Anat Rec, 13*, 69–75.

Fournier, G. R., Jr., Juenemann, K.-P., Lue, T. F., & Tanagho, E. (1987). Mechanisms of venous occlusion during canine penile erection: an anatomic demonstration. *J Urol, 137*, 163–167.

Francois-Franck, C. A. (1895). Recherches sur l'innervation vasomotrice du penis; topographie des nerfs constricteurs et dilatateurs. *Arch Physiol Norm Pathol, 19*, 122–138, 744–816.

Freeman, S. (1990). The evolution of the scrotum: a new hypothesis. *J Theor Biol, 145*, 429–445.

Fuller, P. M., & Heulke, D. F. (1973). Kidney vascular supply in the rat, cat, and dog. *Acta Anat, 84*, 516–522.

Gersh, I. (1937). The correlation of structure and function in the developing mesonephros and metanephros. *Contr Embryol Carnegie Inst, 26*, 33–58.

Giuliano, F., & Rampin, O. (2004). Neural control of erection. *Physiol Behav, 83*, 189–201. doi:10.1016/j.physbeh.2004.08.014.

Gordon, N. (1960). Surgical anatomy of the bladder, prostate gland and urethra in the male dog. *J Am Vet Med Assoc, 136*, 215–221.

Gordon, N. (1961). The position of the canine prostate gland. *Am J Vet Res, 22*, 142–146.

Grandage, J. (1972). The erect dog penis: a paradox of flexible rigidity. *Vet Rec, 91*, 141–147.

Grandage, J. (1975). Some effects of posture on the radiographic appearance of the kidneys of the dog. *J Am Vet Med Assoc, 166*, 165–166.

Grandage, J., & Robertson, B. (1971). An os clitoridis in a bitch. *Aust Vet J, 47*, 346.

Greiner, T. P., & Betts, C. W. (1975). Diseases of the prostate gland. In S. J. Ettinger (Ed.), *Textbook of veterinary internal medicine* (Vol. 2). Philadelphia: Saunders.

Grieco, V., Riccardi, E., Greppi, G. F., et al. (2008). Canine testicular tumours: a study on 232 dogs. *J Comp Pathol, 138*, 86–93.

Griffiths, W. F. B., & Amoroso, E. C. (1939). Proestrus, oestrus, ovulation and mating in the greyhound bitch. *Vet Rec, 57*, 1279–1284.

Gruber, C. M. (1933). The autonomic innervation of the genitourinary system. *Physiol Rev, 13*, 497–609.

Hansel, W., & McEntee, K. (1977). Male reproductive processes. In M. Swensen (Ed.), *Dukes' physiology of domestic animals*. Ithaca, NY: Cornell University Press.

Hanyu, S. (1988). Morphological changes in penile vessels during erection: the mechanism of obstruction of arteries and veins at the tunica albuginea in dog corpora cavernosa. *Urol Int, 43*, 219–224.

Hare, W. C. D. (1976). Intersexuality in the dog. *Can Vet J, 17*, 7–15.

Harrison, R. G. (1949). The comparative anatomy of the blood supply of the mammalian testis. *Proc Zool Soc London, 119*, 325–344.

Hart, B. L. (1972). The action of extrinsic penile muscles during copulation in the male dog. *Anat Rec, 173*, 1–5.

Hart, B. L., & Kitchell, R. L. (1965). External morphology of the erect glans of the dog. *Anat Rec, 152*, 193–198.

Hart, B. L., & Kitchell, R. L. (1966). Penile erection and contraction of penile muscles in the spinal and intact dog. *Am J Physiol, 210*, 257–262.

Hayes, H. M., Wilson, G. P., Pendergrass, T. W., et al. (1985). Canine cryptorchidism and subsequent testicular neoplasia: case-control study with epidemiologic update. *Teratology, 32*, 51–56.

Hayssen, V., & van Tienhoven, A. (1993). *Asdell's patterns of mammalian reproduction: a compendium of species-specific data*. Ithaca, NY: Cornell University Press.

Heape, W. (1900). The sexual season of mammals. *Q J Microp Sci, 44*, 1–70.

Hildebrand, M. (1954). Comparative morphology of the body skeleton in recent canidae. *Univ Calif Pub Zool, 52*, 399–470.

Hodson, N. (1968). On the intrinsic blood supply to the prostate and pelvic urethra in the dog. *Res Vet Sci, 9*, 274–280.

Hofliger, H. (1971). Zur kenntnis der kongenitalen unilateralen nierenagenesie bei haustieren. *Schweiz Arch Tierheilkd, 113*, 330–337.

Holst, P. A., & Phemister, R. D. (1971). The prenatal development of the dog: preimplantation events. *Biol Reprod, 5*, 194–206.

Holst, P. A., & Phemister, R. D. (1974). Onset of diestrus in the beagle bitch: definition and significance. *Am J Vet Res, 35*, 401–406.

Hook, S. J., & Hafez, E. S. E. (1968). A comparative anatomical study of the mammalian uterotubal junction. *J Morphol, 125*, 159–184.

Johnson, A. D., Gomes, W. R., & Vandemark, N. L. (1970). *The testis, vol I, Development, anatomy, and physiology, vol II, Biochemistry, vol III. Influencing factors*. New York: Academic Press.

Kiss, F. (1921). Anatomisch-histologische untersuchungen uber die erektion. *Z Ges Anat, 61*, 455–521.

Konig, H. E., & Liebich, H.-G. (2004). *Veterinary anatomy of domestic mammals*. Schattauer: Stuttgart.

Kumar, M. S. A. (2015). *Clinically oriented anatomy of the dog and cat* (2nd ed.). Ronkakoma, NY: Linus Learning.

Kuntz, A. (1919a). The innervation of the gonads in the dog. *Anat Rec, 17*, 203–219.

Kuntz, A. (1919b). Experimental degeneration in the testis of the dog. *Anat Rec, 17*, 221–234.

Lamming, G. E. (1990-1992). *Marshall's physiology of reproduction, 4th ed, vol I, Reproductive cycles of vertebrates, vol II, Reproduction in the male, vol III, Pregnancy and lactation*. London: Churchill Livingstone.

Langley, J. N. (1896). The innervation of the pelvic and adjoining viscera. *J Physiol, 20*, 372–406.

Larson, B. L. (1974). *Lactation: a comprehensive treatise, vol I, The mammary gland: development and maintenance*. New York: Academic Press.

Latshaw, W. K. (1987). *Veterinary developmental anatomy: a clinically oriented approach*. Philadelphia: BC Decker.

Leav, L., & Ling, G. V. (1968). Adenocarcinoma of the canine prostate. *Cancer, 22*, 1329–1345.

Lee, D. G., & Allam, M. W. (1952). True unilateral hermaphroditism in a dog. *Univ Penn Bull, Vet Ext Quart, (128)*, 142–147.

Liao, A. T., Chu, P. Y., Yeh, L. S., et al. (2009). A 12-year retrospective study of canine testicular tumors. *J Vet Med Sci, 71*, 919–923.

Lindsay, F. E. F. (1983). The normal endoscopic appearance of the caudal reproductive tract of the cyclic and non-cyclic bitch: post-uterine endoscopy. *J Small Anim Pract, 24*, 1–15.

Marshall, F. H. A., & Halnan, E. T. (1917). On the post-oestrous changes occurring in the generative organs and mammary glands of the non-pregnant dog. *Proc R Soc B, 89*, 546–559.

Mason, K. E., & Shaver, S. L. (1952). Some functions of the caput epididymis. *Ann NY Acad Sci, 55*, 585–593.

McCarthy, P. H. (1976). The anatomy of the superficial inguinal ring and its contained and adjacent structures in the live greyhound—a study by palpation. *J Small Anim Pract, 17*, 507–518.

McEntee, K. (1990). *Reproductive pathology of domestic mammals*. Orlando, FL: Academic Press.

McEntee, K., & Zepp, C. P., Jr. (1953). *A study of canine and bovine ovarian tumors (abst), Ann rep NY state vet coll*. Ithaca, NY: Cornell University.

McGeady, T. A., Quinn, P. J., FitzPatrick, E. S., et al. (2009). *Veterinary embryology*. Ames, IA: Blackwell Publishing.

Meyers-Wallen, V. N., & Patterson, D. F. (1986). Disorders of sexual development in the dog. In D. A. Morrow (Ed.), *Current therapy in theriogenology*. Philadelphia: Saunders.

Mitchell, G. A. G. (1938). The innervation of the ovary, uterine tube, testis and epididymis. *J Anat (London), 72*, 508–517.

Morison, D. M. (1926). A study of the renal circulation with special reference to its finer distribution. *Am J Anat, 37*, 53–93.

Mossman, H. W., & Duke, K. L. (1973). *Comparative morphology of the mammalian ovary*. Madison: University of Wisconsin Press.

Naaktgeboren, C., & Slijper, E. J. (1970). *Biologie der geburt*. Berlin: Paul Parey.

Neville, M. C., & Daniel, C. W. (1987). *The mammary gland: development, regulation, and function*. New York: Academic Press.

Ninomiya, H. (1980). The penile cavernous system and its morphological changes in the erected state in the dog. *Jpn J Vet Sci, 42*, 187–195.

Ninomiya, H., & Nakamura, T. (1981a). Vascular architecture of the canine prepuce. *Zbl Vet Med C, 10*, 351–360.

Ninomiya, H., & Nakamura, T. (1981b). The capillary circulation in the penile skin of the dog. *Zbl Vet Med C, 10*, 361–369.

Ninomiya, H., Nakamura, T., Niizuma, I., et al. (1989). Penile vascular system of the dog: an injection-corrosion and histological study. *Jpn J Vet Sci, 51*, 765–773.

Nitschke, T. (1966). Der m. compressor venae dorsalis penis s. Clitoridis des hundes. *Anat Anz, 118*, 193–208.

Nitschke, T. (1970). Diaphragma pelvis. Clitoris and vestibulum vaginae der hundin. *Anat Anz, 127*, 76–125.

Noden, D. M., & de Lahunta, A. (1985). *The embryology of domestic animals: developmental mechanisms and malformations*. Baltimore, MD: Williams & Wilkins.

Olson, P. N., Seim, H. B., Park, R. D., et al. (1989). Female pseudohermaphroditism in three sibling greyhounds. *J Am Vet Med Assoc, 194*, 1747–1749.

O'Morchoe, C. C. C., & Albertine, K. H. (1980). The renal cortical lymphatic system in dogs with unimpeded lymph and urine flow. *Anat Rec, 198*, 427–438.

O'Shea, J. D. (1962). Studies on the canine prostate gland. 1. Factors influencing its size and weight. *J Comp Pathol, 72*, 321–331.

Patsikas, M. N., & Dessiris, A.: *The lymph drainage of the mammary glands in the bitch, Athens*, 1992, Third Hellenic Veterinary Symposium of Small Animal Medicine and PhD thesis, Aristotelian Univ., Thessaloniki, Greece.

Patsikas, M. N., & Dessiris, A. (1996). The lymph drainage of the mammary glands of the bitch: a lymphographic study. Part 1: The 1st, 2nd, 4th, and 5th glands. *Anat Histol Embryol, 25*, 131–138.

Pearson, H., & Gibbs, C. (1971). Urinary tract abnormalities in the dog. *J Small Anim Pract, 12*, 67–84.

Peirce, E. C. (1944). Renal lymphatics. *Anat Rec, 90*, 315–335.
Perry, J. S. (1972). *The ovarian cycle of mammals*. New York: Hafner.
Petras, J. M., & Cummings, J. F. (1978). Sympathetic and parasympathetic innervation of the urinary bladder and urethra. *Brain Res, 153*, 363–369.
Pineda, M. H., Kainer, R. A., & Faulkner, L. C. (1973). Dorsal median postcervical fold in the canine vagina. *Am J Vet Res, 34*, 1487–1491.
Pohl, L. (1911). Das os penis der carnivoren einschliesslich der pinnepedia. *Jena Ztschr Naturw, 47*, 115–160.
Polano, O. (1903). Beitrage zur anatomie der lymphbahnen im menschlichen eierstock. *Mschr Geburstch Gynak, 17*, 281–295, 466–496.
Pond, C. M. (1984). Physiological and ecological importance of energy storage in the evolution of lactation: evidence for a common pattern of anatomical organization of adipose tissue in mammals. *Symp Zool Soc London, 51*, 1–32.
Price, D. (1963). Comparative aspects of development and structure in the prostate. In *Biology of the prostate and related tissues*. *Natl Cancer Inst Monogr, 12*, 1–27.
Purohit, R. C., & Beckett, S. D. (1976). Penile pressures and muscle activity associated with erection and ejaculation in the dog. *Am J Physiol, 231*, 1343–1348.
Ramsey, A. J. (1946). Lymphatic vessels of the fallopian tube. *Anat Rec, 94*, 524.
Raps, G. (1948). The development of the dog ovary from birth to six months of age. *J Am Vet Med Assoc, 9*, 61–64.
Reese, W. O. (1991). *Physiology of domestic animals*. Philadelphia: Lea & Febiger.
Reynolds, S. R. M. (1937). The nature of uterine contractility: a survey of recent trends. *Physiol Rev, 17*, 304–334.
Reynolds, S. R. M. (1949). Adaptation of uterine blood vessels and accommodation of the products of conception. *Contr Embryol Carnegie Inst, 33*, 1–19.
Roszel, J. F. (1975). Genital cytology of the bitch. *Vet Scope, 19*, 2–15.
Rouiller, C., & Muller, A. F. (1969-1971). *The kidney* (4 vols.). New York: Academic Press.
Ruberte, J., Sautet, J. Y., Gine, J. M., et al. (1990). Topographic des collecteurs lymphatique mammaires de la chienne. *Anat Hist Embryol, 19*, 347–358.
Rudolph, L., & Ivy, A. C. (1930). Physiology of the uterus in labor: experimental study of the dog and rabbit. *Am J Obstet Gynecol, 19*, 317–335.
Runnells, R. A. (1954). *Animal pathology* (5th ed.). Ames: Iowa State College Press.
Ruth, E. B. (1934). The os priapi: a study in bone development. *Anat Rec, 60*, 231–249.
Rytand, D. A. (1938). The number and size of mammalian glomeruli as related to kidney and to body weight with methods for their enumeration and measurement. *Am J Anat, 62*, 507–520.
Sampson, J. A. (1937). The lymphatics of the mucosa of the fimbriae of the fallopian tube. *Am J Obstet Gynecol, 33*, 911–930.
Sawyer, H. R., Olson, P. N., & Gorell, T. A. (1984). Effects of progesterone on the oviductal epithelium in estrogen-primed prepubertal beagles: light and electron microscopic observations. *Am J Anat, 169*, 75–87.
Schlotthauer, C. F. (1952). The mammary glands. In J. V. Lacroix & H. P. Hoskins (Eds.), *Canine surgery* (3rd ed.). Evanston, IL: American Veterinary Publications.
Schlotthauer, C. F., & Bollman, J. L. (1936). The prostate gland of the dog. *Cornell Vet, 26*, 342–349.
Segal, S. J., Crozier, R., Corfman, P. A., et al. (1973). *The regulation of mammalian reproduction*. Springfield, IL: Charles C Thomas.
Setchell, B. P. (1978). *The mammalian testis*. Ithaca, NY: Cornell University Press.
Shane, B. S., Dunn, H. O., Kenney, R. M., et al. (1969). Methyltestosterone-induced female pseudohermaphroditism in dogs. *Biol Reprod, 1*, 41–48.
Smith, H. W. (1951). *The kidney*. New York: Oxford University Press.
Sokolowski, J. H., Stover, D. G., & Van Ravenswaay, F. (1977). Seasonal incidence of estrus and interestrus interval for bitches of seven breeds. *J Am Vet Med Assoc, 171*, 271–273.
Spurgeon, T. L., & Kitchell, R. L. (1982). Electrophysiological studies of the cutaneous innervation of the external genitalia of the male dog. *Anat Histol Embryol, 11*, 289–306.
Spurgeon, T. L., & Reddy, V. K. (1986). Electrophysiological studies of the cutaneous innervation of the external genitalia of the female dog. *Anat Histol Embryol, 15*, 249–258.
Stalker, L. K., & Schlotthauer, C. F. (1936). Neoplasms of the mammary gland in the dog. *North Am Vet, 17*, 33–43.
Stead, A. C. (1972). Fracture of the os penis in the dog: two case reports. *J Small Anim Pract, 13*, 19–22.
Stewart, R. W., Menges, R. W., Selby, L. A., et al. (1972). Canine intersexuality in a pug breeding kennel. *Cornell Vet, 62*, 464–473.
Szabo, K. T. (1989). *Congenital malformations in laboratory and farm animals*. Orlando, FL: Academic Press.
Trentin, J. J., DeVita, J., & Gardner, W. U. (1952). Effect of moderate doses of estrogen and progesterone on mammary growth and hair growth in dogs. *Anat Rec, 113*, 163–177.
Turner, C. W. (1939). *The comparative anatomy of the mammary glands*. Columbia, MO: University Coop. Store.
Turner, C. W., & Gomez, E. T. (1934). The normal and experimental development of the mammary gland. II. The male and female dog. *Mo Agr Exp Sta Res Bui, 207*.
Urgel, J. C., & Lacalle, L. P. (1970). Desarrollo pre y postnatal del os penis en canis familiaris. *An Fac Vet Catedra Anat Embry*, 47–54.
Vaerst, L. (1938). Uber die blutversorgung des hundepenis. *Morph Jb, 81*, 307–352.
van Tienhoven, A. (1983). *Reproductive physiology of vertebrates*. Ithaca, NY: Cornell University Press.
Verma, O. P., & Chibuzo, G. A. (1974). Hormonal influences on motility of canine uterine horns. *Am J Vet Res, 35*, 23–26.
Vimtrup, B. J. (1928). On the number, shape, structure, and surface area of the glomeruli in the kidneys of man and mammals. *Am J Anat, 41*, 123–151.
Wakuri, H. (1966a). Embryological and anatomical studies on the mammary formula of mongrel dogs: on the newborn and adult dog. *J Mamm Soc Jpn, 3*, 19–23.
Wakuri, H. (1966b). Embryological and anatomical studies on the mammary formula of mongrel dogs: report 1: the canine fetus. *J Mamm Soc Jpn, 2*, 147–150.
Wensing, C. J. G. (1968). Testicular descent in some domestic mammals. I. anatomical aspects of testicular descent. *Proc K Ned Akad Wet Ser C, 71*, 423–434.
Wensing, C. J. G. (1973a). Testicular descent in some domestic mammals. II. The nature of the gubernacular changes during the process of testicular descent in the pig. *Proc K Ned Akad Wet Ser C, 76*, 190–195.
Wensing, C. J. G. (1973b). Testicular descent in some domestic mammals. III. Search for the factors that regulate the gubernacular reaction. *Proc K Ned Akad Wet Ser C, 76*, 196–202.

Wensing, C. J. G. (1980). Developmental anomalies including cryptorchidism. In D. A. Morrow (Ed.), *Current therapy in theriogenology*. Philadelphia: Saunders.

Wensing, C. J. G., & Colenbrander, B. (1986). Normal and abnormal testicular descent. In *Oxford review of reproductive biology* (Vol. 8). Oxford: Clarendon Press.

Wensing, C. J. G., & Van Straten, H. W. M. (1980). Normal and abnormal testicular descent in some mammals. In E. S. E. Hafez (Ed.), *Descended and cryptorehid testis* Nijhoff. Boston.

Wenzel, J. G. W., & Odend'hal, S. (1985). The mammalian rete ovarii: a literature review. *Cornell Vet, 75*, 411–425.

Wildt, D. E., Levin, C. J., & Seager, S. W. J. (1977). Laparoscopic exposure and sequential observation of the ovary of the cycling bitch. *Anat Rec, 189*, 443–450.

Willis, R. A. (1962). *The borderland of embryology and pathology* (2nd ed.). London: Butterworth.

Woodburne, R. T., & Lapides, J. (1972). The ureteral lumen during peristalsis. *Am J Anat, 133*, 255–258.

Yeager, A. E., & Concannon, P. W. (1990). Association between the preovulatory luteinizing hormone surge and the early ultrasonic detection of pregnancy and fetal heartbeats in beagle dogs. *Theriogenology, 34*, 655–665.

Yeager, A. E., Mohammed, H. O., Meyers-Wallen, V., et al. (1992). Ultrasonic appearance of the uterus, placenta, fetus, and fetal membranes throughout accurately timed pregnancy in beagles. *Am J Vet Res, 53*, 342–351.

Zietzsehmann, O. (1928). Uber den processus vaginalis der hundin. *Dtsch Tieraerztl Wochenschr, 36*, 20–22.

Zuckerman, S. (1971). *The ovary* (2nd ed.). New York: Academic Press.

10
The Endocrine System
RONALD L. HULLINGER

General Features of the Endocrine Glands

The endocrine system contrasts with other body systems in that component organs, tissues, and cells are distributed throughout the body, typically in widely separated locations. Hormone synthesis is the principal function shared by all components of the system. The various components of the endocrine system are linked functionally by the circulatory system: blood vessels, lymphatic vessels, and interstitial fluids. There are morphologic similarities in these organs and tissues: a general sparsity of stromal connective tissue; an abundant blood and lymph vasculature; epithelioid cell types, composing parenchymal units (e.g., racemi, follicles); and an absence of secretory ducts. The specific structural features vary with the endocrine gland. Accordingly, *endocrine system* refers to a functional relationship of various cells, tissues, and organs, not to a structurally contiguous set of component organs. The name *endocrine* has a derivational meaning taken from the Greek words *endon,* meaning "within," and *krinein,* meaning "to separate"—thus released internally. The study of the structure and functioning of this system of units that secrete internally is termed *endocrinology.*

Endocrine glands exercise a major regulation of the organism. They supplement and augment the function of the nervous system in response to signal from both internal and external environments. These signals directly or indirectly affect the specific metabolism of epithelioid cells of the endocrine tissues and organs and cells of some nervous system tissues, causing them to release into the intercellular space relatively small quantities of substances termed *hormones.* Hormones are the secretory products of parenchymal cells found singly or, more often, in aggregates as endocrine tissues and organs. Hormones (*ligands*) released by endocrine cells may diffuse directly to other loci via the interstitial fluids or enter into blood or lymphatic vessels and are distributed to more distant *receptor* molecules. These receptors are on or within cells of target sites. These target cells are modulated in activity by the hormone. The hormones are considered *trophic* or *-tropic* substances (meaning they *feed* or *cause turning*).

Tissues and glands organized from these endocrine cells are without ducts and, accordingly, have been called *glandulae sine ductibus,* the ductless glands. Tissue fluids immediately surrounding the secretory cells become the initial transport media for secretions of the glandular parenchyma. Nearly all cells, and therefore nearly all tissues and organs of the body, are commonly within humoral or fluid secretions, that is products and byproducts of their metabolism. Many of these secretions do not function as hormones, but some of these metabolites diffuse into the organism and, as hormones, bind to receptors and modulate specific target sites. Some excite and others suppress the activity of these target organs, tissues, or cells.

Components of the endocrine system are classified according to their major functional activity. Primary endocrine organs are the **hypophysis** (*glandula pituitaria* [pituitary]); **thyroid gland**; **parathyroid gland**; **pineal gland** (*glandula pinealis*), formerly *epiphysis*; and **adrenal gland**. Their exclusive function is production of hormones. The **testis**, **ovary**, and **pancreas** have both endocrine and exocrine functions. Other organs (e.g., **kidney**, **liver**, and **placenta**) have a secondary (no less important) endocrine function. Still other tissues and cells—the gastric and intestinal mucosal epithelium, granulated cardiac myocytes, thymic epithelioreticular cells, and cells of the general connective tissues—also produce hormones.

The size of endocrine structures singly or as a group is generally unimpressive, as is the extent of their distribution. However, these endocrine foci integrate information from exteroceptive and interoceptive portions of the nervous system. By chemoreceptive and chemostimulative means, these ductless glands exert functional and structural regulation of the organism.

The significant and enduring role of the endocrine secretions also affects normal development, differentiation, and functioning of the immune system (Kelley et al., 1988); subtleties of sexual differentiation (Aumuller, 1983); and dimorphism, fertility control, alimentation, and normal growth and aging.

Most endocrine parenchyma develop in the embryo and fetus from cells derived from one of the three germ layers; the adrenal gland, however, develops from two germ layers. Prior to birth, the endocrine structures of the fetus are under the influence of the maternal endocrine system.

Although the endocrine system is significantly developed at birth, major differentiation of structural and functional relationships are affected postnatally. Once established, this system regulates normal growth, propels the organism to sexual maturity, controls metabolism and homeostasis, and precipitates senescent change.

A normal endocrine regulatory system is essential for integration of functioning body systems. A malfunctioning endocrine system often causes dramatic change in body form, function, and behavior. Diabetes insipidus, hypophyseal adenoma, diabetes mellitus, hypothyroidism, hyperthyroidism, interstitial cell tumor, and hyperadrenocorticoidism are examples of endocrine disturbances affecting the dog. Bloom (1959) and Feldman et al. (2015) present a general discussion of endocrine diseases of the dog.

Endocrine organs vary in structure and function among the breeds (Stockard, 1941), among individuals, seasonally, and, at a cellular level, diurnally. The morphologic characteristics of some endocrine organs can change rapidly in response to variations in normal physiologic activity. In many of the endocrine tissues there is a storage of substrate or products of cellular synthesis leading to the eventual formation of active hormone. The adrenal cortex, interstitial endocrine cells of the testis, and the corpus luteum store neutral fats and cholesterol in large quantities. The thyroid produces great amounts of iodinated thyroglobulin that is initially exocytosed into a follicular lumen. In light of this "reserve capacity" and a normal variation in cell numbers or percentages within the same individual, abnormal changes leading to or resulting from disease of the endocrine system are very difficult to assess by morphologic means. Laboratory findings suggestive of hyper- or hypofunctioning must be correlated with case history, clinical signs, as well as assays for hormone production. Hormonal assay is accomplished primarily by direct measurement of blood hormone levels or urinary excretion of hormone metabolites.

The dog continues to serve as a model for endocrine research and, as such, has provided much comparative information relating to functions of this system. The term *hormone* was first applied by Bayliss and Starling (1902) in their observations of the mechanisms of pancreatic secretion in the dog. In 1922, when Banting and Best made medical history (Banting was co-recipient of the 1923 Nobel Prize in medicine) by discovering the effects of pancreatic extract in reducing blood sugar, the dog was the experimental animal. The dog was also the test animal used for the demonstration of secretin (Ivy & Oldberg, 1928; Kosaka & Lim, 1930).

Initially endocrine cells and organs were often identified based on their morphologic characteristics (i.e., epithelioid cells, accumulated secretory products, no exocrine ducts, extensive blood capillaries, and little interstitial stroma). The presumed endocrine functions were often confirmed by clinical signs following hyperplasia, neoplasia, surgical removal, histochemistry of secretory product, and enzyme histochemistry. Immunofluorescence now makes accurate assessment of endocrine cell function more feasible.

Michaelson (1970) presented a review of the general anatomic features of the endocrine glands of the dog, along with an account of specific functional and clinical parameters. Much of the structural and functional detail relative to the endocrine system of the dog has been inferred from work with other mammals, including humans, and specific information about morphology of the dog endocrines is still widely scattered in the literature. Stockard (1941) presented detailed information on the morphologic characteristics of the endocrines in many breeds of dogs. Venzke (1976) discussed the macroscopic anatomy of selected endocrine organs of the dog. Compendia have been edited by Harris and Donovan (1966) for the pituitary gland; Pitt-Rivers and Trotter (1964) for the thyroid gland; Chester-Jones (1957), Nussdorfer (1986), and Chester-Jones et al. (1986) for the adrenal cortex; and Chester-Jones (1976) and Epple et al. (1990) for comparative endocrinology.

Endocrine morphology varies with breed and with the individual, often depending on age, nutrition, environment, and general health. Most endocrine research in dogs is conducted using the medium-sized, mesaticephalic breeds.

The Hypophysis

A terminology appropriate to this gland follows and is based upon the *Nomina Anatomica Veterinaria* (2017), *Nomina Histologica* (1992), and *Nomina Anatomica* (1989) (Figs. 10.1 and 10.2).

Hypophysis (*Glandula pituitaria*)
Adenohypophysis
    Pars tuberalis
    Pars intermedia
    Cavum hypophysis
    Pars distalis
Neurohypophysis
    Infundibulum
    Lobus nervosus
    Pars cava

The **hypophysis**, or **pituitary gland** (*glandula pituitaria*), is a reddish appendage attached at the ventral midline to the diencephalon (Fig. 10.1). The Greek term *hypophysis cerebri* conveys this positional meaning, *hypo* meaning under and *physis* meaning growth—thus the growth on the undersurface of the brain. The Latin term *pituitary* is derived from a historical interpretation by Vesalius concerning the function of this gland as the source of nasal exudate, *pituita*, or phlegm (Field & Harrison, 1957).

The size of the hypophysis varies greatly among breeds of dogs and among individuals of the same breed (Hanström, 1966; Hewitt, 1950; Latimer, 1941, 1965; Stockard, 1941; White & Foust, 1944). In the adult of the mesaticephalic breeds, the size of the unpreserved gland is approximately 1 cm in length, 0.7 cm in width, and 0.5 cm in depth. Its weight is approximately 0.06 g in the male. The hypophysis of the larger dog shows an absolute increase in size, but a relative decrease in proportion to body weight. When other factors such as breed and nutrition are constant, the hypophysis of the female is somewhat larger than that of the male. It is also larger in the gravid versus nongravid female (Latimer, 1941; White & Foust, 1944).

Although small, this organ plays a major regulatory role for much of the endocrine system. The close structural positioning of glandular and nervous parts of this gland is symbolic of its function in interrelating nervous and endocrine systems. So extensive are influences of the hypophysis on cells, tissues, and organs that it has been referred to as *master gland* of the body. The early work of Putnam et al. (1929), reporting effects of injecting extracts of the gland to young dogs, demonstrated widespread changes in multiple body tissues and indicated the significance of this endocrine gland. The works of Crowe et al. (1910) and Dandy and Reichert (1925) established the hypophysis cerebri as essential for maintenance of life.

Macroscopic Features

The hypophysis occupies a bony recess in the basisphenoid (*os basisphenoidale*) (Fig. 4.18). The recess is a shallow, oval depression, the **hypophyseal fossa** (*fossa hypophysials*). The rostral and caudal margins of the fossa are formed by the rostral clinoid processes and the dorsum sella, respectively. When the fossa is viewed dorsally, the rostral and caudal clinoid processes accentuate the boundaries of the fossa on the dorsal surface of the basisphenoid bone, referred to as the *sella turcica*. In the dog the fossa is quite shallow and is lined by the external, or endosteal, layer of dura mater. The inner, or meningeal, layer of the dura forms the *diaphragma sellae*. The latter does not pass directly into the fossa with the external dural layer but extends partially over the dorsal aspect of the fossa to provide an incomplete septum. The primary attachments of this septum, or diaphragm, are by way of the clinoid processes. A large oval foramen is present in the center of the diaphragm, which loosely encircles the stalklike connection of the hypothalamus to the hypophysis, as it extends into the fossa. This thin meningeal layer then continues around the main portion of the gland as a delicate capsule. Schwartz (1936) demonstrated that the subarachnoid space does not invest the hypophysis.

The space created by the separation between the inner and outer dural layers contains prominent cavernous and intercavernous sinuses. Large cavernous sinuses bound the hypophysis laterally and are connected by intercavernous sinuses. The larger intercavernous sinus passes just caudal to the hypophysis (Figs. 12.22 and 12.24). The smaller intercavernous sinus is variably present, and, when present, it passes rostral to the hypophysis. The proximal portion of the middle meningeal artery and the anastomotic ramus of the external ophthalmic artery pass through each of the cavernous sinuses. The internal carotid artery also courses through each of the cavernous sinuses lateral to the hypophysis, from the dorsum sella rostral to the region of the optic chiasm (Figs. 10.3, and 11.28). The oculomotor, trochlear, and abducent nerves and the ophthalmic nerve from the trigeminal nerve pass in close proximity to the hypophysis. The interpeduncular cistern is adjacent to the caudal aspect of the attachment of the infundibulum to the hypothalamus and within the cistern lies the caudal part of the cerebral arterial circle (*circulus arteriosus cerebri*). A bony wall separates the hypophyseal fossa from the sphenoid sinus, lying rostroventrally. Positional relations of these structures to the hypophysis create some surgical risk and, as reported by Harrison (1964) and emphasized by Farrow (1969), may account for many of the signs accompanying hypophyseal disease.

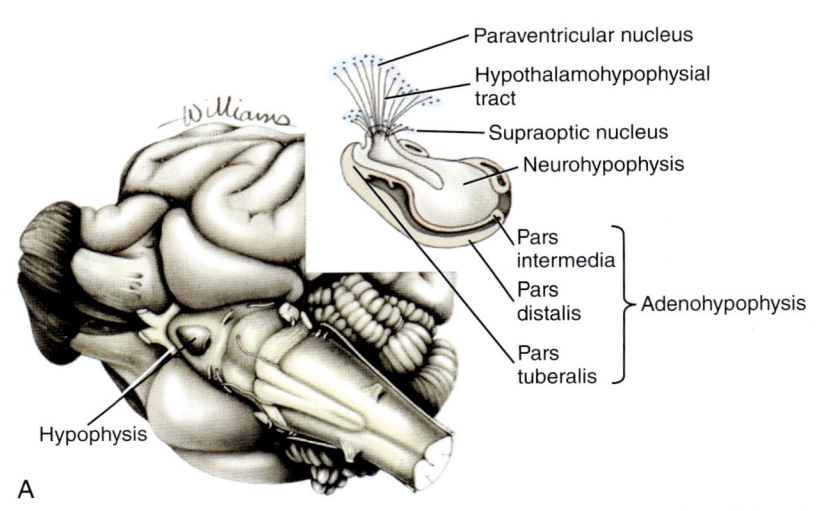

• **Fig. 10.1 A**, Hypophysis attached to ventral midline of brain, left caudoventrolateral view. Inset is a schematic representation of the midsagittally sectioned hypophysis and the extension into the neurohypophysis of axons from cell bodies found in the supraoptic and paraventricular nuclei of the hypothalamus.

Continued

472 CHAPTER 10 The Endocrine System

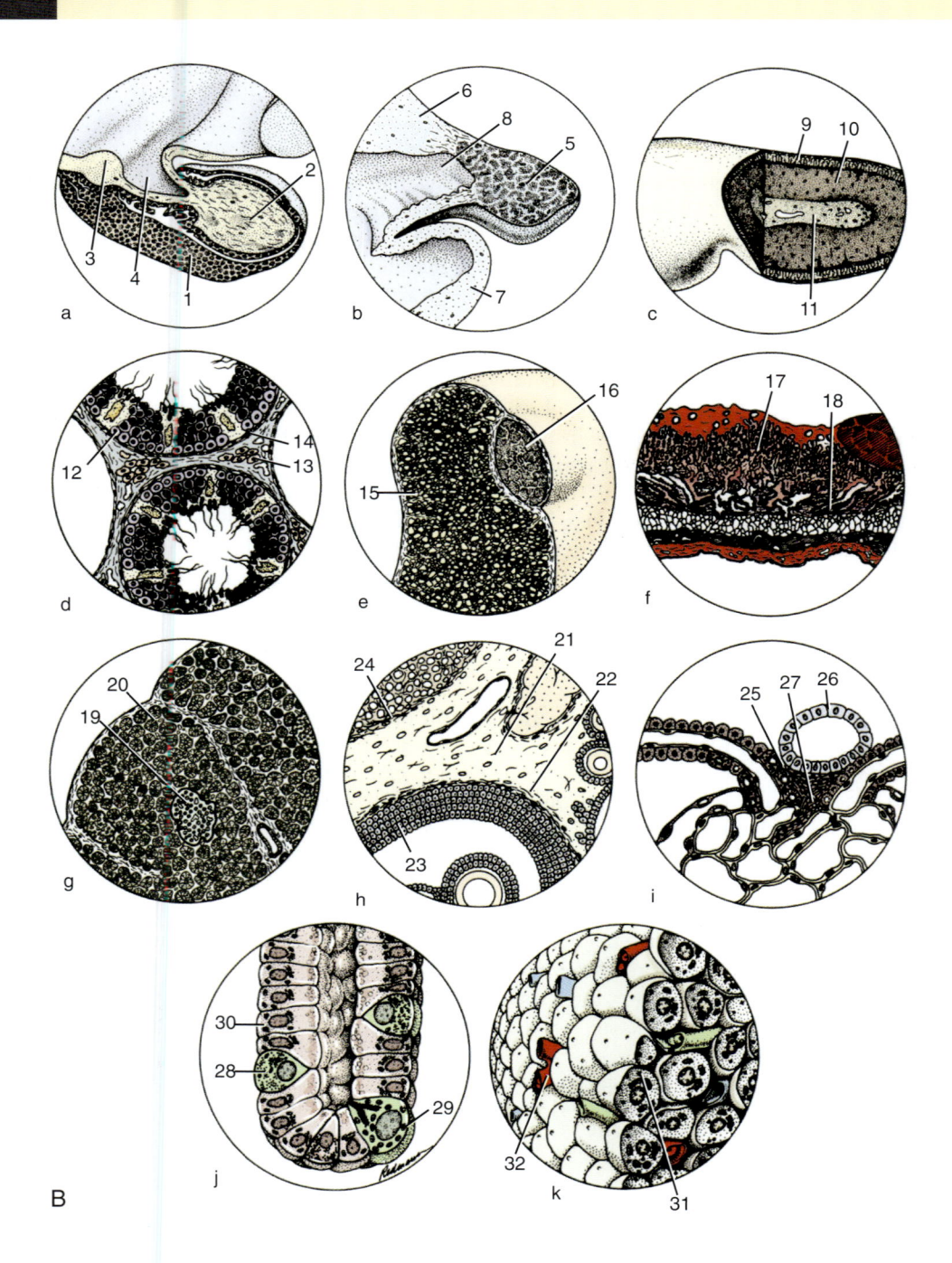

a. Hypophysis and hypothalamus
  1. Adenohypophysis
  2. Neurohypophysis
  3. Hypothalamic nuclei
  4. Third ventricle
b. Glandula pinealis
  5. Parenchyma
  6. Habenular commissure
  7. Caudal commissure
  8. Third ventricle
c. Adrenal gland
  9. Outer cortex
  10. Inner cortex
  11. Medulla
d. Testis
  12. Seminiferous tubule
  13. Interstitial cells
  14. Sustentacular cell
e. Thyroid and parathyroid
  15. Thyroid follicle
  16. Parathyroid
f. Placental labyrinth
  17. Fetal syncytiotrophoblast
  18. Maternal glands
g. Pancreas
  19. Endocrine islet
  20. Exocrine acinus
h. Ovary
  21. Interstitial cells
  22. Thecal cells
  23. Follicular epithelium
  24. Corpus luteum
i. Kidney
  25. Juxtaglomerular cells
  26. Macula densa
  27. Mesangium
j. Enteric mucosa
  28. Enteroendocrine cell
  29. Parietal cell
  30. Zymogenic cell
k. Generalized endocrine parenchyma
  31. Epithelioid cells
  32. Blood and lymph capillaries

• **Fig. 10.1, cont'd B**, Mesoscopic and microscopic organization of endocrine tissues from a variety of organs. (After Budras KD, Fricke W: *Atlas der Anatomie des Hundes,* 3rd ed., Hannover, 1991, Schlütersche Verlaganstalt und Druckerei.)

Mesoscopic Features

As noted by Hanström (1966), much of the literature demonstrates individual and breed differences in morphologic characteristics of the hypophysis. The hypophysis of the adult (Figs. 10.1 and 10.2) has grossly visible rounded protuberances, *adenohypophysis* and *neurohypophysis*. The adenohypophysis, composed of glandular parenchyma and having an extensive blood supply, appears reddened and friable in comparison to the pallor and the brainlike texture of the neurohypophysis. A median section of hypophysis and hypothalamus, when examined with slight magnification, reveals further subdivisions of the organ (Fig. 10.1). The gland is suspended from the midline of the hypothalamus by a cylindrical stalk. This stalk is an extension from the *tuber cinereum* of the hypothalamus (Figs. 11.27 and 18.3). This stalk is the proximal portion of the neurohypophysis, the *infundibulum*. In most dogs the third ventricle continues as an invagination into the infundibulum, a recess called the **pars cava**, but it rarely passes into the more distal portion of the infundibulum. The distal compact infundibulum is continuous with the distal enlargement, **neural lobe** (*lobus nervosus*) of the neurohypophysis, a modest expansion at the distal end of the infundibulum, constituting the major portion of the neurohypophysis.

The principal axis of the gland is in a median plane and extends caudally, nearly parallel to the floor of the diencephalon. The largest portion of the adenohypophysis lies ventrorostral to the neural lobe and invests nearly all of the surface of the neurohypophysis, forming three major subdivisions (see following description). The adenohypophysis contains a large, funnel-shaped vesicle and, when seen in sagittal slices of the gland, appears as a cleft. It is termed **hypophyseal cavity** (*cavum hypophysis*) and is a remnant of development of the stomodeal adenohypophyseal sac (see following). The dorsal portion of the adenohypophysis is in direct contact with the neural lobe and is termed *pars intermedia adenohypophysis*, owing to its location between the two major parts of the adenohypophysis. The largest portion of the adenohypophysis remains separated from the pars intermedia by the hypophyseal cavity (Fig. 10.2), forming the distal portion of the adenohypophysis, *pars distalis adenohypophysis*. The adenohypophysis also extends as a cuff or collar around the infundibulum, enveloping the tuber cinereum. This is the *pars tuberalis adenohypophysis*.

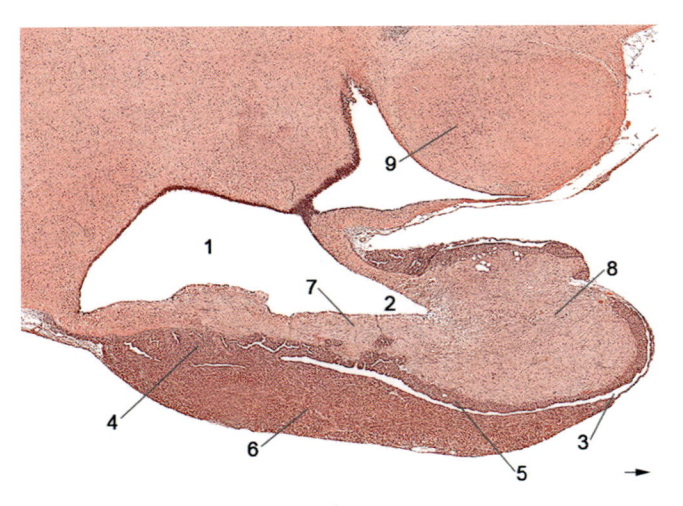

1. Ventriculus tertius
2. Recessus infundibuli
3. Cavum hypophysis
4. Pars tuberalis adenohypophysis
5. Pars intermedia adenohypophysis
6. Pars distalis adenohypophysis
7. Infundibulum
8. Lobus nervosus
9. Corpus mamillare

• **Fig. 10.2** Mesoscopic features of adult hypophysis, sagittal section. (Pentachromic staining, 15×.)

Developmental Anatomy

By the 7-mm stage of development in the dog, a small portion of oral ectoderm lining the dorsum of the stomodeum contacts the ventral surface of the neural tube. This positioning between oral and neural ectoderm is maintained while differential growth and resultant proliferation

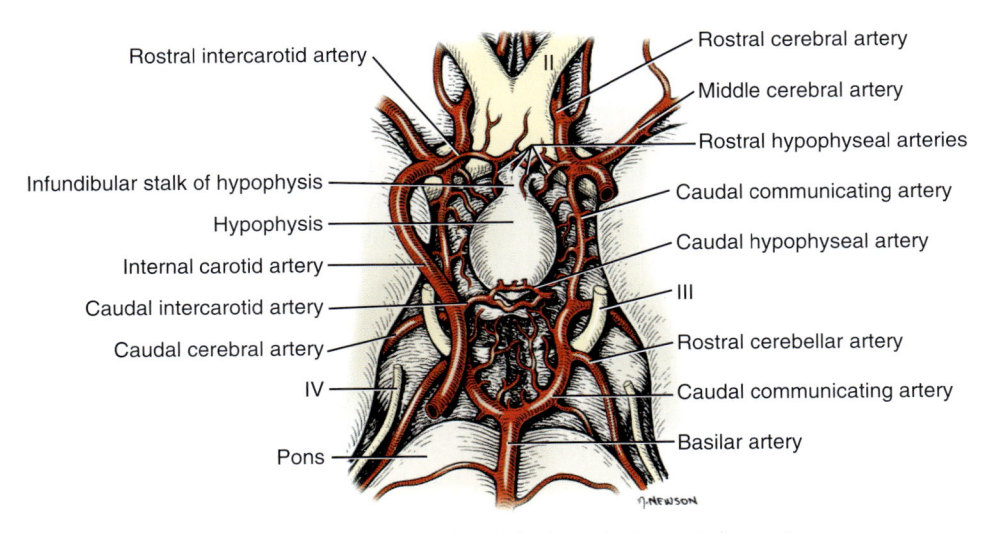

• **Fig. 10.3** The vascularization of the hypophysis, ventral aspect.

of mesoderm continues in the head region. The neural ectoderm retains its relative position, and the adjacent portion of oral ectoderm is drawn from the stomodeum, first as a cul-de-sac and then as a closed vesicle, *saccus adenohypophysialis,* separated from the developing oral cavity. With continued differentiation of the neural ectoderm, a small projection or evagination develops at the midline of the ventral surface of diencephalon at the point of contact with the oral ectodermal vesicle. This structure, the *sacculus infundibuli,* is surrounded by the collapsing vesicle of oral ectoderm. The adjoining mesenchyme develops the stroma and vascularization for this parenchymal primordium, the adenohypophysis (Kingsbury & Roemer, 1940; Latimer, 1965; Stockard, 1941).

This duality of origin, both oral and neural ectoderm, results in an organ having differing structures as well as functions. Neural ectoderm forms the neurohypophysis, comprised of infundibulum and neural lobe. The vesicle of oral ectoderm invests the neurohypophyseal primordium on all of its surfaces except a small area at the distal, caudal extremity. Surfaces of the vesicle of oral ectoderm contacting the neural lobe of the neurohypophysis develop into the pars intermedia adenohypophysis. The vesicle also extends toward the tuber cinereum, enveloping the infundibulum and forming the pars tuberalis adenohypophysis. The portion of the vesicle not contacting any of the neurohypophysis becomes pars distalis adenohypophysis.

Microscopic Features

General microscopic features of this gland are those of an endocrine gland and a segment of central nervous system tissue. A description of the microscopy of the hypophysis cerebri is presented by Hullinger and Andrisani (2006). The stroma is formed by a capsule of delicate pial connective tissue forming around the neurohypophysis during development and remaining as a boundary between it and the adenohypophyseal subdivisions. The adenohypophysis is enveloped by a delicate investment of collagenous connective tissue of the arachnoid that binds the adenohypophysis to the adjoining inner layer of dura mater. At a point representing the original connection to the oral ectoderm, on the midventral surface of the adenohypophysis, the adenohypophysis is attached to the inner dural layer and fused to the outer layer. This attachment is easily broken and usually accounts for some separation artifact in preparations of the pars distalis adenohypophysis. When a small remnant of development called the *parahypophysis* is present, it is attached at this location (Kingsbury & Roemer, 1940). The stroma forming a capsule for both neurohypophysis and adenohypophysis is originally quite delicate and increases in amount only slightly with advancing age. Blood vessels are invested by small amounts of adventitial connective tissues, and the parenchymal cells of the adenohypophysis are supported by a delicate interstitium of reticular fibers.

The **pars distalis adenohypophysis** is comprised of epithelioid cell types arranged in small, interconnected clusters, *racemi endocrinocyti,* permeated by numerous sinusoids. These aggregates of cells are quite varied in size and shape and arranged three-dimensionally as anastomosing lattices. The close proximity of nearly all parenchymal cells to a sinusoid is maintained throughout. By immunohistochemistry specific hormonal secretions of these cells have been identified. With routine staining there is a separation of three distinctive cell populations: *endocrinocytus acidophilus, endocrinocytus basophilus,* and *endocrinocytus chromophobus.* The frequency of occurrence of each cell type varies according to age, sex, breed, and physiologic state. Francis and Mulligan (1949) reported in the adult male dog acidophilic cells outnumbered basophilic cells approximately five to one and chromophobic cells occurred with three times the frequency of basophilic cells. Stockard (1941) reported basophilic cells were outnumbered 30 to 1 by acidophilic cells. White and Foust (1944) reported no significant sex differences and a ratio of 11 to 1 in acidophilic to basophilic cells.

The **acidophilic endocrine cells** have an affinity for acidic dyes, staining well with the acid dyes of bichromic and trichromic procedures. The dye is taken up by cytoplasmic granules which are stored secretory products. These cells are smaller than the basophilic cells, measuring approximately 15 μm in diameter. The acidophilic cells are located adjacent to sinusoids, in most cases being displaced only by basophilic cells from that site. Their distribution within the pars distalis adenohypophysis is generally uniform, with only a slight increase in their numbers near the inner aspect. During pregnancy the proportion of acidophilic cells increases and remains elevated, constituting approximately 65% of cells, until the end of lactation, when their numbers return to prepregnancy levels. These cells are of two types: one that produces a somatotrophin protein and another that produces a lactotrophin protein.

Basophilic endocrine cells possess cytoplasmic granules that have a moderate affinity for the basic component of routine laboratory stains. The granules are composed of glycoprotein and react positively when stained with dyes specific for that component. The cells are larger than the acidophilic cells, measuring approximately 20 μm in diameter, and are more elongated. Like acidophilic cells, these cells are generally observed along a sinusoid. They occur in greater numbers at the periphery of the pars distalis adenohypophysis. Stockard (1941) has reported that basophilic cells proliferate during proestrus. Thyrotrophin and gonadotrophins are the hormones produced by a subset of specific basophilic cell types, respectively.

Chromophobic cells do not stain well with routine dyes. They occur in moderate numbers near the central region of a racemose. Their nuclei are easily visible, but their cytoplasmic boundaries are difficult to determine. There is equivocal evidence that some of these cells, which lack marked staining affinity, produce adrenocorticotrophin (Goldberg & Chaikoff, 1952; Mikami, 1956; Purves, 1966). Ricci and Russolo (1973) present immunocytologic evidence that suggests this hormone is produced by the chromophils.

Many investigators have described a fourth cell type in the dog. Most believe it to be a functional variant (Hartman et al., 1946; Purves & Griesbach, 1957; Smith et al., 1953; Wolf & Cleveland, 1932). Kagayama (1965) and Gale (1972) term this cell a *stellate*, or *follicular cell*. Goldberg and Chaikoff (1952), Carlon (1967), and Gale (1972) describe six cell types based on specific histochemistry or structural features.

The **pars tuberalis adenohypophysis** is composed of epithelioid cells packed between sinusoids in anastomosing walls or *muralia*. Occasionally, small follicles bounded by epithelia are seen. The cells are uniform in size, being low columnar, and in staining characteristics, being largely chromophobic. There are often a few cells typical of the chromophobic cells of the pars distalis adenohypophysis mixed among cells of the pars tuberalis adenohypophysis, near that segment. Their cytoplasm is finely granular and reacts slightly positive with dyes for glycogen. When follicles occur, they are filled with a homogeneous glycoprotein and typically lined by a simple columnar epithelium. The tissues of the pars tuberalis are also continuous with those of the pars intermedia adenohypophysis, with which it shares many structural and cytochemical features.

Parenchyma of the **pars intermedia adenohypophysis** is a complexly folded pseudostratified columnar epithelium. It envelops nearly all of the neural lobe of the neurohypophysis and is separated from it by only a delicate band of vascularized, pial connective tissue. The remnant of the vesicular space, the hypophyseal cavity, separates the pars intermedia from the pars distalis adenohypophysis. The pars intermedia adenohypophysis blends with the pars distalis adenohypophysis as it reflects distally to merge with that part. Where it is continuous with the pars tuberalis adenohypophysis, the folded epithelium projects into the lumen of the hypophyseal cavity. These folds are more prominent in the brachycephalic breeds. Infrequently, there are villus-like projections extending for short distances into the neurohypophyseal tissues. The parenchyma is normally devoid of sinusoids, but has access to numerous pial capillaries at the neurohypophyseal surface. Often these vessels can be seen projecting into the connective tissue septa of the folds. The epithelioid parenchymal cells stain faintly. Melanocyte-stimulating hormone and adrenocorticotropin are secreted by these cells (Halmi et al., 1981).

Cells of the neural lobe and the infundibulum are chiefly glial cells, termed *gliocyti centrales* (*pituicytes*), supporting axons in an extensive neuropil. The axons are processes of neuronal cell bodies found in specific nuclei of the hypothalamus and compose the supraopticohypophyseal and paraventriculohypophysial tracts (Fig. 10.1). These axonal processes store and release neurohumors produced in the hypothalamic nuclei, vasopressin and oxytocin. These neurohumors enter capillaries of the neural lobe and, by veins exiting at the caudal aspect of the lobe, enter the systemic circulation. The tuberohypophysial tracts convey releasing factors from numerous hypothalamic nuclei, to the tuber cinereum and infundibulum where they enter the capillary loops that circulate to the adenohypophysis.

Vascularization

Blood supply and venous drainage of all the hypophyseal regions are structurally interrelated. The functional interdependence of the hypophyseal subdivisions is facilitated by their common vascularization.

The arterial supply of the hypophysis arises from two major sources, the **internal carotid arteries** and the **caudal communicating arteries** (Figs. 10.3, 11.27, and 11.28). Several branches passing directly to the region of the gland arise from the rostral and caudal intercarotid arteries and the caudal communicating arteries. The number of vessels from these sources that converge on the hypophysis is extensive and was described by Dandy and Goetsch (1910) as appearing "like spokes to the hub of a wheel." The **rostral intercarotid artery** provides a variable number of branches, 4 to 10, to the region of the infundibulum (Basir, 1932). An equally extensive group of vessels arises from the **rostral communicating arteries** (Fig. 11.27). In addition, a vessel arises from each of the internal carotids and proceeds toward the infundibulum. Less prominent vessels may also originate from the caudal aspect of the arterial circle. All of these vessels pass centripetally toward the infundibulum where they join in forming a plexus, the **mantle plexus** (Green, 1951). The plexus is incorporated into the meningeal investment of the hypophysis.

From this mantle plexus many arterioles enter the tuber cinereum and continue as capillaries to the **primary blood capillary network** (*rete hemocapillare primarium*). On the rostral and lateral surfaces of the tuber cinereum major vessels arise from the mantle plexus or as direct branches of the intercarotid vessels that are termed the **rostral hypophyseal arteries**. Several of these also provide capillaries to the tuber cinereum and the initial portion of the infundibulum and join in the primary blood capillary network (Akmayev, 1971a). These capillaries receive neurohumoral secretions called *releasing factors*, which are subsequently carried from this region of the hypothalamus, called the *median eminence gland* by Reichlin (1974), to the hypophysis via a portal blood vascular system (Campbell, 1970; Green, 1966). Akmayev (1971b) reported that those nuclei of the tuber cinereum that have the greatest vascularity have the smallest caliber capillaries. A major portion of the venous drainage from this capillary network returns to the surface of the infundibulum and is collected by veins that run parallel to its outer surface. These veins supply the sinusoids of the adenohypophysis. The capillaries (sinusoids) of the adenohypophysis form the **secondary blood capillary network** (*rete hemocapillare secundus*). The veins that connect these two capillary networks are the **hypophyseal portal vessels** (*venulae portis hypophysis*), meaning the *gateway vessels* to the adenohypophysis. This portal circulation in the dog is less obvious than in some other species owing to the relatively short infundibulum in the dog. Green (1966) and Bergland

and Page (1979) suggest a less direct influence of the circulation.

From the caudal rim of the mantle plexus a few arterioles pass directly to the neurohypophysis at its distal extremity. In this region the adenohypophysis does not completely invest the neural lobe. At this position these arterioles, termed the **caudal hypophyseal arteries**, enter the parenchyma of the neural lobe and distribute as capillaries. A few small branches may pass to the pars distalis adenohypophysis.

The pars tuberalis adenohypophysis receives its blood supply from the hypophyseal portal vessels and sinusoids of the pars distalis adenohypophysis; the latter also receives its supply from the portal vessels. The pars intermedia adenohypophysis lacks an intraepithelial vascular network. Instead, the epithelial cells rest on a basement membrane in close proximity to capillaries, the *rete intermedius,* in the stromal tissues coursing between the pars intermedia adenohypophysis and the neural lobe.

The neurohypophysis receives a blood vascular supply from the rostral hypophyseal arteries supplying the tuber cinereum and the infundibulum. The neural lobe also receives some small number of caudal hypophyseal arteries. Unlike in the adenohypophysis, within the neural tissue there are profiles of arterioles and a few muscular arteries.

Regulation of the adenohypophysis by the hypothalamus is made possible by the architecture of the portal system. Structural and functional data suggest that blood entering the hypophysis from these multiple sources will eventually percolate through the sinusoids of the pars distalis adenohypophysis. From these sinusoids venous drainage is by way of vessels that exit from the gland parenchyma to empty into the cavernous and intercavernous sinuses (Dandy & Goetsch, 1910; Flerko, 1980; Green, 1951; 1966; Morato, 1939).

Innervation

Parenchyma of the neurohypophysis is primarily composed of axons extending from cell bodies in the hypothalamic regions (Dandy, 1913; Watkins, 1975). The majority of these cell bodies are located in the supraoptic and paraventricular nuclei and, to a lesser degree, in other hypothalamic regions (Green, 1951). These axons extend into the neural lobe in the supraopticohypophyseal and paraventriculohypophysial tracts. The unmyelinated axons transport, store, and release neurosecretory product. The nerve supply to the hypophysis passes primarily to the neurohypophysis. Sympathetic axons arising from the cranial cervical ganglion pass by way of the tunica externa of the internal carotid artery and its branches to the vessels of the hypophysis (Dandy, 1913; Green, 1951; Truscott, 1944). A parasympathetic innervation has not been described. The results of ablation experiments suggest that hormonal output from the adenohypophysis is not under direct autonomic control. Yamada et al. (1956) and Green (1966) review the literature on innervation to portions of the adenohypophysis. Castel et al. (1984) provide a comprehensive review of neurosecretory systems and of the neurohypophyseal tracts, specifically.

Thyroid Gland

Thyroid tissue in most dogs forms paired structures, each gland, *glandula thyroidea,* is also referred to as a *lobe*. Each lobe is an elongated, dark red mass attached to the external surface of the proximal portion of the trachea (Fig. 10.4). Lobes are positioned laterally and somewhat ventrally on the trachea, spanning the initial five to eight tracheal rings on its respective side. The size of the thyroid is variable, depending on breed and individual (Marine, 1907; Stockard, 1941). In the adult of the medium-sized breeds, the fresh gland is approximately 5 cm in length, 1.5 cm in width, and 0.5 cm in thickness, with the dorsal margin of the gland being somewhat thicker than its ventral counterpart.

The thyroid is the largest of the ductless endocrine glands, performing only an endocrine function. By virtue of its size and position, the thyroid is unique among the exclusively endocrine organs in that it can be palpated during a physical examination, especially when enlarged. The mass of the fresh gland of the adult is quite variable. Data comparing the thyroid mass to body mass revealed a ratio of approximately 0.1 g thyroid per kg body mass (Gilmore et al., 1940; Mulligan & Francis, 1951).

Thyroids exert major control of metabolic processes of the body and affect most body systems. The thyroid hormone is synthesized by the glandular parenchyma, stored intercellularly in a follicle, resorbed by the parenchymal cell, and released from the gland into circulation. Foster et al. (1964a, b) demonstrated the presence of a second hormone produced by the thyroid called *thyrocalcitonin,* or *calcitonin,* which lowers blood calcium by stimulating calcium uptake by the bony skeleton.

Macroscopic Features

Each gland is embedded in the deep cervical fascia and is closely adherent to the trachea (Fig. 10.4). The sternocephalicus muscle passes immediately lateral to the convex surface of each gland, and the sternothyroideus covers each thyroid on its ventral surface.

The cranial pole of the right thyroid lobe lies at the level of the caudal border of the cricoid cartilage of the larynx. Caudally it extends to the region of the fifth tracheal ring. It is bounded dorsolaterally by the carotid sheath containing the common carotid artery, the internal jugular vein, the tracheal duct, and the vagosympathetic trunk. Axons of the recurrent laryngeal nerve pass cranially, in close association with the right thyroid lobe. The stroma of the thyroid is continuous with and tightly bound within the pretracheal lamina of the cervical fascia and blends with the fascia of the carotid sheath.

The left thyroid lobe is generally indistinguishable from its counterpart in size and shape. It does differ in positional relationships, being further caudal, extending from the third through the eighth tracheal rings. Its dorsolateral boundary is formed by the esophagus. The caudal laryngeal nerve passes dorsal to the gland, and the trachea provides its medial boundary. The components of the carotid sheath on the left side are displaced by the esophagus and therefore are not in contact with the gland.

Mesoscopic Features

The thyroid gland of the adult has an organization of tissues based primarily upon follicles. The stromal connective tissues are best developed at the dorsal aspect, where many of the main vessels enter and leave the gland. From this dorsal median mass of stroma extend the septa, which incompletely subdivide the gland into lobules. The larger parenchymal follicles can be resolved with only slight magnification.

In some dogs there is a narrow connection between the two lobes. When present, this bridge, *isthmus glandularis*, composed of glandular parenchyma, passes horizontally as a band on the ventral surface of the trachea, connecting the caudoventral aspects of each lobe (Figs. 10.4B and C). The isthmus is more frequently observed in the brachycephalic breeds but can also be found in individuals of most other breeds.

The thyroid glands are intimately related structurally to the parathyroid glands. Each thyroid lobe is typically related to a pair of these endocrine glands. One parathyroid is usually found near the cranial dorsolateral margin of the gland, but the positional relationship of the thyroid and the

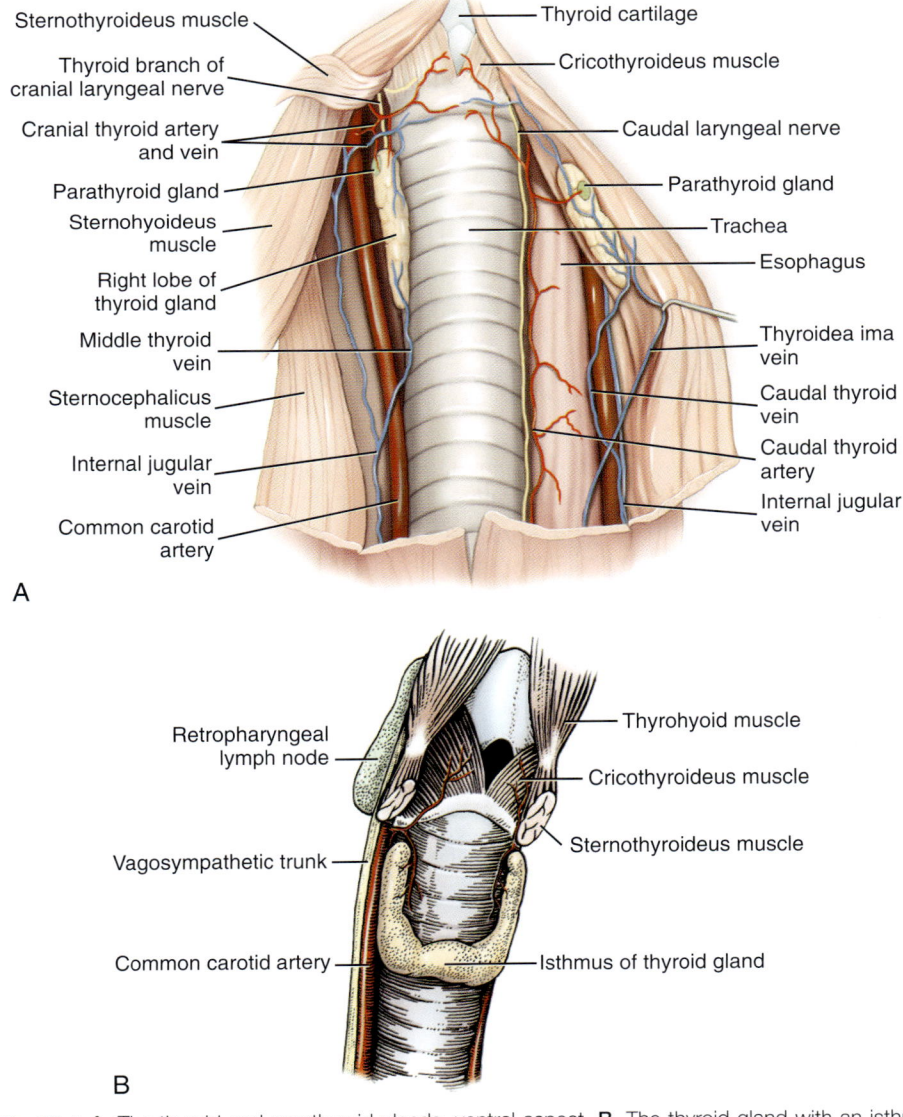

• **Fig. 10.4** A, The thyroid and parathyroid glands, ventral aspect. B, The thyroid gland with an isthmus connecting the lobes. Of infrequent occurrence in the dog. *Continued*

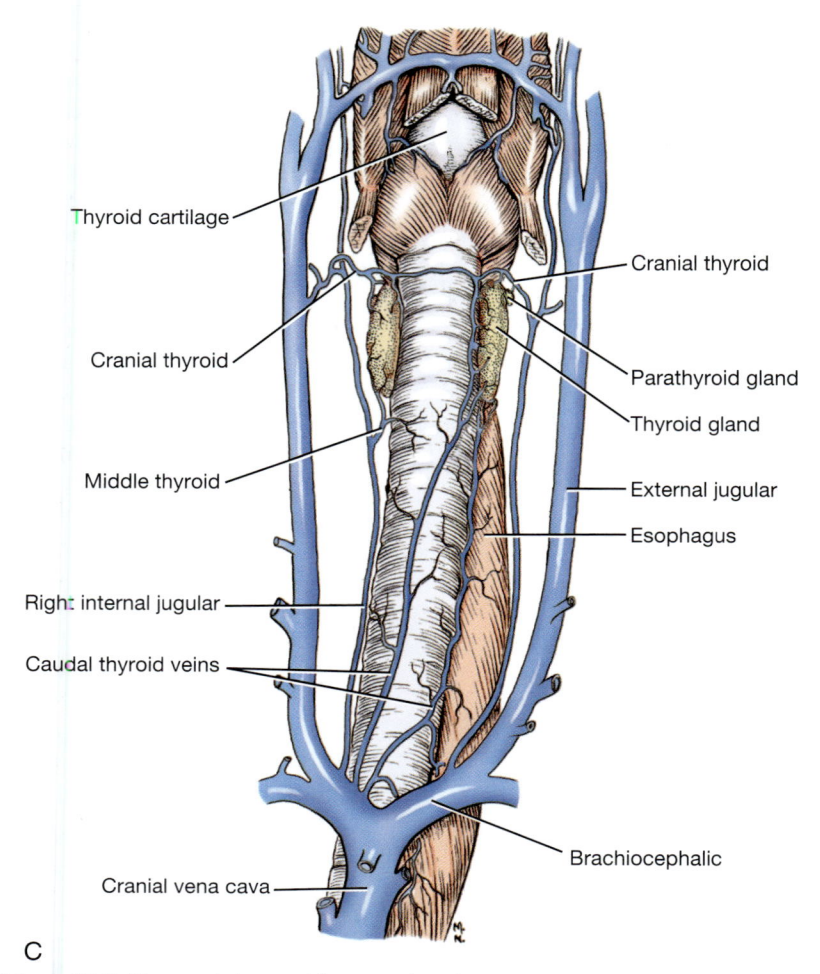

Fig. 10.4, cont'd C, Venous drainage of the ventral neck including the thyroid and parathyroid glands.

cranial parathyroid varies. This parathyroid (*glandula parathyroidea externa [III]*) in some individuals is a satellite only; in others it indents into surface of the thyroid and is enveloped by thyroid fascia, and in others may be embedded within the thyroid parenchyma (Figs. 10.4A and Fig. 10.4C). The second parathyroid (*glandula parathyroidea interna [IV]*) is more often not "para" in position but is embedded within the thyroid at a variable depth, generally in the caudal portion of the gland.

Developmental Anatomy

Parenchyma of the thyroid develops from pharyngeal endoderm. Beginning at the 4-mm stage, the midventral surface of the pharynx gives rise to a thickening and evagination, the **thyroid diverticulum** (Godwin, 1936). Further growth in size occurs predominantly at the distal aspect of the diverticulum, the **thyroglossal duct**. The duct narrows as a stalk before regressing completely. Occasionally, portions of the duct may persists in the subcutaneous fascia as nodules and cysts of functional glandular tissue.

After separating from its attachment to the **pharynx**, the median thyroid diverticulum forms a two lobes connected by a broad isthmus, on the ventral aspect of the trachea. As these thyroid primordia shift caudally with morphogenesis of the head and neck, they pass near the developing pairs of pharyngeal pouches. A dorsal portion of the third and ventral portion of the fourth of the pharyngeal pouch epithelium migrate from the pouches and associate with the adjacent thyroid lobe, eventually differentiating as parathyroid III and IV, respectively (Boyd, 1964; Godwin, 1937a; Latshaw, 1987). Nilsson and Williams (2016) propose that genetic lineage tracing data support endodermal epithelium of ultimobranchial bodies of the fifth pharyngeal pouch merging with the thyroid lobes and giving rise to the parafollicular (calcitonin) cells. The isthmus narrows and, in many cases, remains only as a fibrous band linking the caudal aspect of each gland. The orientation of each gland eventually parallels the trachea. The stroma of the glands develops from the adjacent mesoderm.

An outstanding feature of thyroid development in the dog is frequent occurrence of **accessory thyroid** tissue (*glandula thyroidea accessoria*). Islets of cells of the thyroid primordia may separate from the main mass and become incorporated in developing structures of the neck and thorax. Functional accessory thyroid tissue is frequently found along the trachea, at the thoracic inlet, within the mediastinum, or along the thoracic portion of the descending aorta. Swarts and Thompson (1911) reported accessory thyroid tissue in the pericardial sac of 24 of 30 dogs examined. Halsted (1896), French (1901), Godwin (1936), and Kameda (1972) reported on the occurrence of numerous accessory thyroid tissues in the dog, and Smithcors (1964) reported some accessory tissues in all embryos and nearly one-half of adults examined.

As the main mass of developing thyroid parenchyma extends first ventrocaudally and then laterally, it also incorporates cells that will eventually function to produce calcitonin. According to Nilsson and Williams (2016), the origin of these cells is pharyngeal endoderm of the fifth pharyngeal pouch. These cell groups, **ultimobranchial bodies**, fuse with and become dispersed between the developing thyroid follicles (Godwin, 1937a; Latshaw, 1987). As thyroid development proceeds, these cells occupy positions satellite to or within the epithelium of thyroid follicles (Nonidez, 1932a, b), differentiating to form **parafollicular endocrine cells** (*endocrinocyti parafolliculares*, "C cells"). The developing cords of the thyroid analogue, solid initially, branch and separate forming isolated groupings that differentiate into small follicles prior to birth.

Microscopic Features

The thyroid gland is delineated from adjacent tissues and organs by a delicate *capsula thyroideae*. Septa and trabeculae, conveying arteries, veins, and lymphatic vessels, subdivide each gland (lobe) into lobules, *lobulae thyroideae*. From this stroma the fine reticular fibers pass to form the interstitium that supports the follicles and conveys an extensive capillary network.

Follicles, *folliculae thyroideae*, are the principal parenchymal units. These spheres vary in size from 50 to 900 μm in diameter. Sectional geometry makes the determination of maximum and minimum diameters difficult (Wissig, 1964). Venzke (1940) reported that, for puppies younger than 3 months of age, follicular diameter varies from 30 to 160 μm. The follicles accumulate a homogeneous mass of glycoprotein termed *colloid*. Each follicle is lined by a simple epithelium, the **follicular endocrine cells** (*endocrinocyti folliculares*) which vary in shape (from high columnar to squamous) from one follicle to another, depending on functional status of the follicle. These cells secrete thyroglobulin (colloid) into the lumen, and, following proteolysis of the colloid, the hormones tetraiodothyronine (thyroxin) and triiodothyronine diffuse from the basolateral surfaces of the cell into the interstitium. The follicular epithelial cell is the most numerous of the parenchymal cells (Nunez et al., 1972).

The *endocrinocytus parafollicularis* (also "C cell" for calcitonin), named for its commonly close position to the follicle, is larger and lighter staining than the follicular endocrine cell (Kameda, 1971, 1973; Vicari, 1937). Roediger (1973) distinguished between "intrafollicular" and "parafollicular" cells. The former being within the lining epithelium of the follicle; the latter are adjacent to it. As demonstrated by Kalina and Pearse (1971), these cells secrete calcitonin (thyrocalcitonin). Parafollicular endocrine cells are commonly seen bordering the follicle, often displacing follicular epithelial cells. They may also occur singly or in groupings between follicles as *endocrinocyti interfolliculares*. Hedhammar et al. (1974) reported that these cells decrease markedly with aging. Teitelbaum et al. (1970) demonstrated follicle profiles of parenchyma composed entirely of the "C cells."

Vascularization

The principal vascular supply arises from two vessels: the **cranial** and **caudal thyroid arteries** (*arteria thyroidea cranialis, arteria thyroidea caudalis*). The cranial thyroid artery commonly arises from the common carotid at the caudal aspect of the larynx. This artery terminates in branches supplying the larynx and associated structures and supplies a major vessel to the thyroid. As it approaches the cranial pole of the thyroid, it passes parallel to the dorsal surface of the gland to anastomose with the caudal thyroid artery. The caudal thyroid artery has a variable origin but most commonly arises from the brachiocephalic trunk by a common trunk with the opposite vessel and courses along the lateral surface of the trachea on both sides to join with the respective cranial thyroid artery. In other dogs it arises from the caudal portion of the common carotid (Fig. 10.4A,B).

From the vessel formed by anastomosis of the thyroid arteries dorsal to each gland/lobe arise vessels in various numbers and patterns that approach the dorsal surface. Some smaller vessels may pass to the ventral aspect of the gland. These branches, both dorsal and ventral, bifurcate before entering the gland and supply the lateral and medial surfaces. From this branching of the cranial thyroid artery a small vessel continues directly to the cranial parathyroid.

At the surface of the gland and within the delicate capsule these vessels anastomose freely across the surface to form a blood vascular network (*rete arteriosum*) (Major, 1909). Passing via septa and trabeculae into the gland, the distributing arteries possess marked valvelike tunica media tissue, the arterial cushions (Modell, 1933). These vessels subdivide to the capillary level. Each follicle is enveloped by an extensive, fenestrated sinusoidal network, and the tissues between follicles are equally well supplied with these channels (*rete hemocapillare perifolliculare*) (Fujita & Murakami, 1974).

Modell (1933) described arteriovenous anastomoses within the gland and noted large and small vessels he hypothesized shunted blood past parenchyma, indirectly regulating secretion from the gland. Venous output is via venules and veins that generally parallel the arterial system. Numerous valves are reported in the veins of the thyroid (Modell, 1933). Venous flow from the thyroid is primarily from **cranial and caudal thyroid veins** (Figs. 10.4C and

12.5), which exit from the respective poles of the gland. At the caudal margin of the larynx the cranial thyroid vein joins the internal jugular vein and, as it passes to the caudal neck region, receives the middle thyroid vein if present. The caudal thyroid vein is unpaired, passes caudally on the ventral surface of the trachea, and enters the brachiocephalic vein. Smithcors (1964) reported many cases of an unpaired vessel near the midline of the trachea receiving a large tributary from the middle segment of the left thyroid and passing to enter the brachiocephalic vein.

Satellite to the follicles and from within the interfollicular region arise numerous lymphatic capillaries (*plexus lymphocapillaris perifollicularis.*) These beginnings as dilated cul-de-sacs have been reported by Rienhoff (1938), who called them *bursella*. He observed that each follicle was only partially enveloped by these endothelial capillaries. The lymphatic vessels do not pass as closely to the follicles as do the blood sinusoids. They merge and flow as larger vessels toward the surface of the gland. In the septa these lymphatic vessels become quite large and run parallel to the blood vessels. Valves are numerous in these thin-walled channels (Baber, 1877). At the surface and beneath the capsule they join a lymphatic plexus. Rienhoff (1938) demonstrated large lymphatic trunks draining the cranial aspect of the gland toward the cranial deep cervical lymph node. He suggested that in 10% of cases a collateral circulation of lymph may occur via lymphatics communicating between glands at a point corresponding to the location of the isthmus. Lymphatics draining the caudal aspect of the gland pass to the caudal deep cervical lymph nodes. Mahorner et al. (1927) described these draining lymphatics and veins of the caudal aspect of the neck. In the majority of cases efferents are ultimately drained on the right side by the right lymphatic duct and on the left by the left tracheal duct (see Fig. 13.8).

Innervation

Innervation to the thyroid is via the **cranial laryngeal nerve**, joined by postganglionic sympathetic axons from the cranial cervical ganglion. This nerve runs in close association with the cranial thyroid artery (Nonidez, 1931; Ross & Moorhouse, 1938). Sympathetic postganglionic axons are distributed as a plexus in the adventitia of the interfollicular blood vessels (Mikhail, 1971). Ganglionic cells in the interfollicular space suggest the presence of a preganglionic parasympathetic supply. It has been proposed that both types of autonomics might regulate secretion by controlling the rate of blood flow to major portions or to the gland (Cunliffe, 1961; Nonidez, 1935). Other axons may pass to the gland from the middle cervical ganglion via the perivascular plexuses. Terminal endings have not been demonstrated in association with the follicles. Prolonged stimulation of the cranial laryngeal nerve or denervation via transplantation of the thyroid does not produce secretory or histologic change in the follicular parenchyma (Mason et al., 1930; Ross and Moorhouse, 1938).

Parathyroid Glands

The **parathyroid glands** (*glandulae parathyroideae*), which are closely related to the thyroid and parathyroid tissue, are generally circumscribed, occurring as small ellipsoid discs, measuring 2 to 5 mm in diameter and 0.5 to 1 mm in thickness. Mulligan and Francis (1951) were unable to demonstrate a correlation between body weight and parathyroid weight. As a result of an extensive blood supply and small, compact parenchymal cells that do not store significant amounts of precursors or products, the glands have a purplish coloration.

As noted in the preceding discussion of the thyroid, parathyroids usually occur as four structurally independent glands in close association with the thyroid—one applied to the surface and one embedded within each lobe. The Greek term *parathyroid*, meaning "applied to the shield," applies only for parathyroid III, which is normally found on the cranial dorsolateral surface of the respective thyroid. Parathyroid gland III is referred to as the **external parathyroid** (*glandula parathyroidea externs - III*) because of its most common location on the surface of the gland, deep to the capsule. Parathyroid gland IV is embedded within the thyroid at various depths, most often within the caudal portion of each gland and is referred to as the **internal parathyroid gland** (*glandula parathyroidea interna - IV*). Those that are beside the thyroid can be visualized readily. Those deeply embedded within the thyroid can be seen upon fresh dissection.

Like the hypophysis and adrenal gland, this composite of thyroid and parathyroid brings together tissues of different functions and different origins. Mulligan and Francis (1951) reported frequent variations in the relationship of thyroid and parathyroids and in the number and distribution of parathyroids. Liles et al. (2010) studied 10 dog cadavers using ultrasound and histopathology and found that two dogs had extra parathyroids on one or the other side, and three of the 10 dogs had less than two parathyroids on each side. They noted this variation and concluded that there are several structures and ultrasound artifacts that can be incorrectly identified as parathyroids using only ultrasonography. The parathyroids produce parathyroid hormone, which acts to mobilize body stores of calcium from bone, increase kidney tubule resorption of calcium, and enhance calcium absorption from the intestine.

Mesoscopic Features

The position of parathyroid bodies is generally in close relation to the thyroid (see Fig. 10.4). Consequently, removal of the thyroid without regard for the preservation of the parathyroid and its support tissues is fatal for the dog owing to the precipitous loss of blood calcium. The external parathyroid gland is most frequently located at the cranial dorsolateral edge of the thyroid, occupying a shallow indentation in this gland. The profile and curvature of the thyroid gland is generally unaltered by the presence of the parathyroid.

The internal parathyroid is frequently found embedded within the caudal portion of the thyroid (Vicari, 1937) but has been reported with greatest frequency on the dorsolateral surface (Godwin, 1937b).

Developmental Anatomy

The four most commonly occurring parathyroids are named parathyroid III and IV, indicating the external and internal glands, respectively. This number designation refers to their pharyngeal pouch origin. At approximately the 7-mm stage in the dog embryo there is a proliferation of cells on the dorsorostral aspect of the third pharyngeal pouch. This budding of pharyngeal endoderm gives rise to a short projection of cells that invades the branchial mesenchyme. From a similar location on the fourth pharyngeal pouch there develops a second evagination of endoderm. At first the growth is as a solid cord of cells followed by a hollowing out to form a duct, as in the case of an exocrine duct development. With differential growth of the branchial region, these connections are lost, and the remaining islets of endoderm associate with the developing thyroid endoderm. Cells from pouch III associate with the cranial pole of the thyroid, and those from pouch IV become associated with and frequently embedded within the caudal portion of the developing thyroid (Godwin, 1937b).

Microscopic Anatomy

The parenchyma of the parathyroid gland is arranged as an anastomosing reticulum of epithelioid cell types. In two dimensions these cells are arranged in coils or glomeruli. The cells have little cytoplasm and thus are compactly arranged. Syncytial cells are occasionally present (Meuten et al., 1984). Numerous sinusoids separate the parenchyma into racemi and provide secretory channels (Bensley, 1947; Godwin, 1937a; Vicari, 1938; Wild & Manser, 1980).

A delicate stroma of collagenous connective tissues envelops the gland as a capsule (*capsula parathyroideae*) and from this project trabeculae carrying vascular and nervous tissues into the gland. The parenchymal cells (*endocrinocyti parathyroidea*) are supported by fine reticular fibers, which are barely visible in a routine preparation. Bergdahl and Boquist (1973) describe light, dark, and oxyphilic parenchymal cells in the glands of both young and adult dogs.

Accessory parathyroid tissue (*glandula parathyroidea accessoria*) was reported by Marine (1914). Following parathyroidectomy 5% to 6% of the dogs did not show signs of tetany, and Marine attributed his observations to the presence of accessory parathyroid tissue. In similar studies, Reed et al. (1928) concluded that the incidence of accessory parathyroid tissue was only approximately 3%. Routine serial sections of the thyroid frequently reveal accessory parathyroids (Godwin, 1937a). Such accessory tissues may also migrate caudally into the thorax with the thymus (Godwin, 1937b; Mulligan & Francis, 1951).

Vascularization and Innervation

The blood supply to the parathyroids is directly related to that of the thyroid. The external parathyroid receives its vascular supply by one or more small branches that are direct continuations of the cranial thyroid artery. The internal parathyroid receives its supply from vessels of the adjacent thyroid parenchyma. In the peripheral stroma there are small arteriolar networks that supply the sinusoids, which in turn perfuse the parenchyma.

Venous and lymphatic drainage of these small glands is accomplished by the corresponding structures in the thyroid. The innervation to the parathyroid is likewise related to that of the thyroid. Mikhail (1971) and Atwal (1981) described nerves ending in close association with the parenchymal cells and terminal ganglion cell bodies in the substance of the gland. Yeghiayan et al. (1972) reported a well-developed adrenergic innervation to the blood vessels of the parathyroid.

Pineal Gland

The **pineal gland** (*glandula pinealis*), formerly *epiphysis,* is an unpaired, cream-colored, wedge-shaped, small excrescence on the dorsal midline surface of the diencephalon (Figs. 10.5, 18.4, and 18.22) where it is part of the epithalamus.

Mesoscopic Features

The pineal gland forms the caudal boundary demarcation of the roof of the third ventricle. The polyp-like growth extends into the potential space between the cerebellum caudally and the approximation of the two cerebral hemispheres dorsally and laterally. Its size in the dog, approximately 3 by 1.5 by 1 mm, requires that one intending to observe the gland use care to preserve this organ in these

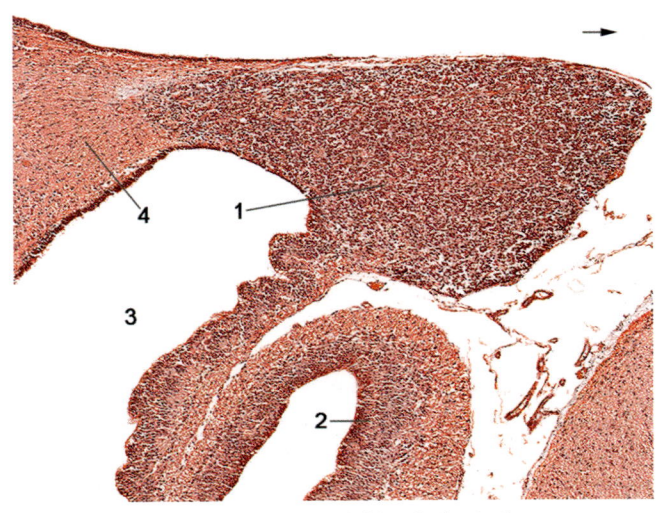

1. Pineal gland
2. Commissura caudalis
3. Ventriculus tertius
4. Commissura habenularum

• **Fig. 10.5** Mesoscopic features of adult pineal gland, sagittal section. (Pentachromic staining, 15×.)

relationships (Ellsworth et al., 1985; Oksche, 1965; Venzke & Gilmore, 1940; Zach, 1960).

The antigonadotrophic influences of the pineal gland have been established by observation of precocious sexual development subsequent to tumor formation in the pineal, reducing the functional parenchyma, or following pinealectomy. Research into the function of the pineal explores its role as a photoreceptor-photointegrator of the endocrine system and its relationship to the sympathetic nervous system (Wurtman & Cardinali, 1974).

Developmental Anatomy

Except for a small amount of stroma derived from mesoderm, the pineal develops from neural ectoderm. In the developing pineal, the ependymal layer proliferates, forming an expanded mantle layer. This focal proliferation just dorsal to the caudal commissure forms the parenchyma of the pineal. The pial investment is at first an encapsulation, but, with continued growth, the parenchyma becomes folded and the gland is subdivided by septa. Primary support for the parenchyma is provided by the glial cell population. The gland is small at birth, even difficult to observe. Postnatal growth and differentiation continues until sexual maturation, when growth subsides and the gland begins a slow regression. In older dogs there may occasionally appear intercellular concretions termed "brain sand" (*acervulus cerebri*).

Microscopic Anatomy

Parenchyma of the pineal gland is composed of pinealocytes (endocrinocytus pinealis), which are large acidophilic epithelioid cells, and astrocytes (gliocytus centralis), which compose the neuropil. The pia mater provides an outer limit of the gland, and small amounts of connective tissues extend from the periphery as a delicate capsule, septa, and trabeculae. Through these stromal structures course the blood vessels with accompanying postganglionic sympathetic axons.

Vascularization and Innervation

The blood vascular supply arises from the pia, providing the septa and trabeculae and numerous arterioles. These vessels penetrate into the parenchyma, forming sinusoids that are fenestrated as in the hypophysis. A lymphatic drainage for this organ has not been described.

The innervation of the pineal is of principal importance. The efferent axons are of postganglionic sympathetics, having their origin at the **cranial cervical ganglion**. These axons enter the adventitia of the internal carotid arteries and follow its branches to the pineal. Hartmann (1957) and Zach (1960) described axons of cerebral origin that enter the pineal from the habenular commissure but, for the most part, return to the habenular commissure without synapsing on endocrine cells of the pineal. Calvo et al. (1988) describe the electron microcopy of the pineal. An occasional neuron cell body can be seen within the parenchyma. Ariëns-Kappers (1965) has presented evidence for a contact termination of sympathetic axons on the pinealocytes.

Adrenal Gland

The **adrenal gland** (*glandula suprarenalis*) is composed of two structurally and functionally different tissues that have unique developmental histories. Each adrenal gland is composed of an outer cortex and an inner medulla. Each adrenal gland is located near the craniomedial border of the kidney. In man the topographic relationship of the adrenal gland in the standing position led to the use of the term "suprarenal gland" for humans and other primates. The sixth edition of *Nomina Anatomica* retains *glandula adrenalis* as an alternate term.

The adrenal cortex is a major steroid-producing organ, the secretions of which are essential for regulating mineral balance via normal kidney function and augmenting carbohydrate metabolism. The adrenal cortex is essential for the maintenance of life. Together with the nervous system, the adrenal medulla augments the general adaptation of the body to stress. The cortex and medulla combine to markedly influence the organism's response to both acute and chronic stress.

Macroscopic Features

The left adrenal gland is the larger of the two glands (Fig. 10.6). Its cranial aspect is somewhat flattened dorsoventrally and oval in outline; its caudal projection is cylindrical. The right adrenal gland is triangular in transverse profile with an acute angular bend, its vortex projecting cranially. Positioned near the kidney, its longer segment projects caudally along the caudal vena cava, and the shorter segment projects toward the cranial pole of the right kidney. This left adrenal gland, lying ventral to the transverse process of the second lumbar vertebra, is not as cranial in position as the right, which lies ventral to the transverse process of the last thoracic vertebra. Baker (1936) reported that adult males of mixed breeds have adrenal tissue mass of approximately 1.14 g. The female in diestrus has glandular tissue mass of approximately 1.24 g. This slight difference in mass is not statistically significant.

The left adrenal gland is retroperitoneally positioned near the craniomedial border of the left kidney. This adrenal gland is bound in the loose collagenous connective tissue of the fascia. Thus, it is more structurally related by position to the abdominal aorta than to the left kidney. Its dorsal border is applied closely to the body of the psoas minor muscle and the transverse process of the second lumbar vertebra. Medially it is bounded by the abdominal aorta at a position just caudal to the origin of the cranial mesenteric artery and adjacent to the origin of the common trunk for the caudal phrenic and cranial abdominal arteries. This latter vessel courses over its dorsal surface at the midpoint of the gland. The caudal border of the left adrenal gland is

CHAPTER 10 The Endocrine System   483

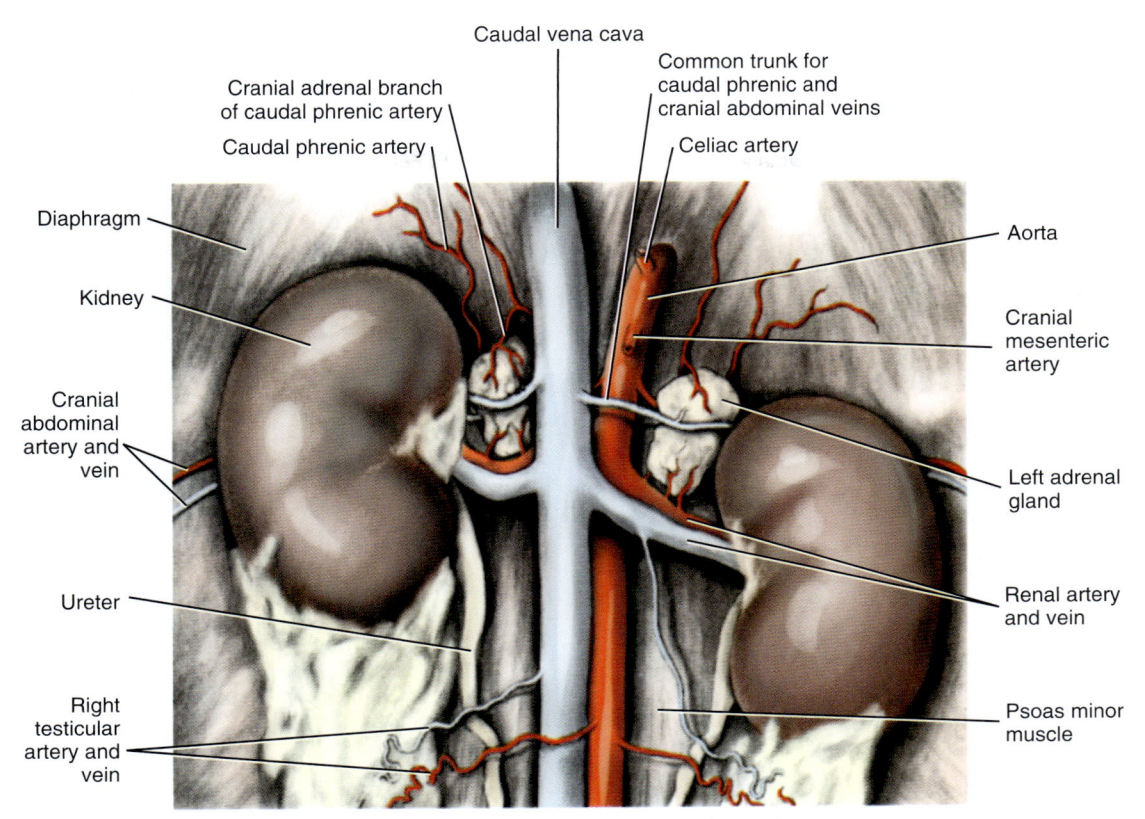

• **Fig. 10.6** The adrenal glands, ventral aspect.

formed by the renal artery and vein. Its ventral surface is bisected by the common venous trunk accompanying the above artery and is covered to varying degrees by the spleen. Laterally its boundary is formed by the kidney.

The right adrenal gland is also retroperitoneal, but it lies near the hilus of the right kidney. Its firm connective tissue attachments bring it into close proximity with the caudal vena cava at its immediate medial boundary. Often, the capsule of the right adrenal gland is continuous with the tunica externa/adventitia of the caudal vena cava. This presents a special challenge for surgical removal of the right gland when indicated. The psoas minor and the crus of the diaphragm form its dorsal border. The right common trunk for the caudal phrenic and cranial abdominal arteries crosses its dorsal surface, and the mass of the right kidney covers this adrenal gland on the ventrolateral surface. As a result of these organ relationships, this gland presents a triangular or wedge shape in transverse profile. Its ventral surface is bisected by the common venous trunk accompanying the cranial abdominal artery, and the cranial two-thirds of this adrenal gland is covered by the caudal extension of the right lateral hepatic lobe of the liver. Both adrenals lie within retroperitoneal fat.

The adrenal cortex usually completely invests the adrenal medulla. The medulla comes closest to the outer surface at the hilus of each gland. Subtle and easily overlooked, the hilus is located near the midpoint of the medial surface and serves as the exit point for the adrenal vein or veins; no artery enters at the hilus.

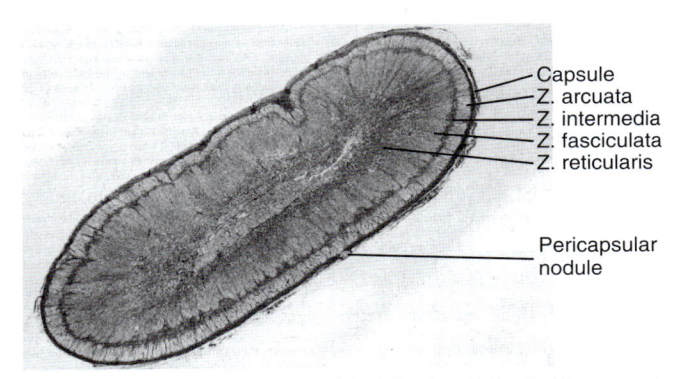

• **Fig. 10.7** Mesoscopic features of the left adrenal gland of the normal, mature dog. Two-year-old female Beagle, transverse section. (Mallory's triple staining, 15×.)

As with the hypophysis, the major subdivisions of the adrenal cortical parenchyma can be resolved with the unaided eye (Figs. 10.7 and 10.8). In a fresh preparation, the cortex is white or faintly yellow owing to the relative amount of lipid storage in the cortical parenchyma; the medulla is dark brown or black.

Developmental Anatomy

The adrenal cortex and adrenal medulla have different developmental origins. The cortex is the first to develop, originating from mesenchymal cells of the celomic mesoderm. The initial mass of these mesodermal cells proliferates

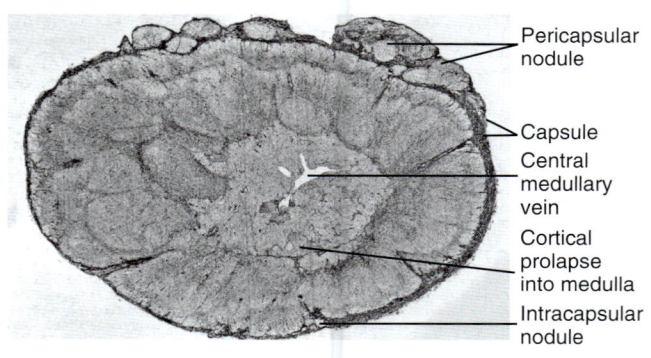

• **Fig. 10.8** Mesoscopic features of the left adrenal gland of the normal, aging dog. Twelve-year-old female Corgi, transverse section. (Mallory's triple staining, 15×.)

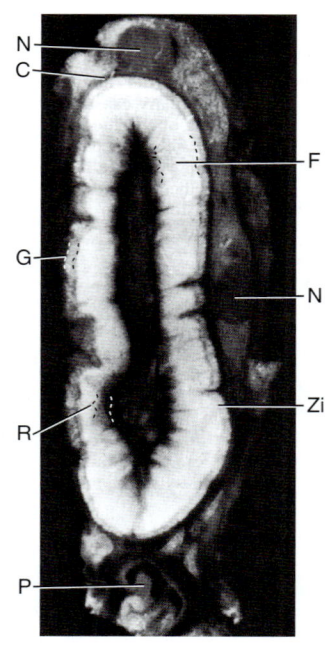

• **Fig. 10.9** Mesoscopic features of the right adrenal gland of a 1-year-old female Beagle, transverse section, 5-mm thick, unstained, magnified 25×. Structures indicated include capsula fibrosa (C), zona arcuata (G), zona fasciculata (F), zona reticularis (R), zona intermedia (Zi), sympathetic ganglion (N), caudal vena cava (P). (From Hullinger RL: Adrenal cortex of the dog [*Canis familiaris*]: I. Histomorphologic changes during growth, maturity, and aging, *Zbl Vet Med C Anat Histol Embryol* 7:1–27, 1978.)

near the genital ridge and accumulates to form an elongate, spherical group of cells termed the **fetal cortex**. Soon a second migration of mesenchyme begins, eventually envelops the fetal cortex, and differentiates to form the permanent or **adult cortex** while the fetal cortex regresses. The medullary parenchyma arises from trunk neural crest cells, which migrate into the developing mesodermal mass, penetrate into this mesenchyme, and assume a central position characteristic of the adrenal medulla of the adult. The adrenal medulla is functionally a sympathetic ganglion, and it develops by a process similar to that of the ganglia of the sympathetic trunk. Numerous ganglionic cells can be seen in the medulla at birth, but their number decreases with age. This migration of ectodermal cells of the neural crest is not completed until after birth, and often, even in the adult, islets of medullary tissue can be found intermixed within the cortical parenchyma, within the capsule, or as satellite structures of the adrenal glands (Appleby & Sohrabi-Haghdoost, 1980; Hullinger, 1978; Saleh et al., 1974).

The **adrenal capsule** (*capsula adrenalis*) develops as a condensation of mesenchyme at the periphery of the cortex. The outer portion, *pars fibrosa*, becomes a fibrous supportive stroma. The inner portion of the capsule at birth and in the young remains quite cellular and during that period is termed the *pars cellulosa*. Until the development in the perinatal period, of the outer cortical zone, the *zona arcuata*, this inner cellular layer of the adrenal capsule serves as the stem cell population for the generation of additional adrenal cortical parenchyma (Hullinger, 1978).

Masses of neural cells develop elsewhere in the abdomen as sympathetic ganglia. These so-called paraganglia and the adrenal medulla react histochemically to reduce salts of chromium and other heavy metals and, because of that property, are called *chromaffin tissues*.

Adrenal cortical tissue also occurs randomly as accessory aggregates, satellite to or incorporated within various abdominal organs. Those aggregates associated with the gland occur as nodules, owing to compensatory hyperplasia and they increase in size and number with advancing age.

Mesoscopic Features

The mesoscopic organization of the adrenal gland is based on concentric lamellae of cortical parenchyma enveloping a central medulla (Figs. 10.7 to 10.9). The medulla, or heart of the gland, is separated from the cortex by a delicate network of reticular and loose collagenous connective tissues, the *septum corticomedullae*. Like the cortex, the parenchyma of the medulla can be partitioned into zones according to cellular or tissue morphology. The innermost cortical layer is applied to all surfaces of the undulating medullary contour. The parenchyma of this inner zone is disposed in a relatively random and loose network and is termed the *zona reticularis*. In most dogs this zone composes the innermost 25% of the cortex. Upon examination with the unaided eye, the zona reticularis appears the darker zone of the cortex. This appearance is due to the relatively greater numbers and size of the sinusoids in the parenchyma of this zone and a correspondingly lesser amount of lipid storage in the cytoplasm of these cells.

The next cortical zone, moving inner to outer cortex, is the largest. It typically composes 50% or more of the cortex. This *zona fasciculata* is so named because of its appearance in two dimensions. In three dimensions it is composed of anastomosing plates (*muralia*) of cells that radiate toward the periphery (Elias & Pauly, 1956). This zone appears white to yellow in a fresh specimen. Parenchymal cells of the outer one-third of this zona fasciculata store more lipid and are somewhat larger than those of the inner two-thirds. These regions are called *pars externa* and *pars interna*, respectively.

A narrow *zona intermedia corticalis* is at the outer surface of the zona fasciculata. This small, dark-appearing region composes less than 5% of the total cortex and, in the dog, functions as a blastemic region for replacement cells of the zonae arcuate and fasciculata (Hullinger, 1978; Hullinger & Getty, 1971; Nussdorfer, 1986).

The outermost cortical zone is the *zona arcuata*. This zone, constituting approximately 25% of the adrenal cortex, is composed of cells arranged in arches nestled into a stromal template provided by the inner surface of the capsule.

Microscopic Features

A cursory view of the microscopic features of this endocrine organ suggests a homogeneity of component cell types (*endocrinocyti corticales* and *endocrinocyti medullares*) and the extensive vascularity (*rete hemocapillare sinusoideum*).

The stroma of the adrenal gland, *stroma glandulae adrenalis,* varies considerably in amount and kind. It ranges from the thick fibrous capsule found in the aged adult to the fine reticular support fibers of the parenchymal cells in the medulla. When compared with other endocrine organs, the capsule of the adrenal gland is especially prominent. In the adult it is composed, for the most part, of dense, irregular collagenous connective tissue with some scattered elastic fibers. Smooth muscle fibers found in some other species have not been demonstrated in the dog's adrenal capsule (Bloodworth & Powers, 1968). On the capsular surface the fibrous portion is continuous with the fascia and periadrenal adipose tissue. Its inner aspect is extended as septa and a few trabeculae into the cortical parenchyma. These septa become confluent and, as thin walls or sheets, envelop the parenchyma of the zona arcuata. At the inner margins of the zona arcuata these stromal elements send delicate fibrous branches laterally compartmentalize the zona arcuata. From this connective tissue boundary that has formed within the zona intermedia, trabeculae and numerous fine reticular fibers project into the inner aspects of the adrenal cortex. Coursing through the parenchyma of the zonae fasciculata and reticularis, these fibers provide support for the cortical parenchymal cells and the network of sinusoids. Most fibers terminate at the corticomedullary boundary and become a part of the moderate connective tissue investment of the medulla. In comparison with the cortex, the medulla contains only moderate amounts of connective tissue as reticular fibers for support of the parenchyma and vascular channels. The stroma increases in amount with age.

The zona arcuata is composed of vermiform whorls of columnar epithelioid cells that, to a degree, resemble the arrangement of columnar cells on the villi of the small intestine. The structural differentiation of this zone occurs for the most part after birth. The cellular groupings are initially in coils or glomeruli, as in the *zona glomerulosa* of other species, but by 6 weeks of age most dogs have adrenal cortices with distinct zona arcuata morphologic features. These columnar epithelial cells are oriented as a simple or a pseudostratified epithelium as if they composed an epithelium on a free surface. Thus it is likely that two surfaces or poles of these cells may bound a loose collagenous connective tissue rich in sinusoids. The nucleus is centrally located, and neutral lipids and cholesterol precursors for steroidogenesis are stored in large quantities toward the poles of the cell. These cells produce the mineralocorticoids essential for the regulation of electrolyte balance and of life.

Cells of the zona intermedia appear between the parenchyma of the zona arcuata and zona fasciculata (Figs. 10.7 and 10.9). These are observed as small, polygonal cells with only small amounts of cytoplasm. There is little cytoplasmic lipid stored in these cells, and the nuclei suggest that the cells are still undifferentiated. The cells appear to be compressed tightly into the network of collagenous and reticular fibers found here at the junction of the two major cortical zones that bound it. Its location and cytologic appearance have led others to refer to this zone as the *zone of compression, zone of transition,* and *intermediate zone.* The cells of this zone are not prominent in most other species. Hullinger (1968) and Hullinger and Getty (1971) hypothesized that these were a blastemic population of cells developing as the zona arcuata forms and that this cell group is, in effect, a displaced inner cellular layer from the capsule. The cells of this zone are continuous with those of the zona arcuata and zona fasciculata, and there is not a sharp morphologic boundary separating these zones. In acute adrenal cortical failure, the entire adrenal cortex can regenerate from the zona intermedia (Hullinger et al., 1983).

The cells of the zona fasciculata are polygonal, arranged in plates, forming a *murus complexus,* as shown by Elias and Pauly (1956), that radiates from the zona reticularis. These plates or walls compose anastomosing networks of labyrinths that are separated by an equally complex system of sinusoids and delicate reticular connective tissue. The functional parenchymal units of this zone communicate via the intercellular space with a sinusoid on multiple surfaces. Histochemical staining affinities reveal that these cells are rich in neutral fats and cholesterol, in accordance with their functional status. This cell population produces glucocorticoids.

The zona reticularis is composed of cells similar in appearance to those of the zona fasciculata. Their cytoplasm contains a lesser amount of lipid, which in some cells is stored as large droplets. The plates of this zone are direct continuations of the zona fasciculata but differ in that they are quite randomly arranged; the overall arrangement is much looser, and the intervening sinusoids are larger. These cells produce sex steroids.

Sinusoids of the cortex form a continuous network throughout the cortex and provide a venous drainage passing centripetally to the corticomedullary boundary. These sinusoids penetrate the moderate amount of stroma at the corticomedullary capsule to become confluent with the sinusoids of the medulla. The number and specific distribution of these channels have been investigated in an attempt to link these features to functional specificity of the cortical zones. The medullary sinusoids anastomose to form larger venous sinuses.

Endocrine cells of the medullary parenchyma are larger than those of the cortex and are polygonal; those bordering the medullary sinusoids are columnar. Most stain darkly, and a heterogeneity of affinities for dye suggests a functional difference. The occasional ganglionic cell can be found dispersed among the epithelioid parenchyma. The function of the medullary cells is synthesis, storage, and release of the catecholamines epinephrine (columnar cells) and norepinephrine (polygonal cells), which are termed *endocrinocytus lucidus* and *endocrinocytus densus,* respectively. This reference to density describes the known content and numerous stored secretory vesicles stored within the respective cell type.

Vascularization

As with the hypophysis, the blood supply and venous drainage of the adrenal cortex and medulla are structurally and functionally interrelated (Vinson et al., 1985). All blood flowing in the cortex passes into the medulla before leaving the adrenal gland.

The arterial supply of the adrenal gland arises from multiple major vessels (Figs. 10.6, 11.60, and 11.61) (Flint, 1900; Ljubomudrov, 1939). Branches from these vessels to the gland are numerous and of smaller caliber (Fig. 10.10). They include cranial adrenal branches from the caudal phrenic and cranial abdominal arteries or their common trunk, middle adrenal branches from the abdominal aorta, and caudal adrenal branches from the lumbar and renal arteries. These provide 20 to 30 contributing arterioles that approach the gland from all surfaces, enter the fibrous portion of the capsule, and anastomose to form a network (*rete arteriosum capsulare*). Numerous vessels plunge from the capsular network into the cortex. Some of these—according to Flint (1900), approximately 50—pass as small muscular arteries and arterioles in the trabeculae and septa and descend directly to the corticomedullary boundary. Here they supply oxygen-rich blood to the medullary parenchyma. The supply to the sinusoids of the cortex is via small arterioles from the capsular network that pass in the smaller trabeculae and septa that separate the arches of the zona arcuata. These vessels pass to the zona intermedia and form a second network in the connective tissues there (*rete arteriosum subcapsulare*). From this network arise sinusoids of the zona arcuata and the inner zones of the cortex (*rete hemocapillare sinusoideum*).

The sinusoids of the cortex and medulla become confluent, as outlined previously, and join to forming the large medullary sinuses and a *plexus venosus medullae*. These sinuses, which may mediate cortical control of epinephrine synthesis (Pohorecky & Wurtman, 1971), pass toward the hilus of the adrenal gland and are drained via the adrenal vein. Smithcors (1964) described a venous tree in the medulla that is independent of the medullary sinuses and that joins with the sinuses to form the adrenal vein. Arteriovenous anastomoses have been observed in the connective tissues around the adrenal gland (Brondi & Castorina, 1953). The adrenal veins of each gland terminate differently due to their position relative to the caudal vena cava. The right adrenal vein joins directly the caudal vena cava; the left adrenal vein enters the left renal vein.

According to Verhofstad and Lensen (1973), lymphatic vessels in the adrenal gland form extensive plexuses in the capsule, cortex, corticomedullary boundary, and medulla. There is also a well-developed lymphatic plexus surrounding the central vein of the medulla.

Innervation

The innervation of the adrenal cortex has been difficult to demonstrate (Wilkinson, 1961). Saleh et al. (1974) reported multipolar neurons in all regions of the adrenal cortex. They propose a hypothalamic control of cortical secretion by nervous as well as humoral means. The parenchyma of the adrenal medulla is essentially a modified sympathetic ganglion, specialized for neurohumoral release. Axons passing to the medulla travel through the cortex, accompanying the medullary arteries in the major cortical trabeculae and septa. These fibers are, for the most part, preganglionic sympathetic axons that can be traced from the splanchnic supply through the celiac, splanchnic, and adrenal ganglia (Fig. 10.10). The medullary cells are the modified neuronal cell bodies of postganglionic axons, but lacking axons. These cells release their neurotransmitters directly into the perivascular space; the neurotransmitters are distributed systemically to bind receptors.

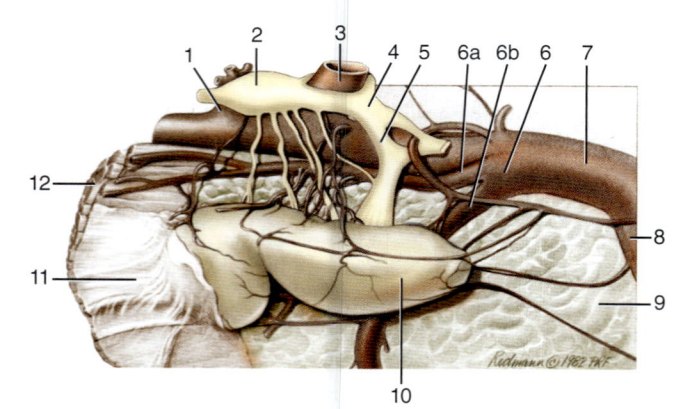

1. Celiac artery
2. Celiac ganglion
3. Cranial mesenteric a.
4. Cranial mesenteric *ganglion*
5. Splanchnic ganglion
6. Common trunk
   a. Caudal phrenic
   b. Cranial abdominal a
7. Aorta
8. Renal a
9. Perirenal fat
10. Adrenal gland
11. Peritoneum
12. Crus of diaphragm

• **Fig. 10.10** Blood supply and innervation, right adrenal gland. Adrenal receives multiple arterioles variously from aorta, renal a., phrenic a., and abdominal a.

Pars Endocrina Pancreatis

The endocrine pancreas of the dog has served as the classic model for the exploration of insulin-deficiency diabetes by Banting and Best (1922).

The endocrine pancreas is a composite of thousands of small endocrine racemi (*insulae pancreaticae*) seemingly scattered randomly among the exocrine pancreatic acini. Each racemus is composed of several endocrinocyti of multiple cell types, the normal functioning of which is essential for homeostatic regulation of blood sugar. The endocrine pancreas is essential for maintaining life.

Developmental and Mesoscopic Anatomy

The exocrine and endocrine portions of the pancreas develop from the same epithelial outgrowths of foregut endoderm. Some endodermal cells eventually lose contact with the branching cords of cells that eventually become the exocrine ducts of the pancreas. Cells of these isolated clusters differentiate to form the typical heterogeneous cell population constituting the endocrine islet. This hypothesized origin is supported by much experimental embryology and by clonal proliferation results of oncogenesis studies of endodermal tissues and epithelial regeneration studies of the enteric mucosa (Asa et al., 1980; Hawkins et al., 1987; Peranzi and Lehy, 1984; Sidhu, 1979). More recent studies dissecting the molecular mechanisms of pancreas and islet cell differentiation from pluripotent stem cells show potential for signaling stem cell differentiation toward islet cell phenotypes (Yang et al., 2013; Stanger & Hebrok, 2013; Nostro & Keller, 2012; Soggia et al., 2011; McKnight et al., 2010; Liu & Habener, 2009).

The islets are distributed randomly among the exocrine acini, but there are differences in the cellular components of the endocrine islets. The pancreas develops from a dorsal and ventral pancreatic anlage. These two differing sites of origin may play a determining role in the cytogenesis of the alpha endocrine cell (*endocrinocytus alpha*); Bencosme and Liepa (1955a) reported that the ventral pancreas in the dog, the right lobe, is devoid of alpha endocrine cells. Interestingly, Collombat et al. (2009) provide evidence that murine progenitor cells differentiate into alpha endocrine cells and continue differentiation to beta cells; the former produce glucagon and the latter produce insulin.

The endocrine islets vary in size from approximately 1500 to 20,000 μm^2 and are composed of from 10 to 120 epithelioid cells (Acosta et al., 1969; Saladino & Getty, 1972). Davis et al. (1988) reported dogs have an average volume fraction of endocrine parenchyma of 1.8% but that it varies with regions of the pancreas. The number and size of the islets increase progressively from the right lobe to the left lobe of the pancreas. Perfusion of the pancreas with neutral red allows one to observe without magnification the number and distribution of the larger endocrine islets. The volume of islet tissue in the dog differs significantly between individuals without apparent relation to the volume of pancreas or body weight (Acosta et al., 1969).

Microscopic Features

The endocrine islet is a highly vascularized epithelioid cell parenchyma with small amounts of collagenous and reticular connective tissue fibers separating it from the adjoining exocrine acini. The term *islet* is used rather loosely in describing endocrine cell groups. Acosta et al. (1969) considered 10 endocrine cells as the minimum number composing an islet and suggested that it was also necessary to establish the existence of a separate set of blood capillaries to consider such cell groups as pancreatic endocrine islets. Bordi et al. (1972) and Watanabe et al. (1989) reported that all of the intrainsular cell types can be found singly in extrainsular locations. Hellman et al. (1962) described the islets of the pancreatic body as smaller and possessing a different cellular composition from those in the head of the pancreas.

The endocrine cells in small numbers or in islets can be detected by routine staining procedures, whereby they stain faintly in contrast to the exocrine parenchymal cells. Immunocytochemical methods reveal smaller collections of endocrine cells scattered throughout the exocrine part (Atkins et al., 1988). The principal cells of the islet are the *endocrinocytus alpha* and the *endocrinocytus beta*. The cells are closely positioned and somewhat randomly oriented in each racemus. With routine staining, the alpha cells show a marked cytoplasmic granulation, occur in fewer numbers (approximately 20% of the total), and tend to be positioned more peripherally in the islets. The beta cells have only a delicate granulation, compose nearly 75% of the islet cells, and assume a more central position. A delta cell (Kobayashi & Fujita, 1969) and an "F" cell have also been described as additional endocrine cell types of the endocrine islets in the dog (Munger et al., 1965). These investigators also reported that beta and delta cells were found in islets of all regions of the pancreas. In the body, the alpha cells were lacking, and in their place were "F" cells, called *alpha₁ cells* by Hellman et al. (1962). Munger et al. (1965), Forssmann et al. (1977), and Greider et al. (1978) all have suggested that alpha cells might be further limited to only the tail portion of the left lobe of the pancreas. This segregation of the alpha cell population was first described by Bencosme et al. (1955b) and originally provided an excellent model for study of alpha cell function.

Kobayashi and Fujita (1969) and Smith and Madson (1981) emphasized the large number of axons in contact with the islet cells. They described a complex forming between the endocrine cells of the islet and the axons. Radke and Stach (1986a) concluded that they are not of vagal origin. Shimosegawa et al. (1983) demonstrated extensive innervation of the pancreatic parenchyma, whereas others propose that the neuroinsular complex is, in effect, a modified ganglion (Serizawa et al., 1979). Radke and Stach (1986b) demonstrated a simulations nerve contact of endocrine and exocrine cells and correlated this with the coincident release of secretory products. The principal endocrine cells respond to altered blood sugar levels: the alpha cell reacts to a lowered level by releasing glucagon; the beta cell to an elevated level by releasing insulin.

Enteroendocrine Cells

Intraepithelial endocrine cells occur singly in the epithelial lining of the tunica mucosa of the digestive and respiratory tracts. The basal surface of these *entero-endocrine* cells is in contact with the epithelial basement membrane. The cells are positioned quite closely to the lumen of the digestive tract, and, in the pyloric gland region of the stomach and the duodenal segment of the small intestine, some of these cells have an apical projection reaching the lumen. The distribution of organelles and inclusions in these cells, coupled with experimental evidence, suggests that they are releasing their secretions basally (Kobayashi & Fujita, 1974). Such a morphology indicates that these endocrine cells may directly monitor the external (luminal) environment.

In support of the ectodermal origin is the close neural contacts of the enteroendocrine cells populating the epithelium of the respiratory and gastrointestinal mucosa (Fujita & Kobayashi, 1979; Smith & Madson, 1981); the similar origin and structural relationships to cells within paraganglia generally and adrenal medulla in particular (Shimosegawa et al., 1983); the widespread ability of cells to take up and decarboxylate the precursors of bioamines, thus *amine precursor uptake and decarboxylation* (APUD) applied to many (Pearse, 1977); the similarities of these cells to neurosatellite cells, also of neural crest origin (Serizawa et al., 1979); and several reports of structural characteristics of tumor cells from presumed neural crest derivatives (Morrison, 1984).

Andrew (1974) and Pictet et al. (1976) have presented evidence that the precursors of the enteroendocrine cells are present in the gut before the migration of the neural crest cells.

Cells originally described in the pancreatic endocrine islets have now been observed in the gastric, intestinal, and respiratory mucosal epithelium. Solcia et al. (1970), Forssmann (1970), and Polak et al. (1971) reported alpha endocrine cells in the gastric wall and attributed to them the release of enteroglucagon. Fujita and Kobayashi (1974) considered the delta cell of the gastric and intestinal mucosa to be the gastrin-producing cell, but Sasagawa et al. (1974) concluded that the delta cell produced secretin. Inage (1974) reported that "F" cells of the pancreas (Munger et al., 1965) and a structurally similar enterochromaffin cell (Bencosme & Liepa, 1955a) were different cell types.

Endocrine Tissues of the Ovary

In the ovary the gametogenic exocrine function is initiated and regulated by the ovarian endocrine functions. As a sequel to follicular atresia, especially of the secondary and tertiary follicles, thecal luteal cells of the internal thecal layer remain in the dense cellular connective tissue stroma of the ovary as an interstitial parenchymal cell population. In other species these cells have been called the **interstitial gland** tissue (Guraya, 1973).

Guraya and Greenwald (1964) described clusters and single epithelioid cells widely distributed in the stroma and varying in number and distribution between individuals. These investigators reported some of these cells arose from invaginations of surface epithelial cells and others developed from single cells forming from thecal and stromal tissues of normal and atretic follicles. Stott (1974) suggested that the interstitial gland tissue developed from an isolation of granulosal cells from large atretic follicles. Guraya (1973, 1985) outlined the development of the interstitial gland tissue from the hypertrophy of the theca interna and adjoining stromal tissues of medium-sized and maturing atretic follicles. These generally sparsely distributed cells are believed to produce androgens and small amounts of estrogens and progestins.

With the continued maturation of those follicles, some of which will rupture and discharge ovocytes from the ovary, there is the formation of an **internal thecal** (*theca interna*) **layer** adjacent to the follicle. This inner investment or case is composed of epithelioid cells that have differentiated from the mesenchymally derived stromal support tissues of the ovary. The endocrine cells of the theca (*endocrinocyti thecales*) are somewhat elongated or spindle-shaped and are enveloped by a network of fine reticular fibers. Numerous blood capillaries form a network that permeates this tissue. Using cellular morphologic findings and data from other mammals, one might hypothesize that these theca cells produce androgens that are enzymatically converted by the adjacent follicular cells to estrogens (Guraya, 1985; Hsueh et al., 1984).

After ovulation and the formation of a *corpus hemorrhagicum*, cells of the internal theca and of the follicular epithelium accumulate large amounts of lipid and hypertrophy forming the *corpus luteum*. Those cells arising from the internal theca are called **theca lutein endocrine cells** (*thecaluteocytus*) and those arising from the granulosa cells are called **follicular lutein endocrine cells** (*granulosoluteocytes*) (Abel et al., 1975; Hsueh et al., 1984). Angiogenesis of the capillary network of the theca interna vascularizes the corpus luteum. Balboni (1973) noted that, in endocrine tissues of the ovary, blood capillaries have an attenuated and fenestrated wall, as in the sinusoids of the major endocrine organs. The corpus luteum produces progesterone. It is a transient endocrine structure, the corpus luteum cyclium, recurrent with each estrous cycle (most breeds having two cycles per year, one in the spring and one in the fall) and retained in full functional maturity during the gestation period, the corpus luteum graviditatis.

Fetal Membrane Endocrine Tissues

It is inferred from the work done with other species that the fetal membrane of the dog also has an endocrine function. Wynn and Björkman (1968), Anderson (1969), and Lee et al. (1983) provide structural evidence that suggests such a function for carnivores. Kiso and Yamauchi (1984) provide histochemical evidence of this functional capability. During the latter two-thirds of gestation, there is a relatively undifferentiated *cytotrophoblast*, which forms as a simple cuboidal basal layer beneath the outer *syncytiotrophoblast* layer of the fetal epithelium. Both layers are well vascularized with fetal blood capillaries. Extensive decidual cells were reported by Anderson (1969). Sokolowski et al. (1973) described the changes in various endocrine organs during the estrous cycle and pregnancy.

Endocrine Tissues of the Testis

The testis, like the ovary, has both an exocrine and an endocrine function; the gametogenic or holocrine (cytogenic) function results in the production of spermatozoa, and testosterone results from its endocrine function.

With the onset of puberty, in the *interstitium testis* between the developing seminiferous tubules there is a differentiation of islets of epithelioid cells, the *endocrinocyti interstitiales* (Cornell & Christensen, 1975). These cells synthesize large amounts of the male steroid hormones (androgens), the primary active component of which is testosterone (Setoguti et al., 1974). These cells normally compose approximately 15% of the testicular volume, are supported by a delicate connective tissue stroma, and supplied by a rich network of blood and lymphatic capillaries (Kothari et al., 1972). The distribution of these vessels to the parenchyma has not been reported in detail for the dog, but the extent of their distribution may be inferred from observations of several species of domesticated and common laboratory mammals. When comparing the distribution of lymphatics among the endocrine cells of the testis, Fawcett et al. (1973) described an elaborate, varied relationship among the species. On the basis of their work, one would expect to find conspicuous and centrally located lymph capillaries in the dog.

Structural features and histopathologic evidence also suggest an endocrine function for the *epitheliocytus sustentans* (supporting or nurse cell) of the seminiferous epithelium. These cells produce androgen-binding protein and estrogen. The descent of the testes into the scrotal compartment during the perinatal period may involve a response to testis-derived humoral factors (Baumans et al., 1985; Wensing, 1988; see discussion in Chapter 9).

Endocrine Cells of the Kidney

At the vascular pole of the renal glomeruli, the smooth muscle cells of the tunica media of both the afferent and the efferent arterioles are epithelioid in morphology and contain secretory granules. Each of these is an *endocrinocytus myoideus*, or **juxtaglomerular cell** of the **juxtaglomerular complex**, which also includes epithelial cells of the macula densa of the distal tubular portion of the nephron and granulated cells of the extraglomerular mesangium.

The granules of the juxtaglomerular cells, in the dog highly soluble in water, have proved difficult to demonstrate histochemically. These granules have been shown in other species to contain the hormone renin. Renin is released from these cells in response to altered blood volume, blood pressure, and ionic concentration. Renin acts on a blood protein to bring about the formation of angiotensin II. In addition to other functions, angiotensin II increases the release of mineralocorticoids from the zona glomerulosa of the adrenal cortex, which in turn act upon the distal tubule of the kidney nephron to bring about greater resorption of sodium (Spangler, 1979).

The smaller laboratory animals have been used as the model for this important endocrine function. As more is understood of its action and as more sophisticated measurement techniques are developed, the dog may provide a reliable model for investigating this system. For related reading, consult Davis et al. (1961), Rojo-Ortega et al. (1970), and Granger et al. (1971).

Bibliography

Abel, J. H., Verhage, H. G., McClelkn, M. C., et al. (1975). Ultrastructural analysis of the granulosa-lutein cell transition in the ovary of the dog. *Cell Tissue Res, 160*, 155–176.

Acosta, J. M., Buceta, J. C., Pons, J. E., et al. (1969). Distribution and volume of the islets of Langerhans in the canine pancreas. *Acta Physiol Lat Am, 19*, 175–180.

Akmayev, I. G. (1971a). Morphological aspects of the hypothalamic-hypophyseal system. II. Functional morphology of pituitary microcirculation. *Z Zellforsch, 116*, 178–194.

Akmayev, I. G. (1971b). Morphological aspects of the hypothalamic-hypophyseal system. III. Vascularity of hypothalamus, with special reference to its quantitative aspects. *Z Zellforsch, 116*, 195–204.

Anderson, J. W. (1969). Ultrastructure of the placenta and fetal membranes of the dog. I. the placental labyrinth. *Anat Rec, 165*, 15–36.

Andrew, A. (1974). Further evidence that enterochromaffin cells are not delivered from the neural crest. *J Embryol Exp Morphol, 31*, 589–598.

Appleby, E. C., & Sohrabi-Haghdoost, I. (1980). Cortical hyperplasia of the adrenal gland in the dog. *Res Vet Sei, 29*, 190–197.

Ariëns-Kappers, J. (1965). Survey of the innervation of the epiphysis cerebri and the accessory pineal organs of vertebrates. In J. Ariëns-Kappers & J. P. Schade (Eds.), *Progress in brain research* (Vol. 10). New York: Elsevier.

Asa, S. L., Kovacs, K., Killinger, D. W., et al. (1980). Pancreatic islet cell carcinoma producing gastrin, ACTH, alpha-endorphin, somatostatin and calcitonin. *Am J Gastroenterol, 74*, 30–35.

Atkins, C. E., LeCompte, P. M., Hill, J. R., et al. (1988). Morphologic and immunocytochemical study of young dogs with diabetes mellitus associated with pancreatic islet hypoplasia. *Am J Vet Res, 49*, 1577–1581.

Atwal, O. S. (1981). Myelinated nerve fibers in the parathyroid gland of the dog: a light and electron-microscope study. *Acta Anat, 109*, 3–12.

Aumuller, G. (1983). Morphologic and endocrine aspects of prostatic function. *Prostate, 4*, 195–214.

Baber, E. C. (1877). On the lymphatics and parenchyma of the thyroid gland of the dog. *Q J Micr Sc, 17*, 204–212.

Baker, D. D. (1936). Studies on the suprarenal glands of dogs. I. comparison of the weights of suprarenal glands of mature and immature male and female dogs. *Am J Anat, 60,* 231–252.

Balboni, G. C. (1973). The problem of the ovarian stroma. *Arch Ital Anat Embriol, 75,* 37–58.

Banting, F. G., & Best, C. H. (1922). The internal secretion of the pancreas. *J Lab Clin Med, 7,* 251–266.

Basir, M. A. (1932). The vascular supply of the pituitary body in the dog. *J Anat, 66,* 387–397.

Baumans, V., Dielman, S. J., Wouterse, H. S., et al. (1985). Testosterone secretion during gubernacular development and testicular descent in the dog. *J Reprod Fertil, 73,* 21–25.

Bayliss, W. M., & Starling, E. H. (1902). The mechanism of pancreatic secretions. *J Physiol, 28,* 325–353.

Bencosme, S. A., & Liepa, E. (1955a). Regional differences of the pancreatic islet. *Endocrinology, 57,* 588–593.

Bencosme, S. A., Liepa, E., & Lazarus, S. S. (1955b). Glucagon content of pancreatic tissue devoid of alpha cells. *Proc Soc Exp Biol Med, 90,* 387–392.

Bensley, S. H. (1947). The normal mode of secretion of the parathyroid gland of the dog. *Anat Rec, 98,* 361–381.

Bergdahl, L., & Boquist, L. (1973). Parathyroid morphology in normal dogs. *Pathol Eur, 8,* 95–103.

Bergland, R. M., & Page, R. B. (1979). Pituitary-brain vascular relations: a new paradigm. *Science, 204,* 18–24.

Bloodworth, J. M., Jr., & Powers, K. L. (1968). The ultrastructure of the normal dog adrenal. *J Anat, 102,* 457–476.

Bloom, F. (1959). The endocrine glands. In H. D. Hoskins, J. V. LaCroix, & K. Mayer (Eds.), *Canine medicine* (2nd ed.). Santa Barbara, CA: American Veterinary Publications.

Bordi, C., Togni, R., Costa, A., et al. (1972). Extrainsular endocrine cells of the dog pancreas. A light microscopic study. *Endokrinologie, 60,* 39–50.

Boyd, J. D. (1964). Development of the human thyroid gland. In R. Pitt-Rivers & W. R. Trotter (Eds.), *The thyroid gland* (Vol. I). Washington, DC: Butterworths.

Brondi, C., & Castorina, S. (1953). Arterial circulation of the adrenal glands in the dog. *Minerva Chir, 8,* 380–383.

Calvo, J., Boya, J., & Garcia-Maurino, E. (1988). Ultrastructure of the pineal gland in the adult dog. *J Pineal Res, 5,* 479–487.

Campbell, H. J. (1970). Control of the anterior pituitary gland by hypothalamic releasing-factors. In *The scientific basis of medicine annual reviews*. British Postgraduate Federation, London: Athlone Press.

Carlon, N. (1967). Cytologic du lobe antérieur de l'hypophyse du chien. *Z Zellforsch, 78,* 76–91.

Castel, M., Gainer, H., & Dellmann, H. D. (1984). Neuronal secretory systems. *Int Rev Cytol, 88,* 303–459.

Chester-Jones, I. (1957). *The adrenal cortex*. New York: Cambridge University Press.

Chester-Jones, I. (1976). Evolutionary aspects of the adrenal cortex and its homologues. *J Endocrinol, 71,* 1P–31P.

Chester-Jones, I., Ingleton, P. M., & Phillips, J. G. (1986). *Fundamentals of comparative vertebrate endocrinology*. New York: Plenum.

Collombat, P., Xu, X., Ravassard, P., et al. (2009). The ectopic expression of pax4 in the mouse pancreas converts progenitor cells into alpha and subsequently beta cells. *Cell, 138,* 449–462.

Cornell, C. J., & Christensen, K. (1975). The ultrastructure of the canine testicular interstitial tissue. *Biol Reprod, 72,* 368–382.

Crowe, S. J., Cushing, H., & Homans, J. (1910). Experimental hypophysectomy. *Johns Hopkins Hosp Bull, 21,* 127–169.

Cunliffe, W. J. (1961). The innervation of the thyroid gland. *Acta Anat, 46,* 135–141.

Dandy, W. E. (1913). The nerve supply to the pituitary body. *Am J Anat, 15,* 333–343.

Dandy, W. E., & Goetsch, E. (1910). The blood supply of the pituitary body. *Am J Anat, 22,* 137–150.

Dandy, W. E., & Reichert, F. L. (1925). Studies on experimental hypophysectomy: effect on the maintenance of life. *Johns Hopkins Hosp Bull, 37,* 1–13.

Davis, D. J., MacAulay, M. A., MacDonald, A. S., et al. (1988). Islets of Langerhans in dog pancreas: volume fraction and relative distribution of diameters. *Transplantation, 45,* 1099–1103.

Davis, J. O., Ayers, C. R., & Carpenter, C. C. J. (1961). Renal origin of an aldosterone-stimulating hormone in dogs with thoracic caval constriction and in sodium-depleted dogs. *J Clin Invest, 40,* 1466–1474.

Elias, H., & Pauly, J. E. (1956). The structure of the human adrenal cortex. *Endocrinology, 58,* 714–789.

Ellsworth, A. F., Yang, T. J., & Ellsworth, M. L. (1985). The pineal body of the dog. *Acta Anat, 122,* 197–200.

Epple, A., Scanes, C. G., & Stetson, M. H. (1990). *Progress in comparative endocrinology. Proceedings 11th international symposium on comparative endocrinology*. Malaga, Spain, 1989, New York: Wiley-Liss.

Farrow, B. R. H. (1969). Chromophobe adenoma of the pituitary in a dog. *Vet Res, 84,* 609–610.

Fawcett, D. W., Neaves, W. B., & Flores, M. N. (1973). Comparative observations on intertubular lymphatics and the organization of the interstitial tissue of the mammalian testis. *Biol Reprod, 9,* 500–532.

Feldman, E., Nelson, R., & Scott-Moncrieff, J. C. (2015). *Canine & feline endocrinology* (4th ed.). St. Louis, MO: Elsevier.

Field, E. J., & Harrison, R. J. (1957). *Anatomical terms: their origin and derivation* (2nd ed.). Cambridge: W Heifer & Sons.

Flerko, B. (1980). The hypophyseal portal circulation today. *Neuroendocrinol, 30,* 56–63.

Flint, J. M. (1900). The blood-vessels, angiogenesis, organogenesis, reticulum and histology of the adrenal. *Johns Hopkins Hosp Rept, 39,* 153–230.

Forssmann, W. G. (1970). Ultrastructure of hormone-producing cells of the upper gastrointestinal tract. In W. Creutzfeldt (Ed.), *Origin, chemistry, physiology and pathophysiology of the gastrointestinal hormones*. New York: F. K. Schattauer Verlag.

Forssmann, W. G., Helmstaedter, V., Metz, J., et al. (1977). The identification of the F-cell in the dog pancreas as the pancreatic polypeptide producing cell. *Histochemistry, 50,* 281–290.

Foster, G. V., Baghdiantz, A., Kumar, M. A., et al. (1964a). Thyroid origin of calcitonin. *Nature, 202,* 1303–1305.

Foster, G. V., MacIntyre, I., & Pearse, A. G. E. (1964b). Calcitonin production and the mitochondrion-rich cells of the dog thyroid. *Nature, 203,* 1029–1030.

Francis, K. C., & Mulligan, R. M. (1949). The weight of the pituitary gland of the male dog in relation to body weight and age, with a differential cell count of the anterior lobe. *J Morphol, 85,* 141–161.

French, C. (1901). The thyroid gland and thyroid glandules of the dog. *J Comp Med Vet Arch, 22,* 1–14.

Fujita, T., & Kobayashi, S. (1974). The cells and hormones of the GEP endocrine system. In T. Fujita (Ed.), *Gastro-entero-pancreatic endocrine system: a cell-biological approach*. Baltimore, MD: Williams & Wilkins.

Fujita, T., & Kobayashi, S. (1979). Proposal of a neurosecretory system in the pancreas. An electron microscope study in the dog. *Arch Histol Jpn, 42,* 277–295.

Fujita, H., & Murakami, T. (1974). Scanning electron microscopy on the distribution of the minute blood vessels in the thyroid gland of the dog, rat and rhesus monkey. *Arch Histol Jpn, 36*, 181–188.

Gale, T. F. (1972). An electron microscopic study of the pars distalis of the dog adenohypophysis. *Z Anat Entwickl-Gesch, 137*, 188–199.

Gilmore, J. W., Venzke, W. G., & Foust, H. L. (1940). Growth changes in body organs. Part II. Growth changes in the thyroid of the normal dog. *Am J Vet Res, 1*, 66–72.

Godwin, M. C. (1936). The early development of the thyroid gland in the dog with especial reference to the origin and position of accessory thyroid tissue within the thoracic cavity. *Anat Rec, 66*, 233–251.

Godwin, M. C. (1937a). Complex IV in the dog with special emphasis on the relation of the ultimobranchial body to interfollicular cells in the postnatal thyroid gland. *Am J Anat, 60*, 299–330.

Godwin, M. C. (1937b). The development of the parathyroids in the dog with emphasis upon the origin of accessory glands. *Anat Rec, 68*, 305–325.

Goldberg, R. C., & Chaikoff, I. L. (1952). On the occurrence of six cell types in the dog anterior pituitary. *Anat Rec, 112*, 265–274.

Granger, P., Rojo-Ortega, J. M., Pérez, S. C., et al. (1971). The renin-angiotensin system in newborn dogs. *Can J Physiol Pharmacol, 49*, 134–138.

Green, J. D. (1951). The comparative anatomy of the hypophysis, with special reference to its blood supply and innervation. *Am J Anat, 88*, 225–311.

Green, J. D. (1966). The comparative anatomy of the portal vascular system and of the innervation of the hypophysis. In G. W. Harris & B. T. Donovan (Eds.), *The pituitary gland* (Vol. I). Los Angeles: University of California Press.

Greider, M. H., Gersell, D. J., & Gingerich, R. L. (1978). Ultrastructural localization of pancreatic polypeptide in the F cell of the dog pancreas. *J Histochem Cytochem, 26*, 1103–1108.

Guraya, S. S. (1973). Interstitial gland tissue of mammalian ovary. *Acta Endocrinol, 171*(Suppl.), 1–27.

Guraya, S. S. (1985). *Biology of ovarian follicles in mammals*. New York: Springer-Verlag.

Guraya, S. S., & Greenwald, G. S. (1964). A comparative histochemical study of interstitial tissue and follicular atresia in the mammalian ovary. *Anat Rec, 149*, 411–434.

Halmi, N. S., Peterson, M. E., Colurso, G. J., et al. (1981). Pituitary intermediate lobe in dog: two cell types in high bioactive adrenocorticotropin content. *Science, 211*, 72–74.

Halsted, W. S. (1896). An experimental study of the thyroid gland of dogs, with especial consideration of hypertrophy of this gland. *Johns Hopkins Hosp Rep, 12*, 373–409.

Hanström, B. (1966). Gross anatomy of the hypophysis in mammals. In G. W. Harris & B. T. Donovan (Eds.), *The pituitary gland* (Vol. I). Los Angeles: University of California Press.

Harris, G. W., & Donovan, B. T. (Eds.), (1966). *The pituitary gland* (Vol. 3). Los Angeles: University of California Press.

Harrison, R. G. (1964). The ductless glands. In G. J. Romanes (Ed.), *Cunningham's textbook of anatomy* (11th ed.). New York: Oxford University Press.

Hartmann, F. (1957). Uber die innervation der epiphysis cerebri einiger säugetiere. *Z Zellforsch, 46*, 416–429.

Hartman, J. F., Fain, W. R., & Wolfe, J. M. (1946). A cytological study of the anterior hypophysis of the dog with particular reference to the presence of a fourth cell type. *Anat Rec, 95*, 11–27.

Hawkins, K. L., Summers, B. A., Kuhajda, F. P., et al. (1987). Immunochemistry of normal pancreatic islets and spontaneous islet cell tumors in dogs. *Vet Pathol, 24*, 170–179.

Hedhammar, A., Wu, F., Krook, L., et al. (1974). Overnutrition and skeletal disease: an experimental study in growing great dane dogs. *Cornell Vet, 64*(Suppl. 5), 1–160.

Hellman, B., Wallgren, A., & Hellerström, C. (1962). Two types of islet alpha cells in different parts of the pancreas of the dog. *Nature, 294*, 1201–1202.

Hewitt, W. F., Jr. (1950). Age and sex differences in weight of pituitary glands in the dog. *Proc Soc Exp Biol Med, 74*, 781–782.

Hsueh, A. J. W., Adahsi, E. Y., Jones, P. B. C., et al. (1984). Hormonal regulation of the differentiation of cultured ovarian granulosal cells. *Endocr Rev, 5*, 76–127.

Hullinger, R. L. (1968). *A histocytological study of age changes in the canine adrenal gland studied by light and electron microscopy*. Ames, IA: Iowa State University. Ph.D. Thesis.

Hullinger, R. L. (1978). Adrenal cortex of the dog (*Canis familiaris*): i. Histomorphologic changes during growth, maturity, and aging. *Zbl Vet Med C Anat Histol Embryol, 7*, 1–27.

Hullinger, R. L., & Getty, R. (1971). The genesis and maintenance of the canine adrenal cortex from birth to one year of age. *XIX Congreso Mundial de Medicina Veterinaria y Zootecniz, 2*, 563.

Hullinger, R., & Andrisani, O. (2006). The endocrine system. *Dellman's textbook of veterinary histology* (6th ed.). Ames, IA: Blackwell.

Hullinger, R. L., Mershon, J., & Berner, B. (1983). Regeneration of the adrenal cortex flowing o, p'-DDD toxicity. *Anat Rec, 205*, 86A–87A.

Inage, T. (1974). Fluorescence histochemical and electron microscopic observations on the enterochromaffin cells in the dog pancreas. In T. Fujita (Ed.), *Gastro-entero-pancreatic endocrine system: A cell-biological approach*. Baltimore, MD: Williams & Wilkins.

Ivy, A. C., & Oldberg, E. (1928). A hormone mechanism for gallbladder contraction and evacuation. *Am J Physiol, 86*, 599–613.

Kagayama, M. (1965). Follicular cells in the pars distalis of the dog pituitary gland. An electron microscopic study. *Endocrinology, 77*, 1053–1060.

Kalina, M., & Pearse, A. G. E. (1971). Ultrastructural localization of calcitonin in C-cells of dog thyroid: an immunocytochemical study. *Histochemie, 26*, 1–8.

Kameda, Y. (1971). The occurrence of a special parafollicular cell complex in and beside the dog thyroid gland. *Arch Histol Jpn, 33*, 115–132.

Kameda, Y. (1972). The accessory thyroid glands of the dog around the intrapericardial aorta. *Arch Histol Jpn, 34*, 375–391.

Kameda, Y. (1973). Electron microscopic studies on the parafollicular cells and parafollicular cell complexes in the dog. *Arch Histol Jpn, 36*, 89–105.

Kelley, K. W., Davila, D. R., Brief, S., et al. (1988). A pituitary-thymus connection during aging. *Ann NY Acad Sci, 521*, 88–98.

Kingsbury, B. F., & Roemer, F. J. (1940). The development of the hypophysis of the dog. *Am J Anat, 66*, 449–469.

Kiso, Y., & Yamauchi, S. (1984). Histochemical study on hydroxysteroid dehydrogenases in the trophoblast of the dog placenta. *Jpn J Vet Sci, 46*, 219–223.

Kobayashi, S., & Fujita, T. (1969). Fine structure of mammalian and avian pancreatic islets with special reference to d cells and nervous elements. *Z Zellforsch, 100*, 340–363.

Kobayashi, S., & Fujita, T. (1974). Emiocytotic granule release in the basal-granulated cells of the dog induced by intraluminal application of adequate stimuli. In T. Fujita (Ed.), *Gastro-entero-pancreatic* endocrine system: A cell-biological approach. Baltimore, MD: Williams & Wilkins.

Kosaka, T., & Lim, R. K. S. (1930). Demonstration of the humoral agent in fat inhibition of gastric secretion. *Proc Soc Exp Biol Med*, 27, 890–891.

Kothari, L. K., Srivastava, D. K., Mishra, P., et al. (1972). Total Leydig cell volume and its estimation in dogs and in models of testis. *Anat Rec*, 174, 259–264.

Latimer, H. B. (1941). The weight of the hypophysis in the dog. *Growth*, 5, 293–300.

Latimer, H. B. (1965). Changes in relative organ weights in the fetal dog. *Anat Rec*, 153, 421–428.

Latshaw, W. K. (1987). *Veterinary developmental anatomy*. Toronto: B.C. Decker.

Lee, S. Y., Anderson, J. W., Scott, G. L., et al. (1983). Ultrastructure of the placental and fetal membranes of the dog. II. The yolk sac. *Am J Anat*, 166, 313–327.

Liles, S. R., Linder, K. E., Cain, B., & Pease, A. (2010). Ultrasonography of histologically normal parathyroid glands and third lobules in normocalcemic dogs. *Vet Rad Ultrasound*, 51, 447–452. doi:10.1111/j.1740-8261.2010.01686.x.

Liu, Z., & Habener, J. (2009). Alpha cells beget beta cells. *Cell*, 138, 424–426.

Ljubomudrov, A. P. (1939). The blood supply of the suprarenal glands in the dog. *Arkhiv Anat Gistol Embriol*, 20, 220–224. (English Summary, 381–382).

Mahorner, H. R., Caylor, H. D., Schlotthauer, C. F., et al. (1927). Observations on the lymphatic connections of the thyroid gland in man. *Anat Rec*, 36, 341–347.

Major, R. H. (1909). Studies on the vascular system of the thyroid gland. *Am J Anat*, 9, 475–492.

Marine, D. (1907). On the occurrence and physiological nature of glandular hyperplasia of the thyroid (dog and sheep) together with remarks on important clinical problems. *Johns Hopkins Hosp Bull*, 18, 359–364.

Marine, D. (1914). Observations on tetany in dogs. *J Exp Med*, 19, 89–105.

Mason, J. B., Markowitz, J., & Mann, F. C. (1930). A plethysmographie study of the thyroid gland of the dog. *Am J Physiol*, 94, 125–134.

McKnight, K., Wang, P., & Kim, S. (2010). Deconstructing pancreas development to reconstruct human islets from pluripotent stem cells. *Cell*, 6, 300–308. doi:10.1016/j.stem.2010.03.003.

Meuten, D. J., Capen, C. C., Thompson, K. G., et al. (1984). Syncytial cells in the canine parathyroid gland. *Vet Pathol*, 21, 463–468.

Michaelson, S. M. (1970). Endocrine system. In A. C. Andersen (Ed.), *The beagle as an experimental dog*. Ames, IA: Iowa State University Press.

Mikami, S. (1956). Cytological changes in the anterior pituitary of the dog after adrenalectomy. *J Fac Agric Iwate Univ*, 3, 62–68.

Mikhail, Y. (1971). Intrinsic nerve supply of the thyroid and parathyroid glands. *Acta Anat*, 80, 152–159.

Modell, W. (1933). Observations on the structure of the blood vessels within the thyroid gland of the dog. *Anat Rec*, 55, 251–269.

Morato, M. J. X. (1939). The blood supply of the hypophysis. *Anat Rec*, 74, 297–320.

Morrison, W. B. (1984). The clinical relevance of APUD cells. *Compend Cont Educ*, 6, 884–890.

Mulligan, R. M., & Francis, K. C. (1951). Weights of thyroid and parathyroid glands of normal male dogs. *Anat Rec*, 110, 139–143.

Munger, B. L., Caramia, F., & Lacy, P. E. (1965). The ultrastructural basis for the identification of cell types in the pancreatic islets. II. Rabbit, dog and opossum. *Z Zellforsch*, 67, 776–798.

Nilsson, M., & Williams, D. (2016). On the origin of cells and derivation of thyroid cancer: C cell story revisited. *European Thyroid Journal*, 5, 79–93. doi:10.1159/000447333.

Nomina anatomica (1989). (6th ed.). International Committee on Anatomical Nomenclature. London: Churchill Livingstone.

Nomina Anatomica Veterinaria (2017). *International committee on veterinary gross anatomical nomenclature* (6th ed.). Hannover.

Nomina Histologica (1992). *International committee on veterinary histological nomenclature* (2nd ed.). Gent.

Nonidez, F. J. (1931). Innervation of the thyroid gland. II. Origin and course of the thyroid nerves in the dog. *Am J Anat*, 48, 299–329.

Nonidez, F. J. (1932a). The origin of the "parafollicular" cell, a second epithelial component of the thyroid of the dog. *Am J Anat*, 49, 479–495.

Nonidez, F. J. (1932b). Further observations on the parafollicular cells of the mammalian thyroid. *Anat Rec*, 53, 339–347.

Nonidez, F. J. (1935). Innervation of the thyroid gland. III. Distribution and termination of nerve fibers in dogs. *Am J Anat*, 57, 135–170.

Nunez, E. A., Beishaw, B. B., & Gershon, M. D. (1972). A fine structural study of the highly active thyroid follicular cell of the African basenji dog. *Am J Anat*, 133, 463–481.

Nussdorfer, G. G. (1986). Cytophysiology of the adrenal cortex. *Int Rev Cytol*, 98, 319–320.

Oksche, A. (1965). Survey of the development and comparative morphology of the pineal organ. In J. Ariëns-Kappers & J. Schade (Eds.), *Progress in brain research* (Vol. 10). New York: Elsevier.

Nostro, M. C., & Keller, G. (2012). Generation of beta cells from human pluripotent stem cells: potential for regenerative medicine. *Seminars in Cell & Developmental Biology*, 23, 701–710.

Pearse, A. G. E. (1977). The diffuse neuroendocrine system and the APUD concept. *Med Biol*, 55, 115–125.

Peranzi, G., & Lehy, T. (1984). Endocrine cell populations in the colon and rectum of cat, dog, and monkey: fine structure, immunocytochemistry, and distribution. *Anat Rec*, 210, 87–100.

Pictet, R. L., Rail, L. B., Phelps, P., et al. (1976). The neural crest and the origin of the insulin-producing and other gastrointestinal hormone-producing cells. *Science*, 191, 191–192.

Pitt-Rivers, R., & Trotter, W. R. (1964). *The thyroid gland*. Washington, DC: Butterworths.

Pohorecky, L. A., & Wurtman, R. J. (1971). Adrenocortical control of epinephrine synthesis. *Pharmacol Rev*, 23, 1–35.

Polak, J. M., Bloom, S., Coulling, I., et al. (1971). Immunofluorescent localization of enteroglucagon cells in the gastrointestinal tract of the dog. *Gut*, 12, 311–318.

Purves, H. D. (1966). Cytology of the adenohypophysis. In G. W. Harris & B. T. Donovan (Eds.), *The pituitary gland* (Vol. I). Los Angeles: University of California Press.

Purves, H. D., & Griesbach, W. E. (1957). A study on the cytology of the adenohypophysis of the dog. *J Endocrinol*, 14, 361–370.

Putnam, T. J., Benedict, E. B., & Teel, H. M. (1929). Studies in acromegaly, VIII. Experimental canine acromegaly produced by injection of anterior lobe pituitary extract. *Arch Surg*, 18, 1708–1736.

Radke, R., & Stach, W. (1986a). Innervation of the canine pancreas after vagotomy. *Acta Anat*, 127, 88–92.

Radke, R., & Stach, W. (1986b). Do β cells and peri-insular acinar cells of the canine pancreas have nerves in common? *Acta Anat, 127*, 65–68.

Reed, C. I., Lackey, R. W., & Payte, J. I. (1928). Observations on parathyroidectomized dogs, with particular attention to the regional incidence of tetany and to the blood mineral changes in this condition. *Am J Physiol, 84*, 176–188.

Reichlin, S. (1974). Neuroendocrinology. In R. H. Williams (Ed.), *Textbook of endocrinology* (5th ed.). Philadelphia: Saunders.

Ricci, V., & Russolo, M. (1973). Immunocytological observations on the localization of ACTH in the hypophysis of the dog. *Acta Anat, 84*, 10–18.

Rienhoff, W. F. (1938). The lymphatic vessels of the thyroid gland in the dog and in man. *Arch Surg, 23*, 783–804.

Roediger, W. E. W. (1973). A comparative study of the normal human neonatal and the canine thyroid C cell. *J Anat, 115*, 255–276.

Rojo-Ortega, J. M., Granger, P., Boucher, R., et al. (1970). Studies on the distribution of the JGI in the renal cortex of dogs and beavers. *Nephron, 7*, 61–66.

Ross, W. D., & Moorhouse, U. H. K. (1938). The thyroid nerve in the dog and its function. *Q J Exp Physiol, 27*, 209–214.

Saladino, C. F., & Getty, R. (1972). Quantitative study on the islets of Langerhans of the beagle as a function of age. *Exp Gerontol, 7*, 91–97.

Saleh, A. M., Nawar, N. Y. Y., & Kamal, I. (1974). A study on the adrenal ganglion and adrenal gland of the dog. *Anat Rec, 89*, 345–351.

Sasagawa, T., Kobayashi, S., & Fujita, T. (1974). Electron microscope studies on the endocrine cells of the human gut and pancreas. In T. Fujita (Ed.), *Gastro-entero-pancreatic endocrine system: a cell-biological approach*. Baltimore, MD: Williams & Wilkins.

Schwartz, H. G. (1936). The meningeal relations of the hypophysis cerebri. *Anat Rec, 67*, 35–51.

Serizawa, Y., Kobayashi, S., & Fujita, T. (1979). Neuro-insular complex type i in the mouse. Reevaluation of the pancreatic islet as a modified ganglion. *Arch Histol Jpn, 42*, 389–394.

Setoguti, T., Haruhiko, E., & Shimizu, T. (1974). Electron microscopic studies on the testicular interstitial cells. *Arch Histol Jpn, 37*, 97–108.

Shimosegawa, T., Kobayashi, S., Fujita, T., Mochizuki, T., Yanaihara, C., & Yanaihara, N. (1983). Nerve elements containing met-enkephalin-arg-gly-leu immunoreactivity in canine pancreas—A histochemical study. *Neurosci Lett, 42*, 161–165.

Sidhu, G. S. (1979). The endodermal origin of digestive and respiratory tract APUD cells. *Am J Pathol, 96*, 5–16.

Smith, E. M., Calhoun, M. L., & Reineke, E. P. (1953). The histology of the anterior pituitary, thyroid and adrenal of thyroid-stimulated purebred English bulldogs. *Anat Rec, 117*, 221–240.

Smith, P. H., & Madson, K. L. (1981). Interactions between autonomic nerves and endocrine cells of the gastroenteropancreatic system. *Diabetologia, 20*, 314–324.

Smithcors, J. F. (1964). The endocrine system. In M. E. Miller, G. C. Christensen, & H. E. Evans (Eds.), *Anatomy of the dog*. Philadelphia: Saunders.

Sokolowski, J. H., Zimbelman, R. G., & Goyings, L. S. (1973). Canine reproduction: reproductive organs and related structures of the nonparous, parous, and postpartum bitch. *Am J Vet Res, 34*, 1001–1013.

Solcia, E., Vassallo, G., & Capella, C. (1970). Cytology and cytochemistry of hormone producing cells of the upper gastrointestinal tract. In W. Creutzfeldt (Ed.), *Origin, chemistry, physiology and pathophysiology of the gastrointestinal hormones*. New York: FK Schattauer Verlag.

Spangler, W. L. (1979). Pathophysiologic response of the juxtaglomerular apparatus to dietary sodium restriction in the dog. *Am J Vet Res, 40*, 809–819.

Soggia, A., Hoarau, E., Bechetoille, C., Simon, M.-T., Heimis, M., & Duvillie, B. (2011). Cell-based theory of diabetes: what are the new sources of beta cells? *Diabetes, 37*, 371–375.

Stanger, B., & Hebrok, M. (2013). Control of cell identity in pancreas development and regeneration. *Gastroenterology, 144*, 1170–1179.

Stockard, C. R. (1941). *The genetic and endocrine basis for differences in form and behavior*, Am J Anat Memoir 19. Philadelphia: Wistar Institute of Anatomy and Biology.

Stott, G. G. (1974). Granulosal cell islands in the canine ovary: histogenesis, histomorphologic features, and fate. *Am J Vet Res, 35*, 1351–1355.

Swarts, J. L., & Thompson, R. L. (1911). Accessory thyroid tissue within the pericardium of the dog. *J Med Res, 29*, 299–308.

Teitelbaum, S. L., Moore, K. E., & Shieber, W. (1970). C cell follicles in the dog thyroid: demonstrated by in vivo perfusion. *Anat Rec, 168*, 69–78.

Truscott, B. L. (1944). The nerve supply to the pituitary of the rat. *J Comp Neurol, 80*, 235–255.

Venzke, W. G. (1940). Histology of the thyroid glands of dogs 16 weeks of age. *Proc Iowa Acad Sci, 46*, 439–441.

Venzke, W. G. (1976). Carnivore endocrinology. In R. Getty (Ed.), *Sisson and Grossman's anatomy of the domestic animals*. Philadelphia: Saunders.

Venzke, W. G., & Gilmore, J. W. (1940). Histological observations on the epiphysis cerebri. *Proc Iowa Acad Sci, 47*, 409–413.

Verhofstad, A. A. J., & Lensen, W. F. J. (1973). On the occurrence of lymphatic vessels in the adrenal gland of the white rat. *Acta Anat, 84*, 475–483.

Vicari, E. M. (1937). Observations on the nature of the parafollicular cells in the thyroid gland of the dog. *Anat Rec, 68*, 281–285.

Vicari, E. M. (1938). Variations in structure of the parathyroid glands of dogs. *Anat Rec, 70*(Suppl. 3), 80–81.

Vinson, G. P., Pudney, J. A., & Whitehouse, B. J. (1985). The mammalian adrenal circulation and the relationship between adrenal blood flow and steroidogenesis. *J Endocrinol, 105*, 285–294.

Watanabe, S., Wakuri, H., & Mutoh, K. (1989). Histological studies on the endocrine pancreas in the dog. *Zbl Vet Med C Anat Histol Embryol, 28*, 150–156.

Watkins, W. B. (1975). Neurosecretory neurons in the hypothalamus and median eminence of the dog and sheep as revealed by immunohistochemical methods. *Ann NY Acad Sci, 248*, 134–152.

Wensing, C. J. G. (1988). The embryology of testicular descent. *Hormone Res, 30*, 144–152.

White, J. B., & Foust, H. L. (1944). Growth changes in body organs. III. Growth changes in the pituitary of the normal dog. *Am J Vet Res, 5*, 173–178.

Wild, P., & Manser, E. (1980). Morphometric analysis of parathyroid glands in neonatal and growing dogs. *Acta Anat, 108*, 350–360.

Wilkinson, I. M. S. (1961). The intrinsic innervation of the suprarenal gland. *Acta Anat, 46*, 127–134.

Wissig, S. L. (1964). morphology and cytology. In R. Pitt-Rivers & W. R. Trotter (Eds.), *The thyroid gland* (Vol. I). Washington, DC: Butterworths.

Wolf, J. M., & Cleveland, R. (1932). Cell types found in the anterior hypophysis of the dog (abstr.). *Anat Rec, 52*, 43–44.

Wurtman, R. J., & Cardinali, D. P. (1974). The pineal organ. In R. H. Williams (Ed.), *Textbook of endocrinology* (5th ed.). Philadelphia: Saunders.

Wynn, R. M., & Björkman, N. (1968). Ultrastructure of the feline placental membrane. *Am J Obstet Gynecol, 92*, 533–549.

Yang, Y., Akinci, E., Dutton, J., Banga, A., & Slack, J. (2013). Stage specific reprogramming of mouse embryo liver cells to a beta cell-like phenotype. *Science Direct, 130*, 602–612. doi:10.1016/j.mod.2013.08.002.

Yamada, H., Ozama, S., & Endo, R. (1956). Histological studies on the mammalian pituitary gland with special reference to the innervation. *Bull Tokyo Med Dent Univ, 3*, 55–65.

Yeghiayan, E., Rojo-Ortega, J. M., & Genest, J. (1972). Parathyroid vessel innervation: an ultrastructural study. *J Anat, 112*, 137–142.

Zach, B. (1960). Topographie und mikroskopisch-anatomischer feinbau der epiphysis cerebri von hund und katze. *Zentralbl Veterinaermed, 7*, 273–303.

11
The Heart and Arteries

Pericardium and Heart

Pericardium

The **pericardium**, or heart sac, is the fibroserous envelope of the heart. It can be divided into an outer fibrous and an inner serous part. The serous part consists of a parietal and a visceral layer.

The **fibrous pericardium** (*pericardium fibrosum*) (Fig. 11.1) is a thin, tough sac that contains the serous pericardium, a small amount of fluid and the heart. The greater part of its outer surface is covered by and adhered to the pericardial mediastinal pleura. In young dogs the thymus is in contact with a variable portion of its cranial surface. The inner surface of the fibrous pericardium is intimately lined by the parietal layer of the serous pericardium. The base of the fibrous pericardium is continued on the adventitia of the great arteries and veins that leave and enter the heart. It blends with the adventitia of these vessels. Its apex is continued to the ventral part of the muscular periphery of the diaphragm in the form of a dorsoventrally flattened band of yellow elastic fascicles, the **phrenicopericardiac ligament** (*lig. phrenicopericardiacum*). This is nearly 1 cm wide, less than 1 mm thick, and approximately 5 mm long.

The **serous pericardium** (*pericardium serosum*) (Fig. 11.1) forms a closed cavity into which approximately one-half of its wall is invaginated by the heart to form its visceral layer, the smooth, outer covering of the heart also known as the *epicardium*. The uninvaginated part forms the parietal layer as it covers the inner surface of the fibrous pericardium. The **pericardial cavity** (*cavum pericardii*) (see Fig. 11.1) is located between the two layers of the serous pericardium. It is the smallest of the serous body cavities and, unlike the others, contains 0.3 to 1 mL of a clear, light yellow fluid, the *liquor pericardii*.

The **parietal layer** (*lamina parietalis*) of the serous pericardium is so firmly fused to the fibrous pericardium that no separation is possible. It is composed of interlacing collagenous fibers, which are paved on the inside by mesothelium but on the outside are indistinguishable from the tissue of the fibrous pericardium.

The **visceral layer** (*lamina visceralis*) of the serous pericardium, or *epicardium,* is attached firmly to the heart muscle, except primarily along the grooves where fat and the coronary vessels or their branches intervene. Its smooth mesothelial surface is underlaid by a stroma that contains elastic fibers. The division between the parietal and visceral layers of the serous pericardium is marked by an undulating line that follows the highest part of the pericardial cavity around and across the base of the heart. The aorta and pulmonary trunk, the two great arteries leaving the heart, are united by a tube of epicardium and areolar connective tissue at their origins so that, caudal to them, a part of the pericardial cavity curves transversely across the base of the heart. This is the **transverse sinus of the pericardium** (*sinus transversus pericardii*) (Fig. 11.2), a U-shaped passage between the right and left sides of the pericardial cavity. This sinus passes between the aorta and pulmonary trunk cranially and the pulmonary veins caudally.

Heart

The **heart** (*cor*) (Figs. 11.3, 11.4, and 11.5) is the muscular pump of the cardiovascular system. The musculature and conducting system of the heart are spoken of collectively as the **myocardium** (Langer & Brady, 1974). For references on the heart, blood vessels, and circulation, see Chevalier (1976), Cliff (1976), and Abramson (1976). The heart is cone-shaped and obliquely placed in the thorax so that its **base** (*basis cordis*) faces dorsocranially and its **apex** (*apex cordis*) is directed ventrocaudally and to the left side. A small, roughly triangular area of its dorsocaudal surface adjacent to the apex is related to the diaphragm. The large remaining part of its circumference is largely covered by the lungs and faces the sternum and ribs. The left and right ventricles are separated from each other internally by a transverse curved oblique **interventricular septum** (*septum interventriculare*) that extends from a cranioventral position on the left to a caudodorsal position on the right. On the surface of the heart these positions of the septum are marked by the **paraconal interventricular groove** (*sulcus interventricularis paraconalis*) on the left and the **subsinuosal interventricular groove** (*sulcus interventricularis subsinuosus*) on the right. The atria are separated from each other by a thin muscular **interatrial septum** (*septum interatriale*) that is also transversely curved similar to the interventricular septum but has no surface markings. The atria are the blood receiving chambers and the ventricles are the blood pumping chambers. The left dorsal, lateral, and caudal (caudodorsal) parts of the heart consist of the

CHAPTER 11 The Heart and Arteries

• **Fig. 11.1** Transverse computed tomography (CT) scans of thorax at the level of T7. **A**, Lung window imaging, and **B**, soft tissue window showing IV injected contrast within the heart and several vessels. *1*, Aorta; *2*, azygous vein; *3*, right pulmonary artery; *4*, right pulmonary vein; *E*, esophagus; *RB*, right primary bronchus; *LB*, left primary bronchus; *RCd*, right caudal lung lobe; and *LCd*, left caudal lung lobe. **C**, Schamtic tranvserse section of the thorax.

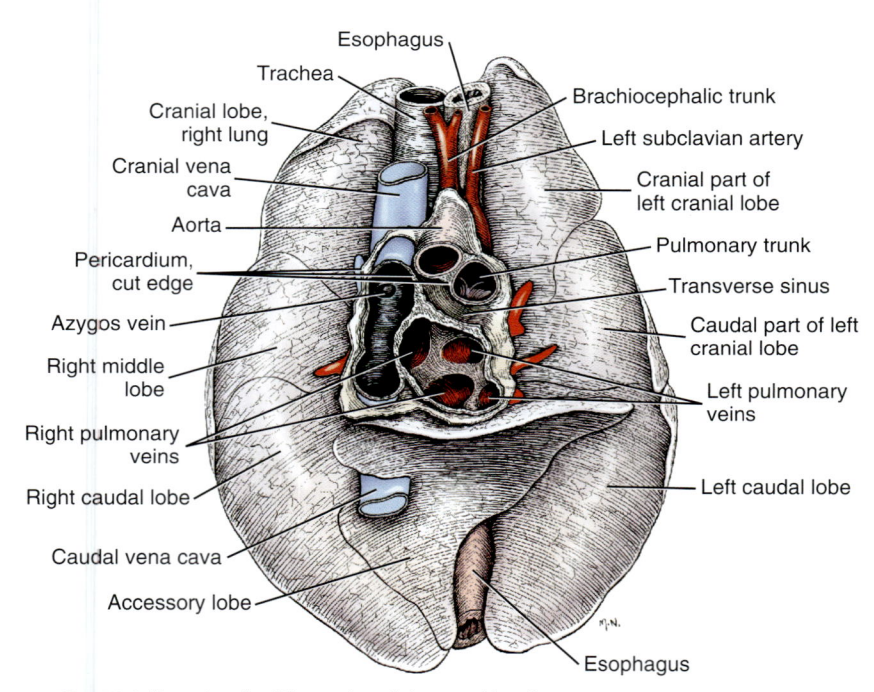

• **Fig. 11.2** Dorsal wall of the pericardial sac, with adjacent structures, ventral aspect.

left atrium (*atrium sinistrum*) and the **left ventricle** (*ventriculus sinister*). The left atrium receives blood from the lungs and the left ventricle pumps it to all parts of the body (systemic circulation). The right dorsal, lateral, and cranial (cranioventral) parts of the heart consist of the **right atrium** (*atrium dextrum*) and **right ventricle** (*ventriculus dexter*). The right atrium receives blood from all parts of the body and the right ventricle pumps it to the lungs (pulmonary circulation).

Orientation

The heart is located in the middle part of the mediastinum, the partition that separates the two pleural cavities (Fig. 11.1). It is the largest organ in this tissue-filled septum located between the walls of the mediastinal pleurae. Covered by its pericardium, the heart extends from the third rib to the caudal border of the sixth rib. Radiographs show that variations in position occur among the breeds and

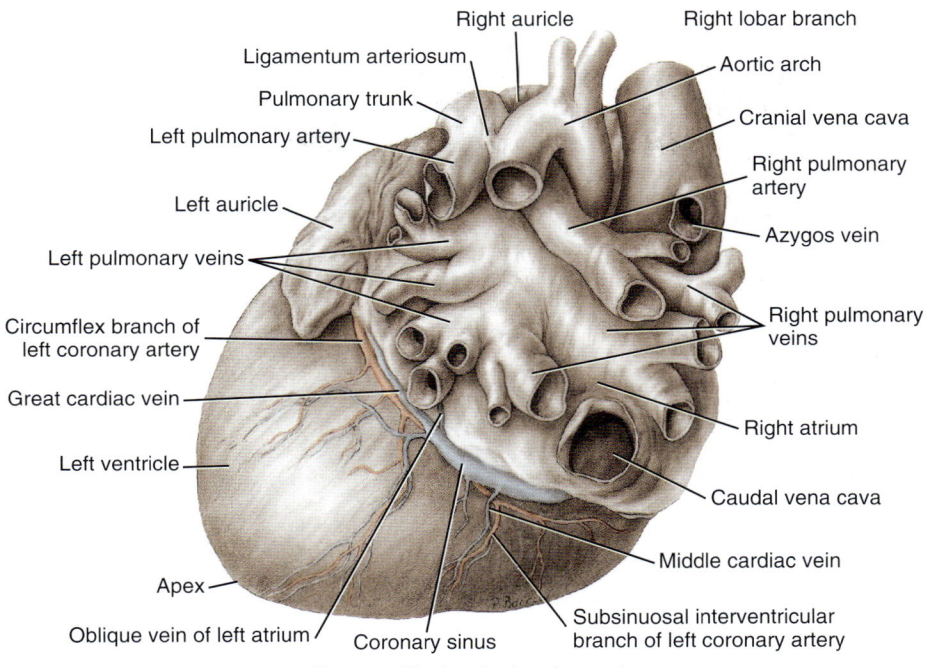

Fig. 11.3 The heart, dorsal aspect.

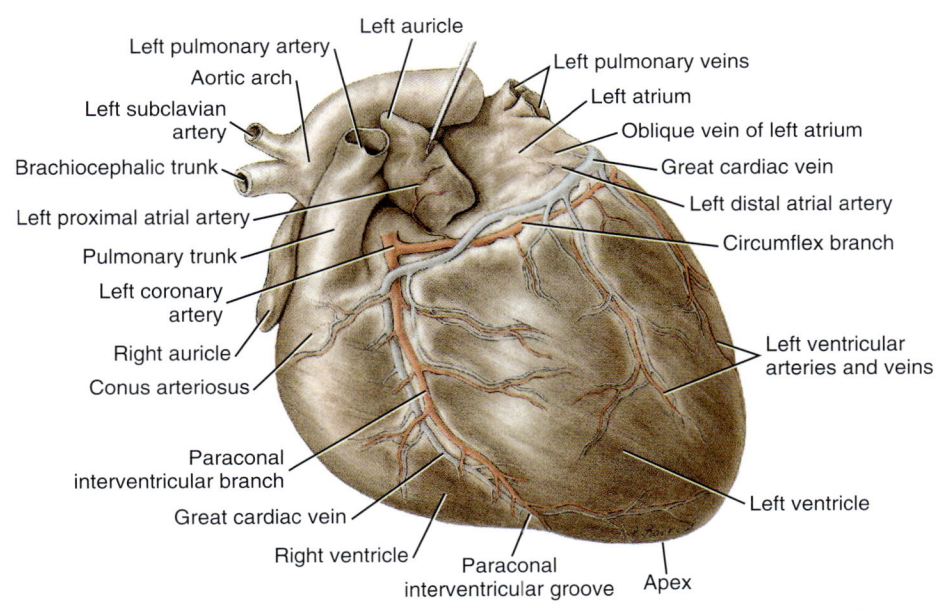

Fig. 11.4 The heart, auricular surface. Left auricle elevated to reveal pulmonary trunk.

individuals, and in the same animal according to age, condition, and the presence of pathologic processes. A longitudinal axis through the heart tips cranially approximately 45 degrees from a vertical plane. The base therefore faces dorsocranially and the bulk of it lies above a dorsal plane dividing the thorax into dorsal and ventral halves. The apex points caudoventrally where it lies slightly to the left and caudal to a transverse plane through the most cranial part of the diaphragm. At this level it touches the cranial surface of a transverse plane through the thorax that bisects the caudal part of the seventh sternebra. Normally the lungs cover most of the surface of the heart. On the right side the cardiac notch of the lung allows a variable area of the heart, covered by its fibrous pericardium and three layers of serosa, to contact the parietal pleura of the lateral thoracic wall. The cardiac notch of the right lung is V-shaped, with the apex directed dorsally. This allows a greater exposure of the heart on the right side than on the left, where the ventral border of the lung is usually not notched. The lung is thin adjacent to the lateral surfaces of the heart so that, in spite of the lung covering it, the beat of the organ can be easily heard and felt through the thoracic wall. The conformation

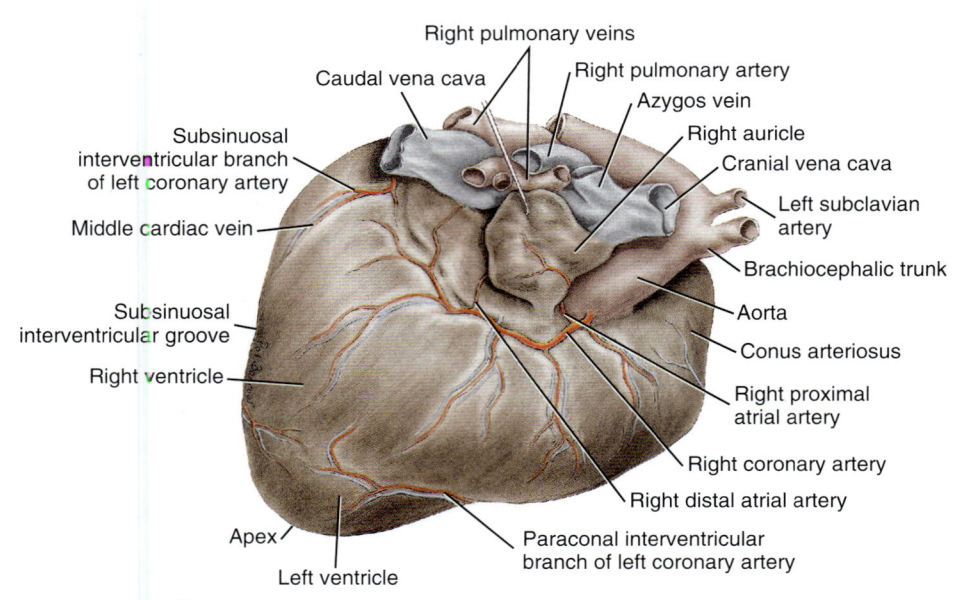

Fig. 11.5 The heart, atrial surface. Right auricle reflected to reveal the base of the aorta.

of the dog has most to do with the ease with which the heartbeat can be felt and heard. The heartbeat is most pronounced in thin, athletic-type animals with a narrow thorax.

Size and Weight

The dog heart is frequently used in studies of cardiac hypertrophy, and several surveys have been made of the normal values. Herrmann (1925) includes data on 200 dogs and cites heart weight-to-body weight ratios averaging 8.10 g per kg of body weight for males and 7.92 g for females. Northup et al. (1957) analyzed Herrmann's data and found that the sex differences were not significant. However, when they studied the heart weight-to-body weight ratios of an additional 346 adult dogs and 135 pups, they found that females have significantly smaller ratios than males. Small adults were found to have higher ratios than large adults, although pups had significantly smaller ratios than those in any adult category. The average ratio for 169 adult males was 7.74 g, and for 177 females it was 7.56 g. The range for 346 adult dogs was 4.53 to 11.13 g per kg. Schoning et al. (1995) found the heart weight-to-body weight ratio to be 1.3% for males and 1.2% for females in the 230 racing and nonracing Greyhounds that they studied. House and Ederstrom (1968) found that heart weight-to-body weight ratios increased during postnatal development from 7.17 g per kg in the newborn to 8.87 g per kg in adults. Latimer (1961) has presented data on the ratios between the weights of the walls of the right and left ventricles in 46 dogs. The right ventricular wall accounted for 22% of the total heart weight, the left ventricular wall for 39%.

In the average young dog the heart weight is approximately 1% of the body weight.

Schneider et al. (1964) compared the hearts of 40 racing Greyhounds with 60 mongrel dogs on heart weight-to-body weight ratios and components of the electrocardiogram. The heart weight-to-body weight ratio of the Greyhounds was 1.25 g, with a heart rate of 115 beats per min. The ratio for mongrel dogs was 0.80, with a heart rate of 86 beats per min. The Greyhound has been bred and trained for speed and endurance, and it would be expected that the heart would be proportionally larger than that of a mongrel.

Radiologists use a vertebral scale system to measure relative heart size on radiographs. Sleeper and Buchanan (2001) used this system to determine relative heart size in 11 clinically normal puppies to assess whether relative heart size changes with growth. They concluded that vertebral heart size measurements in puppies are within the reference range for adult dogs and do not change significantly with growth to 3 years of age.

Surface Topography

The **coronary groove** (*sulcus coronarius*), on the surface of the heart, marks the separation of the atria and ventricles. It contains much fat, which surrounds the coronary vessels. The coronary groove encircles the heart except cranioventrally, where the dorsal part of the right ventricle (conus arteriosus) intervenes.

The **interventricular grooves** are indistinct surface markings of the separation of the right and left ventricles. Because they neither indent the substance of the heart nor contain as much fat as does the coronary groove, vessels are visible in them; however, most vessels stream toward the apex on the surface of the ventricles, rather than following the interventricular grooves. Obliquely traversing the left cranioventral surface of the heart is the **paraconal interventricular groove** (*sulcus interventricularis paraconalis*) (see Fig. 11.4), formerly known as the *left, ventral,* or *cranial longitudinal sulcus* or *groove*. It begins on the caudodorsal side of the conus arteriosus, where it is covered by the auricular portion of the left atrium; it ends before reaching the apex of the heart. The **subsinuosal interventricular groove** (*sulcus interventricularis subsinuosus*) (see Fig. 11.5), formerly known as the *right, dorsal,* or *caudal longitudinal sulcus,* is a short, straight, shallow furrow that marks, on the dorsocaudal surface of the heart, the approximate position of the interventricular septum.

There are two surfaces of the heart. The **auricular surface** (*facies auricularis*) faces the left thoracic wall and the **atrial surface** (*facies atrialis*) faces the right thoracic wall. The **right ventricular margin** (*margo ventricularis dexter*) is the convex cranial border of the heart is comprised of the right ventricle. The **left ventricular margin** (*margo ventricularis sinister*) is the caudal border of the heart facing the diaphragm and comprised of the left ventricle.

In dogs, a line drawn on the left side from the root of the pulmonary trunk to the apex would follow an ill-defined border, known as the **left margin** (*margo ventricularis sinister*). A similar poorly defined border on the right side is known as the **right margin** (*margo ventricularis dexter*). The **base** of the heart (*basis cordis*) is the hilus of the organ. It is the craniodorsal portion and receives the great veins and emits the great arteries. The atria also enter into its formation. The **apex** of the heart (*apex cordis*) is formed by the looping of a swirl of muscle fibers at the apex of the left ventricle. It forms the most ventrocaudal part of the organ.

Atria

The **right atrium** (*atrium dextrum*) (Fig. 11.6) receives the blood from the systemic veins and most of the blood from the heart itself. It lies dorsocranial to the right ventricle. It is divided into a main part, the *sinus venarum cavarum,* and a blind part, which projects cranially, ventrally, and left, the **right auricle** (*auricula dextra*). The main openings of the right atrium are four in number. The **coronary sinus** (*sinus coronarius*) is the smallest of these and enters the atrium caudally from the left. Dorsal to it is the large **caudal vena cava** (*vena cava caudalis*), which enters the heart from caudal. The caudal vena cava returns blood from the abdominal viscera, part of the abdominal wall, and the pelvic limbs. The **cranial vena cava** (*vena cava cranialis*) is approximately the same size as the caudal vena cava. It enters the heart from dorsal and cranial directions. In the dog the azygos vein usually enters the cranial vena cava dorsally at the base of the heart, although occasionally it enters the atrium directly. The azygos vein drains blood back to the heart from part of the lumbar region and the caudal three fourths of the thoracic wall. The cranial vena cava returns blood to the heart from the head, neck, thoracic limbs, the ventral thoracic wall, and the adjacent part of the abdominal wall. The **right atrioventricular orifice** (*ostium atrioventriculare dextrum*) is the large opening from the right atrium into the right ventricle. This opening and the valve that guards it are described with the right ventricle.

Other features of the right atrium are the tuberculum intervenosum, fossa ovalis, limbus fossae ovalis, crista terminalis, right auricle, and the mm. pectinati.

The interatrial septum (*septum interatriale*) extends from the level of the coronary sinus to the opening into the right auricle. On its right side is a transverse ridge of tissue placed between the two caval openings. This is the **intervenous tubercle** (*tuberculum intervenosum*). It diverts the converging inflowing blood from the two caval veins into the right ventricle. Just caudal to the intervenous tubercle on the medial wall of the atrium is a slitlike depression, the **fossa ovalis**, which varies from one to several millimeters in depth. Dias et al. (1979) summarize the appearance of the fossa ovalis in 77 adult dog hearts. All were translucent

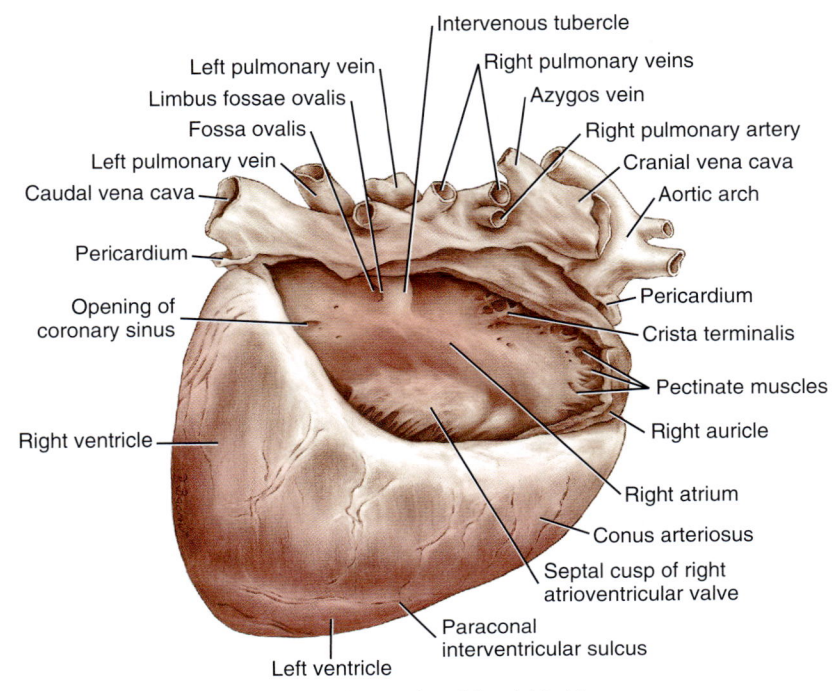

• **Fig. 11.6** The interior of the right atrium.

when illuminated, and the shape varied from piriform, which was most common, through triangular, elliptical, oval, kidney-shaped, and round. The crescent-shaped ridge of muscle that projects from the caudal side of the intervenous tubercle and deepens the fossa is the **limbus fossae ovalis**. In the fetus there is an opening at the site of the fossa, the *foramen ovale*, which allows blood to pass through the interatrial septum from the right to the left atrium. The foramen usually closes during the first few postnatal weeks. Even though a small anatomic opening frequently persists, it is closed physiologically because the obliquity of the foramen and the thin valve of the foramen ovale enable the greater pressure in the left atrium to close the passage. The *sinus venarum cavarum* is the smooth walled portion of the right atrium between the caval openings and the right atrioventricular opening. It is bounded by the interatrial septum and the crista terminalis.

The **right auricle** (*auricula dextra*) is the ear-shaped pouch of the right atrium that extends cranioventrally and to the left. Its apex is cranial to the pulmonary trunk. The internal surface of the wall of the right auricle is strengthened by freely branching, interlacing muscular bands, the pectinate muscles (*mm. pectincti*). These are also found on the lateral wall of the atrium proper. Most of the pectinate muscles radiate from a semilunar crest, a thick ridge of cardiac muscle, which is placed between the entrance of the cranial vena cava and the atrioventricular opening. This is the *crista terminalis*. It is also the dorsal separation of the sinus venarum cavarum and the auricle. On the external surface of a dilated heart, a poorly defined groove, the *sulcus terminalis*, lies opposite the crista terminalis at the ventral part of the junction of the cranial vena cava with the atrium. Small veins empty into the right atrium through openings in the pits between the pectinate muscles. Everywhere, the internal surface of the heart is lined with a thin glistening membrane, the *endocardium*.

The **left atrium** (*atrium sinistrum*) forms the left, dorsocaudal part of the base of the heart. The pectinate muscles are confined to its **left auricle** (*auricula sinistra*), which is similar to the right auricle in shape and structure. It projects ventrally on the midauricular surface and lies caudal to the conus arteriosus and pulmonary trunk. Its apex covers the proximal end of the paraconal interventricular groove. The conus arteriosus and pulmonary trunk separate the right and left auricles. Elsewhere on the surface of the heart there is no distinct indication of the separation of the two atria. Internally, the atria are separated by the **interatrial septum** (*septum interatriale*). Five or six openings (*ostia venarum pulmonalium*) mark the entrance of the pulmonary veins into the left atrium. The two or three veins from the right lung cross dorsal to the right atrium and open into the craniodorsal part of the chamber; the three veins from the left lung usually empty into its caudodorsal part. The veins from the caudal lobes are larger than the others and are most caudal in position. Frequently a thin concave flap of tissue is present on the cranial part of the septal wall. This is the **valve of the foramen ovale** (*valvula foraminis ovalis*). Often an irregularity of the smooth septal surface is the only remnant of where this valve closed and sealed.

Fibrous Base

The fibrous base of the heart, or "cardiac skeleton" (Fig. 11.7B), is the fibrous tissue, containing some cartilage, which separates the thin atrial musculature from the much thicker muscle of the ventricles. Only the special neuromuscular tissue, the atrioventricular bundle, extends continuously through the fibrous base from the atria to the ventricles. Baird and Robb (1950) have reconstructed the principal parts of the conduction system of a puppy's heart. Their dissections and reconstruction show the close spatial relationship that exists between the primary conduction and supporting tissues of the dog's heart. The cardiac skeleton is in the form of four narrow **fibrous rings** (*anuli fibrosi*), one surrounding each atrioventricular orifice, and two scalloped cuffs, or rings, one surrounding each arterial orifice. These provide attachment for the respective valves.

Of the two arterial rings, the **aortic fibrous ring** (*anulus fibrosus aorticus*) is the better developed. Peripherally the collagenous fibers that form it give way to the yellow elastic fibers composing the tunica media of the wall of the ascending aorta. There are three points on its aortic margin, each of which conforms to the attachments of two adjacent semilunar valvulae of the aortic valve. The projections between the attachments of the septal and right and the septal and left semilunar valvulae are best developed and are composed of hyaline cartilage. Between the points, the margin of the aortic fibrous ring is semilunar so that its scalloped circumference is in the form of three arcs. Between the aortic fibrous ring and the fibrous rings of the left and right atrioventricular rings, the fibrous base of the heart forms two triangular-shaped bundles of fibrous tissue. The **left fibrous trigone** (*trigonum fibrosum sinistrum*) is smaller than the right and lies in the triangle between the aortic and left atrioventricular ostia to the left of the right fibrous trigone. The **right fibrous trigone** (*trigonum fibrosum dextrum*) lies between the two atrioventricular ostia. Both trigones contain cartilage and are united through the medium of the opposed aortic and left atrioventricular fibrous rings. In the ox and horse the trigone ossifies in part. Sandusky et al. (1979) found that chondrocytes were common in the central fibrous body and root of the aorta and that bone had formed in the bundle of His in 8 of 40 dogs they examined.

The **pulmonary fibrous ring** (*anulus fibrosus pulmonalis*) is similar to the aortic ring. It serves for the attachment of the pulmonary semilunar valvulae, and distally it blends with the media of the pulmonary trunk. It is thinner than the aortic ring. The muscle fibers of the conus arteriosus attach to its *distal* ventral surface. Between the apposed surfaces of the pulmonary and aortic anuli there is a short mass of collagenous tissue, the **ligament of the conus**, which unites these two structures. Although ligament of the conus is not a term used in the *Nomina Anatomica Veterinaria* (NAV), it is described in human anatomy in reference

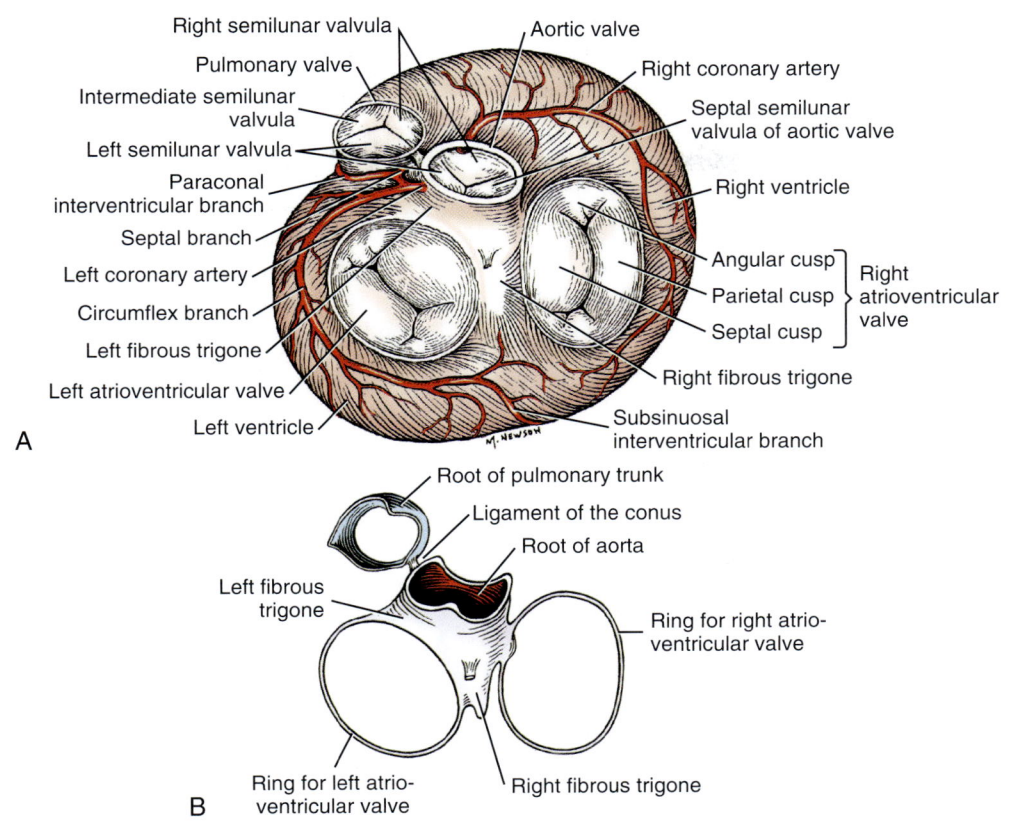

• **Fig. 11.7** The base of the heart. **A,** Atrioventricular, aortic, and pulmonary valves, craniodorsal aspect. **B,** The fibrous base of the heart, craniodorsal aspect.

to connective tissue spanning from the conus arteriosus to the base of the aorta, essentially connecting parts of the fibrous trigone.

The **atrioventricular fibrous rings** (*anuli fibrosi atrioventriculares*) (Fig. 11.7B) are thin rings of collagenous tissue to which the muscle fibers of the atrial and ventricular walls attach. From their endocardial edges emanate the atrioventricular valves. Although the proximal parts of the ventricular musculature attach to their *distal* ventral surfaces, the bulk of the fibers of this muscle at its origin lie peripheral to the rings as the muscle tissue bulges proximally after arising from them. These fibrous rings are so delicate they are best seen in longitudinal sections of the heart cut through the atrioventricular junctions.

Ventricles

The ventricles form the bulk of the heart. Together they form a conical mass, the apex of which is also the apex of the left ventricle. The right ventricle is dextral, ventral, and cranial to the left and arciform in shape (Fig. 11.8).

The **right ventricle** (*ventriculus dexter*) (Fig. 11.9) receives the systemic blood from the right atrium and pumps it to the lungs. Its outline is in the form of a curved triangle, as it is molded on the surface of the caudodorsally lying, conical-shaped left ventricle. It is crescentic in cross-section, and its long axis extends from the subsinuosal interventricular groove to the pulmonary trunk.

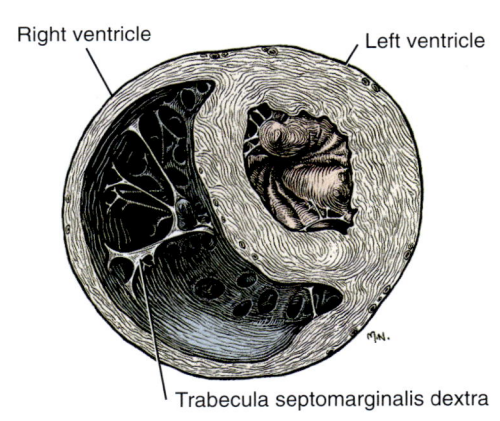

• **Fig. 11.8** Cross-section through the ventricles, craniodorsal aspect.

The large opening through which blood enters the right ventricle is the **right atrioventricular ostium** (*ostium atrioventriculare dextrum*) between the **cusps** of the right atrioventricular valve. Blood leaves the chamber through the **pulmonary trunk ostium** (*ostium trunci pulmonalis*) and is received by the pulmonary trunk. The **conus arteriosus** is the funnel-shaped part of the right ventricle. It is the outflow portion of the right ventricle at its left craniodorsal angle. It is bordered caudally by the left auricle and cranially by the right auricle. The **supraventricular crest** (*crista supraventricularis*) (Fig. 11.9A) is a blunt, obliquely placed ridge

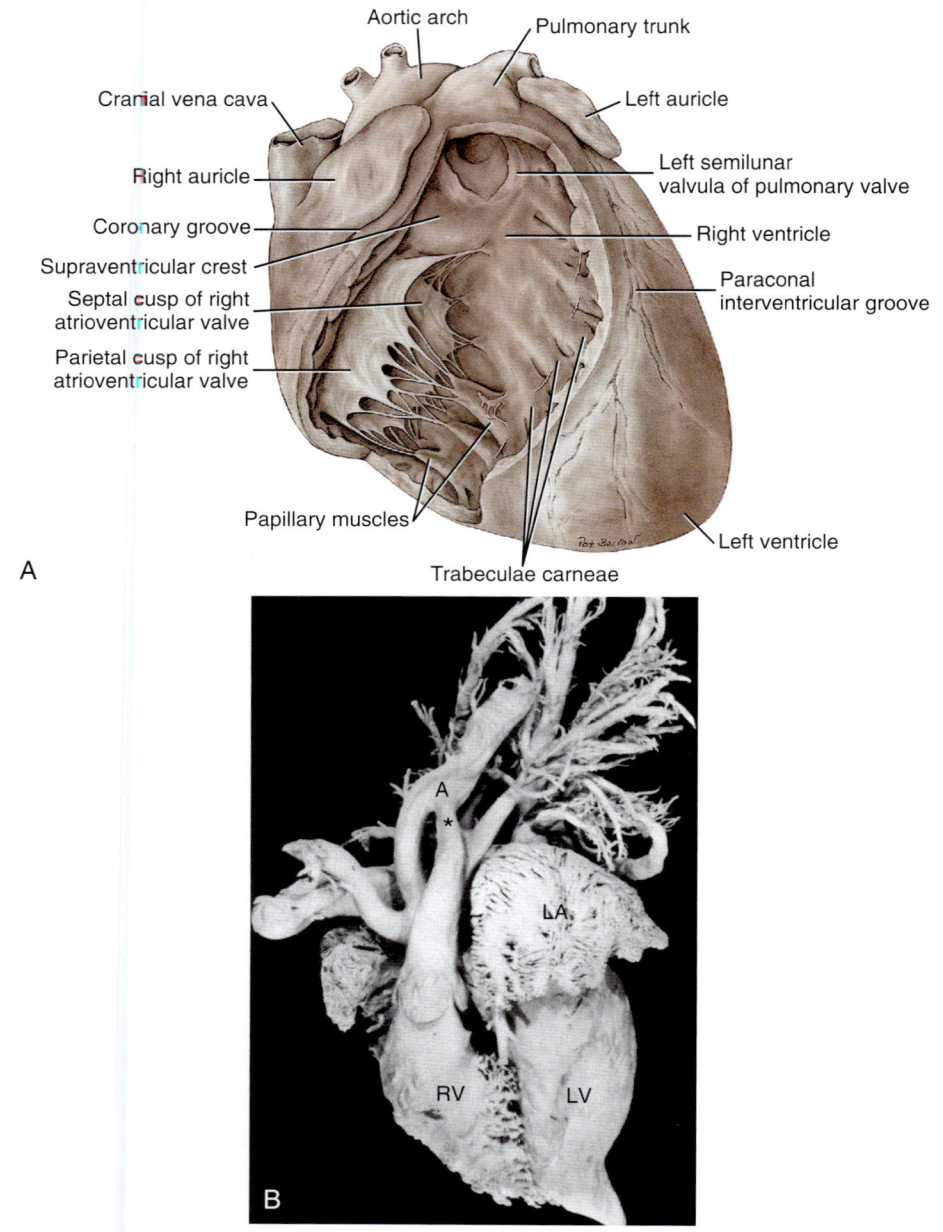

• **Fig. 11.9 A,** A dissection showing the interior of the right ventricle, ventral aspect. **B,** A latex cast of the heart and great vessels to show a patent ductus arteriosus (*) connecting the pulmonary trunk leaving the right ventricle (*RV*) to the aorta (*A*). The tuft of vessels in the upper right are pulmonary arteries. *LV,* Left ventricle; *LA,* left atrium.

of muscle between the origin of the conus arteriosus and the atrioventricular opening.

The interior of both ventricles contains muscular ridges and projections with small, usually deep and oblong depressions between. The conical-shaped muscular projections in each ventricle that give rise to the chordae tendineae are called **papillary muscles** (*musculi papillares*). They are the most conspicuous features of the ventricular walls. There are usually three main papillary muscles in the right ventricle, although great variation exists (see Fig. 11.9A). Typically they arise from the apical third of the septal wall, 1 to 3 cm from its junction with the outer wall. Their branched chordae tendineae, which prevent eversion of the valve, go to the free border and adjacent ventricular surface of the parietal cusp of the right atrioventricular valve. Commonly the papillary muscle that lies farthest cranial is larger than the others, and, when it is, its apex is usually bifid. The papillary muscle that lies farthest caudal may be bifid also. In such specimens the middle muscle is absent. A single compound papillary muscle may replace the three main ones. Other variations are common. Near the angle formed by the septal wall and the outer wall, and caudodorsal to the most caudal large papillary muscle, is a small, blunt to conical papillary muscle that gives rise to chordae tendineae

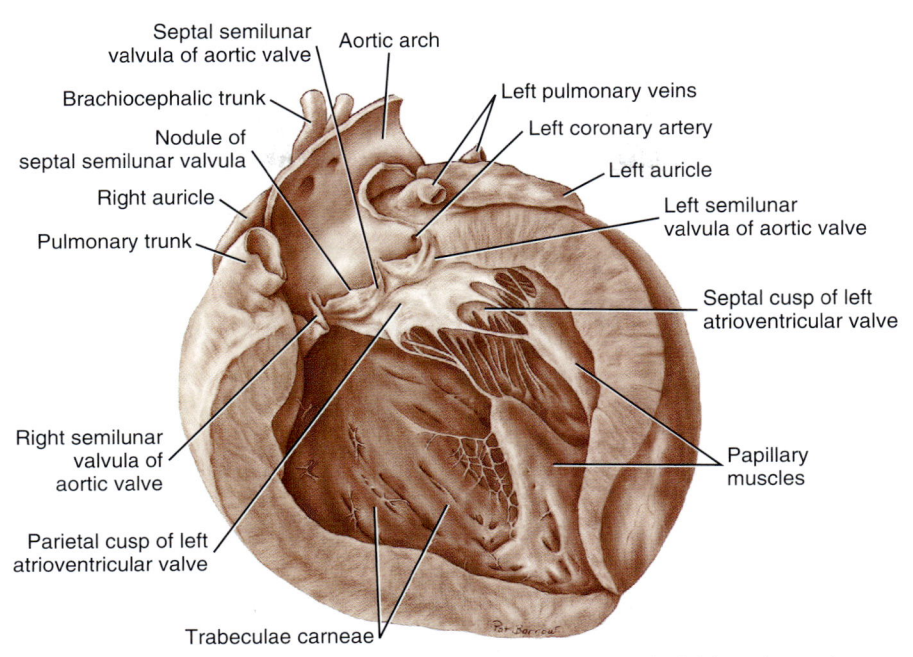

Fig. 11.10 A dissection showing the interior of the left ventricle, left lateral aspect.

going to the most caudodorsal part of the parietal cusp. Truex and Warshaw (1942), in the 12 dogs they studied, found only three large papillary muscles from the septum and a small constant papillary muscle of the conus. The numerous chordae tendineae that go to the septal cusp arise from the septal wall directly or from muscular ridges or papillae located peripheral to the septal cusp, when this valvula lies against the septum.

The *trabeculae carneae* are myocardial ridges that project into the lumen mainly from the outer wall of the ventricle. Because they are endocardial-covered portions of the deepest muscular layer of the right ventricle, their long axes parallel the directions of these fibers. They run from the base and converge toward the apex. Those on the septal wall are largely adjacent to the subsinuosal interventricular groove, and they largely parallel the axis of the heart. Some of the fossae coalesce near the subsinuosal interventricular groove so that muscular columns or pillars are formed.

The *chordae tendineae* are fibromuscular cords that arise from the apices of the papillary muscles or directly from smaller, blunter elevations on the wall. The cords branch, at their valvular extremity, as they approach the free border of the cusps. The smaller cords blend with the tunica media of these cusps at the points of their free borders, and the larger strands fan out on the ventricular surfaces of the cusps.

The *trabecula septomarginalis dextra* (see Fig. 11.8), formerly called *moderator band*, is a branched or single muscular strand that extends across the lumen of the right ventricle. It usually leaves the septal wall of the right ventricle near or from the base of the largest papillary muscle and runs to the outer wall. The extremity of the trabecula usually branches repeatedly as it blends with the muscular ridges of the outer right ventricular wall. It serves for the passage of cardiac conduction fibers from the right branch of the atrioventricular bundle across the lumen of the cavity. Instead of the usual single band, there may be two or more anastomosing strands forming a loose plexus.

The **left ventricle** (*ventriculus sinister*) (Fig. 11.10) is conical in shape, with its apex forming the apex of the heart. It receives the oxygenated blood from the lungs by way of the left atrium and pumps it to the body through the aorta. The **left atrioventricular ostium** (*ostium atrioventriculare sinistrum*) is the large opening between the left atrium and the left ventricle closed by the left atrioventricular valve. The **aortic ostium** (*ostium aortae*), located near the center of the base of the heart, is the opening from the left ventricle into the ascending aorta. The left ventricle is characterized by its thick wall, conical shape and two large papillary muscles. Its wall is three or four times thicker than that of the right ventricle. Truex and Warshaw (1942), in 12 specimens, found the mean thickness of the left and the right ventricle to be 13 and 4.2 mm, respectively.

The two large **papillary muscles** (*musculi papillares*) of the left ventricle come from its outer wall. They are thick, smooth rolls of myocardium, which have compound apices and give rise to the stout chordae tendineae of this chamber. The **subauricular papillary muscle** (*musculus papillaris subauricularis*) lies near the subsinuosal interventricular groove; the **subatrial papillary muscle** (*musculus papillaris subatrialis*) is closer to the paraconal interventricular groove. Adjacent to the subatrial papillary muscle, near its attachment, is a fine network of muscular strands that come from the septal wall. From findings in similar strands from other species (Truex & Warshaw, 1942), it is probable that these contain fascicles of cardiac conduction fibers derived from the left branch of the atrioventricular bundle en route to the subatrial papillary muscle and general ventricular musculature and represent the *trabeculum septomarginalis* *sinistrae.* The strand nearest the atrioventricular opening is larger than the others and extends obliquely to the subatrial papillary muscle from the septal wall. It may be the only one present. Near the apex of the ventricle some of the fine threads that compose this network extend under the endocardium that covers the crests of the muscular ridges. Other threads bridge the sulci between the larger trabeculae carneae in their courses to the subatrial papillary muscle. The chordae tendineae from the subatrial papillary muscle go to both the septal and the parietal cusps of the left atrioventricular valve. Those that go to the septal cusp are shorter and arise closer to the ventricular wall than those that go to the parietal cusp of the valve. The subauricular papillary muscle is separated from the subatrial papillary muscle by a deep cleft. The origin, course, and termination of the chordae tendineae from this muscle are similar to those of the chordae tendineae from the subatrial muscle. Both papillary muscles extend to within a few millimeters of the apex of the ventricle.

The **interventricular septum** (*septum interventriculare*) consists of an inconspicuous, small, proximally located membranous part and a large, thick muscular part. The **membranous part** (*pars membranacea*) of the interventricular septum is the thinnest part and is the last part of the septum to form embryonically. In the dog the membranous part can be seen by transmitted light under the septal cusp of the right atrioventricular valve adjacent to the origin of the aorta. When the foramen fails to close, a subaortic defect or interventricular foramen is left. The **muscular part** (*pars muscularis*), which constitutes the bulk of the interventricular septum, is formed by the myocardium of the combined walls of the two ventricles as they lie adjacent to each other.

Myocardium

The myocardium, or heart muscle of the atria and ventricles, is not divided into distinct layers, except at the interatrial septum. Here the deep fibers of the two chambers fold in and lie adjacent to each other, to form this partition, whereas the superficial fibers are common to both atria. Muscle fibers encircle the ostia of the systemic and the pulmonary veins as they empty into the atria. Between the pectinate muscles the musculature is so thin that the heart wall may be translucent at these places. The fixed point of the atrial musculature, like that of the ventricles, is the fibrous base of the heart. This excludes the atrioventricular bundle.

The musculature of the ventricles in the dog was described by Thomas (1957). There are superficial, middle, and deep layers. All muscle fasciculi of the superficial layer arise from the fibrous base and return to it. The superficial layer is common to both ventricles. When the heart is viewed from the base, these bundles run toward the apex, showing a clockwise twist. At the apex of the heart they turn in and run toward the base in such a manner that they cross, at right angles, the superficial fibers running ventrally. The superficial fibers penetrate the middle layer of the right ventricle to become its deep layer, after which they are disposed as on the left side. They form the papillary muscles. The middle layer forms the bulk of the ventricular walls. These are spiral or circular muscle masses that interdigitate between the two chambers. They primarily decrease the size of the lumen of the ventricles, and the superficial and deep layers shorten and twist the organ. The apex of the heart is quite thin, being formed by muscle fasciculi of the superficial layer of the left ventricle as they swirl in figure-of-eight fashion to form the apex of the chamber.

Atrioventricular Valves

The **atrioventricular valves** (*valvae atrioventriculares*) (Figs. 11.7, 11.9, and 11.10) are irregular, serrated cusps that are located in the atrioventricular ostia. They are the intake valves to the ventricles. They prevent blood from returning to the atria during the systolic phase of the heart beat. Peripherally, they attach to the fibrous rings that separate the musculature of the atria from that of the ventricles. When the ventricles contract, the valves are kept from being pushed into the atria by the chordae tendineae. The chordae tendineae attach to the ventricular surfaces of the valvulae. The largest cords can be followed as ridges under the endocardium to their attached borders, whereas the thinnest cords go to the points of the serrations and disappear. The medium-sized cords go as far as the middle part of the ventricular surfaces of the valvulae before blending with the stratum proprium. Although some blood vessels have been described in the valves adjacent to their attached borders, the bulk of the nutrition of the valves is derived from the free blood in the heart. Smith (1971) found a nerve network in the atrioventricular and semilunar valves of the dog that concentrated near the points of attachment of the chordae tendineae. Nerves composing the atrioventricular valve plexus were derived from the atrial subendocardial network. In general, the right atrioventricular valve was better innervated than the left atrioventricular valve.

The **right atrioventricular valve** (*valva atrioventricularis dextra*) in humans is also known as the *tricuspid valve*. Although Alves et al. (2008) found 2, 4, or 5 cusps in 68% of the 45 dogs they examined, the valve in the dog consists basically of two cusps. The cusp of the right atrioventricular valve that attaches to the fibrous ring adjacent to the septum is called the **septal cusp** (*cuspis septalis*). The cusp that attaches to the fibrous ring adjacent to the lateral or outer wall is the **parietal cusp** (*cuspis parietalis*). The extremities of these two cusps become narrower and merge or, in some specimens, small secondary cusps are formed at these sites. These are the **angular cusps** (*cuspis angularis*).

The **left atrioventricular valve** (*valva atrioventricularis sinistra*), also known in humans as the *bicuspid* or *mitral valve*, is basically similar to the right atrioventricular valve in form and structure, but it is made on a larger scale. The chordae tendineae as well as the papillary muscles from which they arise are several times larger in the left ventricle than they are in the right. This larger construction of the left intake valve, as compared with the right, is necessary, as the blood leaving the left ventricle through the aorta is under approximately four times more pressure than that which leaves the right ventricle through the pulmonary trunk. The division of the left atrioventricular valve into cusps is indistinct. The part that arises from the fibrous ring adjacent to the septum is the **septal cusp** (*cuspis septalis*). This is wider than the **parietal cusp** (*cuspis parietalis*) that comes from the remainder of the ring associated with the outer wall of the ventricle. When the valve is open and viewed from the atrial side it is tricuspid in appearance.

Aortic and Pulmonary Valves

The **aortic valve** (*valva aortae*) (Figs. 11.7 and 11.10) consists of **right**, **left**, and **septal semilunar cusps**, or valvulae (*valvulae semilunares dextra et sinistra et septalis*). These consist of a fibrous tissue stroma covered on each surface by endothelium. Opposite their free borders they are attached to the aortic fibrous ring. In the middle of the free borders of the semilunar cusps are **nodules** (*noduli valvularum semilunarium*). Extending from each nodule toward the periphery of the valvulae are the **lunulae** (*lunulae valvularum semilunarium*). These represent the areas of contact with the adjacent cusps when the valve is closed. The nodules close the space that would otherwise be left open by the coming together of the three contiguous arcs. On the vessel side, or peripheral to each of the semilunar cusps, the wall of the aorta is dilated to form the three **aortic sinuses** (*sinus aortae*). These, like the cusps, are right, left, and septal in position, with the right and left coronary arteries leaving the right and left sinuses. The widening of the base of the ascending aorta, formed by the aortic sinuses, is the **aortic bulb** (*bulbus aortae*). At the end of systole, or ventricular contraction, the pressure in the aorta is greater than that in the left ventricle, and a back pressure is developed that closes the valve and dilates the sinus. The coronary arteries leaving the sinus are affected by the changes in pressure. Boucek et al. (1964) described and illustrated the functional anatomy of the region of the aortic sinus, coronary ostia, and ascending aorta. They correlated their radiographs with different phases of the cardiac cycle and consider the rotation of the aorta during systole.

The **valve of the pulmonary trunk** (*valva trunci pulmonalis*) (Figs. 11.7 and 11.9) lies cranial and to the left of the aortic valve and is similar to it in construction. Because the blood pressure developed in the pulmonary trunk that it guards is not as great as that in the aorta, the development of the cusps and related structures is not as extensive. All parts present in the aortic valve are represented in the pulmonary valve. The valve of the pulmonary trunk consists of **right**, **left**, and **intermediate semilunar cusps**, or valvulae (*valvulae semilunares dextra et sinistra et intermedia*).

Innervation and Conduction System

A three-dimensional description of the distribution and organization of the canine intrinsic cardiac nervous system was developed by Yuan et al. (1994). They consistently found distinct epicardial ganglionated plexuses in four atrial and three ventricular regions, with occasional neurons being located throughout atrial and ventricular tissues in the 67 mongrel dog hearts studied. The first atrial plexus extended from the ventral to the dorsal surface of the right atrium, the second was located in the fat on the ventral surface of the left atrium, the third plexus was located on the mid-dorsal surface of the two atria, and the fourth extended from the base of the cranial vena cava to the dorsal caudal surface of both atria. Ventricular plexuses surrounded the origin of the aorta and extended along the coronary arteries. Pauza et al. (1999, 2002) reported similar results for the 36 mongrel dog hearts they examined. Ursell et al. (1990) showed that the sympathetic innervation of the heart developed progressively after birth and reached maturity by 2 months of age.

No part of the conducting system of a preserved dog's heart can be adequately identified in gross dissection without special preparation. The conducting system consists of three parts, which are closely integrated physiologically: (1) the sinoatrial node, (2) the atrioventricular node, and (3) the atrioventricular bundle. Baerg and Bassett (1963) described a method to stain the conduction tissue with palladium iodide. The sinoatrial and atrioventricular nodes are both associated with the septal wall of the right atrium.

The **sinoatrial node** (*nodus sinuatrialis*) appears to be the center that initiates the heartbeat and also regulates the interval between beats. It is located in the terminal crest at the confluence of the cranial vena cava, sinus venarum cavarum, and right auricular orifice. When it is destroyed experimentally, the heartbeat slows or stops. The sinoatrial node is composed of **cardiac conduction fibers** (*myofibra conducens cardiaca*) formerly known as *Purkinje fibers*. These fibers are little modified from those that compose the atrioventricular conduction system. Nonidez (1943) has shown that both the sinoatrial and the atrioventricular nodes are supplied by postganglionic parasympathetic nerve terminals.

The **atrioventricular bundle** (*fasciculus atrioventricularis*) begins as a mass of cardiac conduction fibers known as the **atrioventricular node** (*nodus atrioventricularis*). This is approximately 1.5 mm in diameter in the dog, according to Baird and Robb (1950), and shows little histologic differentiation from the bundle. Nonidez (1943) demonstrated that the atrioventricular node received a richer parasympathetic innervation than did the sinoatrial node. The atrioventricular node begins in the septal wall of the right atrium approximately 5 mm cranioventral to the opening of the coronary sinus and craniodorsal to the septal cusp of the right atrioventricular valve. From this apparently blind beginning, the atrioventricular bundle runs cranial and ventral through the fibrous base of the heart. As it does so it divides into right and left branches. These lie closely under the endocardium of the septal wall of the right and left ventricles. The right septal branch crosses the cavity of the right ventricle in the septomarginal trabecula of this chamber. It arborizes in the parietal ventricular wall of the right ventricle, where it ends. The left septal branch is more diffuse than the right one and partly traverses the cavity of the left ventricle in the left septomarginal trabeculae to the parietal wall of this chamber in bundles, which are smaller and more branched than those on the right side. The ramification of the conduction system of the heart is more complicated than the previous description indicates. Baird and Robb (1950) found that there were transitions from the atrioventricular node to the atrial muscle and that various parts of the atrioventricular bundle blended with the general ventricular musculature. Abramson and Margolin (1936) wrote that, in the dog, as in other species, the myocardial branches, as they leave the subendothelial plexus, tend to pass perpendicularly to the endocardium in the left ventricular wall and obliquely in the right ventricular wall. They further state that the interventricular septum is traversed by myocardial conduction fibers that arise from the adjacent subendothelial conduction fiber networks.

Racker (1989) was able to demonstrate at least three discrete atrioventricular bundles of myocardium that join the atrial end of the atrioventricular node via a proximal atrioventricular bundle. Her study was to determine the architecture of the atrioventricular junctional region, and she was able to confirm internodal tracts of myocardial fibers.

Halpern (1955) described the blood supply to the atrioventricular system of the dog heart. The interatrial septum is supplied by three arteries: two from the right coronary artery and one from the left. Anastomoses between these branches occur in the septum. The common bundle was supplied by the septal artery and dorsal left atrial artery; both are branches of the left coronary artery. The accessory ventral right atrial branch of the right coronary artery also participates.

Blood Vessels of the Heart

Coronary Arteries

The right and left coronary arteries and their branches supply the muscle of the heart. They arise from the aortic bulb immediately distal to the aortic valve. Higginbotham (1966) investigated the question of variation in coronary artery patterns between closely related pedigreed dogs and mongrels. The conclusion was that there is as much, if not more, variation in purebred dogs.

The **right coronary artery** (*a. coronaria dextra*) (Figs. 11.5 and 11.7A) is smaller than the left coronary artery and measures approximately 1.5 mm in diameter and 5 cm in length. It arises from the right sinus of the aorta and makes a sweeping curve to the right and ventrocranially, lying in the fat of the coronary groove. Its initial part is bounded by the pulmonary trunk and the conus arteriosus cranially and on the left, and dorsally it is covered by the right auricle. The right coronary artery supplies the bulk of the parietal wall of the right ventricle. As a result of ligation studies, Donald and Essex (1954) found that an average of 66% of the parietal right ventricular wall normally receives its blood through the right coronary artery. According to Kazzaz and Shanklin (1950), the right coronary artery rarely extends as far as the borders of the right ventricle and in no case goes beyond them. It also sends branches to the right atrium and small twigs to the initial parts of the aorta and pulmonary trunk. In 20% of specimens, according to Moore (1930), an **accessory right coronary artery** (*a. coronaria dextra accessoria*) arises closely adjacent to the main right coronary artery from the right sinus of the aorta and runs approximately 2 cm distally on the conus arteriosus, where it largely becomes dissipated.

According to Pianetto (1939), there are four to nine ventricular branches of the main right coronary artery. Most of these are small vessels that arborize on and in the right ventricular wall. Tanaka et al. (1999) quantified the branching patterns of intramural and epicardial vessels and found that a typical arterial segment divided into nearly two equivalent branches. They run at right angles to the long axis of the cavity, and none extends as far as the subsinuosal interventricular groove. One of these, the **right marginal branch** (*ramus marginalis dextra*), is larger, longer, and more branched than the others. It supplies the middle part of the right lateral ventricular wall.

The atrial branches from the right coronary artery are variable in development. Kazzaz and Shanklin (1950), Meek et al. (1929), Moore (1930), and Pianetto (1939) all describe an atrial branch, larger than the others, which leaves the distal half of the artery, traverses the sulcus terminalis and, as it does so, supplies the sinoatrial node. This vessel anastomoses with one or more atrial branches that arise from the circumflex branch of the left coronary artery. Usually one or two small atrial rami leave the right coronary artery both proximal and distal to the branch destined for the sinoatrial node. Mitsuoka et al. (1987) present a description of the technique for cannulation of the atrioventricular nodal artery and its anatomical variations in 30 dogs. The distal branches supply the caudal part of the right atrium adjacent to the coronary sulcus. A terminal twig ends on the caudal vena cava. The first branch or two that leave the dorsal surface of the right coronary artery supply the right auricle.

The normal anastomoses between the right coronary artery and adjacent vessels are small. In a corrosion cast study of hearts from normal dogs, Noestelthaller et al. (2005) found inter- and intraarterial anastomoses in 8 out of 31 of the hearts that they studied.

The **left coronary artery** (*a. coronaria sinistra*) (Figs. 11.3 through 11.5, 11.7A, and 11.11) is a short trunk approximately 5 mm long and nearly as wide. It always terminates in the circumflex and paraconal interventricular branches and, in many specimens, in a septal branch also. Noestelthaller et al. (2007) characterize three types of divisions: Type I, in which the short trunk divides into circumflex, paraconal interventricular, and septal branches at the same point; Type II, in which the septal branch comes off the paraconal interventricular branch; and Type III, in which the paraconal interventricular branch originates independently from the aortic sinus.

The **circumflex branch** (*ramus circumflexus*), approximately 1.5 cm in diameter, lies in the coronary groove as it

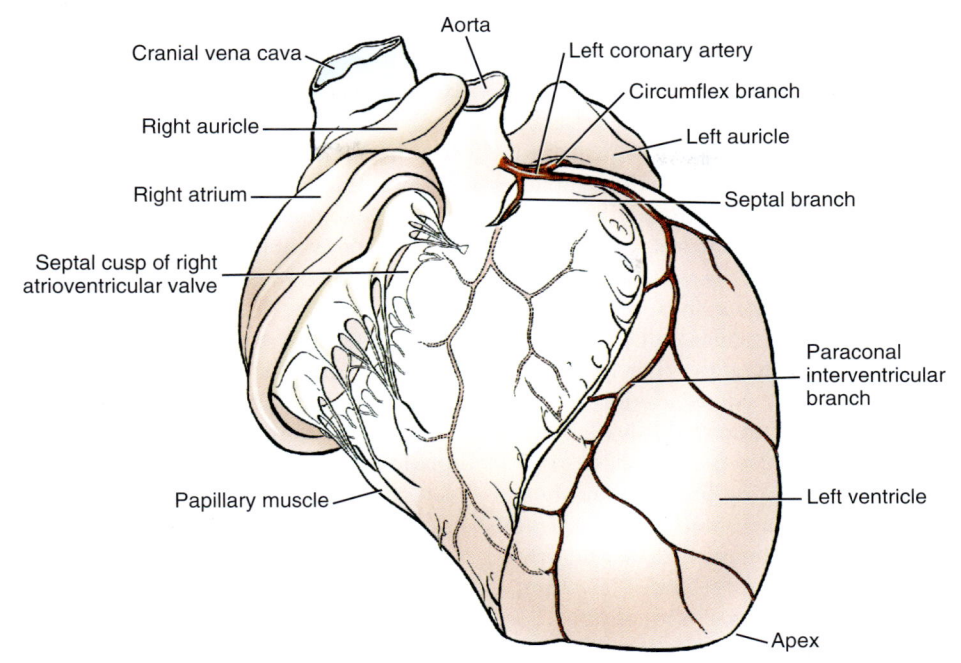

• **Fig. 11.11** Branches of the left coronary artery, ventral aspect. The right ventricle and pulmonary trunk have been removed.

extends to the left, then winds dorsocaudally and to the right across the caudodorsal surface of the heart. On reaching or approaching the subsinuosal interventricular groove, it turns toward the apex of the heart and is known as the *subsinuosal interventricular branch*. The combined length of the circumflex and subsinuosal interventricular branches is approximately 8 cm. The circumflex branch has ventricular and atrial branches.

According to Kazzaz and Shanklin (1950), there are 4 to 11 ventricular branches. Pianetto (1939) found two to six principal ventricular branches. Most of the hearts had five main ventricular branches leaving the circumflex branch, but great variation was found. When the left ventricular branches of the paraconal interventricular branch are well developed, they are a major source of supply to the parietal wall of this chamber, and the ventricular branches of the circumflex branch are confined to a triangular area adjacent to the coronary and subsinuosal interventricular grooves. When the first or first few branches of the circumflex branch cross the superficial muscle fibers of the left ventricle obliquely, they are short; they are much longer when they parallel the superficial muscle fibers as well as the left ventricular branches of the paraconal interventricular vessel. Usually the longest branch leaving the circumflex branch lies adjacent and parallel to the subsinuosal interventricular branch. This is appropriately known as the **left marginal branch** (*ramus marginalis sinister*) as it follows the left border ventrally on the surface of the left ventricle.

The atrial branches of the circumflex branch of the left coronary artery, which supply the left atrium and auricle, are small and variable. The first branch arises deep to the great coronary vein and, extending dorsally and toward the center of the base of the heart, supplies the deep surface of the left atrium and the ventral part of the interatrial septum. It is the largest of the right atrial branches and, according to Meek et al. (1929) its terminal branches may partly encircle the termination of the cranial vena cava, where they anastomose with the right atrial vessel to the sinoauricular node. It may be the main source of supply to this node. At least two other small branches cross the lateral surface of the great cardiac vein or the coronary sinus and supply the right atrium.

The **subsinuosal interventricular branch** (*ramus interventricularis subsinuosus*) is a continuation of the circumflex branch in or near the poorly defined subsinuosal interventricular groove. It is more than 1 mm wide and approximately 3.5 cm long, and has left, right, and septal branches. It is shorter than the paraconal interventricular branch, as its terminal branches usually end at approximately the junction of the middle and distal thirds of the ventricular mass. They may reach to the apex of the heart or even extend beyond around it. Usually three or four branches supply the adjacent musculature of the left ventricle, and usually five or six larger and longer branches arborize in the adjacent part of the right ventricle. The septal branches supply a narrow zone of the interventricular septum adjacent to the subsinuosal interventricular groove.

The **paraconal interventricular branch** (*ramus interventricularis paraconalis*) is approximately the same diameter as the circumflex branch, and averages 1.5 mm in width. It is approximately 7 cm long as it winds obliquely and distally from left to right across the right ventricular border of the heart in the paraconal interventricular groove. It usually extends around the apex of the heart (Christensen, 1962). It has left ventricular, right ventricular, and septal branches.

The **left ventricular branches** are long and large. Usually there are seven, which in general decrease in size toward the apex. As they largely parallel the superficial muscle fibers of the left ventricle, they lie in grooves on its surface. Usually the branch that arises near the end of the proximal third of the parent vessel is longer than the others and supplies the apex of the heart. Most of the left ventricular branches are quite free of superficial collateral branches.

The **right ventricular branches** (*rami ventriculares dextri*), usually five in number, supply a strip, approximately 2 cm wide, of the right parietal ventricular wall adjacent to the paraconal interventricular groove. The first branch is prominent as it partly encircles the conus arteriosus adjacent to the origin of the pulmonary trunk. This is the conal branch. It anastomoses with the conal branch of the right coronary artery. Most of the remaining branches are short and form small anastomoses with the branches of the right coronary artery and the subsinuosal interventricular branch.

The **septal branch** (*ramus septalis*) (Figs. 11.7A and 11.11), as found by Donald and Essex (1954) in the 125 specimens they studied, arose as follows:
1. Paraconal interventricular branch, 48%
2. As one of the three terminal branches of the left coronary artery, 27%
3. Left coronary artery, 19%
4. Aorta, 5%
5. Circumflex branch, 1%

Immediately after entering the interventricular septum, the septal branch usually runs obliquely toward the apex of the heart, giving off major and minor branches along its course. Initially it runs obliquely to the right ventricular side of the septum. In this course it may parallel the right atrioventricular fibrous ring as it lies under the endocardium adjacent to the dorsal half of the septal cusp of the right atrioventricular valve. The first half of the artery lies deep to the endocardium of the right ventricle; the second half penetrates deeply into the septum. It supplies all the main papillary muscles of the right ventricle. Wilson and Scheel (1989), using gradual Ameroid occlusion of the circumflex branch, demonstrated that the septal branch is a significant source of intramyocardial collaterals to other coronary branches in young dogs. According to Donald and Essex (1954), the septal branch supplies 70% to 75% of the interventricular septum. These authors and many others have found that the anastomoses between the septal branch and the adjacent arteries of the canine heart are not sufficiently large or numerous to permit retrograde filling of the septal branch with injected dye. The subsinuosal and paraconal interventricular branches supply the periphery of the interventricular septum. The paraconal vessel contributes much more blood than does the subsinuosal vessel (Christensen & Campeti, 1959).

Hyde and Buss (1986) examined the transmural microvasculature adjacent to the papillary muscles of the left ventricle to address the question of whether a transmural gradient in components of the coronary microvasculature exists in the dog heart. Their results suggest that transmural differences in coronary blood flow are not due to transmural structural differences but rather to physiologic regulatory mechanisms of coronary blood flow.

Cardiac Veins

The **cardiac veins** (*venae cordis*), although in many instances satellites of the arteries to the heart, do not take the names of the comparable vessels. Most of the blood to the heart is returned to the right atrium by a short, wide trunk, the coronary sinus. Some of the ventral cardiac veins and the smallest cardiac veins (Thebesian) open into the cavities of the heart directly. Truex and Angulo (1952) demonstrated that the tributaries of the coronary sinus form an extensive venous plexus in the left ventricle and septum, which is predominant compared with corresponding branches of the left coronary artery. They found that the coronary sinus and cardiac veins provided continuity with the capillary bed of the myocardium. The coronary sinus had anastomoses with cardiac veins, myocardial sinuses, and Thebesian vessels that provided outlets to the lumen of the right atrium. Esperanca-Pina et al. (1981) studied 47 dog hearts using an injection-corrosion-fluorescence technique to visualize the superficial cardiac veins draining the coronary sinus. They noted a large number of Thebesian veins in the subendocardium of the interventricular septum (as imagined by Galen) and all of the cardiac chambers except the internal wall of the left atrium.

The **coronary sinus** (*sinus coronarius*) (Figs. 11.3 and 11.6) is the dilated terminal end of the great coronary vein. It is approximately 2 cm long and 5 to 8 mm in diameter. It lies in the fat of the dorsodextral part of the coronary groove ventral to the caudal vena cava and dorsal to the terminal part of the circumflex branch of the left coronary artery. It opens into the right atrium ventral to the termination of the caudal vena cava. It may be partly covered by a few muscle fibers derived from the left atrium. This small, inefficient semilunar **valve of the coronary sinus** (*valvula sinus coronarii*) is located at the termination of the coronary sinus. Piffer et al. (1994) found a valve between the great cardiac vein and the coronary sinus in 4 out of 34 dog hearts they studied.

In 40 dogs studied, Maric et al. (1996) found the tributaries to the coronary sinus highly variable, with the great and middle cardiac veins the main and constantly present tributaries. The **great cardiac vein** (*v. cordis magna*) (Figs. 11.3 and 11.4) lies in the dorsal part of the coronary groove as it circles the caudal surface of the heart from the left. It arises near the apex of the heart and ascends toward the base in the paraconal interventricular groove, where it is usually paired. Along its course it collects numerous veins from the ventricles and small twigs from the left atrium. Most of those from the ventricles are paired, in that a vein lies on each side of the comparable artery. At its termination in the coronary sinus the diameter of the passage increases threefold, according to Meek et al. (1929). At this place two veins usually enter the great cardiac vein or the coronary sinus. The larger branch, which may not be paired, ascends from near the apex of the heart and is known as the **dorsal**

vein of the left ventricle (*v. dorsalis ventriculi sinistri*). It is the largest vein draining this chamber. Frequently a smaller vein, the **oblique vein of the left atrium** (*v. obliqua atrii sinistri*), can be seen entering the coronary sinus dorsally after emerging from deep to the pulmonary veins (see Fig. 11.3). Its importance lies in the fact that, like the coronary sinus, it is a vestige of the embryonic left common cardinal vein. It may persist as a left cranial vena cava (Fig. 12.3), or it may be nonpatent.

The **middle cardiac vein** (*v. cordis media*) (Fig. 11.5) ascends in the subsinuosal interventricular groove in company with or near the subsinuosal interventricular artery. It is a large paired vessel that collects tributaries from both ventricles and empties into the coronary sinus near its termination. Near the apex of the heart, where the subsinuosal and paraconal interventricular grooves merge, the middle and great coronary veins sometimes anastomose.

The **right cardiac veins** (*vv. cordis dextrae*) consist of several rather long, narrow vessels, which may not be paired as they ascend to the ventral part of the coronary groove from the right ventricle. They usually open into the right atrium directly.

Thebesian Veins

Thebesian veins are microscopic channels of venule size that open into every chamber of the heart and, within the myocardium, anastomose with both the coronary artery branches and other cardiac veins. It is possible that when gradually occluding lesions develop, the blood may flow in a retrograde direction in these valveless veins, which hypertrophy, to provide nourishment for the affected part. Pina et al. (1975) studied the Thebesian veins of the heart in 48 dogs using a corrosion fluorescence method. They found five types of terminations: arborform, sinuous, brushlike, canaliculated, and stellate. Although these small cardiac veins are found in the walls of all chambers of the heart, they are most often found in the right ventricle (81% of dogs) and right atrium (77% of dogs).

Pulmonary Arteries and Veins

Pulmonary Trunk

The **pulmonary trunk** (*truncus pulmonalis*) (Figs. 11.2, 11.3, 11.4, 11.9, and 11.10) and its branches are the only arteries in the body that carry unaerated venous blood. The trunk arises from the pulmonary fibrous ring at the conus arteriosus and, after a course of approximately 4 cm, it divides into the right and left pulmonary arteries. At the conus arteriosus the trunk is flanked by the right and left auricles. Farther out on the trunk, but still within the fibrous pericardium, fat usually masks the true length and position of the intrapericardial part of the vessel. The cranial, lateral, and caudal surfaces of the proximal three-fourths of the vessel are covered by serous pericardium and fat. The distal fourth of the vessel serves for the attachment of the fibrous pericardium and can be examined without opening the pericardial cavity. The pulmonary trunk, along its entire medial surface, contacts the aorta. The two vessels form a slight spiral as they obliquely cross each other. The *ligamentum arteriosum* (Fig. 11.3) is a connective tissue remnant of the fetal ductus arteriosus, which arises from the pulmonary trunk near the bifurcation of the pulmonary trunk and passes to the aorta.

Everett and Johnson (1951) studied the closure of the ductus arteriosus in the dog and found that it remains patent, to a variable degree, for a considerable time after birth. Some reduction in flow occurred 1 to 2 hours after birth, and more marked reduction occurred at 9 hours postpartum. Anatomic obliteration of the slitlike opening was complete at 15 to 18 days postpartum. House and Ederstrom (1968) found that the ductus arteriosus was open in all puppies at less than 4 days of age and did not close anatomically until they were 7 or 8 days of age. For radiographic aspects of patent ductus, see Buchanan (1972). A latex cast of a patent ductus arteriosus in an adult dog is shown in Fig. 11.9B.

The **right pulmonary artery** (*a. pulmonalis dextra*) (Figs. 11.3, 11.5, and 11.6) is approximately 2 cm long and 1 cm in diameter. It leaves the pulmonary trunk at nearly a right angle and runs to the right, where at first it is in contact with the concavity of the arch of the aorta and later with the right bronchus that is dorsal to the artery. It lies obliquely across the base of the heart between the cranial and caudal venae cavae. Its first lobar branch enters the right cranial lobe of the lung, **right cranial lobar branch** (*ramus lobi cranialis*). Approximately 1 cm distal to the origin of this branch the vessel divides into a **middle lobar branch** (*ramus lobi medii*) and a **caudal lobar branch** (*ramus lobi caudalis*) that provide numerous vessels that supply the middle, caudal, and accessory lobes of the right lung.

The **left pulmonary artery** (*a. pulmonalis sinistra*) (Figs. 11.3 and 11.4) is shorter and slightly smaller in diameter than the right artery. It is partly covered dorsally at its origin by the left principal bronchus. The artery then passes obliquely across the pulmonary vein coming from the cranial lobe and divides unevenly into two or more branches. The smaller branch or branches enter the cranial part of the cranial lobe, **left cranial lobar branch** (*rami lobi cranialis*). The large **caudal lobar branch** (*rami lobi caudalis*) enters the bulk of the left lung, where it subdivides and supplies the caudal part of the cranial lobe and the caudal lobe of the lung. The relations of the pulmonary arteries within the lungs are described in Chapter 8, Respiratory System.

Pulmonary Veins

The **pulmonary veins** (*vv. pulmonales*) are valveless and return aerated blood from the lungs to the left atrium. Unlike the pulmonary arteries, the pulmonary veins from each of the lobes of the lungs as a rule retain their separate identity to the heart. An exception to this is frequently found in the veins from the right caudal and accessory lobes, which fuse just before entering the atrium. Often, the vein from the left caudal lobe joins the venous trunk from the right side that results in a single opening in the left atrium, thus serving for the return of the blood from the right and left caudal and accessory lobes. Other variations are common. Frequently, two veins may enter the heart directly from one of the lobes. Usually, however, several veins converge and empty into the heart by a single vessel, which ranges between a few millimeters to approximately 1.5 cm in length. In medium-sized dogs, all pulmonary veins are more than 5 mm in diameter as they enter the heart. The pulmonary veins may be divided into the right pulmonary veins (*vv. pulmonales dextrae*) from the right lung, and the left pulmonary veins (*vv. pulmonales sinistrae*) from the left lung. The pulmonary veins within the lungs are described with the intrinsic structure of the lungs in Chapter 8.

Systemic Arteries

Aorta

The aorta leaves the left ventricle near the center of the base of the heart (Figs. 11.3 and 11.7A). It is a thick-walled vessel through which all the systemic blood of the body passes. All of the large systemic arteries arise directly from it. For descriptive purposes, it may be divided into an ascending and a descending portion, separated by the aortic arch. The initial part attaches to the fibrous base of the heart, is largely located within the pericardium, and is known as the **ascending aorta** (*aorta ascendens*). It is approximately 2 cm long before it makes a U-turn dorsocaudally and to the left as the **aortic arch** (*arcus aortae*). The remainder of the aorta, from the arch to its terminal iliac branches, is the **descending aorta** (*aorta descendens*). The descending aorta may be divided further into a **thoracic part** (*aorta thoracica*) and an **abdominal part** (*aorta abdominalis*).

The ascending aorta, at its origin, is slightly expanded to form the **bulb of the aorta** (*bulbus aortae*). Peripheral to each of the three semilunar cusps that form the aortic valve are the **sinuses of the aorta** (*sinus aortae*). The aggregate of the sinuses forms the bulb of the aorta. The coronary arteries arise from the aortic bulb. Their distribution is described with the heart.

The normal development of the heart and aortic arches in several domestic animals is discussed by Krediet (1962) in a thesis on anomalies of the arterial trunks in the thorax.

Aortic Arch

Arteries of the Head, Neck, and Thorax

The blood supply of the head and neck and the thoracic limbs leaves the aorta through two great vessels arising from the aortic arch, the brachiocephalic trunk and the left subclavian artery.

Brachiocephalic Trunk

The **brachiocephalic trunk** (*truncus brachiocephalicus*) (Fig. 11.12), the first large artery from the aortic arch, passes obliquely to the right and cranially across the ventral surface of the trachea. It is approximately 4 cm long and 8 mm in diameter. The left common carotid artery is the first branch to leave the brachiocephalic trunk. Frequently, a small branch leaves the brachiocephalic trunk close to the heart to aid in the supply of the thymus and pericardium. Jarvis and Nell (1963) have described various origins of a tracheoesophageal branch of the brachiocephalic trunk and a less frequent thymopericardial branch that have caused difficulties in experimental surgery of the great vessels and esophagus. The brachiocephalic trunk terminates in the right common carotid and the right subclavian arteries. This termination is medial to the first rib or first intercostal space of the right side.

Common Carotid Arteries (Box 11.1). The **common carotid arteries** (*aa. carotides communes*) (Figs. 11.12 through 11.14) arise from the brachiocephalic trunk approximately 1 cm apart. Of 123 dogs examined, the right and left common carotids arose from the brachiocephalic trunk by a common trunk in four specimens. The interval between the origins of the common carotids varies from 15 to less than 1 mm. When a **bicarotid trunk** (*truncus bicaroticus*) is formed, it usually arises from the brachiocephalic trunk approximately 2 cm distal to its origin from the aorta opposite the first intercostal space or second rib.

The **left common carotid artery** (*a. carotis communis sinistra*) usually arises opposite the vertebral end of the second rib and ventral to the trachea. Its relations are similar to those of the right vessel as it traverses the neck, except that it is on the left side and is loosely bound to the esophagus dorsomedially by the deep cervical fascia. Its branches and termination are similar to those of the right vessel, which is described here.

The **right common carotid artery** (*a. carotis communis dextra*) diverges from the left and obliquely crosses the ventrolateral surface of the trachea as it runs toward the head. Throughout the neck it lies in the angle formed by the longus colli or longus capitis muscles dorsally, the trachea ventromedially, and the cleidocephalicus and sternocephalicus

---

BOX 11.1 Branches of the Common Carotid, Internal Carotid, and External Carotid Arteries

Common carotid artery:
    Caudal thyroid artery
    Cranial thyroid artery
Internal carotid artery
External carotid artery:
    Occipital artery
    Cranial laryngeal artery
    Ascending pharyngeal artery
    Lingual artery
    Facial artery
    Caudal auricular artery
    Parotid artery
    Superficial temporal artery
    Maxillary artery

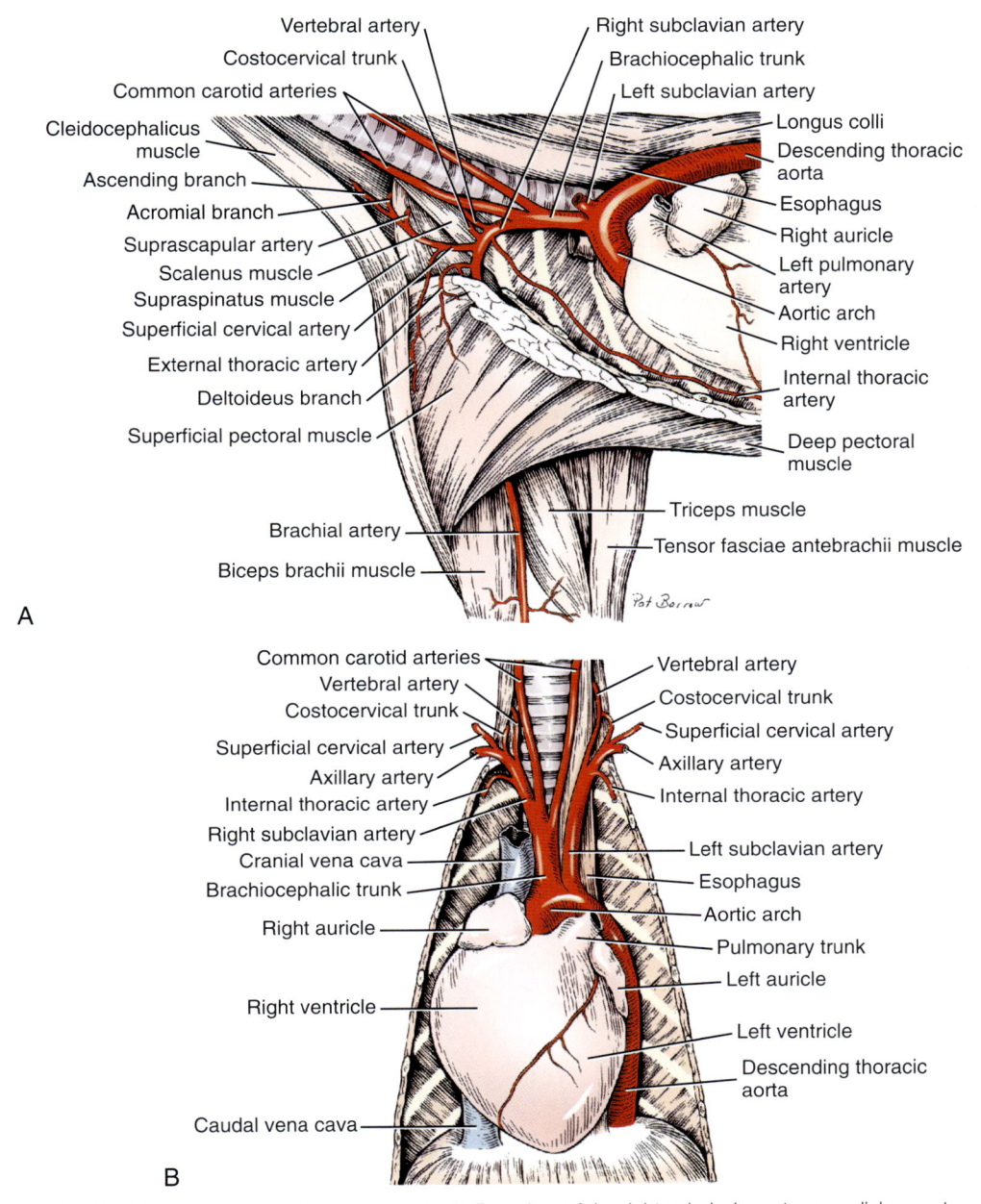

Fig. 11.12 The aortic arch and great vessels. **A**, Branches of the right subclavian artery, medial aspect. **B**, The heart and great vessels, in situ, ventral aspect.

muscles laterally. At the thoracic inlet the vagosympathetic nerve trunk becomes associated with the dorsal surface of the artery and remains bound to it during its course through the neck (Fig. 15.4). The internal jugular vein is also associated with the common carotid artery in the middle half of the neck. The fascia that binds these structures together and attaches them rather loosely to adjoining parts is the **carotid sheath** (*vagina carotica*). It is a part of the loosely developed prevertebral cervical fascia. The common carotid artery terminates at or near a transverse plane through the body of the basihyoid bone by dividing into internal and external carotid arteries. The internal carotid artery, much smaller than the external one, leaves the medial side of the parent vessel and immediately runs through the deep st

ructures of the head to the skull and brain (Fig. 11.14). The external carotid artery is the main supply to either half of the head.

The **caudal thyroid artery** (*a. thyroidea caudalis*) (see Fig. 11.13) is a small vessel that usually arises from the brachiocephalic trunk between the origins of the common carotid arteries. It is not constant in its origin; it may arise from the brachiocephalic trunk, the left subclavian artery, the common carotid arteries or the ascending branch of the superficial cervical artery. It occasionally comes from the costocervical trunk on the right side. The most common origin is in the form of a short trunk from the brachiocephalic trunk, giving rise to the right and left caudal thyroid arteries, which run cranially toward the respective thyroid glands. They lie on the trachea and in contact with the respective borders of the esophagus. Branches from the caudal thyroid arteries are freely supplied to the esophagus, trachea, middle cervical ganglia, and nerves in the region of the thoracic inlet. They anastomose with the larger cranial thyroid arteries.

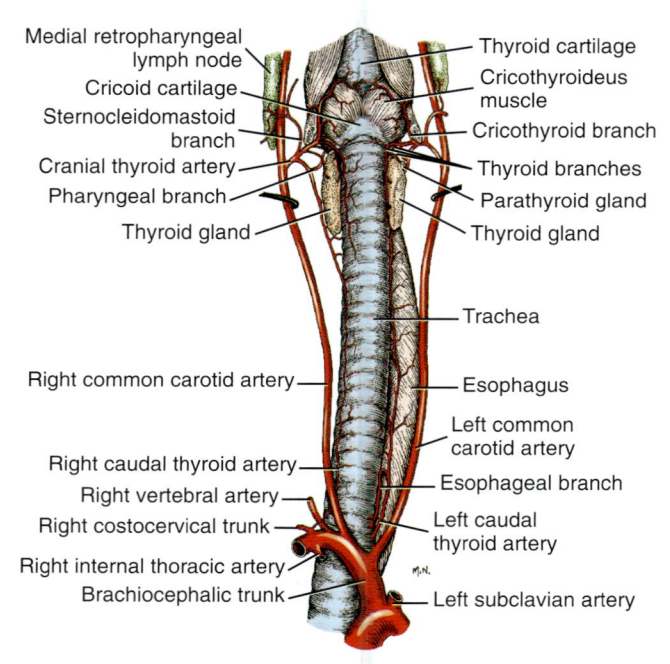

- **Fig. 11.13** The relation of the common carotid arteries to the larynx, trachea, and related structures, ventral aspect.

The **cranial thyroid artery** (*a. thyroidea cranialis*) (Fig. 11.13) is a short vessel that arises from the common carotid artery opposite the caudal part of the larynx. It is the largest and the only constantly present branch of the common carotid artery. In addition to branches that supply the thyroid gland, the cranial thyroid artery has the following branches: pharyngeal, caudal laryngeal, cricothyroid, and sternocleidomastoid. The branches vary in distribution and constancy. Frequently the thyroid branches and the pharyngeal and cricothyroid branches come directly from the common carotid artery as two separate trunks.

The **thyroid branches** (*rr. thyroidei*) are those that run in a caudal direction to the thyroid gland. Their number and location vary; usually, however, several branches enter the dorsal and ventral borders of the gland from its middle to the cranial pole and diverge as they ramify on its lateral and medial surfaces. Thus, the blood supply to the thyroid gland may be divided into dorsal and ventral groups of vessels. One branch, usually from the dorsal group, and more often larger than the others, extends from the cranial pole of the thyroid gland caudally past the dorsal border of the gland. This branch continues caudally in association with the recurrent laryngeal nerve and anastomoses with the caudal thyroid artery, giving off esophageal and tracheal branches along its course. When the caudal thyroid artery is well developed, the cranial vessel is reduced in a reciprocal ratio. In specimens with well-developed caudal thyroid arteries, most of the cervical parts of the trachea and esophagus are supplied by them. The esophageal branches are larger from the left cranial and caudal thyroid arteries.

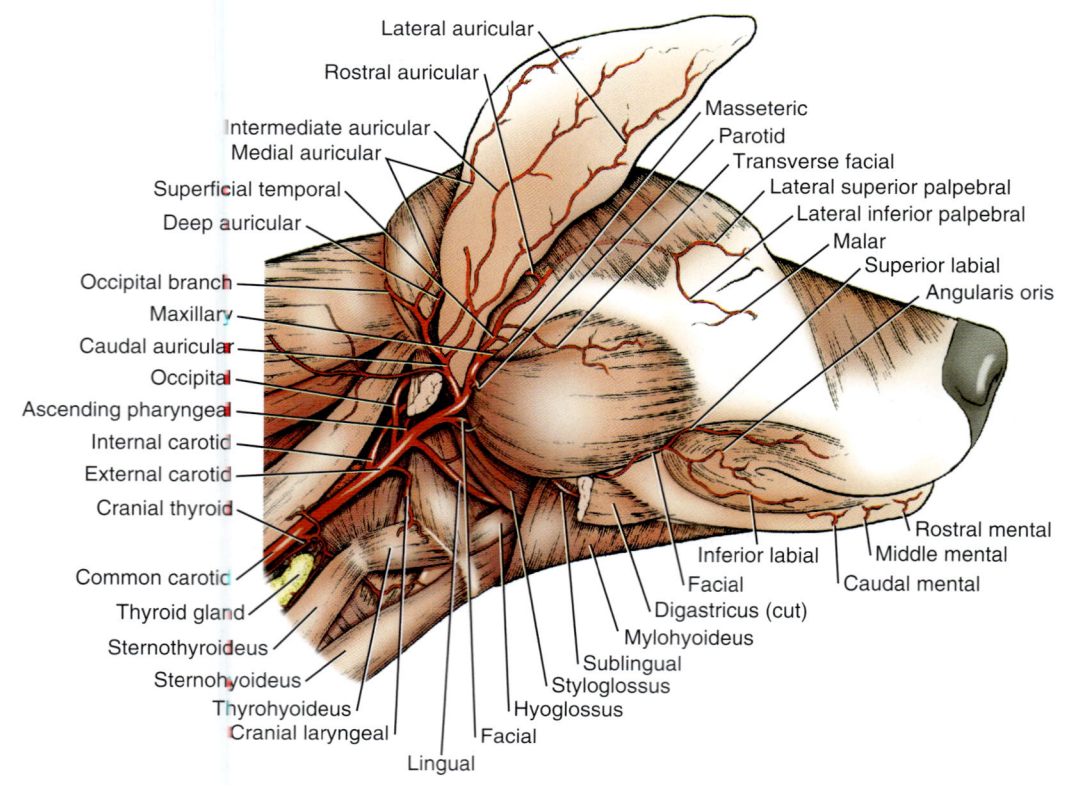

- **Fig. 11.14** Branches of the common carotid artery, lateral aspect.

The **caudal laryngeal branch** (*r. laryngeus caudalis*) runs cranially into the caudal aspect of the larynx with the caudal laryngeal nerve.

The **pharyngeal branch** (*r. pharyngeus*) leaves the cranial side of the cranial thyroid artery, or it may leave in common with one of the thyroid branches. It is the smallest of the branches of the cranial thyroid artery. It runs obliquely dorsocranially and supplies branches to the beginning of the esophagus and continues cranially to supply the constrictor muscles of the pharynx.

The **cricothyroid branch** (*r. cricothyroideus*) is a freely branching vessel that leaves the cranial thyroid artery and runs cranioventrally over the cricothyroid muscle. Branches go to the sternohyoideus, sternothyroideus, thyrohyoideus, and cricothyroideus muscles. End-branches go through the cricothyroid membrane to the mucosa of the caudal compartment of the larynx, where they anastomose with the cranial laryngeal artery. Right and left vessels anastomose on the cricothyroid membrane.

The **sternocleidomastoid branch** (*r. sternocleidomastoideus*) courses dorsolaterally to both parts of the m. sternocephalicus and the mastoid part of the m. cleidocephalicus. Only small parts of these muscles are supplied by these branches. The cranial thyroid artery also sends branches to the capsule of the mandibular salivary gland and mandibular and medial retropharyngeal lymph nodes. A large branch may go to the longus capitis and longus colli muscles. This usually comes from the external carotid vessel near its origin, as described in the discussions of the muscular branches of that vessel.

The common carotid artery terminates in a small internal carotid and large external carotid artery on the dorsolateral surface of the pharyngeal constrictor muscles.

External Carotid Artery. The **external carotid artery** (*a. carotis externa*) (Figs. 11.14 through 11.16) is the main continuation of the common carotid to the head. It is approximately 4 cm long and forms a sigmoid flexure as it winds its way deep to the caudal portion of the hypoglossal nerve, mandibular salivary gland, and digastric muscle. It is bounded deeply by the muscles of the larynx and pharynx.

The **occipital artery** (*a. occipitalis*) (Figs. 11.14 and 11.16) is most frequently the first branch of the external carotid artery. It may, however, arise in the angle formed by the splitting of the common carotid into the external and the internal carotid arteries. In some dogs it arises an appreciable distance distal to the origin of the external carotid artery, and therefore it will be regarded as a branch of this vessel. It is slightly smaller than the internal carotid artery, measuring approximately 1.5 mm in diameter. In general, the vessel takes a tortuous course dorsally, its terminal branches anastomosing with those of its fellow. This occurs caudal to the external occipital protuberance in the epaxial muscles of the neck. The vessel initially runs dorsocranially, being crossed laterally by the hypoglossal nerve and medially by the internal carotid artery. A larger structure, which bears important relations to the initial part of the vessel, is the medial retropharyngeal lymph node, lying caudal and partly lateral to the vessel. The boundary, craniolaterally, is the digastric muscle, and medially the last four cranial nerves, although the accessory nerve may lie lateral to it. Usually the first 15 mm of the occipital artery is free of branches. When it reaches the condyloid fossa, several branches arise. The vessel then forms an arc around the caudal surface of the paracondylar process, courses along the nuchal crest, and runs to the median plane dorsally. In this location it is covered by the occipital part of the sternocephalicus, splenius, obliquus capitis cranialis, and the semispinalis capitis muscles. The branches of the occipital artery are occasionally a ramus to the cranial pole of the medial retropharyngeal lymph node, a condyloid artery, a cervical ramus, a descending ramus, and an occipital ramus with a caudal meningeal artery.

The **condyloid artery** (*a. condylaris*) may arise from the cervical branch of the occipital or directly from the occipital artery. Its branches enter the cranial cavity through the hypoglossal canal and the combined tympanooccipital fissure and jugular foramen. These branches dissipate in the dura at the ventral end of the petrosal part of the temporal bone. It supplies branches to the middle and inner ear. A branch goes to the digastricus before the vessel enters the fissure.

The **cervical branch** is the second branch of the occipital artery. It usually is a short trunk that arises medial to the paracondylar process and dorsolateral to the last four cranial nerves. One branch descends ventral to the wing of the atlas, where it lies close to the bone and supplies the atlantooccipital joint capsule. It also supplies parts of the rectus capitis ventralis, obliquus capitis cranialis, longus capitis, and rectus capitis lateralis muscles. Some branches end by forming a feeble ventral anastomosis with the vertebral artery. Others enter minute foramina on the ventral surface of the atlas in the region of the transverse foramen. An ascending branch runs medial to the last four cranial nerves as they leave the skull. It sends minute branches to these nerves, as well as to the cranial cervical ganglion and the two ganglia on the glossopharyngeal and the vagus nerves. The main muscular branch continues cranially past these ganglia and ends primarily in the longus capitis and rectus capitis ventralis muscles. Some branches go to the mucosa of the roof of the pharynx, where they anastomose with the ascending pharyngeal artery.

The **descending branch** is the largest branch of the occipital artery. It is nearly as large as the continuation of the parent vessel. A branch enters the origin of the m. digastricus from the proximal end of the descending branch or from the occipital artery directly. The descending vessel takes origin approximately 3 mm from the cervical branch and goes directly ventral to the m. obliquus capitis cranialis to the alar notch of the atlas. Here it becomes associated with the ventral division of the first cervical spinal nerve and the vertebral artery and vein. The vertebral artery is several times larger than the descending branch of the occipital artery. An anastomosis between the two vessels occurs. The descending branch continues dorsomedially in the m.

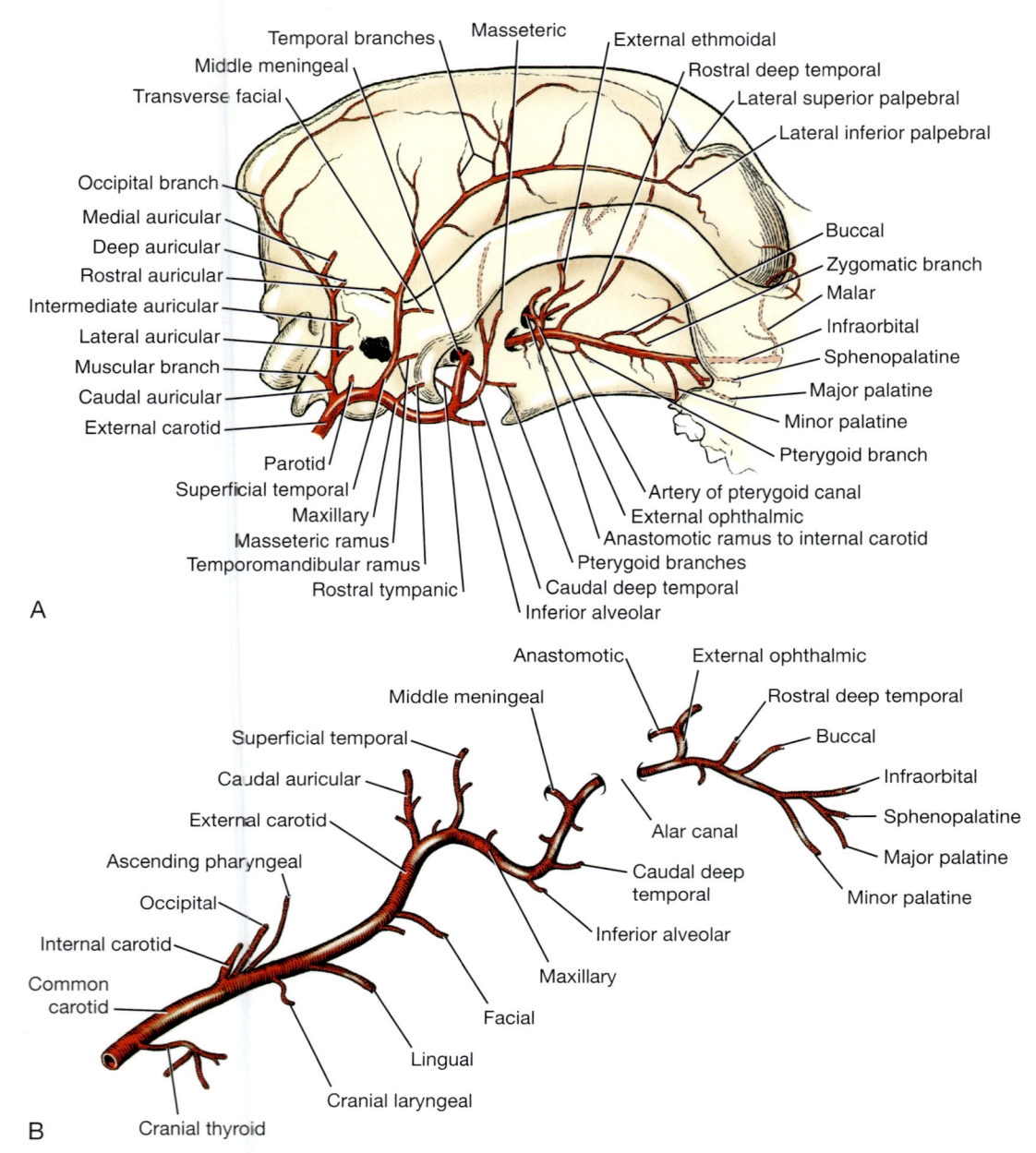

Fig. 11.15 Arteries of the head in relation to lateral aspect of the skull. (Part B from Evans, H.E. & de Lahunta, A. (2017). Guide to the Dissection of the Dog. 8th ed., Elsevier.)

obliquus capitis caudalis, the cranial part of which it supplies. It also supplies the cranial part of the epaxial muscles of the head including the m. semispinalis capitis.

The **occipital branch** (*ramus occipitalis*) is the continuation of the occipital artery beyond the descending branch. The **caudal meningeal artery** (*a. meningea caudalis*) leaves the occipital branch as the occipital courses along the nuchal crest of the occipital bone. This is approximately 1 cm from the base of the paracondylar process. The vessel is approximately 0.7 mm in diameter, and the extracranial part is 5 mm long. It goes through the mastoid foramen and ramifies in the dura of the dorsocaudal cranial cavity. Some branches supply the tentorium cerebelli just dorsal to the petrosal part of the temporal bone.

From the m. digastricus to the mid-dorsal line, where the occipital artery anastomoses with its fellow, numerous branches arise. Most of these are dissipated in the muscles that attach to the caudal surface of the skull. Some, however, ramify in the temporal muscle and the caudal auricular musculature, where they anastomose with branches of the caudal auricular artery.

The **cranial laryngeal artery** (*a. laryngea cranialis*) (Figs. 11.14 and 11.19) is usually the second branch of the external carotid artery, arising ventrally nearly opposite the occipital artery. Sometimes this vessel, which is less than 1 mm in diameter, arises from the common carotid artery at its termination. Near its origin it supplies one or two small branches to the mastoid part of the sternocephalicus

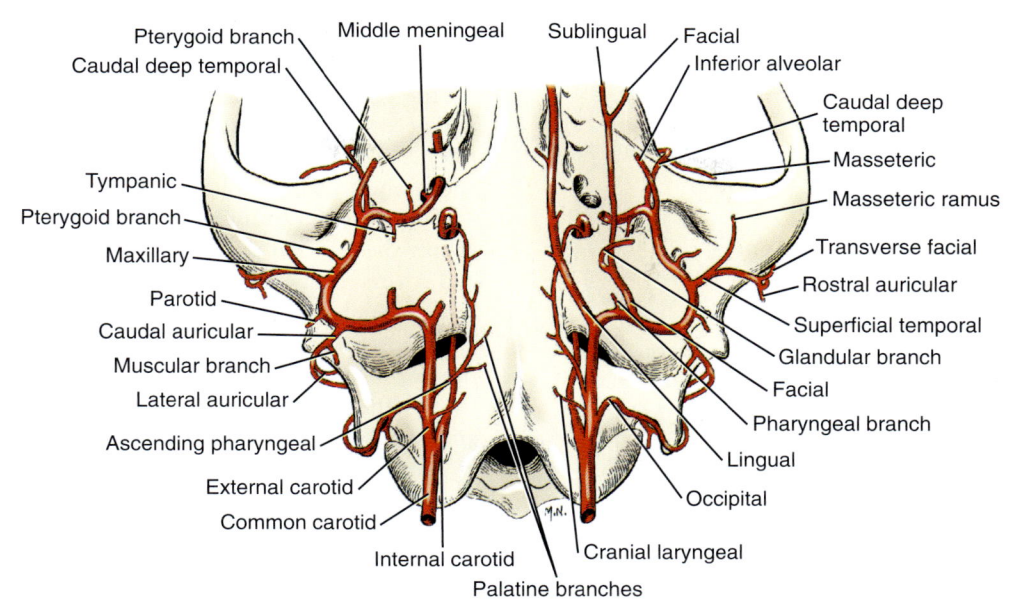

• Fig. 11.16 Branches of the common carotid artery in relation to the ventral aspect of the skull.

muscle. A **pharyngeal branch** (*r. pharyngeus*) runs dorsally and supplies the dorsal portions of the cricopharyngeal, thyropharyngeal, and hypopharyngeal muscles. The main continuation of the vessel, the **laryngeal branch** (*r. laryngeus*), runs ventrally with the cranial laryngeal nerve over the surface of the larynx and disappears in the triangle formed by the mm. thyrohyoideus, thyropharyngeus, and hyopharyngeus. It perforates the thyrohyoid membrane and supplies most of the mucosa and intrinsic muscles of the larynx. Cranial branches have been found that supply the m. hyoglossus in which they may anastomose with the lingual artery. Caudally and ventrally, branches ramify in the m. thyrohyoideus, where an anastomosis occurs with the cricothyroid branch of the cranial thyroid artery.

A **muscular branch**, slightly less than 1 mm in diameter, frequently leaves the dorsal surface of the external carotid artery at its origin. Usually this origin is in the same transverse plane as the origin of the occipital artery. It runs directly to the ventral surface of the m. longus capitis, on which it arborizes. Its most caudal branches also supply the m. longus colli. In many specimens, the branch just described arises from the cranial thyroid artery or by a short trunk with the ascending pharyngeal artery.

The **ascending pharyngeal artery** (*a. pharyngea ascendens*) (Figs. 11.14 and 11.16) is a small, freely branching vessel that arises from the external carotid artery in common with or close to the occipital artery. When the relatively large muscular branch to the m. longus capitis and m. longus colli arises here, instead of from the cranial thyroid artery, it also may be closely related to the ascending pharyngeal artery or arise in common with it. Thus, from a medial origin, the ascending pharyngeal artery runs dorsomedially on the pharyngeal constrictor muscles medial to the tympanic bulla. The pharyngeal branch of the vagus nerve is the only nerve to cross its medial surface. The artery extends as far rostrally as the foramen lacerum, where its terminal branch anastomoses with the loop of the internal carotid artery. Its branches are the palatine and pharyngeal.

The **palatine branches** (*rr. palatini*) are a few small branches that leave the initial part of the ascending pharyngeal artery. They run ventrally in the lateral wall of the pharynx to the soft palate, where they supply the extensive palatine glands, and the palatine mucosa and muscles. These branches anastomose with their fellows, as well as with the tonsillar branch of the lingual artery.

The **pharyngeal branches** (*rr. pharyngei*) are distributed to the musculature and mucosa of the cranial part of the pharynx as well as to the ventral axial muscles, mainly the m. longus capitis. The main ascending pharyngeal artery lies external to the pharyngeal musculature directly against the tympanic bulla. It sends many branches to the cranial part of the roof and sides of the pharynx. After giving origin to these, the artery continues to the foramen lacerum. Here an unusual vascular occurrence takes place. The internal carotid artery, after having traversed the carotid canal, forms a loop that fills the foramen lacerum. The ascending pharyngeal artery ends by anastomosing with the internal carotid loop.

The **lingual artery** (*a. lingualis*) (Figs. 11.14, 11.16, 11.17, and 11.19) is usually the largest collateral branch of the external carotid artery. It leaves the parent trunk just medial to the digastric muscle, runs rostroventrally in company with the hypoglossal nerve, and enters the tongue medial to the hyoglossal muscle, and lateral to the m. genioglossus. The hypoglossal nerve does not accompany the vessel during its initial intramuscular course but runs lateral to the hyoglossal muscle. After a course of approximately 4 cm in this location, the nerve usually crosses the medial surface of the lingual artery and then, in contact with its dorsal surface, extends to the apex of the tongue. At the root of the tongue two or more branches are given off the

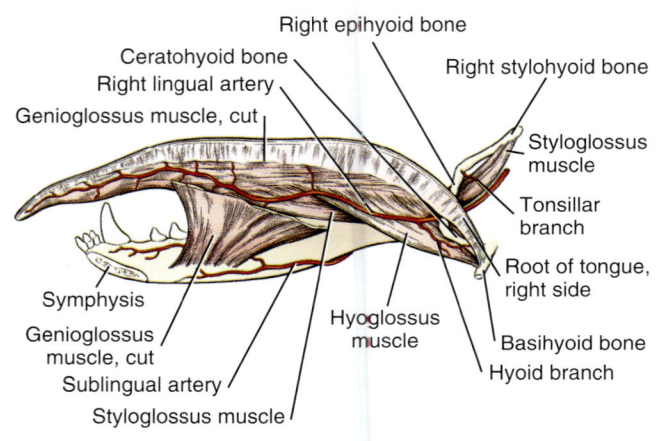

Fig. 11.17 Lingual and sublingual arteries, medial aspect.

lingual artery, which can be traced to the hyoid and pharyngeal muscles and the palatine tonsil. These are the ascending palatine and perihyoid branches. The **ascending palatine artery** (*a. palatina ascendens*) supplies the root of the tongue, the soft palate and the adjacent pharynx. The **perihyoid branches** (*rami perihyoidei*) supply structures around the hyoid bones and the palatine tonsil. The **tonsillar branch** leaves the dorsal surface of the lingual artery opposite the lateral surface of the ceratohyoid bone and runs dorsally rostral to it. In its course dorsocaudally, it perforates the styloglossal muscle to become related medially to the pharyngeal mucosa. The vessel then enters the tonsil near its middle by three or more minute branches. Small branches from the hyoid branches of the lingual artery enter the caudal end of the tonsil and anastomose with the tonsillar branch from the lingual artery. The branches from the caudally lying hyoid branches may be the major supply of the palatine tonsil. The **deep lingual artery** (*a. profunda linguae*) is the rostral continuation of the lingual artery into the tongue on the lateral surface of the genioglossus. Its branches are destined for the supply of the muscles of the tongue. The artery lies near the midline, near the ventral part of the organ. The lingual vein accompanies the artery only in its rostral third. The vein lies in a more ventral and superficial position than the artery in the remainder of the organ. According to Prichard and Daniel (1953), arteriovenous anastomoses occur in the tongue of the dog. The lingual and sublingual arteries anastomose in the tongue.

The **facial artery** (*a. facialis*), (see Figs. 11.14, 11.16, 11.19, and 11.21) is approximately 3 cm long and 1.5 mm in diameter. It arises near the angle of the mandible, 1 cm from the lingual artery, and for the first centimeter is bounded medially by the styloglossal muscle; it then runs rostrally superficial to the stylohyoid muscle. The masseter muscle is related to it dorsally and laterally, and the m. digastricus lies ventral to it. The artery runs rostrally, but its deviation from the horizontal depends on the degree of closure of the mouth. The facial artery gives rise to glandular and muscular branches before its first large collateral branch, the sublingual artery, arises. It terminates in the face as labial arteries. Irifune (1980) has provided a detailed description of the branches and distribution of the facial artery in Japanese dogs.

The **glandular branch** (*r. glandularis*) is the largest but not necessarily the first branch to leave the initial part of the facial artery. It is the main supply to the mandibular and monostomatic sublingual salivary glands.

The **muscular branches** are usually two small vessels that supply the adjacent parts of the digastric, medial pterygoid, and, occasionally, the styloglossal muscles. The largest of these branches is smaller than the glandular branch and arises rostral to it. A branch may supply a small patch of mucosa in the region of the caudal pole of the palatine tonsil. The branch to the mucosa, when present, usually anastomoses with the ascending pharyngeal artery.

The **sublingual artery** (*a. sublingualis*) (Figs. 11.16 and 11.17) arises from the facial artery medial to the ventral part of the body of the mandible, in the depths of a deep cleft that is bounded laterally by the m. masseter, medially by the caudal part of the m. mylohyoideus, and ventrally by the m. digastricus. The sublingual artery parallels the medial surface of the mandible near its ventral border and is distributed largely to the m. mylohyoideus and the rostral belly of the digastric muscle, although some branches perforate the m. mylohyoideus and supply the genioglossus and geniohyoideus muscles. It is accompanied by a satellite vein and the mylohyoid nerve and anastomoses with the lingual and inferior labial arteries. Near the middle of the body of the mandible, the **submental artery** (*a. submentalis*) is given off the sublingual artery or it arises from the facial artery proximal to this. The submental artery runs to the ventral surface of the intermandibular suture, supplying this region and the inferior incisor teeth. Other branches are distributed to the muscles and mucosa in the region of the frenulum of the tongue.

After the origin of the sublingual artery, the facial artery courses ventrally on the medial side of the body of the mandible and crosses its ventral border to the lateral side, where it lies between the m. masseter dorsally and the termination of the m. digastricus ventrally. The facial artery continues rostrally to emerge deep to the m. platysma to give rise to the inferior labial artery, angular artery of the mouth, and superior labial arteries.

The **inferior labial artery** (*a. labialis inferior*) (Fig. 11.21) arises approximately 1 cm from the ventral border of the mandible rostral to the masseter muscle. As it runs rostrally, it lies along the ventral border of the m. orbicularis oris. Some fibers of this muscle may actually cover the artery during its course rostrally. At the caudal mental foramen it anastomoses with the caudal mental branch of the inferior alveolar artery. The inferior labial artery sends branches across the ventral border of the mandible that anastomoses with the sublingual artery.

The **angular artery of the mouth** (*a. angularis oris*) arises from one to several centimeters distal to the origin of the inferior labial artery. It takes a rather tortuous course to the commissure of the lips, where usually one branch extends to the superior and the other to the inferior margin. The angular artery of the mouth supplies in part the m. buccinator, m. orbicularis oris, and the skin and mucosa of this region. It anastomoses with the superior and inferior labial arteries, and may anastomose with mental branches.

The **superior labial artery** (*a. labialis superior*) is the termination of the facial artery and ramifies on the cheek and nose. Small branches may extend dorsally to the orbit and anastomose with the terminal branches of the lateral inferior palpebral and malar arteries; others run rostrally in the m. orbicularis oris and anastomose with the lateral nasal artery. Fine branches that follow the buccal nerves caudally anastomose with those of the masseter artery, a branch of the maxillary artery that runs rostrally. The superior labial artery supplies mainly the orbicularis oris and levator nasolabialis muscles.

The **caudal auricular artery** (*a. auricularis magna*) (Figs. 11.14 through 11.16) arises at the base of the annular cartilage from the dorsocaudal surface of the external carotid artery. In some dogs its origin from the external carotid artery is more proximal near the origin of the lingual artery. It circles around the caudal half of the base of the ear. It is a medium-sized vessel, which at first lies deep to the parotid salivary gland, then is located more dorsally deep to the caudal auricular group of muscles. For convenient exposure of the origin of the caudal auricular artery, it is necessary to remove the digastric muscle that lies lateral to it. Its branches may vary considerably in origin and disposition. They are the stylomastoid, parotid, sternocleidomastoid, lateral auricular, intermediate auricular, medial auricular, occipital, and deep auricular arteries or branches.

The **stylomastoid artery** (*a. stylomastoidea*) is the smallest branch of the caudal auricular artery. It leaves the caudoventral surface of the vessel and runs directly to the stylomastoid foramen in company with the facial nerve, which it supplies. Sometimes the vessel is double. It is located directly caudal to the osseous external acoustic meatus.

The **parotid branch** (*r. parotideus*) goes to the parotid and mandibular salivary glands. It may not arise directly from the caudal auricular artery but from its sternocleidomastoideus or lateral auricular branches. The mandibular branches enter the dorsal surface of the mandibular salivary gland; the parotid branches enter the deep surface of the parotid salivary gland. Some dogs have a parotid branch of the caudal auricular artery to supply the parotid salivary gland and a glandular branch of the sternocleidomastoideus branch for the mandibular salivary gland.

The **sternocleidomastoideus branch** (*r. sternocleidomastoideus*) consists of one or two large vessels that supply the conjoined tendons of the mastoid parts of the cleidocephalic and sternocephalic muscles. They also supply the skin, platysma, and subcutaneous fat, and finally anastomose with the superficial cervical artery. A muscular branch located at a deeper level runs deep to the sternocephalic and cleidocephalic muscles and supplies the cranial end of the splenius muscle. Occasionally, branches supply the medial retropharyngeal lymph node and a **glandular branch** (*ramus glandularis*) supplies the mandibular salivary gland.

The dorsal deep part of the muscular branch anastomoses with the occipital artery.

The **lateral auricular branch** (*r. auricularis lateralis*) arises from the caudal auricular artery or the muscular branch to the m. splenius or from the intermediate auricular branch. It is a large artery that branches as it passes through or in contact with the caudal border of the parotid salivary gland. It extends distally on the caudal surface of the auricular cartilage, near its lateral border. It usually extends beyond the cutaneous pouch 1 cm or more and terminates by anastomosing with the intermediate auricular branch.

The **intermediate auricular branch** (*r. auricularis intermedia*) is the largest artery to the ear. It arises approximately 1 cm distal to the lateral auricular branch deep to the caudal auricular muscles. During its initial course toward the apex of the ear, it sends branches to the caudal auricular muscles. After emerging, it sends many anastomosing branches both laterally and medially over the auricular cartilage. Many small branches pass through foramina in the auricular cartilage to its concave surface.

The **deep auricular artery** (*a. auricularis profunda*) usually arises independently from the caudal auricular artery distal to the origin of the intermediate auricular branch. Occasionally, it arises from the intermediate or medial auricular branch. It is a small vessel that runs distally approximately 2 cm and passes through the space between the tragus and the anthelix to supply part of the dermis of the cartilaginous external acoustic meatus.

The **medial auricular branch** (*r. auricularis medialis*), which is approximately the same size as the lateral auricular branch, arises approximately 1 cm from the considerably larger intermediate auricular branch. It crosses the caudal part of the temporal muscle medial to the external ear. At the scutiform cartilage, it becomes subcutaneous and continues along the medial border of the auricular cartilage to within 2 cm of the apex of the ear. It anastomoses freely with the intermediate auricular branch and the rostral auricular branch of the superficial temporal artery. Branches also perforate the cartilage and extend around its margin to supply the fascia and dermis of the concave surface.

The **occipital branch** (*r. occipitalis*) is the main distal continuation of the caudal auricular artery after the auricular branches are given off. It enters the caudal part of the temporal muscle and at first nearly parallels the nuchal crest. It supplies a large caudal part of the temporal muscle and finally anastomoses with the caudal deep temporal artery. Branches from this or a separate vessel from the caudal auricular artery also supply parts of the caudal auricular muscles and anastomose with the ascending cervical branch of the superficial cervical artery.

The **parotid artery** (*a. parotis*) (Figs. 11.14 through 11.16) is a small vessel that arises 5 to 15 mm distal to the origin of the caudal auricular artery. It arises from the dorsal surface of the external carotid artery as this artery crosses the ventral end of the annular cartilage. The parotid artery may arise from the caudal auricular artery. Thus the vessel arises deep to the parotid gland and immediately enters and freely branches in the gland. Although the periphery of the parotid gland is supplied by parotid rami from adjacent vessels, such as the caudal auricular and superficial temporal arteries, its main supply in the dog is the parotid artery. This vessel sends branches to the facial nerve and the most dorsal mandibular lymph node, and it may supply the skin.

The external carotid artery terminates in the superficial temporal and maxillary arteries.

The **superficial temporal artery** (*a. temporalis superficialis*) (Figs. 11.14 through 11.16) is the smaller of the two terminal branches of the external carotid artery. Its diameter is approximately 1.5 mm, compared with 4 mm for the maxillary artery, the other terminal branch. It arises rostral to the base of the auricular cartilage and at first extends dorsally. As it crosses the zygomatic arch, it makes a sweeping curve rostrally and, approximately 1 cm dorsal to the arch, it dips deep to the thick deep temporal fascia. During part of its subsequent course toward the eye, it actually lies in the temporal muscle. Fahie et al. (1998) describe a subcutaneous location of the artery as it continues rostrally from the caudal aspect of the zygomatic arch. Opposite the orbital ligament the superficial temporal artery perforates the deep temporal fascia and divides into its two terminal branches, which lie in the superficial fascia. The branches of the superficial temporal artery are a masseteric branch and transverse facial, rostral auricular, inferior lateral palpebral, and superior lateral palpebral arteries.

The **masseteric branch** is a relatively large branch, usually more than 1 mm in diameter, which arises from the rostral side of the superficial temporal artery near its origin or from the maxillary artery directly. Hidden by the parotid salivary gland, it runs rostrally and enters the deep surface of the masseter muscle, where it passes rostroventrally between the muscle and the masseteric fossa. Usually several other fine branches arise from the vessel and supply other structures. In approximately half of the specimens, they come off separately from the superficial temporal artery close to the masseteric branch. Some branches enter the parotid salivary gland and parotid lymph node. Others run rostrally on the face with the dorsal and ventral buccal branches of the facial nerve and anastomose with arterial branches of the superior labial artery. Other branches supply the skin and occasionally the temporomandibular joint capsule.

The **transverse facial artery** (*a. transversa faciei*) is no larger than the nutrient branches that accompany the buccal branches of the facial nerve. It usually arises distal to the masseteric branch when present, from the rostral border of the superficial temporal artery. It emerges from deep to the parotid salivary gland, usually after the artery has divided. One branch follows the zygomatic branch of the auriculopalpebral nerve from the facial nerve toward the eyelids. The other runs parallel and ventral to the zygomatic arch in company with the auriculotemporal nerve from the mandibular nerve of the trigeminal nerve.

The **rostral auricular** artery (*a. auricularis rostralis*) arises distal to the transverse facial artery on the opposite or caudal side of the superficial temporal artery. It is larger than the transverse facial artery, but less than 1 mm in diameter. It runs between the dorsorostral part of the parotid salivary gland and the temporal muscle. It supplies both of these and finally ends in the rostral auricular muscles near the tragus of the external ear.

The **temporal branches** arise from the distal half of the superficial temporal artery. These are variable in number, size, and origin. Usually two to five branches leave the dorsal surface of the vessel and are distributed to the substance of the temporal muscle. From the ventral surface of the vessel an average of two dissectible rami are present. These also supply the temporal muscle. Some branches run medial to the zygomatic arch and then ventral to it, to supply the masseter muscle. The larger temporal branches anastomose with the deep temporal arteries of the maxillary artery.

The **lateral inferior palpebral artery** (*a. palpebralis inferior lateralis*) sends branches to the lateral half of the inferior eyelid. Several branches pass ventrally across the zygomatic arch and masseter muscle. Here in the superficial fascia these branches anastomose with the transverse facial and malar arteries.

The **lateral superior palpebral artery** (*a. palpebralis superior lateralis*), approximately 1 mm in diameter, is approximately twice as large as the lateral inferior palpebral artery. It arises opposite the orbital ligament and, by a tortuous course at the junction of the superior eyelid and frontal bone, extends toward the medial canthus of the eye. It freely branches along its course, sending branches to the various structures that form the superior eyelid. Branches also supply the muscles, fascia, and the skin covering the temporal muscle and the subcutaneous part of the frontal bone. It forms an anastomosis with the small arteries that leave the dorsal part of the orbit and with those that perforate the skull through small foramina in the region of the frontonasomaxillary suture. A **dorsocaudal nasal artery** (*a. dorsalis nasi caudalis*) is a branch of the lateral superior palpebral artery that courses rostrally on the nose medial to the orbit to supply the dorsal caudal nasal region. The palpebral arteries are the terminal branches of the superficial temporal artery.

The **maxillary artery** (*a. maxillaris*) (Figs. 11.14 through 11.16 and 11.18 through 11.26) gives off many branches that supply the deep structures of the head lying outside the cranial cavity. It is the larger of the two terminal branches of the external carotid artery and, in a medium-sized dog, measures approximately 4 mm in diameter. It is the main continuation of the external carotid artery. For convenience in describing its branches, it may be divided into three parts: the mandibular portion, the pterygoid portion, and the pterygopalatine portion. The mandibular portion extends to the alar canal. The pterygoid portion lies in the canal, and the pterygopalatine portion extends from the alar canal across the pterygopalatine fossa. No branches arise from the vessel as it passes through the alar canal.

The **first part**, or **mandibular portion**, **of the maxillary artery** includes that part of the artery from the point where the superficial temporal artery leaves the external carotid

CHAPTER 11 The Heart and Arteries 519

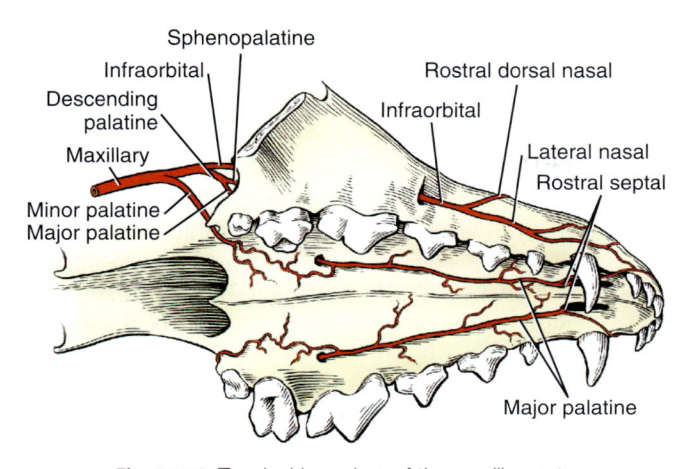

Fig. 11.18 Terminal branches of the maxillary artery.

artery to the alar canal. It begins at the base of the ear, where the vessel reaches its most dorsal level and is covered by the parotid salivary gland. It continues the arch formed by the external carotid artery rostrally and ventrally to the caudal border of the mandible, where it is bounded laterally by the masseter muscle. On reaching the mandible, the artery changes its course and runs medially, lying against the caudomedial part of the temporomandibular joint capsule as it does so. It closely follows the ventral border of the retroarticular process and, because this border is convex, the artery also makes a ventral arch, lying as it makes the arch on the pterygoid muscles. Before entering the alar canal, the vessel is adjacent to the mandibular nerve from the trigeminal nerve dorsally and the chorda tympani ventrally. The first part ends by making a bend rostrally and entering the alar

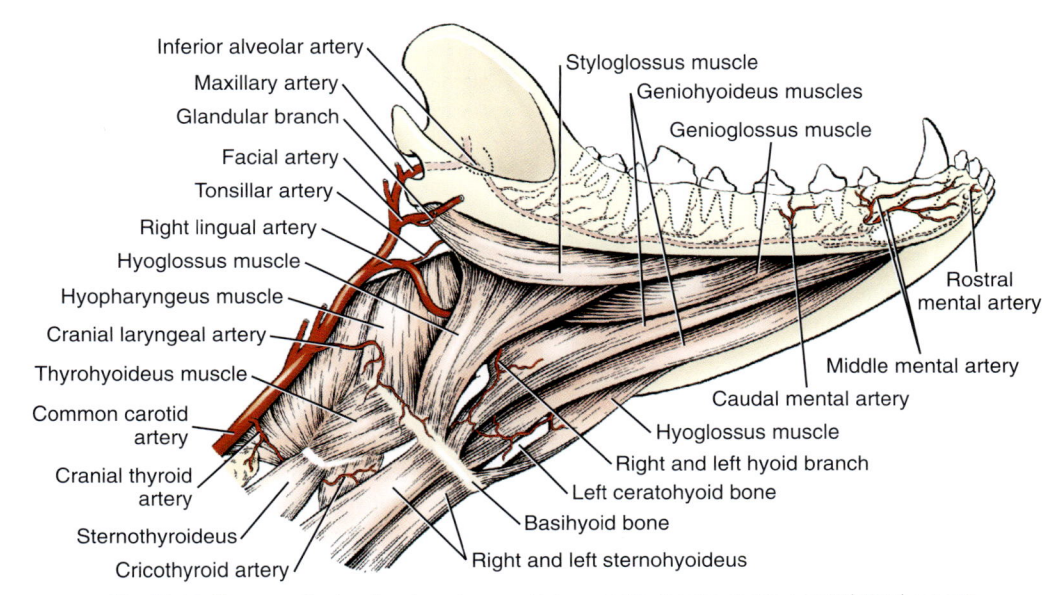

Fig. 11.19 The mandibular alveolar artery and intermandibular structures, ventrolateral aspect.

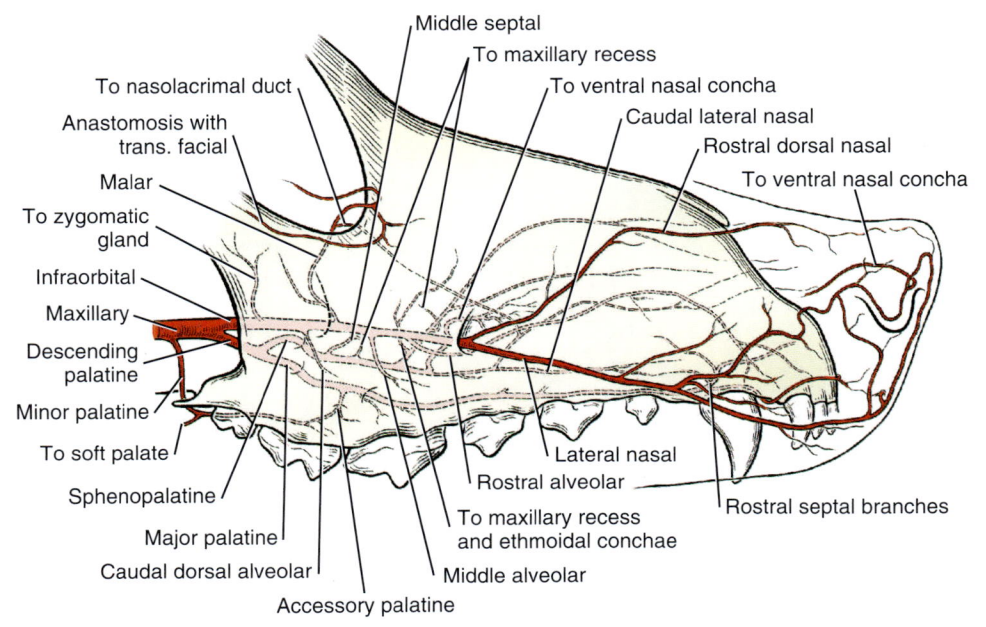

Fig. 11.20 Scheme of the terminal branches of the maxillary artery, lateral aspect.

520 CHAPTER 11 The Heart and Arteries

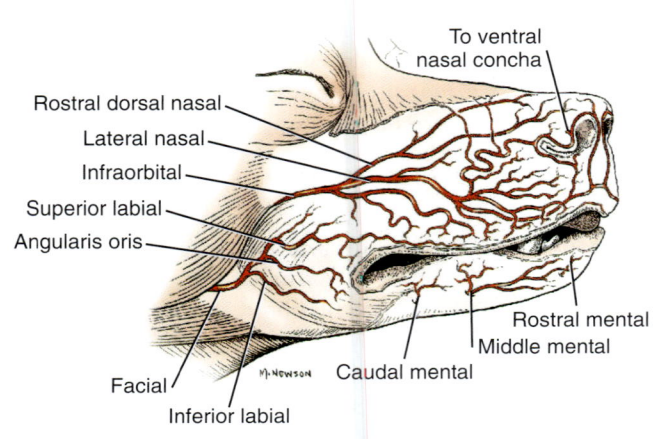

- **Fig. 11.21** Terminal branches of the infraorbital and facial arteries.

canal. The following vessels leave the first part of the maxillary artery: temporomandibular joint branch, inferior alveolar, caudal deep temporal, rostral tympanic, and middle meningeal arteries, and pterygoid branches.

The **temporomandibular joint branch** (*ramus articularis temporomandibularis*) is the main supply to the caudal part of the temporomandibular joint capsule. Sometimes two or three branches are present, instead of one. The branch or branches leave the dorsal surface of the maxillary artery 5 to 15 mm distal to the origin of the superficial temporal artery. When more than a single vessel is present, they are small and threadlike.

The **inferior alveolar artery** (*a. alveolaris inferior*) (see Fig. 11.19) measures slightly more than 1 mm in diameter.

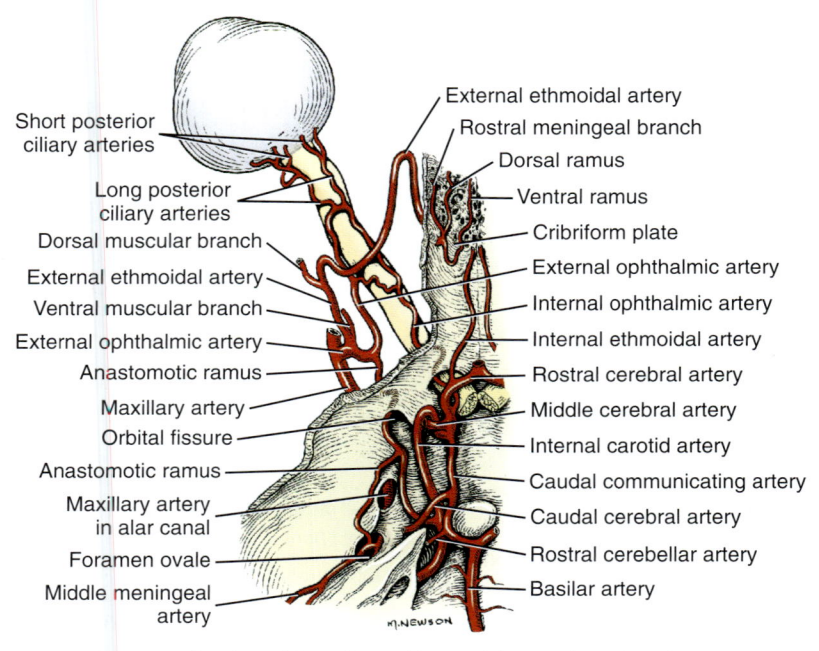

- **Fig. 11.22** Arteries of the orbit and base of the cranium, dorsal aspect.

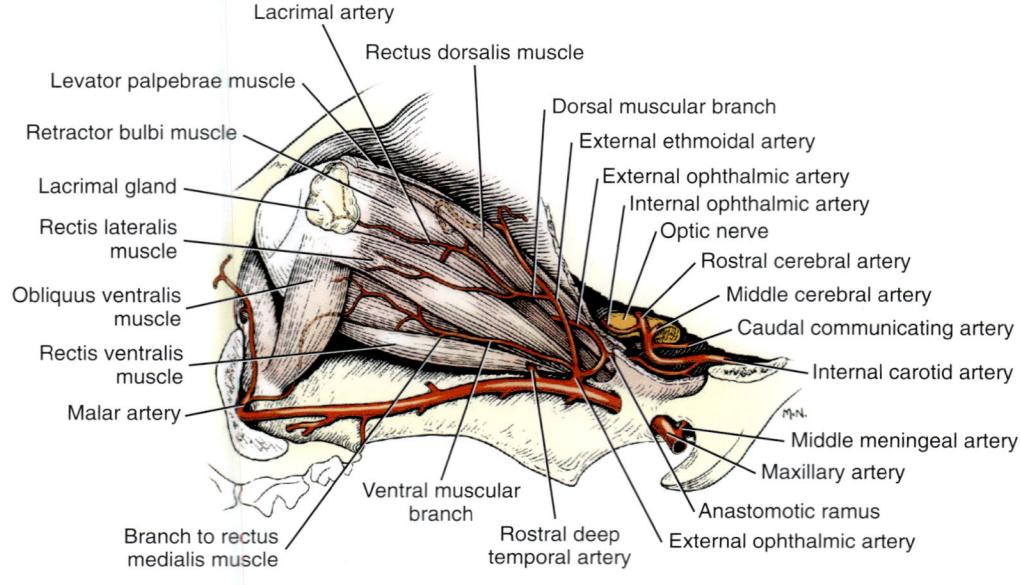

- **Fig. 11.23** Arteries of the orbit and extrinsic ocular muscles, lateral aspect.

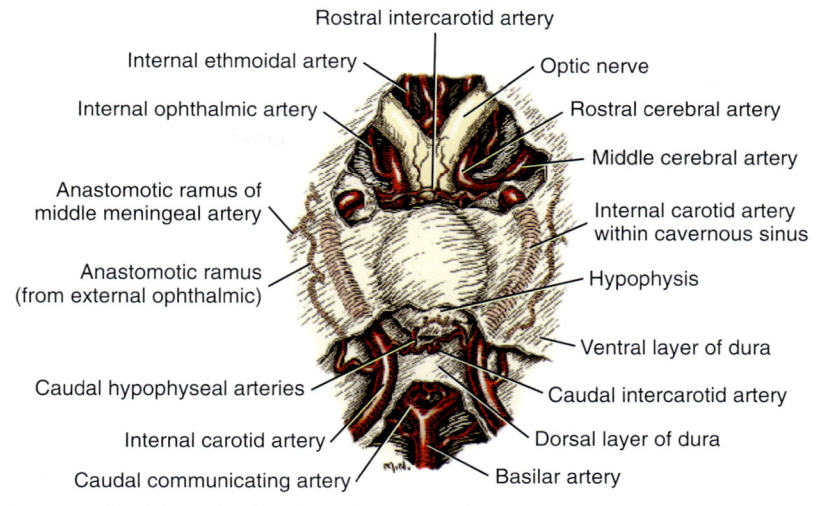

- **Fig. 11.24** Arterial supply of the hypophysis from the internal carotid artery, ventral aspect.

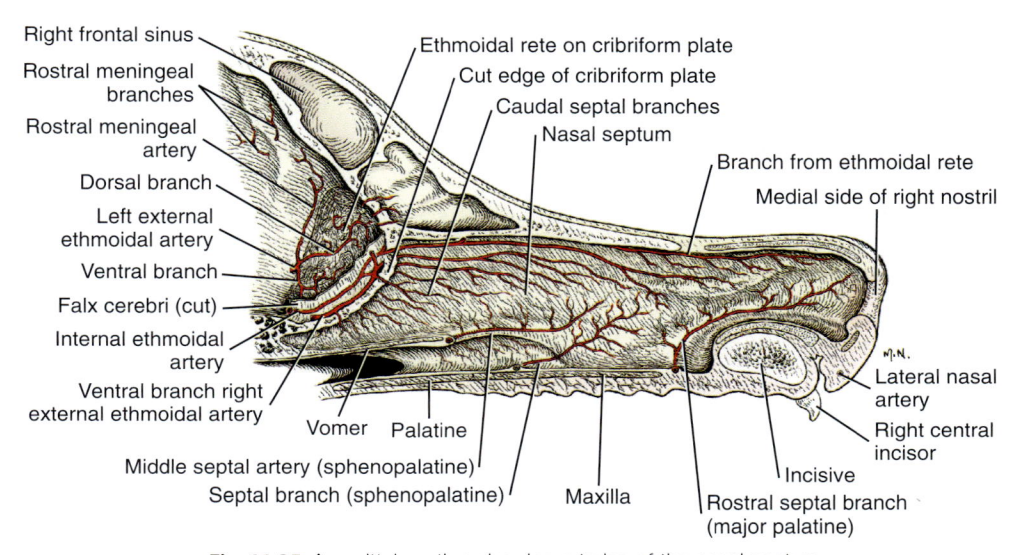

- **Fig. 11.25** A sagittal section showing arteries of the nasal septum.

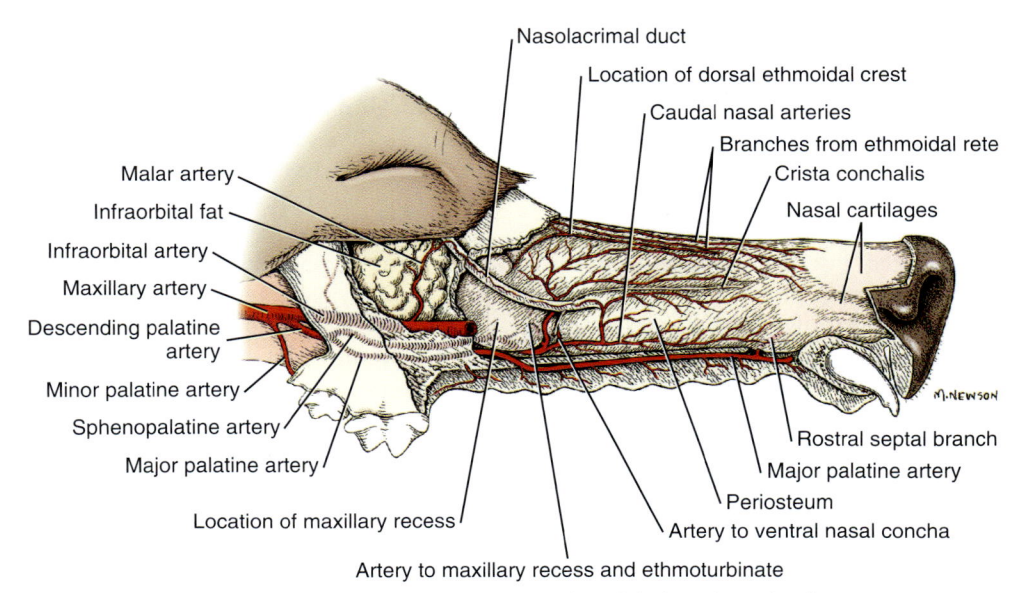

- **Fig. 11.26** A dissection showing arteries of the lateral nasal wall.

It supplies a **mylohyoid branch** (*ramus mylohyoideus*) to the mylohyoideus muscle and enters the mandibular foramen and canal after a course of approximately 1 cm. It arises from the ventral surface of the first part of the maxillary artery. Sometimes a trunk is formed from which the inferior alveolar and caudal deep temporal arteries arise in common. After entering the mandibular canal, the inferior alveolar artery closely follows the ventral border of the bone. It runs from the mandibular foramen to the middle mental foramen. During its course in the mandible, it sends many small **dental branches** (*rami dentales*) through the apical foramina to the roots of the teeth (Boling, 1942) and others to the bone itself. The inferior alveolar nerve is dorsolateral in the mandibular canal. The artery is in the middle, and the vein is ventromedial to the artery. Usually a considerable amount of fat surrounds these structures. Three **mental branches** (*rami mentales*) continue rostrally from the inferior alveolar artery to supply the rostral part of the soft tissues of the mandible. These are the caudal, middle, and rostral mental branches.

The **caudal mental branch** with its satellite nerve and vein, leaves the caudal mental foramen and runs to the inferior lip. It is much smaller than the middle mental branch, with which it anastomoses. It also anastomoses with the inferior labial artery.

The **middle mental branch** (Fig. 11.19) is the largest of the three mental branches and is the main blood supply to the rostral mandibular soft tissues. It leaves the middle mental foramen, which is located in the ventral half of the mandible, ventral to the first two cheek teeth. With its accompanying vein and nerve, it supplies the skin, tactile hair follicles, and other soft structures. It forms an anastomosis with the rostral and caudal mental branches. It is the main continuation of the inferior alveolar artery of the mandible.

The **rostral mental branch** is the smallest of the three mental branches. It leaves the inferior alveolar artery less than 1 cm caudal to the middle mental foramen and, with its satellite vein and nerve, runs in the narrow rostral portion of the mandibular canal, which closely follows the ventral border of the body of the mandible to the rostral mental foramen. It anastomoses with its fellow of the opposite side, as well as with the middle mental branch.

The **caudal deep temporal artery** (*a. temporalis profunda caudalis*) (Figs. 11.15 and 11.16) arises from the ventral surface of the maxillary artery just distal to or in common with the inferior alveolar artery. It immediately crosses the lingual, mylohyoid, and inferior alveolar branches of the trigeminal nerve, as well as the lateral pterygoid muscle. It enters the temporal muscle and extensively arborizes in it. It also sends rami that accompany the mylohyoid and lingual nerves. Most of the branches, however, are confined to that part of the temporal muscle lying medial to the coronoid process. It forms anastomoses with the rostral deep temporal artery, the occipital branches of the caudal auricular artery and the temporal branches of the superficial temporal artery. One branch passes with the masseteric nerve through the mandibular notch to the masseter muscle. This is the **masseteric artery** (*a. masseterica*). It anastomoses with the masseteric branch of the superficial temporal artery, which is the main supply to the masseter, as it runs on its deep surface. The caudal deep temporal artery is accompanied by a satellite nerve and vein or veins.

The **rostral tympanic artery** (*a. tympanica rostralis*) (Fig. 11.15) is a small, inconstant branch of the maxillary artery. It may arise from the caudal deep temporal artery. It usually leaves the maxillary artery medial to the temporomandibular joint and enters one of the small foramina located in a depression medial to the joint. It courses through the temporal bone into the middle ear.

The **middle meningeal artery** (*a. meningea media*) (Figs. 11.15, 11.16, 11.22, 11.23, 11.24, 11.28, and 11.29) leaves the dorsal surface of the maxillary artery before this vessel enters the alar canal. It is approximately 1 mm in diameter and runs through the oval foramen, which is closely adjacent to the maxillary artery. A notch, or still more rarely a foramen (*foramen spinosum*), is formed in the rostral wall of the oval foramen for the passage of the vessel. Within the cranial cavity the middle meningeal artery gives off the *ramus anastomoticus cum a. carotide interna,* which runs medially and is approximately equal in size to the parent artery. This ramus enters the cavernous sinus and makes two to four loops before joining the anastomotic artery from the external ophthalmic artery lateral to the hypophysis. After giving off the ramus anastomoticus, the middle meningeal artery follows the vascular groove on the cerebral surface of the calvaria. It runs in company with two satellite veins along the lateral border of the suture between the petrous and squamous parts of the temporal bone. It then passes almost directly dorsally across the middle part of the calvaria and bifurcates into rostral and caudal branches. At its termination along the mid-dorsal line, it anastomoses with its fellow of the opposite side. The middle meningeal artery is the largest of the meningeal arteries. Its branches leave the parent vessel at right angles and run both rostrally and caudally. They supply the dura and adjacent portions of the calvaria.

Pterygoid branches (*rami pterygoidei*) (Fig. 11.16) leave the ventral surface of the maxillary artery caudal to its entrance into the alar canal and arborize in the medial and lateral pterygoid muscles. Only small caudal portions of the pterygoid muscles are supplied by this source. Branches also supply the origins of the tensor and levator veli palatini, the pterygopharyngeus and palatopharyngeus muscles, and the mucosa of the nasal pharynx.

The **second part**, or **pterygoid portion**, **of the maxillary artery** is approximately 1 cm long, lies in the alar canal, and gives off no branches.

The **third part**, or **pterygopalatine portion**, **of the maxillary artery** emerges from the rostral alar foramen with the maxillary nerve where it lies on the lateral side of the lateral pterygoid muscle and crosses it obliquely. The following vessels leave the pterygopalatine portion of the maxillary artery: external ophthalmic, rostral deep temporal, pterygoid, buccal, minor palatine, terminal infraorbital, and descending palatine arteries. The latter is a trunk that gives rise to the major palatine and sphenopalatine arteries.

The **external ophthalmic artery** (*a. ophthalmica externa*) (Figs. 11.15, 11.22, and 11.23), whose origin was formerly called the *orbital artery*, gives rise to vessels supplying the orbit and anastomoses with vessels inside the cranial cavity. Tandler (1899) originated the term *orbital artery*, which Davis and Story (1943) and Jewell (1952) adopted in their works. Ellenberger and Baum (1943) called it the *external ophthalmic artery* in ruminants and in the horse, and this is now the accepted NAV term for all domestic animals.

The external ophthalmic artery arises from the dorsal surface of the maxillary artery immediately after the latter leaves the alar canal. It is bounded medially by the maxillary nerve and laterally by the zygomatic and lacrimal nerves. The artery penetrates the periorbita with the zygomatic and lacrimal nerves and immediately gives off numerous branches. These include anastomotic branches, muscular branches, lacrimal and external ethmoidal arteries.

An **anastomotic branch** (*ramus anastomoticus cum a. carotide interna*) (Figs. 11.22 and 11.23) leaves the external ophthalmic or even the maxillary artery, according to Jewell (1952), close to the orbital fissure that it traverses. It sends minute branches to the dura and to the nerves that pass through the orbital fissure. Sometimes the vessel is double throughout part or all of its course. It enters the cavernous sinus and receives the ramus anastomoticus from the middle meningeal artery. It continues caudally as a single tortuous vessel and unites with the internal carotid artery at a transverse plane that passes through the dorsum sellae. Thus it is possible for blood to pass from the maxillary artery to the internal carotid artery by the external ophthalmic and anastomotic arteries.

An **anastomotic branch** of the external ophthalmic artery (*ramus anastomoticus cum a. ophthalmica interna*) joins with the smaller internal ophthalmic artery on the surface of the optic nerve (Fig. 11.22). From this union two **long posterior ciliary arteries** (*aa. ciliares posteriores longae*) arise and follow the optic nerve to the eyeball. Here, adjacent to the optic nerve, the long posterior ciliary arteries give rise to a variable number of **short posterior ciliary arteries** (*aa. ciliaris posteriores breves*) that form a ring around the optic nerve. These short arteries pass through the sclera and ramify in the choroid and course anteriorly to supply the ciliary body and adjacent iris. The long posterior ciliary arteries continue anteriorly in the episcleral tissues along the medial and lateral meridians of the eyeball to its equator, where they pass through the sclera and continue anteriorly to the ciliary margin of the iris where they branch to form the **major arterial circle of the iris** (*circulus arteriosus iridis major*).

The **muscular branches** (*rami musculares*) are variable in their origin. Usually there is a ventral and a dorsal muscular branch that arise from a common trunk from the origin of the external ophthalmic artery or by a common trunk or separately from the external ethmoidal artery. Each of their resultant branches dips between adjacent rectus muscles to the fat that lies between these and the mm. retractor bulbi. Many branches are dispersed to the rectus and oblique muscles of the eye and to the eyeball itself. The small lacrimal artery may arise from the dorsal muscular branch.

The **ventral muscular branch** (Fig. 11.23) extends toward the globe of the eye between the ventral and lateral rectus muscles, although some branches pass to the medial side. The muscles it supplies are primarily the lateral and ventral rectus and the ventral portions of the retractor bulbi muscles. It also supplies the medial rectus, the gland of the third eyelid, and the conjunctiva of the inferior eyelid near the fornix. One small arterial branch runs with a branch of the oculomotor nerve to the ventral oblique muscle. It anastomoses with the dorsal muscular branch and the ciliary arteries.

The **dorsal muscular branch** (Fig. 11.23) arises in common with, or 1 cm from, the ventral muscular branch, which it exceeds slightly in size. It crosses the proximal third of the lateral rectus muscle obliquely and passes between the lateral and dorsal rectus muscles toward the globe of the eye. In its course it sends branches to the lateral and dorsal rectus, dorsal oblique, retractor bulbi, and levator palpebrae muscles. In its course to the eyeball it supplies the terminal part of the levator palpebrae muscle and a portion of the lacrimal gland. As the dorsal muscular branch crosses the lateral rectus muscle, it divides into lacrimal and zygomatic branches, which follow the respective nerves. At the equator of the eyeball, the dorsal muscular branch terminates in anterior ciliary, episcleral, and posterior conjunctival arteries. The **anterior ciliary artery** (*a. ciliares anteriores*) courses on the eyeball to the limbus where it pierces the sclera and branches to contribute to an arterial circle that supplies the ciliary body and iris and anastomoses with the long posterior ciliary arteries. **Episcleral arteries** (*aa. episclerales*) are distributed to the surface of the sclera. The **posterior conjunctival artery** (*a. conjunctivalis posterioris*) extends dorsally over the eyeball and ends in the bulbar conjunctiva adjacent to the superior eyelid. The arterial branches supplying the muscles of the orbit are peculiar in that they run centrifugally. The main arteries run deeply in the muscular cone and issue their fine branches peripherally.

The **lacrimal artery** (*a. lacrimalis*), larger than the zygomatic artery, accompanies its satellite nerve and supplies the lacrimal gland. It passes deep to the orbital ligament and terminates in the conjunctiva and skin of the superior eyelid.

The threadlike **zygomatic artery** follows the zygomatic nerve to the lacrimal gland, the skin, the conjunctiva near the lateral canthus of the eye, and the adjacent inferior eyelid. The lacrimal and zygomatic arteries may anastomose with each other. The lacrimal artery occasionally joins the superior palpebral artery; the zygomatic artery usually unites with the inferior palpebral artery.

The **external ethmoidal artery** (*a. ethmoidalis externa*) (Figs. 11.22 through 11.25) is a dorsorostral branch of the external ophthalmic artery that may be the origin of the muscular branches. It makes an initial curve dorsally across the lateral surface of the extraocular muscles, where it runs through the plexus formed by the ophthalmic vein in this location. It sometimes gives off branches to the dorsal oblique muscle and to the frontal bone. It then makes one or two more bends and enters the larger, more dorsally located ethmoidal foramen in company with its small satellite vein. The entrance of the artery into the ethmoidal foramen is unusual in that the vessel enters it from dorsal and rostral and not from the side from which the vessel approaches it. Also unusual is the fact that a separate, smaller, and more ventral ethmoidal foramen conducts the ethmoidal nerve. Usually the dorsal and ventral muscular branches that supply the muscles of the eyeball arise independently from the rostral surface of the external ethmoidal artery, but occasionally they arise by means of a common trunk from the external ethmoidal artery or directly from the external ophthalmic artery. The external ethmoidal artery, after passing through the ethmoidal foramen, reaches the dura. In the dura, between the cribriform plate and the olfactory bulb, it divides into a dorsal and a ventral branch. These branches anastomose rostrally and form an arterial circle on the lateral wall of the cribriform plate. Many small branches leave this arterial circle and reunite, so that an ethmoidal rete is formed. The internal ethmoidal arteries, from the rostral cerebral arteries, run in the falx cerebri to the cribriform plate, where they anastomose and aid in forming the ethmoidal rete. Many branches pass through the cribriform plate from the rete to supply the mucosa of the ethmoturbinates and the nasal septum. Those to the nasal septum are the **caudal nasal septal arteries** (*aa. nasales septales caudales*). Another branch, the **rostral meningeal artery** (*a. meningea rostralis*), runs dorsally in the dura at the caudal margin of the cribriform plate, passes through the inner table of the frontal bone, and enters the mucoperiosteum on the floor of the lateral compartment of the frontal sinus. After running caudally in the frontal sinus, it passes through the inner table of the frontal bone 5 to 10 mm from the median plane and arborizes in the dura ventral to the caudal part of the frontal sinus. It forms a delicate anastomosis with the middle meningeal artery. There is considerable variation in the size and distribution of the branches of the external ethmoidal artery.

After giving off the muscular branches and the external ethmoidal artery, the external ophthalmic artery forms one or two flexures in the fat on the dorsal surface of the optic nerve approximately 15 mm caudal to the eyeball. It runs to the medial side of the optic nerve, where it anastomoses with the smaller internal ophthalmic artery. From the union of the external and internal ophthalmic arteries, two to four **long posterior ciliary arteries** (*aa. ciliares posteriores longae*) arise and run to the eyeball. On reaching the sclera that surrounds the optic nerve, the vessels break up into several branches, **short posterior ciliary arteries** (*aa. ciliares posteriores breves*), which extend through the scleral cribriform area and ramify in the choroid part of the vascular coat as the **choroid arteries**. Other branches do not perforate the sclera in the cribriform area but continue, closely applied to the sclera, toward the cornea and are called the **episcleral arteries** (*aa. episclerales*). The retinal arterioles arise as branches of the short posterior ciliary arteries where the latter penetrate the sclera (see Chapter 21, The Eye). Retinal vessels emerge around the periphery of the optic papilla as nine or more arterioles, which radiate into the retina. According to Catcott (1952), the venules that lie in the retina are three or four in number and converge to the center of the optic papilla. Great variation exists among dogs and between the eyes of the same dog.

The **rostral deep temporal artery** (*a. temporalis profunda rostralis*) (see Fig. 11.15) is a vessel less than 1 mm in diameter that arises close to the external ophthalmic artery. It may be double. From the dorsal surface of the maxillary artery it runs dorsally between the temporal muscle and the caudal part of the frontal bone. The small rostral deep temporal artery enters the temporal muscle near the middle of its rostral border and arborizes in the muscle. Accompanied by two satellite veins, it forms an anastomosis in the temporal muscle with the superficial and caudal deep temporal arteries.

There is a **pterygoid branch** (*r. pterygoideus*) of the maxillary artery rostral to the alar canal (see Fig. 11.15) that supplies the medial and lateral pterygoid muscles. It is approximately 0.5 mm in diameter and arises opposite the origin of the rostral deep temporal artery. Its origin is approximately 2 mm peripheral to the origin of the external ophthalmic artery, but it usually arises from the opposite side. It may arise from the medial side of the external ophthalmic artery. Several branches supply both the lateral and the medial pterygoid muscles. Occasionally, a branch can be traced through the muscle into the pterygoid canal. The pterygoid branch anastomoses with the muscular branch of the buccal artery, which supplies part of the medial pterygoid muscle.

The **buccal artery** (*a. buccalis*) (Fig. 11.15) arises from the ventrolateral surface of the maxillary artery approximately 1 cm distal to the origin of the rostral deep temporal artery. It is nearly 1 mm in diameter as it leaves the maxillary artery at an acute angle and runs toward the cheek. Usually near its origin a small branch is given off to the medial pterygoid muscle. It soon becomes related to the buccal nerve, which accompanies it to the cheek. A tiny branch (*ramus glandularis zygomaticus*) is given off to the ventral portion of the zygomatic salivary gland, and larger branches are distributed to the masseter, temporal, and buccinator muscles. The vessel finally terminates in the region of the soft palate.

The **minor palatine artery** (*a. palatina minor*) (Figs. 11.15, 11.18, 11.20, and 11.26) arises from the ventral surface of the maxillary artery or one of its terminal branches dorsal to the last superior cheek tooth. It is less than 0.5 mm in diameter and passes ventrally through a notch in the caudal part of the palatine bone. It is distributed to the adjacent soft and hard palates. The branch to the soft palate runs nearly the whole length of this part and lies close to the median plane. It supplies the palatine glands, musculature, and mucosa. Fine branches anastomose with the ascending pharyngeal and the major palatine arteries. Occasionally a branch of the minor palatine artery sends a branch to the zygomatic salivary gland.

The infraorbital and descending palatine arteries are the terminal branches of the maxillary artery. The smaller **descending palatine artery** (*a. palatina descendens*) is a common trunk for the sphenopalatine and major palatine arteries (Figs. 11.15, 11.18, 11.20, and 11.26). This termination occurs a few millimeters rostral to the origin of the minor palatine artery. The descending palatine usually has a single, but sometimes a double, muscular ramus to the rostral portion of the medial pterygoid muscle. The muscular ramus may arise from the maxillary or from the descending palatine artery.

The **major palatine artery** (*a. palatina major*) arises from the descending palatine artery as one of its terminal branches. The vessel, which is slightly more than 1 mm in diameter, passes through the caudal palatine foramen and the palatine canal with a delicate vein and relatively large satellite nerve. Within the palatine canal the nerve and artery divide so that two or more sets of major palatine arteries and nerves emerge on the hard palate via the major palatine foramen. Some of the nerve and artery branches pass through the minor palatine foramina located caudal to the major palatine foramen. The arteries anastomose with each other, and the most caudal branch anastomoses with the minor palatine artery. The most rostral branch is the main continuation of the major palatine artery. The palatine groove on the surface of the hard palate, in which the vessels lie, is situated midway between the alveoli and the midline (Fig. 11.18). Anastomoses between the right and left palatine vessels occur throughout their course. The major palatine artery and nerve usually leave the palatine groove midway between the palatine fissure and the major palatine foramen. They extend through the palatine venous plexus in their rostral course so that they lie closely deep to the oral mucosa. The groove rostral to the plane in which the artery and nerve leave it contains a portion of the palatine venous plexus. The major palatine artery supplies the mucosa of the oral surface of the hard palate, the periosteum, and the bone that forms the alveoli. A small branch passes through the palatine fissure and anastomoses with a branch of the sphenopalatine artery, which supplies the mucosa on the nasal side of the hard palate. A small artery extends rostrolaterally, passes through the interdental space between the canine and corner incisor teeth, and anastomoses with the lateral nasal artery. The **rostral septal branches** (Fig. 11.25) from the major palatine artery run dorsomedially through the palatine fissure and supply that part of the septum caudal to the area supplied by septal branches of the lateral nasal and rostral to the area supplied by the middle septal artery from the sphenopalatine artery. By an extensive, fine arterial plexus they anastomose with adjacent vessels. The major palatine artery continues rostral, branching profusely, and caudal to the incisor teeth turns toward the midline and anastomoses with its fellow. At the anastomosis a small vessel runs dorsally through the interincisive canal and joins with the right and left lateral nasal arteries as these anastomose with each other at the median plane. This anastomotic branch is small as it passes dorsally through the interincisive suture.

The **sphenopalatine artery** (*a. sphenopalatine*) (Figs. 11.20 and 11.26), which is the other terminal branch of the descending palatine artery is more than 2 mm in diameter and leaves the pterygopalatine fossa by passing through the sphenopalatine foramen with its satellite nerve and vein. On reaching the nasopharyngeal mucosa, the artery runs rostroventrally in the mucoperiosteum and on the dorsal surface of the palatomaxillary suture to a point ventral to the opening into the maxillary recess. Here the sphenopalatine artery swings dorsorostrally for a few millimeters and divides into a dorsal and a ventral branch and a branch that goes to the ventral nasal concha. The terminal branches of the sphenopalatine artery are collectively known as **caudal**, **lateral**, and **septal nasal arteries** (*aa. nasales caudales, laterales et septales*). As the main sphenopalatine vessel makes its dorsal bend, the ventral branch continues rostrally to supply the mucoperiosteum of the side and floor of the nasal fossa and the adjacent middle portion of the nasal septum. A small artery leaves the dorsal surface of this vessel and, curving dorsocaudally, runs toward the eye on the nasolacrimal duct. This branch supplies blood to the rostral part of the duct and anastomoses with the branch of the malar artery, which supplies its caudal part. Beyond the origin of the small artery to the nasolacrimal duct, the ventral vessel continues rostrally and slightly medially. Its terminal branches anastomose with a branch of the major palatine artery, which ascends through the palatine fissure.

The dorsal branch arises near the opening into the maxillary recess aligned with a transverse plane passing between the third and fourth superior premolar teeth. This vessel runs dorsorostrally and bifurcates: one branch supplies the ventral part of the nasal concha and the mucoperiosteum lateral to it; the other branch goes to the dorsal part of this bone and has an extensive anastomosis with a vessel that runs rostrally in endoturbinate I from the ethmoidal rete.

The branch that goes to the ventral nasal concha is short, medially inclined, and variable in origin. It may come from either the dorsal or the ventral branch previously described. It goes to the caudal part of the conchal crest and divides into five or six small arteries that arborize on the primary scrolls into which the bone is divided. It anastomoses rostrally with a branch of the lateral nasal artery, which curves around the dorsal part of the nostril and extends caudally on the ridge of tissue that is continuous with the conchal crest. In addition to the ventral, dorsal, and ventral conchal branches just described, smaller branches supply the mucosa and bone of the maxillary recess and the rostral parts of the ethmoturbinates and a large part of the middle of the nasal septum. The branches to the maxillary recess arise from the caudal side of the dorsal branch as this vessel runs in the mucoperiosteum that forms the rostroventral and rostrolateral parts of this cavity. A branch to the caudal part of the maxillary recess may leave the sphenopalatine artery shortly after it enters the nasopharyngeal mucosa. Many other branches supply the mucoperiosteum of the floor and sides of the ventral nasal meatus. The **middle septal artery** is the first branch of the sphenopalatine artery after it leaves the sphenopalatine foramen. It runs from the mucoperiosteum and the plate of bone separating the nasopharynx and the nasal fundus to the middle part of the nasal septum. Rostrally it anastomoses with the rostral septal branches from the major palatine artery, and caudally it anastomoses with the caudal septal branches from the ethmoidal rete. All the branches of the sphenopalatine form voluminous arterial plexuses in the mucoperiosteum, which they supply. Numerous anastomoses also occur between adjacent vessels.

The **infraorbital artery** (*a. infraorbitalis*) (Figs. 11.18, 11.20, and 11.21) is the main continuation of the maxillary artery across the medial pterygoid muscle. Accompanied by the maxillary nerve from the trigeminal nerve, it leaves the pterygopalatine fossa, gives off the caudal dorsal alveolar artery, and passes through the maxillary foramen to enter the infraorbital canal. It gives off a branch to the zygomatic gland, caudal dorsal alveolar, malar, middle dorsal alveolar, and rostral dorsal alveolar arteries. These alveolar arteries provide **dental branches** (*rami dentales*) to the superior teeth. The infraorbital artery terminates by dividing into the lateral and rostral dorsal nasal arteries. These terminal arteries arise either before or after the vessel has passed through the infraorbital foramen (Christensen & Toussaint, 1957).

The **caudal dorsal alveolar artery** is a small vessel that may arise from the minor palatine artery or either of the terminal branches of the maxillary artery. It usually arises from the ventral surface of the infraorbital artery before the latter enters the infraorbital canal. The caudal dorsal alveolar artery divides and runs directly to the alveolar canals of the last two molar teeth to provide them with dental branches. These are minute arterial branches accompanied by satellite nerves and veins.

The **malar artery** (*a. malaris*) arises from the dorsal surface of the infraorbital artery prior to its entrance into the maxillary foramen. Near its origin a small branch is given off, which supplies the ventral oblique muscle and passes along its deep surface to anastomose with the ventral muscular branch of the external ophthalmic or external ethmoidal artery. The main trunk runs to the medial canthus of the eye superficial to the periorbita. During its course it gives off a delicate branch that enters the nasal cavity in company with the nasolacrimal duct. The terminal branches go mainly to the inferior eyelid, the medial angle of the eye, and third eyelid (*a. palpebralis inferior medialis, a. palpebralis superior medialis, a. palpebrae tertiae*), where they anastomose with the inferior palpebral and the transverse facial arteries.

The most caudal dental rami to the superior teeth leave the infraorbital artery caudal to the origin of the malar artery. These dental rami enter small alveolar canals that connect with each tooth root. They are accompanied by the satellite vein and nerve. These dental rami continue to arise from the infraorbital artery as it courses through the infraorbital canal. The most rostral dental rami enter alveolar canals that arise from the infraorbital canal near the infraorbital foramen. These course to the rostral premolar teeth, the canine tooth, and the incisive teeth.

The infraorbital artery emerges from the infraorbital canal and terminates in lateral and rostral dorsal nasal arteries. The **lateral nasal artery** (*a. lateralis nasi*) (Figs. 11.18, 11.20, and 11.21) is the larger of the two terminal branches of the infraorbital artery. It measures slightly more than 1 mm in diameter at its origin at the infraorbital foramen. It runs rostrally into the muzzle with many large infraorbital nerve branches and anastomoses with branches of the superior labial and major palatine arteries. It first crosses deep to the levator nasolabialis muscle and then runs among the fibers of the m. orbicularis oris. The vessel branches profusely and supplies the superior lip and snout as well as the follicles of the vibrissae, or tactile hairs. It furnishes blood to the rostral part of the superior lip and the adjacent part of the nose. At the philtrum the vessel anastomoses with its fellow and sends a relatively large branch dorsally between the nostrils and another branch caudally in the mucosa of the nasal cartilage.

The **rostral dorsal nasal artery** (*a. dorsalis nasi rostralis*) travels rostrodorsally across the lateral surface of the nose to its dorsal surface. It runs deep to and supplies the levator nasolabialis muscle, and then it continues to supply the structures of the dorsal surface of the rostral half of the muzzle. It anastomoses with its fellow of the opposite side, as well as with the nasal and septal branches of the sphenopalatine artery and the septal branches of the major palatine artery.

Internal Carotid Artery. The **internal carotid artery** (*a. carotis interna*) (Figs. 11.14, 11.16, 11.22 through 11.24, and 11.27, 11.30 to 11.33) arises with the external carotid artery as the smaller of the two terminal branches of the common carotid artery. Other vessels that arise in close association with this vessel are the occipital and ascending pharyngeal arteries. The termination of the common carotid artery is directly medial to the medial retropharyngeal lymph node, which is bound to the artery and adjacent structures by the fascia that forms the carotid sheath. At a still more lateral level is the sternocephalic muscle. The internal carotid artery at first runs dorsorostrally across the lateral surface of the pharynx. At its origin, from the dorsal surface of the parent artery is a bulbous enlargement, the **carotid sinus** (*sinus caroticus*), which is approximately 3 mm in diameter and 4 mm long and functions as a baroreceptor. Ruiz-Pesini et al. (1995) showed that the carotid sinus receives both sympathetic innervation from the cranial cervical ganglion and sensory innervation from the distal ganglion of the glossopharyngeal nerve. The **carotid body** (*glomus caroticum*), a chemoreceptor, lies at the bifurcation of the carotid arteries or sometimes within the wall of the carotid sinus. The internal carotid artery then narrows to

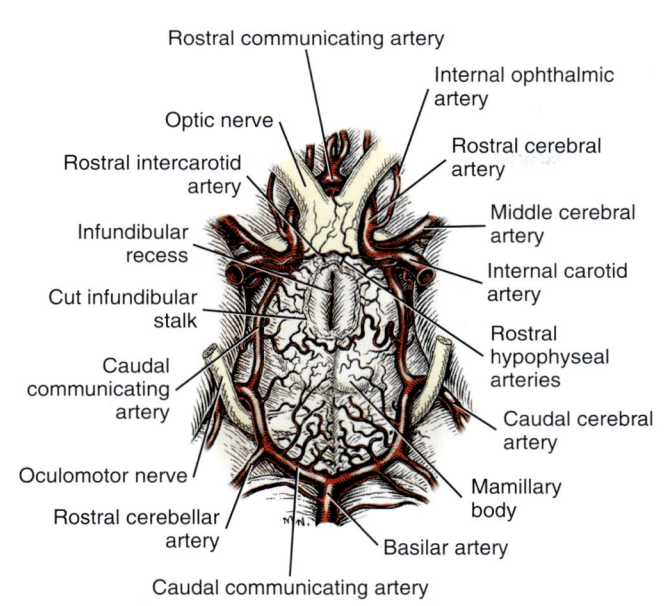

• **Fig. 11.27** The arterial circle of the brain (*circulus arteriosus cerebri*) and the superficial arterial supply of the hypothalamus, ventral aspect.

approximately 1 mm. The internal carotid artery gives off no branches before entering the tympanooccipital fissure. Just before entering this depression, it crosses the lateral surface of the cranial cervical ganglion and the medial surface of the digastric muscle. In the tympanooccipital fissure the artery enters and traverses the carotid canal. On leaving the rostral opening of the carotid canal, it passes ventrally through the *foramen lacerum,* forms a loop, and reenters the cranial cavity through the same foramen. Frequently, a small branch from the ascending pharyngeal artery anastomoses with the loop formed by the internal carotid artery. On reentering the cranial cavity the internal carotid artery perforates a layer of dura to enter the cavernous sinus that is contained within the dura. This is at the level where the cavernous sinus is continuous with the ventral petrosal sinus. The artery courses rostrally within the cavernous sinus, at first obliquely toward the dorsum sellae, then directly rostral to the level of the optic chiasm. Here the artery again perforates the cavernous sinus and the adjacent dura and arachnoid, and comes to lie in the subarachnoid space. On entering this space it trifurcates as the rostral cerebral, middle cerebral, and caudal communicating arteries. A small **rostral intercarotid artery** arises from the trifurcation within the subarachnoid space. While in the cavernous sinus, the internal carotid artery forms an anastomosis with the anastomotic artery of the external ophthalmic.

The **caudal intercarotid artery** (*a. intercarotica caudalis*) (Fig. 11.24) is a small vessel that leaves the first part of the internal carotid as it enters the cavernous sinus. The vessel runs obliquely toward the midline and joins with its fellow, caudal to the hypophysis. It is closely applied to the dura of the cavernous and intercavernous sinuses. It gives off a branch, which perforates the dura surrounding the hypophysis and supplies the neural lobe. This is the **caudal hypophyseal artery**. Occasionally, the caudal intercarotid artery arises from the anastomotic artery.

The **caudal communicating artery** (*a. communicans caudalis*) (Figs. 11.22 through 11.30, and 11.32) leaves the caudal surface of the internal carotid artery after it perforates the dura and arachnoid and enters the subarachnoid space. It forms the lateral and caudal thirds of the arterial circle. Caudally it anastomoses with the basilar artery to complete the arterial circle caudally. It is readily identified by the fact that the third cranial nerve crosses its dorsal surface. It is considered to be the origin of the caudal cerebral artery described later.

The **arterial circle of the brain** (*circulus arteriosus cerebri*) (Figs. 11.22, 11.24, 11.27 through 11.30), formerly the Circle of Willis, is an elongated arterial ring on the ventral surface of the brain, formed by the right and left rostral cerebral arteries and their rostral communicating arteries, the caudal communicating arteries from the internal carotid arteries and the basilar artery. From the arterial circle, on each side, arise three vessels that supply the cerebrum. These are the rostral, middle, and caudal cerebral arteries (Figs. 11.22, 11.30 through 11.33). The rostral cerebellar arteries arise from the caudal part of the arterial circle and the caudal cerebellar arteries from the basilar artery to supply the cerebellum. Pontine and medullary branches of the basilar artery supply the pons and medulla oblongata. All of these vessels form anastomoses with adjacent vessels on the surface of the brain. A rich capillary network is found in the cerebral cortex, whereas the white matter of the brain has a less abundant supply. The arterial circle ensures the maintenance of constant blood pressure in the terminal arteries and provides alternate routes by which blood can reach the brain.

Tanuma (1981) made a morphologic study of the arterial circle and has provided measurements of the components and their variations in 55 dogs. He also described the sympathetic innervation in nine of the dogs and noted that sympathetic axons from the cervicothoracic ganglion that compose the vertebral nerve and accompany the vertebral artery innervate the basilar artery and its branches as far rostral as the rostral cerebellar artery from the arterial circle. Although these axons extended toward the caudal cerebral artery, they did not innervate it. Sympathetic axons from the cranial cervical ganglion supplied all the vessels originating from the internal carotid artery and cerebral arterial circle.

Several **rostral hypophyseal arteries** leave the caudal communicating artery and run over the tuber cinereum to the stalk of the hypophysis. These, with their fellows, supply the major portion of the gland. The pars nervosa, however, is supplied by the **caudal hypophyseal artery**, a branch of the caudal intercarotid artery.

The **middle cerebral artery** (*a. cerebri media*) (Figs. 11.24, 11.27 through 11.31, and 11.33) is the largest vessel that supplies the brain. It leaves the internal carotid artery as a terminal branch approximately 1 mm from the origin of the caudal communicating artery. It lies at first on the

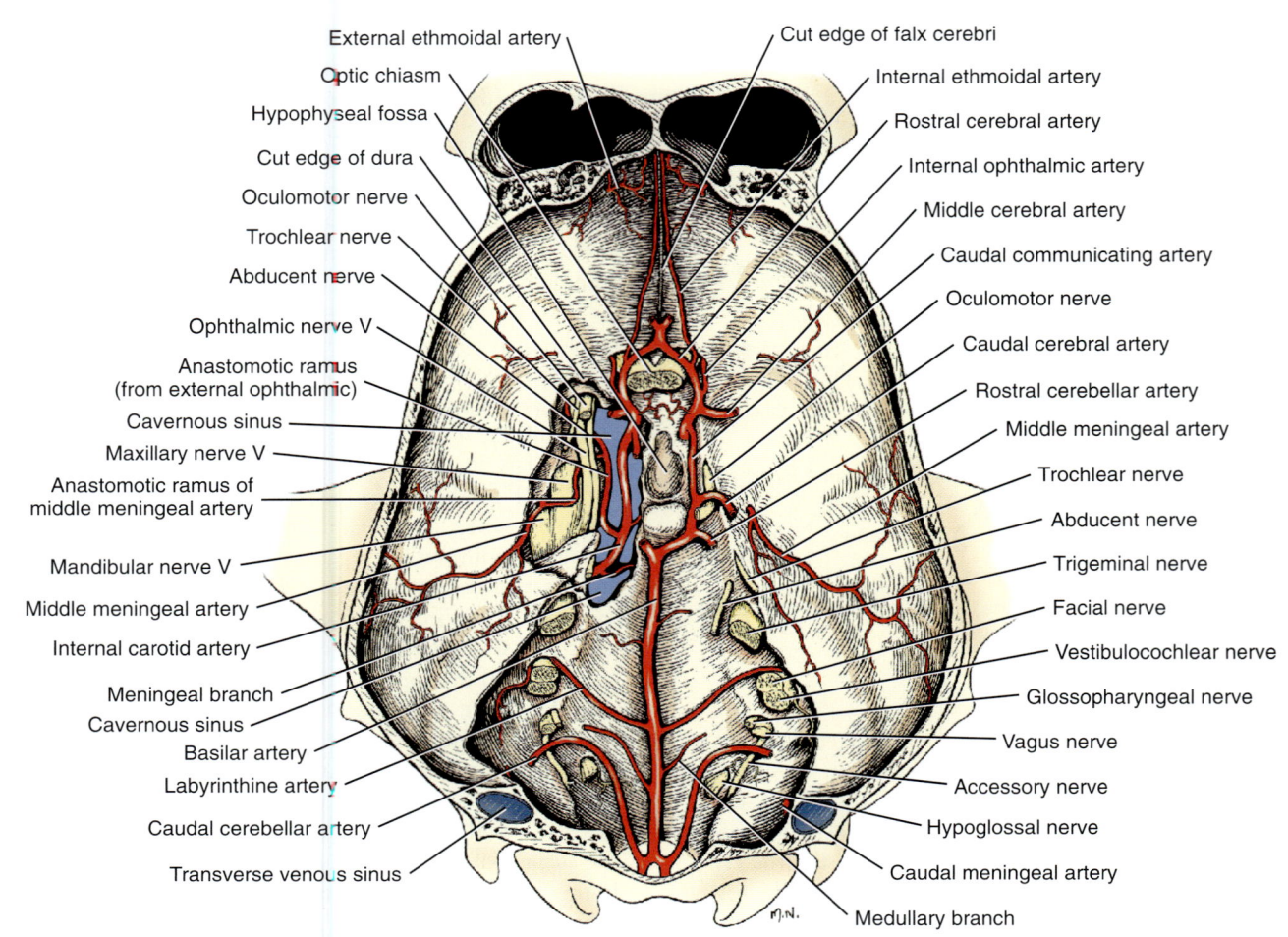

• **Fig. 11.28** Dorsal aspect of the base of the skull showing arteries and nerves. The dura is partially removed on the left side, opening the cavernous sinus.

rostral perforated substance, where it gives rise to the **rostral choroidal artery** (*a. choroidea rostralis*). This reaches the lateral ventricle via the hippocampal sulcus on the medial side of the piriform lobe. It circles around the internal capsule with the hippocampus, and supplies the vessels of the choroid plexus of the lateral ventricle. This rostral choroidal artery may be a direct branch from the arterial circle at the level of the middle cerebral artery. The middle cerebral artery then crosses the ventral surface of the brain rostral to the piriform lobe and divides into at least two large branches that supply the whole cerebral cortex of the lateral surface of the cerebral hemisphere. The vessels follow the sulci in some places and run over the gyri in others. On the dorsal aspect of the cerebral hemisphere, its branches anastomose with the terminal branches of the rostral and caudal cerebral arteries that supply a small area just lateral to the longitudinal cerebral fissure. Minute terminal **cortical branches** (*rami corticales*) of the middle cerebral artery enter the cortex and richly supply it. The **central branches** (*rami centrales*) leave the middle cerebral artery near its origin in the form of several **striate branches** (*rami striati*) that supply the basal nuclei and adjacent tracts.

The **rostral cerebral artery** (*a. cerebri rostralis*) (Figs. 11.24, 11.27 through 11.33) arises lateral to the optic chiasm and runs dorsal to the optic nerve in a rostromedial direction. On reaching the longitudinal fissure, it unites with its fellow. This side-to-side union of right and left rostral cerebral arteries is usually approximately 2 mm long, after which the two vessels separate. In some specimens there is an arterial bridge rather than a broad union connecting the right and left vessels. When an arterial bridge is present, it is called the **rostral communicating artery** (*a. communicans rostralis*). This completes the rostral portion of the arterial circle. The rostral cerebral artery runs dorsally to the genu of the corpus callosum, turns caudally along the corpus callosum, and anastomoses with the caudal cerebral artery, which comes into the longitudinal fissure from caudal. Numerous tortuous and freely branching vessels leave the dorsal and rostral surfaces of the rostral cerebral artery. These extend dorsally over the dorsomedial aspect of the cerebral hemisphere to the level of the marginal sulcus, where they anastomose with the middle cerebral artery laterally and the caudal cerebral artery caudally. The rostral cerebral artery, like the middle vessel, not only supplies the cortex with its cortical branches but also sends branches into the central gray and white matter. Farther ventrally, toward the olfactory bulbs, they are confined to the longitudinal fissure.

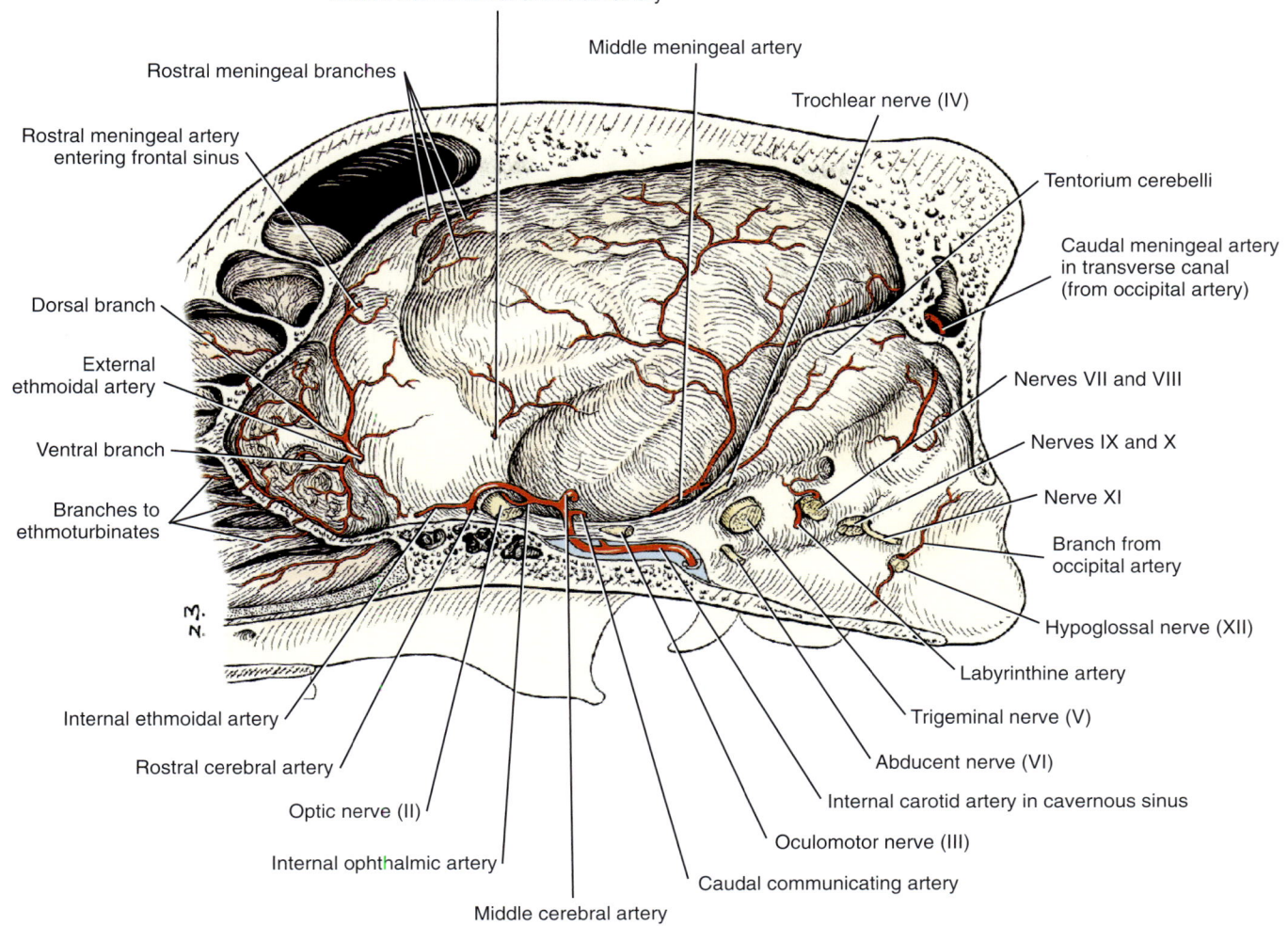

• **Fig. 11.29** A paramedian section of the cranium, showing internal arteries and nerves.

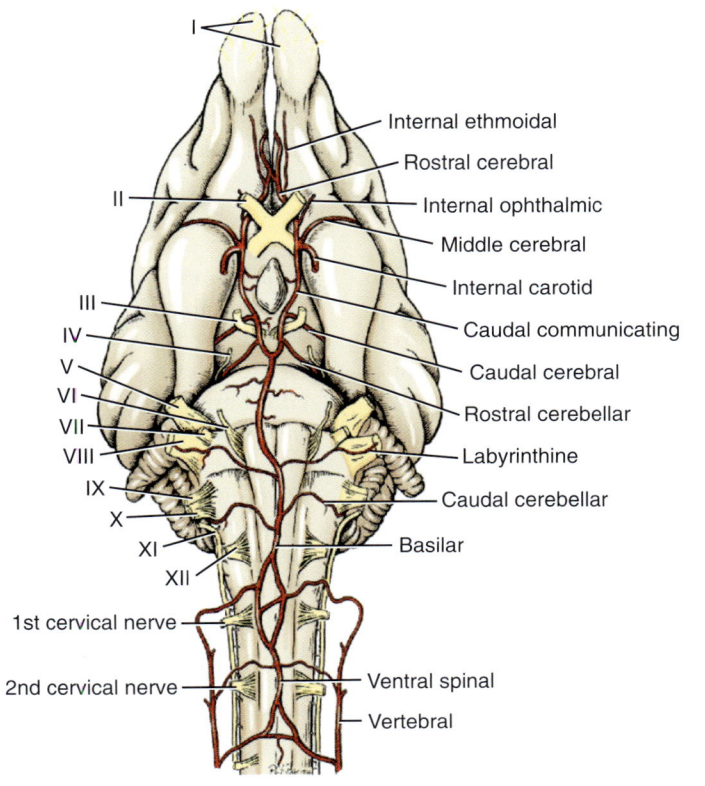

• **Fig. 11.30** Arteries of the brain and cervical spinal cord, ventral aspect.

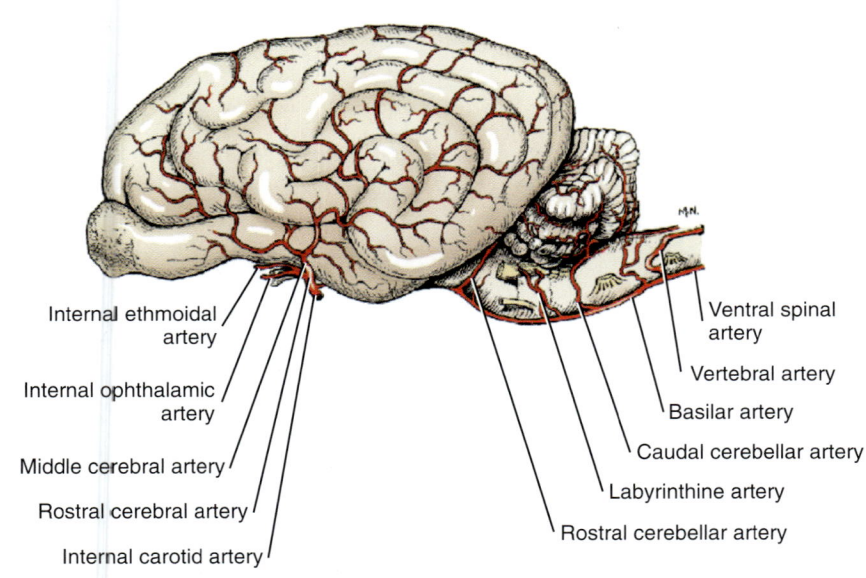

Fig. 11.31 Distribution of the middle cerebral artery, lateral aspect.

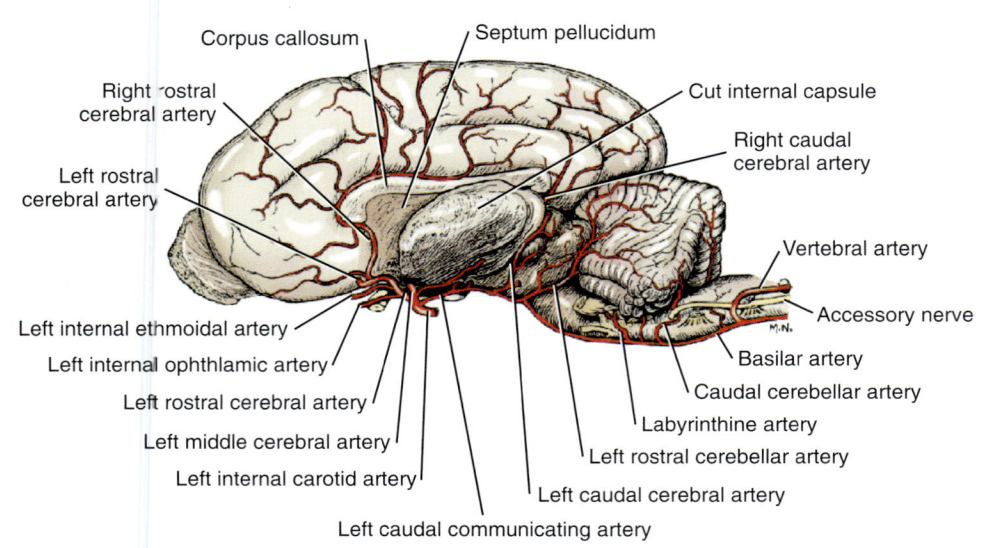

Fig. 11.32 Arteries of the cerebellum and medial surface of the cerebrum. Sagittal section.

The **internal ophthalmic artery** (*a. ophthalmica interna*) (Figs. 11.22, through 11.24, 11.27, and 11.29 through 11.32) is less than 0.5 mm in diameter and leaves the rostral cerebral artery. It follows the dorsal surface of the optic nerve through the optic canal, and may be double. As the artery travels rostrolaterally with the optic nerve, it passes from the dorsal surface to the medial surface of the nerve. At a location approximately 15 mm caudal to the bulbus oculi, the internal ophthalmic artery anastomoses with the external ophthalmic artery. From the anastomosis of the two vessels three or four long posterior ciliary arteries arise and the central artery of the retina, if present. Their distribution is discussed in connection with the description of the external ophthalmic artery.

The **internal ethmoidal artery** (*a. ethmoidalis interna*) (Figs. 11.22, 11.28 through 11.32) is a small artery that arises from the ventral part of the rostral cerebral artery and runs toward the cribriform plate. It lies near the attached portion of the falx cerebri, where it parallels the medial olfactory tract. On reaching the most rostral portion of the cribriform plate, it anastomoses with the ventral branch of the external ethmoidal artery, forming a rete. Most of the branches of the internal ethmoidal artery pass through the cribriform plate to supply the ethmoturbinates and the nasal septum. Branches on the nasal septum anastomose with the middle septal branch of the sphenopalatine as well as with the rostral septal branch of the major palatine arteries.

The **caudal cerebral artery** (*a. cerebri caudalis*) (Figs. 11.27, 11.28, 11.30, 11.32, and 11.33) arises from the caudal communicating artery of the internal carotid when the latter enters the subarachnoid space. This is just rostral to the oculomotor nerve where it crosses the arterial circle.

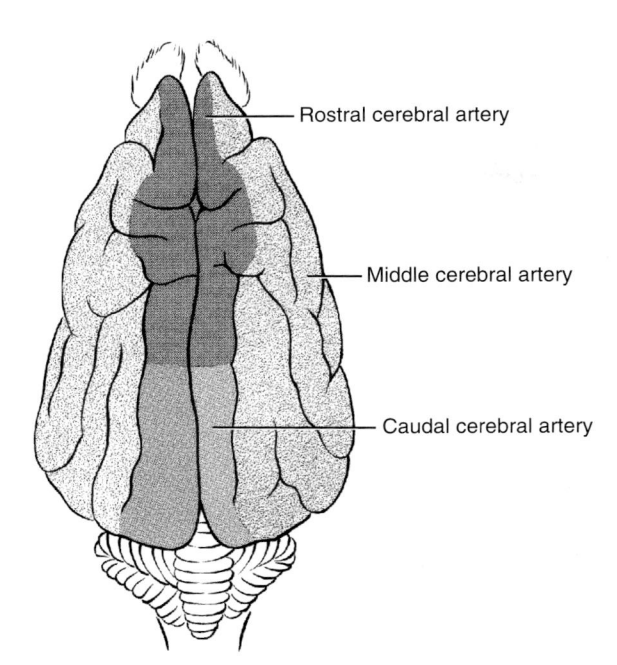

Fig. 11.33 Areas supplied by the cerebral arteries, dorsal aspect.

The caudal cerebral artery courses dorsomedially on the medial aspect of the cerebral hemisphere. It reaches the splenium of the corpus callosum and travels rostrally on its dorsal surface until it meets the rostral cerebral artery coursing caudally where their terminal branches anastomose. The branches of the caudal cerebral artery supply the medial aspect of the occipital lobe as well as the occipital gyrus and caudal aspect of the marginal gyrus. Here the area supplied by the caudal cerebral artery meets the area supplied by the middle cerebral artery where these arteries anastomose.

The caudal cerebral artery and the **rostral cerebellar artery** (*a. cerebelli rostralis*) are branches of the caudal communicating artery. The latter is a terminal branch of the internal carotid that forms the caudolateral portion of the cerebral arterial circle.

Arteries of Thoracic Limb Subclavian Artery

The **subclavian artery** (*a. subclavia*) (Figs. 11.12, 11.34, 11.35, and 11.38) is the intrathoracic portion of the parent vessel to each thoracic limb. It arises on the left side from the arch of the aorta and on the right side as a terminal branch of the brachiocephalic trunk. It is continued at the cranial border of the first rib on each side by the axillary artery. The name *subclavian* implies that the vessel lies deep to the clavicle. This is not the case in quadrupeds because the thorax is laterally compressed so that the clavicle, even when it is well developed, lies ventrolateral to the thoracic inlet associated with the brachiocephalicus muscle. The right subclavian artery arises medial to the first right intercostal space and is approximately 2 cm long. Vitums (1962) noted an anomalous origin of the right subclavian artery in 3 of 275 class dissection specimens. In these dogs the right subclavian artery originated from the aorta caudal to the left subclavian artery and coursed dorsal to the esophagus and then cranially to reach the right thoracic limb. Although there did not appear to be any dilation of the esophagus caused by the constriction, a "partial vascular ring anomaly," there may have been a functional problem as reported by Helphrey (1979), Ellison (1980), and Green (1983).

The left subclavian artery arises medial to the left third intercostal space and is approximately 6 cm long. Because the four arteries that arise from each subclavian artery have similar origins and distributions, only a single description of them is given. All arise medial to the first rib or first intercostal space. These four arteries are the vertebral, costocervical trunk, internal thoracic, and superficial cervical arteries.

The **vertebral artery** (*a. vertebralis*) (Figs. 11.12, 11.30, and Figs. 11.34 through 11.36A, and 11.37) is the first branch of the subclavian artery. It arises from the dorsal surface of the subclavian artery on the ventrolateral side of the trachea. As it ascends to the transverse foramen of the sixth cervical vertebra, it crosses the trachea obliquely on the right side and the trachea and esophagus on the left side. It continues across the m. longus colli and the lateral surface of the transverse process of the sixth cervical vertebra on each side. Near the thoracic inlet, on each side, a small muscular branch supplies the peritracheal fascia and, running cranially, terminates in the caudal part of the longus capitis muscle. Before the vertebral artery enters the transverse foramen at the sixth cervical vertebra and at every intervertebral space cranial to this, it sends dorsal and ventral **muscular branches** (Fig. 11.36A) (see spinal branches for explanation of Fig. 11.36A) into the adjacent musculature. The dorsal branches are distributed to the scalenus, intertransversarius colli, serratus ventralis cervicalis, and omotransversarius muscles. The ventral branch supplies mainly the m. longus capitis and m. longus colli, although some branches go to the cleidocephalicus and sternocephalicus muscles. Arising as a rule separately, but occasionally from a short common trunk, these dorsal and ventral muscular branches follow the distribution of the dorsal and ventral branches of the corresponding cervical spinal nerve. Satellite veins accompany the arteries. According to Whisnant et al. (1956), four or five anastomoses occur between the muscular branches of each vertebral artery and the costocervical artery. These workers indicate that a secondary anastomosis exists between the vertebral and superficial cervical arteries. These combined anastomoses are large enough to sustain life in the majority of dogs when both the vertebral and common carotid arteries are ligated bilaterally at the base of the neck.

From the medial surface of the vertebral artery at each intervertebral foramen, usually opposite the muscular branches, arise the first seven cervical **spinal branches** (*rami spinales*). These enter the vertebral canal at each of the first seven cervical intervertebral foramina and perforate through the dura and arachnoid into the subarachnoid space. Within the subarachnoid space, each divides into a small dorsal and a slightly larger ventral branch. The ventral branches follow the ventral roots to the ventral median

532 CHAPTER 11 The Heart and Arteries

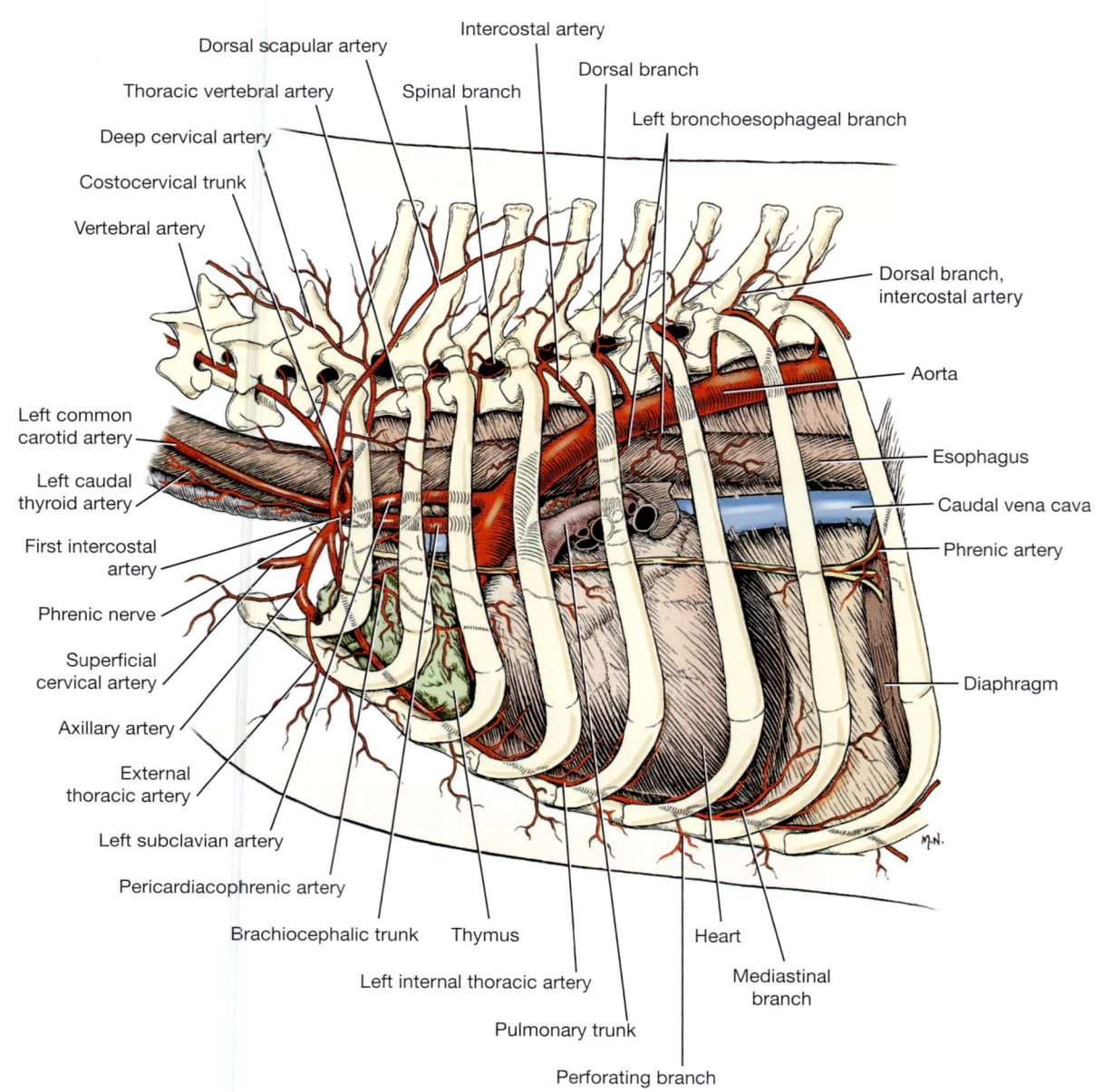

• Fig. 11.34 Arteries of the left thorax.

fissure of the spinal cord. Here, the ventral branches from each side as well as cranially and caudally are all united on the median plane ventral to the spinal cord forming the **ventral spinal artery** (*a. spinalis ventralis*) (Fig. 11.30 and 11.36B). This is an unpaired vessel that lies at the ventral median fissure of the spinal cord and extends along the entire length of the spinal cord. It sends segmental branches dorsally into the ventral median fissure primarily to the gray matter of the spinal cord. Other branches, lying on the pia, partially encircle the spinal cord and supply the ventral and lateral white matter. The dorsal branches of the spinal arteries follow the dorsal nerve root to the spinal cord, where they are dissipated without a continuous dorsolateral trunk being formed. The largest spinal ramus is usually the third cervical, but occasionally the fourth cervical spinal branch equals it in size. After traversing the transverse foramen of the atlas, the vertebral artery divides unequally into a large dorsal and a small ventral branch (see Figs. 11.30 and 11.36A). The ventral branch anastomoses with the small cervical branch of the occipital artery ventral to the wing of the atlas. The larger dorsal branch anastomoses with the descending branch of the occipital artery. The vertebral artery enters the vertebral canal by passing through the lateral vertebral foramen of the atlas. This portion of the vertebral artery was formerly called the *cerebrospinal artery* (see Fig. 11.30). It perforates the dura and arachnoid to the subarachnoid space and divides into cranial and caudal branches, which anastomose with comparable branches from the opposite side. The caudal branches are continuous with the ventral spinal artery, the cranial branches form the basilar artery. The **basilar artery** (*a. basilaris*) (Fig. 11.30) runs cranially through the foramen magnum and rostrally

CHAPTER 11 The Heart and Arteries   533

• **Fig. 11.35** Arteries of the right thorax.

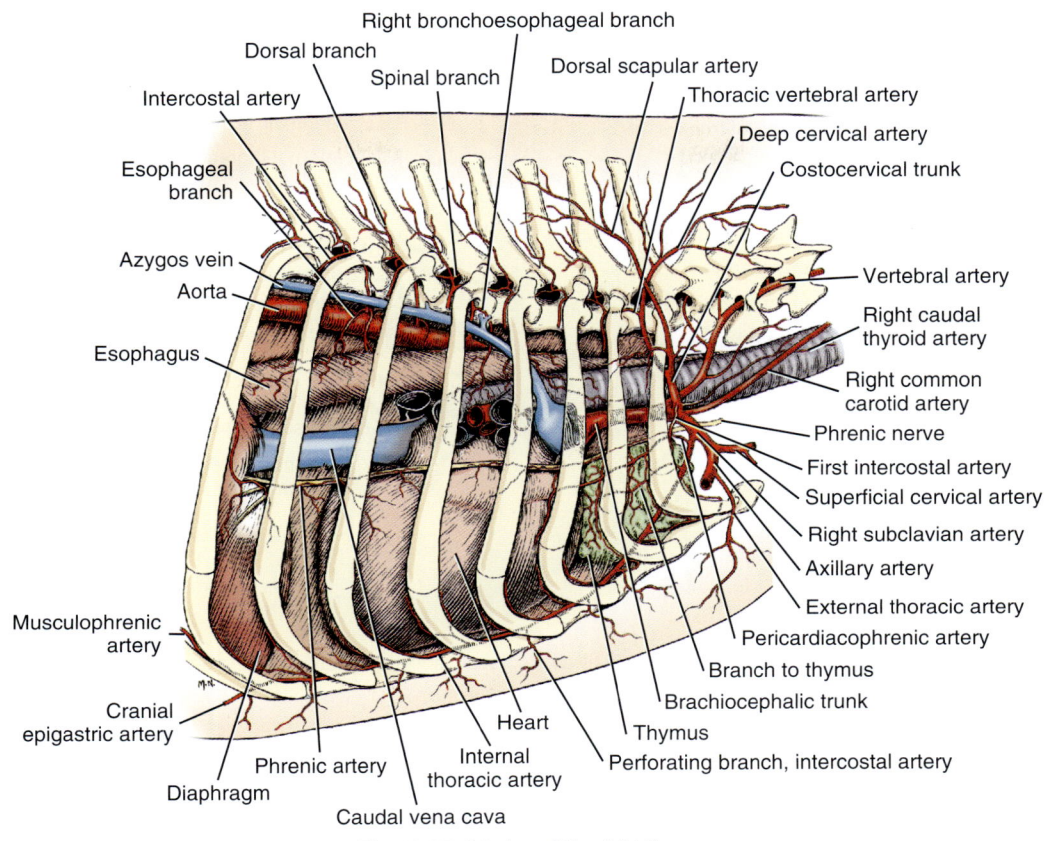

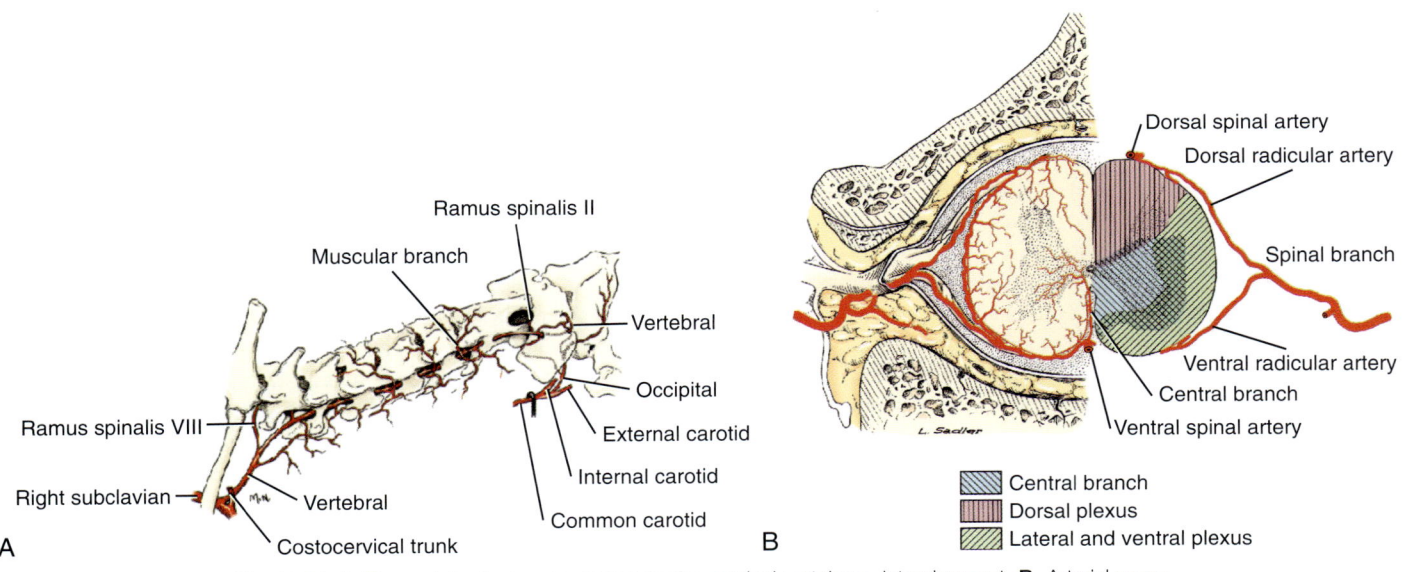

• **Fig. 11.36** A, The vertebral artery in relation to the cervical vertebrae, lateral aspect. B, Arterial vasculature of the canine spinal cord.

along the ventral surface of the brainstem. Along its course it bilaterally gives off **caudal cerebellar arteries** (*a. cerebelli caudalis*) to the caudal aspect of the cerebellum, **labyrinth arteries** (*a. labyrinthi*) that accompany the vestibulocochlear nerves to the inner ear, and **pontine branches** (*rr. ad pontem*) to the pons. Ventral to the mesencephalon the basilar artery divides, and each branch anastomoses with the caudal communicating arteries of the internal carotids to complete the caudal portion of the cerebral arterial circle. The basilar artery is the largest source of blood to the brain via the circulus arteriosus cerebri (Anderson & Kubicek, 1971).

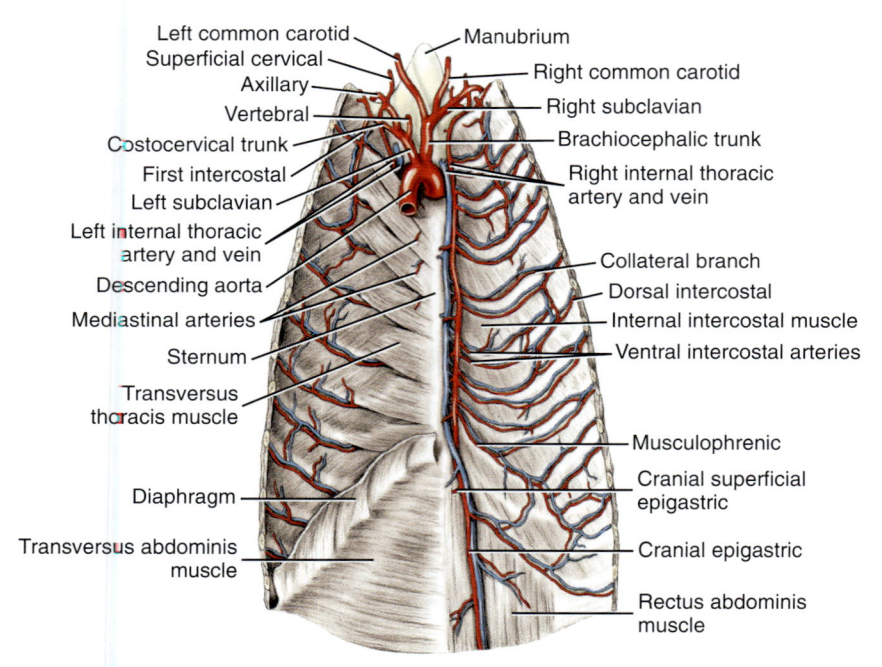

Fig. 11.37 The internal thoracic arteries, dorsal aspect, in relation to the sternum.

The **costocervical trunk** (*truncus costocervicalis*) (Figs. 11.12, 11.34, and 11.35) arises from the subclavian artery 5 to 10 mm peripheral to the origin of the vertebral artery. Because it courses dorsally and the vertebral artery courses cranially, the costocervical trunk on the left side crosses first the lateral surface of the vertebral artery, then the esophagus; on the right it crosses the trachea. On either side, the costocervical trunk crosses the longus capitis muscle and lies largely medial to the first rib. Branches of the costocervical trunk include the small first intercostal artery, large dorsal scapular and deep cervical arteries, and a small thoracic vertebral artery.

The **dorsal scapular artery** (*a. scapularis dorsalis*) (Figs. 11.34 and 11.35), formerly known as the *transverse artery of the neck,* arises from the cranial surface of the costocervical trunk, at an acute angle, at approximately the middle of the medial surface of the first rib. It runs mainly dorsally and leaves the thoracic cavity cranial to the first rib. From its initial part it sends at least one large branch caudally into the thoracic part of the serratus ventralis and mainly two or three smaller branches cranially into the cervical part of the serratus ventralis muscle. The dorsal scapular artery at the proximal end of the first rib inclines dorsocaudally, crosses the lateral surface of the first costotransverse joint, and arborizes extensively in the dorsal part of the thoracic portion of the serratus ventralis muscle. It gives origin to the eighth cervical spinal branch as it passes the intervertebral foramen between the seventh cervical and first thoracic vertebrae. In some specimens this branch arises from that part of the vessel that supplies the thoracic part of the m. serratus ventralis. During its course, it obliquely crosses the deeply lying deep cervical artery.

The **deep cervical artery** (*a. cervicalis profunda*) (Figs. 11.34 and 11.35) extends dorsocranially from the costocervical trunk. It leaves the thorax through the proximal end of the first intercostal space. A medium-sized vessel usually leaves the parent artery here and, extending dorsally, arborizes mainly in the semispinalis capitis muscle in the region of the cranial thorax. The main part of the deep cervical artery runs craniomedially to the median plane, supplying along its course the deep structures of the neck, particularly the semispinalis capitis, multifidus cervicis, longissimus capitis, spinalis and semispinalis thoracis, and cervicis muscles, and the terminal fasciculus of the thoracic portion of the longissimus muscle. It anastomoses with the dorsal muscular branches of the vertebral artery and, in the cranial part of the neck, with the descending branch of the occipital artery. It gives origin to the first thoracic spinal branch.

The **thoracic vertebral artery** (*a. vertebralis thoracica*) (Figs. 11.34 and 11.35) leaves the costocervical trunk in the proximal end of the first intercostal space. It extends caudally to the third and occasionally the fourth intercostal space, where it anastomoses with the dorsal intercostal artery of that space that arises from the aorta. The thoracic vertebral artery passes through the costotransverse foramen dorsal to the neck of the rib and therefore is not homologous to the supreme intercostal artery of other domestic animals, in which it is located ventral to the neck of the rib. However, a supreme intercostal artery (*a. intercostalis suprema*) ventral to the neck of the rib is sometimes seen in the dog together with the thoracic vertebral artery. Caudal to the second and third ribs that it crosses, the thoracic vertebral artery sends a small dorsal intercostal artery (*aa. intercostalis dorsales II et III*) ventrally, which anastomoses

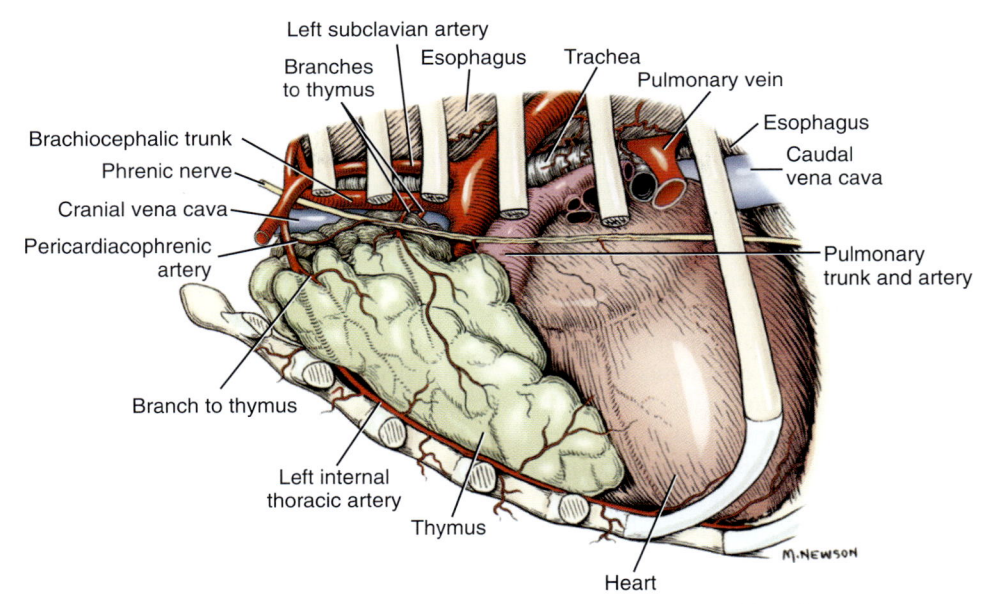

• Fig. 11.38 Arterial supply of the thymus gland in a young dog, left lateral aspect.

with the intercostal branches from the first intercostal artery and the ventral intercostal arteries of the internal thoracic artery in these intercostal spaces when present. The small second and third, and occasionally the fourth, thoracic spinal branches arise from the thoracic vertebral. Variations are common here.

In addition to the three main branches of the costocervical trunk, smaller vessels exist. A constant branch, the **first dorsal intercostal artery** (*a. intercostalis dorsalis I*) leaves the costocervical at its origin and, extending deep to the pleura covering the first two or three intercostal spaces and the intervening ribs, supplies the principal intercostal vessels of these spaces. The dorsal portions of its intercostal branches anastomose with the smaller dorsal intercostal arteries from the thoracic vertebral artery. The ventral portions anastomose with the ventral intercostal arteries from the internal thoracic artery.

Small branches leave the costocervical trunk near its origin and supply the adjacent musculature. Usually a small ramus accompanies the common carotid artery a short distance cranially in the neck. Satellite veins accompany the costocervical trunk and its branches.

The **internal thoracic artery** (*a. thoracica interna*) (Figs. 11.12, 11.34, 11.35, 11.37, 11.38, and 11.49) leaves the caudoventral surface of the subclavian artery opposite the origin of the superficial cervical artery. It runs caudoventrally in a narrow, lateral pleural plica from the cranial mediastinum to the craniomedial border of the m. transversus thoracis. Lying parallel to the sternum, it passes ventral to the m. transversus thoracis and runs caudally dorsal to the sternal ends of the costal cartilages and the intervening interchondral spaces. It ends just medial to the costal arch at the thoracic outlet by dividing into the small musculophrenic and the large cranial epigastric artery. It has numerous branches that include a pericardiophrenic artery, thymic, mediastinal, perforating, and ventral intercostal branches and terminal musculophrenic and cranial epigastric arteries.

The **pericardiacophrenic artery** (*a. pericardiacophrenica*) (Figs. 11.34, 11.35, and 11.38) is a small vessel that leaves the caudal side of the internal thoracic artery near its origin and runs with the phrenic nerve to the pericardium. In addition to supplying the cranial mediastinal and intrathoracic part of the phrenic nerve, the left vessel may send one or more branches to the cranial mediastinum and the thymus, when this is well developed. At the level of the heart on both sides the pericardiacophrenic artery anastomoses with the branch from the musculophrenic artery that courses cranially on the nerve from the diaphragm. Branches leave the vessel to supply the pericardium. A ventral bronchial branch may course to the root of the left lung.

The main **thymic branches** (*rami thymici*) (Figs. 11.35 and 11.38) usually leave the cranial mediastinal part of the internal thoracic artery as it passes through the thymus. Usually a single thymic branch supplies each lobe, but more than one vessel may be present.

Bronchial branches may leave the left pericardiacophrenic artery, or they may come from the internal thoracic arteries directly (Berry et al., 1931). They go to the roots of the lungs and furnish the minor blood supply to the bronchi, bronchial lymph nodes, and connective tissue. They are frequently absent.

The **mediastinal branches** (*rami mediastinales*) (Fig. 11.34) supply the ventral part of the mediastinum. Usually two to four branches run directly into the cranial mediastinum from the internal thoracic arteries. Those to the middle and caudal mediastinum perforate the origin of the overlying transverse thoracic muscle and extend vertically to either the pericardium or the diaphragm. Coming from the various phrenic arteries are mediastinal branches that extend into the ventral part of the mediastinum. Other branches from the phrenic arteries ramify in the plica venae cavae.

The **perforating branches** (*rami perforantes*) (Figs. 11.34 and 11.35) are straight, short, ventrally directed branches that leave the ventral surface of the internal thoracic artery. One is present in each interchondral space except the first and the last (eighth), and occasionally the seventh. These lie close to the lateral surfaces of the sternebrae and give off **sternal branches** (*rami sternales*) to them. The perforating branches also supply the internal intercostal and pectoral musculature adjacent to them. They are continued subcutaneously near the sternum as **ventral cutaneous branches** along with their satellite veins and comparable nerves. The branches that supply the medial portions of the thoracic mammary glands are called **mammary branches** (*rami mammarii*). These come from the fourth, fifth, and sixth vessels and are only evident when the glands are developed.

The **ventral intercostal branches** (*rr. intercostales ventrales*) (Figs. 11.37 and 11.50) usually are double for each of the interchondral spaces, starting with the second and ending with the eighth. Starting with the caudal artery of the eighth space, all remaining ventral intercostal arteries come from the musculophrenic artery. Those from the ventral surface of the internal thoracic artery arise singly, so that a small artery lies on each side of the costal cartilages, except the first, which has a delicate single artery. The artery caudal to the cartilage is slightly larger than the one cranial to it and is accompanied by the intercostal nerve, in addition to the satellite vein. These double arteries anastomose with each other across the medial side of the ribs at a level from one-third to one-half the length of the rib from its sternal attachment. The ventral intercostal artery lying caudal to the rib anastomoses with the dorsal intercostal artery. The ventral intercostal artery lying cranial to the rib anastomoses with the collateral branch of the dorsal intercostal artery. These vessels lie, for the most part, in the endothoracic fascia adjacent to the parietal pleura. Occasionally, some fibers from the internal intercostal muscles cover them. They supply the ventral part of the costal parietal pleura, the adjacent intercostal musculature, and the costal cartilages.

The **musculophrenic artery** (*a. musculophrenica*) (Figs. 11.35, and 11.37) is the smaller, lateral, terminal branch of the internal thoracic artery. It arises deep to the caudal part of the transverse thoracic muscle opposite the eighth interchondral space close to the sternum. It runs caudodorsolaterally, in the angle formed by the diaphragm and the lateral thoracic wall, where it lies in a small amount of fat covered by the pleura. After it has traveled approximately one-fourth of the length of the costal arch, it perforates the diaphragm and comes to lie deep to the peritoneum. It courses dorsally on the inner surface of the costal arch by following the margins of the interlocked digitations of attachments of the diaphragm and the transverse abdominal muscle. Along its course it sends the **ventral intercostal branches** (*rr. intercostales ventrales*) dorsally in the caudal part of the eighth interchondral space, and two each for spaces 9 and 10. The single terminal branch of the musculophrenic artery anastomoses with the eleventh dorsal intercostal artery caudal to the diaphragm. These ventral intercostal branches form feeble anastomoses with the ventral parts of the eighth, ninth, and tenth dorsal intercostal arteries. Numerous small branches leave the musculophrenic artery to supply the muscular periphery of the diaphragm. Some of these end in the caudal mediastinum and plica venae cavae. A small branch runs cranially on both sides with the caudal mediastinal portion of the phrenic nerve and anastomoses with the small pericardiacophrenic artery. Fewer branches ramify in the adjacent abdominal wall. Both sets of branches anastomose with the caudal phrenic and cranial abdominal arteries, and each is accompanied by a satellite vein.

The **cranial epigastric artery** (*a. epigastrica cranialis*) (Figs. 11.35 and 11.37) is the larger, medial terminal branch of the internal thoracic artery. It arises dorsal to the eighth interchondral space lateral to the sternum ventral to the m. transversus thoracis. It perforates the diaphragm, and, in the angle between the costal arch and the xiphoid process, it runs caudally on the dorsal surface of the rectus abdominis muscle as the cranial epigastric artery. This was formerly called the *cranial deep epigastric artery*. At a transverse level through the umbilicus, many of its branches enter the m. rectus abdominis and shortly thereafter the cranial epigastric branches anastomose with the cranially running terminal branches of the caudal epigastric artery. It is the primary blood supply to the middle portion of the m. rectus abdominis. It is accompanied by its laterally lying satellite vein.

The ventral abdominal wall has two arterial channels on each side of the median plane that connect the thoracic circulation with that of the pelvic limbs. One of these is superficial, and the other is deep. The epigastric vessels are deep and always well developed, but the superficial epigastric vessels reach their maximum size only during the height of lactation. The deep vessels anastomose feebly with each other across the linea alba. As each cranial epigastric artery passes through the diaphragm, it may supply a sizable branch.

The **superficial cranial epigastric artery** (*a. epigastrica cranialis superficialis*) is a branch of the cranial epigastric artery and, in a lactating bitch may be larger than the deeply located cranial epigastric artery. It runs through the m. rectus abdominis and its sheath and enters the subcutaneous tissue between the caudal thoracic and the cranial abdominal mammae. It sends most of its branches caudolaterally and is the chief supply of **mammary branches** (*rami mammary*) to the cranial abdominal mamma. Caudal to this gland, several of its many branches anastomose with the end branches of the cranially running superficial caudal epigastric artery.

The **superficial cervical artery** (*a. cervicalis superficialis*) (Figs. 11.12, 11.34, 11.35, 11.37, and 11.39) formerly called the *omocervical trunk*, arises from the cranial surface of the subclavian artery medial to the first rib and opposite the origin of the internal thoracic artery. It is a long, meandering artery that lies in the angle between the shoulder and the neck. It lies deep to the pectoral, brachiocephalic, and

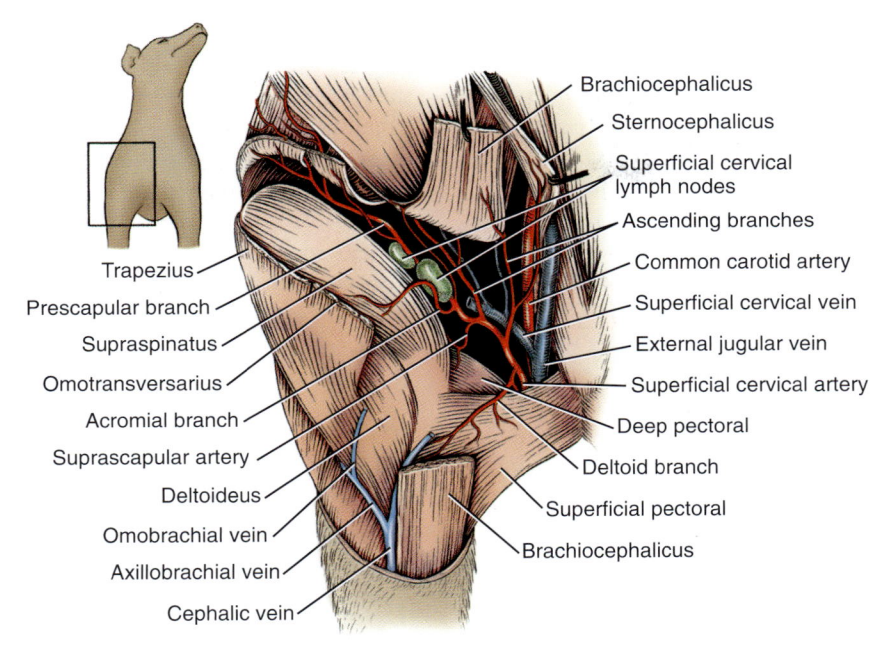

• **Fig. 11.39** Branches of the superficial cervical artery. Cranial aspect.

omotransverse muscles and ventral and medial to the brachial plexus. It has four named branches in addition to several small muscular branches to the muscles that lie adjacent to it. These four named branches are the deltoid, ascending, and prescapular branches, and the suprascapular artery.

The **deltoid branch** (*ramus deltoideus*) (Fig. 11.39), formerly called the *descending branch*, arises from the superficial cervical artery approximately 3 cm from its origin. Occasionally the deltoid branch arises from the internal thoracic instead of from the superficial cervical artery. It runs distolaterally in the brachium in the groove between the pectoral muscles, which bound it caudally, and the m. brachiocephalicus, which bounds it cranially and partly covers it. It ends in the distal third of the brachium in either the superficial pectoral, cleidobrachialis or biceps brachii muscle. Peripheral to the origin of the deltoid branch, the superficial cervical artery sends one or more branches to the muscles that lie ventral to the trachea.

The **ascending branch** (*r. ascendens*) (Fig. 11.39) leaves the superficial cervical artery near the deltoid branch before the origin of the suprascapular artery. Frequently the artery is double. The profusely branching ascending cervical branch is considerably smaller than the suprascapular artery. It courses cranially, medial to the m. cleidocephalicus and lateral to the scalenus muscle. It supplies the sternocephalicus, the occipital portion of the cleidocephalicus, rhomboideus, omotransversarius, and scalenus muscles and the superficial cervical lymph nodes. In the cranial half of the neck, its terminal branches are distributed chiefly to the omotransversarius and cleidocephalicus muscles. Some branches anastomose with the cervical branch of the caudal auricular artery.

The **suprascapular artery** (*a. suprascapularis*) leaves the caudal side of the superficial cervical artery approximately 2 cm distal to the origin of the deltoid and ascending branches. Accompanied by the suprascapular nerve, it goes through the triangular space bounded by the subscapular, supraspinatus, and deep pectoral muscles. On reaching the neck of the scapula, it divides into a large lateral and a small medial branch. The lateral branch passes deep to the m. supraspinatus to the lateral surface of the scapula, on which it ramifies. It supplies the m. supraspinatus and sends one large and several small nutrient arteries into the bone. Passing across the neck of the scapula distal to the spine of the scapula, it sends branches to the infraspinatus and teres minor muscles, and the shoulder joint. Near the caudal border of the scapula, it anastomoses with the circumflex scapular artery, a branch of the subscapular artery. The medial branch of the suprascapular artery passes between the subscapular muscle and the medial surface of the neck of the scapula. It supplies both of these as well as a part of the shoulder joint. It ends in an anastomosis with the circumflex scapular artery.

The **acromial branch** (*r. acromialis*) (Fig. 11.39) is given off the suprascapular artery or the superficial cervical artery 1 cm or less peripheral to the origin of the ascending branch and is usually larger than the latter. The acromial branch circles around the cranial border of the supraspinatus muscle and goes into its lateral surface, being largely distributed by ramifying proximally through it. A few terminal branches, however, reach as far as the infraspinatus muscle. In some specimens a small branch extends distally over the tendon of the supraspinatus muscle and the major tubercle of the humerus, and anastomoses with the deltoid branch. Deep to the m. cleidobrachialis deep branches anastomose with the suprascapular artery.

The **prescapular branch** (*ramus prescapularis*) (Fig. 11.39) is the terminal part of the superficial cervical artery.

It is a continuation of the parent artery after the suprascapular artery has been given off. It runs in the space between the shoulder and neck, caudal to the superficial cervical lymph nodes, which it supplies. It reaches the ventrocranial border of the cervical part of the m. trapezius. At this point it divides into an ascending and a descending branch. The ascending branch usually becomes superficial, sending many branches dorsocranially into the superficial fascia and the cutaneous muscles that cover the occipital part of the m. cleidocephalicus. This branch varies greatly in development. When it is fully developed, it may anastomose with the cervical branch of the caudal auricular artery in the cranial third of the neck. It may remain relatively deep, supplying the superficial muscles of the neck. The descending branch passes deep to the cervical part of the m. trapezius, to which it sends many branches. It terminates in the muscle near the cranial angle of the scapula. The branches of the superficial cervical artery are accompanied by satellite veins.

Axillary Artery

The **axillary artery** (*a. axillaris*) (Figs. 11.12, 11.34, 11.35, 11.37, and 11.40 thru 11.42) is a continuation of the subclavian artery and extends from the cranial border of the first rib to the distal border of the conjoined tendon of the teres major and latissimus dorsi muscles. At first it lies lateral to its satellite vein, then cranial to it. In relation to the axillary vessels, the musculocutaneous nerve is cranial, the radial nerve is lateral, and the median-ulnar nerve trunk is caudal. The axillary vein, at its termination, lies directly medial to the median-ulnar nerve trunk. The axillary artery has four primary branches: the external thoracic, lateral thoracic, subscapular, and cranial circumflex humeral arteries.

The **external thoracic artery** (*a. thoracica externa*) (Figs. 11.34, 11.35, 11.40, and 11.41) is usually the first branch of the axillary artery. It arises approximately 1 cm lateral to the first rib and curves around the craniomedial border of the deep pectoral muscle in company with a nerve and two satellite veins to supply the superficial pectoral muscle.

The **lateral thoracic artery** (*a. thoracica lateralis*) (Figs. 11.40 through 11.42) arises from the axillary artery approximately 2 cm from the cranial border of the first rib. Occasionally its origin is located distal to the large, caudodorsally running subscapular artery. It runs medially in the axillary

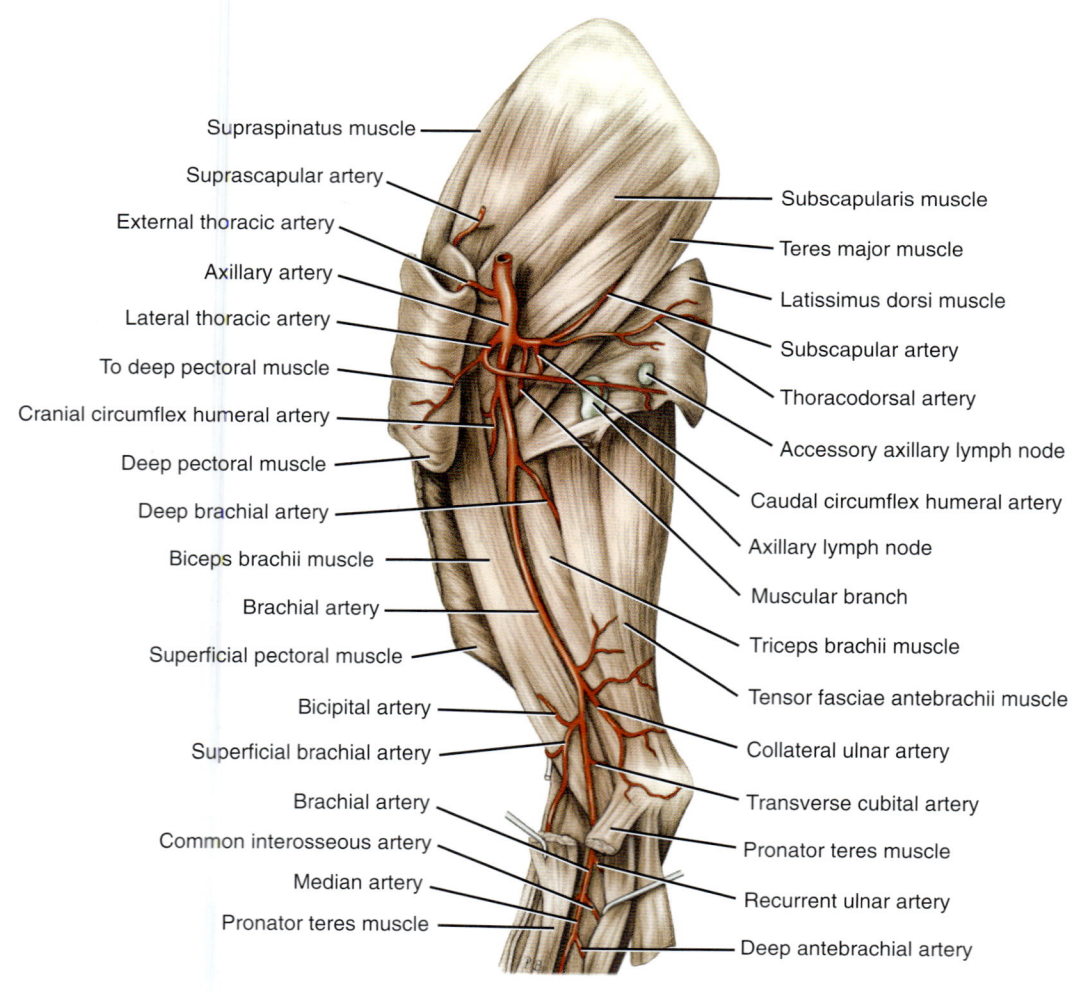

• **Fig. 11.40** Arteries of the right brachium, medial aspect.

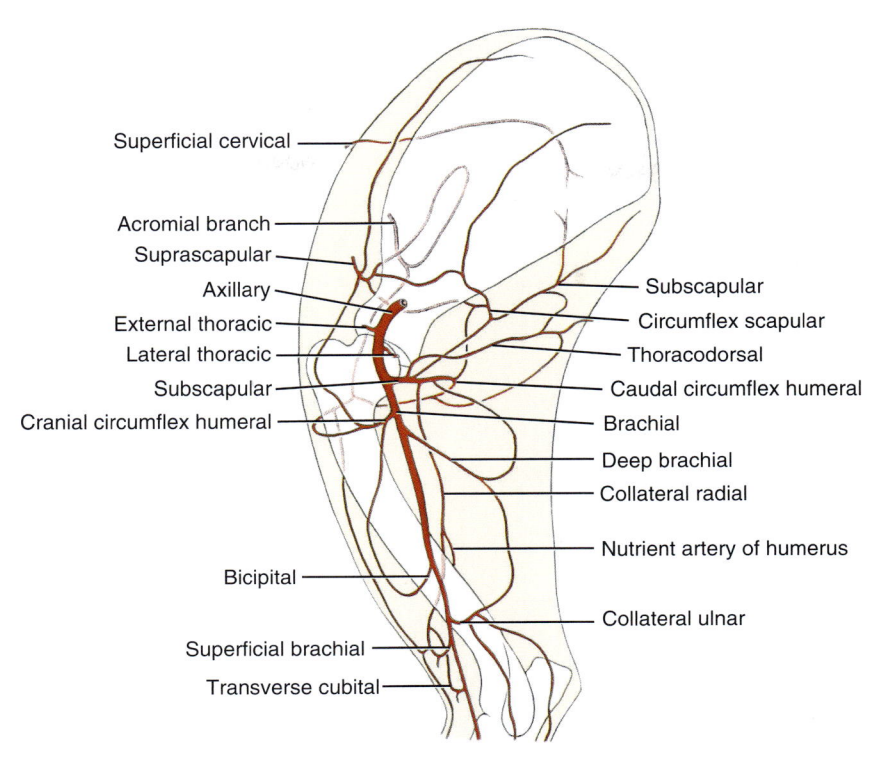

• **Fig. 11.41** Diagram of the arteries of the right brachium, medial aspect.

fat and crosses the lateral surface of the axillary lymph node, which it supplies. It also supplies an area of the m. latissimus dorsi ventral to the area supplied by the thoracodorsal artery. Other branches supply the deep pectoral and cutaneous trunci muscles. Its **lateral mammary branches** (*rami mammarii laterals*) supply the dorsolateral portions of the cranial and caudal thoracic mammary glands when these are fully developed. The lateral thoracic artery is accompanied by a satellite vein and nerve.

The **subscapular artery** (*a. subscapularis*) (Figs. 11.40 to 11.42) may be larger than the continuation of the axillary artery in the brachium. This great size is explained by the fact that the vessel supplies a greater muscle mass in the scapular region and arm than is present in the remainder of the limb. It arises from the caudal surface of the axillary artery usually just peripheral to the origin of the lateral thoracic artery. It runs obliquely in a dorsocaudal direction along the caudal border of the scapula between the subscapularis and teres major muscles and becomes subcutaneous near the caudal angle of the scapula. It has the following principal branches: thoracodorsal, caudal circumflex humeral, and circumflex scapular arteries.

The **thoracodorsal artery** (*a. thoracodorsalis*) is a large artery that leaves the caudal surface of the subscapular artery less than 1 cm from its origin. It runs caudally, usually supplying a part of the teres major muscle as the artery crosses the medial surface of the distal end of the muscle, and terminates in the latissimus dorsi muscle and skin. A satellite vein and nerve accompany the artery.

The **caudal circumflex humeral artery** (*a. circumflexa humeri caudalis*) (Figs. 11.40 and 11.41) leaves the lateral surface of the subscapular artery at approximately the same level as the thoracodorsal artery and immediately courses laterally between the head of the humerus and the teres major muscle. It is the principal source of blood to all four heads of the large triceps muscle. The **collateral radial artery** (*a. collateralis radialis*) leaves the distal surface of the caudal circumflex humeral artery approximately 1 cm from its origin and takes a direct course distally, lateral to the terminal ends of the teres major and latissimus dorsi and the medial head of the triceps muscles. It lies medial to the accessory head and caudal to the brachialis muscle. It may terminate as the **nutrient artery of the humerus** (*a. nutricia humeri*) by entering the nutrient foramen near the middle of the caudal surface of the bone. In most specimens, as Miller (1952) has pointed out, the collateral radial artery, after sending the nutrient artery into the humerus, continues obliquely distocranially on the brachialis muscle and anastomoses with the superficial brachial artery proximal to the flexor angle of the elbow joint. During its course, it supplies branches to the brachialis and heads of the triceps muscles, which lie along its course. This vessel is accompanied by its small satellite vein and the radial nerve.

The main part of the caudal circumflex humeral artery arborizes extensively in the triceps muscle as ascending and descending branches. The caudal part of the shoulder joint capsule, infraspinatus, teres minor, and coracobrachialis muscles also receive branches from this vessel. Some of the proximal branches anastomose with the small circumflex scapular artery, and some of the descending branches anastomose with the deep brachial artery. There is a small anastomosis between the caudal and cranial circumflex humeral

540 CHAPTER 11 The Heart and Arteries

Labels on figure (left side, top to bottom): Teres major, Subscapularis, Subscapular artery, Axillary artery, Lateral thoracic artery, Thoracodorsal artery, Subscapular artery, Cranial circumflex humeral artery, Teres major, Deep brachial artery, Triceps, medial head, Brachial artery, Nutrient artery of humerus, Biceps brachii, Triceps brachii, Anconeus

Labels on figure (right side, top to bottom): Trapezius, Deltoideus, Circumflex scapular artery, Infraspinatus, Triceps, caput longum, Omotransversarius, Caudal circumflex humeral artery, Triceps, accessory head, Triceps, lateral head, Collateral radial artery, Brachialis

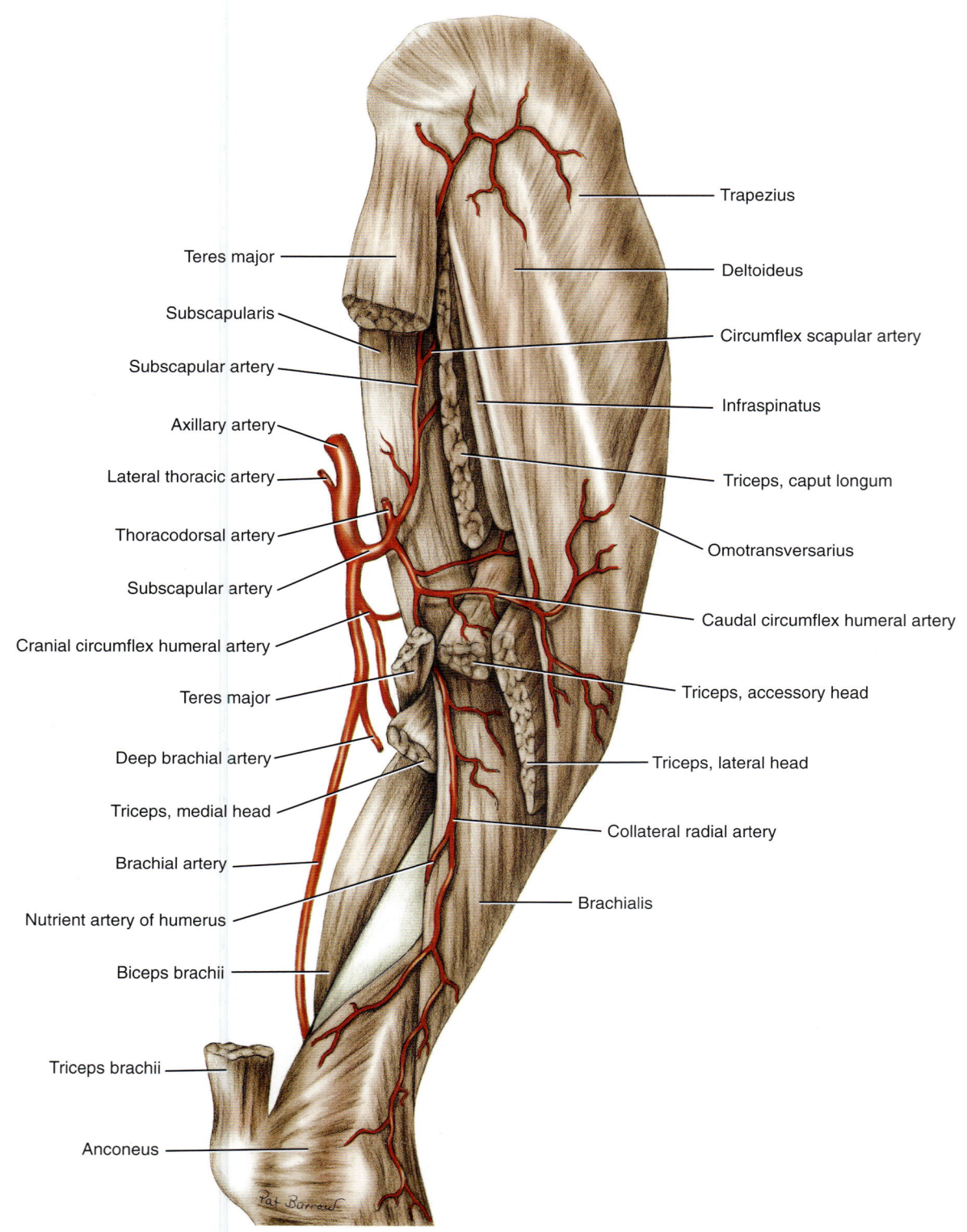

• **Fig. 11.42** Arteries of the right brachium, caudolateral aspect.

arteries. The main stem of the caudal circumflex humeral artery leaves the triceps muscle mass and enters the deep face of the deltoideus muscle. Other branches extend between the deltoid muscle laterally and the long and lateral heads of the triceps muscle medially, to appear subcutaneously near the middle of the lateral surface of the brachium. Some of these branches extend proximally to anastomose with the deltoideus branch of the superficial cervical artery; others run distally and anastomose with the superficial brachial artery. The caudal circumflex humeral artery is accompanied through the fleshy part of the brachium by its satellite vein and the axillary nerve.

The **circumflex scapular artery** (*a. circumflexa scapulae*) is a small vessel that leaves the cranial surface of the subscapular artery and, extending obliquely dorsocranially between the subscapularis muscle medially and the long head of the triceps muscle laterally, reaches the caudal border of the scapula near its middle. Here it divides into a medial and a lateral branch. The medial branch ramifies in the periosteal part of the subscapularis muscle, and the lateral branch arborizes in a similar manner in the infraspinatus muscle. Minute branches enter the bone from both medial and lateral parts.

Distal to the origin of the circumflex scapular artery, the subscapular artery continues along the caudal border of the scapula toward its caudal angle. Muscular branches supply the proximal ends of the teres major, subscapularis, infraspinatus, deltoideus, and latissimus dorsi muscles. A large patch of skin covering the region lateral and caudal to the caudal angle of the scapula is supplied by the terminal cutaneous branches. The subscapular artery and its branches are accompanied by satellite veins.

The **cranial circumflex humeral artery** (*a. circumflexa humeri cranialis*) (Figs. 11.40 to 11.42) is usually the last branch of the axillary artery before the axillary becomes the brachial artery. Usually it arises from the medial surface of the axillary artery distal to the origin of the subscapular artery. It may arise from the axillary artery, proximal to the origin of the subscapular artery, or from the subscapular artery itself. It is a small vessel that curves cranially around the medial aspect of the neck of the humerus deep to the tendon of origin of the m. biceps brachii after crossing the insertion of the coracobrachialis muscle. A relatively large branch supplies the proximal end of the biceps muscle, and smaller branches go to the coracobrachialis and to the conjoined teres major and latissimus dorsi muscles. A branch extends proximally to supply the cranial part of the joint capsule. In the region of the greater tubercle of the humerus, the two circumflex humeral vessels join with each other as well as with the suprascapular artery proximally and with the deltoideus branch of the superficial cervical artery distally. Occasionally the acromial branch of the superficial cervical artery also joins in this anastomosis.

Brachial Artery

The **brachial artery** (*a. brachialis*) (Figs. 11.40 through 11.45) is a continuation of the axillary artery. It begins at the distal border of the conjoined tendons of the teres major and latissimus dorsi muscles and becomes the median artery in the midantebrachium, where it continues into the forepaw as the main blood supply. The brachial artery in the brachium lies caudal to the musculocutaneous nerve and biceps brachii muscle, medial to the medial head of the triceps muscle and humerus, and cranial to the median and ulnar nerves and brachial vein. The deep pectoral muscle and a nerve connecting the musculocutaneous and median nerves form the medial boundary of the brachial artery in the brachium. It crosses the distal half of the humerus obliquely and becomes the median artery as it passes deep to the pronator teres muscle. The collateral branches of the brachial artery as it lies in the arm are the deep brachial, bicipital, collateral ulnar, superficial brachial, transverse cubital, and common interosseus arteries.

The **deep brachial artery** (*a. brachialis profunda*) leaves the caudal side of the brachial artery in the proximal third of the arm. Occasionally the artery is double. The deep brachial artery enters the medial and long heads of the triceps muscle; a smaller branch enters the medial head of the triceps muscle, and a larger one, after a course of more than 1 cm, is distributed to the long head of the triceps muscle. Within the triceps muscle the relatively small deep brachial artery anastomoses with the caudal circumflex humeral artery proximally and with the collateral ulnar artery distally. A satellite vein accompanies the artery. The radial nerve enters the triceps muscle lateral to the artery.

The **bicipital artery** (*a. bicipitalis*) (Figs. 11.40, 11.41, and 11.43) is frequently called the *muscular ramus to the biceps brachii muscle*. It may be double, and usually, when it is double, one branch arises from the superficial brachial artery. The bicipital artery, when it is single, usually arises from the medial surface of the brachial artery at the junction of the middle and distal thirds of the arm. The bicipital artery anastomoses with the muscular branch to the biceps brachii muscle from the cranial circumflex humeral artery. It runs distally and enters the distal end of the biceps brachii muscle. The bicipital artery may arise from the superficial brachial artery. A satellite vein accompanies the artery.

The **collateral ulnar artery** (*a. collateralis ulnaris*) (Figs. 11.40, 11.41, and 11.43) arises from the caudal surface of the brachial artery in the distal third of the arm. Usually the first branch runs proximocaudally to enter the medial surface of the triceps muscle. This may be paired with one branch leaving the brachial artery directly. Another branch runs distally toward the caudal side of the forearm accompanied by the ulnar nerve. Usually a large branch arises from this vessel proximal to the elbow joint and, running deep to the medial head of the triceps and anconeus muscles, courses into the olecranon fossa. It supplies primarily the fat and the pouch of the elbow joint capsule (*rete articulare cubiti*) that are located here. The branch that continues distally arborizes in the proximal parts of the flexor muscles of the antebrachium. An anastomosis exists with a proximally extending branch from the common interosseous artery between the ulnar and humeral heads of the deep digital flexor muscle. Slightly caudal to the branch that runs with the ulnar nerve is a superficial branch that runs distally across the medial surface of the elbow joint and continues in the subcutaneous tissue of the proximal half of the caudal surface of the antebrachium. It supplies the skin here and anastomoses with a proximally extending subcutaneous branch from the caudal interosseous artery. A vein and the caudal cutaneous antebrachial nerve accompany the vessel.

The **superficial brachial artery** (*a. brachialis superficialis*) (Figs. 11.40, 11.41, 11.43, and 11.44), formerly called the *proximal collateral radial artery*, leaves the cranial surface of the brachial artery approximately 3 cm proximal to the

542 CHAPTER 11 The Heart and Arteries

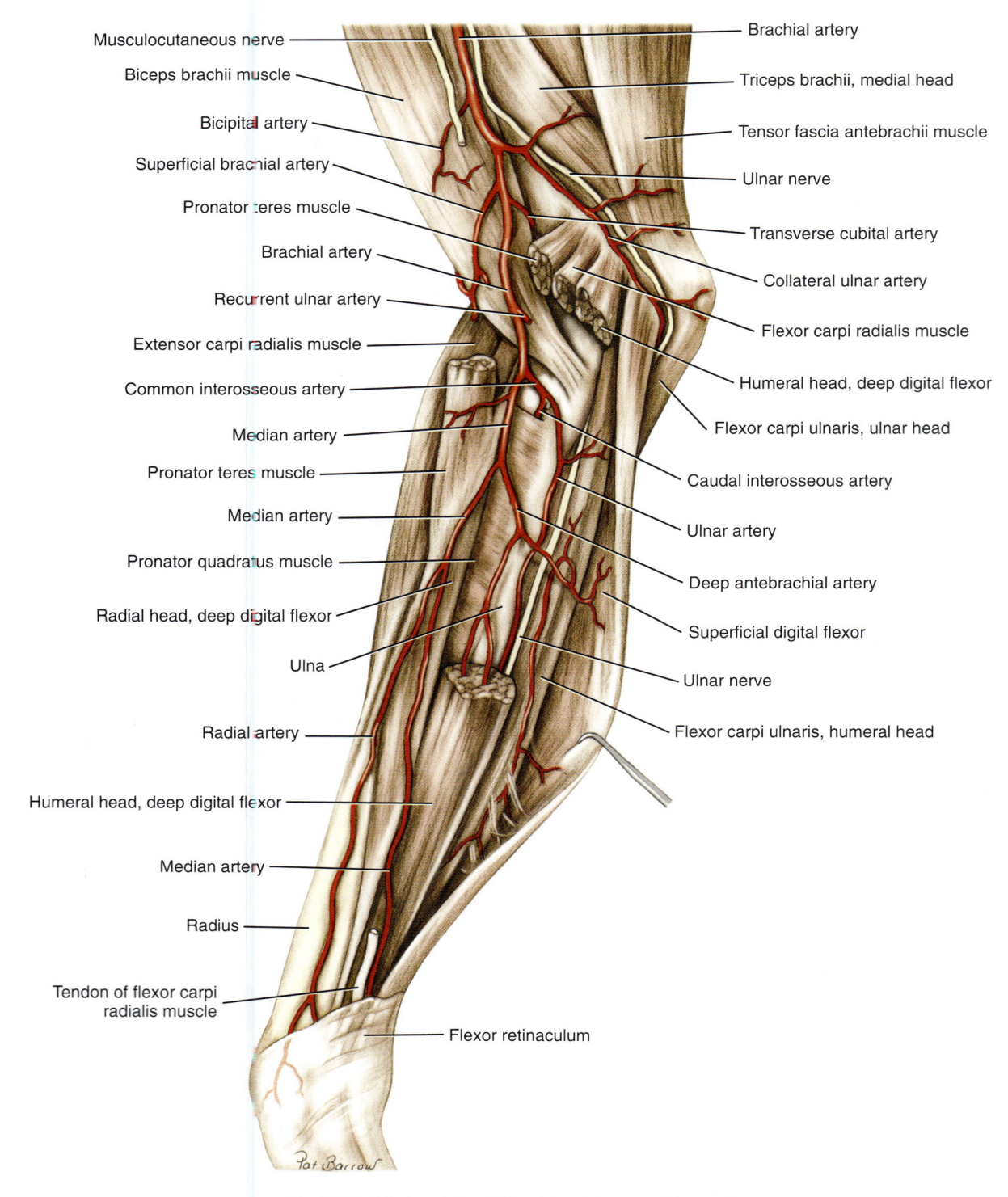

• Fig. 11.43 Arteries of the right antebrachium, medial aspect.

elbow joint and extends obliquely distocraniad to its flexor surface. After it crosses the tendon of the biceps brachii muscle, it gives off a pair of cutaneous branches, **superficial radial arteries** (*aa. radiales superficiales*), that course with the medial cutaneous antebrachial nerve to the skin of the medial surface of the antebrachium. In the region of the cephalic vein, the superficial brachial artery passes deep to it, crosses the cranial surface of the elbow, and becomes the cranial superficial antebrachial artery.

The **cranial superficial antebrachial artery** (*a. antebrachialis superficialis cranialis*) is a short trunk that immediately terminates in medial and lateral branches that continue

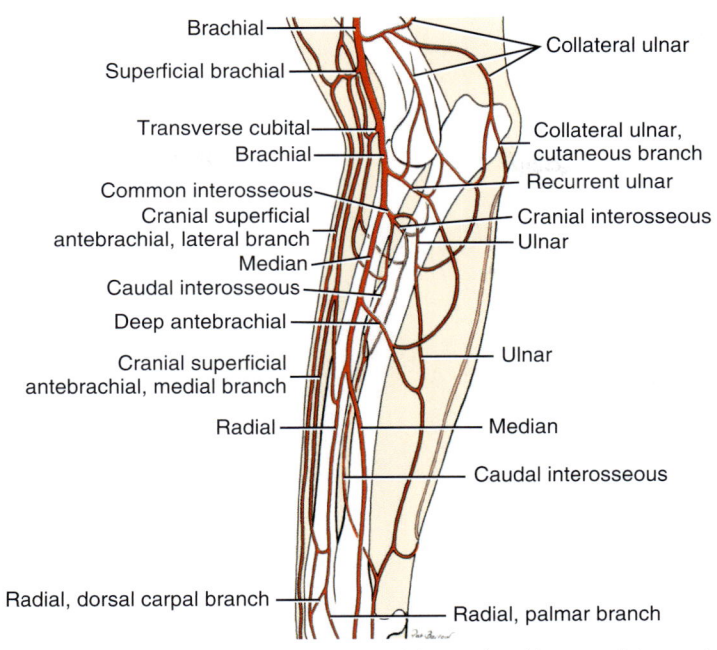

• Fig. 11.44 Diagram of the arteries of the right antebrachium, medial aspect.

into the forepaw to supply the digits. The **medial branch** (*ramus medialis*) of the cranial superficial antebrachial artery extends from the flexor surface of the elbow joint to the medial part of the forepaw. In its course distally in the antebrachium it lies on the extensor carpi radialis muscle, where it is bounded laterally by the large antebrachial part of the cephalic vein and medially by the small medial branch of the superficial radial nerve. Throughout the antebrachium it is accompanied by the medial branch of the superficial radial nerve. At the carpus the medial branch of the cranial superficial antebrachial artery anastomoses with the dorsal branch of the radial artery before continuing to the dorsomedial part of the metacarpus as the **dorsal common digital artery I** (*a. digitalis dorsalis communis*) (Fig. 11.46). The resultant branches of this anastomosis form the medial part of the poorly defined **dorsal rete of the carpus** (*rete carpi dorsale*) (Fig. 11.46B) in the extensor retinaculum on the dorsal surface of the carpus. The lateral part of this rete is formed by the interosseous branch of the caudal interosseous artery and its dorsal carpal branch. The dorsal rete contributes the deep lying dorsal metacarpal arteries to the forepaw, which are described later in this chapter in the section titled "Arteries of the Forepaw."

The **lateral branch** (*ramus lateralis*) of the cranial superficial antebrachial artery runs transversely, laterally across the distal end of the biceps brachii muscle and, on emerging from deep to the cephalic vein, bends distally and accompanies this vein on its lateral side throughout the antebrachium. A small ascending branch, which arises as it turns distally, anastomoses with the deltoid branch of the superficial cervical artery. The lateral branch of the cranial superficial antebrachial artery is somewhat larger than its medial branch, but, like it, is long and sparsely branched in the antebrachium. Throughout its antebrachial course, it is flanked medially by the large cephalic vein of the antebrachium, and laterally by the lateral branch of the superficial radial nerve. On the proximal part of the metacarpus the artery trifurcates. The three resultant dorsal common digital arteries are described later in this chapter in the section titled "Arteries of the Forepaw."

The **transverse cubital artery** (*a. transversa cubiti*) (Figs. 11.40, 11.41, 11.43, and 11.44), formerly called the *distal collateral radial artery*, arises from the lateral surface of the brachial artery, approximately 1 cm before that vessel runs deep to the pronator teres muscle. The transverse cubital artery, which is approximately as large as the superficial brachial artery, runs laterally deep to the distal end of the biceps brachii and brachialis muscles. On reaching the extensor carpi radialis muscle, it breaks up into many branches, most of which supply this muscle. Occasionally a branch runs proximally in company with the radial nerve and anastomoses with that part of the nutrient artery of the humerus, which courses distal to the foramen. Besides the branches that go to the extensor carpi radialis muscle, there are branches that go to the supinator, common digital extensor, and brachialis muscles. Anastomoses with the cranial interosseous and superficial brachial arteries sometimes occur.

The **recurrent ulnar artery** (*a. recurrens ulnaris*) (Figs. 11.40, 11.43, and 11.44) is a small vessel that leaves the caudal side of the brachial artery distal to the elbow or in some dogs the proximal side of the common interosseous artery at the proximal end of the radius. It extends from the caudal border of the pronator teres into the flexor group of muscles. The artery first runs deep to the m. flexor carpi radialis near its origin and contributes to its supply. It continues caudally through the humeral head of the deep digital flexor muscle, which it supplies, and terminates mainly in

544 CHAPTER 11 **The Heart and Arteries**

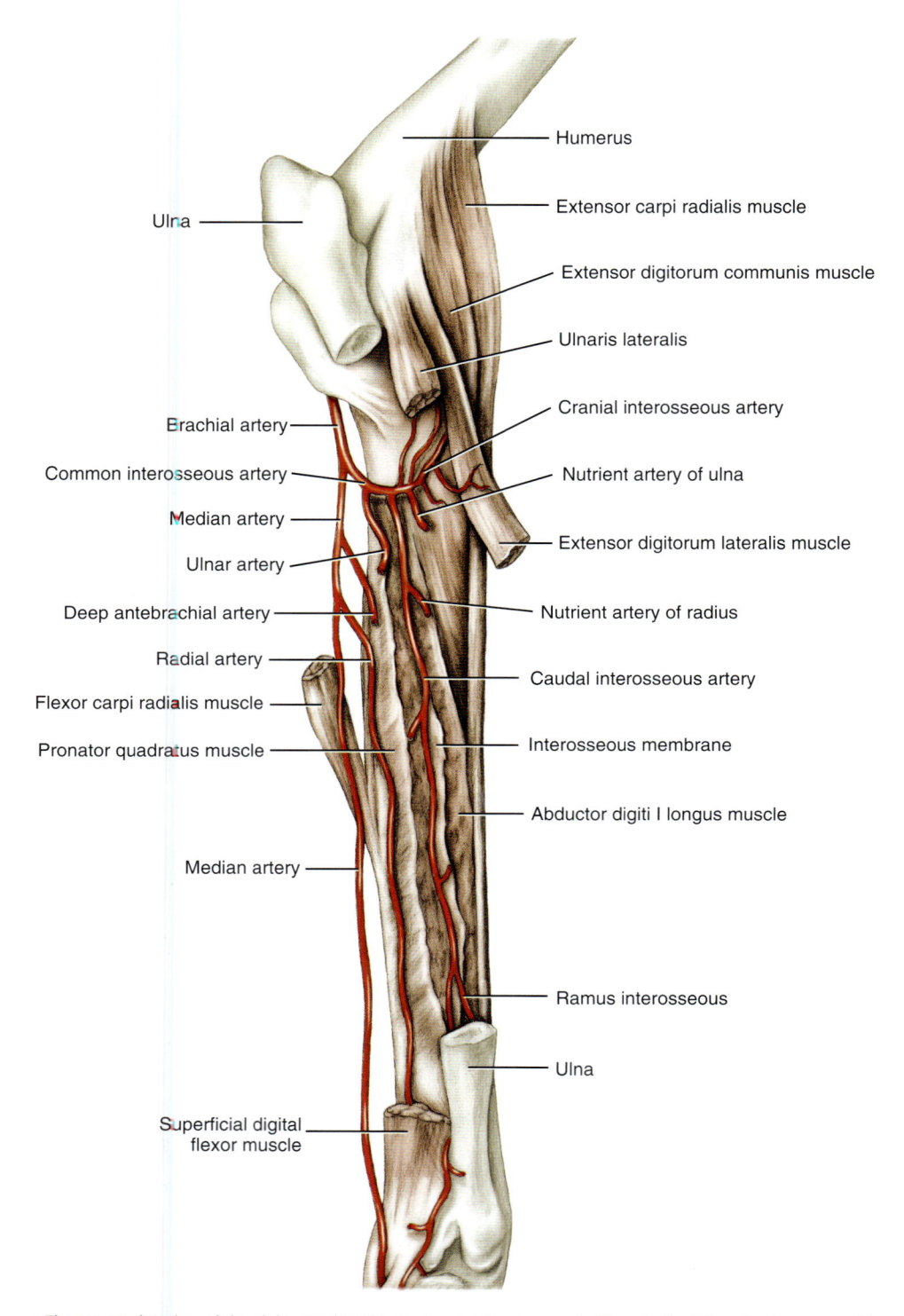

• **Fig. 11.45** Arteries of the right antebrachium, caudolateral aspect. (The shaft of the ulna is removed.)

the superficial digital flexor muscle. Two traceable anastomoses are present. One of these is with the collateral ulnar artery as the recurrent ulnar artery runs proximally over the medial epicondyle of the humerus. The other anastomosis is with the deep antebrachial artery on the deep surface of the superficial digital flexor muscle. Davis (1941) describes two recurrent ulnar arteries in the dog.

The **common interosseous artery** (*a. interossea communis*) (Figs. 11.40, and 11.43 through 11.45) is the largest branch of the brachial artery. It is approximately 3 mm in diameter and 1 cm long, as it runs from the lateral surface of the brachial artery to the interosseous space at the proximal end of the pronator quadratus muscle. This places the artery approximately 1 cm distal to the elbow joint. Before

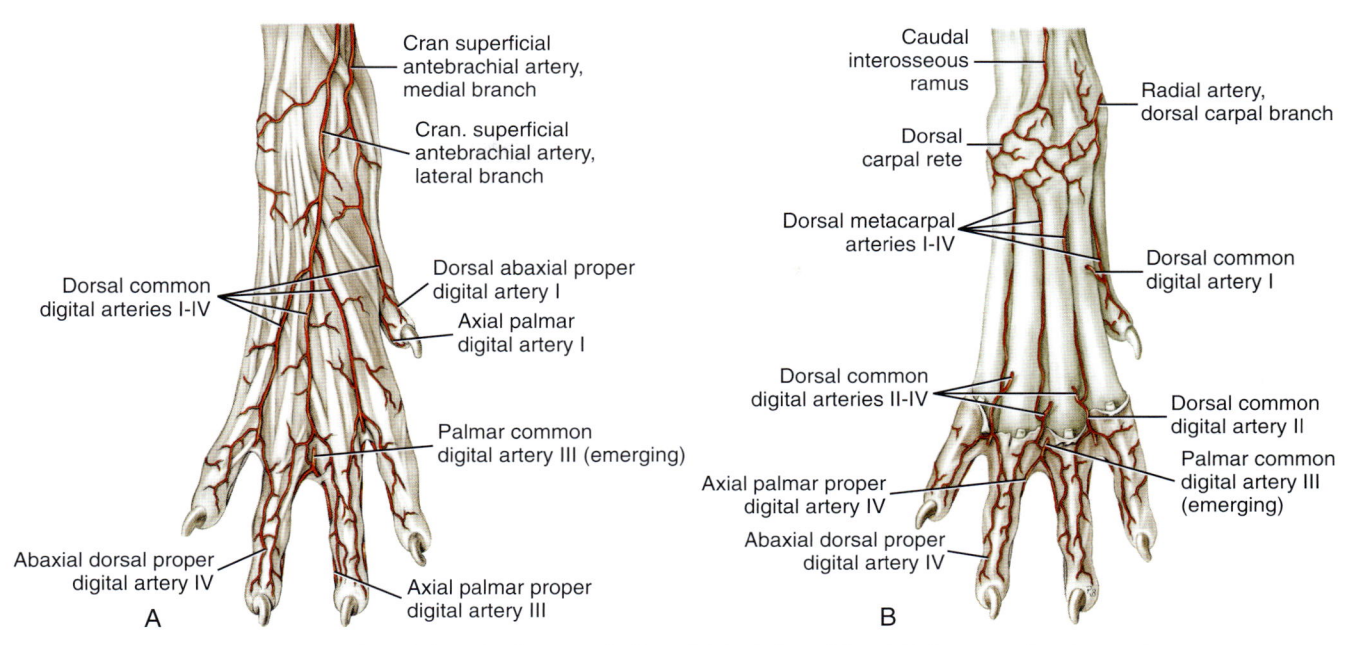

• **Fig. 11.46** Arteries of the right forepaw. **A,** Superficial arteries of the right forepaw, dorsal aspect. **B,** Deep arteries of the right forepaw, dorsal aspect.

entering the interosseous space, it sends one or more muscular branches cranially into the pronator teres muscle and gives off the large caudally running ulnar artery. Within the interosseous space the common interosseous artery terminates by dividing into the caudal interosseous and cranial interosseous arteries.

The **ulnar artery** (*a. ulnaris*) (Figs. 11.43 through 11.45), formerly called the *accessory interosseous artery* in the dog, accompanies the ulnar nerve in the antebrachium (Davis, 1941). It can be exposed by separating the humeral from the ulnar head of the deep digital flexor muscle. The large ulnar nerve, which lies closely applied to the lateral border of the deep digital flexor muscle, largely covers the artery. On leaving the common interosseous artery, the ulnar artery courses obliquely distocaudally across the medial surface of the ulna and enters the deep digital flexor muscle. In some dogs a recurrent branch, *a. recurrens ulnaris,* extends proximally between the radial and ulnar heads of the deep digital flexor muscle and anastomoses with the collateral ulnar artery. This was described earlier. The bulk of the ulnar artery continues distally in association with the deep surface of the humeral head of the m. flexor carpi ulnaris. In the distal third of the antebrachium the ulnar and the deep antebrachial arteries anastomose. The small vessel that results passes distally into the carpal canal, where it usually anastomoses with the caudal interosseous artery. The ulnar artery supplies largely the ulnar and humeral heads of the deep digital flexor and the corresponding heads of the flexor carpi ulnaris muscle. At the carpus a **dorsal branch** (*ramus dorsalis*) of the ulnar artery courses distally on the lateral surface of the carpus, where it contributes a branch to the dorsal carpal rete *ramus carpeus dorsalis,* and continues distally as the abaxial dorsal digital artery V (*a. digitalis dorsalis V abaxialis*).

The **caudal interosseous artery** (*a. interossea caudalis*) (see Figs. 11.43 through 11.45) lies between the apposed surfaces of the radius and ulna. The pronator quadratus muscle lies on the caudolateral side of the artery. In its course distally in the forearm, the artery supplies many small branches to adjacent structures. The m. pronator quadratus and the ulnar and radial heads of the deep digital flexor muscle receive branches on the caudal side of the forearm. The abductor digiti I longus, common digital extensor, lateral digital extensor, and extensor digiti I longus and extensor digiti II muscles receive branches on the craniolateral side of the forearm. In the proximal half of the forearm, it forms a feeble anastomosis with the cranial interosseous artery. At the junction of the proximal and middle thirds of the radius the **nutrient artery of the radius** extends distally into the bone. At a similar location on the ulna, the **nutrient artery of the ulna** extends proximally into the ulna. At the base of the styloid process of the ulna the caudal interosseous artery trifurcates. One of these arteries, the **interosseous ramus** (*r. interosseus*) (Fig. 11.45), leaves the cranial side of the interosseous space proximal to the carpus. From deep to the m. abductor digiti I longus it runs to the extensor retinaculum and aids in the formation of the lateral part of the dorsal carpal rete by contributing a **dorsal carpal branch** (*ramus carpeus dorsalis*). A recurrent branch extends proximally and anastomoses with the ulnar artery on the deep digital flexor. A small **palmar carpal branch** (*ramus carpeus palmaris*) supplies structures on the palmar surface of the carpus. The terminal branch at the trifurcation of the caudal interosseous is the **palmar branch** (*ramus palmaris*) that enters the lateral aspect of the carpal canal where it provides a small superficial branch (*r. superficialis*) that joins the median artery to form the superficial palmar arch. A larger deep branch (*r. profundus*) joins the palmar branch of the radial artery to form the deep palmar arch. The branches of these palmar arches to the digits is described later in this chapter in the section titled "Arteries of the Forepaw."

The **cranial interosseous artery** (*a. interossea cranialis*) (Fig. 11.44) continues in the direction of the common interosseous artery after the caudal interosseous artery arises. It is a small vessel that emerges laterally from the interosseous space, approximately 2 cm distal to the lateral epicondyle of the humerus. It enters the deep surface of the proximal extremities of the extensor carpi ulnaris and the lateral and common digital extensor muscles. Small branches also go to the pronator quadratus, supinator, and the extensor muscles adjacent to the proximal third of the ulna. The caudolateral part of the elbow joint receives branches from deep to the caudal border of the m. extensor carpi ulnaris. Anastomoses exist between the cranial interosseous artery and the collateral ulnar and caudal interosseous arteries.

Median Artery

The **median artery** (*a. mediana*) (Figs. 11.40, and 11.43 to 11.45) is the largest artery of the forearm and was formerly considered to be only an antebrachial part of the brachial artery. It begins after the brachial artery gives rise to the common interosseus artery. The first branch of the median artery is the deep antebrachial artery. The NAV lists the deep antebrachial artery as a branch of the brachial artery proximal to the origin of the common interosseous artery from the brachial artery and the median artery as the continuation of the brachial artery distal to the origin of the common interosseous. In the experience of the authors, the deep antebrachial artery arises in the midantebrachium distal to the origin of the common interosseous and should be considered a branch of the median artery.

The **deep antebrachial artery** (*a. antebrachialis profunda*) (Figs. 11.43 through 11.45) arises from the palmar surface of the median artery approximately 1 cm distal to the origin of the common interosseous artery. It is a branched vessel, approximately 1 mm in diameter, which runs distocaudally deep to the m. flexor carpi radialis into the deep digital flexor muscle. It supplies the flexor carpi radialis, superficial and deep digital flexors muscles, and the m. flexor carpi ulnaris. It anastomoses prominently with the recurrent ulnar artery deep to the superficial digital flexor muscle and with the ulnar artery deep to the humeral head of the m. flexor carpi ulnaris in the distal fourth of the antebrachium. Frequently the small common trunk formed by this anastomosis joins the caudal interosseous artery in the carpal canal. It traverses the antebrachium in such a way that a series of branches leave the vessel, as it lies in the deep digital flexor muscle, and terminates in the superficial digital flexor muscle. These appear in a linear series of approximately eight vessels lying 1 to 2 cm apart. A branch of the median nerve and a satellite vein accompanies the deep antebrachial artery.

The **radial artery** (*a. radialis*) (Figs. 11.43 through 11.45) is a cranial branch of the median artery just proximal to the middle of the forearm. It runs distally deep to the aponeurotic origin of the m. flexor carpi radialis. It closely follows the caudomedial border of the radius in the forearm. At the carpus the radial artery terminates in two carpal branches. The **dorsal carpal branch** (*r. carpeus dorsalis*) supplies the dorsal part of the carpal joint capsule and contributes to the **dorsal carpal rete** (*rete carpi dorsale*) via a branch that joins the medial branch of the cranial superficial antebrachial artery. The dorsal carpal rete is the source of the **dorsal metacarpal arteries I to IV** (*aa. metacarpeae dorsales I to IV*). This dorsal carpal branch continues into the forepaw as the **abaxial dorsal digital artery I** (*a. digitalis dorsalis I abaxialis*). The **palmar carpal branch** (*r. carpeus palmaris*) passes deep to the flexor retinaculum toward the palmar surface of the proximal metacarpus where it joins the terminal deep branch of the caudal interosseous artery to form the **deep palmar arch** (*arcus palmaris profundus*). This arch is the source of the **palmar metacarpal arteries I to IV** (*aa. metacarpae palmares I to IV*).

The distal part of the median artery is the principal source of blood supply to the forepaw. It lies on the medial borders of the radial and humeral heads of the deep digital flexor muscle deep to the antebrachial fascia and tendon of the m. flexor carpi radialis. It obliquely crosses the humeral head of the deep digital flexor muscle, which it grooves. Usually a small branch to the medial surface of the carpus is its only branch in the antebrachium. As it passes through the carpal canal between the tendons of the superficial and deep digital flexor muscles it lies lateral to the median nerve. It emerges from the carpal canal in the palmar groove of the deep digital flexor tendon. A small branch to the carpal pad arises from the median artery just distal to the carpal canal. Lying between the superficial and deep flexor tendons in the proximal part of the metacarpus, the vessel anastomoses with a small branch of the caudal interosseous artery to form the **superficial palmar arch** (*arcus palmaris superficialis*). This arch is not apparent without close inspection and is the source of the palmar **common digital arteries I to IV** (*aa. digitales palmares communes I to IV*). The median artery dominates in the formation of the arch as well as in the supply of blood to the paw. Essentially the median artery terminates as three principal palmar common digital arteries.

Arteries of the Forepaw

The arteries of the forepaw (Figs. 11.46 to 11.48) and hindpaw are divided into a dorsal and a palmar/plantar set, each of which is further divided into a superficial and a deep series. By convention the superficial arteries of the metapodium are named the dorsal or palmar/plantar common digital arteries, whereas the deep arteries are called the *dorsal* or *palmar/plantar metapodial arteries*. The metapodial arteries join the common digital arteries in the distal intermetapodial spaces. Digital arteries that arise from the bifurcation

CHAPTER 11 The Heart and Arteries 547

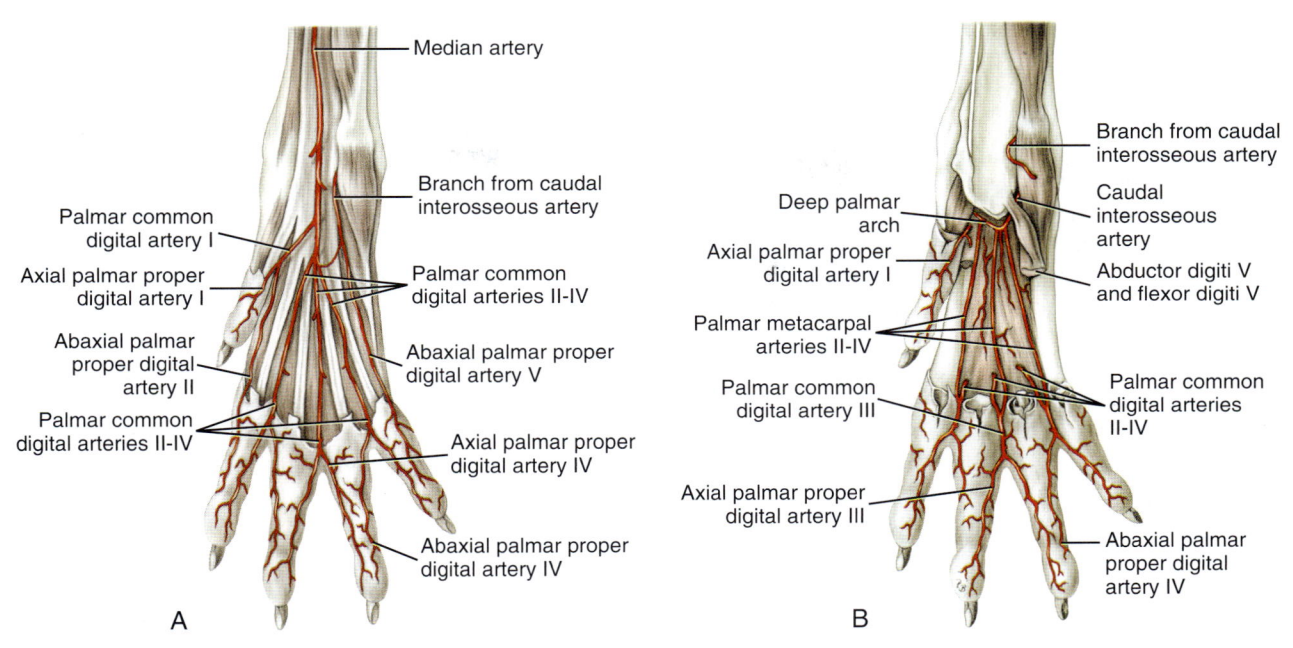

- **Fig. 11.47** Arteries of the right forepaw. **A**, Superficial arteries of the right forepaw, palmar aspect. **B**, Deep arteries of the right forepaw, palmar aspect.

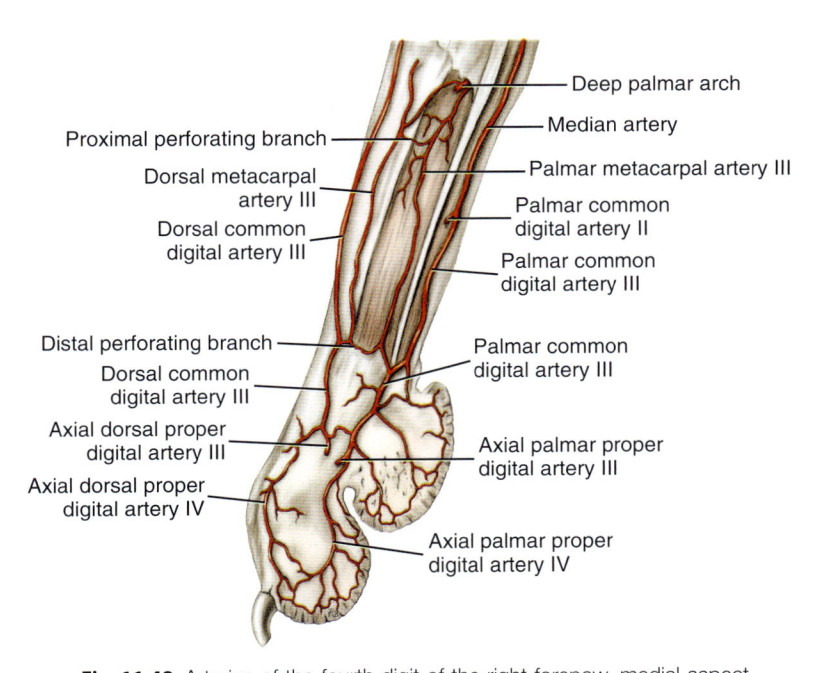

- **Fig. 11.48** Arteries of the fourth digit of the right forepaw, medial aspect.

of the dorsal and palmar/plantar common digital arteries are called *proper digital arteries*. Most common digital arteries terminate by dividing into axial and abaxial dorsal or palmar/plantar proper digital arteries. All are small and of minor importance, except for the superficial series of the palmar set and the deep series of the plantar set, which are the main source of blood supply to the digits and the footpads.

In the forepaw **dorsal common digital artery I** (*a. digitalis dorsalis communis I*) (Fig. 11.46A) arises from the direct continuation of the medial branch of the cranial superficial antebrachial artery. The **dorsal common digital arteries II, III, and IV** (*aa. digitales dorsales communes II to IV*) (Figs. 11.46 and 11.48) are formed by the trifurcation of the lateral branch of the cranial superficial antebrachial artery in the metacarpus. These small vessels first lie on, then between, the tendons of the common digital extensor muscle as both diverge unequally. The distal portions of the main arteries sink into the distal portions of the intermetacarpal spaces and are joined by the dorsal metacarpal arteries. The first artery anastomoses with the corresponding palmar common digital artery.

The **dorsal metacarpal arteries II, III, and IV** (*aa. metacarpeae dorsales II to IV*) (Fig. 11.46B) arise from the distal part of the **dorsal rete of the carpus** (*rete carpi dorsale*). They are the smallest of all the metacarpal arteries, as they lie in the dorsal grooves between adjacent metacarpal bones. Proximally they send branches to the deep palmar arch, and anastomose with perforating branches from the palmar metacarpal arteries proximally (*ramus perforans proximalis*) and distally (*ramus perforans distalis*). They end in the distal metacarpus by anastomosing with the corresponding dorsal common digital arteries. Distal to this union the dorsal common digital arteries II, III, and IV are each approximately 1 cm long as they terminate opposite the metacarpophalangeal joints. Anastomotic branches leave them to go to the corresponding palmar common digital arteries. The dorsal common digital arteries, on reaching the skin that ensheathes the digits, divide into the **axial and abaxial dorsal proper digital arteries II, III, and IV** (*aa. digitales dorsales propriae axialis et abaxialis II, III, et IV*). These go to the dorsal parts of the contiguous sides of adjacent digits and, as branched cutaneous vessels, extend to the claws. The axis of the forepaw and hindpaw passes through the interdigital space between digits III and IV. The axial vessels and nerves are on the sides of the digits that face the axis and the abaxial vessels and nerve are on the side of the digits that face away from the axis. **Abaxial dorsal digital artery V** (*a. digitalis dorsalis V abaxialis*) is the distal continuation of the dorsal branch of the ulnar artery from the lateral side of the carpus.

The palmar set of arteries of the forepaw, like the dorsal set, is divided into a superficial and a deep series of arteries. The palmar set of vessels arises from the superficial and deep palmar arches. The median artery dominates in the formation of the superficial series so completely that the contribution of the caudal interosseous artery, which anastomoses with it to form the **superficial palmar arterial arch** (*arcus palmaris superficialis*), is minor. From this arch arise the relatively large palmar common digital arteries.

The **palmar common digital artery I** (*a. digitalis palmaris communis I*) (Fig. 11.47) runs approximately 1 cm before entering the space between the first digit and the metacarpus. It is the first branch from the metacarpal part of the median artery or the superficial palmar arterial arch. It anastomoses with the dorsal common digital artery I. The main part of the median artery continues as the lateral limb of the superficial palmar arterial arch that gives rise to the **palmar common digital arteries II, III, and IV** (*aa. digitalis palmares communes II to IV*). These run distally deep to the superficial flexor tendons, where, proximal to the large metacarpal footpad, each sends a branch into the proximal part of the pad. At the distal ends of the intermetacarpal spaces, the arteries anastomose with the comparable palmar metacarpal arteries. The palmar common digital arteries are accompanied by small sensory nerve branches from the median nerve. The satellite veins accompany the arteries only in the distal half of the metacarpus.

The **palmar metacarpal arteries II, III, and IV** (*aa. metacarpeae palmares I to IV*) (Fig. 11.47B) arise from the **deep palmar arch** (*arcus palmaris profundus*), which is formed by the palmar branch of the radial artery anastomosing with the terminal part of the caudal interosseous artery. This arch lies distal to the flexor retinaculum, where it is covered by the interosseous muscles. The palmar metacarpal arteries run distally between these muscles, which they supply. The palmar metacarpal arteries terminate by anastomosing with the corresponding palmar common digital arteries. These unions take place more than 1 cm proximal to the metacarpophalangeal joints. The palmar metacarpal arteries send the several nutrient arteries into the proximal third of the palmar surfaces of the four main metacarpal bones. They supply proximal and distal perforating branches to the dorsal metacarpal arteries and are accompanied by satellite veins and companion nerves.

The palmar common digital arteries II, III, and IV continue the superficial vessels after they receive the palmar metacarpal arteries. Each of these three pairs of arteries sends a prominent branch into the center of each of the three parts into which the distal portion of the large metacarpal footpad is divided. After running approximately 1 cm, the palmar common digital arteries divide into **axial** and **abaxial palmar proper digital arteries** (*aa. digitales palmares propriae axialis et abaxialis*), which supply the adjacent palmar sides of contiguous digits. The proper vessels lying on the digits that are closest to the axis through the paw are the chief arteries to the digits. In fact, those that go to the palmar surfaces of the opposite, or abaxial, sides are mainly small cutaneous branches. However, in the palmar vascular canals of the third phalanges, the abaxial and axial proper digital arteries anastomose. Branches given off from these terminal arches nourish the corium of the claws and the third phalanges. **Abaxial palmar digital artery V** (*a. digitalis palmaris V abaxialis*) is a lateral branch from the deep palmar arch or a direct continuation of the caudal interosseous artery distal to the arch.

Daigo et al. (1964a, b) published radiographs and summarized the variations seen in the palmar and dorsal arteries of the forepaw in 100 Japanese Shiba dogs.

Thoracic Aorta

The **thoracic aorta** (*aorta thoracica*) (Figs. 11.34, 11.35, and 11.49) continues from the aortic arch, opposite the fourth thoracic vertebra, and extends to the caudal border of the second lumbar vertebra. There it enters the abdominal cavity by passing between the obliquely placed crura of the diaphragm to become the abdominal aorta. It is accompanied by the azygos vein, thoracic duct, and the cisterna chyli as it passes through the aortic hiatus of the diaphragm. Transverse plane computed tomographic images of the thoracic aorta of 14 German Shepherd dogs showed the widest transverse diameter at the level of T4 to T5, whereas the largest dorsoventral diameter was at T5. The dorsoventral and transversal diameters are smaller in males than in

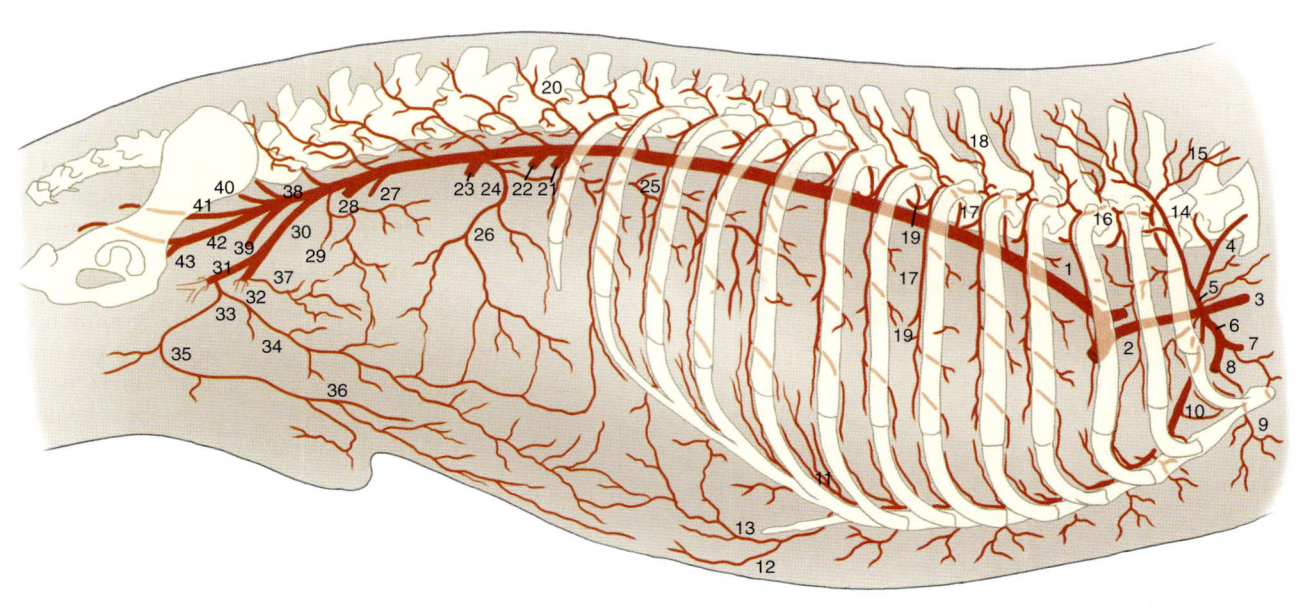

- Fig. 11.49 Parietal branches of the aorta, right lateral aspect.

1. Aorta
2. Brachiocephalic trunk
3. Right common carotid
4. Vertebral
5. Costocervical trunk
6. Right subclavian
7. Superficial cervical
8. Axillary
9. External thoracic
10. Right internal thoracic
11. Musculophrenic
12. Cranial superficial epigastric
13. Cranial epigastric
14. Dorsal scapular
15. Deep cervical
16. Supreme intercostal or thoracic vertebral
17. Intercostal
18. Dorsal branch of intercostal
19. Lateral cutaneous branches of intercostal
20. Lumbar
21. Celiac
22. Cranial mesenteric
23. Right renal
24. Phrenicoabdominal
25. Phrenic
26. Cranial abdominal
27. Right testicular or ovarian
28. Caudal mesenteric
29. Deep circumflex iliac
30. Right external iliac
31. Deep femoral
32. Femoral
33. Pudendoepigastric trunk
34. Caudal epigastric
35. External pudendal
36. Caudal superficial epigastric
37. Caudal abdominal
38. Right internal iliac
39. Right umbilical
40. Median sacral
41. Parietal branch of internal iliac
42. Visceral branch of internal iliac
43. Prostatic/vaginal (formerly urogenital)

females (Dabanoglu, 2007). Small but significant segmental differences in the aortic wall structure were found and characterized by Orsi et al. (2004). At its beginning, the bulk of the thoracic aorta lies to the left of the median plane, being displaced to this position by the esophagus, which crosses the right side of the aorta dorsal to the heart. The aorta lies in the dorsal and caudal mediastinum and inclines slightly to the right and dorsally as it passes to the diaphragm. Caudally it is separated from the bodies of the thoracic vertebrae by a small amount of fat. The thoracic duct lies in this fat as it follows the dorsal surface of the aorta cranially to the midthoracic region.

The branches of the thoracic aorta may be divided into visceral and parietal. The visceral branches are the bronchial and esophageal arteries. The parietal branches include the dorsal intercostal, dorsal costoabdominal, and the first two lumbar arteries.

Visceral Branches

The bronchial and intrathoracic esophageal branches vary in number and origin. The chief nutritional blood supply to the lungs are the right and left **bronchial branches** (*rami bronchiales*) of the **bronchoesophageal artery** (*a. bronchoesophagea*) (Figs. 11.34 and 11.35). This vessel also sends ascending and descending **esophageal branches** (*rami esophagei*) to most of the intrathoracic portion of the esophagus. The bronchoesophageal artery usually arises from the right fifth intercostal artery close to the aorta. Variations in the origin of the bronchial and esophageal branches are common. A common bronchoesophageal artery may arise from dorsal intercostal arteries IV to VI as well as from the aorta. This artery may be single or paired or the bronchial and esophageal arteries may arise independently. Variations described by Berry et al. (1931) include a branch from the right fifth or sixth intercostal artery to the right lung, direct branches from the first part of the descending aorta, and a single branch from the left sixth intercostal artery to the left lung. Aberrant branches of the bronchoesophageal artery to the left pulmonary artery, resembling patent ductus arteriosus, have been reported (Yamane et al., 2001). The esophageal branches come primarily from the bronchoesophageal artery in the form of ascending and descending vessels. The descending branches anastomose with several long esophageal branches that arise from two or more of the right intercostal arteries caudal to the origin of the bronchoesophageal artery. These anastomose with each other, and the last esophageal branch anastomoses with the esophageal branch of the left gastric artery, which ascends through the diaphragm on the esophagus. The ascending branches anastomose with the esophageal branch from the

Fig. 11.50 Scheme of the arteries of the thoracic wall in cross-section, caudal aspect.

caudal thyroid artery. There is a small but definite arterial passage from the caudal thyroid artery to the left gastric artery in or on the wall of the esophagus.

Most bronchial and esophageal branches have satellite veins. Usually the bronchoesophageal vein empties into the azygos vein at the level of the seventh thoracic vertebra. According to Berry et al. (1931) only a capillary anastomosis exists between the bronchial and pulmonary circulations.

Three or four small arteries leave the dorsal part of the thoracic aorta and run ventrally over its sides. Two or more of these are distributed to the dorsal part of the mediastinum as **mediastinal branches** (*rami mediastinales*). In the caudal part of the thorax one or more of these mediastinal vessels may arise from the ventral surface of the aorta. Other branches arise from the bronchoesophageal artery, aorta, or intercostal vessels and run to the fibrous pericardium as the **pericardial branches** (*rami pericardiaci*).

Parietal Branches

The **dorsal intercostal arteries** (*aa. intercostales dorsales*) (Figs. 11.34, 11.35, 11.49 to 11.51) are 12 in number on each side. The first dorsal intercostal artery is a branch of the costocervical trunk. The second and third and occasionally the fourth are branches of the thoracic vertebral artery and the last eight or nine are branches of the aorta. The artery that follows the caudal border of the last (thirteenth) rib is the **dorsal costoabdominal artery** (*a. costoabdominalis dorsalis*). All of the aortic dorsal intercostal arteries arise from

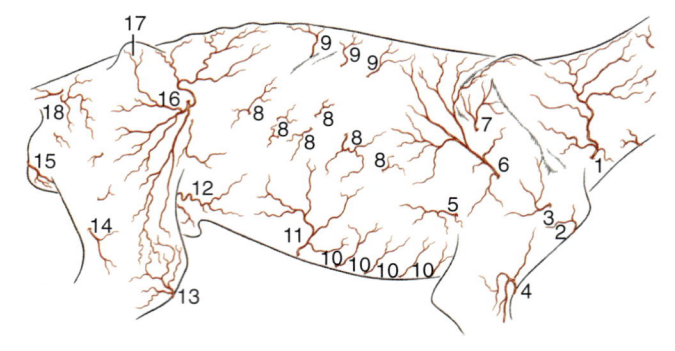

1. Superficial cervical
2. Cranial circumflex humeral
3. Caudal circumflex humeral
4. Superficial brachial
5. Lateral thoracic
6. Cutaneous branch of thoracodorsal
7. Cutaneous branch of subscapular
8. Distal lateral cutaneous branches of intercostals
9. Proximal lateral cutaneous branches of intercostals
10. Ventral cutaneous branches of internal thoracic
11. Cranial superficial epigastric
12. Caudal superficial epigastric
13. Medial genicular
14. Cutaneous branch of caudal femoral
15. Perineal
16. Deep circumflex iliac
17. Tuber coxae
18. Cutaneous branches of superficial lateral caudal

Fig. 11.51 Superficial arteries of the trunk.

the dorsal surface of the aorta and are similar in distribution. The fifth right dorsal intercostal artery may serve as a common trunk for the fourth, occasionally the third, and, in rare instances, for the second dorsal intercostal artery, according to Reichert (1924). The first left aortic dorsal intercostal artery is rarely farther cranial than the fourth intercostal space. Right and left arteries arise close together, and occasionally the first pair comes from a common trunk. In the midthoracic region the paired vessels may be separated by as much as 4 mm at their origins, and this spacing continues throughout the remainder of the thorax. Right and left vessels are not symmetric in their origins; the right vessels usually arise caudal to the left. From the midthoracic region caudally the right dorsal intercostal arteries run directly laterally across the bodies of the vertebrae. Each dorsal intercostal artery gives off a dorsal branch.

The **dorsal branches** (*rami dorsales*) arise from the intercostal arteries lateral to the bodies of the vertebrae. They pass directly dorsally in the medial portion of the m. longissimus, obliquely across the spines of the vertebrae, and end in the epaxial muscles or the skin as small **medial cutaneous branches** (*r. cutaneous medialis*). Each dorsal branch has a **spinal branch** (*ramus spinalis*), which crosses the dorsal surface of the spinal nerve to reach its caudal border. It follows this border medially through the intervertebral foramen, perforates the dura and arachnoid, and follows the nerve roots in the subarachnoid space. It is distributed like the spinal branches of the vertebral artery.

After the dorsal branches arise, the dorsal intercostal arteries extend laterally dorsal to the parietal pleura, sympathetic trunks, azygos vein (on the right side), and hemiazygos vein (at the last two or three intercostal spaces on the left side). The dorsal intercostal arteries supply segmental branches to the overlying epaxial musculature. Some of these branches become cutaneous along the lateral border of the m. iliocostalis. These form a proximal series of **lateral cutaneous branches** (*rami cutanei laterales*). They supply the dorsal part of the latissimus dorsi and cutaneous trunci muscles, which they perforate to reach a paramedian band of skin. On their way to the skin, they are accompanied by the cutaneous branches of the thoracic spinal nerve of their segment. Sometimes a single artery bifurcates, so that each of its branches accompanies intercostal nerves (ventral branches of thoracic spinal nerves) that arise from adjacent segments.

Hughes and Dransfield (1959) have found that in the regions of the body where the skin is covered by hair, there are superficial, middle, and deep arterial and venous plexuses. The deep plexus may be arranged in more than one layer.

A second series of lateral cutaneous branches start usually at the third intercostal space and perforate the intercostal muscles and the thoracic part of the serratus ventralis muscle when it is present. This distal lateral cutaneous series appears along the ventral border of the m. latissimus dorsi. They continue laterally through the cutaneus trunci muscle and subcutaneous fascia to terminate in long ventral and short dorsal branches. In the cranial part of the series, the dorsal and ventral branches usually arise independently from the intercostal arteries. **Mammary branches** (*rami mammarii*) supply adjacent mammary glands in the lactating bitch. Satellite veins and lateral cutaneous nerves accompany the vessels. The nerves are constantly present, although the vessels may be missing in some of the segments.

The **collateral branches** (*rami collaterales*) arise from the dorsal intercostal arteries near the beginning of the ventral half of the thorax. They are the last of four to eight oblique branches that run ventrocranially across the medial surfaces of each of the last 9 or 10 ribs to reach the intercostal spaces cranial to them. They descend to anastomose with the ventral intercostal arteries, which ascend cranial to the costal cartilages. They supply the ventral halves of the intercostal muscles that lie immediately cranial to the ribs. Usually the last three dorsal intercostal arteries (dorsal intercostal arteries 10, 11, and 12) terminate medial to the costal arch and ventrocranial to the intercostal spaces of the same number. After circling the costal margin of the diaphragm, each artery gives a branch to the diaphragm and another to the musculature of the lateral abdominal wall. The phrenic components of these vessels anastomose with the caudal phrenic branches in the muscular periphery of the diaphragm, and the abdominal branches anastomose with the cranial abdominal artery. The end branches of the musculophrenic artery anastomose with the tenth or eleventh dorsal intercostal artery.

The **dorsal costoabdominal artery** (*a. costoabdominalis dorsalis*) is similar to the dorsal intercostal arteries in origin and course, but it is smaller and it courses caudal to the last rib and is therefore not intercostal. It runs dorsolaterally to become related to the caudal border of the last rib. It is covered at first by the pleura, then in succession by the psoas minor and the retractor costae muscles. It is accompanied by a cranially lying vein, but the ventral branch of the last thoracic spinal nerve diverges caudally from the artery and passes ventral to the first lumbar transverse process. The dorsal costoabdominal artery anastomoses with the cranial abdominal artery via the ventral ramus of the costoabdominal artery.

The first two pairs of **lumbar arteries** (*aa. lumbales I et II*) arise as the last branches of the thoracic aorta because of the attachment of the crura of the diaphragm on the third and fourth lumbar vertebrae. They are distributed like other typical lumbar arteries. The first lumbar artery anastomoses with the dorsal costoabdominal and the second lumbar arteries and may have an anastomosis with the cranial abdominal artery.

Abdominal Aorta

The **abdominal aorta** (*aorta abdominalis*) (Figs. 11.49, 11.52 through 11.54, and 11.59) is that portion of the descending aorta that lies in the abdomen. The diaphragm that separates the thoracic from the abdominal cavity is perforated so obliquely by the aorta that the first visceral branch of the abdominal aorta is at a more cranial plane than the origin

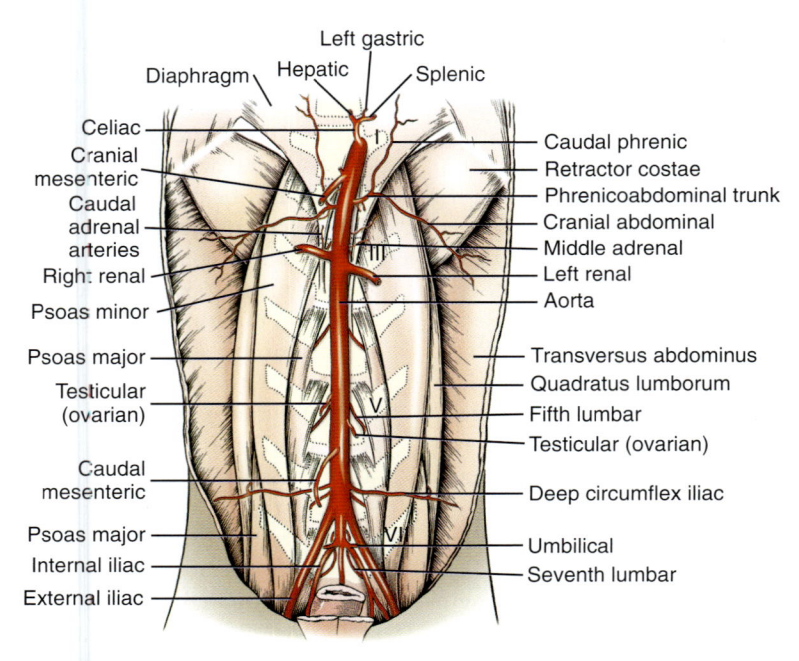

• **Fig. 11.52** Branches of the abdominal aorta, ventral aspect. I to VII are transverse processes of lumbar vertebrae.

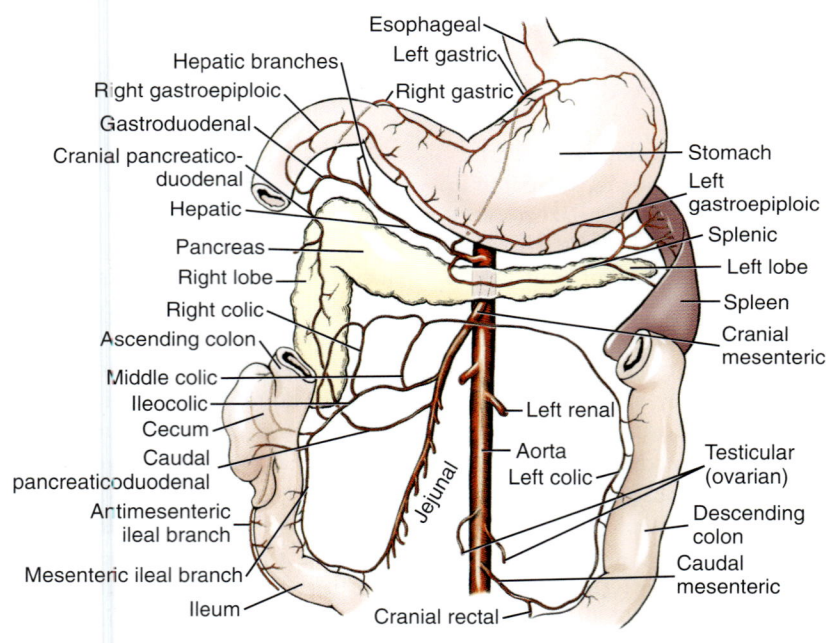

• **Fig. 11.53** Diagram of the visceral branches of the aorta with their principal anastomoses, ventral aspect.

of the second lumbar arteries. The abdominal aorta terminates opposite the seventh lumbar vertebra by bifurcating into right and left internal iliac and median sacral arteries. Cranially it lies in the median plane between the crura of the diaphragm; caudally it is displaced slightly to the left by the caudal vena cava. It lies in the furrow formed by the right and left psoas major muscles. The branches of the abdominal aorta supply both visceral and parietal structures.

The unpaired visceral branches are the celiac, cranial mesenteric, and caudal mesenteric arteries. The paired visceral branches are the adrenal, renal, and testicular or ovarian arteries. The parietal branches are the caudal phrenic, cranial abdominal, lumbar, deep circumflex iliac, external iliac, internal iliac, and median sacral arteries.

Unpaired Visceral Branches of Abdominal Aorta

The **celiac artery** (*a. celiaca*) (Figs. 11.52 through 11.55) arises from the ventral surface of the abdominal aorta as its first visceral branch. This is at the level of the first lumbar vertebra. It is approximately 4 mm in diameter and 2 cm

CHAPTER 11 The Heart and Arteries 553

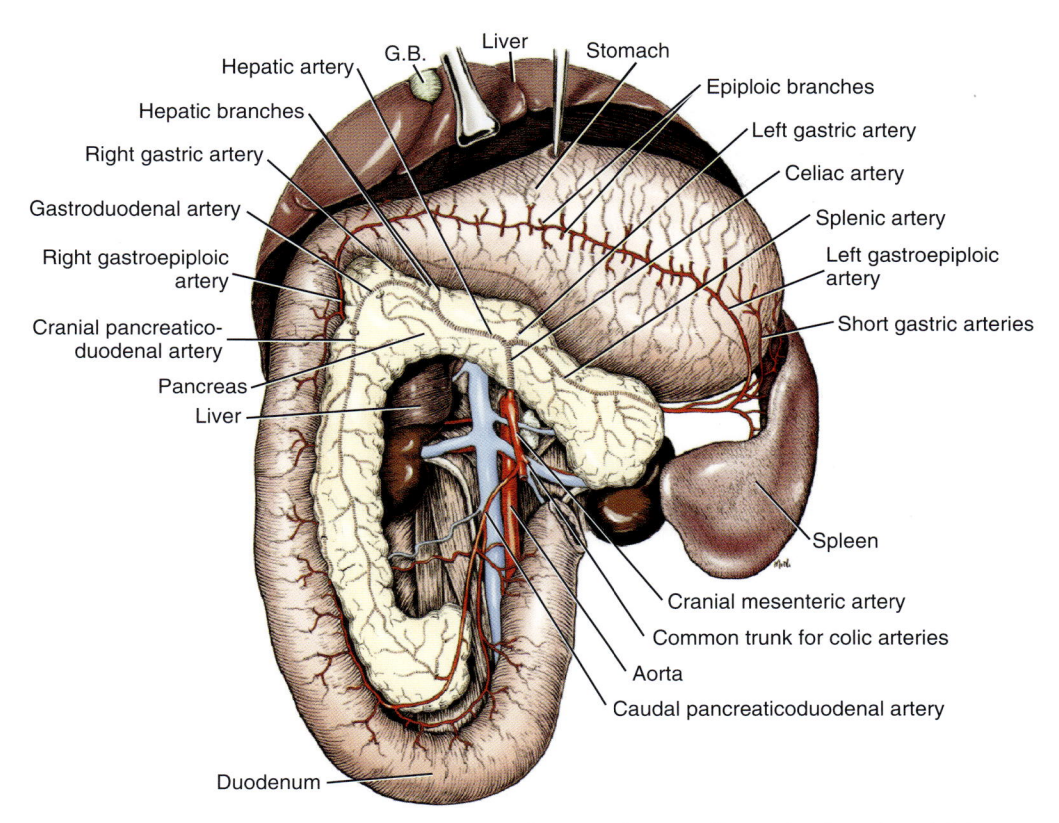

• **Fig. 11.54** Celiac and cranial mesenteric arteries, ventral aspect. (Stomach reflected cranially.)

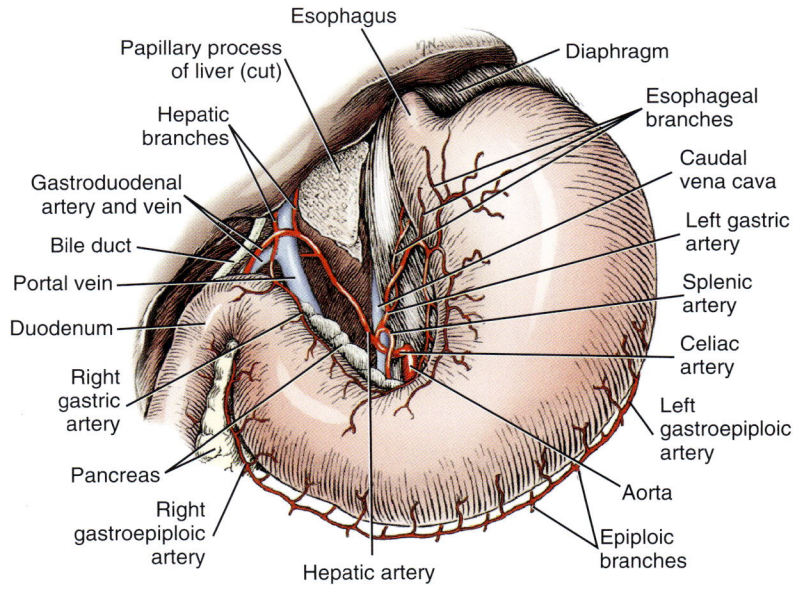

• **Fig. 11.55** Celiac artery, ventral aspect. (Stomach displaced to left.)

long. At its origin it is closely flanked on its lateral sides by the crura of the diaphragm. It is located in the deep leaf of the greater omentum and is related to the stomach on the left and the liver and adrenal gland on the right. The left lobe of the pancreas bounds it caudally. Although the vessel is large, its size is exaggerated by the celiac plexus of nerves and ganglia that surround it. Its terminal branches are the hepatic, splenic, and left gastric arteries. The celiac artery usually trifurcates, although in some specimens the left gastric and splenic arteries arise by a short common trunk. Kennedy and Smith (1930) recorded a case in which the splenic artery arose from the cranial mesenteric artery. Small

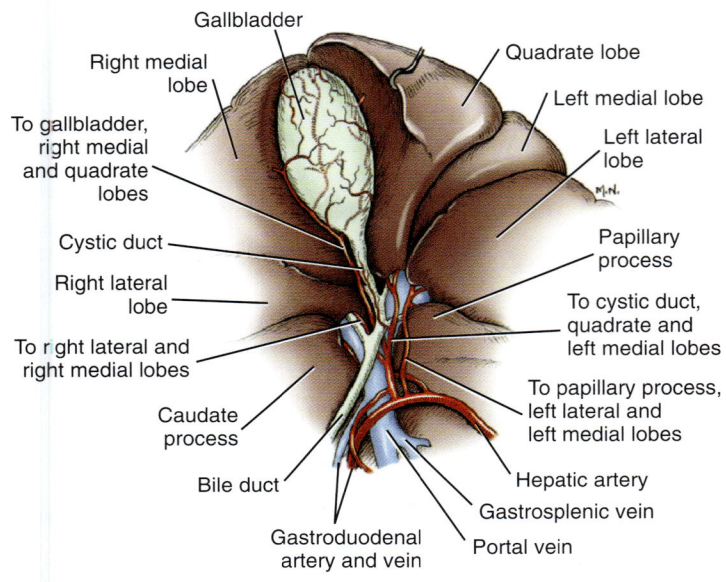

Fig. 11.56 Distribution of the hepatic arteries.

inconstant pancreatic and phrenic branches may arise from the celiac artery.

The **hepatic artery** (*a. hepatica*) (Figs. 11.52 through 11.56) runs cranioventrally and to the right, in a groove of the pancreas. Where the deep leaf of the greater omentum is continuous with the mesoduodenum, the hepatic artery is in the ventral border of the epiploic foramen where it approaches the porta of the liver in the hepatoduodenal ligament. At the porta it sends three to five rather long branches into the hilus of the organ. These furnish the nutritional blood to the liver. When three branches are present, the first branch, the **right lateral branch** (*ramus dexter lateralis*), goes to the right portion of the liver and supplies the caudate and right lateral lobes. The **right medial branch** (*ramus dexter medialis*) goes to the right medial lobe, dorsal part of the quadrate, and part of the left medial lobe; this vessel may be replaced by two or more arteries. The **left branch** (*ramus sinister*), shortest of the three, supplies the large left liver lobes and the quadrate lobe. **Left lateral branches** (*ramis sinistri laterales*) supply the left lateral hepatic lobe. **Left medial branches** (*rami sinister medialis*) of this left branch supply the left medial and quadrate lobes and gives rise to the **cystic artery** (*a. cystica*). This vessel leaves the left medial branch, approximately 1 cm before it enters the liver, and ramifies by two or more branches primarily on that surface of the gallbladder that is attached to the liver. After giving off its hepatic branches, the hepatic artery turns caudally in the lesser omentum and at the region of the pylorus it terminates in the small right gastric and the much larger gastroduodenal artery. Schmidt et al. (1980) studied the branching patterns of the hepatic artery and found three major types in 51 dogs: a single hepatic artery trunk (4 dogs); two separate branches of the hepatic artery (27 dogs); and three, four, or five branches that originated directly from the hepatic artery (20 dogs). Ursic et al. (2007) found the right lateral, right medial, and left branches of the major arteries originating from the hepatic artery.

The **right gastric artery** (*a. gastrica dextra*) (see Figs. 11.53 through 11.55) leaves the hepatic artery at nearly a right angle and, running in the lesser omentum at the pylorus, continues to the left along the lesser curvature of the stomach. It frequently arises from one of the hepatic branches, in which case the hepatic artery becomes the gastroduodenal artery after the last hepatic branch. The right gastric artery sends branches to both the parietal and the visceral surfaces of the pyloric part of the stomach and the lesser omentum. It anastomoses with the much larger left gastric artery along the pyloric antrum as it runs toward the cardia in the lesser omentum.

The **gastroduodenal artery** (*a. gastroduodenalis*) (see Figs. 11.53 through 11.55) runs across the dorsal surface of the pylorus and enters the mesoduodenum adjacent to the body and left part of the left lobe of the pancreas and terminates at the junction of the pylorus and cranial part of the descending duodenum. It may issue delicate branches to the pylorus, and constantly sends one or more larger branches into the body and left lobe of the pancreas. It terminates as the right gastroepiploic and cranial pancreaticoduodenal arteries.

The **right gastroepiploic artery** (*a. gastroepiploica dextra*) (Figs. 11.53 and 11.55) leaves the pancreas at the medial surface of the duodenum and enters the superficial leaf of the greater omentum near its attachment to the greater curvature. It lies approximately 1 cm from the greater curvature of the stomach as it runs to the left in the greater omentum toward the cardia. It sends branches to the stomach at intervals of approximately 5 mm. Most of these **gastric branches** divide on reaching the greater curvature of the stomach into branches that go to the visceral surface.

These anastomose in the musculature of the organ with gastric branches of the right and left gastric arteries that lie on the lesser curvature. Long, freely branching **epiploic branches** leave the opposite or omental side of both gastroepiploic arteries and ramify mainly in the superficial leaf of the greater omentum. Grävenstein (1938) demonstrated that there is a large epiploic branch that leaves the right gastroepiploic artery near its origin and runs caudally in the superficial leaf of the greater omentum near its right border. A second vessel with a similar origin essentially parallels the first, but runs in the deep leaf of the greater omentum near its right border. The comparable vessels near the left border of the greater omentum are continuations of the splenic artery near the apex of the spleen. There are many other smaller epiploic branches that arise at short intervals from the gastroepiploic arteries as they lie in the omentum just peripheral to the greater curvature of the stomach. These vessels anastomose freely with each other. The fat of the omentum is deposited around the epiploic vessels. The right and left gastroepiploic arteries anastomose with each other opposite the beginning of the pyloric antrum. The long left gastroepiploic artery on its way to the stomach supplies most of the epiploic vessels to the greater omentum.

The **cranial pancreaticoduodenal artery** (*a. pancreaticoduodenalis cranialis*) (Figs. 11.53 and 11.54) is the slightly larger terminal branch of the gastroduodenal artery. It continues the parent artery in the mesoduodenum and enters the head of the pancreas at the junction of its right and left lobes. Shortly before entering the right lobe of the pancreas, it sends a small branch to the left lobe, which, after extending a short distance, anastomoses with the pancreatic branch of the splenic artery, which is the chief supply to this part of the gland (Cadete-Leite, 1973). The principal part of the cranial pancreaticoduodenal artery continues caudally in the right lobe of the pancreas, sending **pancreatic branches** to the right lobe of the pancreas and **duodenal branches** through the gland to the descending duodenum. In the caudal half of the right lobe of the pancreas, it anastomoses with one or more pancreatic branches coming from the caudal pancreaticoduodenal artery. The main part of the artery usually leaves the caudal third of the right lobe of the pancreas, traverses a part of the mesoduodenum, and comes to lie on the mesenteric border of the descending duodenum. Near the caudal flexure it anastomoses with the main duodenal branch of the caudal pancreaticoduodenal artery, which is the second branch of the cranial mesenteric artery.

The **splenic artery** (*a. lienalis*) (Figs. 11.52 through 11.55, and 11.57) is that branch of the celiac artery that runs to the left in the deep leaf of the greater omentum along the dorsocranial surface of the left lobe of the pancreas. It is nearly straight throughout its length (Borley et al., 1995) and lies in a groove of the left lobe of the pancreas near its free end. It is usually more than 2 mm in diameter and gives off a variable number of **pancreatic branches** (*rami pancreatici*) to the left lobe of the pancreas. It is the main supply to this lobe of the gland and

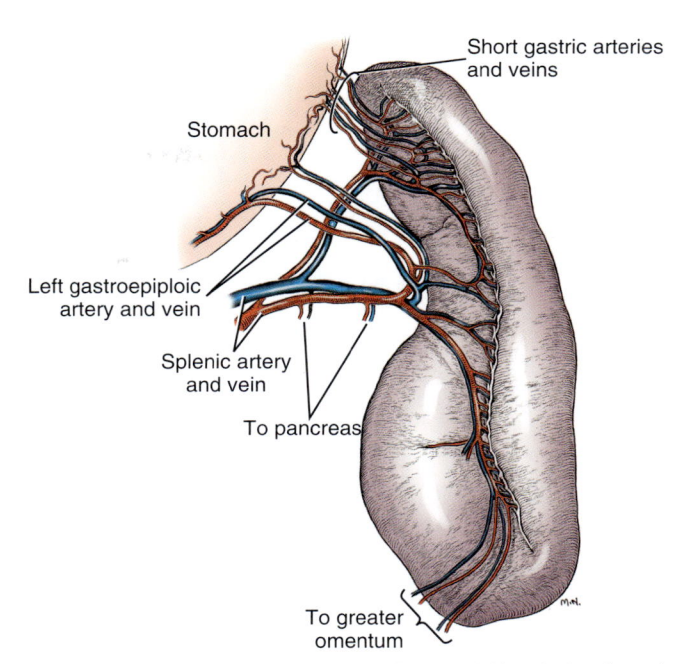

• **Fig. 11.57** Blood supply of the spleen. (The cranial border is reflected laterally.)

anastomoses with the smaller pancreatic branch from the cranial pancreaticoduodenal artery. Arising from the cranial surface of the splenic artery are usually two large long vessels and a smaller intermediate one that run toward the visceral surface of the spleen but variations of this branching pattern are common. They do not enter the spleen directly but pass at right angles to the long hilus of the spleen, where they send **splenic branches** to it. The large dorsal branch divides twice resulting in four branches that give off the short gastric arteries and then enter the hilus of the spleen. The **short gastric arteries** (*aa. gastricae breves*) pass in the gastrosplenic ligament to the dorsal part of the greater curvature of the stomach. These arteries anastomose with the much larger gastric branches from the left gastric artery. The gastric arteries in this region run considerable distances in the subserosa before entering the muscularis. The large ventral branch of the splenic artery provides numerous splenic branches and then is continued by the **left gastroepiploic artery** (*a. gastroepiploica sinistra*) (Figs. 11.53 and 11.55), which follows the gastrosplenic ligament to the greater curvature of the stomach. Here it passes along the greater curvature to the right toward the pyloric part where it anastomoses with the smaller right gastroepiploic artery. The dorsal, ventral, and intermediate branches of the splenic artery provide a plethora of splenic branches that enter the spleen on its visceral surface. All primary branches course along the visceral surface of the spleen. Running through the greater omentum and its gastrosplenic ligament, they give off **omental** (or **epiploic**) **branches** to the omentum. These are disposed like the comparable branches from the right gastroepiploic artery. The vascular pattern in the superficial leaf of the greater omentum is similar to that in the deep leaf.

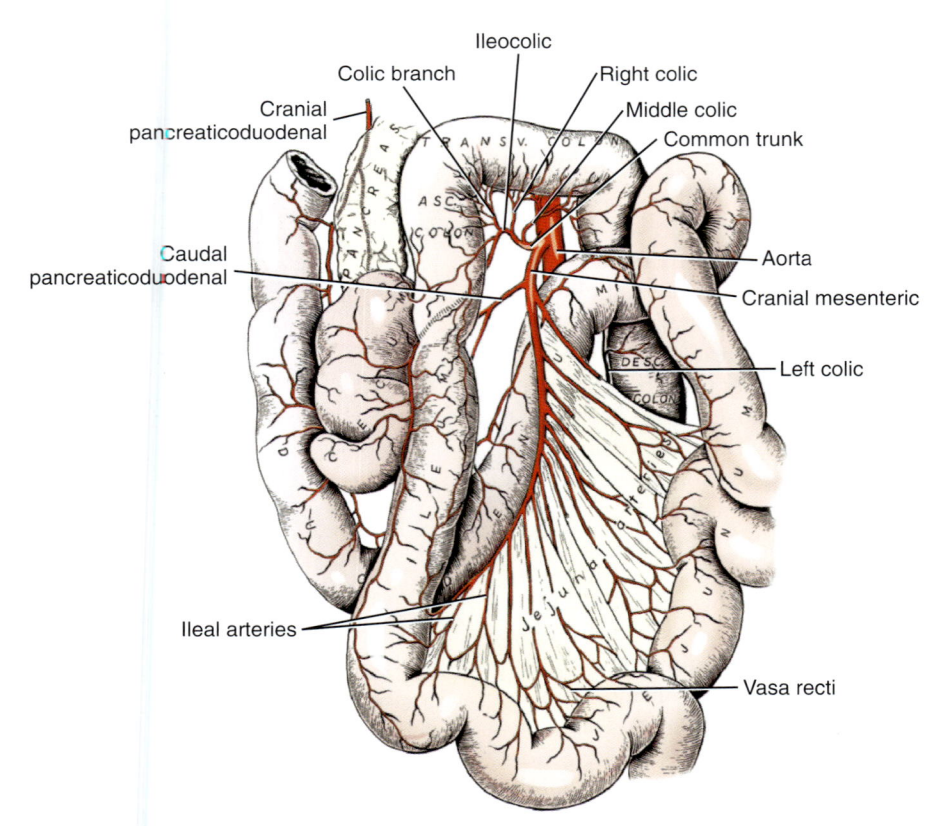

• Fig. 11.58 Branches of the cranial mesenteric artery, ventral aspect.

The **left gastric artery** (*a. gastrica sinistra*) (Figs. 11.52 through 11.55) arises from the cranial surface of the celiac artery as its smallest terminal branch. It may be double. When single, it may form a common trunk with the splenic artery. From its origin, the left gastric artery runs cranially in the deep leaf of the greater omentum and gastrophrenic ligament to the fundus of the stomach adjacent to the cardia of the stomach. It crosses the right surface of the cardia to reach the lesser omentum on the lesser curvature of the stomach. It sends long subserous branches to both surfaces of the organ, with the larger branches going to the parietal surface. It follows the lesser curvature of the stomach to the right where it anastomoses with the right gastric arteries in the lesser omentum. In addition to supplying the fundus, small **epiploic branches** go to the lesser omentum, and one or more **esophageal branches** (*rami esophagei*) run through the esophageal hiatus to supply the caudal part of the esophagus. These branches anastomose with the esophageal rami from the thoracic aorta.

At its origin, the celiac artery is surrounded by the celiac plexus of nerves and the two celiac ganglia, which are intimately connected with both the adrenal and the cranial mesenteric nerve plexuses and ganglia.

Lymph vessels from the stomach, spleen, pancreas, and a portion of the duodenum run dorsally in association with the celiac trunk to the cisterna chyli. The hepatic, splenic, and left gastric arteries and their branches have accompanying lymphatics and satellite veins that are radicles of the portal vein.

The **cranial mesenteric artery** (*a. mesenterica cranialis*) (Figs. 11.52 through 11.54, 11.58, and 11.59) is the largest visceral branch of the aorta. This unpaired artery arises from the ventral surface of the abdominal aorta approximately 5 mm caudal to the origin of the celiac artery opposite the first or second lumbar vertebra. It is approximately 5 mm in diameter and is surrounded by the cranial mesenteric plexus of autonomic nerves and a large sympathetic ganglion. It passes ventrocaudally through the mesentery and acts as an axis around which the whole small and large intestine rotates during development. As it extends into the intestinal mass, it is loosely bounded by the duodenum on the right and caudally. This is followed distally by the colon, which hooks around the artery in such a way that the ascending colon lies to its right, the transverse colon cranial to it, and the descending colon to the left. The cranial mesenteric ganglion and plexus are so intimately associated with the celiac ganglia and plexuses that it is usual to find a combined celiacomesenteric plexus and ganglion, which obscures the origin of both vessels. Peripheral to the plexus are the long jejunal lymph nodes and the portal vein. The first two branches of the cranial mesenteric artery arise from opposite sides of the artery, approximately 2 cm from its origin. One of these, a common trunk for colic and ileocolic arteries, runs cranially in the transverse mesocolon, and the other, the caudal pancreaticoduodenal artery, from a caudal origin runs to the right and cranially. The remaining part of the artery gradually diminishes in size as some 14 jejunal arteries arise

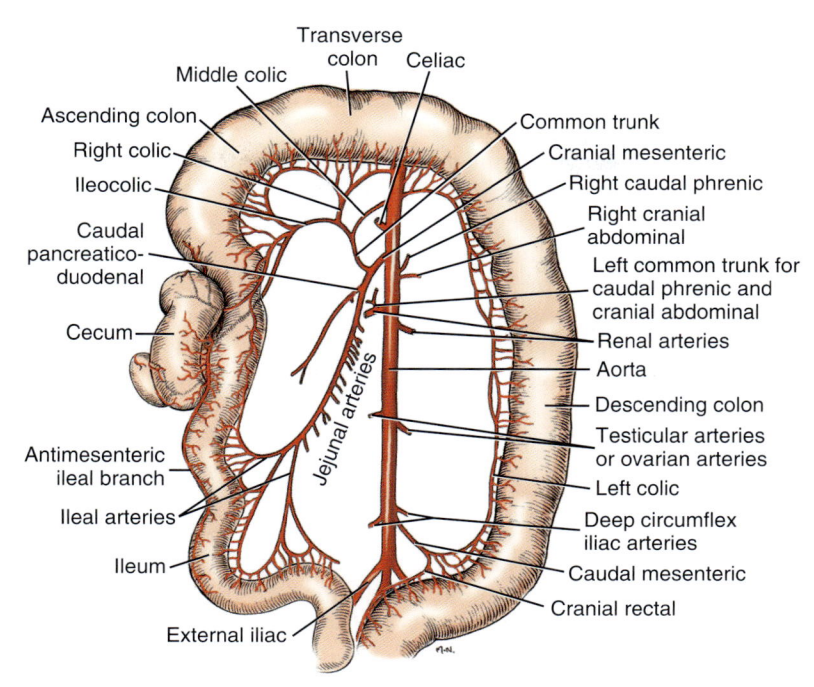

• **Fig. 11.59** Branches of the cranial and caudal mesenteric arteries, ventral aspect.

from it. Ileal arteries terminate the cranial mesenteric artery.

The common trunk for the colic and ileocolic arteries courses cranially and to the right in the transverse mesocolon as it gives origin in succession to the middle colic, right colic, and the terminal ileocolic arteries. The **middle colic artery** (*a. colica media*) (Fig. 11.59) arises from the first few millimeters of the common trunk or from the cranial mesenteric directly. It runs cranially in the transverse mesocolon, where it usually makes one spiral turn. It bifurcates approximately 2 cm from the left colic flexure. One branch runs distally in the descending mesocolon and, after supplying approximately half of the descending (left) colon, anastomoses with the left colic artery, a branch of the caudal mesenteric artery. The other branch swings to the right and forms an arcade with the smaller right colic artery to supply the transverse colon.

The **right colic artery** (*a. colica dextra*) (Figs. 11.53 and 11.59) supplies the distal half of the ascending (right) colon and initial part of the transverse colon. It forms terminal arcades with the middle colic on its left and the colic branch of the ileocolic artery on its right. From these anastomoses vasa recti arise that supply all the transverse colon and the distal part of the ascending colon. This vessel may be absent or double.

The common trunk terminates on the right in the **ileocolic artery** (*a. ileocolica*) (Figs. 11.53, 11.58, and 11.59). This artery supplies the ascending colon, cecum, and ileum. The ileocolic artery was formerly called the *ileocecocolic artery* because it supplies all three structures. The **colic branch** (*ramus colicus*) of the ileocolic artery is a small vessel that arises as the first branch of the ileocolic artery. It runs in the right mesocolon cranially toward the right colic flexure, giving off branches to the middle and distal parts of the ascending colon. It forms a definite arcade with the right colic artery and a smaller anastomosis with the colic branches of the ileocolic artery that supply the proximal part of the ascending colon. After supplying the colic branch and before the ileocolic artery disappears between the ileum and cecum, small **colic branches** (*rami colici*) arise and go to the proximal part of the ascending colon close to the cecum. The **mesenteric ileal branch** (*ramus ilei mesenterialis*) arises near the colic branches and runs to the ventral side of the ileocolic junction. It supplies small branches to the junction and sends a branch proximally along the mesenteric border of the ileum to anastomose with the last intestinal (ileal) artery from the cranial mesenteric artery. Variations in the vascularity of this portion of the digestive tube are extremely common. The **cecal artery** (*a. cecalis*) is a large branch of the ileocolic artery that crosses the dorsal surface of the ileocolic junction. It leaves the subserosa and disappears in the areolar tissue uniting the cecum to the ileum. It supplies branches to the ileum and cecum. The main part of the vessel, after emerging from between the ileum and cecum, continues proximally in the ileocecal fold as the **antimesenteric ileal branch** (*ramus ilei antimesenterialis*). This vessel extends along the ileum and anastomoses with the last jejunal artery in the musculature of the small intestine. The ileocolic artery and its branches are accompanied by plexuses of autonomic nerves that take the names of the vessels they follow, and all have satellite veins and lymphatics.

The **caudal pancreaticoduodenal artery** (*a. pancreaticoduodenalis caudalis*) (Figs. 11.53, 11.54, 11.58, and 11.59) arises from the cranial mesenteric artery opposite the origin of the common trunk for the colic and ileocolic arteries and runs to the right in the mesentery to the descending portion of the duodenum near the caudal flexure. On passing the caudal end of the right lobe of the pancreas, it sends from one to three **pancreatic branches** into the gland, which anastomose in the caudal third of this lobe with similar branches from the cranial pancreaticoduodenal artery. The **duodenal branch**, as it runs obliquely to the mesenteric border of the descending portion of the duodenum, supplies a small branch to the duodenum, which, in the region of the caudal flexure, anastomoses with the first jejunal artery. The main branch anastomoses on the duodenum with the larger duodenal branch of the cranial pancreaticoduodenal artery.

The **jejunal arteries** (*aa. jejunales*) (Figs. 11.53, 11.58, and 11.59) are 12 to 15 in number. Some of these are larger than others, and branch after they have traveled only a few millimeters. They arise from the caudal or convex side of the cranial mesenteric artery. The proximal 8 to 10 vessels are covered on each side by the two large jejunal lymph nodes. Usually the first five to seven arteries arise closely together; rarely are they separated by more than 3 mm. Following this cluster of vessels that go to the proximal part of the jejunum, the artery is free of branches for approximately 1 cm. The cranial mesenteric artery then gives rise to the branches that go to the distal part of the jejunum and finally to the two ileal arteries. The ileal arteries branch on approaching the intestine and join to form primary and secondary arcades, which lie directly adjacent to the intestinal wall. According to Noer (1943), tertiary arcades are rudimentary and, when present, consist of communications between the branchings of the secondary arcades. There is little variation of the vascular pattern throughout the jejunum, ileum, and colon.

The *vasa recti* leave the terminal arcades and go directly to the intestine. They are short and irregular. Numerous lateral branches unite with similar adjacent vessels. Most bifurcate on entering the wall of the intestine; these branches circle the gut on opposite sides and typically anastomose with each other on the antimesenteric border. Eisberg (1924) states that the vasa recti pierce the muscular coats in the mesenteric quarters of the small intestine and the antimesenteric quarters of the large intestine. There is a well-defined arterial anastomosis along the mesenteric border in addition to those between the vasa recti. These anastomoses are small and few in the duodenum. They are moderate in number in the jejunum and occur in large numbers in the ileum and colon. Within the gut there are two arterial networks. The subserous one is well developed as compared with humans and is derived from the mural network. The mural network lies largely in the submucosa and is formed by direct and plexiform anastomoses (Noer, 1943).

Branches are supplied at irregular intervals from the proximal halves of the jejunal arteries to the jejunal lymph nodes, one of which lies on each side of the jejunal mesentery.

The cranial mesenteric artery terminates as jejunal and ileal branches. The cranial mesenteric artery terminates in **ileal arteries** (*aa. ilei*). The first ileal artery forms a terminal arcade with the last jejunal artery and issues vasa recti to the distal part of the jejunum and the proximal part of the ileum. The second and third ileal arteries form anastomotic arcades on the mesenteric border of the ileum and anastomose on the distal ileum with the mesenteric ileal branch of the ileocolic artery. The first jejunal artery anastomoses with the duodenal part of the caudal pancreaticoduodenal artery, and all jejunal and ileal arteries anastomose with each other. Thus a vascular channel is formed along the whole small intestine. The cranial mesenteric artery and its branches are accompanied by the cranial mesenteric plexus of nerves, the intestinal lymph trunk, and the cranial mesenteric vein.

The **caudal mesenteric artery** (*a. mesenterica caudalis*) (Figs. 11.52, 11.53, and 11.59) arises from the ventral surface of the aorta approximately 4 cm cranial to the termination of the aorta or opposite the caudal part of the fifth lumbar vertebra. It runs caudoventrally in the mesocolon to the mesenteric border of the descending colon, where it divides into the proximally running left colic and the distally running cranial rectal arteries. The caudal mesenteric artery is accompanied by the caudal mesenteric plexus and ganglion, which begins approximately 1 cm from the origin of the artery. No veins or lymph vessels accompany the main caudal mesenteric artery.

The **left colic artery** (*a. colica sinistra*) follows the mesenteric border of the descending colon cranially and anastomoses with the middle colic artery at the junction of the proximal and distal halves of the descending colon. No arcade is formed; numerous vasa recti run from it to the descending colon. It is accompanied by the left colic vein and autonomic nerves.

The **cranial rectal artery** (*a. rectalis cranialis*), formerly known as the *cranial hemorrhoidal artery*, descends along the mesenteric border of the descending colon and rectum. It supplies many branches to the rectum and may anastomose with the middle rectal and caudal rectal arteries. The cranial rectal artery supplies most of the blood to the terminal colon and rectum; the middle and caudal rectal arteries supply variable and relatively insignificant amounts (Bellenger et al., 1993).

Paired Visceral Branches of Abdominal Aorta

The **renal arteries** (*aa. renales*) (Figs. 11.52, 11.53, and 11.59; see also Figs. 9.1, 9.3 and 9.5) arise asymmetrically from the lateral surfaces of the abdominal aorta. The right renal artery arises approximately 2 cm cranial to the left renal artery in conformity to the more cranial position of the right kidney. This places it approximately 4 cm caudal to the origin of the cranial mesenteric artery. In a large dog, it is 5 cm long and 4 mm in diameter. The left renal artery is approximately the same diameter as the right, but is only approximately 3 cm long. The fact that the caudal vena cava lies to the right of the aorta accounts for the greater length of the right renal artery, which crosses its dorsal surface. Each renal artery supplies two or three branches to the caudal pole of the adrenal gland (*rami adrenales caudales*) and a small cranial ureteral branch (*ramus uretericus*) to the ureter, although this vessel may arise from the aorta directly. Approximately 1 cm outside the renal hilus, each renal artery divides typically into a dorsal and a ventral branch. According to Christensen (1952), each of these further divides into two, four, or even seven interlobar arteries, or the renal arteries may not divide at all before entering the hilus of the kidney. At the corticomedullary junction, the interlobar arteries give off arcuate arteries laterally. Only in mature or elderly specimens are the arcuate arteries arched toward the cortex. Although the arcuate arteries anastomose, they do not form functional connections. This results in the typical pyramidal infarct of the cortex and medulla seen with thrombosis of arcuate vessels. The arcuate arteries give rise to the numerous interlobular arteries of the cortex. These in turn give rise to the afferent vessels, which are continued as the glomerular arterioles (see Figs. 9.5 and 9.6). The renal arteries may be double in 20% of dogs, particularly on the left side. Christensen (1952) found 29 double renal arteries in 117 specimens. Reis and Tepe (1956) examined 500 dogs and reported that 99.4% had a single right renal artery, whereas 12.8% had double left renal arteries, and in 0.4% the left renal arteries were triple. The renal artery and its larger branches are accompanied by satellite veins and plexuses of autonomic nerves. Both the arteries and the veins have companion lymphatics, according to Peirce (1944).

The **adrenal (suprarenal) arteries** (*aa. adrenales*) in the dog usually arise from the phrenicoabdominal trunk, the aorta, and the renal artery (Fig. 10.6). Usually the **cranial adrenal branches** (*rami adrenales craniales*) arise from the caudal phrenic artery and the **caudal adrenal branches** (*rami adrenalea caudales*) arise from the renal artery. Quite commonly the cranial pole of the adrenal gland receives a branch from the cranial mesenteric artery and occasionally from the celiac also. Ljubomudrov (1939) states that there are 20 to 30 or more fine arteries that supply each gland, and that some of these may arise from the artery to the adipose capsule and from a lumbar artery, unilaterally, in addition to the sources already cited. Flint (1900) gives a classic description of the adrenal gland and details its blood supply. His phrenic and accessory phrenic arteries represent the phrenic part of the phrenicoabdominal of modern terminology, whereas his lumbar artery is the abdominal part. Flint divides the vessels into three groups when they reach the adrenal: capsular, cortical, and medullary. The capsular vessels are represented by a rather poorly defined system of arterioles that arise from all the arteries going to the gland. These form a plexus from which most of its branches, of arteriole size, enter the cortex. The arterioles divide and form capillaries that follow the reticular septa between the coiled columns of cortical cells, which they nourish. The arteries of the medulla, according to Flint, number approximately 50. They come from the capsular plexus and run at right angles to it through the cortex to the corticomedullary junction, where most turn and run short distances in this area as they give off finer vessels that supply the medulla. While traversing the cortex, they neither divide nor supply any branches to it.

The arteries that supply the testes and ovaries arise from the ventral third of the circumference of the aorta in the midlumbar region or opposite the fibrocartilage between the fourth and fifth lumbar vertebrae. The right artery usually arises several millimeters cranial to the left, in conformity with the more cranial location of the right gonad.

The **testicular artery** (*a. testicularis*) (Figs. 9.12, 11.52, 11.53, and 11.59), formerly called the *internal spermatic artery*, is a small vessel, much longer and straighter than its homologue, the ovarian artery. It runs laterally or caudolaterally across the lumbar hypaxial muscles and the ventral surface of the ureter where it makes a sweeping bend caudally to the deep inguinal ring. It lies in a special plica of peritoneum, the **proximal mesorchium** (*mesorchium proximale*) that may be 3 to 4 cm wide. At the deep inguinal ring it becomes a constituent of the spermatic cord and runs to the testis with its companion vein, lymph vessels, and nerve plexuses in the free border of the **distal mesorchium** (*mesorchium distale*). It is the only artery supplying the testis and epididymis.

The **ovarian artery** (*a. ovarica*) (Figs. 9.1, 11.59, 11.61), the homologue of the testicular artery, varies in size and tortuosity, depending on the age and past reproductive activity of the bitch. The ovarian artery (Preuss, 1959) has also been called the *utero-ovarian artery* or the *internal spermatic artery*. The vessel arises from the ventral surface of the aorta at the midlumbar level. Like its homologue, it lies ventral to the caudal vena cava. Each gives a minute branch to the capsule of the kidney. Other branches may go to the periaortic fat, peritoneum, and the adventitia of the caudal vena cava. Medial to the ovary the vessel bifurcates or trifurcates. The resultant branches are very tortuous, even in immature females, as they course in the mesovarium, the cranial part of the broad ligament, on their way to the ovary. Small branches from these supply the peritoneum and fat of the ovarian bursa, and a tubal branch (*ramus tubarius*) supplies the uterine tube. One or more uterine branches (*ramus uterinus*) continue caudally to the ovarian end of the uterine horn and anastomose with the uterine artery, which runs cranially in the mesometrium, the caudal part of the broad ligament. The ovarian artery is accompanied by a plexus of sympathetic nerves, a satellite vein, and lymph vessels. Esperanca-Pina and Reis (1984) describe the vascular pattern of the dog's ovary but do not use NAV terminology (see Constantinescu & Schaller, 2012). The ovarian artery (*a. ovarica*) has a uterine branch (*ramus uterinus*), which formerly was called the *cranial uterine artery*. The uterine artery (*a. uterine*), a branch of the vaginal artery, was formerly termed the *middle uterine artery* (*a. uterina media*) in some textbooks.

Parietal Branches of Abdominal Aorta

The paired **lumbar arteries** (*aa. lumbales*) (Fig. 11.52) are seven in number. The first two pairs arise from the thoracic aorta, and the last five pairs come from the dorsal surface of the abdominal aorta. Those in the cranial part of the series are 4 mm apart at their origins, and usually the right arteries arise 3 to 6 mm caudal to those on the left. The vessels are progressively closer at their origins as they are traced caudally, and the last lumbar arteries may arise from a common trunk. Each pair of vessels runs caudolaterally across the ventrolateral surface of the body of the lumbar vertebra of the same serial number. The first three or four pairs arise opposite the intervertebral disc cranial to the vertebra of the comparable number; the last three or four pairs arise opposite the body of the comparable vertebra. For this reason the last several arteries are less oblique as they run on the side of the vertebral bodies, covered in their courses by the lumbar hypaxial muscles, which they supply. Near their origins each vessel gives off a small, short nutrient branch that enters the body of the vertebra. Brunner and Frewein (1989) examined lumbar intervertebral discs of 21 dogs aged 3 to 14 years. They found that the principal blood supply to nourish the avascular intervertebral disc was from capillary loops that passed from the bone marrow of the vertebral body through the endplate of that body. These loops were most numerous opposite the nucleus pulposus. They reproduce an illustration from a paper by Crock and Goldwasser (1984), which their study confirms.

Lumbar arteries course dorsally along the side of the vertebrae to enter the epaxial muscles caudal to the craniolaterally extending transverse processes. Here each artery divides into a **spinal branch** (*ramus spinalis*), which runs with the nerve into the vertebral canal (see discussion of vertebral artery for description), and a **dorsal branch** (*ramus dorsalis*), which runs dorsocaudally in the longissimus muscle past the lateral surface of the cranially inclined articular process of the vertebra caudal to it. This dorsal branch parallels the dorsal branch of the spinal nerve where it gives off many branches to the epaxial muscles and medial and lateral cutaneous branches (*ramus cutaneous medialis* and *ramus cutaneous lateralis*) to the dorsal subcutaneous fat and skin near and lateral to the midline. Small branches also leave the dorsal branch near the origin of the spinal branch and run laterally on the ventral surfaces of the transverse processes that they supply. The adjacent internal oblique and transversus abdominis muscles receive delicate terminal branches from these. The seventh lumbar arteries differ from the others in that they may arise as a common trunk from the terminal part of the aorta or from the median sacral artery. Each vessel as it courses laterally runs dorsal to the lumbosacral nerve plexus and divides into dorsal and caudal branches at the iliosacral joint. The dorsal branch enters the epaxial muscles by passing through the cranial angle formed by the ilium and the vertebral column. The caudal branch runs into the pelvis in company with the sympathetic trunk. It supplies this, and, at the ganglion impar, continues into the ventral sacrocaudal muscles. The caudal branch may also send a branch laterally to the pelvic surface of the wing of the ilium. The lumbar arteries are accompanied by satellite veins.

The caudal phrenic and cranial abdominal arteries arise from a common trunk in the dog that is referred to as the **phrenicoabdominal trunk** (*truncus phrenicoabdominalis*) (Figs. 11.52, 11.60, and 11.61). It arises from the lateral surface of the aorta between the cranial mesenteric and renal arteries. The right artery occasionally arises from the corresponding renal vessel, and the caudal phrenic and abdominal parts may arise separately. The artery runs caudolaterally, parallel to the ribs, and crosses the ventral surface of the psoas muscles and the dorsal surface of the adrenal gland. The corresponding vein grooves the ventral surface of the adrenal gland. Adjacent to the adrenal gland the phrenicoabdominal trunk terminates in a caudal phrenic and cranial abdominal artery.

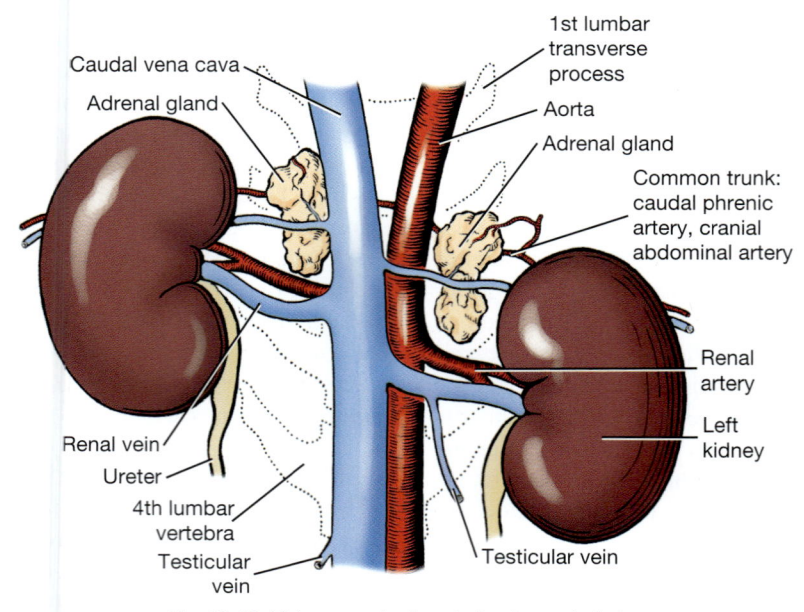

• **Fig. 11.60** Kidneys and adrenal glands, ventral view.

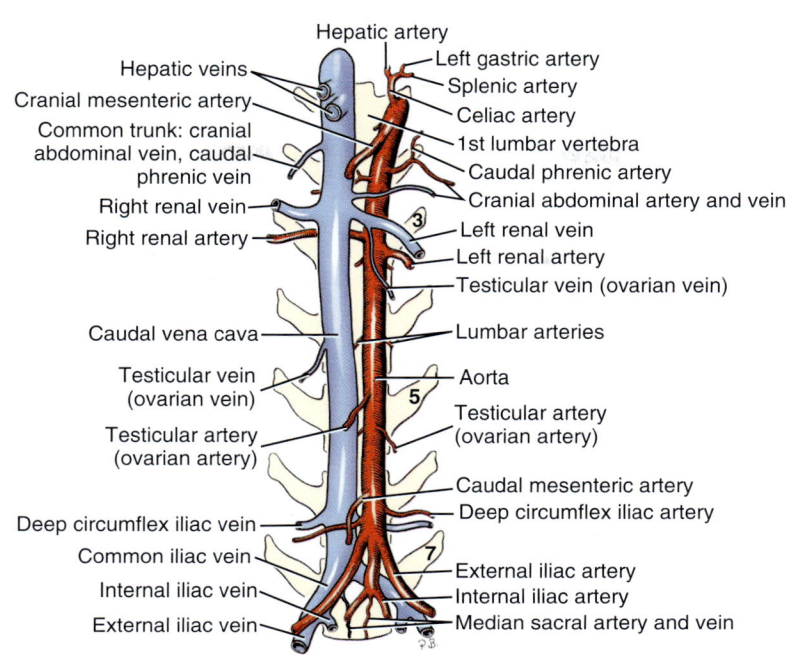

• **Fig. 11.61** Branches of abdominal aorta and tributaries of the caudal vena cava, ventral view.

The main **caudal phrenic artery** (*a. phrenica caudalis*) arises within 1 cm of the origin of the phrenicoabdominal trunk. It supplies branches to the cranial pole of the adrenal (*rami adrenales cranialis*) before it runs cranially to ramify on the ventrocaudolateral surface of the crus of the diaphragm. In its retroperitoneal course along the medial border of the dorsal extension of the tendinous center of the diaphragm, it usually sends two branches ventrolaterally, which redivide laterally as they cross the tendinous part of the diaphragm and enter its muscular periphery. The branches in general follow the course of the muscle fibers peripherally and anastomose within the muscle with the phrenic branches of the tenth, eleventh, and twelfth intercostal arteries.

The **cranial abdominal artery** (*a. abdominalis cranialis*) continues the direction of the common trunk into the abdominal wall after the caudal phrenic vessel arises. It runs medial to the narrow aponeurosis of origin of the transversus abdominis muscle, then perforates the muscle to ramify extensively between it and the internal abdominal oblique muscle. Usually the vessel divides into cranial and caudal branches after perforating the transversus abdominis muscle. The cranial branch runs toward the costal arch; the caudal branch diverges from it and supplies the middle zone of the lateral abdominal wall. The cranial abdominal artery anastomoses cranially with the phrenic vessels, ventrally with the cranial and caudal epigastric arteries, and caudally with the deep branch of the deep circumflex iliac artery. The cranial abdominal artery is accompanied by the cranial iliohypogastric nerve and a satellite vein.

The paired **deep circumflex iliac artery** (*a. circumflexa ilium profunda*) (Figs. 11.52, 11.59, and 11.61) arises from the lateral surface of the aorta approximately 1 cm cranial to the origin of the external iliac artery, ventral to the sixth lumbar vertebra. The right artery usually arises a few millimeters cranial to the left. Its initial part lies between the caudal vena cava dorsally and the cranial pole of the medial iliac lymph node ventrally. It runs laterally across the ventral surface of the lumbar hypaxial muscles and enters the abdominal wall ventral to the tuber coxae. At the lateral border of the psoas major muscle, it usually sends a cranial branch to this muscle and to the overlying m. quadratus lumborum. It terminates as cranial and caudal branches.

The **cranial branch** (*ramus cranialis*) leaves the parent vessel before this perforates the abdominal wall and, running cranioventrally, extends lateral to the transversus abdominis muscle. The main vessel sends branches dorsally, which accompany the lumbar nerves to the lateral surface of the transversus abdominis. The end branches of this vessel anastomose with the cranial and caudal abdominal arteries. It is the main supply of the caudodorsal fourth of the abdominal wall.

The **caudal branch** (*ramus caudalis*) perforates the abdominal wall between the lumbar and inguinal portions of the internal abdominal oblique and the cutaneus trunci muscles to reach subcutaneous structures. It is stellate in form as it subdivides into diverging branches that arborize ventrally and caudally. One or two large branches spray out over the caudal lumbar and pelvic regions to anastomose with their fellows at the mid-dorsal line. The most cranial of the ventral branches ends in the fold of the flank. The cranial branches are smallest as they radiate in the subcutaneous fat of the caudal parts of the lumbar region and abdomen.

The deep circumflex iliac artery is accompanied by a satellite vein that lies caudal to it. At the lateral border of the psoas major muscle it is joined by the lateral cutaneous femoral nerve.

Arteries of the Pelvic Limb

The abdominal aorta gives off the paired external iliac arteries to the pelvic limbs and terminates in the paired internal iliac arteries and the median sacral artery.

External Iliac Artery

The **external iliac artery** (*a. iliaca externa*) (Figs. 11.52, 11.61, and 11.66) is the largest parietal branch of the abdominal aorta. This paired vessel arises from the lateral surface of the aorta ventral to the intervertebral disc between the sixth and seventh lumbar vertebrae. It runs caudoventrally and is related near its origin to the common iliac vein and the psoas minor muscle. Farther distally it lies on the iliopsoas muscle. The ureter and the ductus deferens of the male or the uterine horn of the female, lying in their peritoneal folds, cross the artery ventrally at nearly right angles. Small, slender branches usually leave the vessel to supply the adjacent fat or to run in the broad ligament of the female. The small caudal abdominal artery may arise from it near the pubis, but its only constant branch is the deep femoral artery. It is continued outside the abdominal wall by the femoral artery. Its satellite vein lies caudolaterally.

The **deep femoral artery** (*a. profunda femoris*) (Fig. 11.66) is approximately 3 cm long, with approximately half of it lying within the abdomen and half outside. It arises from the caudomedial surface of the external iliac artery at an angle of approximately 45 degrees, and runs obliquely distocaudally over the medial surface of the external iliac vein to leave the abdominal cavity by passing through the caudal part of the vascular lacuna. It sends a small branch over the pelvic surface of the pubis to the levator ani muscle, where it anastomoses with the obturator branch that ascends through the obturator foramen. Another small branch enters the laterally lying iliopsoas muscle. Its principal intraabdominal branch is the short pudendoepigastric trunk. After leaving the abdomen, the deep femoral artery becomes the medial circumflex femoral artery and passes between the quadriceps femoris and the medially lying pectineus muscles.

The **pudendoepigastric trunk** (*truncus pudendoepigastricus*) (Fig. 11.66) is short and may extend to the deep abdominal inguinal ring before bifurcating terminally. Rarely, it is absent, in which case the terminal caudal epigastric and the external pudendal arteries arise from the deep femoral artery.

The **caudal epigastric artery** (*a. epigastrica caudalis*) runs cranially to lie on the dorsal surface of the rectus abdominis muscle deep to the parietal peritoneum. When it reaches the caudal border of the sheath of the rectus abdominis muscle, it runs ventral to this. It grooves the dorsal surface of the muscle as it parallels the linea alba in its branched, cranial course. At approximately the junction of the cranial and middle thirds of the abdominal part of the rectus abdominis muscle, it anastomoses with the cranial epigastric artery in the substance of the muscle. It sends three or more branches laterally, which anastomose with the terminal abdominal branches of the deep circumflex iliac artery in the middle third of the abdomen and the caudal abdominal branches caudolaterally. Small medial branches supply the relatively avascular linea alba. It is accompanied by a small satellite vein.

The **external pudendal artery** (*a. pudenda externa*) (Figs. 11.62 and 11.63) arises as the ventral terminal branch of the pudendoepigastric trunk. It leaves the abdominal cavity through the caudal part of the inguinal canal. After emerging through the superficial inguinal ring, it continues caudoventrally to the cranial border of the gracilis muscle. It then arches cranially and becomes related to the dorsal surface of the superficial inguinal lymph node. Here, in the fat-laden superficial abdominal fascia, it gives off the small ventral labial in the female or ventral scrotal branch in the male and arches cranially as the caudal superficial epigastric artery. The **ventral labial branch** (*ramus labialis ventralis*) enters the fat ventral to the symphyseal tendon and emerges caudally between the thighs to terminate in the vulva. The comparable **ventral scrotal branch** (*ramus scrotalis ventralis*) may be extremely small or absent. The caudal superficial epigastric artery is the other terminal branch of the external pudendal artery that continues it cranially without any clear demarcation based on the size of the vessels. The external pudendal artery is accompanied by a laterally lying satellite vein.

The **caudal superficial epigastric artery** (*a. epigastrica superficialis caudalis*) (see Figs. 11.62 and 11.63) is small in the male as it runs cranially to supply the prepuce (*rami preputiales*), superficial inguinal lymph node, fascia, fat, and skin. It usually ends before it reaches the umbilicus. In the female it may be the largest artery of the abdominal wall. Its size is in direct proportion to the state of development of the mammary glands it supplies. From its origin, on the convex side of the second arc of the external pudendal artery, it runs cranially deep to the inguinal mammary gland and medial to its papilla, the nipple. It supplies many branches (*rami mammarii*) to this potentially pendulous gland. As it advances cranially, it enters the caudal abdominal mammary gland and divides into several branches, some of which become subcutaneous around the nipple. Many

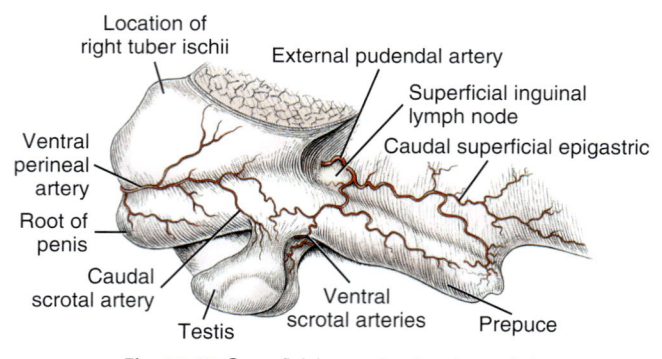

• **Fig. 11.62** Superficial vessels of male genitals.

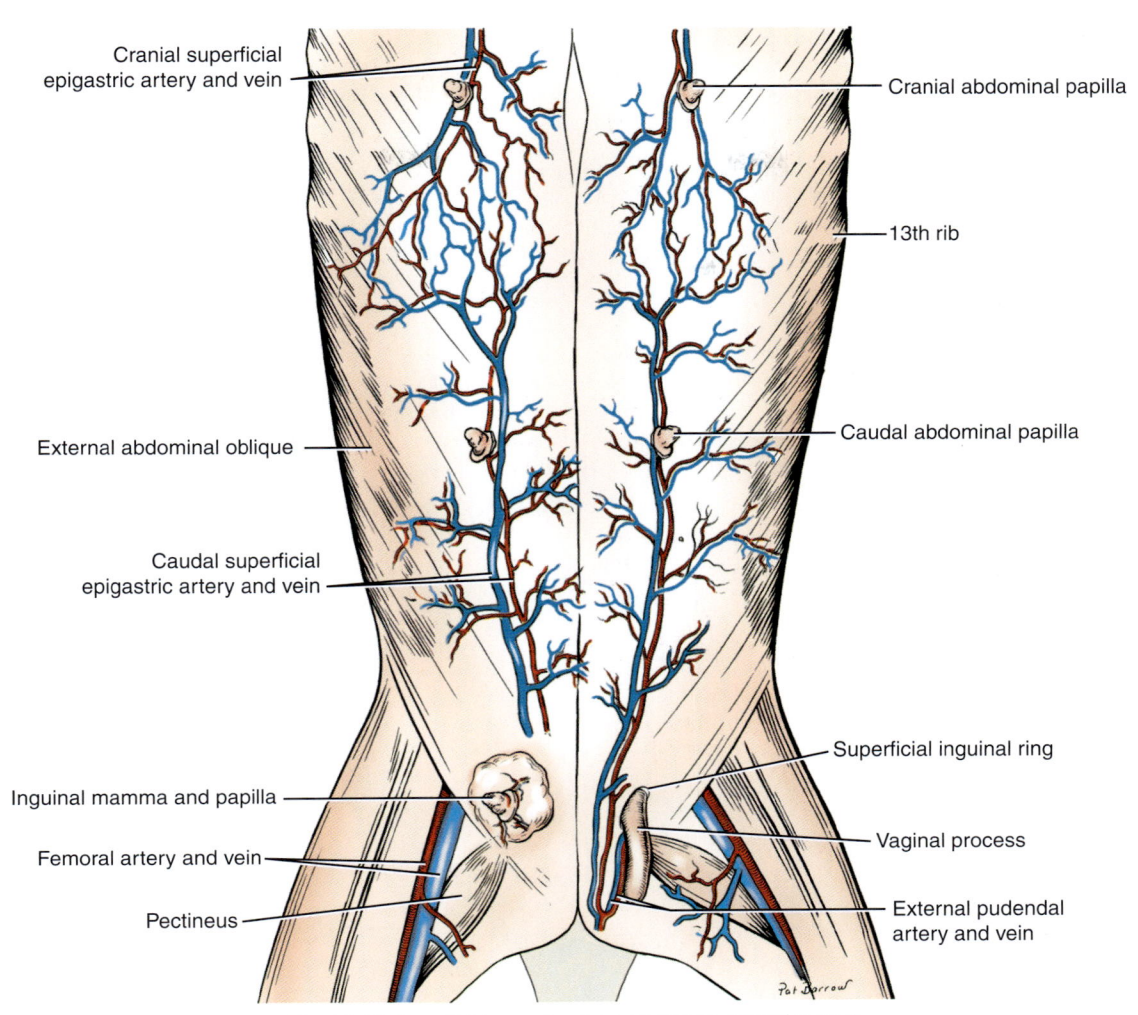

• **Fig. 11.63** Superficial vessels of the abdomen, ventral aspect.

of these branches anastomose with like branches from the cranial superficial epigastric artery between the cranial and caudal abdominal mammary glands. The vessel takes on special significance because of the high incidence of mammary tumors in the dog. It is accompanied by a satellite vein and lymph vessels that drain primarily into the superficial inguinal lymph node.

The **medial circumflex femoral artery** (*a. circumflexa medialis*) (Figs. 11.64 through 11.66) is the continuation of the deep femoral artery beyond the vascular lacuna. It obliquely crosses the surface of the iliopsoas and vastus medialis muscles, sending branches into each, and arborizing extensively in the deep part of the adductor muscle. On the caudal surface of the femur distal to the greater trochanter, a nutrient artery enters the femur at the junction of the proximal and middle thirds. The medial circumflex femoral artery provides obturator, deep, ascending, transverse, and acetabular branches.

Parouti (1962) made a detailed study of the vascularization of the dog's femur and provided illustrations showing the principal supply to be the medial circumflex femoral artery. Cuthbertson and Gilfillan (1964) described variations of the nutrient artery of the diaphysis of the femur and likewise noted that the most common supply (78 of 100 femurs) was from the medial circumflex femoral artery, as described in the literature.

The **obturator branch** (*ramus obturatorius*) (see Fig. 11.66) of the medial circumflex femoral artery, after running a few millimeters caudally, courses dorsally through the cranial part of the obturator foramen, lateral to the obturator nerve. It furnishes branches to the levator ani and coccygeus muscles and the external and internal obturator muscles. On the pelvic surface of the pubis it anastomoses with the small branch from the deep femoral artery that supplies the cranial portion of the levator ani muscle. Most of the intrapelvic portion of the obturator branch terminates in the internal obturator muscle. The **ascending branch** (*ramus ascendens*) (Fig. 11.66) of the medial circumflex femoral artery supplies the proximal end of the massive adductor muscle. It ends in the semimembranosus muscle. Small branches also supply the quadratus femoris, pectineus, external obturator, and semimembranosus muscles. Approximately 5 mm distal to the origin of the branch that ascends through the obturator foramen, a small **acetabular branch** (*ramus acetabularis*)

564 CHAPTER 11 **The Heart and Arteries**

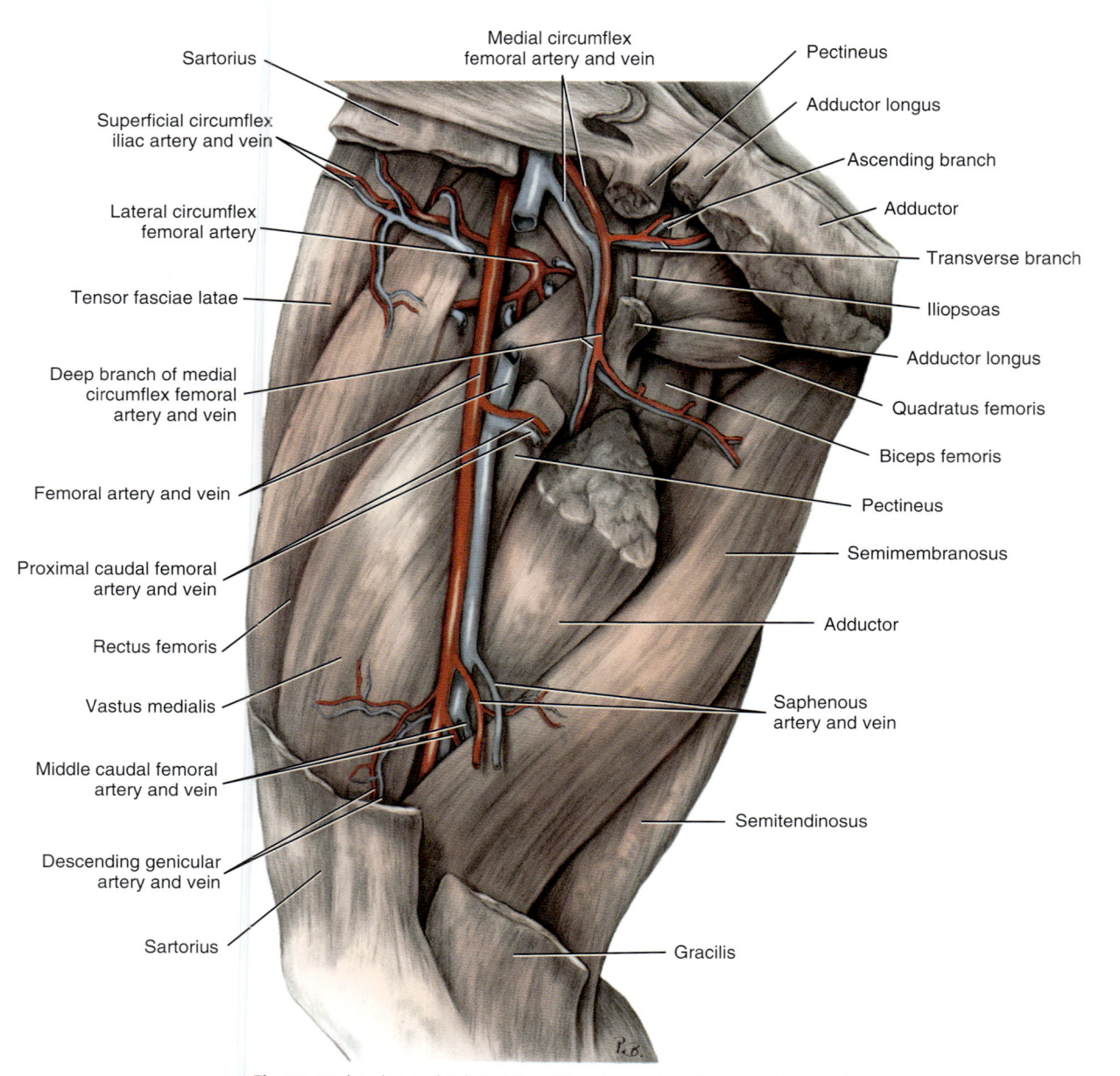

• **Fig. 11.64** Arteries and veins of the thigh, deep dissection, medial aspect.

extends laterally to enter the trochanteric fossa and supply portions of the muscles that insert there. Its chief importance concerns the branches that supply the caudal part of the hip joint capsule and the neck of the femur. Gasse et al. (1999) showed that the arteries supplying the joint capsule enter areas of the joint capsule's wall near its femoral as well as its coxal attachments. These vessels form an intramural vascular network arranged in layers in the fibrous as well as the synovial layers of the joint capsule. The main terminal part of the vessel, the **transverse branch** (*r. transversus*), enters the semimembranosus muscle approximately 3 cm from the tuber ischii and anastomoses with the caudal gluteal artery. A **deep branch** (*ramus profundus*) of the vessel passes distally in the adductor near the femur and anastomoses with the lateral circumflex femoral artery.

The **caudal abdominal artery** (*a. abdominalis caudalis*) (see Fig. 11.66) is a small vessel that usually arises from the cranial surface of the external iliac artery just after the deep femoral artery arises, but it may arise from the deep femoral, the pudendoepigastric trunk, or the caudal epigastric artery (Marthen, 1939). From the region of the vascular lacuna it runs cranially on the deep surface of the internal abdominal oblique muscle and divides typically into dorsal and ventral branches. On reaching the caudal border of the transverse abdominal muscle they arborize on the medial surface of the internal abdominal oblique muscle. Branches perforate this muscle to reach the external abdominal oblique muscle. The ventral branch lies approximately 2 cm from, and parallel to, the lateral border of the m. rectus abdominis. It anastomoses with the caudal epigastric artery. The dorsal

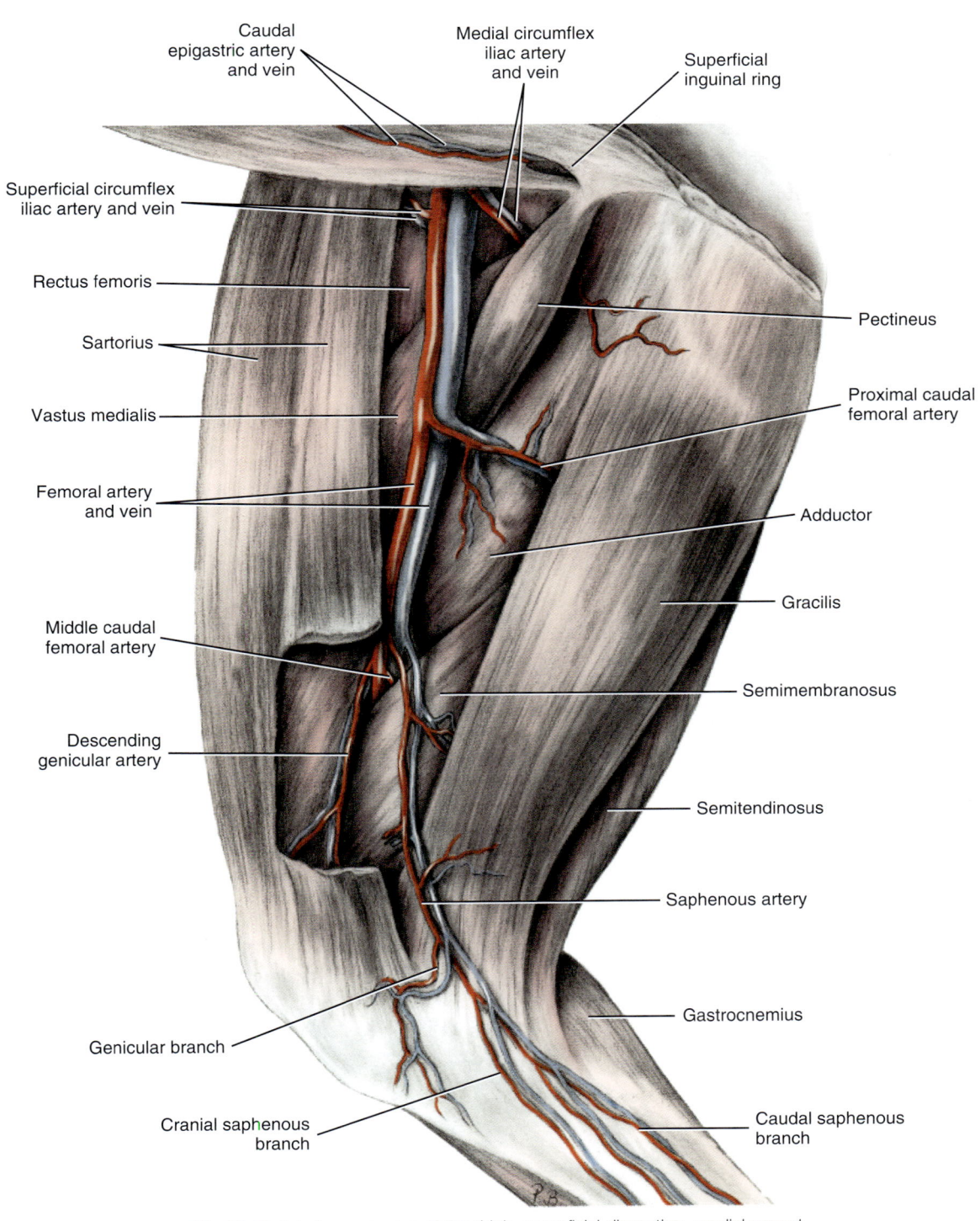

Fig. 11.65 Arteries and veins of the thigh, superficial dissection, medial aspect.

branch passes dorsally and anastomoses with the cranial branch of the deep circumflex iliac artery. The **cremasteric artery** (*a. cremasterica*) is a small branch of the caudal abdominal artery or the pudendoepigastric trunk that runs toward the inguinal canal and supplies the fat lying around the deep inguinal ring. It enters the inguinal canal and supplies the cremaster muscle. According to Joranson et al. (1929) the cremasteric artery, along with the artery of the ductus deferens, continues to the testis. Blood supplied through these vessels is not sufficient to prevent atrophy of the organ when the testicular artery is interrupted.

Femoral Artery

The **femoral artery** (*a. femoralis*) (Figs. 11.63 through 11.67) continues the external iliac artery from the vascular lacuna through the thigh. It in turn is continued caudal

566 CHAPTER 11 The Heart and Arteries

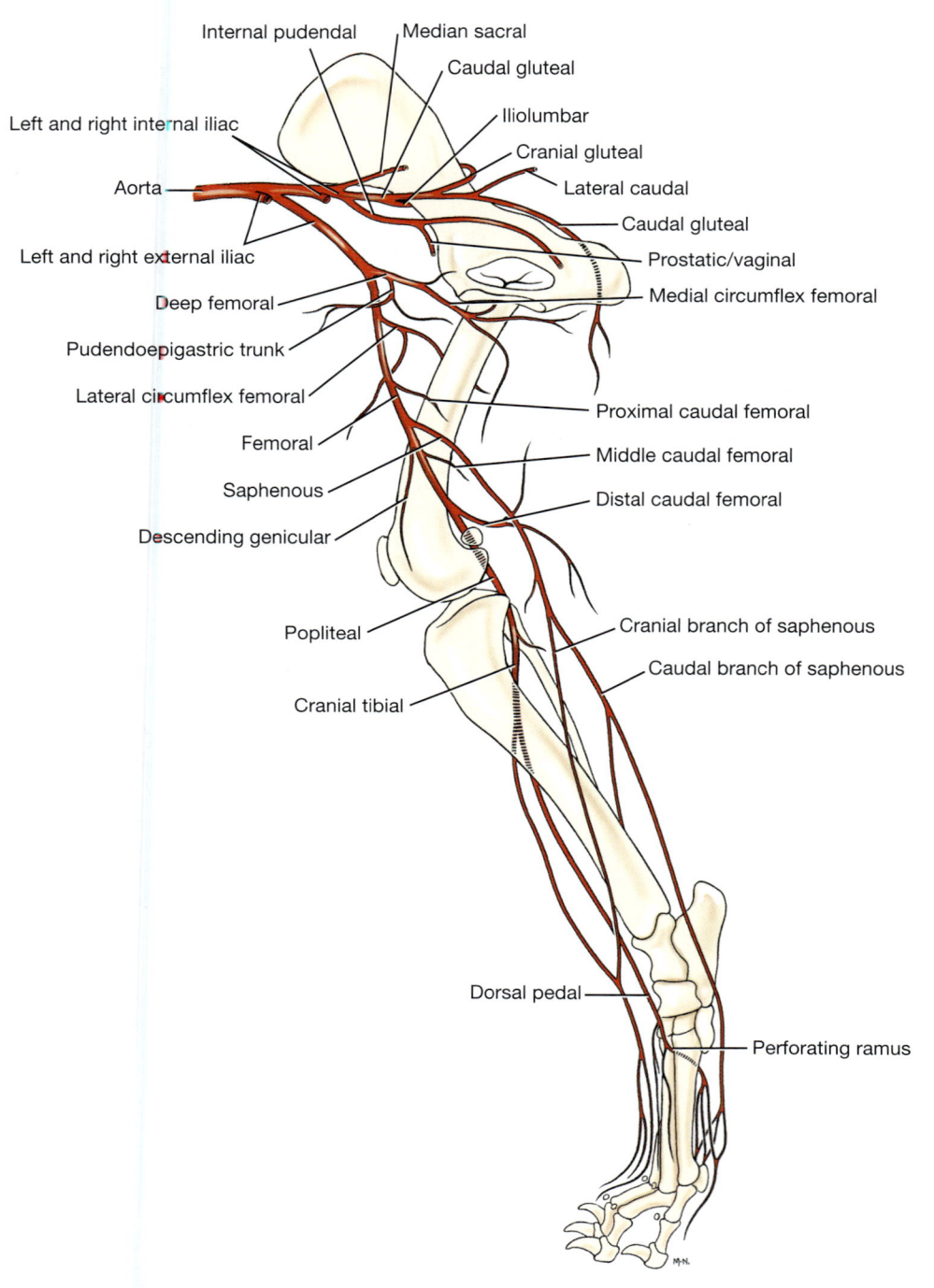

- **Fig. 11.66** Diagram of the arteries of the pelvis and thigh, medial aspect.

to the stifle joint by the popliteal artery. Throughout the proximal half of the thigh, it lies cranial to its satellite vein and either caudal or medial to the saphenous nerve. Here, the artery lies superficially in the **femoral triangle** (*trigonum femorale*), which is the favored site for taking the pulse of the dog. The femoral vein is large and securely placed in the femoral triangle so that venipunctures can be made without compressing it. The femoral vessels are covered only by the thin skin and the deep medial femoral fascia. On leaving the femoral triangle at the middle of the thigh, the femoral artery and vein incline laterally along the medial border of insertion of the adductor muscle, where they are covered by the caudal belly of the m. semimembranosus. On reaching the popliteal surface of the femur, the femoral vessels are continued between the lateral and medial heads of the gastrocnemius muscle as the popliteal artery and veins. The branches of the femoral artery in the order in which they arise are superficial circumflex iliac, lateral circumflex femoral, muscular branches, proximal caudal femoral, saphenous, descending

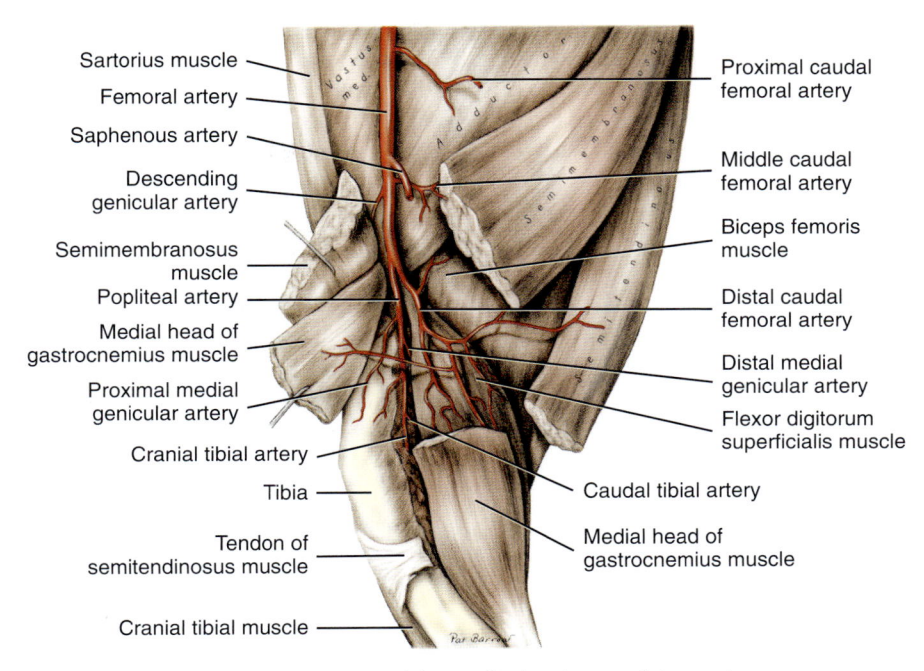

Fig. 11.67 Arteries of the popliteal region, medial aspect.

genicular, middle caudal femoral, and distal caudal femoral arteries.

The **superficial circumflex iliac artery** (*a. circumflexa ilium superficialis*) (Figs. 11.64 and 11.65) is a small artery that runs dorsocranially over the medial surface of the m. rectus femoris to reach the septum between the caudal belly of the sartorius and tensor fascia lata muscles. It arises from the lateral surface of the femoral artery close to the lateral circumflex femoral artery, or it may arise from the latter vessel. Its first branch usually is the principal vessel to the m. tensor fasciae latae. It also sends branches to the underlying rectus femoris muscle. The main vessel then bifurcates into dorsal and ventral branches, deep to the thin, caudal belly of the m. sartorius. The dorsal branch supplies the proximal fourth of the cranial belly of this muscle and becomes subcutaneous at the cranial ventral iliac spine; the ventral branch runs distocranially and supplies the middle portion of the cranial belly of the m. sartorius. It has a satellite vein.

The **lateral circumflex femoral artery** (*a. circumflexa femoris lateralis*) (Fig. 11.64), formerly called the *cranial femoral artery*, leaves the caudolateral surface of the femoral artery approximately 5 mm from the abdominal wall. It immediately disappears between the rectus femoris and vastus medialis muscles. It is approximately 2 mm in diameter at its origin, where it is crossed cranially by the saphenous nerve and caudally by the femoral vein. Usually its first branch is small and enters the m. iliopsoas near its insertion on the trochanter minor. Another small branch may extend lateral to the proximal part of the cranial border of the m. vastus lateralis and enter the caudal, deep part of the m. tensor fasciae latae. As the main artery loses contact with the m. iliopsoas to bend distally in the quadriceps muscle, it sends a large branch caudally, which bifurcates on reaching the neck of the femur. The resultant **ascending branch** (*ramus ascendens*) sends many small branches to the cranial part of the hip joint capsule, then continues dorsally to supply the insertions of the deep and middle gluteal and the tensor fasciae latae muscles. A **transverse branch** (*ramus transversus*) passes laterally to arborize in the proximal portions of the heads of the m. quadriceps femoris. The **descending branch** (*ramus descendens*) bends distolaterally around the caudal surface of the rectus femoris muscle and sends branches to the vasti, rectus femoris, and tensor fasciae latae muscles. It is the principal source of blood to the m. quadriceps. It usually forms a feeble anastomosis with the medial circumflex femoral artery caudal to the femur. It is accompanied by a satellite vein, which lies distal to it, and the large femoral nerve, which lies proximal to it.

The **muscular branches** of the femoral artery are variable in origin, number, size, and distribution. As the femoral artery passes distally from the point where the lateral circumflex femoral artery arises, it lies adjacent to the cranial border of the m. vastus medialis proximally passes over its medial surface and inclines laterally around its caudal border distally. Distal to the origin of the lateral circumflex femoral artery, a muscular branch arises from the lateral surface of the femoral artery, which bifurcates into cranial and caudal vessels. Two separate diverging vessels may arise directly from the femoral artery. The caudal vessel may end in the femoral sheath or terminate in the proximal end of the m. pectineus. The slender cranial branch goes to the deep surface of the caudal belly of the sartorius muscle.

The **proximal caudal femoral artery** (*a. caudalis femoris proximalis*) (Figs. 11.66 and 11.67) leaves the caudal side of the femoral artery, extends distocaudally, and crosses the insertion of the pectineus and then the adductor muscles. On reaching the cranial border of the m. gracilis, at the junction of its proximal and middle thirds, it enters the deep surface of the muscle. It sends one or more branches to the pectineus and the adductor muscles.

Usually three branches go to the adjacent muscles before the femoral artery courses laterally, deep to the m. semimembranosus. Often two of these branches arise from the cranial side of the vessel and, after short courses, disappear into the m. vastus medialis. One or two smaller branches quite regularly leave the caudal side of the femoral artery and disappear into the distal part of the adductor muscle.

The **saphenous artery** (*a. saphena*) (Figs. 11.64 through 11.67), less than 1 mm in diameter, arises from the medial surface of the femoral artery just before the femoral artery disappears deep to the m. semimembranosus. It runs distally across the medial surface of the semimembranosus muscle, where it and its accompanying vein and nerve lie between the converging borders of the caudal belly of the sartorius muscle cranially and the gracilis muscle caudally. It supplies small branches to these muscles. As it passes over the medial surface of the stifle, it sends a single or a paired **genicular branch** (*r. articularis genus*) (Figs. 11.65 and 11.66) to the skin and superficial fascia covering the medial side of the joint. A branch runs proximally and anastomoses with the superficial part of the deep circumflex iliac and the lateral circumflex femoral arteries. Opposite or distal to the tibial condyle the saphenous artery terminates in a small cranial and a larger caudal branch.

The **cranial branch** of the saphenous artery (*r. cranialis*) (see Figs. 11.65 and 11.69) obliquely crosses the subcutaneous medial surface of the tibia in its course distocranially. It then bends around the medial border of the cranial tibial muscle and continues distally in the superficial fascia covering this muscle to traverse the flexor surface of the tarsus. Opposite the tarsus or distal to it, the cranial branch anastomoses with the superficial ramus of the cranial tibial artery. Two or three delicate rami leave the cranial branch in the crus and supply the fascia, periosteum, skin, and cranial tibial muscle. In the proximal part of the metatarsus it terminates in the three dorsal common digital arteries, which are described later in this chapter in the section titled "Arteries of the Hindpaw."

The **caudal branch** of the saphenous artery (*r. caudalis*) (Figs. 11.65, 11.70, and 11.71) is the direct continuation of the saphenous artery in the crus after the cranial branch arises. It lies medial to the tibia opposite the cleft between the medial head of the m. gastrocnemius and the bone. Distally it becomes related to the flexors of the digits, and, with its small accompanying vein and tibial nerve, it crosses the medial surface of the tarsus to enter the metatarsus. It has one prominent branch in the crus. Its distal distribution in the pes is described in the section titled "Arteries of the Hindpaw."

The **descending genicular artery** (*a. genus descendens*) (Figs. 11.64 and 11.65 to 11.67) usually arises from the femoral artery distal to the origin of the saphenous artery, but it may arise in common with it. It runs distally between the vastus medialis and the semimembranosus muscles to the medial surface of the stifle joint. In this course it sends two or more small, short branches into the m. vastus medialis. It lies at a deeper level than does the genicular branch of the saphenous artery. On reaching the medial epicondyle, it divides into articular branches. End branches supply the medial part of the femoropatellar and the medial division of the femorotibial joint capsules. The descending genicular artery is the main blood supply to the stifle joint. It is accompanied by a satellite vein.

The **middle caudal femoral artery** (*a. caudalis femoris media*) (Figs. 11.64, 11.65, and 11.67) arises from the femoral artery as the latter passes lateral to the m. semimembranosus. It runs caudodistally and ramifies in the adductor and semimembranosus muscles. It anastomoses with the distal caudal femoral artery and is accompanied by a satellite vein.

The **distal caudal femoral artery** (*a. caudalis femoris distalis*) (Figs. 11.66 and 11.67) arises from the caudolateral surface of the femoral artery approximately 1 cm proximal to the entrance of the femoral artery between the heads of the m. gastrocnemius to become the popliteal artery. Usually the distal caudal femoral artery runs caudodistally on the gastrocnemius and sends its first and largest branch laterally into the distal end of the m. biceps femoris, but this branch may come from the femoral artery directly. Most of this vessel courses proximally in the muscle, but one or more branches continue through the muscle to end as cutaneous branches to the caudolateral part of the thigh where they anastomose with cutaneous branches of the caudal branch of the deep circumflex iliac artery. Another branch enters the insertion of the m. adductor. The small artery that crosses the lateral surface of the femur to enter the m. vastus lateralis comes from either the femoral or the distal caudal femoral artery. Several branches run distally and are distributed to both heads of the gastrocnemius muscle. Approximately 2 cm from its origin, the distal caudal femoral artery crosses the lateral surface of the tibial nerve and sends a large branch proximally into the m. semimembranosus. Coming from this muscular ramus, or arising independently distal to it, is a smaller branch to the m. semitendinosus. The terminal part of the vessel becomes subcutaneous in the proximal caudal part of the crural region. The large descending branches of the distal caudal femoral artery supply the m. gastrocnemius; the large ascending branches are the chief supply to the caudal thigh muscles. Their principal anastomoses (see Fig. 11.66) are with the caudal gluteal artery, but there are also anastomoses with branches of the deep femoral and with the muscular branches of the femoral artery that reach the caudal thigh muscles. The distal caudal femoral artery is accompanied by the large proximally lying lateral saphenous vein. This receives the veins that accompany the branches of the artery. The main lymph vessels from the limb distal to the stifle ascend over the gastrocnemius in relation to this artery.

Popliteal Artery

The **popliteal artery** (*a. poplitea*) (Figs. 11.66 and 11.67) is the continuation of the femoral artery through the popliteal fossa. It begins by passing between the heads of the gastrocnemius muscle and terminates in the interosseous space between the tibia and fibula distal to their heads. It divides into the small caudal tibial and the much larger cranial tibial artery. Passing between the two heads of the gastrocnemius, it crosses the medial surface of the superficial digital flexor muscle and over the flexor surface of the stifle joint. It inclines laterally deep to the popliteus muscle and, on leaving it, perforates the origin of the m. flexor digitorum lateralis to reach the interosseous space. It is accompanied by a small satellite vein. It has small genicular and muscular branches.

A number of small genicular arteries branch from the popliteal artery as it courses caudal to the stifle joint capsule. These include a **middle genicular artery** (*a. genus media*) and **medial** and **lateral proximal**, and **distal genicular arteries** (*a. genus proximalis medialis, a. genus proximalis lateralis, a. genus distalis medialis, a. genus distalis lateralis*). They supply the joint capsule including the cruciate and collateral ligaments (Tirgari, 1978). These caudal vessels provide the largest blood supply to the stifle joint.

The **sural arteries** (*aa. surales*) are muscular branches to the muscles on the caudal aspect of the crus. These are represented by two branches to the m. gastrocnemius, which also go to the collateral ligaments and by a branch that leaves the caudal surface of the popliteal artery and runs to the caudal surface of the popliteal muscle. Before the popliteal artery terminates, it gives a branch to the small, proximal tibiofibular joint capsule, which continues beyond this to descend in the m. flexor digitorum lateralis.

The small **caudal tibial artery** (*a. tibialis caudalis*) leaves the caudal surface of the popliteal artery at the interosseous space and enters the m. flexor digitorum lateralis. It runs distally in this muscle, giving off medial and lateral branches. It supplies the **nutrient artery of the tibia** (*a. nutriciae tibiae*), which enters the nutrient foramen on the caudal surface near the lateral border at the junction of the proximal and middle thirds of the tibia.

The **cranial tibial artery** (*a. tibialis cranialis*) (Figs. 11.67 through 11.69) continues the popliteal artery between the tibia and fibula after the caudal tibial artery arises. It is larger than the caudal tibial artery and inclines laterally as it runs distally. It crosses deep to the m. fibularis longus to gain the deep surface of the long digital extensor muscle. Here it is partly separated from the bone by the small, flat m. extensor digiti I longus, which lies lateral to the artery. A **recurrent cranial tibial artery** (*a. recurrens tibialis cranialis*) supplies the stifle joint capsule. The superficially lying cranial tibial muscle and the lateral digital extensor muscle receive almost their entire blood supply from branches of the cranial tibial artery. The largest three or four muscular branches arise from the first 2 cm of the artery. The first branch runs proximally and supplies the long digital extensor muscle as it lies in the extensor groove of the tibia, and smaller branches are distributed to the stifle joint capsule. The second muscular branch runs deep to the long extensor muscle and is distributed to the cranial tibial muscle. Nutrient arteries are supplied to the tibia and fibula (*a. nutricia tibiae et fibulae*). Small anastomoses exist between the cranial tibial and the distal caudal femoral and the cranial branch of the saphenous arteries. The **superficial branch** (*ramus superficialis*) is very small in diameter, but long. It reaches the superficial crural fascia between the m. fibularis longus and the long digital extensor muscle at the beginning of the distal third of the crus. Here, it is associated with the superficial fibular nerve and sends a small branch to the lateral malleolus. The artery continues to the flexor surface of the tarsus, where it anastomoses with the cranial branch of the saphenous artery. If this does not occur, the superficial branch continues into the hindpaw as the **abaxial dorsal digital artery V** (*a. digitalis dorsalis V abaxialis*).

Arteries of the Hindpaw

The cranial tibial artery is continued opposite the talocrural joint as the **dorsal pedal artery** (*a. dorsalis pedis*) (Figs. 11.68 and 11.69). Several small branches arise from it to supply adjacent structures. The **medial and lateral tarsal arteries** (*a. tarsea medialis* and *a. tarsea lateralis*) run deeply to the sides of the tarsus and end in the collateral ligaments. The dorsal pedal artery terminates in the proximal metatarsus by forming an **arcuate artery** (*a. arcuata*) (Fig. 11.68), which runs transversely to disappear in the ligamentous tissue of the lateral and plantar sides of the proximal end of the metatarsus. It sends two or three branches proximally to be distributed to the deep structures of the flexor surface of the tarsus. Distally, the arcuate artery gives rise to **dorsal metatarsal arteries II to IV** (*aa. metatarseae*

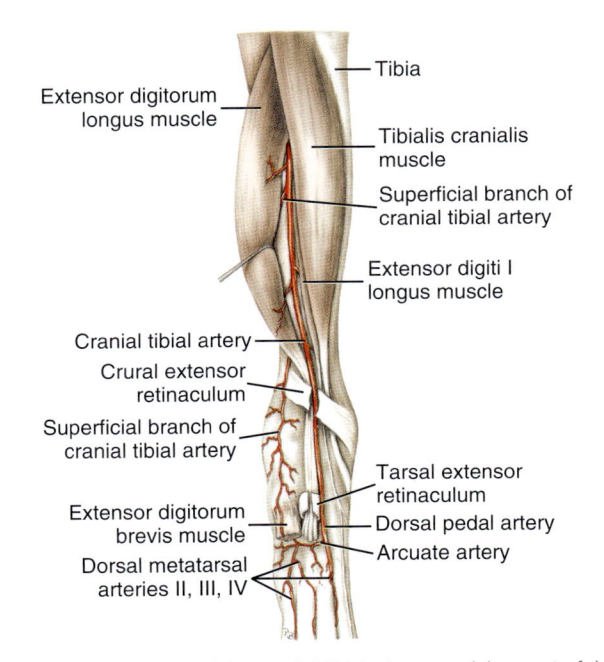

• **Fig. 11.68** Branches of the cranial tibial artery, cranial aspect of right pelvic limb.

570 CHAPTER 11 The Heart and Arteries

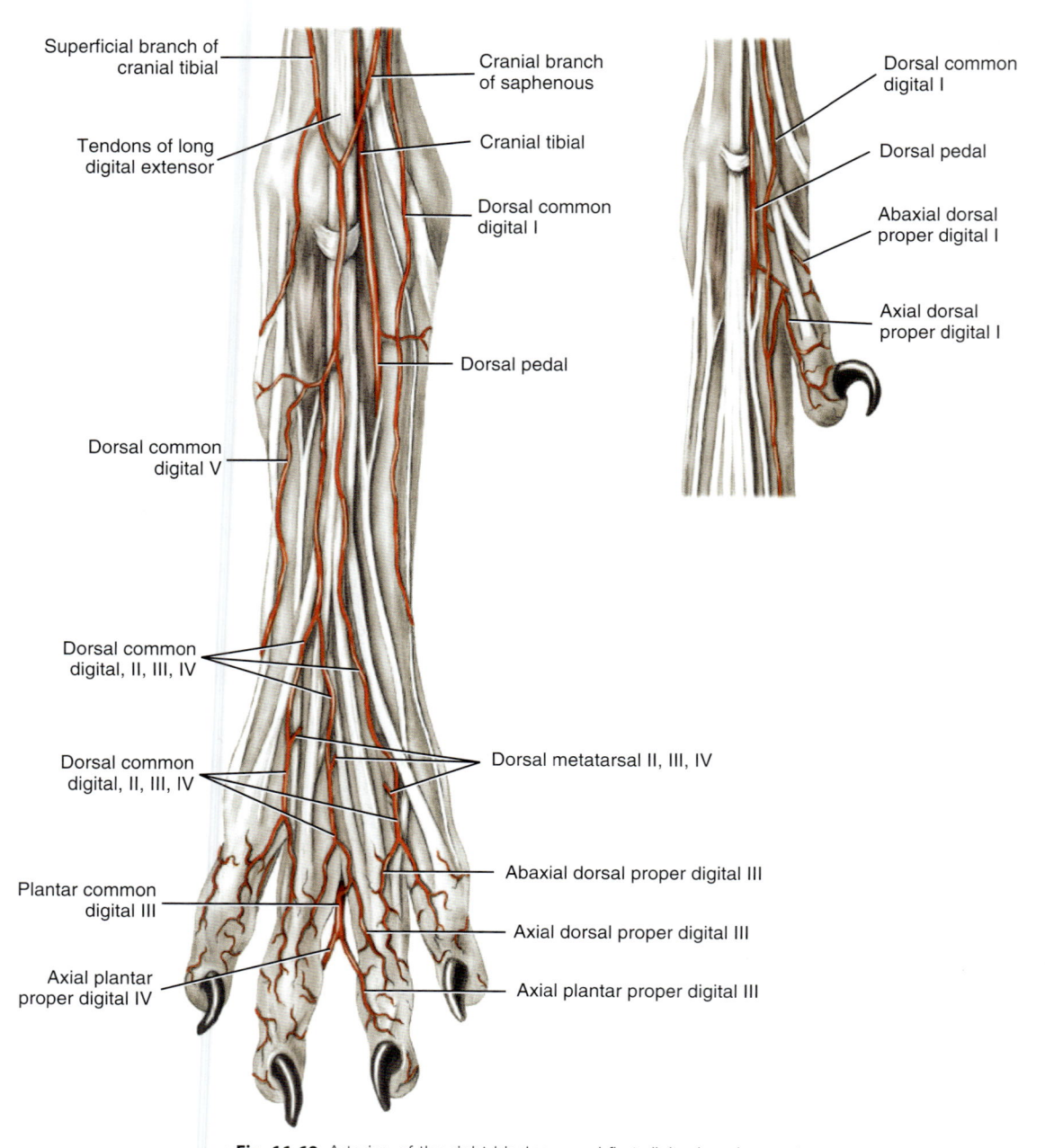

• **Fig. 11.69** Arteries of the right hindpaw and first digit, dorsal aspect.

dorsalis II to IV) (Fig. 11.64). A large **proximal perforating branch** (*ramus perforans proximalis II*) arises from **dorsal metatarsal artery II** (*a. metatarseae dorsalis II*), enters the proximal interosseous space between metatarsal II and III, and passes through it into the interosseous muscles to form the **deep plantar arterial arch** (*arcus plantaris profundus*) by joining with the **medial and lateral plantar arteries** (*aa. plantaris medialis et lateralis*) from the caudal branch of the saphenous artery as it crosses the plantar surface of the tarsus.

The arteries of the metatarsus and digits are similar to those of the metacarpus and digits. Forepaws and hindpaws are similar also in that the main arteries supplying them lie on their flexor sides. In accordance with the NAV, the superficial arteries of the metapodium are designated *aa. digitales communes*, and the deep arteries are termed *aa. metatarsea or metacarpea*. Digital arteries that originate from the bifurcation of *aa. digitales communes* are called *aa. digitales propriae*.

The **dorsal common digital arteries II, III, and IV** (*aa. digitales dorsales communes II, III, et IV*) (Fig. 11.69) arise subcutaneously, over the tendon of the long digital extensor muscle, from a small trunk formed by the anastomosis of the cranial branch of the saphenous and the superficial branch of the cranial tibial arteries. Typically this bifurcates into medial and lateral branches at the proximal end of the metatarsus. The medial branch becomes the second dorsal common digital artery, and the lateral branch divides into

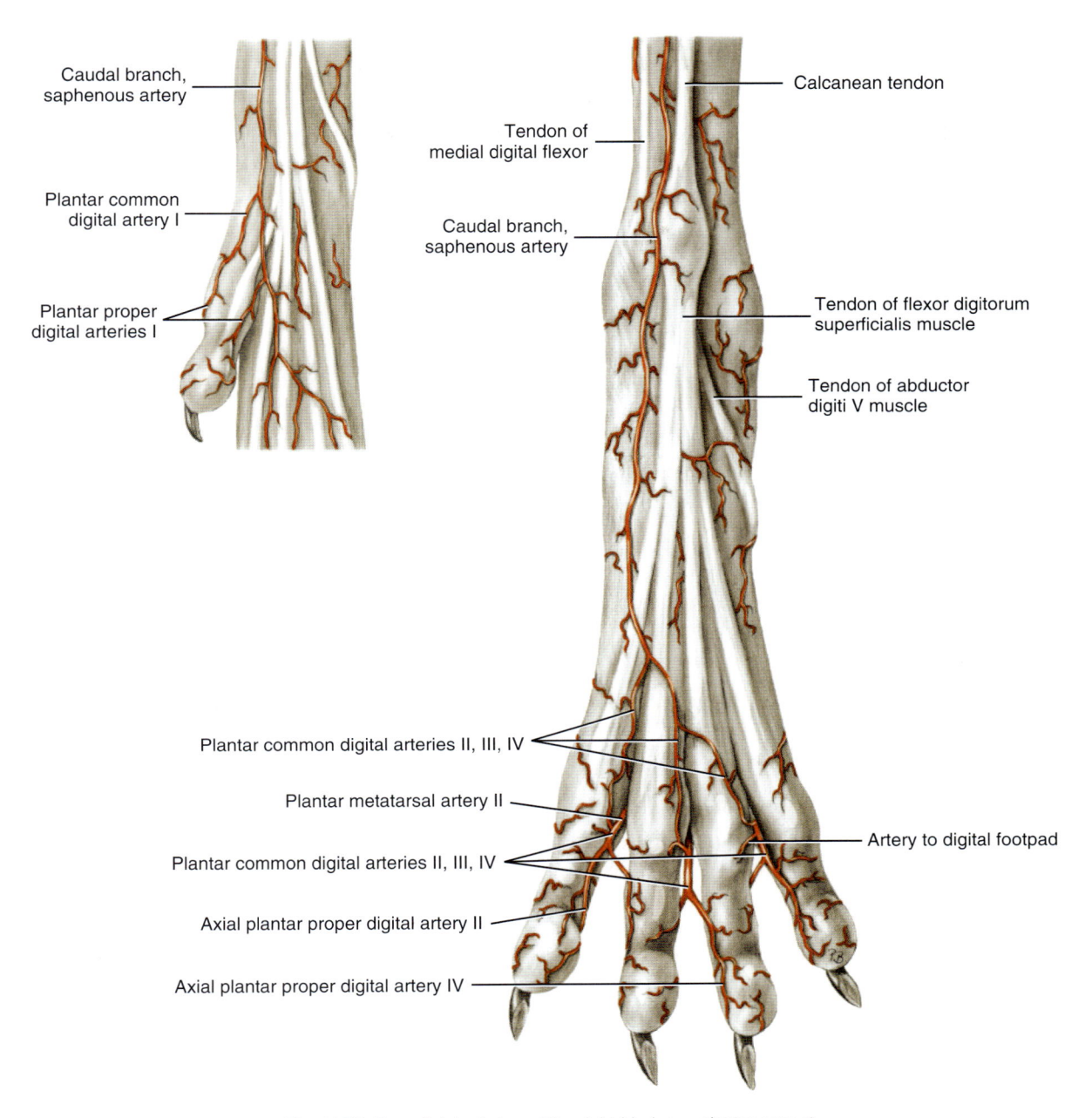

• **Fig. 11.70** Superficial arteries of the right hindpaw, plantar aspect.

the third and fourth common digital arteries. Occasionally an arch formed by the anastomoses of the medial and lateral branches gives off the superficial set. The superficial branch of the cranial tibial and the cranial branch of the saphenous arteries may continue independently to form the dorsal superficial set of arteries. When a first digit or dewclaw is present (Fig. 11.69), its dorsal part is supplied by the **abaxial and axial dorsal proper digital arteries I** (*aa. digitales dorsales propriae I*). These vessels arise from the **dorsal common digital artery I** (*a. digitalis dorsalis communis I*) that comes from the cranial branch of the saphenous artery. When the first digit is missing, as it usually is, the first dorsal common digital artery becomes dissipated on the medial part of the metatarsus. The dorsal common digital arteries II, III, and IV are joined by the dorsal metatarsal arteries in the distal ends of the intermetatarsal spaces.

The **dorsal metatarsal arteries II, III, and IV** (*aa. metatarseae dorsales*) (Figs. 11.68 and 11.69) are similar to the comparable arteries of the forepaw. (No first dorsal metatarsal artery is present, even when a first digit exists.) The dorsal metatarsal arteries II to IV arise from the arcuate artery, the terminal branch of the dorsal pedal artery in the proximal metatarsus. A **proximal perforating ramus** (*ramus perforans proximalis II*) arises from dorsal metatarsal artery II and passes between the proximal ends of the second and third metatarsal bones to contribute to the formation of the

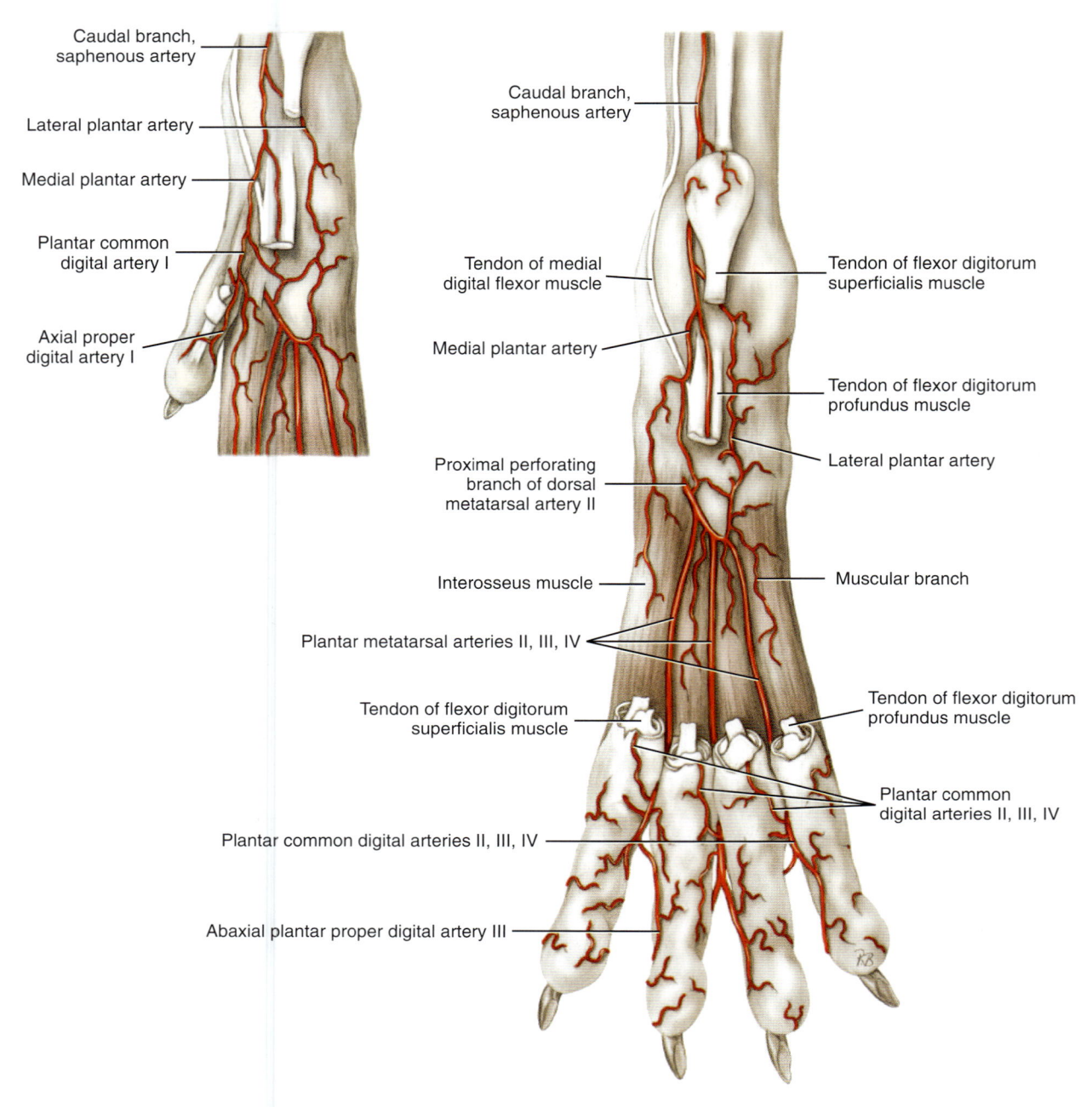

• **Fig. 11.71** Deep arteries of the right hindpaw, plantar aspect.

deep plantar arch. The three dorsal metatarsal arteries anastomose with their respective dorsal common digital arteries in the distal intermetatarsal space. Distal to this the continuing dorsal common digital arteries II, III, and IV are short vessels that give off **axial and abaxial dorsal proper digital arteries II, III, and IV** (*aa. digitales dorsales propriae II, III, et IV*). Each dorsal common digital artery, or one of its proper branches, anastomoses by a short connection deeply in the interdigital cleft with the comparable plantar common digital artery.

As the caudal branch of the saphenous artery approaches the tarsus, it gives off several **tarsal branches** (rami tarsi) to the skin and fascia of the medial side of the tarsus. Distal to the tarsal branches, it terminates in medial and lateral plantar arteries (Fig. 11.71). The **lateral plantar artery** (*a. plantaris lateralis*) runs between the superficial and deep digital flexor muscles and continues along the lateral aspect of the deep digital flexor tendon. It joins the larger **proximal perforating branch of dorsal metatarsal artery II** (*ramus perforans proximalis II*) to form the deep plantar arch. The **medial plantar artery** (*a. plantaris medialis*) terminates in a superficial and a deep branch. The small deep branch also contributes to the deep plantar arch. The larger superficial branch follows along the tendon of the superficial digital flexor muscle. In the metatarsus the superficial branch terminates in the **plantar common digital arteries**

II to IV (*aa. digitales plantares communes II to IV*). If a first digit is present, the **plantar common digital artery I** arises from the medial side of this superficial branch. In the distal intermetatarsal or proximal interdigital spaces the plantar common digital arteries anastomose with the plantar metatarsal arteries.

The **plantar metatarsal arteries II, III, and IV** (*aa. metatarseae plantares II, III, et IV*) (Fig. 11.71) arise from the deep plantar arch. Between their origins, branches arise that supply interosseous muscles. The plantar metatarsal arteries are the chief blood supply to the hindpaw distal to the tarsus. As they run distally, they lie between adjacent interosseous muscles. They anastomose with the corresponding members of the plantar common digital arteries near the distal ends of the intermetatarsal spaces or the proximal interdigital spaces. One or two small anastomotic branches extend dorsally from approximately the last centimeter of each of these arteries and anastomose with either the dorsal metatarsal arteries or the dorsal common digital arteries.

The plantar common digital arteries II, III, and IV are continued distal to these anastomoses. These and their branches are similar to the palmar common digital arteries. Branches supply the metatarsal and digital pads. The plantar common digital arteries terminate by dividing into the **axial and abaxial plantar proper digital arteries** (*aa. digitales plantares propriae*). The superficial and deep dorsal and plantar arteries of the hindpaw are accompanied by corresponding nerves. With the exception of the plantar metatarsal arteries, all are accompanied by satellite veins.

Internal Iliac Artery

The **internal iliac artery** (*a. iliaca interna*) (Figs. 11.66, 11.72, 11.73, and 11.76), with its fellow and the smaller, unpaired median sacral artery, terminate the aorta at the level of the seventh lumbar vertebra (Fig. 11.52). It is approximately half the diameter of the external iliac artery, or 2.5 mm in a medium-sized male or nongravid female. The internal iliac artery has an umbilical branch and terminates as the caudal gluteal artery and the internal pudendal artery.

The **umbilical artery** (*a. umbilicalis*)(Figs. 11.72, 11.73, and 11.76) arises from the internal iliac artery approximately 0.5 cm from its origin, but it may arise from the terminal portion of the aorta. In the fetus it carries blood to the placenta and is the main artery of the pelvis. In approximately half of the specimens, it sends one or more branches to the cranial end of the bladder as the **cranial vesical arteries** (*aa. vesicales craniales*). In the adult dog the lumen of the artery is usually obliterated distal to the origin of these arteries. The vestige of the umbilical artery that courses in the lateral ligament of the bladder forms the **round ligament of the bladder** (*lig. teres vesicae*). Ellenberger and Baum (1943) and Sisson and Grossman (1953) call the prostatic or vaginal artery (formerly urogenital artery) that supplies much of the pelvic parts of the urinary and genital systems the *umbilical artery*. Because this artery never formed a part of the vascular path from the fetus to the placenta, the term is a misnomer.

The **internal pudendal artery** (*a. pudenda interna*) (Figs. 11.72 to 11.74) is the smaller, more ventral terminal branch of the internal iliac artery, formerly referred to as the *visceral branch*. It lies in contact ventrolaterally with its satellite vein as it runs caudally on the terminal tendon of the psoas minor muscle. On reaching the origin of the m. levator ani, it gives rise to the prostatic artery in the male or the vaginal artery in the female. The prostatic and vaginal arteries were

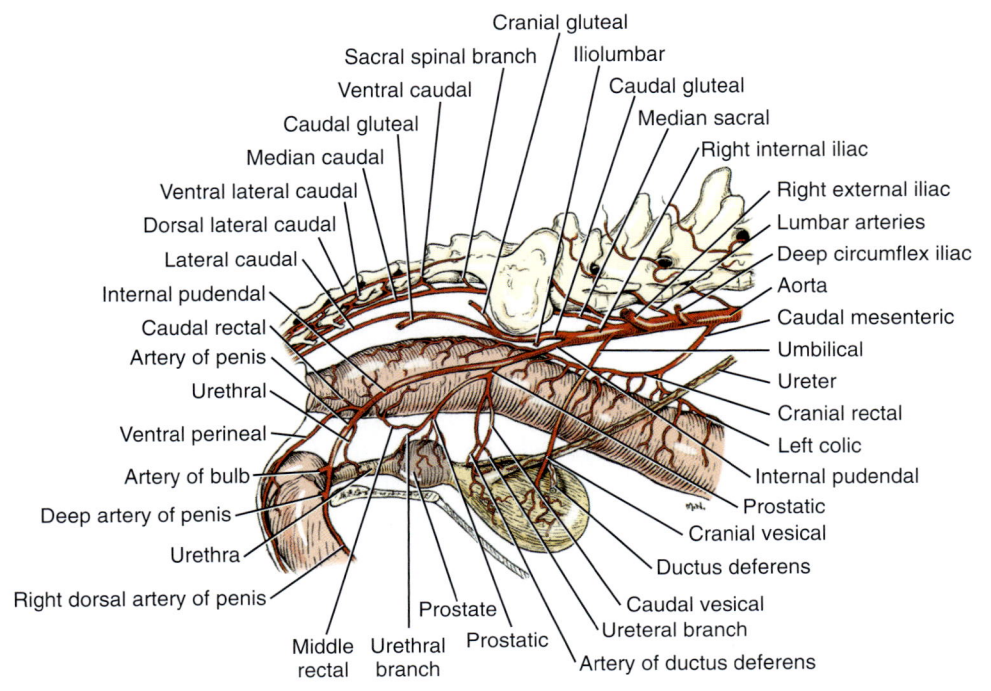

- **Fig. 11.72** Arteries of the male pelvic viscera, right lateral aspect.

574 CHAPTER 11 The Heart and Arteries

• **Fig. 11.73** Arteries of the female pelvis, right lateral aspect.

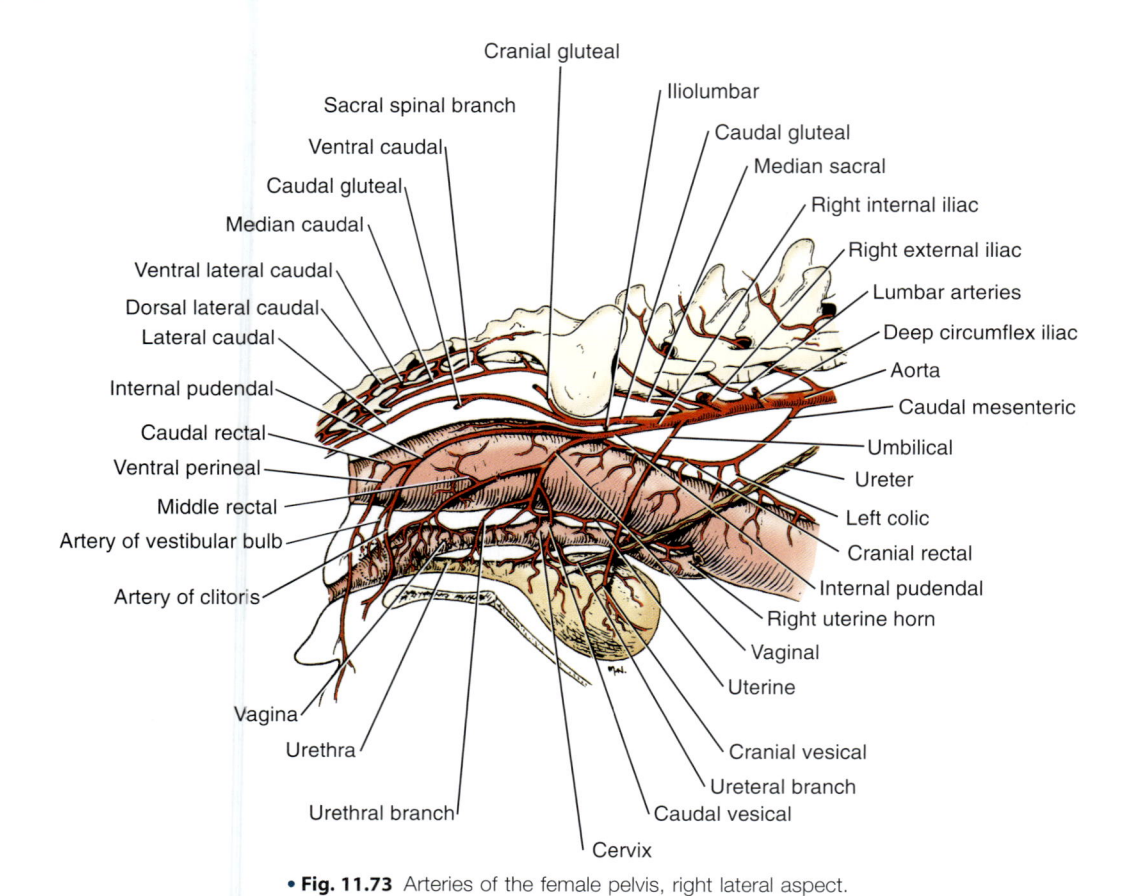

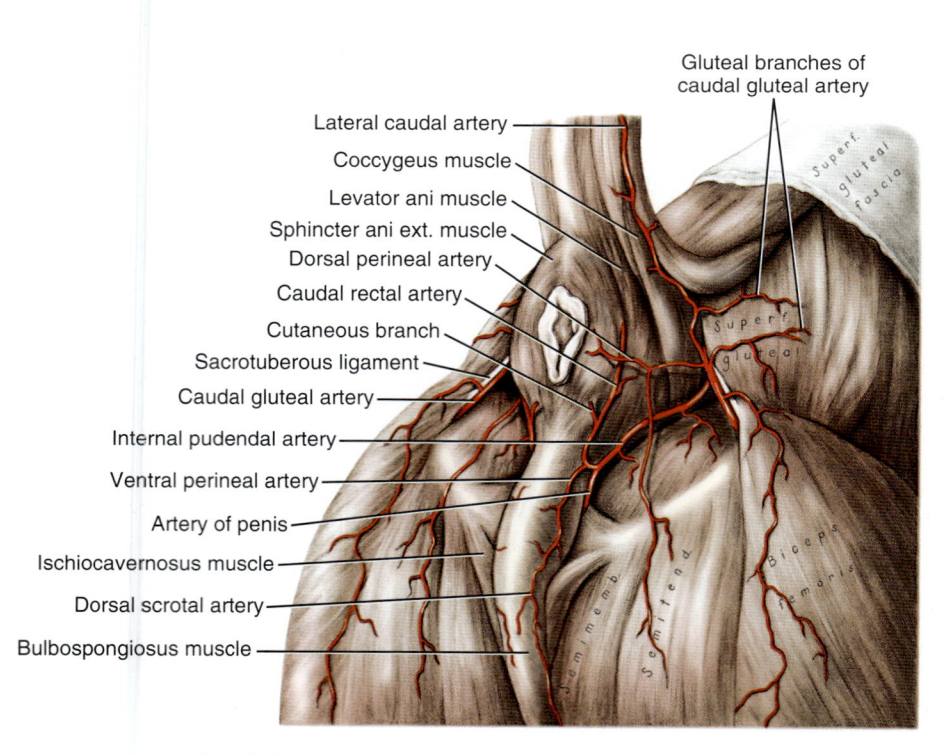

• **Fig. 11.74** Arteries of the male perineum, caudolateral aspect.

formerly known as the urogenital or urethrogenital artery. Campos et al. (1984) found that these arteries arise from the internal iliac artery 85% of the time.

The **prostatic artery** (*a. prostatica*) of the male (Fig. 11.72) is homologous with the **vaginal artery** of the female (see Fig. 11.73). It lies in the pelvic fascia with the pelvic plexus of nerves. As the prostatic artery passes ventrally across the rectum, it gives origin to the caudal vesicle artery of the bladder, with its ureteral and urethral branches, and to the artery of the ductus deferens. Before reaching the prostate gland, the prostatic artery gives rise to the middle rectal artery.

The **caudal vesical artery** (*a. vesicalis caudalis*) is a branched vessel that contacts the bladder at its neck and ramifies over its caudolateral surface. Its medial branches anastomose with their fellows both dorsally and ventrally on the organ. Cranially the caudal vesical artery may anastomose with the cranial vesical artery. If the cranial vesical artery is lacking, the paired caudal vesical artery supplies the whole organ. It is accompanied by a satellite vein and lymph vessels. Sometimes two caudal vesical arteries are present on each side.

In the male the small **artery of the ductus deferens** (*a. ductus deferentis*) is homologous with the uterine artery of the female. On reaching the ductus deferens at the point where it enters the dorsum of the prostate, it runs toward the testis and anastomoses in the epididymis with the testicular artery. It is accompanied by a satellite vein, lymphatics, and a nerve component from the pelvic plexus.

When the prostate is hypertrophied to the extent that it is an abdominal organ, the prostatic artery and related structures are carried cranially with the gland. Two or more branches pass over the lateral surface of the prostate, and others enter the parenchyma of the organ. Some of these extend through the gland to supply the prostatic portion of the pelvic urethra and the colliculus seminalis. The **urethral branches** (*rami urethrales*) are the several branches that arise from the caudal extension of the prostatic artery. The first branch supplies the caudal part of the prostate, as well as the urethra. The remaining branches arborize on the caudal part of the pelvic urethra and its surrounding urethral muscle and, bending distally around the ischial arch, enter the root of the penis to supply the penile urethra and anastomose with the artery of the bulb of the penis. The caudal portion of the prostatic artery and its branches are accompanied by satellite veins, lymphatics, and autonomic nerves.

The **middle rectal artery** (*a. rectalis media*) leaves the dorsal side of the prostatic artery in the male. Wakui et al. (1993) found the middle rectal artery to be the first branch of the prostatic artery in approximately half, and the second branch in approximately one-third of the 50 dogs they studied. In the remainder, the middle rectal artery arose from the ramifications of the prostatic artery on the surface of the prostate. The middle rectal artery arborizes on the wall of the rectum and anastomoses with the cranial and caudal rectal arteries.

The **vaginal artery** (*a. vaginalis*) of the female (Fig. 11.73) courses ventrally across the rectum and divides into two primary branches. The more cranial branch gives rise to a urethral artery, a uterine artery, vaginal branches, and a caudal vesicle artery with ureteral and urethral branches. The caudal branch of the vaginal artery gives rise to a middle rectal artery and terminates by ramifying on the vagina.

The **uterine artery** (*a. uterina*) is the main artery to the uterus in all species and has formerly been called the *middle uterine artery, caudal uterine artery* (Ellenberger & Baum, 1943), or *cervicouterine artery* (Barone & Pavaux, 1962). It is variable in size, depending on the reproductive state. The artery enters the mesometrial portion of the broad ligament at the level of the cervix and passes cranially on the lateral side of the body of the uterus. Shortly after the uterine horns diverge, the uterine artery lies 1 to 4 cm from the uterine horn in the mesometrium and sends branches onto the mesometrial surface of the uterus. Cranially the uterine artery anastomoses with uterine branches of the ovarian artery. Near the origin of the uterine artery, a branch arises that supplies the cranial end of the vagina. The uterine artery has a satellite vein and accompanying autonomic nerve plexuses and lymphatics.

The **caudal vesical artery** (*a. vesicalis caudalis*) contacts the neck of the bladder, as in the male, and ramifies over the caudolateral surface of the bladder. It has a **ureteral branch** extending cranially along the ureter and a **urethral branch** coursing caudally over the neck of the bladder.

The **middle rectal artery** (*a. rectalis media*) leaves the dorsal surface of the vaginal artery and ramifies in the wall of the rectum, where it forms anastomoses with both cranial and caudal rectal arteries.

The terminal portion of the vaginal artery arborizes in the wall of the vagina.

The internal pudendal artery continues along the dorsal border of the ischiatic spine, where it lies lateral to the coccygeus muscle and medial to the gluteal and piriform muscles. The internal pudendal artery is free of branches until it reaches the ischiorectal fossa, where it gives off urethral, ventral perineal, and caudal rectal arteries. Their origins are variable. The internal pudendal artery terminates opposite the paranal sinus or caudal to the caudal border of the m. levator ani as the artery of the penis or clitoris.

The **caudal rectal artery** (*a. rectalis caudalis*) (Figs. 11.73 and 11.74) may arise from the internal pudendal artery cranial to the ventral perineal artery. However, the two usually arise from a common trunk. The caudal rectal artery runs medially and divides into dorsal and ventral branches as it reaches the anal canal just cranioventral to the paranal sinus. In its course medially it gives off a lateral branch to this sinus. Its dorsal part lies deep to the external anal sphincter and anastomoses with the opposite artery middorsally. It sends branches to and through the external anal sphincter to supply the circumanal glands. It anastomoses in a plexiform manner with both the middle and cranial rectal arteries on the dorsal part of the anal canal. The ventral branch anastomoses with its fellow so that an arterial circle is formed around the anal opening. This is frequently plexiform in nature. In some specimens the caudal rectal artery arises as an unpaired vessel from the middle caudal artery opposite the sixth caudal vertebra.

The **ventral perineal artery** (*a. perinealis ventralis*) (Figs. 11.62, and 11.72 through 11.74) usually arises from the internal pudendal artery in common with the caudal rectal artery. It courses superficially and supplies the skin and fat at the pelvic outlet. Ventrally its deeper branches may aid in forming the arterial ring around the anus, after which it leaves the pelvic outlet and runs distally to supply the caudal part of the scrotum as the **dorsal scrotal branch** (*ramus scrotalis dorsalis*). In the female it sends a long branched vessel distally, which ends in the vulva as the **dorsal labial branch** (*r. labialis dorsalis*). The internal pudendal artery is accompanied by the pudendal nerve, and its branches have satellite veins and lymphatics.

The **artery of the penis** (*a. penis*) (Fig. 11.72) terminates the internal pudendal artery in the male (Christensen, 1954). It begins where the ventral perineal artery leaves the internal pudendal artery, or if this vessel should arise by a common trunk with the caudal rectal artery, then the origin of the trunk marks the beginning of the artery of the penis. It is approximately 2 cm long and devoid of collateral branches. It terminates at the medial aspect of the ischial arch by bifurcating or, more commonly, giving off in succession the artery of the bulb of the penis, deep artery of the penis, and the dorsal artery of the penis.

The **artery of the bulb of the penis** (*a. bulbi penis*) is a short artery that divides initially into two or three branches, which then redivide within the bulb of the penis. The penile bulb, corpus spongiosum, penile urethra, and bulbus glandis receive blood through the artery of the bulb.

The **deep artery of the penis** (*a. profunda penis*) divides into two to five branches and passes through the tunica albuginea to supply the corpus cavernosum penis and os penis.

The **dorsal artery of the penis** (*a. dorsalis penis*) runs on the dorsal surface of the body of the penis and on the dorsal surface of the os penis distally to the pars longa glandis. It anastomoses with the deep artery of the penis and the artery of the bulb of the penis. According to Christensen (1954), the artery trifurcates into deep, superficial, and preputial branches. For a discussion of the finer distribution of the arteries and veins of the penis and the mechanism of erection, refer to Chapter 9, The Urogenital System.

The **artery of the clitoris** (*a. clitoridis*) (Fig. 11.73) is homologous with the artery of the penis. It is a minute vessel that supplies the fat, erectile tissue, and integument that compose the clitoris. It is the terminal part of the internal pudendal artery. A branch, the **artery of the vestibular bulb** (*a. bulbi vestibuli*), is homologous to the artery of the bulb of the penis in the male.

The **caudal gluteal artery** (*a. glutea caudalis*) (Figs. 11.66, and 11.72 through 11.76) is the larger terminal branch of the internal iliac artery. Its proximal portion was formerly called the *parietal branch of the internal iliac artery*. The caudal gluteal artery lies ventral to the base of the sacrum caudomedial to the iliopsoas muscle and gives off an iliolumbar and cranial gluteal artery before continuing toward the ischiatic spine parallel to the internal pudendal artery. Before reaching the muscles of the hip, the caudal gluteal artery gives rise to a lateral caudal artery to the tail and a dorsal perineal artery to the anus.

The **iliolumbar artery** (*a. iliolumbalis*) (Figs. 11.66, 11.75, and 11.76), less than 1 mm in diameter, leaves the

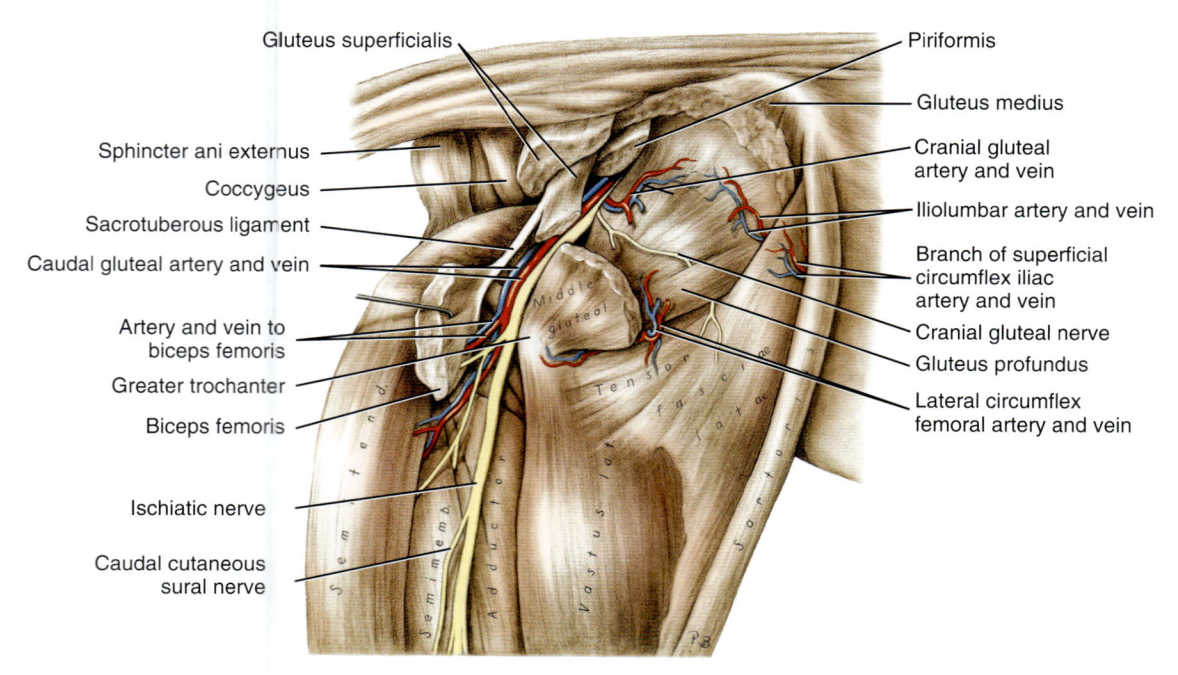

• **Fig. 11.75** Arteries and veins of the gluteal region, lateral aspect.

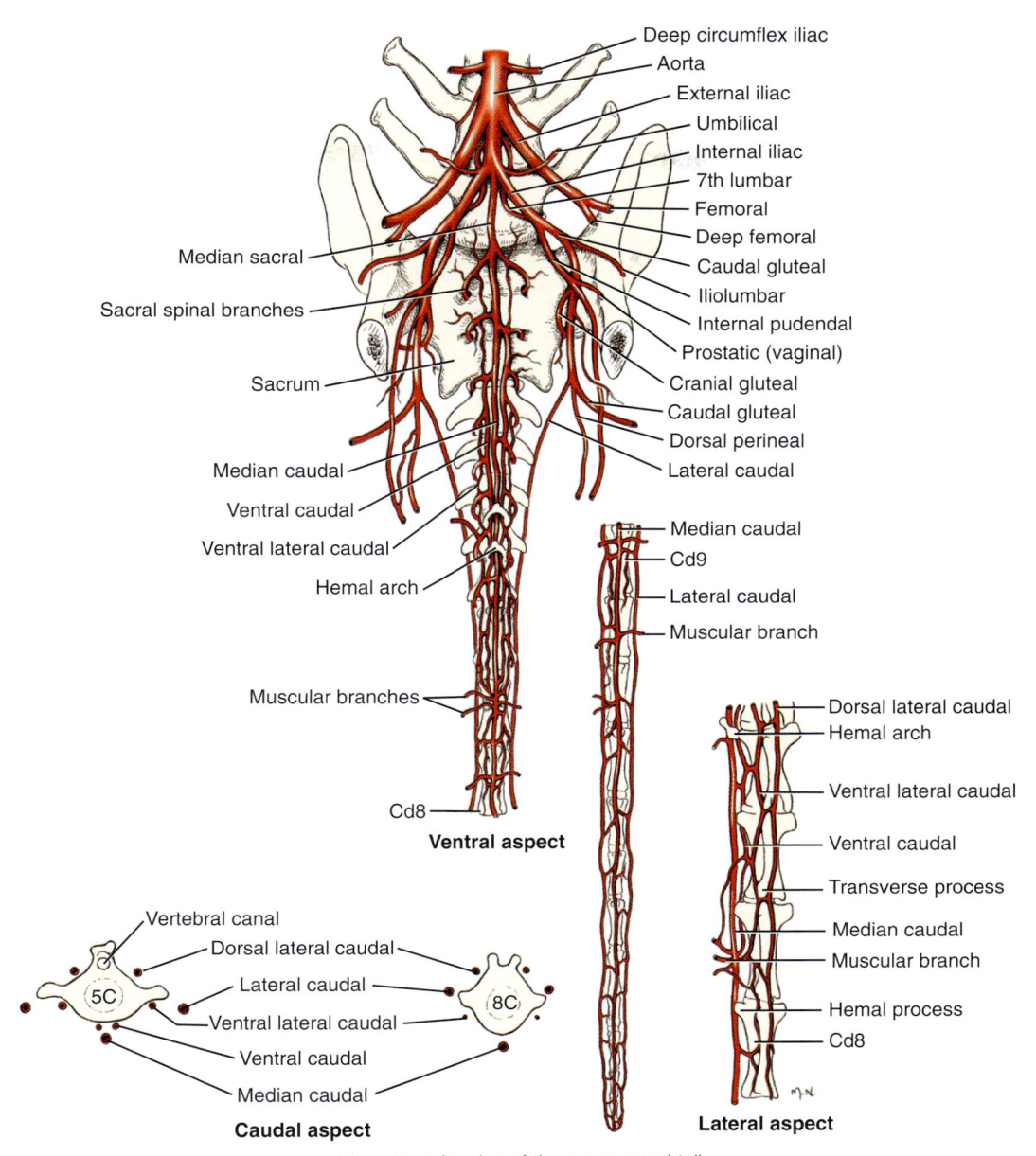

• **Fig. 11.76** Arteries of the sacrum and tail.

pelvic cavity between the iliopsoas muscle and the base of the sacrum. It arises from the caudal gluteal artery or from the internal iliac artery directly. A small branch leaves its caudal side to run with the lumbosacral plexus of nerves. As it crosses the cranioventral border of the ilium, it sends the **nutrient artery of the ilium** caudoventrally to enter the nutrient foramen. The main part of the vessel crosses the cranioventral border of the wing of the ilium at the alar spine and enters the craniolateral muscles of the pelvis and thigh. Branches are supplied to the m. iliopsoas and m. quadratus lumborum as they cross the artery. The principal branches go to the proximal parts of the middle gluteal muscle, and other branches supply the abdominal wall. The iliolumbar artery anastomoses caudally with the cranial gluteal and cranially with the superficial circumflex iliac arteries. It is accompanied by a small satellite vein.

The **cranial gluteal artery** (*a. glutea cranialis*) (Figs. 11.66, 11.75, and 11.76), approximately 1.5 mm in diameter, runs dorsocaudally from its caudal gluteal artery origin across the lateral surface of the lumbosacral trunk and enters the overlying middle gluteal muscle after passing over the cranial part of the greater ischiatic incisure near the caudal dorsal iliac spine. On reaching the deep surface of the middle gluteal muscle, it divides. A small branch extends dorsally between the middle gluteal and the piriformis muscles, both of which it supplies, and becomes superficial at the sacrocaudal junction. The main part of the vessel, with the cranial gluteal nerve and a satellite vein, runs craniolaterally between the deep and middle gluteal muscles. It is the main supply to the middle gluteal muscle and anastomoses with the iliolumbar artery, which enters the muscle cranially. It also anastomoses with the lateral circumflex femoral artery, which enters the middle gluteal muscle after crossing the cranial surface of the hip joint.

The **lateral caudal artery** (*a. caudalis lateralis*) (Figs. 11.72 through 11.74, and 11.76) leaves the caudal gluteal artery approximately 4 cm caudal to the origin of the cranial gluteal artery. It leaves the pelvis by passing caudodorsally between the tail and the superficial gluteal muscle. A cutaneous branch arises at this level and, curving around the sacrotuberous ligament and superficial gluteal muscle, enters the superficial gluteal fascia. It supplies the skin and fascia of the pelvis as far cranial as the crest of the ilium. Branches leave both the dorsal and the ventral surface of the lateral caudal vessel at irregular intervals and supply the skin and adjacent fascia of the tail. At approximately the sixth caudal vertebra, it inclines dorsally and, lying on the deep caudal fascia dorsal to the transverse processes, runs to the end of the tail. In the distal two-thirds of the tail it sends many branches to the skin and muscles along its dorsolateral aspect. Other branches run across the intervertebral discs and anastomose with the median caudal artery; shorter branches run deeply to anastomose with the deep lateral caudal arteries. Arteriovenous anastomoses exist in the caudal third of the tail. The large satellite vein lies ventral to the lateral caudal artery.

The **dorsal perineal artery** (*a. perinealis dorsalis*) (Figs. 11.74 and 11.76) is a long cutaneous branch that originates from the ventral surface of the caudal gluteal artery. It leaves the pelvic outlet at the ischiorectal fossa to course toward the root of the penis in the fat of the pelvic outlet. It supplies the external anal sphincter and fat and skin that cover the dorsal part of the caudal surface of the thigh and perineum. It may anastomose with the ventral perineal artery or may replace it functionally.

The continuation of the caudal gluteal artery distal to the origin of the lateral caudal artery passes toward the tuber ischii in relation to the sacrotuberous ligament caudolaterally, the ischiatic nerve cranioventrally, and its satellite vein medially. It gives a muscular branch to the superficial gluteal muscle, and sends branches to the m. piriformis, m. obturatorius internus, and m. gluteus medius. It anastomoses with the cranial gluteal artery in the m. gluteus medius. The main caudal gluteal artery passes over the greater ischiatic notch and lateral to the origin of the coccygeus muscle from the ischiatic spine along with the ischiatic nerve and satellite vein, and divides into several branches as it enters the biceps femoris muscle. One branch enters the proximal end of the m. semitendinosus, and another enters the m. semimembranosus. The **satellite artery of the ischiatic nerve** (*a. comitans n. ischiadicus*), a branch of the caudal gluteal artery, joins the nerve caudal to the trochanter major and runs distally with it. The quadratus femoris, obturator internus, and gemelli muscles may also receive branches from the proximal part of the artery. The caudal gluteal artery is the main supply to the biceps femoris and semitendinosus muscles, although an extensive anastomosis with the distal caudal femoral and deep femoral arteries exists within these muscles.

Chambers et al. (1989) studied the vascular patterns of 15 pelvic limb muscles to identify those most suitable for transposition in the treatment of large wound closures. The best-suited muscles for transfer in the dog were the cranial part of the m. sartorius, supplied by the superficial circumflex iliac artery; the m. gracilis, supplied by the proximal caudal femoral artery; the m. semitendinosus, vascularized by the caudal gluteal artery proximally and the distal caudal femoral artery distally; and the m. rectus femoris, which was unique among the quadriceps group because it did not share its lateral circumflex femoral artery with any other muscle. The authors classified the muscles by vascular pattern and illustrate the patterns with angiographs.

Median Sacral Artery

The **median sacral artery** (*a. sacralis mediana*) (Figs. 11.66, 11.72, 11.73, and 11.76) is the direct continuation of the aorta caudally, after the internal iliac arteries arise. It usually arises opposite the body of the seventh lumbar vertebra as an unpaired median vessel that is slightly less than 2 mm in diameter. It crosses ventral to the promontory of the sacrum with its dextrally lying satellite vein and enters the fat-filled furrow between the right and left medial ventral sacrocaudal muscles. In this region it usually gives off two pairs of **sacral branches** (*rami sacrales*), which enter the ventral sacral foramina. Arising from these sacral branches are branches to the adjacent ventral sacrocaudal muscles. Within the sacral vertebral canal a **spinal branch** (*ramus spinalis*) joins the ventral spinal artery and a **dorsal branch** (*ramus dorsalis*) passes through the dorsal sacral foramen to supply the adjacent epaxial muscles.

Variations of the arteries to the tail are numerous. Typically, there are seven longitudinal arterial trunks in the proximal third of the tail as follows: one (unpaired) median caudal artery, two (paired) lateral caudal arteries, two (paired) dorsal lateral caudal arteries, and two (paired) ventrolateral caudal arteries.

The **median caudal artery** (*a. caudalis mediana*) is a direct continuation caudally of the median sacral artery at the first caudal vertebra. It runs midventrally on the caudal vertebrae, where it lies between the right and left medial ventral sacrocaudal muscles. It passes through the fourth, fifth, and sixth (if present) hemal arches, and then between the successive hemal processes. Throughout most of its course, segmental arteries that run caudolaterally arise opposite the bodies of the vertebrae. They pass ventral to the transverse processes of the corresponding vertebra and give small branches to the adjacent structures. At irregular intervals, usually the length of two or three segments, there are ventral branches that supply the skin. Other branches successively leave the median caudal artery from alternate sides, starting at the eighth caudal vertebra, each anastomosing with the lateral caudal artery of the same side. Only the two lateral caudal arteries and the median caudal artery reach the end of the tail, where they anastomose. They lose their segmental character in the last few segments and anastomose with each other in a plexiform manner. The right and left ventral caudal arteries may be the first branches to leave the median caudal.

The paired **ventral caudal artery** (*a. caudalis ventralis*) (Fig. 11.76), if present, arises asymmetrically with its fellow as the first branches of the median caudal or the last branches of the median sacral artery. They may be important collateral branches that give rise to the segmental arteries that supply the vertebrae and surrounding soft tissue. Typically, they rejoin the median caudal artery beyond the pelvic outlet after passing through or around the hemal arches.

Delicate bilateral or unilateral longitudinal arterial connections may exist caudal to the pelvic outlet, extending over three to five segments. These closely resemble the ventral caudal arteries that are located cranial to them.

More constant are the paired **dorsal** and **ventral lateral caudal arteries** (*aa. caudales dorsolaterales et ventrolaterales*). Less than 1 mm in diameter, these vessels are joined by the segmental arteries at each caudal vertebra. The segmental arteries, on reaching the transverse processes, bifurcate into dorsal and ventral branches. The resultant ventral branches arch medially and anastomose with the next segmental arteries caudal to them. In this way a small segmental arterial channel is formed, which consists of a series of lateral arches lying ventral to the transverse processes. Collectively this segmental arterial passage is known as the *ventrolateral caudal artery*. It ends at approximately the eighth caudal vertebra. The dorsal branches pass directly dorsally on the lateral surfaces of the intervertebral discs and anastomose at right angles with the dorsolateral caudal artery. This artery begins as a continuation caudally of the last sacral segmental artery. This longitudinal arterial channel is straighter than the ventrolateral caudal artery but, like it, is joined by all the caudal segmental arteries of its side. It passes deep to the dorsal caudal musculature and lies ventral to the articular processes. Each sends branches at every three to six segments into the skin and more numerous and irregular branches into the dorsal tail musculature. As the muscles and vertebrae decrease in size toward the end of the tail, the dorsolateral caudal artery decreases in size also, so that it can no longer be followed caudal to the ninth caudal vertebra. The dorsal and ventral lateral caudal arteries are accompanied by the dorsal and ventral caudal nerve trunks. The only recognizable veins from the tail are the right and left lateral caudal veins.

Located along the tail may be small arteriovenous anastomoses called *corpora caudalia*.

Bibliography

Abramson, D. I. (1976). *Circulation in the extremities*. New York: Academic Press.

Abramson, D. I., & Margolin, S. (1936). A Purkinje conduction network in the myocardium of the mammalian ventricles. *J Anat, 70*, 250–259.

Alves, J. R., Wafae, N., Beu, C. C., et al. (2008). Morphometric study of the tricuspid valve in dogs. *Anat Hist Embry, 37*(6), 427–429.

Anderson, W. D., & Kubicek, W. (1971). The vertebral-basilar system of dog in relation to man and other mammals. *Am J Anat, 132*, 179–188.

Baerg, R. D., & Bassett, D. L. (1963). Permanent gross demonstration of the conduction tissue in the dog heart with palladium iodide. *Anat Rec, 146*, 313–317.

Baird, J. A., & Robb, J. S. (1950). Study, reconstruction and gross dissection of the atrioventricular conducting system of the dog heart. *Anat Rec, 108*, 747–763.

Barone, R., & Pavaux, C. (1962). Les vaisseaux sanguins du tractus génital chez les femelles domestiques. *Bull Soc Sc Vet Lyon, 64*, 33–51.

Bellenger, C. R., Hopwood, P. R., & Rothwell, J. T. (1993). Colorectal blood supply in dogs. *Am J Vet Res, 54*(11), 1948–1953.

Berry, J. L., Brailsford, J. F., & de Burgh Daly, I. (1931). The bronchial vascular system in the dog. *Proc R Soc London Series B, 109*, 214–228.

Boling, L. R. (1942). Blood vessels to the dental pulp. *Anat Rec, 82*, 25–34.

Borley, N. R., McFarlane, J. M., & Ellis, H. (1995). A comparative study of the tortuosity of the splenic artery. *Clin Anat, 8*(3), 219–221.

Boucek, R. J., Takashita, R., & Fojaco, R. (1964). Functional anatomy of the ascending aorta and the coronary ostia (dog). *Am J Anat, 114*, 273–282.

Brunner, K., & Frewein, J. (1989). Untersuchungen der vaskularisation der disci intervertebrales des erwachsenen hundes. *Zbl Vet Met C Anat Histol Embryol, 18*, 76–86.

Buchanan, J. W. (1972). Radiographic aspects of patent ductus arteriosus in dogs before and after surgery. *Acta Radiol Suppl, 319*, 271–278.

Cadete-Leite, A. (1973). The arteries of the pancreas of the dog. An injection corrosion and microangiographic study. *Am J Anat, 137*, 151–157.

Campos, V. J. M., Pinto Silva, P., & Mello Dias, S. (1984). Contribution a l'étude de artere urogenital du chien adulte. *Anat Anz, 155*, 31–37.

Catcott, E. J. (1952). Ophthalmoscopy in canine practice. *J Am Vet Med Assoc, 121*, 35–37.

Chambers, J. N., Purinton, P. T., Allen, S. W., et al. (1989). Identification and anatomic categorization of the vascular patterns to the pelvic limb muscles of dogs. *Am J Vet Res, 51*, 305–313.

Chevalier, P. A. (1976). *The heart and circulation*. Stroudsburg, PA: Dowden, Hutchinger and Ross.

Christensen, G. C. (1952). Circulation of blood through the canine kidney. *Am J Vet Res, 13*, 236–245.

Christensen, G. C. (1954). Angioarchitecture of the canine penis and the process of erection. *Am J Anat, 95*, 227–262.

Christensen, G. C. (1962). The blood supply to the interventricular septum of the heart—a comparative study. *Am J Vet Res, 23*, 869–874.

Christensen, G. C., & Campeti, F. L. (1959). Anatomic and functional studies of the coronary circulation in the dog and pig. *Am J Vet Res, 20*, 18–26.

Christensen, G. C., & Toussaint, S. (1957). Vasculature of external nares and related areas in the dog. *J Am Vet Med Assoc, 131*, 504–509.

Cliff, W. J. (1976). *Blood vessels*. London: Cambridge University Press.

Constantinescu, G. M., & Schaller, O. (2012). *Illustrated veterinary anatomical nomenclature* (3rd ed.). Stuttgart: Enke Verlag.

Crock, H. V., & Goldwasser, M. (1984). Anatomic studies of the circulation in the region of the vertebral end-plate in adult Greyhound dogs. *Spine, 9*, 702–706.

Cuthbertson, E. M., & Gilfillan, R. S. (1964). Variations in the anatomic origin of the nutrient artery of the canine femur. *Anat Rec, 148*, 547–552.

Dabanoglu, I. (2007). Normal morphometry of the thoracic aorta in the German shepherd dog: a computed tomographic study. *Anat Hist Embry, 36*(3), 163–167.

Daigo, M., Morita, S., & Kagami, A. (1964a). Stereoroentgenographic and topographical studies on the anatomy of peripheral blood vessels in domestic animals and domestic fowls. 10. Palmar arteries in the dog. *Bull Nippon Vet Zootec Coll, 13*, 63–80.

Daigo, M., Morita, S., & Kagami, A. (1964b). Stereoroentgenographic and topographical studies on the anatomy of peripheral blood vessels in domestic animals and domestic fowls. 11. Dorsal arteries of the hand in the dog. *Bult Nippon Vet Zootech Coll, 13*, 81–95.

Davis, D. D. (1941). The arteries of the forearm in carnivores. *Zool Series Field Museum of Natural History, 27*, 137–227.

Davis, D. D., & Story, H. H. E. (1943). The carotid circulation in the domestic cat. *Zool Series Field Museum of Natural History, 28*, 3–47.

Dias, S. M., Orsi, A. M., Oliveira, M. C., et al. (1979). Sur la morphologie de la fosse ovale du coeur chez le chien adulte (Canis familiaris). *Anat Hist Embryol, 8*, 168–171.

Donald, D. E., & Essex, H. E. (1954). Pressure studies after inactivation of the major portion of the canine right ventricle. *Am J Physiol, 176*, 155–161.

Eisberg, H. B. (1924). Intestinal arteries. *Anat Rec, 28*, 227–242.

Ellenberger, W., & Baum, H. (1943). *Handbuch der vergleichenden anatomie der haustiere* (18th ed.). Berlin: Springer.

Ellison, G. W. (1980). Vascular ring anomalies in the dog and cat. *Compend Contin Ed, 2*, 693–706.

Esperanca-Pina, J. A., Correia, M., O'Neill, J. G., et al. (1981). Morphology of the veins draining the coronary sinus of the dog. *Acta Anat, 109*, 122–128.

Esperanca-Pina, J. A., & Reis, A. M. (1984). Arterial component of the angioarchitecture of the canine ovary. *Acta Anat, 120*, 112.

Everett, N. B., & Johnson, R. J. (1951). A physiological and anatomical study of the closure of the ductus arteriosus in the dog. *Anat Rec, 110*, 103–111.

Fahie, M. A., Smith, B. J., Ballard, J. B., et al. (1998). Regional peripheral vascular supply based on the superficial temporal artery in dogs and cats. *Anat Hist Embry, 27*(3), 205–208.

Flint, J. M. (1900). The blood-vessels, angiogenesis, organogenesis, reticulum, and histology, of the adrenal. In *Contribution to the science of medicine*. Baltimore MD: The Johns Hopkins Press.

Gasse, H., Godynicki, S., Engelke, E., et al. (1999). The course of blood vessels in the hip joint capsule of the dog. *Ann Anat Anz, 181*(6), 577–579.

Grävenstein, H. (1938). Über die arterien des grossen netzes beim hunde. *Morph Jahrb, 82*, 1–26.

Green, J. A. (1983). Surgical correction of persistent right aortic arch. In M. J. Bojrab (Ed.), *Current techniques in small animal surgery* (2nd ed.). Philadelphia: Lea & Febiger.

Halpern, M. H. (1955). Blood supply to the atrioventricular system of the dog. *Anat Rec, 121*, 753–762.

Helphrey, M. L. (1979). Vascular ring anomalies in the dog. *Vet Clin North Am, 9*, 207–218.

Herrmann, G. R. (1925). Experimental heart disease; I. methods of dividing hearts, with sectional and proportional weights and ratios for two hundred normal dogs' hearts. *Am Heart J, 1*, 213–231.

Higginbotham, F. H. (1966). Ventricular coronary arteries of beagles. *J Atheroscler Res (Amst), 5*, 474–488.

House, E. W., & Ederstrom, H. E. (1968). Anatomical changes with age in the heart and ductus arteriosus in the dog after birth. *Anat Rec, 160*, 289–295.

Hughes, H. V., & Dransfield, J. W. (1959). Blood supply to the skin of the dog. *Br Vet J, 115*, 299–310.

Hyde, D. M., & Buss, D. D. (1986). Morphometry of the coronary microvasculature of the canine left ventricle. *Am J Anat, 177*, 415–425.

Irifune, M. (1980). The facial artery of the dog. *Okajimas Folia Anat Jpn, 57*, 55–78.

Jarvis, J. F., & Nell, A. M. H. (1963). The brachiocephalic artery in the dog with special reference to the arterial supply of the esophagus. *Anat Rec, 145*, 1–5.

Jewell, P. A. (1952). Anastomoses between internal and external carotid circulation in the dog. *J Anat, 86*, 83–94.

Joranson, Y., Emmel, V. E., & Pilka, H. J. (1929). Factors controlling the arterial supply of the testis under experimental conditions. *Anat Rec, 41*, 157–176.

Kazzaz, D., & Shanklin, W. M. (1950). The coronary vessels of the dog demonstrated by colored plastic (vinyl acetate) injection and corrosion. *Anat Rec, 107*, 43–59.

Kennedy, H. N., & Smith, A. W. (1930). An abnormal celiac artery in the dog. *Vet Rec (London)*, 751.

Krediet, P.: *Anomalies of the arterial trunks in the thorax and their relation to normal development*. Thesis, Utrecht, 1962.

Langer, G. A., & Brady, A. J. (1974). *The mammalian myocardium*. New York: John Wiley & Sons.

Latimer, H. B. (1961). Weights of the ventricular walls of the heart in the adult dog. *University Kansas Sci Bull, XLII*, 3–11.

Ljubomudrov, A. P. (1939). The blood supply of the suprarenal glands in the dog. *Arkhiv Anat Grist i Embryol, 20*, 220–224, (English summary 381–382).

Maric, I., Bobinac, D., Ostojic, L., et al. (1996). Tributaries of the human and canine coronary sinus. *Acta Anat (Basel), 156*(1), 61–69.

Marthen, G. (1939). Über die arterien der korpenvand des hundes. *Morph Jahrb, 84*, 187–219.

Meek, W. J., Keenan, M., & Theisen, H. J. (1929). The auricular blood supply in the dog: i. General auricular supply with special reference to the sinoauricular node. *Am Heart J, 4*, 591–599.

Miller, M. E. (1952). *Guide to the dissection of the dog* (3rd ed.). Ithaca, NY: Published by author.

Mitsuoka, T., Pelleg, A., Michelson, E. L., et al. (1987). Canine AV nodal artery: anatomical variations and a detailed description of cannulation technique. *Am J Physiol, 22*, 968–973.

Moore, R. A. (1930). The coronary arteries of the dog. *Am Heart J, 5*, 743–749.

Noer, R. (1943). The blood vessels of the jejunum and ileum: a comparative study of man and certain laboratory animals. *Am J Anat, 73*, 293–334.

Noestelthaller, A., Probst, A., & Koenig, H. E. (2005). Use of corrosion casting techniques to evaluate coronary collateral vessels and anastomoses in hearts of canine cadavers. *Am J Vet Res, 66*(10), 1724–1728.

Noestelthaller, A., Probst, A., & König, H. E. (2007). Branching patterns of the left main coronary artery in the dog demonstrated by the use of corrosion casting technique. *Anat Hist Embry, 36*(1), 33–37.

Nonidez, J. F. (1943). The structure and innervation of the conductive system of the heart of the dog and rhesus monkey as seen with a silver impregnation technique. *Am Heart J, 26*, 577–597.

Northup, D. W., Van Liere, E. J., & Stickney, J. C. (1957). The effect of age, sex, and body size on the heart weight-body weight ratio in the dog. *Anat Rec, 128*, 411–417.

Orsi, A. M., Stefanini, M. A., Crocci, A. J., et al. (2004). Some segmental features on the structure of the aortic wall of the dog. *Anat Hist Embry, 33*(3), 131–134.

Parouti, J. P.: *Contribution a l'etude de la vascularization interne du femur du chien*. DVM Thesis, Toulouse, 1962.

Pauza, D. H., Skripka, V., & Pauziene, N. (2002). Morphology of the intrinsic cardiac nervous system in the dog: a whole-mount study employing histochemical staining with acetylcholinesterase. *Cell Tiss Org, 172*, 297–320. doi:10.1159/000067198.

Pauza, D. H., Skripka, V., Pauziene, N., et al. (1999). Anatomical study of the neural ganglionated plexus in the canine right atrium: implications for selective denervation and electrophysiology of the sinoatrial node in dog. *Anat Rec, 255*, 271–294.

Peirce, E. C. (1944). Renal lymphatics. *Anat Rec, 90*, 315–335.

Pianetto, M. B. (1939). The coronary arteries of the dog. *Am Heart J, 18*, 403–410.

Piffer, C. R., Piffer, M. I. S., Santi, F. P., et al. (1994). Anatomic observations of the coronary sinus in the dog (canis familiaris). *Anat Hist Embry, 23*(4), 301–308.

Pina, J. A. E., Correia, M., & O'Neill, J. G. (1975). Morphological study on the thebesian veins of the right cavities of the heart in the dog. *Acta Anat, 92*, 310–320.

Preuss, F. (1959). Die a. vaginalis der haussäugetiere. *Tierärzt Wchnschr, 72*, 403–416.

Prichard, M. M. L., & Daniel, P. M. (1953). Arteriovenous anastomoses in the tongue of the dog. *J Anat, 87*, 66–74.

Racker, D. K. (1989). Atrioventricular node and input pathways: a correlated gross anatomical and histological study of the canine atrioventricular junctional region. *Anat Rec, 224*, 336–354.

Reichert, F. L. (1924). An experimental study of the anastomotic circulation in the dog. *Bull Johns Hopkins Hosp, 35*, 385–390.

Reis, R. H., & Tepe, P. (1956). Variations in the pattern of renal vessels and their relation to the type of posterior vena cava in the dog (*Canis familiaris*). *Am J Anat, 99*, 1–15.

Ruiz-Pesini, P., Tomé, E., Balaguer, L., et al. (1995). The localization of neurons innervating the carotid sinus in the dog. *J Auton Nev Syst, 50*(3), 291–297.

Sandusky, G. E., Kerr, K. M., & Capen, C. C. (1979). Morphologic variations and aging in the atrioventricular conduction system of large breed dogs. *Anat Rec, 193*, 883–902.

Schmidt, S., Lohse, C. L., & Suter, P. F. (1980). Branching patterns of the hepatic artery in the dog: arteriographic and anatomic study. *Am J Vet Res, 41*, 1090–1097.

Schneider, H. P., Truex, R. C., & Knowles, J. O. (1964). Comparative observations of the hearts of mongrel and greyhound dogs. *Anat Rec, 149*, 173–180.

Schoning, P., Erickson, H., & Milliken, G. A. (1995). Body weight, heart weight, and heart to body weight ratio in greyhounds. *Am J Vet Res, 56*(4), 420–422.

Sisson, S., & Grossman, J. D. (1953). *Anatomy of the domestic animals* (4th ed.). Philadelphia: Saunders.

Sleeper, M. M., & Buchanan, J. W. (2001). Vertebral scale system to measure heart size in growing puppies. *J Am Vet Med Ass, 219*, 57–59.

Smith, R. B. (1971). Intrinsic innervation of the atrioventricular and semilunar valves in various mammals. *J Anat, 108*, 115–121.

Tanaka, A., Mori, H., Tanaka, E., et al. (1999). Branching patterns of intramural coronary vessels determined by microangiography using synchotron radiation. *Am J Physiol, 276*, H2262–H2267.

Tandler, J. (1899). Zur vergleichenden anatomie der kopfarterien bei den mammalia. *Denkschr Akad Wiss Wien Math-Natunviss Kl, 67*, 677–784.

Tanuma, K. (1981). A morphological study on the Circle of Willis in the dog. *Okajimas Folia Anat Jpn, 58*, 155–176.

Thomas, C. E. (1957). The muscular architecture of the ventricles of hog and dog hearts. *Am J Anat, 101*, 17–58.

Tirgari, M. (1978). The surgical significance of the blood supply of the canine stifle joint. *J Small Anim Pract, 19*, 451–462.

Truex, R. C., & Angulo, A. W. (1952). Comparative study of the arterial and venous systems of the ventricular myocardium with special reference to the coronary sinus. *Anat Rec, 113*, 467–492.

Truex, R. C., & Warshaw, L. J. (1942). The incidence and size of the moderator band in man and mammals. *Anat Rec, 82*, 361–372.

Ursic, M., Ravnik, D., Hribernik, M., et al. (2007). Gross anatomy of the portal vein and hepatic artery ramifications in dogs: corrosion study. *Anat Hist Embry, 36*(2), 83–87.

Ursell, P. C., Ren, C. L., & Danilo, P. (1990). Anatomic distribution of autonomic neural tissue in the developing dog heart: i. Sympathetic innervation. *Anat Rec, 226*, 71–80.

Vitums, A. (1962). Anomalous origin of the right subclavian and common carotid arteries in the dog. *Cornell Vet, 52*, 5–15.

Wakui, S., Matsuda, M., Furusato, M., et al. (1993). Branching mode of the middle rectal artery from the prostatic artery in the dog. *Anat Hist Embry, 22*(4), 376–380.

Whisnant, J. P., Millikan, C. H., Wakim, K. G., et al. (1956). Collateral circulation of the brain of the dog following bilateral ligation of the carotid and vertebral arteries. *Am J Physiol, 186*, 275–277.

Wilson, J. L., & Scheel, K. W. (1989). Septa1 collateralization: demonstration of canine intramyocardial collaterals. *Am J Anat, 184*, 62–65.

Yamane, T., Awazu, T., Fujii, T., et al. (2001). Aberrant branch of the bronchoesophageal artery resembling patent ductus arteriosus in a dog. *J Vet Med Sci, 63*(7), 819–822.

Yuan, B. X., Ardell, J. L., Hopkins, D. A., et al. (1994). Gross and microscopic anatomy of the canine intrinsic cardiac nervous system. *Anat Rec, 239*, 75–87.

12
The Veins

General Considerations

Veins follow the same general course as arteries, although variations in their number, size, and course are more frequent than in arteries. The accompanying veins are known as *satellite veins,* or *venae comitantes,* and often take the same name as the artery they accompany (Fig. 12.1). Although the smaller satellite veins are frequently double, the larger veins are single, as are most of the deep veins. All systemic veins have thin walls, and most have a large lumen in comparison with the arteries. The pressure in the veins is low, and the blood flows much more slowly in them than in the arteries. Stone and Stewart (1988) discussed the architecture and structure of canine veins, with special reference to confluences. Because there is generally no pulse in the venous system, the movement of blood depends primarily on pressure relations in the thorax and on muscular activity. The contraction of muscles results in compression of the veins, thus propelling the contained blood toward the heart. Negative pressure in the thorax during inspiration and the presence in most veins of semilunar valves that prevent backflow augment this effect of the skeletal and visceral muscles. Veins farthest from the heart contain the most valves. For an overview, see Shepherd and Vanhoutte (1975), as well as the older classic work by Franklin (1937). Simoens et al. (1984) have illustrated, characterized, and referenced the 963 veins of domestic animals (including the dog) that were listed in the 1973 edition of *Nomina Anatomica Veterinaria* (NAV).

The venous passages in the dura mater of the central nervous system are known as *sinuses.* In the extremities, the veins may be divided into superficial and deep sets. The veins of the superficial set are large and are clinically important because of the frequent necessity of making venipunctures for drawing blood or injecting fluids. In this location they act in cooling the blood as they communicate not only with the deep veins but also with extensive subcutaneous, interconnecting venous plexuses. When the animal is cooled, these plexuses and the larger superficial veins contract so that most of the blood from the extremities must be returned to the heart via the deep veins; this prevents heat loss. When the animal is warmed, and during work, the superficial veins and their connecting plexuses dilate and are plainly visible beneath the skin in short-haired specimens. This dilation provides a means of heat dissipation.

Cardiac and pulmonary veins are discussed with the heart in Chapter 11.

Cranial Vena Cava

The **cranial vena cava** (*v. cava cranialis*), formerly called *precava* (Figs. 12.1 through 12.5, and 12.9), is an unpaired vessel, 1.5 to 2 cm in diameter and 8 to 12 cm long. It lies in the cranial mediastinum ventral to the trachea and is in contact with the esophagus on its left side. It is also in contact with the thymus when this gland is fully developed. It runs through the cranial mediastinum and is the most ventral of the several structures that course through the thoracic inlet. It is formed, at a level just cranial to the thoracic inlet, by the convergence of the right and left brachiocephalic veins. These form an angle, open cranially, of approximately 90 degrees, so that each vein enters the cranial vena cava at an angle of approximately 45 degrees with the median plane. The cranial vena cava empties into the cranial part of the right atrium. Some mammals, such as the rabbit, retain the embryonic pattern of paired cranial venae cavae draining into the sinus venarum of the right atrium. As would be expected, this condition (see Fig. 12.3) is often seen as an anomaly in other animals, including the dog (Fig. 12.3). Cox et al. (1991) describe an example in a horse and make reference to reports in the dog. Sekeles (1982), in his case report for a cow, referred to literature citing 21 reported instances of persistent left venae cavae in the dog. For other reports of this anomaly in the dog see Stoland and Latimer (1947), Schaller (1955), Buchanan (1963), Gomerčič (1967), Hutton (1969), Buergelt and Wheaton (1970), and Larcher et al. (2006).

The **azygos vein** (*vena azygos*), with its tributaries, is discussed after the description of the other tributaries of the cranial vena cava.

The **costocervical vein** (*v. costocervicalis*) (Figs. 12.2 and 12.4) is medial to the proximal end of the first rib. The left vein runs lateral to the left subclavian artery and empties into the dorsolateral surface of the cranial part of the cranial vena cava. It may terminate in the left brachiocephalic vein. The right costocervical vein, approximately 1 cm caudal to the left at its termination, crosses the lateral surface of the trachea and enters the cranial vena cava ventral to the brachiocephalic trunk and vagus nerve. The right costocervical vein is approximately 3 cm long; that of the left side is

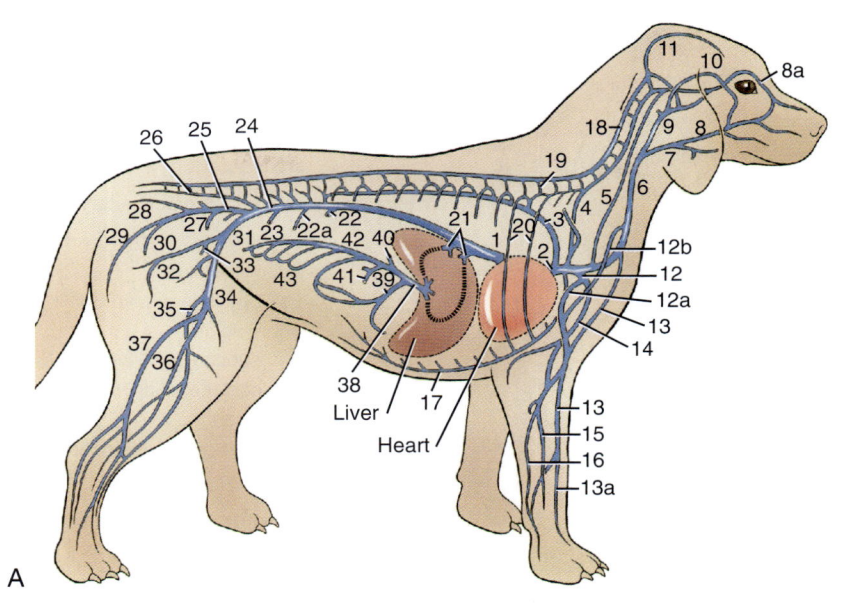

CHAPTER 12 The Veins 583

• Fig. 12.1 A, Schema of the venous system in an adult dog. B, The veins of a 41-day Beagle fetus injected with India ink and then cleared and stained with alizarine red by Evans. (From Evans HE, de Lahunta A: *Guide to the dissection of the dog,* 8th ed., Philadelphia, 2017, Elsevier.)

1. Caudal vena cava
2. Cranial vena cava
3. Azygos
4. Vertebral
5. Internal jugular
6. External jugular
7. Linguofacial
8. Facial
8a. Angularis oculi
9. Maxillary
10. Superficial temporal
11. Dorsal sagittal sinus
12. Axillary
12a. Axillobrachial
12b. Omobrachial
13. Cephalic
13a. Accessory cephalic
14. Brachial
15. Median
16. Ulnar
17. Internal thoracic
18. Right ventral internal vertebral venous plexus
19. Intervertebral
20. Intercostal
21. Hepatic
22. Renal
22a. Testicular or ovarian
23. Deep circumflex iliac
24. Common iliac
25. Right internal iliac
26. Median sacral
27. Prostatic or vaginal
28. Lateral caudal
29. Caudal gluteal
30. Internal pudendal
31. Right external iliac
32. Deep femoral
33. Pudendoepigastric trunk
34. Femoral
35. Medial saphenous
36. Cranial tibial
37. Lateral saphenous
38. Portal
39. Gastroduodenal
40. Splenic
41. Caudal mesenteric
42. Cranial mesenteric
43. Jejunal

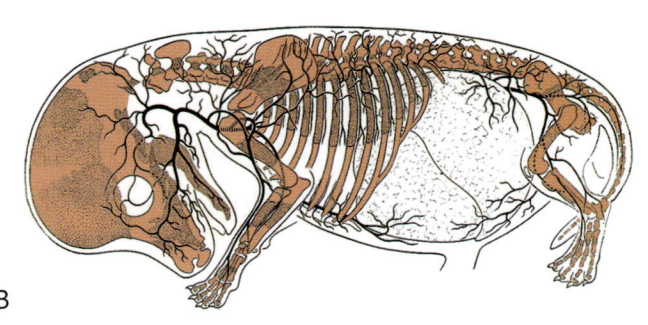

approximately 4 cm. Both vessels are approximately 5 mm in diameter.

In addition to the frequent union of the **vertebral vein** (*v. vertebralis*), there are four main tributaries to the costocervical vein in the dog. All are satellites of arteries, although they are less constant in position. They include the **dorsal scapular vein** (*v. scapularis dorsalis*), formerly called the *transverse colli*; the **first dorsal intercostal vein** (*v. intercostalis dorsalis I*); the **deep cervical vein** (*v. cervicalis profunda*), of which the thoracic vertebral vein is a tributary; and the **supreme intercostal vein** (*v. intercostalis suprema*).

Intervertebral veins (*vv. intervertebrales*) (Figs. 12.26 through 12.28) pass through the intervertebral foramen and connect the ventral internal vertebral venous plexus with the ventral external vertebral venous plexus. The last or eighth cervical intervertebral vein regularly bifurcates into a cranial communicating vein that joins the vertebral vein and a caudal communicating vein that empties into the deep cervical vein. According to Worthman (1956), the supreme intercostal vein receives the second and third thoracic intervertebral veins on each side. In almost half of his specimens, the fourth thoracic intervertebral vein on the left also emptied into the supreme intercostal vein of the same side.

The **vertebral vein** (*v. vertebralis*) (Figs. 12.1, 12.8, 12.22, 12.23, and 12.26) begins by the confluence of the

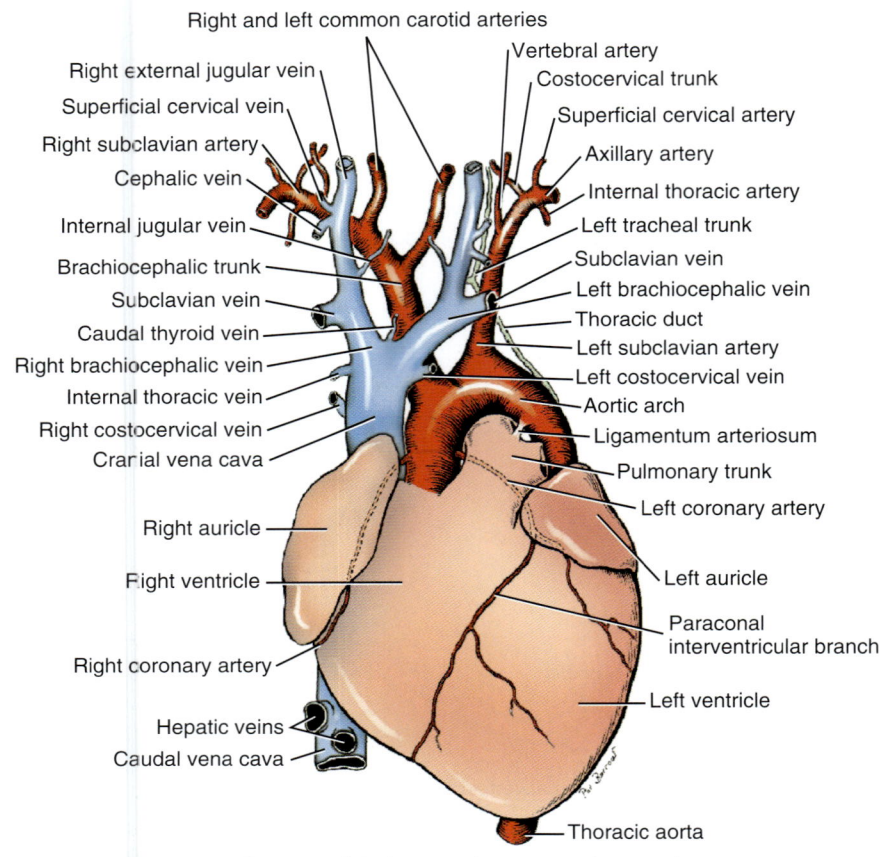

Fig. 12.2 Diagram of the heart and great vessels, ventral aspect.

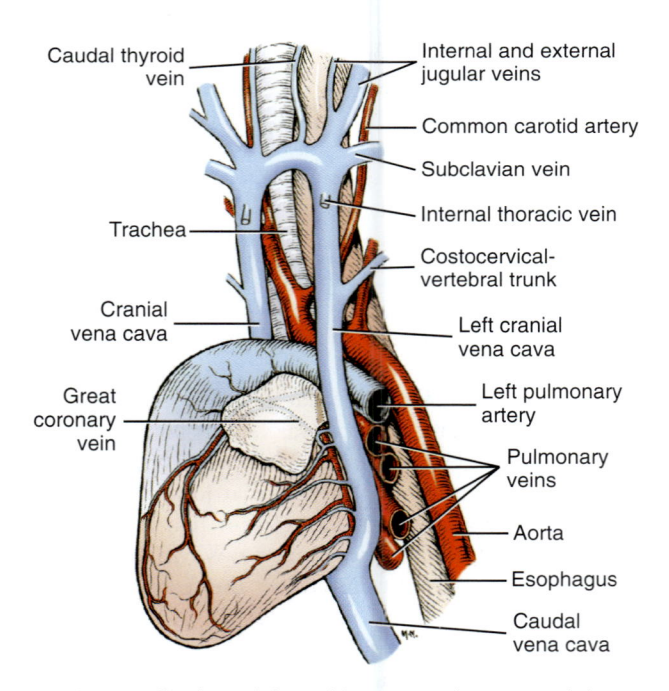

Fig. 12.3 Persistent left cranial vena cava in a mongrel dog.

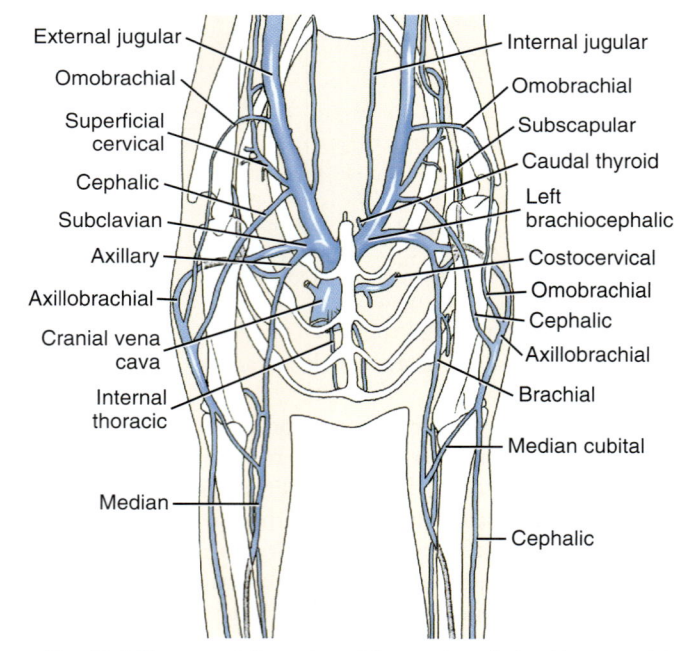

Fig. 12.4 Diagram of the veins of the neck and shoulders, cranial aspect.

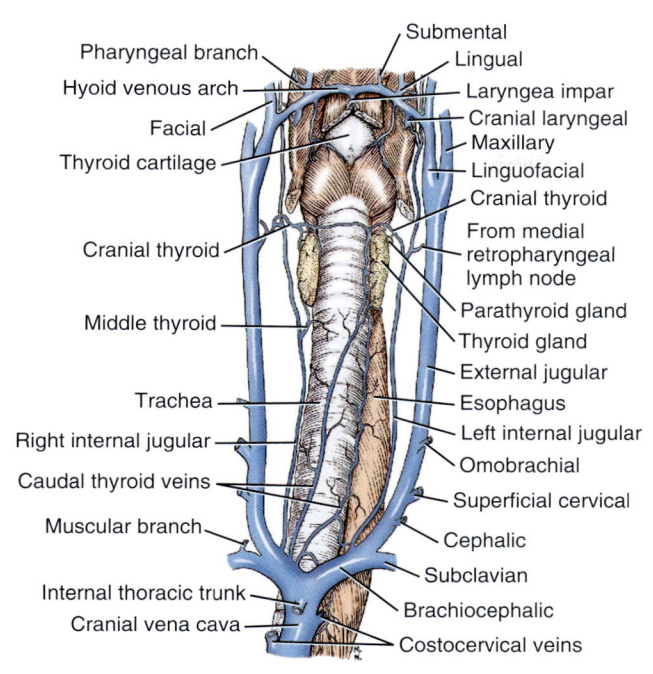

Fig. 12.5 Veins of the neck, ventral aspect.

emissary vein of the hypoglossal canal, if present, and the sigmoid sinus and ventral petrosal sinus in the space between the jugular foramen and the tympanooccipital fissure. The small internal jugular vein also arises wholly or partly at this confluence. The vertebral vein is approximately 1.5 mm in diameter as it runs caudally across the ventrolateral part of the atlantooccipital joint, then ventral to the wing of the atlas to the transverse foramen. It receives the first intervertebral vein, which leaves the ventral internal vertebral venous plexus, passes through the lateral vertebral foramen of the atlas and then through the alar notch, and joins the vertebral vein in the atlantal fossa. Worthman (1956) and Dräger (1937) call the initial portion of the vertebral vein the *occipital vein,* although only a segment of it parallels the occipital artery. The dog, however, may be regarded as not having a true occipital vein (*v. occipitalis*) because the dorsal nuchal area supplied by the occipital artery is drained by the occipital emissary vein and the ventral portion supplied by the occipital artery is drained by the vertebral vein.

After passing through the transverse foramen of the atlas from the atlantal fossa, the vertebral vein receives a small muscular tributary and a slightly larger communication from the caudal portion of the first intervertebral vein and the large second intervertebral vein. The portion of the vertebral vein that passes through the transverse foramen of the axis is its smallest part. There is usually a small anastomotic vein between the second and third intervertebral veins. Most of the blood is conveyed caudally by way of the large vertebral venous plexuses. The remaining portion of the vertebral vein and its tributaries are satellites of the comparable portions of the vertebral artery and its branches.

The **internal thoracic vein** (*v. thoracica interna*) (Figs. 12.1 through 12.4) is unpaired at its termination in the middle of the ventral surface of the cranial vena cava in approximately half of all specimens. In such instances it usually ranges from 1 to 4 cm in length. In the specimens in which it is paired, the right vein usually enters the cranial vena cava, whereas the left enters the left brachiocephalic vein. The peripheral part of the internal thoracic vein and its branches are prominent satellites of the comparable parts of the internal thoracic artery. Tributaries of the internal thoracic vein parallel the arteries and include pericardiacophrenic, thymic, mediastinal, ventral intercostal, perforating, and musculophrenic veins. The cranial epigastric vein of the abdomen is an extension of the internal thoracic vein.

The **brachiocephalic vein** (*v. brachiocephalica*) (Figs. 12.2, 12.4, and 12.5) merges with its fellow of the opposite side cranial to the thoracic inlet to form the cranial vena cava. Each is approximately 1 cm in diameter, and is formed by the joining of the caudally coursing external jugular and the medially coursing subclavian vein. Unlike the comparable artery, no part of the venous channel coming from the thoracic limb normally lies within the thorax. There is therefore no basis for naming a portion of the channel for venous return from the thoracic limb the subclavian vein. The subclavian vein has no tributaries and only consists of the very short vein connecting the axillary vein at the first rib to the external jugular vein to form the brachiocephalic vein. The merging brachiocephalic veins lie ventral to the trachea and esophagus as the most ventral structures in this region. The left brachiocephalic vein is longer than the right as it must cross the median plane to reach the right brachiocephalic vein to form cranial vena cava on the right. The caudal thyroid vein and the internal jugular veins enter the brachiocephalic as well as the left costocervical vein in some dogs.

The **caudal thyroid vein** (*v. thyroidea caudalis*) (Figs. 12.2 through 12.5) is an unpaired vein, approximately 1 mm in diameter, which arises primarily from the deep surfaces of the sternothyrohyoid muscles, but on one or both sides its most cranial tributary may arise in the thyroid lobe or lobes. It terminates usually in the cranial angle formed by the merging brachiocephalic veins. This was formerly known as the *v. thyroidea ima.*

The **internal jugular vein** (*v. jugularis interna*) (Figs. 12.3 through 12.6, 12.8, 12.22, and 12.23), approximately 1 mm in diameter, is formed in the tympanooccipital fissure by the confluence of the ventral petrosal and sigmoid sinuses, and, occasionally, the vein of the hypoglossal canal. Its initial portion may be double. The internal jugular vein lies at first in association with the internal carotid artery and then in the sheath of the common carotid artery. In the vicinity of the larynx, it receives an anastomotic branch from the laryngeal or pharyngeal tributary of the lingual vein. Caudal to the larynx it receives the **cranial thyroid vein** (*v. thyroidea cranialis*) from the cranial pole of the thyroid lobe. Opposite this tributary there is occasionally a second anastomotic connection with the external jugular vein. A branch from the medial retropharyngeal lymph node is also received here. Frequently, it receives the small

586 CHAPTER 12 The Veins

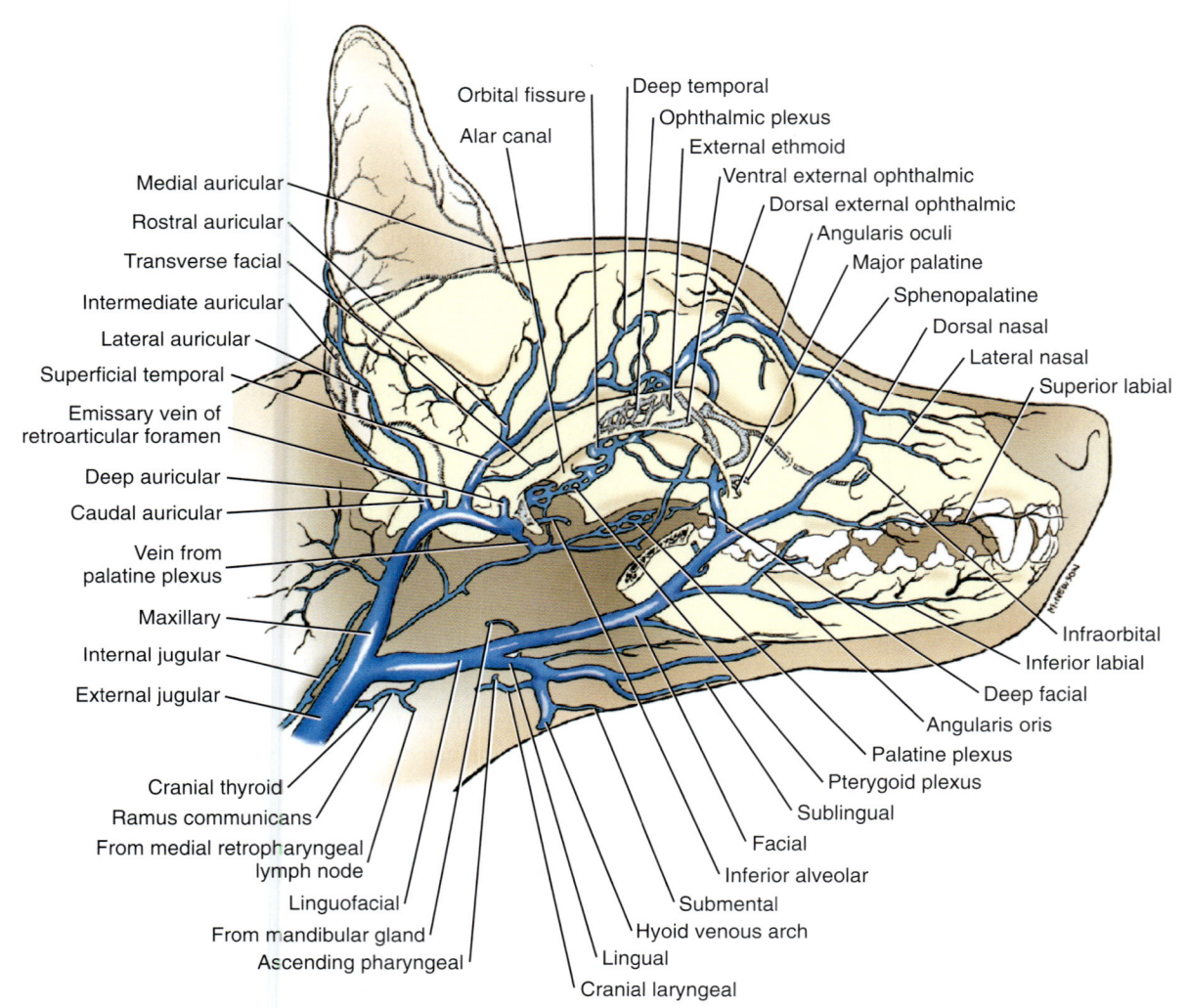

• **Fig. 12.6** Superficial veins of the head, lateral aspect.

middle thyroid vein (*v. thyroidea media*), which comes from the caudal pole of one or both thyroid lobes. On either or both sides, this vein may terminate in the brachiocephalic vein rather than the internal jugular vein, in which case it is considered to be the caudal thyroid vein. The internal jugular vein usually terminates in the caudal portion of the external jugular vein; rarely it terminates in the brachiocephalic vein.

The **external jugular vein** (*v. jugularis externa*) (Figs. 12.1 through 12.6, 12.8, and 12.10) is the main channel for return of venous blood from the head. It begins by the union of the linguofacial and maxillary veins, caudal to the mandibular salivary gland or at a transverse plane through the cricoid cartilage and the axis. It is approximately 1 cm in diameter and 12 cm long. In the adult it contains a few nonfunctional valves, which are irregular in their spacing. As the external jugular vein runs caudally in the superficial fascia, it crosses the lateral surface of the cleidocephalic muscle obliquely. The external jugular vein lies directly deep to the skin and is commonly used for venipuncture in dogs that are too small for the procedure to be feasible in the smaller veins of the extremities. At the cranial border of the shoulder, it receives the omobrachial and cephalic veins that course proximally from the brachium. Approximately 2 cm caudal to the termination of the omobrachial vein, the external jugular receives the **superficial cervical vein** (*v. cervicalis superficialis*), but this is variable. At its termination, the external jugular vein usually receives the internal jugular vein on its medial side.

The **linguofacial vein** (*v. linguofacialis*) (Figs. 12.1, 12.5, 12.6, and 12.8) begins by the confluence of the lingual and facial veins ventral to the mandibular salivary gland. It may have one or more tributaries from the capsule of the mandibular gland, and regularly receives the **glandular vein** (*v. glandularis*), which leaves the caudal pole of the gland. It contains a valve at its termination.

The **facial vein** (*v. facialis*) (Figs. 12.6 and 12.7) begins on the dorsolateral surface of the muzzle, covered by the m. levator nasolabialis. It is formed by the confluence of the smaller **dorsal nasal vein** (*v. nasalis dorsalis*), which drains the dorsolateral surface of the nose, and the larger angular vein of the eye.

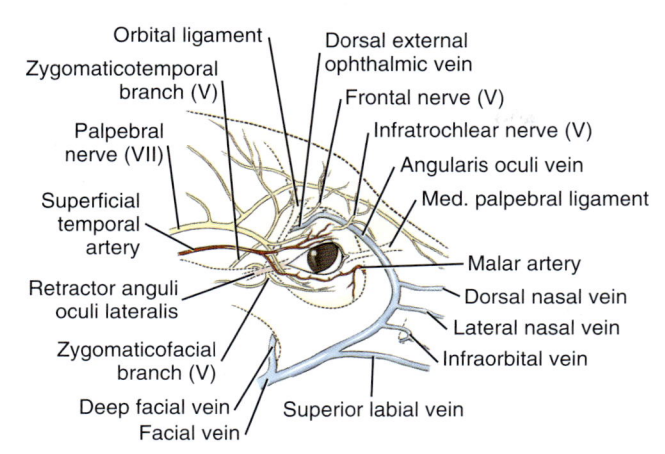

• Fig. 12.7 Schema of the vessels and nerves in the region of the eye.

The **angular vein of the eye** (*v. angularis oculi*) (Figs. 12.6 and 12.7) is approximately 3 mm in diameter and 2 cm long. Blood may flow in either direction in it as it lacks valves. It receives a tributary from the surface of the frontal bone. The angular vein of the eye may anastomose with the superficial temporal vein. It disappears from the surface of the face by curving caudally along the dorsomedial border of the orbit to anastomose with the dorsal external ophthalmic vein. It usually receives an emissary vein from the superficial surfaces of the frontal and nasal bones.

The **dorsal external ophthalmic vein** (*v. ophthalmica externa dorsalis*) (Figs. 12.6, 12.7, and 12.22) runs approximately 2 cm caudally into the orbit and forms the **ophthalmic plexus** (*plexus ophthalmicus*) (see Figs. 12.6 and 12.22). The plexus lies within the periorbita. It extends to the orbital fissure, and therefore lies in the caudal two-thirds of the orbit. The plexus becomes consolidated at the orbital fissure and, after traversing it, joins the cavernous sinus. Dorsally a small branch runs through the optic canal to join its fellow and the dorsal petrosal sinus of its side (Fig. 12.24). Ventrally the plexus is continued caudally outside the alar canal and is to be regarded as the beginning of the maxillary vein. A second connection between the ophthalmic system and the maxillary vein exists here in the form of a vein that runs through the alar canal. This vein also communicates with the cavernous sinus by an **emissary vein** that traverses the round foramen (*v. emissaria foraminis rotundi*). The **ventral external ophthalmic vein** (*v. ophthalmica externa ventralis*) (see Fig. 12.6) joins the dorsal external ophthalmic vein as well as the ophthalmic plexus caudally. Caudal to the eyeball an anastomotic branch unites the dorsal and ventral external ophthalmic veins. At the eyeball, the ventral external ophthalmic vein turns ventrally and receives the ventral vorticose veins and a branch from the third eyelid before anastomosing with the deep facial vein.

Two emissary veins join the ophthalmic plexus. One of these is the **external ethmoidal vein** (*v. ethmoidalis externa*) (see Fig. 12.6), a satellite of the like-named artery, which passes through the ethmoidal foramen. The other emissary vein is the **frontal diploic vein** (*v. diploica frontalis*), from the diploë of the frontal bone, which passes through a small supraorbital foramen in the zygomatic process of the frontal bone. The latter vein may join the dorsal external ophthalmic vein before the plexus is formed. The nasal venous vascular bed has been investigated by Lung and Wang (1989).

The **lateral nasal vein** (*v. lateralis nasi*) (see Figs. 12.6 and 12.7) is a satellite of the lateral nasal artery. It is a tributary that enters the facial vein.

The **infraorbital vein** (*v. infraorbitalis*) (Fig. 12.6 and 12.7) is approximately 1 mm in diameter and 1 cm long. It communicates with the ventral side of the facial vein, which lies dorsal to the infraorbital foramen. It has tributaries from the infraorbital nerve and adjacent musculature. Caudally it passes through the infraorbital canal and unites with the deep facial vein in the rostral part of the pterygopalatine fossa.

The **malar vein** (*v. malaris*) is a small tributary that arises mainly in the skin of the inferior eyelid and terminates in the infraorbital vein or deep facial vein.

The **inferior palpebral vein** (*v. palpebralis inferior*) from the inferior eyelid at the lateral commissure enters the dorsal surface of the facial vein on the side of the maxilla just rostral to the entrance of the superior labial vein.

The **superior labial vein** (*v. labialis superior*) runs caudally along the dorsal margin of attachment of the buccinator muscle and enters the facial vein lateral to the rostral end of the zygomatic arch. It drains blood from the superior lip and the dorsal part of the cheek.

The **angular vein of the mouth** (*v. angularis oris*) is a small tributary from the commissure of the lips that enters the facial vein caudal to the commissure.

The **deep facial vein** (*v. faciei profunda*) (Figs. 12.6 through 12.8) has no companion artery and is significant for its deep course and many anastomoses. A former name was *vena reflexa* (Preuss, 1954). It is 2 to 4 mm in diameter at its terminal end, which lies in the fascia cranial to the masseter muscle, approximately 1.5 cm ventral to the zygomatic arch. It arises in the ventral part of the orbit and the adjacent pterygopalatine fossa. The main portion of the vein arches dorsomedially and anastomoses with the ventral external ophthalmic vein on the floor of the orbit. An anastomosis with the superficial temporal vein frequently occurs as a small vein that obliquely crosses the lateral surface of the zygomatic arch. A small vein unites the deep facial with the maxillary vein by running across the lateral surfaces of the pterygoid muscles.

Union of the sphenopalatine, infraorbital, and occasionally the major palatine veins may form a short venous trunk that enters the deep facial vein. The major palatine vein is small, if it is present at all. These veins are satellites of the comparable arteries. The main venous drainage of the hard palate is by a poorly formed venous plexus that is continuous with the much more salient venous plexus of the soft palate. Therefore the venous drainage of the hard and soft palates is not chiefly through satellites of the arteries

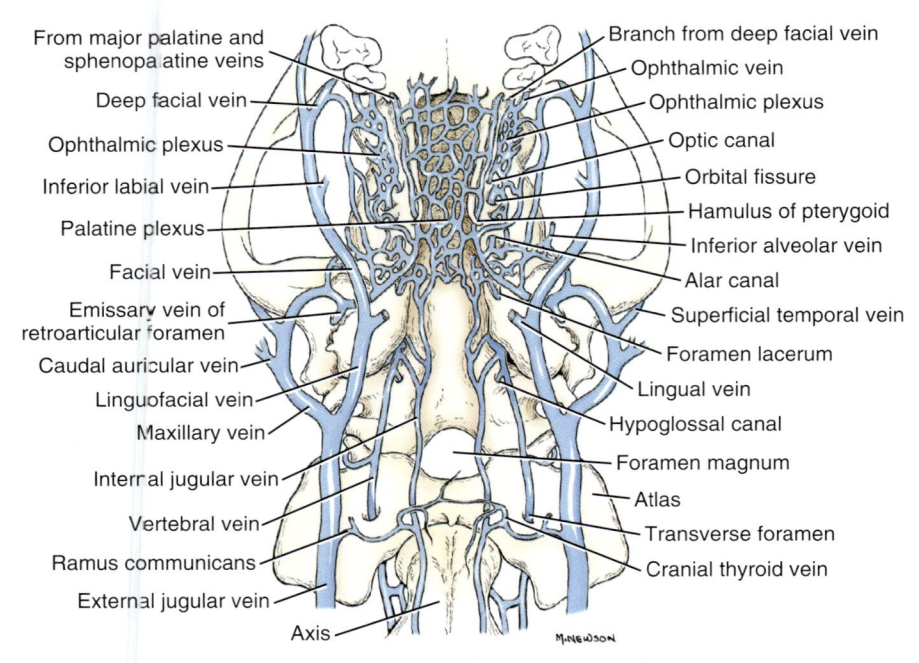

• Fig. 12.8 Veins of the head and neck, ventral aspect.

supplying them, but by means of the veins of the palatine plexuses that drain into the right and left maxillary veins (Figs. 12.6 and 12.8). One or two veins consistently leave the ventral part of the ocular muscles to enter the deep facial vein. It also receives dental rami from superior cheek teeth and tributaries from the maxilla as it curves from the deep surface of the masseter muscle before entering the facial vein.

The **inferior labial vein** (*v. labialis inferior*) (Fig. 12.6), a satellite of its artery, runs along the ventral border of attachment of the buccinator muscle. It receives an anastomosis from the submental vein and at its termination a vein that arises in the intermandibular space. This vessel runs along the margin of insertion of the digastric muscle, then over the lateral surface of the mandible. It may terminate in the facial vein. Throughout the course of the facial vein, small branches from the skin and fascia enter it. Ellenberger and Baum (1943) illustrate a small anastomotic vein located between the facial and the superficial temporal veins, as well as small branches coming from the mandibular lymph nodes.

The **submental vein** (*v. submentalis*) (Figs. 12.5 and 12.6) receives tributaries from the mylohyoid and geniohyoid muscles as it courses caudally along the ventral portion of the body of the mandible. Its termination is variable as it may terminate in the facial vein, inferior labial vein, or the hyoid venous arch.

The **lingual vein** (*v. lingualis*) (Figs. 12.5, 12.6, and 12.8) is the ventral tributary that joins the facial vein to form the linguofacial vein. It begins in the apex of the tongue, and, as it courses caudally, it is augmented by numerous deep lingual tributaries from this organ. It lies in areolar tissue in association with the lingual artery and hypoglossal nerve, lateral to the genioglossal and medial to the hyoglossal muscles. Approximately 1 cm rostral to the body of the basihyoid bone it crosses the dorsal border of the hyoglossus muscle and comes to lie dorsal to the mylohyoid muscle. As it courses caudally from deep to the caudal border of the mylohyoid muscle it is joined by the **sublingual vein** (*v. sublingualis*). This vein begins in the rostral part of the lingual frenulum and runs caudally on the dorsal surface of the mylohyoid muscle. It lies directly deep to the thin mucosa between the lingual frenulum and the sublingual fold that lies lateral to the frenulum. It is occasionally used for venipuncture, but this is ill advised as the exceedingly loose tissue that surrounds the vessel allows considerable hemorrhage to occur. Rostrally, this vein is accompanied by its satellite artery and the lingual branch of the mandibular nerve (V). It carries blood from the frenulum and the closely adjacent major sublingual and mandibular salivary ducts and the polystomatic part of the sublingual salivary gland.

The **hyoid venous arch** (*arcus hyoideus*) (Figs. 12.5 and 12.6) is a constant, large, unpaired vein, approximately 3 mm in diameter and 3 to 4 cm long, which lies ventral to the basihyoid bone. It usually connects right and left lingual veins approximately 1 cm caudal to the termination of the sublingual veins. Petit (1929) illustrates this vessel as extending between the two sublingual veins. It may be double. It may receive the submental vein, and, on each side of the midline, it receives the caudally running small **submental branch** (*ramus submentalis*), which usually begins as a single vessel in the midline between the fellow mylohyoid muscles. It receives delicate tributaries from both the mylohyoid and the geniohyoid muscles. Entering the caudal surface of the hyoid venous arch at the midline is the small unpaired laryngeal vein, *v. laryngea impar*. It anastomoses with the cranial laryngeal vein and usually with end tributaries of the thyroid veins.

The last tributary to the lingual vein is usually the **ascending pharyngeal vein** (*v. pharyngeal ascendens*) (Fig. 12.6) that receives tributaries from a pharyngeal plexus in the lateral wall of the pharynx between the vagosympathetic trunk and the internal carotid artery. The ascending pharyngeal vein may terminate in the hyoid venous arch. It may send a communicating branch to the internal jugular vein.

The **cranial laryngeal vein** (*v. laryngea cranialis*) (Figs. 12.5 and 12.6), a satellite of the like-named artery, leaves the larynx ventral to the cranial corner of the thyroid cartilage in company with the artery and cranial laryngeal nerve. It is usually a tributary of the ascending pharyngeal vein but may join the lingual vein approximately 1 cm from its termination. It may send a communicating branch to the internal jugular vein.

The **maxillary vein** (*v. maxillaris*) (Figs. 12.5, 12.6, 12.8, and 12.22) begins ventral to the alar canal by a continuation and later a consolidation of the extension of the ophthalmic plexus. The formation and anatomy of the venation in this location are complicated and variable. Usually a small vein lies in the alar canal and receives an **emissary vein of the round foramen** (*v. emissaria foraminis rotundi*) from the cavernous sinus through the round foramen. Rostrally the vein in the alar canal joins the ophthalmic plexus, whereas caudally it joins the maxillary vein. Here also the maxillary vein receives an **emissary vein from the oval foramen** (*v. emissaria foraminis ovalis*) and the **middle meningeal vein** (*v. meningea media*) that is a satellite, usually double, of the corresponding artery. Approximately 5 mm caudal to the oval foramen, two more veins join the maxillary vein. One of these is small and comes from the pterygoid canal; the second is the larger emissary vein from the foramen lacerum (*v. emissaria foraminis laceri*) that passes through the foramen lacerum, and connects internally at the confluence of the ventral petrosal and cavernous sinuses. The maxillary vein winds laterally, caudal to the retroarticular process, and receives the vein of the palatine plexus.

The **venous palatine plexus** (*plexus venosus palatinus*) (see Figs. 12.6 and 12.8) is a rather loose network of veins in the soft palate. The largest elements of this plexus are 0.5 mm in diameter. Rostrally the plexus anastomoses with the sphenopalatine and deep facial veins.

The **emissary vein of the retroarticular foramen** (*v. emissaria foraminis retroarticularis*) (Figs. 12.6, 12.8, and 12.22) was formerly called the *retroglenoid* or *retroarticular vein*. It is a continuation of the temporal sinus that leaves the skull through the retroarticular foramen and more than doubles the size of the maxillary vein by joining it caudal to the temporomandibular joint. The intracranial formation of this vein is described with the veins of the central nervous system.

The **inferior alveolar vein** (*v. alveolaris inferior*) (Fig. 12.6), formerly *mandibular vein*, is the satellite of the comparable artery. It leaves the mandibular foramen and at once receives a branch from the musculature medial to the mandible. Entering the maxillary vein approximately 5 mm caudal to the entry of the inferior alveolar vein is the **masseteric vein** (*v. masseterica*). This small tributary comes from the dorsal caudal border of the masseter muscle and curves medial to the caudal border of the mandible before it terminates.

The **superficial temporal vein** (*v. temporalis superficialis*) (Fig. 12.6) is approximately 2.5 mm in diameter as it terminates in the dorsal surface of the maxillary vein. The vein crosses ventral to the base of the ear, deep to the parotid salivary gland. A dorsal tributary arises dorsomedial to the orbit by occasionally anastomosing with the small frontal vein, a tributary of the *v. angularis oculi*. A ventral tributary takes a dorsal course in the caudal part of the orbit. It runs deep to the deep temporal fascia, crosses medial to the orbital ligament, and continues medial to the zygomatic arch to anastomose with a branch of the deep facial vein. This anastomotic channel is more than 1 mm in diameter. A small, third anastomotic channel between the superficial temporal vein and the veins of the orbit is formed by a branch that runs through the rostral portion of the temporal muscle to enter the orbit and anastomoses with the ophthalmic plexus.

The superficial temporal vein, after its formation by the three anastomotic branches, runs caudally deep to the temporal fascia. It receives numerous tributaries from the temporal muscle in its course toward the base of the ear. The **rostral auricular vein** (*v. auricularis rostralis*) is a small vein that begins in the interauricular musculature and skin and runs transversely, deep to the rostroauricular muscles, rostral to the base of the ear. It receives small branches from the skin and auricular muscles and the base of the pinna itself. The **medial auricular vein** (*v. auricularis medialis*) is a tributary to it. The rostral auricular vein terminates in the superficial temporal vein. The **transverse facial vein** (*v. transversa faciei*) is a small tributary that arises in the fascia ventral to the zygomatic arch. It empties into the superficial temporal vein approximately 1 cm ventral to the termination of the much larger rostral auricular vein. According to Ellenberger and Baum (1943), the rostral auricular vein terminates in the caudal auricular vein 50% of the time. As the superficial temporal vein grooves the rostral border of the parotid salivary gland, it receives one or more parotid branches from it.

The **caudal auricular vein** (*v. auricularis caudalis*) (Figs.12.6 and 12.8) is formed by the **lateral and intermediate auricular veins** (*vv. auricularis medialis et lateralis*). The marginal medial and lateral auricular veins anastomose with each other near the apex of the pinna on the caudal, or convex, side. Unlike the caudal auricular artery, the caudal auricular vein anastomoses with the rostral auricular vein by means of a venous circle that lies on the cervicoauricular and interauricular muscles. This venous circle receives tributaries from the adjacent muscles. The caudal auricular vein receives the **deep auricular vein** (*v. auricularis profunda*) near the base of the ear and terminates in the maxillary vein caudal to the termination of the superficial temporal vein. A portion of the caudal auricular vein is bridged superficially by parotid salivary gland tissue and receives **parotid branches** (*rami parotidei*) from the gland. The deep auricular vein may enter the maxillary vein directly between the entry of the superficial temporal and caudal auricular veins.

One or two veins enter the maxillary vein near its termination. These come from the dorsally lying skin and underlying cleidocephalic and sternocephalic muscles. Occasionally one of these ends in the external jugular vein. A communicating vein may be located between the internal jugular and the maxillary veins.

Azygos System of Veins

The **right azygos vein** (*v. azygos dextra*) (Figs. 12.1 and 12.9) develops in the dog. It is approximately 8 mm wide at its junction with the cranial vena cava where the latter terminates in the right atrium opposite the right third intercostal space. It begins on the median plane ventral to the body of the third lumbar vertebra by anastomosing with the single trunk formed by the merging of the right and left third lumbar intervertebral veins. Lying in the fat with the lumbar lymphatic trunk, it runs cranially through the aortic hiatus, flanked by the tendons of the crura of the diaphragm and the psoas major muscles. In the caudal third of the thorax it inclines slightly to the right, where it lies in the angle formed by the vertebral bodies and the aorta. Here, covered only by mediastinal pleura, it passes cranially to the base of the heart, hooks ventrally around the root of the right lung, and empties into the termination of the cranial vena cava at a right angle. It has the following tributaries: lumbar, dorsal costoabdominal, dorsal intercostal, and bronchoesophageal veins.

The **dorsal intercostal veins** (*vv. intercostales dorsales*), except the first three dorsal intercostal veins on the right side and the first three or four dorsal intercostal veins on the left side; the **dorsal costoabdominal veins** (*vv. costoabdominales dorsales*); and the first two **lumbar veins** (*vv. lumbales I et II*) are received by the azygos or the hemiazygos vein. The (third) fourth and fifth dorsal intercostal veins anastomose with each other so that a longitudinal venous trunk is formed adjacent to the necks of the associated ribs. This trunk usually terminates at the terminal end of the sixth dorsal intercostal vein where it drains into the azygos vein. This pattern is usually bilaterally symmetric in its formation, but the left venous trunk is longer than the right because it crosses ventral to the body of the fifth thoracic vertebra to reach the azygos vein.

The first two lumbar veins are smaller than the others. They are received by the initial part of the azygos vein as it extends cranially from an anastomosis with the stem, which receives the right and left third lumbar intervertebral veins. The initial part of the azygos vein may be double as it forms this union. The azygos vein carries most of the blood from the vertebral venous plexus via the dorsal intercostal and lumbar veins to the cranial vena cava (Bowsher, 1954). The intervertebral veins of the thorax are single vessels that join the dorsal intercostal veins at the highest points of the several intercostal spaces. The lumbar intervertebral veins are double as they traverse the intervertebral foramina. They then quickly unite to form the several lumbar veins (Worthman, 1956).

The **hemiazygos vein** (*v. hemiazygos*) is approximately 2 mm in diameter and is extremely variable. It is an

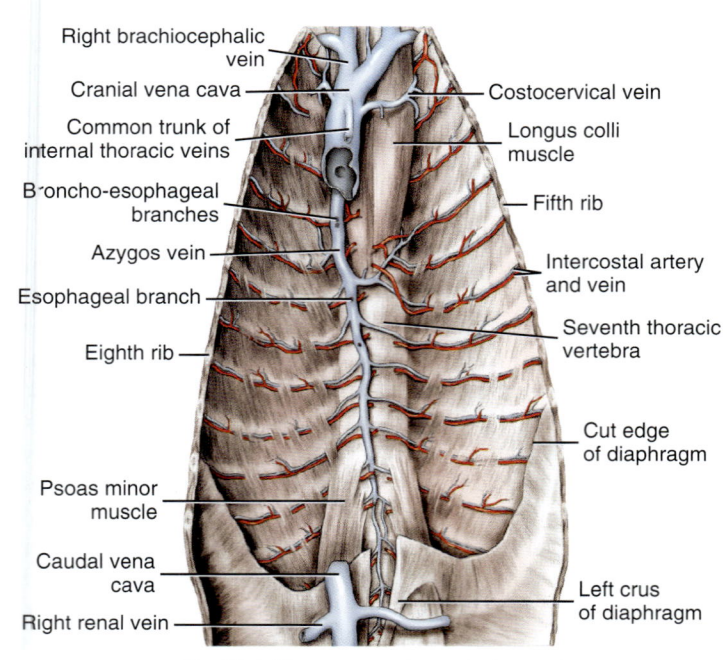

• **Fig. 12.9** The azygos vein, ventral aspect.

unpaired complement or replacement of the caudal portion of the right azygos vein. It lies on the left side of the aorta and connects the caudal vena cava with the azygos vein. It runs from the left phrenicoabdominal venous trunk near its termination in the caudal vena cava through the aortic hiatus and usually anastomoses cranially with the ninth or tenth left dorsal intercostal vein close to the vertebral bodies. The hemiazygos vein receives the left costoabdominal vein and the last two or three left dorsal intercostal veins and terminates in the right azygos vein in the caudal half of the thorax. Occasionally there is an anastomosis between the left phrenicoabdominal venous trunk and the left costoabdominal vein. In such specimens the hemiazygos vein is absent. Occasionally, there is an anastomosis between the azygos or hemiazygos vein and the deep circumflex iliac vein.

The **esophageal** and **bronchoesophageal veins** (*vv. esophageae et bronchoesophageae*) are variable and small. They are satellites of the comparable arteries. The bronchoesophageal veins, larger and more constant than the others, terminate in the azygos vein, usually at the level of the seventh thoracic vertebra. The esophageal veins, with delicate mediastinal tributaries, terminate in the azygos vein caudal to the termination of the bronchoesophageal vein. There are usually two of these, 1 to 3 cm apart, that cross the right face of the aorta to empty into the ventral surface of the azygos vein.

Veins of the Thoracic Limb

The veins of the thoracic limb may be divided into superficial and deep sets.

Superficial Veins of the Thoracic Limb

The **cephalic vein** (*v. cephalica*) (Figs. 12.1, 12.4, 12.10 through 12.12) is a tributary of the external jugular vein. It is the only large superficial vein of the thoracic limb. It begins on the mediopalmar surface of the carpus where it is a continuation of the radial vein. Distal to this the radial vein arises from the **superficial palmar arch** (*arcus palmaris superficialis*) that crosses the palmar side of the distal third of the second to fifth metacarpal bones and drains the **palmar common digital veins** (*vv. digitales palmares communes*). Here this arch is well protected by the heavy metacarpal pad.

The radial vein (*v. radialis*) (Fig. 12.12) leaves the deep palmar venous arch and runs proximally on the

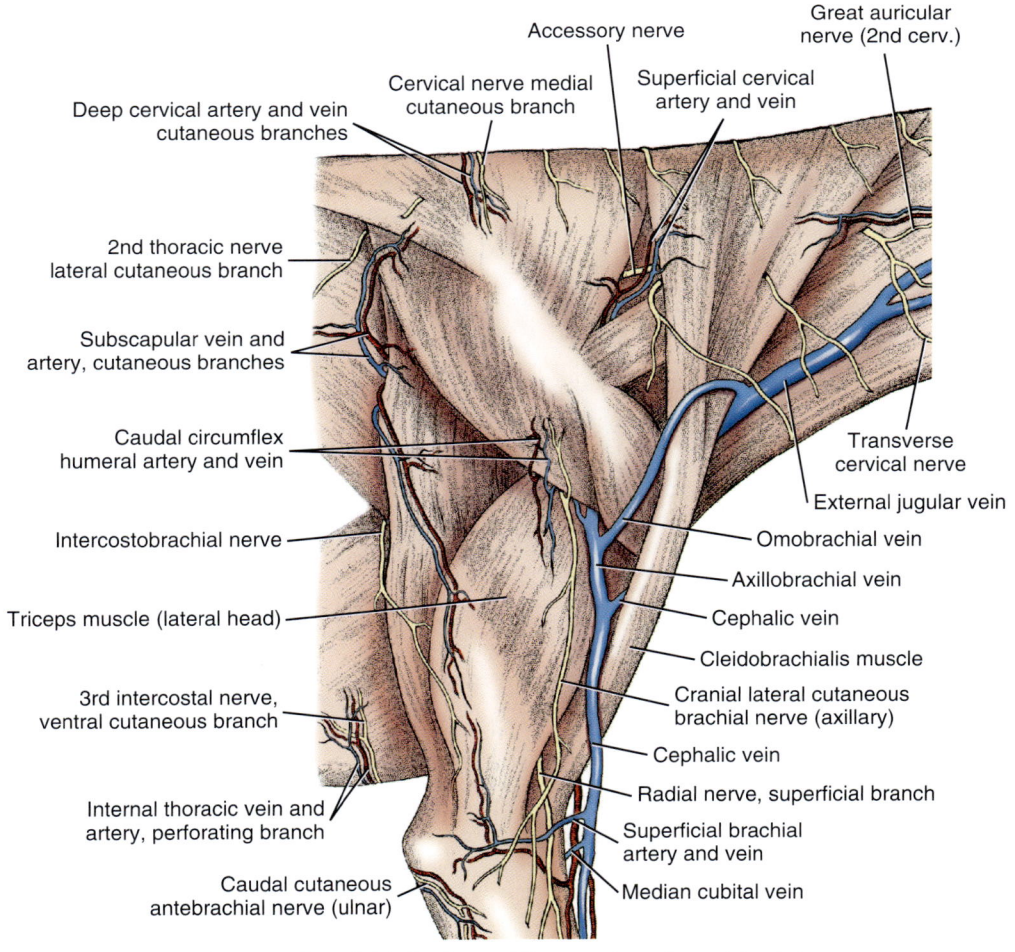

• **Fig. 12.10** Superficial structures of the scapula and arm, lateral view.

palmaromedial side of the interosseous muscles directly caudal to the carpus (Kumar, 2017). The cephalic vein arises near here with the radial vein as a conduit of venous blood from the palmar surface of the paw. The radial vein may join the ulnar vein. The cephalic vein usually receives three tributaries in the antebrachium. On gaining the cranial surface of the antebrachium, it is known as the antebrachial part of the cephalic vein. From the carpus it runs proximally until it reaches the cranial surface of the m. extensor carpi radialis, and then it follows this muscle to the flexor angle of the elbow joint. One of these tributaries comes from a band of skin extending to the elbow, whereas the other two are tributaries from the flexor muscles of the antebrachium. It is flanked on its medial and lateral sides by the medial and lateral branches of the superficial antebrachial artery as well as by the medial and lateral branches of the superficial radial nerve. It is 3 to 5 mm in diameter and lies directly deep to the skin, loosely surrounded by the superficial fascia. Because of its size, location, and ease of compressibility, it is the favored site for venipuncture in the dog. The antebrachial part of the cephalic vein is augmented by receiving the **accessory cephalic vein** (*v. cephalica accessoria*) at the beginning of the distal fourth of the antebrachium. This vein, approximately 2 mm in diameter at its termination, begins on the dorsum of the metacarpus where it receives **dorsal common digital veins II, III, and IV** (*vv. digitales dorsales communes II to IV*) and passes proximally over the carpus and the cranial aspect of the distal portion of the antebrachium before joining the cephalic vein. It is joined by **dorsal common digital vein I** (*v. digitalis dorsalis communis I*) from the first digit and skin of the second metacarpal bone at the distal end of the antebrachium.

The **median cubital vein** (*v. mediana cubiti*) (Figs. 12.4, 12.10, and 12.11) extends between the brachial or superficial brachial vein at the flexor angle of the elbow joint and the cephalic vein of the arm. It is approximately 2 mm in diameter and 2 cm long. It crosses the distal end of the m. biceps brachii obliquely as it runs proximolaterally to anastomose with the cephalic vein near the lateral border of the biceps muscle.

The **brachial part of the cephalic vein** continues the antebrachial part from the flexor angle of the elbow joint. It runs proximally, crosses the cleidobrachialis muscle, and joins the axillobrachial vein on the lateral surface of the triceps muscle. The cephalic vein runs proximomedially deep to the cleidobrachialis muscle at the junction of the middle and distal thirds of the brachium. It enters the

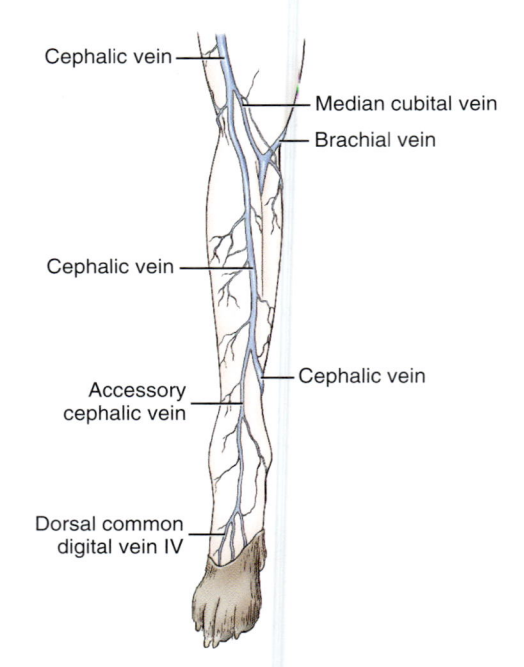

• Fig. 12.11 Veins of the right antebrachium, cranial aspect.

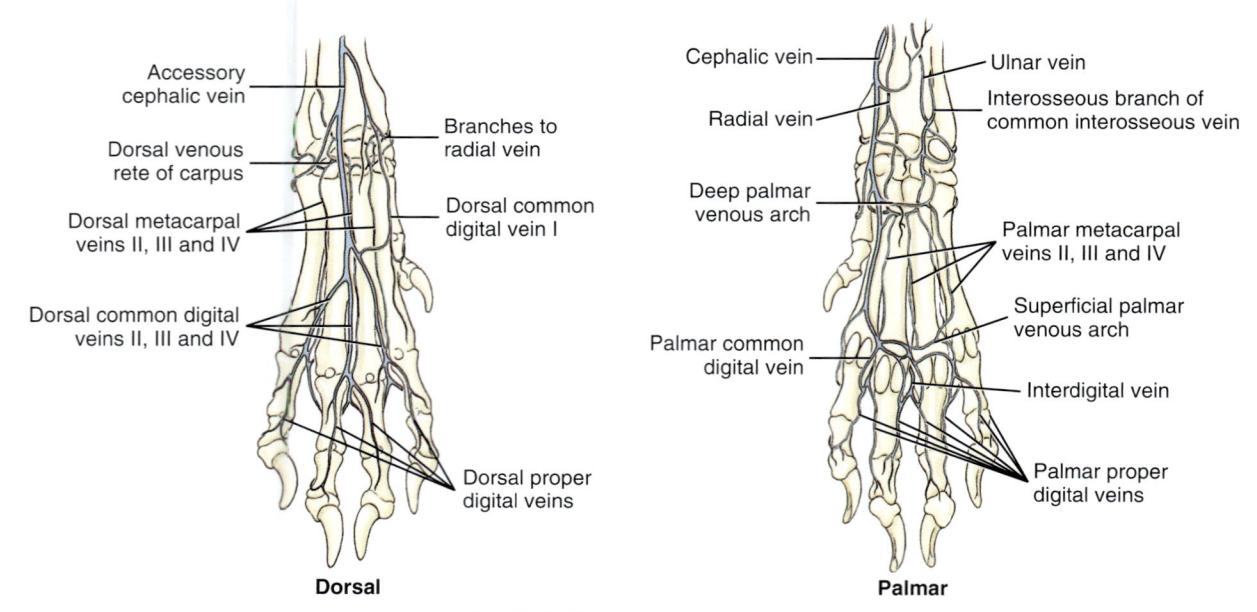

• Fig. 12.12 Veins of the right forepaw.

external jugular vein between the omobrachial and the axillary veins and receives a tributary from the major tubercle of the humerus and two or three more from the brachiocephalicus and pectoral musculature. This connection of the cephalic vein to the external jugular vein was formerly known as the distal communicating branch. Gómez et al. (2007) describe the bilateral absence of the brachial part of the cephalic vein in one dog and the bilateral absence of the omobrachial vein in two dogs.

The **axillobrachial vein** (*v. axillobrachialis*) (Figs. 12.1, 12.4, and 12.10), formerly considered a continuation of the cephalic vein, courses over the lateral head of the triceps muscle and at the distal border of the m. deltoideus passes caudal to the humerus. Caudal to the shoulder joint, the axillobrachial vein anastomoses with both the axillary and the subscapular veins. It receives large tributaries from the triceps muscle in its course through it and terminates in the axillary vein.

The **omobrachial vein** (*v. omobrachialis*), formerly called the *proximal communicating vein of the cephalic vein*, leaves the axillobrachial vein approximately 2 cm proximal to the cephalic vein and runs superficially at first on the m. deltoideus. It then arches cranially and medially, crosses the m. brachiocephalicus, and enters the lateral surface of the external jugular vein approximately 3 cm cranial to the termination of the cephalic vein. The omobrachial vein has no muscular tributaries and receives only small vessels from the skin and fascia.

Deep Veins of the Thoracic Limb

The radial vein (*v. radialis*) (Fig. 12.12) arises from the superficial and deep palmar venous arches (*arcus palmaris superficialis* and *arcus palmaris profundus*). The majority of the venous blood from the superficial arch flows through the anastomosis of the radial vein with the cephalic vein. The small radial vein follows the mediocaudal border of the radius covered by antebrachial fascia. It joins the median vein distal to the deep antebrachial vein.

The ulnar vein (*v. ulnaris*) (Figs. 12.1 and 12.12) accompanies its corresponding artery and arises from its union with the palmar branch of the caudal interosseous vein in the carpal canal. It passes proximally in the deep digital flexor muscle, receiving tributaries from most of the caudal antebrachial muscles. It joins the brachial or common interosseous vein in the proximal antebrachium.

The small median vein (*v. mediana*) (Figs. 12.1 and 12.4) accompanies the corresponding artery. It arises from the superficial palmar venous arch, passes proximally through the carpal canal and in the middle to proximal antebrachium is joined by the radial vein and deep antebrachial vein (*v. profunda antebrachii*). Proximal to this, it is continued by the brachial vein.

The brachial vein (*v. brachialis*) (Figs. 12.1 and 12.4) receives the relatively large common interosseous vein (*v. interossea communis*) with its ulnar and cranial and caudal interosseous branches. At the elbow the large median cubital vein connects the brachial vein or superficial brachial vein with the cephalic vein. In the brachium, the brachial vein receives the transverse cubital (*v. transversa cubiti*), superficial brachial (*v. brachialis superficialis*), collateral ulnar (*v. collateralis ulnaris*), bicipital (*v. bicipitalis*), and deep brachial (*v. profunda brachii*) veins. Proximal to this the brachial vein is continued by the axillary vein.

The axillary vein (*v. axillaries*) (Figs. 12.1, 12.2, 12.4, 12.13) receives the small cranial circumflex humeral vein

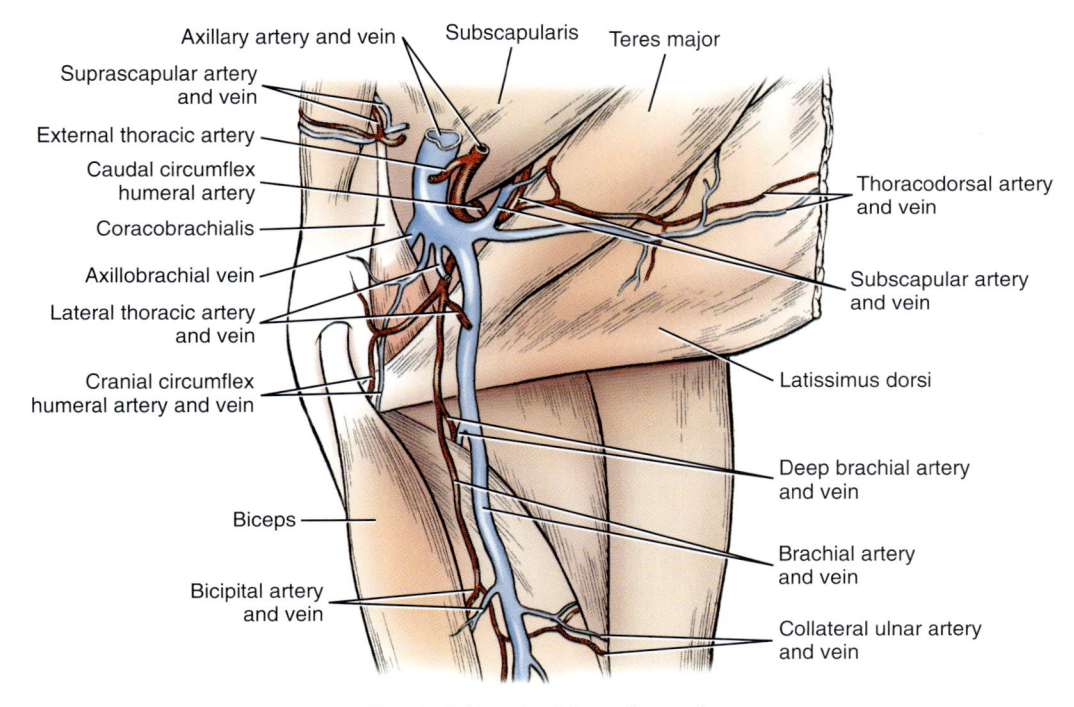

• **Fig. 12.13** Vessels of the axillary region.

(*v. circumflexa humeri cranialis*) cranially and the thoracodorsal vein (*v. thoracodorsalis*) caudally. A large subscapular vein (*v. subscapularis*) with its caudal circumflex humeral vein (*v. circumflexa humeri caudalis*) joins the axillary vein caudal to the shoulder. Proximal to this, a small lateral thoracic vein (*v. thoracica lateralis*) enters caudally and an external thoracic vein (*v. thoracica externa*) enters cranially. The axillobrachial vein connects the cephalic vein superficially with the axillary or caudal circumflex humeral vein caudal to the shoulder joint. At the first rib the axillary vein becomes the subclavian vein and joins the external jugular vein to form the brachiocephalic vein.

Veins of the Forepaw

The veins of the forepaw (*manus*) (Fig. 12.12), like the arteries, nerves, and lymphatic vessels, are divided into a dorsal and a palmar set. These are not as completely divided into superficial and deep series as are the arteries in the metacarpus, and only a single series exist dorsally and palmarly in the digits.

Axial and abaxial **dorsal proper digital veins II, III, IV, and V** (*vv. digitales dorsales propriae*) begin in the *arcus venosus digitales* formed by the anastomoses of the dorsal and palmar sets of proper digital veins. They occur on the axial aspects of digits II and III and on the abaxial aspects of digits IV and V. These digital arches collect small tributaries from the digital pads and the corium of the claws. The dorsal proper digital veins run proximally on the dorsum of the digits and receive communicating branches from the palmar proper digital veins.

The **dorsal common digital veins I, II, III, and IV** (*vv. digitales dorsales communes I to IV*) continue proximally on the extensor tendons from their formation by the confluence of the dorsal digital veins and the palmar communicating branches. The lateral dorsal common digital vein IV runs proximally and joins dorsal common digital vein III. The trunk formed by this union continues the axis of the fourth vessel and in turn is joined by the dorsal common digital vein II to form the **accessory cephalic vein** (*v. cephalica accessoria*). At the level of the first digit a small anastomosis usually occurs between the dorsal common digital vein I and the termination of dorsal common digital vein II on the abaxial surface of the second metacarpal bone.

The **dorsal metacarpal veins I, II, III, and IV** (*vv. metacarpeae dorsales I, II, III, et IV*) are delicate veins that lie in the dorsal grooves between the main metacarpal bones. They anastomose distally with the corresponding dorsal common digital veins at the junction of the middle and distal thirds of the metacarpus and proximally with the poorly formed dorsal rete of the carpus. The blood from the dorsal part of the first digit and the abaxial surface of the second metacarpal drains into the accessory cephalic vein some 4 cm proximal to the carpus via the **dorsal common digital vein I** (*v. digitalis dorsalis communis I*). This vein collects a tributary from the dorsal venous rete of the carpus.

The **dorsal venous rete of the carpus** (*rete carpi dorsale*) is a minute, poorly defined plexus of veins on the dorsal surface of the distal row of carpal bones. The dorsal metacarpal veins drain into it, and the accessory cephalic, dorsal common digital vein I, and the palmar set of veins carry blood from it. The latter include the radial and interosseous veins.

The palmar set of veins of the forepaw begins usually as the single but occasionally double axial and abaxial **palmar proper digital veins II, III, IV, and V** (*vv. digitales palmares propriae*). These commence at the palmar extremities of the sagittally placed digital venous arches and run proximally on the palmar surfaces of the proximal interphalangeal joint and the adjacent phalanges. Usually the middle two veins (III and IV) divide on the first phalanges into axial and abaxial branches. The apposed (axial) branches converge toward the axis through the paw and anastomose with the communicating veins from the dorsal set and with each other or extend singly to the superficial palmar venous arch and anastomose with it. The abaxial branches anastomose with the palmar proper digital veins nearest them. Thus the abaxial branch of palmar proper digital vein III anastomoses with palmar proper digital vein II, and the abaxial branch of palmar proper digital vein IV anastomoses with palmar proper digital vein V. In this way the **palmar common digital veins II, III, and IV** (*vv. digitales palmares communes II to IV*) are formed. These immediately anastomose with veins of the dorsal set and then continue to anastomose with the **superficial palmar venous arch** (*arcus palmaris superficialis*). This arch is formed by an anastomosis of the radial vein, medially, and the fourth palmar metacarpal vein, laterally. It lies deep to the metacarpal pad, on the palmar surfaces of the metacarpophalangeal joints. Occasionally the arch is double, and other irregularities exist. Because of this distal location of the superficial palmar venous arch, the palmar common digital veins may be absent.

The **palmar metacarpal veins II, III, and IV** (*vv. metacarpeae palmares II to IV*) are small satellites of the palmar metacarpal arteries. They lie between the fleshy interosseous muscles and run from the superficial palmar venous arch at the level of the metacarpophalangeal joints proximally to anastomose with the deep palmar venous arch.

The **deep palmar venous arch** (*arcus palmaris profundus*) lies deep to the origins of the interosseous muscles and follows the distal border of the thick palmar carpal ligaments. Medially it connects with the radial vein and laterally it anastomoses deeply with both the ulnar and the interosseous branches of the common interosseous vein. Usually a second venous arch exists here, connecting the radial vein with the interosseous branch across the superficial surface of the superficial flexor tendon. It lies subcutaneously, just distal to the carpal pad. The palmar skin and small carpal pad and the skin on the abaxial surface of the second metacarpal bone and digit are frequently drained by a single vein that terminates in the medial surface of the radial vein opposite the carpus. In some specimens a communicating vein connects the radial vein with the dorsal common digital vein I near the level of the metacarpophalangeal joint (Fig. 12.12A).

Caudal Vena Cava

The **caudal vena cava** (*v. cava caudalis*), formerly postcava (Figs. 12.9, 12.14, 12.16, 12.19, and 12.28), begins in contact with the ventral surface of the seventh lumbar vertebra by convergence of the common iliac veins. It is approximately 1 cm in diameter in large dogs and lies in the furrow formed by the right and left psoas major and minor muscles. At its beginning the aorta lies to the left of it because the aorta terminates ventral to the left common iliac vein. In its course cranially the caudal vena cava

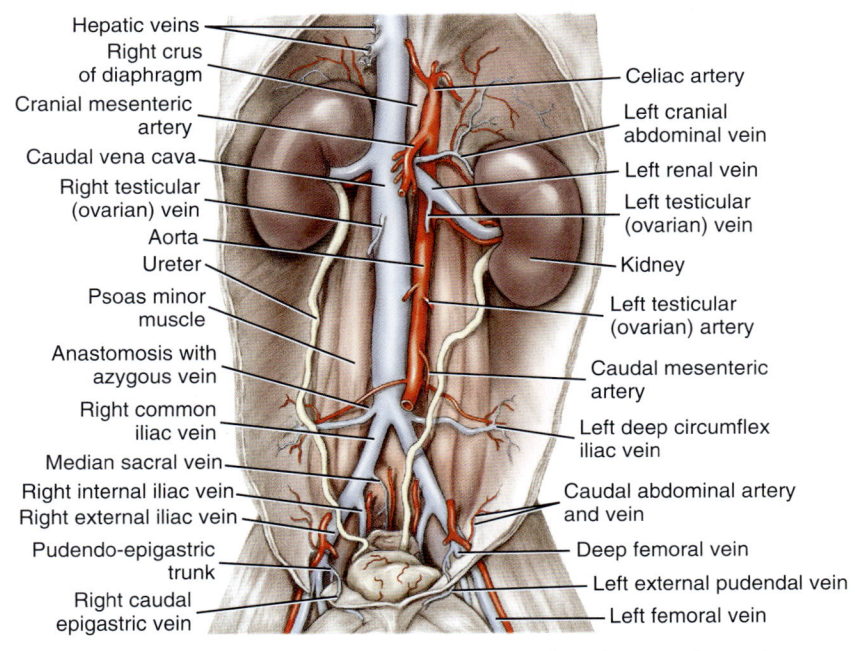

• Fig. 12.14 The caudal vena cava and its main tributaries, ventral aspect.

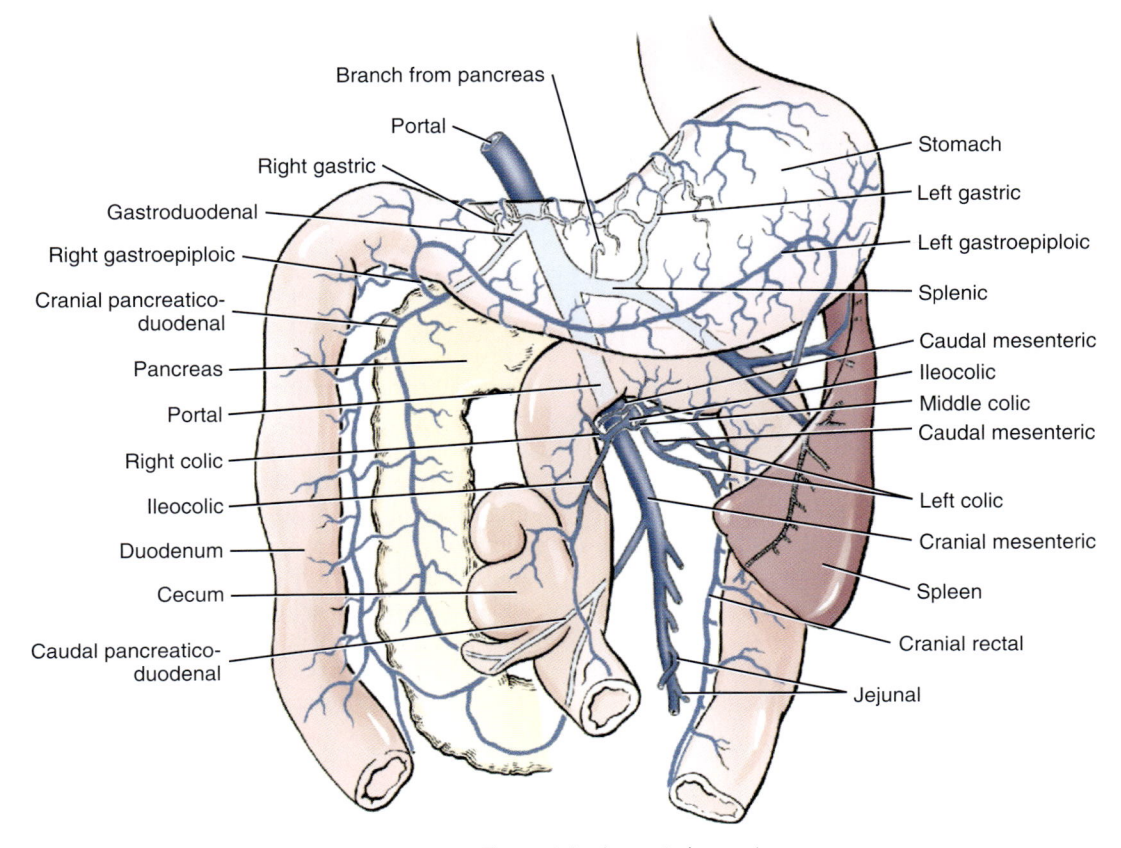

• Fig. 12.15 The portal vein, ventral aspect.

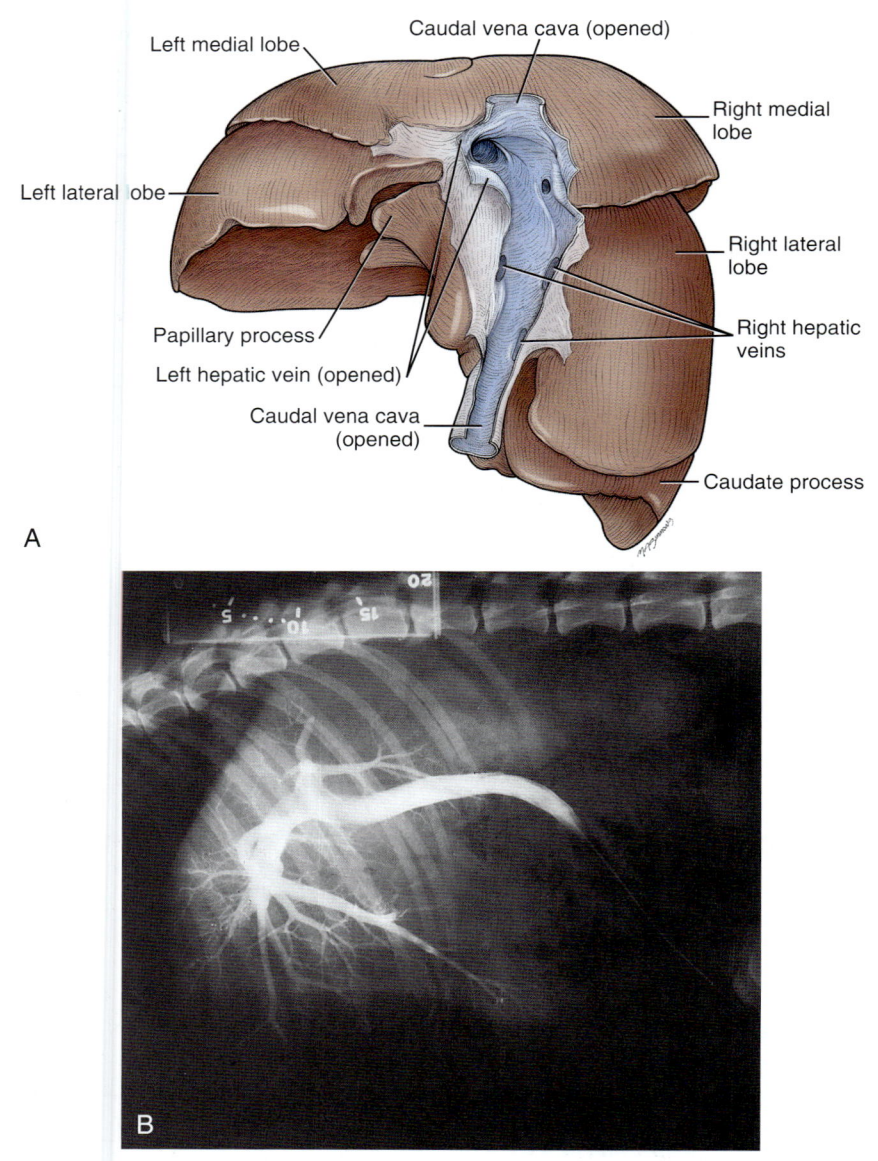

Fig. 12.16 A, Dorsal view of the liver to show hepatic veins. B, Normal portogram highlighting the portal vein (caudally) and the hepatic veins within the liver. Lateral view. (From Evans, H.E. & de Lahunta, A. (2017). Guide to the Dissection of the Dog. 8th ed. Elsevier.)

gradually inclines ventrally until it reaches the medial part of the caudate lobe of the liver. It then inclines ventrally and to the right at a slightly sharper angle and deeply grooves or tunnels the caudate lobe of the liver as it passes in it before reaching the diaphragm. It passes through the obliquely placed foramen venae cavae of the diaphragm, which is approximately 3 cm to the right of the median plane. The intrathoracic portion of the caudal vena cava, approximately 4 cm long, lies in a special mediastinal pleural fold, the plica venae cavae, in company with the right phrenic nerve. Here both the nerve and vessel lie in a deep groove of the accessory lobe of the right lung before the vein terminates in the caudal part of the right atrium.

Reis and Tepe (1956), after examining 500 dogs for variations in the renal veins, list only two variants. One of these had been described previously by Kadletz (1928) and represented a circumaortic venous ring at the level of the renal veins. The other aberration was a persistence of the left supracardinal vein of the fetus. This was found in 2.6% of the 500 dogs examined. Several items of the development of the caudal vena cava, in particular the lumbar segment, are still controversial (Cornillie & Simoens, 2005). In the fetus there are four bilateral venous systems from which a single caudal vena cava is formed. Thus abnormalities are common. Reis and Tepe (1956) described 15 different anomalies of this vessel. We have identified by portography and necropsy a unique malformation of the abdominal venous system in a young dog that was presented for clinical signs of hepatic encephalopathy. The caudal vena cava was normal from its origin at the fusion of the two common iliac veins. Just cranial to the renal veins the caudal vena cava totally anastomosed with the azygos vein. There was no caudal vena cava from this level to the right atrium. In addition, there was a large anastomosis between the cranial mesenteric vein and the point where the caudal vena cava drained into the azygos vein. Only a small portal vein entered the liver. This malformation of the caudal vena cava has been referred to as *azygos continuation of the caudal vena cava*, which can be diagnosed by angiography or ultrasonography (Barthez et al., 1996). If this is the only venous malformation there will be no clinical dysfunction. The caudal vena cava in the dog is essentially devoid of smooth muscle or the *tunica muscularis* is quite slight (Franklin, 1937). It has the following tributaries, in addition to the formative common iliac veins: lumbar, deep circumflex iliac, right testicular or right ovarian, renal, hepatic, and phrenic veins, and phrenicoabdominal trunk.

The **lumbar veins I to VII** (*vv. lumbales*) (see Fig. 12.28) are satellites of the corresponding arteries. The first two lumbar veins are tributaries of the azygos vein on the right side and of the hemiazygos on the left. The third pair of lumbar intervertebral veins anastomose with each other directly ventral to the body of the third lumbar vertebra (see azygos vein). From this small venous yoke a small, median, unpaired vein runs cranially to become the azygos vein. In a similar manner a larger unpaired median vessel runs caudoventrally from the anastomosed third lumbar veins and enters the common trunk formed by the anastomoses of the right and left fourth lumbar veins. This trunk vein is the largest vessel entering the caudal vena cava from the lumbar vertebrae. Because of these venous anastomoses in the middle of the lumbar region, blood can flow cranially to the heart either by the azygos vein or by the caudal vena cava. The members of the fifth and sixth pairs of lumbar veins anastomose with each other to form common trunks that enter the dorsal surface of the caudal part of the caudal vena cava. The right and left seventh lumbar veins empty into the right and left common iliac veins, respectively.

The **deep circumflex iliac vein** (*v. circumflexa ilium profunda*) (Figs. 12.1 and 12.14) is a satellite of the corresponding artery and lies caudal to it. The superficial and deep tributaries have the same anastomoses as do the comparable arteries.

The **right testicular vein** (*v. testicularis dextra*) (Figs. 12.1 and 12.14) enters the ventral surface of the caudal vena cava approximately 2 cm caudal to the termination of the right renal vein. It collects tributaries from the testis and epididymis and becomes greatly coiled as it continues in the free border of the mesorchium. This coiled and flexuous arrangement of the testicular vein is known as the **pampiniform plexus** (*plexus pampiniformis*). The plexus is intertwined with the testicular lymph vessels, artery, and nerve plexus as they form a funiculus that is located cranial to the ductus deferens and its blood vessels as they all traverse the inguinal canal. The vein straightens on approaching the vaginal ring. Throughout its oblique intraabdominal course to the caudal vena cava, it lies in a fold of peritoneum, the **proximal mesorchium** (*mesorchium proximale*), which may be 4 cm wide near the inguinal canal. The testicular vein is joined by one or two small tributaries from the adipose and fibrous renal capsules a few centimeters before its termination. It is accompanied, except at its termination, by the testicular artery, nerves, and lymphatics.

The **right ovarian vein** (*v. ovarica dextra*) (Figs. 12.1 and 12.14) is shorter and less tortuous than the homologous right testicular vein. It begins by two or three tributaries from the right ovary and surrounding fat. These are tortuous and plexiform. The ovarian vein anastomoses with the uterine vein in the mesometrium opposite the cranial third of the uterine horn.

The **renal veins** (*vv. renales*) (Figs. 12.1 and 12.14) are approximately 8 mm in diameter.

The right renal vein is approximately 3 cm long, whereas the left is 4 cm long. Each begins at the hilus of the respective kidney by convergence of the two veins that arise near the poles of the kidney by collecting the interlobar veins. Christensen (1952) described the intrarenal morphologic features of the renal veins of the dog. According to Kazzaz and Shanklin (1951), the dog has a system of stellate veins on the surface of its kidney. Those on the lateral side drain into the interlobar veins; those on the medial side go directly into the renal vein. The renal veins may take an oblique course cranially to reach the caudal vena cava. The left renal vein, like the right renal artery, is longer than its fellow and usually empties into the caudal vena cava more caudally than does the opposite vessel. The renal veins contain valves at their terminations. The left renal vein receives the left gonadal vein, the **left testicular vein** (*v. testicularis sinistra*) or the **left ovarian vein** (*v. ovarica sinistra*). Except for the difference in termination, the left gonadal vein closely resembles its fellow on the right, which empties directly into the caudal vena cava. The left gonadal vein or the left renal vein receives the **left cranial ureteric vein** several centimeters before its termination, whereas the right renal vein usually receives the **right cranial ureteric vein** near the hilus of the kidney. In the 500 dogs examined by Reis and Tepe (1956), double renal veins were found five times on the right side but never on the left.

A **common trunk**, formerly known as the phrenicoabdominal vein, receives the **caudal phrenic vein** (*v. phrenica caudalis*) and the **cranial abdominal vein** (*v. abdominalis cranialis*). This phrenicoabdominal trunk is approximately 4 mm in diameter as each terminates in the lateral surface of the caudal vena cava approximately 1 cm cranial to the renal vein of the same side. Each trunk grooves the ventral surface of the corresponding adrenal gland as the terminal 1 cm of the venous trunk passes ventral to the gland. Here it receives the **adrenal veins** (*vv. adrenales*), which, unlike the arteries, drain entirely into this trunk as it lies in the groove of the gland (Flint, 1900). These veins are short and inconspicuous. The formative caudal phrenic and cranial abdominal veins are satellites of the arteries of the same names.

The **hepatic veins** (*vv. hepaticae*) (Figs. 12.1) are embedded, wholly or in part, in the liver parenchyma. They are therefore short and receive numerous tributaries from within the hepatic parenchyma. They terminate along the lateral and ventral surfaces of the last 4 cm of the intraabdominal portion of the caudal vena cava (Fig. 12.16). The largest hepatic vein serves the left lateral, left medial, quadrate, and part of the right medial lobe. It enters the left ventral part of the caudal vena cava at the foramen venae cavae of the diaphragm and is the most cranially located of all the hepatic veins. A small portion of this hepatic vein can be identified between the cranial surface of the liver and the caudal vena cava. From the right, usually two major hepatic veins enter the caudal vena cava, approximately 2 cm apart. The cranial tributary comes from the right lateral and partly from the right medial lobe. The caudal tributary comes mostly from the caudate lobe. These vessels are approximately 3 mm in diameter. There are a score or more of hepatic tributaries, ranging to less than 1 mm in diameter, which drain into the caudal vena cava at various places as it courses through the liver. These hepatic veins are best seen where they open into the caudal vena cava after incising the caudal vena cava dorsally as it traverses the liver.

The **cranial phrenic veins** (*rv. phrenicae craniales*) are represented by a single tributary on each side, beginning in the ventral part of the muscular periphery of the diaphragm. At the lateral junction of the muscular and tendinous parts, each empties into the caudal vena cava as it passes through the foramen venae cavae. There is usually a small trunk vein that empties into the caudal vena cava on the thoracic side of the foramen venae cavae. This is formed by two or more tributaries that drain the extensive but thin plica venae cavae.

Portal Vein

The **portal vein** (*v. portae*) (Figs. 7.51, 12.1, 12.15 and 12.16) with its tributaries from the abdominal viscera that are not drained by the caudal vena cava forms a portal system within the liver. It arises from capillaries in the viscera and ends in capillaries in the liver. It collects blood from the pancreas, spleen, and the entire gastrointestinal tract except the caudal rectum and anal canal. It is approximately 1.2 cm in diameter at the porta of the liver, where it terminates. It lies deeply buried among the abdominal viscera. It runs cranially from its formation in the root of the mesojejunum, dorsal to the junction of the right and left lobes of the pancreas. The vein continues cranially from the pancreas and cranial duodenum in association with the hepatic artery and plexus of autonomic nerves to form the ventral boundary of the epiploic foramen. At this boundary these structures are all enclosed in the right free border of the lesser omentum that forms the hepatoduodenal ligament. The portal vein is formed by the confluence of the cranial and caudal mesenteric veins. Its large tributaries are the gastroduodenal, splenic, and right gastric veins (Kalt & Stump, 1993). Variations are common in the patterns of formation of these veins. The cranial mesenteric vein is always the largest vessel. Valves have been reported in the canine hepatic portal system. In the fetus the umbilical vein from the placenta enters the liver between the quadrate and left medial lobes and is shunted into the caudal vena cava via a **ductus venosus**. In a study of 84 neonatal dogs, Tisdall et al. (1997) describe the duct as a straight conduit 1 to 3 mm wide and 4 to 12 mm long in pups with a crown-rump length of 80 to 200 mm. The duct enters the caudal vena cava with the large left hepatic vein. Lohse and Suter (1977) found that closure of the ductus venosus began within 48 hours after birth. Olivera et al. (1979), in a larger series of pups, confirmed that the ductus venosus began to close at approximately 2 days of age and, by 6 days postpartum, was closed in all pups. The remnant of the ductus venosus is the **ligamentum venosum**.

The **cranial mesenteric vein** (*v. mesenterica cranialis*) is 8 to 10 mm in diameter at its termination. It collects the ileocolic vein, approximately 12 **jejunal** and **ileal veins** (*vv. jejunales et ilei*), which are satellites of the corresponding arteries and, like them, are divided into a proximal and a distal series. There are only primary formative arcades, and these are largest in the middle of the series and smaller at each end. Some of the vasa recta are double as they flank the straight arteries. The most distal ileal vein anastomoses with the ileal branch of the ileocolic vein, whereas the most proximal jejunal vein forms an arcade with the **caudal pancreaticoduodenal vein** (*v. pancreaticoduodenalis caudalis*). The ileocolic vein is the last tributary to enter the cranial mesenteric vein. The **ileocolic vein** (*v. ileocolica*) enters the cranial mesenteric vein after receiving ileal veins, a colic branch, and cecal, right colic, and middle colic veins. **Ileal veins** (*vv. ilei*) and the **cecal vein** (*v. cecalis*) accompany the corresponding arteries. The cecal vein receives ileal branches from the mesenteric and antimesenteric sides of the ileum. The cecal vein passes across the dorsal surface of the initial portion of the ascending colon. The **colic branch** (*ramus colicus*) drains the most proximal right colon. The **right colic vein** (*v. colica dextra*) drains the distal part of the right colon, the adjacent right colic flexure, and the beginning of the transverse colon. The right colic vein anastomoses with the colic tributary of the ileocolic vein by the formation of a weak arcade. The **middle colic vein** (*v. colica media*) enters the ileocolic vein less than 1 cm from its termination. It is formed by the vasa recta from the transverse colon and the proximal and distal anastomotic arcades, which are also partly formed by the right and left colic veins, respectively. Occasionally the right and middle colic veins form a common terminal trunk.

The **caudal mesenteric vein** (*v. mesenterica caudalis*) is not a satellite of the like-named artery. It begins in the pelvic cavity as the **cranial rectal vein** (*v. rectalis cranialis*), which is a satellite of the cranial rectal artery. In the rectal plexus of veins at the pelvic outlet, it anastomoses with the caudal rectal vein, which drains blood into the caval system of veins. The cranial rectal vein continues cranially from the pelvic inlet in the left mesocolon to the place where the cranial rectal artery becomes associated with it. Here it is continued as the **left colic vein** (*v. colica sinistra*) and collects approximately 25 left colic branches, which are satellites of the vasa recta of the left colic artery. Some of these may be double. The last tributary to enter the left colic vein is larger than the others because it collects blood from the left colic flexure as well as from the adjacent middle and left parts of the colon. Its middle colic tributary anastomoses in an arcade with the middle colic vein. At the left colic flexure, the caudal mesenteric vein enters the mesojejunum, in which it crosses the left face of the cranial mesenteric artery and associated structures. It joins the cranial mesenteric vein to the right of the left lobe of the pancreas to contribute to the portal vein. Zahner and Wille (1996) examined the vascular system of the large intestine of the dog and describe a deep and superficial submucosal vascular plexus. Within the plexus the subepithelial capillaries are predominantly fenestrated, whereas the capillaries of the pericryptal areas show a continuous endothelium.

The **splenic vein** (*v. lienalis*) is one-half to two-thirds as large as the cranial mesenteric vein. It is approximately 5 mm in diameter and 1.5 cm long. It is formed at the entrance into the portal vein by the confluence of the smaller caudally running left gastric vein and the larger splenic vein. Yoshioka et al. (1988) have reported on the distinctive characteristics of the splenic vein in the dog. The **left gastric vein** (*v. gastrica sinistra*) is formed by several veins that come from the lesser curvature of the stomach adjacent to the cardia. Like the corresponding artery, it anastomoses with the **right gastric vein**. The splenic vein receives tributaries from the long hilus of the spleen. The **pancreatic veins** (*vv. pancreaticae*) are represented by two tributaries from the left lobe of the pancreas; they may terminate separately in the last 2 cm of the splenic vein. The **left gastroepiploic vein** (*v. gastroepiploica sinistra*) is a satellite of the left gastroepiploic artery; it comes from the greater curvature of the stomach and collects many epiploic tributaries along its course. The splenic vein enters the left side of the portal vein.

The **gastroduodenal vein** (*v. gastroduodenalis*) is 3 to 4 mm in diameter and empties into the right side of the portal vein approximately 1.5 cm from the hilus of the liver. Its chief formative tributary is the **cranial pancreaticoduodenal vein** (*v. pancreaticoduodenalis cranialis*). Its pancreatic and duodenal tributaries begin as small anastomoses with the pancreatic and duodenal parts of the **caudal pancreaticoduodenal vein** (*v. pancreaticoduodenalis caudalis*) near the caudal flexure of the duodenum. At its termination it receives a small tributary from the left lobe of the pancreas. The **right gastroepiploic vein** (*v. gastroepiploica dextra*) and the **right gastric vein** (*v. gastrica dextra*) are satellites of their companion arteries. They sometimes unite before blending with the larger cranial pancreaticoduodenal vein to form the gastroduodenal vein. They anastomose with the left gastroepiploic and left gastric veins, respectively. Vitums (1959b) reexamined the entire extrahepatic part of the portal system, with special attention to the radicles of the portal vein that might be involved in portosystemic communications.

Ursic et al. (2007) examined the distribution of the portal vein and hepatic artery within the liver in 20 dogs. The portal vein consistently divides, on entering the liver, into a small right branch, which is dispersed in the caudate process and right lateral and the right medial lobes, and a large left branch, which courses ventrally and to the left to supply the remainder of the liver. Vitums (1959a) reviewed the literature on portosystemic communications in the dog and made detailed observations on 10 normal dogs with well-injected portal systems. He also studied the azygos vein and its tributaries in 48 normal dogs, and the effect of gradual constriction of the portal vein in 6 dogs. The two major groups of portosystemic anastomoses he found were portoazygos and portocaval communications. The most common types of anastomoses were between the portal vein and the caudal vena cava. Included in this group were gastrophrenic, duodenal, velar omental, left colic, and rectal vein anastomoses. The cardioesophageal and the velar omental venous connections were regarded as the primary emergency pathways that, in case of emergency, might shunt portal blood into the systemic circulation. Additional reports on portacaval shunts can be found in Audell et al. (1974), Barrett et al. (1976), and Payne et al. (1990). This is a very common malformation in many breeds of dogs.

Veins of the Pelvic Limb

Superficial Veins of the Pelvic Limb

The large superficial veins of the pelvic limb, exclusive of the hindpaw, are the lateral saphenous vein and the superficial branch of the deep circumflex iliac vein on the lateral side, and the medial saphenous vein and proximal part of the femoral vein on the medial side. All of these veins, except the deep circumflex iliac vein, are commonly used for venipuncture.

The **lateral saphenous vein** (*v. saphena lateralis*) (Figs. 12.17, 12.19, and 12.20A) begins by collecting its cranial branch from the flexor surface of the tarsus and its caudal

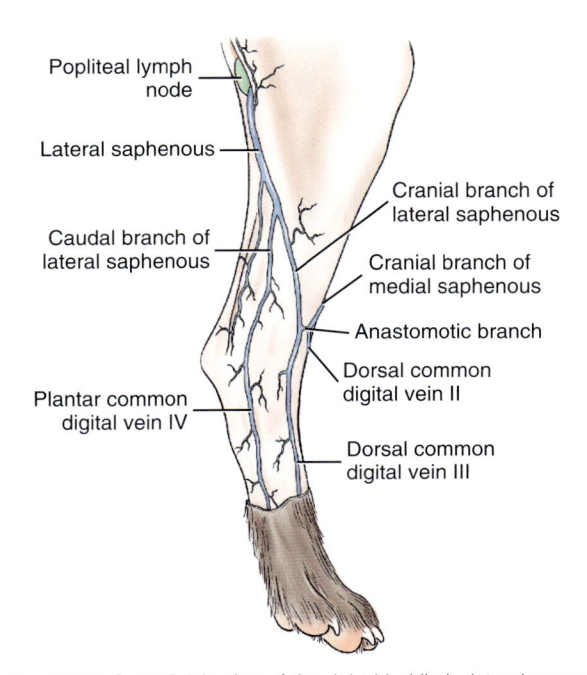

• **Fig. 12.17** Superficial veins of the right hind limb, lateral aspect.

branch from the lateral surface. The **cranial branch** (*ramus cranialis*) is 2 to 4 mm in diameter as it inclines caudally in its proximal course in the distal crus. It obliquely crosses the lateral surface of the distal end of the tibia and is here frequently used for venipuncture. At the space between the deep caudal crural muscles and the beginning of the common calcanean tendon, it receives the smaller **caudal branch** (*ramus caudalis*) and becomes the lateral saphenous vein. This crosses the origin of the common calcanean tendon and receives a small tributary from the skin covering the calcanean tuberosity. The lateral saphenous vein continues its subcutaneous course proximally on the caudal surface of the m. gastrocnemius to the level of the popliteal lymph node caudal to the stifle joint. It runs deep to the node and follows the intermuscular septum between the m. biceps femoris and the m. semitendinosus to terminate in the distal caudal femoral vein in the popliteal fossa.

The **medial saphenous vein** (*v. saphena medialis*) (Figs. 12.18 and 12.19) begins by the confluence of its cranial and caudal branches medial to the stifle joint. The **cranial branch** (*ramus cranialis*), traced from the cranial aspect of the distal crus where it anastomoses with the cranial branch of the lateral saphenous vein, runs proximally across the tibialis cranialis muscle and the tibia. It is approximately 1 mm in diameter. The medial saphenous vein and its main tributaries are satellites of the saphenous artery and its main branches. A prominent **medial genicular vein** from the stifle joint joins the medial saphenous vein proximal to the confluence of the cranial and caudal branches. In most specimens a tributary from the m. gracilis is received by the medial saphenous vein approximately 1 cm before its termination in the femoral vein. It lies deep to the thin but dense medial femoral fascia between the caudal belly of the m. sartorius and the m. gracilis. It is firmly anchored by fascia between these muscles and is a common site for venipuncture. It joins the femoral vein at the apex of the femoral triangle.

The **femoral vein** (*v. femoralis*) (Figs. 12.1, 12.14, 12.18, and 12.19) is accessible for venipuncture as it lies in the femoral triangle. This segment of the vessel is approximately 8 cm long and 5 mm in diameter. It lies caudal to the femoral artery and cranial to the small saphenous nerve. It is sufficiently large and well attached to permit injections without compression.

The **superficial branch** of the **deep circumflex iliac vein** (*v. circumflexa ilium profunda*) drains the caudal half of the dorsal two-thirds of the skin of the abdominal wall and the cranial half of the pelvic region and proximal part of the thigh.

The cutaneous veins of the pelvic limb, exclusive of the hindpaw, are largely tributaries of the superficial veins. However, the skin of the caudal part of the sacropelvic region, the region of the pelvic outlet, and the caudolateral part of the thigh are drained by deeply lying veins. A cutaneous area over the caudal part of the middle gluteal muscle drains into the cranial gluteal vein, whereas a cutaneous tributary that drains into the terminal part of the lateral caudal vein and perineal veins serves the skin of the pelvic outlet. A wide caudolateral zone of skin of the thigh is drained by three or more tributaries of a large vein that descends in the biceps femoris muscle and empties into the terminal part of the lateral saphenous vein. Others are formative tributaries of the caudal and deep femoral veins.

Deep Veins of the Pelvic Limb

The deep veins of the pelvic limb, exclusive of the hindpaw, are largely satellites of the neighboring arteries. The **cranial tibial vein** (*v. tibialis cranialis*) (Fig. 12.19) lies medial to its companion artery, which it approaches in size. It begins on the flexor surface of the tarsus as a continuation of the dorsal pedal vein and its union with the cranial branch of the medial saphenous vein. It receives tributaries from the cranial crural group of muscles mainly at their proximal ends. The cranial tibial vein passes between the tibia and fibula, runs deep to the m. popliteus, and unites with the delicate **caudal tibial vein** (*v. tibialis caudalis*) to form the **popliteal vein** (*v. poplitea*). The popliteal vein (Fig. 12.19) traverses the popliteal notch of the tibia to enter the popliteal fossa. Here it receives a medial and a lateral tributary from the sides of the stifle joint (*vv. genus*). These enter the popliteal vein proximal to the joint. A cluster of veins enters this venous channel at the proximal end of the m. gastrocnemius, where the popliteal vein becomes the femoral vein. The most distal branch of the femoral vein is the **distal caudal femoral vein** (*v. caudalis femoralis distalis*) (Fig. 12.19) that receives tributaries from the distal caudal thigh and proximal caudal crural muscles. The distal caudal femoral vein receives the lateral saphenous vein that is three times larger than any other vein distal to the stifle.

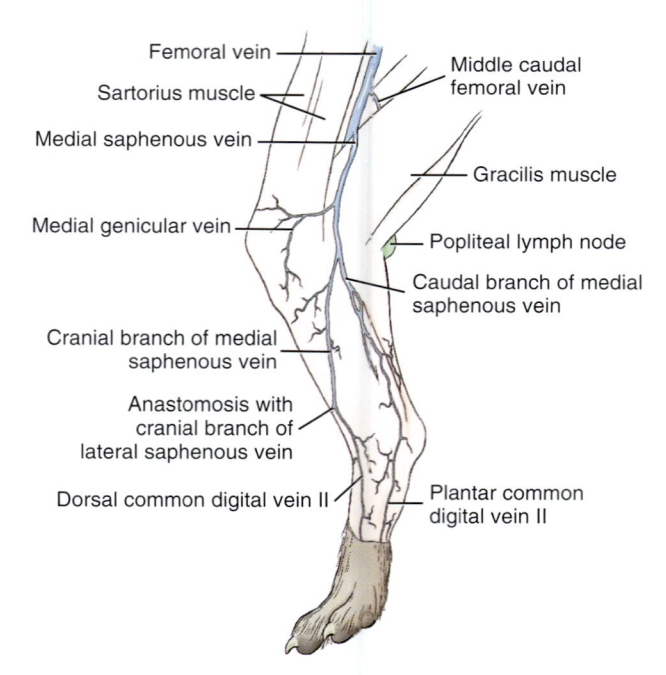

• **Fig. 12.18** Superficial veins of the right hind limb, medial aspect.

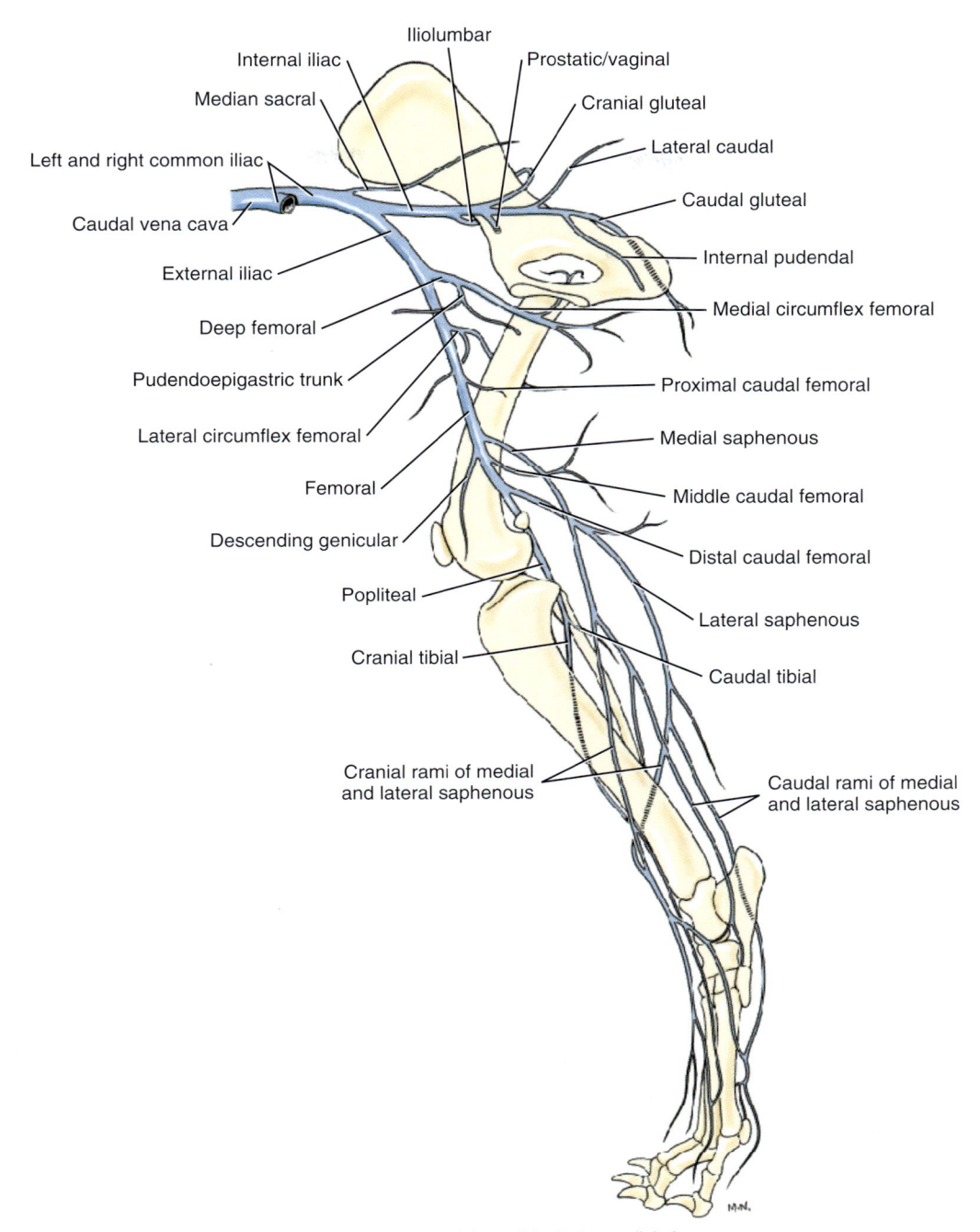

• Fig. 12.19 Veins of the pelvic limb, medial view.

The large **middle caudal femoral vein** (*v. caudalis femoris media*) (Figs. 12.18 and 12.19), 3 mm in diameter, drains the m. biceps femoris. It begins as cutaneous branches from the caudolateral surface of the thigh. Muscular tributaries project proximally to it from the gastrocnemius muscle. Others enter it from cranially and medially from the quadriceps, adductors, and caudal thigh muscles. At the distal end of the femoral triangle, in the vicinity of entry of the medial saphenous vein into it, the femoral vein receives a tributary from the adductor and semimembranosus muscles. In its course through the femoral triangle, the femoral vein receives the **proximal caudal femoral vein** (*v. caudalis femoralis proximalis*) (Fig. 12.19) that is the satellite of the most proximal muscular branch of the femoral artery. This vein arises from the medial surface of the proximal half of the m. gracilis and receives a large tributary from the proximal part of the adductor muscles. Entering the cranial side of the femoral vein, 1 or 2 cm from the abdominal wall, is a long vein that begins in the distal part of the cranial belly of the m. sartorius. It runs proximally on the m. vastus medialis and, after receiving a large tributary from the m. rectus femoris, passes deep to the femoral artery and unites with the **superficial circumflex iliac vein** (*v. circumflexa ilium superficialis*).

602 CHAPTER 12 The Veins

The **lateral circumflex femoral vein** (*v. circumflexa femoris lateralis*) (Figs. 12.19 and 12.20), formerly known as the *cranial femoral vein,* is the largest and the last tributary of the femoral vein, which it enters laterally. As a satellite of the lateral circumflex femoral artery, it begins in the skin of the proximal, lateral surface of the thigh and the adjacent dorsally lying gluteal region. Its formative tributaries cross ventral to the middle gluteal muscle near its insertion, deep to the m. tensor fasciae latae, and then unite and pass the cranial aspect of the neck of the femur and the caudal surface of the origin of the m. rectus femoris to enter the lateral surface of the femoral vein at the vascular lacuna. It may receive the superficial circumflex iliac vein at its termination when this vein does not enter the femoral vein directly.

The femoral vein lies ventromedial to the m. iliopsoas as it passes through the vascular lacuna caudal to the abdominal wall to become the **external iliac vein** (*v. iliaca externa*) (Figs. 12.14 and 12.19). The external iliac vein is approximately 6 mm in diameter and 3 cm long. It arches dorsocranially across the medial surface of the m. iliopsoas and ventral to the promontory of the sacrum and unites with the internal iliac vein to form the **common iliac vein** (*v. iliaca communis*). There are three branches of the external iliac vein, the largest of which is the **deep femoral vein** (*v.*

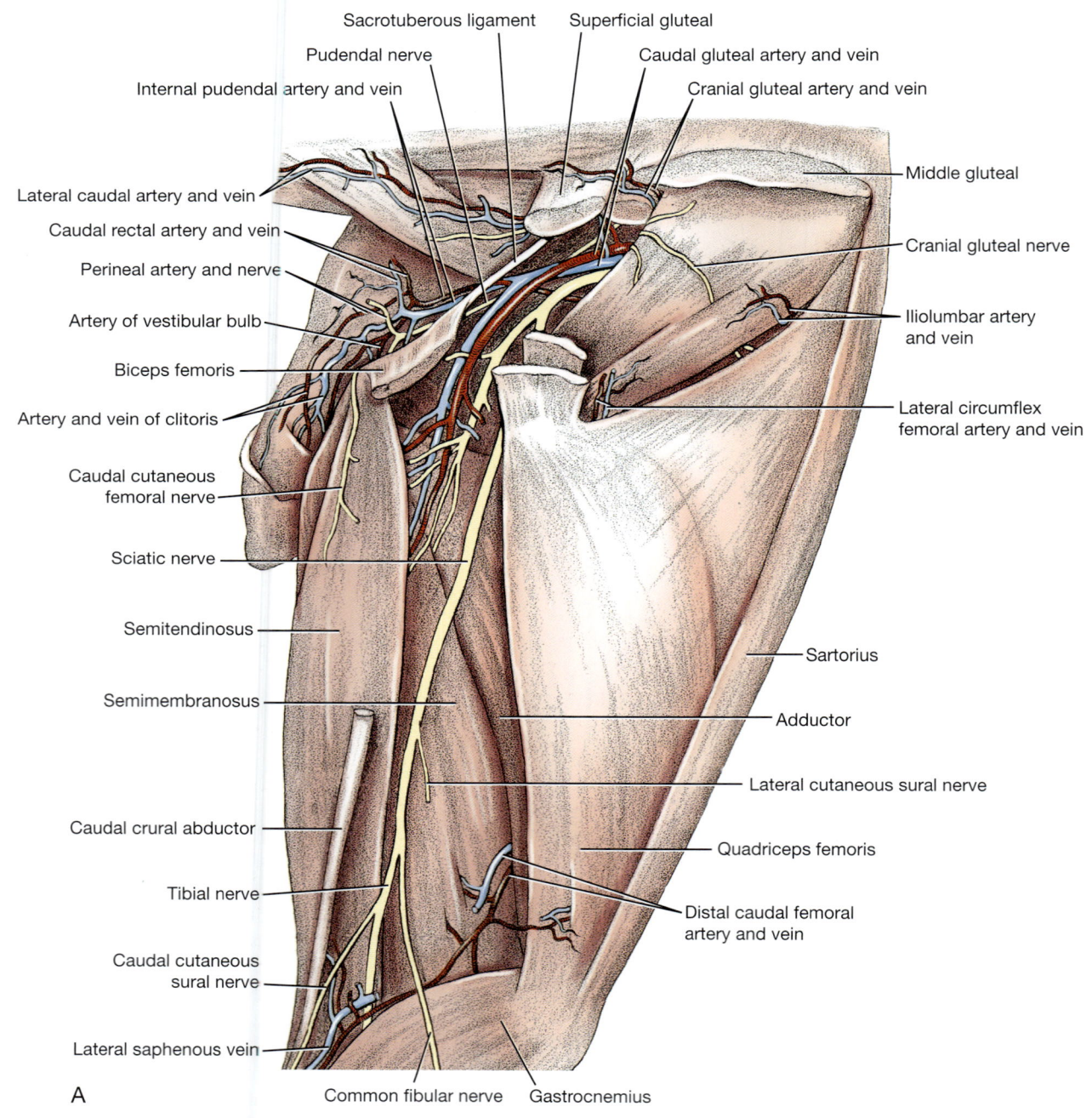

• Fig. 12.20 **A,** Deep structures of the gluteal and femoral regions, lateral aspect.

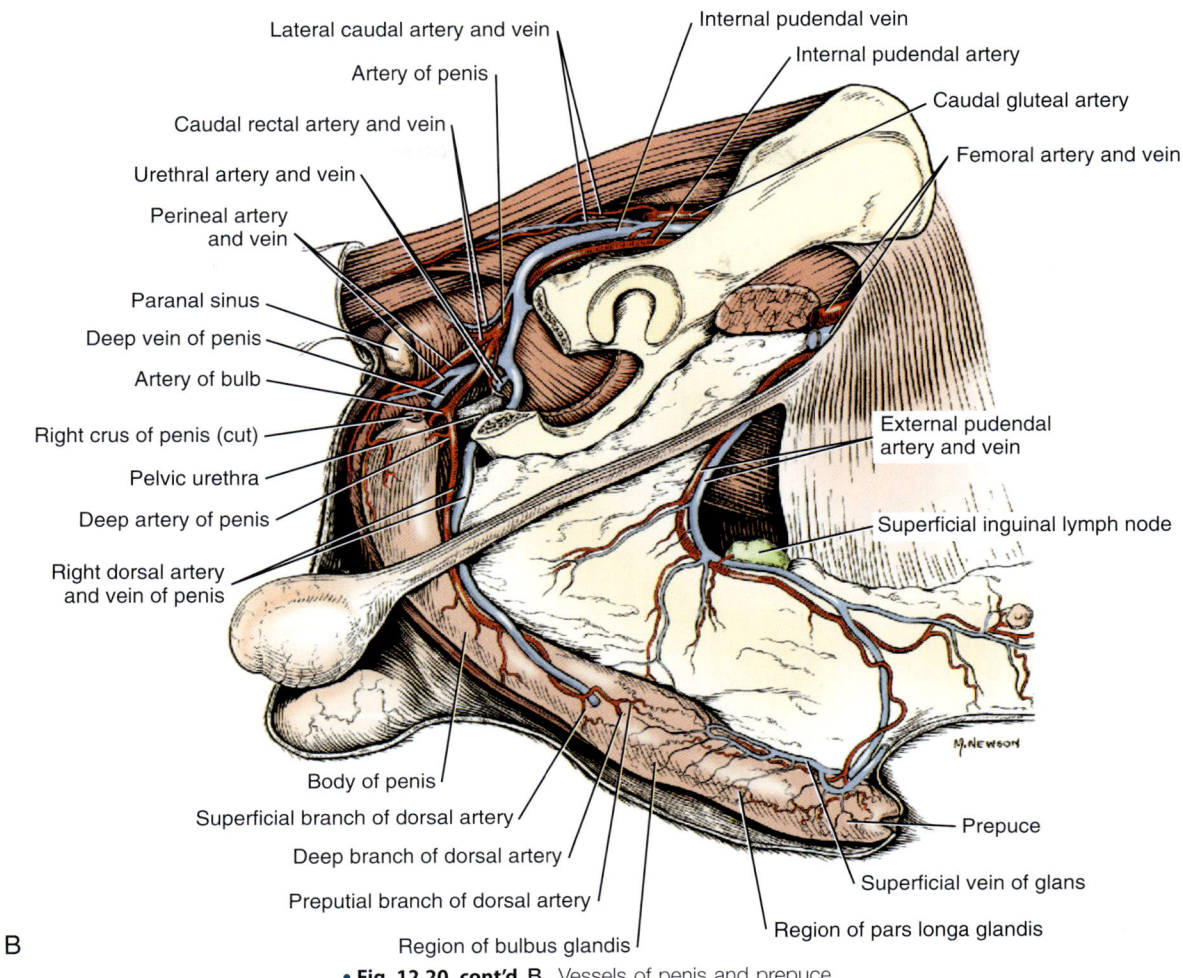

• Fig. 12.20, cont'd B, Vessels of penis and prepuce.

femoris profunda) that enters the caudal side of the external iliac vein on the abdominal side of the vascular lacuna. Its most caudal tributaries, like those of its accompanying artery, are cutaneous branches from the skin of the proximal caudal part of the thigh. These enter the proximal part of the caudal thigh musculature and merge with the large muscular branches of the **medial circumflex femoral vein** (*v. circumflexa femoris medialis*) (Fig. 12.19). The medial circumflex femoral vein emerges from between the m. pectineus medially and the m. iliopsoas laterally where it is continued by the deep femoral vein to the external iliac vein. At its termination the deep femoral vein receives the large **pudendoepigastric vein** (*v. pudendoepigastricus*). This vein is a common trunk for the **caudal epigastric vein** (*v. epigastrica caudalis*) and **external pudendal vein** (*v. pudenda externa*), which follow their satellite arteries. The **caudal abdominal vein** (*v. abdominalis caudalis*) enters the external iliac vein prior to its union with the internal iliac vein and drains the caudal abdominal wall. Two small veins enter the external iliac or deep femoral vein. One enters caudally from the adipose tissue within the pelvic inlet, and the other enters cranially from the m. rectus abdominis.

Veins of the Pelvis

The **internal iliac vein** (*v. iliaca interna*) (Figs. 12.1, 12.14, and 12.19), unlike the internal iliac artery, is not divided into visceral and parietal parts. As a single vein it lies between these two arteries. Its tributaries are satellites of the branches of the two parts of the internal iliac artery. It is formed caudally by the merging of the internal pudendal and caudal gluteal veins.

The **caudal gluteal vein** (*v. glutea caudalis*) (Figs. 12.19 and 12.20) arises mainly in the m. biceps femoris, with smaller tributaries coming from the mm. semimembranosus and semitendinosus. It courses proximally across the greater ischiatic notch lateral to the ischiatic spine and the internal obturator muscle, medial to its companion artery, and caudodorsal to the sciatic nerve. At the pelvic outlet it collects the **dorsal perineal vein** (*v. perinealis dorsalis*) from the proximal perineum and caudal half of the thigh and another branch from the internal obturator muscle. Lateral to the m. coccygeus a branch from the fat of the ischiorectal fossa and the first (with, occasionally, the second) sacral intervertebral vein enter the caudal gluteal vein.

In the male the **internal pudendal vein** (*v. pudenda interna*) (Figs. 12.19 and 12.20) is formed at the root of the penis by the convergence of the **dorsal vein of the penis** (*v. dorsalis penis*) and the **vein of the penis** (*v. penis*). The latter is the common trunk for the **vein of the bulb of the penis** (*v. bulbi penis*) and the **deep vein of the penis** (*v. profunda penis*). These are satellites of the comparable arteries. The vein of the penis usually receives the perineal vein. (For a complete description of the veins of the penis and male perineum, the reader is referred to Chapter 9.) The internal pudendal vein receives the third and sometimes the second sacral intervertebral vein. In the female the vein of the clitoris takes the place of the three veins from the penis.

In the female the **vein of the clitoris** (*v. clitoridis*) is a common trunk for the **vein of the vestibular bulb** (*v. bulbi vestibuli*) and the **deep vein of the clitoris** (*v. profunda clitoridis*) that drains the corpus cavernosum clitoris. The vein of the vestibular bulb is closely associated with the vestibular venous plexus. The **vestibular plexus** is a closely knit venous plexus that completely surrounds the external vulvar opening. It extends approximately 1 cm cranially from the dorsal commissure of the vulva on its dorsal wall. Ventrally it widens to such an extent that it runs proximally on the urethra. This network, the **urethral venous plexus**, surrounds the female urethra and splays out on the neck of the bladder, between the heavy muscular coat and the mucosa. Both the vestibular bulbs and the plexus lie deep to the thick, partly divided constrictor vestibuli muscle. Between the vestibular bulbs ventrally, the vestibular venous plexus reflects the division that occurs in the constrictor vestibuli muscle in such a way that the plexus caudal to the division is thick and annular in nature, whereas that cranial to the division is thin and longitudinal. Opposite the ventral part of the external anal sphincter, the proximal part of the internal pudendal vein or the ventral perineal vein receives the **caudal rectal vein** (*v. rectalis caudalis*), which comes directly from the external anal sphincter, anal sac, and the wall of the anal canal. It anastomoses with the cranial rectal vein via the rectal plexus of veins. Because the cranial rectal vein is indirectly a tributary of the portal vein and the caudal rectal vein is a like tributary of the caudal vena cava, the rectal plexus serves to unite the two systems. The **rectal venous plexus** is poorly developed. It lies on and in the musculature of the rectum just cranial to the anal canal. It is partly covered by the paranal sinuses when these are large. The **ventral perineal vein** (*v. perinealis ventralis*) from the cutaneous anal structures ends in the termination of the internal pudendal vein. The **dorsal scrotal vein** (*v. scrotalis dorsalis*) and **dorsal labial vein** (*v. labialis dorsalis*) usually enter the ventral perineal vein.

The **lateral caudal vein** (*v. caudalis lateralis*) (Fig. 12.20A) is the main venous drainage from the tail. It is approximately 3 mm in diameter at the ischiorectal fossa, through which it runs to enter the internal iliac vein. It receives segmental branches as it runs cranially from the free end of the tail. At the pelvic outlet it receives a large tributary from the skin of the tail and the adjacent part of the pelvic region. It contains valves at intervals of approximately 1 cm.

The **prostatic vein** (*v. prostatica*) of the male is homologous with the **vaginal vein** (*v. vaginalis*) of the female. They were formerly known as the *urogenital veins*. Both veins enter the internal iliac vein at a level cranial to the ventral border of the pelvic inlet.

The prostatic vein originates on the prostate gland and receives tributaries from the **caudal vesicle vein** (*v. vesicalis caudalis*) of the bladder, including ureteral and urethral branches, and from the **vein of the ductus deferens** (*v. ductus deferentis*) as well as from the **middle rectal vein** (*v. rectalis media*).

The vaginal vein originates in the wall of the vagina and receives the **uterine vein** (*v. uterina*), the caudal vesicle vein with a ureteral branch, and the middle rectal vein.

In the female the development of the vaginal vein is directly proportional to the genital activity of the bitch. In late pregnancy and immediately after parturition the uterine tributary is larger than all the others together. In the nongravid bitch the cranial and caudal tributaries are similar to those in the male. The cranial tributary is formed by the caudally running uterine vein, meeting at a right angle with the caudal vesical vein. The caudal ureteral vein ends in the proximal part of the caudal vesical vein. The cranial and caudal ureteral veins anastomose. The caudal vesical vein anastomoses with the cranial vesical vein, if one is present. The uterine vein begins cranially in an anastomosis with the uterine tributary of the ovarian vein. This anastomosis takes place opposite the cranial third of the uterine horn. The main vessel follows the companion artery and therefore lies as much as 3 to 4 cm from the uterus in the mesometrium caudally. There is, however, a smaller venous channel that lies in the uterine wall opposite the attached border of the uterine horn and extends throughout its length. This intramural vein is connected by approximately five communicating veins with the main uterine vein that lies in the mesometrium. From both sides of the uterine wall it receives many tortuous tributaries that anastomose with each other but do not form a definite uterine plexus.

The vaginal vein arises in the submucosa of the wall of the vagina as a fine **vaginal venous plexus**. Unlike the comparable artery, it does not serve the urethra. Caudally it anastomoses with the vestibular plexus of veins.

The prostatic and vaginal veins empty into the medial surface of the internal iliac vein opposite the cranial gluteal vein.

The **cranial gluteal vein** (*v. glutea cranialis*) (Figs. 12.19 and 12.20) is a satellite of the like artery and therefore drains most of the proximal part of the middle gluteal muscle. It usually has a prominent cutaneous tributary that drains the skin over the proximal dorsal part of the pelvic region and also receives the first and occasionally the second sacral intervertebral vein.

The **iliolumbar vein** (*v. iliolumbalis*) (Figs. 12.19 and 12.20) is a satellite of the iliolumbar artery. It crosses the cranial border of the wing of the ilium and drains into the lateral side of the internal iliac vein at its termination. It receives the seventh lumbar intervertebral vein (Worthman, 1956).

The **common iliac vein** (*v. iliaca communis*) (Fig. 12.19) is approximately 8 mm in diameter and 5 cm long. It is formed by the confluence of the external and internal iliac veins on the tendon of the psoas minor muscle approximately 2 cm cranial to its insertion. From their origins the right and left common iliac veins converge and merge, usually ventral to the sixth lumbar vertebra, to form the caudal vena cava. Occasionally, the union of the common iliac veins is unusually far cranial, but this anomaly is more common in the cat than in the dog, according to Darrach (1907) and Huntington and McClure (1920).

The **median sacral vein** (*v. sacralis mediana*) (Figs. 12.14 and 12.19) is the unpaired median vein that receives the middle caudal vein from the tail. It runs cranially between the right and left ventral sacrocaudal muscles and terminates, according to Worthman (1956), in both the right and the left common iliac vein or in only one of them. It is a small vein, approximately 1 mm in diameter, usually devoid of significant tributaries. In one specimen it was large and collected as single short tributaries the first two right and left sacral intervertebral veins and the last pair of lumbar intervertebral veins, after they had united in a common trunk.

Veins of the Hindpaw

The veins of the hindpaw (*pes*) (Figs. 12.17 through 12.19, and 12.21) are divided into a dorsal and a plantar set. In the metatarsus these are further divided into dorsal and plantar common digital veins lying superficially, with dorsal and plantar metatarsal veins lying deeply. Anastomoses occur between the dorsal and plantar series at both the proximal and the distal ends of the intermetatarsal spaces. The veins of the hindpaw in the dog have been described by Preuss (1942).

The **dorsal proper digital veins II, III, IV, and V** (*vv. digitales dorsales propriae*) arise from the axial and abaxial sides of the digits. They arise from the digital venous arches which are located on the abaxial sides of the distal ends of the second phalanges. These digital venous arches are formed by anastomoses between the dorsal and plantar proper digital veins at that level, and these arches receive tributaries from the claws, digital pads, and terminal phalanges. The dorsal proper digital veins also receive anastomoses from the plantar proper digital veins at the level of the metatarsophalangeal joints.

The **dorsal common digital vein III** (*v. digitalis dorsalis communis III*) is formed by the axial dorsal proper digital veins of the third and fourth digits. The **dorsal common digital veins II and IV** (*vv. digitales dorsales communes II et*

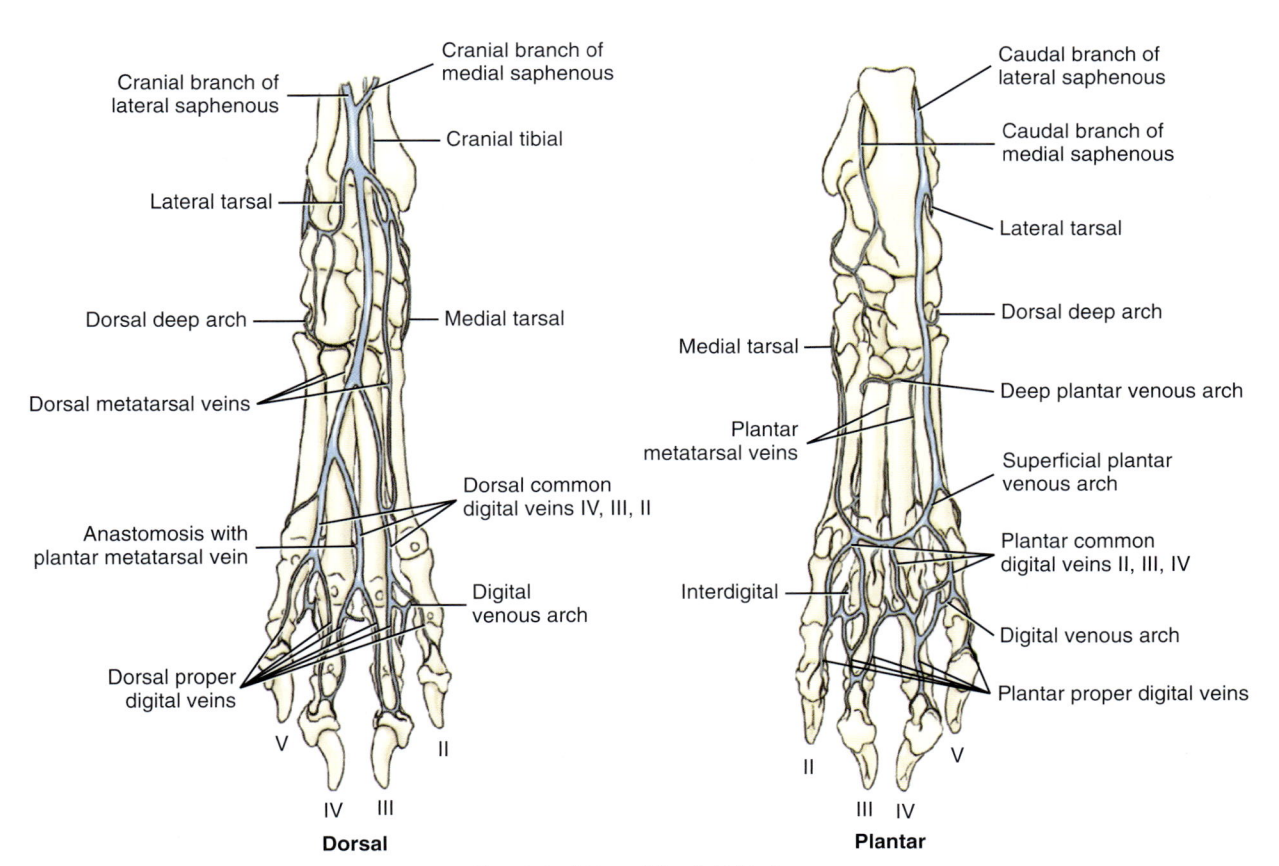

• Fig. 12.21 Veins of the right hindpaw.

IV) are formed by the second and fifth dorsal proper digital veins, which anastomose with the abaxial dorsal branches of the third and fourth dorsal proper digital veins, respectively. The dorsal common digital veins anastomose with the plantar metatarsal veins near the distal ends of the metatarsal bones. The third and fourth dorsal common digital veins anastomose with each other at the middle of the metatarsus, and the resultant common trunk is joined near the proximal end of the metatarsus by the second dorsal common digital vein. The common venous trunk formed by the three dorsal common digital veins is the **cranial branch of the lateral saphenous vein** (*ramus cranialis v. saphenae lateralis*). The cranial branches of the lateral and medial saphenous veins are either confluent or joined by a short anastomosis at the level of the distal end of the tibia. Fig. 12.21 represents confluent saphenous veins. This confluence is also referred to as the **superficial dorsal arch** (*arcus dorsalis superficialis*).

The cranial branch of the lateral saphenous vein continues proximally on the long digital extensor tendon to the distal end of the crus. Opposite the talocrural joint it receives the **lateral tarsal vein** (*v. tarsea lateralis*). The lateral tarsal vein also connects with the caudal branch of the lateral saphenous vein and receives tributaries from the joint capsule, skin, and arcuate vein.

The **dorsal metatarsal veins II, III, and IV** (*vv. metatarseae dorsales II to IV*) are small veins that lie in the grooves between adjacent metatarsal bones. They enter the dorsal deep venous arch proximally. The **dorsal deep venous arch** (*arcus dorsalis profundus*) crosses the dorsal surfaces of the proximal ends of the metatarsal bones where it is formed by small branches of the cranial branches of the medial and lateral saphenous veins. The deep arch receives the threadlike dorsal metatarsal veins and anastomoses with the caudal branch of the lateral saphenous vein and with the more proximal lateral tarsal vein.

The **cranial branch of the medial saphenous vein** (*ramus cranialis*) parallels the tendon of the m. tibialis cranialis as it runs proximally over the flexor surface of the tarsus. On leaving the tarsus, it receives the **medial tarsal vein** (*v. tarsea medialis*) from the plantar surface of the tarsus. At the talocrural joint the cranial branch of the medial saphenous vein receives a long anastomotic branch from the second dorsal common digital vein. It receives an anastomotic branch from the deep plantar venous arch that passes between metatarsal bones II and III.

The plantar set of veins of the hindpaw begins as single or paired **plantar proper digital veins** (*vv. digitales plantares propriae*) and collect tributaries from the digital pads, skin, and terminal phalanges. They connect proximally with the digital venous arches located at the level of the first phalanges. These arches are continued proximally by the plantar common digital veins.

The **plantar common digital veins II to IV** (*vv. digitales plantares communes II to IV*) are short and drain into the **superficial plantar venous arch** (*arcus plantaris superficialis*) that is located distally in the metatarsus. The arch is formed laterally by the large caudal branch of the lateral saphenous vein and medially by a small continuation of the medial tarsal vein proximally with the cranial branch of the medial saphenous vein. The **caudal branch of the lateral saphenous vein** (*ramus caudalis*) passes proximally in the superficial metatarsal fascia along the lateral surface of the metatarsus. At the proximal end of the metatarsus it is joined by the **deep plantar venous arch** (*arcus plantaris profundus*), formed in the proximal metatarsus by the union of the plantar metatarsal veins.

The two or three **plantar metatarsal veins** (*vv. metatarseae plantares II to IV*) are small and lie in the intermetatarsal grooves or on the plantar surface of the third and fourth metatarsal bones. Near the middle of the metatarsus they anastomose with the dorsal common digital veins by passing between the respective metatarsal bones.

The **caudal branch of the medial saphenous vein** (*ramus caudalis*) is the smallest of the main saphenous branches. It begins from the larger medial tarsal vein, distal to the medial malleolus. In the crus it is related to the caudal branch of the saphenous artery and joins the larger cranial branch of the medial saphenous vein opposite the proximal end of the tibia.

The medial and lateral saphenous veins are the main vessels that return blood from the hindpaw. The lateral saphenous vein is appreciably larger than the medial saphenous vein. As its cranial tributary obliquely crosses the distal lateral surface of the tibia, it may be used for venipuncture.

Veins of the Central Nervous System

Venous Sinuses of the Cranial Dura Mater

Within the dura mater, usually between its periosteal (external) and meningeal (internal) layers, and in certain places within large osseous canals, there are venous passages into which drain the veins of the brain and its encasing bone. These passages, known as the **sinuses of the dura mater** (*sinus durae matris*), in the dog are not confined exclusively to the dura mater. By means of these passages the blood is conveyed from the brain and skull to the paired maxillary, internal jugular, and vertebral veins and to the ventral internal vertebral venous plexuses. They lack a tunica media and tunica adventitia in their walls, and they do not have valves in their lumens. They are divided into dorsal and ventral sets, which freely intercommunicate. The dorsal set consists of the unpaired dorsal sagittal and straight sinuses and the paired transverse sinus. The ventral set consists of the double, unpaired intercavernous, and the paired cavernous, sigmoid, basilar, and dorsal and ventral petrosal sinuses. The cranial venous sinuses have been studied in a variety of vertebrates by Hofmann (1901), and in the dog by Zimmermann (1936) and Reinhard et al. (1962). A comparative developmental study of the cranial venous system in man and dog was made by Padget (1957).

The **dorsal sagittal sinus** (*sinus sagittalis dorsalis*) (Figs. 12.22, 12.23, and 12.25) begins by the confluence of the

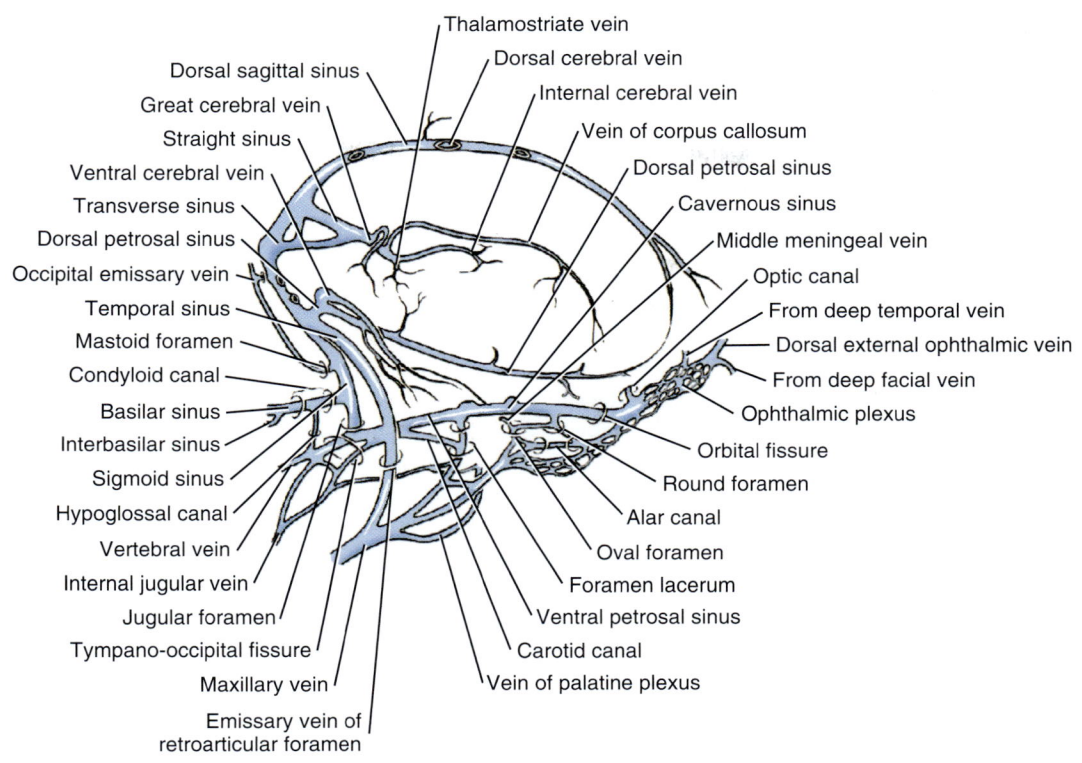

• **Fig. 12.22** Diagram of the cranial venous sinuses, lateral aspect. (From Reinhard KR, Miller ME, Evans HE: The craniovertebral veins and sinuses of the dog, *Am J Anat* 111:67–87, 1962.)

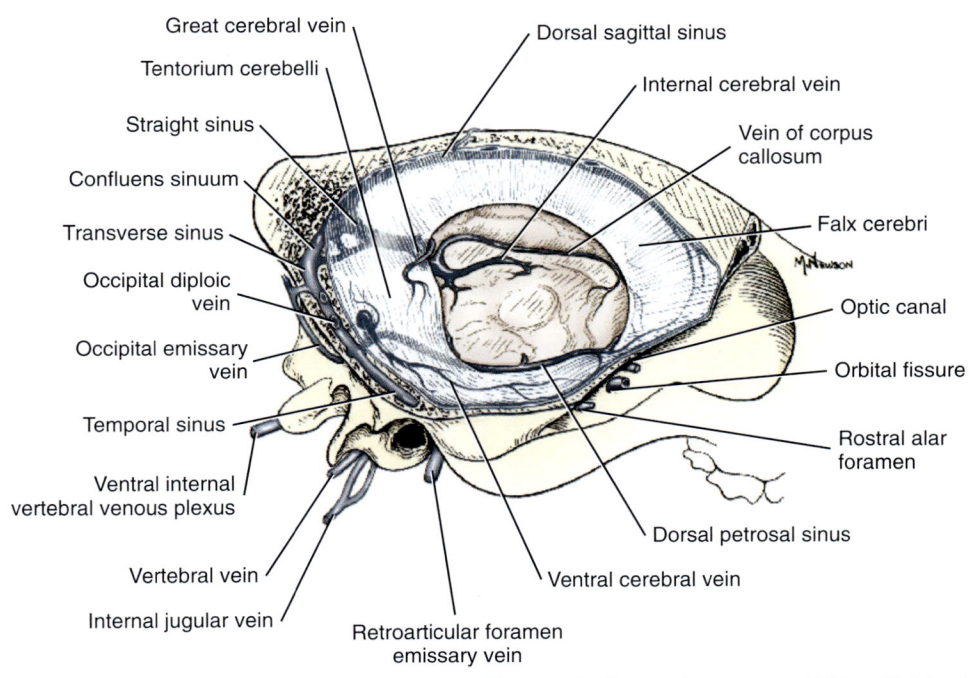

• **Fig. 12.23** Cranial venous sinuses, lateral aspect. (Right cerebral hemisphere removed.) (From Reinhard KR, Miller ME, Evans HE: The craniovertebral veins and sinuses of the dog, *Am J Anat* 111:67–87, 1962.)

right and left veins from the nasal cavity that come from the osseous nasal septum and its covering mucosa, and the olfactory bulbs and their meningeal coverings. From near the middle of the cribriform plate, where the dorsal sagittal sinus is formed, it runs caudally in the attached edge of the falx cerebri. It therefore lies directly ventral to the sagittal suture and the interparietal process of the occipital bone. The dorsal sagittal sinus collects the dorsal cerebral and most of the diploic veins and is usually joined by the straight sinus near its termination. It measures approximately 3 mm in diameter at the foramen for the dorsal sagittal sinus that it traverses to form a junction with the right and left transverse sinuses.

The **straight sinus** (*sinus rectus*) (Figs. 12.22 and 12.23) usually drains into the caudal part of the dorsal sagittal sinus before it enters the foramen for the dorsal sagittal sinus, but it may pursue an independent course through an adjacent accessory foramen and join the confluence of the sinuses within the occipital bone. Another frequent variation is for the dorsal sagittal sinus to bifurcate after the straight sinus has entered it. The straight sinus is approximately 1.5 mm in diameter and 5 mm long. It begins at the free caudal margin of the falx cerebri by the merging of the **great cerebral vein** (*v. cerebri magna*) ventrally and the **vein of the corpus callosum** (*v. corporis callosi*) dorsally. The straight sinus courses through the caudal aspect of the falx cerebri where the right and left parts of the tentorium cerebelli membranaceum join it. It lies rostrodorsal to the tentorium cerebelli osseum.

The **transverse sinus** (*sinus transversus*) (Figs. 12.22 through 12.25) is paired. Each begins mid-dorsally by receiving the dorsal sagittal and occasionally the straight sinuses, and merges with its fellow to form the **confluence of the sinuses** (*confluens sinuum*). This triple or even quadruple merging of sinuses is located within the dorsal part of the occipital bone and may be asymmetric. From the confluens sinuum the transverse sinus runs laterally in the transverse canal for approximately the proximal two-thirds of its length and then continues in the transverse groove. It terminates at the distal end of the transverse groove by dividing into the temporal and sigmoid sinuses. The temporal sinus, larger than the sigmoid sinus, continues in the direction of the transverse sinus through the temporal meatus, whereas the sigmoid sinus bends ventromedially and caudally on its way to the jugular foramen.

Both the transverse and the sigmoid sinus have a connection with the **occipital emissary vein** (*v. emissaria occipitalis*). This vein lies on the caudal surface of the skull and drains blood from the deep muscles on the cranial part of the neck. Right and left veins lie ventral to the ventral nuchal crest as they form a prominent anastomosis with each other dorsally. The occipital emissary vein drains the area supplied by the dorsal part of the occipital artery. The smaller linkage with the transverse sinus occurs lateral to the confluence of the sinuses. The larger connection between this vein and the sinus system passes through the mastoid foramen as it joins the first bend of the sigmoid sinus. The rostral side of the proximal third of the transverse sinus receives an occipital diploic vein, and a second such vessel may enter the sinus as it leaves the transverse canal. The caudally running dorsal petrosal sinus enters the transverse sinus near the ventral end of the transverse groove.

The **temporal sinus** (*sinus temporalis*) (Figs. 12.22 through 12.24) is the rostroventral continuation of the transverse sinus. It lies in the temporal meatus and therefore is placed between the petrous and squamous parts of the temporal bone. It receives no tributaries. At the retroarticular foramen it becomes the emissary vein of the retroarticular foramen (*v. emissaria foraminis retroarticularis*), which, after a course of approximately 1 cm, empties into the maxillary vein as one of its largest tributaries. This emissary vein forms a shallow vertical groove on the caudal side of the retroarticular process. It is joined by a small plexus of veins that lies between the cartilaginous external acoustic meatus and the ventral part of the squamous temporal bone. The plexus receives one or two tributaries from the musculature of the cranial part of the neck.

The **sigmoid sinus** (*sinus sigmoideus*) (Figs. 12.22 and 12.24) is the roughly S-shaped medial and caudoventral continuation from the transverse sinus. It begins by forming

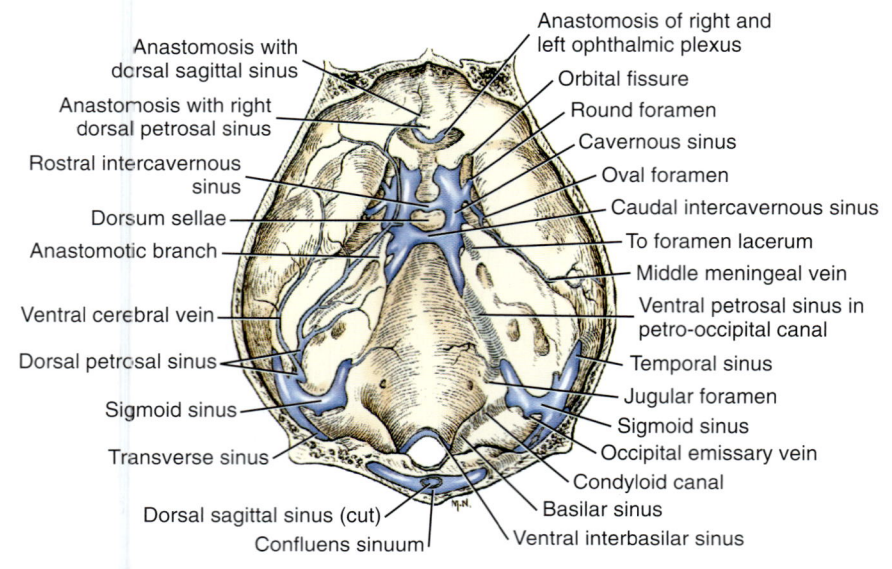

• **Fig. 12.24** Cranial venous sinuses, dorsal aspect. (Calvaria removed.) (From Reinhard KR, Miller ME, Evans HE: The craniovertebral veins and sinuses of the dog, *Am J Anat* 111:67–87, 1962.)

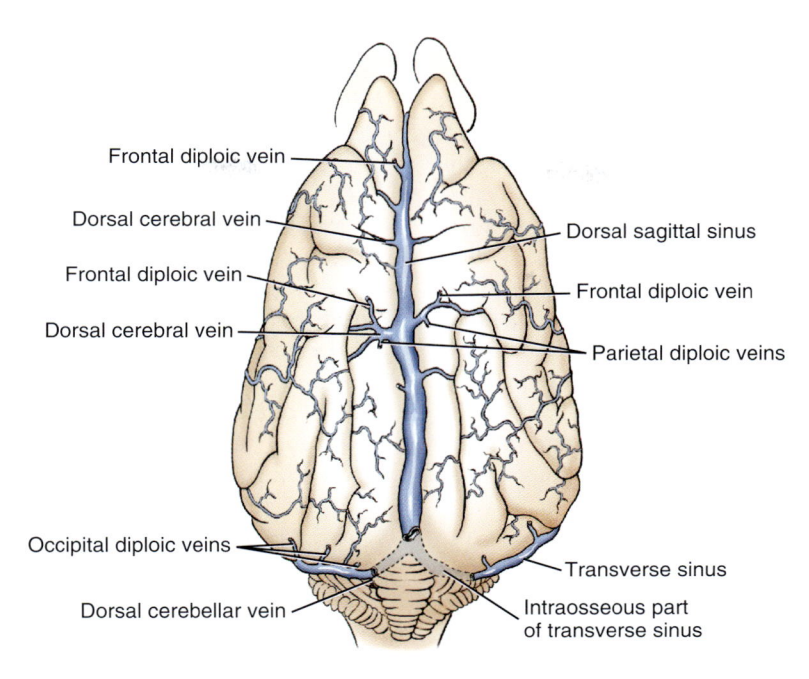

• Fig. 12.25 Veins of the brain, dorsal aspect.

an arc around the caudal end of the petrous portion of the temporal bone. The first arc is continued by the second arc, which lies medial to the vertical portion of the petrooccipital synchondrosis. The sigmoid sinus terminates after traversing the jugular foramen by merging with the ventral petrosal sinus. This merger occurs in the small space between the jugular foramen and the tympanooccipital fissure. It gives rise to the internal jugular vein rostrally and the vertebral vein caudally that emerge from the tympanooccipital fissure. At this merger the ventral petrosal sinus enters from the petrooccipital canal rostrally. The sigmoid sinus receives one or two delicate meningeal veins from the medulla oblongata. Before the sigmoid sinus enters the jugular foramen, a large branch passes though the condyloid canal to emerge as the **basilar sinus** (*sinus basilaris*) that is continued caudally with the ventral internal vertebral venous plexus. Pilcher (1930), by means of dye injections into the dorsal sagittal sinus, demonstrated that the dorsal sagittal, transverse, sigmoid, and basilar sinuses and the vertebral plexus system are the main venous drainage from the brain. Occasionally, there is an osseous canal between the condyloid canal and the hypoglossal canal. This canal conducts the **emissary vein of the hypoglossal canal** (*v. emissaria canalis n. hypoglossi*), which extends from the basilar sinus to the dorsal surface of the initial part of the vertebral vein.

The **dorsal petrosal sinus** (*sinus petrosus dorsalis*) (Figs. 12.22 through 12.24) begins rostroventrally where it anastomoses with the rostral end of the dorsal sagittal sinus. It passes ventrocaudally to the petrosal portion of the temporal bone where it receives a branch from the vein that runs with the trigeminal nerve. It continues caudodorsally along the petrosal crest associated with the free border of the tentorium cerebelli membranaceum. The sinus lies on the lateral surface of the petrosal portion of the temporal bone that it grooves. Approximately 6 mm from its junction with the transverse sinus, it receives the ventral cerebral vein. This vein is 1 mm in diameter and is as large as the sinus it enters. The confluence of the dorsal petrosal and transverse sinuses forms an acute angle ventrally, medial to the temporal meatus.

The **ventral petrosal sinus** (*sinus petrosus ventralis*) (Figs. 12.22 and 12.24) extends between the caudal end of the cavernous sinus and the ventral end of the sigmoid sinus. It lies in the petrooccipital canal and is an intraosseous caudolateral extension of the cavernous sinus. A smaller venous channel, the **emissary vein of the carotid canal** (*v. emissaria canalis carotici*) lies in the laterally adjacent and parallel carotid canal. It connects the same parent sinuses as does the ventral petrosal sinus; this canal contains the internal carotid artery.

The paired **cavernous sinus** (*sinus cavernosus*) (Figs. 12.22 and 12.24) plays a key role in the ventral venation of the brain. The right and left sinuses lie on the respective sides of the floor of the middle cranial fossa and extend from the orbital fissure to the petrooccipital canals. Rostrally each communicates through the orbital fissure with the ophthalmic plexus of veins. Laterally each gives off emissary veins that run through the round and oval foramina and the foramen lacerum to enter the maxillary vein. Caudally each is continued by the ventral petrosal sinus and indirectly is connected with the internal ventral vertebral venous plexus. Laterally the middle meningeal vein, a satellite of the middle meningeal artery, enters the cavernous sinus opposite the round foramen. The two cavernous sinuses are connected medially by means of the large but short rostral and caudal **intercavernous sinuses** (*sinus intercavernosi*), rostral and caudal to the stalk of the dorsum sellae. The expanded dorsal part of the dorsum sellae covers the middle portion of the usually larger rostral intercavernous sinus, which lies directly caudal to the hypophysis. The usually smaller caudal intercavernous sinus runs across the caudal surface of the base of the dorsum sellae and is only approximately 2 mm long. It unites the right and left cavernous sinuses where they lie closest together. This sinus may be absent. A third delicate intercavernous connection may exist rostral to the hypophysis. The cavernous sinus contains, free in its lumen, the internal carotid artery and the anastomotic branches of the middle meningeal and external ophthalmic arteries. The cavernous sinuses contain no trabeculae, but a few stabilizing threads attach to the arteries as they perforate the wall of the sinus (Zimmermann, 1936). The rostral intercavernous sinus contains a small caudal intercarotid artery.

The **basilar sinus** (*sinus basilaris*) (Fig. 12.22) is the venous link between the sigmoid sinus and the internal ventral vertebral venous plexus formerly called the *condyloid vein* or the *ventral occipital sinus*. This sinus is transversely compressed and converges toward the opposite sinus as it lies on the medial surface of the lateral part of the occipital bone. The basilar sinus becomes the **internal ventral vertebral venous plexus** (*plexus vertebralis internus ventralis*) as it leaves the foramen magnum to run across the medial surface of the lateral mass of the atlas. It is always connected to its fellow sinus ventrally by the transversely running, flat ventral interbasilar sinus, and there may be a dorsal connection also. The caudal part of the medulla lies between the right and the left basilar sinuses.

The **ventral interbasilar sinus** (*sinus interbasilaris ventralis*) (Fig. 12.24) is a stout, flat transverse venous passage that connects the right and left basilar sinuses at the foramen magnum. It lies on the floor and adjacent sides of the occipital bone. Its rostral border is irregular, as it apparently sends small, fingerlike processes between the two layers of the dura.

The **dorsal interbasilar sinus** (*sinus interbasilaris dorsalis*) may be absent. It is a dorsal transverse channel or plexus that unites the right and left basilar sinuses. It may be coextensive with the internal ventral vertebral venous plexus, which lies deep to the cranial lip of the arch of the atlas. These plexuses, which are lateral to the junction of the brain stem and spinal cord, might be entered in cisternal puncture at the atlantooccipital joint.

Veins of the Brain

The **veins of the brain** (*venae cerebri*) (Figs. 12.22, 12.23 and 12.25), like the dural sinuses into which they drain, do not contain valves, and their walls contain no muscular coat. They empty into the sinuses in a direction usually opposite to the flow of blood in the sinuses. Those from the cerebral hemispheres may be divided into cortical and central veins. The cortical veins may be divided further into dorsal and ventral cerebral veins. The central veins, which drain into the great cerebral vein, are the corpus callosal, basal, internal cerebral, and thalamostriate veins. The cerebellar veins are divided into dorsal and ventral veins. The veins of the caudal brainstem are the medullary and pontine veins.

The **dorsal cerebral veins** (*vv. cerebri dorsales*) (Figs. 12.22 and 12.25) are paired but are not bilaterally symmetric. All enter the dorsal sagittal sinus. They drain the cortex of nearly the whole cerebrum. Although for the most part they lie in the sulci, they often run across the gyri. From one to four dorsal cerebral veins enter the rostral half of the dorsal sagittal sinus. These come primarily from the cortex of the frontal lobe. Usually the largest and longest dorsal cerebral vein arises in and on the gyri dorsal to the rhinal fissure. It runs over numerous gyri to reach the cruciate sulcus. It collects many tributaries from neighboring gyri and sulci along its course. The last tributary to enter it is the parietal diploic vein just before it enters the dorsal sagittal sinus. One or two small dorsal cerebral veins enter the caudal half of the dorsal sagittal sinus from each hemisphere.

The **ventral cerebral vein** (*v. cerebri ventralis*) (Figs. 12.23 and 12.24) drains most of the cortex of the temporal lobe. One branch arises from the dorsolateral portion of the lobe, and the other branch comes from the piriform area. This branch forms a groove on the lateral surface of the petrosal portion of the temporal bone as it runs dorsocaudally to unite with the more dorsal branch before entering the dorsal petrosal sinus. Sometimes this union is absent, and the branches terminate independently in the dorsal petrosal sinus.

The **great cerebral vein** (*v. cerebri magna*) (Figs. 12.22 and 12.23) is the sole channel for return of venous blood from all the deep or central nuclear veins of the cerebrum. It is an unpaired trunk formed by the confluence of the vein of the corpus callosum located dorsal to the corpus callosum and the paired internal cerebral veins on the dorsal surface of the thalamus. The latter receives the thalamostriate vein from nuclei in the diencephalon and cerebral hemispheres. The great cerebral vein runs caudodorsally in the triangle formed by the cerebral hemispheres and the vermis of the cerebellum. At its termination it receives a tributary from the occipital lobe. Bedford (1934) experimentally produced occlusions of the great cerebral vein in the dog and noted the rapid establishment of a collateral circulation.

The **vein of the corpus callosum** (*v. corporis callosi*) (Figs. 12.22 and 12.23), unpaired, begins by collecting a small tributary from the medial surface of each hemisphere, rostral to the corpus callosum. It runs caudally, dorsal to the corpus callosum, where it is connected to the free margin of the falx cerebri by arachnoid trabeculations. During this course it receives minute tributaries from the medial surfaces of the hemispheres.

The **internal cerebral veins** (*vv. cerebri internae*) (Figs. 12.22 and 12.23) are in the subarachnoid space on the dorsal surface of the thalamus ventral to the corpus callosum. Each vein receives blood from the diencephalon and the dorsal mesencephalon. At the splenium of the corpus callosum it receives the **choroidal vein** (*v. choroidea*), which is a caudal continuation from the choroid plexus of the third ventricle. At necropsy, when the calvaria is reflected caudally to expose the brain, the choroid plexuses of the third ventricle are often removed with the calvaria because of the continuous connection from the choroidal vein to the internal cerebral vein, great cerebral vein and the straight sinus in the falx cerebri. The **thalamostriate vein** (*v. thalamostriata*) is another tributary that enters the caudal end of the internal cerebral vein. It curves from rostral to caudal along the medial border of the caudate nucleus and drains the thalamus medially and corpus striatum laterally. Dorsal to the mesencephalon, right and left vessels anastomose with each other and join the unpaired vein of the corpus callosum. The latter is continued caudally by the great cerebral vein that enters the falx cerebri as the straight sinus.

The cerebellar veins, like the cerebral veins, lie on the pia mater in the subarachnoid space and tend to follow the sulci. They are divided into dorsal and ventral sets.

The **dorsal cerebellar veins** (*vv. cerebelli dorsales*) (Fig. 12.25) are right and left vessels that drain into the right and left transverse sinuses by one or two stems adjacent to the confluence of the sinuses. They arise and lie on either side in the fissure between the two lateral hemispheres and the central vermis. The numerous fine tributaries that enter them lie mostly in the fine sulci between the thin, closely packed folia. Two or more venous threads run across the folia of the vermis from origins in the caudal colliculi.

The **ventral cerebellar veins** (*vv. cerebelli ventrales*) are one or two minute vessels, on each side, that lie between the hemisphere and the medulla. They primarily collect veins from the brainstem including the choroid plexus of the fourth ventricle, but also from the cerebellar hemispheres, and drain into the sigmoid or basilar sinuses.

The **medullary** and **pontine veins** lie on the ventral and lateral surfaces of the medulla oblongata and pons. Those from the pons are transverse, whereas the medullary veins lie lateral to the pyramids. They are approximately 0.2 mm in diameter and lie approximately 4 mm from the basilar artery. They are moderately sinuous and collect many fine branches from each side of the ventral median fissure. The lateral tributaries may also come from a longitudinal vessel that crosses the olive. It receives fine tributaries from the cerebellar hemispheres. The medullary veins empty laterally into the basilar sinuses. The pontine veins, one on each side, arise midventrally and run laterally over the pons or between the pons and the trapezoid body to drain into the sigmoid sinus.

Veins of the Diploë

The **diploic veins** (*vv. diploicae*) (Fig. 12.25) are present only in those places where there is cancellous or spongy bone (diploë) uniting the two tables of the calvarial bones. There are thus no diploic veins in the lateral wall of the cranial cavity, where the two tables are fused, or rostrally, where the two tables of the frontal bone are widely separated to form the frontal paranasal sinuses. The dog has frontal, parietal, and occipital diploic veins.

The **frontal diploic vein** (*v. diploica frontalis*) drains into the angular vein of the eye from the diploë located in the frontal bone caudal to the frontal sinus. It runs rostrolaterally, and leaves the skull by the small foramen to enter the angular vein of the eye ventral to the zygomatic process of the frontal bone. Caudally it anastomoses with either the rostral part of the dorsal sagittal sinus or a large dorsal cerebral vein by a single or a double vessel.

The **parietal diploic vein** (*v. diploica parietalis*) arises in the diploë of the medial part of the parietal bone 1 to 2 cm from the midline by anastomosing with the occipital diploic vein or veins. It terminates in the mid-dorsal part of the dorsal sagittal sinus or in the adjacent large dorsal cerebral vein. When single, it lies in the diploë of the cerebral juga opposite the ectomarginal sulcus. When it is double, the two parts are connected by a dense rete.

The **occipital diploic vein** (*v. diploica occipitalis*) arises from an anastomosis with the parietal diploic vein and enters the transverse sinus approximately 2 cm from the midline. It is frequently double or triple: when it is triple, the second vessel enters the sinus close to the midline, and the third enters the proximal part of the middle third. Zimmermann (1936) illustrates a small diploic vein in the interparietal process that enters the confluence of the sinuses.

Meningeal Veins

The **meningeal veins** lie in and drain the dura mater. The **rostral meningeal vein** is a delicate vessel that begins in the dura covering the frontal lobe. It frequently leaves a faint shallow groove on the cerebral surface of the frontal bone. It perforates the inner table of the frontal bone and joins the frontal diploic vein in the region of the cribriform plate. The **middle meningeal vein** is more extensive in its ramifications within the dura. After the major tributaries converge over the lateral surface of the brain, the vein courses ventrorostrally along the petrous part of the temporal bone. Within the cranium, at the foramen ovale, it joins the emissary vein of the oval foramen that connects the cavernous sinus with the maxillary vein.

Veins of the Spinal Cord and Vertebrae

The vertebral venous system constitutes an alternate route for the return of blood from the body to the heart via anastomoses with rostral systemic veins and the azygos vein, which in effect bypasses the caudal caval system. The ventral internal vertebral venous plexus is in direct communication with the cranial venous sinuses and, because no valves exist in either, blood may flow cranially or caudally, depending on pressure relations. Batson (1940, 1957), in discussing the concept of the vertebral venous system and its active physiologic role, makes reference to anatomic and clinical observations in both humans and animals. Dräger (1937), Worthman (1956), and Reinhard et al. (1962) have

612　CHAPTER 12　The Veins

described and illustrated the vertebral sinuses (now *vertebral venous plexuses*) in the dog. The vertebral venous system is complex and consists of internal and external components. The internal vertebral venous plexus is within the vertebral canal surrounding the spinal cord. Its largest component is the ventral internal vertebral venous plexus. The ventral internal vertebral venous plexus drains laterally via intervertebral veins and dorsally or dorsolaterally through interarcuate branches and ventrally via basivertebral veins. The external vertebral plexus is most developed dorsally.

The **ventral internal vertebral venous plexus** (*plexus vertebralis internus ventralis*) (Figs. 12.26 to 12.28) was formerly called the *sinus vertebrales*. It consists of left and right thin-walled, flattened, valveless vessels that extend from the skull to the caudal vertebrae. They lie on the floor of the vertebral canal covered by epidural fat. As paired trunks coursing through the vertebral canal, they diverge from each other at the intervertebral foramina and approach each other over the vertebral bodies. They are largest in the cervical region. Within the arch of the atlas, where they originate

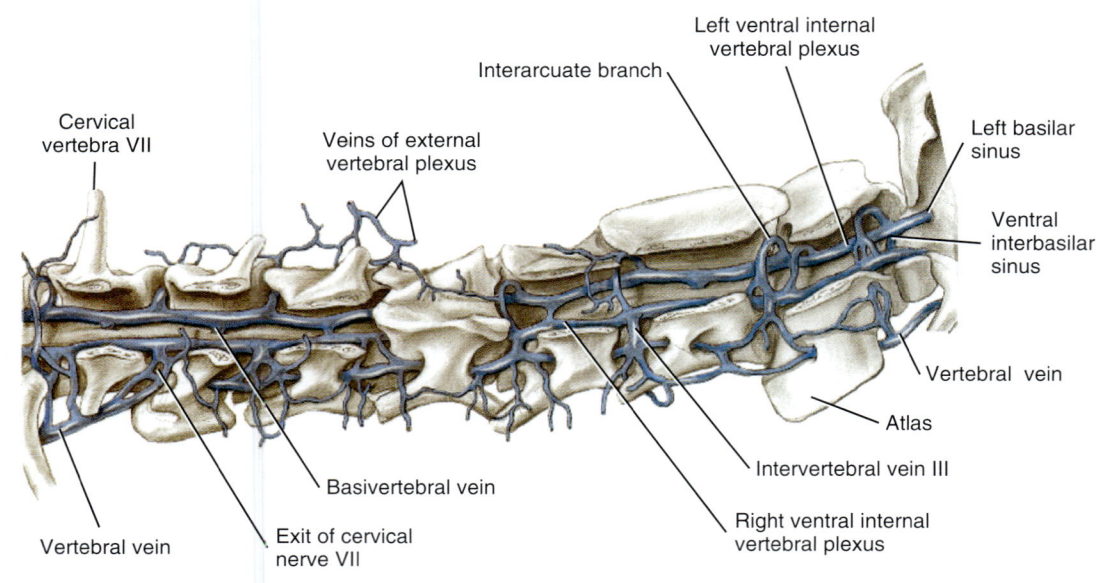

• **Fig. 12.26** Cervical vertebral veins, right lateral aspect. (From Reinhard KR, Miller ME, Evans HE: The craniovertebral veins and sinuses of the dog, *Am J Anat* 111:67–87, 1962.)

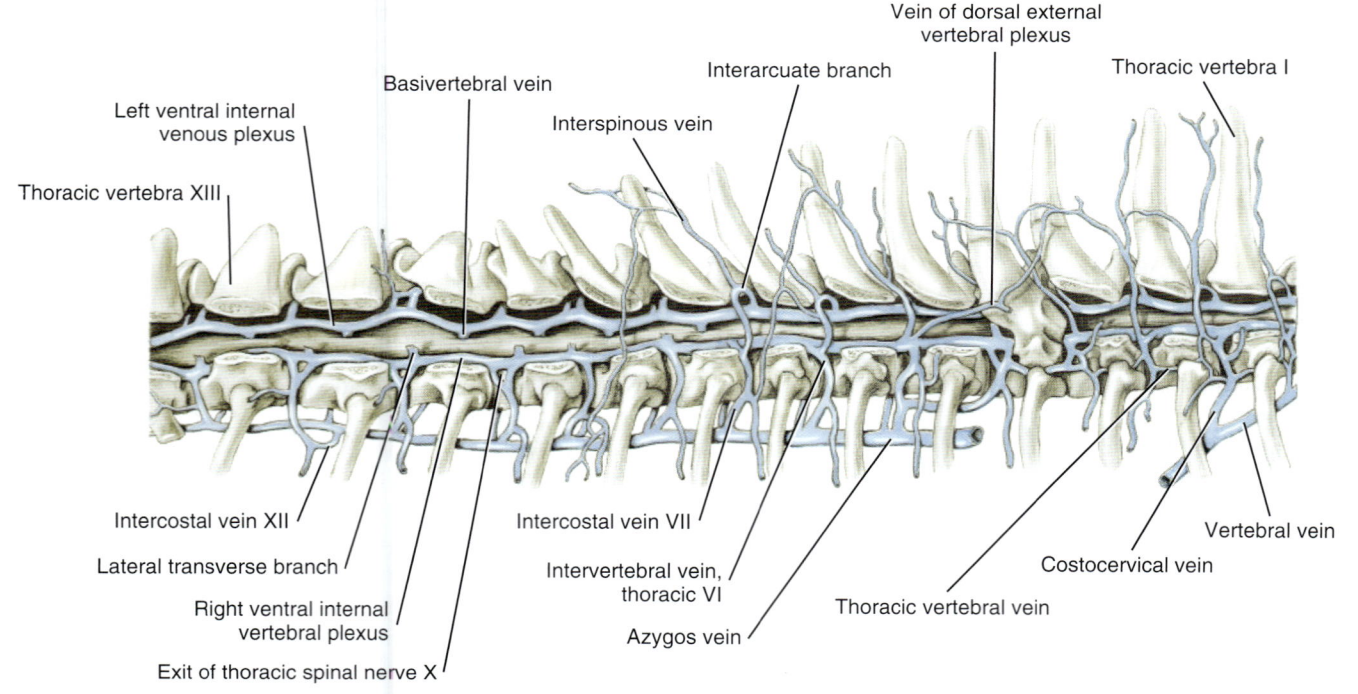

• **Fig. 12.27** Thoracic vertebral veins, right lateral aspect. (From Reinhard KR, Miller ME, Evans HE: The craniovertebral veins and sinuses of the dog, *Am J Anat* 111:67–87, 1962.)

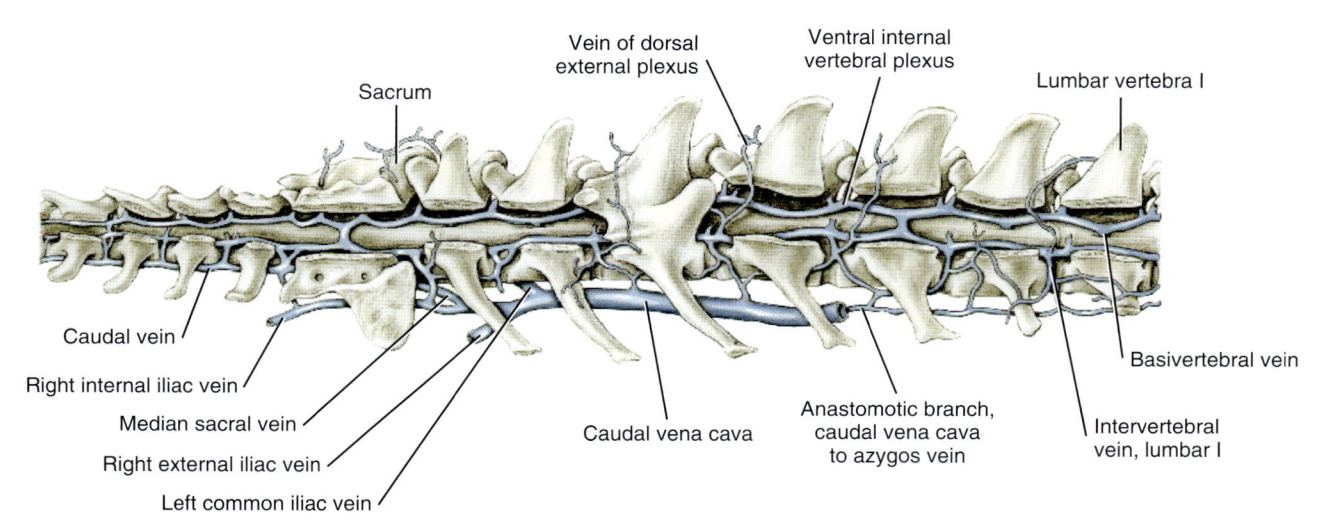

Fig. 12.28 Lumbar, sacral, and caudal vertebral veins, right lateral aspect. (From Reinhard KR, Miller ME, Evans HE: The craniovertebral veins and sinuses of the dog, *Am J Anat* 111:67–87, 1962.)

as continuations of the basilar sinuses, they may appear ampullated (Worthman, 1956). Their diameter is reduced at the junction of the last cervical and first thoracic vertebrae and remains constant from there to the level of the fourth or fifth lumbar vertebra. Caudal to this level the ventral internal venous vertebral plexus vessels decrease in size, and they may fuse within the fourth to sixth caudal vertebrae or terminate as fine venules in the tail musculature. Along the course of this part of the ventral internal vertebral plexus, there are frequent anastomoses between the right and left channels. Some of these anastomoses are superficial, whereas others are ventral to the dorsal longitudinal ligament or within the vertebral body. Within the vertebral canal the ventral internal vertebral venous plexus receives both dorsal and ventral anastomosing tributaries from the spinal cord. It is segmentally drained by the **intervertebral veins** (*vv. intervertebrales*), which follow the nerve roots through the intervertebral foramina on each side. This plexus communicates with the dorsal external vertebral venous plexuses by interarcuate branches that are often incomplete between the fifth and seventh cervical vertebrae, as well as between the ninth thoracic and seventh lumbar vertebrae. The plexus is best developed in the first two cervical segments. At the atlantooccipital joint it is coextensive with the interbasilar and basilar sinuses.

The **basivertebral veins** (*vv. basivertebrales*) are usually paired tributaries that arise within the vertebral bodies or from the soft tissues ventral to the vertebrae or from anastomoses with paravertebral veins. They project dorsally through osseous canals in the vertebral bodies and join the longitudinal ventral internal vertebral venous plexuses. In the cervical region they begin in the ventral external vertebral venous plexuses by an anastomosis with muscular tributaries of the vertebral veins within the longus colli muscle. In some cranial segments of the thoracic region no basivertebral veins are evident; more caudally, single basivertebral veins, at their beginnings, anastomose with intercostal veins. In the lumbar region the basivertebral veins are largest. They are usually paired and connect with the lumbar veins by means of the ventral internal venous plexuses. The sacral and caudal vertebrae usually have no basivertebral veins.

The **intervertebral veins** (*vv. intervertebrales*) are present at every intervertebral foramen, providing communication between the internal vertebral venous plexuses and extravertebral veins. The first few are single on each side, but most are double with one part lying in the caudal and the other in the cranial notch of the contiguous vertebrae. When they are double, the emerging roots of the spinal nerve lie between them, or these roots may be ringed at the intervertebral foramen by dorsal and ventral anastomoses between the double veins. In this way, a venous cushion surrounds the nerve roots at their union. This may include the spinal ganglion. Even when the intervertebral veins are single, they may arise as paired veins. This arrangement is regularly found in the caudal few segments of both the cervical and the thoracic region. The intervertebral veins take the names and numbers of the intervertebral foramina through which they pass, except for the first two sacral intervertebral veins, which pass through the two ventral sacral foramina on each side. They have major extravertebral anastomoses as follows:

Cervical I through VIII, with the vertebral vein

Thoracic I, II, and III, with the costocervical and thoracic vertebral veins

Thoracic IV (left side), approximately 50% with the thoracic vertebral vein

Thoracic IV or V (left side) through left thoracic IX or X, with the azygos vein

Thoracic IX or X (left side) through left thoracic XIII, with the hemiazygos vein

Thoracic IV (right side) through right lumbar III, with the azygos vein

Lumbar IV (V) and V (VI), with the caudal vena cava

Lumbar VI and VII, with the internal iliac vein, the common iliac vein or the caudal vena cava
Lumbar VII with the internal iliac vein
Sacral I (II), with cranial gluteal vein
Sacral II (III), with internal pudendal vein
Caudal I through IV, with the median sacral vein and the internal iliac vein

In the thoracic and lumbar regions the intervertebral veins empty into the intercostal vein before joining the larger channels.

The **interarcuate branches** (*rami interarcuales*) of the internal vertebral venous plexus were called *arcuate veins* by Ellenberger and Baum (1943) and Reinhard et al. (1962). Dräger (1937) and Worthman (1956) called them *interarcuate veins*. As a main contributor to the ventral internal vertebral venous plexus, the interarcuate branches are most prominent in the cervical and thoracic regions. They arise in the epaxial musculature as interspinous veins or veins of the dorsal external vertebral venous plexus. These veins approach the interarcuate spaces, pierce the ligamenta flava, and enter the vertebral canal. Within the vertebral canal the interarcuate branches of the right and left sides frequently join each other dorsally at the apex of the vertebral arch. Longitudinal anastomoses between successive interarcuate branches are also present. The first five pairs of cervical interarcuate branches, of which the third pair is the largest, join the ventral internal vertebral venous plexuses. Those from the fifth cervical to the fifth or sixth thoracic join the intervertebral veins and are lacking between the ninth thoracic and the seventh lumbar vertebrae, and in the caudal region.

The **dorsal external vertebral venous plexus** (*plexus vertebralis externus dorsalis*) is formed by anastomoses between adjacent intervertebral and interspinous veins of the same and of the opposite side, being best developed in the cervical and cranial thoracic regions. Tributaries from superficial and deep epaxial veins also participate in the anastomoses.

The **ventral external vertebral venous plexus** (*plexus vertebralis externus ventralis*) is not very extensive in the dog. Some ventral tributaries of the intervertebral veins are formed by anastomoses ventral to the vertebral bodies. In the cervical and lumbar regions several subvertebral tributaries join to form a long, median vessel that enters an intervertebral vein. Several radicles from the vertebral bodies join the ventral external vertebral venous plexus.

Bibliography

Audell, L., Jönsson, L., & Lannek, B. (1974). Congenital portacaval shunts in the dog. A description of three cases. *Zentralbl Veterinaermed [A]*, *21*, 797–805.

Barrett, R. E., de Lahunta, A., Roenick, W. J., et al. (1976). Four cases of congenital portacaval shunt in the dog. *J Small Anim Pract*, *17*, 71–85.

Barthez, P. Y., Siemens, L. M., & Koblik, P. D. (1996). Azygos continuation of the caudal vena cava in a dog: radiographic and ultrasonographic diagnosis. *Vet Rad Ultras*, *37*(5), 354–356.

Batson, O. V. (1940). The function of the vertebral veins and their role in the spread of metastases. *Ann Surg*, *112*, 138–149.

Batson, O. V. (1957). The vertebral vein system, Caldwell lecture, 1956. *Am J Roentgenol*, *78*, 195–212.

Bedford, T. H. B. (1934). The great vein of Galen and the syndrome of increased intracranial pressure. *Brain*, *57*, 1–24.

Bowsher, D. (1954). A comparative study of the azygos venous system in man, monkey, dog, cat, rat and rabbit. *J Anat*, *88*, 400–407.

Buchanan, J. W. (1963). Persistent left cranial vena cava in dogs: angiocardiography, significance and co-existing anomalies. *J Am Vet Radiol Soc*, *4*, 1–8.

Buergelt, C. D., & Wheaton, L. D. (1970). Dextroaorta, atopic left subclavian artery, and persistent left cephalic vena cava in a dog. *J Am Vet Med Assoc*, *156*, 1026–1029.

Christensen, G. C. (1952). Circulation of blood through the canine kidney. *Am J Vet Res*, *13*, 236–245.

Cornillie, P., & Simoens, P. (2005). Prenatal development of the caudal vena cava in mammals: review of the different theories with special reference to the dog. *Anat Histol Embryol*, *34*(6), 364–372.

Cox, V., Weber, A. F., & de Lima, A. (1991). Left cranial vena cava in a horse. *Anat Histol Embryol*, *20*, 37–43.

Darrach, W. (1907). Variations in the postcava and its tributaries as observed in 605 examples in the domestic cat. *Anat Rec*, *1*, 30–33.

Dräger, K. (1937). Über die sinus columnae vertebralis des hundes und ihre verbindungen zu venen du nachbarschaft. *Morph Jahrb*, *80*, 579–598.

Ellenberger, W., & Baum, H. (1943). *Handbuch der vergleichenden anatomie der haustiere* (ed. 8). Berlin: Springer.

Evans, H. E., & de Lahunta, A. (2017). *Guide to the dissection of the dog* (8th ed.). Philadelphia: Elsevier.

Flint, J. M. (1900). The blood-vessels, angiogenesis, organogenesis, reticulum, and histology of the adrenal. Contributions to the science of medicine. Baltimore, MD: The Johns Hopkins Press.

Franklin, K. J. (1937). *A monograph on veins*. Springfield, IL: Charles C Thomas.

Gomerčič, W. H. (1967). Vena cardinalis sinistra persistens in a dog. *Vet Archiv*, *37*, 307–334.

Gómez, O., Giner, M., & Terrado, J. (2007). Anatomical variations in the cephalic and omobrachial veins in the dog. *Vet J*, *174*(2), 407–409.

Hofmann, M. (1901). Zur vergleichenden anatomie der gehirnund rückenmarksvenen der vertebraten. *Ztschr Morph u Anthropol*, *3*, 239–299.

Huntington, G. S., & McClure, C. F. W. (1920). The development of the veins in the domestic cat (*Felis domestica*) with especial reference (1) to the share taken by the supracardinal veins in the development of the postcava and azygos veins and (2) to the interpretation of the variant conditions of the postcava and its tributaries as found in the adult. *Anat Rec*, *20*, 1–30.

Hutton, P. H. (1969). The presence of a left cranial vena cava in a dog. *Br Vet J*, *125*, xxi–xxii.

Kadletz, M. (1928). Über eine missbildung im bereiche der vena cava caudalis beim hunde. *Ztschr Anat u Entw*, *88*, 385–396.

Kalt, D. J., & Stump, J. E. (1993). Gross anatomy of the canine portal vein. *Anat Hist Embry*, *22*(2), 191–197.

Kazzaz, D., & Shanklin, W. M. (1951). Comparative anatomy of the superficial vessels of the mammalian kidney demonstrated by plastic (vinyl acetate) injection and corrosion. *J Anat*, *85*, 163–165.

Kumar, M. S. A. (2017). *Clinically oriented anatomy of the dog & cat* (2nd ed.). Ronkonkoma, NY: Linus Learning.

Larcher, T., Abadie, J., Roux, F. A., et al. (2006). Persistent left cranial vena cava causing oesophageal obstruction and consequent megaoesophagus in a dog. *J Comp Pathol, 135*(2–3), 150–152.

Lohse, C. L., & Suter, P. F. (1977). Functional closure of the ductus venosus during early postnatal life in the dog. *Am J Vet Res, 38*, 839–844.

Lung, M. A., & Wang, J. C. C. (1989). An anatomical investigation of the nasal venous vascular bed in the dog. *J Anat, 166*, 113–119.

Olivera, M. C., Pinto, P., Silva, E., et al. (1979). Anatomical observations about the closure of the ductus venosus in the dog (*Canis familiaris*). *Anat Anz, 145*, 353–358.

Padget, D. H. (1957). The development of the cranial venous system in man from the viewpoint of comparative anatomy. *Contr to Embryol, 36*, 81–140.

Payne, J. T., Martin, R. A., & Constantinescu, G. M. (1990). The anatomy and embryology of portosystemic shunts in dogs and cats. *Semin Vet Med Surg (Small Anim), 5*, 76–82.

Petit, M. (1929). Les veins superficielles du chien. *Rév Vét et J Méd Vét, 81*, 425–437.

Pilcher, C. (1930). A note on the occipito-vertebral sinus of the dog. *Anat Rec, 44*, 363–367.

Preuss, F. (1942). *Arterien und venen des hinterfusses vom hund, vorzüglich ihre topographie*. Dissertation, Hanover.

Preuss, F. (1954). Gibt es eine v. reflexa? *Tierärztl Umschau, 9*, 388–389.

Reinhard, K. R., Miller, M. E., & Evans, H. E. (1962). The craniovertebral veins and sinuses of the dog. *Am J Anat, 111*, 67–87.

Reis, R. H., & Tepe, P. (1956). Variations in the pattern of renal vessels and their relation to the type of posterior vena cava in the dog (*Canis familiaris*). *Am J Anat, 99*, 1–15.

Schaller, O. (1955). Persistent left vena cava cranialis in domestic mammals especially carnivores. *Z Anat Entwicklungsgesch, 119*, 131–155.

Sekeles, E. (1982). Double cranial vena cava in a cow: a case report and review of the literature. *Zentrabl Veterinaermed [A], 29*, 494–504.

Shepherd, J. T., & Vanhoutte, P. M. (1975). *Veins and their control*. Philadelphia: Saunders.

Simoens, P., De Vos, N. R., & Lauwers, H. (1984). Illustrated anatomical nomenclature of the venous system in the domestic animals. *Gent Mededelingen, 26*, 1–91.

Stoland, O. O., & Latimer, H. B. (1947). A persistent left superior vena cava in the dog. *Trans Kansas Acad Sci, 50*, 84–86.

Stone, E. A., & Stewart, G. J. (1988). Architecture and structure of canine veins with special reference to confluences. *Anat Rec, 222*, 154–163.

Tisdall, P. L., Hunt, G. B., Borg, R. P., & Malik, R. (1997). Anatomy of the ductus venosus in neonatal dogs (canis familiaris). *Anat Hist Embry, 26*(1), 35–38.

Ursic, M., Ravnik, D., Hribernik, M., et al. (2007). Gross anatomy of the portal vein and hepatic artery ramifications in dogs: corrosion study. *Anat Hist Embry, 36*(2), 83–87.

Vitums, A. (1959a). Portal vein in the dog. *Zbl Vet Med, 7*, 723–741.

Vitums, A. (1959b). Portosystemic communications in the dog. *Acta Anat, 39*, 2271–2299.

Worthman, R. P. (1956). The longitudinal vertebral venous sinuses of the dog: i. Anatomy; II. Functional aspects. *Am J Vet Res, 17*, 341–363.

Yoshioka, K., Hayakawa, A., Furuta, T., et al. (1988). Distinctive characteristics of the splenic vein in the dog. Its morphological and pharmacological discontinuities with the portal vein and splenic capsule. *Blood Vessels, 25*, 273–284.

Zahner, M., & Wille, K. H. (1996). Vascular system in the large intestine of the dog (canis lupus f. familiaris). *Anat Histol Embryol, 25*(2), 101–108.

Zimmermann, G. (1936). Uber die dura mater encephali und die sinus der schädelhöhle des hundes. *Ztschr Anat u Entw, 106*, 107–137.

13
The Lymphatic System

Our knowledge of the structure and function of the lymphatic system has increased substantially during recent decades. This is equally true of those aspects of the system that are of practical importance in veterinary medicine. The lymphatic system can be divided into a cellular and a vascular component. Lymphatic tissue found in all organs and lymph nodes represents the cellular component, whereas the vascular component is represented by the lymph vessel and lymph duct systems. The function of lymphatic tissue is drainage of excess tissue fluid and defense. Fixed cells found in lymph nodes, the spleen, the thymus, the tonsils, and aggregated lymph nodules are phagocytic and extract substances foreign to the body from percolating tissue fluid (Fig. 13.1). Furthermore, mobile cells (lymphocytes, monocytes, and plasma cells) that circulate among lymphatic organs, blood, tissue spaces, and the lymph stream are responsible for the immune response of the body. The lymphatic vascular system includes lymph capillaries, lymph vessels, and lymph collecting ducts. For a detailed histologic description of the cells, organs, and vessels of the lymphatic system, see De Wolf-Peeters et al. (2001). Excellent descriptions and depictions of lymph nodes are provided by Boes and Durham (2017).

General Considerations

The lymphatic system serves as an adjunct to the venous part of the circulation. While blood is flowing through the arterial capillary bed, fluid, nutrients, electrolytes, and small proteins escape from it into the tissue spaces. Most of this tissue fluid is reabsorbed into the venous capillaries, but a small amount of a clear, colorless fluid remains. This excess tissue fluid readily enters the lymphatic capillaries as lymph and is returned slowly to the heart and general circulation via lymphatic ducts that enter mainly into the external jugular vein or cranial vena cava. Lymph, like blood, is both fluid and corpuscular. It contains a few red blood cells, some polymorphonuclear cells, and mononuclear cells.

Lymph from each region of the body has a characteristic composition. Garber et al. (1980) have shown that afferent renal hilar lymph contains more lymphoid cells than could be accounted for by random movement of cells from the blood to the lymph. Thus they concluded that lymphoid cells have a preferential pathway from the blood to the lymphatic system and that, in the course of this journey, they undergo a change that is consistent with an active immunologic role. The lymph capillaries in the villi of the intestine absorb and transport emulsified fat or chyle and therefore appear milky. They are known as **lacteals**. Lymph vessels of the liver (Drinker, 1946) carry proteinized lymph to the thoracic duct and, hence, to the blood, thus providing a route for stored or newly formed protein to reach the general circulation. According to Yoffey and Courtice (1956) as much as 50% of the total circulating protein escapes from the blood vessels in the course of a day. This extravascular protein and tissue fluid, which is used in part for cell nutrition, readily enters the lymphatic capillaries, along with foreign particles, if any are present. Blalock et al. (1937) attempted complete blockage of the lymph return in 52 dogs and were apparently successful in three instances. Threefoot (1968) demonstrated lymphaticovenous communications to nearly all veins of the body, but they were most common in the region of the renal veins. Zajac (1972) reported communications between the cisterna chyli and the caudal vena cava. Furthermore, Kagan and Breznock (1979) and Griaznova (1962) created a complete obstruction of the thoracic duct and found that the lymphatic system responded by opening lymphaticovenous anastomoses proximal to the site of obstruction. Anastomoses exist between lymph vessels and veins in several organs (Clark & Clark, 1937), in addition to the main connections at the base of the neck. Pina and Tavares (1980) also demonstrated that the caliber of lymph vessels in the heart increased during the first week after ligation of the superficial veins and decreased thereafter as effective collateral venous drainage was established.

Ontogenesis of the Lymphatic System

Lymph capillaries are simple, transparent endothelial tubes. Huntington (1908, 1910, 1914), McClure (1915), and Kampmeier (1969) reviewed the existing literature and concluded that the lymphatic system arises by confluence of perivenous mesenchymal spaces to form larger spaces, these in turn becoming confluent to form continuous vessels that eventually open into the venous system. The cells lining the spaces at first are undifferentiated mesenchyme but later become flattened to form the endothelium of the lymph vessels. The consecutive development of blood vascular endothelium and lymph vessel endothelium led to the hypothesis that lymph vessel endothelium is derived from neighboring blood vascular endothelium (Sabin, 1911). Töndury and Kubik (1972) suggested that both processes are important in the development of the lymph vessels. First, endothelial buds appear on certain parts of the venous system, and these generally lose their connections with their parent vessel. Second, the lymph vascular system can develop from endothelium-lined perivenous mesenchymal spaces that at first consist of lacunae, which then coalesce and form a secondary link with the venous system. The dual origin of the lymphatic system is supported on the basis of the expression pattern of homeobox transcription factor Prox 1 (Oliver & Harvey, 2002) and by the combination of the expression pattern of Prox 1 and grafting experiments (Wilting et al., 2006). By this means a primitive lymphovascular system develops along all major blood vessels that consist of paired jugular sacs in the neck region, a caudal sac that is made up of paired lumbar sacs and a reticulate iliac part, an inguinal sac that goes to the inguinal region, an unpaired retroperitoneal sac, and a cisterna chyli. The original connections with the veins may be retained as the definitive connections of the adult lymphatic system, or they may disappear entirely or be reestablished later. Except for the cisterna chyli, most sacs do not persist as such in the adult. In mammals the sacs ultimately become primary lymph nodes, whereas secondary nodes develop along the course of the lymph ducts (Yoffey & Courtice, 1956).

The larger lymph collecting vessels are surrounded by smooth muscle and a fibrous adventitia. Although segments of the lymph vessels are contractile, the musculature is poorly organized (Threefoot, 1968). The vessels occasionally exhibit intrinsic pulsations, although the flow of lymph depends mainly on the movement of adjacent muscles.

Lymphatic vessels in specific organs have been shown to be derived from nonvenous cell lineages such that the lymphatic drainage from an organ such as the heart may arise from primordial venous tissues as well as from yolk sac–derived endothelial cells (Semo et al., 2016). It is beyond the scope of this book to detail all of these pathways, but the student should be aware of the complexity of the lymphatic system in terms of origins and function.

Lymph Drainage

Lymph vessels are not necessarily present wherever there are veins. The pattern and distribution of the lymph capillaries and lymph vessels are determined largely by the function of the organ. Baum devoted a large part of his work on the lymphatic system to a systematic description of the lymph drainage of various tissues. For a detailed description of the lymph drainage of the various tissues and organs of the dog, see Baum (1918) (Fig. 13.2). The following is a brief summary of the lymph drainage of various tissues of the body.

Locomotor system: Sparse networks of lymph capillaries are present in the periosteum and endosteum of bone, and lymph capillaries follow the pattern of the Haversian

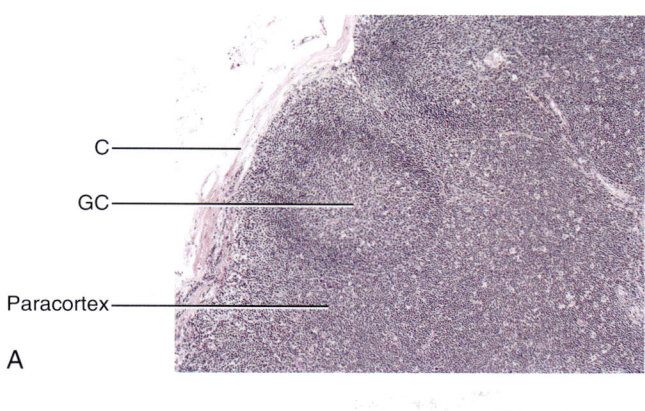

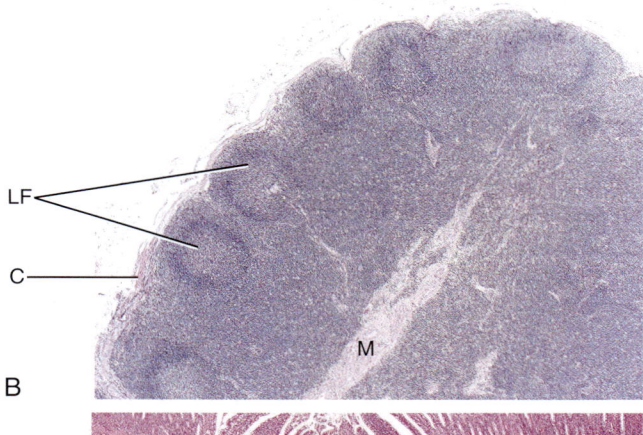

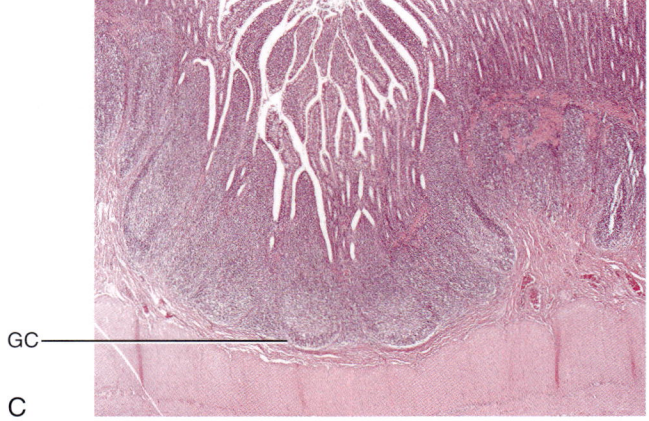

• **Fig. 13.1** Microscopic appearance of two lymphatic structures. **A**, Lymph node illustrating a surface capsule *(C)*, a germinal center or follicle containing lymphocytes *(GC)*, and paracortex *(PC)*. Lymph enters the lymph node via afferent lymphatics through the cortex and exits the lymph node via efferent lymphatics. **B**, Lower magnification view of the same lymph node showing several circular lymph follicles *(LF)* in the cortex and the medulla *(M)*. **C**, Aggregated lymph nodes (Peyer's patch of the canine ileum, also showing a deeply placed germinal center close to the interface of the tunic muscularis and the tunica mucosa.) The internal lumen of the ileum is viewed at the top of this image. There is an abundance of connective tissue (pink) within the Peyer's patch as compared to the lymph node. These aggregated lymph nodes have only efferent lymphatics, and no afferent lymphatics. (Provided by Dr. Andrew Miller, Cornell University)

618 CHAPTER 13 The Lymphatic System

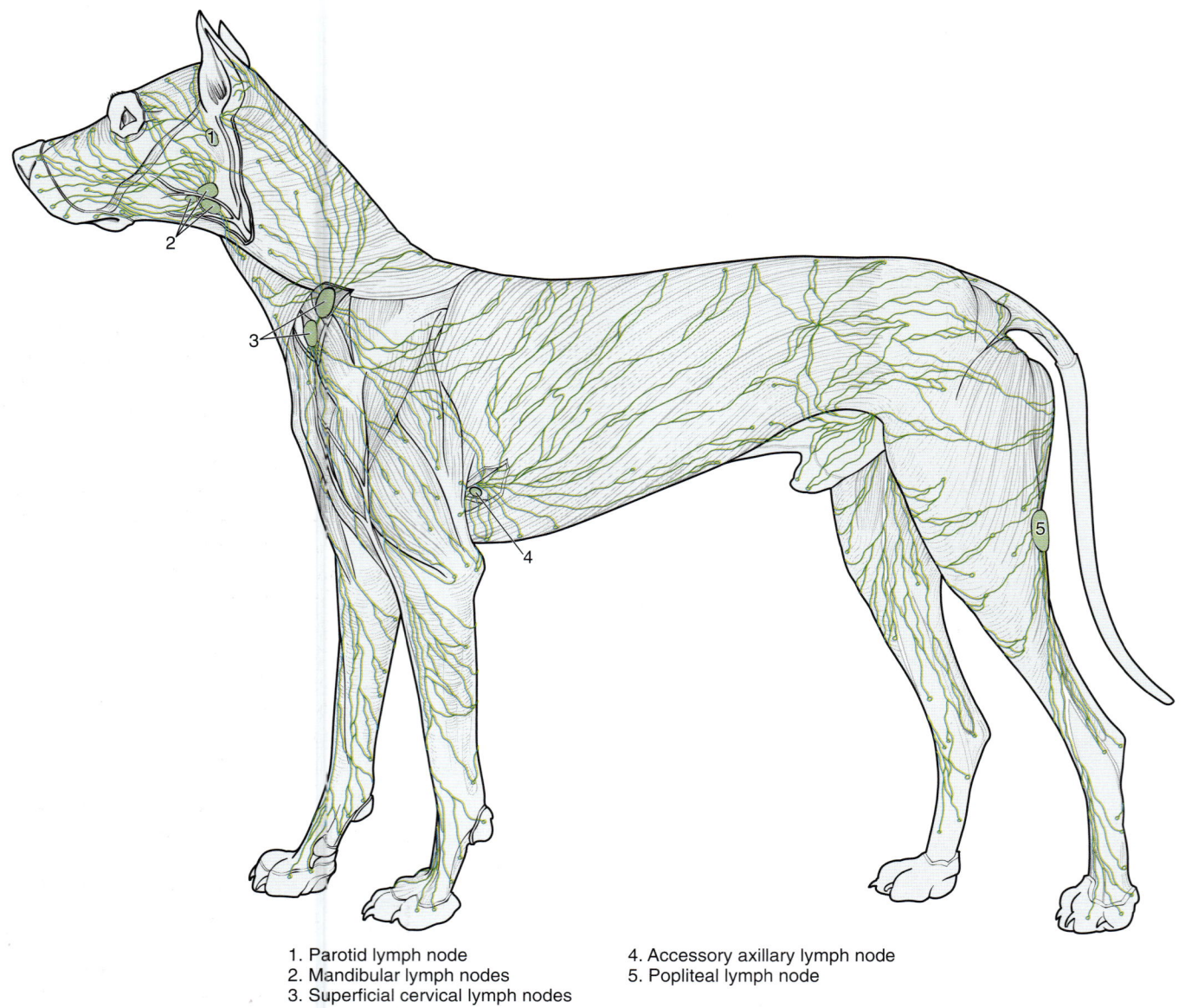

1. Parotid lymph node
2. Mandibular lymph nodes
3. Superficial cervical lymph nodes
4. Accessory axillary lymph node
5. Popliteal lymph node

• **Fig. 13.2** Superficial lymph vessels of the dog showing palpable lymph nodes. (Drawn after Baum, H: Das Lymphgefässystem des Hundes, *Arch wiss prakt Tierheilk Bd* 44:521-650, 1918.)

canals in compact bone. Bone marrow and cartilage do not have lymph capillaries or lymph vessels. Lymph capillaries are present in the endomysium between individual muscle fibers, between tendon fibers, and subsynovially in tendon sheaths and synovial bursae. Yoffey and Courtice (1956) described lymph vessels in the fascial planes between muscles.

Endocrine system: The presence and characteristics of lymph capillaries in the thyroid gland are reviewed by Rienhoff (1931) and Luciano and Koch (1975). Netlike perivascular and capsular plexuses are found in the adrenal gland.

Central nervous system: The central nervous system and the meninges do not have lymph capillaries, although lymph vessels have been described in the perivascular connective tissue of the parenchyma, the intervertebral foramina and epidural fat tissue. Földi et al. (1966) have shown that lymph vessels are present in the substance of the dura mater at the base of the skull and that these vessels have connections to the lymph vessels in the neck. Drainage of cerebrospinal fluid via lymph passages that accompany the olfactory nerves from the nasal cavity, as well as lymph vessels in the perineural and perivascular connective tissue, is of special functional significance.

Skin: The epidermis of skin does not have lymph capillaries, but the dermis has an extensive lymphatic network. The density of the lymphatic network varies from area to area, depending on the amount of mechanical stress exerted on the specific area.

Serous membranes: Serous membranes also have a very rich lymph capillary network that plays an important role in reabsorption of serous fluid from the body cavities. Lymph from the peritoneal cavity drains into the lymph vessels of the diaphragm and from there travels via five different routes (of which the ventral sternal and pulmonary routes are the most important) back to the general circulation (Higgins & Graham, 1929).

Digestive tract: Subserous and submucosal lymph plexuses are present in the digestive tract, although their arrangement is different in the various segments of the digestive tract (Durovičová & Munka, 1974; Hirashima et al., 1984; Tanigawa, 1978; Unthank & Bohlen, 1988; Womack et al., 1988). The lymph capillaries of the liver, pancreas, and salivary glands lie in the perilobular or periacinar interstitial connective tissue. They do not arise within the liver lobules or acini of the pancreas and salivary glands. Pissas (1984) described two different lymph channels draining the pancreas, one draining the left lobe and one draining the right lobe.

Respiratory system: The alveoli of the lungs do not have any lymph capillaries, but peribronchial, perivascular, and subpleural networks are present (Rodrigues-Grande et al., 1983). The lymph vessels of the lung have recently attracted much attention because of their role in the development of lung edema caused by positive end-expiratory pressure and lung damage (Bethune et al., 1979; Drake et al., 1987; Frostell et al., 1987; Haider et al., 1987; Oberdörster et al., 1978; Rodrigues-Grande et al., 1983). On average, half of lung external lymph drainage goes into the right lymph duct and thoracic duct. Furthermore, in experimentally induced pulmonary edema 70% to 100% of lung lymph enters the right lymph duct (Martin et al., 1983; Pieper et al. 1986; Vreim et al., 1977)

Urinary system: Two sets of lymph vessels drain the dog kidney, namely, a smaller capsular and a larger hilar system. Connections between the two systems exist (Holmes et al., 1977). Although earlier workers state that there are no lymph passages in the parenchyma of the renal cortex or medulla, Nordquist et al. (1973) and Eliska (1984) confirmed that the renal cortex contains large numbers of fenestrated lymph capillaries that are distributed among arteries, veins, tubules, and renal corpuscles. Albertine and O'Morchoe (1981) describe four types of lymph vessels in the kidney of the dog. The ureter has lymph vessels in its tunica adventitia, whereas the urinary bladder has submucosal, intermuscular, and subserosal lymph plexuses.

Genital system: In the testis the lymph capillaries begin in the septa, from where they pass either to the tunica albuginea or to the rete testis. In the ovary the lymph capillaries arise below the tunica albuginea and pass into the parenchyma surrounding the follicles and corpora lutea. Mucosal and subserosal lymph plexuses of the uterine tubes and uterus are linked to each other by lymph capillaries in the myometrium. The fetal membranes of the placenta do not have any lymph capillaries. The lymph drainage of the mammary glands is discussed later in this chapter in the section titled "Lymph Nodes and Vessels of the Genital Organs."

Circulatory system: Subendocardial, myocardial, and subepicardial lymph capillary plexuses drain the heart (Eliska & Elišková, 1980; Elišková & Eliska, 1974; Kerestanová & Slezák, 1983; Schmidtova et al., 1974; Shimada et al., 1989), and lymph from the pericardial space drains into the coronary lymph vessels (Miller et al., 1988). Eliska et al. (1999) found that the coronary arteries are drained by adventitial lymph vessels that do not penetrate to the tunica media and via periadventitial lymph vessels consisting of a subepicardial lymph plexus overlying the arteries. Smaller arterioles in the ventricular muscle have many more accompanying lymph vessels than do epicardial coronary arteries. The parietal pericardium has a complicated network of lymph vessels that is different from the lymph vessels that drain the pericardial cavity (Elišková et al. 1994). The dorsal area of the pericardium drains directly into cranial mediastinal lymph nodes; the cranial and lateral areas drain into lymph vessels that pass cranially and caudally along the phrenic nerves. Those that pass cranially drain into cranial mediastinal lymph nodes. Those that pass caudally drain to the lymph vessels from the area of the diaphragm.

The pulp of the spleen does not have lymph vessels, although lymph capillaries and lymph vessels are present in the trabeculae and capsule. Lymph capillaries surround thymic (Hassall) corpuscles in the thymus, whereas lymph vessels are present in the capsular, interlobar, and perivascular connective tissue.

Lymph Vessels

The large **lymph vessels** (*vasa lymphatica*) have walls thinner than those of similar sized veins but contain more valves. (For a comparison of the viscoelastic properties of the walls and functional characteristics of the valves in lymph vessels and veins, see Ohhashi [1987].) Furthermore, central and peripheral lymph vessels have subsurface and surface morphologic features distinct from either arteries or veins (Gnepp & Green, 1979). When the flow of lymph is obstructed, the vessels become distended, and, owing to constrictions at the valves, they often resemble a string of beads in appearance. (For a discussion of the structure of lymph vessels and their valves see Gnepp and Green [1980], Albertine et al. [1982], and Todd and Bernard [1974].) Blockage of lymph vessels results in an accumulation of tissue fluid and consequent swelling, known as lymphedema. Lymph vessels, when cut, remain open longer than do comparable blood vessels, but they have remarkable regenerative capacities (Danese et al., 1962; Reichert, 1926). Reichert (1926) found that the lymph vessels of the thigh of the dog regenerated rapidly after being transected. The cutaneous lymph vessels began to regenerate after 4 days, and the deep lymph vessels after 8 days. Meyer (1906), however, found no regeneration after ligating and resecting 3 to 5 mm of the large lymph trunks in the pelvic limb of the dog.

Because lymph vessels contain numerous valves, they are difficult to inject in a retrograde direction. The valves are usually bicuspid, although occasional tricuspid and monocuspid valves are found (Albertine et al., 1982). They may best be observed by producing congestion after ligation, by injecting dye particles peripherally, or in edematous tissue. Prier et al. (1962) and Kagan and Breznock (1979) performed direct lymphangiography in the dog, using a radiopaque medium injected into the metatarsal and intestinal lymph vessels, respectively. Mulshine et al. (1987) developed an immunolymphoscintigraphic technique to study pulmonary and mediastinal lymph nodes as a new approach to lung cancer images. Clinical applications of lymphography include identification of lymph node lesions, evaluation of lymph vessel blockage, and visualization of the progress of therapy on lymphatic lesions (Fischer, 1959; Fischer & Zimmerman, 1959; Skelley et al., 1964; Suter, 1969).

Research on the anatomy and physiology of the lymphatic system has resulted in a considerable body of knowledge, although many questions remain unanswered. Drinker (1942) commented on the observations of Gaspar Asellius (1581–1626) and of Pecquet (in 1651) on the lymph vessels and nodes in the dog. Asellius described and illustrated the mesenteric lacteals and mesenteric lymph node ("pancreas of Aselli"); Pecquet described the receptaculum chyli ("cistern of Pecquet") and the thoracic duct, including its termination. Rusznyak et al. (1967) credit Rudbeck (1652) and Bartholinus (1653) for having recognized the lymphatic system as an entity. The English edition of the monograph on lymph vessels and lymph circulation by Rusznyak, Földi, and Szabo (1967), revised and enlarged from the Hungarian, German, and Russian editions, contains an extensive bibliography (more than 1700 citations). Frequent reference is also made therein to the morphologic features and experimental physiologic characteristics of the lymphatic system in the dog. Chretien et al. (1967) described the distribution of lymph nodes in the dog and discussed the effects of surgical excision of the thymus, spleen, and all gross lymph nodes on the survival of skin allografts. They injected Pontamine Blue intravenously 3 or more days prior to dissection and found that all lymphoid tissue was stained a deep blue. Excision of lymphoid tissue did not significantly alter the allograft response.

A classic topographic description of the lymph nodes and vessels in the dog was written by Hermann Baum in 1918. Most of the illustrations used in this chapter have been reproduced or redrawn from that work, *Das Lymphgefässystem des Hundes*, through the kind permission of Springer-Verlag, Berlin. Others have provided "lymphosomes" to map the superficial lymphatic system and drainage pathways that may be applicable to therapy following damage to major lymph flow following surgery in canine models (Suami et al., 2013). The homologic characteristics of the lymphatic system of the dog and other domestic animals is discussed by, among others, Wilkens and Munster (1972) and Spira (1962), and Shdanow (1962) attempts to answer some of the contentious questions of his time on the functional morphology of the lymphatic system. The terminology of the present text conforms to the *Nomina Anatomica Veterinaria* (2017).

Innervation of Lymph Vessels and Lymph Nodes

The innervation of lymph nodes and lymph vessels is well established. (For a review see Vajda [1966].) In addition to the findings of earlier works, Vajda (1966) established that the adventitia of lymph vessels is supplied by large-caliber, myelinated axons; that the muscular coat is supplied by a circular plexus of unmyelinated axons; and that lymph capillaries lack a nerve supply. However, Todd and Bernard (1974) could demonstrate only a loose network of sympathetic axons in the adventitia of the thoracic duct. In a study on the effect of vasoactive agents on hemorrhage, Dobbins et al. (1986) and Dabney et al. (1988) found that lymphatic pressure was significantly increased following hemorrhage, carotid occlusion, or the injection of vasoactive agents. This indicated that prenodal lymph vessels actively constrict in response to the neural or hormonal consequences of hemorrhage on lymph vessels or to the introduction of vasoactive substances, and that lymphatic function is subject to neural or hormonal regulation. Volik (1962) studied the inguinal lymph nodes and found that they were innervated by sympathetic and somatic axons. The central nervous system can modulate the immune response through the sympathetic and sensory innervation of lymphoid organs. Results of a study by Popper et al. (1988) indicate that sympathetic and sensory innervation of lymph nodes is involved with the regulation of their blood and lymph flow and that the neuropeptide receptor binding sites in lymph node germinal centers may be expressed by lymphocytes on activation by antigens. The effect of hormonal control over lymph nodes was also demonstrated by Korovina (1985), who states that extirpation of the pancreas resulted in progressive involution of the immunocompetent tissue in the inguinal lymph nodes.

Lymphoid Tissue

Lymphoid tissue is present in all classes of vertebrates but reaches its highest development in mammals. Bryant (1975) used lymph node structure as an ontogenic explanation of divergence in *Eutheria*, *Metatheria*, and *Prototheria*. Under normal physiologic conditions lymphocyte accumulations occur in the lamina propria of mucous membranes of the digestive, respiratory, and urogenital tracts. Spherical lymphoid colonies are known as **lymph nodules** (*nodulus lymphaticus*) and are seen only in specific pathogen-free and newborn animals. On exposure to foreign substances, the **primary nodules** (*nodulus primarius*) change into **secondary nodules** (*nodulus secondarius*) characterized by reaction centers. Some secondary nodules lying in the lamina propria of the mucosa and extending into the submucosa are known as **solitary nodules** (*nodulus lymphaticus solitarius*). They occur in the digestive, respiratory, and urogenital tracts as well as in the conjunctiva and in the mucous membranes of all natural body orifices. Secondary nodules in the intestine also occur as large, connected accumulations and are then known as **aggregated lymph nodules** (*noduli lymphatici aggregati*) or Peyer's patches. In the spleen, thymus, lymph nodes, hemal nodes, and tonsils the lymph nodules develop into circumscribed organs. Lymphocytes are produced mainly by hematopoietic tissue of bone marrow. Yoffey and Courtice (1956) estimate that the total amount of lymphoid tissue in the mammalian body is approximately 1% of the body mass. The proportional distribution and form of the lymphoid tissue in the various species of mammals vary greatly. The dog has but one or two large nodes at each nodal station.

Lymph Nodes

Lymph nodes (*lymphonodi*) are always located in the course of lymph vessels. The vessels that enter the node are known as **afferent lymph vessels** (*vasa lymphatica afferentia*). They break up into many minute vessels before perforating the capsule of the lymph node. After passing through subcapsular, cortical, and medullary lymph spaces or sinuses within the lymph node, they unite and leave the lymph node at the hilus as one or more **efferent lymph vessels** (*vasa lymphatica efferentia*). Probably all lymph vessels pass through at least one lymph node (Yoffey & Courtice, 1956). Some pass through several lymph nodes. The lymph vessels therefore form portal systems comparable to the venous portal system of the mammalian liver and the arterial portal system of the kidney in lower vertebrates.

Certain lymphoid organs have only efferent lymph vessels. Examples of these are the tonsillar masses of the pharynx and the solitary and aggregated lymph nodules in the mucous membrane of the digestive system. The spleen, thymus, and bone marrow are interposed not in the lymphatic system but rather in the blood vascular system. Lymphoid tissue, wherever found, probably reaches its greatest development at sexual maturity. Endocrine and sex differences affect lymphoid tissue. Although Korovina (1985) has shown that the inguinal lymph nodes undergo involution after extirpation of the pancreas, investigators are not in agreement about the effects of endocrine and sex differences on lymphoid tissue (Yoffey & Courtice, 1956).

The **lymph node** (*lymphonodus*) is the structural and functional unit of the lymphatic system. It serves two important functions. It acts as a filter of the lymph and as a germinal center for lymphocytes. Lymph nodes are located in the places where they are afforded maximum protection yet produce minimal interference with the functioning of the skeletal, muscular, and blood vascular systems. They are thus found in the adipose tissue at the flexor angles of joints, in the mediastinum and mesentery, and in the angles formed by the origin of many of the larger blood vessels. Each lymph node consists of a capsule containing elastic and smooth muscle fibers and an internal framework consisting of septa and trabeculae. There is a convex surface and a small flat or concave area, the **hilus**, which is usually not prominent. Internally the node contains a poorly defined **cortex** and **medulla**. The structural unit of the lymph node is the secondary lymph nodule. Each nodule contains light-colored central areas (germinal centers). Most nodules are located in the cortex, where they are partly surrounded by subcapsular and cortical lymph sinuses. The lymphoid tissue of the medulla is in the form of anastomosing cords of lymphocytes with few lymph nodules.

Hemal Nodes

Hemal nodes (*lymphonodus hemalis*) differ from lymph nodes in that their sinuses do not contain lymph, but blood. The occurrence of true hemal nodes in the dog is quite rare. Fitzgerald (1961) described three hemal nodes in the root of the mesentery of a Greyhound.

Lymph Nodules

Solitary and aggregated lymph nodules are found mainly in the wall of the digestive tube. They differ from lymph nodes in that lymph vessels arise in, rather than pass through them; thus, they contain only efferent lymph vessels. These aggregated lymph nodules, or Peyer's patches, originate in the lamina propria, extend into the submucosa, and are often seen in the ileum (Ross & Pawlina, 2016). Lymph nodules of the large intestine can be seen clearly in the cadaver under proper lighting conditions if the intestine is inflated. The various tonsils and the aggregated lymph nodules are described with the digestive system.

The solitary and small aggregated lymph nodules are particularly abundant in the cecum, rectum, anal canal, prepuce, and third eyelid. The lymphoid tissue of the third eyelid is located on its bulbar side. It occasionally becomes infected and hypertrophied, causing nodular conjunctivitis. It may protrude around its free border in the form of a reddened tumor and require excision.

The lymph nodules of the prepuce are commonly infected in old male dogs, and an almost continuous purulent exudate is discharged from the sheath.

Regional Anatomy of the Lymphatic System

The larger lymph vessels and the lymph nodes of the body are described regionally, according to the following categories: head and neck, thoracic limb, thorax, abdominal and pelvic walls, genital organs, abdominal viscera, and pelvic limb. The spleen and thymus are discussed separately.

A **lymphocentrum**, as defined in the Nomina Veterinaria Anatomica (2017), is "a lymph node or group of lymph nodes that occurs in the same region of the body and receives afferent vessels from approximately the same region in most species."

Regional lymph node is the term that refers to a lymph filtration point that receives the *primary lymph* of an organ or body region. Conversely, the *drainage area* of such a

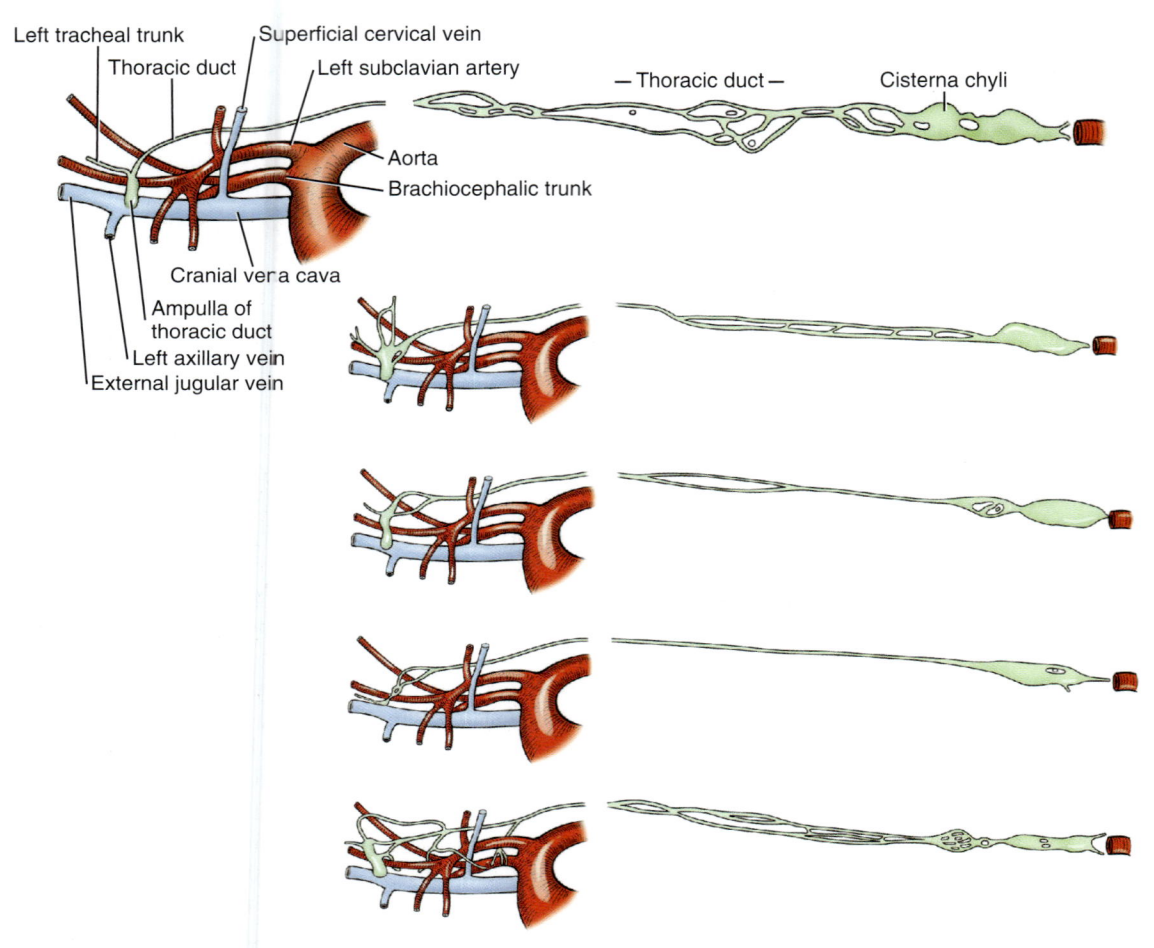

• **Fig. 13.3** Some variations of the thoracic duct and its entrance into the cranial vena cava. (Modified from Huber F: *Der Ductus thoracicus,* Inaugural dissertation, Dresden, 1909.)

regional lymph node is the tributary region from which it receives its primary lymph. This lymph flows from the lymph capillary region via **afferent lymph vessels** to the regional lymph node. **Efferent lymph vessels** leave the lymph node, carrying lymph that is filtered and enriched with lymphocytes. In contrast with primary lymph, this lymph is referred to as *secondary lymph.*

The nomenclature of lymph nodes is based on location. The location is surprisingly constant, and one should remember that in dogs there are usually only one or two lymph nodes at each site. Furthermore, there is such great variation in the number and size of lymph nodes that even in the same individual differences occur between one side of the body and the other.

Large Lymph Vessels

The **thoracic duct** (*ductus thoracicus*) (Figs. 13.3 through 13.5, and Figs. 13.10A through 13.14) is the chief channel for return of the lymph of the body. Lymph from the right thoracic limb and the right side of the neck and head is returned via the **right lymphatic duct** (*ductus lymphaticus dexter*). Normally the lymph vessel system joins the venous system at the "venous angle," that is, the point of confluence of the external and internal jugular veins or the junction of the jugular and subclavian veins.

The thoracic duct begins in the sublumbar region or between the crura of the diaphragm as a cranial continuation of the *cisterna chyli* (see Figs. 13.3, 13.18, and 13.24). This cistern is a dilated, bipartite portion of the lymph channel that lies retroperitoneally in association with the cranial abdominal aorta. The dorsal part is saccular and lies dorsal

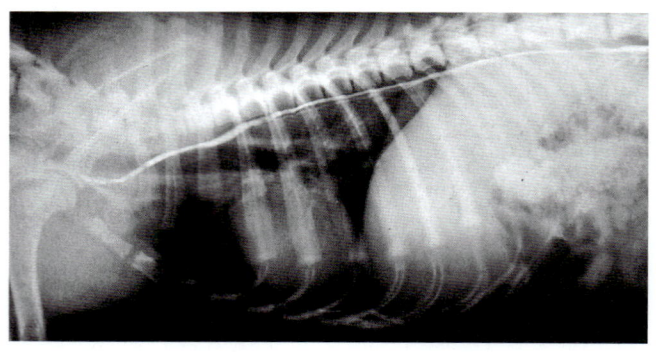

• **Fig. 13.4** Lateral lymphangiogram of the thorax showing the course of the thoracic duct.

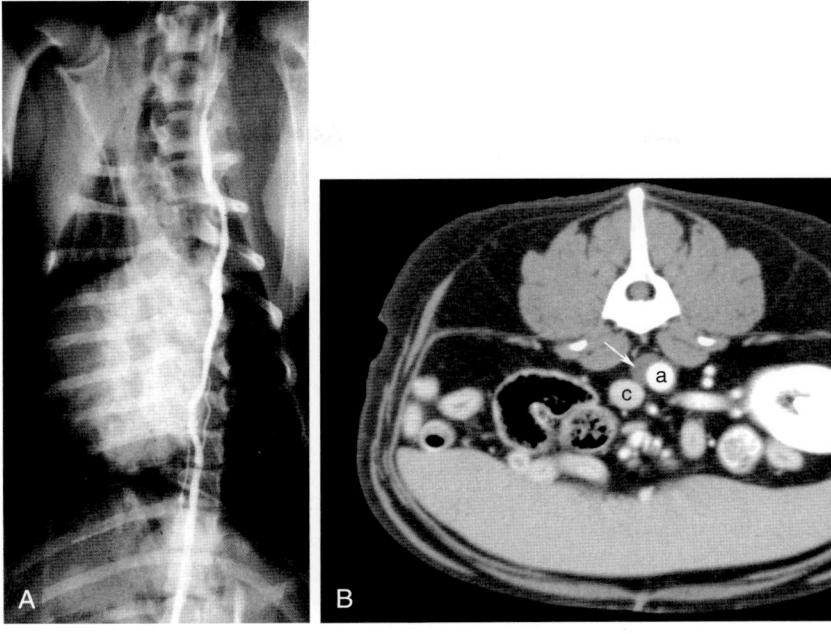

• **Fig. 13.5 A.** Dorsoventral lymphangiogram of the thorax showing the thoracic duct inclining to the left at the level of the fifth thoracic vertebra. **B.** Transverse computed tomorgraphy (CT) scan of the dog abdomen at the level of the left kidney. The cisterna chyli (arrow) is shown alongside the aorta (A) and caudal vena cava (C).

to the aorta from the level of the origin of the celiac artery to approximately the level of the left renal hilus. Cranially it continues through the aortic hiatus of the diaphragm as the thoracic duct. The ventral part of the cistern lies on the ventral surface of the aorta, concealed in part by the caudal vena cava, and extends from the level of origin of the cranial mesenteric artery to just caudal to the caudal pole of the left kidney. The ventral part of the cistern is frequently plexiform and commonly receives paired **visceral lymph trunks** (*truncus visceralis*) from the abdominal viscera, and **lumbar lymph trunks** (*trunci lumbales*) that are the cranial continuations of the lymph vessels from the pelvis and pelvic limbs via efferent lymph vessels from the iliac lymph nodes. The ventral part of the cistern has a variable number of connections around the aorta to the dorsal part of the cistern (Lindsay, 1974). The afferent lymph vessels that drain into the cistern are covered by a fold of endothelium, and lack valves where they enter the cistern (Marais & Fossum, 1988). Magnetic resonance imaging in 30 dogs found that the cisterna chyli always wrapped around the aorta but varied in size and shape (Johnson & Seiler, 2006).

The exact origin of the thoracic duct is somewhat arbitrarily assigned because the morphologic characteristics of the cisterna chyli are so erratic. The thoracic duct is considered to begin mostly as a single duct between the crura of the diaphragm, where the cistern attains its minimum width (de Freitas et al., 1981). Johnson and Seiler (2006) showed that the thoracic duct formed from multiple small branches around the aorta cranial to the diaphragmatic crura, which united to become one tubular structure. The initial part of the thoracic duct is plexiform and variable in form, whereas the distal part is more constant. Detailed descriptions of the variations in morphologic characteristics and topography of the thoracic duct are given by de Freitas et al. (1981), Kagan and Breznock (1979), and Threefoot (1968). Huber (1909) compared the thoracic ducts of the horse, ox, dog, and pig and illustrated 20 variations in the origin, course, or termination of the thoracic duct of the dog (see Fig. 13.3). The thoracic duct runs cranially from a point opposite the first lumbar vertebra on the right dorsal border of the thoracic aorta and the ventral border of the azygos vein to the sixth thoracic vertebrae. Here it inclines to the left, running between the azygos vein and the aorta, and then obliquely crosses the ventral surface of the fifth thoracic vertebra to enter the cranial mediastinum. It continues cranioventrally in the cranial mediastinum, and, in approximately one-half of specimens, it terminates singly at the junction of the left external jugular vein with the left subclavian vein (Baum, 1918). In many specimens the cranial portion of the thoracic duct bifurcates or trifurcates. These branches are usually connected by cross branches so that a coarse, widespread plexus is formed. The termination of the end parts of the thoracic duct varies regarding both the veins they empty into and the places on the vessels at which they empty. When the thoracic duct is single, it usually presents a terminal dilatation immediately before it becomes constricted to perforate the venous wall. Similar ampulla-like dilatations may be present on each of the branches when the thoracic duct terminates in multiple vessels. A monocuspid valve is present at the thoracic duct opening into the venous system. Immediately distally, the lymphaticovenous junction is closed by an extensive, convoluted, bicuspid valve (Marais & Fossum, 1988). Freeman (1942), who examined the termination of the thoracic duct in 25 dogs, found that it had no branches in three and was divided in five and that it sent branches to the right side in eight, to the azygos vein in five, and to both the right side and the azygos vein in four. Suter and Greene (1971) describe a case of chylothorax in a dog with an abnormal termination of the thoracic duct. There is a connection between the thoracic duct and the right lymphatic duct in 50% of the dogs (Martin et al., 1983; Pieper et al., 1986; Vreim et al., 1977).

The **right** and **left tracheal trunks** (*truncus trachealis*), 2 to 4 mm wide, arise from the caudal pole of the ipsilateral medial retropharyngeal lymph node or its efferent lymph ducts. The tracheal trunk is usually single as it leaves the caudal pole of the lymph node, but it may be double or in the form of a plexus. As it runs caudally in the neck, it lies in or adjacent to the medial wall of the carotid sheath. Although it has been reported that no additional nodes are found along the course of the tracheal trunk (Yoffey & Drinker, 1938), others have found middle and caudal deep cervical lymph nodes along and draining into the tracheal trunk. The left tracheal trunk usually terminates in the thoracic duct. The right tracheal trunk usually terminates in the right lymphatic duct (Fig. 13.3).

The **right lymphatic duct** (*ductus lymphaticus dexter*) is located in the right caudal part of the neck. It receives efferent lymph vessels from the right superficial cervical, axillary and thoracic lymph nodes. The right tracheal trunk drains into the right lymphatic duct 20 to 30 mm from the first rib, doubling the size of it (Baum, 1918). After a course of approximately 15 mm, the right lymphatic duct empties into the right subclavian vein or the angle formed by the merging of the right subclavian and right external jugular veins. Commonly, the right lymphatic duct bifurcates and then reunites, forming a circle before it terminates. Sometimes the forked condition persists, so that the right lymphatic duct enters the venous system, cranial to the first rib, by two channels. The right lymphatic duct drains into the thoracic duct in 50% of dogs (Martin et al. 1983; Pieper et al., 1986; Vreim et al., 1977).

Although these ducts are among the larger lymph ducts of the body, the smooth muscle cell component is sparse. A network of sympathetic axons coming from the plexus on blood vessels outside the carotid sheath are present on the surface of the cervical lymph ducts in dogs (Todd & Bernard, 1973). The paucity of contractile cells would however indicate that intrinsic contraction is not a prime mechanism in the propulsion of lymph (Todd & Bernard, 1974).

Lymph Nodes and Vessels of the Head and Neck

There are three lymph centers in the head: lymphocentrum parotideum, lymphocentrum mandibulare, and lymphocentrum retropharyngeum; and two centers in the neck: lymphocentrum cervicale superficiale and lymphocentrum cervicale profundum.

Parotid Lymph Center

The parotid lymph center (*lymphocentrum parotideum*) consists of the **parotid lymph nodes** (*lymphonodi parotidei superficiales*) (Figs. 13.2, 13.6, and 13.7) at the rostral base of the ear. They are bean-shaped nodes located deep to the rostrodorsal border of the parotid salivary gland on the caudal parts of the zygomatic arch and adjacent masseter muscle. In a medium-sized dog they are approximately 10 mm long, 5 mm wide, and 3 mm thick. Occasionally, a second or even a third node may be present (Baum, 1918). They are palpable in this position when enlarged.

Drainage Area. The afferent lymph vessels to the parotid lymph node come from the cutaneous area of the caudal half of the dorsum of the muzzle and the side of the cranium, including the eyelids and associated glands, the external ear, the temporomandibular joint, and the parotid salivary gland. The parotid lymph center also drains the temporal, masseter, and zygomatic muscles; the muscles of the ear; the lacrimal apparatus; the nasal, frontal, parietal, zygomatic, and temporal bones; and the mandible. Its two or three efferent lymph vessels run between the digastric muscle and the parotid salivary gland to the large medial retropharyngeal lymph node. This flow can also drain into the lateral retropharyngeal lymph node, if the latter is present.

Mandibular Lymph Center

The mandibular lymph center (*lymphocentrum mandibulare*) consists of the mandibular and buccal lymph nodes.

The **mandibular lymph nodes** (*lymphonodi mandibulares*) (see Figs. 13.2, 13.6, and 13.7) form a group of two or three nodes or, rarely, as many as five that lie ventral to the angle of the mandible. A flattened, three-sided node, with borders approximately 10 mm long, lying dorsal to the linguofacial vein and a long, ovoid node lying ventral to the linguofacial vein constitute what is probably the most common arrangement. The node lying ventral to the linguofacial vein usually is more than 20 mm long and approximately 10 mm wide. It is flattened transversely. In more than one-third of the specimens examined by Baum (1918), two or more nodes replaced this single node on one or both sides. In only 16 of 36 specimens was the grouping of the mandibular nodes on the two sides similar. The dorsal node may be double, but this condition is rare.

Drainage Area. The afferent lymph vessels to the mandibular lymph nodes come from all parts of the head not drained by the afferent lymph vessels of the parotid lymph node. There is overlapping in the areas of drainage, so that the eyelids and their glands and the skin of the dorsum of the cranium and the temporomandibular joint drain into both nodal centers. Maher (1986) found that a mucosal and submucosal lymphatic network drained the palate. The afferent lymph vessels exit the palatal area and subsequently join lymphatic networks intrinsic to the tongue and pharynx. Maher (1985) and Kostiuk (1986) have shown that superficial and deep lymph capillary networks drained the tongue. Furthermore, Ossoff et al. (1980) and Ossoff and Sisson

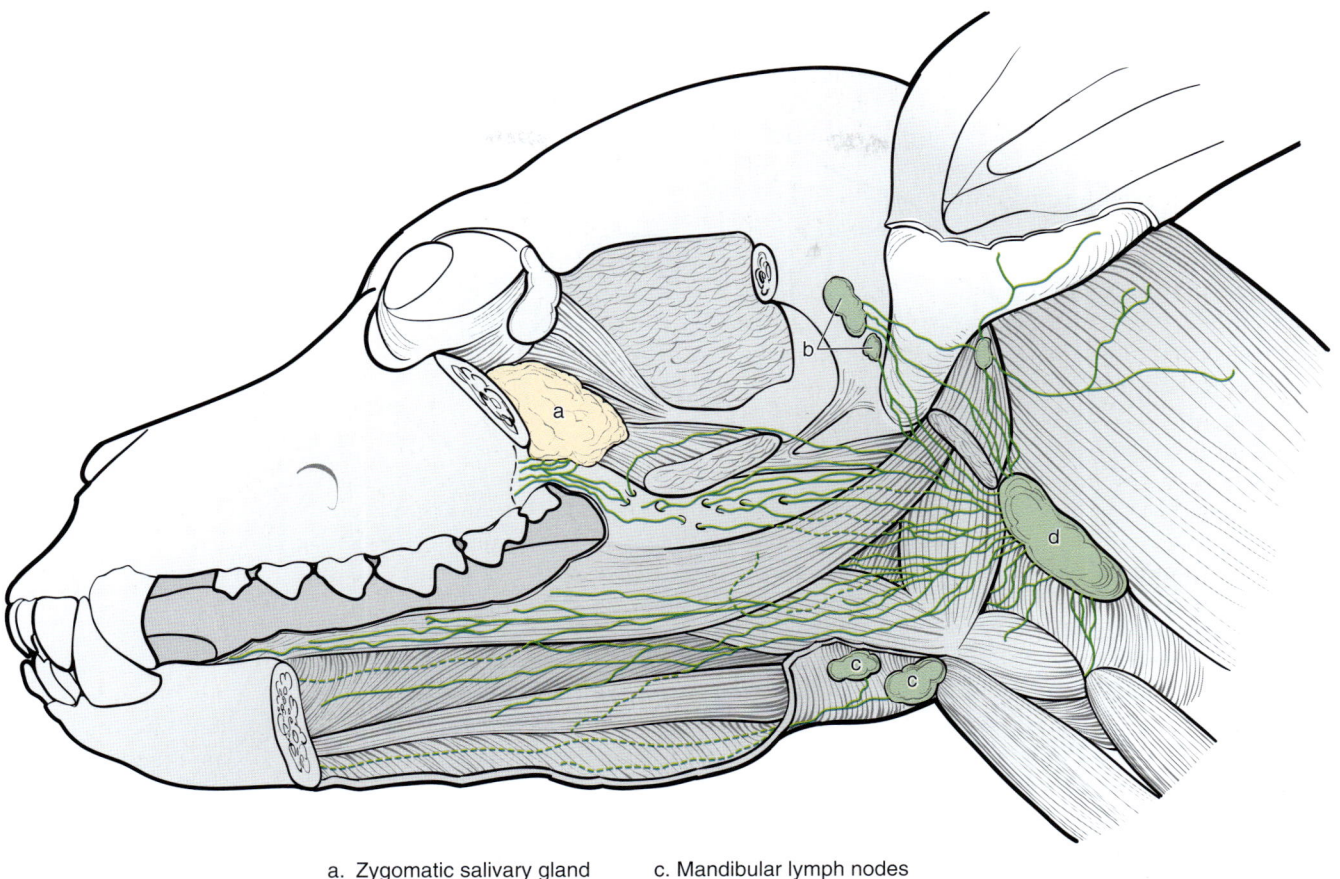

a. Zygomatic salivary gland
b. Parotid lymph nodes
c. Mandibular lymph nodes
d. Medial retropharyngeal lymph node

• **Fig. 13.6** Lymph vessels of the tongue, the tongue muscles, the soft palate, and the larynx of the dog. Left mandible and zygomatic arch removed. (Drawn after Baum H: Das Lymphgefässystem des Hundes, *Arch wiss prakt Tierheilk Bd* 44:521–650, 1918.)

(1981) have shown that a superficial and a deep lymph capillary network drained the floor of the oral cavity. The superficial lymph vessels randomly crossed the midline and drained into either the ipsilateral or the contralateral mandibular lymph nodes. However, the deep lymph vessels drained through the periosteum of the mandible and then into the mandibular lymph nodes, or along the medial surface of the mandible and then into the medial retropharyngeal lymph nodes.

The efferent lymph vessels of the mandibular lymph nodes go primarily to the ipsilateral medial retropharyngeal lymph node. The lymph nodes composing the group are connected with each other as well as with the contralateral medial retropharyngeal lymph node. The 8 to 10 efferent lymph vessels anastomose with each other and form a plexus as they pass over the pharynx. Before reaching the medial retropharyngeal node, they unite to form three to five small trunks that enter the ventrolateral surface of the medial retropharyngeal lymph node. According to Battezzati and Donini (1973), Bronzini in 1935 injected India ink into the cerebellomedullary cistern of a dog and observed the ink in the nasal mucosa, pharynx, and mandibular lymph nodes. This communication between the subarachnoid spaces and the lymph vessels of the nasal mucosa and pharynx may be of considerable importance in disease processes.

The **buccal lymph nodes** (*lymphonodi buccales*) are situated dorsal, ventral, or rostral to the angle of confluence of the facial and superior labial veins, dorsal to the buccinator muscle. The flattened nodes are approximately 10 mm long and 5 mm wide and can be bilateral, unilateral, or absent. Shelton and Forsythe (1979) examined 250 dogs of various breeds and found unilateral lymph nodes in 11 dogs, and bilateral lymph nodes in 11 dogs. Rumph et al. (1980) examined 171 Greyhounds and found lymph nodes to be present in 15 of them, and Casteleyn et al. (2008) found 6 bilateral and 7 unilateral buccal lymph nodes in 150 dogs that they examined.

Retropharyngeal Lymph Center

The retropharyngeal lymph center (*lymphocentrum retropharyngeum*) consists of a medial and sometimes a lateral retropharyngeal lymph node.

The **medial retropharyngeal lymph node** (*lymphonodi retropharyngei mediales*) (Figs. 7.2, and 13.6 through 13.9) is the largest node found in the head and neck. It is an

a. Zygomatic salivary gland
b. Monostomatic sublingual salivary gland
c. Parotid salivary gland
d. Mandibular salivary gland
e. Parotid lymph node
f. Mandibular lymph nodes
g. Lateral retropharyngeal lymph node
h. Medial retropharyngeal lymph node
i. Genioglossus muscle
j. Geniohyoideus muscle

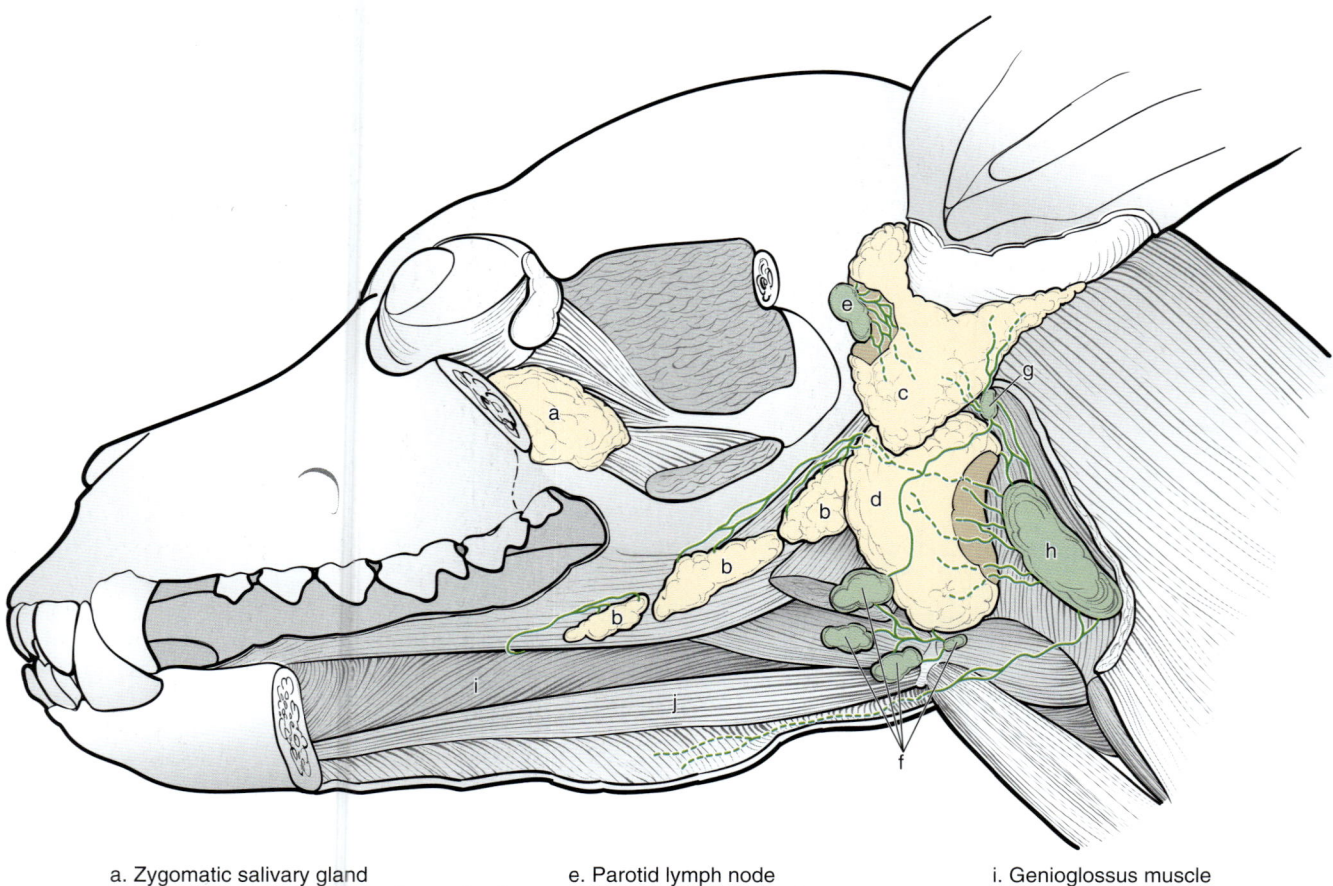

• **Fig. 13.7** Lymph vessels and nodes associated with the salivary glands of the dog. Left mandible and zygomatic arch removed. (Drawn after Baum H: Das Lymphgefässystem des Hundes, *Arch wiss prakt Tierheilk* Bd 44:521–650, 1918.)

elongated, transversely compressed node, with a more pointed caudal end, and is approximately 50 mm long and nearly 20 mm wide. Burns et al. (2008) found that the node increased in size with increased body weight but decreased in size with increased age. The medial retropharyngeal lymph node lies ventral to the wing of the atlas in the triangle bounded by the m. digastricus cranially, the m. longus colli dorsally, and the pharynx and larynx ventromedially. The mastoid parts of both the m. cleidocephalicus and the m. sternocephalicus largely cover the lymph node laterally, although its cranioventral part is related to the mandibular salivary gland. Coursing along its medial surface is the hypoglossal nerve and the terminal portion of the carotid sheath with its common carotid artery, vagus and sympathetic nerves, and the internal jugular vein. In 10 of 47 specimens, Baum (1918) found two medial retropharyngeal lymph nodes present on one or both sides. The afferent lymph vessels of the medial retropharyngeal lymph node come from all the deep structures of the head that have lymph vessels. Thus the tongue; the walls of the oral, nasal, and pharyngeal passages; the salivary glands; and the deep parts of the external ear drain into this lymph node. It also receives afferent lymph vessels from the larynx, esophagus, and the noncutaneous, nonmucous structures of the neck that have lymph vessels. The efferent lymph vessels from the parotid, mandibular, and lateral retropharyngeal lymph nodes drain into the medial retropharyngeal lymph node. Belz and Heath (1995) showed that efferent lymph vessels from the mandibular lymph nodes convey lymph to defined areas in the medial retropharyngeal lymph nodes. Yoffey and Drinker (1938) found four or five lymph vessels, lying between the hamulus of the pterygoid bone and the pharyngeal opening of the auditory tube, that came from the floor and sidewalls of the nasal cavity. The deep lymph vessels of the nasal cavity drain into the retropharyngeal lymph nodes and pass via the tracheal trunks to the region of the thoracic inlet veins. Some of the tracheal lymph vessels of the neck communicate with bronchial lymph vessels and reach the bronchial lymph nodes. Thus it is possible for lymph from the nasal cavity to reach the lung area.

Lateral retropharyngeal lymph nodes (*lymphonodi retropharyngei laterales*) are present in approximately 30% of dogs (Baum, 1918) (Figs. 13.6 and 13.7). This lymph node is less than 10 mm in diameter and lies at the dorsal border

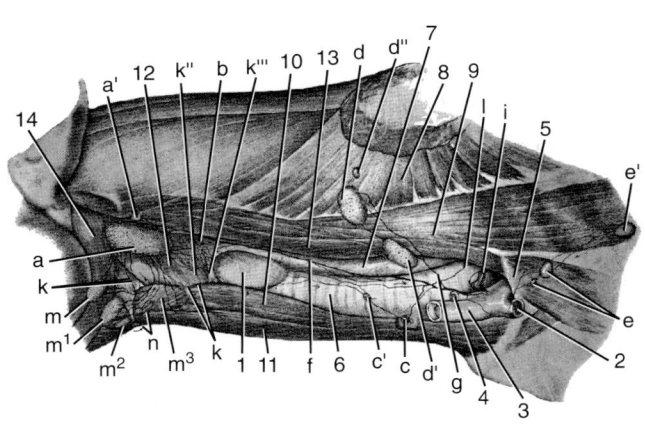

a, a'. Medial retropharyngeal lymph nodes
b. Cranial deep cervical lymph node
c, c'. Caudal deep cervical lymph nodes
d, d', d". Superficial cervical lymph nodes
e. Axillary lymph nodes
e'. Accessory axillary lymph node
f. Left tracheal trunk
g. Efferent vessel of the superficial cervical lymph nodes
i. Thoracic duct with terminal branches
k-k'". Lymph vessels of the larynx
l. Lymph vessel that runs to a cranial mediastinal lymph node
m to m³. Mandibular lymph nodes
n. Efferent vessels of the mandibular lymph nodes that go to the medial retropharyngeal lymph node of the opposite side
1. Thyroid gland
2. Axillary vein (cut)
3. External jugular vein
4. Internal jugular vein
5. First rib
6. Trachea
7. Esophagus
8. M. serratus ventralis
9. M. scalenus
10. M. sternothyroideus
11. M. sternohyoideus
12. Muscles of the pharynx
13. M. longus capitis
14. M. digastricus

• **Fig. 13.8** Lymph nodes and vessels of the neck of the dog. (From Baum H: Das Lymphgefässystem des Hundes, *Arch wiss prakt Tierheilk Bd* 44:521–650, 1918.)

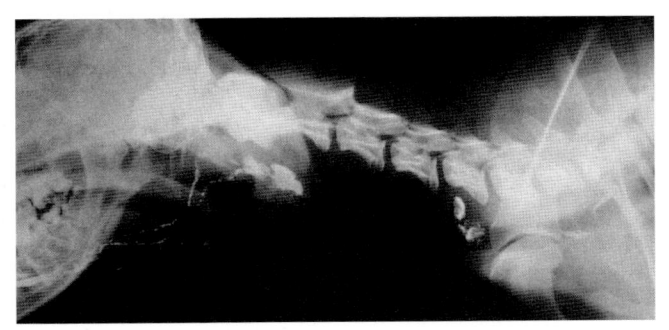

• **Fig. 13.9** Lateral lymphangiogram of the cervical region showing the medial retropharyngeal and superficial cervical lymph nodes.

of the horizontal part of the cartilaginous external acoustic meatus. It is completely or partially covered by the caudal part of the parotid salivary gland.

Drainage Area. The afferent lymph vessels of the lateral retropharyngeal nodes come from the structures lying adjacent to them. Their efferent vessels drain into the medial retropharyngeal lymph node.

Superficial Cervical Lymph Center

The superficial cervical lymph center (*lymphocentrum cervicale superficiale*) consists of the **superficial cervical lymph nodes** (*lymphonodi cervicales superficiales*) (Figs. 13.2, 13.8, and 13.9). They usually consist of two nodes, one lying dorsal to the other in the adipose tissue on the lateral surface of the serratus ventralis and scalenus muscles, cranial to the supraspinatus muscle. They are covered superficially by the thin cleidocephalicus, omotransversarius, and, at their dorsal end, the trapezius muscles. The superficial cervical artery and vein lie medial to the caudal parts of the lymph nodes as they course cranial to the shoulder in the groove between the shoulder and the neck. The more ventral superficial cervical lymph node may encroach on the trachea on the right side and the esophagus and trachea on the left side. Occasionally, a single node is present on each side, but more commonly three or more nodes replace the usual two. Most of the nodes are oval and somewhat flattened. They are collectively approximately 30 mm long and less than 10 mm thick.

Drainage Area. The afferent lymph vessels come mainly from the skin of the caudal part of the head, including the pharyngeal region, a part of the pinna, the lateral surface of the neck, and the whole thoracic limb, except a variable region on the medial side of the brachium and antebrachium, the shoulder, and the cranial part of the thoracic wall. Yang (1986) found that one or occasionally both nodes showed green coloration after tattooing the ear. Mahorner et al. (1927), by making injections into the thyroid gland of humans, revealed efferent connections with the superficial cervical lymph nodes, the tracheal trunks, and the veins at the base of the neck. The efferent lymph ducts connect members of the group when more than one node is present, and, as one to three trunks, they descend over the serratus ventralis and scalenus muscles to merge with the tracheal trunk on the right side, contributing to the right lymphatic duct. On the left side the superficial cervical lymph nodes empty into the thoracic duct. On either or each side they may empty into the external jugular vein directly. Efferent lymph vessels from the first thoracic mammary gland usually enter the axillary lymph node, but may also enter the superficial cervical lymph nodes (Patsikas & Dessiris, 1992).

Deep Cervical Lymph Center

The deep cervical lymph center (*lymphocentrum cervicale profundum*) consists of cranial, middle, and caudal **deep cervical lymph nodes** (*lymphonodi cervicales profundi*) (Fig. 13.8) located along the cervical portion of the trachea on each side. They are exceedingly small and vary in number. In the dog one or more of these nodes are frequently absent. They range considerably in size; they may be barely visible or several millimeters long. The smaller nodes are spherical to ovoid; the larger ones are usually elongated and parallel to the long axis of the trachea.

Cranial deep cervical lymph nodes (*lymphonodi cervicales profundi craniales*) are present in approximately 30% of dogs and are located between the caudal end of the medial retropharyngeal lymph node and the thyroid gland. It lies either dorsomedial to the thyroid gland along the carotid sheath, or on the pharynx cranial to the thyroid gland. **Middle deep cervical lymph nodes** (*lymphonodi cervicales profundi medii*) are present in approximately 6% of dogs, and are rarely found on both sides. They usually lie along the carotid sheath but may lie ventral to the trachea in the middle third of the neck. **Caudal deep cervical lymph nodes** (*lymphonodi cervicales profundi caudales*) are present in approximately 26% of dogs and, similar to the middle deep cervical lymph nodes, are rarely found bilaterally (Baum, 1918). In 11 of 17 specimens dissected by Baum, a single node was located on the ventral surface of the trachea, and in others there were 2 or more nodes lying on the ventral surface of the caudal third of the cervical part of the trachea.

Drainage Area. The afferent lymph vessels to the deep cervical lymph nodes come from the larynx, thyroid gland, trachea, esophagus, and the last five or six cervical vertebrae. The efferent lymph vessels of each cranially located node become a part of the afferent lymph vessels of the node located next caudally. In this way the cranial deep cervical node receives lymph from the medial retropharyngeal node. Those from the caudal deep cervical lymph nodes empty into the right lymphatic duct on the right or into the thoracic duct on the left. On either side they may empty into the tracheal trunk or into a cranial mediastinal node.

Lymph Nodes and Vessels of the Thoracic Limb

Axillary Lymph Center

The axillary lymph center (*lymphocentrum axillare*) drains the thoracic limb and consists of the axillary and accessory axillary lymph nodes.

The **axillary lymph node** (*lymphonodus axillaris proprius*) (Fig. 13.8) usually is the only lymph node of the thoracic limb. In a series of 43 specimens, double nodes were found in 10, and in 6 of these the double nodes occurred on both sides (Baum, 1918). The main axillary lymph node is usually in the form of a disc approximately 2 cm in diameter, although the diameter may range from 3 to 50 mm. It lies 20 to 50 mm caudal to the shoulder joint, in the angle formed by the diverging brachial and subscapular blood vessels. It is bounded laterally by the teres major muscle, medially by the rectus thoracis muscle, and ventrally by the dorsal border of the deep pectoral muscle. The **accessory axillary lymph node** (*lymphonodus axillaris accessorius*) (see Fig. 13.8), when present, lies caudal to the principal node in the fascia between the adjacent borders of the deep pectoral and latissimus dorsi muscles, caudal to the muscles of the brachium. It varies in size from less than 1 mm to 15 mm. When it is large, the axillary lymph node is correspondingly reduced in size. In 4 of 29 specimens a third node in close relation to the axillary node was present (Baum, 1918). In only one of his specimens was it present on both sides.

Drainage Area. The afferent lymph vessels of the axillary lymph node or nodes come mainly from the mammary glands, thoracic and cranioventral abdominal walls, and the deep structures of the thoracic limb. Both the thoracic and the cranial abdominal mammary glands of each side have lymph vessels that drain into the axillary nodes (Fig. 13.10B). An anastomosis between the afferent lymph vessels of the axillary nodes and those of the superficial inguinal lymph nodes sometimes occurs between the cranial and the caudal abdominal mammary glands. Only the cranial abdominal mammary gland has direct drainage to both the axillary and the superficial inguinal lymph nodes (Patsikas & Dessiris, 1992; Ruberte et al., 1990). Afferent lymph vessels from the right and left mammary glands do not cross the midline and are independent of each other. Contrary to this, the axillary lymph nodes are connected with each other by lymph vessels. The efferent lymph vessels from the axillary nodes of each side course cranially and unite with each other to form one or more anastomosing larger trunks that lie on the m. rectus thoracis. The efferent trunks pass medial to the axillary vein, curve around the first rib, and empty by one or several branches on the left side into the thoracic duct, left tracheal trunk, left external jugular vein, or into all of these. On the right side the axillary efferent lymph vessels empty into the right tracheal trunk, the right lymphatic duct, the right external jugular vein, or into all three of these.

Lymph Nodes and Vessels of the Thorax

The lymph nodes of the thorax may be divided into parietal and visceral groups. The parietal group includes the lymph nodes of the ventral and dorsal thoracic lymph centers; the visceral group includes the nodes of the mediastinal and bronchial lymph centers. The parietal lymph nodes are smaller and less constant in number and location than are the visceral lymph nodes.

Ventral Thoracic Lymph Center

The ventral thoracic lymph center (*lymphocentrum thoracicum ventrale*) is only represented by the **cranial sternal lymph nodes** (*lymphonodi sternales craniales*) (Figs. 13.10A, 13.12 through 13.15). On each side it is usually represented by a single lymph node. In others a single median lymph node, which may be located either right or left of the median plane, serves both sides. The lymph node may be lacking completely, or, in rare instances, a double lymph node may be present on one side.

When one lymph node is present on each side, it lies immediately cranial to the m. transversus thoracis and medial to the second costal cartilage or second interchondral space, cranioventral to the internal thoracic blood vessels. Typically, the lymph node is ellipsoidal and 2 to 20 mm in length. If a single node is present, it may be dumbbell-shaped. When two nodes are present on one side, they may lie close together and may be mistaken for a single node.

CHAPTER 13 The Lymphatic System 629

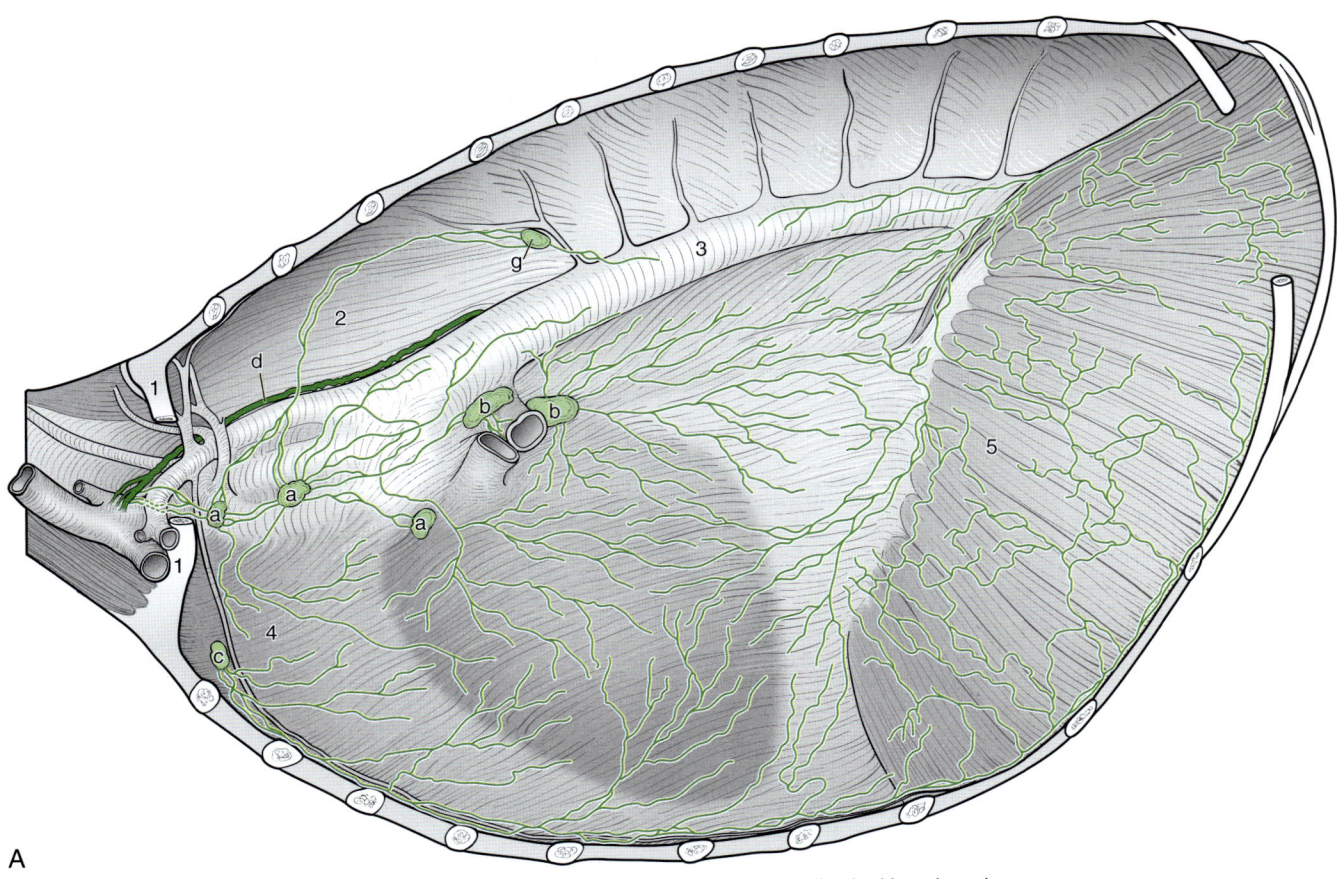

1. First rib (cut)
2. Splenius (epaxial muscles)
3. Aorta
4. Cranial mediastinum
5. Diaphragm

a. Cranial mediastinal lymph nodes
b. Left tracheobronchial lymph node
g. Aortic thoracic lymph node

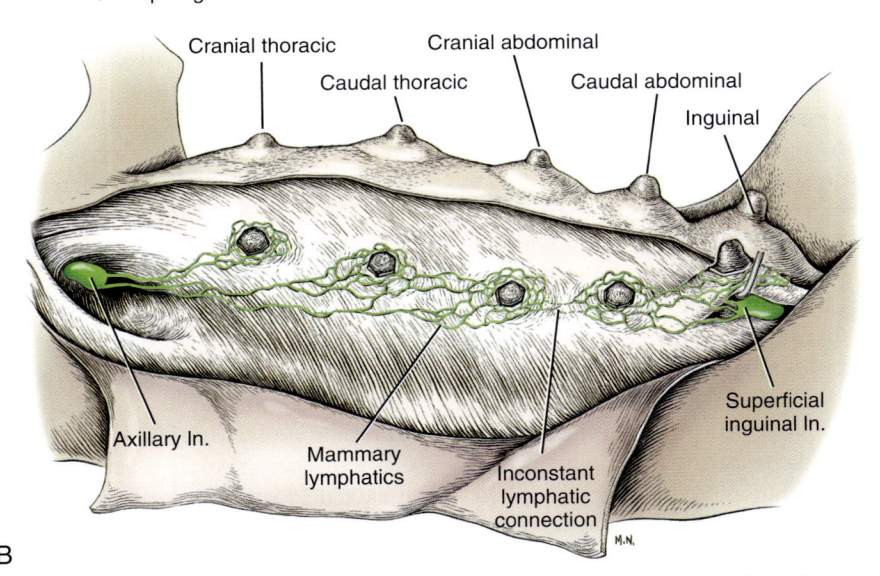

• **Fig. 13.10** A, Lymph vessels of the mediastinum, pericardium, diaphragm, aorta, and esophagus of the dog; the left lung is removed, and the left wall of the thorax is almost completely removed, as is the m. transversus thoracis. B, Lymph drainage of the mammary glands. (Drawn after Baum H: Das Lymphgefässystem des Hundes, *Arch wiss prakt Tierheilk Bd* 44:521–650, 1918.)

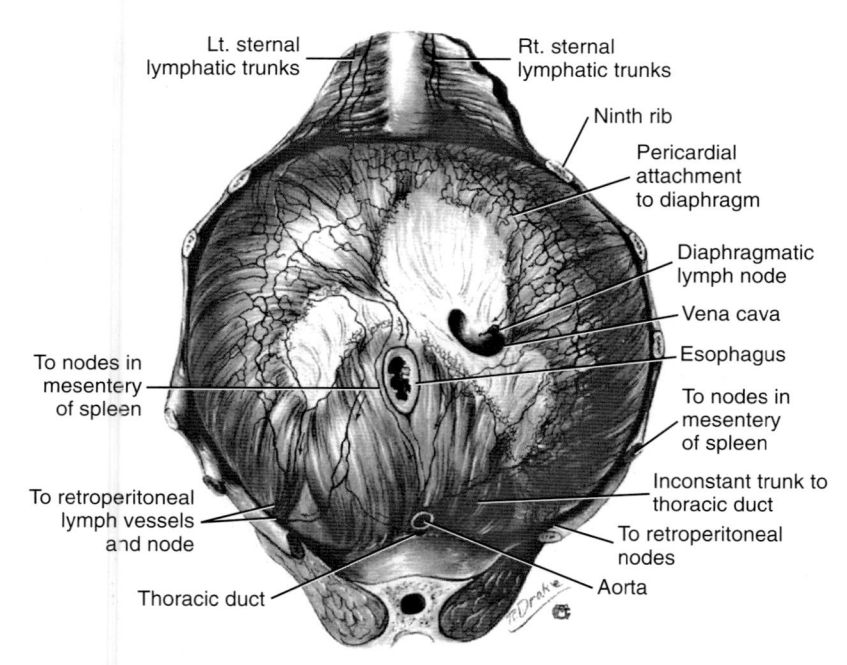

• **Fig. 13.11** The pleural surface of the diaphragm in a dog after the intraperitoneal injection of a graphite preparation. (From Higgins GM, Graham AS: Lymph drainage from the peritoneal cavity in the dog, *Arch Surg* 19:453–465, 1929. Copyright 1929, American Medical Association.)

Drainage Area. The afferent lymph vessels of the cranial sternal lymph node on each side lie deep to the transverse muscle of the thorax in the fat lying between this muscle and the dorsal surfaces of the sternal ends of the costal cartilages. Occasionally, a single afferent lymph vessel is present. It arises in the abdominal wall, perforates the diaphragm near the middle of the costal arch, and, running deep to the pleura in the costodiaphragmatic recess, extends cranially and ventrally to course deep to the m. transversus thoracis. The cranial sternal lymph node receives tributaries from the ribs, sternum, serous membranes, thymus, adjacent muscles, and mammary glands (Baum, 1918). According to Stalker and Schlotthauer (1936) lymph vessels do not penetrate the thoracic or abdominal walls. Experimental observations by Patsikas and Dessiris (1992) using Lipiodol indicate that the cranial sternal lymph nodes receive no direct afferent lymph vessels from the mammary glands, although Baum (1918) states that there are connections. In the absence of the cranial sternal lymph nodes, the afferent lymph vessels that would otherwise drain into them drain into the mediastinal lymph nodes. The one to three efferent lymph vessels from the cranial sternal lymph node on each side run cranial to the internal thoracic blood vessels, where they form a plexus. The right efferent lymph vessels terminate in the right lymphatic duct, the left in the thoracic duct. Many variations exist.

Higgins and Graham (1929) introduced 40 to 50 mL of graphite preparation into the peritoneal cavity of dogs to trace the lymph drainage routes. Within 20 minutes to 1 hour the lymph channels on the surface of the diaphragm were completely delineated. Muscular activity hastened the absorptive process. The major lymph drainage from the peritoneal cavity appeared to be via the diaphragm to the cranial sternal lymph vessels. A group of lymph channels course cranially from the diaphragm (Figs. 13.11, 13.12, and 13.14) onto the sternum parallel to the internal thoracic artery and vein. Occasionally, plexuses are formed. These sternal lymph channels continue into the cranial sternal lymph nodes that lie near the ventral ends of the second costal cartilage or second intercostal space. In the region of the cranial sternal lymph nodes, numerous collecting ducts unite the afferent lymph vessels of the right and left sides. In general, the drainage of the right cranial sternal efferent lymph vessels is to the right lymphatic duct, and drainage from the left efferent lymph vessels is toward the thoracic duct. Thus it appears that the thoracic duct plays a relatively insignificant part in the drainage of the peritoneal cavity.

Dorsal Thoracic Lymph Center

The dorsal thoracic lymph center (*lymphocentrum thoracicum dorsale*) of the dog is only represented by the **aortic thoracic nodes** (*lymphonodi intercostales*) (Figs. 13.10 and 13.13). They are present in approximately 25% of dogs and bilateral in only 4% of animals (Baum, 1918). This small spherical node lies in the vertebral end of either the fifth or the sixth intercostal space deep to the sympathetic trunk, caudal to the intercostal artery.

Drainage Area. The aortic thoracic lymph node receives a portion of the lymph vessels that pass into the thoracic cavity through the last six to eight intercostal spaces with afferent lymph vessels from the axial, shoulder, thoracic, and abdominal musculature (Baum, 1918). It probably also receives afferent lymph vessels from the ribs, vertebrae,

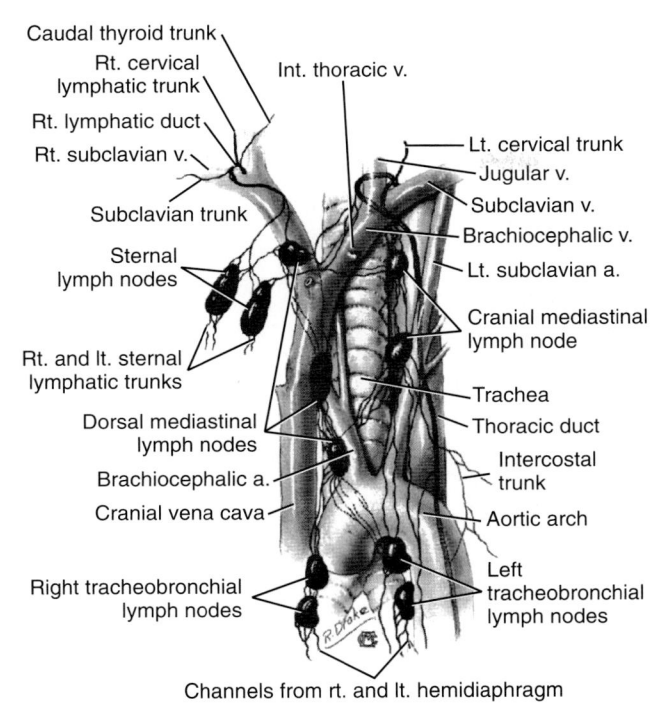

• **Fig. 13.12** The arch of the aorta and mediastinum, showing lymph channels in a dog given an intraperitoneal injection of a graphite solution. (From Higgins GM, Graham AS: Lymph drainage from the peritoneal cavity in the dog, *Arch Surg* 19:453–465, 1929. Copyright 1929, American Medical Association.)

pleura, aorta, and spinal cord meninges. These afferent lymph vessels lie on the thoracic vertebrae and m. longus colli. The efferent vessels go to the mediastinal lymph nodes.

Mediastinal Lymph Center

The mediastinal lymph center (*lymphocentrum mediastinale*) of the dog is only represented by the **cranial mediastinal lymph nodes** (*lymphonodi mediastinales craniales*) (Figs. 13.10 through 13.17). They vary in number and shape and most of them are associated with the large vessels of the heart that run through the dorsal part of the cranial mediastinum. Unlike in most other animals, the mediastinal lymph nodes in the dog are confined to the cranial mediastinum or the surface of the heart. Although they lie in the cranial mediastinal septum, most lymph nodes are not visible through the pleura from both sides, even in emaciated specimens. For this reason right and left lymph nodes are described. In young animals some of these lymph nodes are partly embedded in the thymus.

On the left side, the cranial mediastinal lymph nodes vary in number from one to six and in length from less than 1 mm to 3 mm. Most of these lymph nodes are oblong, and they lie along the cranial vena cava, the brachiocephalic trunk, left subclavian artery, and costocervical trunk. When several lymph nodes are present on the left side, one of these is located opposite the first intercostal space either cranial or caudal to the left costocervical vein. Small, kernel-like lymph nodes lying between the dorsally lying left subclavian artery and the ventrally lying brachiocephalic trunk or in the left groove between the trachea and the esophagus, are not apparent unless they are exposed by removal of the overlying mediastinal pleura and fat.

On the right side, the cranial mediastinal lymph nodes usually number two or three, with a maximum of six. The disc-shaped lymph node lying between the right costocervical vein and the cranial vena cava is most constant. It may be double. In large dogs it measures more than 10 mm in diameter and may partly cover both veins between which it lies. Additional lymph nodes are frequently found along the dorsolateral surface of the trachea, between the costocervical and the azygos veins. A lymph node may lie between the cranial vena cava and the brachiocephalic trunk ventral to the trachea.

Drainage Area. The afferent lymph vessels come from the muscles of the neck, thorax, and abdomen and the peritoneal cavity, the scapula, the last six cervical vertebrae, the thoracic vertebrae, ribs, trachea, esophagus, thyroid gland, thymus, mediastinum, costal pleura, heart, aorta, and spinal cord meninges (Baum, 1918). Lymph vessels do not invade the central nervous system or the contractile elements of skeletal muscles. The mediastinal lymph nodes also receive efferent vessels from the intercostal, sternal, middle, and caudal deep cervical, tracheobronchial, and pulmonary lymph nodes. The efferent lymph vessels of all lymph nodes caudal to the relatively constant lymph node located cranial to the costocervical vein on each side drain into it. From this node on the left side, efferent lymph vessels that empty into either the thoracic duct or the left tracheal trunk or into both. On the right side similar efferent lymph vessels go to the right lymphatic duct, the right tracheal trunk, or to both.

Bronchial Lymph Center

The bronchial lymph center (*lymphocentrum bronchale*) is represented by the pulmonary and tracheobronchial lymph nodes. It includes all nodes that lie on the initial parts of the bronchi at the bifurcation of the trachea.

The **pulmonary lymph nodes** (*lymphonodi pulmonales*) (Fig. 13.16) are often absent. They were present on one side in only 14 of 41 specimens examined by Baum (1918) and were never present on both sides. They are small lymph nodes that lie on the dorsal surfaces of the principal bronchi between the right and left tracheobronchial nodes and the parenchyma of the lungs.

Drainage Area. They receive lymph from the lungs. Their efferent vessels go to the tracheobronchial lymph nodes.

The **tracheobronchial lymph nodes** (*lymphonodi tracheobronchiales*) (Figs. 13.10, 13.12 through 13.14, 13.16, and 13.17) are constantly present and are known as the *right, left,* and *middle tracheobronchial lymph nodes.*

The **right** and **left tracheobronchial lymph nodes** (*lymphonodi tracheobronchales dextri et sinistri*) are similar in size and location. Each lies on the lateral side of its respective principal bronchus, but also on the trachea, to a small

632 CHAPTER 13 The Lymphatic System

a. Thoracic duct
b. Aortic thoracic lymph node
c. Tracheobronchial lymph nodes
d. Cranial mediastinal lymph nodes
e. Cranial sternal lymph nodes
f. Right lymphatic duct
g. Right tracheal duct

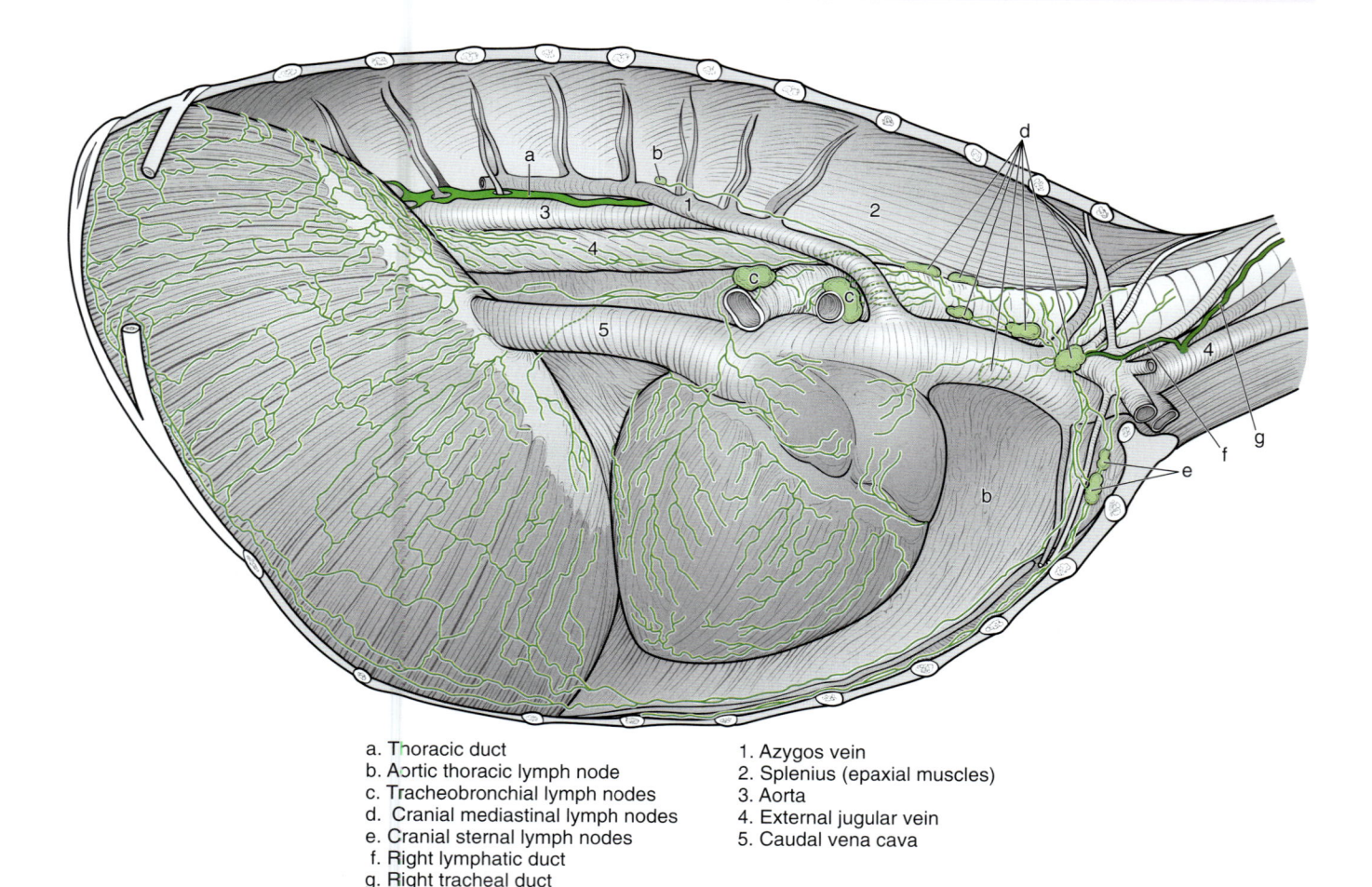

1. Azygos vein
2. Splenius (epaxial muscles)
3. Aorta
4. External jugular vein
5. Caudal vena cava

• **Fig. 13.13** Right side of the thoracic cavity of the dog, lung removed. (Redrawn after Baum H: Das Lymphgefässystem des Hundes, *Arch wiss prakt Tierheilk* Bd 44:521–650, 1918.)

extent. Dorsally the right tracheobronchial lymph node is located ventral to the azygos vein; the left tracheobronchial lymph node has a similar relation to the beginning of the thoracic aorta. These lymph nodes are 5 to 30 mm long and are ellipsoidal, with truncated caudal extremities. The left lymph node is more angular as it is wedged in the space bounded medially by the left principal bronchus and trachea, dorsally by the aorta, and ventrally by the pulmonary vein from the left cranial lung lobe.

The **middle tracheobronchial lymph node** (*lymphonodi tracheobronchales medii*) is always the largest node of this group. It is in the form of a V as it lies in the angle formed by the origin of the principal bronchi from the trachea. The left limb of the V lies on the dorsal surface of pulmonary vein of the left caudal lung lobe; the right limb lies along the right cranial surface of the pulmonary vein from the right caudal lung lobe. The lymph node is related to the esophagus dorsally. Its apex fits snugly into the angle formed by the bifurcation of the trachea. The vagus nerves lie in contact with the limbs of the lymph node as these nerves become intimately related to the ventrolateral surfaces of the esophagus. Sometimes the tracheobronchial group of lymph nodes includes a fourth lymph node just cranial to the right tracheobronchial lymph node, in the angle formed by the azygos vein at its entrance into the cranial vena cava. In other specimens the middle tracheobronchial lymph node and either the right or the left lymph node form one confluent mass.

Drainage Area. The afferent lymph vessels to the tracheobronchial lymph nodes come primarily from the pulmonary lymph nodes, bronchi, and lungs, but also from the thoracic parts of the aorta, esophagus, trachea, heart, mediastinum, and diaphragm. The two to four efferent lymph vessels from each tracheobronchial lymph node go partly to another node of this group and partly to the mediastinal lymph nodes. Dogs that have lived in dusty or smoky environments have deeply pigmented tracheobronchial lymph nodes. Inhaled foreign materials, regardless of their nature, are filtered out of the lymph as it passes through these lymph nodes; this accounts for the markedly dark color of both the tracheobronchial and the pulmonary lymph nodes in some specimens.

Lymph from the cranial lung lobes drains into the right and left tracheobronchial lymph nodes, and lymph from the caudal lung lobes drains into the middle tracheobronchial lymph node. Lymph from the middle lobe drains into all the tracheobronchial lymph nodes (Kubik et al., 1956; Kubik & Tömböl, 1958). Miller (1937) has also described the lymph vessels of the dog's lung.

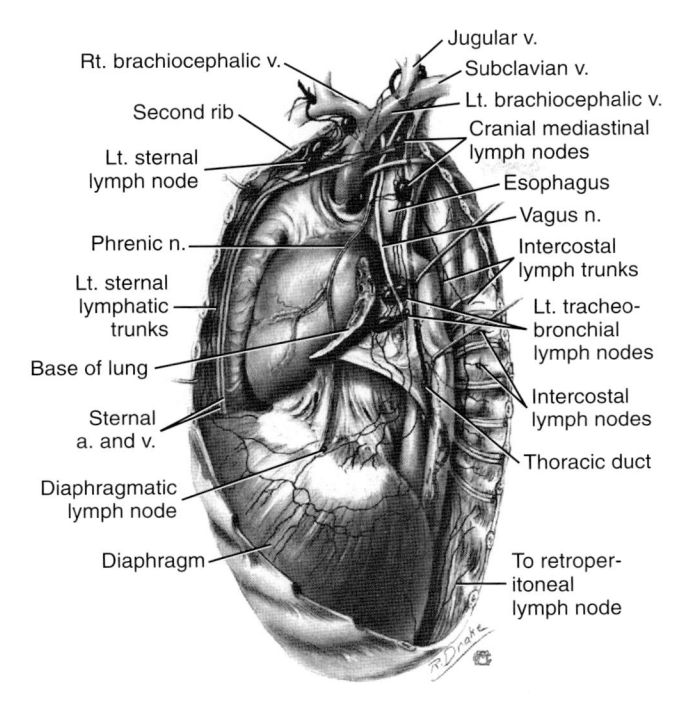

Lymph Nodes and Vessels of the Abdominal and Pelvic Walls

These lymph nodes, like those of the thorax, can be divided into parietal and visceral groups (Grau & Barone, 1970). The parietal group includes the lymph centers of the abdominal and pelvic walls: lumbar, iliosacral, and iliofemoral lymph centers. The visceral group is divided largely into subgroups that serve specific organs.

Lumbar Lymph Center

The lumbar lymph center (*lymphocentrum lumbale*) consists of the lumbar aortic and renal lymph nodes.

The **lumbar aortic lymph nodes** (*lymphonodi lumbales aortici*) (Figs. 13.18, and 13.24 through 13.27) are small nodes that lie along the aorta and caudal vena cava, from the diaphragm to the deep circumflex iliac arteries. Except for a paired node near the diaphragm, they are erratic in their development and are often absent. In some specimens as many as 17 individual nodes are present (Baum, 1918). Because of their small size and their similarity in color to

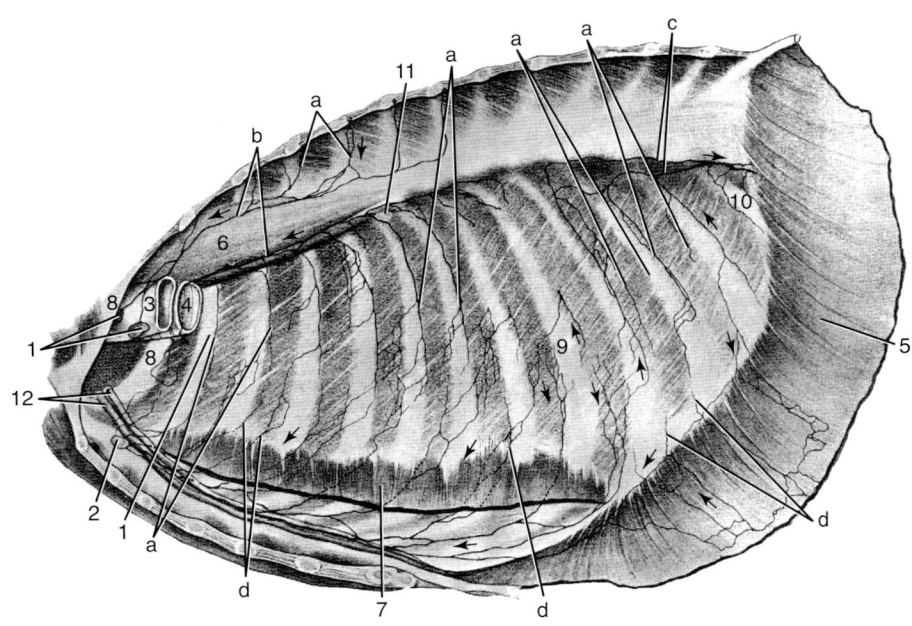

- **Fig. 13.14** The left thoracic cavity, lung removed, after the intraperitoneal injection of a graphite preparation. (From Higgins GM, Graham AS: Lymph drainage from the peritoneal cavity in the dog, *Arch Surg* 19:453–465, 1929. Copyright 1929, American Medical Association.)

a. Dorsally running lymph vessels; they form various small branches that run in part (b) cranially to the cranial mediastinal lymph nodes (1,1′) and in part (c) caudally to the cranial lumbar aortic lymph node

d. Ventrally running lymph vessels that empty into the cranial sternal lymph node (2). Some of them (d′) first run on the diaphragm

1. Cranial mediastinal lymph nodes
2. Cranial sternal lymph node
3. Esophagus (cut)
4. Trachea (cut)
5. Diaphragm (cut and reflected)
6. M. longus colli
7. M. transversus thoracis (cut)
8. 8′. Left and right first ribs
9. Ninth rib
10. Thirteenth rib
11. Intercostal lymph node
12. Internal thoracic artery and vein

- **Fig. 13.15** Lymph vessels of the pleura of the dog. (From Baum H: Das Lymphgefässystem des Hundes, *Arch wiss prakt Tierheilk Bd* 44:521–650, 1918.)

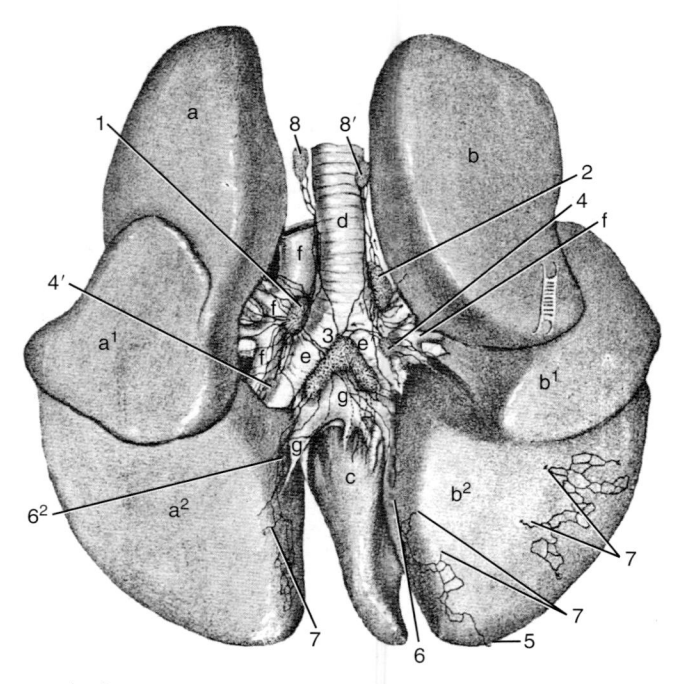

634 CHAPTER 13 The Lymphatic System

a, a¹, a². Cranial and caudal parts of cranial lobe and caudal lobe of the left lung
b, b¹, b². Cranial, middle, and caudal lobes of the right lung
c. Accessory lobe
d. Trachea
e, e'. Left and right principal bronchus
f. Pulmonary trunk and its branches
g. Pulmonary veins
1, 2, 3. Left, right, and middle tracheobronchial lymph nodes
4, 4'. Pulmonary lymph nodes
5. Subserosal lymph vessels that pass around the acute margin to the diaphragmatic surface and there pass deeply
6. Subserosal lymph vessels that course along the attachment of the pulmonary ligament
7. Subserosal lymph vessels that pass deeply
8, 8'. A left and a right cranial mediastinal lymph node

• **Fig. 13.16** Lymph nodes and vessels of the lungs and bronchi of the dog. (From Baum H: Das Lymphgefässystem des Hundes, *Arch wiss prakt Tierheilk Bd* 44:521–650, 1918.)

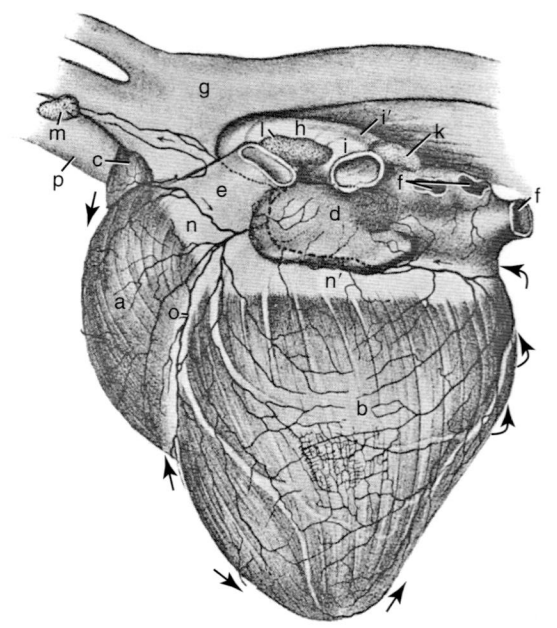

a. Right ventricle
b. Left ventricle
c. Right auricle
d. Left auricle
e. Pulmonary trunk (cut)
f. Pulmonary veins (cut)
g. Aorta
h. Trachea
i, i'. Left and right principal bronchus
k. Middle tracheobronchial lymph node
l. Left tracheobronchial lymph node
m. Cranial mediastinal lymph node
n, n'. Coronary sulcus
o. Paraconal interventricular sulcus
p. Cranial vena cava

• **Fig. 13.17** Left side of the heart of the dog with injected lymph vessels. (From Baum H: Das Lymphgefässystem des Hundes, *Arch wiss prakt Tierheilk Bd* 44:521–650, 1918.)

the fat in which they are embedded, they are easily overlooked. The most constant in size and position is the paired lumbar aortic node, which has somewhat different relations on either side. The left lymph node is occasionally double. It is 10 to 20 mm long and lies between the left crus of the diaphragm and the left lumbar hypaxial muscles, dorsal or caudal to the left renal artery. Its cranial pole usually touches or extends dorsal to the left phrenicoabdominal common trunk. The right member of this pair, usually smaller than the left, lies on the right crus of the diaphragm, dorsal to the right renal vein, and may have its cranial pole located dorsal to the right common trunk for the caudal phrenic and cranial abdominal arteries and veins just after these vessels have crossed the respective dorsal and ventral surfaces of the right adrenal gland.

Drainage Area. The afferent lymph vessels to the lumbar aortic lymph nodes come from the lumbar vertebrae; last ribs; lumbar, intercostal, and abdominal muscles; aorta; spinal cord meninges; and parietal pleura; diaphragm and parietal peritoneum; the adrenal glands; and the abdominal portions of the urogenital system. Suami et al. (2008) found perforating lymph vessels in the lumbar and gluteal regions that originate in the skin, penetrate the abdominal wall, and then drain into lumbar aortic lymph nodes instead of the axillary and inguinal lymph nodes.

They receive efferent vessels from more caudally located nodes. Testicular lymph vessels drain primarily to lumbar aortic lymph nodes at the level of L2 to L4, medial to the opening of the testicular vein (Yeh et al., 1986). Similarly, lymph from the ovaries drains into the lumbar aortic lymph nodes (Kocisova & Munka, 1974). The latter authors also describe the location and frequency of various lumbar aortic lymph nodes in 50 mongrel dogs. Efferent vessels from these nodes empty directly into the lumbar lymphatic trunks; those from the more constant, cranially located nodes drain directly into the cisterna chyli.

Renal lymph nodes (*lymphonodi renales*) are small, inconstant lymph nodes associated with the renal vessels. They receive afferent lymph vessels from the kidneys and drain into lumbar aortic lymph nodes or the lumbar lymph trunks.

wide, and 5 mm thick. It is irregular in outline, and more often its cranial end extends ventral or dorsal to the deep circumflex iliac vessels rather than caudal to the external iliac artery. This lymph node is bounded deeply on the right side by the caudal vena cava, which lies dorsal and to the right of the aorta. Each lymph node lies in the furrow between the m. psoas major and the aorta and caudal vena cava, ventral to the bodies of the fifth and sixth lumbar vertebrae. Caudally it more often bends laterally and follows along the cranial border of the external iliac artery rather than running ventral to it.

Drainage Area. The medial iliac lymph node or nodes receive afferent lymph vessels from the skin of the dorsal abdominal wall caudal to the last rib, the skin in the region of the pelvis, the tail root, the craniolateral aspect of the thigh and stifle, abdominal muscles, muscles and bones of the pelvic limb, pelvic and lumbar muscles, colon, rectum, anus, vagina, vulva, testis, epididymis, spermatic cord, vaginal tunic and cremaster muscle, prostate gland, ureter, bladder and urethra, aorta, and spinal cord meninges, as well as from efferent vessels from the deep and superficial inguinal, left colic, sacral, and internal iliac lymph nodes. The efferent vessels from the medial iliac lymph node or nodes drain cranially to form the lumbar lymph trunks or drain into the caudal members of the lumbar aortic lymph nodes if these nodes are present.

The **internal iliac lymph nodes** (*lymphonodi iliaci interni*) (Figs. 13.22 and 13.24 through 13.27) were formerly called the *hypogastric lymph nodes*. They are usually small, paired nodes that lie in the angle between the internal iliac and the median sacral artery, ventral to the body of the sixth or seventh lumbar vertebra on the ventral sacrocaudal muscle. There may be three nodes, one caudal to another, on one side, or the nodes may be double on each side. In six of Baum's specimens only a single node served both sides. It can extend cranially as far as the external iliac artery (Baum, 1918).

Drainage Area. The afferent lymph vessels come from the mm. psoas minor, quadratus lumborum, gluteus medius and profundus, biceps femoris, semitendinosus, semimembranosus, quadratus femoris, and obturator externus; tail muscles; pelvis; femur; lumbar, sacral, and caudal vertebrae; colon; rectum and anus; uterus, vagina, vestibule, vulva, and clitoris of the female; testis, epididymis, ductus deferens, prostate, and penis of the male; ureters; bladder and urethra; accessory genital glands; and nervous system. The internal iliac lymph nodes also receive lymph from the sacral and iliofemoral lymph nodes. The efferent lymph vessels drain into the medial iliac lymph nodes.

The **sacral lymph nodes** (*lymphonodi sacrales*) (Figs. 13.18, 13.20, 13.24, 13.25, and 13.27) are not present approximately half of the time. They are not sharply differentiated from the internal iliac lymph nodes when more than one internal iliac lymph node is present. Baum (1918) divides the sacral lymph nodes into a medial group along the dorsal wall and a lateral group along the dorsolateral wall of the pelvic cavity. The sacral lymph nodes lie ventral

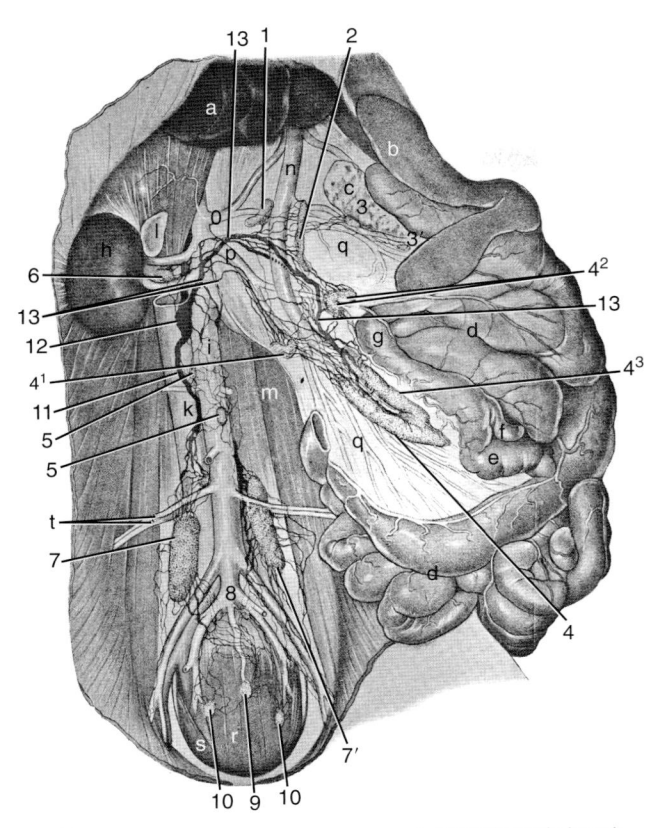

a. Liver
b. Spleen
c. Pancreas
d. Jejunum
e. Ileum
f. Cecum
g. Colon
h. Right kidney
i. Aorta
k. Caudal vena cava
l. Right adrenal gland
m. Psoas muscles
n. Portal vein
o. Celiac artery
p. Cranial mesenteric artery
q. Mesentery with blood vessels
r, s. Muscles of the tail
t. Deep circumflex iliac artery and vein

1. Right hepatic lymph node
2. Left hepatic lymph node
3, 3′. Splenic lymph nodes
4 to 4³. Jejunal lymph nodes
5. Lumbar aortic lymph nodes
6. Right cranial lumbar aortic lymph node
7, 7′. Medial iliac lymph nodes
8. Internal iliac lymph nodes
9. Sacral lymph nodes
10. Sacral lymph nodes
11. Lumbar trunk
12. Ventral part of the cisterna chyli
13. Intestinal lymph trunk

• **Fig. 13.18** Lymph vessels and lymph nodes of the abdominal cavity of the dog. (From Baum H: Das Lymphgefässystem des Hundes, *Arch wiss prakt Tierheilk Bd* 44:521–650, 1918.)

Iliosacral Lymph Center

The iliosacral lymph center (*lymphocentrum iliosacrale*) consists of the medial iliac, internal iliac and sacral lymph nodes.

The **medial iliac lymph node** (*lymphonodi iliaci mediales*) (see Figs. 13.18 through 13.20, 13.22, 13.24 through 13.27), formerly known as the *external iliac lymph node*, is a large, constant lymph node located between the deep circumflex iliac and the external iliac arteries. It is usually single but may be double on one or both sides. The medial iliac lymph node is approximately 40 mm long, 20 mm

- **Fig. 13.19** Lateral volume rendered computed tomography (CT) lymphangiogram. Contrast material (blue) was injected into the left popliteal lymph node and is seen passing through lymphatic vessels of the pelvis, abdomen, and thorax. The region of the medial iliac lymph nodes *(MI)*, cisterna chyli *(CC)*, and the thoracic duct *(TD)* are indicated. The contrast material is seen diffusely entering the cranial vena cava.

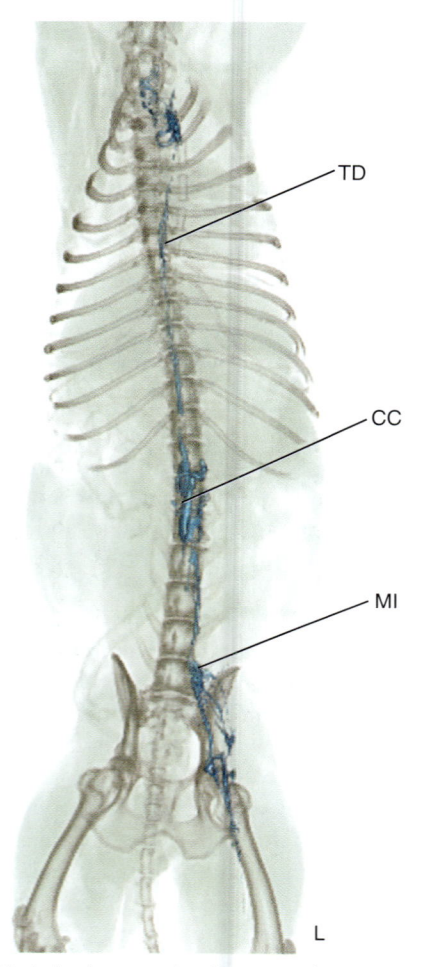

- **Fig. 13.20** Ventral volume rendered computed tomography (CT) lymphangiogram. Contrast material (blue) was injected into the left popliteal lymph node. The contrast material is seen in lymphatic vessels of the abdomen and thorax and includes the medial iliac lymph nodes *(MI)*, cisterna chyli *(CC)*, and the thoracic duct *(TD)*. Cranially the lymph flow breaks into a variable number of small tributaries before entering the cranial vena cava.

to the body of the sacrum or ventral to the ventral sacrocaudal muscle. Small nodes, when present, lie on each side of the median sacral artery. Occasionally, there is a single small lymph node, located in the fat ventral to the artery; in other dogs one or two lymph nodes are present on one side. Baum (1918) occasionally found a small sacral lymph node located between the mm. piriformis and sacrocaudalis ventralis, closely associated with the internal iliac artery and vein.

Drainage Area. The afferent lymph vessels come from the mm. gemelli; muscles of the tail; pelvic bones; caudal vertebrae; femur; sacrum; the uterus, vagina, vestibule, vulva, and clitoris of the female; the prostate and penis of the male; and the urethra. The efferent vessels go as a plexus to the internal iliac and medial iliac lymph nodes.

Lymph Nodes and Vessels of the Abdominal and Pelvic Viscera

The lymph nodes of the viscera are divided largely into subgroups that serve specific organs.

Lymph Nodes and Vessels of the Genital Organs

The lymph vessels of the female genital organs (Fig. 13.25) empty into the lumbar, medial iliac, internal iliac, superficial inguinal, and sacral lymph nodes. A fine lymphatic network in the mesosalpinx and fat surrounding the ovary drains into lumbar lymph nodes in the region of the renal artery and vein (Baum, 1918; Kocisova & Munka, 1974). The lymph vessels of the cranial half of the uterus empty into the lumbar and medial iliac lymph nodes, whereas vessels of the caudal half of the uterus drain into internal iliac, medial iliac, and sacral lymph nodes. Lymph vessels of the vagina enter the internal iliac lymph nodes, whereas those from the vestibule, in addition to entering the internal iliac and sacral lymph nodes, also pass to the superficial inguinal node. Occasionally lymph vessels from the vagina or vestibule bypass the internal iliac and sacral lymph nodes and empty directly into the medial iliac lymph node. The lymph vessels of the vulva and clitoris pass, for the most part, into the superficial inguinal lymph node.

The lymph vessels of the male genital organs (Figs. 13.26 and 13.27) empty into the same lymph nodes as do those of the female (Baum, 1918; Yeh et al., 1986). A coarse network of lymph vessels that drain the scrotum enters the superficial inguinal node. The lymph vessels of the testis and epididymis extend in the spermatic cord into the abdominal cavity to enter the medial iliac and lumbar aortic lymph nodes. For the most part they accompany the blood vessels of the spermatic cord. Lymph vessels of the prostate gland form a coarse network on the surface of the gland, from which several vessels on each side drain into the medial iliac and internal iliac lymph nodes. Lymph vessels of the prepuce and penis enter the superficial inguinal lymph node. Lymph vessels from the urinary bladder (Fig. 13.27) were found to drain into the lumbar and internal iliac lymph nodes (Milroy & Cockett, 1973).

Mammary tumors are fairly common in the bitch and frequently metastasize; therefore the lymph drainage from the glands is clinically significant. In clinically normal dogs lymph from the cranial thoracic mammary gland generally drains into lymph nodes of the axillary lymph center, and less commonly also into lymph nodes of the superficial cervical and ventral thoracic lymph centers. Lymph from the caudal thoracic mammary gland normally drains into lymph nodes of the axillary lymph center. Pereira et al. (2003) found that drainage into lymph nodes of the superficial cervical and ventral thoracic lymph centers is more common in neoplasia of the thoracic mammary glands.

Lymph from the cranial abdominal mammary gland is unique in that it can drain both cranially into lymph nodes of the axillary lymph center, as well as caudally into lymph nodes of the inguinofemoral lymph center. Lymph from the caudal abdominal mammary gland drains into lymph nodes of the inguinofemoral and popliteal lymph centers (Pereira et al., 2003). The latter authors also found that lymph from neoplastic cranial and caudal abdominal mammary glands may drain into lymph nodes of the axillary and inguinofemoral lymph centers and that the popliteal lymph center receives lymph only from healthy caudal abdominal mammary gland.

The inguinal mammary gland can by drained by both inguinofemoral and popliteal lymph centers in both normal and neoplastic conditions (Pereira et al., 2003).

According to Pereira et al. (2003) mammary neoplasia presents more types of anastomosis compared with healthy glands and an increase in contralateral anastomosis. This can change the lymph drainage patten in terms of lymph centers and vascular arborization, thus forming new drainage channels and recruiting a larger number of lymph nodes.

Lymph Nodes and Vessels of the Abdominal Viscera

The lymph nodes of the abdominal viscera of the dog are not numerous, in comparison with those of other species. They, like the lymph nodes of the abdominal wall, can be grouped into various lymph centers. The following lymph centers serve the abdominal viscera: (1) celiac, (2) cranial mesenteric, and (3) caudal mesenteric lymph centers.

Celiac Lymph Center

The celiac lymph center (*lymphocentrum celiacum*) consists of the lymph nodes associated with the organs supplied by the celiac artery. In the dog the lymph nodes in this center are usually the hepatic, splenic, gastric, and pancreaticoduodenal lymph nodes.

The **hepatic lymph nodes** (*lymphonodi hepatici*) (Figs. 13.18 and 13.21 through 13.23) usually consist of right and left lymph nodes, lying one on each side of the portal vein, 1 or 2 cm from the hilus of the liver. They may, however, vary greatly in number, form, and size. The lymph node on

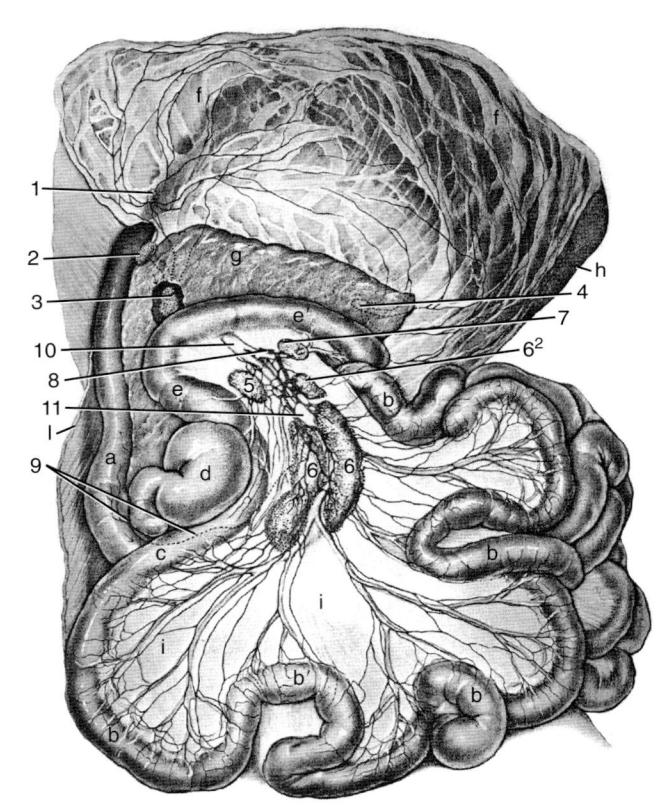

a. Duodenum
b, b'. Jejunum
c. Ileum
d. Cecum
e, e'. Colon
f. Dorsal wall (deep leaf) of omentum through which the stomach can be seen
g. Pancreas
h. Spleen (covered in part by omentum)
i. Intestinal mesentery
l. Cut edge of abdominal wall

1, 2. Pancreaticoduodenal lymph nodes
3. Right hepatic lymph node
4. Splenic lymph node
5. Right colic lymph node
6, 6^2. Jejunal lymph nodes
7. Middle colic lymph node
8. Intestinal trunk
9. Lymph vessel of the duodenum that goes to the right jejunal lymph node (6)
10. Cranial mesenteric artery
11. Jejunal lymph trunk

• **Fig. 13.21** Lymph vessels of the small intestine and omentum of a dog lying on its back. (From Baum H: Das Lymphgefässystem des Hundes, *Arch wiss prakt Tierheilk* Bd 44:521–650, 1918.)

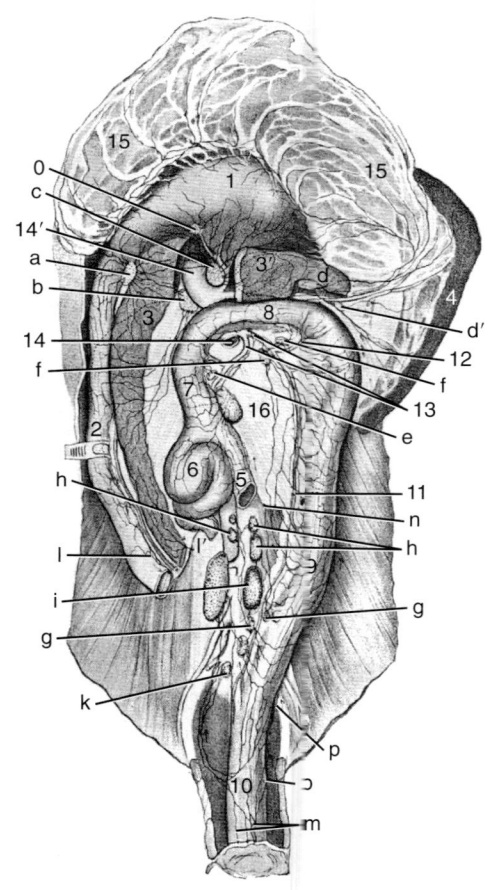

a. Pancreaticoduodenal lymph node
b. Right hepatic lymph node
c. Left hepatic lymph node
d, d'. Splenic lymph nodes
e. Right colic lymph node
f. Middle colic lymph nodes
g. Left colic lymph nodes
h. Lumbar aortic lymph nodes
i. Medial iliac lymph nodes
k. Internal iliac lymph nodes
l, l'. Lymph vessel of the duodenum and lymph vessel of the pancreas that go to the jejunal lymph nodes (removed)
m. Lymph vessels of the anus and rectum
n. Lymph vessels that go directly to the lumbar cistern
o. Gastric lymph node
p. Lymph vessels of the rectum that course over the dorsal surface of the rectum to the internal iliac and medial iliac lymph nodes

1. Stomach
2. Duodenum (cut)
3, 3'. Pancreas
4. Spleen (with splenic veins displaced)
5. Ileum (cut)
6. Cecum
7, 8, 9. Colon
10. Rectum
11. Left colic vein
12. Middle colic vein
13. Ileocolic vein
14, 14'. Portal vein
15. Superficial leaf of the omental sac (reflected) —deep leaf removed.
16. Mesentery of the colon

• **Fig. 13.22** Lymph vessels and lymph nodes of the stomach, spleen, pancreas, duodenum, and large intestine of the dog. (From Baum H: Das Lymphgefässystem des Hundes, *Arch wiss prakt Tierheilk* Bd 44:521–650, 1918.)

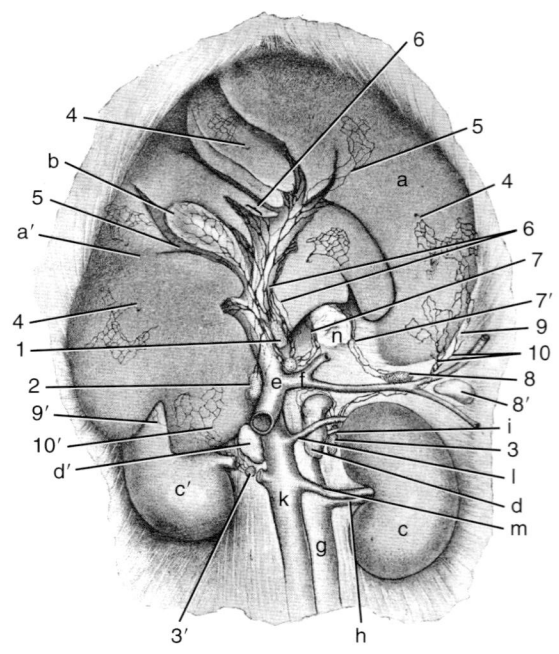

1, 2. Left and right hepatic lymph nodes
3, 3'. Cranial lumbar aortic lymph nodes
4. Subserosal lymph vessels that course deeply
5. Subserosal lymph vessels that can be followed to the hepatic lymph nodes
6. Deep lymph vessels of the liver
7, 7'. Lymph vessels that leave the distal end of the esophagus
8, 8'. Splenic lymph nodes
9, 9'. Subserosal lymph vessels that originate from the parietal surface of the liver
10, 10'. Subserosal lymph vessels from the visceral surface of the liver that course to the cranial lumbar aortic lymph nodes (3, 3')

a, a'. Liver
b. Gallbladder
c, c'. Left and right kidneys
d, d'. Left and right adrenal glands
e. Portal vein
f. Splenic vein
g. Aorta
h. Renal artery
i. Phrenicoabdominal trunk
k. Caudal vena cava
l. Cranial abdominal vein
m. Renal vein
n. Esophagus (cut)

• **Fig. 13.23** Lymph vessels of the liver of the dog. (From Baum H: Das Lymphgefässystem des Hundes, *Arch wiss prakt Tierheilk* Bd 44:521–650, 1918.)

the left is longer and larger than that on the right. It lies in the lesser omentum, dorsal to the bile duct. It is approximately 30 mm long and irregular in form; the caudal part that reaches to, extends along, or even extends beyond the splenic vein may be separated from the main lymphoid mass and may form one or two additional lymph nodes. When single, the left node is approximately 30 mm long. On the right there may be one to five lymph nodes of various sizes and forms. They lie on the right side of the portal vein opposite the left hepatic lymph node and to the right of the splenic vein at its termination. They are closely related to the body of the pancreas and may be flattened as they lie between the layers of peritoneum. Occasionally, the two nodal masses are joined cranially.

Drainage Area. The afferent lymph vessels of the hepatic lymph nodes come from the stomach, duodenum, pancreas, and liver. Kahlenberg et al. (2001) injected isosulfan blue dye directly into the right medial lobe of the liver and found that it drained into a portal lymph node in all cases, without any adverse affects to liver function. Lymph vessels connect several of the nodes. The efferent lymph vessels from the right hepatic lymph node unite into four to eight vessels that run over both surfaces of the portal vein to the cranial mesenteric artery, where they help form the intestinal trunk or the network of lymph vessels that represents this trunk.

The **splenic lymph nodes** (*lymphonodi lienales*) (Figs. 13.18 and 13.21 through 13.23) are a group of three to five nodes that lie along the course of the splenic artery and vein and their terminal branches in the deep leaf of the greater omentum (Mall, 1903). Most are small lymph nodes that can be more easily palpated than seen in obese specimens. Usually the largest lymph node lies on the cranial side of the splenic vessels or in the angle of their division, approximately 20 mm from the termination of the splenic vein. This lymph node may be as long as 40 mm, but it is more commonly 15 mm in length.

Drainage Area. The afferent lymph vessels to the splenic lymph nodes come from the esophagus, stomach, pancreas, spleen, liver, omentum, and diaphragm. Their efferent lymph vessels help form the intestinal trunk or the lymphatic plexus that frequently replaces it.

The **gastric lymph nodes** (*lymphonodi gastrici*) (Fig. 13.22) lie in the lesser omentum, close to the lesser curvature of the stomach, near the pylorus. Occasionally, they are absent or double.

Drainage Area. The afferent lymph vessels to the gastric lymph node(s) come from the esophagus, stomach, diaphragm, and lesser omentum. Their efferent lymph vessels drain into the left hepatic or splenic lymph nodes, or both.

The **pancreaticoduodenal lymph nodes** (*lymphonodi pancreaticoduodenales*) (Figs. 13.21 and 13.22) lie along the initial portion of the duodenum and include the nodes formerly called *duodenal* and *omental lymph nodes* by Baum (1918). A small, constant lymph node that may be double (duodenal) lies between the pylorus and the right lobe of the pancreas. An inconstant, even smaller lymph node (omental) may be present in the superficial leaf of the greater omentum a few centimeters from the pylorus.

Drainage Area. The afferent lymph vessels to the pancreaticoduodenal lymph nodes come from the duodenum, pancreas, and greater omentum. The efferent lymph vessels from the pancreaticoduodenal lymph node go into the right hepatic or right colic node.

Cranial Mesenteric Lymph Center

The cranial mesenteric lymph center (*lymphocentrum mesentericum craniale*) of the dog consists of the jejunal and colic lymph nodes.

The **jejunal lymph nodes** (*lymphonodi jejunales*) (Figs. 13.18 and 13.21), previously called the *cranial mesenteric lymph nodes,* are the largest lymph nodes of the abdomen. There are usually two, occasionally more, which are present along both sides of the vascular "tree" of the mesentery and cover the proximal branches of the cranial mesenteric artery. In medium-sized dogs they average 60 mm long, 20 mm wide, and 5 mm thick. They are irregular in form. Frequently, their distal ends are knobbed or even lobated. The middle parts of jejunal lymph nodes may be roughly triangular in cross-section. They lie between the leaves of the long jejunal mesentery, along the cranial mesenteric artery and vein. The initial parts of some 12 jejunal arteries are sandwiched between the two jejunal lymph nodes. The right jejunal lymph node lies between the cranial mesenteric vein and the ileum and is seen more easily from the dorsal aspect. This lymph node may be double or even triple. When it is double, the distal member is the larger. In 20 of 25 specimens examined by Baum (1918) the jejunal lymph node on the right was single. In one specimen as many as five lymph nodes were present on the left. There was no constant grouping of smaller jejunal lymph nodes.

Drainage Area. The afferent lymph vessels to the jejunal lymph nodes come from the jejunum, ileum, and pancreas. The efferent vessels from these nodes are the chief formative tributaries of the **intestinal trunk** (*truncus intestinalis*) or of the lymphatic plexus that replaces it.

The **colic lymph nodes** (*lymphonodi colici*) (Figs. 13.21 and 13.22) are found between the peritoneal laminae of the mesocolon. They usually lie close to the ascending and transverse colon.

Sterns and Vaughan (1970) studied the lymph drainage patterns of the colon under normal and abnormal conditions by means of indirect lymphography and confirmed the specific segmental distribution of lymph vessels of the dog colon. On the mucosal surface of the cecum, there are smooth, rounded elevations approximately 3 mm in diameter that can be seen on the mucosal folds and between them. These elevations are sites of lymphoglandular complexes that penetrate the muscularis mucosae (Atkins & Schofield, 1972). There are approximately three nodules per cm^2. Similar structures were seen in the colon adjacent to the cecum but not elsewhere in the colon. These submucosal lymphoid nodules are invaginated by extensions of the overlying intestinal glands and thus are called *lymphoglandular* complexes. The structure and development of these complexes in the dog indicate that they have a secondary rather than a primary role as a lymphoid organ. The colic lymph nodes can be divided into a right group along the ascending colon, a middle group along the transverse colon, and a left group along the descending colon (Baum, 1918).

The **right colic lymph node** is disc-shaped and usually more than 10 mm in diameter and lies dorsomedial to the ascending colon at the ileocolic junction. It is usually single, but as many as five lymph nodes may be present. The largest lymph node is located in the angle formed by the converging veins that form the ileocolic vein.

The **middle colic lymph node** is a spherical or oval lymph node, usually less than 10 mm long, that lies 50 to 57 mm from the transverse colon, near the attachment of the transverse mesocolon to the mesentery. It is located near or on the junction of the middle colic tributary with the caudal mesenteric vein. If two lymph nodes are present, one lies on either side of the caudal mesenteric vein. The incidence of multiple lymph nodes in this location is the same as for the right side. The dorsocranial pole of the left jejunal lymph node may be in apposition to the most proximal part of the middle colic lymph node or the most proximal lymph node of this group.

The **left colic lymph nodes** number two to five and lie in the caudal part of the descending mesocolon near the pelvic inlet. The largest member of the group is usually located in the angle formed by the terminal branches of the caudal mesenteric artery. The others are mostly located between the cranial rectal artery and its satellite vein, which lies on the intestine. They form an interconnected chain of oval lymph nodes that do not extend further caudally than the pelvic inlet. Each lymph node is not more than a few millimeters long.

Drainage Area. The afferent lymph vessels to the colic lymph nodes come from the ileum, cecum, and colon. The middle colic lymph node receives efferent lymph vessels from the left colic lymph nodes. The efferent lymph vessels from the right and middle colic lymph nodes empty into the intestinal trunks. Those from the left colic lymph nodes go as groups of one to three efferent vessels from each node and either enter the medial iliac, the lumbar, or the middle colic lymph node, or empty into the intestinal trunk directly.

Lymph Trunks

A number of lymphatic trunks from the abdominal viscera provide routes of lymph drainage to the cisterna chyli. The **visceral trunk** (*truncus visceralis*) is the largest, unpaired, and it collects lymph from the celiac and intestinal lymph trunks. The **celiac trunk** (*truncus celiacus*) drains the lymph nodes of the celiac lymph center. The **intestinal trunk** (*truncus intestinalis*) drains the lymph nodes of the cranial mesenteric lymph center and receives the **colic trunk** (*truncus colicus*) from the colic lymph nodes.

Lymph Nodes and Vessels of the Pelvic Limb
Superficial Lymph Vessels

Schacher and Sulahian (1972) recognized two systems of superficial lymph vessels in the pelvic limb. However, Pflug and Calnan (1969) and Satjukova et al. (1977) describe three separate systems of lymph vessels in the pelvic limb of the dog that they believe function independently to counter any occlusion of lymph drainage. Communications between these systems were located at the paw, at mid-crus, and in the inguinal region. In no instance were any lymphaticovenous anastomoses observed at peripheral sites. The three collecting systems are a superficial lateral system, a superficial medial system, and a deep medial system.

The superficial lateral system begins on the dorsum of the paw, parallels the dorsal metatarsal veins, and then crosses to the caudolateral surface at mid-crus, following the lateral saphenous vein. After accompanying the calcanean tendon, the superficial lateral lymph vessels pass over the belly of the gastrocnemius muscle and enter the popliteal lymph node.

The superficial medial lymph vessels begin in the crus proximal to the tarsus and are closely associated with the skin. They continue over the gracilis muscle to the level of midthigh, where they run between the gracilis and vastus medialis muscles before passing into the superficial inguinal lymph node.

The deep medial afferent lymph vessels begin just proximal to the level of the tarsus between the distal end of the tibia and the calcanean tendon. They pass proximally toward the belly of the gastrocnemius muscle and bypass the popliteal lymph node. At the level of the stifle, they cross the insertion of the adductor muscle and run along the gracilis muscle, where they are joined by deep lymph vessels before passing to the medial iliac lymph nodes.

The pelvic limb of the dog is drained by the popliteal, iliofemoral, and inguinofemoral lymph centers.

Popliteal Lymph Center

The popliteal lymph center (*lymphocentrum popliteum*) consists of the popliteal lymph nodes. The dog only has a **superficial popliteal lymph node** (*lymphonodus popliteus superficiales*) (Figs. 13.2, 13.19, and 13.20) The superficial popliteal lymph node is the largest lymph node of the pelvic limb, is rarely double, and is constant in location. It is an oval lymph node, approximately 20 mm long, that lies in the fat depot between the medial border of the m. biceps femoris and the lateral border of the m. semitendinosus as these muscles diverge from each other. The node and its surrounding fat are subcutaneous caudally as they lie in the popliteal space caudal to the stifle joint. There is no deep popliteal lymph node in the dog (Constantinescu & Schaller, 2012).

Drainage Area. The afferent lymph vessels to the popliteal lymph node come from all parts of the pelvic limb distal to the location of the node. The 8 to 10 efferent lymph vessels accompany the medial saphenous vein in the popliteal space and unite to form two to four trunks proximal to the origin of the m. gastrocnemius. They continue proximally, close to the femur, where they lie between the m. semimembranosus and the m. adductor, to reach the apex of the femoral triangle. The efferent lymph vessels traverse the femoral triangle and the vascular lacuna and, after crossing the medial surface of the pelvis, empty into the medial iliac lymph node.

Iliofemoral Lymph Center

The iliofemoral lymph center (*lymphocentrum iliofemorale*) in the dog consists of an inconstant distal femoral lymph node and the external iliac lymph node. These nodes may be spaced widely.

The **distal femoral lymph node** (*lymphonodus femoralis distalis*) is a small, inconstant lymph node present in approximately 10% of dogs (Baum, 1918). It is never more than a few millimeters in diameter and lies in the fat deep to the deep medial femoral fascia at the distal part of the femoral triangle. The femoral vessels lie cranial to it. Mayer et al. (2013) reported finding a "femoral lymph node" in two dogs, a part of the iliofemoral lymph center. Constantinescu and Schaller (2012) illustrate the distal femoral lymph node at a position more than halfway along the length of the femur.

Drainage Area. The distal femoral lymph node drains the skin lying medially over the stifle joint, crus, and pes; the stifle and tarsal joints; the patella and bones of the crus and pes; and tendons of the muscles of the crus and pes. It also receives efferent vessels from the popliteal lymph node (Baum, 1918; Schacher & Sulahian, 1972).

The **external iliac lymph node** (*lymphonodus iliaci externi*) (Fig. 13.24), formerly called the *iliofemoral* or *deep inguinal lymph node,* is an inconstant, small node present in approximately 30% of dogs (Baum, 1918). It lies on the ventral surface of the tendon of the psoas minor muscle at its insertion on the ilium, and caudal to the external iliac vein.

Drainage area. The lymph node receives afferent lymph vessels from the muscles and bones of the crus and thigh, gluteal muscles, as well as efferent lymph vessels from the popliteal and superficial inguinal lymph nodes. The efferent lymph vessels from the external iliac lymph node unite to form 1 or 2 lymph trunks that cross the surface of the external iliac blood vessels and drain into the medial iliac lymph nodes.

Inguinofemoral Lymph Center

The **inguinofemoral lymph center** (*lymphocentrum inguinofemorale*) of the dog consists of the superficial inguinal lymph nodes. These are specified as the **scrotal lymph nodes** (*lymphonodi scrotales*) of the male and the **mammary lymph nodes** (*lymphonodi mammarii*) of the female animal.

The **superficial inguinal lymph nodes** (*lymphonodi inguinales superficiales*) (Figs. 13.25 through 13.27), usually two in number, begin a few millimeters cranial to the vaginal process or vaginal tunic and lie in the fat that fills the furrow between the abdominal wall and the medial surface of the thigh. In the male, right and left lymph nodes lie along the dorsolateral borders of the penis cranial to the vaginal tunic at approximately the level of the bulbus glandis. In the female these lymph nodes are located deep to the inguinal mammary gland. When a single lymph node is present, the external pudendal vessels lie lateral to it. However, when two lymph nodes are present, these vessels usually run between the cranial and the caudal poles of the lymph nodes, or the cranial lymph node lies medial to the vessels in a location deeper than that of the caudal lymph node. The lymph nodes are usually oval in shape and approximately 20 mm long, but can vary between wide extremes.

Drainage Area. The afferent vessels to the superficial inguinal lymph nodes come from the ventral half of the abdominal wall, including the abdominal and inguinal mammary glands. In the male, the afferent vessels come from the penis and the skin of the prepuce and scrotum. Other afferent vessels come from the ventral part of the pelvis, the tail, and the medial side of the thigh, stifle joint, and crus. The superficial inguinal lymph nodes receive the efferent vessels from the popliteal lymph node and thus serve as one of the nodal stations for the whole pelvic limb. However, Mayer et al. (2013) found no direct connection

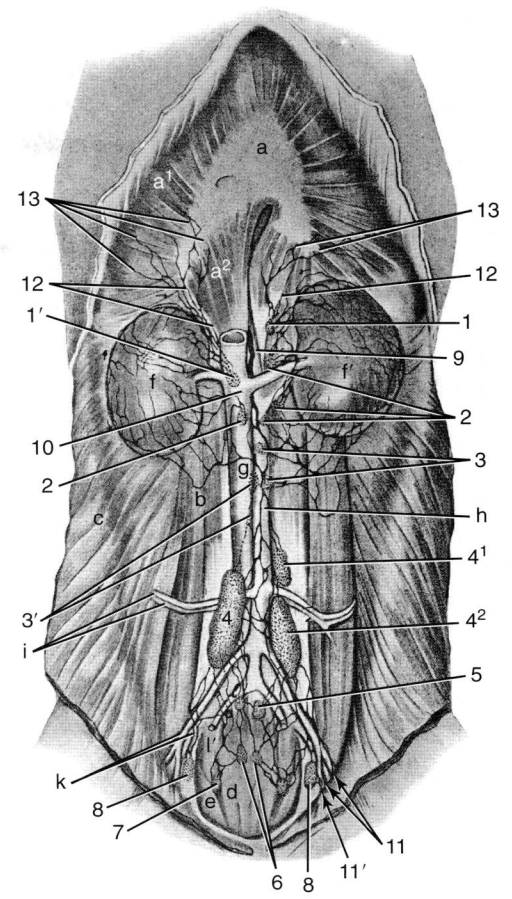

a, a^1, a^2. Diaphragm
b. Psoas muscles
c. Lateral abdominal wall
d, e. Muscles of the tail
f, f'. Kidneys
g. Caudal vena cava
h. Abdominal aorta
i. Right deep circumflex iliac artery and vein
k. Right external iliac artery and vein
l, l'. Right internal iliac artery and vein
1, 1'. Left and right lumbar aortic lymph nodes (the right node is covered by the caudal vena cava)
2. Lumbar lymph nodes that are located near the renal artery and vein
3. Lumbar lymph nodes
4, 4^1, 4^2. Medial iliac lymph nodes
5. Internal iliac lymph nodes
6, 7. Sacral lymph nodes
8. External iliac lymph nodes
9. Cisterna chyli
10. Lumbar trunk
11. Efferent vessels of the superficial inguinal and femoral lymph nodes (from them a part [11'] enters the external iliac lymph nodes [8])
12. Lymph vessels that enter the abdominal cavity from the thorax with the major splanchnic nerve and sympathetic trunk
13. Lymph vessels of the diaphragm

• **Fig. 13.24** Lymph vessels of the kidney of the dog; the lymph nodes lying ventral to the aorta and its terminal branches. (The right kidney [f] is displaced toward the pelvis.) (From Baum H: *Das Lymphgefässystem des Hundes*, *Arch wiss prakt Tierheilk Bd* 44:521–650, 1918.)

642 CHAPTER 13 The Lymphatic System

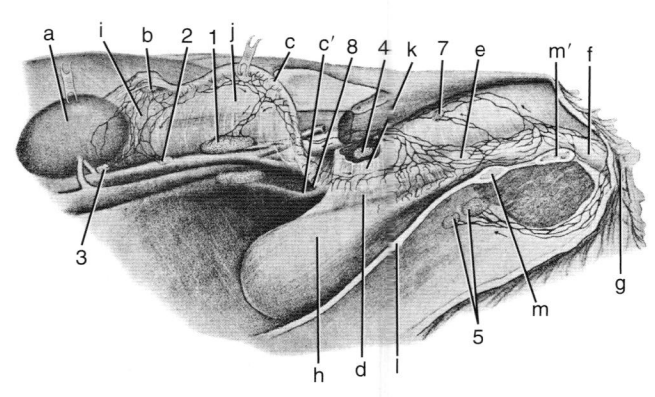

1. Medial iliac lymph node
2, 3. Lumbar aortic lymph nodes
4. Internal iliac lymph node
5. Superficial inguinal lymph nodes
7. Sacral lymph node
8. Lymph vessel that courses to the other surface of the uterine horn
a. Left kidney (reflected)
b. Left ovary (reflected)
c. Left uterine horn (reflected)
c′. Right uterine horn
d. Body of the uterus
e. Vagina
f. Vestibule
g. Vulva
h. Bladder
i. Mesosalpinx
j. Broad ligament of the uterus
k. Lateral ligament of the bladder
l. Ventral abdominal wall
m, m′. Pelvis, transected

• **Fig. 13.25** Lymph vessels of the female genital organs of the dog. (From Baum H: Das Lymphgefässystem des Hundes, *Arch wiss prakt Tierheilk* Bd 44:521–650, 1918.)

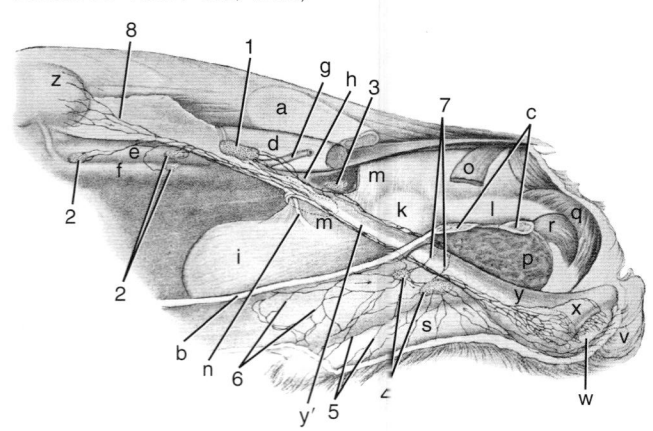

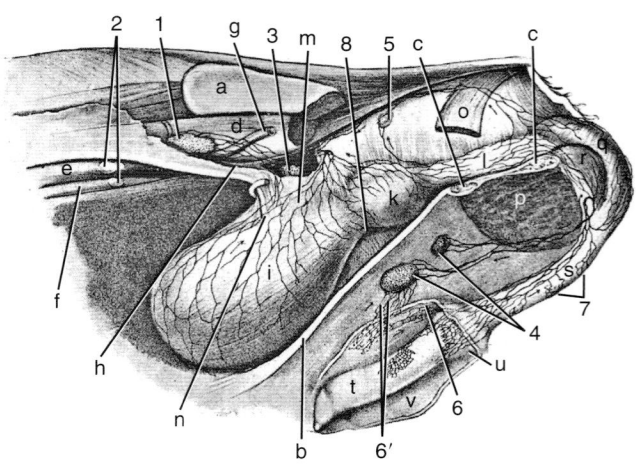

1. Medial iliac lymph node
2. Lumbar aortic lymph nodes
3. Internal iliac lymph node
4. Superficial inguinal lymph nodes
5, 6. Lymph vessels of the preputial fold
7. Efferent vessels of the superficial inguinal lymph nodes
8. Lymph vessels of the testicles, which can be followed to the capsule of the kidney
a. Ilium
b. Ventral abdominal wall
c. Pelvis, transected
d. Lumbar muscles
e. Aorta
f. Caudal vena cava
g. Left external iliac artery
h. Internal iliac artery
i. Bladder
k. Prostate
l. Urethra
m. Lateral ligament of the bladder
n. Ureter
o. M. coccygeus (cut)
p. Cut surface of m. adductor
q. M. bulbospongiosus
r. M. ischiocavernosus
s. Penis
u. Prepuce
v. Scrotum
w. Testicle
x. Epididymis
y. Vaginal tunic
z. Left kidney

• **Fig. 13.26** Lymph vessels of the bladder and the male genital organs of the dog. (From Baum H: Das Lymphgefässystem des Hundes, *Arch wiss prakt Tierheilk* Bd 44:521–650, 1918.)

1. Medial iliac lymph node
2. Lumbar aortic lymph nodes
3. Internal iliac lymph node
4. Superficial inguinal lymph nodes
5. Sacral lymph node
6, 6′. Lymph vessels of the preputial folds
7. Lymph vessels of the urethra
8. Lymph vessel of the bladder
a. Ilium
b. Ventral abdominal wall (cut)
c. Pelvis, transected
d. Lumbar hypaxial muscles
e. Aorta
f. Caudal vena cava
g. Left external iliac artery
h. Internal iliac artery
i. Bladder
k. Prostate
l. Urethra
m. Lateral ligament of the bladder
n. Ureter
o. M. coccygeus (cut)
p. Cut surface of m. adductor
q. M. bulbospongiosus
r. M. ischiocavernosus
s. Penis
t. Glans penis—pars longa
u. Bulbus glandis
v. Prepuce (opened and reflected)

• **Fig. 13.27** Lymph vessels of the urinary and male genital organs of the dog. (From Baum H: Das Lymphgefässystem des Hundes, *Arch wiss prakt Tierheilk* Bd 44:521–650, 1918.)

from the popliteal lymph nodes to the superficial inguinal lymph nodes in 16 dogs studied. There are lymph vessel connections between the right and the left superficial inguinal lymph nodes (Patsikas & Dessiris, 1992). The efferent lymph vessels unite to form one or two trunks that pass through the inguinal canal together with the external pudendal vessels and finally drain into the medial iliac lymph nodes.

Spleen

The **spleen** (*lien*) (Figs. 13.18, 13.21, 13.22, and 13.28) is situated in the left hypogastric region, approximately parallel to the greater curvature of the stomach. It is reddish-brown and often has a purple cast. The spleen is rather firm in consistency, especially when contracted, and has a thick trabecular framework. It is roughly tongue-shaped, is considerably longer than it is wide, and is slightly constricted in the middle. The spleen presents two extremities, two surfaces, and two borders. In cross-section it is triangular. Its longest surface is the lateral, or parietal, surface. The location of the organ depends on the size and position of the other abdominal organs. Its position depends largely on the fullness of the stomach. When the stomach is empty, the spleen is entirely cranial to the left costal arch. However,

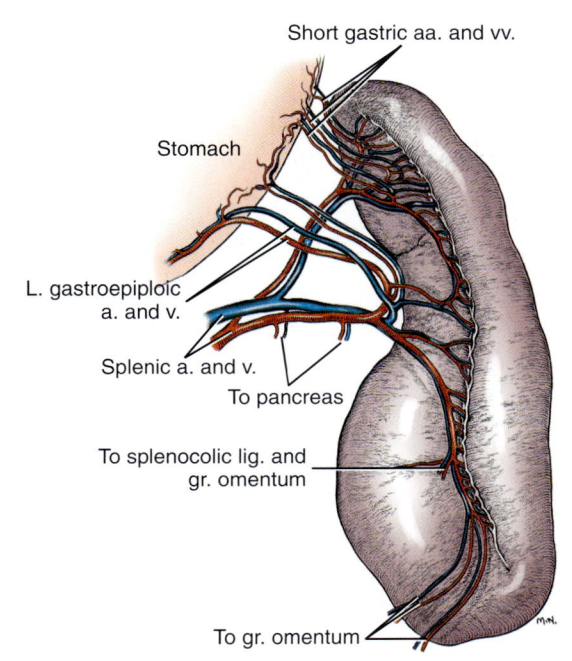

Fig. 13.28 The spleen, showing its blood supply. (The cranial border is reflected laterally.)

when the stomach is greatly distended, the spleen is displaced fully into the flank and may reach the pelvic inlet.

The **dorsal extremity**, *extremitas dorsalis*, is rounded and wedge-shaped. It lies ventral to the left crus of the diaphragm, between the fundus of the stomach and the cranial pole of the left kidney. Because of the relatively fixed position of the left kidney, the position of this part of the spleen is the least variable. In a dog with a moderately full stomach, the last two ribs cover the dorsal extremity of the spleen. A three-dimensional stereoroentgenographic analysis of the spleen showed that the dorsal extremity lies between T13 and L2 in the dorsal half of the abdominal cavity (Ogawa et al., 1976).

The **ventral extremity**, *extremitas ventralis*, is most variable, in both position and shape. When the spleen is maximally contracted, it is completely hidden deep to the middle of the caudal border of the rib cage. When it is maximally distended, not only does most of the organ extend beyond the rib cage, but also the ventral extremity moves beyond the midventral line to the right side of the floor of the abdomen. Depending on the fullness of the stomach, this may reach any level from the caudal sternum to a transverse plane caudal to the umbilicus. In a dog with a moderately full stomach, the ventral extremity projects beyond the costal arch and reaches ventrally as far as the level of the ventral ends of the seventh to the tenth ribs and caudally to a transverse plane through the second to the fourth lumbar vertebrae. Ogawa et al. (1976) found the ventral extremity between T13 and L2 in the ventral half to the ventral third of the abdominal cavity. The ventral extremity may be uniformly rounded and approximately twice as wide as the dorsal half of the organ. Usually the most cranial portion of this extremity is pointed in a direction that ranges from cranioventral to craniodorsal.

The **parietal surface** (*facies parietalis*) is convex and lateral and faces the diaphragm and the lateral abdominal body wall on the left side. It extends from the vertebral ends of the last two ribs ventrolaterally, mainly opposite the left eleventh intercostal space. As the distal portions of the last few costal cartilages bend cranially and ventrally to form the costal arch, the spleen continues tangentially across the medial surface of the costal arch and obliquely ventrally along the medial surface of the cranial part of the abdominal wall. It is at first related to the diaphragm and then to the m. transversus abdominis. The parietal surface is slightly convex transversely. The proximal part is most convex longitudinally as it bends medially toward the median plane.

The **visceral surface** (*facies visceralis*) of the spleen is concave, faces medially, and is divided into two nearly equal longitudinal parts by the long **hilus** (*hilus lienis*) of the organ. The area cranial to the hilus is related to the greater curvature of the stomach (*facies gastrica*); that caudal to the hilus is related to the left kidney proximally (*facies renalis*) and distally is related to the colon at its middle and to the mass of the small intestine ventrally (*facies intestinalis*). Even in hardened specimens, the organs related to the spleen do not make clear-cut impressions on it as the fatty omentum prevents direct contact of the visceral surface with the adjacent viscera.

The **cranial** and **caudal borders** (*margo cranialis* and *margo caudalis*) of the spleen are thin and irregular in contour. They may contain shallow or deep fissures. There is always a concavity of the cranial border proximal to the expanded ventral extremity. This concavity may involve the whole border, or it may be replaced by an angular depression. In such instances, the dorsal two-thirds of the cranial border is usually sigmoid in shape. This is masked by a sweeping cranial concavity involving the middle half of the organ. The cranial border may be infolded.

The spleen is suspended by the part of the greater omentum that leaves the left crus of the diaphragm between the esophageal hiatus and the celiac artery. This is the **phrenicosplenic ligament** (*lig. phrenicolienale*). Caudally this part of the omentum is wide and passes first to the hilus of the spleen and then to the greater curvature of the stomach, forming an extensive **gastrosplenic ligament** (*ligamentum gastrolienale*).

The spleen consists of a **capsule** (*capsula*) that is rich in elastic and smooth muscle fibers, **trabeculae** (*trabeculae lienis*) that are large and fibromuscular, and the **parenchyma**, that consists of the **red** and **white splenic pulp** (*pulpa lienis rubra et alba*). The trabeculae form a complicated network within the organ. Some trabeculae join the veins, strengthening their walls, and others are independent of them (Trautmann & Fiebiger, 1952). The larger intrasplenic arteries lie mainly in the trabeculae. The collagenous fibers of the trabeculae continue directly into the reticular fibers of the splenic pulp. There is no cortex and medulla in the organization of the spleen.

The **white pulp** in the dog consists of diffuse and nodular lymphoid tissue, mostly lymphocytes. The **nodules** (*lymphonoduli lienales*) are usually less than 1 mm in diameter and are not grossly visible. The germinal centers of these nodules are lighter in color than the surrounding pulp. Lymphatic tissue is also elaborated along the central arteries (diffuse lymphatic tissue, or periarterial lymphatic sheaths, PALS: Ross & Pawlina, 2016). The **red pulp** consists of splenic cords that form a spongy network with venous sinuses filling the spaces between them. The cells of the cords include many lymphocytes, megakaryocytes, free and fixed macrophages, and all the elements of the circulating blood. The agranular leukocytes are the most numerous among these free cells (Bloom & Fawcett, 1986). Large numbers of erythrocytes are in the red pulp where they are filtered and where senescent cells are degraded (Ross & Pawlina, 2016). The splenic cords gradually merge into the tissue of the white pulp.

The blood vessels of the spleen are the splenic artery from the celiac artery and the splenic vein, which drains into the gastrosplenic vein. However, Cardinet and Hartke (1972) examined the blood supply to the spleen in 38 Beagle dogs and found that the splenic artery was a branch of the cranial mesenteric artery in three dogs. Furthermore, Gupta et al. (1978) have shown that the arterial supply to the spleen revealed the presence of two segments, a dorsal and a ventral one. According to them there is no connection between the vessels of the two segments. A further study by Gupta et al. (1981) on the venous drainage of the spleen also revealed the same segmentation. Blood enters the organ by way of approximately up to 25 **splenic branches** (*rami lienales*), which pass through the long hilus. Once through the capsule, they course in the trabeculae, branching repeatedly and becoming smaller. When they reach a diameter of 0.2 mm, they leave the trabeculae and become surrounded by lymphoid tissue (white pulp), in which they continue to divide. According to Bloom and Fawcett (1986), when they reach the caliber of 40 to 50 µm they leave the lymphatic tissue and enter the red pulp. Here they branch into small, straight vessels, called *penicilli*. After these have divided and become smaller, their walls become greatly thickened. Further divisions reduce the arterial capillary to a caliber of not more than 10 µm (Bloom & Fawcett, 1986).

The venous side of the vascular pathway through the spleen begins in the venous sinuses. These **sinuses** (*sinus lienis*) play an active role as a part of the reticuloendothelial system (mononuclear phagocyte system). They occupy more space than does the solid part of the red pulp, among which they profusely anastomose. They range from 12 to 40 µm in width and have walls that are composed of long, narrow reticuloendothelial cells. The sinuses coalesce into veins of the red pulp, and these finally merge to become the trabecular veins. The venous pathway through the splenic capsule parallels the arterial inflow.

The exact method by which blood passes from the arterial to the venous side of the capillary bed is still in doubt. (For a review of the existing literature see Blue and Weiss [1981] and Schmidt et al. [1983]). Schmidt et al. (1982) obtained clear evidence for abundant connections between arterial capillaries and venous sinuses. However, they have also shown that the majority of capillaries end in the marginal zone around lymphatic nodules. Their findings are also supported by the work of Takubo et al. (1986). The salient observations of Kniseley's experiments (1936) were that the sinuses become filled with whole blood by the closing of a physiologic sphincter at the venous or efferent end of the sinus. As more blood is allowed to pass into the sinus, the fluid of the blood diffuses through the sinus wall, bringing about a great concentration of the cellular residue. Apparently the fluid of the blood reenters adjacent capillaries because these have been observed to contain relatively cell-free blood. One stage merges into the next, and, at the same time, other capillary–sinus units are not undergoing cyclic changes at all. In one animal the time interval for each cycle varied from a few minutes to as long 10 hours.

True accessory spleens are rare in the dog.

The nerve supply to the spleen is from the celiac plexus and consists chiefly of nonmyelinated postganglionic sympathetic axons. The few myelinated axons present are probably afferent axons. The vagi also send axons to the spleen. The nerves to the spleen form the splenic plexus of nerves that entwine the spleen of the dog.

Several diverse functions have been attributed to the spleen of the dog:

1. It stores and concentrates the erythrocytes and releases them during times of need.
2. It filters the blood, as the lymph nodes filter the lymph, and removes the worn-out erythrocytes from the circulation. From these cells it produces bilirubin, which is collected by the liver. From the hemoglobin, it extracts iron, which is released here, and is again used by the red bone marrow in the production of new erythrocytes.
3. It produces many of the lymphocytes and probably most of the monocytes and has an important function in the production of antibodies.
4. The spleen of the dog also contains megakaryocytes responsible for the formation of blood platelets.

Whereas lymph nodes filter lymph, the spleen is a lymphatic organ filtering the blood. The spleen is not essential to life or even to health as most of its normal functions are taken over by other tissues in its absence.

Thymus

The thymus (Figs. 13.29 and 13.30) is a light-gray, distinctly lobulated organ with a pink tinge in fresh material. It is laterally compressed and lies in the cranial ventral part of the thoracic cavity. Because it is predominantly lymphoid in structure and hormone production is questionable, it is described under the vascular rather than the endocrine system.

The organ, relatively large at birth, grows rapidly during the first few postnatal months and reaches its maximum development before sexual maturity, or between the fourth

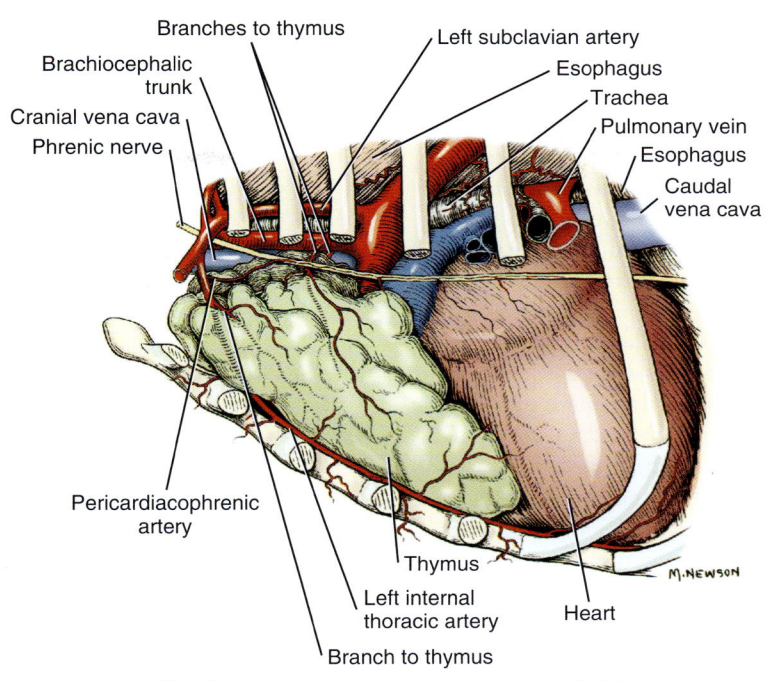

- **Fig. 13.29** The thymus gland of a young dog, showing its blood supply.

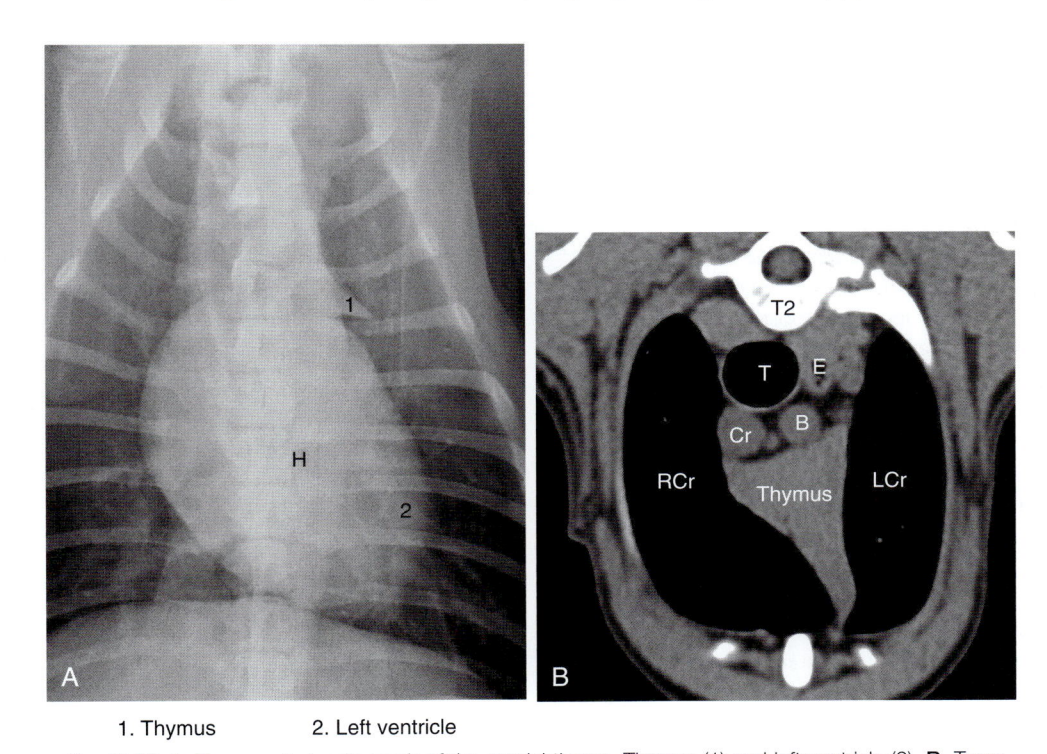

- **Fig. 13.30** A, Dorsoventral radiograph of the cranial thorax. Thymus (1) and left ventricle (2). B, Transverse computed tomography (CT) image of a young dog at the level of T2 vertebra highlighting the size and position of the thymus. *1*, Aorta; *2*, azygous vein; *3*, right pulmonary artery; *4*, right pulmonary vein; *E*, esophagus; *RB*, right primary bronchus; *LB*, left primary bronchus; *RCd*, right caudal lung lobe; and *LCd*, left caudal lung lobe.

1. Thymus   2. Left ventricle

and fifth postnatal months, just before the shedding of the deciduous incisor teeth. The thymus begins to involute at the same time as changing of the teeth from deciduous to permanent generations. Although the process is rapid at first, the organ usually does not atrophy completely, even in old age. As it decreases in size and loses its lymphoid structure, it is replaced by fat. However, evidence of a thymus can be seen in most dogs regardless of age.

The canine **thymus** is represented by the thoracic part (*lobus thoracicus*) only and is located almost entirely in the cranial mediastinal septum. When maximally developed, it lies against the sternum ventrally with its cranial pole ventral to the trachea, where it extends beyond the first rib by some 5 mm. Its caudal limit extends to approximately the fifth or sixth costal cartilage.

Each polygonal lobule (*lobuli thymi*), which may measure more than 10 mm in length, is separated from adjacent lobules by delicate but distinct connective tissue septae. The whole organ is further divided into right and left lobes (*lobi dexter et sinister*) although the compressed lobes are difficult to separate from one another. The division between the two lobes is distinct caudally, but cranially it is not always possible to determine to which lobe the adjacent lobules belong because the lobes are united here by essentially the same amount and kind of connective tissue that unites the lobules.

The **left lobe** extends farther caudally than the right. It occupies a special outpocketing of the cranial mediastinal portion of the pleura of the left pleural sac. It covers the right ventricle, and its caudal border is gently curved and thin as it lies between the left thoracic wall and the cranial aspect of the left ventricle. In a small dog this portion of the left lobe may have a dorsoventral dimension of 50 mm and may be 5 mm thick. The left lobe becomes slightly narrower cranially as it lies in the mediastinal septum, loosely fused to the right lobe.

The **right lobe** of the thymus usually abuts the cranial surface of the pericardial sac and is expanded laterally. The thickest part of the thymus is located here. When maximally developed in the Beagle, the thymus is 12 cm long by 6 cm wide by 3 cm high. When fully developed in this breed, the thymus weighs approximately 50 g. The right lobe accounts for 60% of the weight and the left lobe for 40%. Variations in size and form are common. Latimer (1954) has studied the fetal development of the thymus in the dog, and Schneebeli (1958) studied the prenatal and postnatal development of the thymus in various breeds of dogs. Dorsally the thymus is related to the phrenic nerves, cranial vena cava, and trachea. The cranial lobes of the lungs produce large, smooth impressions on its lateral sides when it is maximally developed. The internal thoracic vessels form deep clefts or even run through the cranioventral portion of the gland. The thymus receives its chief blood supply from one or two thymic branches that go to each lobe from the ipsilateral internal thoracic artery. Occasionally, an additional thymic branch leaves the brachiocephalic trunk on the right side and the subclavian artery on the left side.

The veins from the thymus are satellites of the thymic arteries. The efferent lymph vessels from the thymus form four to six vessels that empty into the cranial mediastinal and cranial sternal lymph nodes. Both parasympathetic (vagal) and sympathetic axons supply the thymus. The basic cell unit of the thymus is a small lymphocyte, sometimes referred to as a *thymocyte*. These cells do not differ from small lymphocytes found in other organs of the body. The thymic corpuscles (Hassall bodies) are spherical or oval structures in the medulla of the gland, composed of concentrically arranged cells. The centers of many thymic corpuscles consist of degenerated cells that may be hyalinized, cystic, or calcified.

Bibliography

Albertine, K. H., & O'Morchoe, C. C. (1981). An ultrastructural study of the transport pathways across arcuate, interlobar, hilar, and capsular lymphatics in the dog kidney. *Microvasc Res, 351*, 3–61.

Albertine, K. H., Fox, L. M., & O'Morchoe, C. C. (1982). The morphology of canine lymphatic valves. *Anat Rec, 202*, 453–461.

Atkins, A. M., & Schofield, G. C. (1972). Lymphoglandular complexes in the large intestine of the dog. *J Anat, 113*, 169–178.

Battezzati, M., & Donini, I. (1973). *The lymphatic system*, revised edition translated from Italian by V. Cameron-Curry. New York: J. Wiley and Sons.

Baum, H. (1918). Das Lymphgefassystem des Hundes. *Arch Wiss Prakt Tierheilk, 44*, 521–650.

Belz, G. T., & Heath, T. J. (1995). Lymph pathways of the medial retropharyngeal lymph node in dogs. *J Anat, 186*(3), 517–526.

Bethune, D. C. G., Chu, R. C. J., Mulder, D. S., et al. (1979). In vivo mapping of pulmonary lymphatic pathways: a new technique. *J Surg Res, 26*, 513–518.

Blalock, A., Robinson, C. S., Cunningham, R. S., et al. (1937). Experimental studies on lymphatic blockage. *Arch Surg, 34*, 1049–1071.

Bloom, E., & Fawcett, D. W. (1986). *A textbook of histology* (8th ed.). Philadelphia: Saunders.

Blue, J., & Weiss, L. (1981). Electron microscopy of the red pulp of the dog spleen, including vascular arrangements, periarterial macrophage sheaths (ellipsoids) and the contractile, innervated reticular meshwork. *Am J Anat, 161*, 189–218.

Boes, K. M., & Durham, A. C. (2017). Bone marrow, blood cells, and the lymphoid/lymphatic system. In J. F. Zachary (Ed.), *Pathologic basis of veterinary disease* (7th ed.). St Louis, MO: Elsevier.

Bryant, B. J. (1975). Lymph node structure: an ontogenetic explanation for divergence in Eutheria, Metatheria, and Prototheria. *Am Zool, 15*, 147–153.

Burns, G. O., Scrivani, P. V., & Thompson, M. S. (2008). Relation between age, body weight, and medial retropharyngeal lymph node size in apparently healthy dog. *Vet Radiol Ultrasound, 49*(3), 277–281.

Casteleyn, C. R., van der Steen, M., Declercq, J., et al. (2008). The buccal lymph node (*lymphonodus buccalis*) in dogs: occurrence, anatomical localization, histological characteristics and clinical implications. *Vet J, 175*, 379–383.

Cardinet, G. H., & Hartke, G. T. (1972). Variation in the origin of the splenic artery in the dog. *Anat Rec, 172*, 449.

Chretien, P. B., Behar, R. J., Kohn, S., et al. (1967). The canine lymphoid system: a study of the effect of surgical excision. *Anat Rec, 159*, 5–15.

Clark, E. R., & Clark, E. L. (1937). Observations on living mammalian lymphatic capillaries-their relation to the blood vessels. *Am J Anat, 60*, 253–298.

Constantinescu, G. M., & Schaller, O. (2012). *Illustrated veterinary anatomical nomenclature* (3rd ed.). Stuttgart: Enke Verlag.

Dabney, J. M., Buehn, M. J., & Dobbins, D. E. (1988). Constriction of lymphatics by catecholamines, carotid occlusion, or hemorrhage. *Am J Physiol, 255*, 514–524.

Danese, A. R., Brower, R., & Howard, J. M. (1962). Experimental anastomoses of lymphatics. *Arch Surg, 84*, 6–9.

de Freitas, V., Piffer, C. R., Zorzetto, N. L., et al. (1981). On the topography of the ductus thoracicus in the dog. *Anat Anz, 149*, 451–454.

De Wolf-Peeters, C., Tierens, A., & Achten, R. (2001). Normal histology and immunoarchitecture of the lymphohematopoietic system. In D. Knowles (Ed.), *Neoplastic hematopathology* (2nd ed.). Philadelphia: Lippincott Williams & Wilkins.

Dobbins, D. E., Buehn, M. J., & Dabney, J. M. (1986). Constriction of canine prenodal lymphatic vessels following the intra-arterial injection of vasoactive agents and hemorrhage. *Microcirc Endothelium Lymphatics, 87,* 297–310.

Drake, R. E., Allen, J., Williams, J. P., et al. (1987). Lymph flow from edematous dog lungs. *J Appl Physiol, 62,* 2416–2420.

Drinker, C. K. (1942). The lymphatic system, Lane Medical Lectures. *Stanford Univ Pub Med Sci, 4,* 137–235.

Drinker, C. K. (1946). Extravascular protein and the lymphatic system. *Ann NY Acad Sci, 46,* 807–821.

Durovičová, J., & Munka, V. (1974). Stages of lymph drainage from the stomach in the dog. *Folia Morphol (Praha), 22,* 353–355.

Eliska, O. (1984). Topography of intrarenal lymphatics. *Lymphology, 17,* 135–141.

Eliska, O., & Elišková, M. (1980). Lymphatic drainage of the ventricular conduction system in man and in the dog. *Acta Anat, 107,* 205–213.

Eliska, O., Elišková, M., & Miller, A. J. (1999). The morphology of the lymphatics of the coronary arteries in the dog. *Lymphology, 32*(2), 45–57.

Elišková, M., & Eliska, O. (1974). Lymph drainage of the dog heart. *Morphologica, 22,* 320–323.

Elišková, M., Eliska, O., & Miller, A. J. (1994). The lymphatics of the canine parietal pericardium. *Lymphology, 27*(4), 181–188.

Fischer, H. W. (1959). A critique of experimental lymphography. *Acta Radiol, 52,* 448–454.

Fischer, H. W., & Zimmerman, G. R. (1959). Roentgenographic visualization of lymph nodes and lymphatic channels. *Am J Roentgenol, 81,* 517–534.

Fitzgerald, D. V. M. (1961). Hemal lymph nodes in a dog. *Vet Med, 56,* 256–257.

Földi, M., Gellert, A., Kozma, M., et al. (1966). Neue Beitrage zu den anatomischen Verhindungen zwischen Gehirn und Lymphsystem. *Acta Anat, 64,* 498–505.

Freeman, L. W. (1942). Lymphatic pathways from the intestine in the dog. *Anat Rec, 82,* 543–550.

Frostell, C., Blomqvist, H., Hedenstierna, G., et al. (1987). Thoracic and abdominal lymph drainage in relation to mechanical ventilation and PEEP. *Acta Anaesthesiol Scand, 31,* 405–412.

Garber, S. L., O'Morchoe, P. J., & O'Morchoe, C. C. (1980). A simultaneous comparison of the cells of blood, renal hilar, and thoracic duct lymph in the dog. *Anat Rec, 198,* 255–261.

Gnepp, D. R., & Green, F. H. Y. (1979). Scanning electron microscopy of collecting lymphatic vessels and their comparison to arteries and veins. *Scanning Microsc, 3,* 757–762.

Gnepp, D. R., & Green, F. H. Y. (1980). Scanning electron microscopic study of canine lymphatic vessels and their valves. *Lymphology, 13,* 91–99.

Grau, H., & Barone, R. (1970). Sur la topographie comparee et la nomenclature des nodules lymphatiques du bassin et du membre pelvien. *Rev Med Vet NS, 33,* 649–659.

Griaznova, A. V. (1962). On ligation of thoracic lymphatic duct in dog. *Arkh Anat, 42,* 90–97.

Gupta, S. G., Gupta, C. D., & Gupta, S. B. (1978). Segmentation in the dog spleen. *Acta Anat, 101,* 380–382.

Gupta, S. G., Gupta, C. D., & Gupta, S. B. (1981). Study of venous segments in the spleens of buffalo and dog. *Acta Anat, 111,* 204–206.

Haider, M., Schad, H., & Mendler, N. (1987). Thoracic duct lymph and PEEP studies in anaesthetized dogs. I. Lymph formation and the effect of a thoracic duct fistula on lymph flow. *Intensive Care Med, 13,* 183–191.

Higgins, G. M., & Graham, A. S. (1929). Lymphatic drainage from the peritoneal cavity in the dog. *Arch Surg, 19,* 453–465.

Hirashima, T., Kuwahara, D., & Nishi, M. (1984). Morphology of lymphatics in the canine large intestine. *Lymphology, 17,* 69–72.

Holmes, M. J., O'Morchoe, P. J., & O'Morchoe, C. C. (1977). Morphology of the intrarenal lymphatic system: capsular and hilar communications. *Am J Anat, 149,* 333–352.

Huber, F. (1909). *Der Ductus thoracicus.* Inaugural dissertation, Dresden.

Huntington, G. S. (1908). The genetic interpretation of the development of the mammalian lymphatic system. *Anat Rec, 2,* 19–45.

Huntington, G. S. (1910). The genetic principles of the development of the systemic lymphatic vessels in the mammalian embryo. *Anat Rec, 4,* 399–449.

Huntington, G. S. (1914). The development of the mammalian jugular lymph sac, of the tributary primitive ulnar lymphatic, and of the thoracic ducts from the viewpoint of the recent investigations of vertebrate lymphatic ontogeny, together with a consideration of the genetic relations of lymphatic and haemal vascular channels in the embryos of amniotes. *Am J Anat, 16,* 259–317.

Johnson, V. S., & Seiler, G. (2006). Magnetic resonance imaging appearance of the cisterna chyli. *Vet Rad Ultras, 47*(5), 461–464.

Kagan, K. G., & Breznock, E. M. (1979). Variations in the canine thoracic duct system and the effects of surgical occlusion demonstrated by rapid aqueous lymphography, using an intestinal lymphatic trunk. *Am J Vet Res, 40,* 948–958.

Kahlenberg, A. S., Kane, J. M., Kanter, P. M., et al. (2001). Hepatic lymphatic mapping: a pilot study for porta hepatis lymph node identification. *Cancer Invest, 19*(3), 256–260.

Kampmeier, O. F. (1969). *Evolution and comparative morphology of the lymphatic system.* Springfield, IL: Charles C Thomas.

Kerestanová, M., & Slezák, J. (1983). [Morphologic study of the lymphatic vessels of the heart in an experiment]. (Slovak) *Rozhl Chir, 62,* 513–520.

Kniseley, M. H. (1936). Spleen studies: I. Microscopic observations of the circulatory system of living unstimulated mammalian spleens. *Anat Rec, 65,* 23–50.

Kocisova, M., & Munka, V. (1974). Comparative anatomical study of the lymph vessels and nodes of the human and dog ovary. *Folia Morphol, 22,* 282–285.

Korovina, A. M. (1985). Structure of the inguinal lymph nodes after extirpation of the pancreas. *Arkh Anat Histol Embriol, 88,* 51–56.

Kostiuk, V. K. (1986). The intraorganic lymphatic bed of the mucous membrane of the tongue. *Arkh Anat Histol Embriol, 90,* 14–18.

Kubik, I., & Tömböl, T. (1958). Uber die Abflussfolge der regionaren Lymphknoten der Lunge des Hundes. *Acta Anat, 33,* 116–121.

Kubik, I., Vizkelety, T., & Balint, J. (1956). Die Lokalisation der Lnngensegmente in den regionalen Lymphknoten. *Anat Anz, 104,* 104–121.

Latimer, H. B. (1954). The prenatal growth of the thymus in the dog. *Growth, 18,* 71–77.

Lindsay, F. E. F. (1974). The cisterna chyli as a source of lymph samples in the cat and dog. *Res Vet Sci, 17,* 256–258.

Luciano, L., & Koch, A. (1975). Feinstruktur von Venolen und Lymphgefässen in der Schilddrüse des Hundes. *Acta Anat, 92,* 101–109.

Maher, W. P. (1985). Arterial, venous and lymphatic pathways in dorsal mucosa of dog tongue (implicated routes for metastatic lesions). *Microcirc Endothelium Lymphatics, 2*, 161–184.

Maher, W. P. (1986). Arterial venous and lymphatic pathways intrinsic to the palate and fauces. *Microcirc Endothelium Lymphatics, 3*, 129–162.

Mahorner, H. R., Caylor, H. D., Schlotthauer, C. F., et al. (1927). Observations on the lymphatic connections of the thyroid gland in man. *Anat Rec, 36*, 341–347.

Mall, F. P. (1903). On circulation through the pulp of the dog's spleen. *Am J Anat, 2*, 315–332.

Marais, J., & Fossum, T. W. (1988). Ultrastructural morphology of the canine thoracic duct and cisterna chyli. *Acta Anat, 133*, 309–312.

Martin, D. J., Parker, J. C., & Taylor, A. (1983). Simultaneous comparison of tracheobronchial and right duct lymph dynamics in dogs. *J Appl Physiol, 54*, 199.

Mayer, M. N., Silver, T. I., Lowe, C. K., & Anthony, J. M. (2013). Radiographic lymphangiography in the dog using iodized oil. *Vet Comp Oncol, 11*, 151–161. doi:10.1111/j.1476-5829.2012.00334.x.

McClure, C. F. W. (1915). On the provisional arrangement of the embryonic lymphatic system. *Anat Rec, 9*, 281–297.

Meyer, A. W. (1906). An experimental study on the recurrence of lymphatic gland and regeneration of lymphatic vessels in the dog. *Johns Hopkins Hosp Bull, 17*, 185–192.

Miller, A. J., De Boer, A., Pick, R., et al. (1988). The lymphatic drainage of the pericardial space in the dog. *Lymphology, 21*, 227–233.

Miller, W. S. (1937). *The lung*. Springfield, IL: Charles C Thomas.

Milroy, E. J., & Cockett, A. T. (1973). Lymphatic system of the canine bladder. An anatomical study. *Urology, 23*, 75–377.

Mulshine, J. L., Keenan, A. M., Carrasquillo, J. A., et al. (1987). Immunolymphoscintigraphy of pulmonary and mediastinal lymph nodes in dogs: a new approach to lung cancer imaging. *Cancer Res, 47*, 3572–3576.

Nomina Anatomica Veterinaria. (2017). 8th ed. International Committee on Veterinary Gross Anatomical Nomenclature. Hanover.

Nordquist, R. E., Bell, R. D., Sinclair, R. J., et al. (1973). The distribution and ultrastructural morphology of lymphatic vessels in the canine renal cortex. *Lymphology, 6*, 13–19.

Oberdörster, G., Gihb, F. R., Beiter, H., et al. (1978). Studies of the lymphatic drainage of dog lungs. *J Toxicol Environ Health, 4*, 571–586.

Ogawa, Y., Daigo, M., & Sato, Y. (1976). Stereoroentgenographical and dimensional studies on the physical structure of the dog. *Bull Nippon Vet Zootech Coll, 25*, 74–122.

Ohhashi, T. (1987). Comparison of viscoelastic properties of walls and functional characteristics of valves in lymphatic and venous vessels. *Lymphology, 20*, 219–223.

Oliver, G., & Harvey, N. (2002). A stepwise model of the development of lymphatic vasculature. *Ann NY Acad Sci, 979*, 159–165.

Ossoff, R. H., & Sisson, G. A. (1981). Lymphatics of the floor of the mouth and neck: anatomical studies related to contralateral drainage pathways. *Laryngoscope, 91*, 1847–1850.

Ossoff, R. H., Bytell, D. E., Hast, M. H., et al. (1980). Lymphatics of the floor of the mouth and periosteum: anatomic studies with possible clinical correlations. *Otolaryngol Head Neck Surg, 88*, 652–657.

Patsikas, M. N., & Dessiris, A. (1992). *The lymph drainage of the mammary glands in the bitch*, Third Hellenic Veterinary Symposium of Small Animal Medicine, Athens.

Pereira, C. T., Rahal, R. C., de Carvalho Balieiroa, J. C., et al. (2003). Lymphatic drainage on healthy and neoplastic mammary glands in female dogs: can it really be altered? *Anat Hist Embryol, 32*(5), 282–290.

Pflug, J. J., & Calnan, J. S. (1969). Lymphatics: normal anatomy in the dog hind leg. *J Anat, 105*, 457–465.

Pieper, R., Frostel, C., Blomqvist, H., et al. (1986). An experimental model for the separate sampling of thoracic and abdominal lymph. *Acta Chir Scand, 530*, 1–3.

Pina, J. A. E., & Tavares, A. S. (1980). Comparative morphological study of the epicardial ventricular lymphatics in the dog before and after ligature of the superficial veins. *Acta Anat., 107*, 72–79.

Pissas, A. (1984). Anatomoclinical and anatomosurgical essay on the lymphatic circulation of the pancreas. *Anat Clin, 6*, 255–280.

Popper, P., Mantyh, C. R., Vigna, S. R., et al. (1988). The localization of sensory nerve fibers and receptor binding sites for sensory neuropeptides in canine mesenteric lymph nodes. *Peptides, 99*, 257–267.

Prier, J. E., Schaffer, B., & Skelley, J. F. (1962). Direct lymphangiography in the dog. *J Am Vet Med Assoc, 140*, 943–947.

Reichert, F. L. (1926). The regeneration of the lymphatics. *Arch Surg, 13*, 871–881.

Rienhoff, W. F. (1931). The lymphatic vessels of the thyroid gland in the dog and in man. *Arch Surg, 23*, 783–804.

Rodrigues-Grande, N., Ribeiro, J., Soares, M., et al. (1983). The lymphatic vessels of the lung: morphological study. *Acta Anat, 115*, 302–309.

Ross, M. H., & Pawlina, W. (2016). *Histology, a text and atlas* (7th ed.). Philadelphia: Wolters Kluwer.

Ruberte, J., Sautet, J. Y., Gine, J. M., et al. (1990). Topographie des Collecteurs lymphatique Mammaires de la Chienne. *Anat Histol Embryol, 19*, 347–358.

Rumph, P. F., Garret, P. D., & Gray, B. W. (1980). Facial lymph nodes in dogs. *J Am Vet Med Assoc, 176*, 342–344.

Rusznyak, I., Földi, M., & Szabo, G. (1967). In: L. Youlten (Ed.), *Lymphatics and lymph circulation* (2nd ed.). New York: Pergamon Press.

Sabin, F. R. (1911). A critical study of the evidence presented in several recent articles on the development of the lymphatic system. *Anat Rec, 5*, 417–446.

Satjukova, G. S., Kirpatowski, I. D., & Kiprenski, J. W. (1977). Enige neue Angaben znm Lymphbett der Extremitt des Hundes. *Verh Anat Ges, 71*, S793–S800.

Schacher, J. F., & Sulahian, A. (1972). Lymphatic drainage patterns and experimental filariasis in dogs. *Ann Trop Med Parasitol, 66*, 209–217.

Schmidt, E. E., MacDonald, I. C., & Groom, A. C. (1982). Direct arteriovenous connections and the intermediate circulation in dog spleen, studies by scanning electron microscopy of microcorrosion casts. *Cell Tissue Res, 225*, 542–555.

Schmidt, E. E., MacDonald, I. C., & Groom, A. C. (1983). Circulatory pathways in the sinousal spleen of the dog, studied by scanning electron microscopy of microcorrosion casts. *J Morphol, 178*, 111–123.

Schmidtova, K., Gregor, A., & Munka, V. (1974). Note on lymph drainage of the heart in the dog. *Folia Morphol, 22*, 405–407.

Schneebeli, S. (1958). Zur Anatomie des Hundes im Welpenalter. 2. Beitrag: Form un Grossenverhaltnisse innerer Organe, Dissertation. *Med Vet Zurich*.

Semo, J., Nicenboim, J., & Yaniv, K. (2016). Development of the lymphatic system: new questions and paradigms. *Development, 143*, 924–935. doi:10.1242/dev.132431.

Shdanow, D. A. (1962). Zur Lösung der Streitfragen über die funktionelle Morphologie des Lymphgehsystems. *Anat Anz, 111*, 17–50.

Shelton, M. E., & Forsythe, W. B. (1979). Buccal lymph node in the dog. *Am J Vet Res, 40*, 1638–1639.

Shimada, T., Noguchi, T., Takita, K., et al. (1989). Morphology of lymphatics of the mammalian heart with special reference to the architecture and distribution of the subepicardial lymphatic system. *Acta Anat, 136*, 16–20.

Skelley, J. F., Prier, J. E., & Koehler, R. (1964). Applications of direct lymphangiography in the dog. *Am J Vet Res, 24*, 747–755.

Spira, A. (1962). Die Lymphknotengruppen (Lymphocentra) bei den Sugern-ein Homologisierungesversuch. *Anat Anz, 111*, 294–364.

Stalker, L. K., & Schlotthauer, C. F. (1936). Neoplasms of the mammary gland in the dog. *North Am Vet*, 1733–1743.

Sterns, E. E., & Vaughan, G. E. (1970). The lymphatics of the dog colon. A study of the lymph drainage patterns by indirect lymphography in the dog under normal and abnormal conditions. *Cancer, 26*, 218–231.

Suami, H., O'Neil, J. K., Pan, W. R., et al. (2008). Perforating lymph vessels in the canine torso: direct lymph pathway from skin to the deep lymphatics. *Plast Reconstr Surg, 121*(1), 31–36.

Suami, H., Yamashita, S., Soto-Miranda, M. A., et al. (2013). Lymphatic territories (lymphosomes) in a canine: an animal model for investigation of postoperative lymphatic alterations. *PLoS ONE, 8*, e69222. doi:10.1371/journal.pone0069222.

Suter, P. (1969). *Die lymphographie beim Hund, eine rontgenologische methode zur diagnose von veranderungen am lymphsystem*. Zurich, Juris-Verlag.

Suter, P. F., & Greene, R. W. (1971). Chylothorax in a dog with abnormal termination of the thoracic duct. *J Am Vet Med Assoc, 159*, 302–309.

Takubo, K., Miyamoto, H., Imamura, M., et al. (1986). Morphology of the human and dog spleen with special reference to intrasplenic microcirculation. *Jpn J Surg, 16*, 29–35.

Tanigawa, N. (1978). Experimental studies on surgical problems concerning lymphatics. I. Microlymphangiography of canine intestine and microlymphangiographic study of lymphatic regeneration following intestinal anastomosis (author's trans). *Nippon Geka Hokan, 47*, 563–574.

Threefoot, S. A. (1968). Gross and microscopic anatomy of the lymphatic vessels and lymphaticovenous communications. *Cancer Chemother Rep, 52*, 1–20.

Todd, G. L., & Bernard, G. R. (1973). The sympathetic innervation of the cervical lymphatic duct of the dog. *Anat Rec, 177*, 303–316.

Todd, G. L., & Bernard, G. R. (1974). The cervical lymphatic ducts of the dog: structure and function of the endothelial lining. *Microvasc Res, 8*, 139–150.

Töndury, G., & Kubik, S. (1972). *Zur ontogenese des lymphatischen systems. handhuch der allgemeinen patologie* (Vol. 3). Berlin: Springer-Verlag.

Trautmann, A., & Fiebiger, J. (1952). *Fundamentals of the histology of domestic animals* (translated and revised from 8th and 9th German eds., 1949, by RE Habel and EL Biberstein). Ithaca, NY: Comstock.

Unthank, J. L., & Bohlen, H. G. (1988). Lymphatic pathways and role of valves in lymph propulsion from small intestine. *Am J Physiol, 254*, 389–398.

Vajda, J. (1966). Innervation of lymph vessels. *Acta Morphol Acad Sci Hung, 14*, 197–208.

Volik, U. Y. (1962). Experimental morphological investigation of the innervation of the inguinal lymph nodes in dogs. *Bull Exp Biol Med (USSR), 53*, 111–114, (in Russian).

Vreim, C. E., Ohkuda, K., & Staub, N. C. (1977). Proportions of dog lymph in the thoracic and right lymph ducts. *J Appl Physiol, 43*, 894.

Wilkens, H., & Munster, W. (1972). Eine vergleichende Darstellung des Lymphsystems bei den Haussaugetieren (Hund, Schwein, Rind, Pferd). *Dtsch Tieraerztl Wochenschr, 79*, 573–612.

Wilting, J., Aref, Y., Huang, R., et al. (2006). Dual origin of avian lymphatics. *Dev Biol, 292*, 165–173.

Womack, W. A., Tygart, P. K., Mailman, D., et al. (1988). Villous motility: relationship to lymph flow and blood flow in the dog jejunum. *Gastroenterology, 94*, 977–983.

Yang, T. J. (1986). Green coloration of superficial cervical lymph nodes in dogs tattooed in the ear. *J Vet Med A, 33*, 788–790.

Yeh, S. D. J., Morse, M. J., Granda, R., et al. (1986). Lymphoscintigraphic studies of lymphatic drainage from the testes. *Clin Nucl Med, 11*, 823–827.

Yoffey, J. M., & Courtice, F. C. (1956). *Lymphatics, lymph, and lymphoid tissue*. Cambridge, MA: Harvard University Press.

Yoffey, J. M., & Drinker, C. K. (1938). The lymphatic pathways from the nose and pharynx. *J Exp Med, 68*, 629–640.

Zajac, S. (1972). Natural lympho-venous communication between the cisterna chyli and inferior vena cava. *Pol Med J, 11*, 1271–1277.

14

Introduction to the Nervous System

MARNIE FITZMAURICE

General

The nervous system (*systema nervosum*) informs an animal about its environment, both internal and external, and initiates responses to that environment. Other body systems are specialized to perform various life-sustaining functions, such as locomotion, digestion, respiration, and circulation, and it is essential that these functions be regulated and coordinated by the nervous system. The most extensive treatment of the nervous system can be found in Nieuwenhuys, Donaklaar, and Nicholson (1998) *The Central Nervous System of Vertebrates*, and the best source for standard terms is to be found in *Nomina Anatomica Veterinaria* (NAV).

The cells constituting the nervous system are highly specialized for receiving stimuli, by means of receptors and highly specialized sense organs, for transmitting and storing information, and for coordinating and initiating responses to stimuli (Fig. 14.1). Cells composing the nervous system are of two types: neurons (*neurona*), which receive and transmit impulses, and neuroglial cells, which facilitate conduction of axonal impulses; provide mechanical, immunological, developmental, and metabolic support for nervous tissue; regulate CNS blood flow, capillary permeability, and synaptic function; and contribute to scar formation in response to disease (Sofroniew & Winters, 2010).

The gross nervous system, formed by these two types of cells and connective and vascular tissue, is subdivided into the central nervous system (CNS) (*systema nervosum centrale*), consisting of the brain (*encephalon*) and spinal cord (*medulla spinalis*), and the peripheral nervous system (PNS) (*systema nervosum periphericum*), composed of cranial and spinal nerves. The divisions are arbitrary because, as we shall see in this chapter, parts of the same neuron can be in both the CNS and the PNS.

The term nerve (*nervus*) is applied to a collection of neuronal processes, axons, located in the PNS external to the CNS. In addition to the axons, a nerve contains their supporting Schwann cells (lemmocytes) and connective tissue arranged as endoneurium, perineurium, and epineurium. These nerves connect the CNS with the structures in the other systems that compose the body. Most nerves are grossly visible. A ganglion is a collection of neuronal cell bodies (*corpora neurona*) in the PNS and their surrounding supporting cells and connective tissue. A nucleus is a collection of neuronal cell bodies in the CNS.

Structure of Neurons

The basic anatomic, genetic, and functional unit of the nervous system is the neuron, a highly specialized cell. A neuronal cell (*neurocytus*), whether in the CNS or PNS, consists of a cell body (*corpus neurona*), an axon (*neuritum*), and dendrites. The dendrites, or dendritic zone or receptive segment, are located where a neuron receives a stimulus from another neuron in the CNS or from its environment in the PNS. The axon, or conductive segment, conducts the impulse that is generated from the dendritic zone to the terminal portion of the axon referred to as the *telodendron* or *transmissive segment*. This will be at a synapse with another neuron in the CNS or with an effector organ in the PNS. The cell body contains the nucleus and organelles and is located at the origin of the axon or at some point along its course. Neurons are classified on the basis of the shape of the cell body and the number, shape, and ramifications of the processes into unipolar (*neuronum unipolare*), pseudounipolar (*neuronum pseudounipolare*), bipolar (*neuronum bipolare*), or multipolar (*neuronum multipolare*) cells.

The processes of a neuron are classified on a structural basis as an axon (*axon*) or as dendrites (*dendriti*), based on their shape, length, and cytoplasmic contents. Dendrites have a tapered shape, are relatively short, and contain large amounts of endoplasmic reticulum. Axons are narrow, do not taper, and have little endoplasmic reticulum. Traditionally, some histology texts refer to dendrites as conducting nerve impulses toward the cell body and axons as conducting impulses away from the cell body. Thus, these texts classify the peripheral processes of pseudounipolar and bipolar sensory neurons as dendrites because they conduct nerve impulses toward the cell body. This is not acceptable because this process structurally is an axon. In addition, the dendrites of multipolar neurons do not conduct nerve impulses because their function is to initiate the bioelectrical change at the synapse on the neuron.

Pseudounipolar cells embryologically start out as bipolar cells, but the cell body grows out on one side, and the two processes emerge from a tortuous neck of the cell

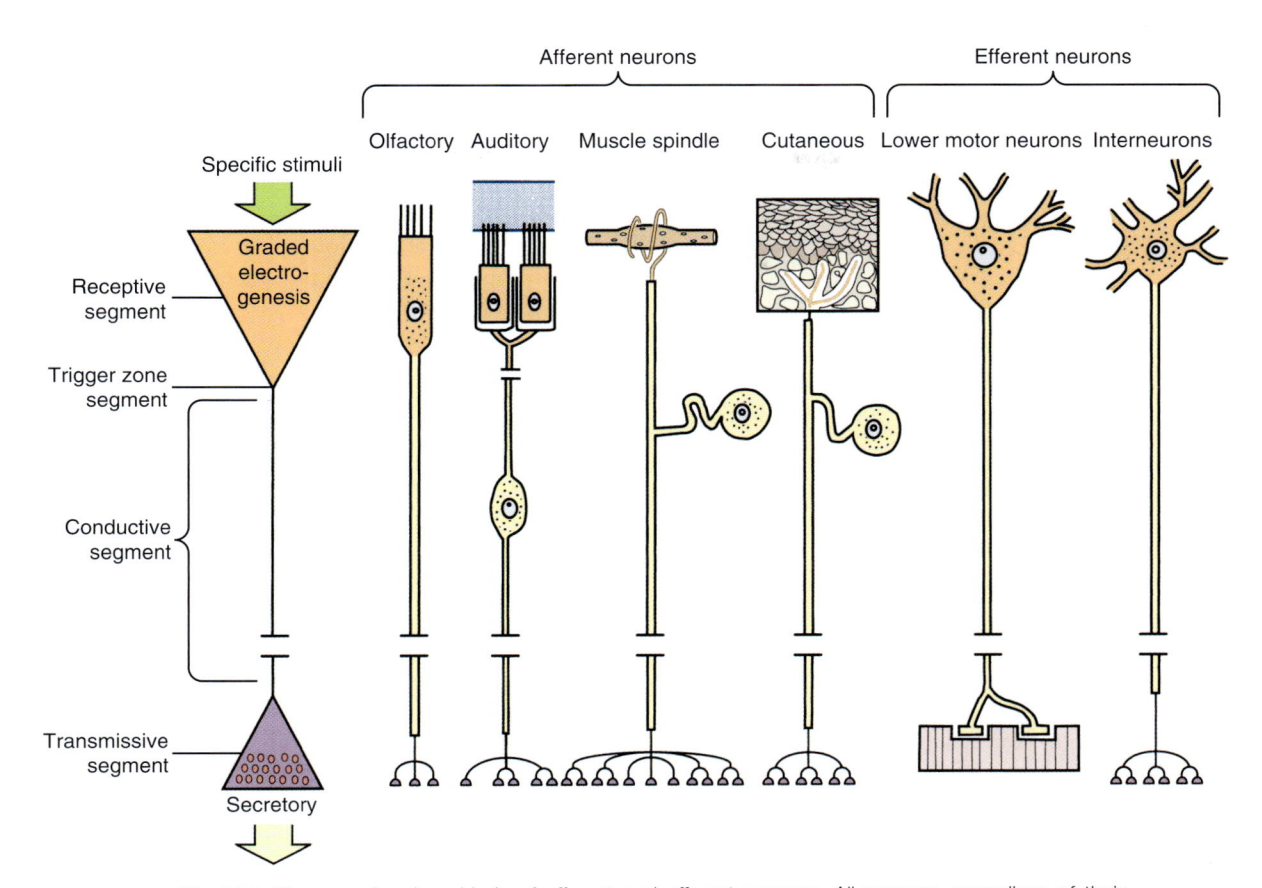

• **Fig. 14.1** Diagram of various kinds of afferent and efferent neurons. All neurons, regardless of their shape, have receptive segments (dendritic zones), trigger zones, conductile (axons) and transmissive segments (telodendrons), and trophic areas (cell bodies). Olfactory neurons are unipolar, auditory neurons are bipolar, muscle spindle and cutaneous afferents are pseudounipolar, and lower motor neurons and interneurons are multipolar in shape. The location of the cell body is not critical to the functioning of the various neurons. The cell body may be in the receptive segment (olfactory afferent neurons; motor and interneurons), in the conductile segment (auditory and vestibular afferent neurons), or branching off of the conductile segment (all other afferent neurons). The transmissive segments end on other neurons or on muscle or gland cells in the case of motor neurons.

(Fig. 14.2). Both processes are structurally axons. Bipolar cells have two processes, classified structurally as axons. Multipolar cells have many processes, one axon and the rest classified as dendrites (Figs. 14.1 and 14.3). Olfactory neurons are unipolar; auditory, visual, and vestibular neurons are bipolar; muscle spindles and cutaneous afferents are pseudounipolar; and **lower motor neurons** (LMNs) and interneurons are multipolar. The location of the cell body is not critical to the functioning of the various neurons. The cell body may be in the receptive segment such as olfactory afferent neurons, LMNs, and interneurons. The cell body may be in the conductive segment such as auditory and vestibular afferent neurons, or the cell body may branch off the conductive segment such as all other afferent neurons. The transmission segments end on other neurons, or on muscle or gland cells in the case of motor neurons.

The endoplasmic reticulum (*reticulum endoplasmicum*), or cytoplasmic chromidial substance, of neurons is concentrated in the cell body and in parts of dendrites close to the cell body (see Fig. 14.3). The endoplasmic reticulum is sparse in one region of the cell body, called the *axon*

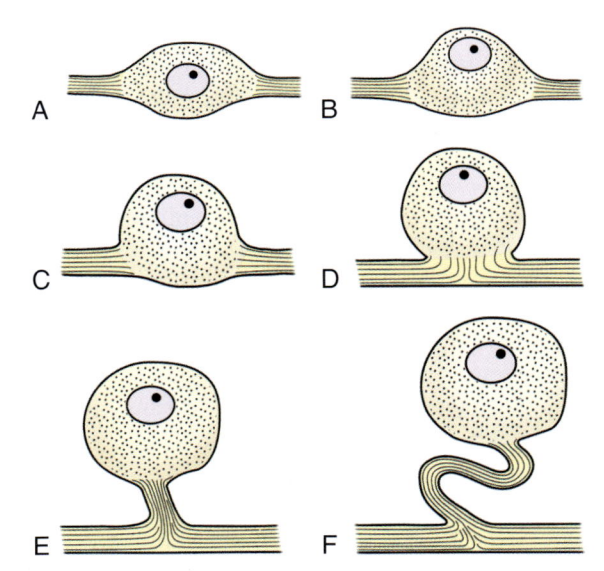

• **Fig. 14.2** Schematic illustration of how eccentric growth transforms a primitive bipolar cell into a pseudounipolar cell (an afferent ganglion cell). A through F represent successive stages of this transformation.

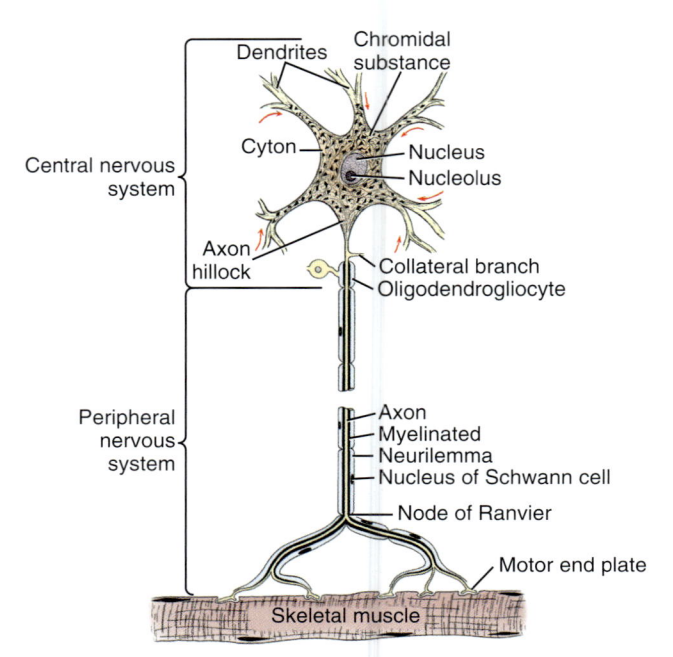

• Fig. 14.3 A schematic drawing of a lower motor (alpha) neuron showing intracellular constituents and the myelinated axon. The myelin within the central nervous system is formed by the oligodendroglia, whereas the myelin outside the central nervous system is formed by neurilemma (Schwann) cells.

hillock (*colliculus axonis*), where the axon arises, and in the axon and in the distal branches of dendrites. Because the endoplasmic reticulum of the cell body is so densely packed and is highly organized, it appears in microscopic sections as basophilic clusters, called *Nissl substance* (*substantia chromatophilia*) or *Nissl bodies*. The Nissl substance stains blue with basic dyes, such as thionin, cresyl violet, toluidine blue, and methylene blue.

Electron microscopy shows Nissl substance to be a highly developed and organized endoplasmic reticulum consisting of densely packed, narrow tubes with fine granules associated with the tubes. Histochemical and other studies have demonstrated that the granules consist primarily of ribonucleic acid. The cytoplasm of the cell body also contains *mitochondria* and Golgi substance. Mitochondria are present in the dendrites and are concentrated in specialized regions of the axon, such as nodes or terminals (end bulbs or receptors). Neurofibrillae (*neurofilamenta*) run in all directions within the cell body and longitudinally to the long axis of dendrites and axons. Microtubules (*microfilamentae*), prominent in dendrites and axons, are involved in the rapid transport of molecules away from and toward the cell bodies.

Functional Segments of Neurons

Based on both structure and function, every neuron can be divided into five segments (see Fig. 14.1): cell body, receptive segment, trigger zone segment, conductile segment, and transmissive segment.

Cell Body Segment

The cell body segment (perikaryon) is the trophic or metabolic center of the neuron. It consists of the nucleus and the cytoplasm with its organelles around the nucleus. The location of the cell body is not critical to the functioning of neurons that are pseudounipolar in shape because the cell body is not involved in the generation, conduction, or transmission of nerve impulses.

Receptive Segment

The receptive segment of the neuron, also referred to as the *dendritic zone*, varies in shape and location. It is the site on a neuron where a stimulus results in a change in the cell membrane potential that will generate a nerve impulse in the trigger zone. In primary afferent neurons the receptive segment is in the receptor (the ending in a sense organ). In the olfactory system, the receptive segment is the distal end of the cell body of the neuron that is acted on by the chemical odor. In interneurons and LMNs the dendrites and cell bodies are the receptive segment and are acted on by chemical neurotransmitters released by synaptic terminals of other neurons. In some instances, the receptive segments may be on the synaptic end bulbs (the transmissive segment) of a neuron (axoaxonic synapses; see Fig. 14.7D). Receptive segments of neurons function by developing a nonpropagated change in the membrane potential of the neuron that is spread decrementally along the neuron to affect the trigger zone segment of the neuron (see Fig. 14.1).

The peripheral terminal ends of somatosensory afferent axons are modified to form specialized structures, called *receptors* (*receptori*) (Figs. 14.5 and 14.6). These may, or may not, have connective tissue capsules (*corpusculi nervosi capsulata*) surrounding them. Receptors are specialized to generate neuronal impulses in their axons when a specific stimulus or sensory modality is applied to them. These include chemical, mechanical, thermal, or electromagnetic energy. In humans, each receptor type has a low threshold for a specific modality thus is most sensitive to that modality. Free nerve endings (*terminationes nervi libera*) (see Fig. 14.6A) are responsive to warm or cold temperatures, intense mechanical stimulation that is potentially or actually damaging to tissue, and ions and cytokines in the interstitium. End bulbs of Krause (*corpora bulboidei*) (Fig. 14.6B and C) respond to slow movement (flutter). Pacinian corpuscles (*corpusculi nervosi capsulata*) (Fig. 14.6D) respond to rapid vibration. Muscle spindles (*fusi neuromusculari*) (Fig. 14.6E) detect muscle length and the velocity at which a muscle is being stretched. Golgi tendon organs (*fusi neurotendini*) (Fig. 14.6F) detect muscle tension. Ruffini corpuscles (*corpora tacti*) (Fig. 14.6G) respond to tangential stretching. Hair follicle receptors (*terminationes folliculi pili*) (Fig. 14.6H) respond to movement but not to continual pressure and thus are referred to as *mechanical motion detectors*. Merkel discs (*epithelioidocyti tacti*) (Fig. 14.5) and Meissner's corpuscles (*toruli tactiles*) (Fig. 14.5) respond continuously to sustained perpendicular pressure.

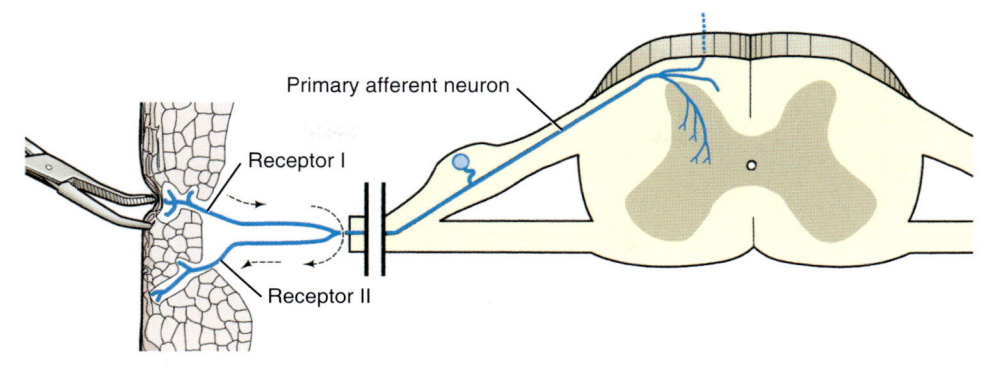

• **Fig. 14.4** A multiple sensory receptor unit. (Compare with Fig. 14.8, which shows a single sensory receptor unit.) In a multiple sensory unit, excitation of only one receptor (one unit, receptor I) gives rise to a neuronal impulse that travels along the axon in the usual direction, *orthodromic conduction.* When the neuronal impulse reaches the point where the afferent axon has branches, it excites the distal part of the branch, which conducts the neuronal impulse in the direction of receptor II (another unit), which is opposite to the usual direction the nerve impulse travels. This is referred to as *antidromic conduction.* Efferent axons can also conduct nerve impulses in both directions if they are artificially stimulated.

Trigger Zone

The trigger zone segment is the site of generation of nerve impulses in the conductile segments of the neuron. The trigger zone of receptor cells of the olfactory system, interneurons, and LMNs is the initial segment of the axon just distal to the axon hillock of the cell body. The trigger zone of primary afferent neurons is the part of an axon that is the closest to the receptive segment of the neuron (the receptor).

Conductile Segment

The conductile segment of the neuron is commonly referred to as the *neuronal fiber* or *axon.* In the case of bipolar or pseudounipolar neurons the conductile segment is divided into two parts, depending on the relationship of the segment to the cell body. The conductile segment of a primary afferent neuron that begins at a receptor in the periphery is referred to as the *peripheral conductile segment.* (As stated earlier, in many histology textbooks this is erroneously called a *dendrite.*) The conductile segment of these cells that carries the nerve impulses away from the cell bodies and into (and within) the CNS is called the *central conductile segment.* The conductile segments of olfactory neurons, interneurons, and LMNs begin at a specialized part of the cell body referred to as the *axon hillock,* and the conductile segments (axons) extend away from the cell bodies to their termination at the transmissive segments, which are the location of the synapses with other neurons or effector organs. In alpha, beta, and gamma LMNs, the axon begins at the axon hillock and has a long peripheral conductile segment within the PNS that conducts nerve impulses to the transmissive segment. Spinal cord autonomic lower motor neurons have preganglionic axons that have synapses with ganglionic autonomic neurons (only the axon is postganglionic) (see Fig. 14.11). Ganglionic autonomic neurons have postganglionic axons that activate smooth or cardiac muscle or glands or, in the case of the adrenal medulla, release the neurotransmitter directly into the bloodstream.

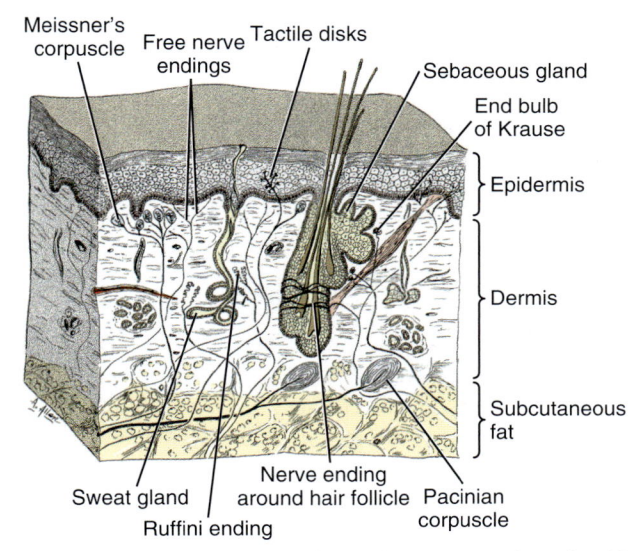

• **Fig. 14.5** Schematic representation of the nerve supply to the skin. (Modified with permission from Woolard HH, Weddell G, Harpman JA: *J Anat [London]* 74:413–440, 1940; and Gardner E: *Fundamentals of neurology,* 3rd ed., Philadelphia, 1940, Saunders.)

The conductile segments of all neurons are capable of conducting impulses in either direction, depending on the site on the neuron where the neuronal impulses are generated (see Fig. 14.4). In some primary afferent neurons that have branching peripheral conductile segments, each with a receptor associated with them, a nerve impulse generated at the trigger zone of one branch can travel toward the CNS via the conductile segment, then travel away from the CNS via another branch of the conductile segment. Those nerve impulses traveling away from the trigger zone are referred to as being conducted *orthodromically;* those traveling away from the CNS are referred to as being conducted *antidromically* (in human primary afferents, *anterograde*).

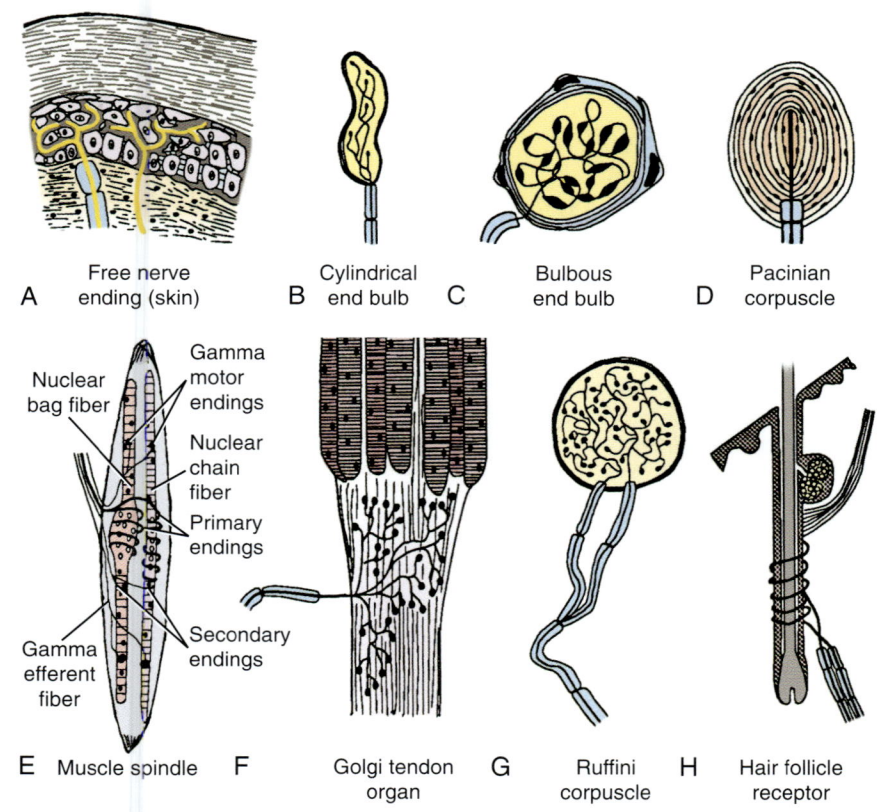

• **Fig. 14.6** Examples of the histologic features of various sensory receptors. Some free nerve endings are responsive to mechanical stimuli, others to warmth, others to cold, and others to noxious stimuli. All the other receptors are responsive only to mechanical stimuli.

Dendrites of interneurons and LMNs are not included in the conductile segments of these neurons because dendrites of these neurons do not conduct nerve impulses, but the bioelectrical change initiated in them by synapses spreads decrementally (not regenerated as a neuronal impulse) to the cell body (orthodromically) or away from the cell body (antidromically).

Transmissive Segment

The transmissive segment of a neuron is located at the terminal end of the conductile segment, or axon, called the *telodendron* of the neuron. The transmissive segment of primary afferent neurons, interneurons, LMNs, and projection neurons of the CNS is modified to form synaptic end bulbs (terminal boutons, see Fig. 14.7), in which synaptic vesicles (*vesicula synaptica*) containing a neurotransmitter are concentrated. The synaptic end bulbs contact and release neurotransmitter on another neuron (dendrites, cell body, or occasionally an axon) or on an effector (muscle or gland). The transmissive segments of alpha, beta, and gamma motor neurons are modified to form neuroeffector junctions called *motor end plates* (*terminationes neuromusculi*), where neurotransmitters are released to act on the effector (skeletal muscle fibers). Along the length of autonomic telodendria are swellings called *varicosities*, where neurotransmitter vesicles accumulate and are released in variable proximity to effectors (Burnstock, 2008).

Groups of Neurons

The function of the nervous system is carried out by the interaction of neurons with one another, which involves a plethora of neurotransmitters. Four general groups of neurons are recognized. These are primary afferent neurons, interneurons, projection neurons, and final efferent neurons referred to as *LMNs*. In simple terms, a primary afferent neuron conducts impulses into the CNS. Projection pathways conduct this afferent (sensory) information cranially to higher centers of the brain where neurons located there are activated. When a motor response results, projection pathways referred to as *upper motor neurons* (UMNs) course caudally from these higher centers in the prosencephalon and brainstem to activate LMNs located in the brainstem and spinal cord. These efferent neurons are distributed in the PNS to the effector organ (muscle or gland) where a response occurs. Interneurons are activated at various levels of this pathway.

Primary afferent neurons are the only neurons that conduct nerve impulses from the periphery into the CNS (Fig. 14.9). Primary afferent neurons have their cell bodies located largely outside the CNS in connective tissue, in encapsulated structures called *craniospinal (afferent) ganglia*. They have receptors located in the periphery that are stimulated to produce neuronal impulses by the various kinds of energies (mechanical, chemical, thermal, or electromagnetic) applied

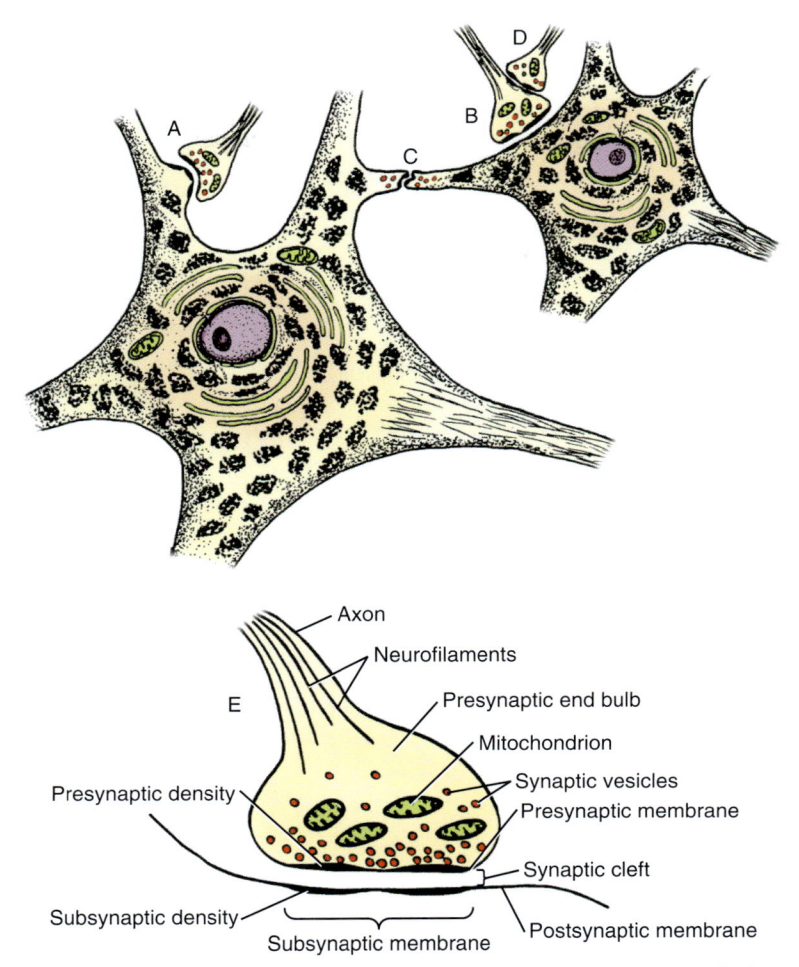

• **Fig. 14.7** Drawing showing various locations of synapses. **A**, An axodendritic synapse. **B**, An axosomatic synapse. **C**, A reciprocal dendrodendritic synapse. **D**, An axoaxonic synapse. **E**, Essential morphologic elements of a synapse. The subsynaptic densities, subsynaptic membrane, and postsynaptic membrane are parts of the second neuron in the series (the postsynaptic neuron).

to them. Most primary afferent neurons are pseudounipolar or bipolar in shape. Primary afferent neurons send their central processes into the CNS, where they branch into a longer cranial branch and a shorter caudal branch that give off many additional branches (collaterals) that terminate by synapsing with many interneurons, with cranial projection neurons, and, in some instances, also with LMNs.

Interneurons (Figs. 14.8 to 14.10) are short neurons that have their cell bodies and all their processes located entirely within the CNS. They are stimulated to generate nerve impulses by a neurotransmitter released at synapses made by primary afferent axons, by other interneurons, by projection neurons, and, in one specific instance, by axon collaterals of LMNs. Interneurons send their axons to synapse with another interneuron, a projection neuron, or a LMN. Interneurons are of two general classes: excitatory interneurons, if they release excitatory neurotransmitters at their synaptic end bulbs, or inhibitory interneurons, if they release inhibitory neurotransmitters at their synaptic end bulbs (Fig. 14.8). Many interneurons function as a part of a spinal cord or brainstem reflex.

Projection neurons send their axons long distances before terminating. If their cell body is in the spinal cord, most project cranially to terminate in a neuronal population (nucleus or cortex) in the brain. These form tracts that are named by their origin and termination (i.e., *spinocerebellar, spinothalamic,* and *spinovestibular*). If the projection pathway begins in a nucleus or cortex of the brain, its axon extends caudally to terminate in the brainstem or spinal cord on an interneuron that in turn synapses on a final efferent neuron. This is an upper motor neuron or UMN, pathway that forms tracts that are also named by their origin and termination (i.e., *corticospinal, reticulospinal,* and *vestibulospinal*). In humans the cranially projecting pathways are referred to as *ascending pathways* and the caudally projecting pathways are *descending pathways.*

Lower motor neurons (LMNs) are of four categories, alpha (*neuronum somaticum*), beta, gamma LMNs (*neuronum fusi neuromuscularis*), and autonomic nervous system LMNs (*neuronum autonomicum*) (Fig. 14.11). All LMNs are stimulated to generate nerve impulses by a neurotransmitter released at a synapse by an interneuron, by a projection neuron, or

Introduction to the Nervous System

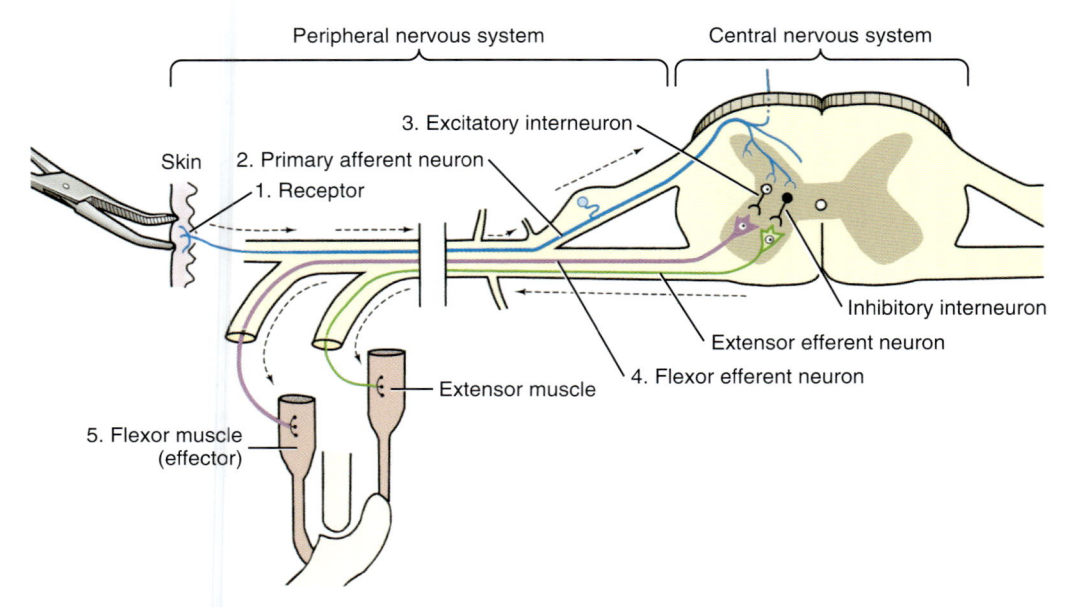

Fig. 14.8 Five essential elements of a simple reflex arc. The peripheral receptor (*1*) transmits impulses via the afferent axon (*2*) to the central nervous system. Within the central nervous system the afferent axon synapses with many other neurons in the integrating area (*3*). The efferent neuron (*4*), called the *lower motor neuron,* carries impulses away from the central nervous system. The effector in this diagram is striated muscle. (In the autonomic nervous system, it may be smooth muscle or gland.) In the withdrawal reflex illustrated here, the flexor lower motor neurons are excited, and the extensor motor neurons are inhibited. The size of all nerve axons is exaggerated for clarity.

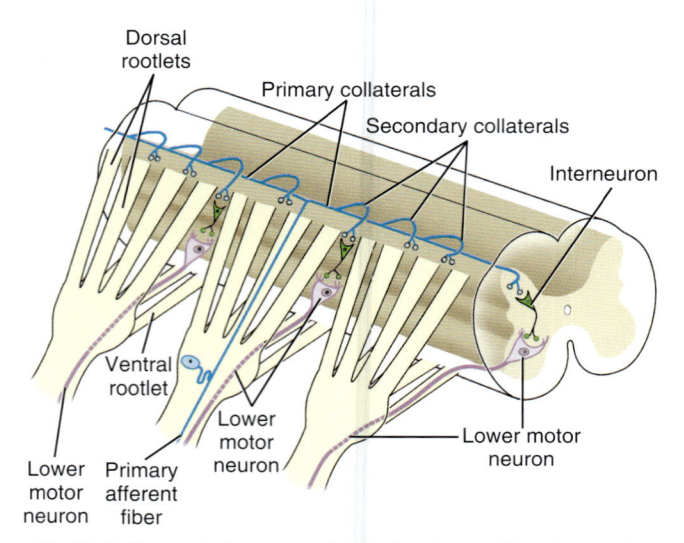

Fig. 14.9 The central process of a single primary afferent axon does not end in one segment but extends three or more segments (usually only one segment caudally) and synapses with many interneurons.

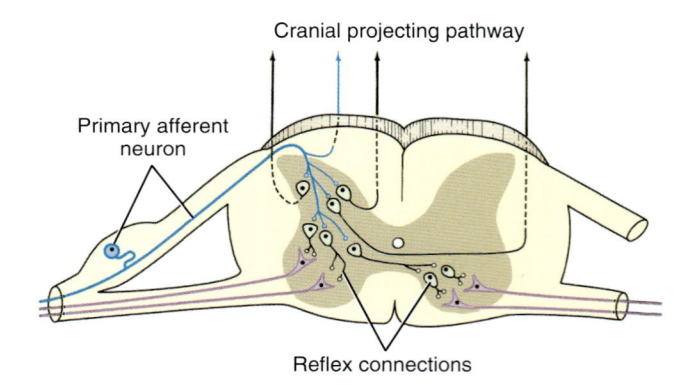

Fig. 14.10 Central connections of a primary afferent axon. One primary afferent axon may have synapses with numerous reflex pathways (arcs) and many projection neurons that form pathways that project cranially.

by a primary afferent neuron. Alpha motor neurons (most commonly referred to simply as *lower motor neurons*) have their cell bodies located in the gray matter of the CNS and transmit nerve impulses to the periphery to release a neurotransmitter at neuromuscular junctions located on skeletal voluntary (extrafusal) striated muscle fibers. Gamma efferent neurons have their cell bodies located in the gray matter of the CNS and send their axons to the periphery to release a neurotransmitter on small striated muscle fibers (called *intrafusal fibers*) located in an encapsulated stretch receptor called a *muscle spindle* (Figs. 14.6 and 14.11). Beta efferent neurons are of lesser importance and branch to end on both extrafusal and intrafusal muscle fibers. The autonomic nervous system has two neurons classified as LMNs. The first autonomic LMN has its cell body located in the CNS and has its axon (preganglionic) extending peripherally to synapse with a number of ganglionic neurons that have their cell bodies located in an autonomic ganglion. The ganglionic neuron is the second LMN, which has its axon (postganglionic) terminating on, or near, an effector cell (smooth muscle, cardiac muscle or a gland cell), or it secretes a neurotransmitter directly into the blood stream. In reality, only the axon of the second neuron is actually postganglionic, although these are often referred to as *postganglionic neurons*.

Supporting Cells

Supporting cells within the CNS are referred to as *neuroglia* (for details consult a histology textbook). There are four general classes of neuroglia. Three are ectodermal in origin and one is mesodermal. The ectodermal include the astrocytes (*astrocytus*), which bind neurons together; the oligodendroglia (*oligodendrocytus*) cells, which form myelin sheaths for the conductile segments; the axons; and ependymal (*ependymocytus*) cells, which line the cavities within the CNS. The microglia (*microglia*) are mesodermal cells that are part of the macrophage phagocytic system and are scattered throughout the gray and white matter. In the PNS, neurolemma (Schwann) cells (*neurolemmocytus*) ensheathe the axons. Many nonmyelinated (unmyelinated) axons are enveloped by one neurolemma (or in the CNS, oligodendroglial) sheath. If the neurolemma cell (or the oligodendroglia) is wound around the axon to form myelin, the axon is referred to as a *myelinated axon* (Fig. 14.12). The larger the axon and its myelin sheath the more rapidly it will conduct an impulse. The relationship of the axon and its neurolemma or oligodendroglial sheath is critical to the conduction of a neuronal impulse along the axon. If either the axon or its sheath are damaged or absent, no conduction, or altered conduction, of neuronal impulses will occur.

The Central Nervous System (CNS)

The CNS consists of the brain (*encephalon*) and the spinal cord (*medulla spinalis*) (see Chapters 16 and 19). The structures contained within the CNS are those located within the pial-glial membrane of the brain or spinal cord; thus the roots and ganglia usually illustrated with the CNS belong to the PNS, not the CNS.

CNS tissue is divided into white and gray matter based on the gross appearance of freshly sectioned CNS parts. The gray matter consists primarily of cell bodies of neuronal cells, neuroglia, and intertwined dendrites and both myelinated and nonmyelinated axons. The white matter consists

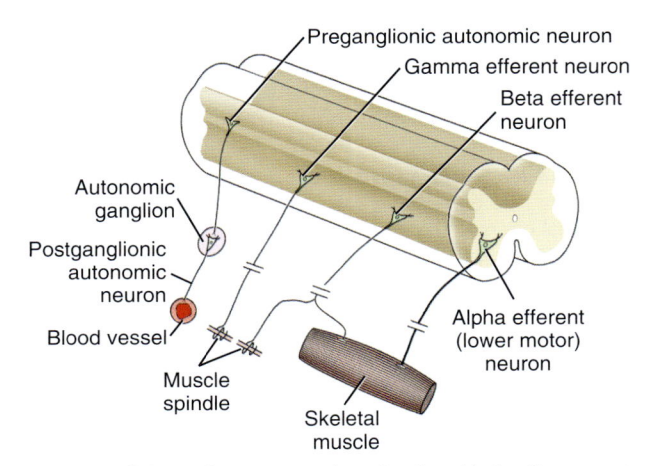

• **Fig. 14.11** Schematic representation of various kinds of lower motor neurons. Alpha motor neurons supplying striated muscle are the most commonly recognized lower motor neurons. Both preganglionic and postganglionic sympathetic and parasympathetic neurons are considered lower motor neurons because damage to either one of them produces paralysis characteristic of lower motor neuron disease. In this figure the postganglionic axon is supplying smooth muscle of a peripheral blood vessel. Gamma efferent fibers supply intrafusal muscle fibers in muscle spindles. Damage to gamma efferent axons produces a loss of muscle tone (atonia).

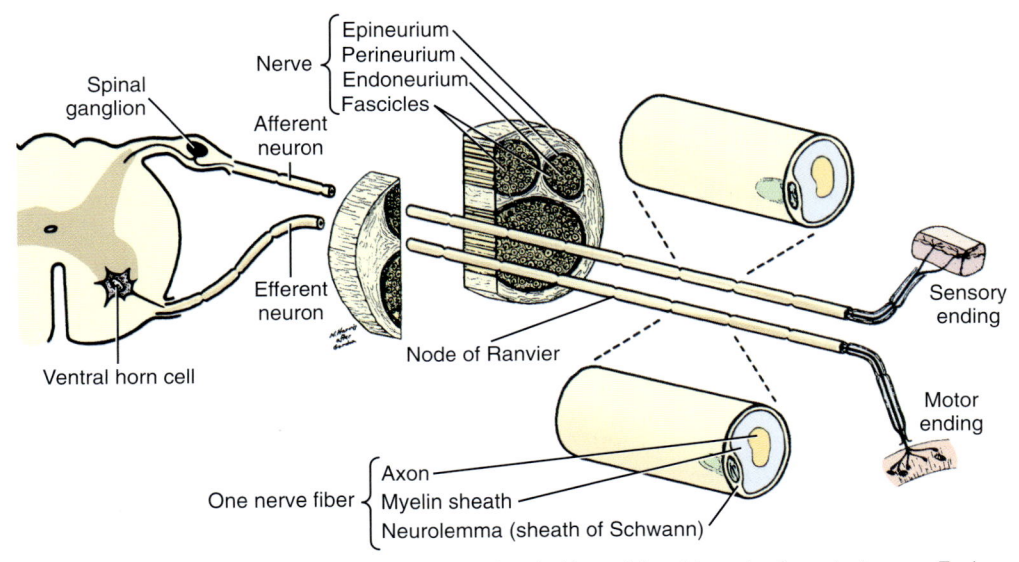

• **Fig. 14.12** Diagram showing the various parts of a sizable peripheral branch of a spinal nerve. Each fascicle contains large numbers of variously sized, myelinated axons and even larger numbers of nonmyelinated axons (not shown). Afferent axons can be myelinated and nonmyelinated (unmyelinated). Efferent axons going to striated muscle are always myelinated. The only nonmyelinated, efferent axons are postganglionic sympathetic axons supplying smooth muscle of blood vessels, mm. arrectores pilorum, and sweat glands. (Modified with permission from Ham AW, Leeson TS: *Histology,* 4th ed. Philadelphia: JB Lippincott, 1961.)

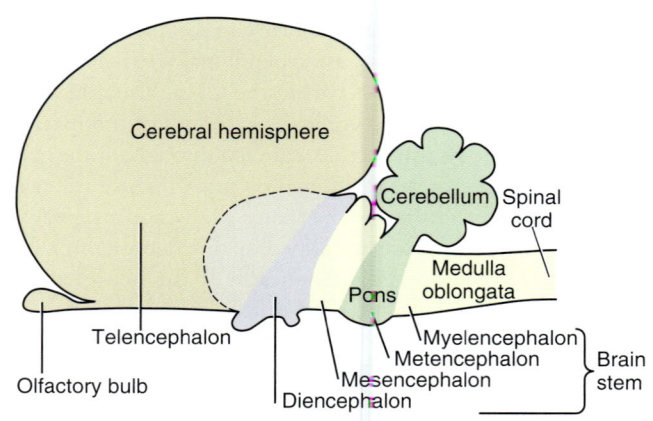

• **Fig. 14.13** Schematic representation of the major parts of the brain. The telencephalon consists of the cerebral hemispheres with their basal nuclei. The brain stem consists of the diencephalon, mesencephalon, the ventral part of the metencephalon (the pons), and the myelencephalon.

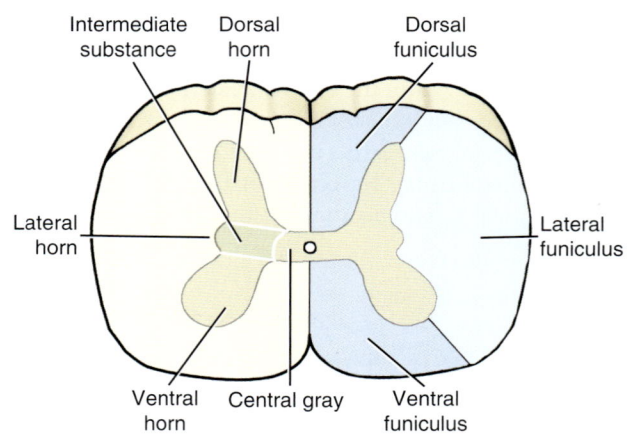

• **Fig. 14.14** Major subdivisions of the gray and white matter of the spinal cord. The gray matter (*horn* or *column*) consists primarily of longitudinal columns of cells, which when transected are referred to as *horns*. Within each horn are collections of cell bodies with similar functions that are called *nuclei*. The white matter of the spinal cord is divided by the entrance or exit of dorsal and ventral spinal nerve roots, respectively, and into columns of myelinated axons called *funiculi*. Within each funiculus, bundles of axons with similar functions are referred to as *fasciculi*, or *tracts*.

of myelinated axons and the neuroglia associated with the white matter.

The brain is subdivided into five major parts based on its development from the rostral part of the neural tube (Fig. 14.13). These subdivisions include the telencephalon, diencephalon, mesencephalon, metencephalon, and myelencephalon. The term *brainstem* refers to the diencephalon, mesencephalon, the pons part of the metencephalon, and the myelencephalon.

In the cerebrum and cerebellum, neuronal cell bodies compose the external layer, the cortex, and nuclei that are deep to the surface cortex. In the cerebrum, these nuclei are the basal nuclei, and, in the cerebellum, these are the cerebellar nuclei. In the cerebrum the major white matter pathways compose the projection pathways, the commissural pathways, and the association pathways. White matter in three cerebellar peduncles attach the brainstem to the cerebellum. The brainstem consists of a mixture of gray matter and white matter, some of which is clearly defined as nuclei and tracts, but much of which is less clearly organized. The reticular formation is a mixture of gray and white matter that composes the core of the brainstem.

In the spinal cord the neuronal cell bodies of the gray matter of the spinal cord are arranged in longitudinal columns that in cross-section give the appearance of horns, named dorsal, lateral, and ventral horns (also referred to as *gray columns*) (Fig. 14.14). The cell bodies of somatic LMNs are grouped together in motor nuclei in the ventral horns.

The white matter of the spinal cord surrounds the gray matter and is organized in tracts that compose the funiculi (Fig. 14.14). The dorsal funiculus is separated from the lateral funiculus by the entrance of dorsal root axons that are the central processes of primary afferent axons. The lateral funiculus is separated from the ventral funiculus by the exit of the efferent axons.

The central conductile portions of primary afferent axons in the dorsal roots enter the spinal cord (or the brainstem) and branch to run cranially (rostrally in the brainstem) and caudally varying distances (i.e., they never end in just one segment) (see Fig. 14.9). As they pass cranially and caudally, they give off many collateral branches that enter the gray matter of the dorsal horn. These collaterals of afferent axons form many thousands of synapses with interneurons, with projection neurons, and, in some instances, with efferent neurons. The segmental interneurons establish multisynaptic reflex arcs (Fig. 14.8). The central conductile segments of some muscle afferents have synapses with interneurons to form multisynaptic arcs (Fig. 14.8) as well as directly with LMNs to form monosynaptic arcs. The reference to multisynaptic and monosynaptic connections means synapses between one or two (or more) neurons connected *in series* like a chain. All afferent axons have many thousands of synapses *in parallel*.

The cell bodies of alpha efferent neurons (commonly called *LMNs*) (Figs. 14.3 and 14.15) are grouped together to form nuclei in the gray matter of the brainstem or as nuclei located in the ventral horn of the spinal cord. The axons of these neurons often give off a collateral branch, called a *recurrent collateral*, within the gray matter near the origin of the axon, and then the axon leaves the CNS to form the ventral root, a part of the PNS. This axon is the general somatic efferent axon found in nerves. It terminates by branching and forming motor end plates on a number of muscle fibers (called *extrafusal muscle fibers*), constituting a motor unit.

The cell bodies of gamma efferent neurons are found in locations similar to those of the alpha LMNs (Fig. 14.11). Gamma efferent neurons supply small muscle fibers, called *intrafusal muscle fibers*, located in connective tissue-encapsulated, specialized stretch receptors called **muscle spindles** (Fig. 14.6E).

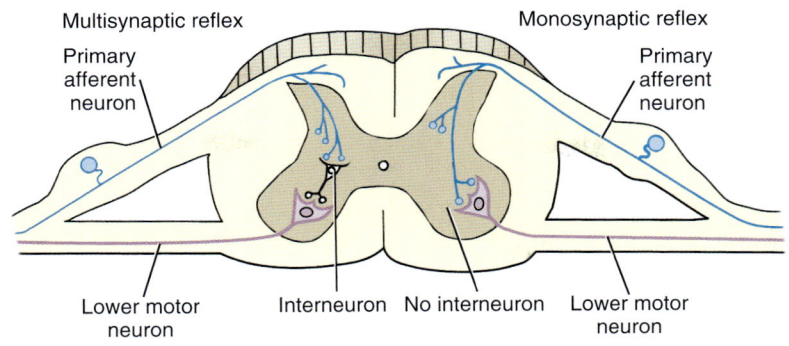

• **Fig. 14.15** Illustration of monosynaptic and multisynaptic reflex arcs. The primary afferent axons extend cranially and caudally, synapsing with many interneurons (or directly with lower motor neurons). The only monosynaptic arc involves a primary afferent axon from a muscle spindle synapsing with a lower motor neuron supplying extrafusal fibers in the same muscle that the muscle spindle is located.

The autonomic LMNs are linked together in series (Fig. 14.11). The first neuron in the series is referred to as a *preganglionic neuron,* with its small, multipolar cell body located in the CNS and its peripheral conductile process (preganglionic axon) extending out peripherally to synapse in an autonomic ganglia with varying numbers of neuronal dendrites of neuronal cell bodies of postganglionic axons. The cell body of the preganglionic neuron may be located in a cranial nerve nucleus or in the intermediate gray substance/lateral horn of the spinal cord. The autonomic ganglionic neurons are discussed with the PNS.

The Peripheral Nervous System

The PNS is subdivided into spinal nerves (*nervi spinales*) and cranial nerves (*nervi craniales*).

Functional Components of Nerves

A grossly visible nerve is made up of many axons (in the tens of thousands) (Fig. 14.12). Each axon may have a function distinctly different from that of the axon lying next to it. Histologically, the axons having differing functions cannot be distinguished from each other in the PNS. The functional classification of neurons in the PNS can be organized by the direction of the impulses within neurons (i.e., afferent or efferent or by the region of the body supplied by the neurons—somatic or visceral). Based on the former organization, afferent axons conduct impulses toward the CNS and efferent axons conduct impulses away from the CNS. Using the term *sensory* for afferent axons is misleading as the majority of activity in afferent neurons is never "sensed" because it never reaches a level in the brain for perception. Using the term *motor* for efferent axons may also be misleading as *motor* suggests movement, and the activity of many efferent neurons never results in movement because they innervate smooth muscle of blood vessels that regulates the vessel size or glands for secretion.

There are two general regions of the body supplied by afferent or efferent neurons. Neurons that originate or terminate in the body wall or limbs are referred to as *somatic*. Those that originate or terminate in the body organs (viscera) are visceral. Note that smooth muscle and glands, regardless of their location, are classified as visceral structures. Thus a nerve supplying the body wall or limb (bone, muscle, connective tissue, skin) can contain somatic afferent and efferent axons as well as visceral afferent and efferent axons. Special categories are used when the area supplied is limited to a small portion of the body (Table 14.1). Some texts include proprioception in the general somatic afferent (GSA) classification. In this text we consider it as a separate system because of its clinical significance. Disorders of proprioception express clinical signs very different from disorders that affect the GSA system.

Each cranial or spinal nerve consists of thousands of individual axons (Fig. 14.12). In this text, the term *nerve* is used to designate a grossly visible collection of axons in the PNS. A collection of cell bodies of neurons located outside the CNS is a ganglion. Two types of ganglia are found. Afferent (sensory) ganglia consist of collections of cell bodies of pseudounipolar neurons (bipolar neurons for the vestibulocochlear or eighth cranial nerve). Efferent ganglia are part of the autonomic nervous system and consist of cell bodies of postganglionic sympathetic or parasympathetic axons. Although it is customary to describe these second neurons as *postganglionic,* in reality only the axons of these neurons are truly postganglionic. Their cell bodies compose the ganglion. These autonomic ganglia consist of collections of many multipolar cells that have many synapses located on them.

Most nerves are composed of a mixture of afferent and efferent axons. Those distributed to the organs of the body cavities contain only visceral afferent and visceral efferent axons. Those distributed to the body wall, its surface, and the limbs are a mixture of general somatic afferent and efferent axons as well as general visceral afferent and efferent axons as previously described.

The cranial nerves connect to specific divisions of the brain. Cranial nerve I, the olfactory nerve, is associated with each cerebral hemisphere, the telencephalon. Cranial nerve II is a tract of the brain associated predominantly with the diencephalon. Cranial nerves III and IV are associated with

660 CHAPTER 14 Introduction to the Nervous System

TABLE 14.1 Functional Classification of Peripheral Neurons

System	Function and Anatomic Location
1. Afferent (A): Sensory	
Somatic (S)	
General (GSA)	Temperature, touch, noxious stimuli All spinal nerves, cranial nerve V
Special (SSA)	Vision: cranial nerve II Hearing: cranial nerve VIII
Visceral (V)	
General (GVA)	Organ content, distention, chemicals Spinal nerve splanchnic branches Cranial nerves VII, IX, X
Special (SVA)	Taste: cranial nerves VII, IX, X Olfaction: cranial nerve I
Proprioception (P)	
General (GP)	Muscle and joint movement All spinal nerves, cranial nerve V
Special (SP)	Vestibular system: cranial nerve VIII
2. Efferent (E) Motor:	
Somatic (S)	
General (GSE)	Striated skeletal muscle All spinal nerves Cranial nerves III, IV, V, VI, VII, IX, X, XI, XII
Visceral (V)	
General (GVE)	Smooth muscle, cardiac muscle, glands Sympathetic: all spinal nerves, splanchnic nerves Parasympathetic: sacral spinal nerves Cranial nerves III, VII, IX, X

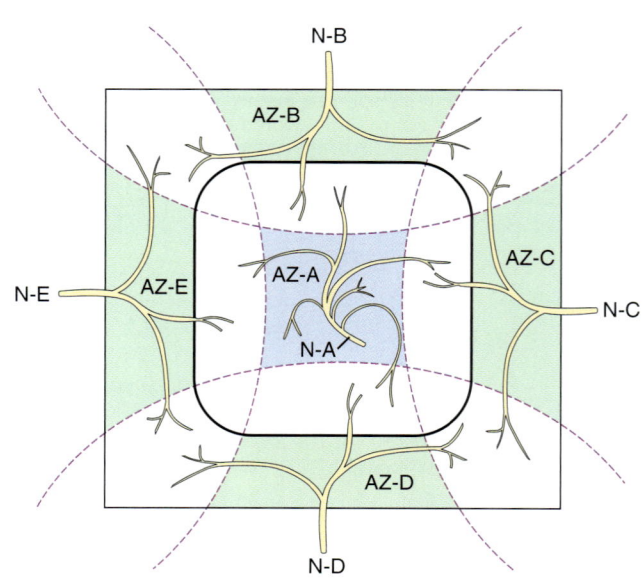

• **Fig. 14.16** Schematic illustration of the innervation of a cutaneous area. The central shaded area (*AZ–A*) is the autonomous zone of innervation of nerve "A" (*N–A*). The surrounding clear areas are zones of overlap with other nerves. Thus, each of the other nerves (*N–B, N–C, N–D,* and *N–E*) has an autonomous (*shaded*) zone (*AZ–B, AZ–C, AZ–D, AZ–E*) as well as overlapping zones (*clear areas*) of cutaneous innervation.

the mesencephalon, cranial nerve V with the ventral metencephalon, and cranial nerves VI through XII with the myelencephalon. Cranial nerves vary in the functional types of axons that they contain. Cranial nerves I and II only contain afferent axons. Cranial nerve II in reality is not a nerve but is a tract of the brain and therefore a CNS structure. All the remaining cranial nerves contain a varying amount of afferent and efferent axons that will be described in detail in Chapter 19. For most of the cranial nerves there is no distinct separation into afferent and efferent roots as in the spinal cord.

Nerves often intermingle to form plexuses wherein bundles of axons from different nerves intermingle and form new peripheral branches. These plexuses may largely supply body wall structures (**somatic plexuses**) or may supply the internal organs of the body (**visceral plexuses**). Somatic plexuses do not contain any or contain only very few cell bodies (ganglia) and thus have no or few synapses. Visceral plexuses commonly have cell bodies, general visceral efferent autonomic ganglion cells, scattered in the plexus, and thus may have many synapses occurring in them. The two large somatic plexuses of the body are the brachial plexus, which supplies the thoracic limb, and the lumbosacral plexus, which supplies the abdominal wall, pelvis, and the pelvic limb (for details see Chapter 17).

Nerves that supply only the skin are referred to as *cutaneous nerves*. They contain general somatic afferent, general visceral afferent, and general visceral efferent (postganglionic sympathetic) axons. The area of skin supplied by a cutaneous nerve is referred to as its **cutaneous area** (**CA**) (Fig. 14.16). The CA consists of two zones: a peripheral area, called the **overlap zone**, which is supplied by two or more cutaneous nerves, and a central zone, called the **autonomous zone** (**AZ**), which is supplied by only that one cutaneous nerve. Knowledge of the general location of the AZs of nerves is important because if a given cutaneous nerve, or the nerve giving rise to a cutaneous nerve, is damaged, an area of anesthesia (loss of any sensation) will result. The area of anesthesia will correspond to the AZ of a cutaneous nerve.

The general visceral efferent LMN differs from the general somatic efferent LMN in that it is a two-neuron system with one neuronal cell body in the CNS and the other located in the PNS. The first neuron in the chain has its cell body in the CNS and is referred to as a *preganglionic neuron*. Its preganglionic axon is myelinated and 2 to 7 µm in diameter in the dog. The cell bodies of the preganglionic axons are located in collections in the CNS called *nuclei* or *cell columns*. The cell body of the second neuron in the chain is located in a autonomic ganglion. Its axon is nonmyelinated and is referred to as the *postganglionic axon*.

The general visceral efferent LMN is subdivided into two parts, parasympathetic (*pars parasympathica*) and sympathetic (*pars sympathica*), on anatomic, physiologic, and pharmacologic bases (Fig. 14.17). The parasympathetic division has the cell bodies of its preganglionic neurons located in the cranial and sacral regions of the CNS, whereas the sympathetic system has the cell bodies of its preganglionic neurons located in the lateral horn regions of the thoracic and cranial lumbar regions of the spinal cord. As a result, these divisions may be referred to as the *craniosacral division* and the *thoracolumbar division* respectively. The neurotransmitter at the preganglionic neuronal transmitter segment synapses of both systems is acetylcholine. The neurotransmitter at the postganglionic neuronal transmitter segment–effector junction of the parasympathetic nervous system is acetylcholine. Thus, this is called the *cholinergic system*. In the sympathetic nervous system, the neurotransmitter is norepinephrine (or epinephrine). Thus, this is called the *adrenergic system*. An exception is that in most sweat glands, the sympathetic neurotransmitter is acetylcholine. Activation of the sympathetic nervous system, in general, produces a "mass" effect, whereas activation of the parasympathetic system produces more "localized" effects. Stimulation of the parasympathetic nervous system produces catabolic effects, or maintains the "status quo," whereas stimulation of the sympathetic nervous system produces anabolic effects—the "flight-or-fight" effects.

Postganglionic sympathetic axons supply smooth muscle of the vascular beds throughout the body, except within the CNS. To reach these vascular beds, the postganglionic axons "hitchhike" by running various distances in almost every nerve (including its branches) and along blood vessels, forming plexuses around the vessels. Any time that a nerve is severed (except olfactory, optic, and vestibulocochlear nerves) the neural control of a vascular bed will be lost.

The **intramural** or **enteric** nervous system is a network of afferent and efferent neurons that are found in the walls of abdominal organs. Many of the afferent neurons in this part of the nervous system have been shown to never reach the CNS, but instead they synapse on cell bodies of postganglionic axons in the walls of the intestine (terminal ganglia) or, in some instances, in the abdominal autonomic ganglia of both the sympathetic and the parasympathetic parts of the autonomic general visceral efferent LMN (Drake, 2007).

Reflexes

A reflex is an inherent, relatively consistent response to a particular stimulus. A reflex may or may not be perceived. A reflex involves a small component of a local area of the nervous system and occurs without the participation of projection pathways to and from the higher centers of the brain. The afferent component of the reflex may not be significant enough to recruit a projection pathway to result in perception of the stimulus that elicited the reflex. Most reflexes that regularly occur in the body are not perceived. In contrast to this, in clinical neurology, recognizing the ability to elicit a reflex without the patient being able to perceive a noxious stimulus is critical to determining the location of the lesion (the anatomic diagnosis) and to contributing to the prognosis for the patient.

In conducting a neurologic examination in animals, the understanding of reflexes is critical to establishing an anatomic diagnosis. Reflexes have five components: (1) a receptor, (2) an afferent limb, (3) an integration component, (4) an efferent limb, and (5) an effector (see Fig. 14.8).

The afferent limb of a reflex must involve nerves that contain primary afferent axons. The central conductile segment enters the spinal cord or the brainstem via primary afferent nerves. In the spinal cord these are the dorsal roots. Within the spinal cord or the brainstem, the primary afferent axons branch and run cranially (rostrally) and caudally and thus are not restricted to one spinal cord segment or to a small region of the brainstem. In the spinal cord these axons extend at least three segments cranially and two

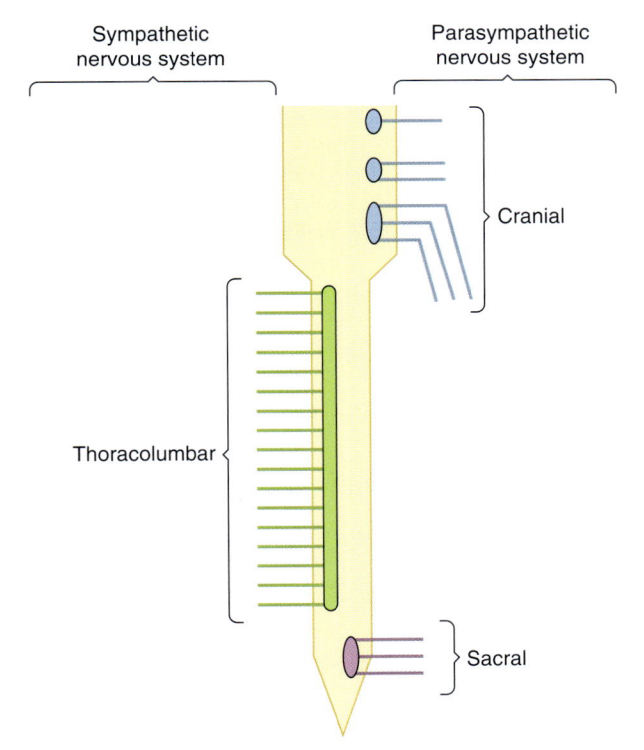

• **Fig. 14.17** Schematic illustration showing that the preganglionic axons of the parasympathetic system originate in the cranial and sacral regions of the central nervous system, whereas the preganglionic axons of the sympathetic nervous system originate in the thoracolumbar region of the spinal cord. The fibers must project into other regions of the body to supply visceral structures located there.

segments caudally, giving off numerous collaterals and making thousands of synapses (Fig. 14.9).

The integrating area, which is located in the gray matter of the spinal cord or the brainstem, consists of interneurons and the cell bodies of LMNs. The interneurons are of two types, excitatory and inhibitory interneurons (Fig. 14.8). Excitatory interneurons release neurotransmitters on other interneurons or directly on efferent neurons that either lower the threshold (facilitate) of these neurons and make them more easily excited by other axonal impulses or result in efferent neurons generating nerve impulses in their trigger zones. Inhibitory interneurons release neurotransmitters that raise the threshold (inhibit) of the next neuron, making it more difficult to elicit a reflex from the LMNs on which they act. Inhibitory interneurons are not directly involved in causing movement in a reflex pathway, but act to raise the thresholds of motor neurons supplying muscles that are antagonistic in action to reduce opposition to the reflex movement elicited. Both excitatory and inhibitory interneurons as well as the LMNs have their level of excitation influenced by a convergence of excitatory and inhibitory axons synapsing on them from segmental and suprasegmental (more cranial) sources. Conceptually, it is important to realize that inhibitory activity always accompanies the motor response that characterizes a reflex.

The efferent limb of a reflex consists of efferent axons from LMNs running in a nerve to supply motor units in striated muscle or, in the case of general visceral efferent axons, to supply smooth muscle, cardiac muscle, or glands.

The functional components involved in a reflex may be any combination of somatic and visceral axons; that is, general somatic afferents–general somatic efferents (muscle stretch reflexes); general somatic afferents–general visceral efferents (constriction of visceral blood vessels when cold is applied to the body); general visceral afferents–general visceral efferents (reflex dilation of peripheral blood vessels when the blood pressure rises); general visceral afferents–general somatic efferents (increase in muscle tension when the viscera is strongly stretched); or special visceral afferents (e.g., taste)–general visceral efferents (salivation reflex). The most obvious reflexes are the somatic afferents–somatic efferents because they result in gross movement of body parts. Visceral reflexes are less obvious because they result in changes in gastrointestinal movement or in vasoconstriction or vasodilation, which are seldom perceived or noticed.

The afferent and efferent limbs of a reflex can involve axons in the same nerve, or the afferent and efferent limbs can be in widely separated nerves. As each cranial and spinal nerve is studied, emphasis should be placed on recognizing which reflex functions will be lost if the nerve involved is damaged.

Most of the major peripheral branches of spinal nerves contain both afferent and efferent limbs of some reflex arc, either a somatic reflex or a visceral reflex. In some reflexes involving spinal nerves, cranial nerves, or both, the afferent limb may be in a spinal or cranial nerve different from that of the efferent limb.

Bibliography

Burnstock, G. (2008). Non-synaptic transmission at autonomic neuroeffector junctions. *Neurochem Int*, *52*, 14–25. doi:10.1016/j.neuint.2007.03.007.

Drake, M. J. (2007). The integrative physiology of the bladder. *Ann R Coll Surg Engl*, *89*, 580–585. doi:10.1308/003588407X205585.

Gardner, E. D. (1958). Fundamentals of neurology (3rd ed.). Philadelphia: Saunders.

Ham, A. W., & Leeson, T. S. (1961). Histology (4th ed.). Philadelphia: Lippincott.

Sofroniew, M. V., & Winters, H. V. (2010). Astrocytes: biology and pathology. *Acta Neuropathol*, *119*, 7–35.

15

The Autonomic Nervous System

MARNIE FITZMAURICE

The **autonomic nervous system** (ANS) is primarily concerned with the innervation of the smooth muscle of the viscera of the body. The anatomic components of the autonomic nervous system are controversial. Some consider that the ANS only consists of the **general visceral efferent** (GVE) **lower motor neuron** (LMN) and its parasympathetic and sympathetic components. Others, prefer a more expansive definition that correlates its function with its anatomy and consider that the ANS has a plethora of components in the **central nervous system** (CNS) as well as in the **peripheral nervous system** (PNS). Its primary afferents are the **general visceral afferent** (GVA) system and its efferent LMN is the GVE system with its parasympathetic and sympathetic components.

In this text the ANS is considered to be an anatomic and physiologic system with central and peripheral components. It includes higher centers in the hypothalamus, midbrain, pons, and medulla as well as tracts and nuclei in the spinal cord. The hypothalamus is the primary integrating center of the ANS. Nuclei in its rostral portion subserve the parasympathetic division of the GVE-LMN. Nuclei in its caudal portion subserve the sympathetic division of the GVE-LMN. These hypothalamic nuclei receive afferents from the cerebrum by way of numerous pathways, from thalamic nuclei and from GVA projection pathways. The hypothalamus influences the activity of the autonomic regulatory centers in the reticular formation of the midbrain, pons, and medulla. These centers control the activity of visceral smooth muscle, glands, and cardiac muscle by means of the GVE-LMN, which is located in specific cranial nerves and all spinal nerves. The hypothalamus also regulates homeostasis by controlling activity in endocrine systems and in skeletal muscles through the GSE system. Thus visceral efferent, somatic efferent, and endocrine output of the CNS is coordinated.

The ANS is concerned with activating emergency mechanisms and with the repair and preservation of the internal environment of the body. It maintains a steady state in the internal environment for the continuous efficient function of the body, which is called *homeostasis*. In order to carry out these functions, the ANS must receive information from the body via sensory neurons in the GVA system, then process this information in centers in the brain and send responses back to the body by brainstem and spinal cord pathways that activate LMNs in the GVE system.

Despite efforts to simplify the anatomy of this system and especially its GVE component, the complexity of it continues to defy simple organizational principles (Baumann & Gajisin, 1975). Exceptions to the rules that we have set are continually disclosed, and this chapter makes no attempt to document all of these.

General Visceral Efferent System

The GVE system is grouped anatomically and physiologically into two components: the parasympathetic and sympathetic systems. The LMN pathway involves two or more neurons between the CNS and the effector organ innervated. These two neurons are historically referred to as the *preganglionic* and *postganglionic neurons.* Only the axon of the second neuron is postganglionic. Therefore, in this text, the second LMN in this system will be referred to as the *ganglionic neuron.* The cell body of the preganglionic neuron is in the gray matter of the CNS and the cell body of the ganglionic neuron is in an autonomic ganglion in the PNS. The telodendron of the preganglionic neuron synapses on the dendritic zone of the ganglionic neuron. The primary neurotransmitter released at the synapse between these two neurons in the autonomic ganglion is acetylcholine.

The sympathetic system is referred to as the *thoracolumbar system* based on the location of the cell body of the first neuron, the preganglionic neuron, which is in the lateral gray horn from spinal cord segments T1 to approximately L4 or L5. As a general rule the sympathetic ganglia are located relatively close to the CNS, and the postganglionic axons are fairly long. With a few exceptions the neurotransmitter released at the telodendron of the sympathetic postganglionic axon is norepinephrine. Thus the sympathetic system is referred to as the *adrenergic system.*

The parasympathetic system is referred to as the *craniosacral system* because the cell bodies of the preganglionic neurons are located in the brainstem nuclei of cranial nerves III, VII, IX, or X, or in the sacral spinal cord segments. As a general rule the ganglia of this parasympathetic system are located in or fairly close to the effector organ, and the postganglionic axons are short. Acetylcholine is the neurotransmitter released at the telodendron of the postganglionic axon. Thus this parasympathetic system is called the *cholinergic system*.

Most structures innervated by the GVE system receive both parasympathetic and sympathetic axons with functions that are not always antagonistic. The activity of the parasympathetic and sympathetic GVE systems is integrated for neurologic regulation of normal body functions as well as its response to stress.

Parasympathetic Division

Parasympathetic preganglionic axons leave the brainstem as part of cranial nerves III, VII, IX, and X (Figs. 15.1 and 15.2). The axons in nerves III, VII, and IX are distributed to the head region, whereas the vagus nerve distributes autonomic axons to the cervical, thoracic, and abdominal viscera as far caudally as the left colic flexure. Parasympathetic preganglionic axons also leave the spinal cord as part of the ventral roots of the sacral nerves and become part of the pelvic plexus. Because the preganglionic neurons are located in the brainstem and sacral spinal cord, the parasympathetic nervous system is referred to as the *craniosacral division* of the ANS. Other routes of parasympathetic distribution may exist. For example, a rich and widely distributed cholinergic innervation of cerebral blood vessels has been described in the dog (Amenta et al., 1980).

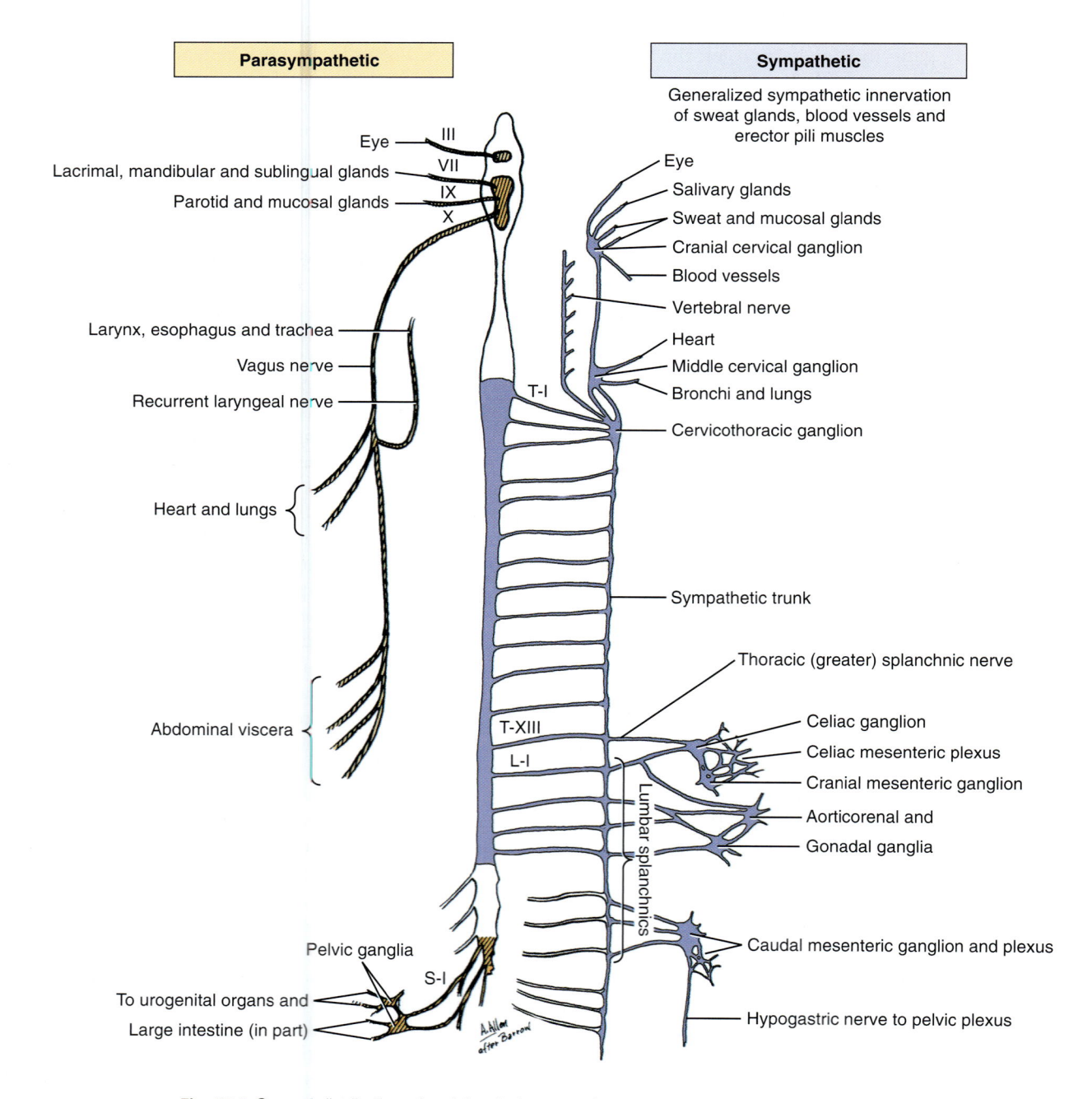

• Fig. 15.1 General distribution of peripheral elements of sympathetic and parasympathetic divisions.

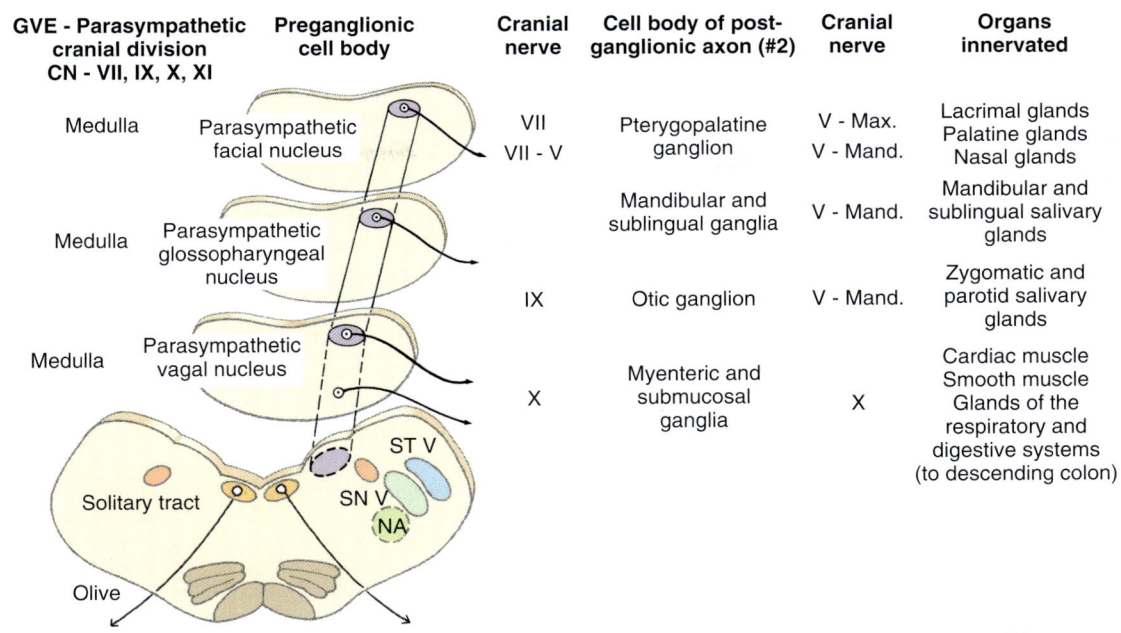

GVE - Parasympathetic cranial division CN - VII, IX, X, XI	Preganglionic cell body	Cranial nerve	Cell body of postganglionic axon (#2)	Cranial nerve	Organs innervated
Medulla	Parasympathetic facial nucleus	VII / VII - V	Pterygopalatine ganglion	V - Max. / V - Mand.	Lacrimal glands Palatine glands Nasal glands
			Mandibular and sublingual ganglia	V - Mand.	Mandibular and sublingual salivary glands
Medulla	Parasympathetic glossopharyngeal nucleus	IX	Otic ganglion	V - Mand.	Zygomatic and parotid salivary glands
Medulla	Parasympathetic vagal nucleus	X	Myenteric and submucosal ganglia	X	Cardiac muscle Smooth muscle Glands of the respiratory and digestive systems (to descending colon)

- **Fig. 15.2** Parasympathetic general visceral efferent nuclear column in the medulla. *NA*, Nucleus ambiguus; *SN V*, spinal nucleus of V; *ST V*, spinal tract of V.

The nerves are restricted mainly to the adventitia, are more prominent in arteries, remain intact after removal of the cranial cervical ganglia, and are therefore assumed to be parasympathetic.

Oculomotor (III)

Preganglionic neurons lie in the parasympathetic nucleus of the oculomotor nerve (*nucleus parasympathici oculomotorii*), which is unpaired in the dog and is located on the median plane just ventral to the central gray substance of the rostral mesencephalon (Fig. 15.1). The axons run as part of the third cranial nerve through the middle cranial fossa to leave the cranial cavity via the orbital fissure. Within the periorbita, they leave the oculomotor nerve by a short root and terminate in the **ciliary ganglion** (*ganglion ciliare*). Synapse occurs in the ciliary ganglion, and the postganglionic axons leave as the short ciliary nerves. They supply the ciliary muscle, which regulates lens curvature, and the sphincter of the iris, which, when activated, reduces pupillary diameter. Distribution of cholinergic as well as adrenergic innervation in the eye is described (Gwin et al., 1979). An accessory ciliary ganglion has been described in 13 mammalian species, including canines, in which it is located approximately 4 mm from the ciliary ganglion on one of the short ciliary nerves (Kuchiiwa et al., 1989).

Facial (VII)

The cell bodies of the preganglionic parasympathetic neurons associated with the facial nerve form two small nuclei in the medulla, the parasympathetic nuclei of the facial and intermediate nerves (Figs. 15.1 and 15.2). The **parasympathetic nucleus of the facial nerve** (*nucleus parasympatheticus n. facialis*) is closely associated with the somatic motor facial nucleus (Azuma et al., 1983). The preganglionic axons of these small cell bodies emerge from the medulla in the pars intermedia of the facial nerve, the **intermediate nerve** (*n. intermedius*) which immediately follows the facial nerve. Within the facial canal of the petrosal portion of the temporal bone, these preganglionic axons leave the facial nerve in the **major petrosal nerve** (*n. petrosus major*) and continue into the orbit in the **nerve of the pterygoid canal** (*n. canalis pterygoidei*) (Wakata, 1975) to terminate in synapses in the **pterygopalatine ganglion** (*ganglion pterygopalatinum*) located medial to the sphenopalatine nerve on the surface of the medial pterygoid muscle. Postganglionic axonal distribution to the lacrimal gland is not well defined. Apparently, some axons may go directly as small branches, and some may run with the lacrimal and zygomatic nerves. Other postganglionic axons go to glands and smooth muscle of the nasal and oral cavities via branches of the fifth cranial nerve (Jung et al., 1926; Nitschke, 1976).

The **parasympathetic nucleus of the intermediate nerve** (*nucleus parasympatheticus n. intermedii*) is located in the medulla dorsomedial to the somatic motor nucleus. These preganglionic axons leave the brainstem with the pars intermedia of the facial nerve. They join the main trunk of the facial nerve (Van Buskirk, 1945), and, as they traverse the facial canal of the petrosal part of the temporal bone, they leave as part of the chorda tympani nerve (Foley, 1945). The latter traverses the tympanic cavity and joins the lingual branch of the mandibular nerve. Synapse occurs in the **mandibular ganglion** (*ganglion mandibulare*) and the **sublingual ganglion** (*ganglion sublinguale*) and the postganglionic axons innervate the sublingual and mandibular salivary glands. The parasympathetic nucleus of the intermediate nerve also supplies glands of the tongue (see Chapter 7, The Tongue).

Glossopharyngeal (IX)

See Figs. 15.1 and 15.2. The cell bodies of the preganglionic neurons that initially travel with the glossopharyngeal nerve are located in the medulla in the **parasympathetic nucleus of the glossopharyngeal nerve** (*nucleus parasympatheticus n. glossopharyngei*). This nucleus is located at the rostral end of the parasympathetic nucleus of the vagus nerve lateral to the hypoglossal nucleus and adjacent to the floor of the fourth ventricle. The preganglionic axons leave the medulla in the rootlets of the glossopharyngeal nerve, which enters the jugular foramen. These preganglionic axons branch from the glossopharyngeal nerve and become part of the **tympanic plexus** (*plexus tympanicus*) on the ventral surface of the petrosal portion of the temporal bone within the tympanic cavity. They leave the plexus in the **minor petrosal nerve** (*n. petrosal minor*) to synapse in the **otic ganglion** (*ganglion oticum*), which is adjacent to the external opening of the oval foramen and the origin of the mandibular nerve from the trigeminal nerve. The postganglionic axons run with the auriculotemporal nerve, a branch of the mandibular nerve to their destination on the gland cells of the parotid salivary gland. A large number of these postganglionic axons also run in the adventitia of the maxillary artery and a small number of axons run in the facial nerve (Holmberg, 1971). The zygomatic salivary gland also receives parasympathetic postganglionic axons from the otic ganglion. The otic ganglion is a plexiform structure containing a number of small ganglia and having close contact with the maxillary artery (Gienc & Kuder, 1983).

Vagus (X)

The **vagus nerve** contains a number of functional components that include a large component of GVA axons and a smaller component of preganglionic parasympathetic GVE axons (Figs. 15.1, 15.3, 15.4, and 15.6).

The cervical portion of the vagus nerve is said to contain more than 80% "C" axons, with the balance myelinated (Fussey et al., 1973). The majority of the "C" axons are assumed to be afferent and the rest efferent, including parasympathetic fibers and somatic efferent fibers to skeletal muscle in the pharynx, larynx and esophagus. The parasympathetic fibers originate in the **parasympathetic nucleus of the vagus nerve** (*nucleus parasympatheticus vagi*), located in the dorsal part of the caudal medulla oblongata lateral to the hypoglossal nucleus ventral to the floor of the fourth ventricle, and the **nucleus ambiguus**, located in the ventrolateral medulla (Hopkins & Armour, 1984). Various

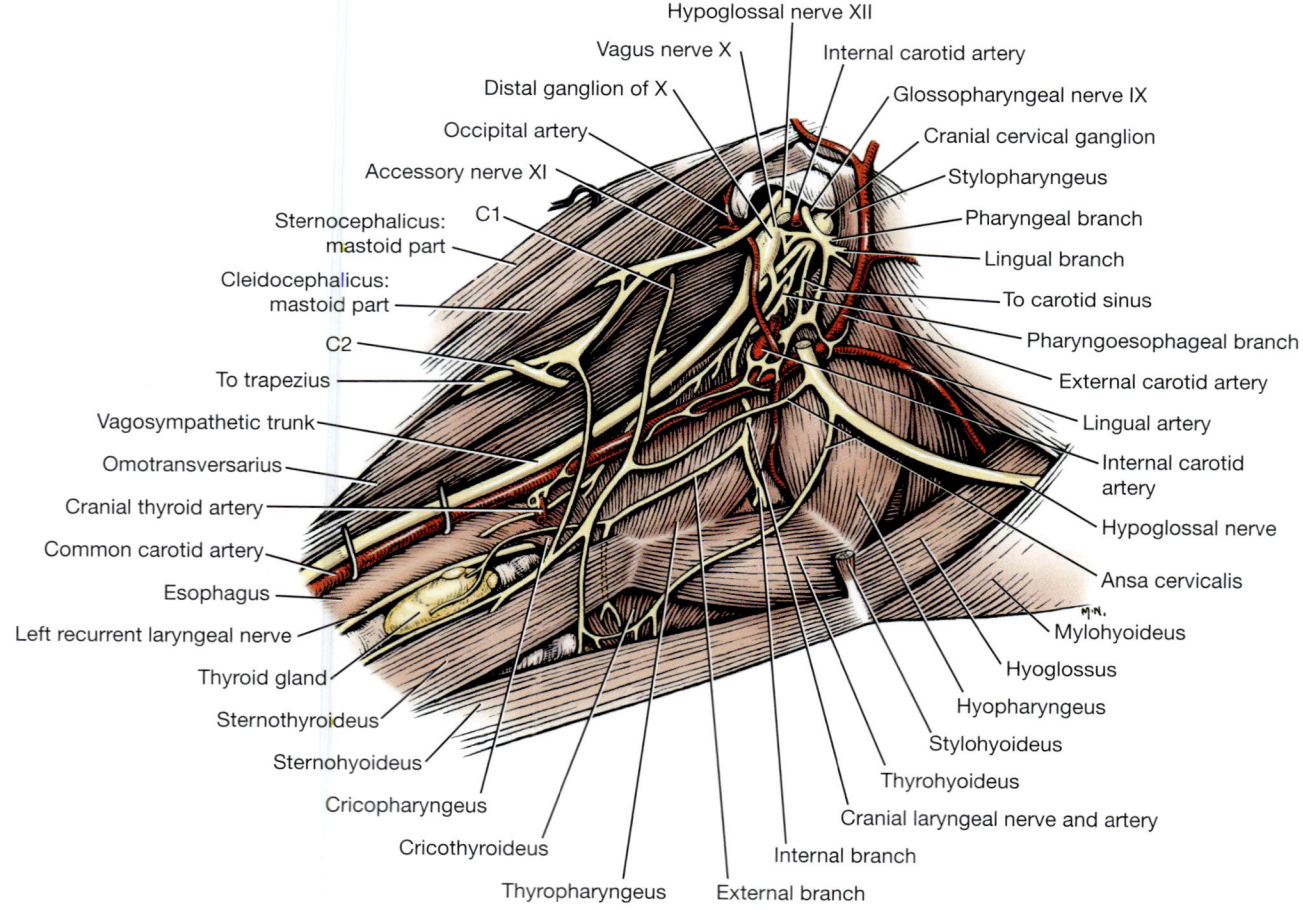

• **Fig. 15.3** Nerves of the pharyngeal region, lateral aspect. (The digastric muscle and superficial structures have been removed.)

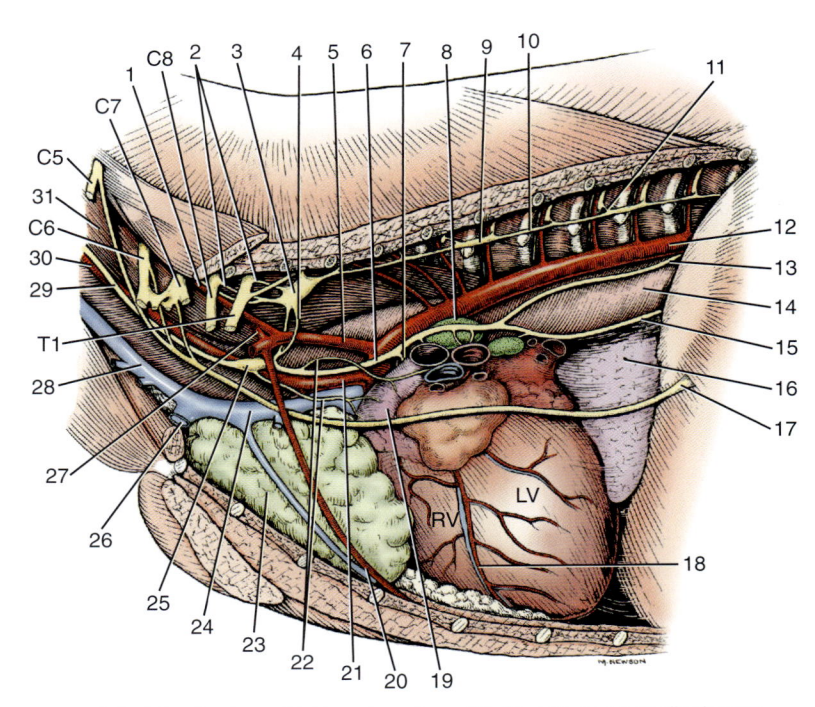

1. Vertebral artery and nerve
2. Communicating rami from cervicothoracic ganglion to ventral branches of cervical and thoracic nerves
3. Left cervicothoracic ganglion
4. Ansa subclavia
5. Left subclavian artery
6. Left vagus nerve
7. Left recurrent laryngeal nerve
8. Left tracheobronchial lymph node
9. Sympathetic trunk ganglion
10. Sympathetic trunk
11. Ramus communicans
12. Aorta
13. Dorsal branch of vagus nerve
14. Esophagus
15. Ventral trunk of vagus nerve
16. Accessory lobe of lung (through caudal mediastinum)
17. Phrenic nerve to diaphragm
18. Paraconal interventricular a., v., and groove
19. Pulmonary trunk
20. Internal thoracic artery and vein
21. Brachiocephalic trunk
22. Cardiac autonomic nerves
23. Thymus
24. Cranial vena cava
25. Middle cervical ganglion
26. Left subclavian vein
27. Costocervical trunk
28. External jugular vein
29. Vagosympathetic trunk
30. Common carotid artery
31. Longus colli muscle

• Fig. 15.4 Dissection of the thoracic region, right side.

branches of the vagus are discussed in this section, but distribution of the branches other than preganglionic parasympathetic GVE axons is described in the section on cranial nerves. The vagal rootlets leave the brain along the dorsolateral sulcus of the medulla oblongata in series with the rootlets of cranial nerves IX and XI. Close association of some of the vagal axons with those of the accessory (XI) nerve for a very short distance has led to the description of these vagal axons as part of the cranial root of the accessory nerve in some species.

A few millimeters distal to the origin of the vagus is located the small **proximal vagal ganglion** (*ganglion proximale n. vagi*). It is located at the level of the tympanooccipital fissure and contains unipolar general somatic afferent neurons whose axons are distributed with the **auricular branch** (*r. auricularis*) of the vagus. This branch leaves the vagus at approximately the level of the proximal vagal ganglion and has been shown to be distributed in part via branches of the seventh cranial nerve. There are also some branches in the tongue of the dog that have their cell bodies in the proximal ganglion of the vagus.

The **pharyngeal branch** (*r. pharyngeus*) of the vagus is given off between the proximal and **distal vagal ganglia** (*ganglion distale n. vagi*). The latter ganglion is primarily composed of unipolar GVA neurons that have their peripheral distribution in the viscera.

The **cranial laryngeal nerve** (*n. laryngeus cranialis*) leaves the vagus at the level of the distal ganglion. The sympathetic cranial cervical ganglion is located rostral and medial to the distal vagal ganglion. The epineurial sheaths of the two ganglia may be separate or may show variable degrees of fusion. By careful dissection, it is possible to peel the epineurial sheath away from the vagus and its ganglia, thereby clearly demonstrating the branches that leave the vagus. In some specimens a small, unnamed bundle of vagal axons may be seen to bypass the distal ganglion.

Distal to the distal vagal ganglion, the vagus joins the sympathetic trunk, and the two are bound in a common sheath along the entire cervical region. The sympathetic trunk may retain a rounded contour (in cross-section) or may assume a crescent shape where it is closely applied to the vagus. In some specimens it is nevertheless possible to easily separate the two by dissection.

At the level of the middle cervical ganglion (Fig. 15.5) the **right recurrent laryngeal nerve** (*n. laryngeus recurrens*) leaves the right vagus and passes dorsally around the caudal side of the right subclavian artery. As it runs cranially on the trachea, it lies deep to the common carotid artery in the

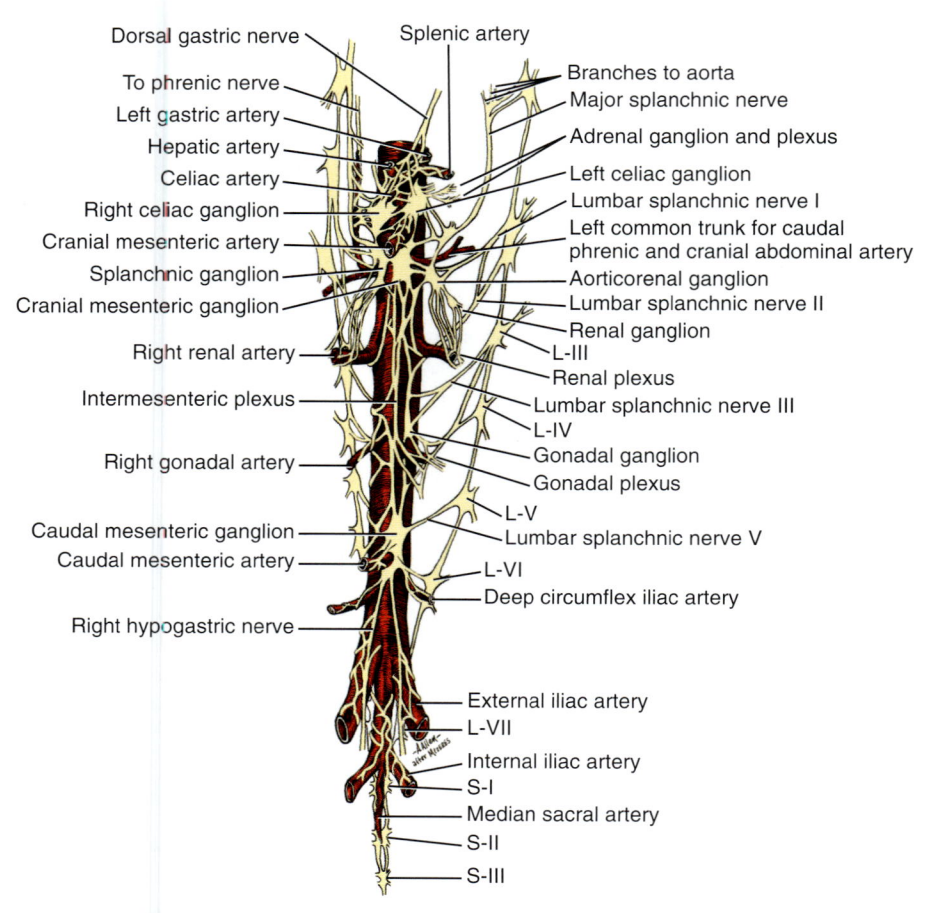

Fig. 15.5 Ganglia and plexuses of the abdominal cavity.

angle between the longus colli muscle and the trachea. Near its origin, the right recurrent laryngeal nerve gives off a fairly large branch, the **cervical cardiac nerve** (*n. cardiacus cervicalis*), which receives contributions from the middle cervical ganglion, the vagal trunk, and the left recurrent laryngeal nerve. It is distributed mainly to plexuses along the right and left coronary arteries. The cervical cardiac nerve contains postganglionic sympathetic, preganglionic parasympathetic, and visceral afferent axons for the heart.

Terminal parasympathetic ganglia in the heart contain neuronal cell bodies that differ markedly in size (Nonidez, 1939). As a consequence, the postganglionic axons also vary in diameter. These axons lie in the walls of the atria and the interatrial septum and form extensive cardiac plexuses. Smaller branches leave the plexuses and end as ring-shaped, club-shaped, or reticulated enlargements, which contact the surface of the cardiac muscle fibers. Similar enlargements may also occur along the course of the finer branchings. Terminations are especially abundant among the specialized muscle fibers of the sinoatrial (SA) and atrioventricular (AV) node. These nodes are also richly supplied with adrenergic fibers (Dahlström et al., 1965). Postganglionic parasympathetic axons of the cardiac ganglia are also distributed via nerve plexuses along branches of the coronary arteries. These axons form plexuses in the adventitia and finally end in relation to the smooth muscle cells of the outer media. Primarily, these axons innervate the arteries of the atrium and proximal part of the ventricles. Most of the parasympathetic distribution is to structures dorsal to the coronary sulcus, whereas sympathetic axons innervate the ventricles. Further information on intrinsic innervation of the heart may be found in Tcheng (1950, 1951), Holmes (1956, 1957), Uchizono (1964), Hirsch et al. (1964, 1965), Napolitano et al. (1965), Ehinger (1967), Kent et al. (1974), Kyösola et al. (1976), Denn and Stone (1976), Geis et al. (1973), Martin et al. (1977), Coleridge et al. (1973), Mizeres (1955b), and Hopkins and Armour (1984).

The right vagus nerve, having usually separated from the sympathetic trunk a short distance cranial to the level of the middle cervical ganglion, runs ventral to the right subclavian artery and continues caudally along the lateral surface of the trachea. At the level of the subclavian artery, the ansa subclavia may be intimately attached to the vagus for a short distance. Also in this region the vagus and recurrent laryngeal nerves may receive branches from the middle cervical ganglion or ansa subclavia. Distal to the origin of the recurrent laryngeal nerve, the vagus gives off two or more fine cardiac branches. The cranial branches go mainly to the pretracheal plexus. The caudal cardiac branches distribute to the dorsal wall of the right atrium.

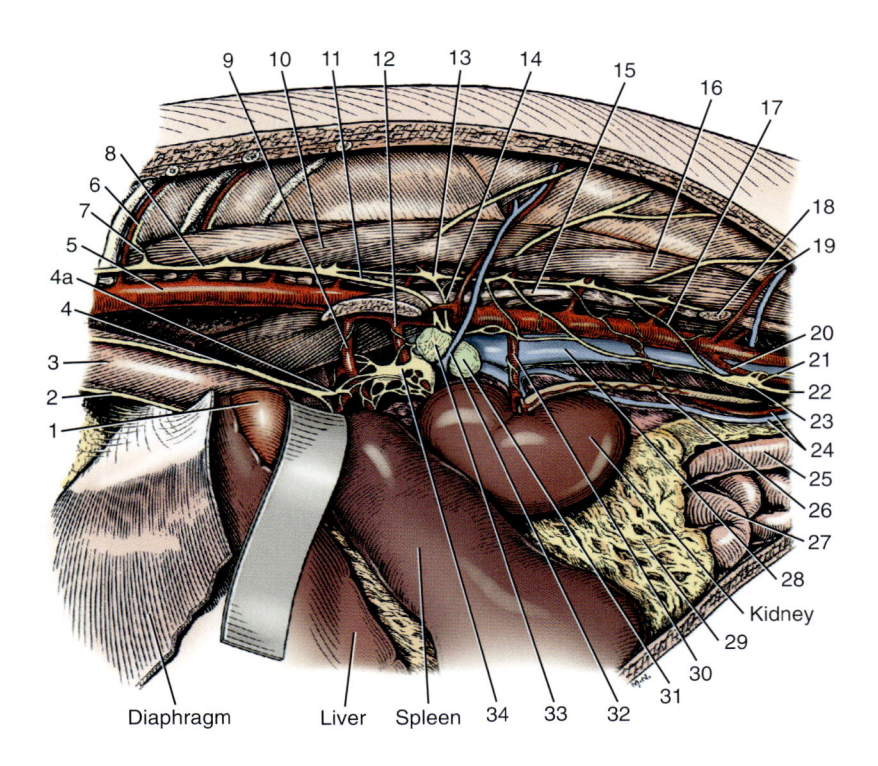

- Fig. 15.6 Exposure of abdominal autonomic nervous system on left side.

1. Stomach
2. Ventral trunk of vagus n.
3. Esophagus
4. Dorsal trunk of vagus n.
4a. Celiac br. of dorsal vagal trunk
5. Aorta
6. Intercostal a. and n.
7. Ramus communicans
8. Sympathetic trunk
9. Celiac a.
10. Quadratus lumborum
11. Major splanchnic n.
12. Cranial mesenteric a.
13. Lumbar sympathetic ganglion at L2
14. Minor splanchnic n.
15. Tendon of left crus of diaphragm
16. Psoas major
17. Lumbar splanchnic n.
18. Transected psoas minor
19. Deep circumflex iliac a.
20. Caudal mesenteric a.
21. Caudal mesenteric plexus
22. Left hypogastric n.
23. Caudal mesenteric ganglion
24. Testicular a. and v.
25. Descending colon
26. Cranial ureteral a.
27. Jejunum
28. Caudal vena cava
29. Greater omentum
30. Renal a. and plexus
31. Adrenal gland
32. Common trunk for caudal phrenic and cranial abdominal v.
33. Adrenal plexus
34. Celiac and cranial mesenteric ganglia and plexus

The main trunk of the right vagus continues caudally dorsal to the root of the lung. At this level it gives off several prominent branches along the bronchi (Ziemianski et al., 1967). Parasympathetic ganglia are found in the lung, and postganglionic parasympathetic axons have been traced to smooth muscle and glandular structures. The lung is also richly innervated with a wide variety of receptor structures as far distally as the alveoli. Receptors have been described in smooth muscle, tracheal and bronchial epithelium, respiratory bronchioles, alveolar ducts, and alveolar walls (Elftman, 1943). The vagus supplies branches directly to the trachea and esophagus and also via the recurrent laryngeal nerve.

Immediately caudal to the root of the lung, both right and left vagi split into dorsal and ventral branches. The ventral branch of the right fuses with its left counterpart to form the **ventral vagal trunk** (*truncua vaglis ventralis*). A similar anastomosis occurs between right and left dorsal vagal branches more distally near the diaphragm to form the **dorsal vagal trunk** (*truncus vagalis dorsalis*).

Both dorsal and ventral vagal trunks supply branches to the esophagus before passing through the diaphragm at the esophageal hiatus. On reaching the abdominal cavity, the ventral vagus becomes plexiform for a short distance. Branches from this plexus supply mainly the liver and stomach. The hepatic branches (usually two or three) originate from both vagal trunks and run in the lesser omentum to the liver (Chiu, 1943). These pass between the caudate and left lateral lobe of the liver to form a simple plexus just rostral to the porta hepatis. Autonomic nerve branches are distributed from the plexuses to the cystic duct, gallbladder, left lateral lobe of the liver, and bile duct. Groups of axons also pass along the right gastric and cranial pancreaticoduodenal arteries to the pancreas and along the right gastric artery to the pylorus. A small filament may go directly to the duodenum.

The second group of three or four gastric branches from the ventral vagus supply the parietal surface of the stomach. Some parasympathetic axons join the sympathetic plexus on the branches of the left gastric artery (Mizeres, 1955a).

The dorsal vagal trunk supplies the cardiac region of the stomach and then forms a plexus on its visceral surface. Distribution is mainly to the lesser curvature and pyloric regions of the stomach. Branches of the dorsal vagal trunk may also join the celiac, left gastric, hepatic, and cranial mesenteric nerve plexuses associated with the corresponding arteries. Further references on abdominal distribution of the vagus nerve are those of Obrebowski (1965), Kapellar (1965), Mizeres (1955a), and Kemp (1973).

Information on vagal parasympathetic distribution caudal to the stomach is sparse, but there seems to be general agreement that these fibers reach as far caudally as the left colic flexure.

Branching and distribution of the left vagus are similar to the right as far distally as the level of the middle cervical ganglion. Here a branch leaves the vagus to join a branch from the middle cervical ganglion, resulting in formation of a cervical cardiac nerve. This is distributed to the base of the brachiocephalic trunk and ventral surface of the aortic arch.

It must be emphasized that details of autonomic nerve distribution to the heart are extremely variable, particularly with respect to origin of axons. Many of the nerves to the heart are mixed in the sense that they carry sympathetic, parasympathetic, and visceral afferent fibers. Terminology is varied and often confusing. In general it can be said that impulses propagated in sympathetic axons tend to accelerate heart rate and force of contraction, whereas parasympathetic stimulation reduces heart rate. Branches leave the left recurrent laryngeal nerve near its origin and go to the left atrium or plexuses that supply it. Other branches to the left atrium leave the vagus distal to the origin of the recurrent nerve. The vagus also contributes axons to certain other cardiac nerves, which is discussed with the sympathetic system.

Axons that make up the left recurrent laryngeal nerve leave the vagus at the level of the aortic arch and loop around the arch caudal to the ligamentum arteriosum. The recurrent laryngeal nerve then proceeds cranially along the left ventrolateral surface of the trachea adjacent to the ventromedial side of the esophagus. Branches are supplied to the trachea and esophagus as the nerve passes to its termination in the larynx (Hwang et al., 1948; Watson, 1974). In the cervical region the left recurrent laryngeal supplies more branches to the esophagus than it does to the trachea. The opposite is true of the right recurrent laryngeal nerve. In dogs whose esophagus lies to the right of the midline in the cervical region, there is a more even distribution of branches of right and left recurrent laryngeal nerves to both trachea and esophagus.

Cranial to the root of the lung, the left vagus may contribute a variable number of axons to the cardiac nerves, as previously noted. Several branches leave the left vagus for distribution along the bronchi much as occurs on the right side. Distal to the root of the lung, the left vagus divides into dorsal and ventral branches, each of which joins its counterpart of the right side to result in dorsal and ventral vagal trunks. Their distribution has been discussed.

Parasympathetic ganglionic neurons may be found scattered in the walls of structures that they supply or else as part of well-defined plexuses in similar regions. These intramural nerve plexuses are most prominent in the digestive tract (Filogamo, 1950; Lawrentjew, 1931; Richardson, 1960; Schofield, 1961). The **myenteric plexus** (*plexus myentericus*) is located between the longitudinal and circular muscle layers, and the **submucosal plexus** (*plexus submucosus*) lies in the submucosa of the digestive tube (El'bert, 1956; Leaming & Cauna, 1961). Ganglia are common in these enteric plexuses (*plexus entericus*). Prominent ganglionated plexuses are also found in the atria of the heart. Much of their regulating effect is thought to be mediated by way of the SA and AV nodes.

Sacral Parasympathetics

Parasympathetic preganglionic neurons are located in the sacral spinal cord segments. The preganglionic cell bodies are not confined to the substantia intermedia lateralis, but extend medially throughout the broad substantia intermedia, laterally to the adjoining part of the lateral funiculus, and ventrally among the somatic motor neurons of the ventral gray horn (Petras & Cummings, 1978). Preganglionic axons leave as part of the ventral roots of the sacral segments (Gaskell, 1886; Mizeres, 1955a; Schnitzlein et al., 1963; Wozniak & Skowronska, 1967). These axons continue in the ventral branches of the sacral spinal nerves and form separate branches that join more distally as the **pelvic nerve** (*nn. pelvini*), located on the lateral wall of the caudal portion of the rectum (Fig. 15.7). The pelvic nerve is supplied with preganglionic axons originating mainly from cell bodies in sacral segments 1, 2, and 3 (Samson & Reddy, 1982). On both sides the pelvic nerve expands into a plexus that also receives the hypogastric nerves with their postganglionic sympathetic axons. This plexus is associated with the vaginal or prostatic artery. One or more ganglia, primarily parasympathetic, are located within the plexus (Jayle, 1935). Distribution of postganglionic axons is via branches and plexuses to the pelvic viscera and reproductive organs. Parasympathetic axons from the sacral region have been traced through the length of the large intestine (Schmidt, 1933). Parasympathetic ganglia are found in the wall of the rectum and urinary bladder (Iljina & Lawrentjew, 1932a, b). Spinal cord origin of parasympathetic axons influencing the urinary bladder is in segments S1 to Cd1 (Purinton & Oliver, 1979). Visceral afferent activity from urethra, rectum, and genitalia reaches the spinal cord via the pelvic nerve and is then relayed through projection pathways to the cerebral cortex. Afferent activity from the urinary bladder reaches the spinal cord via both pelvic and hypogastric nerves, but only neural activity via the latter is relayed to the cerebral cortex (Purinton et al., 1981).

Based on molecular and developmental characterization of autonomic nerves and ganglia, it has recently been proposed that the sacral parasympathetic pathways are actually part of the sympathetic system (Espinosa-Medina et al., 2016; Fritzsch et al., 2017; Neuhuber et al., 2017). Such a restructuring of conceptual organization better explains some features of lumbar and sacral innervation, including the predominance of trisynaptic innervation of pelvic viscera. However, it ignores the functional and neurochemical organization of these systems, which form the basis for the distinction between the sympathetic and parasympathetic systems (Horn, 2018).

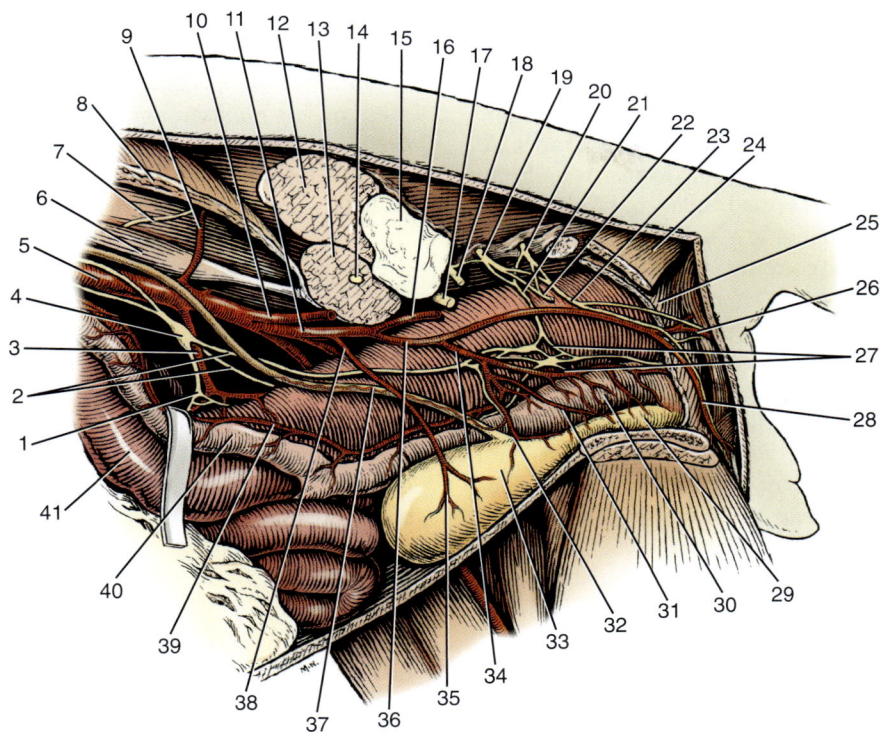

- Fig. 15.7 Autonomic nerves and vessels of pelvic region, left lateral view.

1. Caudal mesenteric plexus
2. Right and left hypogastric nerves
3. Caudal mesenteric artery
4. Caudal mesenteric ganglion
5. Aorta
6. Psoas minor
7. Lateral cutaneous femoral nerve
8. Abdominal oblique muscles
9. Deep circumflex iliac artery
10. External iliac artery
11. Internal iliac artery
12. Quadratus lumborum
13. Iliopsoas
14. Femoral nerve
15. Sacroiliac articulation
16. Caudal gluteal artery
17. Lumbar nerves 6 and 7
18. First sacral nerve
19. Second sacral nerve
20. Third sacral nerve
21. Pelvic nerve
22. Caudal cutaneous femoral nerve
23. Pudendal nerve
24. Coccygeus
25. Levator ani
26. Perineal nerve and artery
27. Pelvic plexus
28. Artery and nerve to clitoris
29. Urethra
30. Vagina
31. Urethral branch of vaginal artery
32. Caudal vesical artery
33. Bladder
34. Vaginal artery
35. Cranial vesical artery
36. Internal pudendal artery
37. Ureter and ureteral branch of vaginal artery
38. Umbilical artery
39. Uterine artery
40. Uterine horn
41. Descending colon

Sympathetic Division

The sympathetic preganglionic cell bodies in the dog are located in the lateral horn (substantia intermedia lateralis) of the spinal cord gray matter from C8 or T1 through the L4 or L5 segments. Most of the preganglionic neurons are contained in the triangular cell nests of this region of gray matter. However, substantial numbers also extend across the substantia intermedia toward the central canal (Cummings, 1969; Petras & Faden, 1978). Sympathetic preganglionic axons may sometimes appear in the ventral roots of the more caudal cervical segments. The myelinated small-diameter preganglionic axons leave in the ventral roots of the previously named segments and for a short distance are part of the corresponding spinal nerves. These axons then leave each spinal nerve in one or more communicating rami (*rami communicantes*) that attach to the sympathetic trunk. The sympathetic trunk (*truncus sympathicus*) is a paired strand of preganglionic and postganglionic sympathetic and visceral afferent axons located ventrolateral to the bodies of the vertebrae in the thoracic and lumbar regions. Continuations of the two trunks caudally into the sacral and caudal region may be partially fused and lie ventral to the bodies of the vertebrae. Both sympathetic trunks are continued cranially into the cervical region, where each is no longer adjacent to the vertebral bodies and is located in a common sheath with the vagus nerve. Each trunk then terminates in the cranial cervical ganglion, which is just external to the tympanooccipital fissure. Except for the cervical region, sympathetic trunk ganglia (*ganglia trunci sympathici*) are located at segmental intervals along the sympathetic trunk. In reality these cell bodies can be found by microscopic examination throughout the sympathetic trunk, but they accumulate in these ganglia.

The ganglia are numbered according to the spinal nerve to which the communicating branches attach. The part of the sympathetic trunk that joins adjacent ganglia is the interganglionic segment. The ganglia contain the multipolar neurons that give rise to the predominantly nonmyelinated postganglionic axons. Synapses may occur, for example, between preganglionic axons of the T12 ramus communicans and cells in the T12 sympathetic trunk ganglion, or the preganglionic axons may proceed cranially or caudally in the sympathetic trunk to synapse in ganglia at other segmental levels. Preganglionic axons in the dog may project cranially or caudally over a number of segments within the spinal cord before exiting in the ventral roots (Faden & Petras, 1978). In general, preganglionic axons from T1 to T5 are directed cranially, whereas caudal to T5 the axons pass caudally. Thus preganglionic axons from a given segmental level of the spinal cord are distributed to sympathetic trunk ganglia at many different levels. For example, sympathetic preganglionic vasoconstrictor fibers to the pelvic limb leave the spinal cord through the ventral roots of segments T10 through L4, whereas the postganglionic axons leave the sympathetic trunk at and caudal to the L4 spinal nerve level (Donald & Ferguson, 1970). The rami communicans from T1 to L4 or L5 contain both preganglionic as well as postganglionic axons. However, those rami caudal to L4 or L5 only contain postganglionic axons.

Preganglionic axons may also leave the caudal thoracic and lumbar sympathetic trunk in splanchnic nerves and synapse in autonomic plexus ganglia such as the celiac, cranial, and caudal mesenteric ganglia.

Postganglionic axons may be distributed in a number of different ways:

1. Axons leave the sympathetic trunk ganglia via the communicating rami to return to the spinal nerve at the same level. These are distributed to smooth muscle (vasomotor and pilomotor fibers) and glands by way of the spinal nerve.
2. Axons run either rostrally or caudally in the sympathetic trunk and join the adjacent spinal nerves via their respective communicating rami.
3. Axons leave sympathetic trunk ganglia such as the cervicothoracic or middle cervical to go directly to a visceral structure such as the heart via a cardiac nerve or to the thoracic limb by branches that join the ventral branches of the spinal nerves that contribute to the brachial plexus.
4. Axons leave the cranial cervical ganglion for distribution as plexuses along arteries of the head region.
5. Axons leave autonomic plexus ganglia such as the celiac for distribution as plexuses along arteries to the abdominal viscera.

Reference is sometimes made to gray versus white rami communicans, the gray being made up mainly of non-myelinated postganglionic axons and the white mainly of myelinated preganglionic axons. At most segmental levels of the thoracic and cranial lumbar regions of the dog, the rami are mixed in the sense that they contain both preganglionic and postganglionic axons. Cranial to the thoracic, and caudal to the cranial lumbar levels, the communicating rami are made up mostly of nonmyelinated axons because usually no preganglionic contributions to the sympathetic trunk arise from the cervical, caudal lumbar, and sacral regions. The comparatively few myelinated fibers that may be present in these "gray" rami are probably visceral afferent.

The small size of the sympathetic nerves that are grossly dissectible belies their extensive distribution. In general it appears that sympathetic postganglionic axons are as widely distributed as the arterial system.

Both microscopic and macroscopic ganglia may be found more or less randomly scattered along the peripheral portions of the sympathetic system. These are for the most part unnamed ganglia either proximal or distal to ganglia such as celiac, cranial mesenteric, or those of the sympathetic trunk chain. For this reason any given segment of sympathetic nerve cannot be considered to carry all preganglionic or all postganglionic axons. Microscopic examination of a sympathetic nerve could not be expected to enable one to identify completely the nature of the axons because not all preganglionic axons are universally myelinated throughout their length. Postganglionic axons usually have no myelin sheath, but this also is probably not a constant characteristic. Apparently, sympathetic axons acquire myelin sheaths after birth, whereas myelinization of vagal axons begins before birth (Diamare & de Mennato, 1930).

Sympathetic Distribution to Head and Neck

See Figs. 15.3 and 15.4. In the dog, preganglionic cell bodies from the C8 through the T7 spinal segments give rise to axons that run as part of the vagosympathetic trunk to synapse in the cranial cervical ganglion (Petras & Faden, 1978). The cervical sympathetic trunk of the dog has been shown to contain approximately 5000 to 13,000 axons, of which approximately half appear to be myelinated (Foley & Du Bois, 1940). The cranial cervical ganglion (*ganglion cervicale craniale*) lies medial to the tympanic bulla and the proximal portions of cranial nerves IX, X, XI, and XII. A large portion of the postganglionic axons leaving the ganglion continue as plexuses along the arteries of the head region. For example, rather prominent bundles of axons can be seen going to both external and internal carotid arteries. The external carotid nerves (*nn. carotici externi*) form a plexus (*plexus caroticus externus*) around the external carotid artery. The internal carotid nerve (*n. carotici internus*) forms a plexus (*plexus caroticus internus*) around the internal carotid artery to supply postganglionic axons to the cerebral arteries and structures in the orbit. Sympathetic postganglionic axons also follow the common carotid artery. In general, the arterially distributed sympathetic axons supply sweat and salivary glands, nasal glands, and smooth muscle such as that of vascular walls, nictitating membrane, dilator pupillae, and erector pili (Ehinger, 1967; Esterhuizen et al., 1967; Franke & Bramante, 1964; Malmfors, 1968). In addition, adrenergic axons to the eye appear to have a wide distribution, including the iris stroma, cornea, trabeculae of the iridocorneal angle, ciliary body, ciliary processes, and retina (Ehinger, 1966). Some adrenergic fibers to the sphincter pupillae have also been seen, but their function is unknown. A similar "double innervation" (sympathetic and parasympathetic) of the dilator pupillae of the cat has also been described (Ehinger, 1967). Those sympathetic nerves that follow the arteries may be fairly discrete bundles or plexiform (Billingsley & Ranson, 1918a, b).

Axons from the cranial cervical ganglion may in some specimens be seen to join the ninth, tenth, eleventh, and twelfth cranial nerves, the connection to the tenth being most common. A fairly constant branch to the first cervical nerve occurs (see Fig. 15.3), and this may also supply axons to the second and third cervical nerves. Other branches may join the pharyngeal and cranial laryngeal branches of the vagus. In some dogs a pharyngeal plexus is formed by contributions from cranial nerves IX and X and the cranial cervical ganglion. Axons also attach the cranial cervical ganglion to the region of the carotid sinus and carotid body (glomus). A larger branch (see Fig. 15.3) leaves the caudal end of the cranial cervical ganglion, contributes to the pharyngeal plexus, and sends axons along the cranial thyroid artery to the thyroid gland. The rest of the nerve continues caudally in the connective tissue membrane that joins the vagosympathetic trunk to the common carotid artery. It is joined by small branches of the cranial laryngeal and glossopharyngeal nerves and continues caudally as an esophageal branch. The thyroid gland receives sympathetic postganglionic axons that are distributed as interfollicular nerves and plexuses along arteries. The vascular nerve plexuses lie in the tunica media and tunica adventitia. It may be assumed that other visceral structures of the head and neck region as well as the rest of the body are also supplied with afferent innervation.

The adventitia of the cervical lymphatic tracheal duct is innervated by a loose, interrupted network that appears to arise from plexuses of sympathetic axons surrounding the vasa vasorum of the ducts.

Sympathetic innervation, arising at least in part from the cranial cervical and cervicothoracic ganglia and terminating on cochlear and vestibular blood vessels, ganglia, and structural elements has been demonstrated in several species. This innervation plays a role in blood flow and possibly in auditory and vestibular processing (Densert & Flock, 1974; for guinea pigs see Hozawa & Takasak, 2009).

Sympathetic Distribution in Thoracic Region

See Fig. 15.4. Fusion of sympathetic trunk ganglia in the cranial thoracic and caudal cervical regions has resulted in formation of the **cervicothoracic** (*ganglion cervicothoracicum*) and **middle cervical ganglia** (*ganglion cervicale medium*). The cervicothoracic is the largest autonomic ganglion in the dog and is located on the lateral surface of the longus colli muscle at the level of the first intercostal space. It receives mixed rami from T1, T2, and T3 spinal nerves and sometimes from T4. Preganglionic axons ending in the cervicothoracic ganglion may originate as far caudally as the T5 spinal cord segment. Postganglionic axons in communicating rami connect to the C8 and C7 spinal nerves. Some of the rami attached to the cervicothoracic ganglion may be double. The ramus to C7 may be fused with the **vertebral nerve** (*n. vertebralis*), and both may be fused with a third nerve, the branch of the seventh cervical nerve to the longus colli muscle. For this reason the vertebral nerve may appear deceptively large. Actually, the vertebral nerve is comparatively small. Supposedly the nerve plexus that runs along the vertebral artery supplies postganglionic axons to spinal nerves cranial to C7 as far as C3. In some instances the vertebral nerve leaves the cervicothoracic ganglion as a separate entity (Fukuyama & Yabuki, 1958). The nerve enters the transverse foramen of the sixth cervical vertebra along with the vertebral artery and usually continues as a plexus along the artery.

Cranioventral to the cervicothoracic ganglion, the sympathetic trunk splits to pass around the subclavian artery as the ansa subclavia. One or both sides of this loop may be double. At the junction of the vagosympathetic trunk with the ansa subclavia medial to the subclavian artery lies the middle cervical ganglion of the sympathetic division (Fig. 15.4). It lies in the path of the sympathetic trunk and may be variably fused with the vagal trunk.

The ansa contains largely preganglionic sympathetic axons but also large- and medium-diameter visceral afferent axons. The sympathetic axons may synapse in the middle cervical ganglion or else proceed cranially as part of the cervical sympathetic trunk. Other preganglionic axons may leave with cervical cardiac nerves and synapse in small unnamed ganglia along their course. The ansa subclavia may contain scattered ganglion cells, or some may be grouped as a small ganglion. On the left side, nerve branches may join this ganglion to the subclavian artery. On the right these branches, if present, go to the base of the cranial vena cava and the right atrium.

Cardiac nerves are named by their origin. Cervical cardiac nerves arise from the middle cervical ganglia and the cervicothoracic ganglia or the adjacent nerves. The cervical cardiac nerves contain primarily postganglionic sympathetic axons, preganglionic parasympathetic axons, and GVA axons.

Sympathetic Distribution in the Abdominal Region

See Figs. 15.5 and 15.6. Branches of the thoracic and abdominal sympathetic trunk supply preganglionic axons to the abdominal and pelvic regions. In addition, these branches also carry a few postganglionic axons and a considerable number of visceral afferent axons. As is true of other areas of autonomic nerve distribution in the body, the specific nerve branching in this region may vary considerably from one animal to the next (Table 15.1).

The **major splanchnic nerve** (*n. splanchnicus major*) leaves the thoracic sympathetic trunk approximately at the level of the thirteenth thoracic ganglion. The nerve is larger in diameter than the continuation of the sympathetic trunk. Both pass dorsal to the lumbocostal arch to enter the abdominal cavity. Other branches designated as **minor splanchnic nerves** (*nn. splanchnicus minor*) may leave the sympathetic trunk just caudal to the major splanchnic nerve. The major splanchnic nerve supplies axons to the thoracic aorta and the adrenal gland. It terminates mainly as several branches to the celiacomesenteric plexus. The minor splanchnic nerves, if present, distribute to the same

TABLE 15.1 Autonomic Plexuses of the Abdominal Region

Plexus	Main Arterial Branches Continuing the Plexus	Grossly Dissectible Source (Need Not Imply Synapse)	Structures Supplied
Celiaco-mesenteric	Celiac and cranial mesenteric	Dorsal vagus, thoracic splanchnic nerves	See structures supplied by branches of celiac and cranial mesenteric arteries
Hepatic	Right gastric Proper Hepatic Gastroduodenal (also direct branches to pancreas, common bile duct, and pyloric region of stomach)	Right celiac ganglion, dorsal vagus	Pancreas Duodenum Stomach Cystic duct Gallbladder Liver Bile duct
Splenic	Left gastroepiploic Continuation of splenic artery to spleen and pancreas	Left celiac ganglion	Spleen, pancreas, greater curvature of stomach
Left gastric		Celiac ganglia Dorsal vagus	Lesser curvature, cardiac and fundic regions of stomach
Phrenico-abdominal	Phrenic (may arise directly from aorta) Branches to adrenal gland and abdominal wall	Celiac ganglion Adrenal ganglia	Diaphragm, part of abdominal wall Adrenal gland
Adrenal (paired)		Celiac ganglion Thoracic splanchnic nerve Adrenal ganglia Splanchnic ganglia	Adrenal gland
Renal (paired)	Phrenicoabdominal artery may arise from renal	Splanchnic ganglia Aorticorenal ganglia Renal ganglia	Kidney
Cranial mesenteric	Common colic Caudal pancreaticoduodenal Intestinal	Cranial mesenteric ganglion Celiac ganglia Dorsal vagus Lumbar splanchnic nerves	Large intestine Small intestine Cecum
Aortic (intermesenteric)		Cranial mesenteric ganglion, lumbar splanchnic nerves	Caudal mesenteric ganglion Pelvic plexus
Testicular		Aortic plexus Gonadal ganglion (not constant) Lumbar splanchnic nerves	Testis Epididymis
Utero-ovarian	Cranial uterine Ovarian	Same as previous	Ovary Uterine tube Uterus
Caudal mesenteric	Left colic Cranial rectal	Lumbar splanchnic nerves (caudal group) Aortic plexus	Hypogastric nerves (paired) Distal colon (left) Rectum Pelvic plexus

general area. Branches may sometimes be found joining the major splanchnic nerve to the first lumbar splanchnic nerve.

Immediately after the major splanchnic nerve branches off, the lumbar sympathetic trunk is small, but becomes larger as it proceeds caudally. Ganglia may be present for each of the seven lumbar segments, or variable fusion of adjacent ganglia may occur. Preganglionic contributions to the lumbar sympathetic trunk usually do not occur caudal to the L4 or L5 contributions.

Lumbar splanchnic nerves (*nn. splanchnici lumbales*) may arise from each of the lumbar sympathetic segmental levels, those from the first five being most constant. They are named according to the level from which they arise. Most originate as grossly dissectible single branches, but some may be double, and anastomotic branches may join adjacent nerves. Origin may be from a lumbar ganglion or from interganglionic segments of the sympathetic trunk. As noted earlier, the first lumbar splanchnic nerve may have connections with the major splanchnic nerve. In general, the first four lumbar splanchnic nerves distribute to one or more of the following: aorticorenal, cranial mesenteric, and gonadal ganglia; intermesenteric, renal, and gonadal plexuses. Axons arising from the aorticorenal ganglion provide adrenergic terminals found on the glomerular afferent and efferent arterioles and close to the macula densa cells of the kidney. These nerves also supply the vasa recta and adjacent cortical veins (Dolezel et al., 1976). Adrenergic axons innervating the loops of Henle in the dog kidney have been described (Ohgushi et al., 1969). It should be remembered that veins in general are well innervated and play an active role in circulatory regulation. The fifth through seventh lumbar splanchnic nerves go to the caudal mesenteric ganglion. Branches also go to the caudal vena cava and iliac arteries. Correspondingly named plexuses of variable complexity are found along the arteries of the abdominal region. Those at the root of the celiac and cranial mesenteric arteries form a dense mat or sheath called the *celiacomesenteric plexus*. This is continuous with the plexuses that are distributed with the branches of these two arteries. Interwoven in the celiacomesenteric plexus are the paired **celiac** (*ganglia celiaca*) and unpaired **cranial mesenteric ganglia** (*ganglion mesentericum craniale*).

Small sympathetic ganglia each containing approximately 25 to 100 neurons have been demonstrated along the course of the larger arteries of the abdominal cavity. Because these lie distal to the large ganglia such as celiac and cranial mesenteric, it follows that the nerve plexuses along the arteries can be expected to contain some sympathetic preganglionic axons in addition to the preponderance of sympathetic postganglionic axons. These plexuses also include parasympathetic preganglionic and visceral afferent fibers.

The cellular makeup of the adrenal medulla and the chemical mediators involved indicate that this portion of the adrenal glands is much like a sympathetic ganglion. The medulla is richly innervated by preganglionic axons that originate from T4 or T5 through L1 or L2 spinal cord segments in the dog (Cummings, 1969). This is in contrast to the sparsely innervated adrenal cortex (Arikhbayev, 1957; Teitlebaum, 1942; Wilkinson, 1961).

Branches that follow the external and internal iliac arteries apparently may arise from the more caudally located lumbar splanchnic nerves, the hypogastric nerves, and as continuations of the aortic plexus.

The right and left **hypogastric nerves** (*n. hypogastricus*) represent largely postganglionic connections between the caudal mesenteric ganglion and the pelvic plexuses. They are usually grossly dissectible nerves. The caudal part of the ureter is innervated by hypogastric and pelvic nerves, whereas the cranial part is innervated by the vagus nerve and sympathetic axons under the control of cells in spinal cord segments T10 to T12.

Sympathetic Distribution in the Pelvic Region

See Figs. 15.5 and 15.7. Both sympathetic trunks lie in close apposition in the sacral region. Variable fusion between corresponding ganglia of the two sides usually occurs. Disagreement exists as to whether or not a **ganglion impar** is present in the dog. Fusion of right and left L7 or S1 or both sympathetic ganglia results in a structure that has been interpreted as an impar ganglion, but both sympathetic trunks continue caudal to this level and may contain one or more additional pairs of sacral ganglia (Mizeres, 1955a; Wozniak, 1966). Rami communicans containing postganglionic axons join the sympathetic trunk to each of the sacral spinal nerves.

The hypogastric nerves carry sympathetic postganglionic axons to the pelvic viscera via the pelvic plexus (Purinton & Oliver, 1979). The preganglionic axons that terminate in the caudal mesenteric ganglia have their origin in L1 to L4 segments of the spinal cord. Sympathetic inhibition of parasympathetic activity may occur at the level of the pelvic ganglia.

The pelvic plexus is located on the lateral surface of the rectum associated with the vaginal or prostatic artery and receives a large contribution of parasympathetic preganglionic axons via the pelvic nerve.

An intact parasympathetic and sympathetic nerve supply is essential to normal regulation of physiologic activities such as urination, defecation, erection, and ejaculation. It must be remembered that afferent pathways must also be intact for normal control of these functions. The spinal nuclei for control of erection are located in the lateral horn of spinal cord segments T12 to L3 and S1 to S3 (Lue et al., 1984).

There is a vascular, interstitial, and peritubular innervation of the epididymis. This consists of both adrenergic and cholinergic fibers, with the former being dominant (El-Badawi & Schenk, 1967). The distal third of the tail of the epididymis is especially richly innervated with intricate interstitial and peritubular plexuses.

Sympathetic Distribution to Somatic Vasculature

Vasomotor fibers present in the lumbar sympathetic trunk reach the vessels of the distal pelvic limb muscles via the sciatic and femoral nerves and also along the femoral artery (Cloninger & Green, 1955). As might be expected when considering the corresponding field of somatic innervation, the sciatic nerve is the main route for these axons.

The perivascular nerve plexuses of an intramuscular artery consist of a plexus of axons in the adventitia and perivascular connective tissue. Here are located terminations of sensory fibers that are distributed with the segmental somatic innervation to the muscle. A deep plexus of small-diameter axons is located in the outer media and inner adventitia. These are postganglionic sympathetic axons that end as small nets and varicosities among and on the smooth muscle cells. (Borodulia & Plechkowa, 1977; Derom, 1945; Hassin, 1929; Polley, 1955; Shepherd & Vanhoutte, 1975; White, 1963).

Enteric Nervous System

The majority of parasympathetic innervation in the body is reflexly controlled without activation of a pathway for conscious perception. This is especially true for the autonomic innervation of the viscera of the thoracic, abdominal and pelvic cavities. During development, the neural crest populated the enteric viscera with a plethora of neurons, many of which reflexly function independent of sympathetic and parasympathetic neurons. This enteric nervous system consists of ganglionated plexuses located in the wall of the gastrointestinal tract that are responsible for contraction of the muscular tunic, glandular secretion, intestinal transport, and mucosal blood flow. Although these enteric neurons have complex interactions with the sympathetic and parasympathetic innervation and are a source of GVA stimuli, this enteric nervous system can sustain local reflex activity independent of the CNS. Complete sectioning of the extrinsic innervation of all or part of a body organ does not result in a loss of function of that portion of an organ. Thus transplanted organs are not functionally denervated (Schofield, 1961, 1962). An intramural plexus with associated ganglia has also been demonstrated in the bladder wall of several species (Drake, 2007).

Bibliography

Amenta, F., Sancesario, G., & Ferrante, F. (1980). Cholinergic nerves in dog cerebral vessels. *Neurosci Lett, 16*, 171–174.

Arikhbayev, K. P. (1957). On the problem of innervation of the adrenal glands. *Tr Stalingrad Med Inst, 25*, 55–64.

Azuma, E., Asakura, K., & Kataura, A. (1983). Central origin of canine vidian nerve studied by the HRP method. *Acta Otolaryngol, 96*, 131–137.

Baumann, J. A., & Gajisin, S. (1975). Multiplicity and dispersion of the parasympathetic ganglia of the head. *Bull Assoc Anat (Nancy), 59*, 329–332.

Billingsley, P. R., & Ranson, S. W. (1918a). On the number of nerve cells in the ganglion cervicale superius and of nerve fibers in the cephalic end of the truncus sympathicus in the cat and on the numerical relations of preganglionic and postganglionic neurones. *J Comp Neurol, 29*, 359–366.

Billingsley, P. R., & Ranson, S. W. (1918b). Branches of the ganglion cervicale superius. *J Comp Neurol, 29*, 367–384.

Borodulia, A. V., & Plechkowa, E. K. (1977). [Adrenergic–sympathetic nervous apparatus of the cerebral arteries and its role in regulating cerebral circulation]. *Zh Nevropatol Psikhiatr Im S S Korsakova, 77*, 975–980.

Chiu, S. L. (1943). The superficial hepatic branches of the vagi and their distribution to the extrahepatic biliary tract in certain mammals. *Anat Rec, 86*, 149–155.

Cloninger, G. L., & Green, H. D. (1955). Pathways taken by the sympathetic vasomotor nerves from the sympathetic chain to the vasculature of the hind leg muscles of the dog. *Am J Physiol, 181*, 258–262.

Coleridge, H. M., Coleridge, J. C. G., Dangel, A., et al. (1973). Impulses in slowly conducting vagal fibers from afferent endings in the veins, atria and arteries of dogs and cats. *Circ Res, 33*, 87–97.

Cummings, J. F. (1969). Thoracolumbar preganglionic neurons and adrenal innervation in the dog. *Acta Anat (Basel), 73*, 27–37.

Dahlström, A., Mya-Tu, M., & Fuxe, K. (1965). Observations on adrenergic innervation of dog heart. *Am J Physiol, 209*, 689–692.

Denn, M. J., & Stone, H. L. (1976). Autonomic innervation of dog coronary arteries. *J Appl Physiol, 41*, 30–35.

Densert, O., & Flock, A. (1974). An electron microscopic study of adrenergic innervation in the cochlea. *Acta Otolaryngol, 77*, 185–197.

Derom, E. (1945). Experimental researches on the vasomotor innervation of the dog's front paw. *Bull Acad R Med Belg, 10*, 427–459.

Diamare, V., & de Mennato, M. (1930). Contributo all' anatomia ed allo sviluppo del sistema nervoso simpatico. *Atti R Accad Sci Fis e Mat (Naples), 18*, 1–115.

Dolezel, S., Edvinsson, L., Owman, C., et al. (1976). Fluorescence histochemistry and autoradiography of adrenergic nerves in the renal juxtaglomerular complex of mammals and man with special regard to the efferent arteriole. *Cell Tissue Res, 169*, 211–220.

Donald, D. E., & Ferguson, D. A. (1970). Study of the sympathetic vasoconstrictor nerves to the vessels of the dog hind limb. *Circ Res, 26*, 171–184.

Drake, M. J. (2007). The integrative physiology of the bladder. *Ann R Coll Surg Engl, 89*, 580–585. doi:10.1308/003588407X205585.

Ehinger, B. (1966). Distribution of adrenergic nerves in the eye and some related structures in the cat. *Acta Physiol Scand, 66*, 123–128.

Ehinger, B. (1967). Double innervation of the feline iris dilator. *Arch Ophthalmol, 77*, 541–545.

El-Badawi, A., & Schenk, E. A. (1967). The distribution of cholinergic and adrenergic nerves in the mammalian epididymis: a comparative histochemical study. *Am J Anat, 121*, 1–14.

El'bert, M. E. (1956). On the problem of the cytoarchitecture of Auerbach's plexus of the small intestines in the cat and dog. *Tr Mosk Vet Akad, 18*, 35–38.

Elftman, A. G. (1943). The afferent and parasympathetic innervation of the lungs and trachea of the dog. *Am J Anat, 72*, 1–23.

Espinosa-Medina, I., Saha, O., Boismoreau, F., et al. (2016). The sacral autonomic outflow is sympathetic. *Science, 354*, 893–897. doi:10.1126/science.aah5454.

Esterhuizen, A. C., Graham, J. D., & Lever, J. D. (1967). The innervation of the smooth muscle of the nictitating membrane of the cat. *J Physiol (Lond), 192*, 41P–42P.

Faden, A. I., & Petras, J. M. (1978). An intraspinal sympathetic preganglionic pathway: anatomic evidence in the dog. *Brain Res, 144*, 358–362.

Filogamo, G. (1950). Ricerche sul plesso mienterico. *Arch Ital Anat Embriol, 54*, 401–412.

Foley, J. O. (1945). The sensory and motor axons of the chorda tympani. *Proc Soc Exp Biol Med, 60*, 262–267.

Foley, J. O., & Du Bois, F. S. (1940). A quantitative and experimental study of the cervical sympathetic trunk. *J Comp Neurol, 72*, 587–601.

Franke, F. E., & Bramante, P. O. (1964). Spinal origin of nasal vasoconstrictor innervation in the dog. *Proc Soc Exp Biol Med, 117*, 769–771.

Fritzsch, B., Elliot, K. L., & Glover, J. C. (2017). Gaskell revisited: new insights into spinal autonomics necessitate a revised motor neuron nomenclature. *Cell Tissue Res, 370*, 195–209. doi:10.1007/s004441-017-2676-y.

Fukuyama, U., & Yabuki, M. (1958). On the vertebral nerve and the communicating rami connecting with the inferior cervical ganglion in the dog. *Fukushima J Med Sci, 5*, 63–88.

Fussey, I. F., Kidd, C., & Whitwam, J. G. (1973). Activity evoked in the brainstem by stimulation of C fibers in the cervical vagus nerve of the dog. *Brain Res, 49*, 436–440.

Gaskell, W. H. (1886). On the distribution and function of the nerves which innervate the visceral and vascular systems. *J Physiol, 7,* 1–80.

Geis, W. P., Kaye, M. P., & Randall, W. C. (1973). Major autonomic pathways to the atria and s-A and A-v nodes of the canine heart. *Am J Physiol, 224,* 202–208.

Gienc, J., & Kuder, T. (1983). Otic ganglion in dog: topography and macroscopic structure. *Folia Morphol (Warsz), 42,* 31–40.

Gwin, R. M., Gelatt, K. N., & Chiou, C. V. (1979). Adrenergic and cholinergic innervation of the anterior segment of the normal and glaucomatous dog. *Invest Ophthalmol Vis Sci, 18,* 674–682.

Hassin, G. B. (1929). The nerve supply of the cerebral blood vessels: a histologic study. *Arch Neurol Psychiatry, 22,* 375–391.

Hirsch, E. F. G., Kaiser, C., & Cooper, T. (1964). Experimental heart block in the dog. I. The distribution of nerves, their ganglia, and terminals of septal myocardium of the dog and human heart. *Arch Pathol, 75,* 523–532.

Hirsch, E. F. G., Kaiser, C., & Cooper, T. (1965). Experimental heart block in the dog. III distribution of the vagus and sympathetic nerves in the septum. *Arch Pathol, 79,* 441–451.

Hirsch, E. F. C., Nigh, A., Kaye, M. P., et al. (1964). II studies of the perimysial innervation apparatus and of sensory receptors in the rabbit and in the dog with the techniques of total extrinsic denervation, bilateral cervical vagotomy and bilateral thoracic sympathectomy. *Arch Pathol, 77,* 172–187.

Holmberg, J. (1971). The secretory nerves of the parotid gland of the dog. *J Physiol (Lond), 219,* 463–476.

Holmes, R. L. (1956). Further observations on the nerve endings in the adult dog heart. *J Anat (London), 90,* 600.

Holmes, R. L. (1957). Structures in the atrial endocardium of the dog which stain with methylene blue, and the effects of unilateral vagotomy. *J Anat (London), 91,* 259–266.

Hopkins, D. A., & Armour, J. A. (1984). Localization of sympathetic postganglionic and parasympathetic preganglionic neurons which innervate different regions of the dog heart. *J Comp Neurol, 229,* 186–198.

Horn, J. P. (2018). The sacral autonomic outflow is parasympathetic: Langley got it right. *Clin Auton Res*, epub. doi:10.1007/s10286-018-0510-6.

Hozawa, K., & Takasak, T. (2009). Catecholaminergic innervation in the vestibular labyrinth and vestibular nucleus of Guinea pigs. *Acta Otolaryngol Case Rep, 113,* sup503, 111–113. doi:10.3109/00016489309128089.

Hwang, K., Grossman, M. I., & Joy, A. C. (1948). Nervous control of the cervical portion of the esophagus. *Am J Physiol, 154,* 343–357.

Iljina, W. J., & Lawrentjew, B. J. (1932a). Zur lehre von der cytoarchitektonik des peripherischen autonomen nervensystems; Ganglien des rektums und ihre beziehungen zu dem sakralen parasympathikus. *Z Mikrosk Anat Forsch, 30,* 530–542.

Iljina, W. J., & Lawrentjew, B. J. (1932b). Experimentell-morphologische studien über den feineren bau des autonomen nervensystems; über die innervation der harnblase. *Z Mikrosk Anat Forsch, 30,* 543–550.

Jayle, G. E. (1935). Le centre hypogastrique du chien. *Arch Anat (Strasbourg), 19,* 357–367.

Jung, L., Tagand, R., & Chavanne, F. (1926). Sur l'innervation excito-sécrétoire de la muqueuse nasale. *C R Soc Biol (Paris), 95,* 835–837.

Kapellar, K. (1965). The origin and the course of nerves leading to the liver of the dog. *Folia Morphol (Praha), 13,* 12–14.

Kemp, D. R. (1973). A histological and functional study of the gastric mucosal innervation in the dog. Part I: the quantification of the fibre content of the normal supradiaphragmatic vagal trunks and their abdominal branches. *Aust N Z J Surg, 43,* 288–294.

Kent, K. M., Epstein, S. E., Cooper, T., et al. (1974). Cholinergic innervation of the canine and human ventricular conducting system: anatomic and electrophysiologic correlations. *Circulation, 50,* 948–955.

Kuchiiwa, S., Kuchiiwa, T., & Suzuki, T. (1989). Comparative anatomy of the accessory ciliary ganglion in mammals. *Anat Embryol, 180,* 199–205.

Kyösola, K., Partanen, S., Korkala, O., et al. (1976). Fluorescence histochemical and electron-microscopical observations on the innervation of the atrial myocardium of the adult human heart. *Virchows Arch A Pathol Anat Histol, 371,* 101–119.

Lawrentjew, B. J. (1931). Zur lehre von der cytoarchitektonik des peripherischen autonomen nervensystems: die cytoarchitektonik der ganglien des verdauungskanals beitn hunde. *Z Mikrosk Anat Forsch, 23,* 527–551.

Leaming, D. B., & Cauna, N. (1961). A qualitative and quantitative study of the myenteric plexus of the small intestine of the cat. *J Anat (London), 95,* 160–169.

Lue, T. F., Zeineh, S., Schmidt, R. A., et al. (1984). Neuroanatomy of penile erection: its relevance to iatrogenic impotence. *J Urol, 131,* 273–280.

Malmfors, T. (1968). Histochemical studies on the adrenergic innervation of the nictitating membrane of the cat. *Histochemie, 13,* 203–206.

Martin, P. (1977). The influence of the parasympathetic nervous system on atrioventricular conduction. *Circ Res, 41,* 593–599.

Mizeres, N. J. (1955a). The anatomy of the autonomic nervous system in the dog. *Am J Anat, 96,* 285–318.

Mizeres, N. J. (1955b). Isolation of the cardioinhibitory branches of the right vagus nerve in the dog. *Anat Rec, 123,* 437–446.

Napolitano, L. M., Willman, V. L., Hanlon, C. R., et al. (1965). Intrinsic innervation of the heart. *Am J Physiol, 208,* 455–458.

Neuhuber, W., McLachlan, E., & Janig, W. (2017). The sacral autonomic outflow is spinal, but not "sympathetic." *Anat Rec, 300,* 1369–1370. doi:10.1002/ar.23600.

Nitschke, T. (1976). Die rami orbitales des ganglion pterygopalatinum des hundes: zugleich ein beitrag über die innervation der tränendrüse. *Anat Anz, 139,* 58–70.

Nonidez, J. F. (1939). Studies on the innervation of the heart: distribution of the cardiac nerves with special reference to the identification of the sympathetic and parasympathetic postganglionics. *Am J Anat, 65,* 361–407.

Obrebowski, A. (1965). Subdiaphragmatic segments of the vagus nerve in dogs. *Folia Morphol (Warsz), 24,* 295–301 (trans).

Ohgushi, N., Mohri, K., Sato, M., et al. (1969). Histochemical demonstration of adrenergic fibers in the renal tubules in dog. *Experientia, 26,* 401.

Petras, J. M., & Cummings, J. F. (1978). Sympathetic and parasympathetic innervation of the urinary bladder and urethra. *Brain Res, 153,* 363–369.

Petras, J. M., & Faden, A. I. (1978). The origin of sympathetic preganglionic neurons in the dog. *Brain Res, 144,* 353–357.

Polley, E. H. (1955). The innervation of blood vessels in striated muscle and skin. *J Comp Neurol, 103,* 253–268.

Purinton, P. T., & Oliver, J. E., Jr. (1979). Spinal cord origin of innervation to the bladder and urethra of the dog. *Exp Neurol, 65,* 422–434.

Purinton, P. T., Oliver, J. E., Jr., & Bradley, W. E. (1981). Differences in routing of pelvic visceral afferent fibers in the dog and cat. *Exp Neurol, 73*, 725–731.

Richardson, K. C. (1960). Studies on the structure of autonomic nerves in the small intestine, correlating the silver impregnated image in light microscopy with the permanganate fixed ultrastructure in electron microscopy. *J Anat (London), 94*, 457–472.

Samson, M. D., & Reddy, K. (1982). Localization of the sacral parasympathetic nucleus in the dog. *Am J Vet Res, 43*, 1833–1836.

Schmidt, C. A. (1933). Distribution of vagus and sacral nerves to the large intestine. *Proc Soc Exp Biol Med, 30*, 739–740.

Schnitzlein, H. N., Hoffman, H. H., Hamlett, D. M., et al. (1963). A study of the sacral parasympathetic nucleus. *J Comp Neurol, 120*, 477–493.

Schofield, G. C. (1961). Experimental studies on the innervation of the mucous membrane of the gut. *Brain, 83*, 490–514.

Schofield, G. C. (1962). Experimental studies on the myenteric plexus in mammals. *J Comp Neurol, 119*, 159–185.

Shepherd, J. T., & Vanhoutte, P. M. (1975). *Veins and their control.* Philadelphia: Saunders.

Tcheng, K. T. (1950). Étude histologique de l'innervation cardiaque chez le chien. *C R Soc Biol (Paris), 144*, 882–883.

Tcheng, K. T. (1951). Innervation of the dog's heart. *Am Heart J, 41*, 512–524.

Teitlebaum, H. (1942). The innervation of the adrenal gland. *Q Rev Biol, 17*, 135.

Uchizono, K. (1964). Innervation of the blood capillary in the heart of dog and rabbit. *Jpn J Physiol, 14*, 587–598.

Van Buskirk, C. (1945). The seventh nerve complex. *J Comp Neurol, 82*, 303–330.

Wakata, S. (1975). Studies on the inflowing and outflowing myelinated nerve fibers of the pterygopalatine ganglion in the dog. *Chin Med J, 51*, 133–142.

Watson, A. G. (1974). *Some aspects of the vagal innervation of the canine esophagus, an anatomical study.* Masters Thesis, New Zealand: Massey University.

White, J. C. (1963). Nervous control of the cerebral vascular system. *Clin Neurosurg, 9*, 67–87.

Wilkinson, I. M. S. (1961). The intrinsic innervation of the suprarenal gland. *Acta Anat (Basel), 46*, 127–134.

Wozniak, W. (1966). Sacral segments of the sympathetic trunks in the dog, cat, and man. *Folia Morphol (Warsz), 25*, 407–414.

Wozniak, W., & Skowronska, U. (1967). Comparative anatomy of pelvic plexus in cat, dog, rabbit, macaque and man. *Anat Anz, 120*, 457–473.

Ziemianski, A., Orebowski, A., & Kampf, A. (1967). Participation of the vagus nerve in the innervation of the sites of division of the bronchi in the dog. *Folia Morphol (Warsz), 26*, 471–478.

16

The Spinal Cord and Meninges

The Spinal Cord

The spinal cord and the brain constitute the central nervous system. The spinal cord is enclosed within the vertebral canal, as are dorsal and ventral spinal roots that belong to the peripheral nervous system (Fig. 16.1). By means of spinal roots and spinal nerves, the spinal cord innervates the neck, trunk and tail, the limbs, and the caudal and dorsal surfaces of the head. Dorsal roots convey sensory (afferent) input to the spinal cord, whereas ventral roots carry motor (efferent) output from the spinal cord to muscles and glands.

The spinal cord performs three general functions:
1. Via spinal nerve connections, it processes afferent information from muscles, tendons, joints, ligaments, blood vessels, skin, and viscera, and it discharges efferent commands that control muscles and regulate glands.
2. The spinal cord is a reflex center, producing subconscious responses of muscles and glands to particular stimuli.
3. The spinal cord conducts information to and from the brain through a system of axonal tracts, by which the brain receives status information about the neck, trunk, and limbs while dispensing commands that control posture, movement, and the visceral aspects of behavior.

Morphologic Features of the Spinal Cord

Within the vertebral canal, the spinal cord and spinal roots are enveloped by three protective layers termed *meninges* (Fig. 16.2). The *dura mater*, the most superficial meningeal coat, is fibrous and thick. It forms a cylinder surrounding the spinal cord, and through lateral extensions it and the other meningeal layers ensheathe spinal roots. The thin *arachnoid membrane* lines the inner surface of the dura mater. A subarachnoid space containing cerebrospinal fluid is located deep to the arachnoid membrane. Arachnoid trabeculations traverse this space to attach to the pia mater.

The *pia mater*, the deepest, most vascular meninx, is bound to glial cells concentrated at the spinal cord surface (glial limiting membrane) (Uehara & Ueshima, 1988). The pia mater is thickened bilaterally along the lateral margin of the spinal cord, forming *denticulate ligaments*. Each denticulate ligament has periodic lateral extensions midway between adjacent spinal nerve roots, that attach to dura mater, thereby suspending the spinal cord such that it is surrounded by cerebrospinal fluid (Fig. 16.3). In many areas of the vertebral canal, there is a fibrous fascial connection between the ventral median surface of the spinal cord dura mater and the adjacent dorsal longitudinal ligament on the ventral surface of the vertebral canal. This may play a role in the pattern of disease processes seen in some veterinary patients that is easily recognized with magnetic resonance imaging. This tissue, a leptomeningeal ligament, must be cut to free the spinal cord for its removal during necropsy.

The center of the spinal cord features a **central canal** (*canalis centralis*) that is filled with cerebrospinal fluid and lined by ependymal cells. The canal is slightly enlarged at the caudal termination of the spinal cord, forming a **terminal ventricle** (*ventriculus terminalis*).

Immediately surrounding the central canal, gray matter forms the core of the spinal cord. **Gray matter** (*substantia grisea*) is composed of cell bodies and processes of neurons and glial cells. It has a relatively rich capillary supply but contains only sparse myelinated axons.

In transverse sections, gray matter appears butterfly-shaped, having bilateral wings connected across the midline by central intermediate substance (Fig. 16.3). The **central intermediate substance** (*substantia intermedia centralis*) surrounds the central canal and includes the *gray commissure* (*commissura grisea*), which traverses the midline dorsal and ventral to the central canal. The bilateral extension of intermediate substance into each gray matter "wing" is called **lateral intermediate substance** (*substantia intermedia lateralis*).

Lateral intermediate substance projects into surrounding white matter as a **lateral horn** (*cornu laterale*) in thoracic and cranial lumbar segments of the spinal cord. Gray matter extending dorsal to the lateral intermediate substance is designated **dorsal horn** (*cornu dorsale*), whereas that extending ventrally is termed **ventral horn** (*cornu ventrale*). The term *horn* refers to the two-dimensional profile that can be seen when the respective column of gray matter is transected.

The **white matter** (*substantia alba*) is positioned superficially in the spinal cord. It features packed myelinated axons. Concentrated myelin lipid is responsible for the pale appearance of unstained white matter. Nonmyelinated axons are also present in white matter, as are oligodendrocytes, astrocytes, and blood vessels (these vessels are less dense than those in gray matter). The white matter of each half of the spinal cord is divided into three funiculi (white matter bundles or columns).

The **dorsal funiculus** (*funiculus dorsalis*) includes all of the white matter located medial to the dorsolateral sulcus, where dorsal rootlets enter the spinal cord. The **ventral funiculus** (*funiculus ventralis*) is medial to where ventral rootlets exit from the spinal cord. The white matter located between dorsal and ventral root attachments is **lateral funiculus** (*funiculus lateralis*). Myelinated axons crossing from one-half of the spinal cord to the other constitute the **white commissure** (*commissura alba*). It is ventral to the gray commissure and connects right and left ventral funiculi.

The spinal cord features septae, sulci, and fissures, which are useful as landmarks (Fig. 16.3). A septum is a thin barrier formed principally by astrocytes in white matter. A sulcus is a shallow groove on the spinal cord surface. A fissure is a midline cleft typically lined by pia mater.

The spinal cord is divided into symmetric right and left halves by a **ventral median fissure** (*fissura mediana ventralis*), into which central blood vessels project, and a **dorsal median fissure**. In cervical and thoracic segments, the cleft of the dorsal median fissure is generally obliterated, resulting in a **dorsal median sulcus** (*sulcus medianus dorsalis*) at the surface and a **dorsal median septum** (*septum medianum dorsale*) that extends from the sulcus to the gray commissure.

A **dorsolateral sulcus** (*sulcus lateralis dorsalis*) is evident where dorsal roots enter the spinal cord. A corresponding ventrolateral sulcus (*sulcus lateralis ventralis*) where ventral

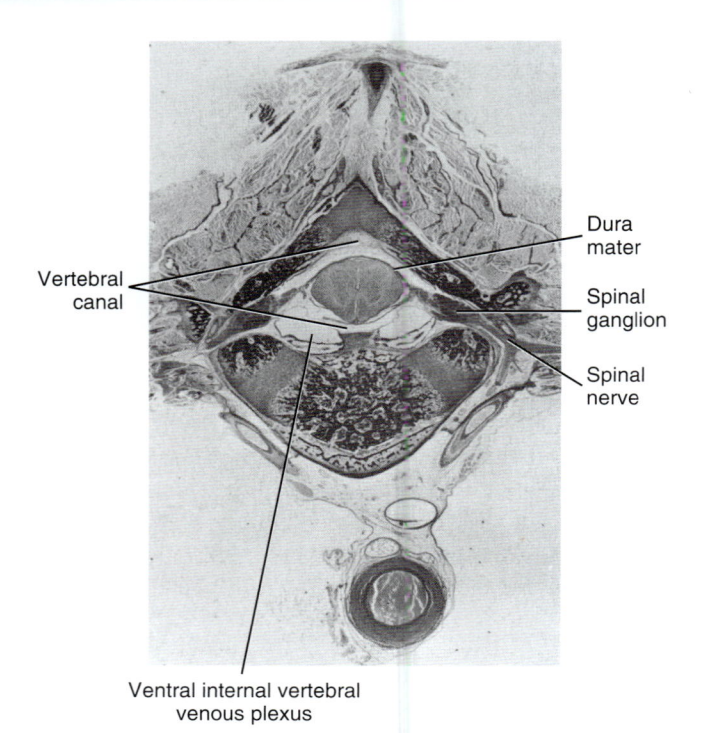

• **Fig. 16.1** Transverse section through the vertebral column of a canine fetus. The vertebral canal contains the spinal cord and dorsal and ventral spinal roots, which bilaterally join to form a spinal nerve at an intervertebral foramen. A spinal ganglion is present on each dorsal root, near the spinal nerve. The spinal cord and roots are enclosed by meninges. Internal ventral vertebral venous plexus is evident bilaterally at the floor of the vertebral canal.

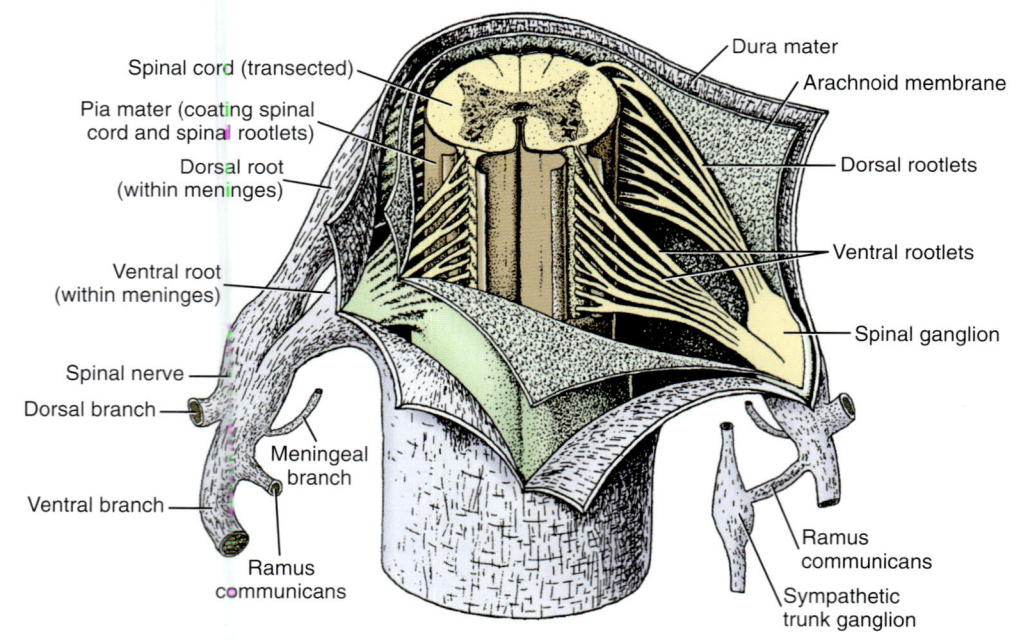

• **Fig. 16.2** Schematic illustration of a transected spinal cord with meninges incised to reveal a spinal cord segment and spinal roots (ventral view). Spinal cord roots attach to the spinal cord as a series of rootlets. Bilaterally, dorsal and ventral roots join to form a spinal nerve that immediately divides into four primary branches (dorsal, ventral, meningeal, and ramus communicans). A spinal ganglion is located on the dorsal root, and the ramus communicans joins a sympathetic trunk ganglion. The meninges (dura mater, arachnoid membrane, and pia mater) enclose the spinal cord and on the left separately ensheathe dorsal and ventral roots to the level of the spinal nerve, where meninges blend with connective tissue surrounding spinal nerves. On the right only the pia mater ensheathes the spinal roots. (Modified from Krstic RV: *General histology of the mammal*, Berlin, 1985, Springer-Verlag.)

CHAPTER 16 The Spinal Cord and Meninges **681**

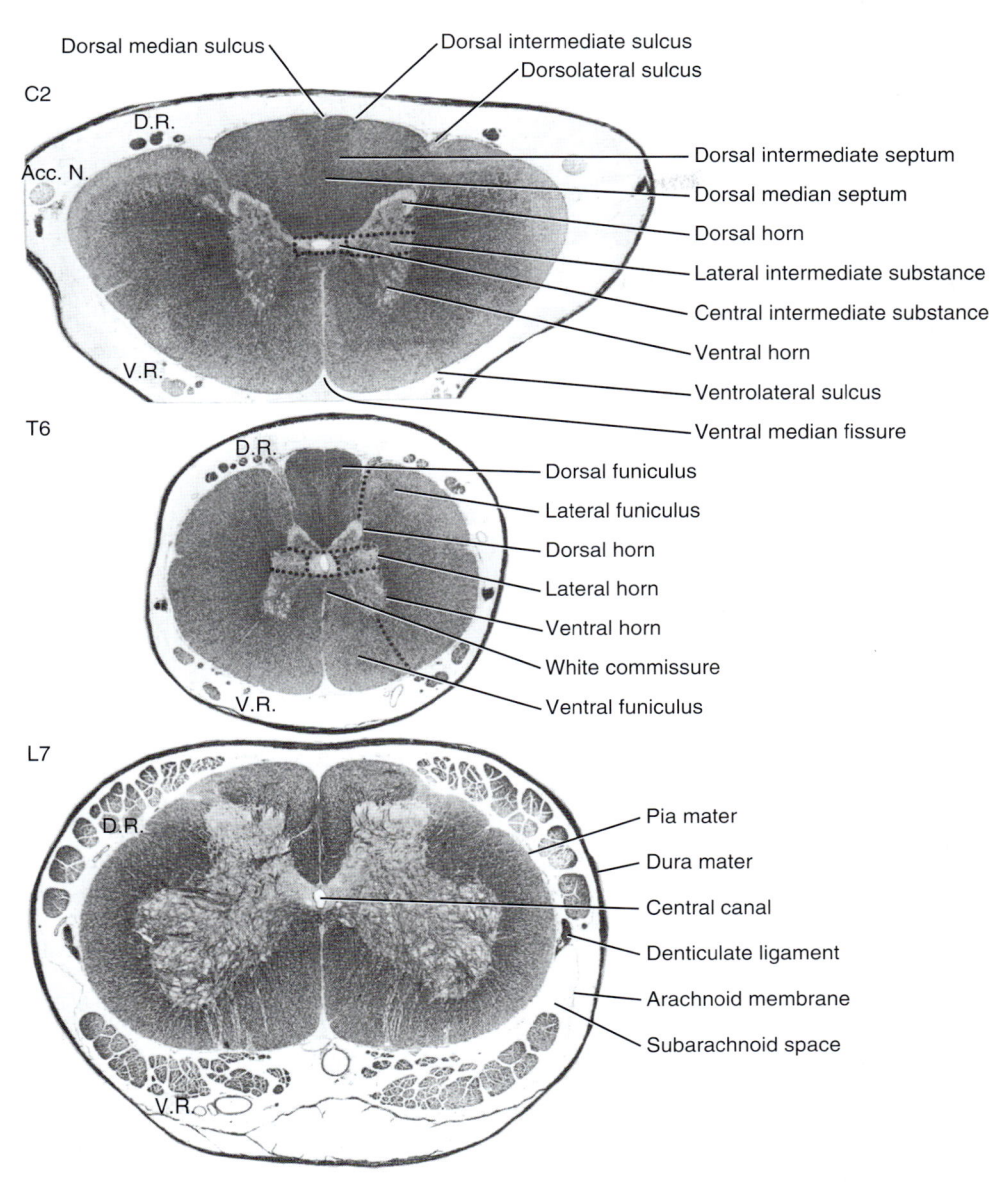

• **Fig. 16.3** Morphologic features of the spinal cord illustrated in transverse sections of second cervical, sixth thoracic, and seventh lumbar segments (Luxol fast blue and hematoxylin stain). Surface features and gray and white matter regions are labeled in C2 and T6 segments. Gray matter has a "butterfly" shape and is surrounded by darker-staining white matter. Meninges are labeled in the L7 segment. The ventral split in the dura mater is artifact. Escape of cerebrospinal fluid has allowed arachnoid membrane to separate from dura mater. A process of denticulate ligament can be seen extending from pia mater toward dura mater. *Acc. N.,* Spinal root of the accessory nerve; *DR,* dorsal rootlets; *VR,* ventral rootlets.

rootlets leave the spinal cord is typically imperceptible. A **dorsal intermediate sulcus** (*sulcus intermedius dorsalis*) and, extending from it, a **dorsal intermediate septum** (*septum intermedium*) can often be distinguished in cervical segments.

Spinal Cord Segments

The basis for dividing the spinal cord into segments is the attachments of dorsal (or ventral) roots. Each dorsal or ventral **spinal root** (*radix dorsalis*; *radix ventralis*) is composed of thousands of axons with varying amounts of Schwann cell myelin and enveloped by meninges. The axons of each root are bound together laterally where dorsal and ventral roots join to form the spinal nerve, but as roots approach the spinal cord, their axons regroup into separate bundles called **rootlets** (*fila radicularia*). The rootlets attach serially along the spinal cord (Fig. 16.4). Caudal, formerly *coccygeal,* roots may have only 1 or 2 rootlets, whereas segments innervating limbs may have 12 or more rootlets per dorsal or ventral root (Fletcher & Kitchell, 1966a).

In addition to dorsal and ventral roots, the first seven (sometimes eight) cervical segments have rootlets that emerge midlaterally from the spinal cord and join to form

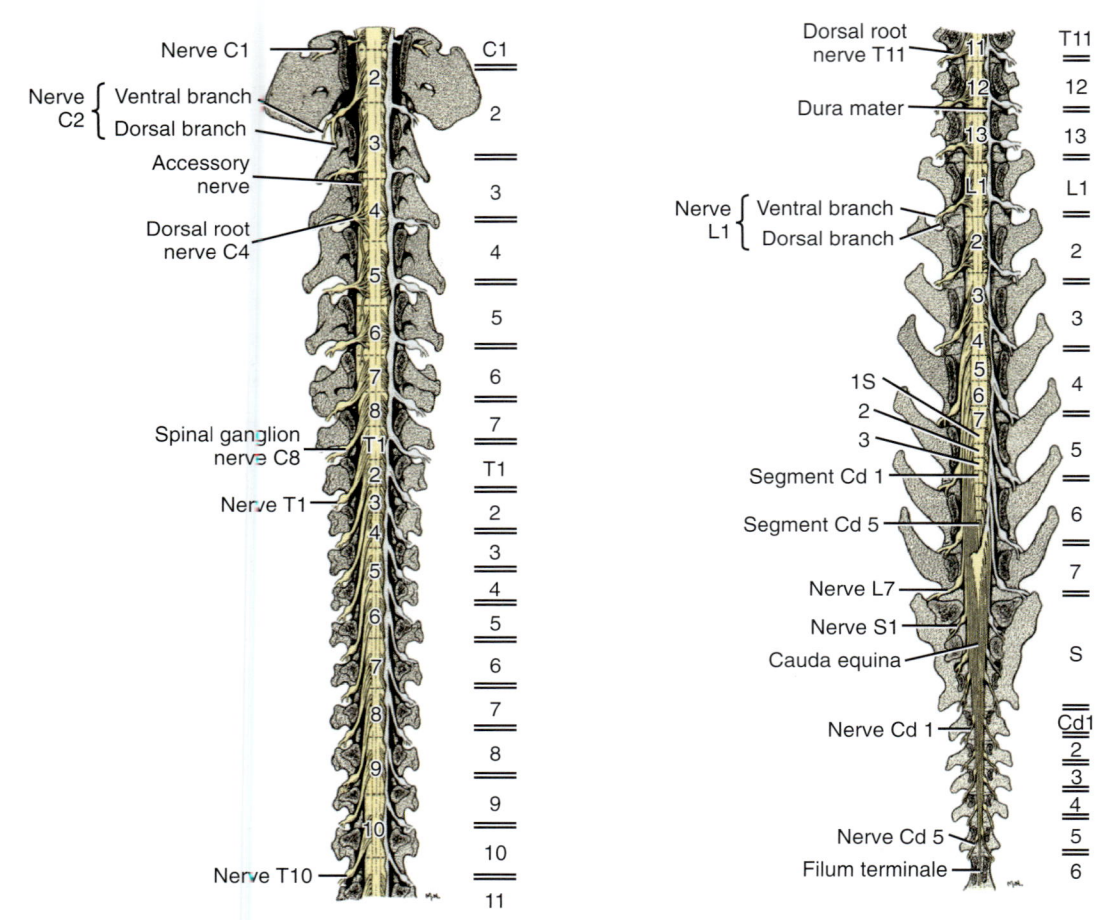

• **Fig. 16.4** Typical relationship between spinal cord segments and vertebrae for medium-sized and large dogs. A laminectomy and removal of dura mater except along the right side reveals root attachments in the cranial (*left*) and caudal (*right*) halves of the spinal cord. Boundaries between spinal cord segments are indicated by *dashed lines*; boundaries between vertebral bodies are shown to the right of the vertebral column. *Note:* accessory nerve = spinal root of accessory nerve. (With permission from Fletcher TF, Kitchell RL: Anatomical studies on the spinal cord segments of the dog, *Am J Vet Res* 27:1759–1767, 1966a.)

the **spinal root of the accessory nerve** (*radices spinales n. accessorius*), which runs cranially through the foramen magnum to join the cranial roots of the accessory cranial nerve that emerge from the medulla.

Boundaries between **spinal cord segments** are conventionally placed midway between attachments of, respectively, most caudal and most cranial rootlets of adjacent dorsal roots. Spinal cord segments, spinal roots, and spinal nerves are identified numerically according to region: cervical, 1 to 8; thoracic, 1 to 13; lumbar, 1 to 7; sacral, 1 to 3; and caudal, 1 to 5. Thus segments are named like vertebrae, except that there is an extra (eighth) cervical segment and only five caudal segments.

At the two locations, where nerves to the limbs arise, the relative diameter of the spinal cord is increased. The **cervical enlargement** (*intumescentia cervicalis*) gives rise to spinal nerves that form the brachial plexus that innervates the thoracic limb. The cervical enlargement involves part of segment C6, segments C7 and C8, and part of segment T1. The **lumbar (lumbosacral) enlargement** (*intumescentia lumbalis*), which innervates the pelvic cavity and pelvic limbs, involves part of segment L5, segments L6 and L7, and part of segment S1 (Fletcher & Kitchell, 1966a).

Caudal to the lumbar enlargement, the spinal cord tapers into an elongate cone, designated **conus medullaris**. This region consists of segments S2, 3, and Ca1 to Ca5. These segments appear successively smaller, and they are surrounded by caudally directed spinal roots (Fig. 16.5).

Approximately 1 cm caudal to the last segment (spinal cord termination), the spinal cord is reduced to a uniform strand of glial and ependymal cells called the **terminal filament** (*filum terminale*) encased in a layer of pia mater. A caudal extension of dura mater that envelops the filum terminale is called the **spinal dura mater filament** (*filum durae matris spinalis*). This filament extends caudally in the vertebral canal where it attaches to a sacral or caudal vertebra. A dura-arachnoid sac, enclosing subarachnoid space and cerebrospinal fluid in a lumbar cistern, extends approximately 2 cm caudal to the end of the spinal cord neural parenchyma. Caudal to this the dura mater constricts

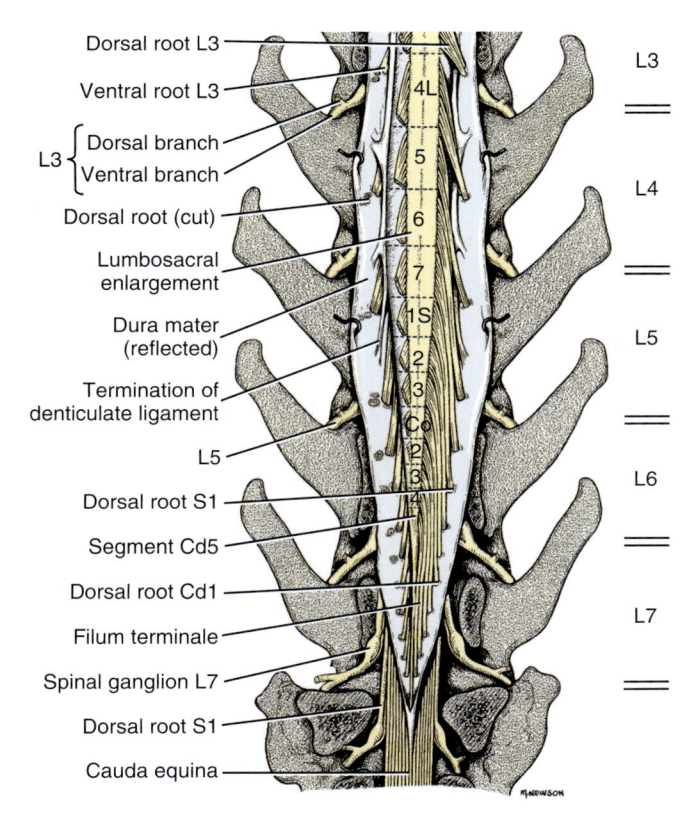

- **Fig. 16.5** Enlarged view of the terminal spinal cord, shown with dura mater reflected. Dorsal roots are partially removed on the left side to show ventral roots and the denticulate ligament, which terminates in a process that attaches to dura mater between the entrances of L5 and L6 roots into dural sheaths. (With permission from Fletcher TF, Kitchell RL: Anatomical studies on the spinal cord segments of the dog, *Am J Vet Res* 27:1759–1767, 1966a.)

Spinal cord segments alternately lengthen, shorten, lengthen, and shorten again along the extent of the spinal cord (Fig. 16.4). The longest spinal cord segment is C3; caudal to it, segment length declines, reaching a minimum at the level of segment T2. Caudal to this, thoracic segments lengthen, particularly by increased distance between adjacent roots. Segments of the thoracolumbar junction are relatively long. Caudal to these, segments become progressively shorter. Thus spinal cord segments display considerable differential growth relative to more subtle changes in vertebral length.

With respect to position within the vertebral column, four spinal cord regions can be distinguished (Fig. 16.4): (1) an initial cervical region, where at least the first cervical segment lies within its corresponding vertebra; (2) a caudal cervical through cranial thoracic region, where segments are positioned cranial to their respective vertebrae; (3) a thoracolumbar junction, where segments again lie within their corresponding vertebrae; and (4) a caudal lumbar, sacral, caudal region, where segments lie progressively cranial to their respective vertebrae (Fletcher & Kitchell, 1966a).

Positions of spinal cord segments relative to vertebrae may vary by half a vertebral length cranial or caudal to the typical relationship for medium-sized and large dogs, depicted in Fig. 16.4. In these dogs, the conus medullaris ends approximately at the level of the L6 to L7 intervertebral disc. Small dogs (weighing less than 7 kg) have relatively longer spinal cords, particularly evident in the lumbosacral and caudal regions, where segments may be one vertebra caudal to the relationship illustrated in Fig. 16.5.

Because spinal roots always travel to intervertebral foramina formed by corresponding vertebrae, spinal root length reflects the location of a spinal cord segment relative to its numerically corresponding vertebra. Spinal roots are short in initial cervical and thoracolumbar junction regions where segments lie near to or their corresponding vertebrae. Roots are longer where segments are displaced cranial to corresponding vertebrae as a result of segment shortening and differential growth between the spinal cord segments and the vertebrae (Fig. 16.6).

The first spinal nerve exits the vertebral canal through a lateral vertebral foramen, located in the dorsal arch of the atlas. Spinal nerves C2 through C7 exit through intervertebral foramina formed by cranial margins of corresponding (C2 to C7) vertebrae. Because it lacks a corresponding vertebra, the C8 spinal nerve exits through the intervertebral foramen formed by the cranial margin of vertebra T1. The remaining spinal nerves, T1 to Ca5, exit through intervertebral foramina formed by caudal margins of their corresponding vertebrae (Fig. 16.4).

The relationship between the spinal cord dorsoventral diameter to the dorsoventral diameter of the vertebral canal is important in assessing lesions that have the potential of compressing the spinal cord. Based on measurements made on cervical myelograms, small breeds have a higher spinal cord-to-vertebral canal ratio than do large breeds (Fourie & Kirberger, 1999).

around the filum terminale. At the level of the filum terminale, leakage may occur between the central canal and the narrowed subarachnoid space (Marin-Garcia et al., 1995).

Within the vertebral canal, sacral and caudal spinal roots stream caudally, beyond the conus medullaris, to exit at their respective intervertebral foramina. Collectively, these roots are designated **cauda equina**. In the dog, most of the cauda equina lies caudal to the lumbar cistern; the roots are individually enveloped by meningeal sheaths (Fletcher & Kitchell, 1966a).

Segmental Relationships to Vertebrae

At birth, the canine spinal cord extends into the sacrum. Following postnatal development, the spinal cord terminates in the caudal lumbar region. Overall, the vertebral column outgrows the spinal cord in length; however, the degree of elongate growth of spinal cord segments is regionally variable (Fletcher & Kitchell, 1966a). As a result, the positional relationship between spinal cord segments and vertebrae is regionally variable. In certain experimental and clinical situations, it is necessary to locate spinal cord segments with respect to more readily identifiable vertebrae.

684 CHAPTER 16 Spinal Cord and Meninges

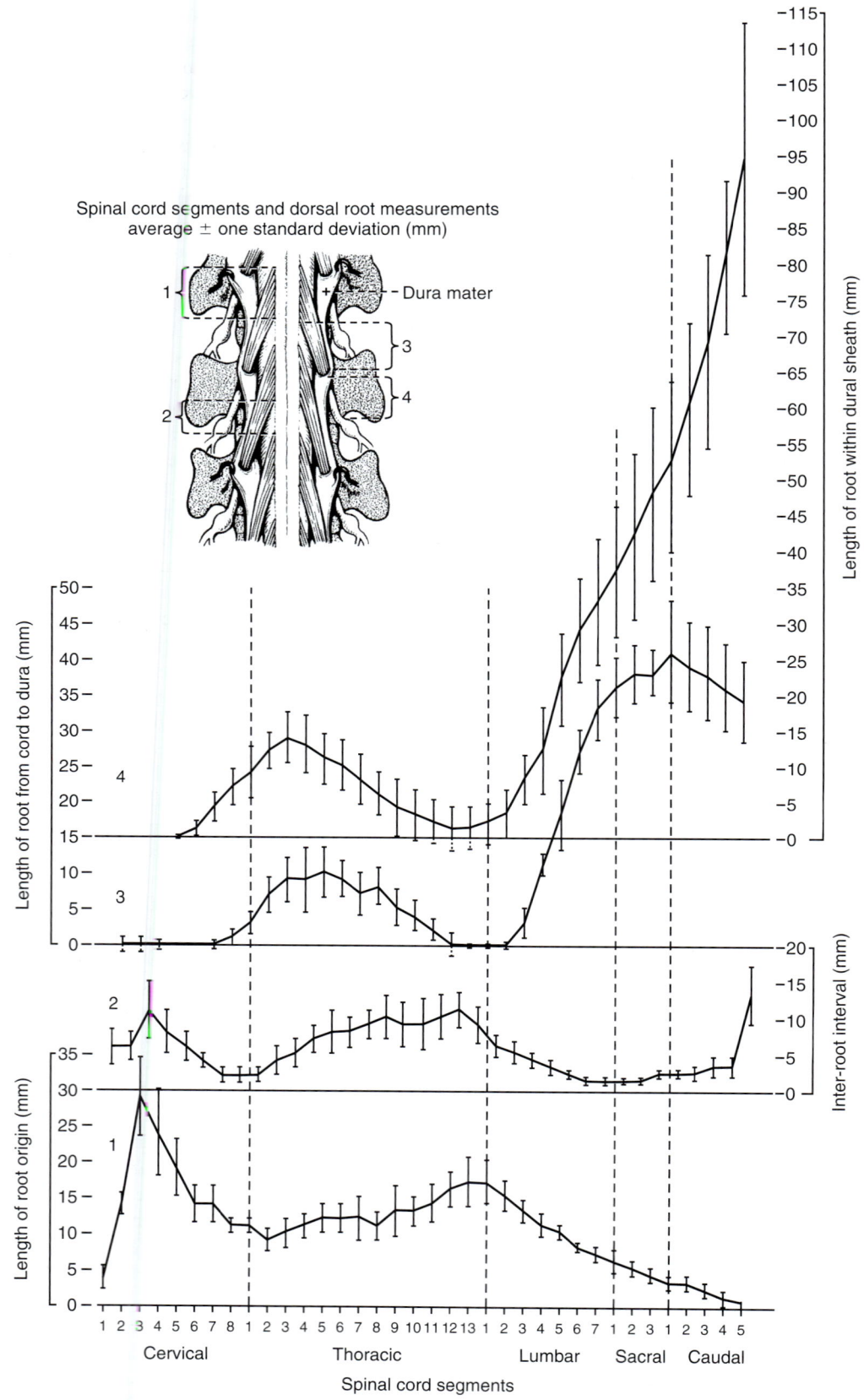

- **Fig. 16.6** Segment and root length along the spinal cord. Four measurements (*shown on the insert*) were made unilaterally in 20 dogs. Means for each measurement are graphed; vertical bars show one standard deviation above and one below each mean. Segment length is represented by length of root origin (*1*) and interroot interval (*2*). Root length is represented by craniocaudal length to the dural sheath (*3*) and length within a dural sheath (*4*). Segments lengthen, shorten, lengthen, and shorten again along the spinal cord. Root length increases following segment shortening and decreases when segments lengthen because short segments shift cranially in the vertebral column, whereas long segments shift caudally. (With permission from Fletcher TF, Kitchell RL: Anatomical studies on the spinal cord segments of the dog, *Am J Vet Res* 27:1759–1767, 1966a.)

Gray Matter of the Spinal Cord

Gray matter* consists of neurons, neuroglia (mainly astrocytes and oligodendrocytes), and a relatively rich blood supply. All of the neuronal cell bodies located in spinal cord gray matter are multipolar. Thus, each cell body gives rise to multiple dendrites and usually a single axon. The location of the cell body indicates the neuron's dendritic (receptive) zone, where other neurons synapse to influence excitability of the target neuron. Spinal cord neurons can be categorized as interneurons, projection neurons, or efferent neurons.

Spinal cord interneurons are interposed between a particular input and the resulting output from the spinal cord. In the process of "wiring" connections between input and output, interneurons establish elementary patterns of motor neuron output that can be used in such activities as spinal reflexes, locomotion, and other voluntary movement. Interneurons may be activated by synaptic input arriving from primary afferent neurons, from caudally projecting pathways (coming from the brain), from other interneurons, and from axonal branches of efferent neurons. Different reflexes and caudally projecting paths may share the same interneurons (Hongo et al., 1989).

Interneurons exhibit a variety of features. Some have short axons, others have long axons. Some remain ipsilateral, others cross to the contralateral side. Some are inhibitory, others excitatory. Some are spontaneously active, others are quiescent until they are synaptically activated. Some discharge in bursts, others discharge in a graded fashion proportional to factors such as synaptic input.

Spinal cord projection neurons send axons into white matter to form, generally, cranial projecting pathways to the brain. The projection neurons are activated by primary afferent neurons that become excited in response to stimulation of viscera, muscles, joints, or skin. Primary afferent neurons influence the excitability of projection neurons directly or through interneurons or other projection neurons (Willis, 1985, 1986; Yaksh, 1986). The excitability of spinal cord projection neurons is also modified, directly or through interneurons, by caudally projecting axons from brain projection neurons (Noble & Riddell, 1989).

Spinal cord projection neurons may be characterized by the nature of the peripheral stimulation that ultimately activates them. Some neurons respond specifically to noxious stimuli, or specifically to touch and pressure stimuli, or specifically to thermal stimuli. Neurons that respond to a specific stimulus function in modality identification and precise localization of the stimulus (Yaksh, 1986).

Many projection neurons respond nonspecifically to both mild mechanical stimulation and mechanical or thermal noxious stimulation (Willis, 1986). Nonspecific neurons have a wide dynamic range of responses and appear specialized to code the intensity of stimulation. These multireceptive neurons have relatively large receptive fields. Commonly, the nociceptive sensitivity and receptive field size of multireceptive neurons are subject to modification by caudally projecting tracts.

The majority of spinal cord projection neurons respond just to somatic stimulation (skin or muscles and joints), but others respond to both somatic and visceral stimulation (Cervero & Lumb, 1988).

Spinal cord efferent neurons send axons through ventral roots to innervate muscles and glands. They may be classified as somatic or autonomic (visceral). Cell bodies of preganglionic autonomic neurons are located in the lateral intermediate substance and lateral horn. Their axons synapse on cell bodies of postganglionic axons located in autonomic ganglia along nerves or in the wall of organs. Neurons in autonomic ganglia innervate cardiac or smooth muscle or glands.

Somatic efferent neurons innervate skeletal muscles. Cell bodies of the neurons are located in the ventral horn, grouped into motor nuclei. Somatic neurons that innervate typical muscle fibers responsible for producing muscle tension are referred to as **alpha motor neurons**. In a clinical context, these neurons are referred to as **lower motor neurons**—the motor neuron with an axon that leaves the central nervous system to innervate the target organ. Their destruction results in flaccid paralysis of the muscles innervated (Brooks, 1986).

The smallest somatic efferent neurons are designated fusimotor or **gamma motor neurons**. They innervate intrafusal muscle fibers located within muscle spindles. A few somatic efferent neurons, called **beta motor neurons**, innervate both intrafusal and extrafusal muscle fibers.

A motor neuron and all of the muscle fibers it innervates constitute a **motor unit**. All motor units of a particular skeletal muscle have their neuronal cell bodies grouped together, forming a motor neuron pool within a motor nucleus within the ventral horn. Motor units vary in their properties. Small motor units (relatively small alpha motor neurons innervating relatively few muscle fibers) are typically activated earliest during muscle contraction; they produce small degrees of tension and contract relatively slowly, and their muscle fibers are highly resistant to fatigue. At the other extreme, the largest motor units are recruited only during maximal muscle contraction; their muscle fibers contract rapidly and are easily fatigued (Binder & Mendell, 1990; Henneman et al., 1965).

In addition to the conventional organization of neuronal cell bodies in the core of the spinal cord, a very small population of neuronal cell bodies and their processes have been found in a subpial position primarily in the segments of the spinal cord enlargements. Here they predominate on the dorsolateral surface of the white matter where the processes form a subpial plexus (Fedorets, 2001).

---

*In sections of gray matter, white matter, and spinal reflexes, much of the information presented is based on experimental work involving cats because the dog is not used for current neuroscience research, and the cat seems to be an adequate neurologic model for the dog.

Gray Matter Organization

Spinal cord neurons having similar function tend to have their cell bodies grouped together, forming longitudinal columns of cells. Some neuronal cell columns extend the entire length of the spinal cord; others are restricted to certain segments. Columns of cell bodies are termed *nuclei* when they are viewed as clusters of cell bodies in transverse sections of the spinal cord.

Two schemes are currently used for categorizing spinal cord neurons into functionally significant groups (Fig. 16.7). One approach involves identification of cell columns (nuclei). This scheme works for some functionally specific nuclei; however, it omits many neurons that are morphologically dispersed.

The other approach involves dividing spinal cord gray matter into ten laminae (Rexed, 1952, 1954). The laminar classification scheme accounts for all spinal cord neurons;

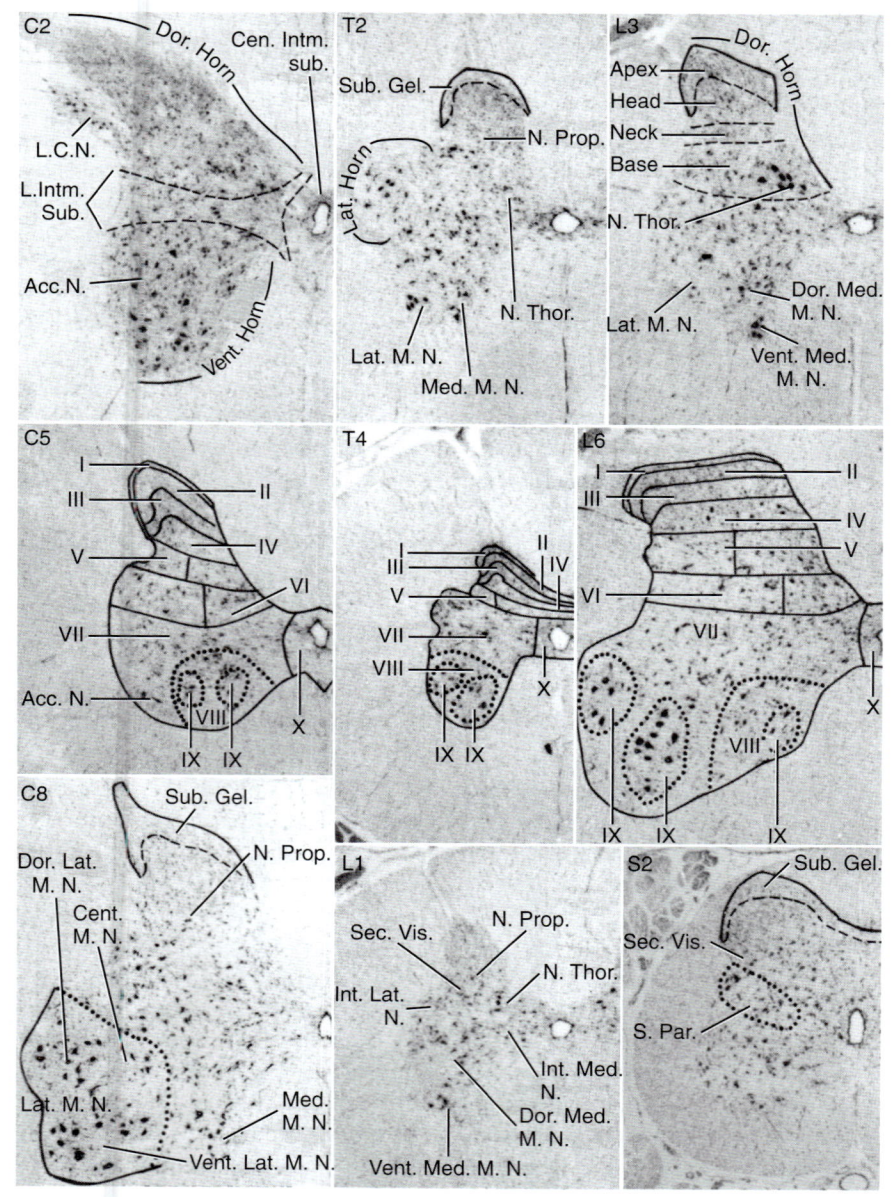

• **Fig. 16.7** Features of spinal cord gray matter. Photomicrographs of gray matter in transverse sections (Nissl stain, 12 μm thick) from various levels of the canine spinal cord are labeled to show regions, nuclei, and laminae. Spinal cord laminae are illustrated at the middle for a cervical, thoracic, and lumbar segment. (*Note:* It is customary to identify laminae by Roman numerals.) *Acc. N.*, Spinal nucleus of the accessory nerve; *Cen. Intm. Sub.*, central intermediate substance; *Cent. M. N.*, central lateral motor nucleus; *Dor. Lat. M. N.*, dorsal lateral motor nucleus; *Int. Lat. N.*, intermediolateral nucleus; *Int. Med. N.*, intermediomedial nucleus; *LCN*, lateral cervical nucleus; *L. Intm. Sub.*, lateral intermediate substance; *Lat. M. N.*, lateral motor nucleus; *Med. M. N.*, medial motor nucleus; *N. Prop.*, nucleus proprius; *N. Thor.*, nucleus thoracicus; *S. Par.*, sacral parasympathetic nucleus; *Sec. Vis.*, location where some visceral afferents terminate; *Sub. Gel.*, substantia gelatinosa; *Vent. Lat. M. N.*, ventral lateral motor nucleus.

however, it is usually difficult to distinguish individual lamina in routine preparations. In general, both laminar and nuclear schemes are used, depending on which applies best to a specific situation.

Gray Matter Nuclei

Dorsal Horn Nuclei

The **lateral cervical nucleus** (*nucleus cervicalis lateralis*) is found in the first two cervical segments of the spinal cord (Brodal & Rexed, 1953; Ha & Liu, 1966). Lateral to the dorsal horn, the profile of the nucleus forms a peninsula or island surrounded by white matter. The nucleus consists of projection neurons (third-order neurons of the spinocervicothalamic pathway). The nucleus relays cutaneous noxious stimuli and touch to conscious centers (Lu & Yang, 1989). In this text nociception is the response of an animal to a noxious stimulus, one that causes injury or has the potential to cause injury. This response indicates a patient's discomfort or pain caused by the noxious stimulus. Pain is not a sensory modality. It is the conscious response to a noxious stimulus.

Marginal nucleus (dorsomarginal nucleus) refers to flattened neurons located at the dorsal surface of the dorsal horn along the entire length of the spinal cord. Although the nucleus is not morphologically prominent, it is important as a site of nociceptive projection neurons (Craig et al., 1988; Yaksh, 1986).

The **substantia gelatinosa**, a concentration of small neurons, forms a homogeneous crown at the apex of the dorsal horn, deep to the marginal nucleus. It extends the entire length of the spinal cord and blends cranially with the nucleus of the spinal tract of the trigeminal nerve. Most substantia gelatinosa cells are interneurons that project to the remainder of the dorsal horn, but a few larger cells are spinothalamic tract projection neurons. The substantia gelatinosa receives cutaneous input from axons activated by noxious, tactile, or thermal stimulation (Light & Kavookjian, 1988; Rethelyi et al., 1989).

Nucleus proprius is a term applied to dorsal horn neurons located deep to substantia gelatinosa. The nucleus extends the entire length of the spinal cord. It receives input from dorsal root afferent axons, substantia gelatinosa interneurons, and caudally projecting spinal cord tracts. Neurons of the nucleus proprius are either interneurons or projection neurons. The latter contribute to a variety of cranially projecting tracts.

The **nucleus thoracicus** (*nucleus dorsalis*; nucleus of the dorsal spinocerebellar tract; Clarke column) consists of sparse, large cell bodies located medially at the base of the dorsal horn of T1 through L4 spinal cord segments. The nucleus thoracicus receives input from muscles caudal to the thoracic limbs. The nucleus is composed of projection neurons that give rise to the ipsilateral dorsal spinocerebellar tract, which projects to the cerebellum and to nucleus Z of the medulla oblongata (McIntyre et al., 1989).

Intermediate Substance Nuclei

The **intermediomedial nucleus** is located along the medial margin of the lateral intermediate substance. The nucleus contains predominantly interneurons that synapse on autonomic efferent neurons.

The **intermediolateral nucleus** is located at the lateral margin of the lateral intermediate substance of thoracic and cranial lumbar levels of the spinal cord. The nucleus forms the lateral horn of segments T1 through L3. The nucleus contains preganglionic sympathetic neurons (Cummings, 1969). Embryologically, the neurons occupy a medial position, but subsequent migration positions the majority of cell bodies laterally.

The **sacral parasympathetic nucleus** is found in the sacral spinal cord segments, chiefly S2 and S3 (Oliver et al., 1969; Purinton & Oliver, 1979). It consists of parasympathetic preganglionic neurons that form a mediolateral band in the lateral intermediate substance. The dorsal portion of the nucleus is concerned with bowel control, the lateral portion with urinary bladder contraction (Leedy et al., 1988).

Ventral Horn Nuclei

The cell bodies of alpha and gamma efferent neurons that innervate a particular skeletal muscle are grouped together, forming a motor neuron pool. Related skeletal muscles have their motor neuron pools grouped into longitudinal columns that extend over one or more spinal cord segments (Horcholle-Bossavit et al., 1988). These columns are designated *motor nuclei* when viewed in spinal cord sections. From one to seven motor nuclei are evident in the different segments along the length of the spinal cord (Romanes, 1951).

A **medial motor nucleus** is recognized at most levels of the spinal cord; however, it is reduced in segments that innervate the limbs, and it is absent in segments L7 and S1. The nucleus innervates axial muscles of the neck and trunk,

Clusters of neuronal cell bodies located laterally in the ventral horn are designated **lateral motor nuclei**. They innervate limb musculature. In cervical segments, a lateral **motor nucleus of the accessory nerve** (*nucleus motorius n. accessorii*) gives rise to the spinal roots of the accessory nerve. Lateral motor nuclei are best developed in the enlargement segments, which innervate limbs. In these segments, the nuclei are somatotopically arranged, relative to the locations of the muscles they innervate. For example, proximal to distal muscles of the pelvic limb are innervated by ventral to dorsal nuclei, and the most lateral nuclei supply cranial limb muscles, whereas the more medial nuclei innervate caudal muscles of the limb (Fig. 16.8).

Gray Matter Laminae

Lamina I, also known as the *marginal (dorsomarginal) nucleus (zone)*, is located superficial to the substantia gelatinosa. It contains scattered, flattened neuron cell bodies that

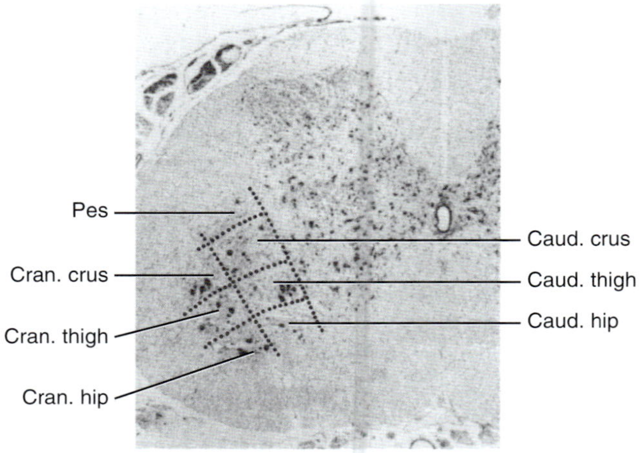

• **Fig. 16.8** Somatotopic organization of lateral motor nuclei. A transverse section through L7 is labeled to show which lateral motor nuclei innervate the different regional muscles of the pelvic limb (based on Romanes, 1951). Ventral nuclei innervate proximal muscles, and dorsal nuclei innervate distal muscles. Cranial muscles are innervated by lateral nuclei and caudal muscles by medial nuclei within the group of the lateral motor nuclei. (Actually, cranial thigh motor neurons do not extend to the level of L7, and those so labeled really innervate the crus.)

have dendrites oriented mediolaterally. The neurons are predominantly nociception-specific projection neurons, excited by noxious cutaneous (mechanical or thermal), proprioceptive, and visceral input. They send axons to spinothalamic, spinoreticular, and spinomesencephalic tracts. Thermoreceptive projection neurons, responding to mild warming or cooling, are also reported to be present.

Lamina II, also known as *substantia gelatinosa*, has a homogeneous population of small neurons activated by cutaneous afferents. Although some of the lamina neurons send axons to the spinothalamic tract, most are interneurons that project to laminae **I**, **III**, **IV**, and **V**.

Lamina III, the dorsal extent of the nucleus proprius, features cutaneous, mechanoreceptive projection neurons that contribute to spinocervicothalamic, dorsal column postsynaptic, and spinoreticular tracts. Dendrites of the neurons are oriented mediolaterally within the lamina.

Lamina IV has cutaneous, mechanoreceptive projection neurons, as described for lamina III, nociception-specific neurons, and multireceptive neurons, activated by both noxious and tactile somatic stimulation. The projection neurons contribute to spinocervicothalamic and dorsal column postsynaptic tracts. The lamina also contains interneurons that send axons to laminae V and VI.

Lamina V contains projection neurons that are excited by cutaneous, proprioceptive, and visceral input. The neurons send axons to spinomesencephalic, spinoreticular, spinothalamic, and long propriospinal tracts. A majority of the projection neurons are multireceptive, activated by both noxious and tactile somatic stimulation, but some are nociception-specific. Interneurons that project to lamina VI are also present. Lamina V can be divided into medial and lateral zones. The lateral border of the lateral zone has an irregular contour and has been designated the **spinal cord reticular formation** (*formatio reticularis*).

Lamina VI is the base of the dorsal horn, and, like lamina V, it can be divided into medial and lateral zones. The latter has larger neurons and a lower neuron density than does the medial zone. The lamina is largest in spinal cord segments that innervate the limbs, and it is absent in segments T3 through L1. It has a preponderance of interneurons, but it does have projection neurons that contribute to the spinoreticular tract.

Lamina VII occupies the lateral intermediate substance and extends a variable distance into the ventral horn, particularly in cervical and lumbosacral enlargement segments. The lamina contains viscerosomatic-responsive neurons that receive bilateral visceral input. Lamina VII has spinoreticular and spinothalamic tract projection neurons as well as projection neurons that form the nucleus thoracicus. Within the lamina, autonomic preganglionic efferent neurons are present in the sympathetic intermediolateral nucleus and sacral parasympathetic nucleus. In thoracic and cranial lumbar segments, lamina VII forms a lateral horn.

Lamina VIII occupies the medial part of the ventral horn in cervical and lumbosacral enlargement segments and most of the ventral horn in the remaining spinal cord segments. The lamina contains viscerosomatic-responsive neurons that receive bilateral visceral input. Lamina VIII has spinoreticular and spinothalamic tract projection neurons and commissural interneurons, which are believed to play a role in coordinating motor neurons in the right and left ventral horns.

Lamina IX consists of individual columns of alpha and gamma motor neurons that send axons through ventral roots to innervate skeletal muscles. The columns are embedded in lamina VII or VIII in the ventral horn. In spinal cord sections, the cell columns are recognized as medial and lateral motor nuclei.

Lamina X is the central intermediate substance that surrounds the central canal. Neurons are sparse and responsive to noxious stimulation.

White Matter of the Spinal Cord

Spinal cord white matter is formed by concentrations of myelinated and nonmyelinated axons. Within white matter, there are *afferent axons,* which enter the spinal cord through dorsal roots; *efferent axons,* which exit the spinal cord through ventral roots; and axons that compose pathways that convey information cranially and caudally in the spinal cord.

Cranially and caudally projecting axons conveying information from one location to another typically have a common function and travel together in the white matter. Collectively, the related axons are identified as a *tract* or *fasciculus*. Tracts are named for their origin and termination (e.g., *spinothalamic* and *vestibulospinal*).

Dorsal root afferent axons enter the spinal cord by penetrating the dorsolateral sulcus, which marks the separation

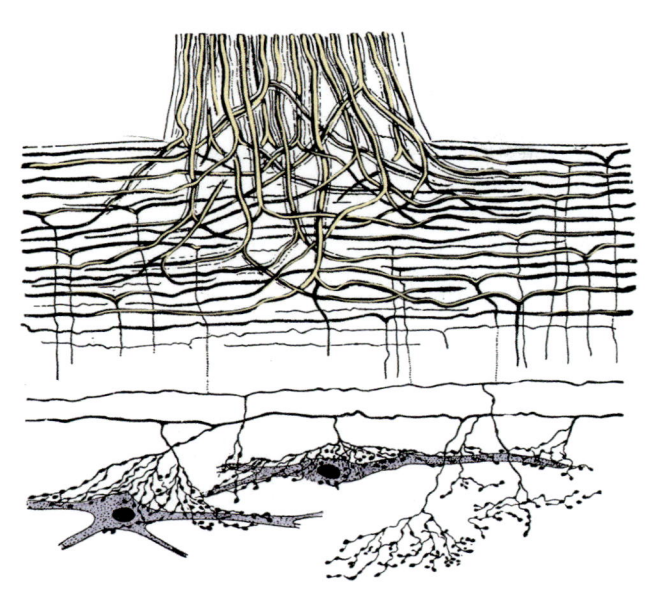

• **Fig. 16.9** Schematic illustration of a dorsal rootlet entering the spinal cord. From the rootlet (*top*), axons enter spinal cord white matter and bifurcate into cranial and caudal branches. Collaterals of the branches enter the gray matter to synapse on neuron cell bodies and dendrites. Cranial and caudal branches of nonmyelinated and small myelinated fibers collect separately from those of large myelinated fibers. (From Ranson SW, Clark Sl: *The anatomy of the nervous system,* 10th ed., Philadelphia, 1959, Saunders.)

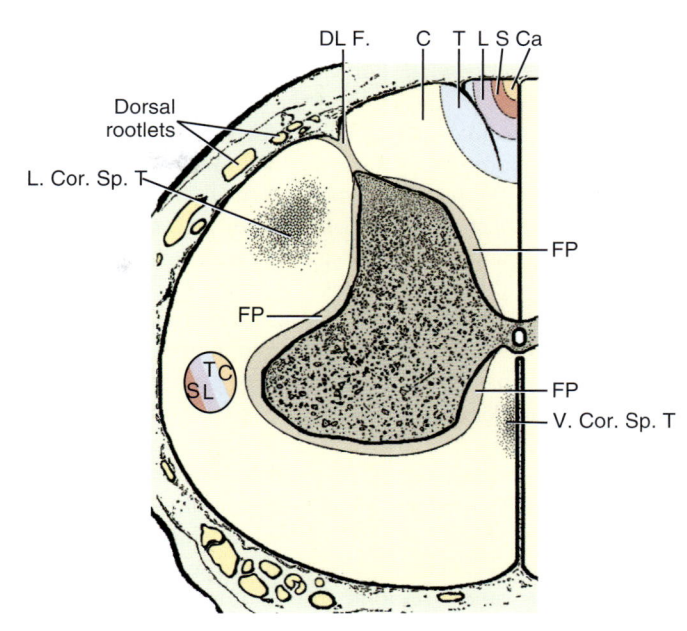

• **Fig. 16.10** Features of white matter organization illustrated in a cervical spinal cord segment. White matter immediately adjacent to gray matter is termed *fasciculus proprius (FP)*. It consists of relatively short axons that run from one spinal cord segment to another. As dorsal rootlet axons enter the spinal cord, cranial and caudal branches of nonmyelinated and small myelinated axons collect in the dorsolateral fasciculus *(DL F.)*, which extends between the dorsolateral sulcus and the dorsal horn. Cranial branches of large myelinated fibers that project cranially to the brain in fasciculus gracilis and fasciculus cuneatus are somatotopically organized, so are axons of other cranial and caudal projecting tracts, as shown to the left of the ventral horn. Locations of lateral *(L)* and ventral *(V)* corticospinal tracts *(Cor. Sp. T.)* are shown. Generally, tracts have a dense core surrounded by a zone of decreasing axon density. *C*, Cervical; *Ca*, caudal; *L*, lumbar; *S*, sacral; *T*, thoracic.

between dorsal and lateral funiculi. Within the dorsal funiculus, afferent axons typically bifurcate into longer cranial and shorter caudal branches (Fig. 16.9). These branches, in turn, give off collateral branches that penetrate gray matter to synapse on projection neurons, interneurons, and, in some cases, motor neurons. The number of segments (generally two to eight) over which cranial and caudal branches extend and give off collaterals is proportional to the size of the receptive field of the primary afferent neuron.

Afferent axons within a dorsal rootlet segregate by size as they enter the spinal cord. Larger myelinated axons, which conduct urgent information from muscles, joints, and skin, are positioned medially as the rootlet enters the spinal cord. Nonmyelinated (C fibers) and small myelinated (A_{delta}) axons collect laterally within the dorsal rootlet; these axons conduct excitation from nociceptors, thermoreceptors, and certain mechanoreceptors.

Small afferent axons gather laterally, immediately deep to the dorsolateral sulcus, and their overlapping cranial and caudal branches form a relatively nonmyelinated band called the *tractus dorsolateralis* (Fig. 16.10), formerly dorsolateral fasciculus. In cranial cervical segments, the dorsolateral tract blends with the spinal tract of the trigeminal nerve.

In all projection pathways, shorter axons (e.g., to or from the cervical region) lie closer to the gray matter than do longer axons (e.g., to or from the sacral region). Thus axons within individual tracts exhibit a somatotopic organization. As well, spinal tracts that travel to or from the brain are located more peripherally in white matter than are shorter

axons that originate in one spinal segment and terminate at another level of the spinal cord.

Intersegmental axons that arise and terminate within the spinal cord are known collectively as **fasciculus proprii**. They can be found bordering gray matter in all funiculi. These fasciculi convey intersegmental reflexes (e.g., scratch reflex, reflex twitch of the cutaneous trunci muscle, inhibition of phrenic and intercostal motor neurons by cervical inspiratory neurons) (Hoskin et al., 1988).

Typically, axonal tracts are not sharply circumscribed. A relatively localized tract may have axons densely grouped at its center, but axons become dispersed at the tract margin, mingling with margins and centers of other tracts. Some functionally recognized tracts have axons scattered widely over the white matter with no distinct center of high axon density.

Spinal Cord Cranial Projecting Tracts

Cranial projecting pathways begin with primary afferent neurons that activate spinal cord projection neurons that ultimately terminate in the brain. Spinal cord projection neurons have cell bodies in spinal cord gray matter and axons that travel craniad in a white matter *tract*. The name of the tract is often the same as the name of the pathway (e.g., spinothalamic; ventral spinocerebellar).

For some pathways, it is the cranial branches of primary afferent axons that project cranially to the brain, where they synapse on projection neurons located in brainstem nuclei. Such cranial branches form fasciculus gracilis and fasciculus cuneatus in the dorsal funiculus.

The information that cranial projecting tracts relay to the brain can be defined in terms of the responses of the projection neurons that give rise to the tracts. Some spinal cord projection neurons are activated specifically by noxious stimuli (mechanical or thermal). Others are activated specifically by nonnoxious mechanical or thermal stimuli. Still other projection neurons are activated nonspecifically by both noxious and mild mechanical stimuli. Some projection neurons are activated by both visceral and somatic stimulation, whereas others respond just to somatic stimulation (i.e., skin, muscle, or joint receptors). In general, each of the aforementioned varieties of projection neurons has multiple destinations in the brain and contributes to multiple cranial projecting tracts.

How information conveyed by cranial projecting tracts is interpreted by the brain is a matter of speculation. Some of the tracts relay information that presumably is discriminated as noxious, touch, pressure, warmth, coolness, and so forth. Other tracts convey information that is not discriminated but is sensed to the extent that it affects such functions as behavior, mood, motivation, and alertness. The response to a noxious stimulus, nociception, reflects widespread activation of neurons in the cerebrum that results in a behavior that we interpret as "pain." Finally, some tract information is entirely subconscious, functioning only as feedback for movement control adjustments.

In the presentation that follows, cranial projecting tracts are organized by funiculus (Fig. 16.11, Box 16.1). The presumed functions of these tracts are listed in Box 16.2.

Dorsal Funiculus

The dorsal funiculus differs from lateral and ventral funiculi, which almost exclusively contain axons of projection neurons. Instead, the dorsal funiculus is composed of axons of primary afferent neurons except for relatively few axons from spinal cord projection neurons and a negligible number of caudally projecting tract axons. Most of the dorsal funiculus is formed by overlapping cranial and caudal primary afferent branches that terminate after extending over several segments. However, a minority of the cranial branches travel all the way to the brainstem. These cranial branches form two fasciculi, each named for the nucleus in which the cranial branch terminates.

Fasciculus gracilis is formed by cranial branches of primary afferent neurons that innervate the caudal half of the body, particularly the pes. The cranial branches project medially in the dorsal funiculus to terminate on neurons of the nucleus gracilis in the medulla oblongata. The

---

• BOX 16.1 Summary of Projection Pathways in the Three Funiculi

Dorsal Funiculus

Cranial Projections	Caudal Projections
Fasciculus gracilis	Corticospinal tract
Fasciculus cuneatus	
Dorsal postsynaptic tract	

Lateral Funiculus

Cranial Projections	Caudal Projections
Spinothalamic tract	Lateral corticospinal tract
Spinocervicothalamic tract	Rubrospinal tract
Dorsal spinocerebellar tract	Lateral tectotegmentospinal tract
Spinomedullary tract	
Ventral spinocerebellar tract	Medial reticulospinal tract
Cranial spinocerebellar tract	Other reticulospinal projections
Spinopontine projections	Locus ceruleus projections
	Raphe nuclei projections
	Diencephalic projections

Ventral Funiculus

Cranial Projections	Caudal Projections
Spinoreticular tract	Ventral corticospinal tract
Spinovestibular tract	Medial tectospinal tract
Spinomesencephalic tract	Lateral vestibulospinal tract
Spinoolivary tract	Medial vestibulospinal tract
	Pontine reticulospinal tract

---

branches convey information predominantly from cutaneous mechanoreceptors that have small receptive fields and are rapidly adaptive (e.g., encapsulated tactile and lamellar corpuscles). The information is referred to as discriminative touch.

Approximately 20% to 25% of axons composing the dorsal funiculus of lumbar segments continue to the brainstem as fasciculus gracilis. The axons have a dermatome organization when they first enter the white matter and reorganize somatotopically as they project cranially (Willis, 1986).

Fasciculus cuneatus consists of cranial projecting branches of primary afferent neurons that innervate the thoracic limb and neck. The cranial branches synapse in medial or lateral cuneate nuclei of the medulla oblongata. The fasciculus contains axons that serve three general functions:

1. Cutaneous mechanoreceptor afferents synapse in the dorsal portion of the medial cuneate nucleus and function in discriminative touch, particularly from the manus analogous to fasciculus gracilis for the pelvic limb.
2. Muscle spindle and joint proprioceptive afferents synapse in the ventral part of the medial cuneate nucleus and function in thoracic limb kinesthesia (like the spinomedullary tract to nucleus Z functions for the pelvic limb).

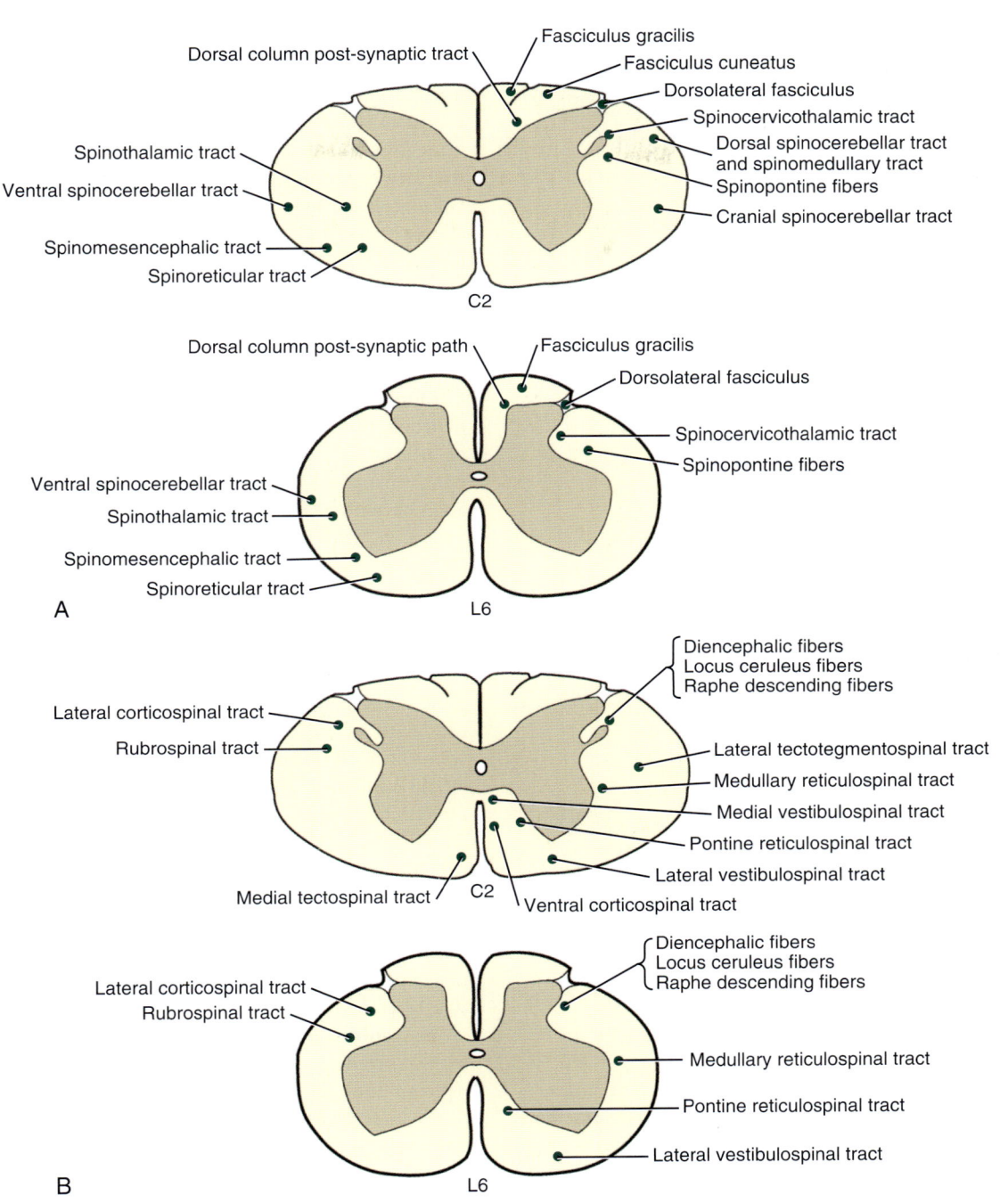

• **Fig. 16.11** A, Approximate locations of major cranial projecting tracts are labeled in white matter of cervical (*C2*) and lumbar (*L6*) segments of the spinal cord. (A lateral cervical nucleus projects laterally from the dorsal horn in C2.) All tracts are labeled relative to afferent input entering on the right side. Thus tracts labeled on the right are predominantly ipsilateral; tracts shown on the left project cranially mainly contralaterally (axons decussate in the white commissure). Some cranial projecting tracts have large bilateral contributions (e.g., the spinoreticular tract). Notice that the cervical segment has more tracts than the lumbar segment. **B**, Approximate locations of major caudal projecting tracts are labeled in white matter of cervical (*C2*) and lumbar (*L6*) segments of the spinal cord. The tracts are labeled relative to projection neurons located on the right side of the brain. Thus tracts labeled on the right project caudally ipsilaterally (or bilaterally); those shown on the left project caudally contralaterally (axons having decussated in the brain). Notice that the cervical segment has more tracts than the lumbar segment.

• **BOX 16.2** **Cranial Projecting Spinal Cord Tracts Categorized According to Their Presumed Information Content**[a]

Stimulus Discrimination (e.g., pain, warmth, coolness, touch)
Pain
    Spinocervicothalamic tract (mainly skin)
    Spinothalamic tract (visceral and somatic)
    Dorsal column postsynaptic tract (skin)
Warmth and Coolness
    Spinothalamic tract (visceral and somatic)
Tactile Stimuli and Pressure
    Dorsal column postsynaptic tract (skin)
    Spinocervicothalamic tract (skin)
    Spinothalamic tract (visceral and somatic)
Discriminative Touch
    Fasciculus cuneatus (manus)
    Fasciculus gracilis (pes)
Kinesthesia
    Fasciculus cuneatus (thoracic limb)
    Spinomedullary tract—to nucleus Z (pelvic limb)
Alertness, Motivation, and Affective Behavior
    Spinothalamic tract
    Spinoreticular tract
    Spinomesencephalic tract
Subconscious Sensory Feedback for Movement Control
    Dorsal spinocerebellar tract
    Ventral spinocerebellar tract and cranial spinocerebellar tract
    Fasciculus cuneatus (spinocuneocerebellar path)
    Spinoreticular tract
    Spinoolivary fiber
    Spinopontine fibers

[a]The information content of a pathway is determined first by the stimuli to which the primary afferent neurons and projection neurons of the pathway respond. Then the significance of the information depends on the destination in the brain to which it is delivered. Because individual spinal projection neurons may receive different kinds of sensory input and individual tracts may synapse in multiple brain locations, a given tract may have multiple sensory roles.

3. Muscle spindle, tendon organ, joint, and some cutaneous afferents synapse in the lateral cuneate nucleus that projects to medial and intermediate regions of the cerebellum. The axons constitute a *spinocuneocerebellar pathway* that is analogous to the dorsal spinocerebellar pathway for the pelvic limb. Collateral branches are sent to lateral vestibular nucleus, nucleus of the lateral funiculus (lateral reticular nucleus), and olivary nucleus, all of which project to the cerebellum.

The **dorsal column postsynaptic tract** arises from projection neurons of laminae III and IV. Typical projection neurons are multireceptive, responsive to both noxious and mechanical nonnoxious stimulation of the skin, although some neurons respond only to cutaneous tactile stimuli. Axons of the projection neurons run ipsilaterally in fasciculus gracilis or fasciculus cuneatus or, to a lesser extent, in the dorsal half of the lateral funiculus. The axons terminate in nucleus gracilis or the medial cuneate nucleus (some go to nucleus Z) in the medulla oblongata.

Lateral Funiculus

The **dorsolateral tract** (*tractus dorsolateralis*) (fasciculus of Lissauer) is situated at the junction of the dorsal and lateral funiculi, deep to the dorsolateral sulcus and superficial to the apex of the dorsal horn. The fasciculus consists of overlapping cranial and caudal axonal branches of small, primary afferent neurons. The neurons, which respond to noxious, thermal, or tactile stimuli, have nonmyelinated or small myelinated axons.

The **spinothalamic tract** (*tractus spinothalamicus*) is heterogeneous, conveying noxious stimuli, touch, and temperature sense from viscera, skin, muscles, and joints. Through modality-specific and multireceptive projection neurons, the tract functions in sensory discrimination and in arousal-affective behavior. Tract axons come predominantly from projection neurons of laminae VII and VIII, augmented by fibers from laminae I, II, and V (Bessen & Chaouch, 1987; Craig et al., 1989). Contributions from other laminae are variously reported.

The majority of tract axons immediately decussate in the white commissure and then project cranially contralaterally in the ventral region of the lateral funiculus. They send collaterals to reticular formation nuclei and periaqueductal gray matter and terminate in the thalamus (rostral and caudal to where the medial lemniscus terminates). Some spinothalamic axons that travel in the dorsal half of the lateral funiculus are referred to as a *dorsolateral spinothalamic tract* (Stevens et al., 1989).

With respect to noxious stimuli discrimination, the spinothalamic tract is apparently less important in carnivores than in other species (rodents, primates). Spinocervicothalamic and dorsal column postsynaptic pathways, along with multisynaptic, bilateral cranial projecting axons, all convey nociceptive information to the thalamus in carnivores (Casey & Morrow, 1988).

The **spinocervicothalamic tract** (spinocervical tract), which originates from cutaneously activated projection neurons located in laminae III and IV, is regarded as the dominant nociceptive pathway in carnivores (Bessen & Chaouch, 1987). Individual projection neurons respond to both mild mechanical and noxious mechanical stimulation. Axons of the projection neurons travel ipsilaterally in the dorsal half of the lateral funiculus and synapse on neurons of the lateral cervical nucleus. Axons from this nucleus decussate and travel through the medial lemniscus to the thalamus (and midbrain). Some spinal projection neurons send axonal branches to both the dorsal column postsynaptic tract and the spinocervicothalamic tract (Willis, 1985).

The **dorsal spinocerebellar tract** (*tractus spinocerebellaris dorsalis*) originates from the ipsilateral nucleus thoracicus, which receives input from spinal nerves caudal to the thoracic limb. Afferent activity arises from muscle spindles, tendon organs, slowly adapting joint receptors, and skin. Some of the tract projection neurons are located outside of the nucleus thoracicus, ipsilaterally in laminae IV to VI and contralaterally in laminae VIII and IX (Aoyama et al., 1988; Grant & Xu, 1988). Tract axons run along the lateral margin of the dorsal half of the lateral funiculus, join the caudal cerebellar peduncle, and terminate in medial and intermediate regions of the cerebellum. Axon collaterals terminate in nucleus Z in the medulla oblongata.

The **spinomedullary tract** to nucleus Z is formed by collateral branches of the dorsal spinocerebellar tract and by projection neurons located ventral to the nucleus thoracicus (McIntyre et al., 1989). Tract axons terminate in nucleus Z, which are neurons at the rostral margin of the nucleus gracilis in the medulla oblongata. The tract is activated by primary afferents from muscle spindles, tendon organs, and joints located caudal to thoracic limbs. Axons from neurons of nucleus Z decussate and join the medial lemniscus to reach the thalamus, thereby conveying conscious kinesthesia for the pelvic limb.

The **ventral spinocerebellar tract** (*tractus spinocerebellaris ventralis*) arises from projection neurons located in the lateral margin of the ventral horn. Many axons of the projection neurons decussate in the white commissure, but some axons remain ipsilateral. The tract projects cranially along the lateral margin of the ventral half of the lateral funiculus and joins the rostral cerebellar peduncle (Grant & Xu, 1988; Ha & Liu, 1968). Previously crossed axons decussate again in the cerebellum, and the tract terminates in the medial and intermediate cerebellar regions.

The projection neurons receive input similar to that impinging on motor neurons; thus they are able to convey information about the status of motor neurons directly to the cerebellum as well as indirectly via collateral branches to the nucleus of the lateral funiculus (lateral reticular nucleus) and the olivary nucleus (Orsal et al., 1988).

Medial axons of the ventral spinocerebellar tract that originate from projection neurons receiving input from thoracic limbs and neck may be designated the **cranial spinocerebellar tract**. The axons ascend ipsilaterally and enter the cerebellum through both rostral and caudal cerebellar peduncles.

The **spinopontine axons** run in the dorsal half of the lateral funiculus and convey sensory feedback to pontine nuclei neurons that project to the cerebellum through the middle cerebellar peduncle.

Ventral Funiculus

The **spinoreticular tract** arises from projection neurons that receive visceral and various somatic inputs. The neurons are located predominantly in laminae VII and VIII, but the tract includes noxious stimuli-specific axons from lamina I, multireceptive axons from laminae V and VI, and mechanical stimulation-specific axons from lamina III. The fibers project cranially bilaterally in the lateral region of the ventral funiculus and terminate in multiple nuclei of the pons and medulla oblongata.

Some of the target nuclei process sensory information for alerting and motivational purposes, and other nuclei (nucleus of the lateral funiculus and olivary nucleus) process sensory feedback for integration in the cerebellum. Some spinoreticular axons send branches to the thalamus.

The **spinovestibular tract** relays proprioceptive information from the cervical spinal cord to the caudal vestibular nucleus. Axons of the tract run in the ventral funiculus mingled with axons of the lateral vestibulospinal tract (Pompeiano & Brodal, 1957).

The **spinomesencephalic tract** (formerly named *spinotectal tract* [*tractus spinotectalis*]) originates from nociceptive and mechanoreceptive projection neurons located in laminae I and V. Their axons decussate and project cranially in the lateral region of the ventral funiculus (or ventral region of the lateral funiculus; *Nomina Anatomica Veterinaria*, 2017) to terminate in various midbrain nuclei, including rostral colliculus, red nucleus, cuneiform nucleus, interstitial nucleus, reticular formation, and periaqueductal gray matter (Boivie, 1988; Vinay & Padel, 1990; Yezierski, 1988). Many of the axons continue on to the thalamus. The tract may activate a caudally projecting analgesia system involving neurons in the periaqueductal gray matter.

The **spinoolivary tract axons** (*tractus spinoolivaris*) convey sensory feedback for integration in the olivary nucleus, which, in turn, activates localized zones of cerebellar cortex. These sensory axons reach the olivary nucleus by traveling in different tracts; namely, the spinoolivary and spinoreticular tracts in the ventral funiculus, the ventral spinocerebellar tract in the lateral funiculus, and the fasciculus cuneatus (spinocuneocerebellar pathway) in the dorsal funiculus.

Spinal Cord Caudal Projecting Tracts

Caudally projecting pathways are formed by projection neurons located in brainstem nuclei or in the cerebral cortex (Petras, 1967; Tunturi, 1982). The projection neurons send their axons caudally, forming named tracts in spinal white matter (e.g., vestibulospinal, corticospinal) (see Fig. 16.11). Caudally projecting tracts generally terminate on interneurons, although some axons contact motor neurons directly (Staal & Verhaart, 1963). The tracts modify autonomic and somatic reflexes and control muscle tone, posture, and movement. They also modify excitability of spinal projection neurons and synaptic effectiveness of primary afferent neurons (presynaptic inhibition) to regulate traffic in cranial projecting pathways. As noted earlier, there are few studies of these tracts on dogs so one may gain insights from work conducted on mice to elucidate pathways and their distribution of various mammals (see, for example, Watson & Harrison, 2012; Liang et al., 2012).

Particularly in regard to voluntary movement, caudal projecting tracts are often divided into pyramidal and extrapyramidal systems. Pyramidal (corticospinal) tracts arise from projection neurons in the cerebral cortex that send axons directly to spinal cord gray matter, running in pyramids of the medulla oblongata to reach the spinal cord. The tracts affect particularly muscles that control the manus and pes.

Caudal projecting tracts that originate from brainstem nuclei are termed extrapyramidal because their axons project caudally outside of the medullary pyramids. The cerebral cortex simultaneously drives both pyramidal and extrapyramidal systems to effect voluntary posture and movement.

In the following sections, the caudal projecting tracts are arranged according to site of origin in the brain (i.e., forebrain, midbrain, or hindbrain).

Forebrain Origin

Telencephalic Caudal Projection Axons

The corticospinal tracts arise mainly from the motor area of the cerebral cortex but also from the premotor area, somesthetic area, and related association areas. More than 90% of corticospinal axons are of small diameter and slowly conducting. Corticospinal projection neurons send axons through the ipsilateral medullary pyramid to reach spinal white matter. Via decussations in the caudal medulla, corticospinal axons from one cerebral hemisphere control the contralateral side of the body (Brodal, 1965; Buxton & Goodman, 1967; Lassek et al., 1930; van Crevel & Verhaart, 1963).

Corticospinal axons that arise from the somesthetic area of the cerebral cortex terminate in the dorsal horn on interneurons that, in turn, synapse on spinal projection neurons and on terminating branches of primary afferent axons (presynaptic inhibition). Through such axons, the cerebral cortex can regulate sensory input to the brain.

Corticospinal axons from the motor cortex terminate in the intermediate substance and ventral horn. These corticospinal axons are concerned with voluntary control of muscles, particularly those in the antebrachium and crus. Corticospinal axons are important for learning movements. Through interneurons, both alpha and gamma motor neurons are activated to produce muscle contraction (alpha) while maintaining spindle sensitivity (gamma). As well, spinal reflexes are inhibited to minimize their interference with cerebral cortex control of posture and movement.

At the brain–spinal cord junction, more than three-fourths of the pyramidal axons turn dorsally, decussate, and continue throughout the spinal cord in the dorsal half of the contralateral lateral funiculus as the lateral corticospinal tract (**tractus pyramidalis lateralis**). A small population of corticospinal axons does not decussate but continues ipsilaterally in the lateral corticospinal tract, eventually decussating at the level of their termination in gray matter.

Some pyramidal axons proceed directly into the ventral funiculus, forming an ipsilateral ventral corticospinal tract (**tractus pyramidalis ventralis**). The axons course along the medial margin of the ventral funiculus to the level of segments that innervate the thoracic limb. The axons decussate in the segments where they terminate.

In the cervical region, a small number of axons descend in the dorsal funiculus along the medial edge of the dorsal gray horn (Satomi et al., 1989). These constitute a *dorsal corticospinal tract* (which is well developed in rodents).

Diencephalic Caudal Projecting Axons

Lateral and medial hypothalamic regions and periventricular gray matter send axons through the dorsal portion of the lateral funiculus to terminate in laminae I and II. The paraventricular nucleus of the hypothalamus releases vasopressin and oxytocin into superficial laminae of the spinal cord. Other diencephalic nuclei also project to the spinal cord, including those of the caudal commissure and pretectal region (Spence & Saint-Cyr, 1988).

Mesencephalic Caudal Projecting Axons

The **rubrospinal tract** (*tractus rubrospinalis*) arises from the magnocellular portion of the red nucleus. The tract axons decussate immediately and ultimately project caudally in the contralateral lateral funiculus. The tract is positioned just ventral to, and overlapping with, the lateral corticospinal tract. Individual rubrospinal axons distribute collateral branches to multiple segments of the spinal cord (Shinoda et al., 1988). The tract is distributed to all segments of the spinal cord, terminating on interneurons located in the base of the dorsal horn (laminae V and VI) and in the lateral intermediate substance (lamina VII) (Holstege & Tan, 1988).

The red nucleus receives input from the motor cortex (typically collateral branches of corticospinal axons) and the cerebellar interpositus nucleus. The rubrospinal tract is the most important of the pathways through which a dog executes voluntary movement. Preservation of the red nucleus following decerebration (removal of the forebrain) allows a dog to sit, crouch, walk, climb, and spontaneously right itself when prodded (Henneman, 1980).

The **medial tectospinal tract** (*tractus tectospinalis*) originates mainly from neurons in the rostral colliculus. The axons decussate in the midbrain and descend in the ventral funiculus. They are distributed to cervical segments of the spinal cord, where they terminate on interneurons in the ventral horn. The tract is concerned with turning the head toward sudden auditory or visual stimuli.

The **lateral tectotegmentospinal tract** (*tractus tectospinalis lateralis*) travels in the lateral funiculus just ventral to the rubrospinal tract. It terminates in the ventral horn and lateral intermediate substance of the cervical and first two thoracic segments. The tract originates from neurons in the rostral colliculus and midbrain tegmentum (Holstege & Cowie, 1989). Axons from the tegmentum synapse on preganglionic sympathetic neurons that dilate pupils, among other sympathetic effects. This tract exerts its influence directly or indirectly on the entire thoracolumbar column of preganglionic sympathetic neurons. Dogs with an acute lesion of one cervical spinal cord lateral funiculus exhibit hyperthermia of the entire ipsilateral body surface (de Lahunta, Glass & Kent, 2015). Axons from the colliculus are involved in orienting the head toward sudden auditory or visual stimuli.

Rhombencephalic Caudal Projecting Axons

The **lateral vestibulospinal tract** arises primarily from neurons of the lateral vestibular nucleus (Erulkar et al.,

1966). These neurons are responsive to linear acceleration (detected by the utricle and saccule), and they receive spinal and cerebellar input. Tract axons travel through the ipsilateral ventral funiculus and terminate medially in the ventral horn on interneurons that excite alpha and gamma motor neurons of extensor muscles. Some tract axons synapse directly on motor neurons. Because of spontaneous activity in vestibular nerve axons, the lateral vestibulospinal tract contributes significantly to maintenance of normal standing posture as well as providing sudden activation of extensor tone to preclude stumbling or falling.

The **medial vestibulospinal tract** originates from neurons of rostral, medial, and caudal vestibular nuclei. The neurons are activated by angular acceleration (detected by semicircular ducts), and their axons project caudally mainly ipsilaterally to cervical and cranial thoracic spinal cord segments. The axons travel in the medial longitudinal fasciculus of the brainstem and the ventral funiculus of the spinal cord to terminate, via interneurons, on motor neurons of neck muscles (Nyberg-Hansen, 1964). The tract maintains head position by activating motor units that oppose potential head displacement.

The **pontine reticulospinal tract** arises from neurons of the pontine reticular formation (nucleus reticularis pontis). The axons project caudally ipsilaterally in the ventral funiculus along the medial border of the ventral horn and terminate, some decussating, on alpha and gamma motor neurons of extensor muscles. The tract provides excitatory drive to antigravity muscles for standing posture (Brooks, 1986).

The **medullary reticulospinal tract** (*tractus reticulospinalis lateralis*) arises from neurons located centrally in the reticular formation (nucleus gigantocellularis) of the medulla oblongata. The axons project caudally bilaterally in the lateral funiculus along the lateral border of the ventral horn and terminate, some decussating, on interneurons in the ventral horn (lamina VII). The tract suppresses standing and other motor activities by inhibiting alpha and gamma motor neurons (Henneman, 1980).

Other **reticulospinal fibers** are numerous and dispersed in lateral and ventral funiculi. Brainstem medullary neurons give rise to a multisynaptic dorsal reticulospinal pathway that travels in the dorsal part of the lateral funiculus and is known to inhibit flexor reflex interneurons in the dorsal horn. Some reticulospinal axons regulate visceral reflex activity by activating preganglionic autonomic neurons in the lateral intermediate substance. Axons from respiratory bulbospinal neurons that travel in the lateral funiculus and synapse on motor neurons in the ventral horn generate breathing movements. Caudally projecting axons from the nucleus of the solitary tract inhibit nociceptive neurons that receive visceral input (Du & Zhou, 1990; Kuypers & Maisky, 1977).

The locus ceruleus is a nucleus located in the pons beside the fourth ventricle. Axons from the nucleus project caudally in the lateral funiculus. They synapse in the dorsal horn and also in the ventral horn directly on motor neurons.

The axons release norepinephrine as a neurotransmitter molecule that produces inhibition of neuronal responses, particularly to noxious stimulation (Massari et al., 1988). Age-related declines in the function of the locus ceruleus may be related to cognitive dysfunction in dogs, comparable to Alzheimer's disease in humans (Insua et al., 2010).

Raphe nuclei, particularly the nucleus raphe magnus located at the midline of the rostral medulla oblongata, project axons caudally through the dorsal half of the lateral funiculus to synapse especially in lamina I. The axons synaptically release serotonin, which increases the threshold of projection neurons to noxious stimulation. Raphe nuclei can also alter the excitability of alpha motor neurons (Fung & Barnes, 1989).

Spinal Reflexes

A reflex is an inherent, subconscious, relatively consistent response to a particular stimulus, and a spinal reflex is one that involves only the spinal cord and spinal nerves. The reflex response is predetermined by the interneuronal circuitry interposed between primary afferent neurons and efferent neurons (Fig. 16.12). Reflexes exhibit some inconsistency because the involved neurons are subject to brain regulation via caudal projecting tracts. The following is a synopsis of three typical spinal reflexes.

The **myotatic reflex** (muscle stretch reflex) is the basis for muscle tone (the resistance a muscle offers to being stretched). The reflex can be demonstrated by tapping the tendon of a muscle (abruptly stretching the muscle) and observing its immediate contraction.

Receptors for the reflex are *annulospiral endings,* which surround central nuclear regions of intrafusal muscle fibers

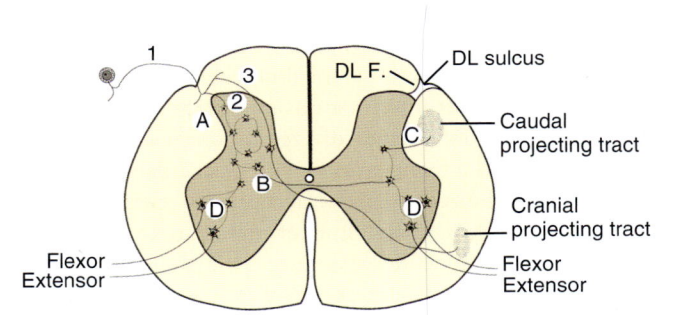

• **Fig. 16.12** Hypothetical wiring diagram for neurons involved in the withdrawal (flexor-crossed extensor) reflex. *(1)* The axon of a nociceptive afferent neuron penetrates the dorsolateral sulcus *(DL Sulcus)* and bifurcates into cranial and caudal branches in the dorsolateral fasciculus *(DL F)*. *(2)* A collateral branch activates the beginning of an interneuronal circuit that diverges to affect motor units of most muscles of both limbs. *(A)* A positive-feedback loop enables the reflex to persist beyond the duration of the stimulus. *(B)* A commissural interneuron activates extensor motor neurons in the contralateral limb. *(C)* Caudal projecting tracts can inhibit the contralateral limb extension. *(D)* Inhibitory interneurons *(black)* impinge on alpha motor neurons to ensure that antagonist muscles are inhibited (reciprocal innervation). *(3)* Independent of the reflex, another collateral branch activates a projection neuron that decussates in the white commissure and joins a cranial projecting tract to reach the brain.

within muscle spindles. The receptors are associated with the fastest-conducting, largest myelinated fibers (type Ia). The type Ia axons bifurcate into cranial and caudal branches in the dorsal funiculus. Collaterals of these branches go to the ventral horn and excite nearly all the alpha motor neurons that innervate the muscle being stretched. The collateral branches also synapse on motor neurons of synergist muscles, and, via interneurons, they inhibit motor neurons of antagonist muscles (Binder & Mendell, 1990).

The myotatic reflex is unique in that it has a monosynaptic component, that is, primary afferent neurons synapsing directly on efferent neurons, bypassing interneurons. Thus this reflex is the fastest, and it is relatively resistant to fatigue and other insults to which synapses are susceptible (e.g., hypoxia, anesthetic agents). The same primary afferent neuron that elicits a myotatic reflex can simultaneously be part of one or more cranial projecting pathways via a continuing cranial branch or synapses on spinal projection neurons. The most reliable example of this reflex in dogs is the patellar reflex and involves the femoral nerve and spinal cord segments L4 and L5. It is performed in the recumbent animal with its limb relaxed.

The **withdrawal reflex** is usually elicited by applying a noxious stimulus to the distal part of the limb (e.g., toe pinch) and observing withdrawal (flexion) of the entire limb. The reflex is typically evoked with the animal recumbent. Under these circumstances a corresponding extension of the contralateral limb is seen in neonatal pups and again in certain neurologically impaired dogs. The contralateral limb extension, which is dictated by interneuronal circuitry, is inhibited by caudal projecting tracts when they mature and remains suppressed unless the tracts are damaged.

The reflex is initiated by free nerve endings associated with small myelinated and nonmyelinated axons. The axons enter the dorsolateral fasciculus, where they bifurcate into cranial and caudal branches that extend over several segments. These give off collateral branches that enter gray matter to synapse on interneurons and projection neurons.

The interneurons provide divergence of excitability from a few stimulated afferent axons to all of the flexor muscles of the limb. The interneurons account for persistence of limb flexion beyond the time of stimulation, and they ensure reciprocal inhibition of antagonistic extensor muscles. The multisynaptic withdrawal reflex is often used by clinicians to assess depth of anesthesia.

The **cutaneous trunci reflex** is elicited by pricking the skin along the dorsum of the trunk and observing it twitch owing to contraction of cutaneous trunci muscle. It is an *intersegmental reflex* because a number of segments intervene between the afferent input and the efferent output. From cranial and caudal branches in the dorsolateral fasciculus, collateral branches enter gray matter to activate projection interneurons that send their axons predominantly in the contralateral fasciculus proprius to motor neurons in the contralateral cervical enlargement spinal cord segments that innervate the cutaneous trunci muscle via the lateral thoracic nerve

Transverse Sections of the Spinal Cord

The appearance of spinal cord segments, as viewed in transverse section, varies along the length of the spinal cord. The 14 sections illustrated in Fig. 16.13 depict the variety of spinal cord appearance. Spinal cord segments omitted from the figure appeared similar to preceding segments in the figure; that is, C4 and C5 were similar to C3, C8 and T1 were similar to C7, and so on. The one exception is that the omitted L6 segment appeared similar to L7 rather than to L4. Segments in the figure are represented by midlevel transections. However, at abrupt transitions (e.g., enlargements) the center of a segment may not be representative of the entire segment.

At the first cervical segment, the transition from medulla oblongata to spinal cord is evident. Pyramidal fibers can be seen coursing dorsally and decussating to form lateral corticospinal tracts. Gray matter is beginning to assume the typical butterfly shape of the spinal cord.

In cervical segments, the ratio of white matter to gray matter is greatest. As one progresses caudally along the spinal cord, the white matter to gray matter ratio gradually declines as caudal and cranial projecting axons to and from more cranial segments are eliminated from white matter tracts. However, both white matter and gray matter are augmented at segments that innervate limbs.

In the cranial cervical region, the spinal cord perimeter is quite oval in transverse section. In thoracic segments, between the enlargements, the spinal cord appears circular in transverse section.

In the cranial half of the spinal cord, a dorsal intermediate sulcus and septum is often evident in the dorsal funiculus. The dorsolateral sulcus is most prominent in the thoracic region. In lumbar and sacral segments, a dorsal median fissure is consistent, whereas a dorsal median septum is present in cervical and thoracic segments.

The apex of the dorsal gray horn tends to be pointed in the cervical region, blunted in the thoracic region, and rectangular in the lumbosacral region. A lateral gray horn is evident in thoracic and cranial lumbar segments of the spinal cord. The ventral gray horn is considerably enlarged by expansion of lateral motor nuclei in segments that innervate the limbs.

Meninges, Brain Ventricles, and Cerebrospinal Fluid

The central nervous system is protected by bones of the cranium and vertebral canal (Fig. 16.14). Within the bone, the central nervous system is enveloped by protective membranes termed *meninges* (singular is *meninx*). **Meninges** differentiate into three layers: dura mater, arachnoid membrane, and pia mater.

The dura mater (pachymeninx) is relatively thick and fibrous. It is the most superficial of the meningeal layers. Arachnoid membrane and pia mater are collectively designated

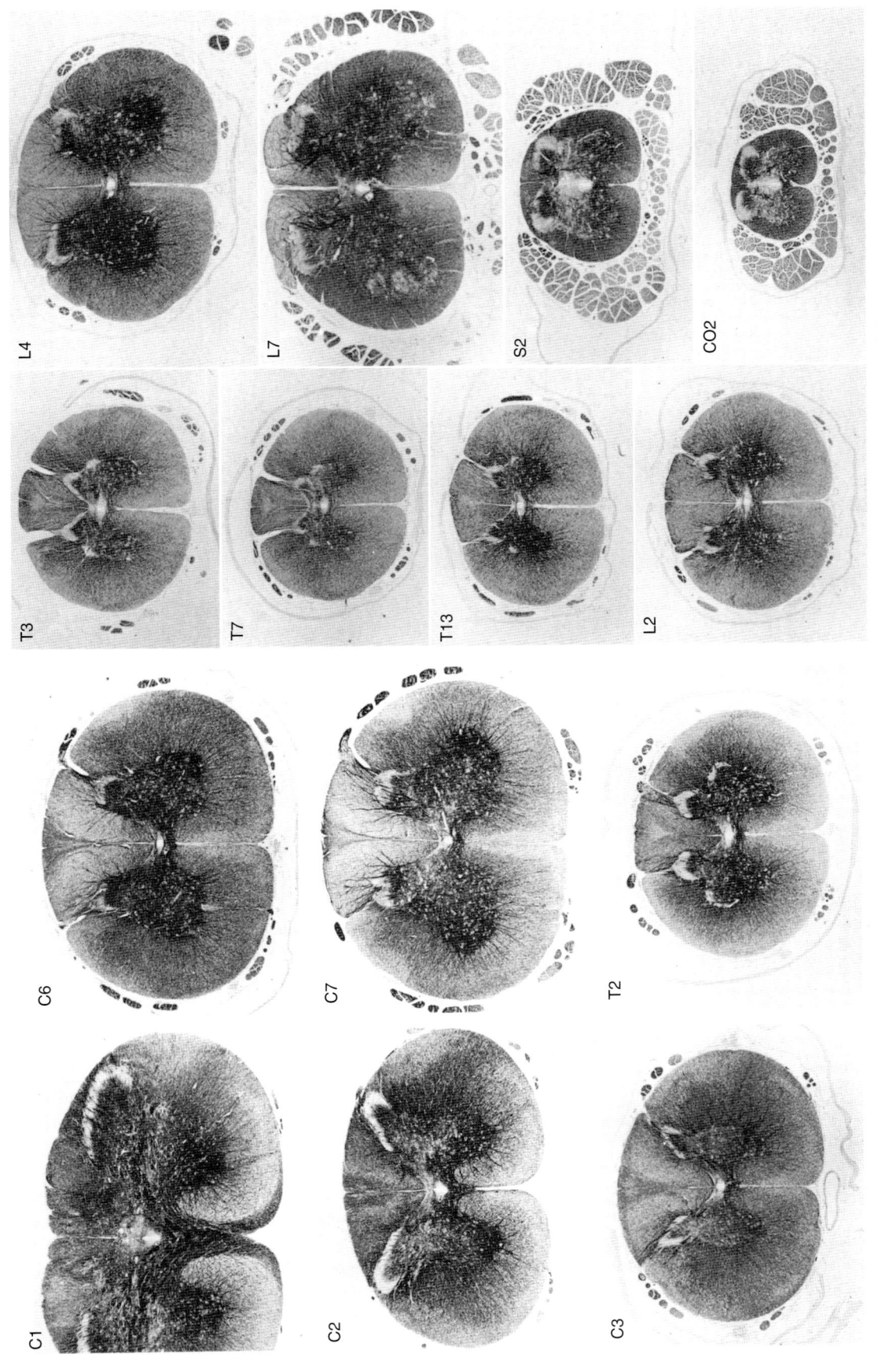

Fig. 16.13 Transected segments at different levels of the spinal cord (modified Holmes silver stain, 6.5× magnification). Transections were made at the middle of each segment. Omitted segments appeared similar to the preceding illustrated segment, except that L6 was more similar to L7 than to L4.

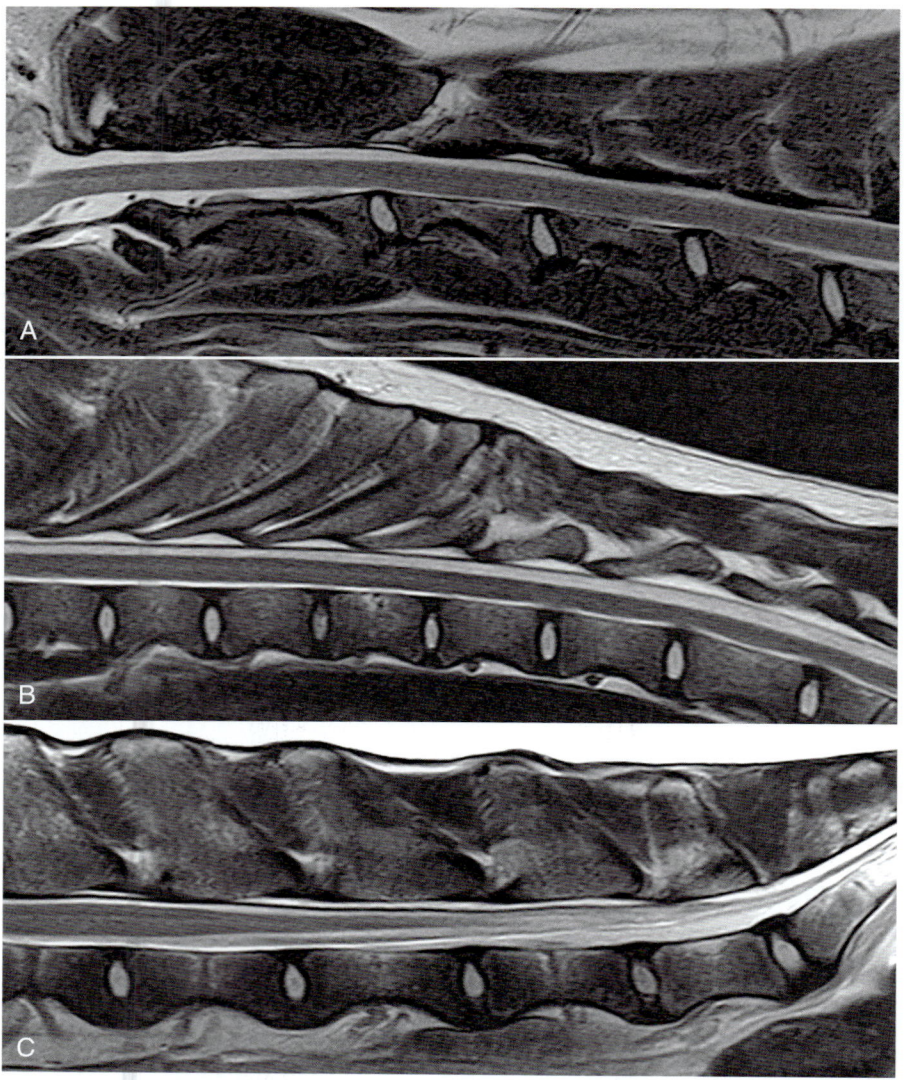

Fig. 16.14 T2-weighted MRI scans illustrating the sagittal plane of the vertebral column. **A,** Cranial cervical region. **B,** Thoracolumbar region. **C,** Lumbosacral region. In all images, the subarachnoid space has high signal intensity (white) and surrounds the spinal cord, which has an intermediate signal intensity. The conus medullaris (caudal termination of spinal cord) is at the L4 to L5 vertebral junction. The cauda equina, dura mater, and subarachnoid space extend caudally into the sacrum. Between successive vertebral bodies, the nucleus pulposus of the intervertebral disks also has a high signal intensity (white).

leptomeninges because they are delicate relative to dura mater. Arachnoid membrane lines the deep surface of the dura mater to which it is attached. It is joined to pia mater by arachnoid trabeculae that traverse a subarachnoid space filled with cerebrospinal fluid. Pia mater coats the surface of the brain, the spinal cord, nerve roots, and the optic nerve. It is bound to the surface of the central nervous system, where astrocyte processes form a glial limiting membrane.

Major vessels bringing blood to the brain and spinal cord run through the subarachnoid space and along the pia mater surface. Some arachnoid trabeculae connect to the vessels, which are thus coated by leptomeningeal tissue that is continuous with arachnoid membrane and pia mater. Branches of vessels penetrate pia mater and tunnel through the central nervous system.

The brain contains ventricles, which are cavities derived from the embryonic neural tube. The ventricles are lined by ependymal epithelium and filled with cerebrospinal fluid. In each ventricle, modified ependymal cells and vascular proliferations of pia mater vessels form a choroid plexus that produces cerebrospinal fluid. From the ventricular system, cerebrospinal fluid flows into the subarachnoid space that surrounds the brain, the spinal cord, nerve roots, and the optic nerves.

Thus the central nervous system is buoyed by fluid that is present within ventricles and between leptomeninges. It is enveloped by protective dura mater and encased in bone. Without such precautions, many of the inconsequential traumas sustained daily by an average dog would be fatal.

The Meninges

The **dura mater** is composed mainly of collagen bundles arranged in variably oriented planes. Fibroblasts, some elastic fibers, occasional vessels, and sensory nerves are also present. The inner surface of dura mater features layers of flattened fibroblasts, to which flattened fibroblasts of the arachnoid membrane adhere by desmosomes. Under pathologic conditions, hemorrhage can produce an apparent separation between dura mater and arachnoid membrane. Blood accumulates in an acquired "subdural space" that is normally nonexistent (Orlin et al., 1991).

The **spinal cord dura mater** (*dura mater spinalis*) forms a long tube. It is continuous with cranial dura mater at the foramen magnum, where it fuses with periosteum lining the foramen and with periosteum along the floor of the vertebral canal within vertebrae C1 and C2. Caudally spinal cord dura mater tapers to a slender filament, the *filum durae matris spinalis*, which ensheathes the filum terminale (Fig. 16.5). The dural filament can be traced through the vertebral canal to the middle of the tail (Fletcher & Kitchell, 1966a).

Within the vertebral canal, an **epidural space** (*cavum epidurale*) separates spinal cord dura mater from the periosteum lining the canal, except ventrally in the first two cervical vertebrae. The space contains fat and, particularly along the floor of the canal, the internal ventral vertebral venous plexus. There is no epidural space in the cranial cavity because cranial dura mater doubles as periosteum.

As spinal roots traverse the vertebral canal, they are enclosed by lateral extensions of dura mater, which may be designated dural (meningeal) sheaths. Generally, each dorsal root and each ventral root is enclosed in a separate meningeal sheath (see Fig. 16.2). However, dorsal and ventral roots of C1 share a common meningeal sheath, and meningeal sheaths of C2 and C3 dorsal and ventral roots are usually joined by connective tissue. In the caudal lumbar region, two separate meningeal sheaths are provided for each dorsal and each ventral root (Fletcher & Kitchell, 1966a).

At an intervertebral foramen, meningeal sheath fibrous tissue becomes continuous with epineurium and perineurium of spinal nerves. Also, dura mater merges with periosteum.

In the lumbosacral region, fibrous bands extend from the spinal cord dura mater to the floor of the vertebral canal. The bands often accompany spinal roots and attach near intervertebral foramina. Similar bands are given off by the filum durae matris spinalis (Fletcher & Kitchell, 1966a).

Cranial dura mater (*dura mater encephali*) lines the cranial cavity, simultaneously covering the brain and serving as periosteum for the cranial cavity. It originates embryologically as a double layer, and, at certain locations, it splits into an outer periosteal layer and an inner layer that forms partitions between parts of the brain. A venous sinus is generally present where the layers separate (Fig. 16.17). Veins of the brain drain into such dural venous sinuses, which, by virtue of their rigid walls, remain open during periods of increased intracranial pressure.

The largest partition formed by dura mater is the *falx cerebri*, which extends into the longitudinal fissure that separates right and left cerebral hemispheres. The dorsal sagittal venous sinus is present along the dorsal margin of the falx cerebri. Caudally the falx cerebri meets the surface of the *tentorium cerebelli*, a partition inserted into the transverse fissure that separates cerebral hemispheres from cerebellum. The core of the tentorium is osseous (a process of parietal and occipital bones), but a reflection of dura mater encloses the bone and extends beyond it as *tentorium cerebelli membranaceum*. The free edge of the membranous tentorium cerebelli bounds the tentorial notch (*incisura tentorii*) through which the brainstem passes. A straight venous sinus is present along the junction of the falx cerebri and tentorium cerebelli (see Figs. 12.22 and 12.23).

Another partition, the *diaphragma sellae*, separates brain from the hypophysis and the cavernous venous sinuses. It is penetrated by the infundibulum of the hypophysis and by internal carotid arteries.

Leptomeninges

Arachnoid membrane and pia mater, separated by a subarachnoid space but connected by arachnoid trabeculae, constitute the leptomeninges. Embryologically, the arachnoid membrane and pia mater are derived from a common mesenchyme layer predominantly of neural crest origin, that undergoes cavitation to form the subarachnoid space.

Arachnoid membrane (*arachnoidea encephali, arachnoidea spinalis*) is composed of flattened fibroblasts associated with a fine net of collagen fibers. *Arachnoid trabeculae*, which connect arachnoid membrane to pia mater, are formed by thin strands of collagen fibers coated by flattened fibroblasts.

Pia mater consists of collagen fibers and superficial, flattened fibroblasts (Allen & Low, 1975). Flattened leptomeningeal fibroblasts thus line the entire subarachnoid space (fenestrations may occur in the cellular lining). The collagen fibers of pia mater make contact with a basal lamina on the nervous tissue surface (astrocyte processes of a glial limiting membrane contact the deep surface of the basal lamina). Because it is intimately attached to the surface of the central nervous system, the pia mater extends into the depths of various sulci, fissures, and crevices of the central nervous system.

The depth of the **subarachnoid space** (*cavum subarachnoideale*) is variable because arachnoid membrane contacts dura mater and the pia mater follows every irregularity of the brain surface. At certain sites, crevices of the brain surface establish subarachnoid space enlargements known as *cisternae*. Most important is the *cisterna cerebellomedullaris*, formerly *cisterna magna*, which is located where the caudal surface of the cerebellum meets the dorsal surface of the medulla oblongata (Fig. 16.15). It is the largest cisterna and the most common site for obtaining cerebrospinal fluid (de Lahunta, 1983).

CHAPTER 16 Spinal Cord and Meninges

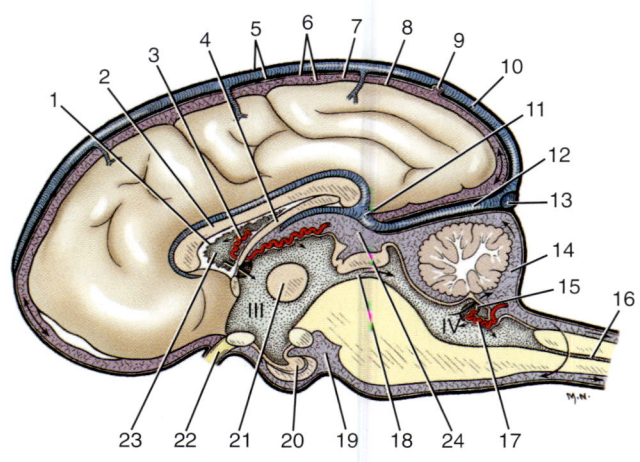

1. Cut edge of septum pellucidum
2. Corpus callosum
3. Choroid plexus in lateral ventricle
4. Fornix of hippocampus
5. Dura mater
6. Arachnoid membrane and trabeculae
7. Subarachnoid space
8. Pia mater
9. Arachnoid villus
10. Dorsal sagittal sinus
11. Great cerebral vein
12. Straight sinus
13. Transverse sinus
14. Cerebellomedullary cistern
15. Lateral aperture of fourth ventricle
16. Central canal
17. Choroid plexus
18. Mesencephalic aqueduct
19. Interpeduncular cistern
20. Hypophysis
21. Interthalamic adhesion
22. Optic nerve
23. Lateral ventricle
24. Quadrigeminal cistern

• **Fig. 16.15** Schema of meninges and ventricles. Arrows indicate the flow of cerebrospinal fluid. (From Evans HE, de Lahunta A: *Guide to the dissection of the dog*, St. Louis, MO, 2017, Elsevier.)

Pia mater collagen is bilaterally thickened along the lateral surface of the spinal cord, forming a **denticulate ligament** (*ligamentum denticulatum*) (Figs. 16.3 and 16.5). Denticulate ligaments have lateral extensions that traverse the subarachnoid space and attach to dura mater, thereby suspending the spinal cord in cerebrospinal fluid within the subarachnoid space. Caudally each denticulate ligament terminates in a process that connects to the dura mater between the entrances of the L5 and L6 spinal roots into dural sheaths; in 25% of dogs, the termination is between the L6 and L7 roots (Fletcher & Kitchell, 1966a).

The pia mater is relatively vascular because all vessels entering and leaving the central nervous system must travel in pia mater. Vessels passing through the subarachnoid space are covered by leptomeningeal fibroblasts, derived from arachnoid trabeculae. Large vessels penetrating central nervous system tissue are surrounded for a short distance by an apparent perivascular extension of the subarachnoid space, although communication between subarachnoid and perivascular spaces may be sealed by merger of the leptomeningeal fibroblast layer covering vessels with that on the pia mater surface (Krahn, 1982).

As a vessel proceeds and divides into smaller branches within the central nervous system, the size of its perivascular space is progressively reduced. Ultimately, capillaries are surrounded only by basal laminae, the outer surface of which is contacted by astrocyte end feet. (Endothelial cells of the central nervous system capillaries lack fenestrations and are united by zonulae occludentes, which is the explanation for the blood–brain barrier to diffusion of hydrophilic molecules.)

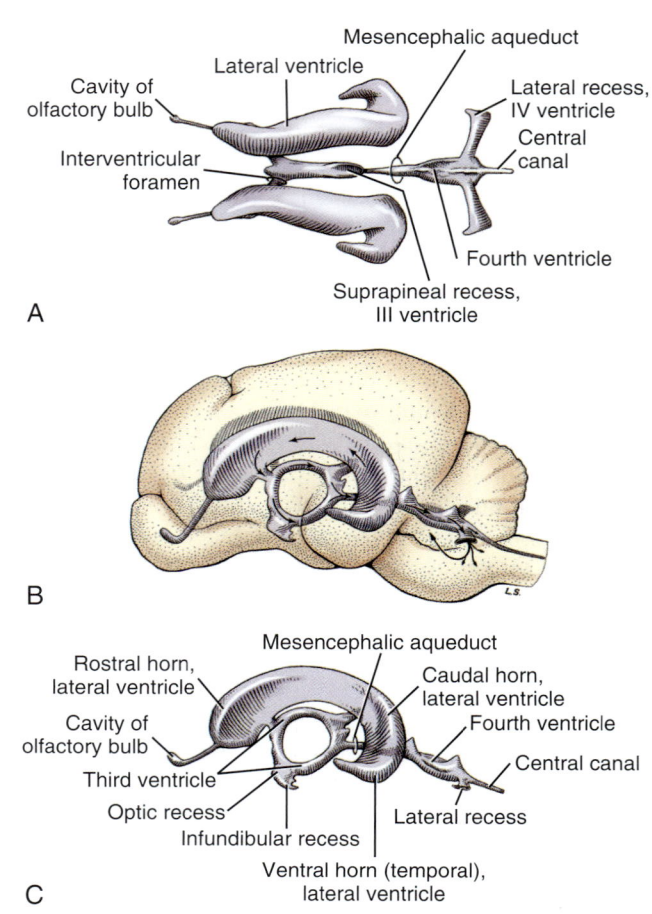

• **Fig. 16.16** Ventricular system of the dog brain. **A**, Dorsal view; **B** and **C**, lateral views. The arrows indicate the direction of flow through the ventricles and, through the lateral recess and aperture, to the subarachnoid space. (From de Lahunta A, Glass E, Kent M: *Veterinary neuroanatomy and clinical neurology*, 4th ed. Philadelphia, 2015, Elsevier.)

The Ventricular System

The lumen of the embryonic neural tube persists as the ventricular system of the brain and the central canal of the spinal cord. These cavities are lined by ependymal epithelium and are filled with cerebrospinal fluid. The chambers of the ventricular system communicate with one another, with the central canal, and with the subarachnoid space (Fig. 16.16).

The brain has one **lateral ventricle** (*ventriculus lateralis*) within each cerebral hemisphere. Through an interventricular foramen, each lateral ventricle communicates with the **third ventricle** (*ventriculus tertius*), a narrow, median plane chamber surrounding the interthalamic adhesion of the diencephalon. The **mesencephalic aqueduct** (*aqueductus mesencephali*) of the midbrain is a canal that connects the third and fourth ventricles. The **fourth ventricle** (*ventriculus quartus*) is located in the pons and medulla of the hindbrain. It communicates with the central canal and, by means of paired lateral recesses and apertures, with the subarachnoid space (see Fig. 16.16).

At one region along the wall of each ventricle, nervous tissue is absent so that pia mater contacts ependyma. The combined tissue, called *tela choroidea,* forms part of the floor of each lateral ventricle and the roof of the third and fourth ventricles. Tela choroidea plus a plexus of capillaries gives rise to *choroid plexus.* Each choroid plexus projects into a ventricle as a band of clustered villi. The linear attachment of tela choroidea to the adjacent brain parenchyma is designated *taenia choroidea.* Each villus of a choroid plexus features microvascular proliferation and cuboidal ependymal cells (choroidal epithelium). Choroid plexus produces cerebrospinal fluid by secretion and ultrafiltration.

The choroid plexus of each lateral ventricle continues into the third ventricle through an interventricular foramen. Consequently, two choroid plexuses are found in the roof of the third ventricle. The roof of the fourth ventricle also contains paired choroid plexuses, and each projects into the subarachnoid space by extending through the lateral recess and aperture of the fourth ventricle.

At selective sites within ventricles, ependymal cells become specialized for secretion (tanycytes). Within the third ventricle, secretory sites are located caudally (subcommissural organ), rostrally (subfornical organ), and ventrally (at the tuberculum cinereum).

Cerebrospinal Fluid

Cerebrospinal fluid (*liquor cerebrospinalis*) is normally a clear, colorless, slightly alkaline liquid. It contains inorganic ions, protein, sugar, and a few cells. The fluid is a few millivolts positive with respect to extracellular fluid of the body.

The rate of cerebrospinal fluid production by choroid plexuses of brain ventricles is approximately 0.05 mL/min (3 mL/hr) in the dog. Cerebrospinal fluid can be secreted against a hydrostatic gradient with sufficient force to produce dilated ventricles (hydrocephalus) in cases of impaired drainage (de Lahunta et al., 2015).

Cerebrospinal fluid is separated from extracellular fluid of nervous tissue by glial limiting membrane and either pia mater or ependyma. Solutes can be exchanged between the two fluid compartments, and cerebrospinal fluid is normally augmented by flow of extracellular fluid from nervous tissue. Large molecules, in particular, flow to cerebrospinal fluid, which thus functions like a lymphatic drainage system for the central nervous system, which lacks lymph vessels.

Flow

Cerebrospinal fluid flows from the lateral ventricles, through interventricular foramina, into the third ventricle, and, through the mesencephalic aqueduct, into the fourth ventricle. From the fourth ventricle, fluid flows into the subarachnoid space, through bilateral recesses and apertures (Fig. 16.16). A small amount of fluid from the fourth ventricle flows into the central canal and, ultimately, the terminal ventricle of the spinal cord.

Flow in the subarachnoid space is variable. During breathing, the alternate changes in thoracic and abdominal pressure cause spinal cord cerebrospinal fluid to shift cranially during inspiration and caudally during expiration. Cerebrospinal fluid currents are generated by such actions as coughing, straining, lying down, sitting up, running, jumping, and stopping owing to regional differences in blood pressure and pressure differentials caused by gravity and other accelerating influences.

Particularly in the cranial cavity, dura mater attached to the bones of the cranium forms a rigid chamber that is completely filled with nervous tissue, cerebrospinal fluid, and blood within vessels. Any volume increment in one intradural component will be opposed and must be balanced by reciprocal volume changes in one or both of the other intradural components. Central nervous system arteries undergoing sudden increased blood pressure are limited in expansion by an opposing increase in cerebrospinal fluid pressure. Pulsations in these intracranial arteries contribute to the flow of cerebrospinal fluid from the intracranial to the spinal cord subarachnoid space.

Drainage

Cerebrospinal fluid is derived from blood, principally that of choroid plexus vessels, and the fluid must ultimately be returned to the circulating blood. Because of return flow, the volume of cerebrospinal fluid remains approximately constant despite continuous fluid production. Two major drainage routes for return of cerebrospinal fluid to blood are arachnoid villi and lymphatics associated with nerves. Specific cerebrospinal fluid drainage pathways were well reviewed with regard to human cerebrospinal fluid by Sakka et al. (2011) and from a comparative perspective by Pollay (2010).

Arachnoid villi (*granulationes arachnoideales*) are projections of arachnoid membrane into dural venous sinuses (Kataoka & Wakuri, 1987) (Fig. 16.17). At a villus, cerebrospinal fluid is separated from blood by flattened fibroblasts and endothelial cells. Each villus functions as a valve regulating flow of cerebrospinal fluid into the venous sinus. When cerebrospinal fluid pressure exceeds venous pressure, villi expand and spaces between cell processes increase, allowing more fluid to flow from the subarachnoid space to the venous sinus. When pressure in the venous sinus exceeds cerebrospinal fluid pressure, the villi collapse, effectively blocking reflux of blood to the subarachnoid space. Arachnoid villi have also been reported in association with veins located at intervertebral foramina.

Cerebrospinal fluid is also drained from the distal recesses of meningeal sheaths surrounding nerve roots. Where roots continue as spinal and cranial nerves, cerebrospinal fluid escapes across the arachnoid membrane into nerve lymphatics. There is considerable fluid drainage associated with the optic (Lüdemann et al., 2005) and olfactory nerves (Leeds et al., 1989).

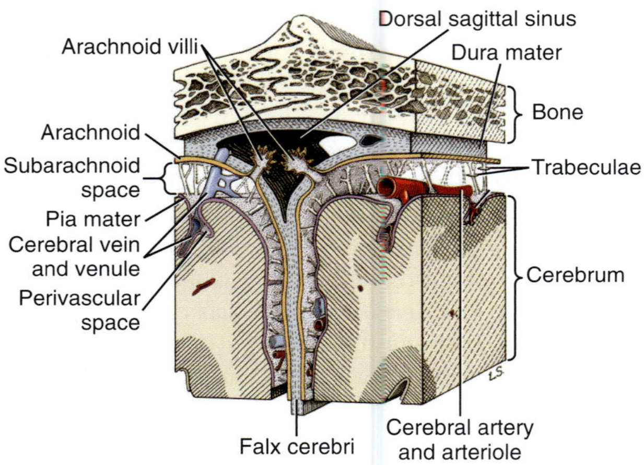

• **Fig. 16.17** Schematic view of arachnoid villi projecting into the dorsal sagittal venous sinus. The sinus is located where dura mater splits into a periosteal layer and a partition, the falx cerebri. Perivascular spaces are also shown, where large vessels penetrate the brain. (From de Lahunta, Glass and Kent: *Veterinary neuroanatomy and clinical neurology,* 4th ed., St Louis, MO, Elsevier, 2015.)

Bibliography

Allen, D. J., & Low, F. N. (1975). Scanning electron microscopy of the subarachnoid space in the dog. III. Cranial levels. *J Comp Neurol, 161,* 515–540.

Aoyama, M., Hongo, T., & Kudo, N. (1988). Sensory input to cells of origin of uncrossed spinocerebellar tract located below Clarke's column in the cat. *J Physiol Lond, 398,* 233–257.

Bessen, J. M., & Chaouch, A. (1987). Peripheral and spinal mechanisms of nociception. *Physiol Rev, 67,* 67–186.

Binder, M. D., & Mendell, L. M. (1990). *The segmental motor system.* New York: Oxford University Press.

Boivie, J. (1988). Projections from the dorsal column nuclei and the spinal cord to the red nucleus in cat. *Behav Brain Res, 28,* 75–79.

Brodal, A. (1965). Experimental anatomical studies of the corticospinal and cortico-rubrospinal connections in the cat. *Symp Biol Hung, 5,* 207–217.

Brodal, A., & Rexed, B. (1953). Spinal afferents to the lateral cervical nucleus in the cat. *J Comp Neurol, 98,* 179–211.

Brooks, V. B. (1986). *The neural basis of motor control.* New York: Oxford University Press.

Buxton, D. F., & Goodman, D. C. (1967). Motor function and the corticospinal tracts in the dog and raccoon. *J Comp Neurol, 129,* 341–360.

Casey, K. L., & Morrow, T. J. (1983). Supraspinal nocifensive responses of cats: spinal cord pathways, monoamines, and modulation. *J Comp Neurol, 270,* 591–605.

Cervero, F., & Lumb, B. M. (1988). Bilateral inputs and supraspinal control of viscerosomatic neurones in the lower thoracic spinal cord of the cat. *J Physiol, 403,* 221–237.

Craig, A. D., Heppelmann, B., & Schaible, H. G. (1988). The projection of the medial and posterior articular nerves of the cat's knee to the spinal cord. *J Comp Neurol, 276,* 279–288.

Craig, A. D., Linington, A. J., & Kniffki, K. D. (1989). Cells of origin of spinothalamic tract projections to the medial and lateral thalamus in the cat. *J Comp Neurol, 289,* 568–585.

Cummings, J. F. (1969). Thoracolumbar preganglionic neurons and adrenal innervation in the dog. *Acta Anat, 73,* 27–37.

de Lahunta, A. (1983). *Veterinary neuroanatomy and clinical neurology* (2nd ed.). Philadelphia: Saunders.

de Lahunta, A., Glass, E., & Kent, M. (2015). *Veterinary neuroanatomy and clinical neurology* (4th ed.). St Louis, MO: Elsevier.

Du, H. J., & Zhou, S. Y. (1990). Involvement of solitary tract nucleus in control of nociceptive transmission in cat spinal cord neurons. *Pain, 40,* 323–331.

Erulkar, S. D., Sprague, J. M., Whitsel, B. L., et al. (1966). Organization of the vestibular projection to the spinal cord of the cat. *J Neurophysiol, 29,* 626–664.

Evans, H. E., & de Lahunta, A. (2017). *Guide to the dissection of the dog* (8th ed.). Philadelphia: Saunders.

Fedorets, V. N. (2001). Subpial nerve plexus in the dog spinal cord [Russian]. *Morfologlia, 120,* 52–55.

Fletcher, T. F., & Kitchell, R. L. (1966a). Anatomical studies on the spinal cord segments of the dog. *Am J Vet Res, 27,* 1759–1767.

Fourie, S. L., & Kirberger, R. M. (1999). Relationship of cervical spinal cord diameter to vertebral dimensions: a radiographic study of normal dogs. *Vet Radiol Ultrasound, 40,* 137–143.

Fung, S. J., & Barnes, C. D. (1989). Raphe-produced excitation of spinal cord motoneurons in the cat. *Neuroscience, 103,* 185–190.

Grant, G., & Xu, Q. (1988). Routes of entry into the cerebellum of spinocerebellar axons from the lower part of the spinal cord: an experimental anatomical study in the cat. *Exp Brain Res, 72,* 543–561.

Ha, H., & Liu, C. (1966). Organization of the spino-cervico-thalamic system. *J Comp Neurol, 127,* 445–470.

Ha, H., & Liu, C. (1968). Cell origin of the ventral spino-cerebellar tract. *J Comp Neurol, 133,* 185–206.

Henneman, E. (1980). Motor functions of the brain stem and basal ganglia. In V. B. Mountcastle (Ed.), *Medical physiology* (14th ed.). St Louis, MO: Mosby.

Henneman, E., Somjen, G., & Carpenter, D. O. (1965). Functional significance of cell size in spinal motor neurons. *J Neurophysiol, 28,* 560–580.

Holstege, G., & Cowie, R. J. (1989). Projections from the rostral autoradiographical tracing study in the cat. *Exp Brain Res, 75,* 265–279.

Holstege, G., & Tan, J. (1988). Projections from the red nucleus and surrounding areas to the brain stem and spinal cord in the cat: an HRP and autoradiographical tracing study. *Behav Brain Res, 28,* 33–57.

Hongo, T., Kitazawa, S., Ohki, Y., & Xi, M. C. (1989). Functional identification of last-order interneurones of skin reflex pathways in the cat forelimb segments. *Brain Res, 505,* 167–170.

Horcholle-Bossavit, G., Jami, L., Thiesson, D., et al. (1988). Motor nuclei of peroneal muscles in the cat spinal cord. *J Comp Neurol, 277,* 430–440.

Hoskin, R. W., Fedorko, L. M., & Duffin, J. (1988). Projections from upper cervical inspiratory neurons to thoracic and lumbar expiratory motor nuclei in the cat. *Exp Neurol, 99,* 544–555.

Insua, D., Suárez, M.-L., & Santamarina, G. (2010). Dogs with canine counterpart of Alzheimer's disease lose noradrenergic neurons. *Neurobiol Aging, 31*(625), 635. doi:10.1016/j.neurobiolaging.2008.05.014.

Kataoka, S., & Wakuri, H. (1987). Anatomical study of canine arachnoid granulation. *Okajimas Folia Anat, 64,* 165–170.

Krahn, V. (1982). The pia mater at the site of the entry of blood vessels in the central nervous system. *Anat Embryol, 164,* 257–263.

Krstic, R. V. (1985). *General histology of the mammal.* Berlin: Springer-Verlag.

Kuypers, H. G., & Maisky, V. A. (1977). Funicular trajectories of descending brain stem pathways in cat. *Brain Res, 136,* 159–165.

Lassek, A. M., Dowd, L. M., & Weil, A. (1930). The quantitative distribution of the pyramidal tract in the dog. *J Comp Neurol, 51,* 153–163.

Leeds, S. E., Kong, A. K., & Wise, B. L. (1989). Alternative pathways for drainage of cerebrospinal fluid in the canine brain. *Lymphology, 22,* 144–146.

Leedy, M. G., Bresnahan, J. C., Mawe, G. M., et al. (1988). Differences in synaptic inputs to preganglionic neurons in the dorsal and lateral band subdivisions of the cat sacral parasympathetic nucleus. *J Comp Neurol, 268,* 84–90.

Liang, H., Paxinos, G., & Watson, C. (2012). Projections from the presumptive midbrain locomotor area to the spinal cord in the mouse. *Brain Struct Funct, 217,* 211–219.

Light, A. R., & Kavookjian, A. M. (1988). Morphology and ultrastructure of physiologically identified substantia gelatinosa (lamina II) neurons with axons that terminate in deeper dorsal horn laminae (III–V). *J Comp Neurol, 267,* 172–189.

Lu, G. W., & Yang, C. T. (1989). The morphology of cat spinal neurons projecting to both the lateral cervical nucleus and the dorsal column nuclei. *Neurosci Lett, 101,* 29–34.

Lüdemann, W., von Rautenfeld, D. B., Samii, M., & Brinker, T. (2005). Ultrastructure of the cerebrospinal fluid outflow along the optic nerve into the lymphatic system. *Child's Nerv Sys, 21,* 96–103. doi:10.1007/s00381-004-1040-1.

Marin-Garcia, P., Gonzalez-Soriano, J., Martinez-Sainz, P., et al. (1995). Spinal cord central canal of the German shepherd dog: morphological, histological and ultrastructural considerations. *J Morphol, 224,* 205–212.

Massari, V. J., Park, C. H., Suyderhoud, J. P., & Tizabi, Y. (1988). Norepinephrine throughout the spinal cord of the cat. I. Normal quantitative laminar and segmental distribution. *Synapse, 2,* 258–265.

McIntyre, A. K., Proske, U., & Rawson, J. A. (1989). Corticofugal action on transmission of group I input from the hind limb to the pericruciate cortex in the cat. *J Physiol Lond, 416,* 19–30.

Noble, R., & Riddell, J. S. (1989). Descending influences on the cutaneous receptive fields of postsynaptic dorsal column neurons in the cat. *J Physiol Lond, 408,* 167–183.

Nomina Anatomica Veterinaria. (2017). International Committee on Veterinary Gross Anatomical Nomenclature (ed. 6), Hanover.

Nyberg-Hansen, R. (1964). Origin and termination of fibers from the vestibular nuclei descending in the medial longitudinal fasciculus. *J Comp Neurol, 124,* 71–100.

Oliver, J. E., Jr., Bradley, W. E., & Fletcher, T. F. (1969). Identification of preganglionic parasympathetic neurons in the sacral spinal cord of the cat. *J Comp Neurol, 137,* 321–328.

Orlin, J. R., Osen, K. K., & Hovig, T. (1991). Subdural compartment in pig: a morphologic study with blood and horseradish peroxidase infused subdurally. *Anat Rec, 230,* 22–37.

Orsal, D., Perret, C., & Cabelguen, J. M. (1988). Comparison between ventral spinocerebellar and rubrospinal activities during locomotion in the cat. *Behav Brain Res, 28,* 159–162.

Petras, J. M. (1967). Cortical, tectal, and tegmental fiber connections in the spinal cord of the cat. *Brain Res, 6,* 275–324.

Pollay, M. (2010). The function and structure of the cerebrospinal fluid outflow system. *Cerebrospinal Fluid Res, 7,* 9. doi:10:1186/1743-8454-7-9.

Pompeiano, O., & Brodal, A. (1957). Spino-vestibular fibers in the cat, an experimental study. *J Comp Neurol, 108,* 353–381.

Purinton, P. T., & Oliver, J. E., Jr. (1979). Spinal cord origin of innervation to the bladder and urethra of the dog. *Exp Neurol, 65,* 422–434.

Rethelyi, M., Light, A. R., & Perl, E. R. (1989). Synaptic ultrastructure of functionally and morphologically characterized neurons of the superficial spinal dorsal horn of cat. *J Neurosci, 9,* 1846–1863.

Rexed, B. (1952). The cytoarchitectonic organization of the spinal cord in the cat. *J Comp Neurol, 96,* 415–495.

Rexed, B. (1954). A cytoarchitectonic atlas of the spinal cord in the cat. *J Comp Neurol, 100,* 297–379.

Romanes, G. J. (1951). The motor cell columns of the lumbosacral spinal cord of the cat. *J Comp Neurol, 94,* 313–363.

Sakka, L., Coll, G., & Chazal, J. (2011). Anatomy and physiology of cerebrospinal fluid. *Eur Ann Otolaryngol Head Neck Dis, 126,* 309–316. doi:10.1016/j.anaorl.2011.03.002.

Satomi, H., Takahashi, K., Kosaka, I., et al. (1989). Reappraisal of projection levels of the corticospinal fibers in the cat, with special reference to the fibers descending through the dorsal funiculus: a WGA-HRP study. *Brain Res, 492,* 255–260.

Shinoda, Y., Futami, T., Mitoma, H., et al. (1988). Morphology of single neurons in the cerebello-rubrospinal system. *Behav Brain Res, 28,* 59–64.

Spence, S. J., & Saint-Cyr, J. A. (1988). Comparative topography of projections from the mesodiencephalic junction to the inferior olive, vestibular nuclei, and upper cervical cord in the cat. *J Comp Neurol, 268,* 357–374.

Staal, A., & Verhaart, W. J. C. (1963). Subcortical projections on the spinal grey matter of the cat. *Acta Anat, 52,* 235–243.

Stevens, R. T., Hodge, C. J., & Apkarian, A. V. (1989). Medial, intralaminar, and lateral terminations of lumbar spinothalamic tract neurons: a fluorescent double-label study. *Somatosens Mot Res, 6,* 285–308.

Tunturi, A. R. (1982). Spinal cord tracts mediating voluntary movement of hind limb in dog. *Brain Res, 240,* 338–340.

Uehara, M., & Ueshima, T. (1988). Scanning electron microscopy of the superficial glial limiting membrane in the cat brain and spinal cord. *Jpn J Vet Sci, 50,* 115–124.

van Crevel, H., & Verhaart, W. J. C. (1963). The "exact" origin of the pyramidal tract: a quantitative study in the cat. *J Anat, 97,* 495–515.

Vinay, L., & Padel, Y. (1990). Spatio-temporal organization of the somesthetic projections in the red nucleus transmitted through the spino-rubral pathway in the cat. *Exp Brain Res, 79,* 412–426.

Watson, C., & Harrison, M. (2012). The location of the major ascending and descending spinal cord tracts in all spinal cord segments in the mouse: actual and extrapolated. *Anat Rec, 295,* 1692–1697. doi:10.1002/ar.22549.

Willis, W. D. (1985). Pain and headache. In P. L. Gildenberg (Ed.), *The pain system* (Vol. 8). New York: S. Karger.

Willis, W. D. (1986). Ascending somatosensory systems. In T. L. Yaksh (Ed.), *Spinal afferent processing.* New York: Plenum Press.

Yaksh, T. L. (1986). *Spinal afferent processing.* New York: Plenum Press.

Yezierski, R. P. (1988). Spino-mesencephalic tract: projections from the lumbosacral spinal cord of the rat, cat, and monkey. *J Comp Neurol, 267,* 131–146.

17
The Spinal Nerves

The **spinal nerves** (*nervi spinales*) (Figs. 17.1 and 17.2) usually number 36 pairs in the dog. Each spinal nerve consists of four segments from proximal to distal: (1) roots, (2) main trunk, (3) four primary branches, and (4) numerous peripheral branches (Fig. 17.3A). The roots lie within the vertebral canal and consist of a **dorsal root** (*radix dorsalis*) with a **spinal ganglion** (*ganglion spinale*), and a **ventral root** (*radix ventralis*). Each root is formed by a variable number of rootlets (*fila radicularia*) that attach to the spinal cord. Union of the dorsal and ventral roots forms the main trunk of the spinal nerve, which is located largely within the intervertebral foramen. Within the intervertebral foramen, the spinal nerve gives off a small and variable **meningeal branch** (*ramus meningeus*). After emerging from the intervertebral foramen, the spinal nerve gives off a **dorsal branch** (*ramus dorsalis*), then a **communicating branch** (*ramus communicans*), and continues as a larger **ventral branch** (*ramus ventralis*). The dorsal and ventral branches usually subdivide into medial and lateral branches, which give rise to numerous smaller branches.

The dorsal and ventral roots are found within the vertebral canal; the **spinal ganglion**, formerly the *dorsal root ganglion,* is located in the dorsal root at the junction of the dorsal and ventral roots, near the intervertebral foramen. Each dorsal and ventral root consists of a varying number of rootlets, or **root filaments** (*fila radicularia*) (Fig. 17.3B). The dorsal rootlets send axons into the spinal cord at the dorsolateral sulcus. The ventral rootlets emerge from the spinal cord at a wide, indistinct, ventrolateral sulcus. Neither the dorsal nor the ventral roots are compact units. They consist of loosely united bundles of axons, root filaments, that are difficult to differentiate from each other because of the transparency of the covering arachnoid membrane that collapses on them after death. The number of dorsal root filaments agrees closely with the number of ventral root filaments for each spinal nerve. The number of dorsal and ventral root filaments averages six each for the first five cervical nerves. They increase in size and in number to an average of seven dorsal and seven ventral filaments from the fifth cervical segment as far caudad as the second thoracic segment. From the second thoracic segment through the thirteenth thoracic segment there are two dorsal and two ventral filaments that form each thoracic nerve root.

Each dorsal and ventral root is surrounded near the spinal cord by pia and arachnoid trabeculae and then by cerebrospinal fluid in the subarachnoid space. This segment of a nerve root is often referred to as the *intradural segment*. More distally, a nerve root enters a meningeal tube formed by the arachnoid membrane and the dura mater (Fig. 16.2). This segment of a spinal nerve in a meningeal tube has been referred to as the *extradural segment* of a spinal nerve root. This is a misleading term because the meningeal tube consists of three layers of meninges, including a small subarachnoid space containing cerebrospinal fluid. If a term is warranted for this section of the roots, the tubular portion describes that component of the roots that is enveloped by all three meningeal layers. At the spinal ganglion, the meninges continue on the main trunk of the spinal nerve and its branches as the epineurium.

Because the vertebral column and the spinal cord continue to grow after birth at different rates (Chapter 16), the total length of the spinal cord is less than the length of the vertebral canal; thus the last several lumbar, the sacral, and the caudal nerves have to run increasingly longer distances before they reach the corresponding intervertebral foramina to exit from the vertebral canal. These roots have much longer intradural as well as tubular segments than do the more cranial roots (Figs. 16.4–16.6). Because the caudal part of the spinal cord (S1 caudally) and the nerves that leave it resemble a horse's tail, this part of the spinal cord (the conus medullaris), with the spinal roots coming from it, is called the *cauda equina* (see Chapter 16). The cauda equina is therefore a part of the peripheral nervous system.

The **spinal ganglia** (*ganglia spinalia*), formerly referred to as *dorsal root ganglia,* are aggregations of pseudounipolar nerve cell bodies that are located in the dorsal root within (rarely external to) the corresponding intervertebral foramen. The axons of the pseudounipolar cells divide into central and peripheral processes. The central processes form the dorsal root filaments, whereas the peripheral processes intermingle with the axons of the ventral root filaments in forming the main trunk of a spinal nerve that thus contains both sensory (afferent) and motor (efferent) fibers, commonly referred to as a *mixed* nerve.

Initial or Primary Branches of a Typical Spinal Nerve

Each spinal nerve usually has three or four primary branches arising from the main trunk. Just peripheral to the spinal ganglion, a variable **meningeal branch** (*ramus meningeus*) may arise from the main trunk and turn back into the vertebral canal. The meningeal branch consists of afferent (sensory) axons and postganglionic sympathetic axons that supply the dura mater, the dorsal longitudinal ligament, the ventral internal vertebral venous plexus, and other blood vessels located in the vertebral canal (Pederson et al., 1956). The meningeal branch in the dog is microscopic in size (Forsythe & Ghoshal, 1984). They also report that each annulus fibrosus of the intervertebral disk is supplied by meningeal branches from two or more spinal nerves.

The **dorsal branch** (*ramus dorsalis*) of a spinal nerve extends dorsad and usually divides into medial and lateral branches to epaxial muscles and the skin near the dorsal midline (Fig. 17.4).

The **ventral branch** (*ramus ventralis*) is the largest of the four primary branches. It divides into medial and lateral branches except where the ventral branches form the large brachial and lumbosacral plexuses or supply the tail. The medial and lateral branches supply hypaxial muscles of the body wall and give off lateral and ventral cutaneous branches that supply the skin of the lateral and ventral aspects of the body wall.

The **communicating branch** (rami communicantes), also called the *visceral branch,* differs from the dorsal and ventral branches in that it carries no somatic afferent or somatic efferent axons. It carries only general visceral

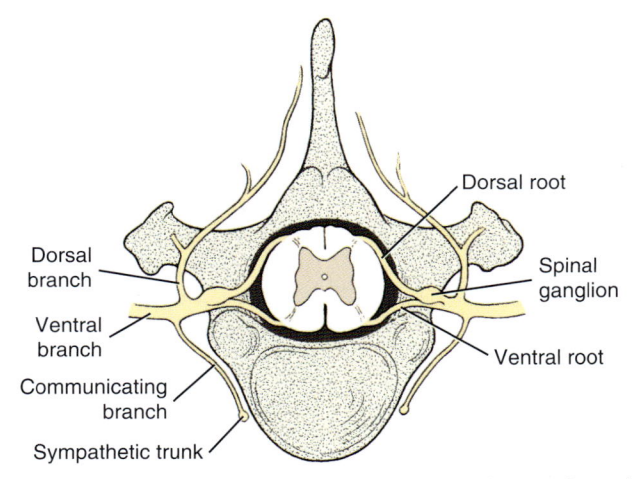

• **Fig. 17.1** Diagram of a spinal nerve. The spinal ganglion was formerly called "dorsal root ganglion."

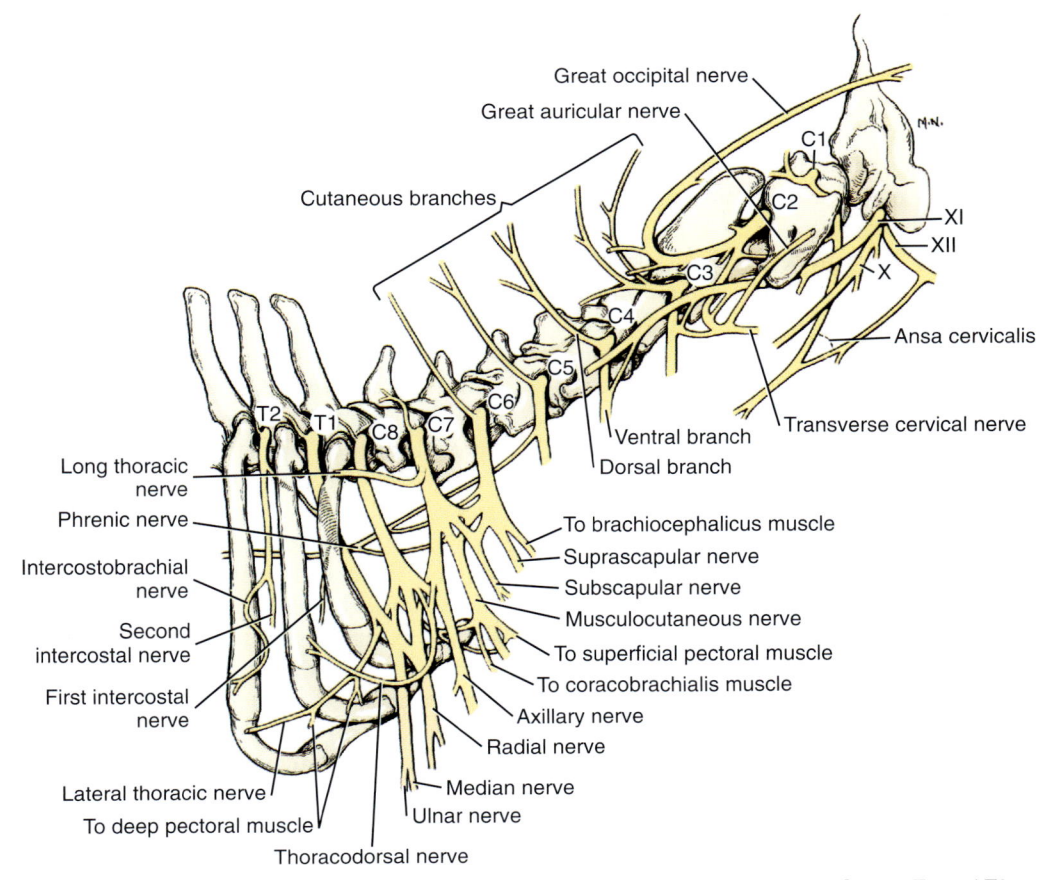

• **Fig. 17.2** Schema of the cervical nerves and brachial plexus. The labels C1 through C8 and T1 and T2 refer to spinal nerves, not vertebrae.

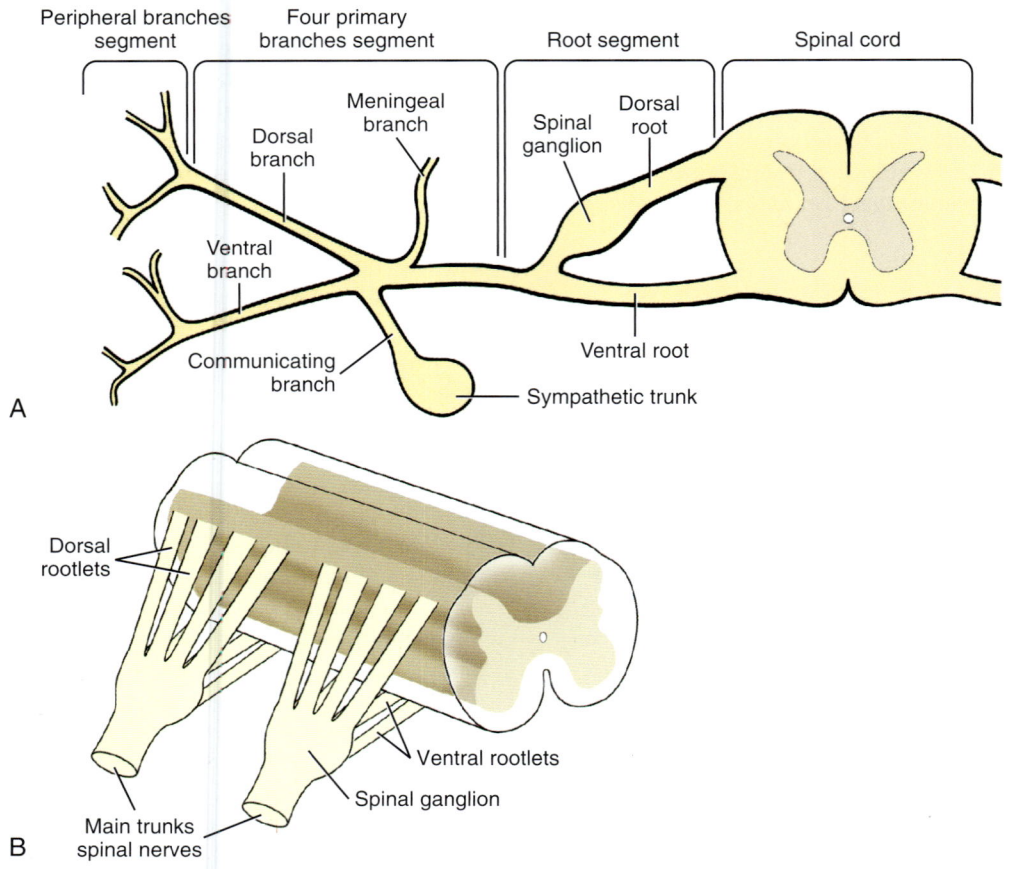

• **Fig. 17.3** **A**, Schematic drawing of the longitudinal segments of a typical spinal nerve. **B**, Schematic drawing of the dorsal and ventral rootlets of a typical spinal nerve.

afferent and efferent axons to and from visceral structures (gland tissue and smooth muscle). The efferent axons are preganglionic sympathetic axons.

The spinal nerves usually leave the vertebral canal through spaces between adjacent vertebrae, the **intervertebral foramina**. The number of vertebrae and the number of spinal nerves for each vertebral region are not always the same. There are eight pairs of cervical nerves, but only seven cervical vertebrae. In most dogs, there are 20 caudal vertebrae, but only the first five pairs of caudal nerves usually develop.

The three sacral vertebrae are fused to form the sacrum, and there are two dorsal and two ventral pairs of sacral foramina for the passage of the dorsal and ventral branches of the first two pairs of sacral nerves. The third pair of sacral nerves pass through intervertebral foramina located between the sacrum and the first caudal vertebra.

General Features of Spinal Nerves

Functionally, peripheral branches of the dorsal and ventral primary branches of spinal nerves can be classified as sensory nerves with axons from the skin (cutaneous branches) or deeper, nonmuscular structures; motor nerves with efferent axons to muscle and afferent axons from receptors in muscle; or mixed, giving off both sensory and motor branches.

Most spinal nerves leave the vertebral canal through intervertebral foramina formed between the pedicles of adjacent vertebrae. The foramina through which the first cervical nerves pass (the lateral vertebral foramina) are not located between the skull and the atlas, but in the craniodorsal portion of the dorsal arch of the atlas (Fig. 17.2). The second pair of cervical nerves leave the vertebral canal through the first pair of intervertebral foramina, which are located between the atlas and the axis. The last, or eighth, pair of cervical nerves passes through the seventh intervertebral foramina, which are located between the seventh cervical and the first thoracic vertebrae. Therefore the cervical nerves leave the vertebral canal via intervertebral foramina cranial to the vertebra of the same number with the exception of the first and last pairs of cervical nerves. Each spinal nerve from the first thoracic nerve caudally leaves the vertebral canal through the intervertebral foramen caudal to the pedicle of same numbered vertebra. For example, the sixth thoracic spinal nerve leaves the vertebral canal through the intervertebral foramen caudal to the sixth thoracic vertebra.

Peripherally, fasciculi from branches of spinal nerves often intermingle to form plexuses. Two types of plexuses exist. Plexuses supplying the body wall and the appendages are referred to as *somatic plexuses*. No cell bodies of neurons are located in somatic plexuses; thus no synapses are found in them. Plexuses found around arteries supplying the viscera and in the walls of visceral organs are called *visceral plexuses*. Visceral plexuses may have associated ganglia with cell bodies of autonomic sympathetic neurons in them and thus have synapses occurring within them (see the section on the autonomic nervous system in Chapter 15). Two major somatic plexuses, and a number of minor somatic plexuses, are recognized. The two major somatic plexuses consist of intermingling axons coming from ventral branches of spinal nerves. The **brachial plexus** (*plexus brachialis*) serves the thoracic limb, and the **lumbosacral plexus** (*plexus lumbosacralis*) serves the pelvic limb.

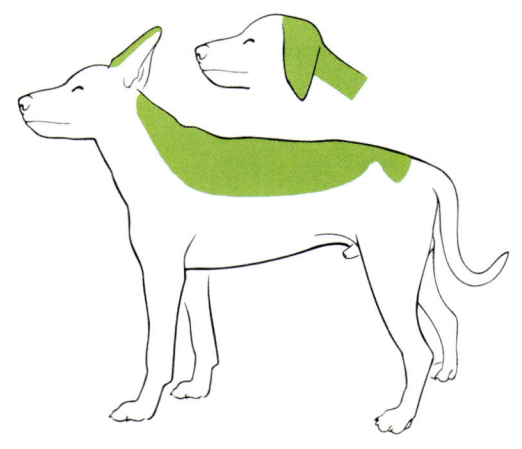

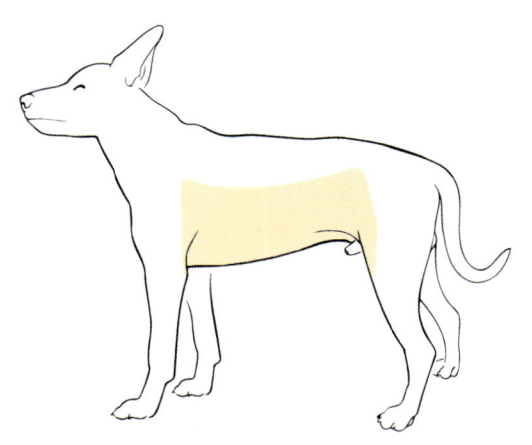

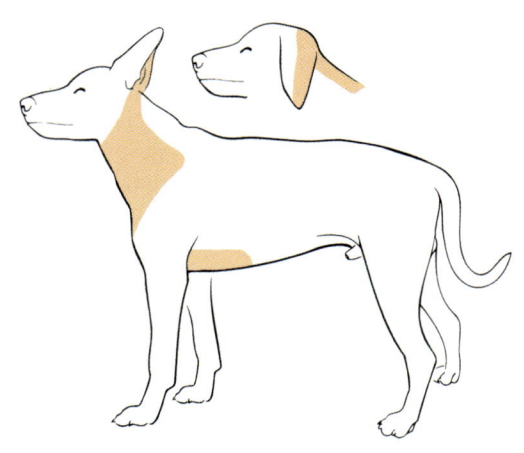

Cutaneous branches of spinal nerves have a definite pattern of origin from the spinal nerves except for cutaneous branches arising from peripheral branches of the brachial and lumbosacral plexuses (Fig. 17.5). **Dorsal cutaneous branches** (*rami cutaneus dorsales*) are only present in cervical nerves 3 through 6. Here they are branches of the medial branch of the dorsal primary branch of the cervical nerves. In the thoracic and lumbar nerves, **medial** and **lateral cutaneous branches** (*rami cutaneus medialis et lateralis*) arise from the lateral branch of the dorsal primary branch of these spinal nerves. Lateral cutaneous branches also arise from the ventral primary branches of thoracic nerves 2 through 8 and the first three lumbar nerves of the lumbar plexus. **Ventral cutaneous branches** (*rami cutaneus ventrales*) arise from the ventral primary branches of thoracic nerves 2 through 10. There are no lateral or ventral cutaneous branches of cervical nerves and no dorsal cutaneous branches of thoracic or lumbar nerves.

A cutaneous region innervated by afferent axons (dorsal root axons) from a single spinal nerve is termed a **dermatome**. Dermatomes usually form continuous fields and are arranged serially on the body from cranial to caudal in an overlapping fashion. Most dermatomes overlap to the extent that most skin areas are innervated by receptors from three spinal nerves. The migration and merging of somites provides multiple innervation of the musculature and deeper structures, but not the skin, especially in the skin over the trunk, where autonomous zones are present. The dermatomes in the dog have not been extensively studied except for the caudal thoracic, lumbar, and sacral spinal nerves (Fletcher & Kitchell, 1966b). These are discussed with the nerve supply to the pelvic limb.

The musculature innervated by a single spinal nerve (general somatic efferents from a single ventral root) is termed a **myotome**. Individual neck and trunk muscles are formed by a merger of adjacent somites; thus muscles are innervated by multiple spinal nerves. This is most readily apparent in long muscles, such as the abdominal muscles. In the limbs, where muscles are supplied by nerves arising from the large somatic plexuses, the regional nerves contain axons from two or more spinal nerves.

• **Fig. 17.4** Schematic illustration of the areas supplied by dorsal, lateral, and ventral branches of spinal nerves. The skin of the limbs is innervated by cutaneous branches of the nerves arising from the brachial and lumbosacral plexuses.

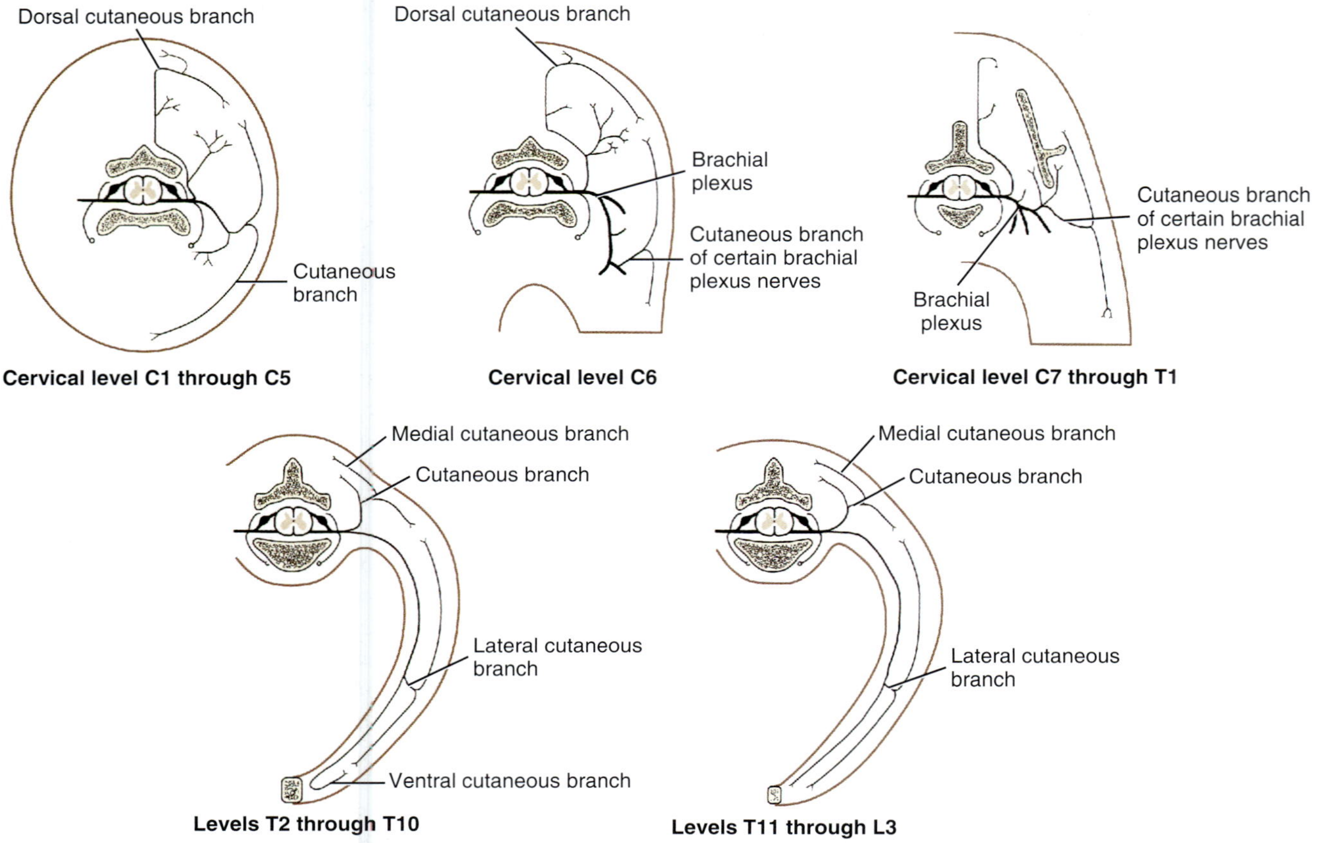

• **Fig. 17.5** Schematic illustration of cutaneous innervation. Note that the dorsal cutaneous branches in the cervical region arise from the medial branches of the dorsal branches, whereas in the thoracic and lumbar areas they arise from the lateral branches. (Modified, with permission, from Kitchell RL, Whalen LR, Bailey CS, et al: Electrophysiologic studies of cutaneous nerves of the thoracic limb of the dog, Am J Vet Res 41:61–76, 1980.)

Cervical Nerves

There are eight pairs of cervical nerves (*nn. cervicales*) (Fig. 17.2), although there are only seven cervical vertebrae. Many ventral branches of cervical nerves communicate with one another and run variable distances in common before joining still other branches. This results in the formation of a variable **cervical plexus** (*plexus cervicalis*) that can include axons of all cervical nerves.

The **first cervical nerve** (*n. cervicalis I*) (Fig. 17.2) arises from the first segment of the spinal cord, which is located just caudal to the foramen magnum, and is surrounded by the cranial portion of the atlas. Both its dorsal and its ventral formative root filaments number from three to five and are approximately equal in size. In most specimens a barely distinguishable spinal ganglion is present, whereas in others it may be 1 mm in diameter. On emerging through the lateral vertebral foramen of the atlas, the first cervical nerve divides into dorsal and ventral branches of equal size, measuring approximately 2 mm in diameter.

The **dorsal branch of the first cervical nerve** (*ramus dorsalis n. cervicalis I*), or the **suboccipital nerve** (*n. suboccipitalis*), does not divide into medial and lateral branches and does not have any cutaneous branches. It lies initially deep to the cranial part of the large obliquus capitis caudalis muscle. It arborizes in the muscles of the cranial portion of the neck. These include the obliquus capitis cranialis, obliquus capitis caudalis, rectus capitis dorsalis major, rectus capitis dorsalia minor, and the cranial ends of the semispinalis capitis and splenius.

The **ventral branch of the first cervical nerve** (*ramus ventralis n. cervicalis I*) initially lies in the osseous groove of the atlas, which runs transversely to the alar notch from the lateral vertebral foramen. The ventral branch passes through the alar notch and continues in a ventrocaudal direction by passing between the mm. rectus capitis lateralis and rectus capitis ventralis. It is initially covered by the medial retropharyngeal lymph node. After running past the caudal border of this lymph node, the ventral branch continues its course caudally in the neck in close relation to the vago-sympathetic nerve trunk. It usually communicates with the smaller descending branch of the hypoglossal nerve to form the **cervical loop** (*ansa cervicalis*) (Fig. 17.2). Variations in the formation of the cervical loop are common (see Benson and Fletcher [1971] regarding the variability of the ansa cervicalis). In approximately 3% of dogs it fails to develop.

The ansa cervicalis may be a long loop measuring 10 cm. Usually the cervical loop extends to a level through the third cervical vertebra, but in some dogs it is short, lying on the carotid sheath approximately 2 cm caudal to the paracondylar process. Several branches arise from the cervical loop. As the sternothyroid and sternohyoid muscles cross the larynx, they each receive a branch from the loop that, according to Benson and Fletcher (1971), comes largely from the hypoglossal nerve. Another branch runs caudad on the trachea and bifurcates near the middle of the neck. The shorter of these branches becomes related to the middle of the lateral border of the m. sternothyroideus before entering its distal portion. The longer branch follows the lateral border of the m. sternohyoideus caudally and enters the muscle approximately 4 cm cranial to the manubrium of the sternum. The ventral branch of the first cervical nerve has no cutaneous branches.

The **second cervical nerve** (*n. cervicalis II*) differs from other typical spinal nerves in three respects. First, its afferent component (number and size of dorsal rootlets) is larger than that of any of the other cervical or thoracic nerves. Second, the dorsal and ventral roots fuse peripheral to the second intervertebral foramen. Third, the large spinal ganglion lies completely outside of the vertebral canal.

The **dorsal branch of the second cervical nerve** (*ramus dorsalis n. cervicalis II*), or the **greater occipital nerve** (*n. occipitalis major*), is approximately the same size as the ventral branch (3 mm in diameter in a large dog). It runs caudodorsally (Figs. 17.2 and 17.7), where it is located deep to the obliquus capitis caudalis. Emerging between this muscle and the spine of the axis, it sends muscular branches into the semispinalis capitis and the splenius. It then turns cranially, perforates the overlying muscles, and gives off cutaneous branches to the skin that cover most of the dorsal aspects of the temporal muscle and the medial border and caudal aspect of the pinna (convex surface), including the apex of the pinna (Fig. 17.8). Rostrally its cutaneous area extends around the medial border of the pinna on to the rostral aspect (concave surface) of the pinna, where it overlaps with the rostral border of the cutaneous area of the auricular branches of the facial nerve dorsally and of the auriculotemporal nerve from the mandibular nerve from the trigeminal nerve ventrally (Whalen & Kitchell, 1983a,b). The rostroventral border of its cutaneous area overlaps the cutaneous area of the frontal nerve, a branch of the ophthalmic nerve from the trigeminal nerve. Caudally the cutaneous area of the greater occipital nerve overlaps dorsomedially with the cutaneous area of the dorsal cutaneous branch of the third cervical nerve and laterally with the cutaneous area of the greater auricular nerve from the ventral branch of the second cervical nerve on the caudal (convex) surface of the pinna.

The **ventral branch of the second cervical nerve** (*ramus ventralis cervicalis II*) runs caudoventrad on the lateral surface of the mastoid part of the cleidocephalicus muscle for 1 or 2 cm and divides into two ventral cutaneous branches, the **transverse cervical** and **great auricular nerves** (Fig. 17.2).

The **transverse cervical nerve** (*n. transversus colli*), formerly the *n. cutaneus colli,* runs cranioventrad deep to the

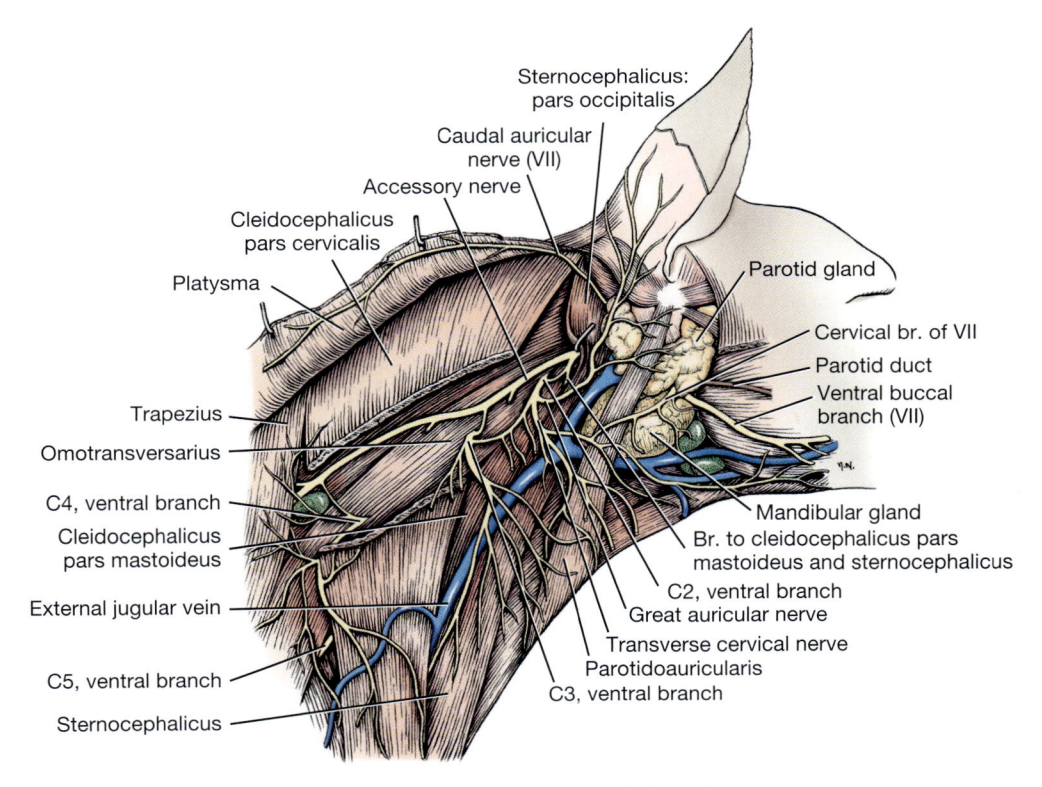

• **Fig. 17.6** Superficial nerves of the neck, lateral aspect.

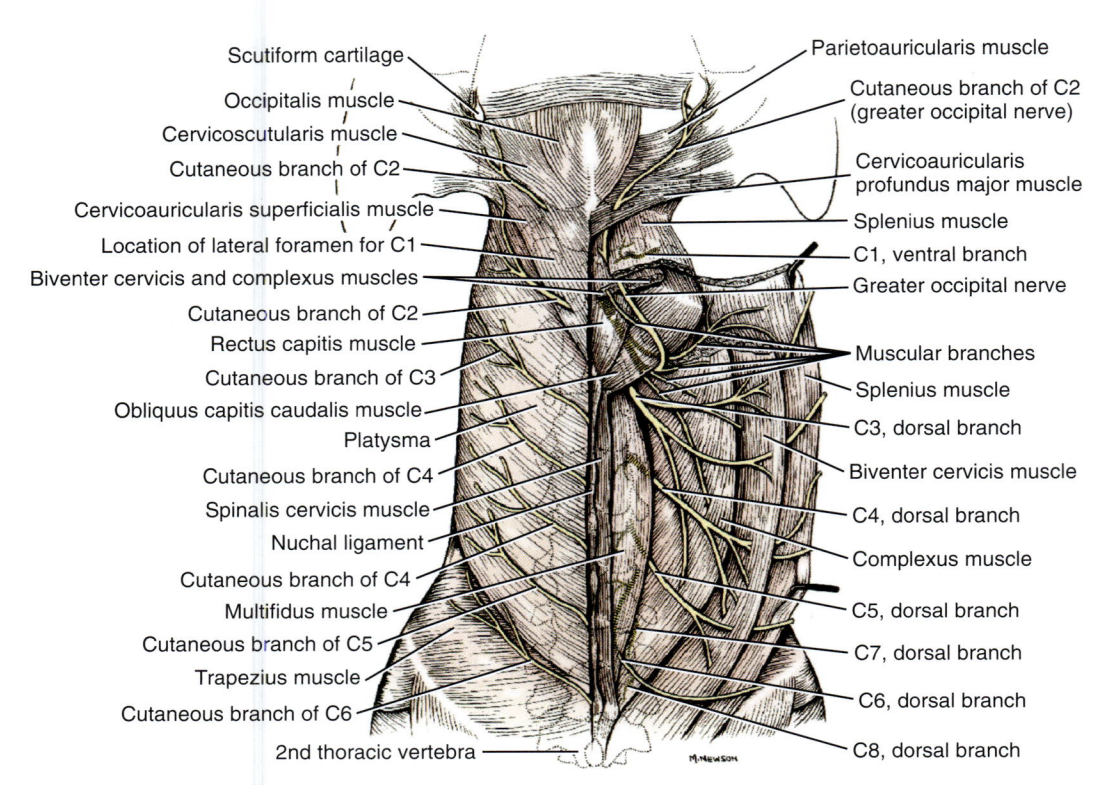

• **Fig. 17.7** Dorsal branches of the cervical nerves, dorsal aspect. (The muscles on the right side are reflected.) Although C6 and C7 nerves appear reversed on the right side of this view, their identity is revealed by deeper dissection demonstrating their point of emergence from the vertebral column.

platysma and crosses the maxillary and linguofacial veins just before they unite to form the external jugular vein. The nerve may branch before crossing these veins. The branches of this nerve arborize in the skin between the mandibles where its cutaneous area (Fig. 17.8) overlaps with the cutaneous areas of the mylohyoid nerve from the mandibular nerve ventrally and the auriculotemporal nerve from the mandibular nerve from the fifth cranial nerve (Whalen & Kitchell, 1983a).

The **great auricular nerve** (*n. auricularis magnus*) is the larger of the two terminal branches of the ventral branch of the second cervical nerve. It runs dorsocranially to the base of the pinna of the ear and divides into at least two branches, which run toward the apex of the ear. Each of these nerves runs approximately midway between the intermediate auricular artery and the peripheral arteries—the lateral and the medial auricular arteries—as they arborize in their course toward the apex of the ear. Variations in both the numbers and the distribution of the arteries and nerves to the pinna are common. The greater auricular nerve has a cutaneous area that covers the lateral two-thirds of the caudal (convex) surface and the lateral border of the pinna. The latter overlaps on the rostral (concave) surface (Fig. 17.8). It overlaps with the cutaneous areas of the greater occipital nerve on the caudal surface of the ear and the auricular branches of the seventh cranial nerve on the rostral surface of the ear (Whalen & Kitchell, 1983a).

The **dorsal branches of cervical nerves 3 through 7** (*rami dorsales nn. cervicales III-VII*) (Fig. 17.7) vary in both their distributions and their form. Each of these branches sends a small branch medially into the m. multifidus cervicis. Only their peripheral portions definitely divide into medial (cutaneous) and lateral (muscular) branches. The dorsal branches of cervical nerves 3 through 7 gradually decrease in size caudally. The seventh dorsal cervical branch is reduced to a small muscular branch that innervates only the deep muscle fibers that lie adjacent to it. The dorsal branch of the eighth cervical nerve may be absent. The dorsal branches of the middle cervical nerves perforate the lateral portion of the multifidus cervicis and run dorsally with a slight caudal inclination. On reaching the ventral portion of the biventer cervicis, they usually bifurcate into medial and lateral branches. The third dorsal branch divides near its origin, and the fourth dorsal branch may also divide deeply.

The **lateral branch** of the ramus dorsalis of cervical nerve 3 is a muscle nerve with no cutaneous branches. It supplies the middle portion of the complexus muscle. The main lateral branches of the rami dorsales of cervical nerves 4 and 5 innervate the middle portion of the biventer muscle. The splenius muscle is innervated by branches that come from the rami dorsales of cervical nerves 3 and 4, which leave near their origins. The branches enter the deep surface of the middle and caudal parts of the muscle. The cranial part

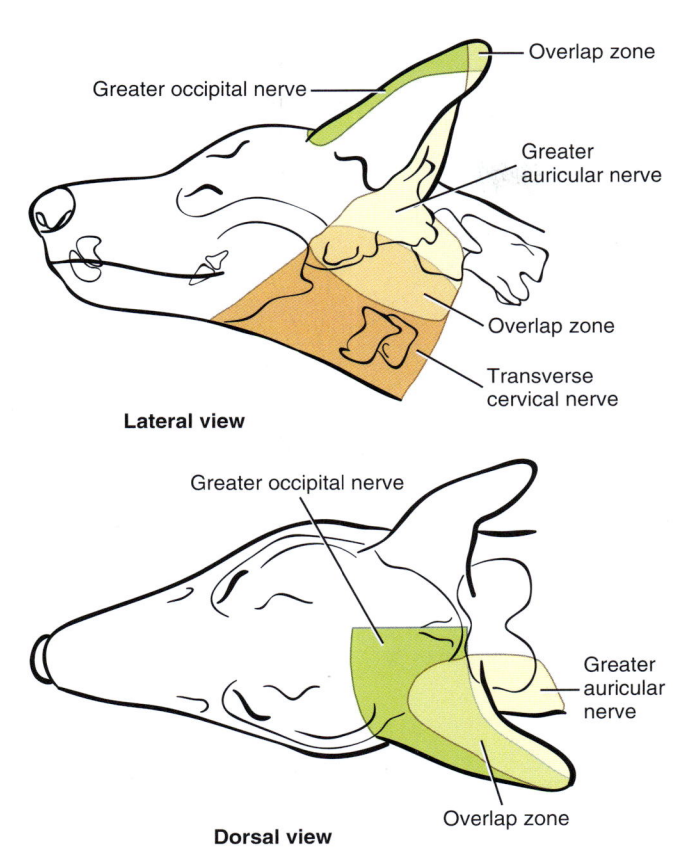

• **Fig. 17.8** Schematic illustration of the cutaneous areas of the cutaneous branch of the dorsal branch of the second cervical nerve (greater occipital) and the cutaneous branch of the ventral branch of the second cervical nerve (greater auricular). Note the extensive overlap zone of these three nerves. (Modified, with permission, from Whalen LR, Kitchell RL: Electrophysiologic studies of the cutaneous nerves of the head of the dog, *Am J Vet Res* 44:615–627, 1983.)

of the splenius muscle is supplied by large muscular branches from the dorsal branch of cervical nerve 2.

The **medial branches** of the rami dorsales of cervical nerves 3 through 7 perforate the m. intertransversarius dorsalis and run almost directly dorsad (Fig. 17.7). In their dorsal courses they lie between the multifidus cervicis and spinalis cervicis muscles located medially and the complexus and biventer muscles (the two portions of the semispinalis capitis) located laterally. The dorsal cutaneous branches are a continuation of these branches of cervical nerves 3 through 6. They run dorsally in the midline to cross the lateral side of the ligamentum nuchae to reach the skin (Kitchell et al., 1980; Whalen & Kitchell, 1983a). In most specimens the third and fourth medial dorsal cervical branches further divide into cranial (dorsal) and caudal (ventral) parts. They thus appear by their spacing in the subcutaneous fascia as if they were branches of separate cervical nerves. Bilaterally these **dorsal cutaneous branches** (*rami cutaneus dorsales*) innervate the loose, thick skin of the dorsal and adjacent sides of the neck. Their cutaneous areas are aligned in a segmental manner along the dorsum of the cervical region (Figs. 17.9 and 17.10). There are no dorsal cutaneous branches for cervical nerves 7 and 8 (Kitchell et al., 1980).

The cutaneous area of the dorsal cutaneous branch of cervical nerve 6 overlaps with the cutaneous area of the medial cutaneous branch of thoracic nerve 2 (Fig. 17.10).

The **ventral branches** of cervical nerves 2 through 5 (Fig. 17.6) pass between the muscle bundles of the intertransversarius cervicis to reach the medial surface of the omotransversarius. The ventral branches of cervical nerves 2, 3, and 4 regularly intermingle with the accessory nerve, however, and a connection between cervical nerves 2 and 3 is frequent. The ventral branch of the large, second cervical nerve has been described. The ventral branches of the third and fourth cervical nerves supply the skin of the ventrolateral part of the neck (Fig. 17.9) via **supraclavicular nerves** (*nn. supraclaviculares*) and smaller medial (muscular) branches (*rami mediales*) that supply the longus capitis, longus colli, intertransversarius cervicis, omotransversarius, and brachiocephalicus muscles. The medial branches appear as loose clusters of nerves that arise just peripheral to the intervertebral foramina and, after short caudoventral courses, enter the several muscles. The size of the ventral branches of the second to the fifth cervical nerves decreases progressively. The ventral branch of the second cervical nerve is approximately three times larger than that of the fifth. The cutaneous areas of the cutaneous branches of the ventral branches of cervical nerves 2 through 5 are quite large (Figs. 17.9 and 17.10). This cutaneous area of cervical nerve 5 extends onto the brachium, supplying the craniolateral and medial surfaces of that region (Fig. 17.10). Caudodorsally it overlaps with the cutaneous area of the cutaneous cranial lateral brachial nerve from the axillary nerve. Caudomedially it overlaps with the cutaneous area of the nerve to the brachiocephalicus and ventromedially with the cutaneous area of the ventral cutaneous branch of the second thoracic nerve.

Nerves to the Diaphragm

The cervical origins of the **phrenic nerve** (*n. phrenicus*) (Fig. 17.2) reflect the fact that the diaphragm that it supplies has a cervical origin. The phrenic nerve regularly arises from the fifth, sixth, and seventh cervical nerves, and occasionally a small branch comes from the fourth.

The branches of origin of the phrenic nerve run caudally, dorsomedial to the brachial plexus. While running in the fascia adjacent to the external jugular vein, these nerve branches converge and unite to form the phrenic nerve just cranial to the thoracic inlet. The nerve on each side then passes through the thoracic inlet ventral to the subclavian artery and dorsal to the superficial cervical artery. At this site it is joined by a fine branch from the middle cervical ganglion or the sympathetic trunk adjacent to the ganglion. Within the thorax the right phrenic nerve lies in a narrow plica of pleura from the right lamina of the cranial and middle mediastinum pleura and the plica venae cavae. The left phrenic nerve lies in a similar plica from the entire left pleural sheet of the mediastinum. Each phrenic nerve spreads out on its respective half of the diaphragm,

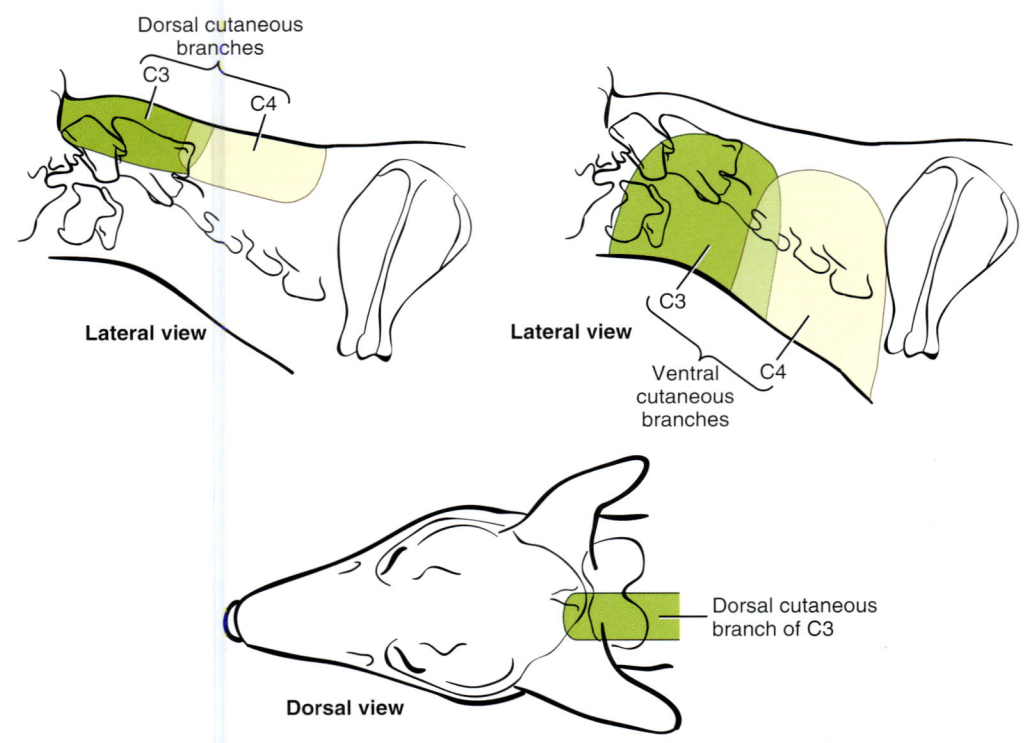

• **Fig. 17.9** Schematic illustration of the cutaneous areas of the cutaneous branches of the third and fourth cervical nerves. (Modified, with permission, from Whalen LR, Kitchell RL: Electrophysiologic studies of the cutaneous nerves of the head of the dog, *Am J Vet Res* 44:615–627, 1983.)

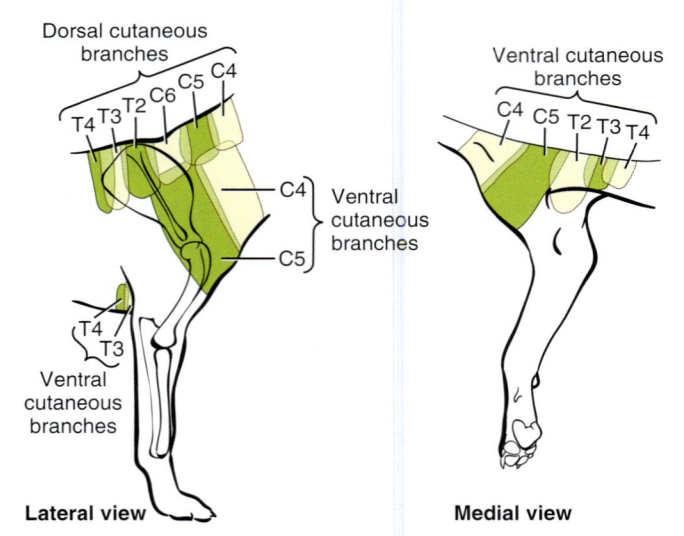

• **Fig. 17.10** Schematic illustration of the cutaneous areas of the caudal cervical, and cranial thoracic nerves. Observe that the cutaneous areas of the dorsal cutaneous branches of the sixth cervical and the second thoracic overlap. (There are no cutaneous branches for the seventh and eighth cervical and the first thoracic spinal nerves.) Also note that the cutaneous area for the ventral cutaneous branch of the fifth cervical nerve overlaps with the cutaneous area of the ventral cutaneous branch of the second thoracic spinal nerve. (Modified, with permission, from Kitchell RL, Whalen LR, Bailey CS, et al: Electrophysiologic studies of cutaneous nerves of the thoracic limb of the dog, *Am J Vet Res* 41:61–76, 1980.)

where it supplies this muscle with motor and sensory fibers. On reaching the diaphragm, each phrenic nerve divides into three main branches: ventral, lateral, and dorsal. This splitting takes place lateral to the middle portion of the tendinous center. Each nerve division supplies its appropriate third of its half of the diaphragm. Each dorsal branch therefore supplies the crus of its side. There usually is a connection between each phrenic nerve and the sympathetic system at the celiac plexus. It is generally agreed that the phrenic nerves are the only motor nerves to the diaphragm (Botha, 1957) and that the left and right portions of the diaphragm are controlled by discrete ipsilateral phrenic nerve bundles (Hammond et al., 1989). De Troyer et al. (1982) reported that C5 portions of the phrenic nerve primarily innervate costal diaphragm while C7 is distributed to the crural diaphragm. The periphery of the diaphragm also receives sensory fibers from the last several intercostal nerves (Lemon, 1928) although afferent feedback from the diaphragm appears poorly understood (Pickering & Jones, 2002). Further review of sensory nerves and their role in the diaphragm may be found in Teitelbaum et al. (1993), Nair et al. (2017), Davenport et al. (1985), and De Troyer (1998).

Brachial Plexus

The **brachial plexus** (*plexus brachialis*) (Figs. 17.11 to 17.13) is a large somatic nerve plexus that gives origin to the nerves that supply the thoracic limb. It is usually formed by the ventral branches of the sixth, seventh, and eighth

CHAPTER 17 The Spinal Nerves   713

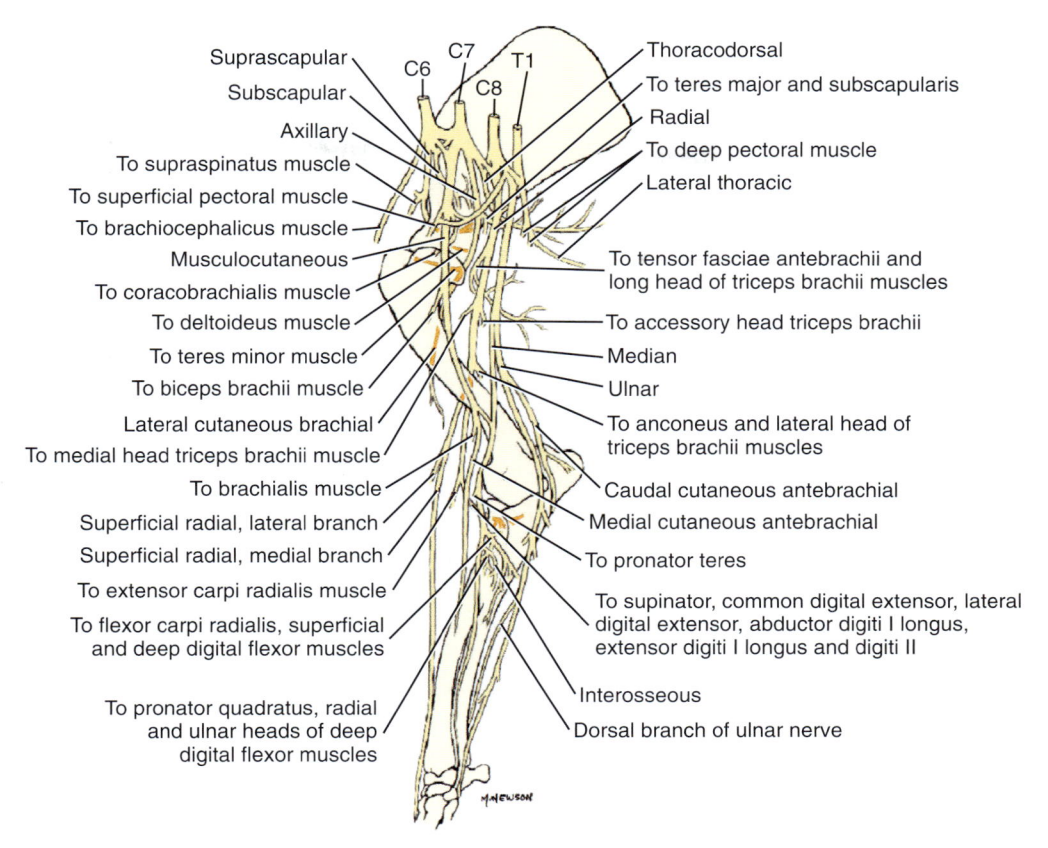

- Fig. 17.11 Schema of the nerves of the right thoracic limb, medial aspect.

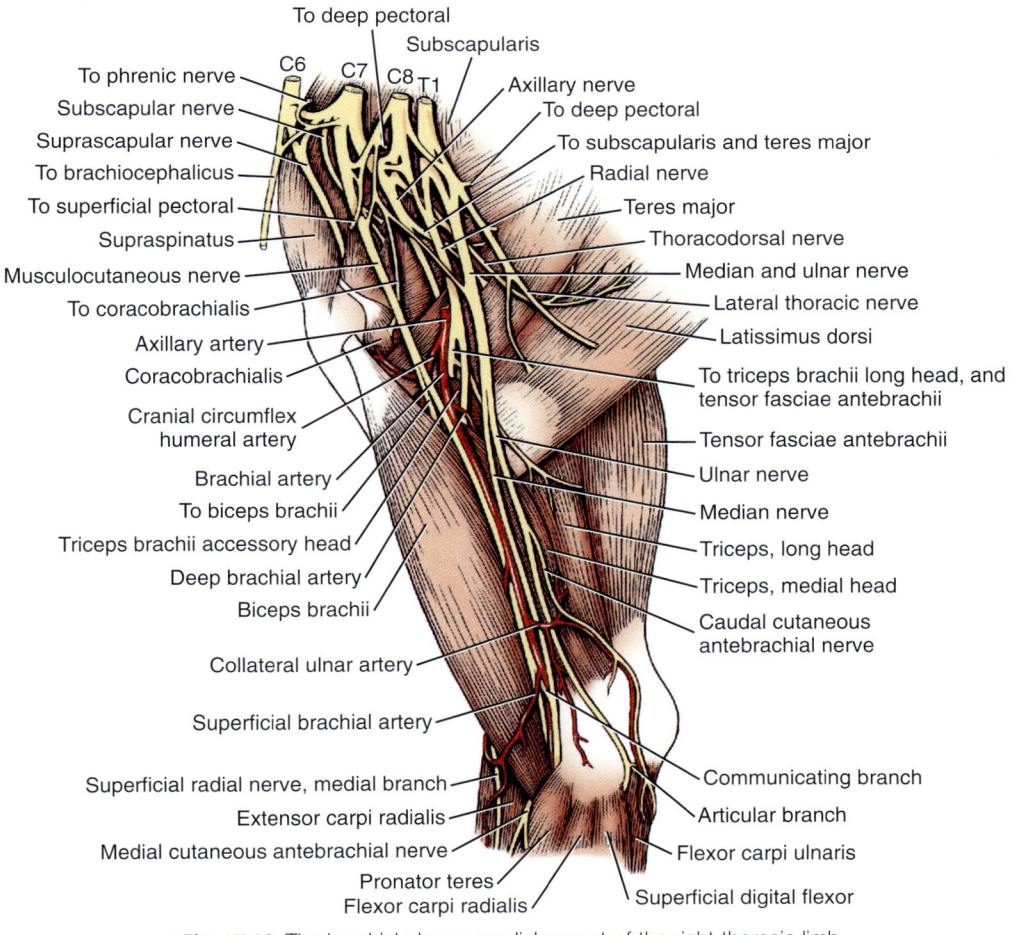

- Fig. 17.12 The brachial plexus, medial aspect of the right thoracic limb.

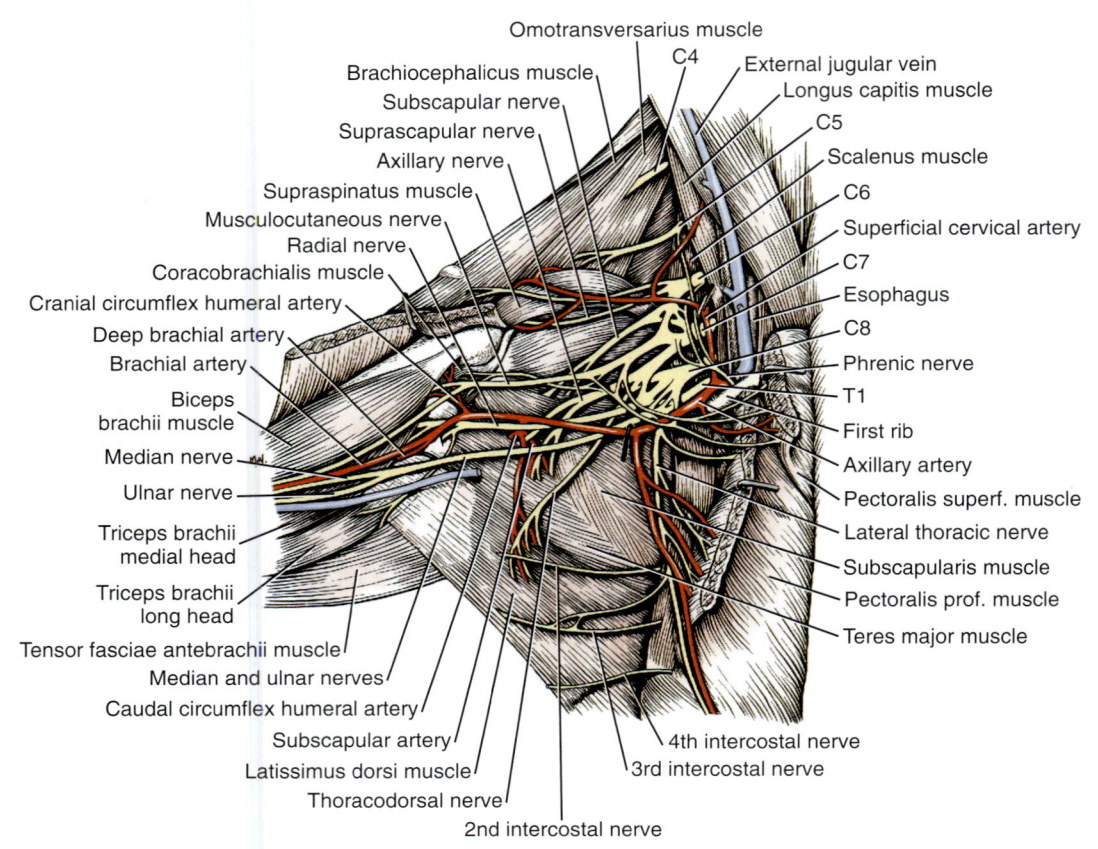

• Fig. 17.13 The right brachial plexus, medial aspect.

cervical and the first and second thoracic spinal nerves. Occasionally, the ventral branch of the fifth cervical nerve also contributes to its formation; frequently, the second thoracic contribution is lacking. When either or both the fifth cervical and the second thoracic spinal nerves send branches that enter into the formation of the brachial plexus, they are exceedingly small compared with the other ventral branches that compose the plexus. In more than 250 dissections, neither one of these nerves was found to be more than 1 mm in diameter. Allam et al. (1952) found in 58 dissections that the fifth cervical and the second thoracic nerve contributions to the brachial plexus are more often absent than present.

Ventral branches of the cervical (C) and thoracic (T) spinal nerves that form the brachial plexus are distributed in a variable manner. They were grouped as follows in dogs studied by Allam et al. (1952): 58.62% formed by C6, C7, C8, and T1; 20.69% formed by C5, C6, C7, C8, and T1; 17.24% formed by C6, C7, C8, T1, and T2; and 3.4% formed by C5, C6, C7, C8, T1, and T2.

In an electrophysiologic study of the dorsal (afferent) roots contributing to the cutaneous branches of the nerves arising from the brachial plexus in 8 of 10 dogs, C6, C7, C8, T1, and T2 contributed axons; in 1 of 10 dogs, C6, C7, C8, and T1 contributed; and in another dog, C5, C6, C7, C8, and T1 contributed (Bailey et al., 1982). In another electrophysiologic study of the ventral (efferent) root contributions in six of six dogs, the ventral roots of C6, C7, C8, T1, and T2 all contributed efferent fibers to the brachial plexus (Sharp et al., 1990, 1991). After the ventral branches of the last three cervical and the first and second thoracic spinal nerves have passed through the intertransverse musculature, they cross the ventral border of the scalenus muscle and extend to the thoracic limb by traversing the axillary space. In this course, parts of these nerves unite with each other and exit the plexus as various specific named nerves that supply the structures of the thoracic limb and adjacent muscles and skin. The axillary artery and vein lie ventromedial to the caudal portion of the brachial plexus. The external jugular vein, after it has been augmented by the proximal tributary of the cephalic vein, crosses the ventral surfaces of the seventh and eighth cervical nerves, from which it is separated by the superficial cervical artery. The axillary artery, after having crossed the cranial margin of the first rib, lies closely applied to the ventral margin of the scalenus ventralis and later follows along the craniomedial margin of the radial nerve as both the artery and the nerve run distad in the brachium. They are crossed ventrally at the first rib by a muscular nerve branch that goes to the deep pectoral muscle.

Allam et al. (1952) described three cords (*trunci plexus*) in the brachial plexus of the dog to assist the exploring surgeon by establishing suitable landmarks for electrical stimulation. These cords lie as intermediate nerve trunks

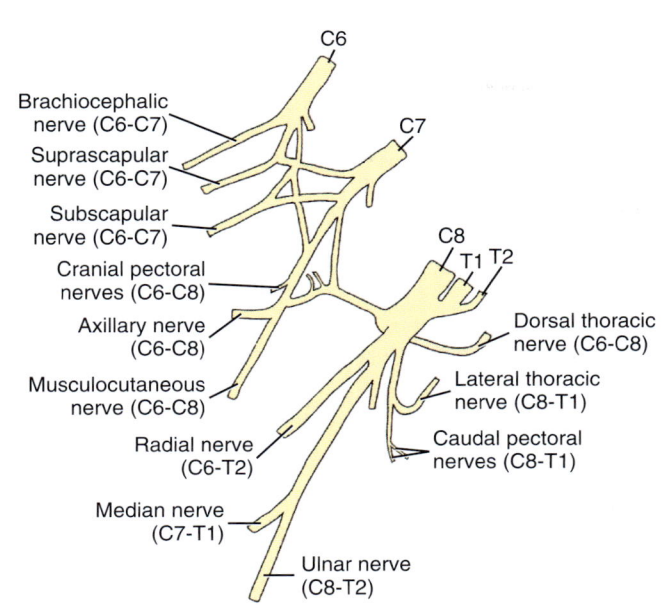

Fig. 17.14 Schematic illustration of the brachial plexus showing the most common spinal root origin of the various nerves arising from the plexus. (Based on the results of Sharp JS, Bailey CS, Johnson RD, et al.: Spinal nerve root origin of the median, ulnar, and musculocutaneous nerves and their muscle nerve branches to the canine forelimb, *Anat Histol Embryol* 19:359–368, 1990; and Sharp JS, Bailey CS, Johnson RD, et al.: Spinal root origin of the radial nerve and of nerves innervating the shoulder muscles of the dog, *Anat Histol Embryol* 20:205–214, 1991.)

between the ventral branches of the spinal nerves that form the plexus and the named nerves that innervate structures of the limb. These trunks vary considerably. For further information on the morphologic features of the brachial plexus of the dog, refer to Russell (1893), Reimers (1925), Miller (1934), and Bowne (1959).

The nerves that are branches of the brachial plexus or are direct continuations of the formative ventral branches include the suprascapular, subscapular, axillary, musculocutaneous, radial, median, ulnar, dorsal thoracic, lateral thoracic, long thoracic, pectoral, and muscular branches. The term *radices plexus* refers to the contributions of the ventral spinal nerves that form the brachial plexus. Some of the radices may form trunks (*trunci plexus*) prior to forming the definitive brachial plexus.

The basic plan of the brachial plexus appears as a variable communication of the last three cervical and first two thoracic nerve ventral primary branches, whose axons run in common for short distances and then segregate in variable combinations to form the extrinsic and intrinsic named nerves of the thoracic limb (Fig. 17.14).

Nerves of the Brachial Plexus That Supply Intrinsic Muscles of the Thoracic Limb

The **suprascapular nerve** (*n. suprascapularis*) arises primarily and occasionally entirely from the sixth cervical nerve (Fig. 17.14). It often has a contribution from the seventh, but rarely from the fifth, cervical nerve. According to Sharp et al. (1991), this nerve arose from both C6 and C7 in six of six dogs. In this nerve, 65% of the efferent axons arise from C6 and 34% from C7. The nerve enters the distal end of the intermuscular space between the mm. supraspinatus and subscapularis from the medial side. It is accompanied by the suprascapular artery and vein. The suprascapular nerve is primarily a muscle nerve to the mm. supraspinatus and infraspinatus. It passes over the scapular notch, innervates the supraspinatus and continues across the neck of the scapula distal to the end of the spine to enter the infraspinatus. Prior to passing distal to the spine the nerve sends a small branch to the lateral part of the shoulder joint (Fig. 17.15). The suprascapular nerve does not have any cutaneous branches in the dog (Kitchell et al., 1980).

The **subscapular nerve** (*n. subscapularis*) is usually a single, but occasionally double, nerve that arises from the union of a branch from the sixth and seventh cervical nerves, or, if the nerve is double, one part usually arises from the seventh cervical nerve directly (Fig. 17.14). A contribution from the sixth cervical nerve may also be present. It may arise completely or nearly completely from either the seventh or the eighth cervical nerve (Allam et al., 1952). According to Sharp et al. (1991), its efferent supply arises from C6 and C7 in six of six dogs; 59% of the efferent axons in this nerve arise from C6 and 41% from C7. It usually divides into cranial and caudal parts on entering the medial surface of the distal fifth of the subscapular muscle. The subscapular nerve is approximately 5 cm long in a medium-sized dog. This permits the extensive sliding movement of the scapula on the thorax during locomotion without nerve injury. The subscapular nerve does not have any cutaneous branches (Kitchell et al., 1980).

The **axillary nerve** (*n. axillaris*), like the subscapular nerve, is much longer than the distance between its origin and its peripheral fixed end. It arises as a branch from the combined seventh and eighth cervical nerves (Fig. 17.14). A contribution from the sixth cervical nerve may also be present. It may arise completely or nearly completely from either the seventh or the eighth cervical nerve (Allam et al., 1952). According to Sharp et al. (1991), its efferent supply included C6 in six of six dogs, C7 in five of six, and C8 in two of six; 59% of the efferent axons in this nerve arise from C6 and 41% from C7, with fewer than 1% from C8. Bailey et al. (1982) report that C6 contributed afferent axons to its cutaneous branches in 8 of 10 dogs; C7, 10 of 10; C8, in 2 of 10 dogs. The axillary nerve leaves the axillary space caudodistal to the subscapular muscle and proximal to the teres major muscle. It supplies mainly the muscles of the shoulder joint as it curves around the caudoventral border of the subscapular muscle near its distal end. In its intermuscular course proximocaudal to the shoulder joint, it divides basically into two portions; one part sends branches to caudal fascicles of the subscapular muscle and completely supplies the m. teres major. The other portion, accompanied by the caudal circumflex humeral vessels, runs laterally to supply the laterally lying teres minor and deltoideus. Before

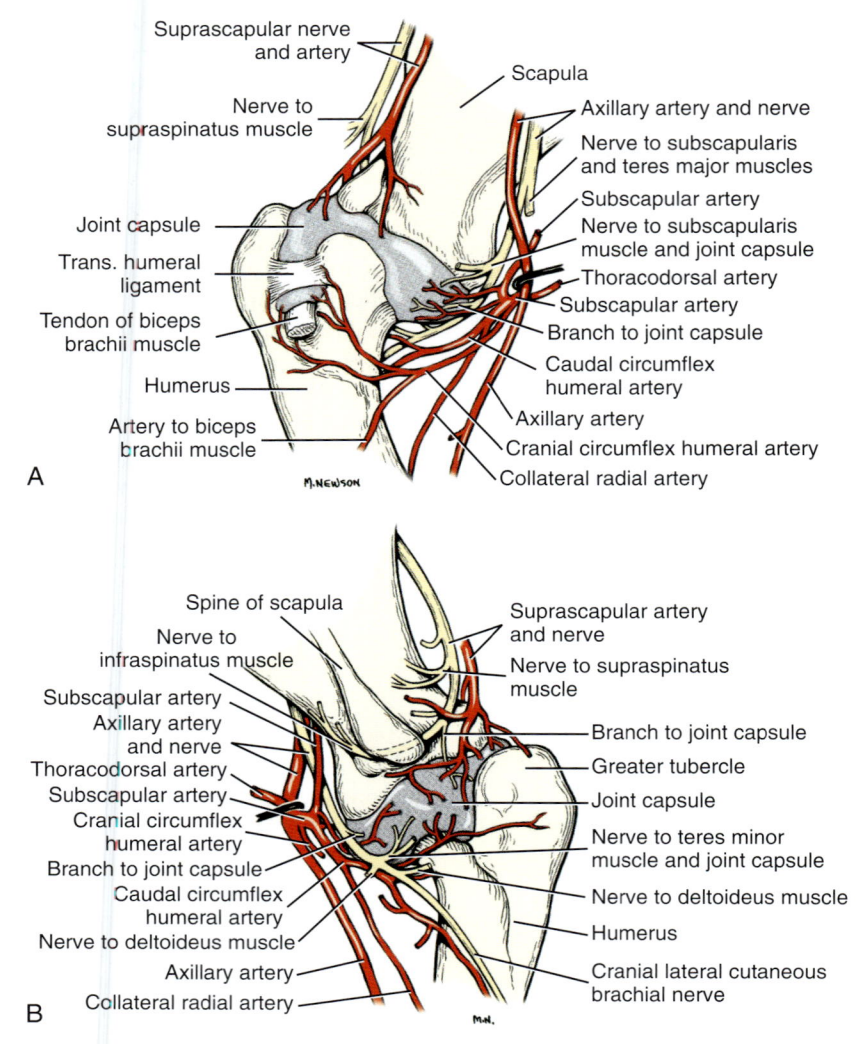

Fig. 17.15 A, Nerves and arteries of the right shoulder joint, medial aspect. B, Nerves and arteries of the right shoulder joint, lateral aspect.

entering the teres minor, a branch enters the caudal part of the shoulder joint capsule (Fig. 17.15).

The **cranial lateral cutaneous brachial nerve** (*n. cutaneus brachii lateralis cranialis*) leaves the axillary nerve just prior to the entry of this nerve into the deltoid muscle. Therefore it arises lateral to the space between the origins of the lateral and long heads of the triceps muscle. It runs distally on the lateral head of the triceps muscle, where it is covered by the deltoid muscle. It appears subcutaneously caudal to the main portion of the cephalic vein, where it is associated with the cutaneous branches of the caudal circumflex humeral artery and vein (Fig. 17.16). The cutaneous area of this nerve lies on the lateral surface of the brachium (Fig. 17.17), overlapping in its distribution cranial aspects of the cutaneous area of the intercostobrachial nerve (lateral cutaneous branch of thoracic spinal nerve II) caudally and overlapping cranially the caudal aspects of the cutaneous areas of the fifth cervical nerve, dorsally, and the cutaneous branch of the brachiocephalicus nerve, ventrally (Kitchell et al., 1980). On entering the forearm, the cranial lateral cutaneous brachial nerve is named the **cranial cutaneous antebrachial nerve** (*n. cutaneus antebrachii cranialis*). It terminates in the skin of the proximocraniolateral aspect of the forearm, where its cutaneous area is completely overlapped by the cutaneous areas of the radial and musculocutaneous nerves (Kitchell et al., 1980). At the elbow joint or just distal to it, it often joins the medial branch of the superficial radial nerve (Fig. 17.16), and by means of this nerve its fibers are carried to the skin of the cranial two-thirds of the length of the antebrachium (Kitchell et al., 1980).

The **musculocutaneous nerve** (*n. musculocutaneus*) gives muscular branches to the coracobrachialis, biceps brachii, and brachialis (Figs. 17.11 and 17.13). It continues in the forearm as the medial cutaneous antebrachial nerve (Figs. 17.18 and 17.19). The musculocutaneous nerve is irregular in its formation, arising mainly from the seventh cervical nerve but also receiving contributions from C6 and C8 (Fig. 17.14). It receives branches from the first and second thoracic nerves in rare instances. According to Sharp et al.

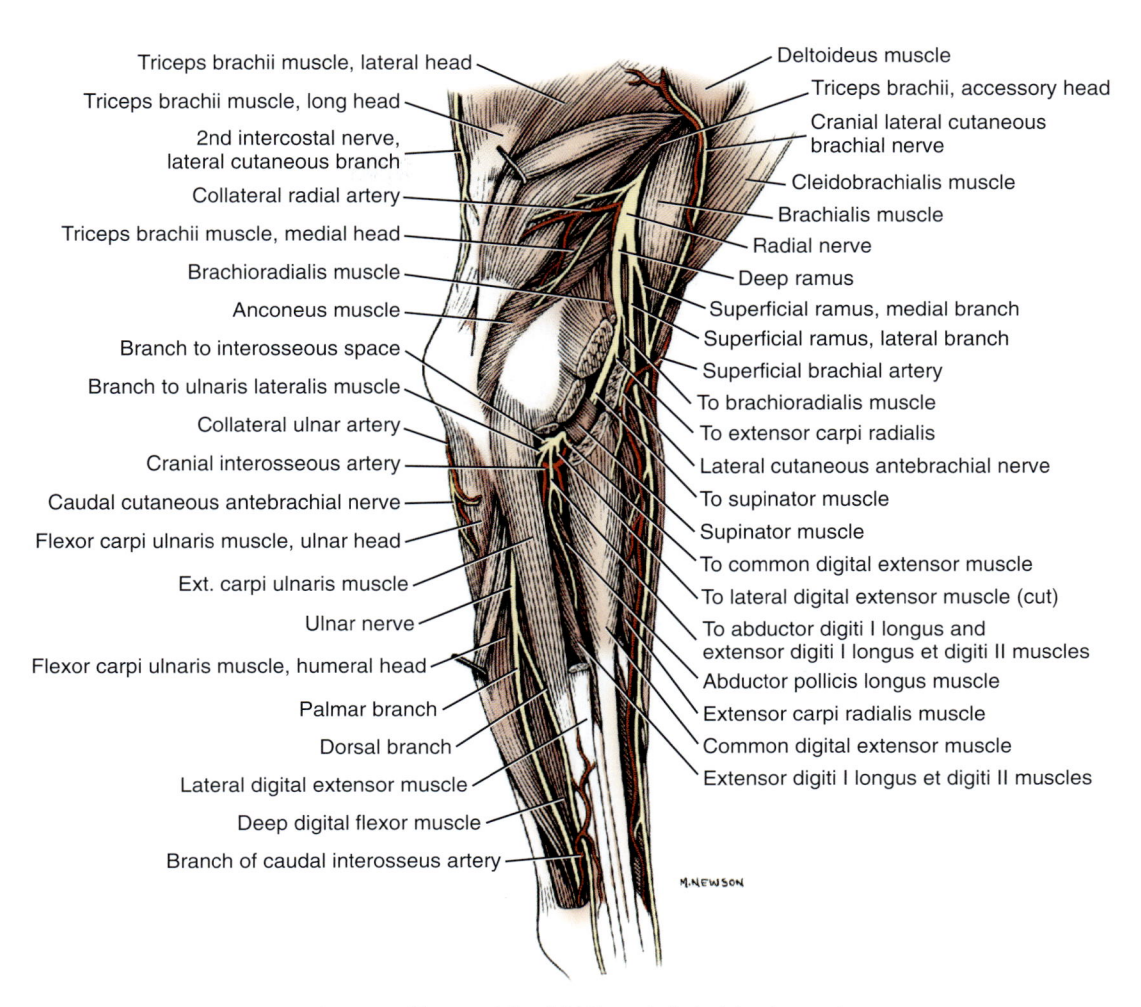

Fig. 17.16 Nerves of the right thoracic limb, lateral aspect.

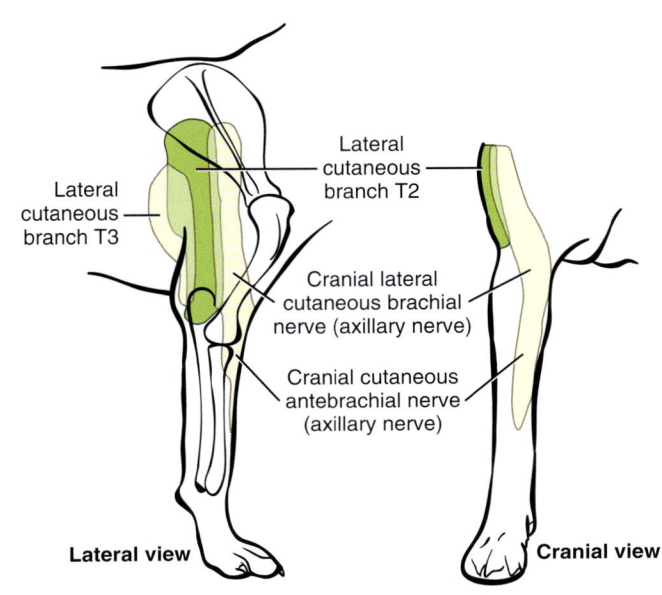

Fig. 17.17 Schematic illustration of the cutaneous areas of the cutaneous nerves supplying the skin of the lateral aspect of the thoracic limb. (Modified, with permission, from Kitchell RL, Whalen LR, Bailey CS, et al.: Electrophysiologic studies of cutaneous nerves of the thoracic limb of the dog, *Am J Vet Res* 41:61–76, 1980.)

(1990) it was formed by contributions from C6, C7, and C8 in six of six dogs and T1 in two of six; 57% of the efferent axons in the nerve came from C7, 26% from C6, and 16% from C8, with fewer than 1% from T1. Bailey et al. (1982) found that its cutaneous nerves have a much wider origin, arising in part from C6 in six of nine dogs, C7 in nine of nine, C8 in six of nine, and T1 in two of nine. Throughout its course in the brachium it lies between or deep to the cranially lying m. biceps brachii and the brachial vessels caudally (Fig. 17.12). There are three muscular branches. Proximally a small branch goes to the coracobrachialis. This branch is small, and often instead of arising from the musculocutaneous nerve directly it may exist as a separate branch that comes from the eighth cervical or first thoracic nerve, or both (Fig. 17.12). In reaching the coracobrachialis, it follows the cranial circumflex humeral vessels over a portion of its course. A large branch, the **proximal muscular branch** (*ramus muscularis proximalis*), often called the muscular nerve to the m. biceps brachii, enters the deep surface of the biceps brachii approximately 4 cm from its origin and near its caudomedial border. In the distal third of the brachium, a **communicating branch** (*ramus communicans cum n. mediano*) passes distocaudad,

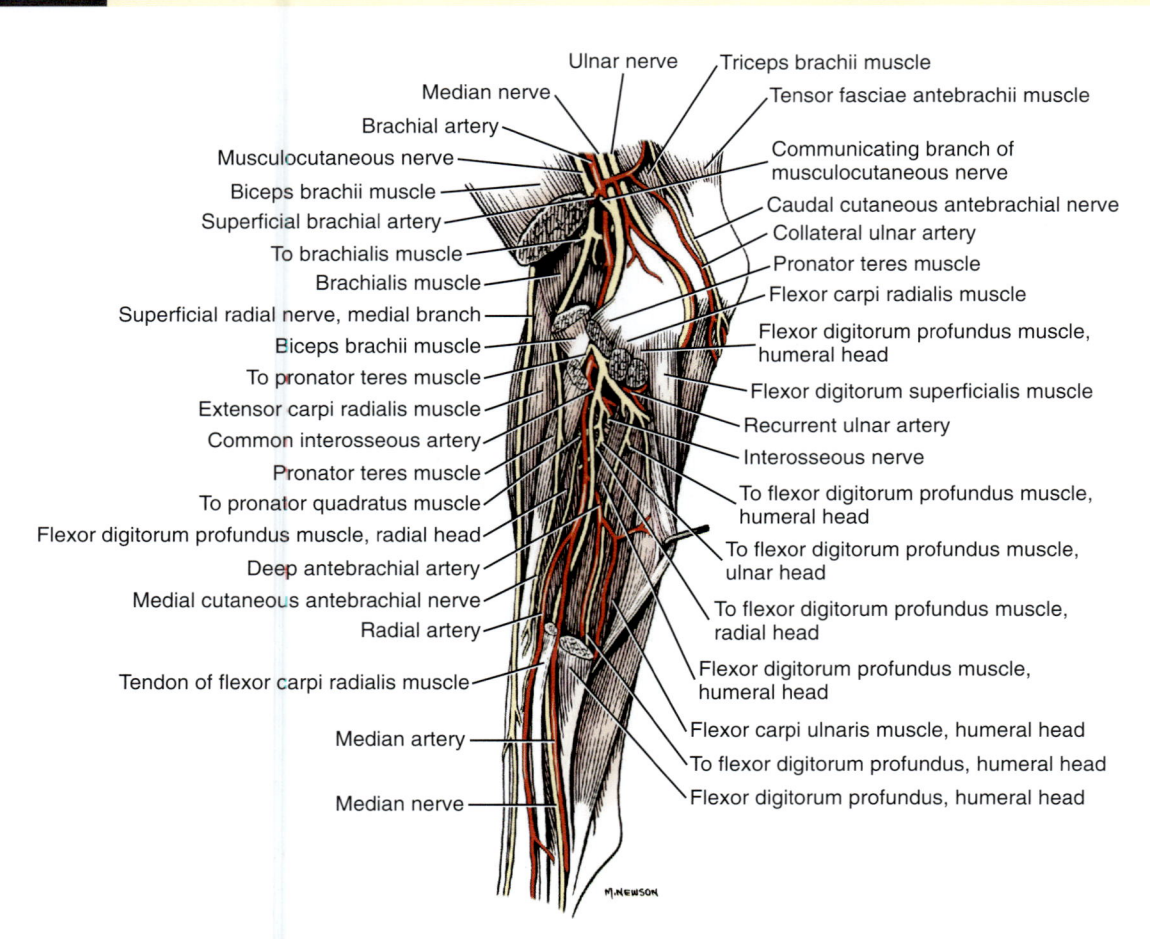

• **Fig. 17.18** Nerves of the right antebrachium, medial aspect. Dissection showing median and musculocutaneous nerves.

usually medial to the brachial vessels, and joins the median nerve, which with the ulnar nerve lies caudal to the brachial vessels (Figs. 17.12, 17.18 to 17.20). The communicating branch carries both cutaneous (afferent) and efferent axons to the median nerve (Kitchell et al., 1980). The cutaneous afferents from the communicating branch supply a cutaneous area located on the palmar aspect of the forepaw (Fig. 17.21). This cutaneous area is also supplied by the median nerve axons (described later). The efferent axons go to some of the antebrachial muscles that are supplied by the median nerve. Sharp et al. (1990) reported that efferent axons from the median nerve also go through the communicating branch to supply the brachial muscle. (This communication between the musculocutaneous and the median nerves in the dog is not homologous to the ansa axillaris, according to the *Nomina Anatomica Veterinaria* [NAV, 2005].) As the musculocutaneous nerve winds deep to the terminal part of the biceps brachii from the medial side, it terminates by dividing into the **distal muscular branch** (*ramus muscularis distalis*), also called the *muscle nerve to the brachialis muscle* (Figs. 17.18 and 17.19), which enters the distal medial portion of the brachialis muscle, and the small **medial cutaneous antebrachial nerve** (*n. cutaneus antebrachii medialis*) (Figs. 17.18 and 17.19). This cutaneous branch crosses the lateral side of the tendon of the biceps brachii

and enters the cranial surface of the antebrachium from the flexor angle of the elbow joint. As the nerve crosses the cranial surface of the elbow joint, it sends a small branch to the craniolateral part of it (Fig. 17.19). It freely branches in its course distad in the forearm. Its cutaneous area lies on the craniomedial portion of the antebrachium (Fig. 17.21). The cutaneous area of the medial cutaneous antebrachial nerve does not extend into the carpus. The cutaneous area that it supplies is overlapped medially by the cutaneous area supplied by the cutaneous branches of the medial branch of the superficial radial nerve and by cutaneous branches of the axillary nerve and laterally by the cutaneous areas of the caudal cutaneous antebrachial nerve proximally and the cutaneous areas of the median and the dorsal branch of the ulnar nerve distally.

The **radial nerve** (*n. radialis*) (Figs. 17.11 to 17.13) arises from the seventh and eighth cervical and the first and second thoracic nerves (Fig. 17.14). According to Sharp et al. (1991) C7, C8, and T1 contributed to the radial nerve in six of six dogs. In five of six, C6 also contributed. In three of six dogs, T2 gave some fibers to this nerve. In the radial nerve, 45% of the efferent axons came from C8, 29% from T1, 21% from C7, and 1% from T2. Bailey et al. (1982) reported that the cutaneous afferent axons in the radial nerve came in part from C6 in 7 of 10 dogs, from C7 in

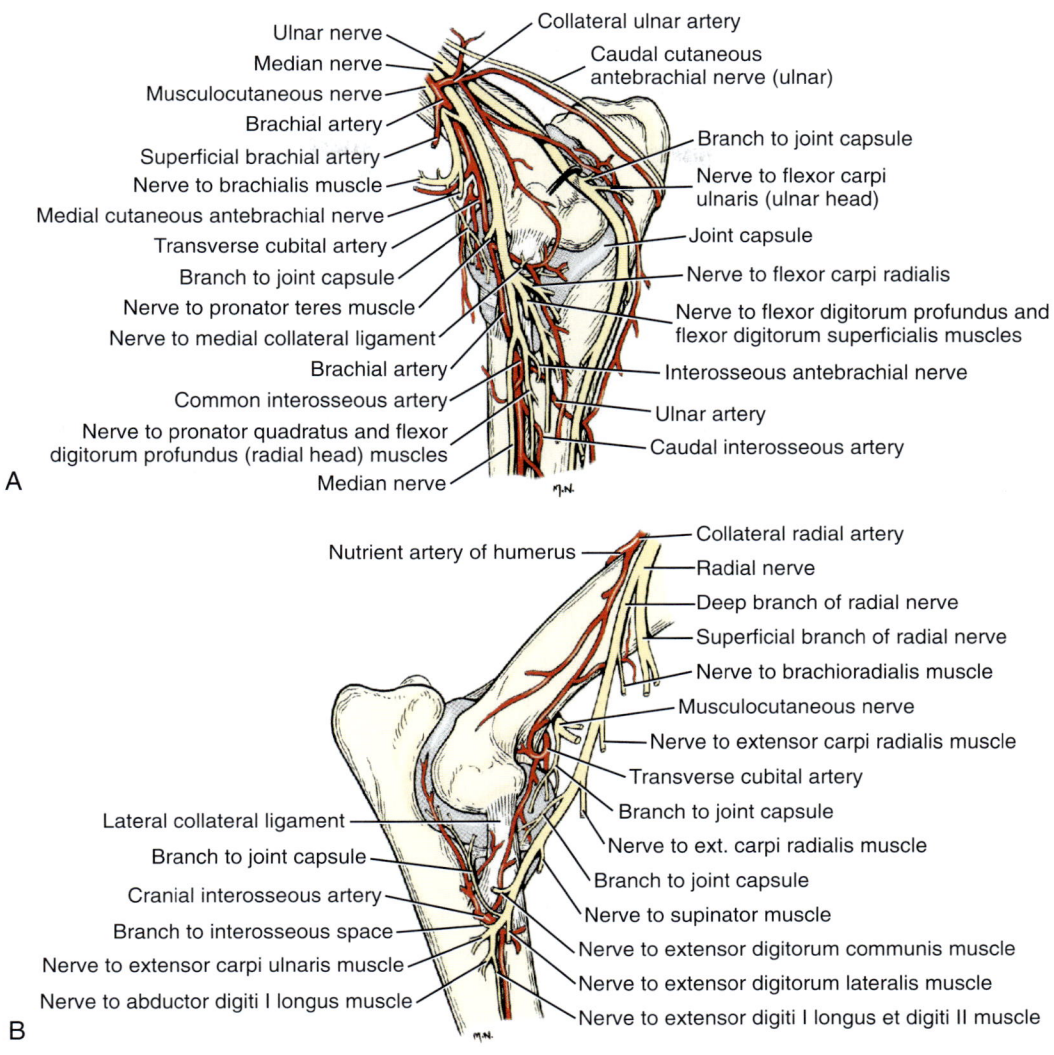

Fig. 17.19 **A**, Nerves and arteries of the right elbow joint, medial aspect. **B**, Nerves and arteries of the right elbow joint, lateral aspect.

10 of 10, from C8 in 10 of 10, and from T1 in only 2 of 10; none came from T2. The radial nerve is the largest nerve of the brachial plexus. It supplies all the extensor muscles of the elbow, carpal, and digital joints and also the supinator, brachioradialis, and abductor digiti I longus muscles. The skin on the cranial portion of the antebrachium and the dorsal surface of the paw is also supplied by axons of the radial nerve (Fig. 17.22). As the radial nerve approaches the brachium by traversing the axillary space, it lies lateral to the axillary vein and medial to the axillary artery. On crossing the medial surface of the conjoined tendons of the teres major and latissimus dorsi, it lies caudal to the brachial vessels that are the continuation of the axillary vessels after these have crossed the conjoined tendon. It exits from the axilla distal to the conjoined tendons of the teres major and the latissimus dorsi. On entering the interval between the medial and the long heads of the triceps muscle, the radial nerve gives off a small branch to the tensor fascia antebrachial muscle, then divides into a branch that runs proximolateral and is distributed to the long head of the triceps.

The second branch runs distolateral and represents the main continuation of the radial nerve. It supplies a branch to the accessory and medial heads of the triceps muscle before it makes contact with the brachialis muscle. Accompanied by the nutrient artery of the humerus, it follows this muscle in a spiral manner around the humerus. On contacting the lateral head of the triceps, it sends a branch to it, and shortly thereafter it bifurcates into deep and superficial branches. Prior to this bifurcation the radial nerve gives off the **caudal lateral brachial cutaneous nerve** (*n. cutaneus brachii lateralis caudalis*), which supplies the skin covering the lateral head of the triceps muscle. The deep branch of the distal radial nerve runs deep to the proximocranial border of the extensor carpi radialis. According to Sharp et al. (1990), the deep branch of the radial has a higher percentage of its efferent axons coming from the more cranial roots of the brachial plexus than do the more proximally located muscles supplied by the radial nerve. At the place of bifurcation of the radial nerve, a minute branch runs to the deep surface of the brachioradialis. The superficial branch pursues a more

720 CHAPTER 17 The Spinal Nerves

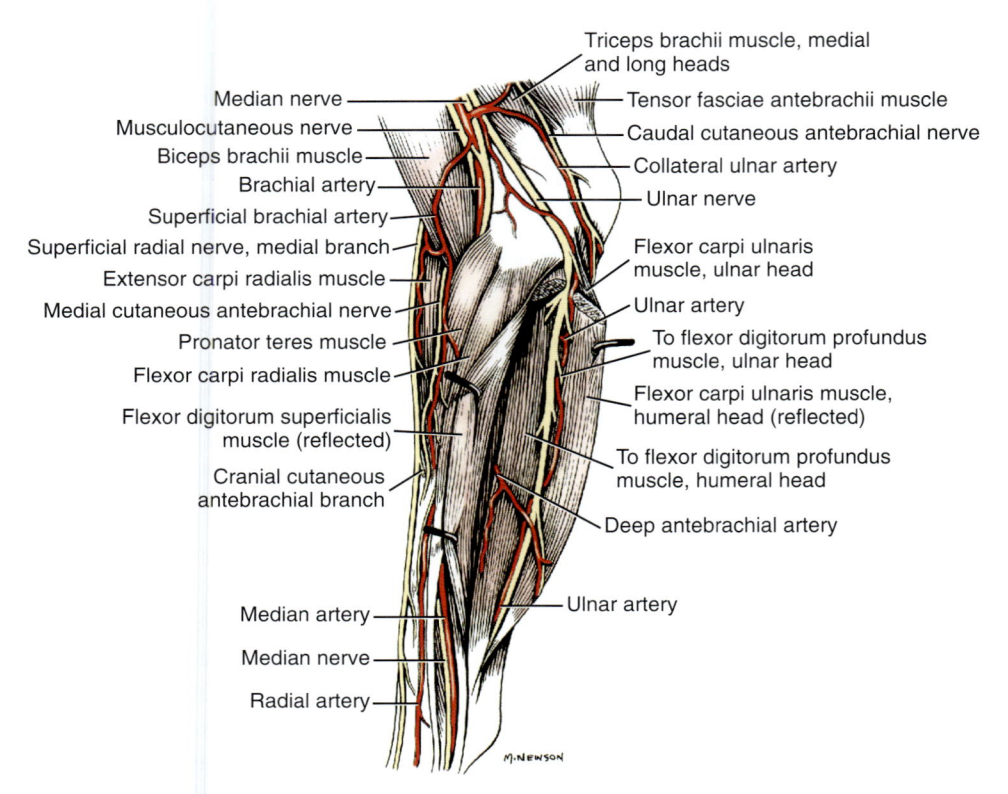

• **Fig. 17.20** Nerves of the right antebrachium, medial aspect. Dissection showing the ulnar nerve.

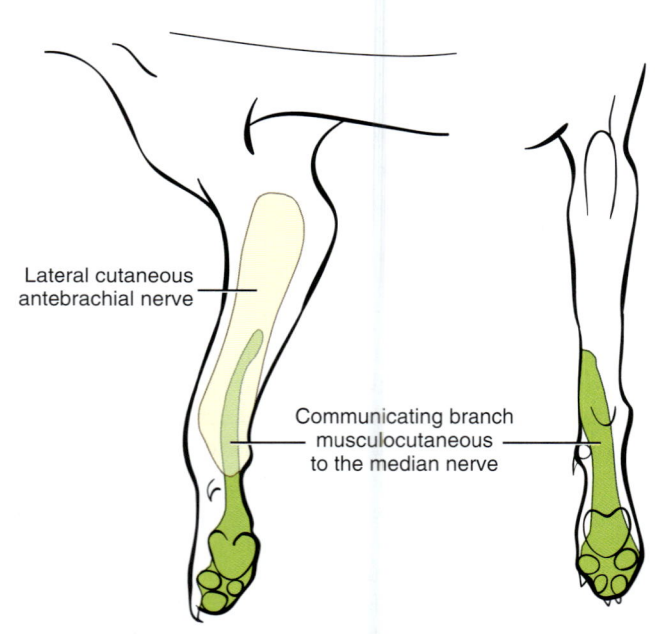

• **Fig. 17.21** Schematic illustration of the cutaneous areas of the peripheral branches of the musculocutaneous nerve. The fibers of the musculocutaneous nerve forming the communicating branch between the musculocutaneous nerve and the median nerve travel in the median nerve in the antebrachium to reach the skin of the forepaw.

cranial course and becomes superficial between the distocranial border of the lateral head of the triceps and the lateral surface of the deeply lying brachialis muscle.

The **deep branch** (*ramus profundus*) supplies all of the extensor muscles of the carpus and the digits (Fig. 17.16). On the lateral aspect of the elbow joint it passes deep to the extensor carpi radialis near its origin from the lateral supracondyloid crest and sends a branch into it (Fig. 17.16). As the deep branch crosses the flexor surface of the elbow joint, it sends an articular branch to the craniolateral part of it (Fig. 17.19A). The remaining part of the deep branch then passes deep to the supinator muscle, which it supplies. On emerging from deep to this muscle, it immediately divides into branches that supply the common and lateral digital extensors and a small branch that closely follows the lateral border of the radius and runs distad to innervate the abductor digiti I longus and extensor digiti I longus et digiti II. The distal end of the deep branch of the radial nerve supplies the antebrachiocarpal joint.

The **superficial branch** (*ramus superficialis*) of the radial nerve is its more cranial branch (Fig. 17.16). On emerging from deep to the cranial part of the distal border of the lateral head of the triceps muscle, it runs obliquely craniodistad on the brachialis muscle, where it is covered by the thick intermuscular fascia. After running approximately 1 cm in this location, it perforates the thick fascia and divides unevenly into a larger **lateral branch** (*ramus lateralis*) and a smaller **medial branch** (*ramus medialis*). These branches continue to the carpus in relation to the lateral and medial branches of the cranial superficial antebrachial arteries, respectively. Thus they closely flank the medial and lateral sides of the cephalic vein as they traverse the antebrachium. From the lateral branch of the superficial branch of the radial nerve the usually double **lateral cutaneous antebrachial nerve** (*n. cutaneus antebrachii lateralis*) arises

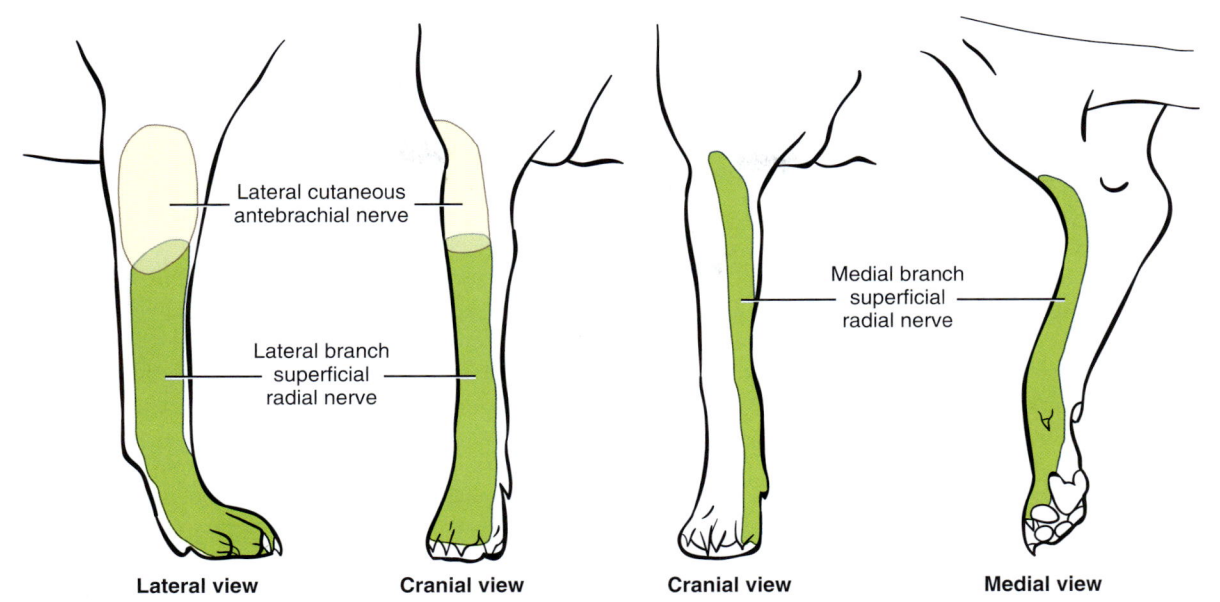

• **Fig. 17.22** Schematic illustration of the cutaneous areas of the peripheral branches of the superficial branch of the radial nerve. The extent of the lateral cutaneous antebrachial branch is quite variable. The nerve is often double. The most common extent is shown here. (Modified, with permission, from Kitchell RL, Whalen LR, Bailey CS, et al.: Electrophysiologic studies of cutaneous nerves of the thoracic limb of the dog, *Am J Vet Res* 41:61–76, 1980.)

(Fig. 17.16). It supplies a variable cutaneous area around and distal to the lateral epicondyle of the humerus (Fig. 17.22). The more proximal branch is the larger and is the branch that is more constantly present. It arises just distal to the flexor surface of the elbow joint, and, associated with relatively large cutaneous branches of the lateral branch of the cranial superficial antebrachial vessels, it supplies the skin of the proximal one-third to two-thirds of the lateral surface of the antebrachium (Fig. 17.22). The more distally located nerve to the skin of the lateral side of the antebrachium, smaller than the more proximally located nerve, also is accompanied by a cutaneous artery and vein, which serve the cutaneous area of the region. Occasionally, more than two lateral cutaneous antebrachial nerves are present.

Small branches leave both the medial and the lateral branches of the superficial radial nerves and innervate the skin on the cranial surface of the antebrachium (Fig. 17.22). The medial branches of the superficial radial often join the cranial cutaneous branches of the axillary nerve, which results in the cutaneous areas extensively overlapping; however, neither cutaneous area completely overlaps that of the other nerve. Because the medial and lateral branches of the superficial radial nerves also innervate the dorsum of the forepaw, they and their cutaneous areas are described under the description of the nerves to the forepaw.

Because the radial nerve supplies all the extensor muscles of the thoracic limb except those of the shoulder joint, injury to the proximal part of the nerve results in the inability to support weight on the thoracic limb. The most common traumatic injury that results in a radial paralysis, usually caused by a moving vehicle, is an avulsion of the spinal nerves or their roots or both that contribute to the brachial plexus. When this is complete, multiple brachial plexus nerves are affected and there is a total flaccid paralysis of the affected thoracic limb and analgesia distal to the elbow. Radial nerve injuries distal to the innervation of the triceps brachii do not result in any permanent gait abnormality. The loss of extension of the carpus and digits is rapidly compensated for by an increase in the length of protraction (swing phase) of the limb so that the forepaw is placed on its palmar surface.

The **median nerve** (*n. medianus*) (Figs. 17.11 to 17.13) arises primarily from the eighth cervical nerve by a lateral root (*radix lateralis*) and first thoracic nerve by a medial root (*radix medialis*), with small contributions from the seventh cervical and the second thoracic spinal nerves (Fig. 17.14). Before its junction with the communicating branch with the musculocutaneous nerve, Sharp et al. (1990) determined that the efferent axons in the median nerve came from C8 and T1 in six of six dogs, from C7 in five of six, and from T1 in four of six. Of the total efferent axons in the nerve, 9% came from C7, 38% from C8, 46% from T1, and 6% from T2. Reimers (1925) did not regard the nerve to be formed until it had received the communicating branch from the musculocutaneous nerve in the distal part of the brachium. He believed that, through this communication, the median nerve is augmented by axons from the sixth and seventh cervical nerves. Sharp et al. (1990) are in agreement with this deduction in that they determined that, of the efferent axons in the communicating branch from the musculocutaneous to the median nerve, 60% came from C7, 22% from C8, 2% from T1, and 17% from T2. Bailey et al. (1982) found the afferent axons in the cutaneous branches of the median nerve to come in part from C7 in five of eight dogs, C8 in eight of eight, and T1 in eight of eight. Mutai et al. (1986), using horseradish peroxidase, found that the median nerve arose from C7 through T1.

The median and ulnar nerves in the forearm lie caudal to the brachial artery and vein, where they are loosely joined by fascia (Fig. 17.12). The median nerve is cranial in relation to the ulnar nerve. The median nerve does not give off any branches proximal to the elbow joint. It crosses the flexor surface of the elbow joint cranial to the medial epicondyle. The median nerve passes deep to the pronator teres and enters the large caudal group of flexor muscles located in the antebrachium (Fig. 17.18). It gives muscular branches to the pronator teres, pronator quadratus, flexor carpi radialis, and flexor digitorum superficialis and the radial head of the flexor digitorum profundus. It also sends axons to the deep part of the humeral head of the flexor digitorum profundus and a small articular branch to the medial aspect of the elbow joint.

On emerging from deep to the pronator teres, to which it sends a small branch, several **muscular branches** (*rami musculares*) leave the caudal portion of the nerve (Fig. 17.18). The shortest and most proximal of these nerves enters the flexor carpi radialis close to its humeral origin. The remaining flattened bundle of muscular branches crosses the medial surface of the brachial vessels at the place where the common interosseous artery arises, and, after running deep to the flexor carpi radialis and through the humeral head of the flexor digitorum profundus, most of them end in the superficially lying, flattened flexor digitorum superficialis. In their path to this muscle, they lie approximately 1 cm proximal and parallel to the deep antebrachial vessels. In this deep location a branch is sent to the radial head of the flexor digitorum profundus, which it completely innervates, and smaller branches enter the humeral head of this muscle, the lateral part of which is also supplied by the ulnar nerve (Sharp et al., 1990). The small **interosseous nerve of the antebrachium** (*n. interosseus antebrachii*) first runs on the proximal part of the delicate interosseous membrane. It then perforates this membrane and runs distally on approximately the proximal half of the pronator quadratus, where it appears as a fine, white streak. It enters this muscle in its distal half and innervates it.

The portion of the median nerve that continues distad in the antebrachium, after the muscular branches have arisen, is at first related to the median artery and vein. At approximately the middle of the antebrachium, the median artery gives off the radial artery. Here, the median nerve continues distad in relation to the larger median artery (Fig. 17.18). This portion of the median nerve is small, measuring approximately 0.5 mm in diameter. The remaining branches of the median nerve will be described with the nerves to the forepaw.

The **ulnar nerve** (*n. ulnaris*) (Figs. 17.11 and 17.12) arises in close association with the radial and median nerves from the eighth cervical and the first and second thoracic nerves (Fig. 17.14). Sharp et al. (1990) determined that C8 and T1 contributed to the ulnar nerve in six of six dogs, C7 in one of six, and T2 in four of the six dogs. Of the total efferent axons in the nerve, 24% came from C8, 65% from T1, 11% from T2, and fewer than 1% from C7. Bailey et al. (1982) found that the cutaneous afferents in the ulnar nerve arose from C8 in 10 of 10 dogs, T1 in 10 of 10, and T2 in 8 of 10. Mutai et al. (1986), using horseradish peroxidase, found that the ulnar nerve arose from C8 through T2. After leaving the caudal part of the brachial plexus, the median and ulnar nerves are flanked by the brachial artery cranially and the brachial vein caudally (Fig. 12.13). They are deep to a thick layer of brachial fascia and bound to each other by areolar tissue until they reach the middle of the brachium, where they diverge. The ulnar nerve, which measures approximately 3 mm in diameter, runs distad along the cranial border of the medial head of the triceps brachii and adjacent to the caudal border of the biceps brachii. It crosses the elbow caudal to the prominent medial epicondyle. On entering the caudomedial part of the antebrachium, the ulnar nerve runs deep to the thick antebrachial fascia. After crossing caudal to the medial epicondyle of the humerus just proximal to the origin of the humeral head of the superficial digital flexor, it runs deep to the ulnar head of the flexor carpi ulnaris (Fig. 17.18). Like the median nerve, no muscular branches leave the ulnar nerve as it traverses the brachium.

The **caudal cutaneous antebrachial nerve** (*n. cutaneus antebrachii caudalis*) leaves the caudal part of the ulnar nerve near the beginning of the distal third of the brachium and passes over the medial surface of the olecranon tuber into the caudomedial part of the antebrachium (Figs. 17.12, 17.18, 17.19A, and 17.20). Bailey et al. (1982) determined that this branch of the ulnar nerve arose from T1 in 1 of 10 dogs, T1 and T2 in 7 of 10, and C8, T1, and T2 in 1 of 10. In its subcutaneous course throughout most of the area it supplies, it is accompanied by the collateral ulnar artery and vein. It freely sends branches to the skin as it winds across the proximal portion of the antebrachium from the medial to the caudolateral aspects. Ascending branches arborize in the skin of the distal part of the brachium. The cutaneous area of the caudal cutaneous antebrachial nerve lies on the proximal two-thirds of the skin of the caudolateral aspect of the antebrachium (Fig. 17.23). The cutaneous area of the lateral cutaneous antebrachial branches of the superficial radial nerve overlaps the cutaneous area of the caudal cutaneous antebrachial nerve caudolaterally, and the cutaneous area of the medial cutaneous antebrachial branch of the musculocutaneous nerve overlaps its cutaneous area caudomedially. Distally the cutaneous area of the proximal branch of the dorsal branch of the ulnar overlaps the cutaneous area of the caudal cutaneous antebrachial nerve. This overlap is described when the innervation of the forepaw is described. The caudal cutaneous antebrachial nerve is an excellent site for testing for avulsions of the caudal roots of the spinal nerves contributing to the brachial plexus because of its origins from T1 and T2 and, seldom, from C8 (Bailey & Kitchell, 1984).

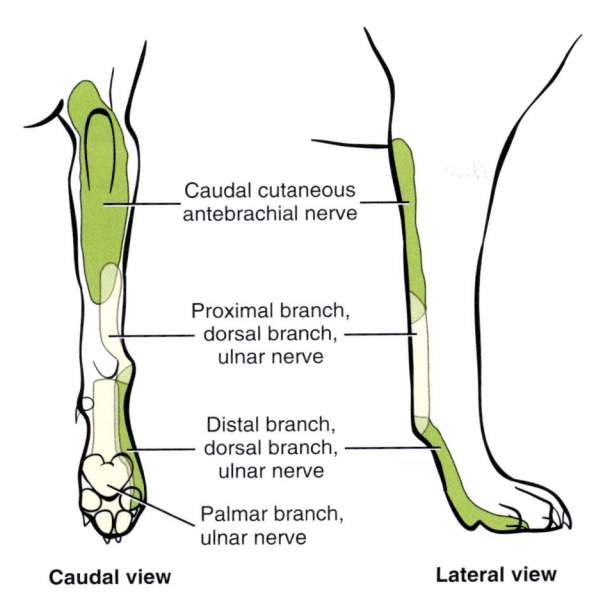

Fig. 17.23 Schematic illustration of the cutaneous areas of the peripheral branches of the ulnar nerve. (Modified, with permission, from Kitchell RL, Whalen LR, Bailey CS, et al.: Electrophysiologic studies of cutaneous nerves of the thoracic limb of the dog, Am J Vet Res 41:61–76, 1980.)

Median Nerve Only	Both Ulnar and Median Nerves	Ulnar Nerve Only
Pronator quadratus Pronator teres Radial head of deep digital flexor Superficial digital flexor	Superficial part of humeral head of deep digital flexor Lateral part of humeral head of deep digital flexor	Ulnar head of deep digital flexor
Flexor carpi radialis Deep part of humeral head of deep digital flexor Medial part of humeral head of deep digital flexor		Flexor carpi ulnaris

TABLE 17.1 Innervation of Muscles of the Caudal Side of the Forearm

The muscular branches (*rami musculares*) of the ulnar nerve, which supply the muscles of the antebrachium, are peripheral branches of a short, stout trunk that leaves the caudal side of the ulnar nerve as it passes caudal to the medial epicondyle of the humerus and plunges into the deep surface of the thin, wide ulnar head of the flexor carpi ulnaris (Fig. 17.20). The ulnar nerve, entering the septum between the ulnar and the humeral heads of the flexor carpi ulnaris, sends a branch approximately 1 mm in diameter and 1.5 cm long distally into the caudal border of the humeral head of the deep digital flexor. In the proximal fifth of the antebrachium, as the ulnar nerve curves around the caudal border of the humeral head of the flexor carpi ulnaris, it sends a stout branch into its lateral surface. Throughout the middle third of the antebrachium the ulnar nerve lies on the caudal border of the deep digital flexor, where it is covered by the humeral head of the flexor carpi ulnaris. At approximately the middle of the antebrachium, the small, cutaneous dorsal branch of the ulnar nerve arises. This branch and the palmar branch arise as terminal branches of the ulnar nerve. Both of these branches are distributed to the structures of the forepaw and are described with the nerves of the forepaw.

Both the ulnar and the median nerves supply muscles on the caudomedial side of the forearm. A summary of these muscles and their innervation is shown in Table 17.1.

Nerves of the Forepaw (Manus)

Like the vessels that serve the forepaw, the nerves may be divided into dorsal and palmar sets. Kopp (1901) described the morphologic features of the nerves of the forepaw of the dog. The radial nerve nearly totally supplies the dorsum of the forepaw, where it forms a single set of dorsal common digital and dorsal proper digital nerves. The median and ulnar nerves supply the palmar aspect of the forepaw and all other parts that are not supplied by the radial nerve. In the palmar part of the metacarpus they form the palmar common digital nerves, which are derived largely from the median nerve, and the palmar metacarpal nerves from the ulnar nerve.

In accordance with NAV (2005), the superficial nerves of the metapodium are designated *nn. digitales communes*, whereas the deep nerves are called *nn. metacarpei* and *metatarsei*. Digital nerves that originate from the bifurcation of nn. digitales communes are called *nn. digitales proprii*. Those that originate from some other source are simply *nn. digitales*. The dog has nn. digitales dorsales communes I, II, III, and IV.

The nn. digitales palmares communes I, II, and III are the terminal branches of the median nerve in the dog. They receive the nn. metacarpei palmares from the deep branch of the ulnar nerve just before they divide into nn. digitales proprii. The n. digitalis palmaris communis IV is formed by the superficial branch of the ulnar nerve and is joined by the n. metacarpeus palmaris IV from the deep branch of the ulnar nerve.

The **radial nerve of the forepaw** (*n. radius manus*) (Fig. 17.24) is represented by the terminal portions into which the medial and lateral branches of the superficial radial nerve divide.

The **medial branch of the superficial radial nerve** (*ramus medialis n. radialis superficialis*) continues into the proximal part of the metacarpus where it gives off the **dorsal abaxial digital nerve I** (*n. digitalis dorsali I abaxialis*) to the skin of the dorsomedial aspect of the first digit and continues into the metacarpus as the **dorsal common digital nerve 1** (*n. digitalis dorsalis communis 1*). This continues on the medial aspect of the second digit as the **dorsal abaxial**

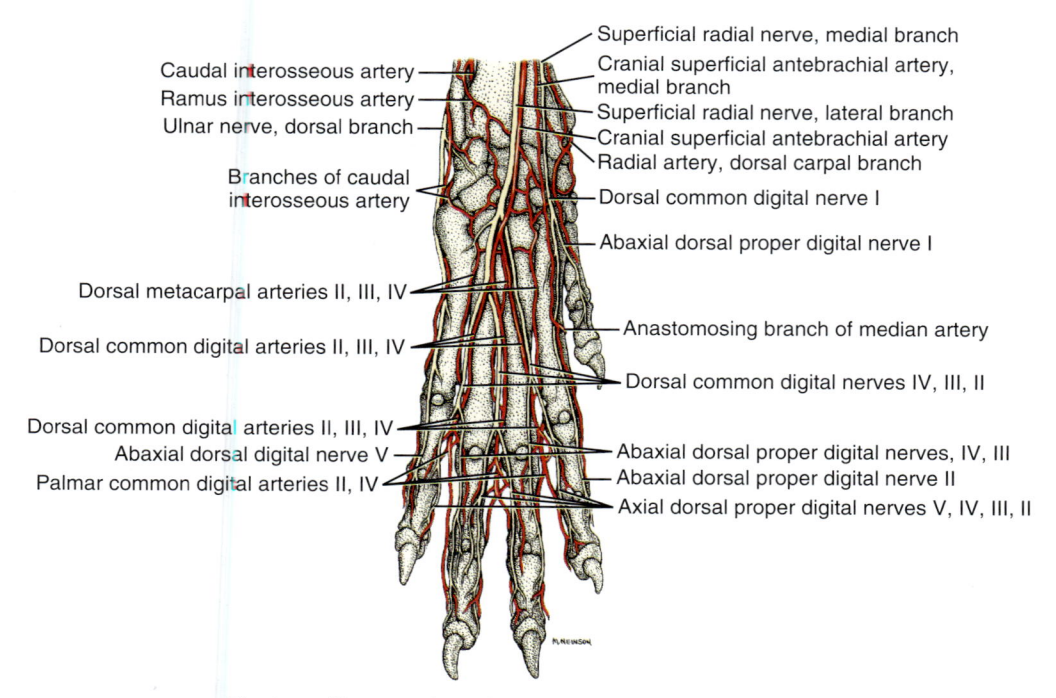

Fig. 17.24 Nerves and arteries of the right forepaw, dorsal aspect.

proper digital nerve II (*n. digitalis dorsalis proprius II abaxialis*). The cutaneous area of the medial branch of the superficial radial nerve is located on the craniomedial surface of the forearm and dorsomedial surface of the paw (Fig. 17.22). It is located on all surfaces of the first digit (including the digital pad) and the dorsal and medial (abaxial) surface (does not include the digital pad) of the second digit. Its medial border is overlapped by the cutaneous area of the cranial cutaneous antebrachial nerve (axillary) proximally and the cutaneous areas of the ulnar and median nerves distally. Its lateral border is overlapped by the cutaneous areas of the caudal cutaneous antebrachial branch of the ulnar nerve proximally and the dorsal branch of the ulnar distally.

The **lateral branch of the superficial radial nerve** (*ramus lateralis n. radialis superficialis*) crosses the dorsal surface of the carpus accompanied by the lateral branch of the cranial superficial antebrachial artery and the accessory cephalic vein (Fig. 17.24). The nerve trifurcates at approximately the carpometacarpal junction into **dorsal common digital nerves II, III, and IV**. Each of the dorsal common digital nerves II, III, and IV bifurcate before reaching the clefts that separate the four main digits, which are proximal to the metacarpophalangeal joints. The resultant branches are either **axial** or **abaxial dorsal proper digital nerves II, III**, and **IV**, depending on which side of the digit they lie. The axis of the limb passes between the third and fourth digits. Thus dorsal common digital nerve III divides into axial dorsal proper digital nerve III and axial proper digital nerve IV. The cutaneous area of the lateral branch of the superficial radial nerve is located on the craniolateral surface of the forearm and the dorsal and lateral surface of the paw (Fig. 17.22). It supplies the dorsolateral and axial surfaces of the second digit, the dorsal surfaces of the webbing of all of the digits, and the dorsomedial and axial surfaces of the fifth digit. Its medial border is overlapped by the cutaneous area of the medial branch of the superficial radial nerve, and its lateral border is overlapped by the caudal cutaneous antebrachial nerve (ulnar) proximally, and the dorsal branch of the ulnar distally.

At the level of the carpus, the median nerve divides into three branches. The medial branch gives off the **abaxial palmar digital nerve I** (*n. digitalis palmaris I abaxialis*) to supply the skin on the abaxial palmar side of the first digit. The medial branch continues into the metacarpus as the **palmar common digital nerve I** (*n. digitalis palmarlis communis I*). At the level of the metacarpophalangeal joint this nerve receives a branch of the palmar metacarpal nerve I from the deep branch of the ulnar nerve and branches into the **axial palmar proper digital nerve I** (*n. digitalis palmaris proprius I axialis*) and **abaxial palmar proper digital nerve II** (*n. digitalis palmaris proprius II abaxialis*). The middle terminal branch of the median nerve courses into the metacarpus as the **palmar common digital nerve II** (*n. digitalis palmaris communis II*). Further description of the distribution of these median nerve branches is provided with the description of the ulnar nerve. The lateral terminal branch of the median nerve becomes the **palmar common digital nerve III** (*n. digitalis palmaris communis III*) in the metacarpus. Communicating branches occur between palmar common digital nerves II and III. The cutaneous area of the median nerve in the forepaw is completely overlapped by the cutaneous area of the palmar branch of the ulnar nerve. It covers the palmar surfaces of the medial half of the second digit, all of the third digit, and the medial half of the fourth digit (Fig. 17.25).

Palmar branches, median nerve

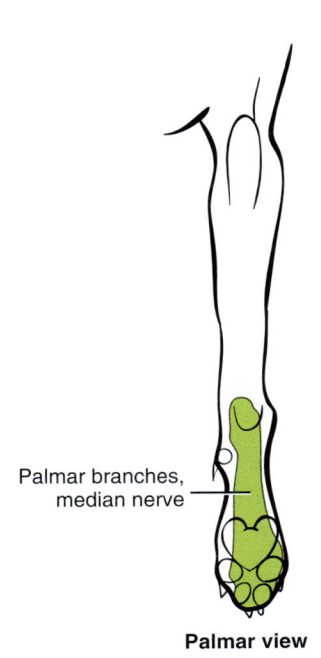

Palmar view

• **Fig. 17.25** Schematic illustration of the cutaneous area of the palmar branches of the median nerve as recorded from the median nerve proximal to the junction of the communicating branch from the musculocutaneous nerve. Compare with Fig. 17.21, and note that the fibers in the median nerve that come from the musculocutaneous nerve via the communicating branch with the median nerve have the same distribution as fibers that run all the way in the median nerve. Compare also with Figs. 17.23 and 17.28, and note that the palmar branches of the median and ulnar nerves completely overlap in the forepaw. (Modified, with permission, from Kitchell RL, Whalen LR, Bailey CS, et al.: Electrophysiologic studies of cutaneous nerves of the thoracic limb of the dog, *Am J Vet Res* 41:61–76, 1980.)

The **ulnar nerve of the forepaw** (*n. ulnaris*) (Fig. 17.26) is represented by the dorsal and palmar branches, which arise as terminal branches of the ulnar nerve at the junction of the proximal and middle thirds of the antebrachium.

The **dorsal branch** (*ramus dorsalis*) passes distad toward the lateral aspect of the carpus by passing obliquely laterad between the caudally lying flexor carpi ulnaris and the cranially lying ulnaris lateralis. It perforates the deep antebrachial fascia from 3 to 8 cm proximocaudal to the styloid process of the ulna. The dorsal branch divides into a proximal branch, which turns and runs proximally, and a distal branch, which is closely applied to the skin. In association with a cutaneous branch of the caudal interosseous artery, the distal branch obliquely crosses the lateral side of the carpus. In its subcutaneous course on the dorsolateral surface of the forepaw, it is called **abaxial dorsal proper digital nerve V** (*n. digitalis proprii dorsalis V abaxialis*), where it supplies the skin of the dorsolateral and abaxial palmar surfaces of the metacarpus and the fifth digit. The cutaneous area of the dorsal branch of the ulnar nerve is located on the lateral aspect of the distal third of the forearm and the dorsolateral and lateral and abaxial palmar surfaces of the fifth digit (Fig. 17.23). Proximally it overlaps with the caudal cutaneous antebrachial nerve. Medially it overlaps with the medial cutaneous antebrachial (musculocutaneous) proximally, and the combined cutaneous areas of the palmar branches of the median and ulnar nerves. Distally the cutaneous area of the dorsal branch of the ulnar is overlapped dorsomedially by the cutaneous area of the lateral branch of the superficial radial nerve. On the palmar

Radial artery
Median nerve
Dorsal carpal branch
Palmar carpal branch
Median artery
Medial branch
Lateral branch
Palmar metacarpal nerve I
Axial palmar proper digital nerve I
Palmar common digital nerves II, III, IV
Abaxial palmar proper digital nerves III, IV
Abaxial palmar proper digital nerve II

Ulnar nerve, palmar branch
Caudal interosseous artery
Ulnar nerve, dorsal branch
Superficial branch
Deep branch
Deep palmar arterial arch
Muscular branches
Superficial palmar arterial arch
Palmar metacarpal nerves, I, II, III, IV
Nerves to metacarpal foot pad
Abaxial palmar proper digital nerve V
Axial palmar proper digital nerves II, III, IV, V
Nerves to digital foot pad

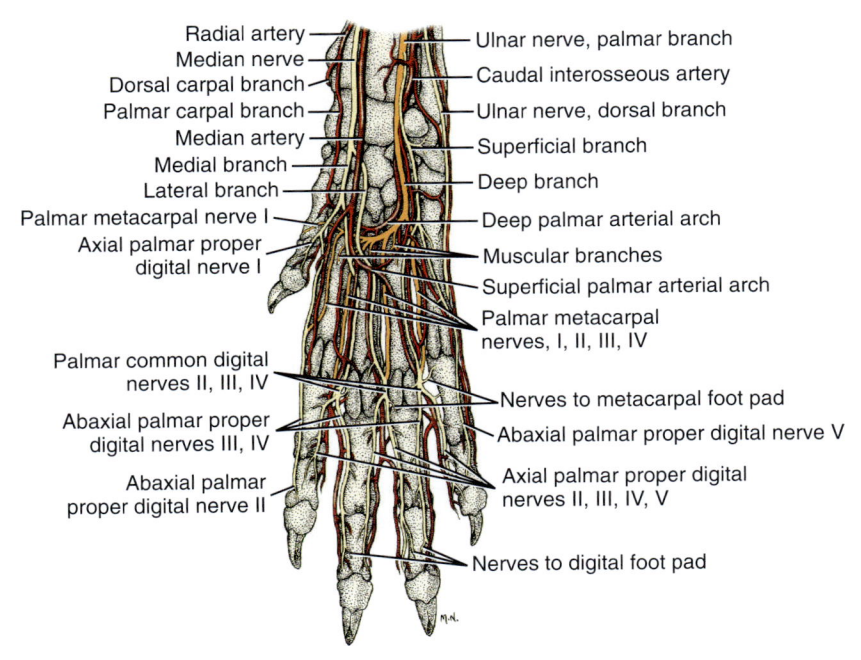

• **Fig. 17.26** Nerves and arteries of the right forepaw, palmar aspect.

aspect of the fifth digit it overlaps the medial half of the cutaneous area of the palmar branch of the ulnar nerve.

The **palmar branch** (*ramus palmaris*) of the ulnar nerve is the main continuation of the ulnar nerve after the dorsal branch has arisen (Fig. 17.26). As it passes through the distal portion of the antebrachium, it lies on the caudomedial surface of the deep digital flexor muscle approximately 1 cm lateral to the ulnar artery. It converges toward the artery distally in the antebrachium. The nerve passes through the deep portion of the carpal canal adjacent to the accessory carpal bone where it is joined by the caudal interosseous artery. Lying medial to the accessory carpal bone, the palmar branch issues a small branch to the carpal pad. A larger branch runs almost directly medially at the distal end of the palmar carpal fibrocartilage and innervates the special muscles of the fifth digit.

In the distal antebrachium the palmar branch of the ulnar nerve gives off a small **superficial branch** that traverses the carpal canal just medial to the accessory carpal bone. In the proximal metacarpus the superficial branch divides into a lateral **abaxial palmar proper digital nerve V** (*n. digitalis proprii palmaris V abaxialis*), which innervates the skin of the fifth digit and a medial **palmar common digital nerve IV** (*n. digitalis palmaris communis IV*).

The **deep branch** of the ulnar nerve traverses the carpal canal on the medial side of the accessory carpal bone closely associated with the caudal interosseous artery. In the proximal metacarpus the deep branch turns from lateral to medial and gives off the **palmar metacarpal nerves I, II, III, and IV** (*nn. metacarpal palmares*). These are the terminal branches of the deep branch of the ulnar nerve located on the palmar surface of the interosseous muscles and the abductors of digits II and V.

The **muscular branches** (*rami musculares*) arise directly from the deep branch of the ulnar or individually from the several palmar metacarpal nerves. They innervate the four interosseous muscles; the three lumbricales; the special muscles of the first, second, and fifth digits; and the single, small m. flexor digitorum brevis.

Proximally the palmar metacarpal nerves lie on the palmar surfaces of the proximal ends of the interosseous muscles. As they run distad toward the digits, they lie between the main interosseous muscles in relatively superficial positions. Communication occurs between the palmar metacarpal nerves and the palmar common digital nerves near or at the distal ends of the metacarpal bones (Fig. 17.27). Communications between the members of the superficial and deep sets of nerves are irregular and, in some instances, multiple. Occasionally, the deep members send slender communicating branches to the palmar digital nerves into which the palmar common digital nerves terminally divide. The palmar common digital nerves are therefore short as they cross the contact surfaces of adjacent metacarpophalangeal joints. From palmar proper common digital nerves II, III, and IV, or occasionally proximal or distal to these nerves, the three sensory nerves arise that innervate the large metacarpal foot pad. Minute branches from the palmar common digital nerves supply the structures of the metacarpophalangeal joints of the four main digits.

Just distal to these communications the palmar common digital nerves I through IV divide into the **axial** and **abaxial palmar proper digital nerves II, III, and IV** (*nn. digitales proprii palmares axiales et abaxiales*). They lie on the contact sides of the four main digits, dorsal to the comparable vessels, and like the vessels the proper nerves that face the

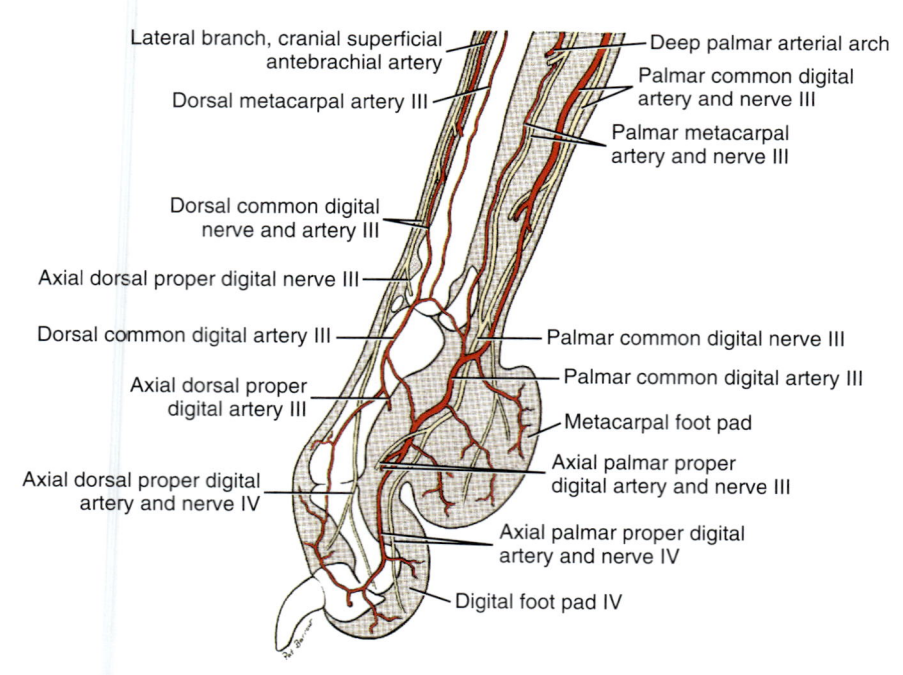

• **Fig. 17.27** Arteries and nerves of the fourth digit and metacarpus, medial aspect.

axis through the paw (axial branches) are larger and longer than are the abaxial proper nerves. They supply the overlying skin and the digital joints that they cross. At the distal interphalangeal joints, sensory branches are supplied to the digital foot pads. Axial and abaxial digital nerves enter the palmar vascular canal of the distal phalanges, and thereby axons reach the corium of the horny claw. The cutaneous areas of the palmar surface of the forepaw are shown in Fig. 17.28. Note that the palmar branch of the ulnar nerve completely overlaps the cutaneous area of the median nerve; thus this nerve and the palmar branches of the ulnar nerve have no autonomous zones that can be tested for loss of skin sensitivity (areas of anesthesia). The distal branch of the dorsal branch of the ulnar nerve can be tested by pinching the skin of the lateral surface of the fifth digit (Bailey & Kitchell, 1984).

Nerves of the Brachial Plexus That Supply Extrinsic Muscles of the Thoracic Limb

The nerves in this group are smaller than the nerves that supply the intrinsic structures of the thoracic limb. They consist of a brachiocephalic nerve, cranial pectoral nerves, long thoracic nerve, dorsal thoracic nerve, lateral thoracic nerve, and caudal pectoral nerves.

The **brachiocephalic nerve** (*n. brachiocephalicus*) (Figs. 17.11, 17.12, and 17.14), not described in the NAV, arises mainly from the sixth cervical nerve, but it may be joined by a branch from the fifth cervical nerve (Allam et al., 1952). According to Sharp et al. (1991) the efferent component of this nerve arose from both C6 and C7 in six of six dogs. The sixth cervical nerve contributed 67% of the axons, and 33% came from the seventh cervical nerve. The brachiocephalic nerve passes directly laterad into the m. cleidobrachialis cranial to the shoulder joint. The **cutaneous branch of the brachiocephalic nerve** (*n. cutaneus*) continues the brachiocephalic nerve through the cleidobrachialis muscle and supplies a cutaneous area around the cranial, craniolateral, and craniomedial aspects of the arm (Fig. 17.29) (Kitchell et al., 1980). Its cutaneous area overlaps the cutaneous area of the ventral branch of the fifth cervical nerve craniolaterally and the cutaneous areas of the ventral cutaneous branch of the second thoracic nerve and the lateral cutaneous branch of the third thoracic nerve caudomedially. The cutaneous branch of the brachiocephalic nerve receives its

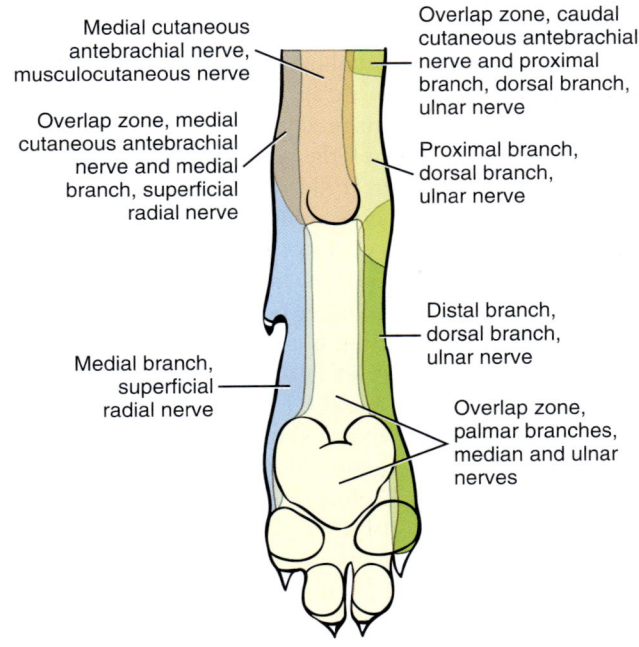

• **Fig. 17.28** Schematic illustration of the cutaneous innervation of the palmar aspect of the forepaw. This shows that the central regions of the forepaw, including the metacarpal and digital pads of the second, third, and fourth digits, are innervated by both the median and the ulnar nerves. The digital pad of the first digit is innervated only by the medial branch of the superficial radial nerve. (Modified, with permission, from Kitchell RL, Whalen LR, Bailey CS, et al.: Electrophysiologic studies of cutaneous nerves of the thoracic limb of the dog, *Am J Vet Res* 41:61–76, 1980.)

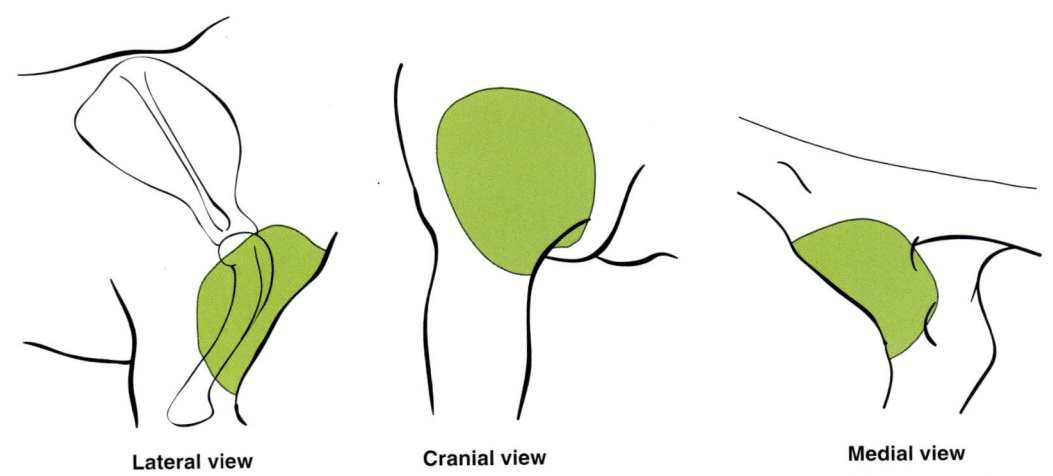

Lateral view   **Cranial view**   **Medial view**

• **Fig. 17.29** Schematic illustration of the cutaneous area of the cutaneous branch of the nerve to the brachiocephalicus. (Modified, with permission, from Kitchell RL, Whalen LR, Bailey CS, et al.: Electrophysiologic studies of cutaneous nerves of the thoracic limb of the dog, *Am J Vet Res* 41:61–76, 1980.)

afferent fibers from C6 in 10 of 10 dogs and C7 in 2 of 10 dogs (Bailey et al., 1982).

The **cranial pectoral nerves** (*nn. pectorales craniales*) (Figs. 17.11 and 17.12) supply the superficial pectoral muscles. They are irregular in number and origin but usually arise as two branches from the sixth, seventh, and eighth cervical nerves (Fig. 17.14). They have formerly been included under the term "ventral thoracic nerves" (Miller et al., 1964). They do not give off any cutaneous branches (Kitchell et al., 1980).

The **long thoracic nerve** (*n. thoracicus longus*) (Fig. 17.2) usually arises from the ventral branch of the seventh cervical nerve before it branches to aid in forming the brachial plexus. It runs largely horizontally on the superficial surface of the thoracic portion of the serratus ventralis cervicis, which it supplies. Miller (1934) regarded a small branch from the fifth cervical nerve as also belonging to the long thoracic nerve. It has no cutaneous branches.

The **thoracodorsal nerve** (*n. thoracodorsalis*) (Figs. 17.2 and 17.11 through 17.13) arises primarily from the eighth cervical nerve with contributions from the first thoracic or the seventh cervical nerve or both (Fig. 17.14). According to Sharp et al. (1991) C6 and C7 contribute axons to it in six of six dogs, C8 contributes in five of six dogs. They also reported that the thoracodorsal nerve gets 51% of its efferent supply from C7, 43% from C8, and 6% from T1. It is the motor nerve to the latissimus dorsi. It runs caudodorsad in close relation to the thoracodorsal vessels on the medial surface of the muscle. The thoracodorsal nerve does not have any cutaneous branches (Kitchell et al., 1980).

The **lateral thoracic nerve** (*n. thoracicus lateralis*) is composed of axons that come primarily from the eighth cervical and the first thoracic nerves (Figs. 17.11 and 17.14). According to Sharp et al. (1991), C8 and T1 contributed to it in six of six dogs, T1 in five of six. It received 38% of its efferent axons from C8, 56% from T1, and 5% from T2. This long nerve gives rise to branches that supply the deep pectoral muscle and is the sole motor supply to the m. cutaneus trunci and, in the male, the cranial preputial muscles. At first the nerve accompanies the lateral thoracic artery and vein (Fig. 17.13). It lies between the adjacent borders of the latissimus dorsi and deep pectoral muscles after passing medial to the axillary lymph nodes. It intermingles with the lateral cutaneous branches of the thoracic and cranial lumbar nerves but does not contain any cutaneous afferent axons from C8, T1, or T2 from the brachial plexus (Kitchell et al., 1980).

The **caudal pectoral nerves** (*nn. pectorales caudales*) are represented by three or four branches that innervate the deep pectoral muscle. They originate from the eighth cervical and the first two thoracic nerves (Fig. 17.14). According to Sharp et al. (1991), C8 contributed to this nerve in six of six dogs, T1 in four of six, and C7 in one of six. They found that 81% of the axons in this nerve come from C8, 17% from T1, and 2% from C6. No axons from T2 were found in this nerve. Some of the branches may appear to originate from the proximal portion of the lateral thoracic nerve. The caudal pectoral nerves have no cutaneous branches (Kitchell et al., 1980).

Thoracic Nerves

The **thoracic nerves** (*nn. thoracici*) (Fig. 17.30) number 13 pairs in the dog, and as a group they retain the simplest segmental form of all the spinal nerves. Each pair of thoracic nerves has the same serial number as the vertebra that lies cranial to their intervertebral foramina of exit. Each thoracic nerve gives off a dorsal and ventral branch. The dorsal branch gives off medial and lateral branches. The **medial branches** (*rami mediales*) run dorsolaterally, essentially parallel and caudal to the first 10 caudally sloping thoracic vertebral spines, with which they correspond in number. Caudal to the eleventh thoracic spine, the thoracic spines slope cranially, and the corresponding nerve branches cross them obliquely because they run caudodorsally. The medial branches supply the multifidus thoracis, rotatores, longissimus dorsi, and spinalis et semispinalis thoracis et cervicis. It is probable that the vertebrae, ligaments, and dura receive branches from these nerves. The medial branches do not end in cutaneous branches (Fig. 17.5).

The **lateral branches** (*rami laterales*) from the dorsal branches of the thoracic nerves run caudolaterally at approximately a 45-degree angle to a sagittal plane. They course between the longissimus dorsi muscle medially and the iliocostal muscle laterally to reach the medial surfaces of the segments of the serratus dorsalis muscles where these are present. They usually perforate these segments as well as the iliocostalis dorsi. As these nerves cross the medial border of the iliocostalis dorsi, they give off medial branches to it and to the levator costae muscle segments. With the exception of the first thoracic nerve, longer lateral branches perforate the cutaneus trunci muscle to reach the skin, where they divide in the superficial fascia into a short **medial cutaneous branch** (*ramus cutaneus medialis*) and a longer **lateral cutaneous branch** (*ramus cutaneus lateralis*) that supply the skin of approximately the dorsal third of the thorax (Figs. 17.30 to 17.33). These cutaneous branches do not communicate with adjacent branches and thus establish a segmental innervation of the dorsal part of the thorax with considerable overlap between adjacent branches, although distinct autonomous zones are present (Figs. 17.10 and 17.33) (Bailey et al., 1984). The cutaneous area of the cutaneous branches of the second thoracic spinal nerve dorsal branch overlap with the cutaneous area of the medial branch of the dorsal branch of the sixth cervical nerve.

The **ventral branches** (*rami ventrales*) of the thoracic nerves, with the exception of most of the first and the thirteenth, are more commonly known as the intercostal nerves (*nn. intercostales*). A typical **intercostal nerve** (*n. intercostalis*) (Figs. 17.30 and 17.31) begins where the main trunk terminates by dividing into the communicating and the ventral branches. For approximately the first centimeter, the intercostal nerve lies embedded in the dorsal border of the cranioventrally running internal intercostal muscle.

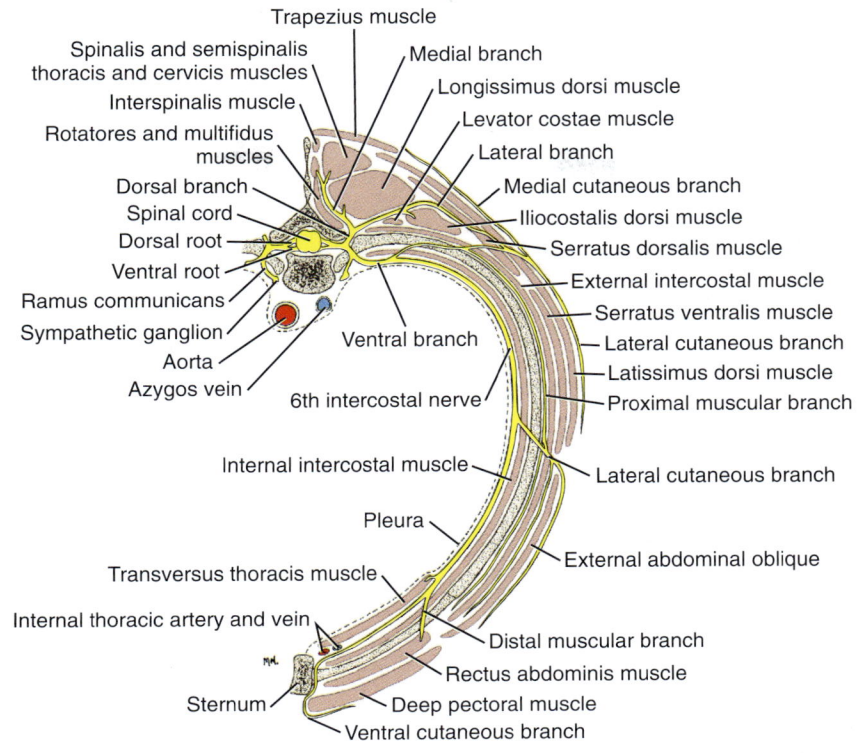

• **Fig. 17.30** Diagram of the sixth thoracic nerve. (Section caudal to the sixth rib.)

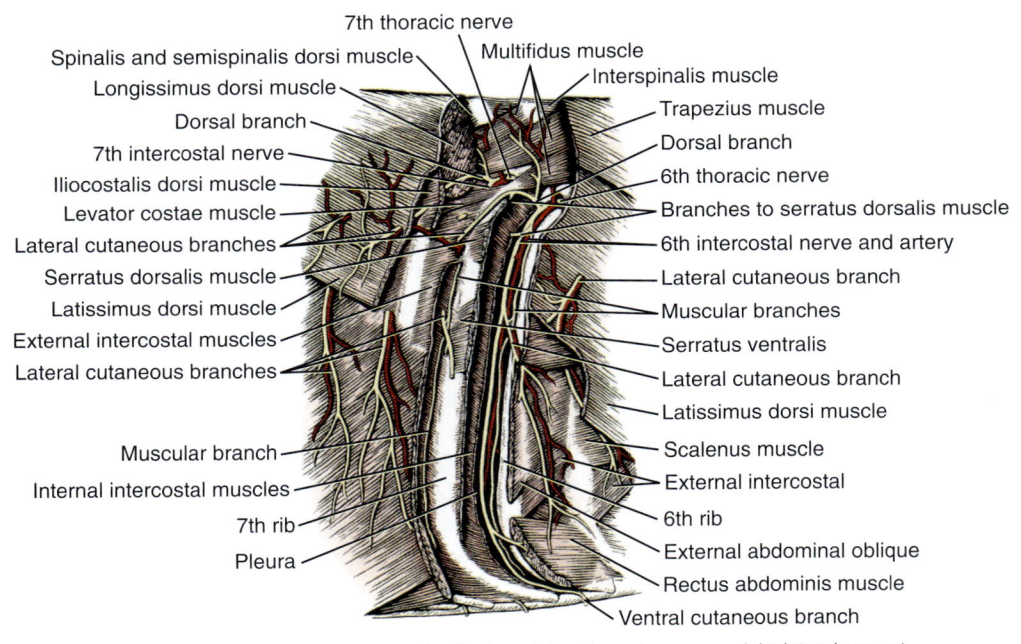

• **Fig. 17.31** Dissection showing distribution of the thoracic nerves, right lateral aspect.

It then turns distad on the medial surface of the internal intercostal muscle, where it is separated from the caudal border of the corresponding rib by the intercostal vein and the intercostal artery. Variations in this order of arrangement occur most frequently in the cranial part of the series. This triad of structures is surrounded by a variable quantity of fat. The nerve lies adjacent to or among the fiber strands of the internal intercostal muscle. In the caudal part of the thorax, fleshy sheets of the internal intercostal muscle from the intercostal space cranial to it extend over the ribs medially and cover the intercostal vessels and nerves that lie caudal to the rib. In most intercostal spaces, the intercostal vessels and nerves are covered medially only by the pleura.

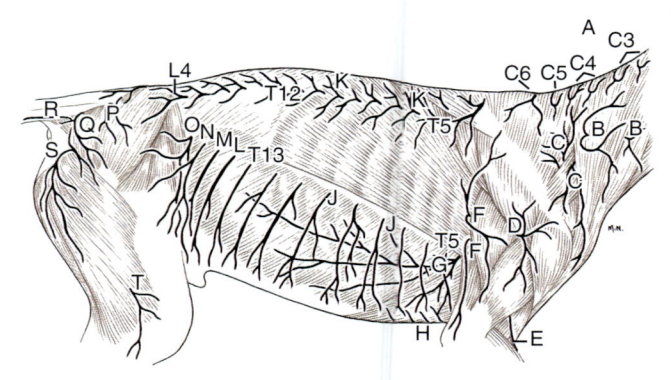

A. Dorsal branches of cervical nerves
B. Ventral branches of C3
C. Ventral branches of C4
D. Cranial lateral cutaneous brachial nerve (from axillary)
E. Radial nerve, superficial branch
F. Intercostobrachial nerve (from T2)
G. Lateral thoracic nerve (from C8 and T1)
H. Ventral cutaneous branches of intercostal nerves
J. Lateral cutaneous branches of intercostal nerves
K. Medial and lateral cutaneous branches of thoracic nerves
L. Cranial iliohypogastric nerve (L1)
M. Caudal iliohypogastric nerve (L2)
N. Ilioinguinal nerve (L3)
O. Lateral cutaneous femoral nerve (L3 and L4)
P. Dorsal cutaneous branch of S1
Q. From ventral branch of S1 and S2
R. From ventral branch of S3
S. Caudal cutaneous femoral nerve
T. Lateral cutaneous sural nerve

• **Fig. 17.32** Cutaneous nerves of the neck and trunk, lateral aspect.

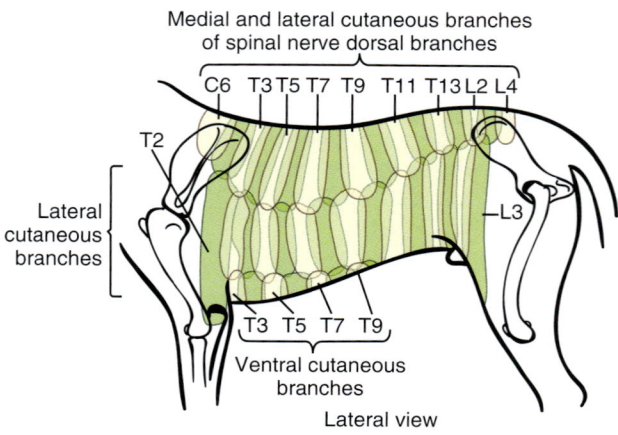

• **Fig. 17.33** Schematic illustration of the cutaneous areas of the cutaneous branches of the thoracic and cranial lumbar spinal nerves, lateral view. (Modified, with permission, from Bailey CS, Kitchell RL, Haghighi SS, et al.: Cutaneous innervation of the thorax and abdomen of the dog, *Am J Vet Res* 45:1689–1698, 1984.)

A typical intercostal nerve has the following muscular and cutaneous branches* (Figs. 17.30 and 17.31). A proximal muscular branch leaves the dorsal (lateral) side of the intercostal nerve 1 or 2 cm from its origin (Fig. 17.30). Before it perforates the external intercostal muscle, it sends a long, slender branch distally on the deep (medial) surface of the external intercostal muscle, which lies only a few millimeters caudal to the corresponding rib. It sends delicate branches to the external intercostal muscle throughout its length. On contact with the external intercostal muscle, a branch leaves the nerve that runs laterally and supplies the serratus dorsalis cranialis. It does not give off any cutaneous branches.

A lateral branch of the intercostal nerve (Fig. 17.30) passes through the midlateral portion of the thoracic wall and runs distad in the superficial fascia with the like-named artery. The lateral branch terminates by dividing into a middle muscular branch that supplies the thoracic parts of dorsal muscles of the abdominal wall and a **lateral cutaneous branch** (*ramus cutaneus lateralis*) (Figs. 17.5, 17.30, and 17.31) that collectively supplies all the skin on the ventrolateral half of the thoracic wall except a narrow, longitudinal ventral strip (Figs. 17.33 and 17.34) (Bailey et al., 1984). In the regions of the thoracic mammary glands, **lateral mammary branches** (*rami mammarii lateralis*) branch from the distal portion of the lateral cutaneous branches and ramify under the skin of the mammary glands.

Two distal muscular branches consist of a short branch that enters the transversus thoracis muscle and a longer branch that passes to the lateral side of the rib cage and enters the rectus abdominis.

The **ventral cutaneous branch** (*ramus cutaneus ventralis*) (Figs. 17.30 through 17.32) is the terminal part of intercostal nerves T2 through T10. The first and last two intercostal nerves have no ventral cutaneous branches. In the superficial thoracic fascia, which lies on the medial portion of the deep pectoral muscle, the ventral cutaneous branch is closely bound to the only slightly larger ventral cutaneous artery. The aggregate of these nerves supplies a zone of skin approximately 5 cm wide that lies adjacent to the midventral line (Figs. 17.4, 17.33, and 17.34) (Kitchell et al., 1980; Bailey et al., 1984). The cutaneous area of the ventral cutaneous branch of the second thoracic intercostal nerve overlaps with the cutaneous area of the cutaneous branch of the ventral branch of the fifth cervical nerve on the medial surface of the arm (Kitchell et al., 1980) (Fig. 17.10). The terminal branches of the ventral cutaneous branches of the fifth and seventh intercostal nerves ramify in the skin covering the medial portions of the two thoracic mammary glands when these glands are functional. They are named the **medial mammary branches** (*rami mammarii mediales*).

---

*A number of authors consider the **communicating branch** (*ramus communicans*) to arise from the intercostal nerve. Others, including these authors, do not consider the intercostal nerve to begin until after the communicating branch is given off the main trunk. The communicating branch consists of general visceral efferent (sympathetic) axons and general visceral afferent axons that are distributed to organs in the body cavities or go back to the main trunk to be distributed via one of the other three primary branches to a visceral structure (smooth muscle or glands) in the body wall. The communicating branches are connections between the initial part of the main trunk of a spinal nerve and the sympathetic trunk, usually at a ganglion. The communicating branches vary in length, averaging approximately 1 mm in diameter and 3 mm in length.

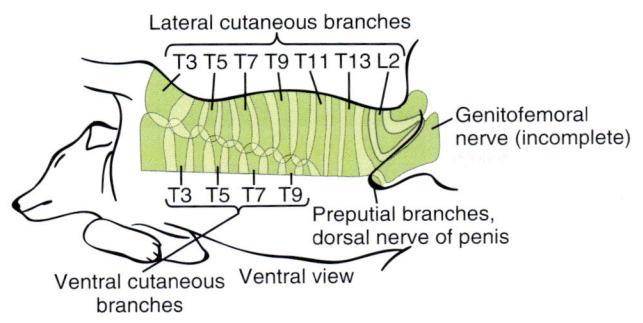

• **Fig. 17.34** Schematic illustration of the cutaneous areas of thoracic and cranial lumbar nerves, ventral view. (Modified, with permission, from Bailey CS, Kitchell RL, Haghighi SS, et al.: Cutaneous innervation of the thorax and abdomen of the dog, *Am J Vet Res* 45:1689–1698, 1984.)

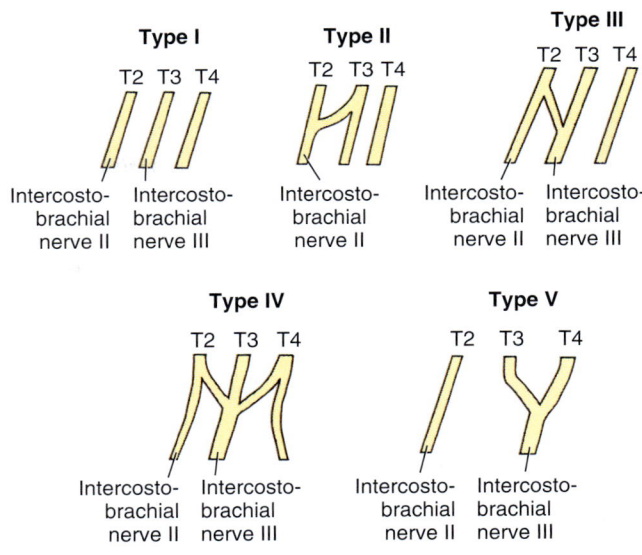

• **Fig. 17.35** Schematic illustration of the five types of contributions to the formation of the intercostobrachial nerves in descending order of frequency. (Modified, with permission, from Bailey CS, Kitchell RL, Haghighi SS, et al.: Cutaneous innervation of the thorax and abdomen of the dog, *Am J Vet Res* 45:1689–1698, 1984.)

The ventral extensions of the last two intercostal nerves leave the intercostal spaces medial to the costal arch and extend toward the linea alba on the superficial surface of the m. transversus abdominis, which they supply before terminating in the rectus abdominis. These nerves fail to send ventral cutaneous branches to the skin (Bailey et al., 1984).

The major portion of the ventral branch of the first thoracic nerve passes cranial medial to the neck of the first rib and contributes appreciably to the formation of the brachial plexus. The intercostal portion of the first thoracic nerve is but a delicate branch that enters the muscles of the first intercostal space. It has no ventral cutaneous branch (Kitchell et al., 1980).

The **second intercostal nerve** (*n. intercostalis II*) differs from the intercostal nerves that lie caudal to it in two respects. First, it usually sends a small communicating branch to the first thoracic nerve, and, second, its **lateral cutaneous branch, intercostal nerve II** (*n. intercostobrachialis II*), is the largest of all these branches. Furthermore, this branch runs to the thoracic limb and supplies the skin overlying the long head of the m. triceps brachii (Figs. 17.17 and 17.33) (Kitchell et al., 1980). This area of innervation is of major significance because in avulsions of the roots of the brachial plexus the roots of the second thoracic nerve are not usually avulsed; thus this cutaneous area retains its sensitivity (Bailey, 1984). The **lateral cutaneous branch of the third intercostal nerve, intercostal nerve III** (*n. intercostobrachialis III*), often intermingles with that of the second intercostal nerve and branches of the lateral thoracic nerve. Five combinations of lateral branches contributing to the formation of intercostobrachial nerves have been described (Fig. 17.35) (Bailey et al., 1984). The cutaneous area of the intercostobrachial nerve III lies caudal to the second and also supplies the caudomedial aspect of the arm overlapping with the ventral cutaneous branches of the second and third thoracic intercostal nerves medially and with the cutaneous area of the cutaneous branch of the brachiocephalic nerve cranially (Figs. 17.17 and 17.33) (Kitchell et al., 1980).

The eleventh and twelfth intercostal nerves have no ventral branches. Instead, their lateral cutaneous branches are much longer, and their cutaneous areas extend ventral to reach the ventral midline (Figs. 17.33 and 17.34) (Bailey et al., 1984).

The **costoabdominal nerve** (*n. costoabdominalis*) is the ventral branch of the last or thirteenth thoracic nerve. It supplies a band of the abdominal wall that lies adjacent to the caudal border of the last rib and then continues tangentially to the last rib and costal arch in the abdominal wall. In its area of distribution it lies cranial but parallel to the bands of the abdominal wall that are supplied by the ventral branches of the first three lumbar nerves. It divides into lateral and medial branches that resemble those of the lumbar nerves lying caudal to it. Its lateral branch gives off a lateral cutaneous branch that has a cutaneous area that reaches the ventral midline (Figs. 17.33 and 17.34) (Bailey et al., 1984).

Lumbar Nerves

The **lumbar nerves** (*nn. lumbales*) (Figs. 17.36 and 17.37) are seven in number on each side. Each member of a pair has the same number as its intervertebral foramen of exit and the vertebra that lies cranial to it. The middle of the first lumbar segment of the spinal cord lies dorsal to intervertebral disc between the first and the second lumbar vertebrae. The nerve roots of the first pair of lumbar nerves therefore lie essentially in the same transverse area as the foramina of exit of these nerves. As traced caudally, the segments of the spinal cord are shorter than the vertebral segments. As a result, the spinal cord ends dorsal to the intervertebral disc between the sixth and the seventh lumbar

732 CHAPTER 17 The Spinal Nerves

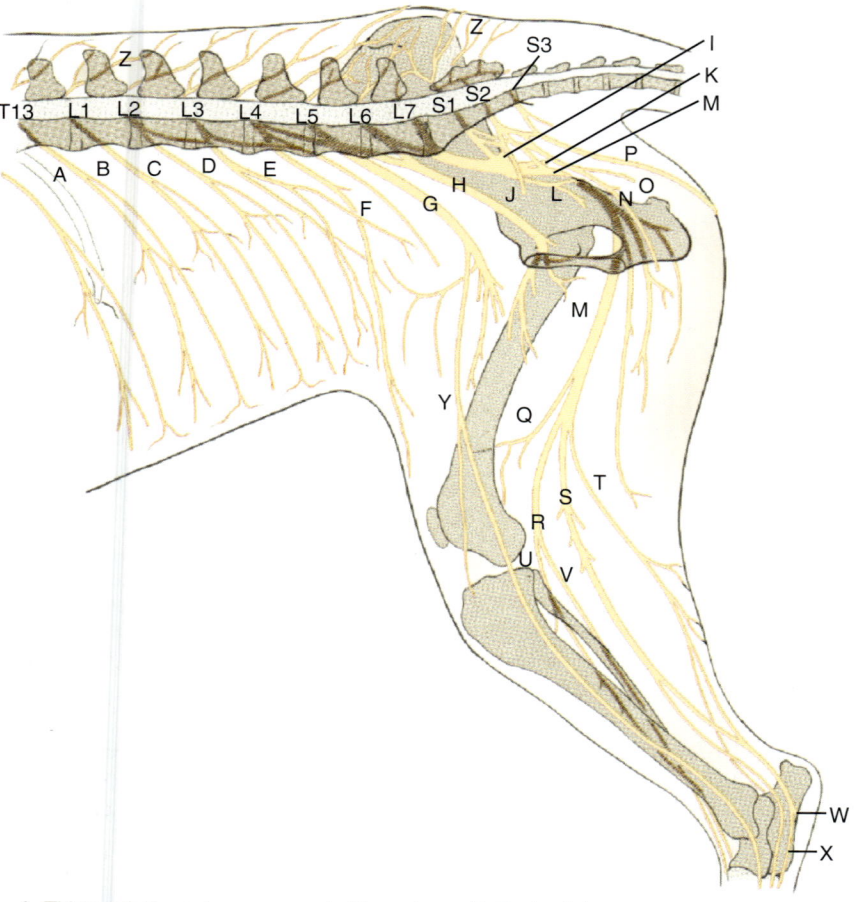

A. Thirteenth thoracic nerve, ventral branch
B. Cranial iliohypogastric nerve
C. Caudal iliohypogastric nerve
D. Ilioinguinal nerve
E. Lateral cutaneous femoral nerve
F. Genitofemoral nerve
G. Femoral nerve
H. Obturator nerve
I. Cranial gluteal nerve
J. Pelvic nerve
K. Caudal gluteal nerve
L. Nerve to mm. obturator internus, gemelli, and quadratus femoris
M. Ischiatic nerve
N. Pudendal nerve
O. Perineal nerve
P. Caudal cutaneous femoral nerve
Q. Lateral cutaneous sural nerve
R. Common fibular nerve
S. Tibial nerve
T. Caudal cutaneous sural nerve
U. Deep fibular nerve
V. Superficial fibular nerve
W. Lateral plantar nerve
X. Medial plantar nerve
Y. Saphenous nerve
Z. Dorsal branches of lumbar and sacral nerves

• **Fig. 17.36** Schematic medial view of lumbar and sacral nerves.

---

vertebrae (Fig. 16.4). Because of this disproportionate length, the dorsal and ventral roots of the last several pairs of spinal nerves run increasingly longer distances within the vertebral canal before leaving their osseous confines by means of the intervertebral foramina. The leash of sacrocaudal nerve roots thus formed is called the *cauda equina*. According to Hopkins (1935), in a 40- to 50-pound dog the intraspinal extent of the lumbar nerves varies from 0.6 cm for the first pair to 3.5 cm for the seventh. This author was undoubtedly measuring the nerve roots rather than the spinal nerves that they form. The reason for this spatial disparity between the length of the spinal cord and the vertebral column is a continuation of the growth of the vertebral column after the spinal cord has stopped growing and a difference in the length of the spinal cord segments of the different regions of the spinal cord (Fletcher & Kitchell, 1966a). Purinton (1982) described considerable variation in the lumbosacral spinal roots in the dog. Variations were found in 11 of 99 dogs. The most frequent variation was a confluence of spinal ganglia (interganglia bridges). Other variations seen were the union of one spinal root to an adjacent root, the formation of a single spinal root from rootlets of adjacent spinal cord segments and dividing into two spinal nerves at the level of the spinal ganglion, and two or more roots bound together in a common connective tissue sheath.

The main trunk of the lumbar spinal nerves is formed by the merging of the dorsal and ventral roots at the

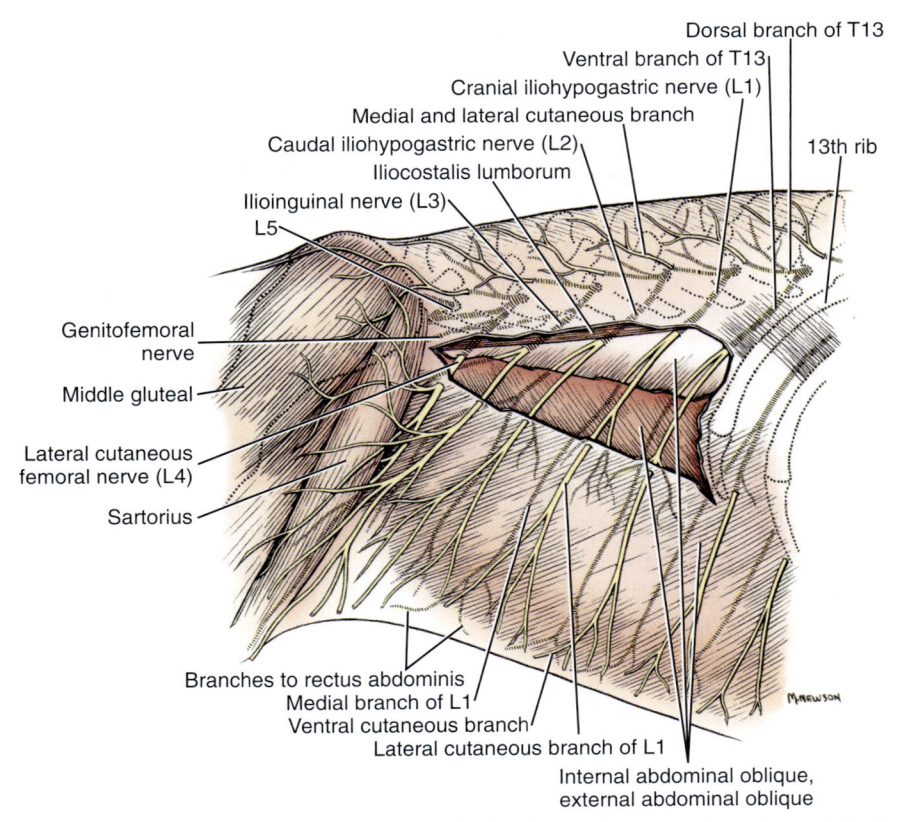

• **Fig. 17.37** Dissection showing the arrangement of the first four lumbar nerves, lateral aspect. A window has been cut into the m. external abdominal oblique to demonstrate the underlying m. internal abdominal oblique and the course of nerves in this area.

intervertebral foramina. As the roots of the several lumbar spinal nerves run caudally, their proximal parts lie within the dural covering of the spinal cord, and their distal parts lie in meningeal tubes in soft epidural fat. Like the typical spinal nerves of the preceding regions, each lumbar spinal nerve divides on leaving the intervertebral foramen into four primary branches: a small and variable meningeal branch, small dorsal and communicating branches, and a larger ventral branch. The actual length of the main trunk of each lumbar spinal nerve is only a few millimeters, and it lies largely in and just lateral to the intervertebral foramen through which it passes.

The **dorsal branches** (*rami dorsales*) of the lumbar nerves are similar throughout most of the region. Like the thoracic nerves, each typically divides into medial and lateral branches (Fig. 17.5). The **medial branches** (*rami mediales*) arborize in the m. longissimus lumborum, which they supply, and send terminal branches to the multifidus lumborum and interspinales lumborum. They run caudodorsad obliquely across the lateral surface of the cranially inclined spinous processes of the vertebrae that are caudal to them. They are separated from the ventral borders of the tendons of the longissimus lumborum that go to the accessory processes of the lumbar vertebrae by the large branches of the dorsal branches of the lumbar segmental arteries. No dorsal cutaneous branches arise from the medial branches of the dorsal branches of the lumbar nerves.

The **lateral branches** (*rami laterales*) of the dorsal branches of the first three or four lumbar nerves are clearly separated from the medial branches (Fig. 17.5). The dorsal branches of the last three or four lumbar nerves do not clearly divide into medial and lateral portions, but they arborize in the caudal lumbar epaxial muscles. The lumbar nerves do not give off any dorsal cutaneous branches (Bailey et al., 1984). The lateral branches of the dorsal branches of the first three or four lumbar nerves run caudolaterad through the mm. longissimus and iliocostalis and perforate the iliocostalis midlaterally in a segmental manner. They supply the lumbar part of the iliocostalis. After continuing in a caudolateral direction in the areolar tissue deep to the thoracolumbar fascia 1 cm or more, they perforate the thoracolumbar fascia and arborize in the skin (Fig. 17.37) of the dorsolateral parts of the lumbar and sacral regions as the **medial and lateral cutaneous branches** (*rami cutanei medialis et lateralis*). These cutaneous branches of the lumbar nerves that innervate the skin of the gluteal region and over the tensor fascia lata are referred to as the **cranial clunial nerves** (*nn. clunium craniales*). The cutaneous branches of the dorsal branches in the lumbar region are variable in that there may or may not be a cutaneous branch from the dorsal branch of the fourth lumbar nerve (Bailey et al., 1984, 1988; Haghighi et al., 1991).

The **clunial nerves** (*nn. clunii*) are cutaneous nerves to the skin of the pelvic region (clunis = buttocks; clunial =

gluteal). The **cranial clunial nerves** (*nn. clunii craniales*) are branches of the medial or lateral branch of the dorsal branch of the caudal lumbar nerves. The **middle clunial nerves** (*nn. clunii medii*) have a similar origin from the sacral nerves. The **caudal clunial nerves** (*nn. clunii caudales*) arise from the sacral plexus.

In some specimens the cutaneous branches of the dorsal branch of the seventh lumbar nerve join the cutaneous branches of the dorsal branches of the sacral spinal nerves to help form the middle clunial nerves (Bailey et al., 1988). In the lumbar nerves that do not have cutaneous branches from their dorsal branches, it is not possible to differentiate medial and lateral branches; instead muscular branches arise that are dissipated in the epaxial musculature without first dividing into medial and lateral parts.

The main trunk of each lumbar nerve is connected to the sympathetic trunk by a ramus communicans, with rare exceptions. The connections are exceedingly variable, as Mehler et al. (1952) have pointed out. In 100 dogs dissected by these investigators, only 23 specimens had symmetrically located bilateral trunk ganglia at every lumbar segment. These 23 specimens also had at least two paired sacral ganglia. The rami communicantes may be double, or the rami from two adjacent nerves may go to the same ganglion. The first four or five rami contain preganglionic as well as postganglionic sympathetic axons. The remaining communicating rami contain only postganglionic sympathetic and visceral afferent axons. The communicating rami, as they run between the lumbar nerves and the sympathetic trunk, lie largely deep to the psoas minor muscle. They are less than 1 mm in diameter and are approximately 5 mm in length. According to Mehler et al. (1952), the fourth lumbar nerve is the most caudal spinal nerve with preganglionic sympathetic axons in the ramus communicans. Rami caudal to the fourth lumbar ramus consist only of postganglionic sympathetic axons and general visceral afferent axons going back to the main trunk, to be distributed via the other three lumbar nerve branches.

The **ventral branches** (*rami ventrales*) of the seven pairs of lumbar nerves are variable, but less so than the dorsal branches. They are usually described as lumbar nerves without specifically referring to them as *ventral branches*. Like the brachial plexus, which gives origin to the nerves that innervate the thoracic limb, the last five lumbar nerve ventral branches and all the sacral nerve ventral branches are joined together to form the **lumbosacral plexus** (*plexus lumbosacralis*), from which the nerves to the pelvic limb originate (Fig. 17.38). This plexus can be divided into lumbar and sacral portions. The first two lumbar nerves are usually not joined to each other or to adjacent nerves but run caudolaterally in the abdominal wall in series with the last several caudal thoracic nerves and are therefore not included in the lumbosacral plexus.

The **cranial** and **caudal iliohypogastric nerves** (*nn. iliohypogastrici craniales et caudales*) (Figs. 17.37 and 17.38) represent the ventral branches of the first and second lumbar nerves, respectively. Both nerves give off medial branches that are muscular branches to the quadratus lumborum and psoas minor. After passing between the two segments of the quadratus lumborum, the cranial iliohypogastric nerve lies in the subserous endothoracic fascia at its origin. It then passes into the subserous transversalis fascia of the abdomen by passing dorsal to the lumbocostal arch. It gives branches to the serosa and to the segments of the quadratus lumborum, against which it lies. After having passed through the aponeurosis of origin of the transversus abdominis, it then runs between two adjacent fleshy bundles of the transversus abdominis as these bundles arise from a narrow aponeurosis that attaches to the ends of the transverse processes of the lumbar vertebrae. Shortly after entering the fascia that separates the transverse abdominal from the internal abdominal oblique

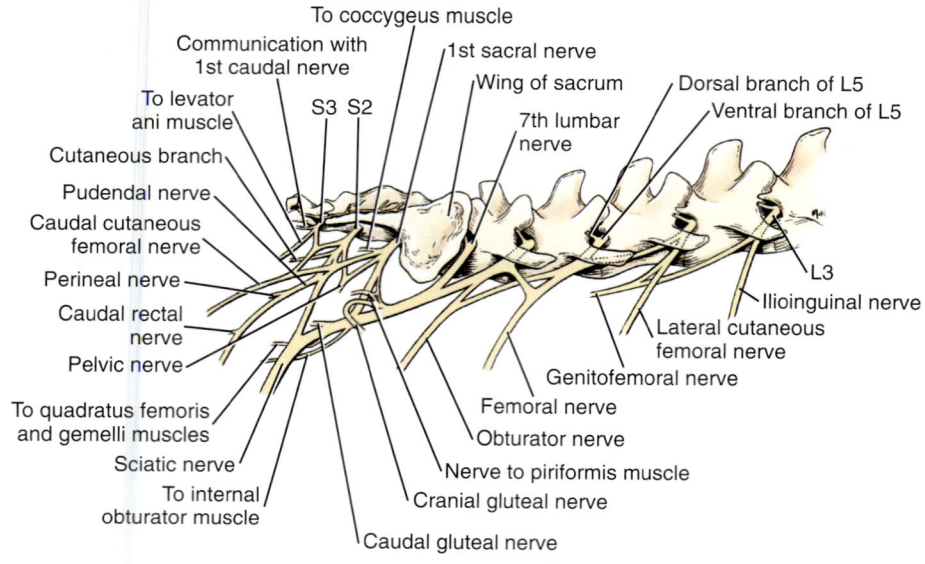

• **Fig. 17.38** Diagram of the lumbosacral plexus, right lateral aspect.

muscle, the cranial iliohypogastric nerve divides into lateral and medial branches.

The **lateral branch** (*ramus lateralis*) passes through the internal abdominal oblique to run in the septum between the two abdominal oblique muscles. In its course ventrocaudally it sends most of its branches to these muscles, and near the middle of the abdomen it perforates the external abdominal oblique muscle to become subcutaneous as the **lateral cutaneous branch** (*ramus cutaneus lateralis*) (Figs. 17.32 and 17.37). It is accompanied by a branch of the cranial abdominal artery and vein. The lateral cutaneous branch is distributed to a ventrolaterally running band of skin that crosses the junction of the cranial and middle thirds of the abdomen caudal to the ribs (Figs. 17.33, 17.34, and 17.39). Its cutaneous area extends ventrally to the ventral midline except in the male, in which it does not supply the prepuce (Spurgeon & Kitchell, 1982) (Fig. 17.39).

The **medial branch** (*ramus medialis*) lies closely applied to the lateral surface of the m. transversus abdominis, where it appears in series with the last five thoracic and the second and third lumbar nerves. Like the lateral branch, it is also accompanied by a small branch of the cranial abdominal artery and vein. It supplies a band of the transversus abdominis and peritoneum along its course. It ends in the first lumbar segment of the rectus abdominis and peritoneum dorsal to it. It has no ventral cutaneous branch (Bailey et al., 1984) (Fig. 17.5).

The ventral branch of the **second lumbar nerve** is the caudal iliohypogastric nerve (Fig. 17.37). This nerve is in all respects similar to the first lumbar nerve except that it supplies the abdominal wall caudal to it and appears at the lateral border of the hypaxial musculature after having passed between the quadratus lumborum and iliopsoas at the lumbocostal arch. Occasionally, one of the iliohypogastric nerves is double, with a reciprocal diminution in size of the nerve caudal to it. Rarely is a single nerve formed by the fusion of the first and second or the second and third lumbar nerves. The lateral cutaneous branch of the caudal iliohypogastric nerve is similar to that of the cranial iliohypogastric except that it does not reach as far ventrally as the ventral midline (Figs. 17.36 and 17.44). The caudal iliohypogastric nerve also does not have any ventral cutaneous branch (Bailey et al., 1984).

The **lumbosacral plexus** (*plexus lumbosacralis*) (Figs. 17.38, 17.40, and 17.41) consists of the intercommunicating ventral branches of the last five lumbar nerves and the three sacral nerves. It may be divided into lumbar and sacral plexuses, although the two always have communications. The **lumbar plexus** (*plexus lumbalis*) provides the nerves that innervate the cranial and medial muscles of the thigh and the skin on the medial aspect of the pelvic limb. The **sacral plexus** (*plexus sacralis*) provides the nerves that innervate the caudal muscles of the thigh and all the muscles of the crus and pes as well as the corresponding skin. There is an overlapping of contributed axons to the named nerves of the plexus so that most pelvic and pelvic limb muscles and structures are innervated from more than one level of the spinal cord. *Lumbar plexus* is a term ordinarily restricted to the interconnected third, fourth, and fifth lumbar nerves (Havelka, 1928). In some specimens the third lumbar nerve is connected to the second by a fine branch (Bradley & Grahame, 1959), and usually the fifth lumbar nerve is connected to the sixth. The division of the lumbosacral plexus into its two components is made primarily because of the location of the plexuses and not its origin. The connection between the third and fourth lumbar nerves gives origin to the genitofemoral nerve, whereas the connection between the fourth and fifth nerves is usually devoid of branches.

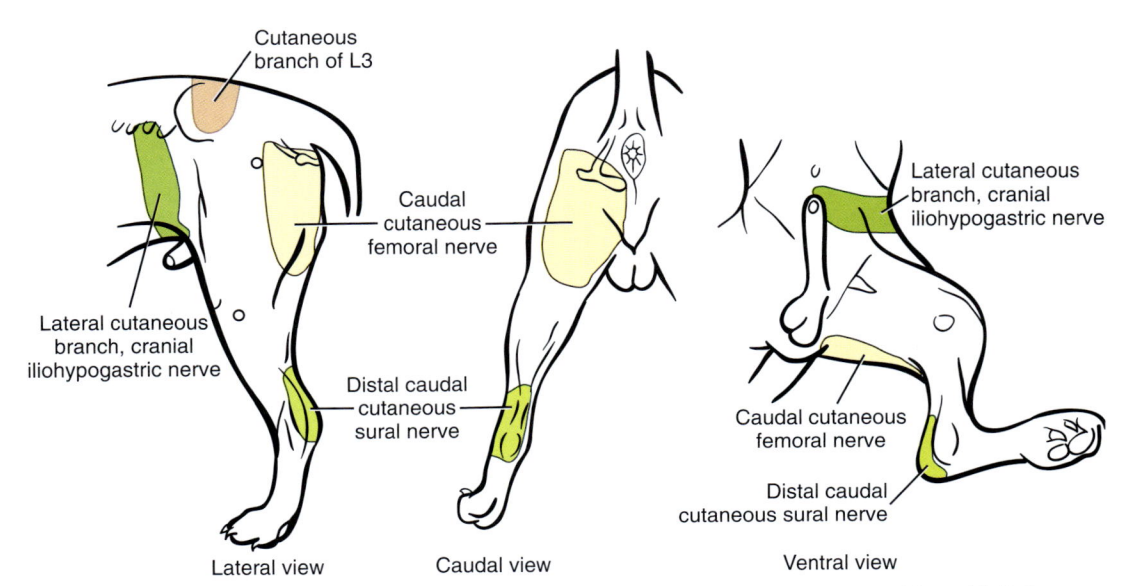

• **Fig. 17.39** Schematic illustration of the cutaneous areas of selected cutaneous nerves of the pelvic limb. (Modified, with permission, from Haghighi SS, Kitchell RL, Johnson RD, et al.: Electrophysiologic studies of the cutaneous innervation of the pelvic limb of male dogs, *Am J Vet Res* 52:352–362, 1991.)

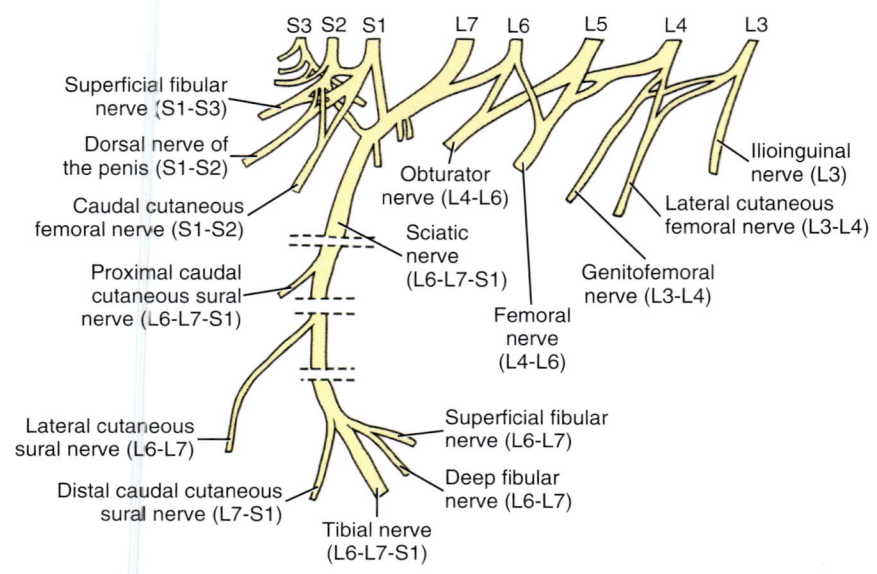

• **Fig. 17.40** Schematic representation of the spinal root origins of the major nerves of the lumbosacral plexus. (Based on the work of Fletcher TF: Lumbosacral plexus and pelvic limb myotomes in the dog, *Am J Vet Res* 31:35–41, 1970; and Bailey CS, Kitchell RL, Haghighi SS, et al.: Spinal root origins of the cutaneous nerves of the canine pelvic limb, *Am J Vet Res* 45:1689–1698, 1984.)

Variability in the segmental origin of nerves arising from the lumbosacral plexus frequently occurs (Fletcher, 1970) (Fig. 17.41). A plexus is said to be **prefixed plexus** when the nerves are formed by rootlets more cranial than is the usual case. In a **postfixed plexus**, axons forming regional nerves originate more caudally from spinal cord segments, compared with a **median fixed plexus**, which is the most common type. In general, the third, fourth, and fifth lumbar nerves contribute to the femoral nerve; L3 and L4 to the genitofemoral; L4, L5, and L6 to the obturator; L6, L7, and S1 to the cranial gluteal; L6, L7, S1, and S2 to the sciatic and its branches; and S1, S2, and S3 to the pudendal nerves (de Lahunta et al., 2015). Fletcher (1970) studied the spinal root origin of the nerves arising from the lumbosacral plexus and the muscles they supplied. The muscles supplied by a spinal nerve constitute a **myotome**. Seldom is a single muscle supplied by only one spinal nerve. Bailey et al. (1988) studied the dorsal root origins of the axons in the cutaneous nerves that are branches of nerves originating from the lumbosacral plexus. The results of these two studies are summarized in Fig. 17.40.

Bennett (1976) studied the gross and histologic features of the sciatic nerve and its branches in the cat and dog and provided a table showing details of the internal funicular structure of the common fibular and tibial nerves. His findings agree with those of Havelka (1928) and others regarding the components of the sciatic nerve. Worthman (1957), Bennett and Vaughan (1976), and Gilmore (1984) studied the results of surgical transection, traumatic injury, or both to the various branches of nerves arising from the lumbosacral plexus. Fletcher and Kitchell (1966a) and Fletcher (1970) studied the cutaneous innervation of the pelvic limb and found variation in the spinal segments involved. The lumbosacral dermatomes overlap considerably (Fig. 17.42).

The **ilioinguinal nerve** (*n. ilioinguinalis*) (Figs. 17.37, 17.38, and 17.44) is the direct ventrolateral continuation of the major part of the ventral branch of the third lumbar nerve. It gives off medial branches that supply the psoas major, psoas minor, and iliacus. The ilioinguinal nerve communicates with the fourth lumbar nerve and divides into medial and lateral branches that resemble those of the lumbar nerves that precede it. The lateral branch extends caudoventrally and terminates as the **lateral cutaneous branch** (*ramus cutaneus lateralis*), which ramifies in the skin of the craniolateral surface of the thigh (Figs. 17.32 to 17.34, and 17.40) (Bailey et al., 1984). Its cutaneous area does not extend to the ventral midline but instead overlaps with the craniodorsal aspects of the cutaneous area of the genitofemoral nerve (Fig. 17.34). The medial branch of the ilioinguinal nerve is small. It runs more caudally than ventrolaterally. It is accompanied by a cranial branch of the ascending branch of the deep circumflex iliac vessels. It has no grossly demonstrable cutaneous branches, and thus no cutaneous area (Bailey et al., 1984).

The **lateral cutaneous femoral nerve** (*n. cutaneus femoralis lateralis*) (Figs. 17.36, 17.37, and 17.48) is formed primarily by the ventral branch of the fourth lumbar nerve, although there are connections with both the third and the fifth lumbar nerves (Fig. 17.40). Bailey et al. (1984) reported that this nerve originated from L3 and L4 in 7 of 12 dogs; L3, L4, and L5 in 4 of 12; and L4 and L5 in 1 of 12. It originated in part from L4 in 12 of 12 dogs and in part from L3 in 11 of 12. As it runs caudolaterad through the substance of the psoas minor muscle, it sends branches to it and to the other hypaxial muscles of the region. The main

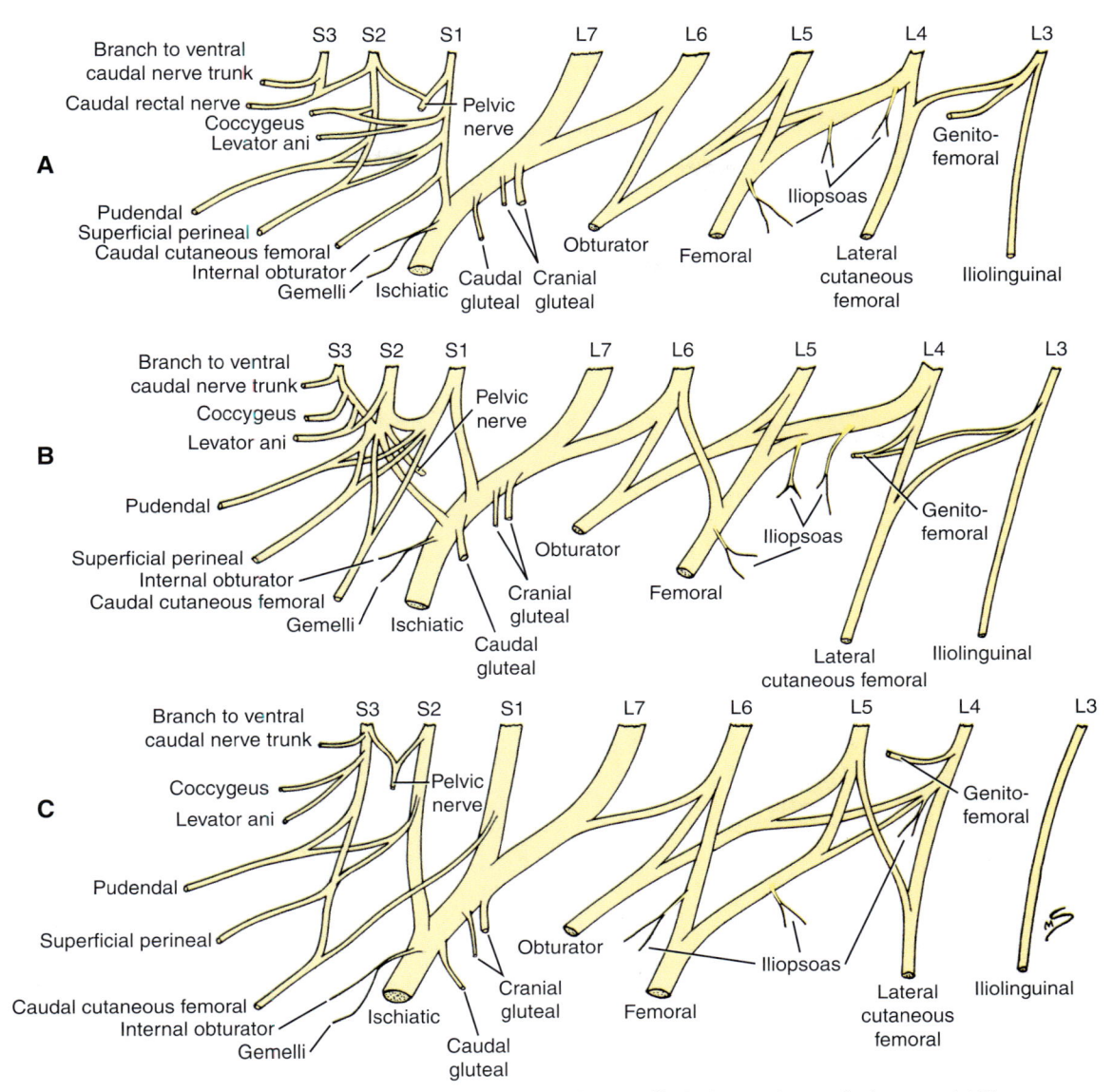

• **Fig. 17.41** Lateral views of canine lumbosacral plexuses illustrate spectrum of plexus variability. **A**, Prefixed type; **B**, median type; **C**, postfixed type. *ca. rect.*, Caudal rectal nerve; *ccf*, caudal cutaneous femoral; *cd.*, branch to ventral caudal nerve trunk; *cr. glu.* and *c. glu.*, cranial and caudal gluteal; *fem.*, femoral; *gen.*, genitofemoral; *il.*, ilioinguinal; *int. obt.* and *gem.*, branches to internal obturator, gemelli, and quadratus femoris muscles; *L3* to *S3* designate ventral rami; *lcf*, lateral cutaneous femoral; *m.*, muscular branches to iliopsoas muscle; *m. lev. ani* and *cocc.*, branches to levator ani and coccygeus muscles; *obt.*, obturator; *pel.*, pelvic nerve. *pud.*, pudendal; *sci.*, ischiatic (sciatic); *sup. perin.*, superficial perineal. (With permission from Fletcher TF: Lumbosacral plexus and pelvic limb myotomes in the dog, *Am J Vet Res* 31:35–41, 1970.)

portion of the nerve passes through the abdominal wall, lying between the deep circumflex iliac artery cranially and the satellite vein caudally. It passes between the lumbar and the inguinal portions of the internal abdominal oblique and over the dorsal margin of the external abdominal oblique muscles. Its terminal cutaneous branches are variable, but in general they follow the accompanying vessels. A branch ramifies in the skin in the region of the tuber coxae and the adjacent cranial part of the pelvic region. Other branches supply the skin over the cranial portion of the thigh, and its longest branch runs distally, supplying the skin over the thigh and the lateral surface of the stifle joint. Kunzel (1957) illustrates this nerve in his work on the topography of the hip joint. The cutaneous area of the lateral cutaneous femoral nerve is very extensive (Fig. 17.45). It reaches to the dorsal midline caudal to the tuber coxae. Laterally it overlaps cranially with cutaneous branches of the dorsal branch of the third (occasionally the fourth) lumbar nerve and ventrally with the cutaneous area of the lateral cutaneous branch of the ilioinguinal nerve (Haghighi et al., 1991).

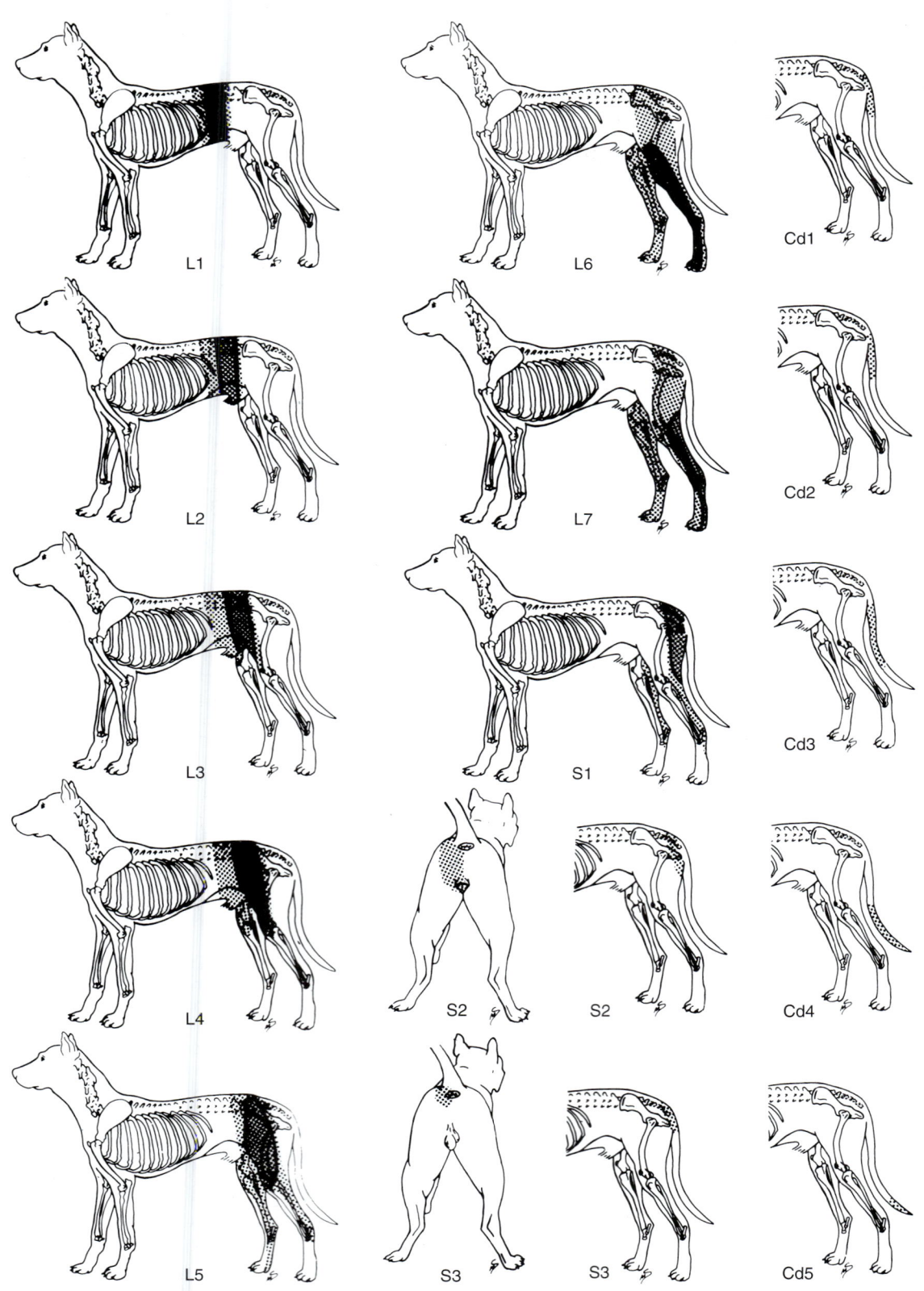

Fig. 17.42 Lumbar, sacral, and caudal tactile dermatomes of the dog are illustrated in relation to skeletal landmarks. Each dotted area represents the entire distribution of a dermatome. The darker zones, shown within L1 to S1, represent regions of denser innervation. Cd, caudal nerves. (With permission from Fletcher TF, Kitchell RL: Anatomical studies on the spinal cord segments of the dog, *Am J Vet Res* 27:1759–1767, 1966b.)

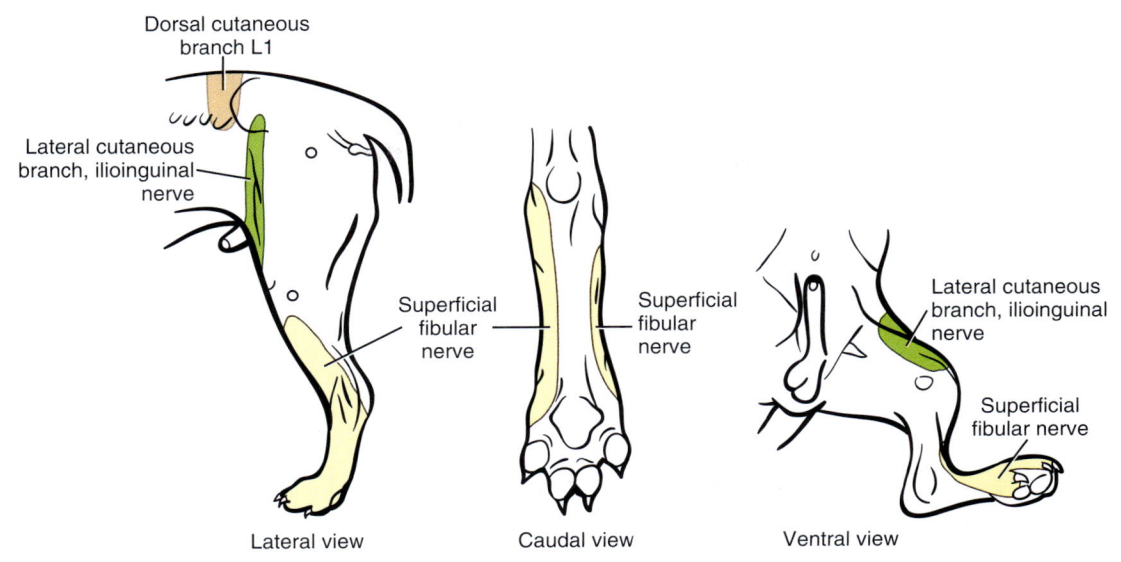

• **Fig. 17.43** Schematic illustration of the cutaneous areas of selected cutaneous nerves of the pelvic limb. (Modified, with permission, from Haghighi SS, Kitchell RL, Johnson RD, et al.: Electrophysiologic studies of the cutaneous innervation of the pelvic limb of male dogs, *Am J Vet Res* 52:352–362, 1991.)

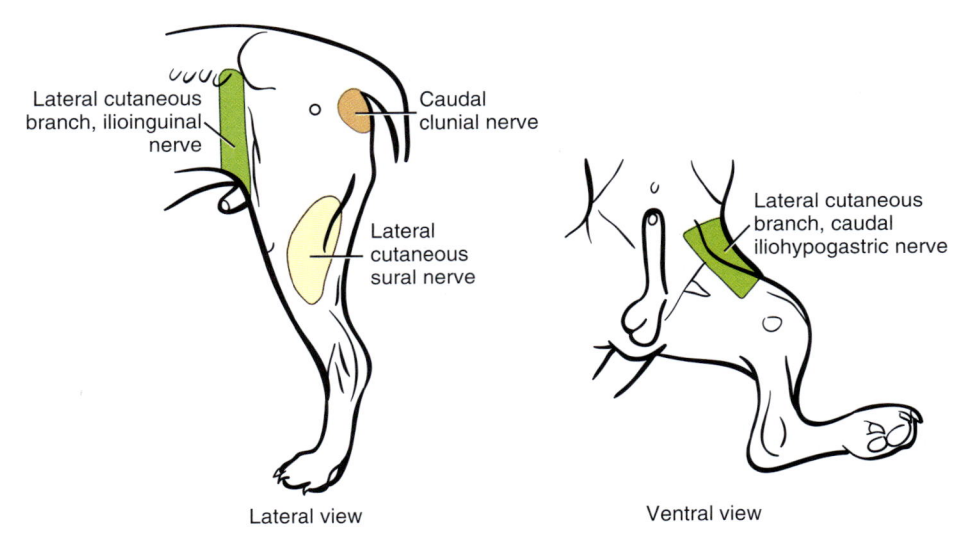

• **Fig. 17.44** Schematic illustration of the cutaneous areas of selected cutaneous nerves of the pelvic limb. (Modified, with permission, from Spurgeon TL, Kitchell RL: Electrophysiological studies of the cutaneous innervation of the external genitalia of the male dog, *Anat Histol Embryol* 11:289–306, 1982; and Haghighi SS, Kitchell RL, Johnson RD, et al.: Electrophysiologic studies of the cutaneous innervation of the pelvic limb of male dogs, *Am J Vet Res* 52:352–362, 1991.)

Caudally it reaches the level of the greater trochanter where it is overlapped by the cutaneous area of the caudal cutaneous femoral nerve.

The **genitofemoral nerve** (*n. genitofemoralis*) (Figs. 17.36, 17.37, and 17.46), formerly the external spermatic nerve, has femoral branches that supply the skin of the proximal aspect of the medial thigh (Figs. 17.46 and 17.47) and a number of genital branches that supply the skin of the pudendal region. The genitofemoral nerve arises from the ventral branches of the third and fourth lumbar nerves, the root from the third being larger than that from the fourth (Fig. 17.40). Bradley and Grahame (1959) state that the contribution from the fourth may be absent. Bailey et al. (1984) found that the nerve arose from L3 and L4 in three of four dogs and L2 and L3 in one of four dogs. Ellenberger and Baum (1891) stated that occasionally the nerve is double, and in some specimens the ilioinguinal nerve joins the genitofemoral nerve and is distributed with it. Usually the nerve is single, small, and long. It is formed in the substance of the medial portion of the psoas major near the body of the fourth lumbar vertebra. As it runs caudally, it leaves the substance of the medial part of the muscle and continues caudally in the fat that fills the irregularities around the caudal vena cava and aorta. After passing dorsal to the medial iliac lymph node, to which it sends a small branch, it becomes related to the distal portion of the

740 CHAPTER 17 The Spinal Nerves

• **Fig. 17.45** Schematic illustration of the cutaneous areas of selected cutaneous nerves of the pelvic limb. (Modified, with permission, from Spurgeon TL, Kitchell RL: Electrophysiological studies of the cutaneous innervation of the external genitalia of the male dog, *Anat Histol Embryol* 11:289–306, 1982; and Haghighi SS, Kitchell RL, Johnson RD, et al.: Electrophysiologic studies of the cutaneous innervation of the pelvic limb of male dogs, *Am J Vet Res* 52:352–362, 1991.)

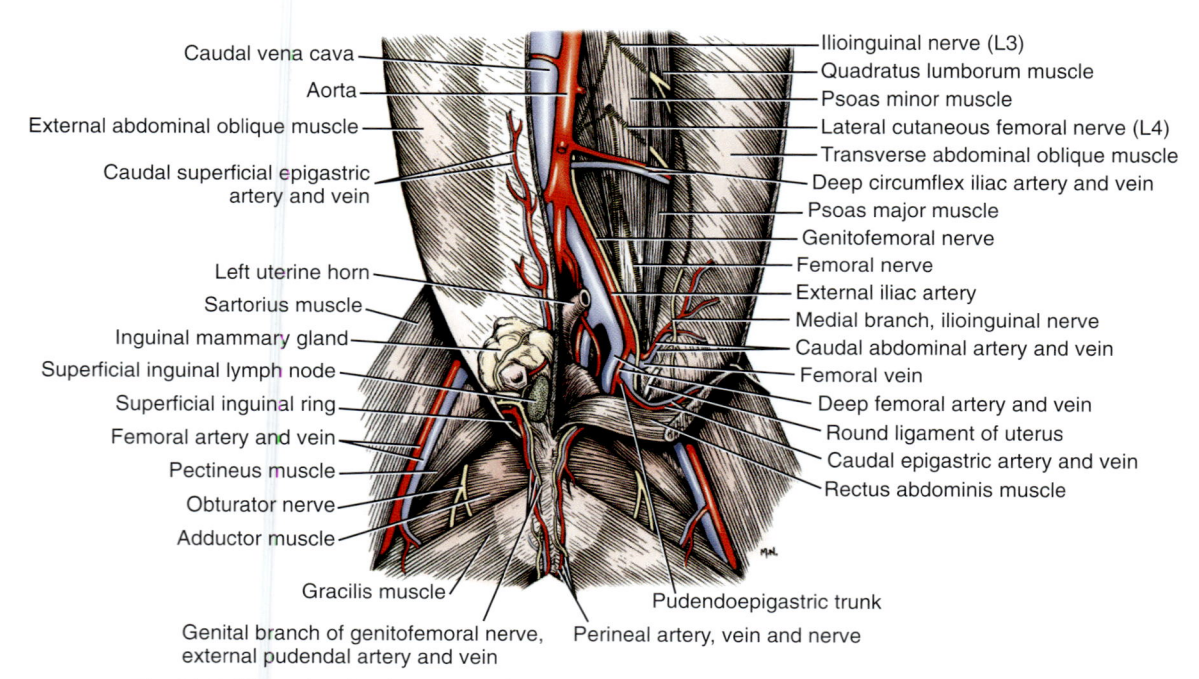

• **Fig. 17.46** Dissection showing course of the genitofemoral nerve and its genital branches in the female, ventral aspect. (The left abdominal wall is reflected.)

external iliac artery, which it crosses medially (Fig. 17.46). It leaves the abdomen by passing through the inguinal canal, where it lies in the spermatic fascia medial to the vaginal tunic in the male or associated with the vaginal process in the female. Minute muscular branches are given off to the cremaster muscle. On passing through the superficial inguinal ring, it provides genital branches to the skin of the prepuce in the male (Figs. 17.34 and 17.47) (Spurgeon & Kitchell, 1982) or to the inguinal mammary gland and its covering skin in the female (Spurgeon & Reddy, 1986). In both sexes the femoral branches of the nerve run caudolaterally and distally and supply a zone of skin on the proximomedial surface of the thigh (Fig. 17.47).

The **femoral nerve** (*n. femoralis*) (Figs. 17.36 and 17.38) arises primarily from the fifth segment of the lumbar plexus, with sizable contributions also coming from the fourth and sixth ventral branches (Fig. 17.40). Bailey et al. (1988) found that the nerve arose from L5 and L6 in 5 of 11 dogs; L4, L5, and L6 in 4 of 11 dogs; L4 and L5 in 1 of 11 dogs; and L5 only in 1 of 11 dogs. After being formed in the substance of the psoas major, it continues caudally in the substance of this muscle and leaves the abdomen along with the iliopsoas muscle. In the proximal extent of its course, it sends muscular branches to the psoas major and iliopsoas. The prominent saphenous nerve arises from its cranial side. Shortly thereafter the femoral nerve enters the quadriceps femoris by passing between the rectus femoris and vastus medialis at the proximal end of the cleft that separates these heads (Fig. 17.48). It supplies all four heads of the quadriceps (rectus femoris, vastus medialis, vastus intermedius, and vastus lateralis) and also sends a small branch to the articularis coxae. The branches to the various parts of the quadriceps accompany largely the lateral circumflex femoral artery, which is the chief source of blood supply to the quadriceps muscle proximally. No cutaneous branches arise directly from the femoral nerve, nor can a branch be found going to the hip joint.

The **saphenous nerve** (*n. saphenus*) (Figs. 17.48 and 17.49) is the only superficial branch of the femoral nerve. Arising from the femoral before this nerve leaves the iliopsoas, the saphenous becomes related to the medial surface of the tensor fasciae latae and immediately divides into muscular and cutaneous branches. This division is lacking in many specimens because the muscular branch arises from the femoral nerve either proximal or distal to the origin of that part of the saphenous nerve that is cutaneous. The **muscular branch** (*ramus muscularis*) bifurcates, one branch going to the cranial belly of the sartorius muscle and the other to the caudal belly (Fig. 17.48). These nerve branches accompany the blood vessels serving the proximal part of the sartorius muscle. The **cutaneous branch** (*ramus cutaneus*) of the saphenous nerve is long and slender (Figs. 17.48 and 17.49). It lies in apposition to the cranial surface of the femoral artery as it runs distally across the medial surface of the quadriceps muscle. It sends branches to the skin of the middle and distal medial surfaces of the thigh. Proximal to the stifle, a small nerve accompanies the descending genicular vessels to the deep structures of the medial surface of the stifle, and a cutaneous branch accompanies the medial genicular vessels to the skin supplied by this vessel (Fig. 17.49A). Distal to the stifle joint, the saphenous nerve continues with the cranial branch of the saphenous vessels and supplies branches to the medial, cranial and craniolateral skin of the crus. A small cutaneous branch also follows

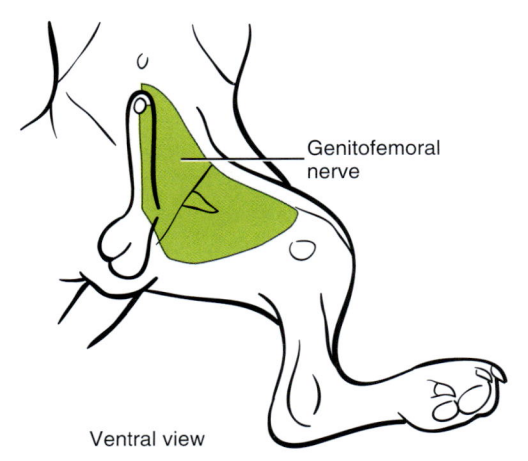

• **Fig. 17.47** Schematic illustration of the cutaneous area of the genitofemoral nerve. (Modified, with permission, from Spurgeon TL, Kitchell RL: Electrophysiological studies of the cutaneous innervation of the external genitalia of the male dog, *Anat Histol Embryol* 11:289–306, 1982; and Haghighi SS, Kitchell RL, Johnson RD, et al.: Electrophysiologic studies of the cutaneous innervation of the pelvic limb of male dogs, *Am J Vet Res* 52:352–362, 1991.)

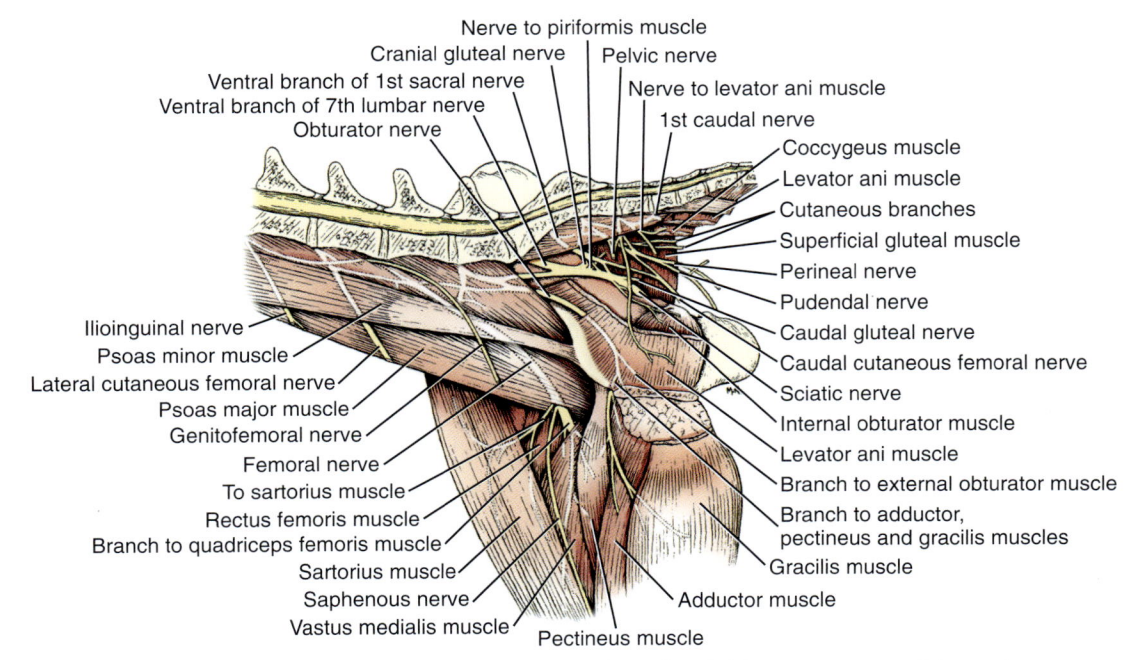

• **Fig. 17.48** Dissection showing distribution of the femoral and obturator nerves, medial aspect.

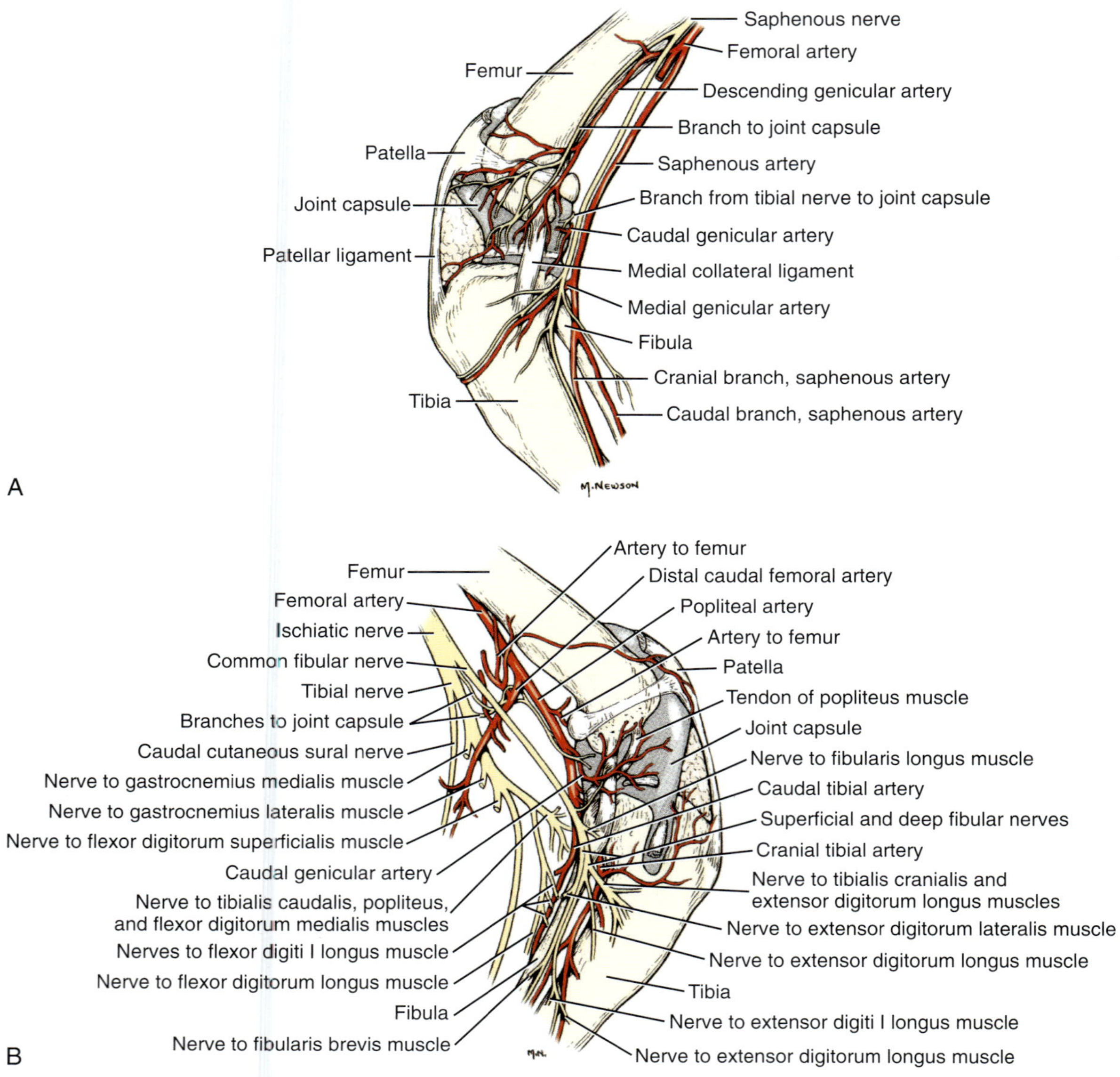

Fig. 17.49 A, Nerves and arteries of the right stifle joint, medial aspect. B, Nerves and arteries of the right stifle joint, lateral aspect.

the caudal branch of the saphenous artery and vein and supplies the skin that overlies them. In the paw it supplies the skin of the dorsomedial part of the tarsus and metatarsus and ends in the skin over the first digit, when a first digit is present (Fig. 17.50, and see Haghighi et al., 1991). The first digit is also supplied by the cutaneous area of the superficial fibular nerve. If a first digit is not present, the cutaneous area extends distally to cover the first phalanx of the second digit. The cutaneous area of the saphenous nerve is very extensive, lying largely on the medial aspect of the pelvic limb, with some extension cranially to supply the craniolateral aspect of the crus (Fig. 17.50). The cutaneous area is overlapped by the cutaneous areas of adjacent nerves. It is important to note that in the hindpaw distal to the tarsus the cutaneous area of the saphenous nerve is completely overlapped by other cutaneous areas and thus no autonomous zone for this nerve is present distal to the tarsus.

The **obturator nerve** (*n. obturatorius*) (Figs. 17.36, 17.38, and 17.51) arises from the fourth, fifth, and sixth lumbar nerves (Langley & Anderson, 1896) (Fig. 17.40 and 17.41). The sixth root of origin is usually the largest, and the fourth smallest or even absent. The roots of origin do not arise close to the intervertebral foramina, but from large nerve trunks of the lumbar plexus that also contribute to other nerves (sciatic for the sixth, and the femoral for the fifth) that are the main continuations of the fifth and sixth lumbar nerves. The obturator nerve is formed within the caudomedial portion of the psoas major muscle. It leaves this muscle dorsomedially and, after crossing the ventrally

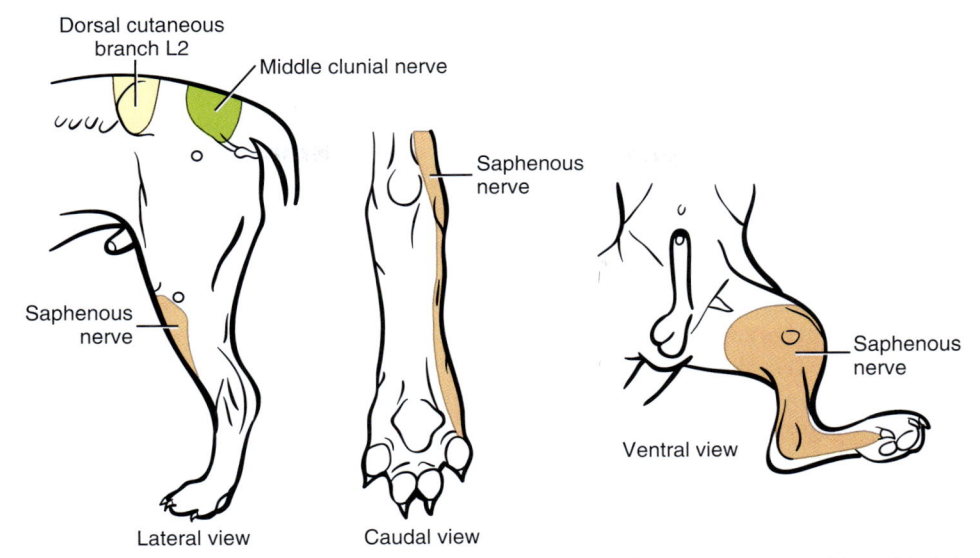

• Fig. 17.50 Schematic illustration of the cutaneous areas of selected cutaneous nerves of the pelvic limb. (Modified, with permission, from Haghighi SS, Kitchell RL, Johnson RD, et al.: Electrophysiologic studies of the cutaneous innervation of the pelvic limb of male dogs, *Am J Vet Res* 52:352–362, 1991.)

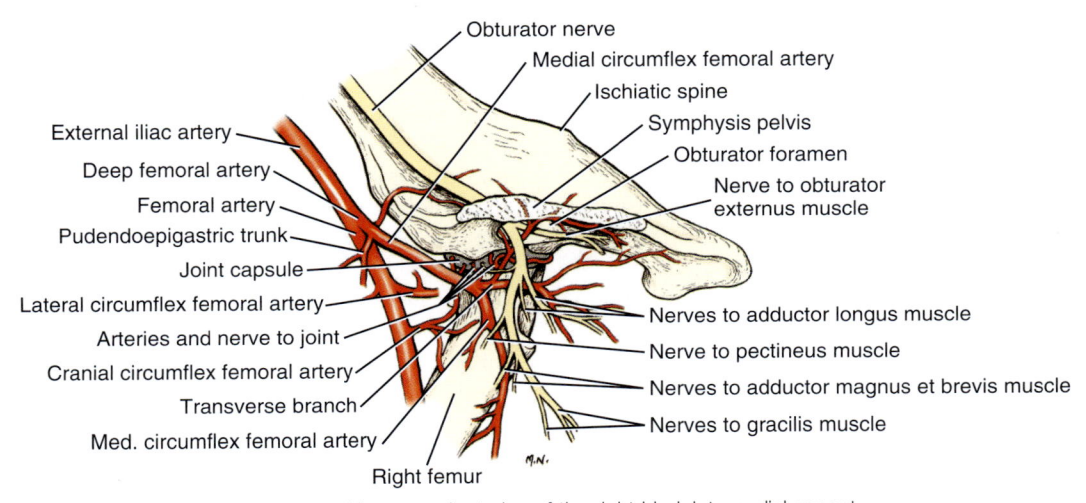

• Fig. 17.51 Nerves and arteries of the right hip joint, medial aspect.

lying common iliac vein, enters the subserosa of the pelvis. After running obliquely caudoventrad across the laterally lying shaft of the ilium, it disappears from view by first passing between the iliopubic and the ischial portions of the levator ani (Fig. 17.48). The obturator nerve leaves the pelvis by passing through the cranial part of the obturator foramen, where it lies in relation to the small obturator ramus of the deep femoral artery that ascends through the opening. It sends branches into the external obturator, pectineus, gracilis, and adductor muscles, innervating all the muscles that primarily adduct the pelvic limb. The obturator nerve does not have any cutaneous branches.

Sacral Nerves

The **sacral nerves** (*nn. sacrales*) (Figs. 17.38 and 17.48) leave the three sacral segments of the spinal cord by means of long dorsal and ventral roots because these spinal cord segments form the part of the conus medullaris that lies in the vertebral foramen of the fifth lumbar vertebra. The three sets of roots merge to form the sacral nerves within the sacral canal prior to their intervertebral foramina of exit. It is usual for the spinal ganglia of the first two sacral nerves to lie within the vertebral canal considerably cranial to the foramina for their exit. The main trunks of the first two sacral nerves give off dorsal branches that leave the sacrum through the two dorsal sacral foramina and the main trunks leave the sacral canal through the ventrally located sacral pelvic foramina. The third pair of sacral nerves leaves the vertebral canal by passing through the intervertebral foramina between the sacrum and the first caudal vertebra, as do the other typical spinal nerves. The intermixing of the ventral branches of these sacral nerves forms the **sacral plexus** (*plexus sacralis*).

The **dorsal branches** (*rami dorsales*) of the three sacral nerves leave the two dorsal sacral foramina and the intervertebral foramen between the sacrum and the first caudal vertebra. External to these foramina, the dorsal branches are connected to each other by communicating strands, forming a small dorsal sacral trunk or plexus. This trunk is usually joined to the dorsal branches of the last lumbar and first caudal nerves. They decrease in size from first to third and, like the dorsal branches of the lumbar nerves, are divided medially, giving off muscular branches, and laterally, giving rise to cutaneous branches. The short medial branches supply the lateral and medial dorsal sacrocaudal muscles. The lateral branches are longer. They run caudodorsolaterad between the dorsal lateral sacrocaudal and the dorsal intertransverse caudal muscles to reach the deep gluteal fascia through which they pass, usually accompanied by the corresponding dorsal sacral vessels. The single lateral branch of the dorsal branch of the first sacral nerve bifurcates on passing through the gluteal fascia so that two cutaneous nerves run caudoventrad on the superficial gluteal muscle. The second and third sacral nerves are similarly disposed, supplying bands of skin caudal to the first. These three nerves, the **middle clunial nerves** (*nn. clunium medii*) of Ellenberger and Baum (1943), supply the piriform muscle (Henning, 1965) and collectively have a cutaneous area that reaches the dorsal midline dorsally and ventrally ends just ventral to the wings of the sacrum (Haghighi et al., 1991) (Fig. 17.50). This area of skin covers the superficial gluteal and the cranial part of the biceps femoris muscles.

The main trunks of the three sacral nerves, after leaving the confines of the sacral canal, are connected to the sympathetic trunk by single rami communicantes. The ventral branches (*rami ventrales*) then continue on the medial wall of the pelvis.

The **ventral branches** (*rami ventrales*) of the sacral nerves divide and redivide shortly after leaving the vertebral canal and interconnect to form the **sacral plexus** (*plexus sacralis*) (Figs. 17.38 and 17.48).

The **lumbosacral trunk** (*truncus lumbosacralis*) (Fig. 17.52) is the largest part of the lumbosacral plexus that is continued external to the pelvis as the sciatic nerve. It arises primarily from the sixth and seventh lumbar nerves, with a small contribution from the first and occasionally the second sacral nerves (Havelka, 1928), and it has a root of origin from the fifth lumbar, according to Ellenberger and Baum (1891). The lumbosacral trunk has two medium-sized branches, the cranial and caudal gluteal nerves. The trunk lies in the pelvic fascia and crosses the shaft of the ilium in nearly a dorsal plane, where it is sandwiched in the space between the origin of the ventral lateral sacrocaudal muscle medially and the thin levator ani muscle laterally. It is covered by peritoneum and is crossed obliquely on its ventral aspect by the caudal gluteal vessels. It becomes the sciatic nerve after the last sacral branch enters it at the greater ischiatic foramen. Each of the five constant, main trunks of spinal nerves contributing to the lumbosacral trunk is usually united to the sympathetic trunk by a single ramus communicans.

The **cranial gluteal nerve** (*n. gluteus cranialis*) (Figs. 17.52 and 17.53) arises from the lumbosacral trunk or its roots mainly from the sixth and seventh lumbar nerves and from the first sacral nerve. It leaves the pelvis by passing immediately through the greater sciatic foramen and plunges into the lateral muscles of the pelvis. It is accompanied by the cranial gluteal artery and vein. It circles craniad across the lateral aspect of the shaft of the ilium at the origin of the caudal bundle of the deep gluteal muscle (Fig. 17.52). The cranial gluteal nerve continues cranioventrad between the middle and deep gluteal muscles, usually perforates the cranial edge of the deep gluteal, and terminates in the tensor

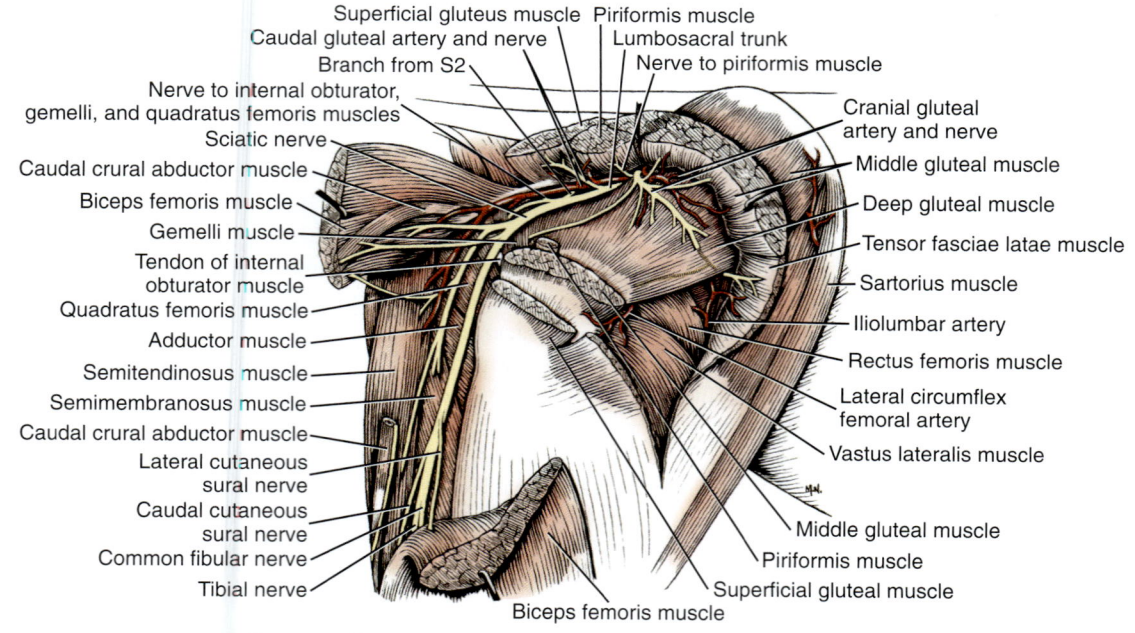

• **Fig. 17.52** Nerves, arteries, and muscles of the right hip, lateral aspect.

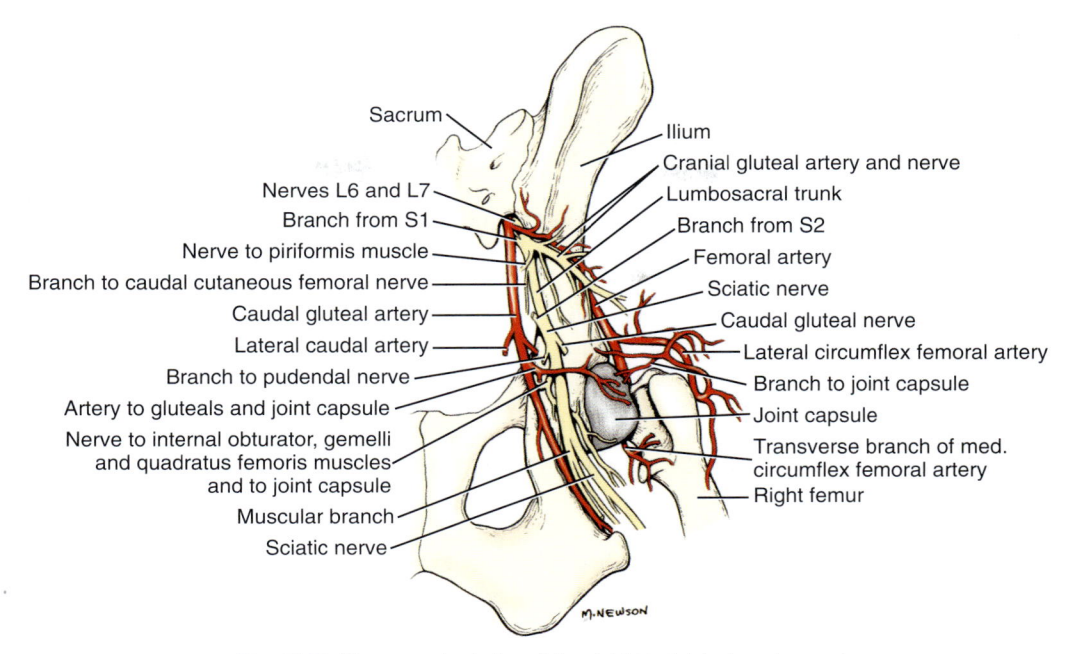

• Fig. 17.53 Nerves and arteries of the right hip joint, dorsal aspect.

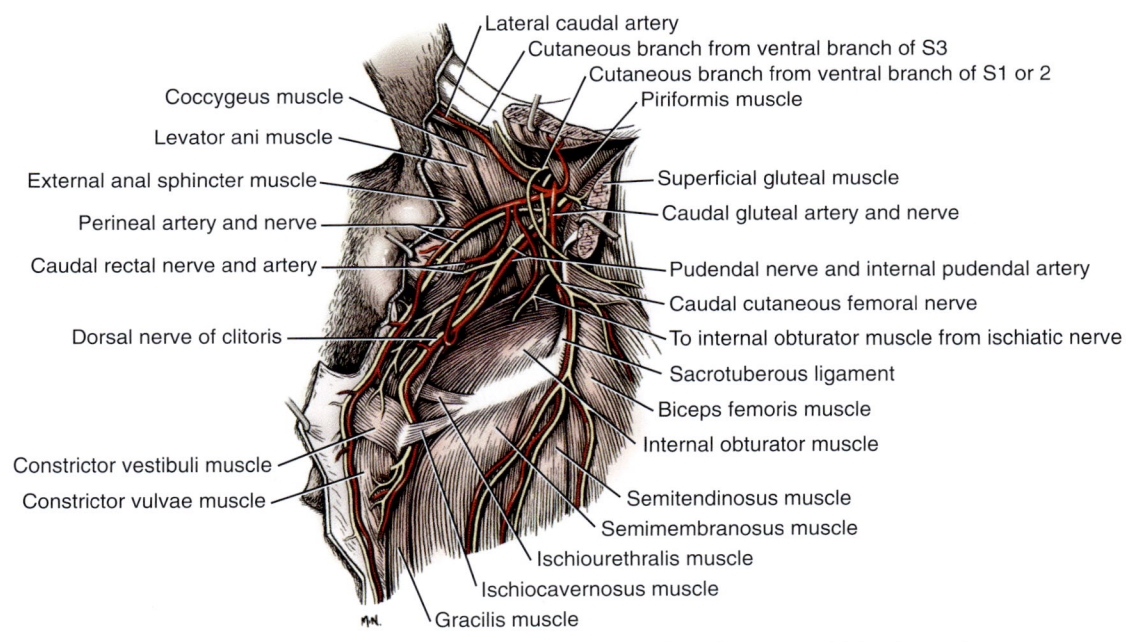

• Fig. 17.54 Nerves, arteries, and muscles of the female perineum, caudolateral aspect.

fasciae latae. It supplies the deep and middle gluteal muscles and the tensor fasciae latae. It has no cutaneous branches (Haghighi et al., 1991).

The **caudal gluteal nerve** (*n. gluteus caudalis*) (Figs. 17.52 and 17.54) is a small nerve that may be double. It usually arises from the caudal margin of the lumbosacral trunk or from its seventh lumbar root. Occasionally the cranial and caudal gluteal nerves arise in common; at the other extreme the caudal gluteal nerve may arise only from the first and second sacral nerves independent of the lumbosacral trunk, as Bradley and Grahame (1959) illustrate. The caudal gluteal nerve runs parallel to the ventrocaudal border of the lumbosacral trunk on the medial surface of the shaft of the ilium, and, after passing through the greater sciatic foramen, it crosses the caudal border of the piriform muscle or passes between the piriform and the middle gluteal muscles to enter the medial surface of the superficial gluteal muscle. It may also send a branch to the middle gluteal muscle. In its course of approximately 2.5 cm, it lies between the sacrotuberous ligament medially and the large caudal gluteal artery and vein laterally. It is distributed to the superficial gluteal muscle. It also supplies the piriform muscle by a delicate branch that enters the proximal third of the muscle. The caudal gluteal nerve has no cutaneous branches (Haghighi et al., 1991).

The **caudal cutaneous femoral nerve** (*n. cutaneus femoris caudalis*) (Figs. 17.54 and 17.55) is nearly as large as the pudendal nerve, to which it is united for most of its intrapelvic course. It arises from the first and second sacral nerves and seldom from the third sacral (Havelka, 1928) (Fig. 17.40 and 17.41). Bradley and Grahame (1959) state that it arises from the seventh lumbar and first sacral nerves, with a possible addition from the sixth lumbar. Bailey et al. (1988) found that it arose from S1 and S2 in 5 of 11 dogs; S1 alone in 2 of 11; L6, L7, and S1 in 1 of 11; L7 and S1 in 1 of 11; L7, S1, and S2 in 1 of 11; and L7, S1, S2, and S3 in 1 of 11. The ventral branch of S1 contributed to the caudal cutaneous femoral nerve in 11 of 11 dogs, S2 in 7 of 11, L7 in 4 of 11, L6 in only 1 of 11, and S3 in only 1 of 11. As the caudal cutaneous femoral nerve passes out of the pelvis dorsal to the ischial arch, it gives off a spray of branches, the **caudal clunial nerves** (*nn. clunium caudales*), that stream out of the ischiorectal fossa in the fat covering the dorsal surface of the internal obturator muscle. The cutaneous area of the caudal clunial nerves is an oval area surrounding and just dorsal to the greater trochanter (Fig. 17.44) (Haghighi et al., 1991). The spinal roots of S1 and S2 were most often the only contributors to the caudal clunial nerves, but occasionally S3 contributed as well.

The caudal cutaneous femoral nerve courses caudally on the caudal attachment of the sacrotuberous ligament where it terminates by dividing into cranial and caudal branches (Spurgeon & Kitchell, 1982; Spurgeon & Reddy, 1986). The caudal branch ran distally over the semitendinosus and semimembranosus, and the cranial branch ran distally in the furrow between the biceps femoris and semitendinosus. The cutaneous area covered much of the caudal and lateral surfaces of the femoral region (Fig. 17.39) (Spurgeon & Kitchell, 1982; Spurgeon & Reddy, 1986). The cranial aspect of the cutaneous area was on a vertical plane through the greater trochanter, where it overlapped with the cutaneous area of the lateral cutaneous femoral nerve. Caudally and medially, the cutaneous area extends to within 2 or 3 cm of the midline, where it overlaps the cutaneous area of the superficial perineal nerve. Distally, the cutaneous area extends to the proximal part of the popliteal fossa, overlapping the cutaneous area of the lateral cutaneous sural nerve cranially, the proximal caudal cutaneous sural nerve caudally, and the cutaneous area of the saphenous nerve medially.

The **pelvic nerves** (*nn. pelvini*) (Figs. 17.38 and 17.48), formerly the *pelvic splanchnic nerves*, usually arise from the ventral branches of the first and second sacral nerves. They may also originate from the pudendal nerve. They may arise as a single nerve or as two separate nerves that may run independently to the pelvic plexus. They are composed of preganglionic parasympathetic and general visceral afferent axons that supply the descending colon as far cranially as the left colic flexure, the viscera of the pelvic cavity, the urinary bladder, and the erectile tissue of the penis or clitoris (Chapter 15).

The **pudendal nerve** (*n. pudendus*) (Figs. 17.36, 17.38, 17.54, and 17.55) usually arises from the ventral branches of all three sacral nerves via the sacral plexus. A prefixed origin of the pudendal by one segment is described by Havelka (1928). Hummel (1965) says that it may originate as far cranially as L5. Bailey et al. (1988) found that it came from S1, S2, and S3 in 5 of 11 dogs; from S2 and S3 in 3 of 11; from S1 and S2 in 2 of 11; and from S1 only in 1 of 11. The ventral branch of S2 contributed to the pudendal nerve in 10 of 11 dogs, S3 in 8 of 11 dogs, and S1 in 7 of 11. As the pudendal nerve runs obliquely caudoventrad to the pelvic outlet, it lies lateral to the coccygeus muscle and appears superficially medial to the superficial gluteal muscle. It lies dorsal to the accompanying internal pudendal vessels. At the pelvic outlet the pudendal nerve gives rise to the caudal rectal and perineal nerves and the nerves to the external genital organs: the dorsal nerve of the penis in the male and the nerve of the clitoris in the female.

The **caudal rectal nerve** (*n. rectalis caudalis*) (Figs. 17.54 and 17.55) is a short nerve that leaves the pudendal at the caudal border of the levator ani muscle or less often may arise from the sacral plexus independent of the pudendal nerve. It enters the external anal sphincter muscle slightly ventral to its middle. It is accompanied by the more deeply lying caudal rectal artery and vein. It, and its companion nerve of the opposite side, are apparently the sole supply to the external sphincter muscle of the anus. Blakely (1957) found that unilateral severance of this nerve in perineal hernia operations could be performed without producing incontinence, but that bilateral severance of the caudal rectal nerve resulted in incontinence of feces.

The **perineal nerves** (*nn. perinei*) (Figs. 17.54 and 17.55) have been divided into superficial (*n. perinealis superficialis*) and deep perineal (*n. perinealis profundus*) branches by Spurgeon and Kitchell (1982) in accordance with the NAV (2005). The deep perineal branches are represented by several long branches that leave the pudendal nerve at the pelvic outlet. The first branch to leave the pudendal nerve goes to the mucosa of the anal canal. It either crosses the external anal sphincter superficially or runs deeply between the dorsal portion of the paranal sinus and the internal sphincter muscle of the anus to reach the mucosa. Other deep perineal branches supply the striated muscle of the external urethral sphincter (Griffin et al., 1989), the ischiourethralis, bulbospongiosus, and ischiocavernous muscles. The superficial perineal nerve leaves the pudendal near or in common with the nerve going to the mucosa and sends several branches to the skin of the perineum as it runs distally in the furrow located between the proximal part of the penis and the gracilis muscle. One of these branches, larger than the others, becomes related to the root of the penis and, as a branched nerve, runs distally on the caudolateral surface of the proximal portion of the penis. The main superficial perineal nerve, however, continues distally and supplies the skin of the perineum and proximal

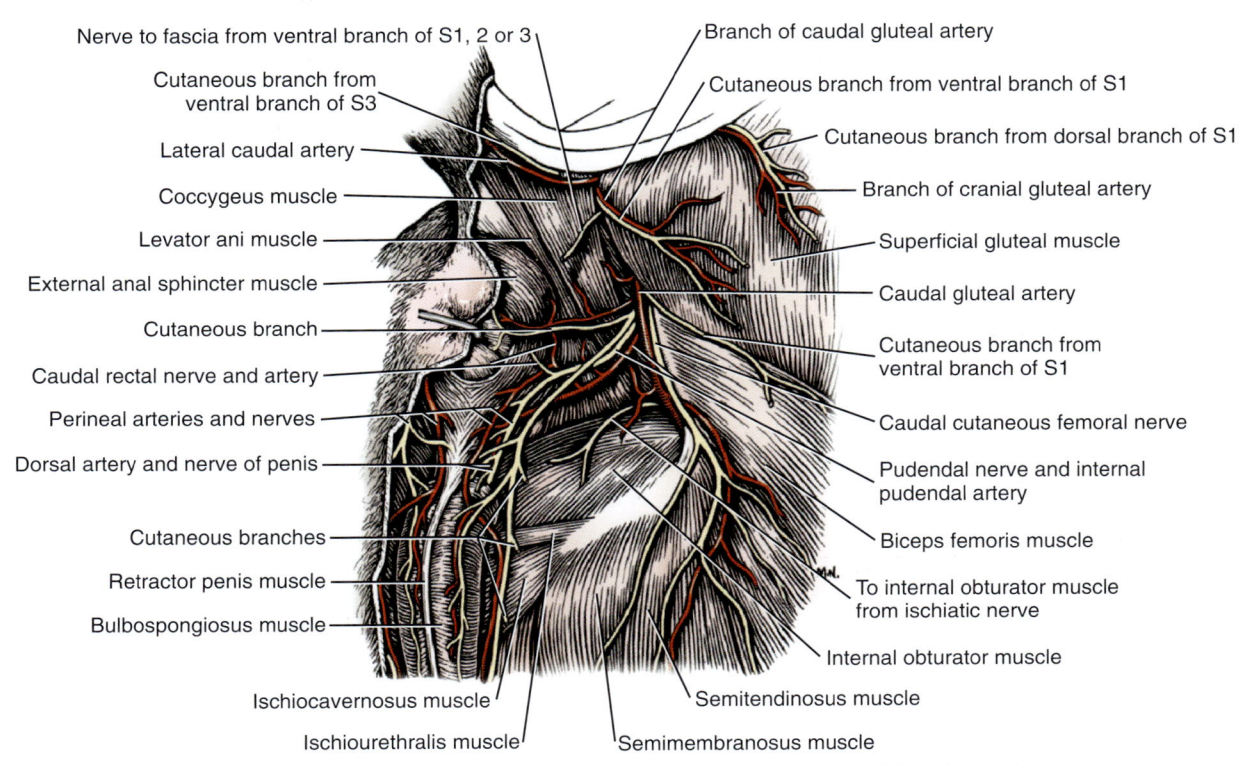

Fig. 17.55 Nerves, arteries, and muscles of the male perineum, caudolateral aspect.

caudomedial thigh with its fellow. Its cutaneous area is located on the perineum around and distal to the anus and on the caudomedial surface of the thigh (Fig. 17.45), where its cranial aspect is overlapped by the branches from the genitofemoral nerve, which passes through the inguinal canal (for the male Spurgeon and Kitchell [1982]; for the female Spurgeon and Reddy [1986]). A terminal spray of branches of this nerve supplies the skin of the scrotum as the **dorsal scrotal nerves** (*nn. scrotales dorsales*) in the male. No comparable branches of the superficial perineal nerve supply the skin of the labia (Spurgeon & Reddy, 1986). The skin of the labia is supplied entirely by branches from the dorsal nerve of the clitoris.

The **dorsal nerve of the penis** (*n. dorsalis penis*) (Fig. 17.55) in the male is the main extrapelvic continuation of the pudendal nerve. It arises from the S1 and S2 spinal nerves, but occasionally S3 contributes (Bailey et al., 1988). It curves around the pelvic outlet near the symphysis ischiadica, where it is separated from the opposite nerve by the paired artery and vein of the penis. At this point it issues a thin but long branch that inclines medially where it comes to lie between the dorsal vein and the tunica albuginea of the penis. It usually communicates with the larger nerve just caudal to the bulbus glandis. On reaching the dorsal surface of the penis, the dorsal nerve of the penis runs cranially on the organ, sending branches to it. It gives off a spray of preputial branches that supply the internal sheath of the prepuce and has a cutaneous area around the preputial orifice (Fig. 17.45) (Spurgeon & Kitchell, 1982) and the rest of the dorsal nerve of the penis enters the caudal part of the bulbus glandis. It continues through the glans along the dorsal surface of the os penis and finally ends in the mucosa of the apex of the glans. It is the chief sensory nerve to the penis, mediating afferent impulses that result in orgasm. The **dorsal nerve of the clitoris** (*n. dorsalis clitoridis*) (Fig. 17.54) in the female is the homologue of the dorsal nerve of the penis of the male and mediates similar impulses. It is much smaller than the comparable nerve of the male and runs to the ventral commissure of the vulva, where it gives off a spray of branches to the vulva before it terminates in the clitoris (Spurgeon & Reddy, 1986).

The **muscular branches** of the ventral sacral nerves (*rami musculares*) are usually two in number. One supplies the levator ani and coccygeus, and the second, larger nerve innervates the lateral rotators of the hip joint. Coming mainly from the second sacral nerve, but also receiving a small branch from the third, usually, is a small single or double nerve that crosses the lateral surface of the lateral ventral sacrocaudal muscle. Its medial branch arborizes largely on the medial, subperitoneal surface of the levator ani. Its lateral branch enters the cranial medial surface of the much narrower, more caudally located coccygeus. The muscular branch from the lumbosacral trunk to the muscles that rotate the hip joint laterally was called the rotator nerve (*n. rotatorius*) by Schmaltz (1914). It is short. As it leaves the caudal margin of the lumbosacral trunk just prior to the passing of this trunk through the caudal part of the greater ischiatic foramen to be continued as the sciatic nerve, a branch runs caudally and arborizes in the dorsal surface of the internal obturator muscle as it lies on the ischiatic table caudomedial to the lesser ischiatic foramen. When this nerve is double, the second branch leaves the caudal border of the lumbosacral trunk or its continuation, the sciatic nerve, approximately 1 cm distal to the origin of the branch to the internal obturator, and curves around the caudal border of the deep gluteal muscle and enters the fascia between the deep gluteal and the cranial gemellus muscles. Sometimes the two parts of this nerve arise in common. After crossing the lateral surface of the shaft of the ischium the second branch supplies both parts of the gemelli and, after passing ventral to the cranial gemellus, terminates in the larger, obliquely running quadratus femoris.

The **sciatic**, or **ischiatic**, **nerve** (*n. ischiadicus*) (Figs. 17.52 and 17.56) is the largest nerve in the body. It arises largely from L6, L7, and S1 (Fig. 17.40), with an occasional contribution from S2 (de Lahunta et al., 2015; Fletcher, 1970). It is a continuation of the lumbosacral trunk. The division between the two is marked by the second sacral nerve, contributing to this nerve complex. Because this contribution is located at the greater ischiatic notch, the extrapelvic part of the trunk is regarded as the sciatic nerve. It consists of two nerves, the tibial and common fibula, which are so closely bound together, proximally, that they appear as one. The two parts, however, can be forcefully separated back to their origins from the spinal nerves. The normal division of the sciatic nerve is variable. Occasionally it is located as far proximally as the hip joint, whereas at other times it may be as far distally as the popliteal space. On leaving the pelvis, the sciatic nerve first lies on the gemelli and the tendon of the internal obturator caudomedial to the hip joint. As it passes distally in the thigh, it lies in succession on the quadratus femoris, adductor, and semimembranosus. It is covered first by the superficial gluteal muscle and then by the biceps femoris muscle and lies in close association with the small abductor cruris caudalis, which crosses it obliquely in the proximal third of the thigh. Its proximal portion is accompanied by the caudal gluteal vessels that lie caudal to it, and it is nourished by the small sciatic artery, which is partly embedded in its caudolateral surface. In addition to the **muscular branch** (*ramus muscularis*) to the lateral rotators, which is usually double and arises from the lumbosacral trunk, the sciatic nerve that continues this trunk external to the pelvis has a single, stout, muscular branch to the caudal thigh muscles and a muscular branch to the m. abductor cruris caudalis. Other main branches of the sciatic nerve include the lateral cutaneous sural nerve, the proximal and distal caudal cutaneous sural nerves, and the terminal common fibular and tibial nerves. See Bennett (1976) for details of their internal funicular structure.

This main **muscular branch** (*ramus muscularis*) of the sciatic nerve (Fig. 17.52) is approximately 1 cm in length and 3 mm in diameter. It leaves the caudomedial border of the sciatic nerve opposite the space between the middle gluteal and the cranial gemellus muscles. It lies cranial and parallel to the sacrotuberous ligament and caudal gluteal artery and vein. After running approximately 1 cm in the furrow (trochanteric fossa) medial to the greater trochanter, it sends a branch into the larger superficial portion of the biceps femoris approximately 3 cm from its main origin on the tuber ischiadicum. The remaining portion of the nerve, which is approximately the same size as the branch to the superficial portion of the biceps muscle, runs distally, and at the distal border of the quadratus femoris branches into usually four parts that arise variably. The most caudal portion regularly bifurcates into a smaller, distolaterally running branch that supplies the smaller, deeper portion of the biceps femoris and a shorter, larger branch that innervates the proximal part of the semitendinosus. The main portion of the muscular branch then continues distally and divides into two or three branches. The more caudal branch enters the middle portion of the semitendinosus distal to the tendinous intersection that partly divides the muscle. The more cranial part of the nerve runs distally and again bifurcates; one branch goes to the caudal belly, and the other to the cranial belly of the semimembranosus. A long, slender, mixed nerve arises from the tibial portion of the sciatic nerve opposite or distal to the trochanteric fossa. After obliquely crossing the caudal surface of the tibial part, it becomes associated with the medial border of the abductor cruris caudalis. In this region it sends a muscular branch to this small abductor. At approximately the middle of the thigh, it leaves the medial border of the abductor cruris caudalis and obliquely crosses the caudal surface of the muscle as it runs distally as the **proximal caudal cutaneous sural nerve** (*n. cutaneus surae caudalis proximalis*) (Haghighi et al., 1991). This nerve has been called the communication between the caudal cutaneous femoral and the caudal cutaneous sural nerve by Nickel et al. (1984). Budras and Fricke (1983) refer to it as the accessory caudal cutaneous sural nerve. The proximal caudal cutaneous sural nerve becomes subcutaneous in the proximal part of the popliteal region, where it supplies the skin on the proximal aspect of the caudal surface of the crus (Fig. 17.45).

The **lateral cutaneous sural nerve** (*n. cutaneus surae lateralis*) (Figs. 17.52 and 17.56) arises from the lateral surface of the common fibular portion of the sciatic nerve at approximately the junction of the middle and distal thirds of the thigh. This is proximal to its muscular branches to the cranial crural muscles. After running a few centimeters distally deep to the biceps femoris, it enters this muscle between its smaller, deep head and its larger, more cranially lying, superficial head. The nerve passes through the biceps femoris without contributing to its supply and appears subcutaneously with cutaneous branches of the caudal femoral vessels in the proximal, lateral portion of the crus. Its cutaneous area is on the lateral aspect of the distal thigh, stifle and crus (Fig. 17.44) (Haghighi et al., 1991).

The **distal caudal cutaneous sural nerve** (*n. cutaneus surae caudalis distalis*) is known as the *n. suralis s. communicans tibialis s. cutan. fem. et tibiae post. long.* by Ellenberger and Baum (1943). It is called the *n. cutaneous surae medialis* by Bradley and Grahame (1959). It is a long, slender nerve that arises from the caudal border of the tibial portion of the sciatic

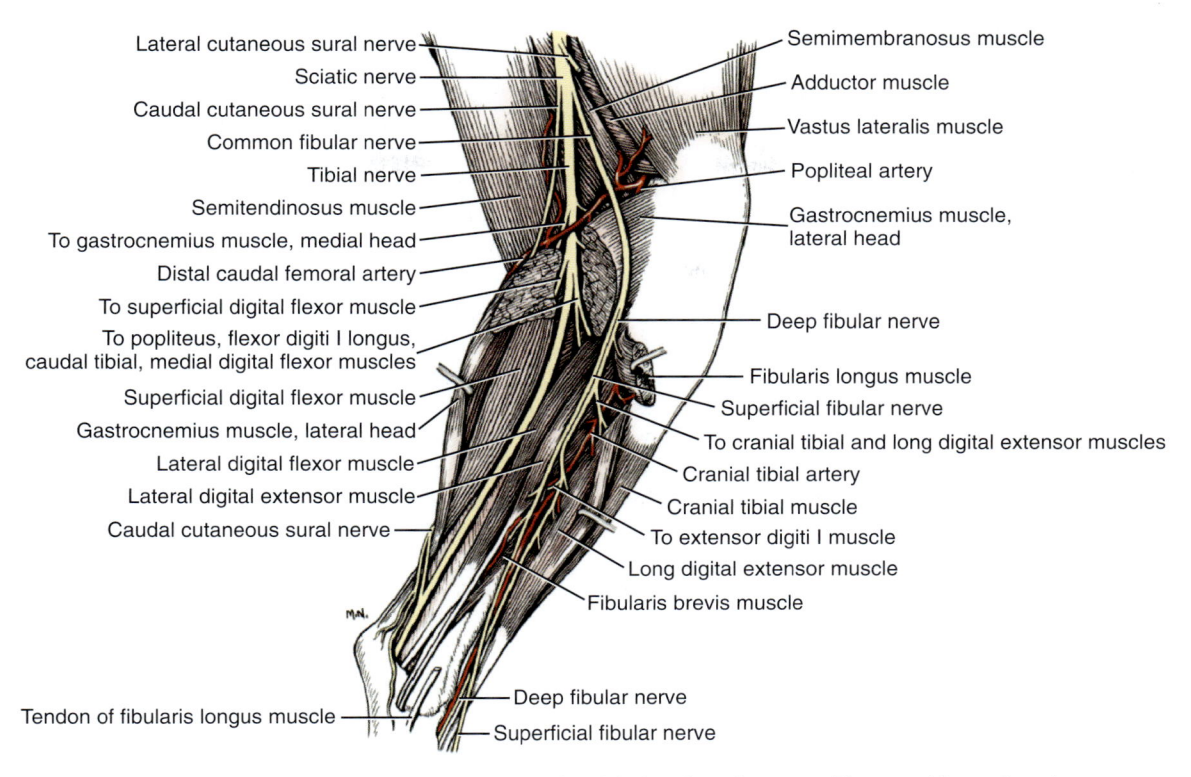

• **Fig. 17.56** Nerves, arteries, and muscles of the right leg, lateral aspect. (The mm. biceps femoris, abductor cruris caudalis and portions of the lateral head of the gastrocnemius and the fibularis longus have been removed.)

nerve, usually approximately 1 cm distal to the origin of the lateral cutaneous sural nerve and proximal to the muscular branches of the tibial nerve to the caudal crural muscles. It runs a short distance distally, bounded laterally by the biceps femoris and medially by the semimembranosus. On entering the popliteal region, it becomes associated with the caudal surface of the gastrocnemius muscle, running distally on the muscle near the fusion of its two heads and in association with the lateral saphenous vein. Throughout its course it sends branches to the skin of the caudal part of the crus. On reaching the calcanean tendon, it usually divides into two branches of unequal size. The smaller branch extends distally. On reaching the tarsus, it usually bifurcates into a small **articular branch** (*ramus articularis*) that runs over the caudal part of the lateral malleolus and supplies the lateral portion of the tarsal joint. The **lateral calcaneal branch** (*ramus calcanei lateralis*) crosses the distolateral surface of the tuber calcanei and ends in the skin of this region. A small branch may innervate the tarsocrural joint capsule. The larger branch of the distal caudal cutaneous sural nerve (communicating ramus between the distal caudal cutaneous sural and the tibial nerves) runs mediad between the calcanean tendon and the tibia and joins the tibial nerve 1 to 3 cm proximal to the tarsal canal. This communicating branch contains somatic efferent fibers that supply the plantar muscles of the hindpaw (Cuddon et al., 1989).

The **common fibular** nerve (*n. fibularis communis*), also referred to as the *common peroneal nerve*) (Figs. 17.49 and 17.56), is the smaller of the two terminal branches of the sciatic. It lies deep to the thin terminal part of the deep portion of the biceps femoris. The nerve runs almost directly distad, obliquely crossing the lateral head of the gastrocnemius muscle. At the level of the stifle joint, it sends an articular branch to the lateral collateral ligament and crosses the head of the fibula. On reaching the thin lateral border of the flexor digitorum lateralis approximately 1.5 cm distal to the stifle joint, it enters between this muscle and the lateral digital extensor on the caudal side, and the fibularis longus that lies cranial to it, and enters the muscles of the cranial part of the crus. The common fibular nerve supplies a small branch to the fibularis longus before dividing into superficial and deep fibular nerves.

The **superficial fibular nerve** (*n. fibularis superficialis*) is the most caudal terminal branch of the common fibular nerve. It leaves the lateral portion of the parent nerve (Fig. 17.56) approximately 3 cm distal to the stifle joint, where it lies in the intermuscular septum between the flexor digitorum lateralis caudally and the fibularis longus cranially. It supplies the fibularis brevis and the lateral digital extensor. As it extends distally, it curves deep to the distal part of the belly of the fibularis longus, which it innervates to enter the septum between this muscle and the long digital extensor. At the beginning of the distal third of the crus, it becomes subfascial, and on approaching the flexor surface of the tarsus, it perforates the crural fascia to become subcutaneous. At this point it sends a recurrent branch proximally to ramify in the skin of the craniolateral aspect of the crus (Haghighi et al., 1991).

In accordance with the NAV, the proper digital nerves and vessels are designated as *axial* or *abaxial,* depending on which side of the digit they lie in regard to the axis of the limb that passes between the third and fourth digits. Thus, the nerves on the lateral side of the third digit and the medial side of the fourth digit are both axial digital nerves. For example, the third dorsal common digital nerve gives origin to axial dorsal proper digital nerve IV and axial dorsal proper digital nerve III, whereas the second dorsal common digital nerve provides axial dorsal proper digital nerve II and abaxial dorsal proper digital nerve III. The fourth dorsal common digital nerve forms abaxial dorsal proper digital nerve IV and axial dorsal proper digital nerve V. The dorsal proper digital nerves, as they run toward the distal ends of the digits, lie plantar to the corresponding arteries and send many branches to the skin of the dorsal and adjacent sides of the digit, finally ending in the corium of the claw.

The superficial fibular nerve continues distally in the subcutaneous tissue. At or just proximal to the tarsus it becomes related to the small, cranial division of the saphenous artery, which it follows into the dorsum of the paw. At or just proximal to the tarsus, it gives off on its lateral surface a long nerve that continues distally on the dorsolateral aspect of metatarsus V to enter digit V, where it is known as **abaxial dorsal proper digital nerve V** (*n. digitalis proprius dorsalis V abaxialis*). The superficial fibular nerve continues to run distally on the dorsal surface of the tarsus, where it becomes related to the continuation of the small, cranial division of the saphenous artery. Like the artery, it bifurcates into medial and lateral terminal parts, the lateral being larger. The lateral branch divides again to form **dorsal common digital nerves III and IV** (*nn. digitalis dorsalis communis III et IV*). These continue distally in the grooves between adjacent metatarsal bones, where they are related to the corresponding arteries and are deep to the corresponding veins. Dorsal common digital nerve IV divides at the level of the metatarsophalangeal joint into **axial dorsal proper digital nerve V** (*n. digitalis dorsalis proprius V axialis*) and **abaxial dorsal proper digital nerve IV** (*n. digitalis dorsalis proprius IV abaxialis*). Dorsal common digital nerve III divides at the level of the metatarsophalangeal joints into **axial proper digital nerves III and II** (*nn. digitalis dorsalis proprius III et II axialis*). The medial branch of the superficial peroneal nerve just distal to the tarsus divides into **dorsal common digital nerve II** (*n. digitalis dorsalis communis II*) and **abaxial dorsal proper digital nerve II** (*n. digitalis dorsalis proprius II abaxialis*). Abaxial dorsal digital nerve II continues on the medial aspect of the full length of the second digit. Dorsal common digital nerve II communicates with dorsal metatarsal nerve II (from the deep fibular) and then divides at the metatarsophalangeal joints of digits II and III into **axial dorsal proper digital nerve II** (*n. digitalis dorsalis proprius II axialis*) and **abaxial dorsal proper digital nerve III** (*digitalis dorsalis proprius III abaxialis*). The cutaneous area of the superficial fibular nerve includes the skin of the cranial and craniolateral surfaces of the distal two-thirds of the crus and the dorsum of the hindpaw, with the exception of the dorsal surface of the webbing between the second and the third digits and the dorsal part of the axial surface of the second digit and the dorsal part of the abaxial surface of the third digit (Figs. 17.43 and 17.58). The cutaneous area in the hindpaw includes the skin around the dorsal surface of the metatarsal region and of digits IV and V, and the dorsal surface of the webbing between digits III and IV and IV and V. If a dewclaw is present, the superficial fibular nerve supplies its dorsal surface and the area around the dorsal aspect of the claw, but not the digital pad of the first digit (Haghighi et al., 1991).

The **deep fibular nerve** (*n. fibularis profundus*) (Fig. 17.56) arises as the cranial terminal branch of the common fibular nerve on the lateral head of the gastrocnemius muscle near its cranial border. In the proximal part of the crus along with the distally lying superficial fibular nerve it passes between the lateral digital flexor and lateral digital extensor muscles caudally and the fibularis longus muscle cranially. From its first 3 cm, there arise in succession usually four branches. The most proximal branch is a **muscular ramus** (*ramus muscularis*) to the deep face, proximal end of the fibularis longus. The next branch crosses deep to the long digital extensor muscle and enters the medial border of the tibialis cranialis. The third branch obliquely crosses the cranial surface of the delicate extensor digiti I longus, which it supplies, and becomes related to the lateral surface of the cranial tibial artery. As it runs to the tarsus, it passes between the artery and the tibia but remains closely united to the artery. In the proximal half of the tarsus, the deep fibular nerve and cranial tibial artery lie in the groove formed by the tendon of the long digital extensor, laterally, and the tendon of the cranial tibial muscle, medially. At the tarsus the deep fibular nerve sends delicate branches to the three heads of the extensor digitorum brevis, which lie on the flexor surface of the tarsus, and the nerve divides into a larger medial and a smaller lateral branch.

Dorsal metatarsal nerve II (*n. metatarseus dorsalis II*) (Fig. 17.57) is the metatarsal continuation of the medial branch of the deep fibular nerve. It joins dorsal common digital nerve II (superficial fibular nerve). Martin (1923), Bradley (1927), Miller et al. (1964), Ghoshal (1975), Budras et al. (2007), and Adams (2004) describe **dorsal metatarsal nerves III and IV** (*n. metatarsus dorsalis III et IV*) as arising from a lateral branch of the deep fibular nerve distal to the tarsus and joining common digital nerves III and IV at the metatarsophalangeal joint. Kitchell et al. (unpublished), using electrophysiologic stimulation of axial dorsal proper digital nerves II, III, IV, and V and abaxial dorsal proper digital nerves II and IV, could not obtain any evoked action potentials in the deep fibular nerve at the level of the tarsus, but they did get large action potentials in the superficial fibular nerve at the tarsus, indicating that dorsal metatarsal nerves III and IV (deep fibular) do not join dorsal common digital nerves II and IV. Large action potentials were elicited in both the superficial and the deep

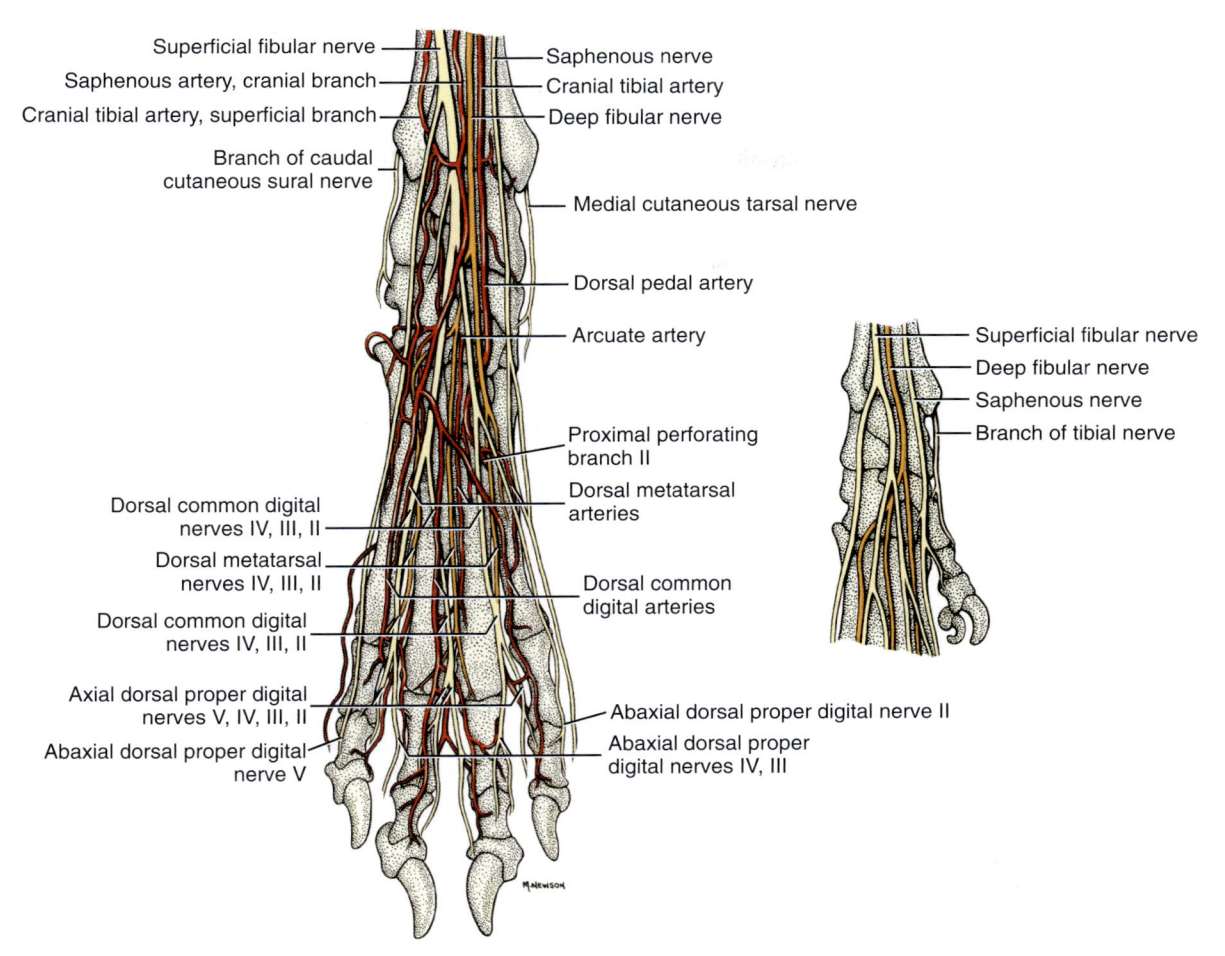

• **Fig. 17.57** Nerves and arteries of the right hindpaw, dorsal aspect. Note that dorsal metatarsal n. II joins dorsal common digital n. II, but dorsal metatarsal nn. III and IV do not join dorsal common digital nn. III and IV.

fibular nerves from stimulating abaxial dorsal proper digital nerve III and axial dorsal proper digital nerve II. Their findings suggest that dorsal metatarsal nerves III and IV supply only the metatarsophalangeal joints. (Fig. 17.56), whereas dorsal metatarsal nerve II does join dorsal common digital nerve II (Kitchell et al., unpublished). Electrophysiologic studies of these dorsal digital nerves have been inconsistent but suggest that in some dogs the dorsal metatarsal nerves do not join the dorsal common digital nerves at all of the metatarsophalangeal joints.

The cutaneous area for the deep fibular nerve is limited to the dorsal interdigital area between digits II and III (Fig. 17.58). The cutaneous areas of the superficial and deep peroneal nerves overlap to supply the dorsal part of the axial surface of digit II and the dorsal part of the abaxial surface of digit III. The deep fibular nerve is the sole supply to the plantar part of the axial surface of digit II, the plantar part of the abaxial surface of digit II, and the webbing between digits II and III (Haghighi et al., 1991).

The **tibial nerve** (*n. tibialis*) (Fig. 17.56), larger than the common fibular, is the more caudal of the two terminal branches of the sciatic nerve. It is approximately 5 mm wide

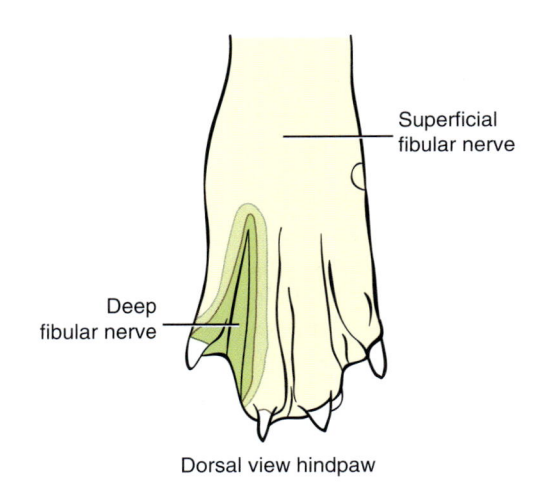

• **Fig. 17.58** Schematic illustration of the cutaneous areas of the dorsal surface of the left hindpaw. (Modified, with permission, from Haghighi SS, Kitchell RL, Johnson RD, et al.: Electrophysiologic studies of the cutaneous innervation of the pelvic limb of male dogs, *Am J Vet Res* 52:352–362, 1991.)

at its origin and is flattened transversely as it lies between the caudal portions of the semimembranosus medially and the biceps femoris laterally. Bennett (1976) found it to arise from S1 and S2 (Fig. 17.40). It separates from the ischiatic nerve gradually in the proximal two-thirds of the thigh. It enters the crus between the two heads of the gastrocnemius muscle. The tibial nerve supplies all the muscles that lie on the caudal aspect of the tibia and fibula and sends branches to the stifle, tarsal, and digital joints (Figs. 17.49 and 17.56). Its terminal portions run to the muscles that lie in the plantar part of the hindpaw and to the skin and foot pads of the plantar surface of the hindpaw.

The **muscular branches** (*rami musculares*) (Fig. 17.56) are numerous. The first two branches arise in common closely bound to the cranial border of the distal caudal cutaneous sural nerve, arising approximately 2 cm before the tibial nerve enters the gastrocnemius muscle. One branch enters the proximal portion of the caudal border of the lateral head, and the other branch enters the medial head of the gastrocnemius muscle at a like place. The muscular branch to the superficial digital flexor enters the muscle at its origin. From the cranial border of the tibial nerve, as it lies between the two heads of the gastrocnemius muscle, arises the muscular branch, which enters the popliteal muscle at approximately the middle of its obliquely running distal border. Arising from this nerve, or separately from the tibial, or from both of these, is the nerve or branches to the deep digital flexor muscle. When single, this nerve soon trifurcates into branches that supply its two constituent bellies, the flexor digitalis lateralis and flexor digitalis medialis. A small branch goes to the tibialis caudalis. After these muscular branches arise, the tibial nerve then runs distad on the flexor digiti I longus, where it is covered by the lateral head of the gastrocnemius muscle. Approximately 2 cm proximal to the tarsus, it receives the caudal cutaneous sural nerve from the lateral side cranial to the common calcanean tendon. At approximately the middle of the crus near the medial surface, the tibial nerve comes into relationship with the caudal branch of the saphenous artery and vein. Just proximal to the tarsus, the tibial nerve gives off one or more **cutaneous branches** (*rami cutanei*), which supply the skin around and slightly distal to the medial aspect of the tuber calcis (Fig. 17.59) (Haghighi et al., 1991). Approximately 1 cm proximal to the tarsocrural joint, the tibial nerve bifurcates into the medial and lateral plantar nerves.

Nerves of the Plantar Surface of the Hindpaw (Pes)

On the plantar surface of the tarsus medial to the calcaneus, the tibial nerve divides into the medial and lateral plantar nerves. The **medial plantar nerve** (*n. plantaris medialis*) (Fig. 17.60) is smaller and more medial and superficial than the lateral plantar nerve. It crosses the medial side of the tarsus in the superficial fascia on the external surface of the extensor retinaculum. At the proximal end of the

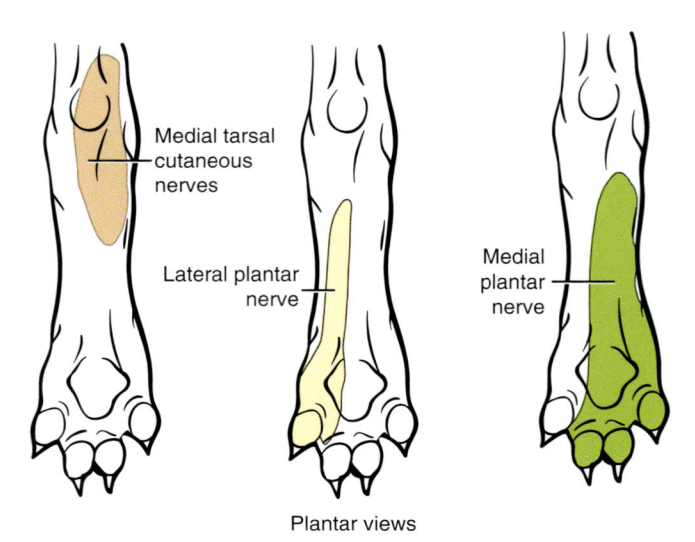

• **Fig. 17.59** Schematic illustration of the cutaneous areas of the plantar surface of the left hindpaw. (Modified, with permission, from Haghighi SS, Kitchell RL, Johnson RD, et al.: Electrophysiologic studies of the cutaneous innervation of the pelvic limb of male dogs, *Am J Vet Res* 52:352–362, 1991.)

metatarsus, it branches irregularly into **plantar common digital nerves II, III,** and **IV** (*nn. digitales plantares communes II, III, et IV*) and **abaxial plantar proper digital nerve II** (*n. digitalis plantaris abaxialis II*), and a **plantar proper digital nerve I** (*n. digitalis plantaris proprius I*) if a first digit is present.

Plantar common digital nerves II, III, and **IV** are formed at the proximal ends of the three main intermetatarsal spaces from the medial plantar nerve. These nerves extend obliquely distolaterad in the fascia covering the four branches of the superficial flexor tendon and send minute branches to the quadratus plantae, lumbricales, and interflexorii. At or near the distal end of the metatarsus, branches are given off their plantar sides to the metatarsal foot pad. Their small continuations communicate with plantar metatarsal nerves II, III, and IV. After running 1 or 2 cm and receiving the communicating branches from the plantar metatarsal nerves, each plantar common digital nerve bifurcates into two **plantar proper digital nerves** (*nn. digiti plantares proprii*) that supply the skin of the axial and abaxial plantar surfaces of contiguous digits. Each nerve terminates as a **dorsal branch**, which innervates the corium of the claw and the distal interphalangeal joint, and a **plantar branch**, which innervates a portion of the digital pad of its side.

The cutaneous area of the medial plantar nerve lies on the plantar surface of metatarsals II, III, and IV (Fig. 17.59) (Haghighi et al., 1991).

The **lateral plantar nerve** (*n. plantaris lateralis*) (Fig. 17.60) is larger, more lateral, and deeper than the medial plantar nerve. Plantar to the distal part of the tarsus, it enters the interval between the superficial and the deep digital flexor tendons and obliquely runs distad between them a short distance before terminating in many muscular branches and plantar metatarsal nerves II, III, and IV. The

CHAPTER 17 The Spinal Nerves 753

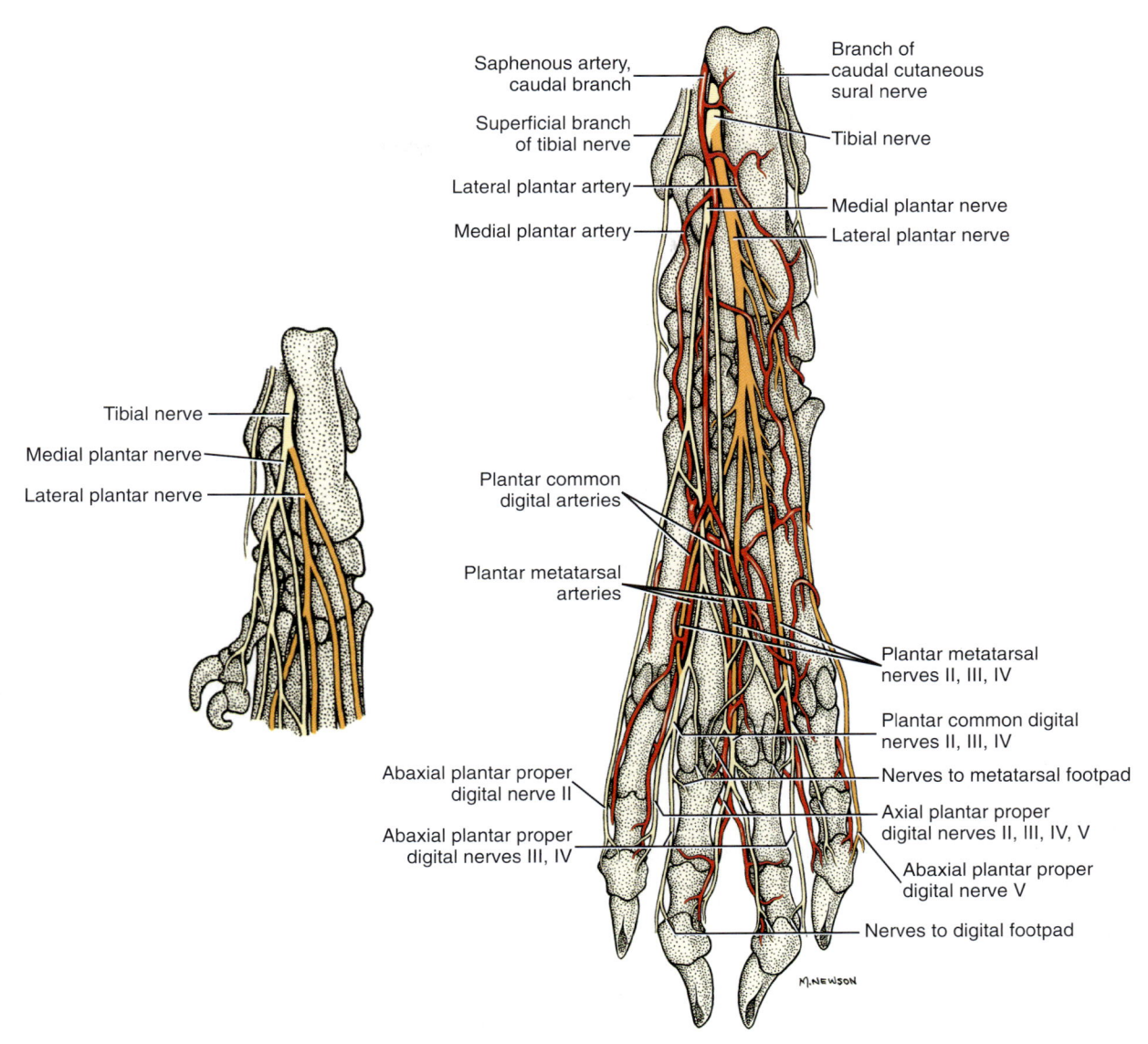

• **Fig. 17.60** Nerves and arteries of the right hindpaw, plantar aspect. Inset of nerve supply to a double dewclaw.

lateral plantar nerve near its origin gives rise to **abaxial plantar proper digital nerve V** (*n. digitalis plantaris abaxialis V*), which runs distad on the lateral surface of the fifth metatarsal bone and digit and terminates by dorsal and plantar branches in the terminal part of the fifth digit. The plantar branch goes to the fifth digital foot pad, and the dorsal branch goes to the dermis of the claw. This nerve sends branches all along its course to the skin of the lateral side of the paw.

The **muscular branches** include a branch proximally that supplies the small quadratus plantae. Remaining branches go to the interosseous muscles and the special muscles of the first, second, and fifth digits, and the quadratus plantae. The first **muscular branch** (*ramus muscularis*) arises from the lateral plantar nerve medial to the distal portion of the calcaneus, it crosses the plantar surface of this bone and enters the small, spindle-shaped belly of the abductor digiti V muscle. Another branch closely associated with it goes to the small, transversely running quadratus plantae. The remaining muscular branches arise rather closely together at the proximal end of the metatarsus. The first branch leaves the lateral border of the lateral plantar nerve and enters the proximal end of the fifth interosseous muscle. Other branches innervate the remaining interosseous muscles. From the second or most medial of the plantar common digital nerves arises the branch that supplies the abductor digiti secundi muscle. When the special muscles of the first digit are developed, they receive their nerve supply from this source also.

The **plantar metatarsal nerves** (**I**), **II**, **III**, and **IV** (*nn. metatarsei plantares [I] II, II, et IV*) are similar in location and termination to the comparable nerves of the forepaw. After running distad under the special muscles of the second and fifth digits and on the interossei, they communicate

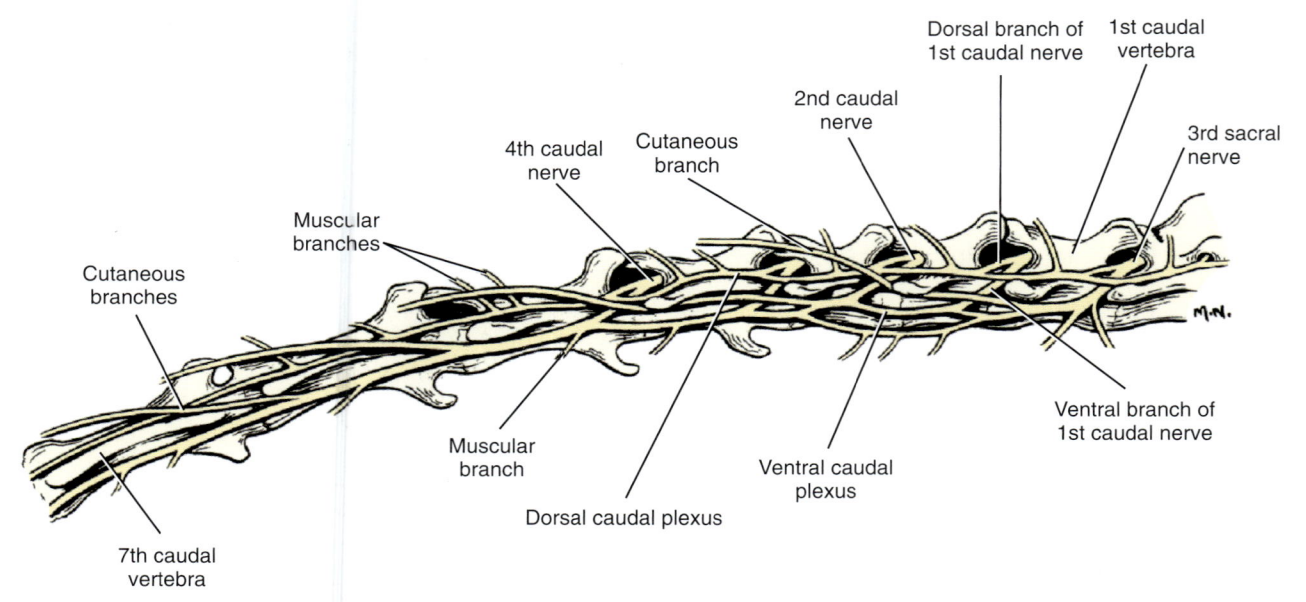

• Fig. 17.61 Diagram of the caudal nerves, lateral aspect.

with the plantar common digital nerves near the metatarsophalangeal joints. Adjacent plantar metatarsal nerves communicate with each other, and cutaneous branches arise from their distal ends and innervate the metatarsal pad.

The cutaneous area of the lateral plantar nerve includes the skin over the plantar surface of metacarpal V, the lateral aspect of the metacarpal pad and the plantar digital surface and pad of digit V (Fig. 17.59) (Haghighi et al., 1991).

Caudal Nerves

The paired **caudal nerves** (*nn. caudales [coccygei]*) (Fig. 17.61) vary in number from four (Havelka, 1928) to seven (Ellenberger & Baum, 1891). Hopkins (1935) found five pairs in each of nine carefully dissected mongrel specimens. Like the other spinal nerves, the caudal nerves branch immediately on leaving their intervertebral foramina into dorsal and ventral branches. Each pair of caudal nerves is numbered according to the vertebra that precedes the intervertebral foramen through which it runs. The **dorsal branch** of the first caudal nerve is joined by the dorsal branch of the third, or last, sacral nerve, and the dorsal branches of the five caudal nerves communicate with each other. In this manner a **dorsal caudal plexus** is formed. In a similar manner the **ventral caudal plexus** is formed. Baum and Zietzschmann (1936) name these plexi the *n. collector caudae dorsalis* and the *n. collector caudae ventralis*, respectively. (Some precedents for the names *dorsal* and *ventral trunks* are found in Sisson and Grossman's text [1953].) Other authors have named these caudal nerve trunks and their branches the *coccygeal plexuses*. The dorsal plexus lies directly dorsal to the transverse processes and the intertransverse muscles that extend only between several of the most proximal transverse processes. The dorsal sacrocaudal muscles lie directly dorsal to the nerve plexus that is accompanied by the dorsolateral caudal artery. The delicate **muscular branches** (*rami musculares*) that leave it extend dorsocaudally into the dorsal lateral and medial sacrocaudal muscles. In some segments there are two muscular branches leaving the plexus between the dorsal caudal nerves that contribute to its formation. In several dissections not more than two of these branches could be traced to terminations in the skin in any single specimen, and these were found near the root of the tail.

The **ventral plexus** is larger than the dorsal plexus. It is united with the ventral branch of the last sacral nerve at its beginning, and thereafter the plexus is augmented by the total volume of each of the ventral branches of the caudal nerves joining it. The plexus reaches its greatest width of approximately 2 mm as it is flattened against the fibrocartilage located between the fifth and the sixth caudal vertebrae. The ventral sacrocaudal muscles cover it ventrally. It lies ventral to the transverse processes and the intertransverse muscles. It is accompanied by the ventrolateral caudal artery; the two structures lie closely lateral to the hemal arches and more distally lateral to the hemal processes. The dorsal and ventral caudal plexi extend to the tip of the tail. **Muscular branches** (*rami musculares*) leave both the dorsal and the ventral surfaces of the plexi. The delicate dorsal branches supply both parts of the intertransverse caudae muscle and the vertebrae. The ventrally running branches innervate the lateral and medial ventral sacrocaudal muscles. The first seven to nine ventral branches terminate in dissectible **cutaneous branches** (*rami cutanei*) that innervate the skin of the tail. Some of these fine nerves can be traced several centimeters distally in the superficial fascia. Their main trunks lie in close association with the large, superficial lateral caudal vein and its small accompanying artery.

Bibliography

Adams, D. R. (2004). Peripheral nervous system: pelvic limb. In *Canine anatomy: a systematic study* (4th ed.). Ames: Iowa State Press.

Allam, M. W., Lee, D. G., Nulsen, F. E., et al. (1952). The anatomy of the brachial plexus of the dog. *Anat Rec, 114,* 173–180.

Bailey, C. S., Kitchell, R. L., & Johnson, R. D. (1982). Spinal nerve root origins of the cutaneous nerves arising from the canine brachial plexus. *Am J Vet Res, 43,* 820–825.

Bailey, C. S. (1984). Patterns of cutaneous anesthesia associated with brachial plexus avulsions in the dog. *J Am Vet Med Assoc, 185,* 889–899.

Bailey, C. S., & Kitchell, R. L. (1984). Clinical evaluation of the cutaneous innervation of the canine thoracic limb. *J Am Anim Hosp Assoc, 20,* 939–950.

Bailey, C. S., Kitchell, R. L., Haghighi, S. S., et al. (1984). Cutaneous innervation of the thorax and abdomen of the dog. *Am J Vet Res, 451,* 689–1698.

Bailey, C. S., Kitchell, R. L., Haghighi, S. S., et al. (1988). Spinal nerve root origins of the cutaneous nerves of the canine pelvic limb. *Am J Vet Res, 49,* 115–119.

Baum, H., & Zietzschmann, O. (1936). *Handbuch der anatomie des hundes.* Berlin: Paul Parey.

Bennett, D. (1976). An anatomical and histological study of the sciatic nerve, relating to peripheral nerve injuries in the dog and cat. *J Small Anim Pract, 17,* 379–386.

Bennett, D., & Vaughan, L. C. (1976). Peroneal nerve paralysis in the cat and dog: an experimental study. *J Small Anim Pract, 17,* 499–506.

Benson, R. O., & Fletcher, T. F. (1971). Variability of the ansa cervicalis in dogs. *Am J Vet Res, 32,* 1163–1168.

Blakely, C. L. (1957). Perineal hernia. In K. Mayer, J. V. Lacroix, & H. P. Hoskins (Eds.), *Canine surgery* (4th ed.). Evanston, IL: American Veterinary Publications.

Botha, G. S. M. (1957). The anatomy of phrenic nerve termination and the motor innervation of the diaphragm. *Thorax, 12,* 50–56.

Bowne, J. G. (1959). *Neuroanatomy of the brachial plexus of the dog.* Thesis, Ames: Iowa State University.

Bradley, O. C. (1927). *Topographical anatomy of the dog* (ed. 2). New York: Macmillan.

Bradley, O. C., & Grahame, T. (1959). *Topographical anatomy of the dog* (6th ed.). New York: Macmillan.

Budras, K. D., & Fricke, W. (1983). *Atlas der anatomie des hundes: kompendium fur tierartze u. Studierende.* Hannover, Germany: Schlütersche.

Budras, K. D., McCarthy, P. H., Fricke, W., et al. (2007). *Anatomy of the dog* (ed. 5). Hannover: Schlütersche.

Cuddon, P. A., Kitchell, R. L., & Johnson, R. D. (1989). Motor fibers in the canine distal caudal cutaneous sural nerve—dual innervation of the hind limb plantar muscles. *Anat Histol Embryol, 18,* 366–373.

Davenport, P. W., Thompson, F. J., Reep, R. L., & Freed, A. N. (1985). Projection of phrenic nerve afferents to the cat sensorimotor cortex. *Brain Res, 328,* 150–153. doi:10.1016/0006-8993(85)91334-4.

de Lahunta, A., Glass, E., & Kent, M. (2015). *Veterinary neuroanatomy and clinical neurology* (4th ed.). St. Louis, MO: Elsevier.

De Troyer, A. (1998). The canine phrenic nerve-to-intercostal reflex. *J Physiol, 508,* 919–927. doi:10.1111/j.1469-7793.1998.919p.x.

De Troyer, A., Sampson, M., Sigrist, S., & MacKlem, P. T. (1982). Action of the costal and crural parts of the diaphragm on the rib cage in dog. *J Appl Physiol, 53,* 30–39.

Ellenberger, W., & Baum, H. (1891). *Systematische und topographische anatomie des hundes.* Berlin: Paul Parey.

Ellenberger, W., & Baum, H. (1943). *Handbuch vergleichenden anatomie der haustiere* (18th ed.). Berlin: Springer.

Fletcher, T. F. (1970). Lumbosacral plexus and pelvic limb myotomes of the dog. *Am J Vet Res, 31,* 35–41.

Fletcher, T. F., & Kitchell, R. L. (1966a). The lumbar, sacral, and coccygeal tactile dermatomes of the dog. *J Comp Neurol, 128,* 171–180.

Fletcher, T. F., & Kitchell, R. L. (1966b). Anatomical studies on the spinal cord segments of the dog. *Am J Vet Res, 27,* 1759–1767.

Forsythe, W. B., & Ghoshal, N. G. (1984). Innervation of the canine thoracolumbar vertebral column. *Anat Rec, 208,* 57–63.

Ghoshal, N. G. (1975). Spinal nerves. In R. Getty (Ed.), *Sisson and Grossman's The anatomy of the domestic animals* (5th ed.). Philadelphia: Saunders.

Gilmore, D. R. (1984). Sciatic nerve injury in twenty-nine dogs. *J Am Anim Hosp Assoc, 20,* 403–407.

Griffin, D. W., Gregory, C. R., & Kitchell, R. L. (1989). Preservation of striated-muscle urethral sphincter function with the use of a surgical technique for perineal urethrostomy in cats. *J Am Vet Med Assoc, 194,* 1057–1060.

Haghighi, S. S., Kitchell, R. L., Johnson, R. D., et al. (1991). Electrophysiologic studies of the cutaneous innervation of the pelvic limb of male dogs. *Am J Vet Res, 52,* 352–362.

Hammond, C. G., Gordon, D. C., Fisher, J. T., & Richmond, F. J. (1989). Motor unit territories supplied by primary branches of the phrenic nerve. *J Appl Physiol, 66,* 61–71. doi:10.1152/jappl.1989.66.1.61.

Havelka, F. (1928). Plexus lumbo-sacralis u psa (in Czech, with a German summary: plexus lumho-sacralis des hundes). *Vysoká skola veterinárni Biologiche spisy, 7,* 1–40. (Pub. hiologiques de l'école des hautes etudes Vet.). Brünn, Czechoslovakia.

Henning, P. (1965). Der m. piriformis und die nn. clunium medii des hundes. *Anat Histol Embryol, 12,* 263–275.

Hopkins, G. S. (1935). The correlation of anatomy and epidural anesthesia in domestic animals. *Cornell Vet, 25,* 263–270.

Hummel, V. P. (1965). Die muskel—und hautnerven des plexus sacralis des hundes. *Anat Anz, 117,* 385–399.

Kitchell, R. L., Whalen, L. R., Bailey, C. S., et al. (1980). Electrophysiologic studies of cutaneous nerves of the thoracic limb of the dog. *Am J Vet Res, 41,* 61–76.

Kopp, P.: *Uber die Verteilung und das topographische Verhalten der Nervens an der Hand der Fleischfresser*, Inaugural dissertation, 1901, Bern.

Kunzel, P. (1957). Die huftgelenkstopographie des hundes und der zugabg zum gelenk. *Zbl Vet Med, 4,* 379–388.

Langley, J. N., & Anderson, H. K. (1896). The innervation of the pelvic and adjoining viscera. III. The external generative organs. *J Physiol (London), 19,* 85–121.

Lemon, W. S. (1928). The function of the diaphragm. *Arch Surg, 17,* 379–388.

Martin, P. (1923). *Lehrbuch der anatomie haustiere.* Stuttgart, Germany: Verlag von Schickhardt and Ebner.

Mehler, W. R., Fischer, J. C., & Alexander, W. F. (1952). The anatomy and variations of the lumbosacral sympathetic trunk in the dog. *Anat Rec, 113,* 421–435.

Miller, M. E., Christensen, G. C., & Evans, H. E. (1964). *Anatomy of the dog.* Philadelphia: Saunders.

Miller, R. A. (1934). Comparative studies upon the morphology and distribution of the brachial plexus in the dog. *Am J Anat, 54,* 143–175.

Mutai, M., Shibati, H., & Suzuki, T. (1986). Somatotopic organization of motoneurons innervating the pronators, carpal and digital flexors, and forepaw muscles in the dog: a retrograde horseradish peroxidase study. *Brain Res, 371,* 90–95.

Nair, J., Streeter, K. A., Turner, S. M. F., et al. (2017). Anatomy and physiology of phrenic afferent neurons. *J Neurophysiol, 118,* 2975–2990. doi:10.1152/jn.00484.2017.

Nickel, R., Schummer, A., & Seiferle, E. (1984). Peripheres nervensystem: legengeflecht, Plexus lumbalis, und nerven der hintergleidmase. In *Lehrbruch der anatomie der haustiere IV. Nervensystem, Endokrine drusen, Sinnesorgane.* Berlin: Paul Parey.

Nomina Anatomica Veterinaria (NAV) (5th ed.). (2005). Inter.Comm. on Veterinary Anatomical Nomenclature (ICVGAN) of World Assoc. of Veterinary Anatomists (WAVA).

Pederson, H. E., Blunck, F. J., & Gardner, E. (1956). The anatomy of lumbosacral posterior rami and meningeal branches of spinal nerves (sinu-vertebral nerves). *J Bone Joint Surg, 38A,* 377–391.

Pickering, M., & Jones, J. F. X. (2002). The diaphragm: two physiological muscles in one. *J Anat, 201,* 305–312. doi:10.1046/j.1469-7580.2002.00095.x.

Purinton, P. T. (1982). Variations in lumbosacral spinal roots in the dog. *Anat Histol Embryol, 11,* 147–151.

Reimers, H. (1925). Der plexus brachialis der haussaugetiere: eine vergleichend-anatomische studie. *Z Anat, 76,* 653–753.

Russell, J. S. (1893). An experimental investigation of the nerve roots which enter into the formation of the brachial plexus. *Phil Trans B, 184,* 39–65.

Schmaltz, R. (1914). *Atlas der anatomie des pferdes* (ed. 3). Berlin: Schoetz.

Sharp, J. W., Bailey, C. S., Johnson, R. D., et al. (1990). Spinal nerve root origin of the median, ulnar, and musculocutaneous nerves and their muscle nerve branches to the canine forelimb. *Anat Histol Embryol, 19,* 359–368.

Sharp, J. W., Bailey, C. S., Johnson, R. D., et al. (1991). Spinal root origin of the radial nerve and of nerves innervating the shoulder muscles of the dog. *Anat Histol Embryol, 20,* 205–214.

Sisson, S., & Grossman, J. D. (1953). *Anatomy of domestic animals* (4th ed.). Philadelphia: Saunders.

Spurgeon, T. L., & Kitchell, R. L. (1982). Electrophysiological studies of the cutaneous innervation of the external genitalia of the male dog. *Anat Histol Embryol, 11,* 289–306.

Spurgeon, T. L., & Reddy, V. K. (1986). Electrophysiological studies of the cutaneous innervation of the external genitalia of the female dog. *Anat Histol Embryol, 15,* 249–258.

Teitelbaum, J., Vanelli, G., & Hussain, S. N. A. (1993). Thin-fiber phrenic afferents mediate the ventilator response to diaphragmatic ischemia. *Respir Physiol, 91,* 195–206. doi:10.1016/0034-5687(93)90099-V.

Whalen, L. R., & Kitchell, R. L. (1983a). Electrophysiologic studies of the cutaneous nerves of the head of the dog. *Am J Vet Res, 44,* 615–627.

Whalen, L. R., & Kitchell, R. L. (1983b). Electrophysiologic and behavioral studies of the cutaneous nerves of the concave surface of the pinna and the external ear canal of the dog. *Am J Vet Res, 44,* 628–634.

Worthman, R. P. (1957). Demonstration of specific nerve paralyses in the dog. *J Am Vet Med Assoc, 131,* 174–178.

18
The Brain

The brain (*encephalon*) and spinal cord (*medulla spinalis*) constitute the central nervous system. Twelve pairs of cranial nerves (*nervi craniales*) emerge from the brain and exit the cranial cavity to innervate the head, certain neck muscles, and viscera of the thoracic and abdominal cavities. Terms such as *body, colliculus, peduncle, pyramid, lobe, gyrus,* and *folium* are used to refer to various elevations of the brain surface.

Brain tissue is composed of billions of neurons and glial cells that form **gray matter** (*substantia grisea*) and **white matter** (*substantia alba*). Localized accumulations of gray matter are designated **nuclei**, and the gray matter covering the surface of the cerebrum or cerebellum is called **cortex**. Concentrations of myelinated axons form white matter, which generally can be subdivided into **tracts** or fasciculi or striae. Regions (in the brainstem) where white and gray matter mix together are designated **reticular formation** (*formatio reticularis*).

The brain develops from three enlargements of the rostral end of the embryonic neural tube (Table 18.1). The enlargements become the **forebrain** (*prosencephalon*), **midbrain** (*mesencephalon*), and **hindbrain** (*rhombencephalon*). Subsequently the forebrain and hindbrain differentiate further, producing five primary divisions of the brain: **telencephalon, diencephalon, mesencephalon, metencephalon,** and **myelencephalon** (Fig. 18.1).

The brain may also be divided into three large regions: **cerebrum, cerebellum,** and **brainstem** (Fig. 18.2). The cerebrum is the telencephalon, the cerebellum is the dorsal part of the metencephalon, and the brain stem encompasses the remaining primary divisions. This chapter is organized to present first the brainstem, then the cerebrum, and finally the cerebellum.

THE BRAINSTEM

The brainstem occupies the fossae of the floor of the cranial cavity, caudal to the optic canals. All of the cranial nerves arise from the brainstem, except for olfactory nerves (including those to the vomeronasal organ). The rostral end of the brainstem is connected to the cerebrum by the internal capsule, a mass of myelinated axons. The brainstem is connected to the cerebellum by axons within three cerebellar peduncles. Caudally the brainstem is continuous with the spinal cord.

A ventral view of the brainstem reveals the primary brain divisions that compose it and the cranial nerves that emerge from it (Fig. 18.3). The **medulla oblongata** (*myelencephalon*) is the most caudal region. It is distinguished by bilateral longitudinal bands of white matter, the *pyramids,* that parallel the ventral midline. Seven cranial nerves (CN VI to XII) arise from the medulla oblongata. A transversely running trapezoid body demarcates the rostral extent of the medulla.

Rostral to medulla oblongata, the **pons** (*ventral metencephalon*) is distinguished by transverse fibers along its ventral surface. The trigeminal nerve (CN V) connects to the pons. Rostral to the pons, the ventral surface of the **midbrain** (*mesencephalon*) features a median interpeduncular fossa between bilateral cerebral peduncles. The ventral surface of each peduncle is capped by the white matter called **crus cerebri**. The oculomotor nerve (CN III) and the trochlear nerve (CN IV) arise from the midbrain; the latter exits from the dorsal surface.

The **diencephalon** is the rostral extent of the brainstem. Its ventral surface features mamillary bodies caudally, **optic chiasm** (*chiasma opticum*) rostrally, and, between these, an infundibulum connecting the brainstem to the hypophysis. Rostral to the optic chiasm, the optic nerve (CN II) runs to the eyeball.

Brain divisions are also evident in a dorsal view of the brainstem (Fig. 18.4). The dorsal surface of the medulla oblongata and pons features a rhomboid fossa (*fossa rhomboidea*), which is the floor of the fourth ventricle. Paired rostral and caudal colliculi mark the dorsal surface of the midbrain. Bilaterally the diencephalon features a prominent thalamus and, more caudally, a metathalamus composed of medial and lateral geniculate bodies.

Cranial Nerve Nuclei Overview

Neurons associated with cranial nerves are found at all levels of the brainstem. Individual cranial nerve nuclei form interrupted longitudinal columns that extend from the midbrain caudally, even entering the spinal cord (Fig. 18.5).

Afferent cranial nerve nuclei contain interneurons and projection neurons and receive synaptic input from primary afferent axons in cranial nerves. General visceral afferent axons collect in the **solitary tract** (*tractus solitarius*) and synapse in the **nucleus of the solitary tract** (*nucleus tractus*

TABLE 18.1 Divisions, Major Components, and Brain Cavities Derived from Primary Embryonic Vesicles That Develop into the Brain

Embryonic Brain Division	Derived Brain Structures	Definitive Brain Cavities
Forebrain		
Telencephalon	Cerebral hemispheres	Lateral ventricles
Diencephalon	Thalamus, hypothalamus, epithalamus, subthalamus, metathalamus	Third ventricle
Midbrain		
Mesencephalon	Cerebral peduncles and tectum	Mesencephalic aqueduct
Hindbrain		
Metencephalon	Pons and cerebellum	Fourth ventricle
Myelencephalon	Medulla oblongata	Fourth ventricle

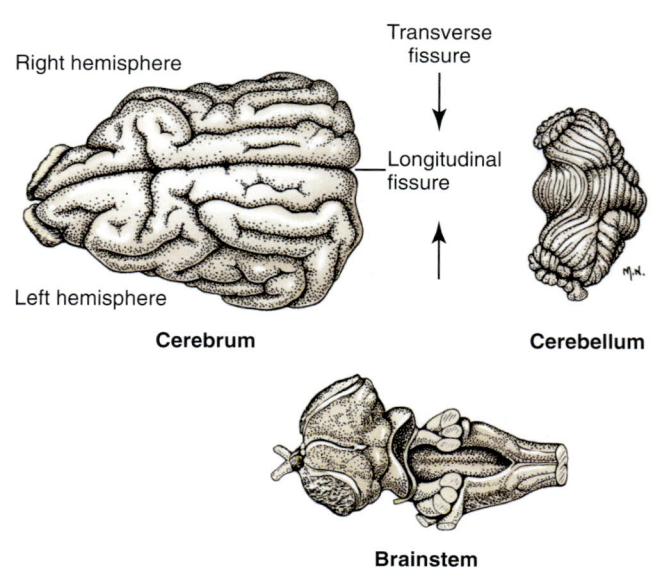

• **Fig. 18.2** Illustration of the cerebrum and cerebellum detached from the brainstem. The longitudinal fissure separates right and left cerebral hemispheres. The transverse fissure separates the cerebrum and cerebellum.

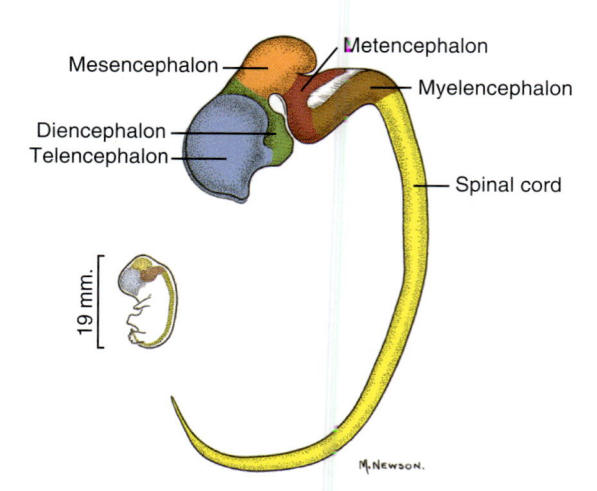

• **Fig. 18.1** Schematic image of the embryonic brain. Early in development, three primary vesicles (prosencephalon, mesencephalon, rhombencephalon) grow at the rostral end of the neural tube (19 mm inset). Subsequently, the three vesicles give rise to the five major divisions of the brain. The telencephalon and diencephalon arise from the forebrain (prosencephalon) and the metencephalon and myelencephalon arise form the hindbrain (rhombencephalon).

solitarii). The rostral end of the nucleus also receives special visceral afferent axons conveying taste.

Somatic afferent axons entering from the trigeminal nerve segregate by modality. Nociceptor and temperature axons form the **spinal tract of the trigeminal nerve** (*tractus spinalis n. trigemini*) and synapse in the **nucleus of the spinal tract of V** (*nucleus tractus spinalis n. trigemini*). Axons conveying touch synapse in the **pontine sensory nucleus of the trigeminal nerve** (*nucleus sensibilis pontinus n. trigemini*). Unipolar cell bodies of proprioceptive primary neurons migrate into the brain and form the **nucleus of the mesencephalic tract of V** (*nucleus tractus mesencephalici n. trigemini*).

Efferent cranial nerve nuclei contain somatic efferent or visceral preganglionic neurons. The somatic and visceral nuclei form separate columns. Also, there are two separate somatic nuclear columns. Eye and tongue muscles are innervated by nuclei found dorsomedially in the brainstem. Striated muscles derived from pharyngeal arch myotomes (jaw, face, pharynx, larynx, esophagus, and some neck muscles) are innervated by somatic efferent nuclei positioned ventrolaterally in the brainstem (previously these somatic efferent nuclei were labeled *special visceral efferent*). Individual cranial nuclei are described in more detail in the discussion of the brainstem region.

Reticular Formation Overview

In addition to distinct regions formed by gray matter nuclei and white matter tracts, the brainstem features extensive areas of **reticular formation** (*formatio reticularis*) where gray and white matter are mixed together. Neurons of the reticular formation give rise to reticulospinal tracts, to thalamic projections that alert the cerebral cortex, to cerebellar relay sites, and to visceral relay and premotor nuclei. Anatomically individual reticular formation nuclei are relatively indistinct but collectively they form three longitudinal zones: lateral and medial zones bilaterally and unpaired raphe nuclei located along the midline (Fig. 18.6).

Many neurons within unpaired **raphe reticular nuclei** (*nuclei raphe*) release serotonin as a neuromodulator that affects mood and sensitivity to noxious stimuli. Raphe nuclei in the pons and midbrain send axons rostrally, influencing the limbic system and affective behavior. The **nucleus**

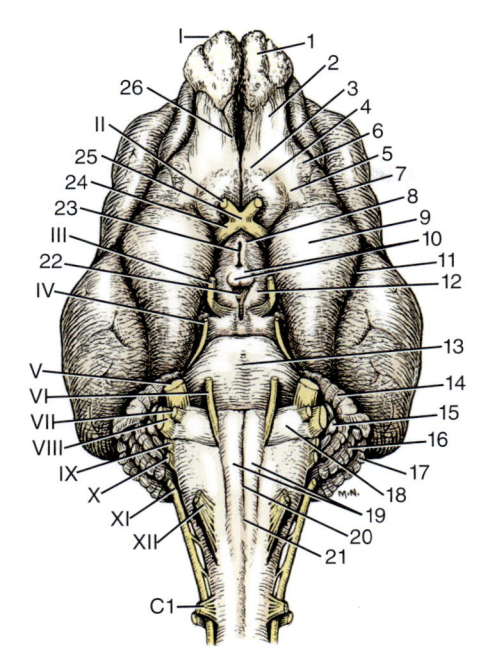

- Fig. 18.3 Ventral view of the brain and the first cervical segment of the spinal cord.

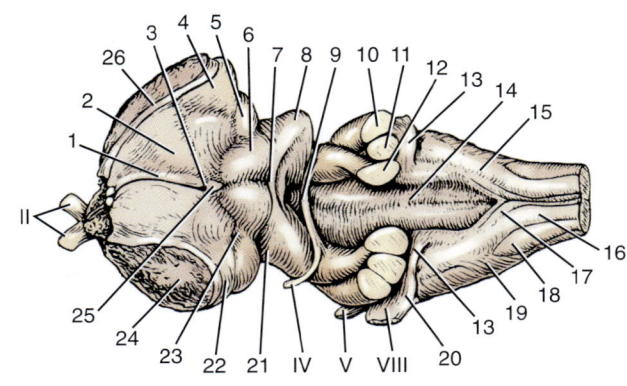

1. Olfactory bulb
2. Olfactory peduncle
3. Medial olfactory tract
4. Olfactory tubercle
5. Lateral olfactory tract
6. Lateral olfactory gyrus
7. Rostral part of lateral rhinal sulcus
8. Tuber cinereum
9. Piriform lobe
10. Mamillary bodies
11. Caudal part of lateral rhinal sulcus
12. Crus cerebri
13. Transverse fibers of pons
14. Ventral paraflocculus
15. Flocculus
16. Cerebellar hemisphere
17. Ansiform lobule
18. Trapezoid body
19. Pyramids
20. Median fissure
21. Decussation of pyramids
22. Interpeduncular fossa
23. Infundibulum
24. Optic tract
25. Optic chiasm
26. Medial rhinal sulcus
II. Optic nerve
III. Oculomotor nerve
IV. Trochlear nerve
V. Trigeminal nerve
VI. Abducent nerve
VII. Facial nerve
VIII. Vestibulocochlear nerve
IX. Glossopharyngeal nerve
X. Vagus nerve
XI. Accessory nerve
XII. Hypoglossal nerve
C1. Spinal ventral root (C1)

1. Stria habenularis thalami
2. Dorsal aspect of thalamus
3. Habenular commissure
4. Lateral geniculate body
5. Medial geniculate body
6. Rostral colliculus
7. Commissure of caudal colliculi
8. Caudal colliculus
9. Decussation of trochlear nerves in rostral medullary velum
10. Middle cerebellar peduncle
11. Caudal cerebellar peduncle
12. Rostral cerebellar peduncle
13. Acoustic stria
14. Median sulcus in fourth ventricle
15. Nucleus cuneatus lateralis
16. Fasciculus cuneatus
17. Fasciculus gracilis
18. Spinal tract of trigeminal nerve
19. Superficial arcuate fibers
20. Cochlear nuclei (dorsal and ventral)
21. Brachium of caudal colliculus
22. Optic tract
23. Brachium of rostral colliculus
24. Cut surface of internal capsule
25. Pineal body
26. Stria terminalis
II. Optic nerve
IV. Trochlear nerve
V. Trigeminal nerve
VIII. Vestibulocochlear nerve

- Fig. 18.4 The brainstem from a dorsolateral perspective.

raphe magnus of the medulla oblongata plays an endogenous analgesia role. Activated by axon input from midbrain periaqueductal gray (PAG) matter, the nucleus directs axons caudally to block nociceptive pathway transmission in the spinal cord dorsal horn via enkephalinergic interneurons (Beitz, 1992).

The medial nuclei of the reticular formation contain large neurons that give rise to reticulospinal tracts. Axons from the *gigantocellular reticular nucleus* of the medulla oblongata form the **lateral (medullary) reticulospinal tract** (*tractus reticulospinalis lateralis*). Magnocellular neurons of the caudal pontine reticular nucleus give rise to the **medial (pontine) reticulospinal tract**.

The lateral nuclei of the reticular formation contain small (parvocellular) neurons. The nuclei are functionally diverse. They receive spinal input and activate reticulospinal neurons. They are involved in forebrain arousal (ascending reticular activating system). They project to the cerebellum. And many of the reticular nuclei scattered along the brainstem are involved processing visceral information (Fig. 18.7). Some visceral nuclei have a relay role, receiving visceral input and projecting their output to other visceral nuclei. Some visceral nuclei have a premotor role, their axons drive preganglionic neurons in visceral efferent nuclei.

The Medulla Oblongata

The **medulla oblongata** (myelencephalon) contains gray matter nuclei, white matter tracts, and mixed gray and white reticular formation. The nuclei may be categorized as *cranial nerve nuclei, relay nuclei for sensory pathways, cerebellar projection nuclei,* and *reticular formation nuclei*. White matter includes cranial nerve axons, axonal connections with the cerebellum, and tract axons traversing or terminating in the medulla oblongata.

The Spinomedullary Junction

The caudal extent of the medulla oblongata has some features resembling the spinal cord, with which it is continuous (Fig. 18.8). In a transverse section, one can see a central canal, superficial white matter, laterally expanded central gray matter, a ventral median fissure, and a dorsal median

760 CHAPTER 18 The Brain

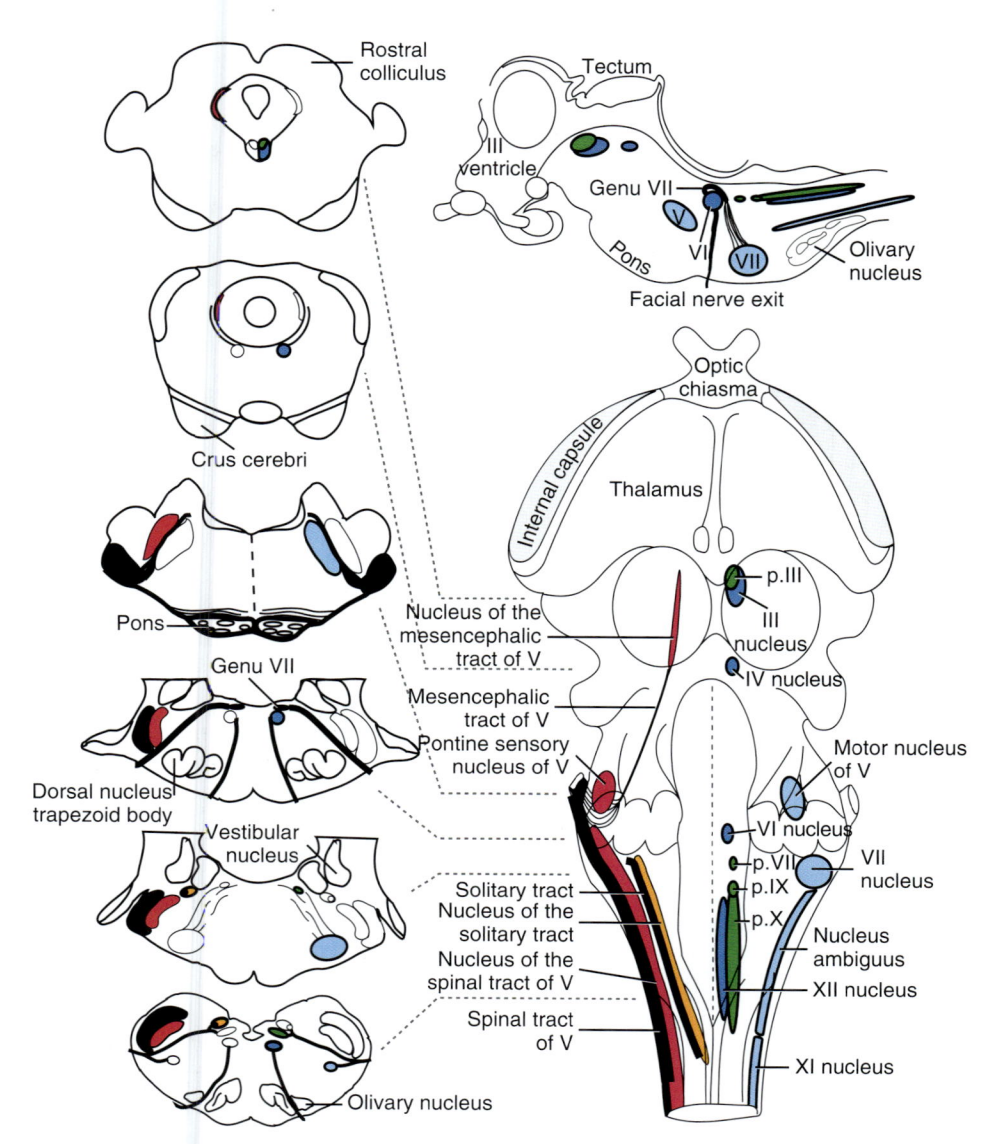

• **Fig. 18.5** Locations of cranial nerve nuclei are shown in transverse sections (*left*), a dorsal view of the brainstem (*lower right*), and a medial view of the right half of the brainstem (*top right*). In all cases, motor nuclei are colored on the right side, and sensory nuclei on the left. Visceral efferent (parasympathetic) nuclei are *green*. Somatic efferent nuclei are *dark blue* and *light blue* (the latter nuclei innervate pharyngeal arch derivatives). The visceral afferent nucleus is *orange*. General somatic afferent nuclei are *red*. Special somatic afferent nuclei (vision, hearing, vestibular sense) are not shown, except as landmarks. The medial view shows the VII genu, formed by axons from facial nucleus hooking dorsal to abducent nucleus before exiting laterally. (*III–XII*, Cranial nerves; *motor V*, motor nucleus of V; *nucl.*, nucleus; *nucl. amb.*, nucleus ambiguus; *nucl. mes. tr. V* and *mes. tr. V*, nucleus of the mesencephalic tract of V and mesencephalic tract of V; *nucl. pon. sen. V*, pontine sensory nucleus of V; *nucl. sp. tr. V* and *sp. tr. V*, nucleus of the spinal tract of V and spinal tract of V; *nucl. sol. tr.* and *sol. tr.*, nucleus of the solitary tract and solitary tract; *p. III, p. VII, p. IX,* and *p. X* = parasympathetic nuclei of the respective cranial nerves. Selected landmarks are labeled.)

sulcus and septum. A dominant feature of the spinomedullary junction is the **pyramidal decussation** (*decussatio pyramidum*).

Each **pyramid** (*pyramis*) consists of myelinated axons that originate from neuronal cell bodies in the cerebral cortex. Axons within the pyramids go to the medulla oblongata (corticonuclear and corticoreticular axons) or to the spinal cord (corticospinal axons). The axons synapse on interneurons that regulate both efferent neurons (motor units) and projection neurons (cranial projecting pathways) (Davidoff, 1990).

Most corticospinal axons turn dorsally and cross the midline (pyramidal decussation) to reach the dorsal half of the contralateral lateral funiculus, where they project caudally as the **lateral corticospinal tract**. A minority of axons delays decussation until they terminate in spinal gray

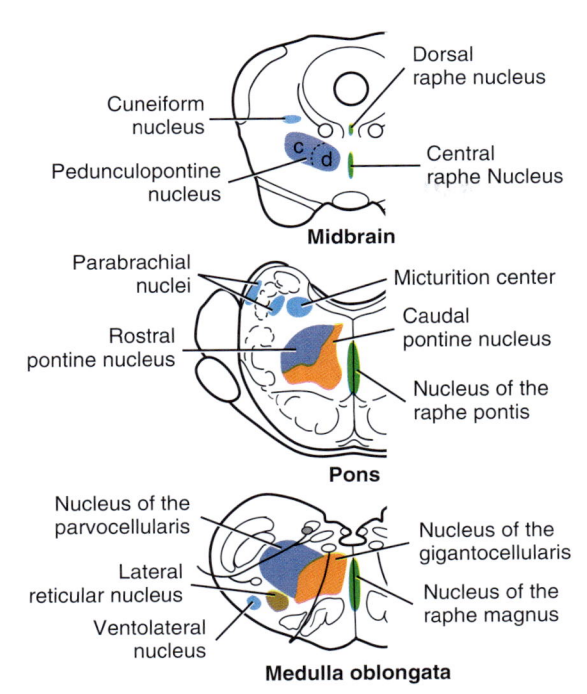

• **Fig. 18.6** Schematic drawing showing selected nuclei of the reticular formation. Reticular formation nuclei are organized into longitudinal columns. Unpaired, midline, raphe nuclei (*green*) contain neurons that release serotonin. Medial column nuclei (*orange*) have large (magnocellular) neurons and give rise to reticulospinal axons. Nuclei composing the lateral column (*dark blue*) generally have small (parvocellular) neurons. The small neurons are activated by collateral branches from sensory tracts; their axons synapse on the large neurons in the medial column. Some lateral reticular nuclei have visceral roles (*pale blue*). Some reticular nuclei project to the cerebellum (*brown*). The pedunculopontine nucleus of the midbrain has compact (*c*) and diffuse (*d*) regions. The former has large cholinergic neurons that project axons to the thalamus. The latter connects to basal nuclei circuits.

The fasciculus and nucleus gracilis are concerned with discriminative touch from the caudal half of the body. Neurons situated medial and rostral to the nucleus gracilis are referred to as **nucleus Z**. Kinesthesia from the caudal half of the body reaches nucleus Z through a spinomedullary tract. Most kinesthetic input is from collateral branches of the dorsal spinocerebellar tract; only scant input arrives via the fasciculus gracilis (Hand, 1966).

Lateral to fasciculus cuneatus, the **spinal tract of the trigeminal nerve** (*tractus spinalis n. trigemini*) is visible (Fig. 18.8). It is superficial to the **nucleus of the spinal tract of the trigeminal nerve** (*nucleus tractus spinalis n. trigemini*). The tract is composed of small, myelinated and nonmyelinated axons from neuronal cell bodies located in the trigeminal ganglion, plus a minority of somatic afferent axons from the vagus, glossopharyngeal, and facial nerves. The nucleus is divisible into rostral, interpolar, and caudal parts. The tract and nucleus extend into the first two cervical segments of the spinal cord overlapping with dorsolateral fasciculus, marginal nucleus, and substantia gelatinosa.

Axons constituting the spinal tract of the trigeminal nerve convey noxious, temperature, and crude touch information from the face and nasal and oral cavities, including the teeth. Within the tract, axons from the dorsal face (ophthalmic division of the trigeminal nerve) travel ventrally, and those from the ventral face (mandibular division) travel dorsally. The nucleus has a comparable somatotopic organization. Additionally, the nasal and oral cavities are represented in rostral regions of the nucleus, while the surrounding perimeter of the face is represented caudally.

Caudal Half of the Medulla Oblongata

The **olivary nucleus** (*nucleus olivaris*) is a prominent feature of the caudal medulla oblongata (Fig. 18.9). It is located dorsolateral to the pyramid and lateral to the medial lemniscus; it presents a distinctive serpentine profile in the ventrolateral medulla. The nucleus receives axonal input from the cerebellum, from the cerebral cortex via the pyramids, and from the red nucleus and PAG via the central tegmental tract. Dorsal and medial accessory olivary nuclei receive afferents from the spinal cord.

Efferent axons from the olivary nuclei decussate and reach the cerebellum via the **caudal cerebellar peduncle** (*pedunculus cerebellaris caudalis*) (Fig. 18.10). Olivocerebellar fibers climb along dendritic trees of Purkinje (piriform) neurons in the cerebellar cortex and intensely activate small, localized regions of cortex for adjusting movement and posture. Other nuclei that project to the cerebellum terminate as mossy endings on granule neurons that diffusely influence the cerebellar cortex.

The **lateral cuneate nucleus** (*nucleus cuneatus lateralis*) is situated most dorsally in the medulla oblongata. It receives proprioceptive input from the thoracic limb and neck via the fasciculus cuneatus. Axons from the nucleus form **superficial arcuate fibers** (*fibrae arcuatae superficiales*). The fibers merge with the dorsal spinocerebellar tract to form the *caudal cerebellar peduncle*, located at the dorsolateral

matter; these run in the ipsilateral lateral corticospinal tract or in the ventral funiculus as the **ventral corticospinal tract**. The decussation of pyramidal axons and other caudally projecting tracts explains why one side of the brain controls voluntary movement on the contralateral side of the body.

Dorsally at the midline, *fasciculus gracilis* axons terminate in the **nucleus gracilis**. Further laterally, *fasciculus cuneatus* axons terminate in the **medial cuneate nucleus** (*nucleus cuneatus medialis*) (Fig. 18.8). The fasciculi are composed of cranial branches of primary afferent axons associated with encapsulated receptors located in skin or in muscles, tendons, and joints. The nuclei relay sensory information from primary afferent neurons to neurons in the thalamus. Axons from the nuclei decussate as **deep arcuate fibers** (*fibrae arcuatae profundae*) and project rostrally as **medial lemniscus** (*lemniscus medialis*).

The fasciculus cuneatus and medial cuneate nucleus are concerned with discriminative touch and kinesthesia (sense of position and movement) from the thoracic limb and neck. Kinesthesia is relayed by neurons located ventrally in the medial cuneate nucleus.

762 CHAPTER 18 The Brain

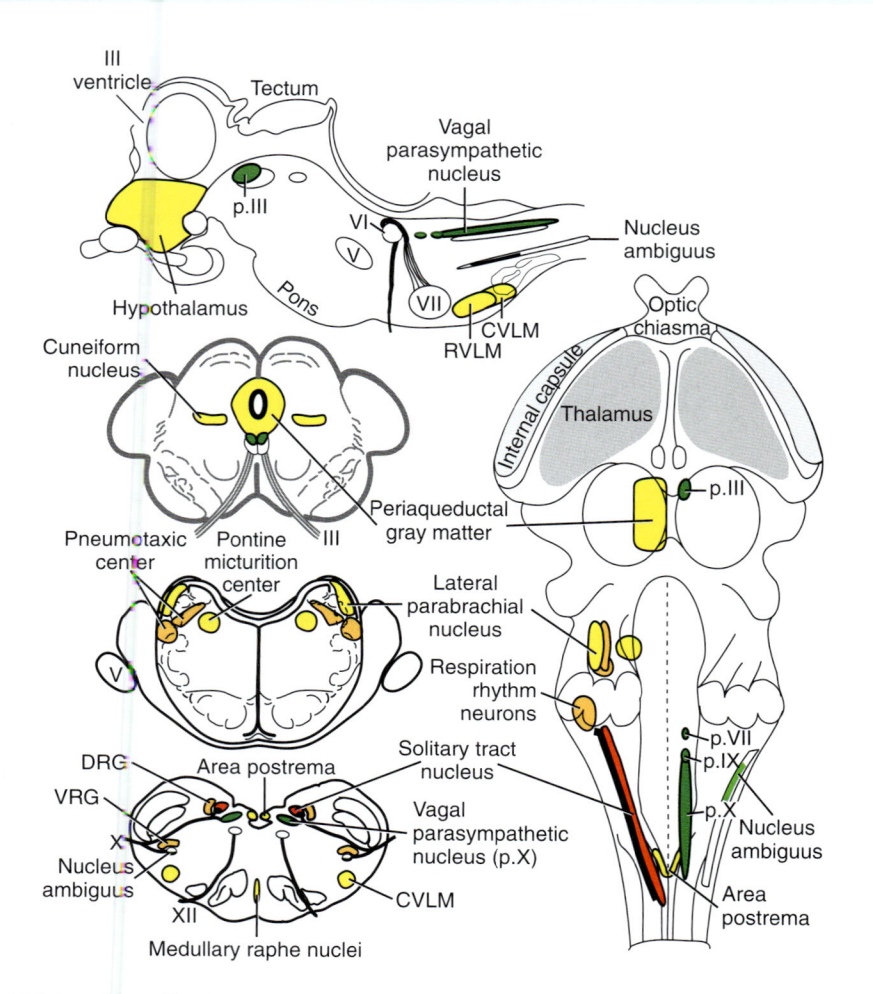

• **Fig. 18.7** Locations of brainstem neurons involved with visceral regulation, including control of breathing and coughing (*orange*), are shown schematically. Selected nuclei and regions are illustrated bilaterally or unilaterally in transverse (*left*), dorsal (*right*), and sagittal (*top*) views of the brainstem. Preganglionic parasympathetic nuclei (*p.*) of cranial nerves III, VII, IX, and X are green, including cardiac visceral efferent neurons within the nucleus ambiguus. The nucleus of the solitary tract (*red*) receives visceral afferent axons from cranial nerves. Locations of selected visceral relay and premotor neurons are shown in *yellow*. *RVLM* and *CVLM*, rostral and caudal ventrolateral medulla (the latter inhibits the former, which elevates blood pressure and receives axons from the midbrain cuneiform nucleus). The lateral parabrachial nucleus relays visceral information to the periaqueductal gray matter and hypothalamus, which send axons to the micturition center to effect urination. *DRG* and *VRG*, Dorsal and ventral respiratory groups, which drive the phrenic nerve.

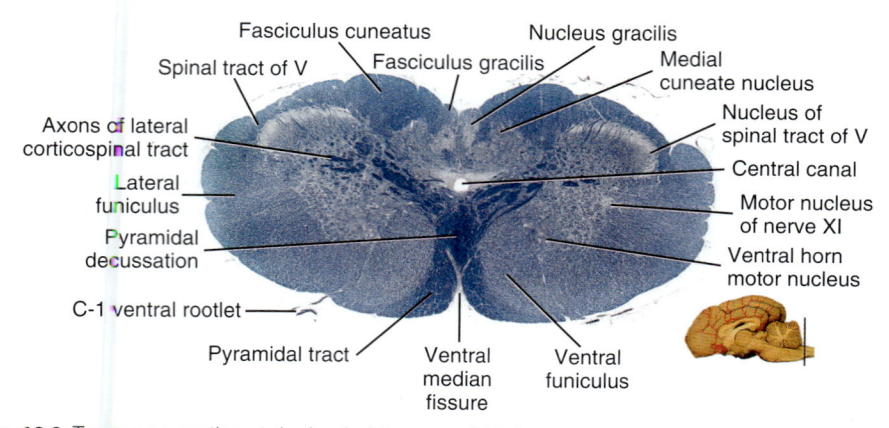

• **Fig. 18.8** Transverse section at the level of the pyramidal decussation, juncture of the canine brain and spinal cord. (Luxol Fast Blue–Cresyl Violet stain.)

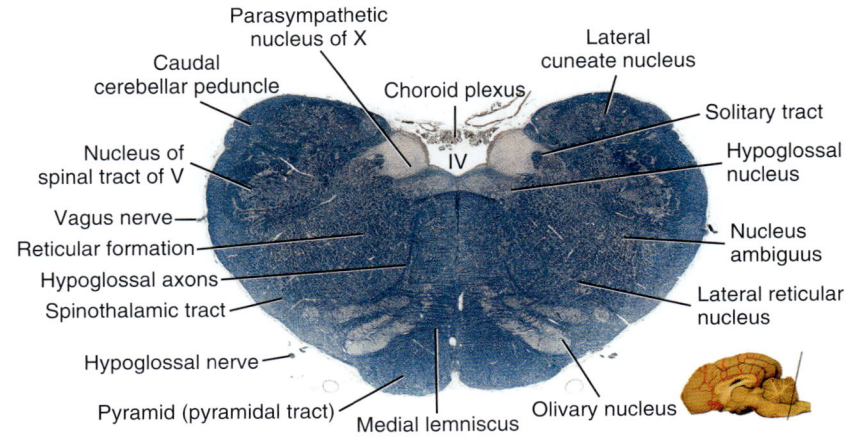

• **Fig. 18.9** Transverse section at the level of the hypoglossal nucleus at the caudal end of a canine medulla oblongata. Choroid plexus is evident in the roof of the fourth ventricle (IV). (Luxol Fast Blue–Cresyl Violet stain.)

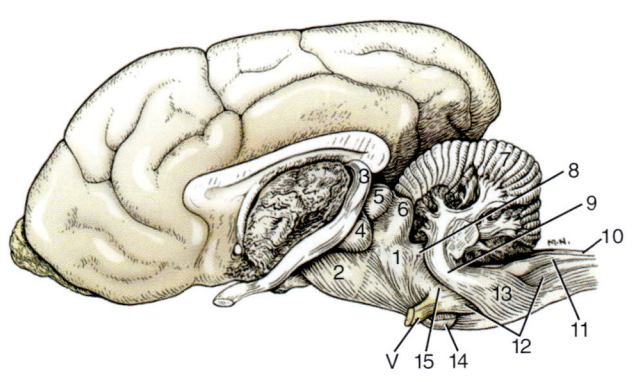

1. Lateral lemniscus
2. Crus cerebri
3. Lateral geniculate body
4. Medial geniculate body
5. Rostral colliculus
6. Caudal colliculus
7. Cerebellum
8. Rostral cerebellar peduncle
9. Caudal cerebellar peduncle
10. Fasciculus gracilis
11. Fasciculus cuneatus
12. Spinal tract of trigeminal nerve
13. Superficial arcuate fibers
14. Trapezoid body (transected)
15. Location of pontine sensory nucleus of trigeminal nerve
V. Trigeminal nerve

• **Fig. 18.10** Lateral view of a brain with the left cerebral hemisphere and middle cerebellar peduncle removed and the pons and cerebellum dissected to show the caudal cerebellar peduncle (9) joining the cerebellum. The spinal tract of the trigeminal nerve is also shown (12).

margin of the medulla oblongata (Fig. 18.9). The dorsal spinocerebellar tract conveys proprioceptive information from the caudal half of the body.

The **fourth ventricle** is located in the medulla oblongata and pons. Caudally the region where the fourth ventricle narrows to a point is called the *obex*. Immediately rostral to the obex, the wall of the ventricle is formed by the *area postrema*, a densely vascularized gray matter that has fenestrated capillaries and serves as an emetic center (activated by apomorphine). As one of the circumventricular organs, it is a region that lacks a blood–brain barrier.

The floor of the fourth ventricle, designated **rhomboid fossa** (*fossa rhomboidea*), has a **median sulcus** (*sulcus medianus*) (Fig. 18.4). Bilaterally, a **sulcus limitans** marks the transition from floor to wall; also, it is the demarcation between the embryonic alar and basal plates. The **roof of the fourth ventricle** (*tegmen ventriculi quarti*) is formed by the **tela choroidea** (*tela choroidea ventriculi quarti*) a layer of ependyma and pia mater that attaches to the medullary wall along a line, called **tenia of the fourth ventricle** (*tenia ventriculi quarti*).

Rostrally tela choroidea that connects to rostral cerebellar peduncles and contains trochlear nerve axons, constitutes **rostral medullary velum** (*velum medullare rostrale*). Caudally the **caudal medullary velum** (*velum medullare caudale*) forms the roof of the fourth ventricle. Tela choroidea of the caudal medullary velum gives rise to two longitudinal proliferations of blood vessels, forming the **choroid plexuses** of the fourth ventricle (*plexus choroideus ventriculi quarti*). The paired choroid plexuses produce cerebrospinal fluid.

Some cerebrospinal fluid enters the central canal, but most of it flows outward to the subarachnoid space, exiting the fourth ventricle bilaterally through a **lateral recess** (*recessus lateralis*) that leads to a **lateral aperture** (*aperturae laterales*). The recess and aperture are located immediately caudal to the caudal cerebellar peduncle. Some choroid plexus extends through the lateral recess and aperture to secrete directly into the subarachnoid space (Fig. 18.11).

The **motor nucleus of the hypoglossal nerve** (*nucleus motorius n. hypoglossi*) is evident dorsally beside the midline (Fig. 18.9). Axons from the nucleus run ventrally and then angle through the lateral region of the olivary nucleus. They leave the medulla oblongata as roots of the hypoglossal nerve and innervate muscles of the tongue (somatic efferent axons).

The **parasympathetic nucleus of the vagus nerve** (*nucleus parasympathicus n. vagi*) is located dorsolateral to the hypoglossal nucleus. Preganglionic parasympathetic visceral efferent axons from the nucleus run laterally to join the vagus nerve and innervate thoracic and abdominal viscera. Rostrally two small nuclei of this cell column contribute axons to the glossopharyngeal and facial nerves

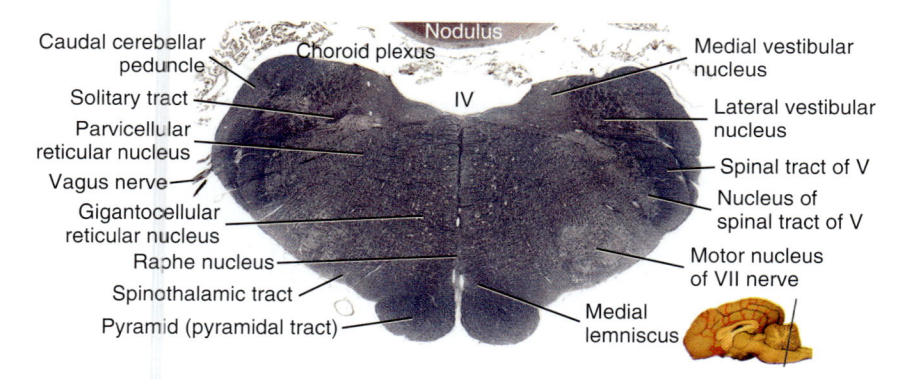

• **Fig. 18.11** Transverse section through a canine medulla oblongata at the level of the motor nucleus of the facial nerve. Choroid plexus is evident bilaterally within the roof of the fourth ventricle *(IV)* and extending into lateral recesses of the fourth ventricle. (Luxol Fast Blue–Cresyl Violet stain.)

(Fig. 18.9). The parasympathetic nucleus of the glossopharyngeal nerve (*nucleus parasympatheticus n. glossopharyngei*) innervates parotid and zygomatic salivary glands. Further rostrally, the parasympathetic nucleus of the facial nerve (*nucleus parasympatheticus n. facialis*) innervates mandibular and sublingual salivary glands and nasal, palatine, and lacrimal glands.

The **nucleus intercalatus**, positioned between the hypoglossal and the parasympathetic nuclei, sends axons to the cerebellum. The nucleus receives input from vestibular nuclei and there is clinical evidence in humans that it is involved in holding vertical gaze position (Munro et al., 1993).

The **solitary tract** (*tractus solitarius*) is distinct dorsolateral to the parasympathetic nucleus of the vagus (Fig. 18.9). The tract contains axons from visceral afferent cell bodies located in distal ganglia of the vagus and glossopharyngeal nerves and the geniculate ganglion of the facial nerve. The axons synapse in the **nucleus of the solitary tract** (*nucleus tractus solitarii*). Caudally right and left nuclei merge dorsal to the central canal, forming a *commissural nucleus*.

The nucleus of the solitary tract contains interneurons and projection neurons concerned with reflexes and sensation from the auditory tube, pharynx, larynx, esophagus, trachea, and other thoracic and abdominal viscera. The rostral end of the nucleus receives taste (special visceral afferent) input from three nerves: vagus (pharynx and larynx), glossopharyngeal (caudal third of tongue), and facial (rostral two-thirds of tongue).

The **nucleus ambiguus** is a column of sparse neurons located ventral to the nucleus of the spinal tract of the trigeminal nerve (Fig. 18.9). Except for some visceral efferent neurons that innervate the heart (Fig. 18.7), the nucleus ambiguus contains somatic efferent neurons. Via vagus and glossopharyngeal nerves, the neurons send axons to striated muscles of the pharynx, larynx, and esophagus.

A caudal continuation of the ambiguus cell column extends through the cervical spinal cord as the **motor nucleus of the accessory nerve** (*nucleus motorius n. accessorii*) (Fig. 18.5). Its axons form the spinal root of the accessory nerve, which innervates certain muscles of the neck (cleidocephalicus, mastoid part of sternocephalicus, omotransversarius, and trapezius). The **accessory nerve** has a cranial root that arises from the caudal pole of the nucleus ambiguus. The root immediately joins the vagus nerve and eventually becomes recurrent laryngeal nerve.

The **lateral reticular nucleus** (*nucleus reticularis lateralis*), also referred to as *nucleus of the lateral funiculus* (*nucleus funiculi lateralis*), is located lateral to the olivary nucleus (Fig. 18.9). It receives input from the red nucleus and the spinal cord. Its axons join superficial arcuate fibers to reach the cerebellum via the caudal cerebellar peduncle.

Level of the Facial Nucleus

The **motor nucleus of the facial nerve** (*nucleus motorius n. facialis*) is located ventrally in the medulla oblongata (Fig. 18.11). The nucleus contains somatic efferent neurons that innervate muscles of facial expression. Neurons are topographically arranged within the nucleus: rostral to caudal positioned neurons innervate rostral to caudal muscles, dorsal neurons innervate ventral muscles, and vice versa (Berman, 1968).

Axons from the facial nucleus stream dorsally and collect in a bundle that arcs, from medial to lateral, dorsally around the abducent nucleus, before proceeding ventrolaterally to exit passing through the trapezoid body (Fig. 18.5). The loop, located dorsal to the abducent nucleus, is referred to as the **genu of the facial nerve** (*genu n. facialis*).

The facial nerve also contains visceral efferent and afferent fibers. The **parasympathetic nucleus of the facial nerve** (*nucleus parasympathicus n. facialis*) is located caudal to the genu of the facial nerve. The nucleus is a rostral satellite of the parasympathetic column that supplies the glossopharyngeal and vagus nerves. Ganglionic cell bodies of the nucleus innervate neuronal cell bodies of postganglionic axons that supply lacrimal, nasal, and palatine glands, and the mandibular and sublingual salivary glands. Special visceral afferent axons in the facial nerve convey taste from the rostral two-thirds of the tongue. The axons join the solitary tract and terminate in the rostral pole of its nucleus.

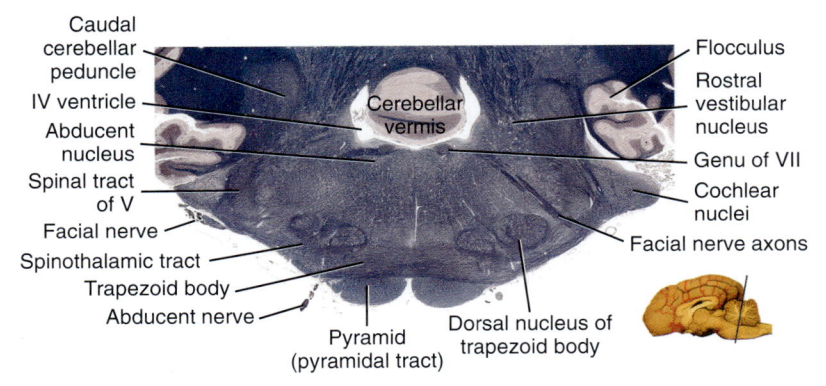

• **Fig. 18.12** Transverse section through a canine rostral medulla oblongata at the level of the trapezoid body. From medial to lateral, three cranial nerves attach at this level: abducent, facial, and vestibulocochlear. The latter joins cochlear nuclei. (Luxol Fast Blue–Cresyl Violet stain.)

The facial nerve has a small contingent of general somatic afferent fibers that supply the concave surface of the auricle of the ear (Whalen & Kitchell, 1983). These axons join the spinal tract of the trigeminal nerve.

White matter at the lateral edge of the medulla oblongata constitutes the **caudal cerebellar peduncle** (*pedunculus cerebellaris caudalis*) (formerly *restiform* and *juxtarestiform bodies*). The axons of the peduncle pass deep to the acoustic stria and turn abruptly dorsad to join the cerebellum (Fig. 18.10). The lateral recess of the fourth ventricle is located immediately caudal to the abrupt turn of the peduncle (Fig. 18.11).

Vestibular nuclei (*nuclei vestibulares*) produce a bulge in the wall of the fourth ventricle. The **caudal vestibular nucleus** (*nucleus vestibularis caudalis*) is situated medial to the caudal cerebellar peduncle, and the **medial vestibular nucleus** (*nucleus vestibularis medialis*) is located medial to the caudal nucleus. More rostrally, the **lateral vestibular nucleus** (*nucleus vestibularis lateralis*) is positioned dorsal to the caudal nucleus, and, further rostrally, the **rostral vestibular nucleus** (*nucleus vestibularis rostralis*) can be found. Both the lateral and the rostral nuclei are shifted dorsally, among axons of merged cerebellar peduncles (Fig. 18.11).

The vestibular nuclei receive axons from the vestibular nerve, cerebellum, and spinal cord. The nuclei project to the cerebellum (via the caudal cerebellar peduncle), to motor nuclei of extrinsic eye muscles for vestibuloocular reflexes (via the medial longitudinal fasciculus), and to the spinal cord for vestibular reflexes concerned with the position of the head and body (via, respectively, ventral and lateral vestibulospinal tracts).

A preposital nucleus (*nucleus prepositus n. hypoglossi*) is located medial to the medial vestibular nucleus. It extends from the nucleus intercalatus to the level of the genu of the facial nerve. The nucleus is functionally involved in eye movement (Berman, 1968).

Rostral End of the Medulla Oblongata

Features of the rostral medulla oblongata include the trapezoid body and attachments of cranial nerves VI, VII, and VIII (Fig. 18.12). The **vestibulocochlear nerve** (CN VIII) is a combined nerve, composed of special proprioceptive axons that innervate the vestibular membranous labyrinth (vestibular nerve) and the special somatic afferent axons that innervate the cochlea duct (cochlear nerve). The vestibular membranous labyrinth responds to linear and angular acceleration of the head, and the vestibular nerve conveys that information to the vestibular nuclei and the cerebellum.

The cochlea duct is the sense organ for hearing. Cochlear nerve axons synapse in both **ventral** and **dorsal cochlear nuclei**. The two nuclei merge into a single mass at the lateral margin of the medulla oblongata, but the dorsal nucleus forms a superficial prominence, the **acoustic tubercle** (*tuberculum acousticum*). Axons from the dorsal cochlear nucleus (and possibly vestibular nerve axons) form a transverse band, the **acoustic stria** (*stria acustica*), on the dorsal surface of the caudal cerebellar peduncle. Axons from the ventral cochlear nucleus form the **trapezoid body** (*corpus trapezoideum*), a large band of transverse fibers at the ventral surface of the rostral medulla oblongata.

Axons from cochlear nuclei project to both sides of the brain; however, the majority of them decussate. Many of the axons terminate in two nuclei that also project to both sides of the brain. The **dorsal nucleus of the trapezoid body** (*nucleus dorsalis corporis trapezoidei*) is prominent immediately dorsal to the trapezoid body. It has a twisted, encapsulated appearance (Fig. 18.12). The nucleus is important in sound localization and it triggers reflex contraction of middle ear muscles. The dorsal nucleus also gives rise to efferent axons that run in the vestibulocochlear nerve to inhibit receptor cells of the cochlear duct. **Ventral nuclei of the trapezoid body** (*nuclei ventrales corporis trapezoidei*) are neuronal cell bodies scattered among the axons of the trapezoid body.

Axons from nuclei of the trapezoid body and from cochlear nuclei project rostrally in the **lateral lemniscus** (*lemniscus lateralis*), toward the caudal colliculus. Some axons of the lemniscus synapse in **nuclei of the lateral lemniscus** (*nucleus menisci lateralis*), located along the lemniscus in the pons and midbrain.

766 CHAPTER 18   The Brain

The **genu of the facial nerve** can be seen in the rostral medulla oblongata (Fig. 18.12). Axons from the genu run ventrolaterally between the dorsal nucleus of the trapezoid body and the nucleus of the spinal tract of V to exit as the facial nerve root. The **motor nucleus of the abducent nerve** (*nucleus motorius n. abducentis*) is located ventral to the genu of the facial nerve. Its somatic efferent axons extend ventrally and exit just lateral to the pyramid (Fig. 18.12). The abducent nerve innervates lateral rectus and retractor bulbi muscles of the eye.

The Pons

The pons (ventral metencephalon) consists of a dorsal part, designated *tegmentum*, and a ventral part that features **transverse pontine fibers** (*fibrae pontis transversae*) (Fig. 18.13). The pontine fibers run along the ventral surface of the pons and form the contralateral **middle cerebellar peduncle** (*pedunculus cerebellaris medius*). The pontine axons arise from contralateral **pontine nuclei** (*nuclei pontis*), gray matter immediately deep to the transverse fibers surrounding longitudinal axons of the ventral pons. The longitudinal axons belong to the **corticopontine tract** (*tractus corticopontinus*) and the **pyramidal tract** (*tractus pyramidalis*). The corticopontine axons and collateral branches of pyramidal axons synapse on neurons of the pontine nuclei.

The **pontine tegmentum** (*tegmentum pontis*) resembles medulla oblongata, including presence of a fourth ventricle. The roof of the fourth ventricle is formed by rostral medullary velum. The walls and floor of the ventricle are lined by a layer of gray matter (Fig. 18.14). This periventricular gray matter contains neuromodulatory cholinergic neurons (tegmental laterodorsal nucleus). **Parabrachial nuclei**, associated with the rostral cerebellar peduncle, are important visceral relay nuclei (Fig. 18.13). The **locus ceruleus** (*nucleus ceruleus*) is a collection of neuromodulatory adrenergic neurons located at the medial border of the rostral cerebellar peduncle (Fig. 18.14). Axons from locus ceruleus are distributed widely within the brain and go to the spinal cord; they release norepinephrine.

The **trigeminal nerve** (CN V) joins the pons (Fig. 18.13). From neuronal cell bodies located in the trigeminal ganglion, central axons of nociceptive and thermoreceptive neurons turn caudally as they enter the pons along the

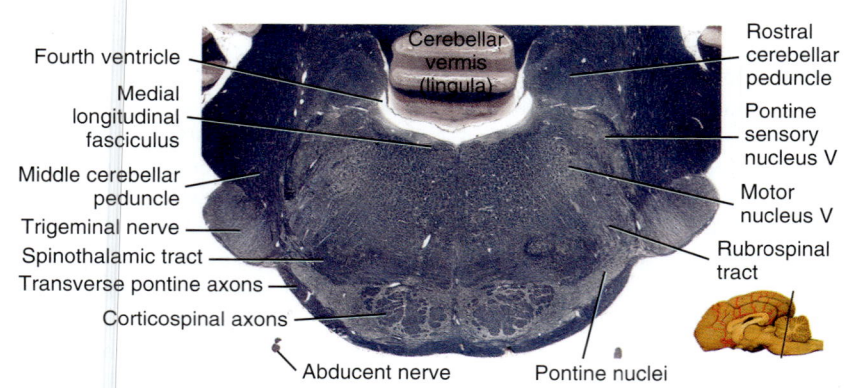

• **Fig. 18.13** Transverse section through the caudal region of the pons. Notice that trigeminal nerve axons join the pons and run toward the pontine sensory nucleus and motor nucleus of the trigeminal nerve. The ventral pons is structurally distinct compared with the pontine tegmentum, which occupies the dorsal two-thirds of the section. (Luxol Fast Blue–Cresyl Violet stain.)

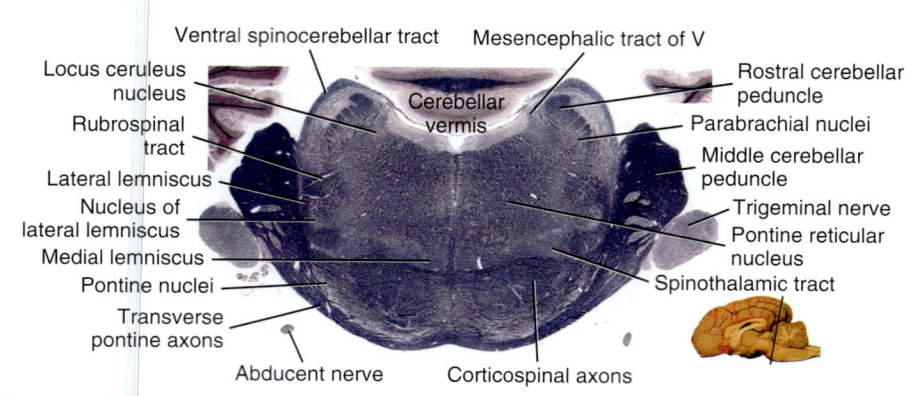

• **Fig. 18.14** Transverse section through the rostral half of the pons. Axons of the rostral cerebellar peduncle are evident dorsally and profiles of the middle cerebellar peduncle and trigeminal nerve are evident bilaterally. Notice that trigeminal nerve axons join the pons and run toward the pontine sensory nucleus and motor nucleus of the trigeminal nerve. The ventral pons is structurally distinct compared with the pontine tegmentum where reticular formation is prominent. (Luxol Fast Blue–Cresyl Violet stain.)

caudal surface of the middle cerebellar peduncle. The axons form the **spinal tract of the trigeminal nerve** (*tractus spinalis n. trigemini*) and synapse in gray matter medial to the tract, in the **nucleus of the spinal tract of V** (*nucleus tractus spinalis n. trigemini*). This tract and nucleus extend caudally the full length of the medulla. Axons from the nucleus go to motor nuclei of cranial nerves for reflex activity, or they decussate and proceed as a trigeminothalamic tract to the thalamus.

Primary afferent axons that convey discriminative touch terminate in the **pontine sensory nucleus of the trigeminal nerve** (*nucleus sensibilis pontinus n. trigemini*). Axons from the nucleus decussate and project rostrally, medial to the medial lemniscus, as the trigeminal lemniscus. For kinesthesia, unipolar cell bodies of proprioceptive primary afferent neurons are located within the midbrain instead of in the trigeminal ganglion (an exception to the rule that primary afferent neuronal cell bodies are found in ganglia in the peripheral nervous system). The unipolar cell bodies form the **nucleus of the mesencephalic tract of V** (*nucleus tractus mesencephalici n. trigemini*). The **mesencephalic tract of V** (*tractus mesencephalicus n. trigemini*) consists of axons traveling between the trigeminal nerve and the nucleus.

The **motor nucleus of the trigeminal nerve** (*nucleus motorius n. trigemini*) contains somatic efferent neurons that innervate chiefly muscles of mastication. It is situated medial to the pontine sensory nucleus, axons of the mesencephalic tract of V pass between the two nuclei (Fig. 18.13). Axons from the motor nucleus form a motor root that joins the mandibular nerve from the trigeminal nerve.

Neuromodulation Overview

Neuromodulation refers to the relatively prolonged influence of acetylcholine, norepinephrine, dopamine, or serotonin on neuronal circuits. Whether the neuromodulation is excitatory or inhibitory depends on the distribution of receptor types on target neurons. The receptors are metabotropic and release second messengers. Most neuromodulation nuclei are found in the midbrain and pons. The nuclei are small but axons from the nuclei are highly branched and widely distributed to broad regions of brain and spinal cord (Fig. 18.15).

For example, the *locus ceruleus* of the pons distributes axons broadly within the brain and spinal cord and releases norepinephrine. In the spinal cord, norepinephrine enhances motor neuron excitability and suppresses spinothalamic synaptic transmission. Locus ceruleus neurons cease firing during rapid eye movement (REM) sleep and during canine narcoleptic episodes, both associated with absence of muscle tone. In the brain, norepinephrine affects mood and enhances arousal. The locus ceruleus receives input from prefrontal cortex, hypothalamus, and raphe nuclei.

The dopamine released by the *substantia nigra pars compacta* of the midbrain impacts basal nuclei circuits that control movement. Dopamine can increase or decrease

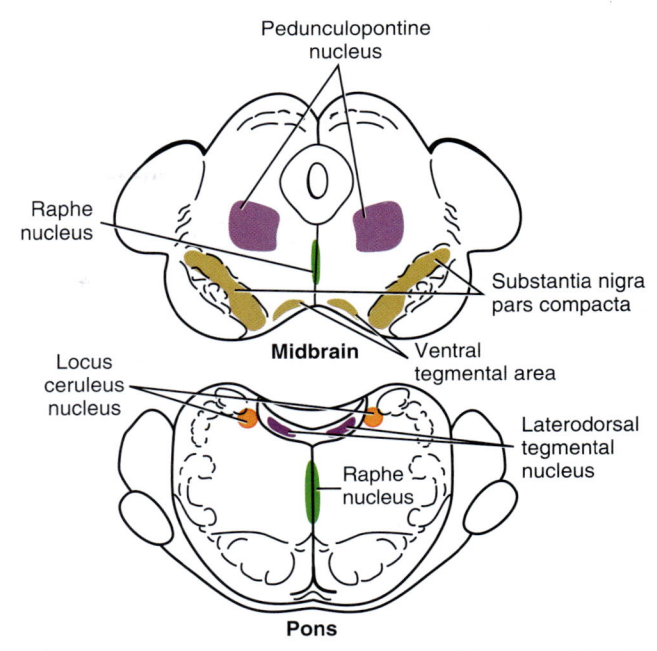

• **Fig. 18.15** Schematic drawing of neuromodulatory nuclei, color coded by the type of neurotransmitter released by neurons composing the nuclei: acetylcholine (*purple*), dopamine (*brown*), serotonin (*green*), and norepinephrine (*orange*). Although their axons are widely distributed to the brain and spinal cord, neuromodulatory nuclei are relatively small and concentrated in the midbrain and pons.

excitability depending on which dopamine receptor is present on the target neuron. The dopamine that is released by neurons of the midbrain *ventral tegmental area* affects brain circuits active during reward conditions.

The serotonin released by *raphe nuclei* generally has an inhibitory effect. It blocks synaptic transmission in nociceptive pathways and it impacts mood (most antidepressive drugs target brain serotonin receptors). The acetylcholine released by midbrain

neurons of the *pedunculopontine nucleus* and *laterodorsal tegmental nucleus* is widely distributed to the thalamus and affects motivation and alertness, including sleep and wakeful status. The *basal nucleus* of the rhinencephalon distributes acetylcholine broadly to alert the cerebral cortex.

The Midbrain

The midbrain (mesencephalon) contains the **mesencephalic aqueduct** (*aqueductus mesencephali*), which links the fourth ventricle of the hindbrain with third ventricle of the diencephalon. PAG surrounds the aqueduct (Fig. 18.16). The tectum (roof) of the midbrain is formed by paired rostral and caudal colliculi. The midbrain region located ventral to the tectum and aqueduct, is composed of paired cerebral peduncles. From dorsal to ventral, each peduncle has three regions: tegmentum, substantia nigra, and crus cerebri. Trochlear and oculomotor cranial nerves emerge from the midbrain.

Periaqueductal gray (PAG) (*substantia grisea centralis*), which surrounds the aqueduct, has a high concentration of

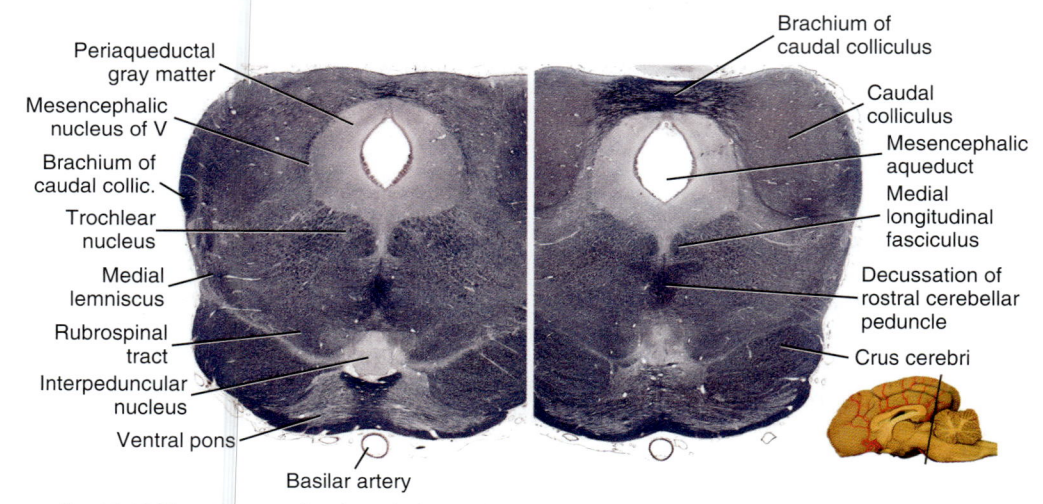

• **Fig. 18.16** Transverse section through the caudal midbrain at two levels: The trochlear nucleus is present on the left. More caudally, on the right, the caudal colliculus is obvious. Mesencephalic aqueduct surrounded by periaqueductal gray matter is a characteristic feature of the midbrain. Overlapping pons is evident ventrally. (Luxol Fast Blue–Cresyl Violet stain.)

opiate receptors. The PAG gives rise to an endogenous analgesia system that enables the brain to suppress nociception. The analgesia is produced by norepinephrine and serotonin release, which blocks synaptic activation of projection neurons by primary afferent neurons. PAG axons go to the spinal cord and to two neuromodulatory nuclei that also project to the spinal cord: locus ceruleus (norepinephrine) and raphe nuclei (serotonin) (Beitz, 1992).

PAG neurons play a role relaying visceral information to and from the forebrain. The **dorsal longitudinal fasciculus** (*fasciculus longitudinalis dorsalis*) courses within the ventral PAG and conveys axons from the hypothalamus to parasympathetic nuclei of cranial nerves. Also, the **dorsal tegmental nucleus** (*nucleus tegmenti dorsalis*) is located within the PAG. It has limbic connections (mamillary, habenular, accumbens, and septum) involving the PAG in affective behavior.

At the lateral margin of the PAG, the **mesencephalic tract of the trigeminal nerve** leads to the **mesencephalic nucleus of the trigeminal nerve**. The nucleus consists of aligned unipolar cell bodies belonging to proprioceptive primary afferent neurons. Further laterally, ventrally directed tectospinal and tectonuclear axons and dorsally directed trochlear nerve axons are evident (Fig. 18.16).

The **tectum** of the midbrain (*tectum mesencephali*) features paired caudal and rostral colliculi and their respective commissures (Fig. 18.17). The commissural axons are inhibitory. Caudal and rostral colliculi reflexly orient the eyes, ears, and head toward the source of a novel auditory and visual stimulus, respectively. A **pretectal region** rostral to the rostral colliculus controls the pupillary light reflex.

The **caudal colliculus** (*colliculus caudalis*) is gray matter situated caudally in the tectum (Fig. 18.16). It receives axons from the **lateral lemniscus** (*lemniscus lateralis*), **commissure of the caudal colliculi** (*commissural colliculorun caudalium*), medial geniculate body, auditory area of the cerebral cortex, and the cerebellum. Axons from the caudal colliculus project to the **medial geniculate body** via the **brachium of the caudal colliculus** (*brachium colliculi caudalis*), located on the lateral surface of the midbrain (Fig. 18.16). Also the caudal colliculus sends axons to **nuclei of the lateral lemniscus** and to the cerebellum. For reflex orientation toward the source of a sound, axons from the caudal colliculus go to the rostral colliculus, where tectospinal and tectonuclear pathways originate.

The **rostral colliculus** (*colliculus rostralis*) has neurons arranged in superficial, intermediate and deep layers (Fig. 18.18). The superficial neurons are organized retinotopically, receiving axons from both the optic tract and visual cortex via the **brachium of the rostral colliculus** (*brachium colliculi rostralis*). The deep neurons, which receive auditory and spinal cord axons (spinomesencephalic tract) are somatotopically organized. The intermediate layer gives rise to the tectonuclear and tectospinal axons that leave the colliculus for orientation reflexes and saccadic eye movements. The rostral colliculus controls eye position by directing horizontal and vertical gaze centers located in reticular formation of the pons and midbrain, respectively.

Tectonuclear tract (*tractus tectonucleares*) axons go to the facial nucleus for ear movements and join the **medial longitudinal fasciculus** (*fasciculus longitudinalis medialis*) for eye movements. Tectospinal fibers (for head movement) join the **medial tectospinal tract** and **lateral tectotegmentospinal tract**.

The **pretectal region** (including pretectal nuclei and nucleus of the optic tract) is located rostral to the rostral colliculus and lateral to the caudal commissure at the mesencephalon-diencephalon junction (Fig. 18.19). The region is involved in reflex regulation of pupil size in response to light. Optic tract axons arrive via the brachium of the rostral colliculus. The parasympathetic oculomotor nucleus constricts pupil size during the pupillary light

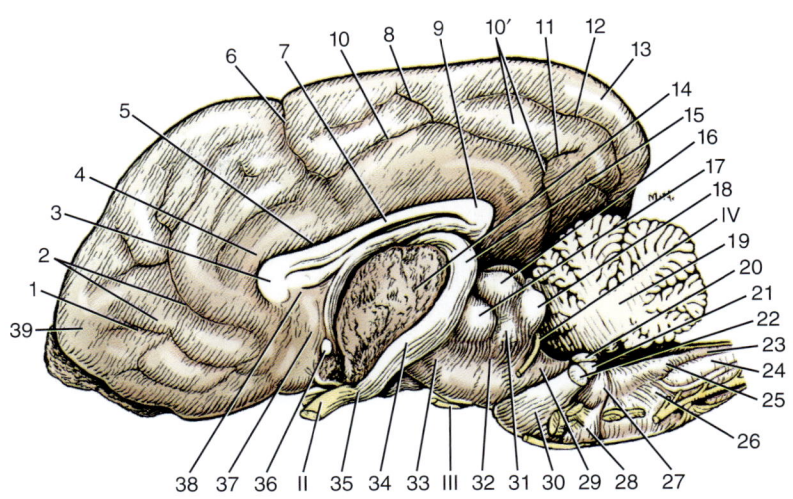

1. Ectogenual sulcus
2. Genual gyrus and sulcus
3. Genu of corpus callosum
4. Cingulate gyrus
5. Callosal sulcus
6. Cruciate sulcus
7. Body of corpus callosum
8. Ramus of splenial sulcus
9. Splenium of corpus callosum
10. Splenial sulcus
10′. Splenial gyrus and sulcus
11. Caudal horizontal ramus of splenial sulcus
12. Suprasplenial sulcus
13. Occipital gyrus
14. Cut surface of internal capsule
15. Optic tract and Lateral geniculate body
16. Rostral colliculus
17. Medial geniculate body
18. Caudal colliculus
19. Cerebellum
20. Rostral cerebellar peduncle
21. Caudal cerebellar peduncle
22. Middle cerebellar peduncle
23. Fasciculus cuneatus
24. Spinal tract of trigeminal nerve
25. Nucleus cuneatus lateralis
26. Superficial arcuate fibers
27. Cochlear nuclei
28. Trapezoid body
29. Lateral lemniscus
30. Transverse fibers of pons
31. Brachium of caudal colliculus
32. Transverse crural tract
33. Crus cerebri
34. Left optic tract
35. Optic chiasm
36. Rostral commissure
37. Septum (paraterminal gyrus)
38. Septum pellucidum
39. Frontal gyrus
II. Optic nerve
III. Oculomotor nerve
IV. Trochlear nerve

• **Fig. 18.17** Lateral view of the brain with the left cerebral hemisphere and the left half of the cerebellum removed from the intact brainstem. Rostral *(16)* and caudal *(18)* colliculi are shown.

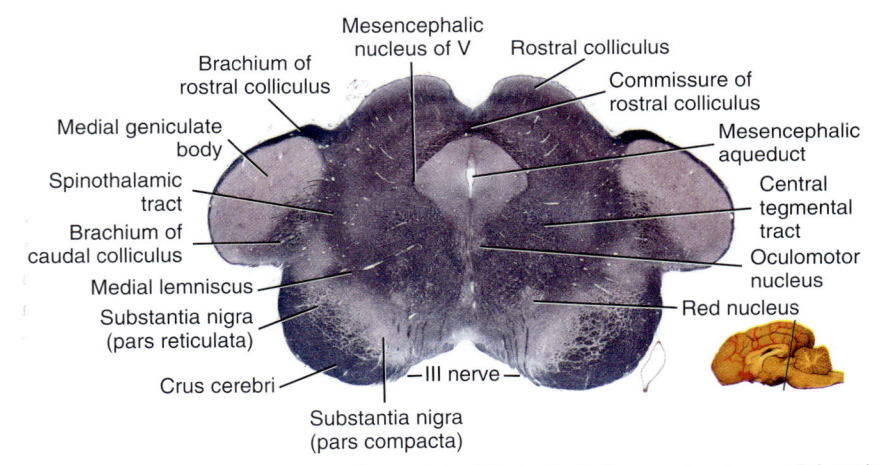

• **Fig. 18.18** Transverse section through the rostral midbrain, including overlapping medial geniculate bodies from the diencephalon. The mesencephalic aqueduct is surrounded by periaqueductal gray matter. Axons from the oculomotor nucleus exit ventrally, medial to the crus cerebri (III nerve). (Luxol Fast Blue–Cresyl Violet stain.)

reflex. Pupillary dilation that is emotionally driven involves the lateral tectotegmentospinal tract that travels to preganglionic sympathetic neurons in the spinal cord.

The **caudal commissure** (*commissura caudalis*) conveys decussating axons between pretectal regions, including the prestitial nucleus (nucleus of the caudal commissure), which also receives optic tract axons. Most decussating axons are concerned with the pupillary light reflex, although some axons in the commissure connect midbrain tegmental nuclei.

Below the tectum, each **cerebral peduncle** (*pedunculus cerebri*) consists of **tegmentum**, **substantia nigra**, and **crus cerebri**. **Crus cerebri** refers to the white matter along the ventral surface of the midbrain (Fig. 18.18). It consists of corticospinal, corticopontine, corticonuclear, and corticoreticular axons that arise from neuronal cell bodies in the cerebral cortex. The axons travel through the internal capsule to reach the crus cerebri. Some axons leave the crus cerebri to terminate in the midbrain and pons. Other axons

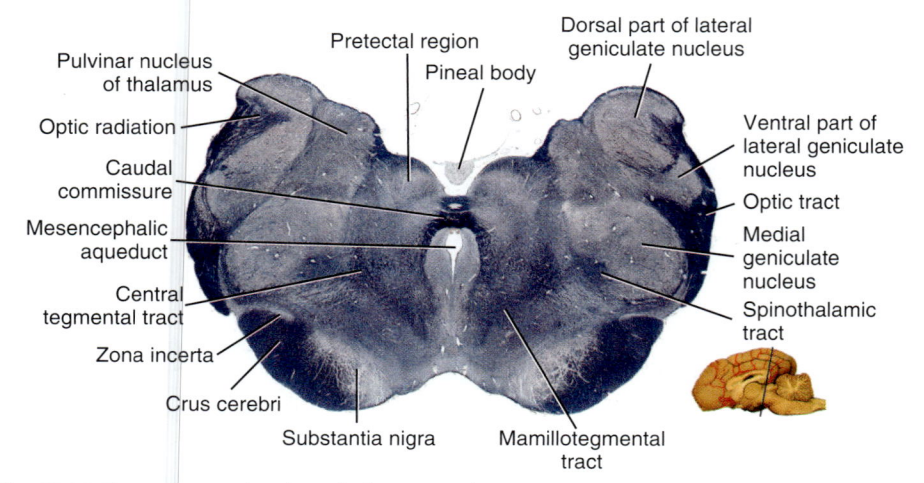

• **Fig. 18.19** Transverse section through the pretectal region at the midbrain-diencephalon junction. The mesencephalic aqueduct is transitioning to third ventricle and subcommissural bodies are evident dorsally in the aqueduct. Midbrain structures are present ventrally. Dorsally the pretectum, thalamus, and metathalamus can be seen. (Luxol Fast Blue–Cresyl Violet stain.)

proceed through the ventral pons and continue within pyramids of the medulla oblongata.

The **fossa interpeduncularis** is the area between bilateral crura on the ventral surface of the midbrain. The **substantia perforata caudalis** refers to the area where vessels enter the fossa. The **sulcus medialis cruris cerebri** runs along the medial margin of each crus. The **transverse crural tract** (*tractus cruralis transversus*), also called **basal optic tract**, refers to the small band of axons from the brachium of the rostral colliculus that cross the surface of the crus cerebri rostral to the oculomotor nerve (Fig. 18.17). The axons terminate in a nucleus located medial to substantia nigra; axons from the nucleus proceed to the oculomotor nucleus and tectum (Berman, 1968).

The gray matter immediately dorsal to the crus cerebri is **substantia nigra**. It has compact and reticulated parts that are functionally quite different (Fig. 18.18). The *pars compacta*, the larger more dorsal component, receives axons from the cerebral cortex, basal nuclei, and thalamus. It projects axons to basal nuclei of the striatum (accumbens, caudate, putamen). The **compact substantia nigra** and the adjacent *ventral tegmental area* contain dopaminergic neurons that neuromodulate basal nuclei circuits by targeting excitatory and inhibitory dopamine receptors. The net effect is movement facilitation. (In humans, Parkinson's disease results from the loss of dopamine neurons in the substantia nigra.)

The **pars reticulata** of the substantia nigra contains spontaneously active, inhibitory, GABAergic neurons that, along with the endopeducular neurons, serve as output for basal nuclei circuits. Pars reticulata axons project to the thalamus, tectum, and red nucleus. In particular, they provide basal nuclei control of saccade eye movements.

The **interpeduncular nucleus** (*nucleus interpeduncularis*) is evident as a round profile located ventrally in the interpeduncular fossa (Fig. 18.16). The nucleus receives input from limbic structures via the medial nucleus of the **habenula** and the **fasciculus retroflexus**. The interpeduncular nucleus projects to midbrain raphe nuclei that release serotonin in connection with forebrain neuromodulation that affects mood.

The **midbrain tegmentum** (*tegmentum mesencephali*) contains the red nucleus and nuclei associated with the reticular formation, cranial nerves, neuromodulation, and the mesencephalic locomotor region. The **mesencephalic reticular formation** receives axonal input from spinoreticular and spinothalamic tracts and gives rise to the ascending axons responsible for maintaining awake status in the ipsilateral cerebral cortex (reticular alerting system). The axons run in the **central tegmental tract** to intralaminar thalamic neurons.

The **pedunculopontine nucleus**, located caudally in the midbrain tegmentum, contains cholinergic neuromodulatory neurons that contribute to forebrain arousal, including electroencephalographic arousal during REM sleep. The nucleus contains other neurons that, along with the adjacent **cuneiform nucleus**, constitute a mesencephalic locomotor region. Stimulation of these neurons evokes stepping locomotor patterns.

The **central tegmental tract** (*tractus tegmenti centralis*) runs through the core of the brainstem (Fig. 18.18). It conveys information rostrally from the reticular formation to the thalamus and subthalamus. It conveys information caudally from the caudal diencephalon and midbrain to the olivary nucleus. The caudally directed axons in the tract arise collectively from zona incerta, parasympathetic oculomotor nucleus, PAG, midbrain reticular formation, and red nucleus.

The **motor nucleus of the trochlear nerve** (*nucleus motorius n. trochlearis*) consists of somatic efferent neurons positioned adjacent to the midline immediately ventral to PAG in the caudal midbrain (Fig. 18.16). Axons from the nucleus course laterally, dorsally, and caudally along the margin of the PAG. They enter the dorsal pons, decussate in the rostral medullary velum, exit dorsal to the rostral cerebellar peduncle, and pass rostroventrally along the side of the mesencephalon. The trochlear neurons innervate only the contralateral dorsal oblique muscle of the eye.

The **motor nucleus of the oculomotor nerve** (*nucleus motorius n. oculomotorii*) is situated rostral to the trochlear nucleus (Fig. 18.18). It consists of somatic efferent neurons that innervate extrinsic muscles of the eye (dorsal rectus, medial rectus, ventral rectus, ventral oblique, and retractor bulbi) and the m. levator palpebrae superioris. Visceral efferent neurons, located dorsomedial to the somatic neurons, constitute the **parasympathetic nucleus of the oculomotor nerve** (*nuclei parasympathici n. oculomotorii*). These preganglionic neurons send axons to the ciliary ganglion, the sources of postganglionic axons to the ciliary body (for lens accommodation) and iris (for pupil constriction). Axons from both somatic and visceral oculomotor nuclei join; they course ventrally and exit medial to the crus cerebri as oculomotor nerve roots.

Certain tegmental nuclei (*nuclei tegmenti*) are referred to as *accessory oculomotor nuclei* because of their proximity and functional relationship to the oculomotor nucleus. These include the interstitial, prestitial, and precommissural nuclei.

The **red nucleus** (*nucleus ruber*) reputedly has a rostral, small-cell region (*pars parvicellularis*) and a caudal, large-cell region (*pars magnocellularis*). In carnivores, the nucleus has small, medium, and large cell regions that overlap, rostral to caudal. The ipsilateral motor cortex projects axons to the red nucleus to drive voluntary movement (Fig. 18.20). Basal nuclei influence the red nucleus via axons from the substantia nigra reticulata.

The population of small neurons located rostrally in the red nucleus receives input from the contralateral lateral nucleus of the cerebellum and from the somatosensory neocortex (Pong et al., 2002). The neurons project ipsilaterally to the ventrolateral thalamic nucleus and to the olivary nucleus via the central tegmental tract (Onodera & Hicks, 2009).

The population of medium cells in the red nucleus also receive axonal input from the contralateral lateral nucleus (formerly the *dentate nucleus*) of the cerebellum (Pong et al., 2008). Axons from these medium projection neurons join the rubrospinal tract and terminate in the cervical spinal cord, for head movement (Fig. 18.20). Also, as rubronuclear tract axons, they innervate cranial nerve nuclei to elicit facial movements (Pong et al., 2002).

The caudal, large-cell region of the red nucleus is somatotopically organized. It receives afferent axons from the contralateral interpositus nucleus of the cerebellum and the ipsilateral motor cortex, including collateral branches of corticospinal axons. Corticorubral projections from the forelimb cortical area are twice as numerous as those from hindlimb area (Ipekchyan, 2008). Axons of the large projections neurons of the red nucleus move limb joints via the rubrospinal tract. Collateral branches of rubrospinal axons synapse in the **lateral reticular nucleus** (*nucleus reticularis lateralis*), which projects to the cerebellum. Also, rubrospinal neurons send reciprocal axons to the interpositus nucleus.

The **rubrospinal tract** (*tractus rubrospinalis*) is the main tract for voluntary movement in the dog (Brooks, 1986). Rubrospinal axons decussate immediately and proceed through the contralateral brainstem and spinal cord, within the dorsal half of the lateral funiculus. The axons terminate at all segments of the spinal cord. Via interneurons, the axons excite flexor and inhibit extensor motor units to the limbs (Massion, 1967). Damage to the red nucleus produces moderate extensor hypertonia in an intact dog.

The Diencephalon

The diencephalon forms the rostral extent of the brainstem. It is connected bilaterally to each cerebral hemisphere by a mass of corticopedal and corticofugal projection axons

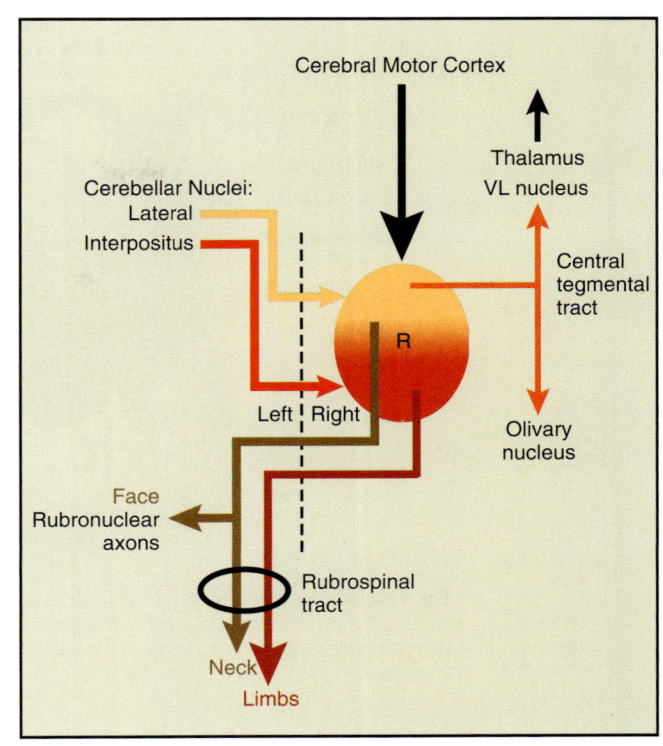

• **Fig. 18.20** Schematic illustration of a right-side red nucleus (*R*), including major projections and input connections. The canine red nucleus exhibits a gradient of cell sizes, ranging from large neurons (magnocellular region) concentrated caudally (*red region*) to small neurons (parvicellular region) concentrated rostrally (*yellow region*). Rubrospinal tract axons that arise from the large projection neurons (*red*) decussate and terminate on interneurons associated with limb motor units. Rubrospinal axons from medium projection neurons (*brown*) decussate and terminate in the cervical spinal cord or in cranial nerve nuclei (*rubronuclear axons*). Small neurons located rostrally in the red nucleus send axons ipsilaterally to the ventrolateral nucleus of the thalamus and the olivary nucleus via the central tegmental tract (*orange*). All projection neurons are driven by the ipsilateral motor cortex. The cerebellar interpositus nucleus excites large neurons. The lateral cerebellar nucleus (formerly the *dentate nucleus*) excites small and medium size neurons. The dashed line indicates the midline.

772 CHAPTER 18 **The Brain**

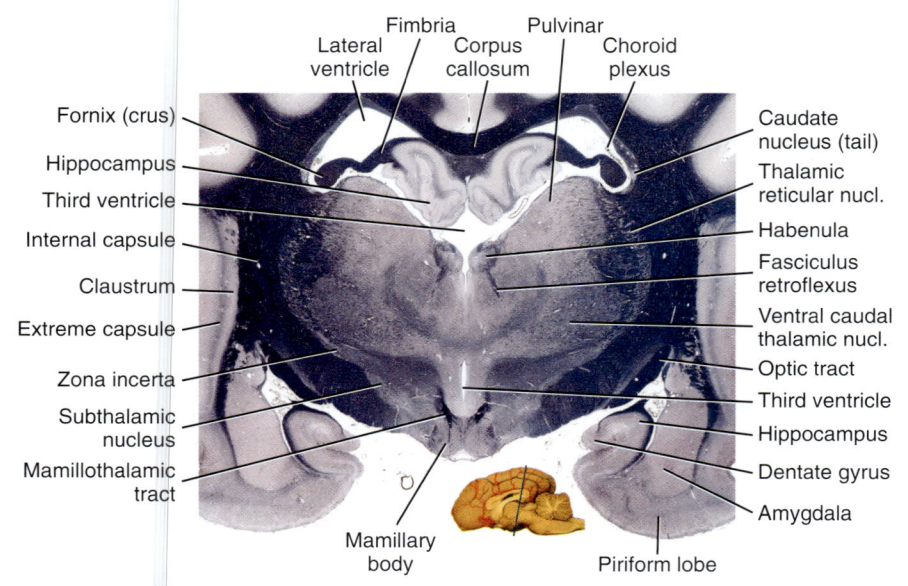

• **Fig. 18.21** Transverse section through the caudal diencephalon, including surrounding telencephalon. The third ventricle surrounds the interthalamic adhesion (*not labeled*) centrally. Within the diencephalon, habenula nuclei are evident dorsally and mamillary nuclei are present ventrally. (Luxol Fast Blue–Cresyl Violet stain.)

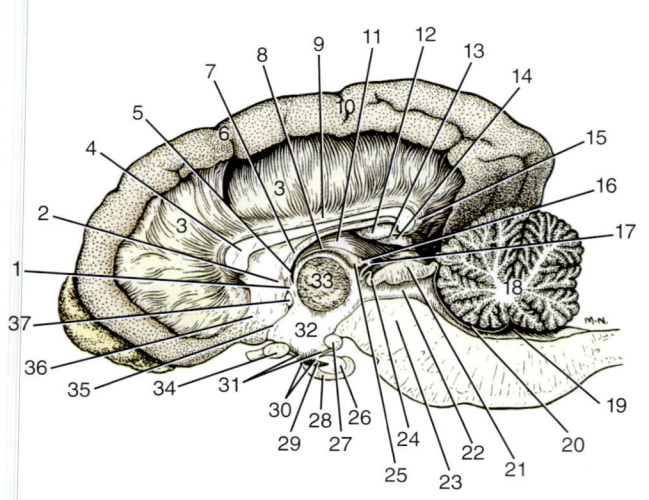

1. Fornix column
2. Precommissural fornix
3. Radiation of corpus callosum
4. Genu of corpus callosum
5. Interventricular foramen
6. Cruciate sulcus
7. Fornix
8. Stria habenularis thalami
9. Indusium griseum
10. Cerebral Cortex
11. Dorsal aspect of thalamus
12. Tubercle of dentate gyrus
13. Subsplenial flexure of dentate gyrus
14. Callosal gyrus
15. Gyrus fasciolaris
16. Habenular commissure
17. Pineal body
18. Arbor vitae of cerebellum
19. Fourth ventricle
20. Rostral medullary velum
21. Tectum of mesencephalon
22. Mesencephalic aqueduct
23. Tegmentum of mesencephalon
24. Caudal commissure
25. Habenular nucleus
26. Neurohypophysis
27. Mamillary body
28. Adenohypophys
29. Infundibular recess of third ventricle.
30. Infundibulum
31. Tuber cinereum
32. Third ventricle
33. Interthalamic adhesion
34. Optic chiasm
35. Lamina terminalis
36. Paraterminal gyrus
37. Rostral commissure

• **Fig. 18.22** A median view of the right half of a brain with cingulate and genual gyri removed to show underlying white matter *(3)*. The mesencephalic aqueduct of the midbrain connects the third *(32)* and fourth *(19)* ventricles.

collectively termed the **internal capsule** (*capsula interna*) (Fig. 18.21). The diencephalon can be divided into five regions: thalamus, metathalamus, hypothalamus, epithalamus, and subthalamus.

The **third ventricle** (*ventriculus tertius*) is a narrow chamber separating right and left halves of the diencephalon, except where the **interthalamic adhesion** (*adhesio interthalamica*) occupies the center of the ventricle (Fig. 18.22). The interthalamic adhesion contains thalamic nuclei but not commissural axons. The third ventricle communicates caudally with the mesencephalic aqueduct. Bilaterally a dorsolateral **interventricular foramen** (*foramen interventriculare*) allows the third ventricle to communicate with the lateral ventricle on each side.

The rostral wall of the third ventricle is formed by **lamina terminalis** (*lamina terminalis grisea*). Combined ependyma and pia mater, constituting **tela choroidea** (*tela choroidea ventriculi tertii*), forms the roof of the third ventricle and gives rise to paired choroid plexuses. Each plexus in the third ventricle continues as the choroid plexus of a lateral ventricle. The lateral attachment of the thin ventricular roof along the thalamus, is referred to as *tenia thalami*. Ventrally the third ventricle exhibits an **optic recess** (*recessus opticus*) between the optic chiasm and the lamina terminalis, a **neurohypophyseal** (**infundibular**) **recess** (*recessus neurohypophysis*) located within the infundibulum of the neurohypophysis, and an **inframammillary recess** (*recesses inframammillaris*) rostroventral to the mamillary bodies.

The third ventricle contains several **circumventricular organs**, areas where the blood supply is enriched, the blood–brain barrier is reduced (fenestrated capillaries), and ependymal cells assume glandular or baroreceptor and chemoreceptor roles. The **subcommissural organ** (*organum subcommissurale*) refers to thickened secretory ependyma located ventral to the caudal commissure (Fig. 18.19). The **subfornical organ** (*organum subfornicale*) is located ventral to the fornix, where the fornix forms columns at the rostral aspect of the third ventricle (Akert et al., 1961); it controls salt intake behavior (Hiyama et al., 2004). Other secretory and sensory cells are found in the lamina terminalis (*organum vasculosum laminae terminalis griseae*) and in the ventricular wall of the hypothalamus (*organum vasculosum hypothalami*). (An additional circumventricular organ [*area postrema*] is located at the caudal end of the fourth ventricle.)

The Thalamus

The thalamus is closely linked to the cerebral cortex, via reciprocal connections. Thalamic projections to the cerebral cortex provide background cortical excitation to maintain wakefulness, convey cranial projecting tract information concerning sensory modalities (except olfaction), and deliver input affecting emotional and affective behavior. Thalamocortical circuits are essential for movement. The circuits involve cerebellar and basal nuclear input to thalamic nuclei that, in turn, project to motor cortices.

Typically, individual thalamic nuclei contain excitatory projection neurons and inhibitory interneurons. In the canine thalamus, eighteen nuclei have been histologically distinguished and arranged into several defined groups (Salazar et al., 1989) (Fig. 18.23).

An **external medullary lamina** (*lamina medullaris thalami externa*) separates the **reticulate thalamic nucleus** (*nucleus reticulatus thalami*) from the other thalamic nuclei (Fig. 18.21). The reticulate nucleus is unusual. Its projection neurons are inhibitory and they target other thalamic nuclei rather than cerebral cortex. Input to the reticulate nucleus comes from collateral branches of thalamic axons projecting to the cerebral cortex, also from collateral branches of reciprocal axons originating in the cerebral cortex (layer VI).

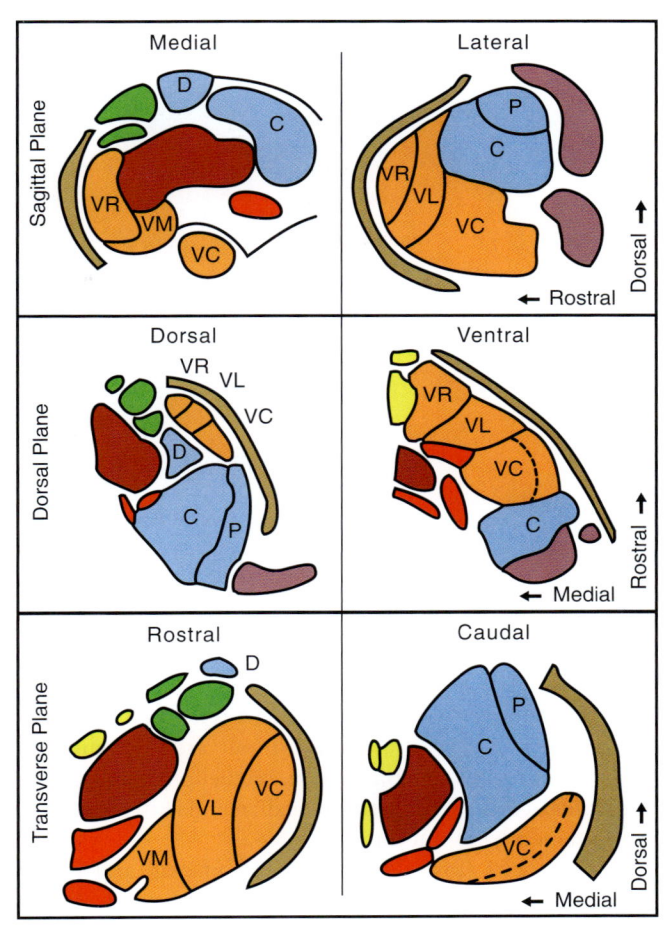

• **Fig. 18.23** Illustration showing profiles of right-side thalamic nuclei in transverse, dorsal, and sagittal planes of view. Per plane, nuclei are drawn at two levels and directions are shown by arrows. Nuclear groups are color-coded: *maroon*, dorsomedial nucleus; *green*, rostral nuclear group; *orange*, ventral group of lateral nuclei; *blue*, dorsocaudal group of lateral nuclei; *red*, intralaminar nuclei; *yellow*, midline nuclei (in contact with the interthalamic adhesion); *brown*, reticular thalamic nucleus; and *purple*, geniculate nuclei (metathalamus). The following abbreviations are used to identify nuclei of the lateral group: *C*, caudal; *D*, dorsal; *P*, pulvinar; *VC*, ventral caudal; *VL*, ventral lateral; *VM*, ventral medial; *VR*, ventral rostral. *Dotted lines* separate medial and lateral parts of the ventral caudal nucleus. Nuclear profiles were copied from Salazar I, et al: The thalamus of the dog: a tridimensional and cytoarchitectonic study, *Anat Anz* 169:101–113, 1989.

The collateral branches excite reticulate neurons that, in turn, inhibit projection neurons within the source thalamic nuclei (Willis, 1985).

An **internal medullary lamina** (*lamina medullaris thalami interna*) divides thalamic nuclei into rostral, lateral, and medial nuclear groups (Berman & Jones, 1982; Salazar et al., 1989). Additionally, the lamina contains **intralaminar thalamic nuclei** (*nuclei intralaminares thalami*) are arranged in a rostral group (central medial, paracentral, and central lateral nuclei) and a caudal group (centrum medianum and parafascicular nuclei). Intralaminar nuclei project axons broadly to superficial layers of cerebral cortex and provide background excitation that keeps the cerebral cortex awake and alert (Steriade & Llinas, 1988). The nuclei are

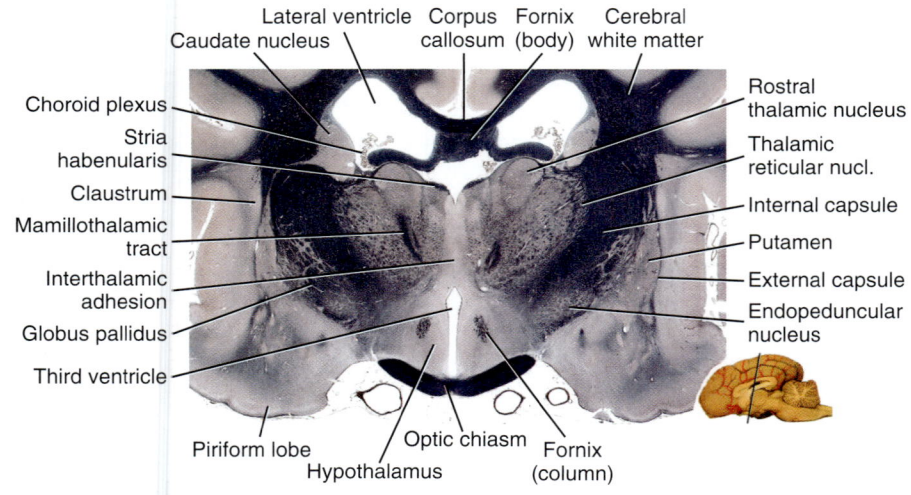

• **Fig. 18.24** Transverse section through the rostral diencephalon, including the optic chiasm. The third ventricle surrounds the interthalamic adhesion centrally. Choroid plexus profiles are evident in the roof of the third ventricle and in both lateral ventricles. Five basal nuclei of the telencephalon are labeled. (Luxol Fast Blue–Cresyl Violet stain.)

activated by axons from the midbrain reticular formation. Intralaminar nuclei also receive input from cholinergic brainstem neurons, cerebral cortex, cerebellum, basal nuclei, and spinal cord. The centrum median nucleus projects to the putamen basal nucleus.

Three nuclei (rostral dorsal, rostral medial, and rostral ventral) compose **rostral thalamic nuclei** (*nuclei rostrales thalami*) (Fig. 18.24). This nuclear group is associated with affective behavior and has reciprocal connections with the cingulate gyrus of the limbic system. Axonal input comes from the hippocampus via the fornix and from the mamillary body via the mamillothalamic tract.

The **lateral thalamic nuclei** (*nuclei laterales thalami*) may be subdivided into dorsocaudal and ventral groups. The dorsocaudal group includes **lateral dorsal nucleus** (*nucleus lateralis dorsalis*), **lateral caudal nucleus** (*nucleus lateralis caudalis*), and the **pulvinar nucleus** (*nucleus pulvinaris*). The lateral dorsal nucleus has connections similar to rostral thalamic nuclei and thus seems to have an affective behavior role. The lateral caudal and pulvinar nuclei are involved in selective visual attention. They receive input from the retina, tectum, and primary visual cortex. They project to visual association areas of the cerebral cortex (Berman & Jones, 1982).

Four nuclei constitute the ventral group of lateral thalamic nuclei. The **ventral rostral nucleus** (*nucleus ventralis rostralis*) receives inhibitory input from basal nuclei circuits (via the endopeduncular nucleus and substantia nigra reticulata). The nucleus projects axons predominantly to the supplementary motor cortex and the premotor cortex. The **ventral lateral nucleus** (*nucleus ventralis lateralis*) receives excitatory input from cerebellar nuclei and projects axons primarily to the motor cortex (Sakai et al., 1993). These two thalamic nuclei participate in voluntary movement selection and execution via circuits involving motor cortices, basal nuclei, and cerebellar nuclei (Brooks, 1986). The **ventral medial nucleus** (*nucleus ventralis medialis*), situated surrounding the mammillothalamic tract, receives axonal input from basal nuclei and the cerebellum and projects axons to superficial laminae of motor-related cortices (Kosmal, 1986; Sakai et al., 1993).

The **ventral caudal nucleus** (*nucleus ventralis caudalis*) relays information from cutaneous and proprioceptive receptors to primary and secondary somesthetic areas of the cerebral cortex. The nucleus is distinguished by the axon bundles that penetrate it. The lateral part of the nucleus (pars lateralis) receives axonal input from the body via the medial lemniscus. The medial part (pars medialis) receives axonal input from the face via the trigeminal lemniscus. Neurons at the medial edge of the nucleus receive taste information. Spinothalamic tract axons terminate within a transition region between the ventral caudal and the ventral lateral thalamic nuclei, on neurons that respond to large receptive fields, multiple modalities, and noxious stimulation (Bessen & Chaouch, 1987; Willis, 1986).

The **dorsomedial thalamic nucleus** (*nucleus dorsomedialis thalami*) receives input from the hypothalamus, amygdala, endopeduncular nucleus, and prefrontal cortex. The nucleus projects output to the prefrontal cortex, which is anatomically defined as cortex receiving projections from the dorsomedial thalamic nucleus. (The prefrontal cortex is essential for planning motivated behavior.)

Paraventricular thalamic nuclei (*nuclei paraventriculares thalami*) are midline nuclei found along the wall of the third ventricle and in the interthalamic adhesion. These nuclei (reuniens, rhomboid, parataenial, and paraventricular nuclei) are functionally diverse (Berman & Jones, 1982). They project to the hypothalamus, hippocampal formation, and nucleus accumbens. Thus they are involved in affective behavior.

The Metathalamus

The metathalamus consists of medial and lateral geniculate bodies (nuclei), which function like thalamus but are specialized for hearing and vision, respectively (Figs. 18.4 and 18.19).

The **medial geniculate body** (*corpus geniculatum mediale*) comprises the caudal extent of the diencephalon (Fig. 18.4). It is attached to the lateral surface of the midbrain and covered dorsally by brachium of the rostral colliculus. When sectioned, the geniculate body presents a round profile, designated **medial geniculate nucleus** (*nucleus geniculatus medialis*). Ventral magnocellular neurons in the nucleus project to primary auditory cortex; dorsal parvocellular neurons project to auditory association cortex. Primary and association auditory areas of the cerebral cortex are essential for pattern recognition and sound-significance interpretation. Projection axons reach the neocortex via the **acoustic radiation** (*radiatio acustica*) of the internal capsule.

The **brachium of the caudal colliculus** conveys auditory axonal input to the medial geniculate nucleus. Most of the axons in the brachium originate from the **caudal colliculus**, the **lateral lemniscus** contributes the remaining axons. Neurons are tonotopically organized within the medial geniculate nucleus (as they are in most nuclei of the auditory pathway). At the level of the medial geniculate nucleus, the intensity of different tones can be distinguished but not temporal relationships (Mountcastle, 1980). Axons from auditory cortex (layer VI axons and layer V collateral branches) reciprocally feed back to the medial geniculate nucleus.

The **lateral geniculate body** (*corpus geniculatum laterale*) is located dorsal, rostral, and slightly lateral to the medial geniculate body (Figs. 18.4 and 18.19). The **lateral geniculate nucleus** (*nucleus geniculatus lateralis*) contains excitatory (glutaminergic) projection neurons and inhibitory (GABAergic) interneurons (typical for thalamic nuclei). The nucleus receives axons from the visual cortex and the optic tract. Retinal axons from large ganglion cells (size and direction vision) and axons from small ganglion cells (detail and color vision) synapse on separate populations of geniculate projection neurons, as does a third type of ganglion cell associated with the *tapetum lucidum* and dim vision.

The lateral geniculate nucleus has dorsal and ventral parts. The *ventral part* (*pars ventralis*) is smaller and has reciprocal connections with the rostral colliculus and pretectal region; it also projects to the suprachiasmatic nucleus of the hypothalamus.

The *dorsal part* (*pars dorsalis*) of the canine lateral geniculate nucleus has neuronal cell bodies arranged in six layers plus a medial interlaminar nucleus (Lee et al., 1999). Right and left optic nerves terminate in alternate cell layers. From superficial to deep, layers 1, 3, and 5 receive axons from the contralateral eye; remaining layers receive ipsilateral eye input. Superficial layers receive axons from both large and small ganglion cells, deeper layers from just large ganglion cells, and deepest layers receive the dim vision axons. The latter also synapse in the medial interlaminar nucleus, which exhibits four vertical layers.

The lateral geniculate nucleus has a rostrolateral "hilus" through which axons of the **optic radiation** (*radiatio optica*) reach the internal capsule and travel to and from the visual cortex. The lateral geniculate nucleus connects mainly with the primary visual cortex (the pulvinar thalamic nucleus connects heavily with visual association cortex).

The **retina** and **optic nerve** (*nervus opticus*) originate from the diencephalon during embryonic development, and, histologically, they are part of the central nervous system. Axons from ganglion cells of the retina compose the optic nerve, which begins at the optic disc of the eye (where the axons become myelinated). Approximately 75% of axons in the canine optic nerves decussate at the **optic chiasm** (de Lahunta et al., 2015). From the chiasm, axons continue as the **optic tract** (*tractus opticus*) and terminate in the *lateral geniculate nucleus* (Fig. 18.17). Some axons leave the optic tract to form the **brachium of the rostral colliculus** (*brachium colliculi rostralis*), which contributes axons to the rostral colliculus, pretectal region, and *transverse crural tract* on the lateral surface of the midbrain.

The Hypothalamus

The hypothalamus is situated ventral to the thalamus and medial to the subthalamus. It occupies the floor and the wall of the third ventricle (Figs. 18.22 and 18.25). A **sulcus hypothalamicus** along the ventricular wall delineates the dorsal boundary of the hypothalamus. The ventral surface of the diencephalon shows only hypothalamic structures: *optic chiasm* rostrally, **tuber cinereum** at the level of the hypophysis, and bilateral **mamillary bodies** caudally (Fig. 18.3).

The *tuber cinereum* is the swollen region of the ventral hypothalamic surface. It gives rise to an **infundibulum** with an attached **neural lobe** (*lobus nervosus*). Together these constitute the **neurohypophysis**. The neurohypophysis and the adenohypophysis that surrounds it compose the **hypophysis** (pituitary gland). The infundibulum itself may be subdivided into a root (*radix*) that arises from the tuber cinereum, a **pars cava** that contains the infundibular recess of the third ventricle, and a distal **pars compacta** that joins the neural lobe.

By controlling the hypophysis, the hypothalamus supervises endocrine secretion. Hypothalamic neurons of two nuclei (paraventricular and supraoptic) send axons directly into the neurohypophysis where they each release vasopressin and oxytocin hormones. Other nuclei send axons to the tuber cinereum where various releasing hormones are secreted and captured by hypothalamic capillaries. Hypothalamic-hypophyseal portal veins convey the releasing hormones to the adenohypophysis where they selectively trigger specific pituitary cells to secrete particular hormones.

The hypothalamus is involved in maintaining homeostasis, including blood electrolytes and osmolarity, body temperature, feeding and drinking behavior, and circadian cycling plus the sleep–awake cycle. Some hypothalamic

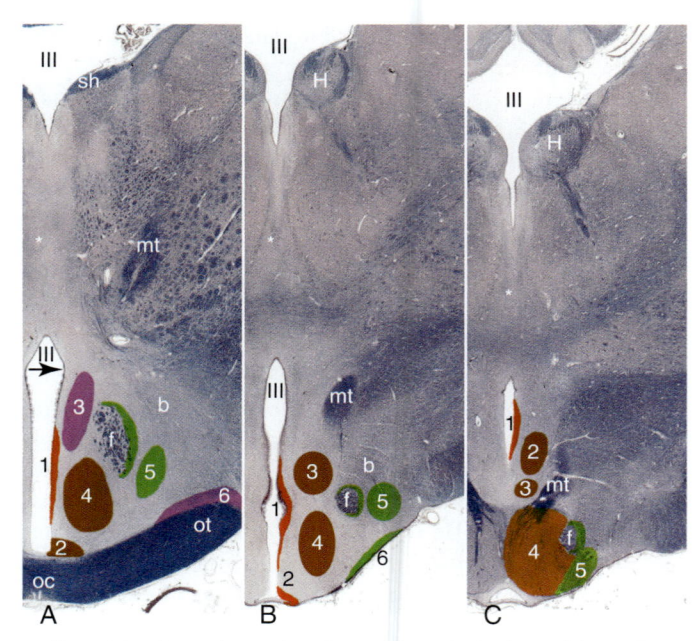

Fig. 18.25 Approximate locations of hypothalamic nuclei are illustrated schematically at three transverse levels (*purple,* axons to neurohypophysis; *red,* periventricular zone; *brown and orange,* medial zone; *green,* lateral zone). **A,** *Rostral level,* through optic chiasm: *1,* periventricular nucleus; *2,* suprachiasmatic nucleus; *3,* paraventricular nucleus; *4,* rostral hypothalamic nucleus; *5,* lateral hypothalamic nucleus; *6,* supraoptic nucleus; *f,* perifornical nucleus (*green*) around the fornix (preoptic nuclei are rostral to this level). The *arrow* indicates the hypothalamic sulcus, ventral to which the hypothalamic vascular organ is evident. **B,** *Intermediate level,* through the tuber cinereum: *1,* periventricular nucleus; *2,* infundibular (arcuate) nucleus; *3,* dorsomedial nucleus; *4,* ventromedial nucleus; *5,* lateral hypothalamic nucleus; *6,* tuberal nuclei; *f,* perifornical nucleus (*green*) around the fornix. **C,** *Caudal level,* through the mamillary body: *1,* periventricular nucleus; *2,* caudal hypothalamic nucleus; *3,* supramammillary nucleus; *4,* medial mamillary nucleus; *5,* lateral mamillary nucleus; *f,* perifornical nucleus (*green*) around the fornix. For all levels: **,* interthalamic adhesion; *III,* third ventricle; *b,* medial forebrain bundle; *f,* column of fornix; *H,* habenula; *mt,* mamillothalamic tract; *oc,* optic chiasm; *ot,* optic tract; *sh,* stria habenularis.

neurons are sensitive to constituents in circulating blood (osmolarity, electrolytes, hormones, glucose, and temperature). Neurons of the rostral hypothalamus are concerned with lowering body temperature, and those in the caudal hypothalamus with conserving heat. Lesions damaging these areas would cause hyperthermia and hypothermia, respectively.

The hypothalamus plays a major role in displaying affective behavior. It contributes to behavioral expressions associated with rage, escape, pleasure, reproductive behavior, and response to stress. The hypothalamus controls the autonomic nervous system. It participates in regulation of cardiovascular, respiratory, gastrointestinal, and urinary organs. Stimulation applied rostrally in the hypothalamus generally produces parasympathetic responses; caudal stimulation evokes sympathetic activity.

The hypothalamus has widespread brain connections. It receives axons from the optic tract. Axons arrive from the limbic system via the ***fornix*** (hippocampus) and ***stria terminalis*** (amygdala). The prefrontal cortex, septal region, and olfactory nuclei contribute axons to the **medial forebrain bundle** (*fasciculus medialis telencephali*), which courses through the lateral hypothalamus and continues caudally, even to the level of the spinal cord. Hypothalamic axons to visceral efferent nuclei in the brainstem travel through the **dorsal longitudinal fasciculus** (*fasciculus longitudinalis dorsalis*). Hypothalamic commissural axons connect right and left sides. Reciprocal hypothalamic connections with the thalamus and midbrain are present, particularly via tracts involving the mamillary body.

The hypothalamus may be divided sagittally into lateral and medial zones, plus a periventricular layer along the ventricular wall. The periventricular layer contains axons that connect the hypothalamus to the thalamus and caudal brainstem. Some periventricular neurons trigger hormone release from the adenohypophysis via axons that run to the tuber cinereum. The majority of hypothalamic nuclei are in the medial sagittal zone. The lateral zone has fewer nuclei but more axon tracts (Fig. 18.25).

The hypothalamus is commonly divided into three transverse regions: a caudal region that includes the mamillary body, an intermediate (tuberal) region at the level of the tuber cinereum, and a rostral region that is dorsal to the optic chiasm and bounded rostrally by lamina terminalis. (The rostral region includes preoptic nuclei derived embryologically from the telencephalon.) Within the hypothalamus, loose collections of neurons are considered an "area" and more dense, discrete neuron clusters are recognized as "nuclei." Hypothalamic nuclei per transverse region include the following (Fig. 18.25).

Preoptic nuclei (*nucleus preopticus lateralis, nucleus preopticus medialis, nucleus preopticus medianis,* and *nucleus preopticus periventricularis*) are the most rostral hypothalamic nuclei (Fig. 18.26). They are associated with parasympathetic activity, including micturition and erection. The **rostral hypothalamic nucleus** (*nucleus hypothalamicus rostralis*) is involved in body temperature reduction (panting, sweating). The **suprachiasmatic nucleus** (*nucleus suprachiasmaticus*), located dorsal to the optic chiasm, beside the midline, receives retinal input and controls circadian rhythms (e.g., body temperature, sleep and wakefulness, hormone levels).

The **paraventricular nucleus** (*nucleus paraventricularis*) and **supraoptic nucleus** (*nucleus supraopticus*) are located at the level of the optic chiasm. Axons from these nuclei form a **paraventriculohypophyseal tract** (*tractus paraventriculohypophsialis*) and a **supraopticohypophyseal tract** (*tractus supraopticohypophysialis*). Axons of both tracts pass through the infundibulum to terminate in the neural lobe of the neurohypophysis. Neurons of both nuclei produce vasopressin (antidiuretic hormone) and oxytocin hormones. The hormones are packaged in secretory vesicles, actively transported along microtubules, and stored in axon terminals. Following secretion in response to arriving action potentials, the hormones are taken up by blood circulating within fenestrated capillaries.

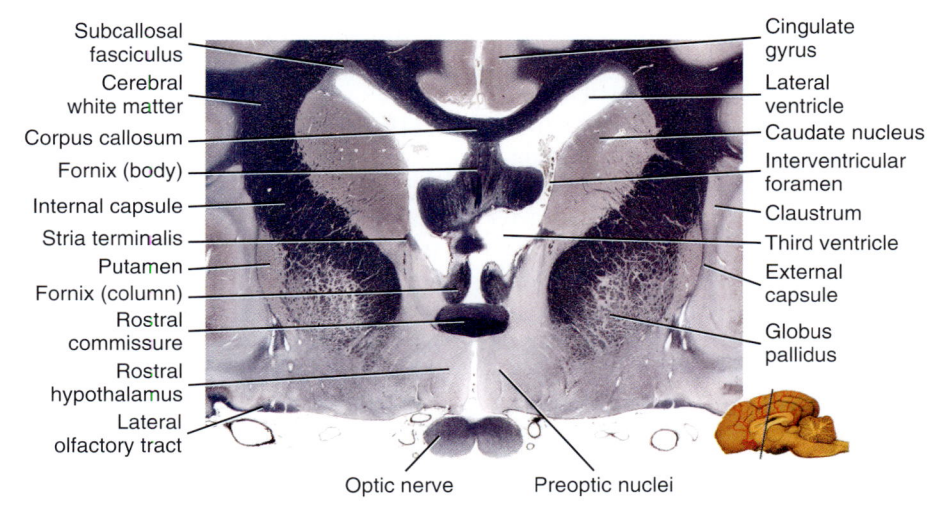

• **Fig. 18.26** Transverse section through the telencephalon at the level of the rostral commissure, including the rostral hypothalamus. The third ventricle communicates with the lateral ventricle via an interventricular foramen. Choroid plexus can be seen passing through the foramen on the right side. (Luxol Fast Blue–Cresyl Violet stain.)

The **intermediate hypothalamic region**, where the tuber cinereum is located, contains the **infundibular** or **arcuate nucleus** (*nucleus infundibularis*), **lateral tuberal nuclei** (*nuclei tuberis laterales*), and **periventricular nuclei**. These nuclei send axons to the tuber cinereum where the axons secrete peptides that are transported by blood to the adenohypophysis where they trigger hormone release. Some of the axons constitute a **tuberohypophysial tract** that secretes releasing hormones within the infundibulum.

The medial zone of the intermediate region contains a **dorsomedial hypothalamic nucleus** (*nucleus hypothalamicus dorsomedialis*) and a **ventromedial hypothalamic nucleus** (*nucleus hypothalamicus ventromedialis*). The latter is concerned with satiety, and lesions affecting it result in voracious appetite leading to hyperphagia and obesity. The adjacent **lateral hypothalamic nucleus** (*nucleus hypothalamicus* laterals) and area act as a feeding center. Damage causes anorexia and weight loss.

The caudal hypothalamic region features the **mamillary body** (*corpus mamillare*), visible at the caudoventral surface of the diencephalon (Fig. 18.21). The body is composed of a large **medial nucleus** (*nucleus mamillaris medialis*) and a small **lateral nucleus** (combined *nucleus mamillaris lateralis and nucleus mamillaris cinereus*). The medial nucleus consists of small neurons organized into several subnuclei; the lateral nucleus has large neurons in two subnuclei.

Mamillary nuclei receive axons from the hippocampus via the fornix, and they project axons to the rostral group of thalamic nuclei via a prominent **mamillothalamic tract** (*tractus mamillothalamicus*). Damage to the tract or to mamillary nuclei results in impaired working memory (diencephalic amnesia) (Vann & Aggleton, 2004). Reciprocal connections with midbrain tegmental nuclei are conveyed by the **mamillotegmental tract** (*tractus mamillotegmentalis*) and the **mamillary peduncle** (*pedunculus mamillaris*).

Additional nuclei of the caudal hypothalamus include several that project to mamillary nuclei: *nucleus periventricularis caudalis, nucleus supramamillaris,* and *nucleus premamillaris*. The *nucleus perifornicalis* refers to neurons surrounding the column of the fornix. The **caudal hypothalamic nucleus** drives sympathetic activity.

The Epithalamus

The epithalamus includes the pineal gland and the habenula with its associated tracts. The **pineal gland** (*glandula pinealis*) is small in the dog (Figs. 18.4 and 18.22). It is a midline endocrine gland situated between the habenular nuclei and the caudal commissure, extending caudally from the pineal recess of the third ventricle. The gland is composed of pinealocytes and glial cells contained within connective tissue trabeculae derived from meninges. The pineal gland has fenestrated capillaries, and therefore lacks a blood–brain barrier.

Pinealocytes secrete melatonin, which promotes sleep and suppresses hypothalamic secretion of gonadotropin-releasing hormone, causing suppression of sexual development. Melatonin production is stimulated by darkness and exhibits circadian rhythm. The gland is innervated by postganglionic sympathetic axons from cell bodies in the cranial cervical ganglion. The sympathetic ganglion neurons are activated in response to optic tract axonal input to the suprachiasmatic nucleus of the hypothalamus. The nucleus projects to the midbrain and, via the tectotegmentospinal tract, it reaches sympathetic preganglionic neurons in the spinal cord. Reciprocal connections between the pineal and habenula also exist.

The **habenula** is located caudally in the diencephalon, on the dorsomedial border of the thalamus (Figs. 18.4, 18.21, and 18.22). Right and left habenulae are connected by a **habenular commissure** (*commissura habenularum*). The habenula is composed of medial and lateral **habenular** nuclei (*nuclei habenulares*), each having four subnuclei (Janklewicz, 1967). The medial nucleus has mainly limbic connections. The lateral nucleus is inhibited by basal nuclei.

The **habenular stria** (*stria habenularis thalami*), which courses along the dorsomedial margin of the thalamus (Fig. 18.24), conveys axons to habenular nuclei from basal nuclei, hypothalamus, and the rhinencephalon (septum, amygdala, and preoptic area). Axons from habenular nuclei travel via the *fasciculus retroflexus* (formerly *habenulointerpeduncular tract*) to the interpeduncular nucleus, to serotonergic raphe nuclei and to dopaminergic nuclei (*substantia nigra compacta* and *ventral tegmental area*).

The habenula suppresses movement via inhibition of dopamine release. During adversity, the habenula exhibits neuronal activity linking the limbic forebrain with serotonergic and dopaminergic brainstem nuclei that neuromodulate brain function in relation to emotional status (pain, stress, reward, sleep). The habenula is involved in threat-induced movement freeze (dopamine effect) and in the movement atonia associated with REM sleep (serotonin effect).

The Subthalamus

The subthalamus is the diencephalic region ventral to the thalamus and lateral to the hypothalamus. It contains the zona incerta, subthalamic nucleus, and white matter fields that border these nuclei (three H fields of Forel). The white matter fields are composed of basal nuclei axons traveling to thalamic nuclei or the red nucleus. Note that the endopeduncular nucleus may be included with the subthalamus (*Nomina Anatomica Veterinaria* [NAV], 2005) or with the cerebrum. In this chapter it is described with the cerebrum.

The **zona incerta** appears as a ventromedial extension of the thalamic reticulate nucleus, bounded dorsally by the axons of field H_1 of Forel and ventrally by field H_2 (Fig. 18.21). Via spontaneously active inhibitory neurons, the zona incerta suppresses activity in ventral caudal thalamic nuclei that relay sensory information to the neocortex. Pain behavior is a consequence of zona incerta damage. Brainstem cholinergic neurons (pedunculopontine nucleus) suppress zona incerta inhibition during activation of brainstem alerting pathways.

The **subthalamic nucleus** (*nucleus subthalamicus*) is situated in the caudal diencephalon, ventromedial to the zona incerta, dorsomedial to the crus cerebri, and rostral to substantia nigra (Fig. 18.21). It contains inhibitory interneurons and excitatory projection neurons. Axons from prefrontal and motor cortices excite subthalamic neurons.

In response to cortical input, the subthalamus suppresses unwanted movements by exciting the inhibitory neurons of endopeduncular nucleus. Premature movements result from damage to the subthalamus. An indirect basal nuclear pathway involving globus pallidus inhibition of subthalamic neurons is sensitive to dopamine and cholinergic neuromodulation. The subthalamic nucleus may play a pacemaker role within movement control circuits because it fires spontaneous bursts of action potentials with regular frequency.

THE CEREBRUM

The **cerebrum** consists of paired cerebral hemispheres, derived from the embryonic telencephalon. A **cerebral transverse fissure** (*fissura transversa cerebri*) separates the cerebrum from the cerebellum. A **cerebral longitudinal fissure** (*fissura longitudinalis cerebri*) (Figs. 18.27 and 18.28) separates right and left hemispheres except where they are connected across the midline by lamina terminalis and commissural axons of the corpus callosum, rostral commissure, hippocampus, and fornix. The **lamina terminalis**, once the rostral end of the embryonic neural tube, forms the rostral wall of the third ventricle (*lamina terminalis grisea*). The rostral commissure decussates in the lamina terminalis (*lamina terminalis alba*).

Cerebral Hemisphere

Each hemisphere is composed of surface gray matter, designated **cerebral cortex** (*cortex cerebri*), underlying **cerebral white matter** (Fig. 18.32), deep accumulations of gray matter called **basal nuclei**, and a **lateral ventricle** filled with cerebrospinal fluid (Fig. 18.29). The ventral region of the hemisphere is called the *rhinencephalon* because of its

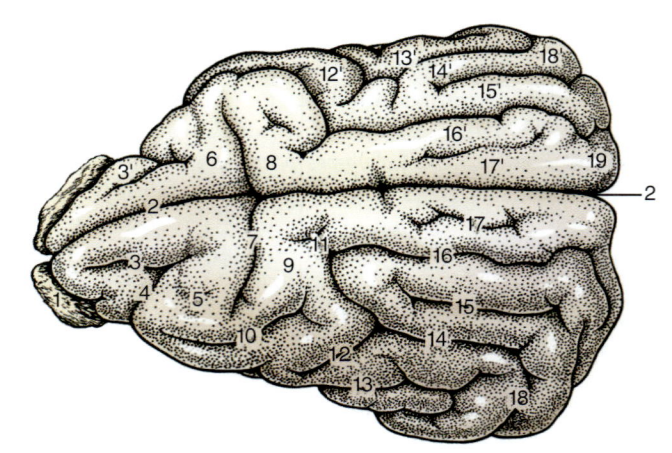

1. Olfactory bulb
2. Longitudinal fissure
3. Prorean sulcus
3'. Prorean gyrus
4. Presylvian sulcus
5. Precruciate sulcus
6. Precruciate gyrus
7. Cruciate sulcus
8. Postcruciate gyrus
9. Postcruciate sulcus
10. Coronal sulcus
11. Ansate sulcus
12. Rostral suprasylvian sulcus
12'. Rostral suprasylvian gyrus
13. Ectosylvian sulcus
13'. Ectosylvian gyrus
14. Middle suprasylvian sulcus
14'. Middle suprasylvian gyrus
15. Ectomarginal sulcus
15'. Ectomarginal gyrus
16. Marginal sulcus
16'. Marginal gyrus
17. Endomarginal sulcus
17'. Endomarginal gyrus
18. Caudal suprasylvian sulcus
18'. Caudal suprasylvian gyrus
19. Occipital gyrus

• **Fig. 18.27** Dorsolateral view of the cerebrum with sulci labeled on left hemisphere and gyri on right. The two hemispheres are separated by a longitudinal fissure (2).

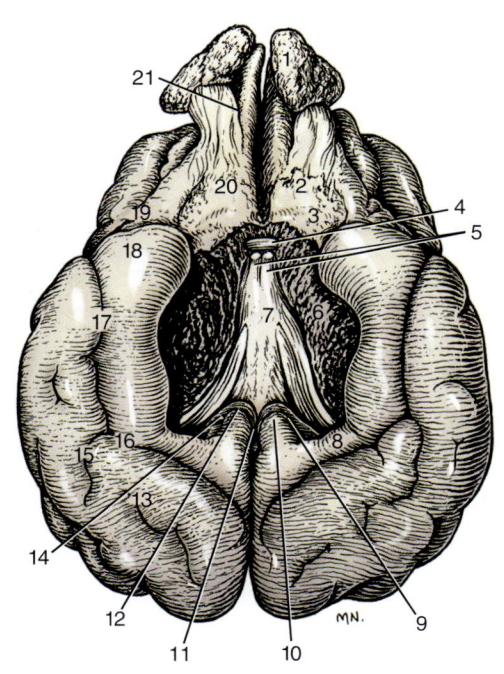

olfactory role (Fig. 18.30). Many **limbic system** structures (emotion and affective behavior components) are within the rhinencephalon.

The surface of each cerebral hemisphere features elevated bands, called gyri (*gyri cerebri*), separated by grooves, called sulci (*sulci cerebri*). Generally the name of a *gyrus* is the same as its adjacent *sulcus* (Figs. 18.30 and 18.31). The rostral end of the hemisphere is called the **frontal pole** (*polus rostralis*), and the caudal end is called the **occipital pole** (*polus caudalis*). The hemispheric region deep to the frontal bone can be referred to as the *frontal lobe*. Lobe terminology could be applied in relation to the parietal, occipital, and temporal bones; however, these lobar designations lack functional utility in the dog.

Three kinds of cerebral cortex (*pallium*) are distinguished per hemisphere. **Archicortex** (*archipallium*) is associated with the hippocampus (a component of the rhinencephalon). **Paleocortex** (*paleopallium*), also found in the rhinencephalon, has three layers. **Neocortex** (*neopallium*), the predominant cortex of the cerebrum, has six layers. The term **isocortex** refers to neocortex and **allocortex** refers to all the other types, including transitions among the above types.

The white matter of each cerebral hemisphere, consists of myelinated axons categorized as association, commissural, or projection axons (Figs. 18.32 through 18.34). **Association axons** connect cortical regions within the same hemisphere. They are differentiated as long versus short. **Commissural axons** cross the midline, connecting the two hemispheres via the corpus callosum for the neocortex and the rostral commissure for the rhinencephalon. Viewed in a bisected brain, the **corpus callosum** presents an elongate trunk region (***truncus corporis callosi***) that has a blunt caudal end (***splenium***) and a rounded rostral end (***genu***) that continues ventrally (***rostrum***) (Fig. 18.35). The divergence of the commissural axons dorsal to the lateral

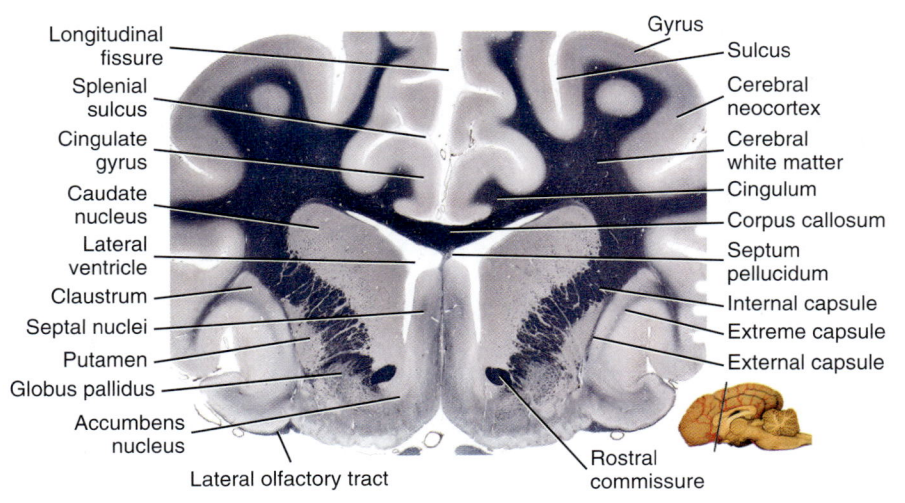

1. Olfactory bulb
2. Olfactory tubercle
3. Diagonal gyrus
4. Rostral commissure
5. Columns of fornix
6. Cut internal capsule
7. Body of fornix
8. Parahippocampal gyrus
9. Hippocampal sulcus
10. Callosal gyrus
11. Subsplenial flexure of dentate gyrus
12. Tubercle of dentate gyrus
13. Occipital lobe
14. Dentate gyrus
15. Ramus of lateral rhinal sulcus
16. Caudal part of lateral rhinal sulcus
17. Caudal part of lateral rhinal sulcus
18. Piriform lobe
19. Rostral part of lateral rhinal sulcus
20. Olfactory peduncle
21. Medial rhinal sulcus

• **Fig. 18.28** A ventral view of the cerebrum. The rhinencephalon is demarcated from the rest of the hemisphere by the lateral rhinal sulcus (*16, 17, 19*).

• **Fig. 18.29** Transverse section through the telencephalon at the level of the septum. Notice that the lateral ventricle is bounded by the corpus callosum, caudate nucleus, and septum. The latter consists of a thick cellular component (nuclei) and a thin septum pellucidum component. (Luxol Fast Blue–Cresyl Violet stain.)

780 CHAPTER 18 The Brain

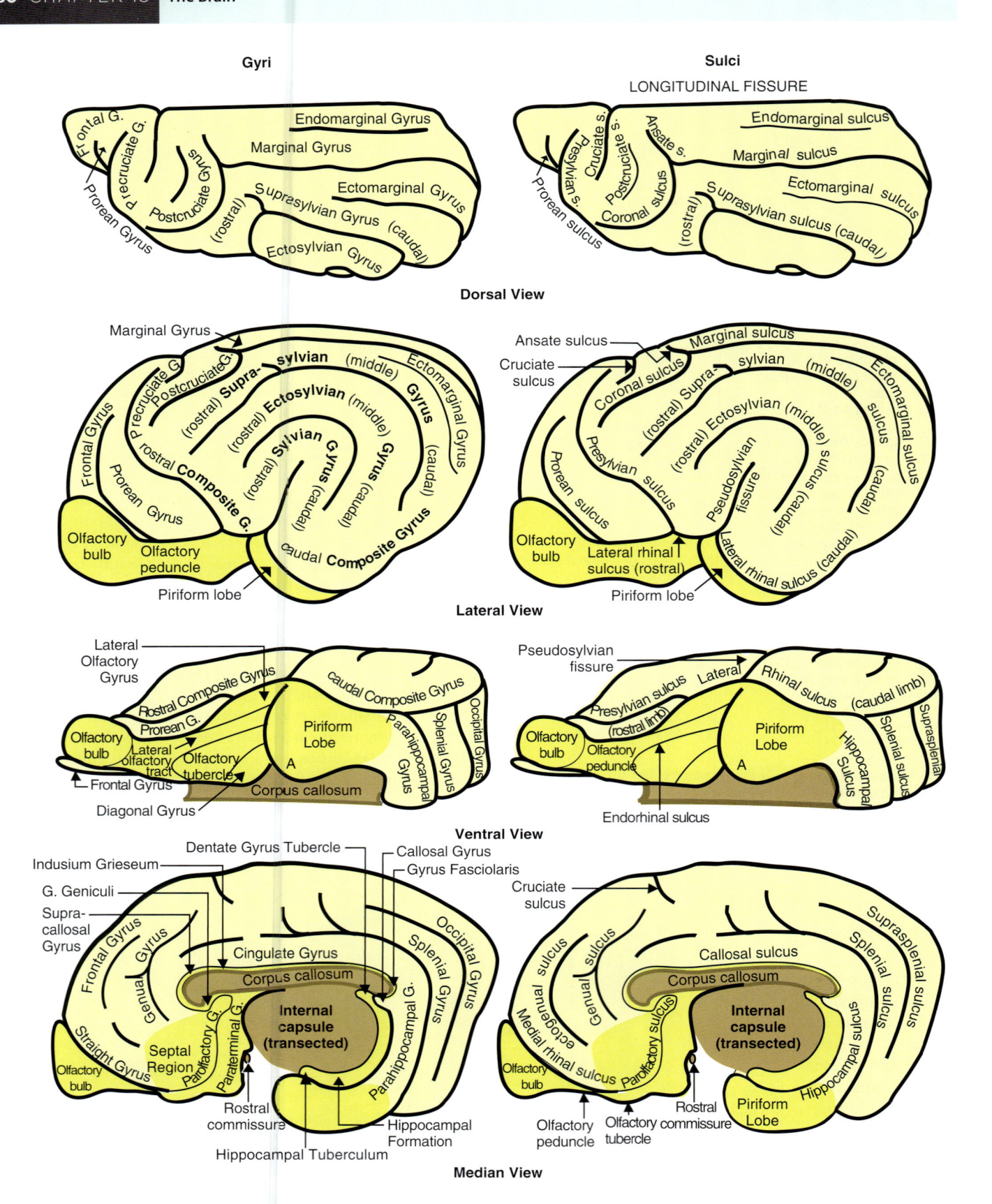

• **Fig. 18.30** Schematic illustration of gyri (*left*) and sulci (*right*) of a canine cerebral hemisphere. Dorsal, lateral, and ventral views are shown for a left hemisphere; the median view is of a right hemisphere. Neocortex is pale yellow, rhinencephalon is brighter yellow, and major white matter bundles are colored brown. In the piriform lobe of the ventral view, *A* marks the location of the amygdala.

CHAPTER 18 The Brain

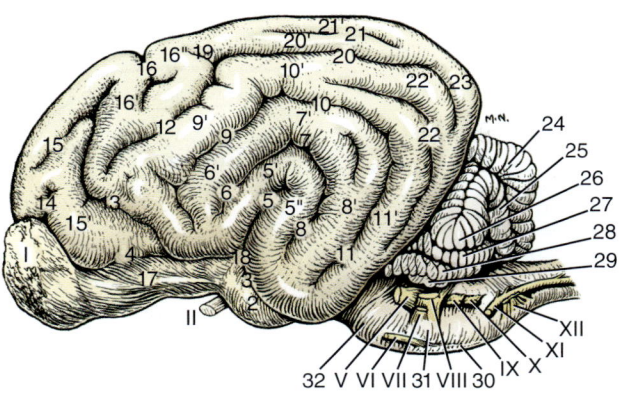

1. Olfactory bulb
2. Piriform lobe
3. Caudal part of lateral rhinal sulcus
4. Rostral part of lateral rhinal sulcus
5. Pseudosylvian fissure
5'. Rostral sylvian gyrus
5". Caudal sylvian gyrus
6. Rostral ectosylvian sulcus
6'. Rostral ectosylvian gyrus
7. Middle ectosylvian sulcus
7'. Middle ectosylvian gyrus
8. Caudal ectosylvian sulcus
8'. Caudal ectosylvian gyrus
9. Rostral suprasylvian sulcus
9'. Rostral suprasylvian gyrus
10. Middle suprasylvian sulcus
10'. Middle suprasylvian gyrus
11. Caudal suprasylvian sulcus
11'. Caudal suprasylvian gyrus
12. Coronal sulcus
13. Presylvian sulcus
14. Prorean sulcus
15. Prorean sulcus
15'. Prorean gyrus
16. Cruciate sulcus
16'. Precruciate gyrus
16". Postcruciate gyrus
17. Olfactory peduncle
18. Insular region
19. Ansate sulcus
20. Marginal sulcus
20'. Marginal gyrus
21. Endomarginal sulcus
21'. Endomarginal gyrus
22. Ectomarginal sulcus
22'. Ectomarginal gyrus
23. Occipital gyrus
24. Vermis of cerebellum
25. Paramedian lobule
26. Ansiform lobule
27. Dorsal paraflocculus
28. Ventral paraflocculus
29. Flocculus
30. Pyramid
31. Trapezoid body
32. Pons
II. Optic nerve
V. Trigeminal nerve
VI. Abducent nerve
VII. Facial nerve
VIII. Vestibulocochlear nerve
IX. Glossopharyngeal nerve
X. Vagus nerve
XI. Accessory nerve
XII. Hypoglossal nerve

• **Fig. 18.31** Lateral view of the brain. The ventral part of the cerebral hemisphere is associated with olfactory axonal input and is designated rhinencephalon.

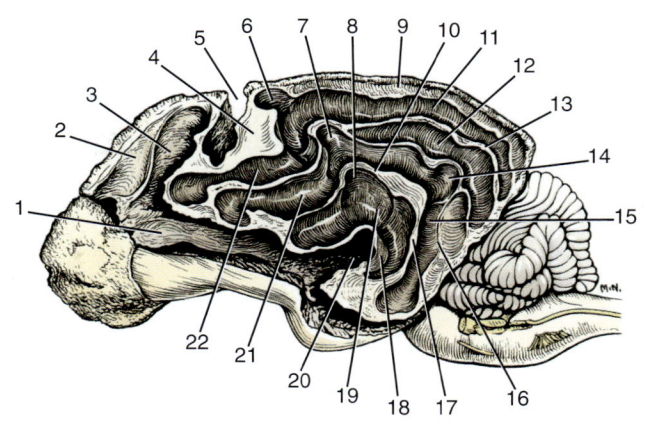

1. Prorean gyrus
2. Prorean sulcus
3. Presylvian sulcus
4. Postcruciate sulcus
5. Cruciate sulcus
6. Ansate sulcus
7. Rostrodorsal branch of middle suprasylvian sulcus
8. Dorsal branch of middle ectosylvian sulcus
9. Endomarginal sulcus
10. Middle ectosylvian gyrus
11. Marginal sulcus
12. Ectomarginal sulcus
13. Ectomarginal gyrus
14. Caudodorsal branch of middle suprasylvian sulcus
15. Caudal suprasylvian sulcus
16. Caudal suprasylvian gyrus
17. Caudal ectosylvian gyrus
18. Caudal sylvian gyrus
19. Middle ectosylvian sulcus
20. Pseudosylvian fissure
21. Rostral suprasylvian sulcus
22. Coronal sulcus

• **Fig. 18.32** Lateral view of a canine brain with cortex removed from the left cerebral hemisphere to show underlying white matter. Locations of sulci are labeled.

ventricle constitutes the *corpus callosum radiation* (*radiatio corporis callosi*).

Projection axons either enter the neocortex (corticopedal), typically from the thalamus, or they exit the neocortex (corticofugal) to terminate in the basal nuclei, brainstem, or spinal cord (Fig. 18.36). Projections axons run in the **internal capsule** (*capsula interna*) or in the **external capsule** (*capsula externa*); the latter also contains rostral commissure axons (Fig. 18.26). The term *centrum semiovale* refers to the region of central white matter where radiations from the corpus callosum and internal capsule converge. *Corona radiata* refers to the collective white matter extensions that radiate from the centrum semiovale into individual cortical gyri.

The **lateral ventricle** (*ventriculus lateralis*) within each cerebral hemisphere communicates with the third ventricle through an *interventricular foramen* (*foramen interventriculare*) (Fig. 18.26). Each lateral ventricle has a choroid plexus that passes through the interventricular foramen and continues along the roof of the third ventricle. Each choroid plexus arises from tela choroidea (combined pia mater and ependyma) having a linear attachment called **tenia choroidea** or **tenia fornicis** (pending attachment location). Choroid plexuses are the source of cerebrospinal fluid.

The lateral ventricle is extended rostroventrally by a **rostral horn** (*cornu rostrale*) and caudoventrally by a **temporal horn** (*cornu temporale*) (Fig. 18.35) Typically the rostral horn loses its connection to the olfactory ventricle (recess) located within the olfactory bulb and olfactory peduncle of the rhinencephalon (Fitzgerald, 1961).

The Rhinencephalon

Rhinencephalon refers to the ventral region of each cerebral hemisphere. It is phylogenetically old and concerned with olfaction, memory formation, and emotional behavior. The rhinencephalon is separated from neocortex by rostral and caudal parts of the **lateral rhinal sulcus** (*sulcus rhinalis lateralis*) along the ventrolateral surface of the cerebral hemisphere (Fig. 18.30). A **medial rhinal sulcus** (*sulcus rhinalis medialis*) separates the olfactory peduncle from the neocortex of the straight gyrus along the ventromedial surface of the hemisphere.

The rhinencephalon has three defined parts: a **basal part** (*pars basalis rhinencephali*) consisting of the olfactory bulb

782 CHAPTER 18 The Brain

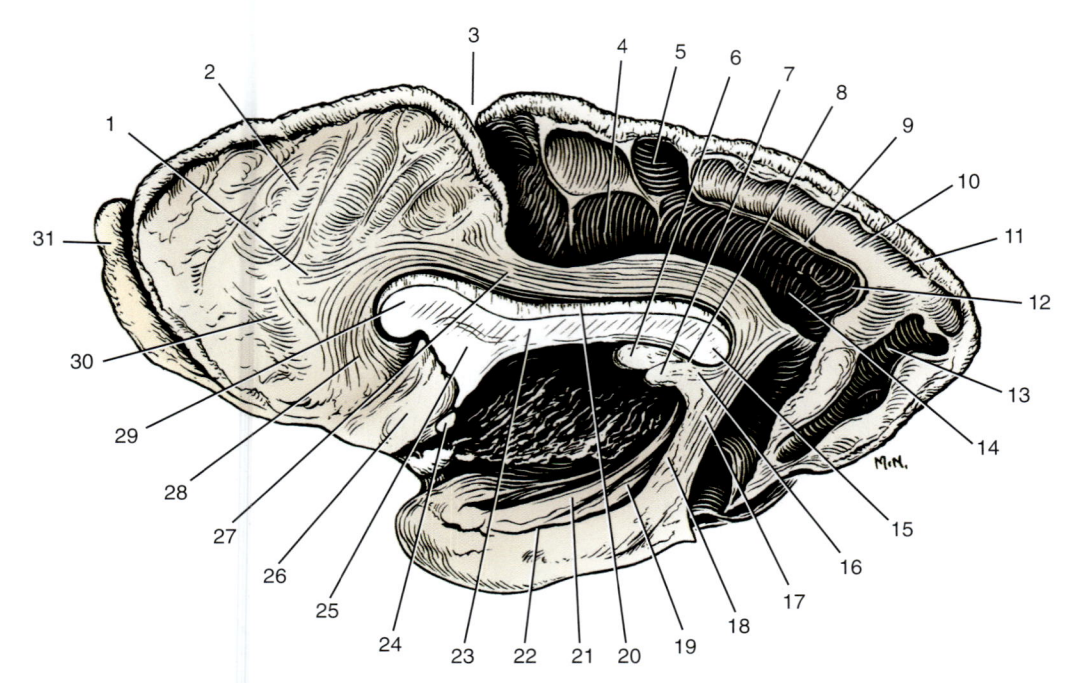

1. Rostral fibers of cingulum
2. Dorsal part of genual sulcus
3. Cruciate sulcus
4. Rostral part of splenial sulcus
5. Ramus of splenial sulcus
6. Tubercle of dentate gyrus
7. Callosal gyrus
8. Subsplenial flexure of dentate gyrus
9. Splenial gyrus
10. Rostral part of suprasplenial sulcus
11. Occipital gyrus
12. Ramus of splenial sulcus
13. Caudal part of suprasplenial sulcus
14. Caudal part of splenial sulcus
15. Splenium of corpus callosum
16. Fibers of cingulum to callosal gyrus
17. Cingulum to parahippocampal gyrus
18. Parahippocampal gyrus
19. Dentate gyrus
20. Callosal sulcus
21. Fimbria of hippocampus
22. Hippocampal sulcus
23. Body of corpus callosum
24. Rostral commissure
25. Septum telencephali
26. Paraterminal gyrus
27. Cingulum
28. Cingulum to paraterminal gyrus
29. Genu of corpus callosum
30. Ventral part of genual sulcus
31. Olfactory bulb

• **Fig. 18.33** Medial view of a right cerebral hemisphere with most of the cortex removed to show underlying white matter. The corpus callosum (*29, 23, 15*) connects right and left hemispheres, as does the rostral commissure (*24*). The cingulum (*28, 27, 17*) is a medial bundle of association fibers.

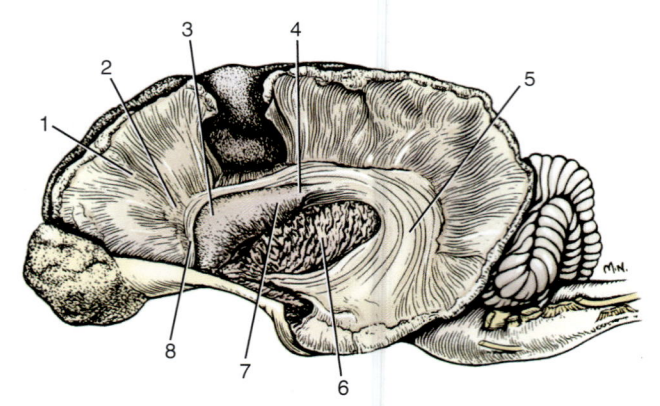

1. Corona radiata
2. Subcallosal fasciculus (rostrodorsal part)
3. Head of caudate nucleus (medial side)
4. Tail of caudate nucleus (medial side)
5. Subcallosal fasciculus (caudoventral part)
6. Cut fibers of internal capsule
7. Body of caudate nucleus
8. Subcallosal fasciculus (rostroventral part)

• **Fig. 18.34** Illustrated lateral view of a brain with much of the left cerebral hemisphere removed. The subcallosal fasciculus (*2, 8, 5*) is a bundle of association fibers that forms the lateral and dorsal wall of the lateral ventricle.

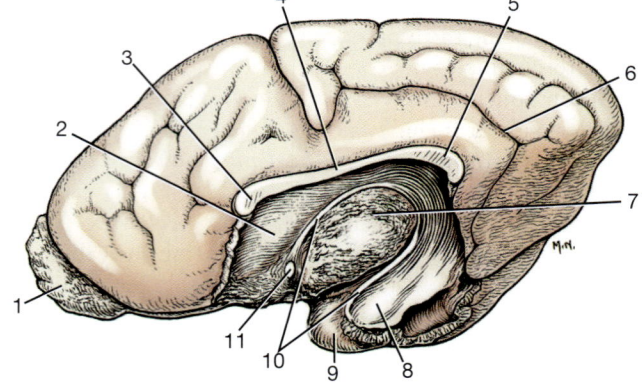

1. Olfactory bulb
2. Caudate nucleus
3. Genu of corpus callosum
4. Body of corpus callosum
5. Splenium of corpus callosum
6. Splenial sulcus
7. Internal capsule
8. Amygdala
9. Piriform lobe
10. Stria terminalis
11. Rostral commissure

• **Fig. 18.35** Medial view of a right cerebral hemisphere with medial structures removed to show the right lateral ventricle. The rostral horn of the ventricle is bounded laterally by the caudate nucleus (*2*), and the distal part of the temporal horn is bounded laterally by the amygdala (*8*); elsewhere, the ventricle is bounded laterally by white matter.

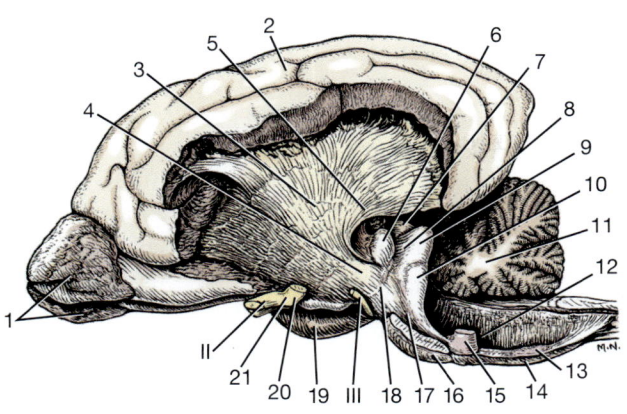

1. Olfactory bulb
2. Left cerebral hemisphere
3. Internal capsule (lateral view)
4. Crus cerebri
5. Acoustic radiation
6. Medial geniculate body
7. Rostral colliculus
8. Brachium of caudal colliculus
9. Caudal colliculus
10. Lateral lemniscus
11. Cerebellum
12. Location of dorsal nucleus of trapezoid body
13. Location of olivary nucleus
14. Pyramid
15. Trapezoid body
16. Transverse fibers of pons
17. Pyramidal and corticopontine tracts
18. Transverse crural tract
19. Piriform lobe
20. Optic tract (cut to show internal capsule)
21. Optic chiasm
II. Optic nerve
III. Oculomotor nerve

- **Fig. 18.36** Lateral view of a brain dissected to show axonal connections between the brainstem and a cerebral hemisphere. The two are connected by internal capsule (*3 and 5*). Corticospinal axons from cerebral cortex travel through the internal capsule (*3*), crus cerebri (*4*), pyramidal and corticopontine tracts (*17*), and pyramid (*14*) to reach the pyramidal decussation and spinal cord.

and the superficial ventral portion of the hemisphere, a **septal part** (*pars septalis rhinencephali*) composed of structures that rostrally form the medial wall of the lateral ventricle, and a **limbic part** (*pars limbica rhinencephali*) strictly defined as being the hippocampus. The term **limbic system** refers to circuits of neocortical, rhinencephalic, and brainstem components involved in memory, emotions, and affective behavior. It includes structures from all three parts of the rhinencephalon.

Olfactory Pathways

The olfactory pathway starts with bipolar special visceral afferent neurons located in the **olfactory mucosa**. The neurons have long cilia embedded in olfactory mucus. The cilia have receptors that are sensitive to odorants trapped by the mucus. Nonmyelinated axons from the bipolar neurons collect into bundles that pass through the cribriform plate as **olfactory nerves**. The nerves terminate in the *olfactory bulb*, which is attached to the cerebral hemisphere by the *olfactory peduncle* (Fig. 18.3). The bulb and peduncle are hollow, containing an *olfactory ventricle* filled with cerebrospinal fluid.

Seven histologic layers compose the wall of the **olfactory bulb** (*bulbus olfactorius*). From superficial to deep, they are (1) an olfactory nerves layer, (2) a layer of glomeruli (multiple olfactory axons synapse with an individual mitral cell within a glomerulus), (3) an external plexiform layer, (4) a mitral cell layer (conical neuron cell bodies aligned in a row), (5) a thin internal plexiform layer, (6) a granule cell layer (granule cells are inhibitory interneurons), and (7) a periventricular layer composed of axons leaving or entering the bulb (Berman & Jones, 1982). Mitral cell axons joining olfactory tracts constitute olfactory bulb output.

Axons from the **vomeronasal organ** accompany those from the olfactory mucosa through the cribriform plate. They terminate in the accessory olfactory bulb, embedded in the dorsomedial surface of the olfactory bulb. The **accessory olfactory bulb** (*bulbus olfactorius accessorius*) is small, but it has a layered structure similar to that of the olfactory bulb. The accessory bulb has reciprocal connections with the amygdala. The vomeronasal organ detects pheromones that influence sexual behavior.

The **olfactory peduncle** (*pedunculus olfactorius*) extends from the olfactory bulb to the level of the *olfactory tubercle* (Fig. 18.30). It is separated from the frontal lobe as medial and lateral rhinal sulci that meet dorsal to the peduncle. The olfactory peduncle contains an olfactory ventricle surrounded by three olfactory tracts and a three-layered paleocortex designated rostral olfactory nucleus.

The **lateral olfactory tract** (*tractus olfactorius lateralis*) conveys mitral axons destined for the rostral olfactory nucleus, olfactory tubercle, nucleus of the lateral olfactory tract, amygdala, and cortices of the lateral olfactory gyrus and piriform lobe. The **medial olfactory tract** (*tractus olfactorius medialis*) conveys axons to the septal region, including septal nuclei and the paraterminal gyrus. The **intermediate olfactory tract** (*tractus olfactorius intermedius*) channels axons through the rostral commissure to the contralateral olfactory bulb, connecting to the rostral limb of the commissure. The tract contains axons that are afferent and efferent per ipsilateral olfactory bulb.

The **olfactory tubercle** (*tuberculum olfactorium*) is a ventral bulge region located caudal to the olfactory peduncle and rostral to the diagonal gyrus (Figs. 18.28 and 18.30). It is separated from the lateral olfactory tract by an *entorhinal sulcus*. The tubercle consists of a three-layered cortex that sends axons to the hypothalamus via the medial forebrain bundle. (Note that the terms *rostral perforated substance* [olfactory tubercle and the diagonal gyrus areas] and *olfactory trigone* are inappropriate for macrosomatic animals such as the dog [Nomina Anatomica Veterinaria (2017)]).

The **diagonal gyrus** (*gyrus diagonalis*) is between the olfactory tubercle and the optic chiasm and tract. It is continuous with the paraterminal gyrus of the septum (Fig. 18.30). The two gyri contain the **diagonal lamella** (*lamella diagonalis*; formerly the diagonal band of Broca). Axons of the lamella join the **medial forebrain bundle** (*fasciculus medialis telencephali*) to convey information from olfactory-related nuclei to the hypothalamus. Also deep to the diagonal gyrus, the **basal nucleus** (of Meynert) contains large cholinergic neurons that project broadly to cerebral cortex to enhance cortical activity via neuromodulation.

The **piriform lobe** (*lobus piriformis*) is concerned with conscious olfaction. It receives mitral axons from the olfactory bulb via the *lateral olfactory tract*. The piriform lobe consists of a flat rostral part demarcated from the swollen caudal part by a fossa (*fossa lateralis cerebri*) (Figs. 18.28 and Fig. 18.30). The rostral part is bounded by the olfactory tubercle. It includes the **lateral olfactory gyrus** (*gyrus olfactorius lateralis*), which is prepiriform paleocortex.

The swollen caudal part of the piriform lobe bulges because of the underlying amygdala, hippocampus, and lateral ventricle. The bulge is covered by different types of cortex. The rostral third of the piriform swelling features prepiriform paleocortex laterally and cortical nuclei of the amygdala medially. The caudal two-thirds is coated by **entorhinal cortex**, identifiable histologically by cell clusters in layer two of approximately six layers (Woznicka et al., 2006). Entorhinal cortex blends medially with subicular and hippocampal archicortex with which it reciprocally communicates (Fig. 18.37). The piriform lobe is continued caudally by the **parahippocampal gyrus** (*gyrus parahippocampalis*), which is also covered by entorhinal cortex. The clustered neurons composing layer two of entorhinal cortex send their axons to the adjacent, attached hippocampus.

The **amygdala** (amygdaloid body) (Fig. 18.35), which is named for its almond shape, is located within the piriform lobe. The amygdaloid complex contains approximately a dozen nuclei, including six major ones arranged in three groups. A basolateral group (*nucleus basalis* and *nucleus lateralis*) receives sensory input. A cortical group (*nucleus corticalis* and *nucleus tractus olfactorii lateralis*) and the ventral tip of the hippocampus occupy the rostromedial surface of the caudal part of the piriform lobe. A centromedial group (*nucleus centralis* and *nucleus medialis*) contains output neurons (Berman & Jones, 1982).

The amygdala assigns emotional reactions, particularly fear-related ones, to sensory information. It is a major component of the limbic system. The amygdala receives axonal input from the lateral olfactory tract, the hippocampus, the rostral hypothalamus, and, via the external capsule, areas of neocortex. Axonal output from the amygdala goes to the piriform cortex, hippocampal formation, dorsomedial thalamic nucleus, nucleus accumbens, and hypothalamus. Also, the amygdala has direct projections to the midbrain and pontomedullary reticular formation. The **stria terminalis** is a slender tract that connects the amygdala to the rostral hypothalamus and septal region (Fig. 18.35) A *nucleus of the stria terminalis* is associated with the rostral end of the stria.

The Septum

The **septal region** is located rostral to the rostral commissure and ventral to the genu and rostrum of the corpus callosum. A thin, variable, septum pellucidum (*septum telencephali pellucidum*) connects the thick cellular septum (*septum telencephali cellulare*) to the corpus callosum and continues caudally to fill the space between the corpus callosum and fornix. The septal region forms a medial wall of the lateral ventricle (Figs. 18.29 and 18.30). The cellular septum is a potent reward site of the limbic system.

The **paraterminal gyrus** (*gyrus paraterminalis*) marks the medial surface of the septal wall and **septal nuclei** (*nuclei septi*) are contained within the wall (Fig. 18.30). The nuclei receive axonal input from the medial olfactory tract. They have reciprocal connections with the amygdala (via the stria terminalis), hippocampus (via the fornix), hypothalamus (via the medial forebrain bundle), and the habenula (via the stria habenularis).

The **rostral commissure** (*commissura rostralis*) traverses the lamina terminalis. Its axons connect the right and left rhinencephalon (Figs. 18.26 and 18.38). The **rostral part** (*pars rostralis*) of the commissure courses rostrally along the ventral edge of the internal capsule and enters the olfactory peduncle, becoming the **intermediate olfactory tract** (*tractus olfactorius intermedius*). The axons reciprocally connect olfactory bulbs and rostral olfactory nuclei of each side; they terminate on granule cells of the olfactory bulb.

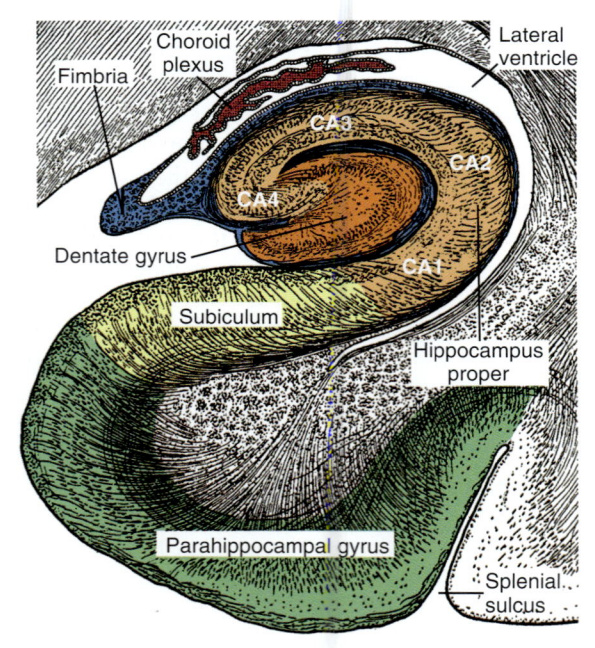

• **Fig. 18.37** Schematic drawing of the hippocampal formation, tucked deep to and continuous with the parahippocampal gyrus. The plane of section is debatable, it could be a dorsal plane section from the right cerebral hemisphere (rostral toward the left and medial toward the bottom) or a transverse section with medial to the left. The hippocampal formation consists of the dentate gyrus (*dark orange*), hippocampus proper (*pale orange*), and subiculum (*yellow*). The latter is continuous with entorhinal cortex covering the parahippocampal gyrus (*green*). The hippocampus proper (cornu ammonis) may be divided into four regions (CA1 to CA4). Output axons (*blue*) from the hippocampal formation run superficially in the alveus and then in the fimbria. The subiculum conveys reciprocal connections between the hippocampus and entorhinal cortex. The hippocampus forms a partial wall of the lateral ventricle, which contains a choroid plexus. (Modified from Ranson SW, Clark SL: *Anatomy of the nervous system*, 10th ed., Philadelphia, 1959, Saunders.)

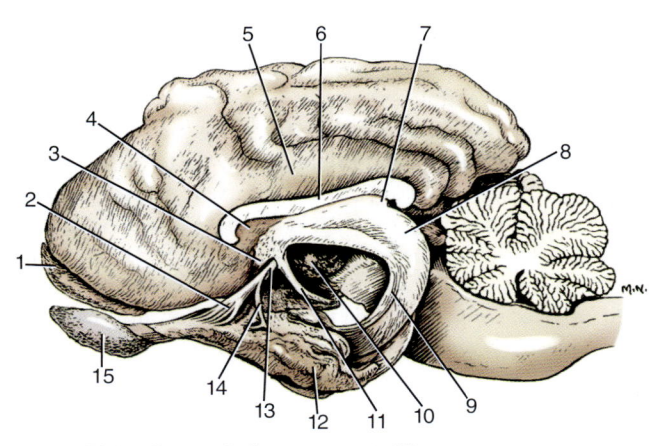

1. Right olfactory bulb
2. Rostral part of rostral commissure
3. Precommissural fornix
4. Septum pellucidum
5. Medial surface of right cerebral hemisphere
6. Corpus callosum
7. Dorsal commissure of fornix
8. Hippocampus
9. Fimbria of hippocampus
10. Interthalamic adhesion
11. Column of fornix
12. Piriform lobe (from dorsal side)
13. Rostral commissure
14. Caudal part of rostral commissure
15. Left olfactory bulb

• **Fig. 18.38** Illustrated lateral view of a brain with the left half removed except for most of the left rhinencephalon. Rostral (*2*) and caudal (*14*) parts of the rostral commissure (*13*) are evident.

Axons of the **caudal part** (*pars caudalis*) of the rostral commissure join the external capsule. They reciprocally connect the amygdala and piriform lobe bilaterally.

Hippocampal Formation

The hippocampal formation (hippocampus) is a principal component of the limbic system. It is necessary for long-term memory formation (though not long-term memory recall). It is essential for spatial memory (e.g., a dog recalling how it got where it is and how to return whence it came).

Phylogenetically and during embryonic development, three parts of the hippocampus can be identified. The *pars precommissuralis*, located rostral to the corpus callosum, blends with the paraterminal gyrus and is not otherwise evident in the mature brain. The *pars supracommissuralis* persists as a thin gray band around the corpus callosum, forming *gyrus geniculi* (ventral to the rostrum), *supracallosal gyrus* (around the genu), and **indusium griseum** (along the dorsal surface of the corpus callosum, within the callosal sulcus) (Fig. 18.30). The *pars retrocommissuralis* becomes the prominent archicortex complex referred to as *hippocampal formation* (Fig. 18.37).

The term **hippocampus** is subject to varying interpretations, but typically it is a synonym for **hippocampal formation**. The **hippocampal formation** consists of the **dentate gyrus**, **hippocampus proper**, and **subiculum**. These are sequential regions joined together as infolded cortex, connected to and tucked deep to the piriform lobe and parahippocampal gyrus (Fig. 18.37).

The **dentate gyrus** (*gyrus dentatus*) is three-layered archicortex (molecular, granular cells, and polymorph cells) embedded into the concavity of the hippocampus proper. The **hippocampus proper** (*pes hippocampi, cornu ammonis*) is a gyrus folded concave medially. It is archicortex composed of three major layers: (1) molecular, (2) double pyramidal cells, and (3) polymorph cell layer. The gyrus is divisible into four zones (CA1 at the subiculum to CA4 at the dentate gyrus) (Fig. 18.37).

The **subiculum** is composed of variable layers. It is a major source of hippocampal output to the adjacent entorhinal cortex of the piriform lobe and parahippocampal gyrus. A transitional gyrus designated *prosubiculum* is situated between the hippocampus proper and the subiculum. The terms *presubiculum* and *parasubiculum* refer to transitional regions between the subiculum and entorhinal cortex.

Grossly, the hippocampal formation makes a rostrally concave semicircle that forms the medial wall of the temporal horn of the lateral ventricle (Fig. 18.38). The ventral tip of the hippocampus, *hippocampal tuberculum* (*tuberculum hippocampi*), is located beside the amygdala deep to the rostromedial surface of the caudal part of the piriform lobe. Dorsally a prominent *tubercle of the dentate gyrus* is evident where the hippocampal formation ends ventral to the splenium of the corpus callosum (Figs. 18.30 and 18.33). The term *gyrus fasciolaris* refers to a continuity between the dentate tubercle and indusium griseum encircling the splenium.

The hippocampal formation has reciprocal connections with entorhinal cortex of the piriform lobe and parahippocampal gyrus with which it is continuous. The hippocampal formation also sends axons to the septum and diencephalon via the fornix. Input to the hippocampal formation includes axons from the septum, amygdala, thalamus, brainstem, and contralateral hippocampus, plus neuromodulatory input from various sources (serotonin, norepinephrine, dopamine, and acetylcholine).

Axons to the fornix arise from double pyramidal cells of the hippocampus proper. They join the **alveus** (*alveus hippocampi*), a surface layer of axons deep to the ependyma of the lateral ventricle. The axons continue, as the **fimbria** (*fimbria hippocampi*), which form a ledge along the lateral surface of the hippocampal formation (Figs. 18.37 and 18.38). At the margin of the fimbria, axons turn rostrally becoming the **crus of the fornix** (*crus fornicis*). The **body of the fornix** (*corpus fornicis*) is formed by merger of the two crura along the midline (Fig. 18.28). Axons of the fornix body continue rostrally. They turn ventrally at the rostral commissure, dividing into a precommissural projection to the septum and rostral hypothalamus and a postcommissural **column of the fornix** (*columna fornicis*) that goes to rostral thalamic nuclei and mamillary nuclei; some axons continue into the midbrain.

A **ventral commissure of the fornix** (*commissura fornicis [hippocampi] ventralis*) is present in the vicinity of the rostral commissure. A **dorsal commissure of the fornix** (*commissura fornicis [hippocampi] dorsalis*) is between the two crura ventral to the splenium of the corpus callosum.

The Limbic System

The term *limbic system* is applied to a collection of brain structures involved with affective (emotional) behavior and memory (Fig. 18.39). Emotional drive ensures that dogs will exert sufficient effort to preserve themselves and their species. Thus self-defense, escape, hunting food, courtship, mating, territory defense, and offspring protection are all emotionally driven. Emotion involves autonomic responses and greatly affects memory and learning.

Emotional drive was a survival requirement early in phylogenetic development, when olfaction was the chief sensory modality; thus much of the rhinencephalon is included in the limbic system. Stimulation or ablation of various limbic system components evokes responses such as docility, apparent pleasure, hypersexuality, irritability, aggression, and rage. A major function of the cerebral neocortex is to keep the limbic system under cognitive control.

Interconnected telencephalic structures bordering the rostral end of the brainstem give the limbic system its name (*limbic* means "border"). The border is composed of two telencephalic rings, separated by the corpus callosum. The outer circle consists of the *piriform lobe, parahippocampal gyrus, cingulate gyrus,* and *septal region* (Fig. 18.39). The inner ring includes the *amygdala, hippocampus,* and *nucleus accumbens*. The limbic system also includes components of the diencephalon: *habenula, hypothalamus* (particularly preoptic and mamillary components), and parts of the *thalamus* (rostral, dorsomedial, lateral dorsal, paraventricular, and intralaminar nuclei) (Fig. 18.40). Related midbrain structures include *interpeduncular* and *tegmental nuclei*.

Structures belong to the limbic system by virtue of their connections with one another. Major limbic highways include *cingulum* within the cingulate gyrus and the *fornix,* which projects hippocampal output to the septum and diencephalon. The *stria terminalis* links the amygdala with the rostral hypothalamus and septal region. The *stria habenularis* connects the septal region to the habenula (Fig. 18.39).

Neocortex surrounding the corpus callosum is part of the limbic system. The **cingulate gyrus**, a transitional isocortex, connects to neocortical association areas, rostral nuclei of the thalamus, and the parahippocampal gyrus. The **septal region** projects to adjacent cortex, to the hippocampus, and to the habenula. The **parahippocampal gyrus** (*gyrus parahippocampalis*) extends from the piriform lobe to the cingulate gyrus. Like the piriform lobe, it is coated by entorhinal cortex and has reciprocal connections with the hippocampal formation, which it conceals. (A short branch of the parahippocampal gyrus, the *callosal gyrus,* is situated ventral to

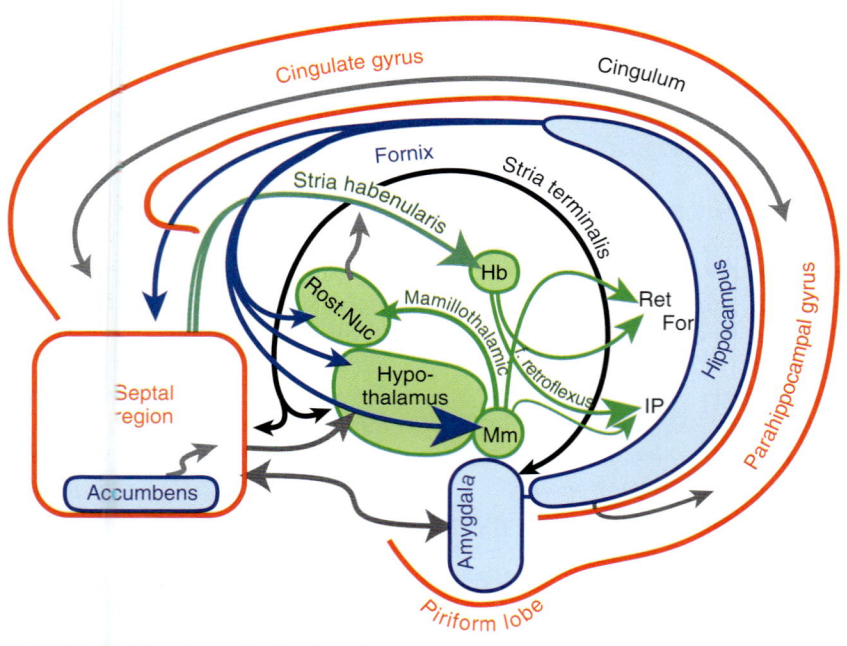

• **Fig. 18.39** Right side schematic drawing of components of the limbic system and their connections from a medial perspective. Cerebral cortex forms the outer rim of the limbic system (shown in *red*). Deeper telencephalic components (basal nuclei and hippocampus) are colored *blue*. Diencephalic nuclei are colored *green* and midbrain components are *black*. Axonal tracts connecting limbic components include cingulum (white matter within the cingulate gyrus), fornix (output from the hippocampus), stria terminalis (a major output of the amygdala), several diencephalic tracts (*green*) and various unlabeled connections. The nucleus accumbens projects to motor nuclei in addition to sharing septal connections and rostral thalamic nuclei project to the cingulate gyrus. (*Rost. Nuc,* Rostral thalamic nuclei; *Mm,* mamillary body; *Hb,* habenula; *IP,* interpeduncular nucleus; *Ret For,* reticular formation; *f.,* fasciculus.)

CHAPTER 18 The Brain   787

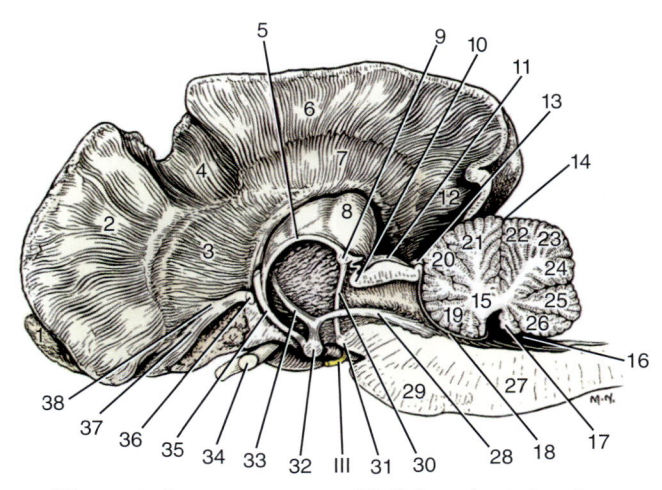

1. Olfactory bulb
2. Corona radiata of frontal lobe
3. Rostral crus of internal capsule
4. Cruciate sulcus
5. Stria habenularis thalami
6. Corona radiata of parietal lobe
7. Fibers in corona radiata derived from caudal crus of internal capsule
8. Dorsal aspect of thalamus
9. Habenular nucleus
10. Caudal commissure
11. Rostral colliculus
12. Corona radiata of occipital lobe
13. Caudal colliculus
14. Fissura prima
15. Cerebellum
16. Caudolateral fissure = uvulonodular fissure
17. Nodulus
18. Rostral medullary velum
19. Lingula
20. Culmen (rostral part)
21. Culmen (caudal part)
22. Declive
23. Folium vermis
24. Tuber vermis
25. Pyramis (vermis)
26. Uvula (vermis)
27. Medulla oblongata
28. Mamillotegmental tract
29. Pons
30. Fasciculus retroflexus
31. Location of interpeduncular nucleus
32. Mamillary body
33. Mamillothalamic tract
34. Optic chiasm
35. Column of fornix
36. Rostral commissure (at median plane)
37. Rostral part of rostral commissure
38. Caudal part of rostral commissure
III. Oculomotor nerve

• **Fig. 18.40** A median view of the right half of a brain with cerebral cortex, corpus callosum, hippocampus, and caudate nucleus removed, showing white matter that forms the lateral wall of the lateral ventricle (3 and 7). Connections of the mamillary body (32) and habenula (9) are shown, as are rostral (37) and caudal (38) components of the rostral commissure.

the splenium of the corpus callosum and caudomedial to the tubercle of the dentate gyrus; Fig. 18.30.)

Cerebral Neocortex

The term *neocortex* refers to surface gray matter covering the dorsal portion of cerebral hemisphere that is not rhinencephalon. Neocortex is composed of six layers, named from superficial to deep: **molecular** (*stratum moleculare*), **outer granular** (*stratum granulare externum*), **outer pyramidal** (*stratum pyramidale externum*), **inner granular** (*stratum granulare internum*), **inner pyramidal** (*stratum pyramidale internum*), and **multiform layer** (*stratum multiforme*) (Fig. 18.41). The molecular layer has relatively few cell bodies.

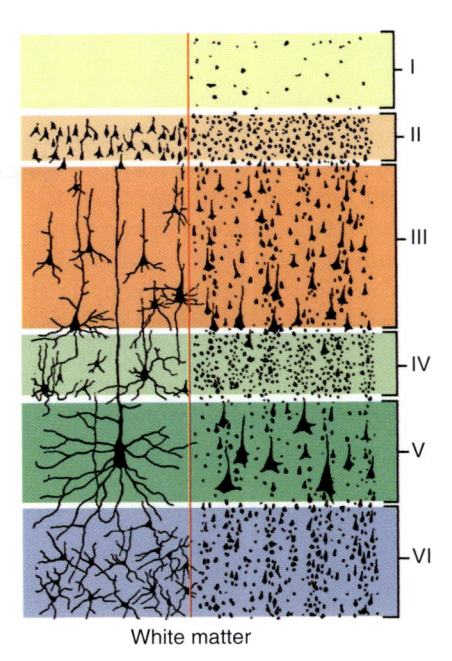

• **Fig. 18.41** Schematic illustration of the six horizontal layers characteristic of the cerebral neocortex. Layers vary in thickness among different regions of cortex. The left side shows individual cell profiles as would be seen in a Golgi stain. The right side shows populations of cell body profiles as would be seen in a Nissl stain. *I*, Molecular layer; *II*, outer granular layer; *III*, outer pyramidal layer; *IV*, inner granular layer; *V*, inner pyramidal layer; *VI*, multiform layer. (Modified from Ranson SW, Clark SL: *Anatomy of the nervous system*, 10th ed., Philadelphia, 1959, Saunders.)

The outer pyramidal neurons are smaller than those in the inner pyramidal layer. Both thickness of the six individual layers and the total depth of the cortex vary across different cortical regions.

Functionally, the cortex is organized into vertical columns (approximately 0.4 mm in diameter), such that all neurons within a column respond to the same specific feature of a particular stimulus. Thalamocortical projections from thalamic nuclei terminate in the internal granular layer, conveying the specific information pertinent to the cortical column. Nonspecific thalamocortical projections from intralaminar thalamic nuclei terminate in superficial cortical layers and function to alert cortical column neurons. Within a cortical column, granule cells serve as excitatory interneurons. Outer pyramidal neurons project axons to adjacent cortex. Inner pyramidal neurons project to distant locations. Multiform layer neurons project to the thalamus (Fig. 18.41).

White Matter Related to Neocortex

Cerebral white matter consists of commissural, projection, or association axons. Relative to the neocortex, axons composing white matter are either corticopedal or corticofugal. Commissural axons are corticofugal from one hemisphere and corticopedal to the other hemisphere. The largest commissure in the brain is the **corpus callosum**, which links corresponding neocortical regions of the two hemispheres, enabling the cerebrum to function coherently as a single cognitive center.

Projection axons travel outside the cerebrum or run from the neocortex to basal nuclei. Corticopedal projection axons typically arise from the thalamus, except for widely distributed axons from neuromodulation cell bodies located in the brainstem or rhinencephalon. Corticopedal axons from the thalamus run in the internal capsule. From lateral and medial geniculate nuclei, respectively, **optic** and **acoustic radiations** (*radiatio optica et acustica*) join the caudal limb of the internal capsule. Although corticofugal projection axons to the thalamus arise from the multiform layer, all other corticofugal axons originate from pyramidal neurons. Projection axons destined for basal nuclei, brainstem, or spinal cord enter the external or internal capsules (Fig. 18.29).

The **internal capsule** (*capsula interna*) is compressed between basal nuclei and thalamus. It exhibits a medially convex angle caudal to the head of the caudate nucleus. The angular region is termed the **genu of the internal capsule** (*genu capsulae internae*), and regions rostral and caudal to the genu are called **rostral crus** (*crus rostrale capsulae internae*) and **caudal crus** (*crus caudale capsuae internae*), respectively. The **external capsule** (*capsula externa*), located between the putamen and claustrum, is composed of projection axons to basal nuclei and axons from the caudal limb of the rostral commissure. An **extreme capsule** (*capsula extrema*) is present between the claustrum and adjacent insular cortex (Fig. 18.29).

Association axons are corticofugal from one cortical region and cortipedal to another region of cortex within the same hemisphere (Figs. 18.33 and 18.34). Association axons may connect adjacent gyri, **arcuate fibers** (*fibrae arcuatae cerebri*), or travel to distant regions, for example, the **superior longitudinal fasciculus** (*fasciculus longitudinalis superior*) from the occipital pole to the frontal pole, the **inferior longitudinal fasciculus** (*fasciculus longitudinalis inferior*) from the occipital pole to the ventral temporal region, and the **uncinate fasciculus** (*fasciculus uncinatus*) from the ventral temporal region to the ventral frontal region. The **cingulum** is a band of association axons that run deep to the cingulate gyrus, connecting the paraterminal gyrus of the septum to the parahippocampal gyrus in the temporal lobe. The *subcallosal fasciculus*, which is distinct in the roof of the lateral ventricle, has connections similar to the cingulum but it includes axons to the caudate nucleus.

Functional Regions of Neocortex

Neocortical regions vary in horizontal layer thicknesses and axonal connections according to their functional role (sensory, association, motor). Axonal connections between neocortical regions are typically reciprocal. Regional connections are made by direct exchange of axonal projections and also via cortico-thalamo-cortical circuits. The circuits involve basal nuclei in the case of motor functions.

Neocortical regions that are designated *primary sensory areas* are the first cortical regions to receive afferent input

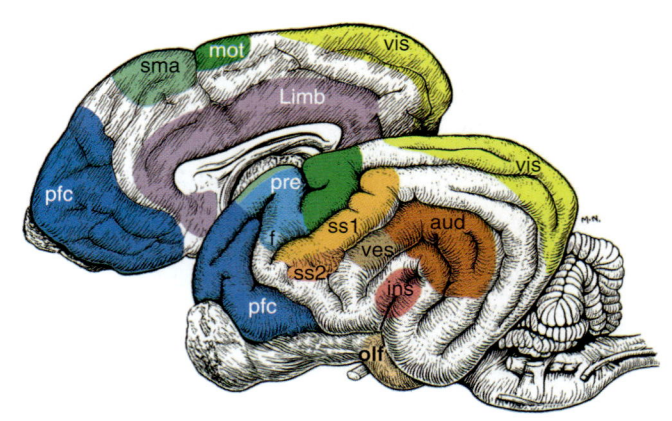

• **Fig. 18.42** Approximate locations of selected functional areas of cerebral cortex are shown in lateral and median views of canine cerebral hemispheres. The following abbreviations are used (*white labels* are movement related and *black labels* are sensory related): *aud*, auditory area; *f*, frontal eye field; *ins*, insular area; *limb*, limbic cortex; *mot*, motor cortex; *olf*, olfactory area; *pfc*, prefrontal cortex; *pre*, premotor cortex; *sma*, supplementary motor area; *ss1*, somatosensory area I; *ss2*, somatosensory area II; *ves*, vestibular area; *vis*, visual area.

for a particular sensory modality (Fig. 18.42). The primary cortical areas are surrounded by zones of *association cortex*, where increasingly complex levels of significance are extracted from the sensation. Ultimate zones of sensory association cortex amalgamate multimodal perception and memory into an ongoing world view. Neocortex of the frontal pole operates as an executive association cortex, deciding behavioral responses and initiating directive cascades to the premotor cortex for movement selection and the motor area for movement execution. Association areas constitute approximately 20% of the canine neocortex (versus 85% of the human neocortex).

The primary **somatosensory area** is located beside the coronal and ansate sulci (Fig. 18.42). The area receives tactile, kinesthetic, and nociceptive axonal projections from ventral caudal thalamic nuclei via the internal capsule. It is somatotopically organized with head representation facing rostrally. Cortical area (number of cortical columns) is proportional to receptor density per region; thus lips and face occupy more cortical area than does the back. Somatosensory cortex is the source of pyramidal tract axons that regulate sensory pathway traffic by altering synaptic transmission between primary afferent and projection neurons. An additional, smaller, somatotopic area is situated ventral to the primary area. It receives bilateral nociceptive input and is called *somatosensory area II*.

A **gustatory** (**taste**) **area** is adjacent to the tongue and pharynx area of the somatosensory cortex. The **insula gyrus** (*gyri insulae*), buried deep to the pseudosylvian fissure, receives sensory information originating from viscera. (The olfactory sensory area is in the piriform lobe of the rhinencephalon.)

The primary **visual area** surrounds the caudal half of the marginal gyrus (Fig. 18.42). The visual area receives axonal input from the lateral geniculate nucleus. Geniculate projections compose the *optic radiation* (*radiatio optica*) of the internal capsule. The visual area is arranged retinotopically. The *area centralis* (visual streak) of the retina, where cones are concentrated, occupies an expanded proportion of the visual area compared with other retinal regions where rods dominate. The two components of visual information (cone-generated detailed vision and rod-generated movement and size detection) reach the same visual area, but the two components are dispersed to separate zones of visual association cortex.

The primary **auditory area** of the dog is centered around the middle ectosylvian gyrus, which receives tonotopic input from the ventral portion of the medial geniculate nucleus (Kowalska, 2000). The caudal ectosylvian and sylvian gyri receive nontonotopic input. Axons from the medial geniculate nucleus arrive via the *acoustic radiation* (*radiatio acustica*) of the internal capsule. Dorsal and rostral regions of the sylvian gyrus are auditory association cortex. A primary **vestibular area** is rostral to the auditory area.

Prefrontal association cortex occupies the frontal pole. It directs goal-oriented behavior, sending projections to premotor cortex for movement selection. The prefrontal cortex processes emotional status and cognitive perception as a prelude to deciding, planning, and temporally organizing behavior directed toward achieving goals. Attention to goal-oriented behavior involves short-term working memory and suppression of distracting influences, including inappropriate emotional behavior.

Prefrontal cortex is identified by corticopedal projections from the dorsomedial thalamic nucleus. The cortex has broad connections to association and premotor neocortex; additionally, it sends axons to the caudate nucleus, cerebellum, and hypothalamus. The medial portion of the prefrontal cortex has abundant limbic connections; the lateral portion has strong somatic (premotor) connections.

The **premotor cortex** is located between the prefrontal cortex and the motor cortex. It receives projections from the former and projects to the latter. Premotor cortex is active particularly during complex movement selection and while learning new movements. Also, patterns of sequential rapid movements are encoded in premotor regions. Premotor cortex drives the motor cortex via circuits involving basal and thalamic nuclei. Premotor projection axons join the pyramidal tract and synapse on pontine nuclei that project to the cerebellum.

The premotor cortex is actually a collection of related cortical regions including a frontal eye field and supplemental motor area. The *frontal eye field* is involved in visual attention and visually tracking objects of interest. The **supplementary motor area** extends onto the medial surface of the hemisphere and features a separate somatotopic arrangement of the entire body. The area is active when movements are being contemplated or observed prior to movement execution. The supplemental cortex receives projections from prefrontal cortex and projects to motor cortex.

The **motor cortex** occupies the postcruciate gyrus; head representation is positioned laterally (Breazile & Thompson, 1967; Buxton & Goodman, 1967). The cortex is somatotopically organized with respect to joint movement (i.e., individual projection neurons activate multiple muscles producing a particular joint movement). The degree of excitation of cortical projection neurons is related to movement force and amplitude. The motor cortex contributes the majority of the pyramidal tract corticospinal and corticonuclear axons. It is also the main driver of movement involving extrapyramidal tracts via projections to the red nucleus and nuclei that give rise to pontine and medullary reticulospinal tracts (Fig. 18.43).

The motor cortex itself can execute movements that are simple, automatic, or habitual in response to trigger stimuli (e.g., from somatosensory cortical input). In the case of movements that are complex or being learned, the motor cortex is driven by the premotor cortex. In either situation, the motor cortex is activated via circuits involving basal and thalamic nuclei, including cerebellar-thalamic circuit involvement.

Basal Nuclei

Anatomically, the term **basal nuclei** refers to noncortical gray matter of the cerebral hemisphere. (Note that the term *basal ganglia* is a commonly used but anatomically improper synonym for *basal nuclei*.) Telencephalic basal nuclei include accumbens, caudate, putamen, pallidum (globus pallidus), endopeduncular, claustrum, and amygdala (Fig. 18.44). The amygdala assigns emotional context to sensory information; it is a major component of the limbic system. The function of the claustrum is unknown. The remaining basal nuclei operate within movement control circuits involving the cerebral cortex, thalamus, and cerebellum. In this context, the term *basal nuclei* is often expanded to include nuclei found in the diencephalon (subthalamic nucleus) and mesencephalon (substantia nigra).

Historical ways of grouping basal nuclei, for example, *corpus striatum* (all telencephalic nuclei), *neostriatum* (caudate and putamen), and *lentiform nucleus* (putamen and pallidum) are not functionally useful. Stripes of gray matter that intersect the internal capsule give rise to the term *striatum*. **Striatum**, including accumbens, caudate, and putamen nuclei, is a useful grouping in the context of movement control.

Telencephalic basal nuclei, which contain inhibitory GABAergic neurons, participate in circuits responsible for movement selection and execution. The overall role of basal nuclei in these circuits is selective inhibition of unwanted movement and release of desired movement, avoiding what otherwise would be a massive uncontrolled motor output (Brooks, 1986). Pending cortical input, basal nuclei selectively suppress thalamocortical circuits and the cerebellum selectively excites thalamocortical circuits. Thus when motivated by limbic drive and decided upon by prefrontal cortex, voluntary movements are then selected and executed via circuits involving basal nuclei (cerebellar circuits monitor ongoing movement progress) (Fig. 18.43).

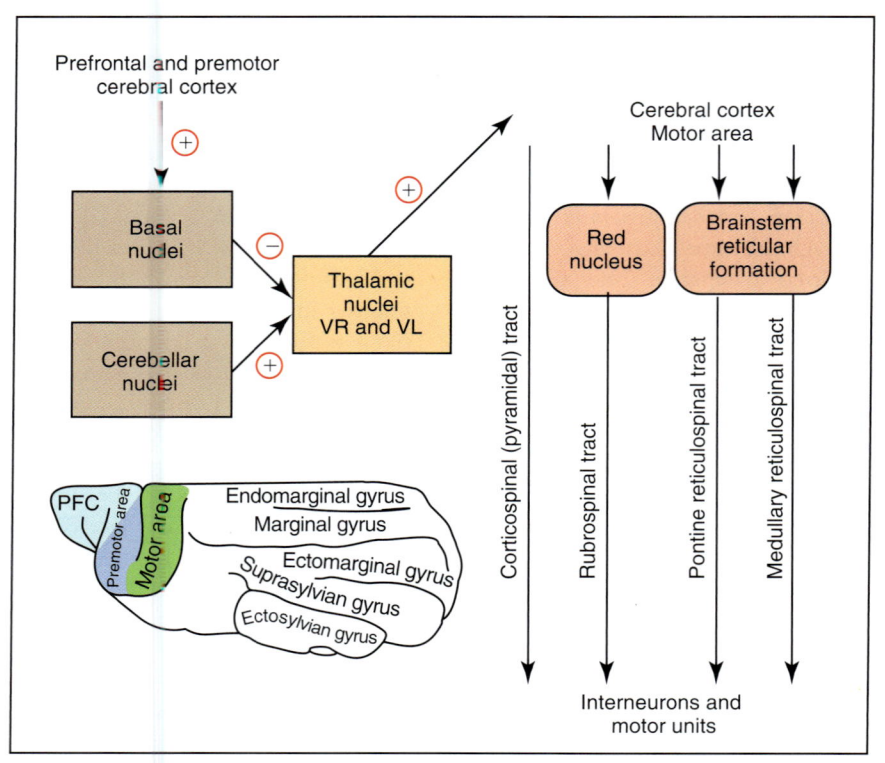

• **Fig. 18.43** Diagram of circuitry involved in voluntary movement. In general, voluntary movements are decided by prefrontal cortex, selected by premotor cortex, and executed by the motor area of the cerebral cortex. The motor area drives voluntary movement via four descending tracts that influence motor units through interneurons. The selection of desired movements and suppression of unwanted movements involve basal nuclei circuits that inhibit thalamic projections to the motor cortex (ventral rostral [*VR*] nucleus). The cerebellum corrects errors in ongoing movements via cerebellar nuclei that excite thalamic projections to the motor cortex (ventral lateral [*VL*] nucleus). The brain image inset shows locations of the motor area, premotor area, and prefrontal cortex (*PFC*).

Individual basal nuclei have input and output roles within movement control circuits (Fig. 18.45). The three basal nuclei of the striatum receive cortical input. Limbic impact is funneled to the *accumbens nucleus*. The *caudate nucleus* is the particular target of association cortex. Control of movement execution is directed to the *putamen*. These striate nuclei project axons to the *globus pallidus* and *endopeduncular nucleus*, both of which contain spontaneously active inhibitory projection neurons. The endopeduncular nucleus provides final output to the thalamus. A *direct path* from input basal nuclei to the endopeduncular nucleus facilitates (disinhibits) desired movement. An *indirect path* suppresses unwanted movement by inhibiting the globus pallidus. Another route for movement suppression is provided by cortical control of the subthalamic nucleus. Net facilitation of movement results from neuromodulation of direct and indirect paths via dopamine released by substantia nigra compacta. (The substantia nigra reticulata tonically inhibits the rostral colliculus and saccadic eye movements.)

The **caudate nucleus** (*nucleus caudatus*) is bounded medially by the lateral ventricle and laterally by the internal capsule (Fig. 18.29). The rostral enlargement of the nucleus is the head (*caput nuclei caudati*). Caudal to the head, the body (*corpus nuclei caudati*) tapers into a tail (*cauda nuclei caudati*), which loops caudal to the internal capsule and terminates near the amygdala (Fig. 18.44). The caudate nucleus receives projections from the prefrontal and premotor cortical regions. It is active particularly during complex movement selection and learning.

The **nucleus accumbens** (*nucleus accumbens*) can be found ventral to the head of the caudate nucleus, interposed between the caudate nucleus and septal region (Fig. 18.44). The accumbens nucleus receives projections from medial prefrontal and limbic (cingulate; parahippocampal) cortex, as well as amygdala, insula cortex, and piriform entorhinal cortex. Accumbens projections go to the hypothalamus and habenula in addition to other basal nuclei.

The **putamen** is situated between internal and external capsules. It is linked to the head of the caudate nucleus by strands of gray matter that penetrate the internal capsule (Fig. 18.29). The putamen receives projections from sensory and motor areas of neocortex. It is active during simple movements, regulating movement amplitude and force.

The **globus pallidus** or **pallidum** (*pallidum* [*globus pallidus*]) is located medial to the putamen and lateroventral to the internal capsule. The nucleus has a reticulated appearance because many white matter bundles penetrate it (Fig. 18.26). A **lateral medullary lamina** (*lamina medullaris*

Basal Nuclei

Lateral View   **Medial View**

1 Accumbens
2 Caudate
3 Endopeduncular
4 Globus pallidus
5 Putamen
6 Amygdala
7 Claustrum

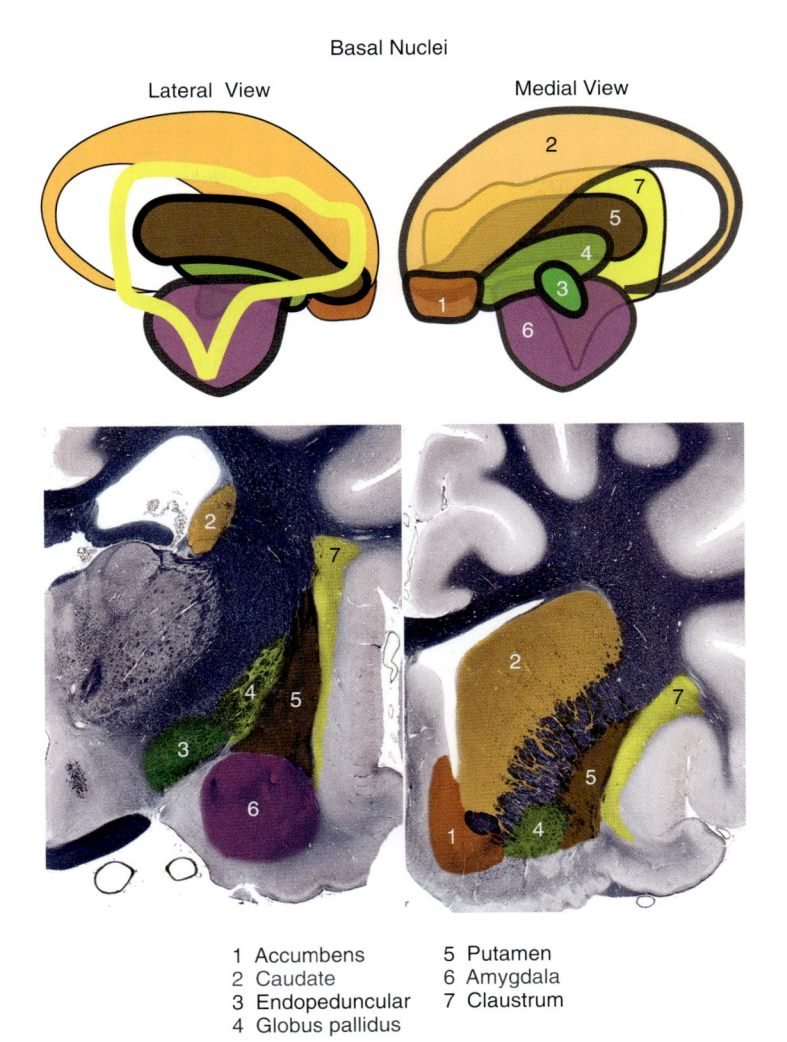

• **Fig. 18.44** *Top,* Schematic drawing of telencephalic basal nuclei of the right cerebral hemisphere, shown in lateral and medial views. Only the outline of the claustrum is shown in the lateral view. Nuclei names are displayed in colors that match their respective nuclear colors. Names and numbers are listed in approximate medial to lateral order. *Bottom,* Approximate transverse sections through the right cerebral hemisphere at the level of the optic chiasm (*left*) and the frontal lobe (*right*). Respective basal nuclei are numbered and shown in colors that correspond to those displayed previously. (*1,* Accumbens; *2,* caudate; *3,* endopeduncular; *4,* globus pallidus; *5,* putamen; *6,* amygdala; *7,* claustrum.) (*Top,* Nuclear topography is based on Vakolyuk NI: *A stereotaxic atlas of subcortical nuclei of the dog's brain,* Kiev, 1974, Academy of Sciences of the Ukrainian SSR.)

lateralis) is located between the globus pallidus and the putamen and a **medial medullary lamina** (*lamina medullaris medialis*) separates globus pallidus from **endopeduncular nucleus** (*nucleus endopeduncularis*) (Fig. 18.24). The globus pallidus inhibits the endopeduncular nucleus, alleviating movement suppression that the endopeduncular nucleus imposes on thalamocortical circuits. Both nuclei are tonically active and controlled by other basal nuclei. (Note that the endopeduncular nucleus of the carnivore corresponds to the internal or medial globus pallidus division of the primate.)

The **claustrum** forms a broad plate between the extreme capsule and insular cortex laterally to the external capsule medially (Fig. 18.26). The function of the claustrum is not understood, but it has broad connections with wide areas of cerebral cortex, including the visual system (Berman & Jones, 1982). The ventral part of the claustrum, which merges with insular cortex, may be related to the limbic system.

The **amygdala** (amygdaloid body) is a rhinencephalic basal nucleus located within the piriform lobe. It is a major component of the limbic system, responsible for implementing emotional reactions. It has reciprocal projections with the prefrontal cortex, but most of its connections are with the limbic components. This was described in detail in the section discussing the rhinencephalon.

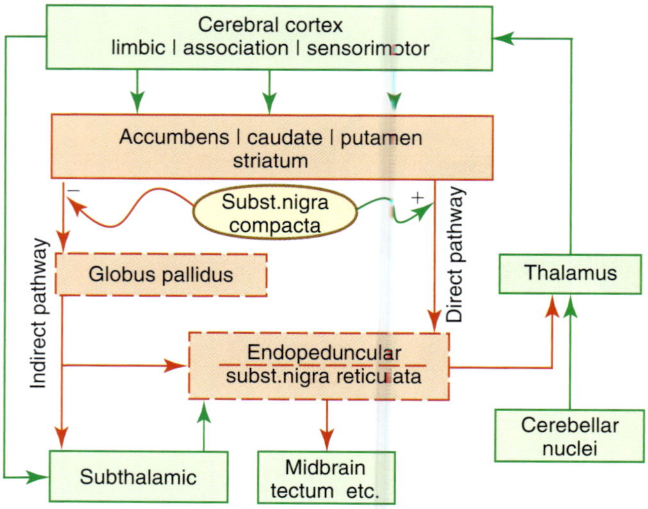

• **Fig. 18.45** Diagram of basal nuclei circuits for selecting and executing movements (*green*, excitatory; *red*, inhibitory; *dotted outline*, spontaneously active). The basal nuclei shown here facilitate desired movements and dampen unwanted movements. Voluntary movements initiated by the cerebral cortex involve thalamocortical circuits propelled by excitation from cerebellar nuclei. Particular regions of cerebral cortex project to three basal nuclei (accumbens, caudate, and putamen) that collectively constitute the striatum. Via two pathways, the striatum controls spontaneously active neurons within basal nuclei that tonically inhibit thalamocortical movement circuits (also midbrain-generated movements). A *direct pathway* facilitates desired movements, via inhibition of the endopeduncular nucleus (and substantia nigra reticulata). An *indirect pathway* suppresses unwanted movement (by inhibiting the globus pallidus, which tonically inhibits endopeduncular and subthalamic nuclei). The cerebral cortex is able to suppress movements directly via input to the subthalamic nucleus, which enhances endopeduncular inhibition. The substantia nigra reticulata tonically inhibits the midbrain tectum, the red nucleus and reticular formation nuclei. Via dopamine release that targets excitatory and inhibitory dopamine receptors on striatal neurons, the substantia nigra compacta modulates the two striatal pathways, favoring movement.

THE CEREBELLUM

The cerebellum coordinates posture and movement by regulating muscle tone and joint action. The cerebellum detects errors in ongoing movement and sends corrective excitatory output to upper motor neurons in the brainstem and thalamocortical circuits that drive voluntary movement. The cerebellar cortex of the flocculonodular lobe corrects vestibular reflex errors. Beyond movement, the cerebellum is crucial for sensorimotor timing, including visual guidance of movement; also, the cerebellum is necessary for judging the distance rate of change of an approaching object or wall. Finally, cerebellar involvement in cognition has been reported, particularly in primates (Salman, 2010).

The cerebellum is the dorsal component of the metencephalon (Fig. 18.46). The entire cerebellum can be partitioned into a median **vermis** and bilateral **cerebellar hemispheres** (*hemispherium cerebelli*). The cerebellum can be further subdivided into lobes and lobules separated by fissures (Table 18.2) (Larsell, 1970). The cerebellar surface features narrow ridges (*folia cerebelli*) separated by grooves (*sulci cerebelli*). Each ridge is called a **folium**, and each groove is a **sulcus**.

A **uvulonodular fissure** (*fissura uvulonodularis*) divides the cerebellum into a small **flocculonodular lobe** (*lobus flocculonodularis*) and a **cerebellar body** (*corpus cerebelli*). The body is divided by the **primary fissure** (*fissura prima*) into a **rostral lobe** (*lobus rostralis*) and a **caudal lobe** (*lobus caudalis*) (Fig. 18.47). These three lobes are phylogenetically and functionally distinct.

The **flocculonodular lobe** (archicerebellum; vestibulocerebellum) functions like a vestibular nucleus (nystagmus and wide-base stance can result when it is damaged). The **rostral lobe** (paleocerebellum; spinocerebellum) has connections with the spinal cord and regulates posture and gait (opisthotonus and ataxia can result when it is damaged). The **caudal lobe** (neocerebellum; cerebrocerebellum) connects to the forebrain and affects voluntary movement, including premovement preparation (dysmetria is one consequence of caudal lobe damage).

The major histological components of the cerebellum are cortex, white matter, and nuclei. The **cerebellar cortex** (*cortex cerebelli*) is surface gray matter. The cortex features large inhibitory Purkinje (piriform) neurons. Their axons are the sole output from the cerebellar cortex. The axons terminate in cerebellar nuclei, or in vestibular nuclei in the case of flocculonodular cortex.

On a median section through the cerebellum, white matter has the appearance of tree branches and is called the **arbor vitae**. The arbor is composed of a **lamina** (*lamina albae*) within each folium and a center mass (*corpus medullare*) referred to as **cerebellar medulla**.

Axons within cerebellar white matter can be categorized as afferent or efferent relative to the cerebellum and as corticopedal or corticofugal relative to the cerebellar cortex. Corticofugal axons are from Purkinje cells. They are inhibitory and terminate in vestibular or cerebellar nuclei. Axons arising from cerebellar nuclei are excitatory. They exit the cerebellum as efferent axons in cerebellar peduncles.

Afferent axons enter the cerebellum through cerebellar peduncles. They are excitatory. All afferent axons send collateral branches to cerebellar nuclei before terminating in the cerebellar cortex. There are two kinds of corticopedal afferent axons based on their terminal endings in the cortex. *Climbing fiber* afferents come from the olivary nucleus, which preprocesses proprioceptor and motor center information. *Mossy endings* are found on all other cerebellar afferents (both proprioception and upper motor neuron input).

Cerebellar Nuclei

Bilaterally, three **cerebellar nuclei** are embedded deeply within cerebellar white matter. From medial to lateral, they are **fastigial nucleus** (*nucleus fastigii*), **interpositus nucleus** (*nucleus interpositus cerebelli*), and **lateral nucleus** (*nucleus lateralis cerebelli*, formerly called the dentate nucleus) (Fig. 18.46). Except for Purkinje axons that are directed to vestibular nuclei, all efferent axons leaving the cerebellum

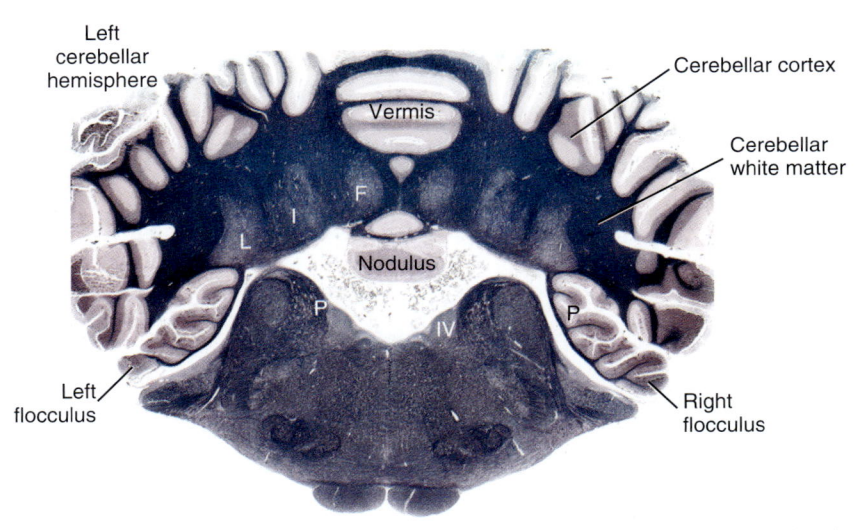

• **Fig. 18.46** Transverse section through the cerebellum and rostral medulla oblongata of a dog. The cerebellum consists of bilateral hemispheres and a midline vermis. The nodulus is the most caudoventral lobule of the vermis. The flocculus is a ventral lobule of each hemisphere. Three cerebellar nuclei, fastigial (F), interpositus (I) and the lateral (L) are located bilaterally within cerebellar white matter. Cerebellar cortex covers the white matter surface. Caudal cerebellar peduncles (P) and medial vestibular nuclei (IV) are evident within the medulla oblongata. (The axons streaming dorsal to each peduncle constitute acoustic stria; they come from dorsal cochlear nucleus and vestibular nerve.) (Luxol Blue–Cresyl Violet stain.)

TABLE 18.2 Equivalents of Descriptive and Numerical Nomenclature of Cerebellar Lobules[a]

VERMIS				HEMISPHERIUM	
		Corpus Cerebelli			
		Lobus Rostralis			
Lingula		Lob. I	Lob. H. I	Vinculum lingulae	
Lob. centralis		Lob. I1	Lob. H. II	Ala lob. centralis	
		Lob. 111	Lob. H. III		
Culmen	P. rostralis	Lob. IV	Lob. H. IV	P. rostralis	Lob. quadrangularis
	P. caudalis	Lob. V	Lob. H. V	P. caudalis	
			Fissura Prima		
			Lobus Caudalis		
Declive		Lob. VI	Lob. H. VI	Lobulus simplex	
Folium vermis		Lob. VII A	Lob. H. VII A	Crus rostrale	Lob. ansiformis
Tuber vermis		Lob. VII B	Lob. H. VII B	Crus caudale	
		Lob. VIII A	Lob. H. VIII A	Lobulus paramedianus	
Pyramis		Lob. VIII B	Lob. H. VIII B	Paraflocculus dorsalis	
Uvula		Lob. IX	Lob. H. IX	Paraflocculus ventralis	
			Fissura Uvulonodularis		
			Lobus Flocculonodularis		
Nodulus		Lob. X	Lob. H. X	Flocculus	

[a]From *Nomina Anatomica Veterinaria*, 2005; for lobule descriptions Larsell (1970).

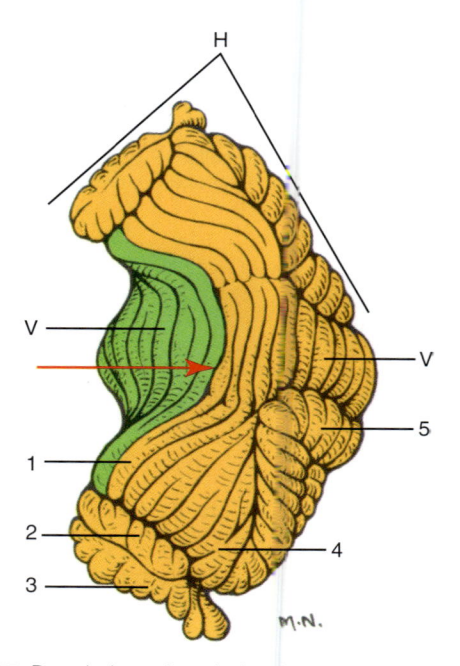

• **Fig. 18.47** Dorsal view of an isolated cerebellum, drawn from a rostrolateral perspective. The primary fissure (arrow) divides the cerebellar body into a rostral lobe (green) and a caudal lobe (orange). The cerebellum is composed of a median vermis (V) and bilateral hemispheres (H). Lobules of the cerebellar hemisphere caudal lobe are lobulus simplex (1), dorsal paraflocculus (2), ventral paraflocculus (3), ansiform lobule (4), and paramedian lobule (5).

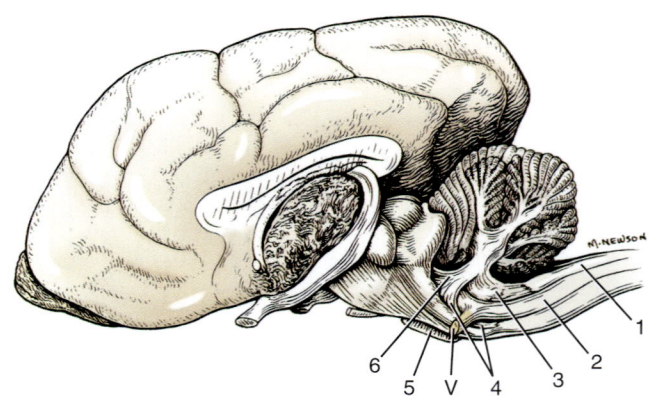

1. Fasciculus cuneatus
2. Spinal tract of trigeminal nerve
3. Caudal cerebellar peduncle
4. Ventral spinocerebellar tract
5. Transverse fibers of pons (transected on midline)
6. Rostral cerebellar peduncle
V. Trigeminal nerve

• **Fig. 18.48** Lateral view of a brain with the left cerebral hemisphere removed and the brainstem and cerebellum dissected to show rostral (6) and caudal (3) cerebellar peduncles. The middle cerebellar peduncle is formed by transverse pontine fibers, shown transected (5).

originate from cerebellar nuclei. All cerebellar afferent axons are excitatory and send excitatory collateral branches to cerebellar nuclei before terminating in the cerebellar cortex. Cerebellar nuclei receive inhibitory input from Purkinje axons of the cortex. Thus, the cerebellar cortex modulates excitatory output from cerebellar nuclei.

Based on direct axonal projections from cerebellar cortex to the nearest cerebellar nuclei, the cerebellum can be functionally partitioned into three bilateral longitudinal zones. The **vermis zone**, located most medially, projects to the fastigial nucleus. This zone activates vestibulospinal and reticulospinal tracts and regulates muscle tone in connection with posture and locomotion. The **paravermis zone**, located immediately lateral to the vermis, projects to the interpositus nucleus, which regulates joints of limbs via the rubrospinal tract. The **lateral** or **hemispheric zone** projects to the lateral nucleus, which projects to the ventral lateral thalamic nucleus to impact motor cortex excitation.

Cerebellar Peduncles

The cerebellum is attached bilaterally to the brainstem by three cerebellar peduncles that convey afferent and efferent cerebellar axons (Figs. 18.4 and 18.48). The **caudal cerebellar peduncle** (*pedunculus cerebellaris caudalis*) contains both afferent and efferent axons. It connects the cerebellum with the pons, medulla oblongata, and spinal cord (Fig. 18.49). The caudal peduncle may be regarded as having two components: a *restiform body* (*corpus restiforme*) and a *juxtarestiform body* (*corpus juxtarestiforme*). The latter refers to the medial part of the peduncle that contains cerebellar efferent axons to reticular formation nuclei, reciprocal connections with vestibular nuclei, and afferent axons from the vestibular nerve. The remaining restiform body conveys cerebellar afferent axons from the brainstem and spinal cord.

The contralateral olivary nucleus sends olivocerebellar climbing axons to the entire cerebellar cortex through the caudal cerebellar peduncle. Spinal proprioceptive and tactile information destined for vermal and paravermal cerebellar zones reaches the caudal peduncle via the dorsal spinocerebellar tract (caudal half of body) and lateral cuneate nucleus (neck and thoracic limb). Via the caudal peduncle, vermal and paravermal zones receive descending tract information from brainstem nuclei (lateral reticular nucleus, paramedian reticular nucleus, and pontine tegmental reticular nucleus). The nucleus of the solitary tract sends visceral axonal input to the vermis via the caudal peduncle.

The **middle cerebellar peduncle** (*pedunculus cerebellaris medius*) is entirely afferent to the cerebellum (Fig. 18.49). The middle peduncle, also called *brachium pontis*, is formed by projections to lateral and paravermal cerebellar zones from cell bodies in contralateral pontine nuclei. The axons travel along the ventral surface of the pons as transverse pontine fibers before becoming the middle cerebellar peduncle. The pontine nuclei receive information from the cerebral cortex via axons that travel through the internal capsule, crus cerebri, and corticopontine tract within the ventral pons. The pontine nuclei also receive axonal input from rostral and caudal colliculi.

The **rostral cerebellar peduncle** (*pedunculus cerebellaris rostralis*) is composed of efferent axons from interpositus and lateral cerebellar nuclei, plus some afferent axons (rubrocerebellar and spinocerebellar). The efferent axons

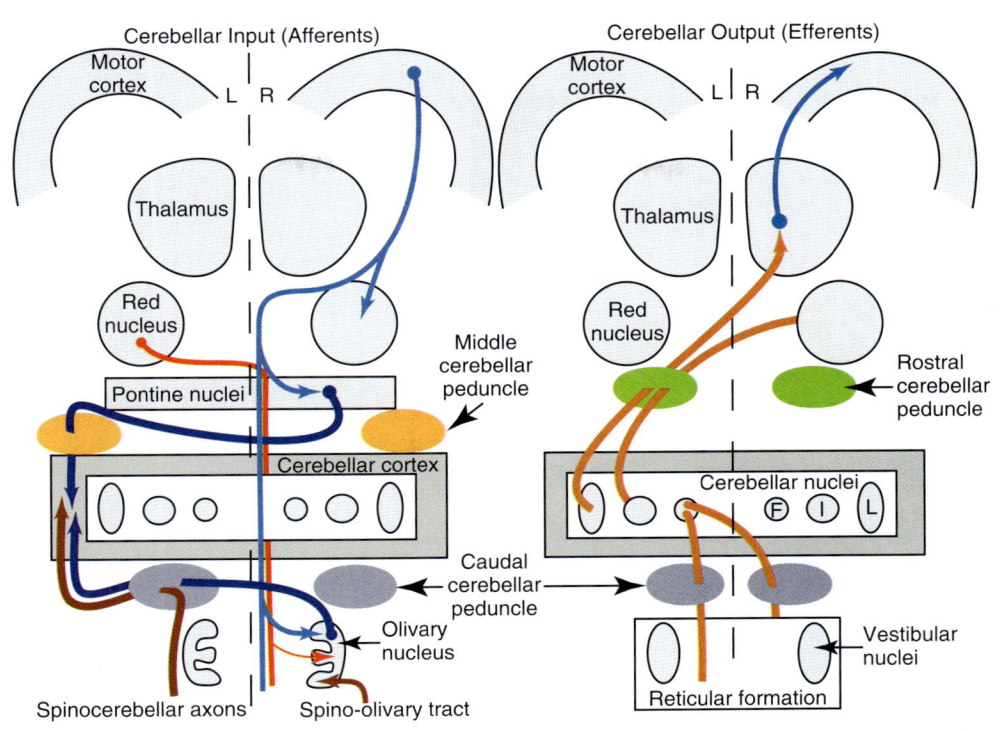

• **Fig. 18.49** Diagram of major axonal input to the cerebellum and output from cerebellar nuclei to the brainstem. *Left,* Afferent axons terminate ultimately in cerebellar cortex. *Right,* Efferent axons originate from cerebellar nuclei (*F,* fastigial; *I,* interpositus; *L,* lateral). The rostral cerebellar peduncle (*green*) conveys output to contralateral motor centers (red nucleus and motor cortex via the thalamus). The middle cerebellar peduncle (*orange*) conveys input from the contralateral motor cortex, via pontine nuclei. The caudal cerebellar peduncle (*blue*) connects to the pons-medulla. The fastigial nucleus sends axons bilaterally to reticular formation and vestibular nuclei. Each caudal peduncle conveys ipsilateral spinal cord input and climbing axons from the contralateral olivary nucleus, which preprocesses spinal and motor content. (Omitted are ventral spinocerebellar tracts that travel through the rostral cerebellar peduncle and cortical output to vestibular nuclei.)

decussate in the caudal midbrain and terminate in contralateral brainstem nuclei (Fig. 18.49). The interpositus nucleus sends axons to the magnocellular part of the red nucleus to modulate activity of the rubrospinal tract. Both interpositus and lateral nuclei project to thalamic nuclei (ventral rostral, ventral lateral, and centrum medianum). The interpositus nucleus innervates thalamic neurons that project to the motor cortex. The lateral nucleus innervates thalamic neurons that project to premotor and supplemental motor areas.

Neuronal cell bodies of the lateral cerebellar nucleus become excited prior to the onset of a movement, whereas interpositus and fastigial neurons become excited during movement execution. The lateral nucleus sends axons to the oculomotor nucleus, to parvicellular neurons of the red nucleus that project to the thalamus, and to the olivary nucleus and reticular nuclei that project to the cerebellum.

The rostral cerebellar peduncle also conveys afferent axons from two spinal tracts. The ventral spinocerebellar tract arises from spinal projection neurons that receive synaptic input similar to that of spinal motor neurons. The axons that decussate in the spinal cord then decussate again within the cerebellum. The ventral spinocerebellar tract is concerned with the caudal half of the body. Comparable axonal input from the thoracic limb and neck is conveyed ipsilaterally in the cranial spinocerebellar tract, which runs with the ventral spinocerebellar tract but contributes axons to both caudal and rostral cerebellar peduncles.

The Cerebellar Cortex

The cerebellar cortex is composed of three layers: a superficial, cell-sparse, **molecular layer** (*stratum moleculare*); a deep **granule cell layer** (*stratum granulosum*); and an intermediate layer (*stratum neuronorum piriformium*) of **Purkinje** (*piriform neuron*) **cells** (Fig. 18.50).

Purkinje (piriform) neuronal cell bodies align in a row at the interface of the superficial and deep cortical layers. Purkinje neurons are inhibitory, as are basket-cell neurons located deep in the molecular layer and the Golgi neurons found within the granule cell layer. Granule neurons are the only excitatory neurons in the cerebellar cortex.

Purkinje neurons have broad, flattened dendritic trees that extend into the molecular layer, oriented with the broad dendritic surface perpendicular to the longitudinal axis of the folium. Axons of Purkinje neurons, the only output from the cerebellar cortex, terminate in cerebellar nuclei (or vestibular nuclei in the case of the flocculonodular lobe).

Granule neurons send axons into the molecular layer. The axons bifurcate and course longitudinally in the folium, synapsing on dendritic trees of numerous Purkinje neurons.

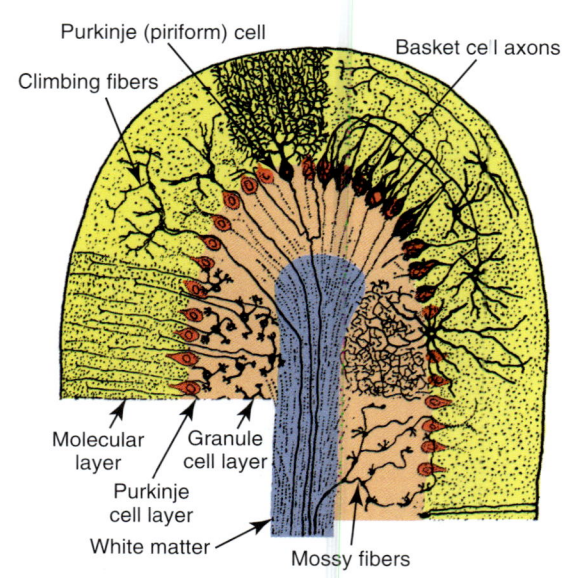

- **Fig. 18.50** Drawing of a transverse section through a cerebellar folium. The folium has a core of white matter (*blue*) surrounded by cerebellar cortex. The white matter is composed of climbing and mossy corticopedal axons and corticofugal axons from Purkinje (piriform) neurons. The cerebellar cortex consists of three layers (labeled sideways). The molecular layer (*yellow*) has relatively few cell bodies. The Purkinje (piriform) cell layer is evident as a row of large cell bodies (*dark orange*). The granule cell layer (*pale orange*) is composed of small neurons that send axons into the molecular layer. The axons course longitudinally in the folium and synapse on dendritic trees of Purkinje cells. Cell bodies of basket cells (generally located deep in the molecular layer) send axons transversely in the folium. The axons terminate in basket arrangements around adjacent Purkinje cell bodies. (From Cajal, modification of Fig. 200, in Ranson SW: Clark SL: *The anatomy of the nervous system,* 10th ed., Philadelphia, 1959, Saunders.)

Granule neurons also excite basket-cell neurons that project transversely in a folium and inhibit laterally positioned Purkinje neurons. Thus granule neurons excite a longitudinal band of Purkinje neurons, and, via basket cells, they inhibit Purkinje neurons positioned bilateral to the band. Purkinje neuronal excitability is translated into inhibition at the level of cerebellar nuclei where Purkinje axons terminate.

Afferent axons to the cerebellar cortex are categorized as **mossy fibers** or **climbing fibers**, based on terminal branch morphology (Fig. 18.50). Climbing axons come from the olivary nucleus. Each axon intensely activates one Purkinje neuron by climbing along its dendritic tree and forming numerous synapses. All other afferent axons to the cerebellar cortex terminate as mossy fibers. Mossy endings terminate within glomerular synaptic complexes, exciting a number of granule cell dendrites. All afferent axons send excitatory collateral branches to cerebellar nuclei before proceeding to the cortex.

To serve its regulatory function, the cerebellum compares axonal input from motor command sites with proprioceptive and tactile information generated by ongoing movements. Cerebellar nuclei project excitatory drive to motor command sites. The cerebellar cortex selectively inhibits ongoing excitatory drive from cerebellar nuclei, via Purkinje axon projections to the nuclei.

The olivary nucleus and the cerebellum are closely related and damage to either structure produces similar deficits of coordination (Brooks, 1986; Murphy & O'Leary, 1971). The olivary nucleus receives and processes motor command and proprioceptive axonal input. Climbing fiber axonal output from the olivary nucleus activates selective microzones within the cerebellar cortex.

Brain Atlas

Appended are 10 plates that represent a sampling of sections through a canine brain (Fig. 18.51). The reader is also directed to an atlas of brain anatomy (Fletcher, 2016).

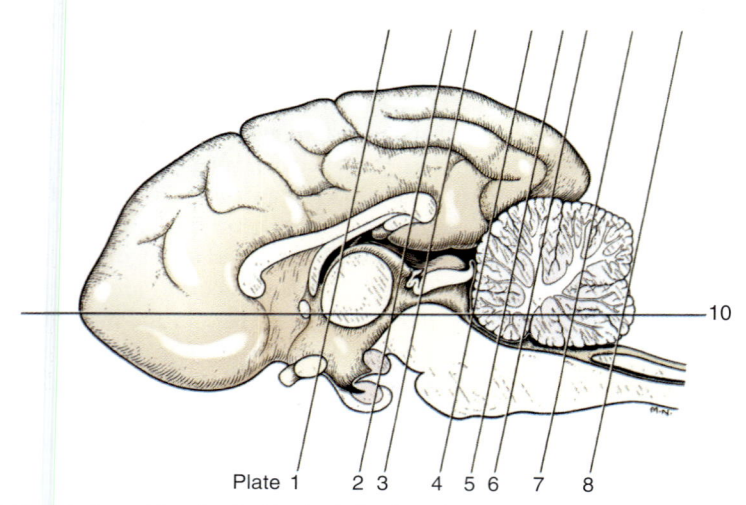

- **Fig. 18.51** Medial view of hemisected brain, indicating planes of transverse and horizontal sections shown in plates 1 through 10. Plate 9 represents a paramedian section.

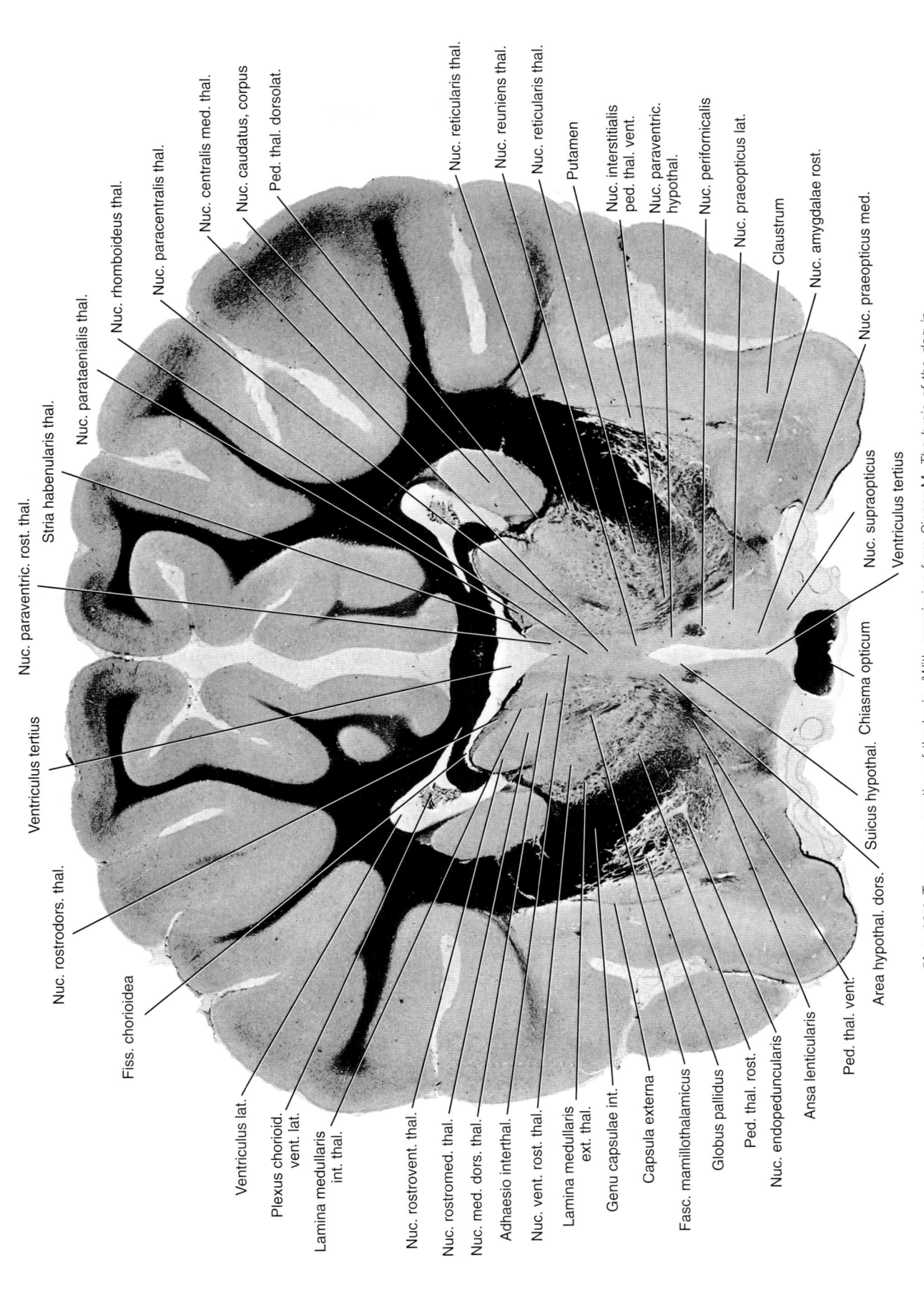

Plate 18.1 Transverse section of the brain. (With permission from Singer M: *The brain of the dog in section*, Philadelphia, 1962, Saunders.)

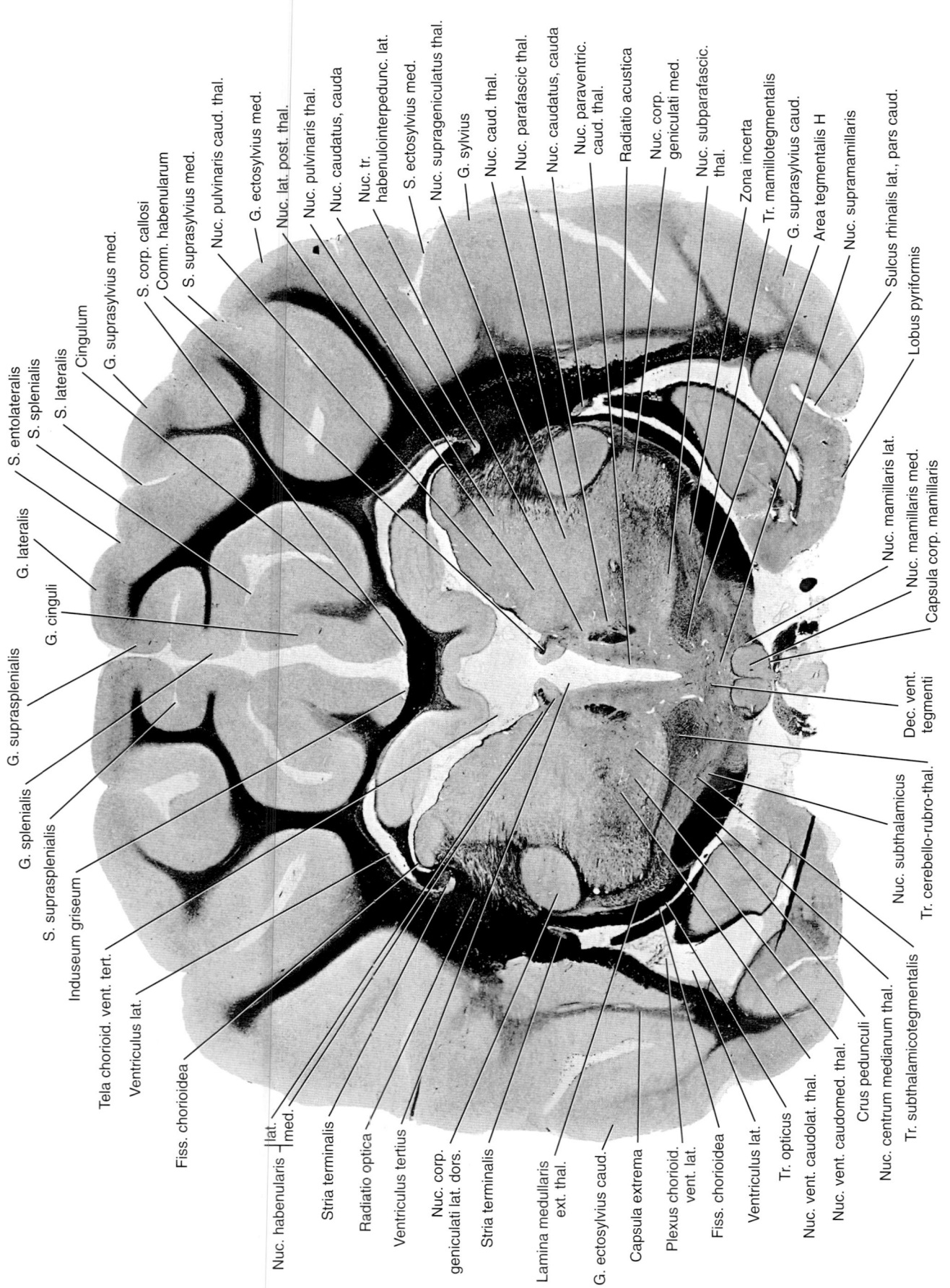

Plate 18.2 Transverse section of the brain. (With permission from Singer M: *The brain of the dog in section*, Philadelphia, 1962, Saunders.)

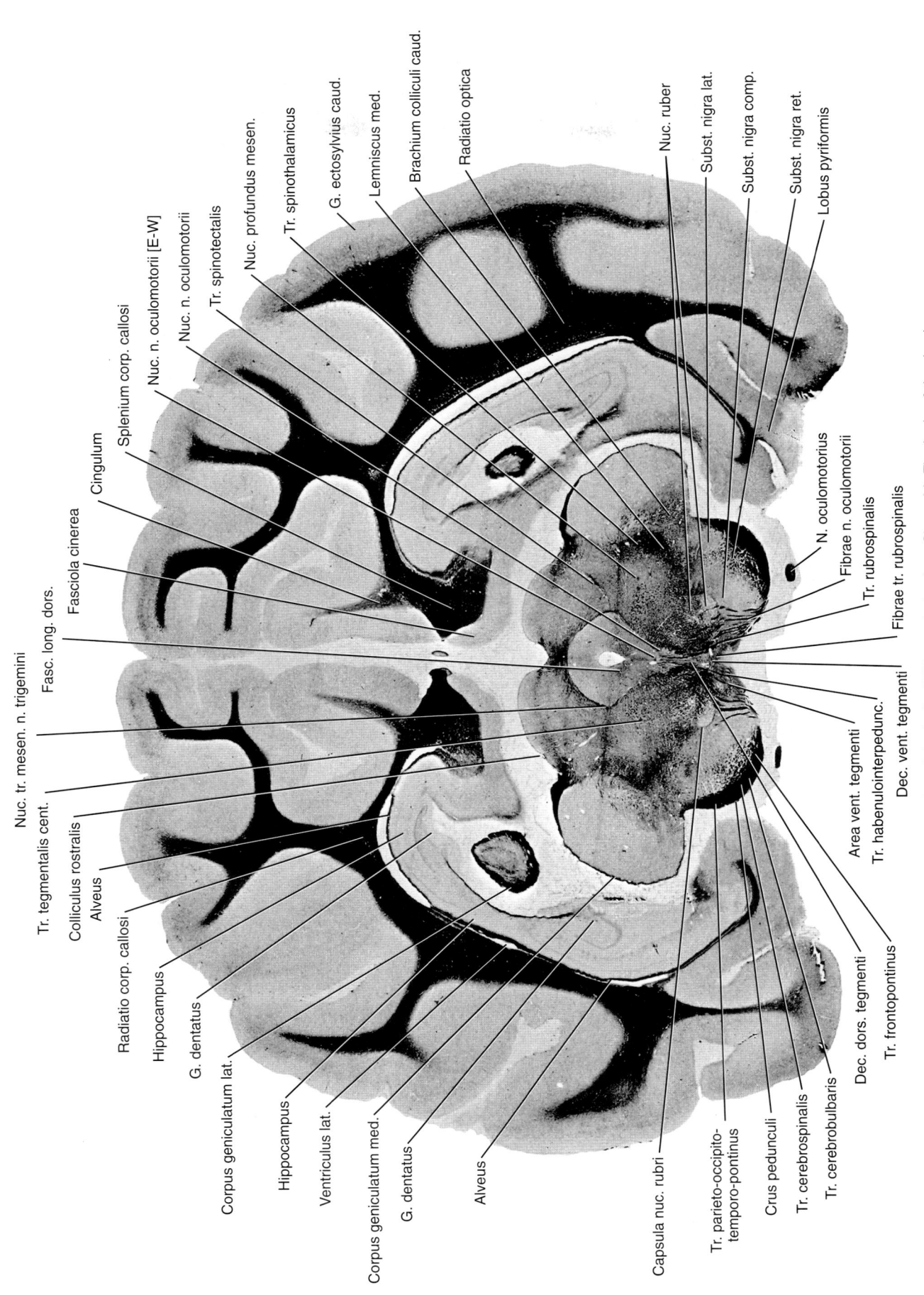

Plate 18.3 Transverse section of the brain. (With permission from Singer M: *The brain of the dog in section*, Philadelphia, 1962, Saunders.)

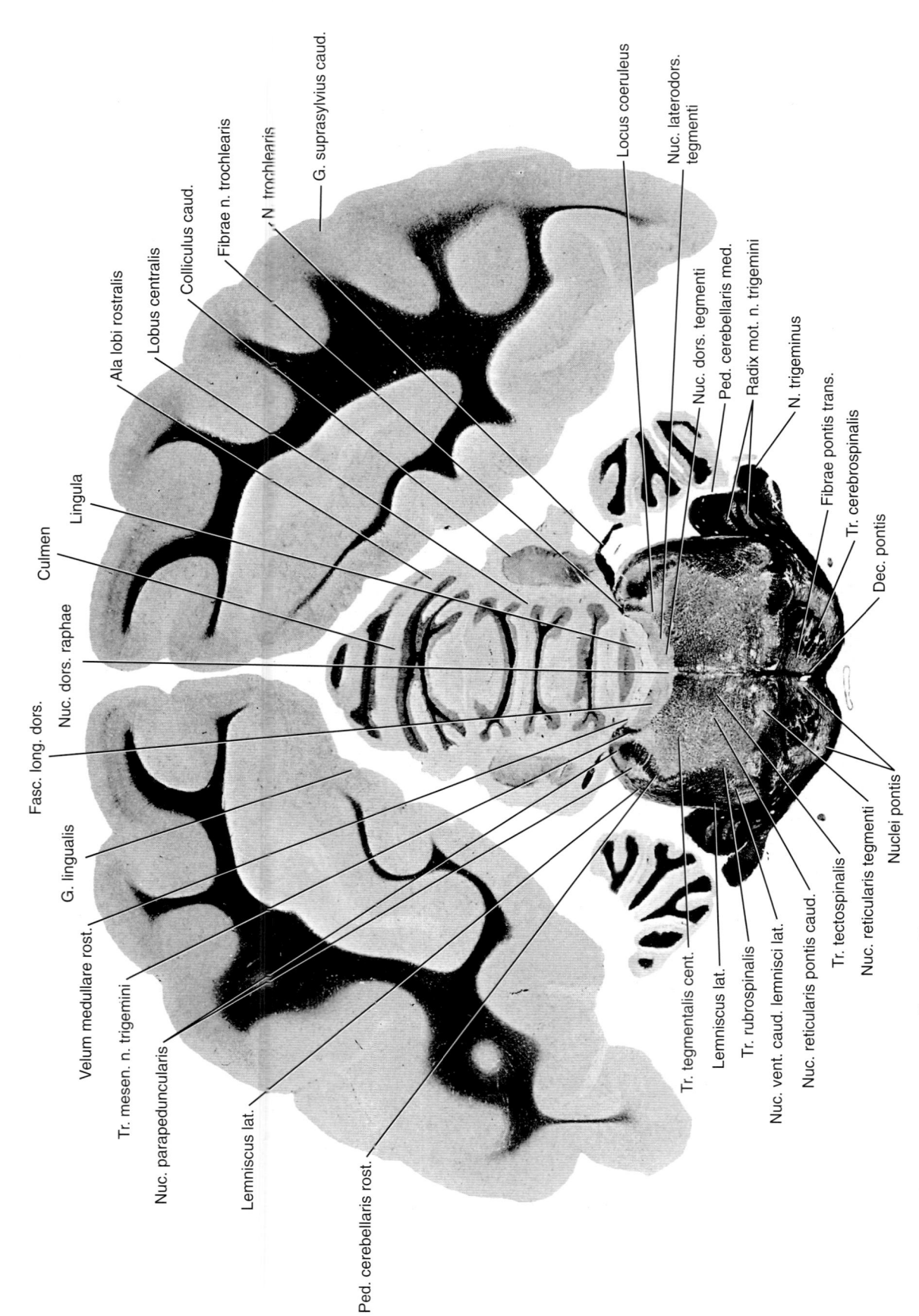

• Plate 18.4 Transverse section of the brain. (With permission from Singer M: *The brain of the dog in section*, Philadelphia, 1962, Saunders.)

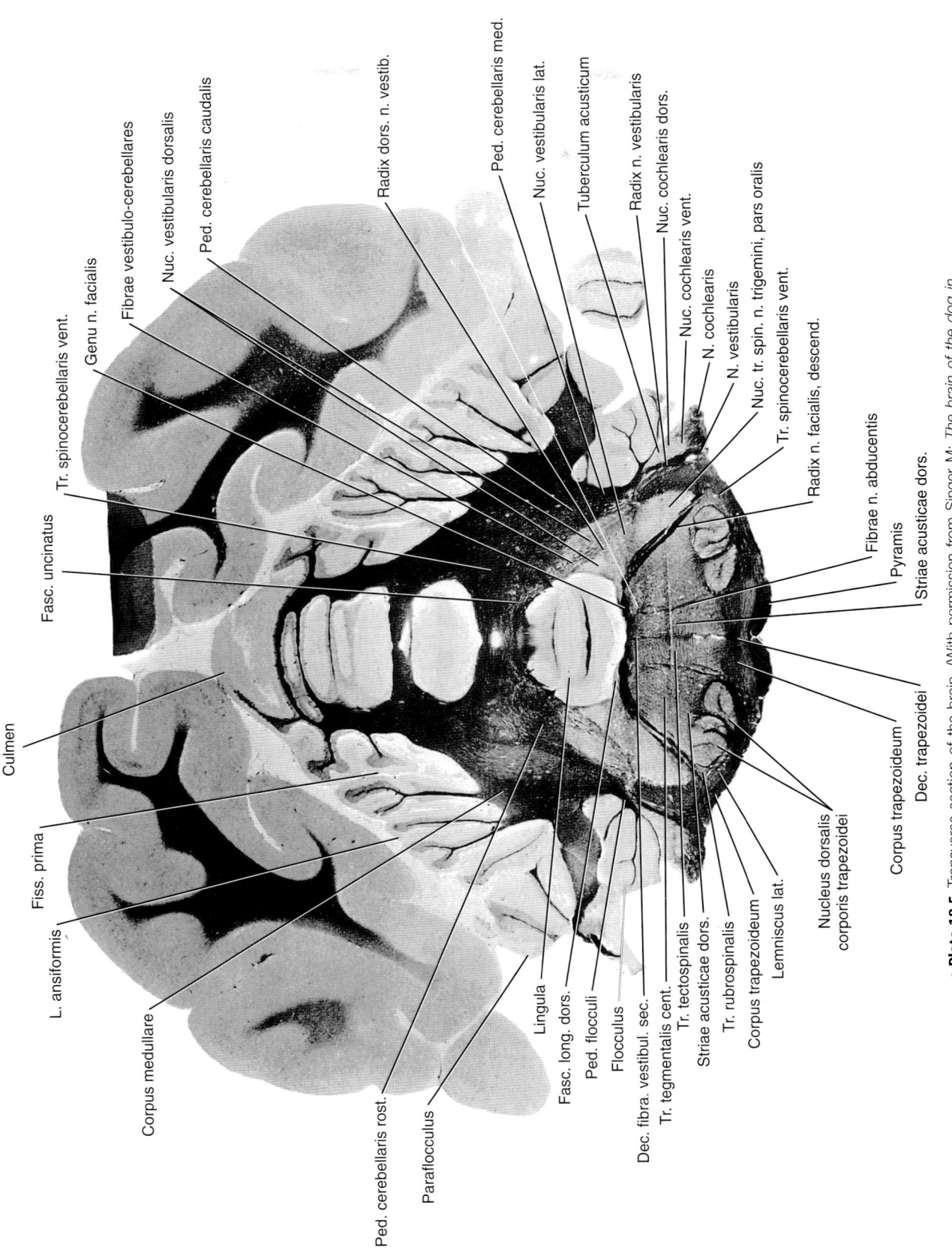

Plate 18.5 Transverse section of the brain. (With permission from Singer M: *The brain of the dog in section*, Philadelphia, 1962, Saunders.)

802 CHAPTER 18   The Brain

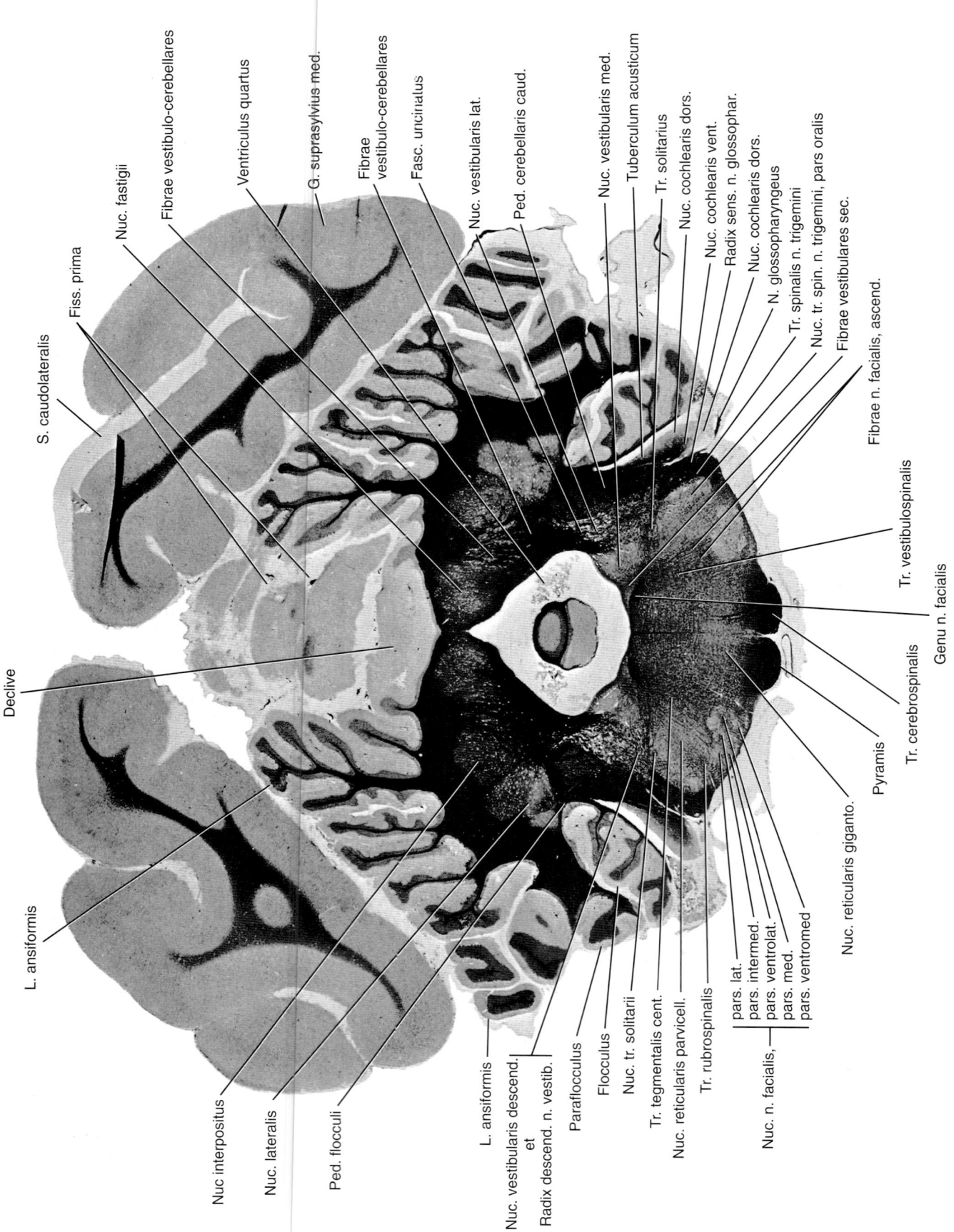

• **Plate 18.6** Transverse section of the brain. (With permission from Singer M: *The brain of the dog in section*, Philadelphia, 1962, Saunders.)

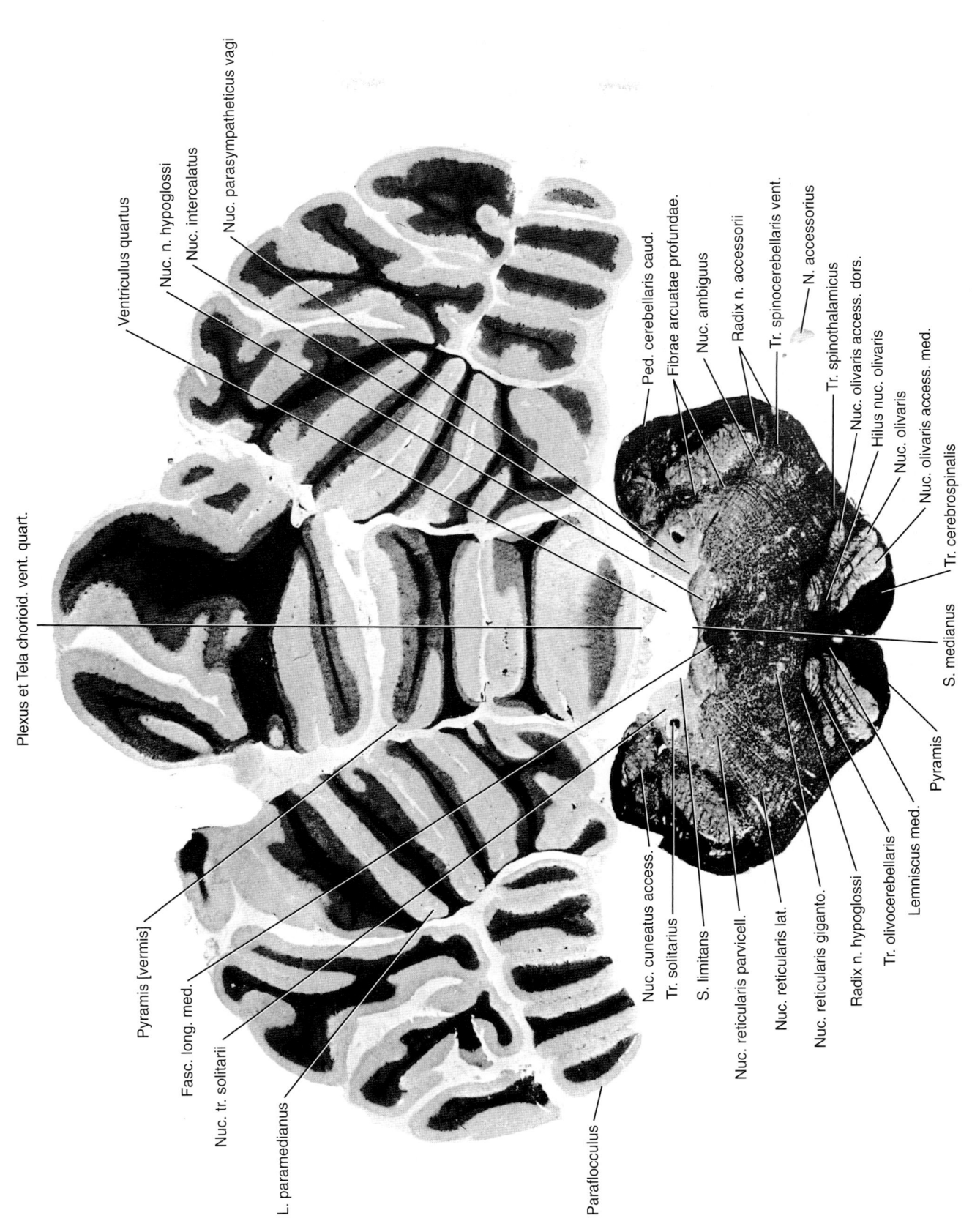

• **Plate 18.7** Transverse section of the brain. (With permission from Singer M: *The brain of the dog in section*, Philadelphia, 1962, Saunders.)

804 CHAPTER 18 The Brain

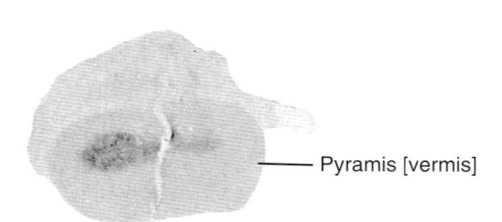

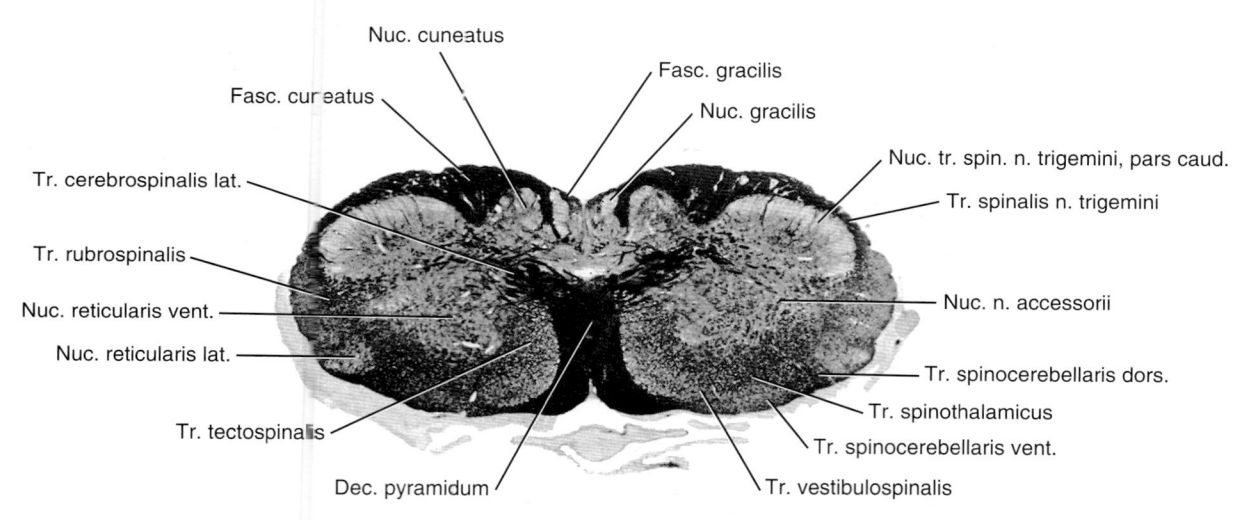

• **Plate 18.8** Transverse section of the brain. (With permission from Singer M: *The brain of the dog in section,* Philadelphia, 1962, Saunders.)

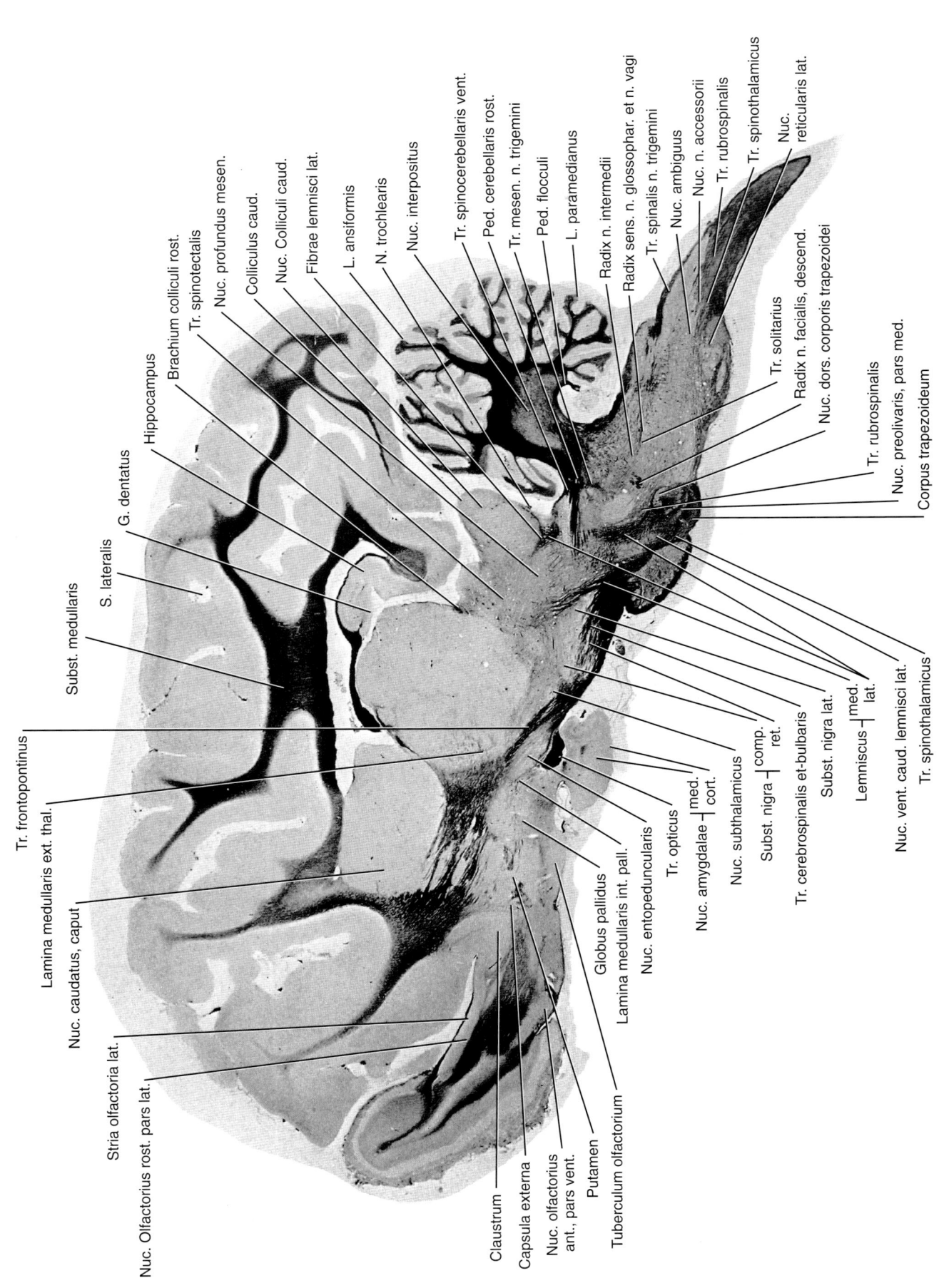

Plate 18.9 Sagittal section of the brain. (With permission from Singer M: *The brain of the dog in section*, Philadelphia, 1962, Saunders.)

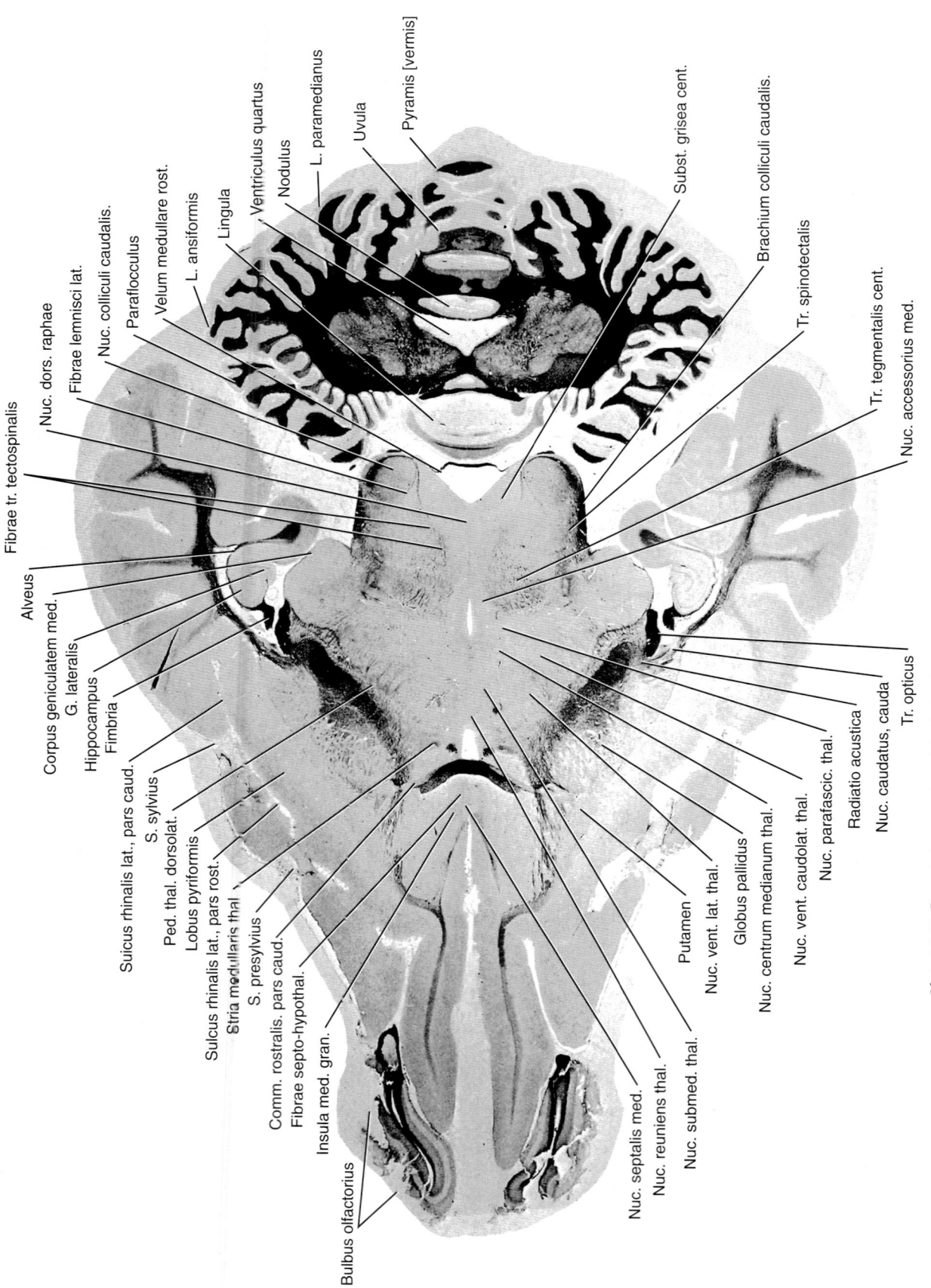

Plate 18.10 Dorsal plane section of the brain. (With permission from Singer M: *The brain of the dog in section,* Philadelphia, 1962, Saunders.)

Bibliography

Adrianov, O. S., & Mering, T. A. (1964). E. F. Domino (Ed.), *Atlas of the canine brain.* Ann Arbor: University of Michigan Press.

Akert, K., Potter, H. D., & Anderson, J. W. (1961). The subfornical organ in mammals. I. Comparative and topographical anatomy. *J Comp Neurol, 116,* 1–13.

Allen, W. F. (1937). Olfactory and trigeminal conditioned reflexes in dogs. *Am J Physiol, 118,* 532–540.

Allen, W. F. (1944). Degeneration in the dog's mamillary body and Ammon's horn following transection of the fornix. *J Comp Neurol, 80,* 283–291.

Allen, W. F. (1945). Effect of destroying three localized cerebral cortical areas for sound on correct conditioned differential responses of the dog's foreleg. *Am J Physiol, 144,* 415–428.

Arey, L. B., & Gore, M. (1942). The numerical relation between the ganglion cells of the retina and the fibers in the optic nerve of the dog. *J Comp Neurol, 77,* 609–617.

Arey, L. B., Bruesch, S. R., & Castanares, S. (1942). The relation between eyeball size and number of optic nerve fibers in the dog. *J Comp Neurol, 76,* 417–422.

Asratian, E. (1935). Motor defensive conditioned reflexes in dogs with extirpated cortical motor areas of the cerebral hemispheres. *C R Acad Sci (USSR), 1,* 159–164. (Quoted from *Biol Abstr* 11:3517, 1937.).

Augustine, J. R., Vidic, B., & Young, P. A. (1971). The intermediate root of the trigeminal nerve in the dog (*Canis familiaris*). *Anat Rec, 169,* 697–703.

Badoni, C. T. (1973). Relationship of sensory and motor cortex to the segments of the dog spinal cord. *Folia Morphol (Praha), 21,* 341–344.

Bahrs, A. M. (1927). Notes on reflexes of puppies in the first six weeks after birth. *Am J Physiol, 82,* 51–55.

Bailey, P., & Haynes, W. (1940). Location of inhibitory respiratory center in cerebral cortex of the dog. *Proc Soc Exp Biol (NY), 45,* 686–687.

Barnes, K. L., & Ferrario, C. M. (1984). Location of the area postrema pressor pathway in the dog brain stem. *Hypertension, 6,* 482–488.

Barstad, K. E., & Bear, M. F. (1990). Basal forebrain projections to somatosensory cortex in the cat. *J Neurophysiol, 64*(4), 1223–1232.

Bartley, S. H., & Newman, E. B. (1931). Studies on the dog's cortex. I. The sensorimotor areas. *Am J Physiol, 99,* 1–8.

Basir, M. A. (1932). The vascular supply of the pituitary body in the dog. *J Anat (London), 66,* 387–398.

Beitz, A. J. (1992). Anatomic and chemical organization of descending pain modulation systems. In C. E. Short & A. V. Poznak (Eds.), *Animal pain.* New York: Churchill Livingstone.

Berman, A. L. (1968). *The brain stem of the cat: a cytoarchitectonic atlas with stereotaxic coordinates.* Madison: University of Wisconsin Press.

Berman, A. L., & Jones, E. G. (1982). *The thalamus and basal telencephalon of the cat: a cytoarchitectonic atlas with stereotaxic coordinates.* Madison: University of Wisconsin Press.

Bessen, J. M., & Chaouch, A. (1987). Peripheral and spinal mechanisms of nociception. *Physiol Rev, 67,* 67–186.

Billenstien, D. C. (1953). The vascularity of the motor cortex of the dog. *Anat Rec, 117,* 129–144.

Binder, M. D., & Mendell, L. M. (1990). *The segmental motor system.* New York: Oxford University Press.

Bleier, R. (1961). *The hypothalamus of the cat.* Baltimore, MD: The Johns Hopkins Press.

Blinkov, S. M., & Ponomarev, V. S. (1965). Quantitative determinations of neurons and glial cells in the nuclei of the facial and vestibular nerves in man, monkey and dog. *J Comp Neurol, 125,* 295–301.

Böhme, G. (1967). Unterschiede am Gehirnventrikelsystem von Hund und Katze nach Untersuchungen an Ausgusspräparaten. *Berl Münch Tierärztl Wochenschr, 80,* 195–196.

Bonvallet, M., & Dell, P. (1949). Stutinsky F: Lésions hypothalamiques et comportement émotional chez le chien. *C R Soc Biol (Paris), 143,* 80–83.

Breazile, J. E., & Thompson, W. D. (1967). Motor cortex of the dog. *Am J Vet Res, 28,* 1483–1486.

Brooks, V. B. (1986). *The neural basis of motor control.* New York: Oxford University Press.

Brown, J. O. (1943a). The nuclear pattern of the non-tectal portions of the midbrain and isthmus in the dog and cat. *J Comp Neurol, 78,* 365–405.

Brown, J. O. (1943b). Pigmentation of the substantia nigra and the locus coeruleus in certain carnivores. *J Comp Neurol, 79,* 393–405.

Brown, J. O. (1944). Pigmentation of certain mesencephalic tegmental nuclei in the dog and cat. *J Comp Neurol, 81,* 249–257.

Brutkowski, S., & Dabrowska, J. (1966). Prefrontal cortex control of differentiation behavior in dogs. *Acta Biol Exp (Warsaw), 26,* 425–439.

Brutkowski, S., Fonberg, E., & Mempel, E. (1961). Angry behavior in dogs following bilateral lesion in the genual portion of the rostral cingulate gyrus. *Acta Biol Exp (Warsaw), 21,* 199–205.

Brutkowski, S., Fonberg, E., Kreiner, J., et al. (1962). Aphagia and adipsia in a dog with bilateral complete lesion of the amygdaloid complex. *Acta Biol Exp (Warsaw), 22,* 43–50.

Burakowska, J. (1966). Extreme capsule in the dog: myeloarchitectonics. *Acta Biol Exp (Warsaw), 26,* 123–133.

Busygina, I. I., Aleksandrov, V. G., Lyubashina, O. A., et al. (2010). Effects of stimulation of the insular cortex on execution of the antrofundal reflex in conscious dogs. *Neursci Behav Physiol, 40*(4), 375–380.

Buxton, D. F. (1967). Function and anatomy of the corticospinal tracts of the dog and raccoon. *Anat Rec, 157,* 222–223.

Buxton, D. F., & Goodman, D. C. (1967). Motor function and the corticospinal tracts in the dog and raccoon. *J Comp Neurol, 129,* 341–360.

Campbell, A. E. (1904–1905). Further histological studies on the localisation of cerebral function—the brains of *Felis, Canis* and *Sus* compared with that of *Homo. Proc R Soc Lond, 74,* 390–392.

Chernicky, C. L., Barnes, K. L., Conomy, J. P., et al. (1980). A morphological characterization of the canine area postrema. *Neurosci Lett, 20,* 37–43.

Chibuzo, G. A., & Cummings, J. F. (1981). The origins of the afferent fibers to the lingual muscles of the dog, a retrograde labeling study with horseradish peroxidase. *Anat Rec, 200,* 95–101.

Chorazyna, H., & Stepien, L. (1961). Impairment of auditory recent memory produced by cortical lesions in dogs. *Acta Biol Exp (Warsaw), 21,* 177–178.

Chusid, J. G., DeGutierrez-Mahoney, C. G., & Robinson, F. (1949). The "motor" cortex of the dog. *Fed Proc, 8,* 25.

Clark, R. (1968). Postnatal myelinization in the central nervous system of the beagle dog. *Anat Rec, 160,* 331.

Cohn, H. A., & Papez, J. W. (1933). The posterior calcarine fissure in dog. *J Comp Neurol, 58,* 593–602.

Corder, R. L., & Latimer, H. B. (1947). The growth of the brain in the fetal dog. *Anat Rec, 97,* 383.

Corder, R. L., & Latimer, H. B. (1949). The prenatal growth of the brain and of its parts and of the spinal cord in the dog. *J Comp Neurol*, *90*, 193–212.

Costa-Llobet, C., Prats-Galino, A., Arroyo-Guijarro, J., et al. (1988). The facial motor nucleus of the dog. II. Morphometric analysis. *Acta Anat (Basel)*, *132*, 280–283.

Crosby, E. C., Humphrey, T., & Lauer, E. W. (1962). *Correlative anatomy of the nervous system*. New York: Macmillan.

Culler, E. A., & Mettler, F. A. (1934). Observations upon conduct of a thalamic dog: hearing and vision in decorticated animals. *Proc Soc Exp Biol (NY)*, *31*, 607–609.

Cummings, J. F., & Petras, J. M. (1977). The origin of spinocerebellar pathways. I. The nucleus cervicalis centralis of the cervical spinal cord. *J Comp Neurol*, *173*, 655–691.

Davidoff, R. A. (1990). The pyramidal tract. *Neurology*, *40*, 332–339.

de Lahunta, A., Glass, E. N., & Kent, M. (2015). *Veterinary neuroanatomy and clinical neurology* (4th ed.). St Louis, MO: Saunders.

Dow, R. S. (1940). Partial agenesis of the cerebellum in the dog. *J Comp Neurol*, *72*, 569–586.

Dua-Sharma, S., Sharma, K. N., & Jacobs, H. L. (1970). *The canine brain in stereotaxic coordinates*. Cambridge, MA: MIT Press.

Dumenko, V. N. (1961). Changes in the electrical activity of the cerebral cortex of dogs during the formation of a stereotype of motor conditional reflexes. *Zhur Vysshei Nervnoi Deiatel' nosti im I P Pavlova (Transl)*, 292–299.

Duvernoya, H. M., & Risold, P. Y. (2007). The circumventricular organs: an atlas of comparative anatomy and vascularization. *Brain Res Rev*, *56*, 119–147.

Dziurdzik, B. (1965). Frontal lobe sulci in the dog. *Acta Biol Exp (Warsaw)*, *25*, 245–261.

Eliasson, S., Lindren, P., & Uvnäs, B. (1952). Representation in the hypothalamus and the motor cortex in the dog of the sympathetic vasodilator outflow to the skeletal muscle. *Acta Physiol Scand*, *27*, 18–37.

Ellenberger, W. (1889). Über die Furchen und Windungen der Grosshirnoberfläche des Hundes. *Arch Wiss Prakt Tierheilkd*, *15*, 263–282.

Ellenberger, W., & Baum, H. (1891). *Systematische und topographische Anatomie des Hundes*. Berlin: Parey.

Ellenberger, W., & Baum, H. (1943). *Handbuch der vergleichenden Anatomie der Haustiere* (18th ed.). Berlin: Springer.

Fike, J. R., LeCouteur, R. A., & Cann, C. E. (1981). Anatomy of the canine brain using high-resolution computed tomography. *Vet Radiol*, *22*, 236–243.

Fitzgerald, T. C. (1961). Anatomy of the cerebral ventricles of domestic animals. *Vet Med*, *56*, 38–45.

Fletcher, T. F. (2016). Canine brain atlas. In C. W. Dewey & R. C. da Costa (Eds.), *Practical guide to canine and feline neurology* (3rd ed.). Hoboken, NJ: Wiley-Blackwell.

Fox, M. W. (1963). Gross structure and development of the canine brain. *Am J Vet Res*, *24*, 1240–1247.

Fox, M. W. (1968). Neuronal development and ontogeny of evoked potentials in auditory and visual cortex of the dog. *Electroencephalography Clin Neurophysiol*, *24*, 213–226.

Fox, M. W., & Inman, O. R. (1966). Persistence of Retzius-Cajal cells in developing dog brain. *Brain Res*, *3*, 192–194.

Fox, M. W., Inman, O. R., & Himwich, W. A. (1966). The postnatal development of the neocortical neurons in the dog. *J Comp Neurol*, *127*, 199–206.

Fujita, H. (1957). Electron microscopic observation on the neurosecretory granules in the pituitary posterior lobe of the dog. *Arch Histol Jpn*, *12*, 165–172.

Gabrawi, A. F., & Tarkhan, A. A. (1967). On the mesencephalic nucleus and root of the fifth cranial nerve (dog, cat). *Acta Anat*, *67*, 550–560.

Gantt, W. H. (1948). Cardiac reaction in partially decorticated dogs. *Trans Am Neurol Assoc*, *73*, 131–133.

Gavelov, A. M., & Badoni, C. T. (1984). Quantitative analysis of synaptic morphology of nucleus gracilis of dog. *Z Mikrosk Anat Forsch*, *98*, 277–283.

Girden, E. (1938). Cerebral mechanisms and auditory localisation in dogs. *Psychol Bull*, *35*, 699–700.

Glorieux, P. (1929). Anatomie et connexions thalamiques chez le chien. *J Neurol (Brux)*, *29*, 525–555.

Goldberg, R. C., & Chaikoff, I. L. (1952). On the occurrence of six cell types in the dog anterior pituitary. *Anat Rec*, *112*, 265–274.

Goldstein, M. H. (1980). The auditory periphery. In V. B. Mountcastle (Ed.), *Medical physiology* (ed. 14, pp. 428–456). St Louis, MO: CV Mosby.

Goldzbrand, M. G., Goldberg, S. E., & Clark, G. (1951). Cessation of walking elicited by stimulation of the forebrain of the unanesthetized dog. *Am J Physiol*, *167*, 127–133.

Gomez, D. G., & Potts, D. G. (1981). The lateral, third, and fourth ventricle choroid plexus of the dog: a structural and ultrastructural study. *Ann Neurol*, *10*, 333–340.

Gorbachevskaia, A. I. (2009). The connections of the zona incerta of the dog diencephalon with the substantia nigra, the ventral tegmental area and the pedunculopontine tegmental nucleus. *Morfologiia*, *135*(3), 24–28.

Gorbachevskaya, A. I., & Chivileva, O. G. (2005). Structural organization of the pedunculopontine nucleus of the tegmentum of the dog midbrain. *Neurosci Behav Physiol*, *35*(8), 793–797.

Gorska, T., & Czarkowska, J. (1978). Motor cortex development in the dog. some cortical stimulation and behavioral data. *Neurosci Behav Physiol*, *3*, 129–131.

Grantyn, A. (1989). How visual inputs to the ponto-bulbar reticular formation are used in the synthesis of premotor signals during orienting. *Prog Brain Res*, *80*, 159–170.

Gröschel, G. (1930). Über die Cytoarchitektonik und Histologie der Zwischenhirnbasis beim Hund. *Dtsch Z Nervenheilk*, *112*, 108–123.

Gross, S. W. (1939). Cerebral arteriography in the dog and in man with a rapidly excreted organic iodide. *Proc Soc Exp Biol (NY)*, *42*, 258–259.

Grünthal, E. (1929). Der Zellaufbau des Hypothalamus beim Hunde. *Z Ges Neurol Psychiat*, *120*, 157–177.

Gurewitsch, M., & Bychowski, G. (1928). Zur Architektonik der Hirnrinde (Isocortex) des Hundes. *J Psychol Neurol*, *35*, 283–300.

Hagen, E. (1957). Morphologische Beobachtungen im Hypothalamus und in der Neurohypophyse des Hundes nach Teilläsion des Infundibulum. *Acta Anat (Basel)*, *31*, 193–219.

Hagg, S., & Ha, H. (1970). Cervicothalamic tract in the dog. *J Comp Neurol*, *139*, 357–373.

Haines, D. E., & Jenkins, T. W. (1968). Studies on the epithalamus. I. Morphology of post-mortem degeneration: the habenular nucleus in dog. *J Comp Neurol*, *132*, 405–417.

Hammond, D. (1986). Control systems for nociceptive afferent processing. The descending inhibitory pathways. In T. L. Yaksh (Ed.), *Spinal afferent processing*. New York: Plenum Press.

Hamuy, T. P., Bromiley, R. B., & Woolsey, C. N. (1950). Somatic afferent areas I and II of the dog's cerebral cortex. *Am J Physiol*, *163*, 719–720.

Hamuy, T. P., Bromiley, R. B., & Woolsey, C. N. (1956). Somatic afferent areas I and II of the dog's cerebral cortex. *J Neurophysiol*, *19*, 485–499.

Hand, P. J. (1966). Lumbosacral dorsal root terminations in the nucleus gracilis of the cat. *J Comp Neurol, 126*, 137–156.

Heinbecker, P., & White, H. L. (1941). Hypothalamico-hypophysial system and its relation to water balance in the dog. *Am J Physiol, 133*, 582–593.

Herre, W., & Stephan, H. (1955). Zur postnatalen Morphogenese des Hirnes verschiedener Haushundrassen. *Morph Jb, 96*, 210–264.

Hikosaka, O. (2010). The habenula: from stress evasion to value-based decision-making. *Neuroscience, 11*, 503–513.

Himwhich, H. E., & Fazekas, J. F. (1941). Comparative studies of the metabolism of the brain of infant and adult dogs. *Am J Physiol, 132*, 454–459.

Hitzig, E. (1900a). Über das corticale Sehen des Hundes. *Arch Psychiat Nervenkr, 33*, 707–720.

Hitzig, E. (1900b). Über den Mechanismus gewisser kortikaler Sehstörungen des Hundes. *Berl klin Wochenschr, 37*, 1001–1003.

Hiyama, T. Y., Watanabe, E., Okado, H., et al. (2004). The subfornical organ is the primary locus of sodium-level sensing by Na$_x$ sodium channels for the control of salt-intake behavior. *J Neuroscience, 24*, 9276–9281.

Hoffmann, G. (1955). *Topographischer und zytologischer Atlas der Medulla oblongata von Schwein und Hund*. Berlin: Deutsche Akademie der Landwirtschaftswissenschaften.

Holbrook, J. R., & Schapiro, H. (1974). The accessory optic tract in the dog: a retino-entopeduncular pathway. *J Hirnforsch, 15*, 365–377.

Holmes, G. M. (1901). The nervous system of the dog without a forebrain. *J Physiol (Lond), 27*, 1–25.

Holstege, G., & Tan, J. (1988). Projections from the red nucleus and surrounding areas to the brainstem and spinal cord in the cat. An HRP and autoradiographical tracing study. *Behav Brain Res, 28*, 33–57.

Houston, M. L. (1968). The early brain development of the dog. *J Comp Neurol, 134*, 371–383.

Howard, D. R., & Breazile, J. E. (1973). Optic fiber projections to dorsal lateral geniculate nucleus in the dog. *Am J Vet Res, 34*, 419–424.

Hukuda, S., Jameson, H. D., & Wilson, C. B. (1973). Experimental cervical myelopathy. 3. The canine corticospinal tract: anatomy and function. *Surg Neurol, 1*, 107–114.

Ipekchyan, N. M. (2008). Quantitative analysis of the distribution of the motor cortex representations of the fore- and hindlimbs in the red nucleus of the cat. *Neurosci Behav Physiol, 38*, 345–347.

Iwai, E. (1961). Visual learning and retention after ablation of inferotemporal cortex in dogs. *Tohoku J Exp Med, 75*, 243–258.

Janklewicz, E. (1967). Habenular complex in the dog's brain. *Acta Biol Exp (Warsaw), 27*, 367–387.

Jasper, H. H., & Ajmone-Marsan, C. (1954). *A stereotaxic atlas of the diencephalon of the cat*. Ottawa, Canada: National Research Council.

Kaada, B. R. (1951). Somato-motor, autonomic and electrocorticographic responses to electrical stimulation of "rhinencephalic" and other structures in primates, cat and dog: a study of responses from the limbic, subcallosal, orbito-insular, piriform and temporal cortex, hippocampus-fornix and amygdala. *Acta Physiol Scand, 24*(Suppl. 83), 1–285.

Kalinina, T. E. (1961). The effects of olfactory stimulations on the higher nervous activity of dogs. *Zhur Vysshei Nervnoi Deiatel'nosti im I P Pavlova (Transl), 11*, 330–333.

Kellogg, W. N. (1949). Locomotor and other disturbances following hemidecortication in the dog. *J Comp Physiol Psychol, 42*, 506–516.

King, A. S. (1987). *Physiological and clinical anatomy of the domestic mammals: volume 1: central nervous system*. New York: Oxford University Press.

Kirk, G. R., & Breazil, J. E. (1972). Maturation of the corticospinal tract in the dog. *Exp Neurol, 35*, 394–407.

Kitchell, R. L., Stromberg, M. W., & Davis, L. H. (1977). Comparative study of the dorsal motor nucleus of the vagus nerve. *Am J Vet Res, 38*, 37–49.

Klempin, D. (1921). Über die Architektonik der Grosshirnrinde des Hundes. *J Psychol Neurol (Lpz), 26*, 229–249.

Knoche, H. (1952). Neurohistologische Untersuchungen am Hypophysenzwischenhirnsystem des Hundes. *Anat Anz (Ergh), 99*, 93.

Knoche, H. (1953). Über das Vorkommen eigenartiger Nervenfasern (Nodulus-Fasern) in Hypophyse und Zwischenhirn von Hund und Mensch. *Acta Anat (Basel), 18*, 208–233.

Kosmal, A. (1986). Topographical organization of frontal association cortex afferents originating in ventral thalamic nuclei in dog brain. *Acta Neurobiol Exp, 46*, 105–117.

Kosmal, A., Malinowskaa, M., Wozniackaa, A., et al. (2004). Cytoarchitecture and thalamic afferents of the sylvian and composite posterior gyri of the canine temporal cortex. *Brain Res, 1023*, 279–301.

Kosaka, K. (1909). Über die Vaguskerne des Hundes. *Neurol Zbl, 28*, 406–410.

Kowalska, D. M. (2000). Cognitive functions of the temporal lobe in the dog: a review. *Prog Neuro-Psychopharmacol Biol Psychiat, 24*, 855–880.

Kreiner, J. (1958). The quantitative myelinization of brains and spinal cords in dogs of various size. *Acta Anat, 33*, 50–64.

Kreiner, J. (1961). The myeloarchitectonics of the frontal cortex of the dog. *J Comp Neurol, 116*, 117–133.

Kreiner, J. (1962a). Myeloarchitectonics of the cingular cortex in dog. *J Comp Neurol, 119*, 255–267.

Kreiner, J. (1962b). The cingular bundle of the dog brain. *Acta Biol Cracoviensia Ser Zool, 5*, 253–261.

Kreiner, J. (1964a). Myeloarchitectonics of the sensorimotor cortex in dog. *J Comp Neurol, 122*, 181–200.

Kreiner, J. (1964b). Myeloarchitectonics of the perisylvian cortex in dog. *J Comp Neurol, 123*, 231–241.

Kreiner, J. (1964c). Myeloarchitectonics of the parietal cortex in dog. *Acta Biol Exp (Warsaw), 24*, 195–212.

Kreiner, J. (1966a). Myeloarchitectonics of the occipital cortex in dog and general remarks on the myeloarchitectonics of the dog. *J Comp Neurol, 127*, 531–557.

Kreiner, J. (1966b). Reconstruction of neocortical lesions within the dog's brain: instructions. *Acta Biol Exp (Warsaw), 26*, 221–243.

Kreiner, J. (1970). Homologies of the fissural patterns of the hemispheres of dog and cat. *Acta Biol Exp (Warsaw), 30*, 295–305.

Kreiner, J., & Maksymowicz, K. (1962). A three-dimensional model of the striatal nuclei in the dog's brain. *Acta Biol Exp (Warsaw), 22*, 69–79.

Kremer, W. F. (1947). Autonomic and somatic reactions induced by stimulation of the cingular gyrus in dogs. *J Neurophysiol, 10*, 371–379.

Kremer, W. F. (1948). Blood pressure changes in response to electrical and chemical (acetyl-beta-methyl choline) stimulation of the cerebral cortex in dogs. *Am J Physiol, 152*, 314–323.

Langley, J. N. (1883–1884). The structure of the dog's brain. *J Physiol (London), 4*, 248–285.

Larsell, O. (1970). J. Jansen (Ed.), *The comparative anatomy and histology of the cerebellum from monotremes through apes*. Minneapolis: University of Minnesota Press.

Lassek, A. M., Dowd, L. W., & Weil, A. (1930). The quantitative distribution of the pyramidal tract in the dog. *J Comp Neurol, 51*, 153–163.

Latimer, H. B. (1942). The weights of the brain and of its parts, and the weight and length of the spinal cord in the dog. *Growth, 6*, 39–57.

Lee, I., Jejoong, K., & Lee, C. (1999). Anatomical characteristics and three-dimensional model of the dog dorsal lateral geniculate body. *Anat Rec, 256*, 29–39.

Lim, R. K. S., Liu, C. N., & Moffitt, R. L. (1960). *A stereotaxic atlas of the dog's brain*. Springfield, IL: Charles C Thomas.

Lindberg, A. A. (1937). The influence of longitudinal transection of the corpus callosum upon locomotion in the dog (in Russian). *Trud Tsentral Psikhonevrol Inst, 8*, 55–60. (Quoted from *Biol Abstr* 13:4020, 1939.).

Lindgren, P., & Borje, U. (1953). Activation of sympathetic vasodilator and vasoconstrictor neurons by electric stimulation in the medulla of the dog and cat. *Circulation Res, 1*, 479–485.

Maksymowicz, K. (1963). Amygdaloid complex of the dog. *Acta Biol Exp (Warsaw), 23*, 63–73.

Marquis, D. G. (1932a). Brightness discrimination in dogs after removal of the striate cortex. *Anat Rec, 52*, 67.

Marquis, D. G. (1932b). Effects of removal of visual cortex in mammals, with observation on the retention of light discrimination in dogs. *Assoc Res Nerv Dis Proc, 13*, 558–592.

Marquis, D. G., & Hilgard, E. R. (1936). Conditioned lid responses to light in dogs after removal of the visual cortex. *J Comp Psychol, 22*, 157–178.

Massion, J. (1967). The mammalian red nucleus. *Physiol Rev, 47*, 383–436.

McCotter, R. E. (1913). The nervus terminalis in the adult dog and cat. *J Comp Neurol, 23*, 145–152.

Mettler, F. A., & Goss, L. J. (1946). Canine chorea due to striocerebellar degeneration of unknown etiology. *J Am Vet Med Assoc, 108*, 377–384.

Meyer, H.: *Zur Anatomie des Hundes in Welpenalter*. 1. Beitrag: Makroskopisches, Zürich, 1952, Veterinary Dissertation.

Meyer, H. (1954). Macroscopic brain dissection in veterinary anatomy. *Am J Vet Res, 15*, 143–146.

Michaels, J. J., & Kraus, W. M. (1930). Measurements of cerebral and cerebellar surfaces. IX. Measurement of cortical areas in cat, dog, and monkey. *Arch Neurol Psychiat (Chic), 24*, 94–101.

Mileykovskiy, B. Y., Kiyashchenko, L. L., Kodama, T., et al. (2000). Activation of pontine and medullary motor inhibitory regions reduces discharge in neurons located in the locus coeruleus and the anatomical equivalent of the midbrain locomotor region. *J Neurosci, 20*(22), 8551–8558.

Miodonski, A. (1962). The nucleus accumbens in the brain of the dog. *Acta Biol Cracoviensia Ser Zool, 5*, 109–115.

Miodonski, A. (1963). Preoptic area of the dog. *Acta Biol Exp (Warsaw), 23*, 209–220.

Miodonski, A. (1967). Myeloarchitectonics of the septum in the brain of the dog. *Acta Biol Exp (Warsaw), 27*, 11–59.

Miodonski, A. (1968a). The myeloarchitectonics of the nuclei of the anterior thalamic group of the dog (*Canis familiaris*). *Acta Biol Cracoviensia Ser Zool, 11*, 77–92.

Miodonski, A. (1968b). The myeloarchitectonics of the nucleus parataenialis in the brain of the dog (*Canis familiaris*). *Acta Biol Cracoviensia Ser Zool, 11*, 111–117.

Miodonski, A. (1974). The angioarchitectonics and cytoarchitectonics (impregnation modo Golgi-Cox) structure of the fissural frontal neocortex in dog. *Folia Biol (Krakow), 22*, 237–279.

Miodonski, R. (1966). Myeloarchitectonics of the stria terminalis in the dog. *Acta Biol Exp (Warsaw), 26*, 135–147.

Miodonski, R. (1967). Myeloarchitectonics and connections of substantia innominata in the dog brain. *Acta Biol Exp (Warsaw), 27*, 61–84.

Miodonski, R. (1968). Bulbus olfactorius of the dog (*Canis familiaris*). *Acta Biol Cracoviensia Ser Zool, 11*, 65–76.

Miodonski, R. (1974). The structure of the posterior piriform cortex in the dog. *Acta Anat (Basel), 88*, 556–573.

Miodonski, R. (1975). The claustrum in the dog brain. *Acta Anat (Basel), 91*, 409–422.

Molliver, M. E., & Van der Loos, H. (1969). The synaptic strata of the somesthetic cortex in neonatal dog. *Anat Rec, 163*, 317–318.

Molliver, M. E., & Van der Loos, H. (1970). The ontogenesis of cortical circuitry: the spatial distribution of synapses in somesthetic cortex of newborn dog. *Erg Anat Entwickl Gesch, 42*, 1–54.

Mountcastle, V. B. (1980). Central nervous mechanism in hearing. In V. B. Mountcastle (Ed.), *Medical Physiology* (14th ed., pp. 457–480). St Louis, MO: Mosby.

Morgan, L. O. (1927). Symptoms and fiber degeneration following experimental lesions in the subthalamic nucleus of Luys in the dog. *J Comp Neurol, 44*, 379–401.

Morgan, L. O. (1930a). Cell groups in the tuber cinereum of the dog with a discussion of their function. *J Comp Neurol, 51*, 271–297.

Morgan, L. O. (1930b). The role of the tuber cinereum and the thyroid gland in experimental fever in the dog. *Anat Rec, 45*, 233.

Morin, G., Donnet, V., & Zwirn, P. (1949). Nature et évolution des troubles consécutifs á la section d'une pyramide bulbaire, chez le chien. *C R Soc Biol (Paris), 143*, 710–712.

Morin, G., Poursines, Y., & Donnet, V. (1949). Pluralité des dégénérescences produites par la cordotomie médullaire postérieure cervicale, chez le chien. *C R Soc Biol (Paris), 243*, 1127–1129.

Morin, G., Poursines, Y., & Maffre, S. (1951). Sur l'origine de la voie pyramidale. Documents obtenus par la méthode des dégénérescences descendants, chez le chien. *J Physiol (Paris), 43*, 75–96.

Mosidze, V. M. (1960). The importance of the cortical auditory area in the conditioned reflex activity of dogs. *Zhur Vysshei Nervnoi Deiatel'nosti im I P Pavlova (Transi), 10*, 923–928.

Munro, N. A., et al. (1993). Upbeat nystagmus in a patient with a small medullary infarct. *J Neurol Neurosurg Psychiatry, 56*, 1126–1128.

Murphy, M. G., & O'Leary, J. L. (1971). Neurological deficit in cats with lesions of the olivocerebellar system. *Arch Neurol, 24*, 145–157.

Narkiewicz, O. (1972). Frontoclaustral interrelations in cats and dogs. *Acta Neurobiol Exp (Warsaw), 32*, 141–150.

Narkiewicz, O., & Brutkowski, S. (1967). The organization of projections from the thalamic mediodorsal nucleus to the prefrontal cortex of the dog. *J Comp Neurol, 129*, 361–374.

Niedzielska, B. (1966). Stria medullaris of the thalamus in the dog. *Acta Biol Exp (Warsaw), 26*, 149–158.

Nigge, K. H. (1944). Die Gewinnung und Untersuchung des Liquor cerebrospinalis beim Hund mit besonderer Berücksichtigung der Liquorbefunde bei der Hundestaupe. *Dtsch tierärztl Wochenschr tierärztl Rundsch, 52*, 26–29.

Nomina Anatomica Veterinaria. (2005). *International Committee on Veterinary Gross Anatomical Nomenclature* (ed. 5). Hannover, Germany.

Nomina Anatomica Veterinaria. (2017). *International Committee on Veterinary Gross Anatomical Nomenclature* (ed. 6). Hanover.

Nowak, A. (1968a). Myeloarchitectonics of the putamen in the dog brain. *Acta Biol Cracoviensia Ser Zool, 11*, 137–147.

Novak, A. (1968b). The myeloarchitectonics of the caudate nucleus in the dog brain. *Acta Biol Cracoviensia Ser Zool, 11,* 227–241.

Oboussier, H. (1950). Über Unterschiede des Hirnfurchenbildes bei Hunden. *Verh Dtsch Zool Mainz Leipzig, 109–114,* 1949.

Oboussier, H. (1950). Zur Frage der Erblichkeit der Hirnfurchen. Untersuchungen an Kreuzungen extremer Rassetypen des Hundes. *Z Menschl Vererb-Konstit-Lehre, 29,* 831–864.

O'Connor, W. J. (1947). Atrophy of the supraoptic and paraventricular nuclei after interruption of the pituitary stalk in dogs. *Q J Exp Physiol, 34,* 29–42.

O'Connor, W. J. (1952). The normal interphase in the polyuria which follows section of the supraopticohypophysial tracts in the dog. *Q J Exp Physiol, 37,* 1–10.

Ogawa, T., & Mitomo, S. (1938). Eine experimentell-anatomische Studie über zwei Faserbahnen im Hirnstamm des Hundes: Tractus mesencephalo-olivaris medialis (Economo, Karplus) und Tractus tectocerebellaris. *Jpn J Med Sci I Anat, 7,* 77–94.

Onodera, S., & Hicks, T. P. (2009). A comparative neuroanatomical study of the red nucleus of the cat, macaque and human. *PLoS ONE, 4,* 1–19. www.plosone.org.

Otten, E. (1943). Umfangsmessungen an der Hypophysis cerebri und ihren Lappen beim Deutschen Schäferhund. *Anat Anz, 94,* 1–25.

Palionis, T.: *Die Nissl-substanz in den Ganglienzellen des Riechkolbens, gyrus olfactorius, lobus piriformis und Ammonshorns des Hundes,* Hannover, Germany, 1950, Veterinary Dissertation.

Pampiglione, G. (1963). *Development of cerebral function in the dog.* London: Butterworths.

Paneth, J. (1885). Uber Lage, Ausdehnung und Bedeutung der absoluten motorischen Felder auf der Hirnoberfläche des Hundes. *Arch Ges Physiol, 37,* 523–561.

Papez, J. W. (1929). *Comparative neurology.* New York: Crowell.

Papez, J. W. (1938). Thalamic connections in a hemidecorticate dog. *J Comp Neurol, 69,* 103–120.

Papez, J. W., & Rundles, R. W. (1938). Thalamus of a dog without a hemisphere due to a unilateral congenital hydrocephalus. *J Comp Neurol, 69,* 89–102.

Petras, J. M., & Cummings, J. F. (1977). The origin of spinocerebellar pathways. II. The nucleus centrobasalis of the cervical enlargement and the nucleus dorsalis of the thoracolumbar spinal cord. *J Comp Neurol, 173,* 693–715.

Phemister, R. D., & Young, S. (1968). The postnatal development of the canine cerebellar cortex. *J Comp Neurol, 134,* 243–254.

Pickford, M., & Ritchie, H. E. (1945). Experiments on the hypothalamic-pituitary control of water excretion in dogs. *J Physiol (London), 105–128.*

Pong, M. K., Horn, K. M., & Gibson, A. R. (2002). Spinal projections of the cat parvicellular red nucleus. *J Neurophysiol, 87,* 453–468.

Pong, M., Horn, K. M., & Gibson, A. R. (2008). Pathways for control of face and neck musculature by the basal ganglia and cerebellum. *Brain Res Rev, 58,* 249–264.

Potts, D. G., Deck, M. D. F., & Deonarine, V. (1971). Measurement of the rate of cerebrospinal fluid formation in the lateral ventricles of the dog. *Radiology, 98,* 605–610.

Radinsky, L. (1978). The evolutionary history of dog brains. *Museologia (Amsterdam), 10,* 25–29.

Ranson, W. S., & Clark, S. L. (1959). *The anatomy of the nervous system.* Philadelphia: Saunders.

Rioch, D. M. (1929a). Studies on the diencephalon of Carnivora. I. The nuclear configuration of the thalamus, epithalamus, and hypothalamus of the dog and cat. *J Comp Neurol, 49,* 1–119.

Rioch, D. M. (1929b). Studies on the diencephalon of Carnivora. II. Certain nuclear configurations and fiber connections of the subthalamus and midbrain of the dog and cat. *J Comp Neurol, 49,* 121–153.

Rioch, D. M. (1931a). Studies on the diencephalon of Carnivora. III. Certain myelinated-fiber connections of the diencephalon of the dog (*Canis familiaris*), cat (*Felis domestica*), and aevisa (*Crossarchus obscurus*). *J Comp Neurol, 53,* 319–388.

Sakai, S. T., Stanton, G. B., & Isaacson, L. G. (1993). Thalamic afferents of area 4 and 6 in the dog: a multiple retrograde fluorescent dye study. *Anat Embryol, 188,* 551–559.

Sakai, S. T., Stanton, G. B., & Tanaka, D., Jr. (1983). The ventral lateral thalamic nucleus in the dog: cytoarchitecture, acetylthiocholinesterase histochemistry, and cerebellar afferents. *Brain Res, 271,* 1–9.

Salazar, I., Ruiz Pesini, P., Fernandez Alvarez, P., et al. (1989). The thalamus of the dog: a tridimensional and cytoarchitectonic study. *Anat Anz, 169,* 101–113.

Salman, M. S. (2010). The cerebellum: It's about time! But timing is not everything–new insights into the role of the cerebellum in timing motor and cognitive tasks. *J Child Neurology, 17,* 1–9.

Scharrer, E. (1954). The maturation of the hypothalamic-hypophyseal neurosecretory system in the dog. *Anat Rec, 118,* 437.

Scharrer, E., & Frandson, R. D. (1954). The mode of release of neurosecretory material in the posterior pituitary of the dog. *Anat Rec, 118,* 350–351.

Scharrer, E., & Wittenstein, G. J. (1952). The effect of the interruption of the hypothalamo-hypophyseal neurosecretory pathway in the dog. *Anat Rec, 112,* 387.

Schneider, A. J. (1928). The histology of the radix mesencephalica n. trigemini in the dog. *Anat Rec, 38,* 321–339.

Seiferle, E. (1966). Zur Topographie des Gehirns bei lang- und kurzköpfigen Hunderassen. *Acta Anat, 63,* 346–362.

Sekita, B. (1931). Über den Faseraustausch zwischen dem nervus hypoglossus und nervus accessorius des Hundes an der Schädelbasis. *Acta Sch Med Univ Kioto, 13,* 239–244.

Sheiman, I. M. (1961). The formation of a conditional reflex to a moving visual stimulus in dogs. *Zhur Vysshei Nervnoi Deiatel'nosti im I P Pavlova (Transl), 22,* 275–283.

Sheinin, J. J. (1930). Typing of the cells of the mesencephalic nucleus of the trigeminal nerve in the dog, based on Nissl-granule arrangement. *J Comp Neurol, 50,* 109–131.

Simpson, R. M. (1930). Adaptive behaviour in circus movements of the dog following brain lesions. *J Comp Psychol, 10,* 67–83.

Singer, M. (1962). *The brain of the dog in section.* Philadelphia: Saunders.

Smialowski, A. (1965). The precommissural hippocampus in the dog. *Acta Biol Exp (Warsaw), 25,* 289–296.

Smialowski, A. (1966). The myeloarchitectonics of the hypothalamus in the dog. I. The anterior nuclei. *Acta Biol Exp (Warsaw), 26,* 99–122.

Smialowski, A. (1967). Magnocellular mammillary nucleus in the dog brain. *Bull Acad Pol Sci Cl II Sér Sc Biol, 15,* 703–705.

Smialowski, A. (1968a). Studies on the hypothalamus of the dog. II. Intermediate (tuberal) part. *Acta Biol Exp (Warsaw), 28,* 121–144.

Smialowski, A. (1968b). Mammillary complex in the dog's brain. *Acta Biol Exp (Warsaw), 28,* 225–243.

Smialowski, A. (1971). Subthalamus in dog brain. *Acta Neurobiol Exp, 31,* 203–212.

Smith, W. K. (1933). A physiological and histological study of the motor cortex of the dog (*Canis familiaris*). *Anat Rec Suppl, 55,* 76.

Smith, W. K. (1935a). The extent and structure of the electrically excitable cerebral cortex in the frontal lobe of the dog. *J Comp Neurol, 62*, 421–442.

Smith, W. K. (1935b). Alterations of respiratory movements induced by electric stimulation of the cerebral cortex in the dog. *Am J Physiol, 115*, 261–267.

Sobusiak, T., Zimny, R., & Matlosz, Z. (1971). Primary glossopharyngeal and vagal afferent projection into the cerebellum in the dog. An experimental study with toluidine blue and silver impregnation methods. *J Hirnforsch, 13*, 117–134.

Sobusiak, T., Zimny, R., Silny, W., et al. (1972). Primary vestibular afferents to the abducens nucleus and accessory cuneate nucleus: an experimental study in the dog with Nauta method. *Anat Anz, 131*, 238–247.

Starck, D. (1954). Die äussere Morphologie des Grosshirns zwergwüchsiger und kurzköpfiger Haushunde. *Gaz Med Port, 7*, 132–146.

Starlinger, J. (1895). Die Durchschneidung beider Pyramiden beim Hunde. *Neurol Zbl, 14*, 390–394.

Steblow, E. M. (1933). Experimentelle Epilepsie der Hunde in atypischen Versuchsbedingungen. Gefrieren des Gehirns nach vorläufig ausgeführter Exstirpation oder Umstechen seiner verschiedenen Gebiete. *Z Ges Neurol Psychiat 149*, 255–265.

Stehr, F. (1963). Fasciculus mammillaris princeps and its branches in the dog. *Acta Biol Exp (Warsaw), 23*, 221–237.

Stella, G., Zatti, P., & Sperti, L. (1955). Decerebrate rigidity in forelegs after deafferentiation and spinal transection in dogs with chronic lesions in different parts of the cerebellum. *Am J Physiol, 181*, 230–234.

Stephan, H. (1954). Die Anwendung der Snellschen Formel h = k₈ •p auf die Hirn-Körpergewichtsbeziehungen verschiedener Hunderassen. *Zool Anz, 153*, 15–27.

Stepien, I., & Stepien, L. (1961). Konorski J: The effect of unilateral and bilateral ablations of sensorimotor cortex on the instrumental (type II) alimentary conditional reflexes in dogs. *Acta Biol Exp (Warsaw), 21*, 121–140.

Stepien, I., Stepien, L., & Sychowa, B. (1966). Disturbances of motor conditioned behavior following bilateral ablations of the precruciate area in dogs and cats. *Acta Biol Exp (Warsaw), 26*, 323–340.

Steriade, M., & Llinas, R. R. (1988). The functional states of the thalamus and the associated neuronal interplay. *Physiol Rev, 68*, 649–742.

Steward, A., Allott, P. R., & Mapleson, W. W. (1975). Organ weights in the dog. *Res Vet Sci, 19*, 341–342.

Ström, G. (1950). Effect of hypothalamic cooling on cutaneous blood flow in the unanesthetized dog. *Acta Physiol Scand, 21*, 271–277.

Suvorov, N. F., Danilova, L. K., & Ermolenko, S. F. (1976). Direct connections of amygdaloid complex nuclei with the caudate nucleus in dogs. *Dokl Akad Nauk SSSR, 229*, 1262–1265.

Swiecimska, Z. (1967). The corpus callosum of the dog. *Acta Biol Exp (Warsaw), 27*, 389–411.

Swiecimska, Z. (1968). Myeloarchitectonics of the medium-long and short association fibers in the frontal region of the dog brain. *Acta Biol Cracoviensia Ser Zool, 11*, 197–211.

Swiecimska, Z. (1970). Cortico-cortical connections in the perisylvian cortex in the dog. *Acta Biol Cracoviensia Ser Zool, 13*, 141–159.

Sych, B. (1976). Architecture of the ventral group of thalamic nuclei in the dog brain. *Folia Biol (Krakow), 24*, 257–276.

Sych, L. (1960). The external capsule in the dog's brain (myeloarchitectonics and topography). *Acta Biol Exp (Warsaw), 20*, 91–101.

Sychowa, B. (1961a). Degenerations after ablations of the anterior and posterior parts of the sylvian gyrus in the dog. *Bull Acad Pol Sci Cl II Ser Sc Biol, 9*, 183–186.

Sychowa, B. (1961b). The morphology and topography of the thalamic nuclei of the dog. *Acta Biol Exp (Warsaw), 21*, 101–120.

Sychowa, B. (1962a). Medial geniculate body of the dog. *J Comp Neurol, 118*, 355–371.

Sychowa, B. (1962b). Degeneration after ablation of the ectosylvian gyrus in dog. *Bull Acad Pol Sci Cl II Ser Sc Biol, 10*, 17–20.

Sychowa, B. (1963). Degenerations of the medial geniculate body following ablations of various temporal regions in the dog. *Acta Biol Exp (Warsaw), 23*, 75–99.

Sychowa, B., Stepien, L., & Stepien, I. (1968). Degeneration in the thalamus following medial frontal lesions in the dog. *Acta Biol Exp (Warsaw), 28*, 383–399.

Tafti, M., Nishino, S., Liao, W., et al. (1997). Mesopontine organization of cholinergic and catecholaminergic cell groups in the normal and narcoleptic dog. *J Comp Neurol, 379*, 185–197.

Takahashi, K. (1951). Experiments on the periamygdaloid cortex of cat and dog. *Folia Psychiat Neurol Jpn, 5*, 147–154.

Tanibuchi, I. (1992). Electrophysiological and anatomical studies on thalamic mediodorsal nucleus projections onto the prefrontal cortex in the cat. *Brain Res, 580*, 137–146.

Tenerowicz, M. (1960). The morphology and topography of the claustrum in the brain of the dog. *Acta Biol Cracoviensia Ser Zool, 3*, 105–113.

Thauer, R., & Stuke, F. (1940). Über die funktionelle Bedeutung der motorischen Region der Grosshirnrinde für den Sehakt des Hundes. *Arch Ges Physiol, 243*, 347–369.

Tryhubczak, A. (1975). Myeloarchitectonics of the hippocampal formation in the dog. *Folia Biol (Krakow), 23*, 177–188.

Tunturi, A. R. (1944). Audio frequency localisation in the acoustic cortex of the dog. *Am J Physiol, 141*, 397–403.

Tunturi, A. R. (1945). Further afferent connections to the acoustic cortex of the dog. *Am J Physiol, 144*, 389–394.

Tunturi, A. R. (1946). A study of the pathway from the medial geniculate body to the acoustic cortex in the dog. *Am J Physiol, 147*, 311–319.

Tunturi, A. R. (1950). Physiological determination of the boundary of the acoustic area in the cerebral cortex of the dog. *Am J Physiol, 160*, 395–401.

Tunturi, A. R. (1952). A difference in the representation of auditory signals for the left and right ears in the iso-frequency contours of the right middle ectosylvian auditory cortex of the dog. *Am J Physiol, 168*, 712–727.

Tunturi, A. R. (1970). The pathway from the medial geniculate body to the ectosylvian auditory cortex in the dog. *J Comp Neurol, 138*, 131–136.

Tunturi, A. R. (1971). Classification of neurons in the ectosylvian auditory cortex of the dog. *J Comp Neurol, 142*, 153–165.

Tunturi, A. R. (1982). Spinal cord tracts mediating voluntary movement of hind limb in dog. *Brain Res, 240*, 338–340.

Vakolyuk, N. I. (1974). *A stereotaxic atlas of subcortical nuclei of the dog's brain.* Kiev: Academy of Sciences of the Ukrainian SSR.

Vann, S. D., & Aggleton, J. P. (2004). The mammillary bodies: two memory systems in one? *Nature Rev Neurosci, 5*, 35–44.

Venzke, W. G., & Gilmore, J. W. (1940). Histological observation on the epiphysis cerebri and the choroid plexus of the third ventricle of the dog. *Proc Iowa Acad Sci, 47*, 409–413.

Wallach, J. H., Rybicki, K. J., & Kaufman, M. P. (1983). Anatomical localization of the cells of origin of efferent fibers in the superior laryngeal and recurrent laryngeal nerves of dogs. *Brain Res, 261*, 307–311.

Whalen, L. R., & Kitchell, R. L. (1983). Electrophysiologic and behavioral studies of the cutaneous nerves of the concave surface of the pinna and the external ear canal of the dog. *Am J Vet Res, 44*, 628–634.

Willis, W. D. (1984). The pain system, vol. 8 of Pain and headache. In P. L. Gildenberg (Ed.), *The Chronic Pain Patient: Evaluation and Management (Pain and Headache)*. New York: S Karger.

Willis, W. D. (1986). Ascending somatosensory systems. In T. L. Yaksh (Ed.), *Spinal afferent processing*. New York: Plenum Press.

Wing, K. G., & Smith, K. U. (1942). The role of the optic cortex in the dog in the determination of the functional properties of conditioned reactions to light. *J Exp Psychol, 31*, 478–496.

Woolsey, C. N. (1933). Postural relations of the frontal and motor cortex of the dog. *Brain, 56*, 353–370.

Woolsey, C. N. (1943). Second" somatic receiving area in the cerebral cortex of cat, dog, and monkey. *Fed Proc, 2*, 55–56.

Woźnicka, A., & Kosmal, A. (2003). Cytoarchitecture of the canine perirhinal and postrhinal cortex. *Acta Neurobiol Exp, 63*, 197–209.

Woźnicka, A., Malinowska, M., & Kosmal, A. (2006). Cytoarchitectonic organization of the entorhinal cortex of the canine brain. *Brain Res Rev, 52*, 346–367.

Yamagishi, Y. (1935). Über die cytoarchitektonische Gliederung des roten Kernes des Hundes. *Z Mikr-Anat Forsch, 37*, 659–672.

Yoda, S. (1941). Beitrag zu den Olivenkernen des Hundes. *Z Mikr Anat Forsch, 49*, 516–524.

Zernicki, B. (1961). The effect of prefrontal lobectomy on water instrumental conditional reflexes in dogs. *Acta Biol Exp, 21*, 157–162.

Zernicki, B., & Santibanez, G. (1961). The effects of ablation of "alimentary area" of the cerebral cortex on salivary conditional and unconditional reflexes in dogs. *Acta Biol Exp (Warsaw), 21*, 163–167.

Zimny, R., Sobusiak, T., & Silny, W. (1972). The pattern of afferent projection from the 8th, 9th, and 10th cranial nerves to the inferior vestibular nucleus: an experimental study in the dog with Nauta method. *Anat Anz, 130*, 285–296.

Zimny, R., Sobusiak, T., Grottel, K., et al. (1973). A bidirectional projection between the gracile nucleus and the cerebellum in the dog? An experimental study with tigrolysis and axonal degeneration methods. *J Hirnforsch, 14*, 89–108.

19
Cranial Nerves

The cranial nerves of vertebrates have been the subject of much study because of their association with the sense organs of the head, their easy accessibility, and their interesting phylogenetic and ontogenetic history (Kappers et al., 1936). From a practical standpoint they have clinical relevance as diagnostic indicators of central nervous system (CNS) disorders (de Lahunta et al., 2015). It is probable that most of the cranial nerves were once associated with a pattern of head segmentation, not unlike dorsal and ventral segmental spinal nerves. In fish and amphibians there are only 10 pairs of cranial nerves because the succeeding nerves are not enclosed by the skull and hence are considered as spinal nerves. The first spinal nerve of fish is large and serves gill and opercular structures that are destined to be incorporated into the skull. Not until reptiles evolved did the development of the skull envelop the first and second spinal nerves, making them cranial nerves XI (accessory nerve) and XII (hypoglossal nerve). The cranial nerve innervation of some ventral neck muscles and the trapezius muscle to the scapula can be understood only in the context of their phylogenetic history beginning as the gill arch levator muscles of fish (Goslow & Hildebrand, 2001; Romer & Parsons, 1986). The ontogenetic sequences of muscle-nerve relations often reflect their phylogenetic history (Noden & de Lahunta, 1985).

The 12 **cranial nerves** of the dog emerge from or enter the brain through foramina of the skull to innervate structures of the head and body. They are sensory, motor, or mixed in function. Some nerves that we usually think of as purely afferent or sensory, such as the optic nerve for vision and the vestibulocochlear nerve for hearing and balance, also have a small component of efferent motor neurons that can modify the function of the end organ by altering transmission at the receptor site. Such efferent neurons have been described in the retina of the eye and the membranous labyrinth of the inner ear. Some of the primarily motor cranial nerves probably have general proprioceptive sensory neurons as well.

Reptiles, birds, and mammals all have 12 pairs of cranial nerves, which by convention are numbered with Roman numerals I to XII. The cranial nerves were named according to early functional interpretations in humans. Long after the present numbering scheme was adopted, an additional, accessory olfactory nerve, the *nervus terminalis*, was recognized as a vomeronasal component of the olfactory system and was sometimes given the numeral designation of cranial nerve "0." Locy (1899), when first describing this nerve, suggested a neural crest and placodal origin. Contrary to statements that sometimes appear in the literature as to the absence of the terminal nerve in humans, it is present and has been described by Johnston (1914), Brookover (1914), and others. It is considered here as a part of cranial nerve I, the olfactory nerve.

Neurons from the autonomic nervous system join and accompany blood vessels and cranial nerves in various ways to reach their effector sites. The cranial nerve components from the parasympathetic system (general visceral efferents from a cranial outflow) have their cell bodies of preganglionic neurons in the brainstem and are associated with cranial nerves III, VII, IX, and X. They function for constriction of the pupil, gland secretion, and smooth muscle contraction of the gastrointestinal system.

Sympathetic neurons that accompany cranial nerves (general visceral efferents from a cranial thoracic outflow) usually have the neuronal cell body for the postganglionic axon located in the cranial cervical ganglion, although there are always some scattered sympathetic second neurons located elsewhere. The preganglionic sympathetic axons that synapse with neuronal cell bodies of postganglionic axons that innervate the iris and smooth muscle of the orbit have their cell bodies in the intermediate gray column of the first three thoracic spinal cord segments. They reach the base of the skull by projecting cranially in the vagosympathetic trunk and synapse with neuronal cell bodies of postganglionic axons in the cranial cervical ganglion. The postganglionic axons then pass through the tympanooccipital fissure with the internal carotid artery and follow the artery through the carotid canal and foramen lacerum to reach the floor of the cranial cavity ventral to the trigeminal ganglion and its three main branches. These postganglionic sympathetic axons join the ophthalmic nerve, a branch from the trigeminal ganglion, which enters the periorbita through the orbital fissure and carries these postganglionic sympathetic axons to the smooth muscle (orbitalis muscle) of the periorbita, and eyelids including the third eyelid and to the dilator pupillae muscle of the iris. Other postganglionic sympathetic axons from the cranial cervical ganglion course with blood vessels or cranial nerves to erector pili muscles associated with hair follicles and sweat glands of the head and face.

For other overall considerations of the cranial nerves and adnexa of the dog, the reader is referred to Jenkins (1972), Meyer (1979), and de Lahunta, Kent, and Glass (2015). The cranial nerves are listed in Box 19.1.

Olfactory Nerve (Cranial Nerve I)

The **olfactory nerves** (*nn. olfactorii*), usually referred to collectively as the *first cranial nerve,* consist of numerous nonmyelinated axons with cell bodies located in the olfactory epithelium covering one-half of the ethmoidal labyrinth and the dorsal part of the nasal septum. Axons from these olfactory cells enter the skull through the cribriform plate of the ethmoid bone (Fig. 19.1), deep in the caudal part of the nasal cavity, to reach the olfactory bulbs of the brain where they synapse. The axons do not form a discrete nerve trunk because they enter the bulbs through many cribriform foramina over the entire contact surface (ventral surface) of the olfactory bulbs. The olfactory nerves are usually torn from the olfactory bulbs when the brain is removed from the skull. Included with the olfactory nerves are the **terminal nerve** (*n. terminalis*) and the **vomeronasal nerve** (*n. vomeronasalis*) both of which arise from the vomeronasal organ (Fig. 19.1) and which enter the olfactory peduncle and bulb, respectively, and form a distinct bundle and tract (Scalia & Winans, 1976).

Read (1908) studied the gross and histologic structure of the olfactory mucosa, vomeronasal organ, and olfactory nerves in the dog, cat, and human. Her historical review points out some of the past controversy involving this relatively simple sensory complex and is followed by an investigation with the techniques of that period. She used 20% nitric acid for 6 to 12 hours to decalcify the bone so that it could be removed from the mucosa to expose the nerves. The nerves appeared white on a dark background of mucosa. Dissection was done under water in bright light, which allowed very small nerves to be seen and photographed. This gross technique is still applicable today but is little used.

The epithelium of the olfactory region shows three kinds of cells: sustentacular cells, which are elongate and cylindrical; olfactory cells, which are fusiform and lie between sustentacular cells; and stellate or basal cells near the basement membrane. In the submucosa there are serous glands. Fresh olfactory mucosa is slightly yellowish in appearance owing to pigment in the sustentacular cells. The olfactory nerve cell bodies are large and numerous, and all of the folds of mucosa in the region of the cribriform plate are olfactory. Read (1908) concluded that the vomeronasal organ was intimately connected with the sense of smell, and we now know that it serves as a pheromone receptor for odors associated with estrus and reproductive functions.

Also seen within the olfactory mucosa is the **ethmoidal nerve** (*n. ethmoidalis*), a branch of the ophthalmic nerve (V), which enters from the orbit through the rostral ethmoidal foramen into the cranial cavity and thence through the cribriform plate into the nasal cavity (Figs. 19.1 and 19.2). The ethmoidal nerve passes along the dorsal border of the nasal septum before dividing into three branches. The **external nasal branches** (*rami nasales externi*) pass to the skin in the vestibule of the nose (Whalen & Kitchell, 1983a). The **medial nasal branch** (*ramus nasalis medialis*) innervates the septum and the **lateral nasal branch** (*ramus*

• BOX 19.1 **Cranial Nerves**

I	Olfactory
II	Optic
III	Oculomotor
IV	Trochlear
V	Trigeminal
VI	Abducent
VII	Facial
VIII	Vestibulocochlear
IX	Glossopharyngeal
X	Vagus
XI	Accessory
XII	Hypoglossal

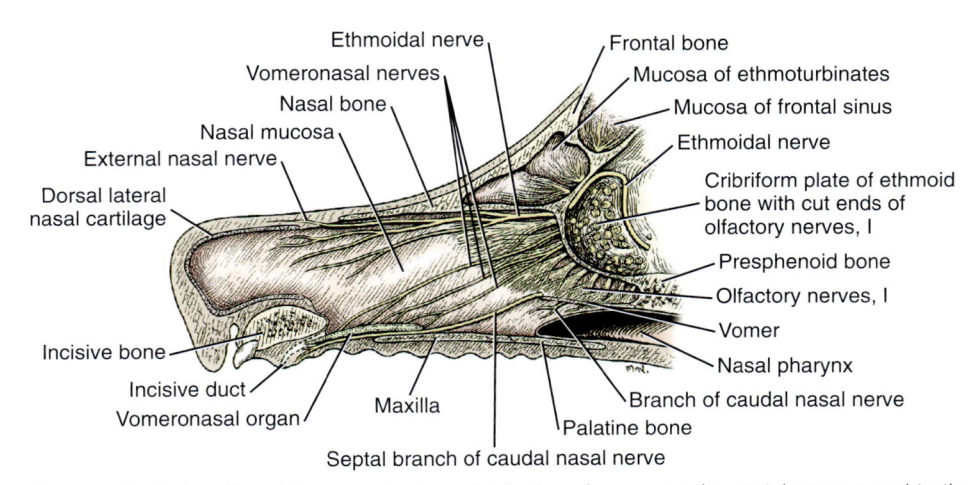

• **Fig. 19.1** Sagittal section of the nose to show distribution of nerves on the septal mucosa and to the vomeronasal organ.

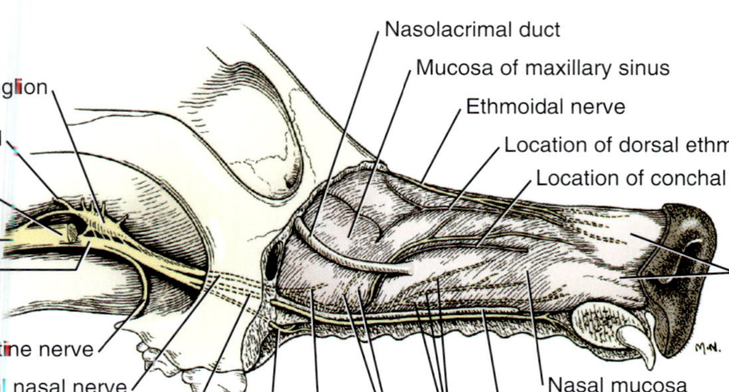

• Fig. 19.2 Nerves of the lateral nasal wall and hard palate.

nasalis lateralis) innervates the nasal conchae. Stimulation of the receptors of this nerve, as well as of the nasal branches of the maxillary (V) nerve, lead to sneezing. The **caudal nasal nerve** (*n. nasalis caudalis*) from the maxillary nerve (V) enters the nasal cavity through the sphenopalatine foramen and innervates the nasal mucosa and maxillary recess rostral to the ethmoidal labyrinth. The **nasopalatine nerve** (*n. nasopalatinus*) from the maxillary (V) is a continuation of the caudal nasal nerve that passes to the incisive canal and vomeronasal organ.

McCotter (1913) described the **terminal nerve** (*n. terminalis*) in the dog and cat and considered the relationship of the vomeronasal nerves to the olfactory nerves in several mammals (McCotter, 1912). Larsell (1920) reviewed the history of the discovery of the terminal nerve and also described its structure in several mammals, including the dog. The nervus terminalis passes through the cribriform plate in company with vomeronasal bundles. Only one small ganglion was found in the dog by Larsell (1920). It was fusiform in shape and located within the cranial cavity on the ventrolateral surface of the olfactory bulb. Barone et al. (1966) in their review of Jacobson's organ noted the difficulty they had observing the terminal nerve. They cited 59 papers relating to the vomeronasal organ and its nerves, several of which refer to the dog.

Optic Nerve (Cranial Nerve II)

The **optic nerve** (*n. opticus*), or second cranial nerve, is actually a tract of the brain and not a nerve by definition, but it is called a nerve by convention. Its developmental origin from ganglion cell axons in the optic vesicle, its neuroglial cells, lack of Schwann cells, myelin produced from oligodendrocytes, and its meninges with a subarachnoid space are evidence of its CNS status. In addition, the optic nerve is involved in diseases of the CNS rather than the PNS. The optic nerve axons collect at the optic disc of the retina, where they are myelinated by oligodendroglial cells, pass through the cribriform area of the sclera, and enter the skull through the optic canals of the presphenoid bone. In all mammals a majority of the axons cross to the opposite side (decussate) at the optic chiasm rostral to the hypophysis (Fig. 19.3) before forming the optic tracts on the lateral aspects of the diencephalon (Fig. 19.4). The axons that cross originate largely from the medial or nasal aspect of each retina. Approximately 75% of the fibers cross in the dog.

The chiasma, or cross-over, is continued by the optic tract (Fig. 19.4), which arches around the diencephalon and terminates in the lateral geniculate nucleus, pretectal region, and rostral colliculus. It would be more anatomically correct to call the optic nerve the prechiasmatic optic tract and the optic tract the postchiasmatic optic tract.

Oculomotor Nerve (Cranial Nerve III)

The **oculomotor nerve** (*n. oculomotorius*), or third cranial nerve, consists primarily of general somatic efferent neurons that innervate several of the striated, voluntary, extraocular muscles that have developed from head somitomeres and parasympathetic general visceral efferent neurons that innervate ocular smooth muscle. The cell bodies of the general somatic efferent neurons are located in the oculomotor nuclei of the rostral mesencephalon, which lie adjacent to the midline on the ventral border of the central gray substance ventral to the mesencephalic aqueduct. The cell bodies of parasympathetic preganglionic general visceral efferent neurons are located in the parasympathetic nucleus of the oculomotor nerve, which lies rostral to the somatic efferent nucleus. As the axons of the oculomotor nerve pass ventrally through the reticular formation of the tegmentum, some fibers cross to the opposite side but most remain uncrossed. The actual proportions are not known for the dog. In the monkey, according to Warwick (1953), the medial and ventral rectus and the ventral oblique muscles are supplied by uncrossed fibers only, the dorsal rectus

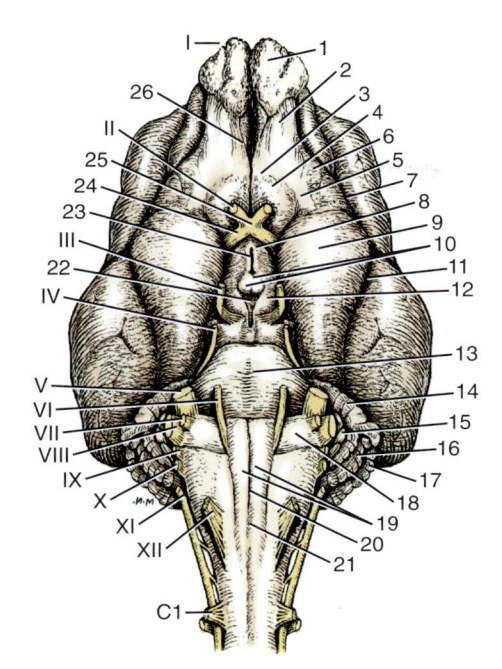

1. Olfactory bulb
2. Olfactory peduncle
3. Medial olfactory tract
4. Rostral perforated substance
5. Lateral olfactory tract
6. Lateral olfactory gyrus
7. Rostral part of lateral rhinal sulcus
8. Tuber cinereum
9. Piriform lobe
10. Mamillary bodies
11. Caudal part of lateral rhinal sulcus
12. Crus cerebri
13. Transverse fibers of pons
14. Ventral paraflocculus
15. Flocculus
16. Dorsal paraflocculus
17. Ansiform lobule
18. Trapezoid body
19. Pyramids
20. Median fissure
21. Decussation of pyramids
22. Caudal perforated substance in interpeduncular fossa
23. Infundibulum
24. Optic tract
25. Optic chiasm
26. Medial rhinal sulcus
I. Olfactory nerves
II. Optic nerve
III. Oculomotor nerve
IV. Trochlear nerve
V. Trigeminal nerve
VI. Abducent nerve
VII. Facial nerve
VIII. Vestibulocochlear nerve
IX. Glossopharyngeal nerve
X. Vagus nerve
XI. Accessory nerve
XII. Hypoglossal nerve
C1. First cervical nerve

• **Fig. 19.3** Ventral view of the brain and cranial nerves.

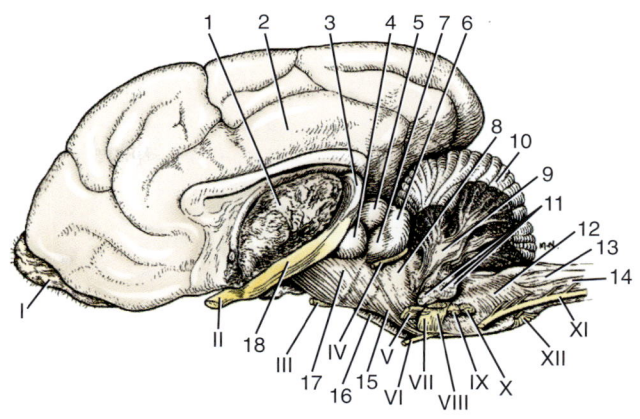

1. Cut surface between cerebrum and brainstem (internal capsule)
2. Medial surface of right cerebral hemisphere
3. Lateral geniculate body
4. Medial geniculate body
5. Rostral colliculus
6. Caudal colliculus
7. Brachium of caudal colliculus
8. Lateral lemniscus
9. Corpus medullare of cerebellum
10. Vermis of cerebellum
11. Flocculus
12. Superficial arcuate fibers
13. Spinal tract of trigeminal nerve
14. Dorsal spinocerebellar tract
15. Longitudinal fibers of pons
16. Transverse fibers of pons
17. Crus cerebri
18. Optic tract
I. Olfactory nerve
II. Optic nerve
III. Oculomotor nerve
IV. Trochlear nerve
V. Trigeminal nerve
VI. Abducent nerve
VII. Facial nerve
VIII. Vestibulocochlear nerve
IX. Glossopharyngeal nerve
X. Vagus nerve
XI. Accessory nerve
XII. Hypoglossal nerve

• **Fig. 19.4** Lateral view of the brain with the left cerebral hemisphere, left transverse fibers of the pons, and left middle cerebellar peduncle removed.

receives only crossed fibers, whereas the levator palpebrae superioris muscle has a bilateral innervation. The oculomotor nerves emerge from the mesencephalon in the interpeduncular fossa (Fig. 19.3) medial to the crus cerebri. Each nerve courses rostrally through the middle cranial fossa, lateral to the hypophysis and dorsal to the cavernous sinus and passes through the orbital fissure (Fig. 19.5). On entering the orbit, the oculomotor nerve divides into a small dorsal branch and a large ventral branch. The **dorsal branch** supplies the dorsal rectus and then penetrates that muscle to go dorsally to supply the levator palpebrae superioris muscle. The **ventral branch** continues rostrally, lateral and slightly ventral, to the optic nerve, where it terminates in a number of branches to the medial rectus, ventral rectus, and ventral oblique muscles. At its termination is the small **ciliary ganglion** (*ganglion ciliare*) (Figs. 19.5 and 19.6) where the preganglionic parasympathetic axons synapse with neuronal cell bodies of postganglionic axons (Fig. 19.6). These postganglionic axons compose the short ciliary nerves that course along the optic nerve to enter the eye and innervate the ciliary muscle (which affect the curvature of the lens) and the sphincter muscle of the iris, the *m. sphincter pupillae*. Neurons in the ciliary ganglion regulate the size of the pupil for the passage of light by stimulation of the sphincter pupillae and inhibition of the dilator pupillae.

Trochlear Nerve (Cranial Nerve IV)

The **trochlear nerve** (*n. trochlearis*), or fourth cranial nerve, provides general somatic efferent innervation to the dorsal oblique muscle of the contralateral side from its cell bodies of origin. It is unique in two ways: It is the only cranial nerve that emerges from the brainstem dorsally (Figs. 18.4 and 19.4), and it is the only cranial nerve to cross entirely to innervate a muscle on the contralateral side. Its cell bodies lie in the trochlear nucleus of the caudal mesencephalon at the level of the caudal colliculi adjacent to the midline on the ventral border of the central gray substance surrounding the mesencephalic aqueduct. The trochlear nucleus is in the caudal part of the mesencephalon, caudal to the oculomotor nucleus.

Fig. 19.5 Schema of the optic, oculomotor, trochlear, trigeminal (ophthalmic nerve) and abducent nerves, dorsal aspect.

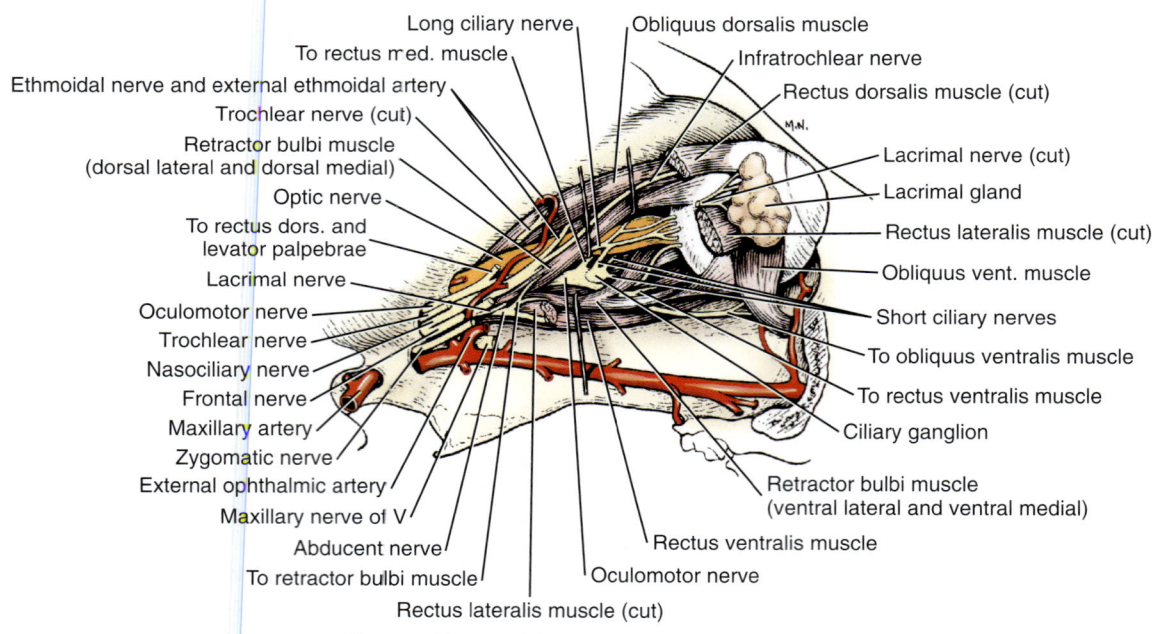

Fig. 19.6 Nerves of the eye and orbit, lateral aspect.

The axons of the trochlear nerve course dorsally around the mesencephalic aqueduct, enter the thin rostral medullary velum caudal to the caudal colliculi, and cross at the trochlear decussation (*decussatio nervorum trochlearium*) in the velum to the opposite side. The nerve emerges from the velum caudal to the contralateral colliculus, passes rostroventrally over the side of the mesencephalon, and leaves the cranial cavity through the orbital fissure to enter the periorbita and innervate the dorsal oblique muscle of the eyeball (Figs. 19.5, 19.6, and 19.8).

Trigeminal Nerve (Cranial Nerve V)

The **trigeminal nerve** (*n. trigeminus*), or fifth cranial nerve, has both motor and sensory components. The sensory portion is larger. The nerve penetrates the pons (Figs. 19.3

and 19.4) just caudal and ventral to where the transverse fibers of the pons are continued dorsally as the middle cerebellar peduncle. This is rostral to the lateral end of the trapezoid body. The trigeminal nerve enters the trigeminal canal (Figs. 19.8 and 19.9) on the rostromedial aspect of the petrosal part of the temporal bone. Within this canal is the large **trigeminal ganglion** (*ganglion trigeminale*) (Figs. 19.5 and 19.9) that contains sensory cell bodies of the general somatic afferent axons found in all three branches of this nerve. As the trigeminal nerve emerges from the trigeminal canal it divides into three nerves: (1) **ophthalmic** (sensory), (2) **maxillary** (sensory), and (3) **mandibular** (sensory and motor). The major branches of these three nerves are shown in Fig. 19.10. Using electrophysiologic techniques, Whalen and Kitchell (1983a, b) determined the cutaneous areas of the head and face innervated by all cutaneous nerves of the head. The cutaneous areas of the three major nerves from the trigeminal nerve, including the autonomous zones (the area innervated by only one nerve) and the overlap zones, are shown in Fig. 19.11.

The Ophthalmic Nerve

The **ophthalmic nerve** (*n. ophthalmicus*) consists of general somatic afferent axons from the eyelids, eyeball, nasal mucosa, and skin of the nose. It passes through the orbital fissure of the skull (Fig. 19.8). Within the periorbita, the ophthalmic nerve divides into three branches—the frontal nerve, lacrimal nerve, and nasociliary nerve.

The **frontal nerve** (*n. frontalis*) is the most dorsal of the three branches of the ophthalmic nerve. It passes rostrally (Figs. 19.5, 19.8, and 19.12) in the periorbita dorsal to the dorsal oblique and dorsal rectus muscles of the eyeball. The frontal nerve becomes subcutaneous just caudal to the orbital ligament to terminate by dividing into **supraorbital** (*n. supraorbitalis*) and **supratrochlear** (*n. supratrochlearis*) nerves. These nerves collectively supply a cutaneous area on the lateral two-thirds of the superior eyelid continuing to the dorsal midline (Fig. 19.13). The cutaneous area overlaps rostrally with the infratrochlear branch of the nasociliary nerve (ophthalmic V) and caudally with branches of the maxillary and mandibular nerves.

The **lacrimal nerve** (*n. lacrimalis*) is smaller than the other two branches and runs along the lateral rectus muscle of the eyeball (Figs. 19.6 and 19.8) to supply the lacrimal gland. It carries postganglionic parasympathetic axons that have their cell bodies in the pterygopalatine ganglion (see discussion of the facial nerve and Fig. 19.7).

The **nasociliary nerve** (*n. nasociliaris*) is the largest and most medial branch of the ophthalmic nerve. It runs medially deep in the orbit across the dorsal surface of the retractor bulbi muscle (Fig. 19.6). The nerve sends a **communicating branch to the ciliary ganglion** (*ramus communicans cum ganglio ciliari*). This branch contains postganglionic sympathetic axons that bypass the ciliary ganglion to enter the short ciliary branches of the oculomotor nerve. These postganglionic axons have their cell bodies located in the cranial cervical ganglion. They reach the ophthalmic nerve by means of an internal carotid plexus around the internal carotid artery, which go with the artery into the carotid canal via the tympanooccipital fissure, then enter the middle cranial fossa of the cranial cavity via the foramen lacerum. Here they join the ophthalmic nerve ventrally as it branches from the trigeminal ganglion. These axons supply the smooth orbitalis muscle in the periorbita and the three eyelids and the dilator of the pupil. The orbitalis muscle tonically retracts the superior, inferior and third eyelids and protrudes the eyeball.

The nasociliary nerve then gives off a number of **long ciliary nerves** (*nn. ciliares longi*) that enter the eyeball dorsal and medial to the optic nerve (Fig. 19.6). These branches are the only general somatic afferent branches to the eyeball, including the corneal epithelium and the bulbar conjunctivum. The nasociliary nerve then terminates by dividing into ethmoidal and infratrochlear branches. The **ethmoidal nerve** (*n. ethmoidalis*) turns medially (Figs. 19.5 and 19.6) to pass through the rostral ethmoidal foramina and the cribriform plate (Fig. 19.1) to enter the nasal cavity, where it divides into medial, lateral, and external branches. The **medial nasal branch** (*ramus nasalis medialis*) supplies the septum and parts of the wall of the nasal cavity (Fig. 19.1). The **lateral nasal branch** (*ramus nasalis lateralis*) innervates the mucosa of the nasal conchae. The **external nasal branches** (*rami nasales externi*) (Fig. 19.1) innervate the skin of the vestibule of the nostril (Whalen & Kitchell, 1983a) (Fig. 19.2). The **infratrochlear nerve** (*n. infratrochlearis*) runs along the medial aspect of the orbit to emerge subcutaneously just ventral to the trochlea of the tendon of the dorsal oblique muscle near the medial canthus of the eye (Figs. 19.10 and 19.12). It supplies an area surrounding the medial canthus (Fig. 19.13). Its cutaneous area overlaps with the frontal nerve dorsally and with branches of the maxillary nerve ventrally.

The Maxillary Nerve

The **maxillary nerve** (*n. maxillaris*) is sensory to the superior eyelid, nasal mucosa, superior teeth, superior lip, and nose (Fig. 19.14), and its distal branches contain postganglionic parasympathetic axons that innervate the lacrimal, nasal, and palatine glands (Fig. 19.7). It leaves the cranial cavity through the round foramen, alar canal, and rostral alar foramen (Figs. 19.5, 19.8, 19.9) and courses rostrally on the dorsal surface of the medial pterygoid muscle to the maxillary foramen (Figs. 19.15 and 19.16). In the orbit on the dorsal surface of the medial pterygoid muscle ventral to the periorbita, the maxillary nerve gives rise to the zygomatic nerve, pterygopalatine nerve, and infraorbital nerve (Fig. 19.10).

The **zygomatic nerve** (*n. zygomaticus*) arises from the maxillary nerve just proximal to the point of entry of the maxillary nerve into the round foramen (Fig. 19.5) or within the alar canal. After the zygomatic nerve exits from the rostral alar foramen (Fig. 19.16), it penetrates the

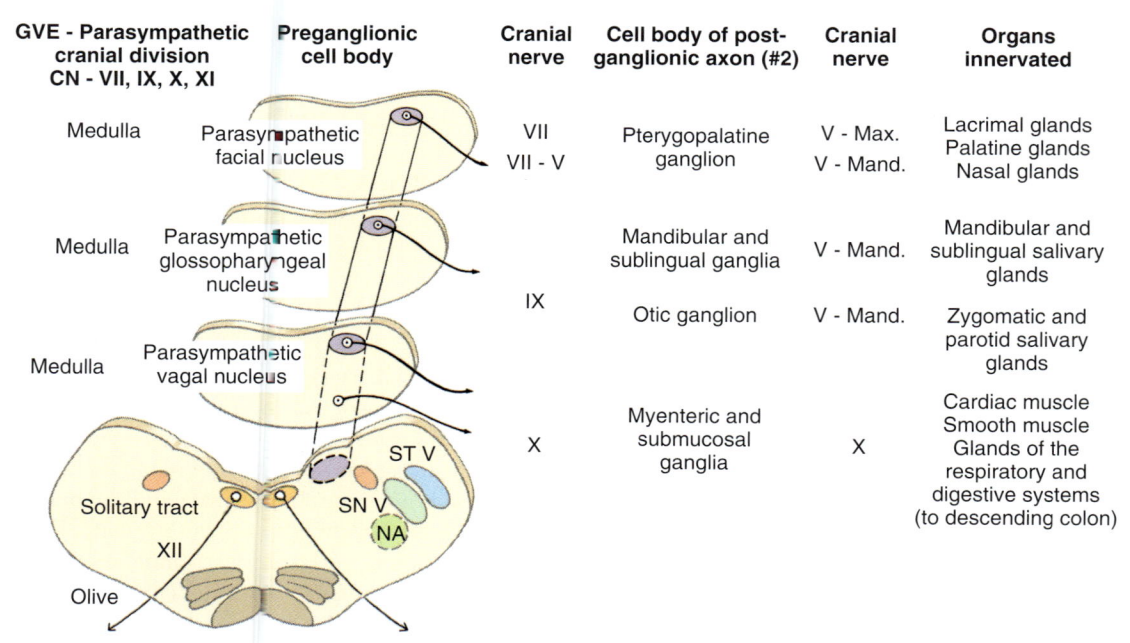

• **Fig. 19.7** Parasympathetic GVE nuclear column in the medulla. *NA*, Nucleus ambiguus; *SN V*, spinal nucleus of V; *ST V*, spinal tract of V.

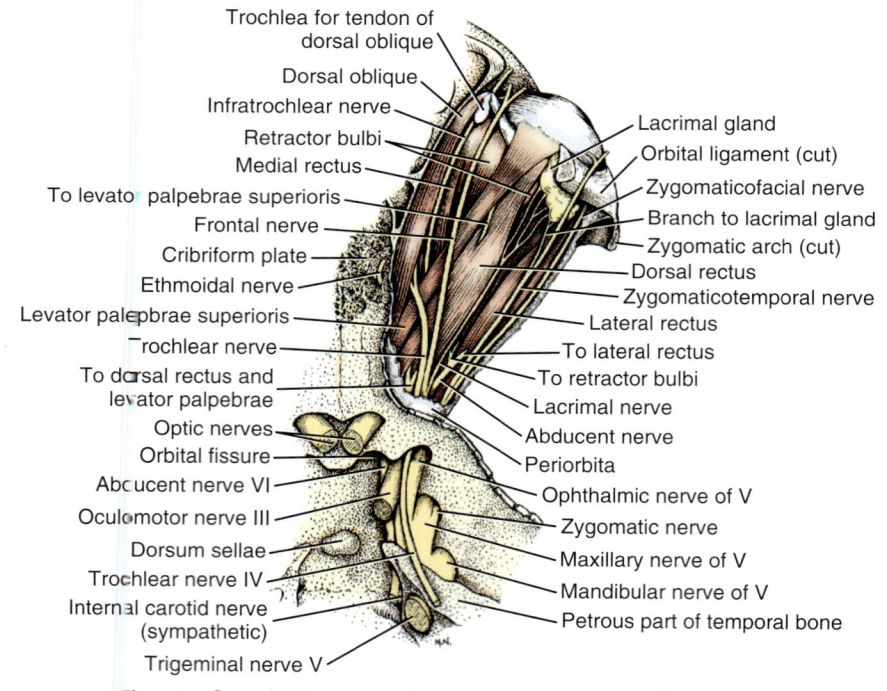

• **Fig. 19.8** Superficial distribution of the nerves of the eye, dorsal aspect.

periorbita and divides into **zygomaticofacial** (*ramus zygomaticofacialis*) and **zygomaticotemporal** (*ramus zygomaticotemporalis*) branches (Figs. 19.5, 19.8, and 19.16). The zygomaticotemporal branch is the more dorsal branch, which runs rostrally in the orbit deep to the periorbita to emerge subcutaneously lateral to the orbital ligament (Fig. 19.8), where it curls ventrally and laterally around the zygomatic arch (Fig. 19.10) to ramify in the skin (Fig. 19.12). It supplies a cutaneous area that includes all of the inferior eyelid (Fig. 19.14). It is overlapped at the lateral canthus of the eye by the frontal nerve (ophthalmic V) (Fig. 19.13) and at the medial canthus by the infratrochlear nerve (ophthalmic V) (Fig. 19.13). The zygomaticofacial nerve is the more ventral branch, which runs rostrally in the orbit deep to the periorbita to emerge medial to the orbital ligament (Fig. 19.8), where it curls dorsally (Fig. 19.12) on the external surface of the temporalis muscle. It supplies a cutaneous area dorsal to the zygomatic arch, over the external surface

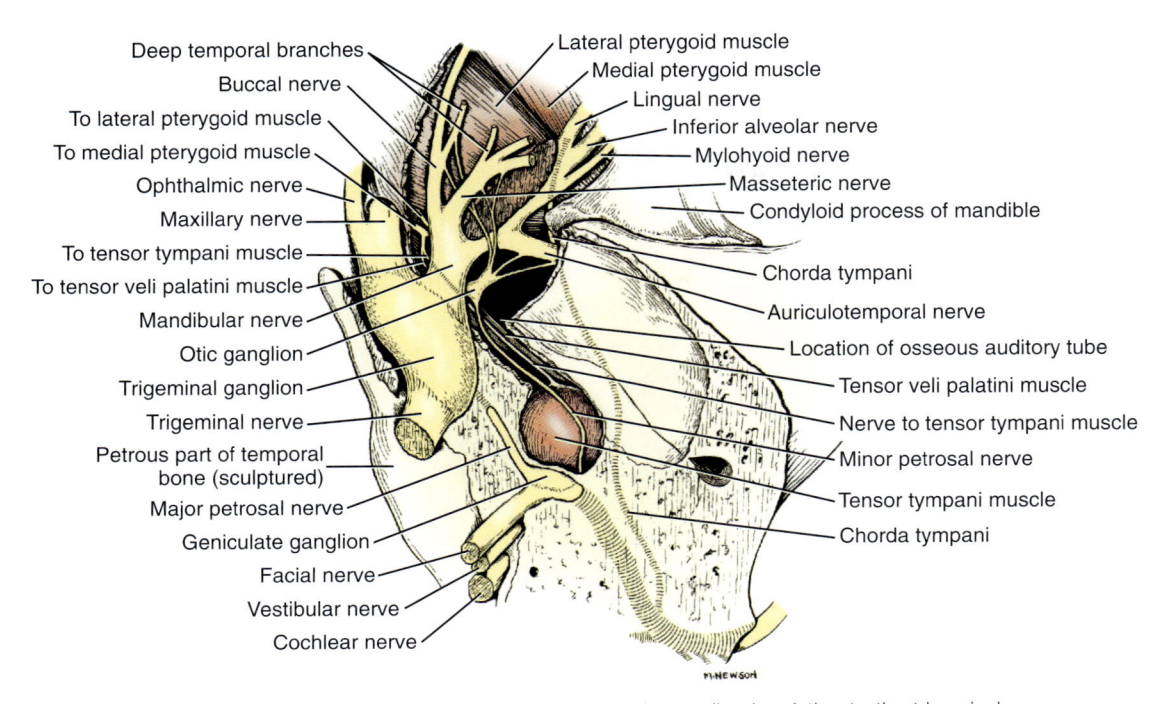

• **Fig. 19.9** The temporal bone sculptured to show the otic ganglion in relation to the trigeminal nerve, dorsal aspect.

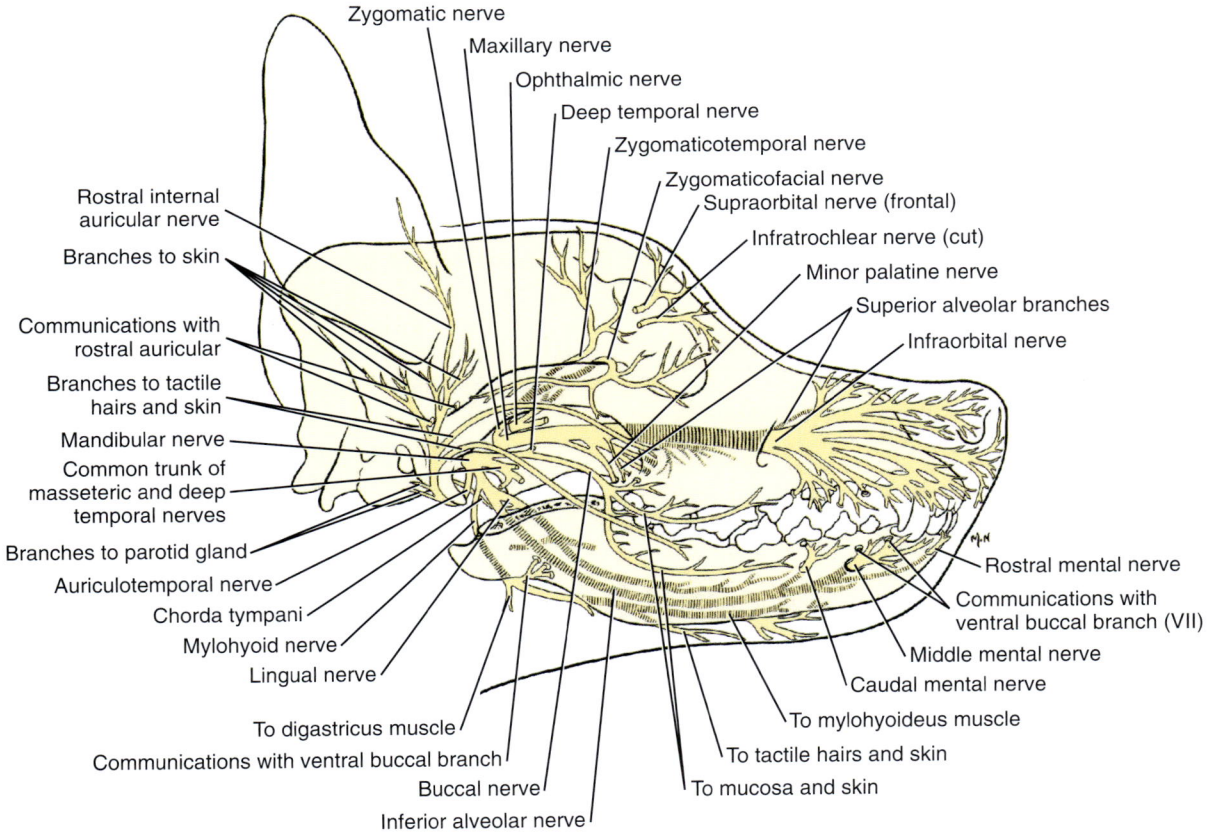

• **Fig. 19.10** Schema of the trigeminal nerve, lateral aspect.

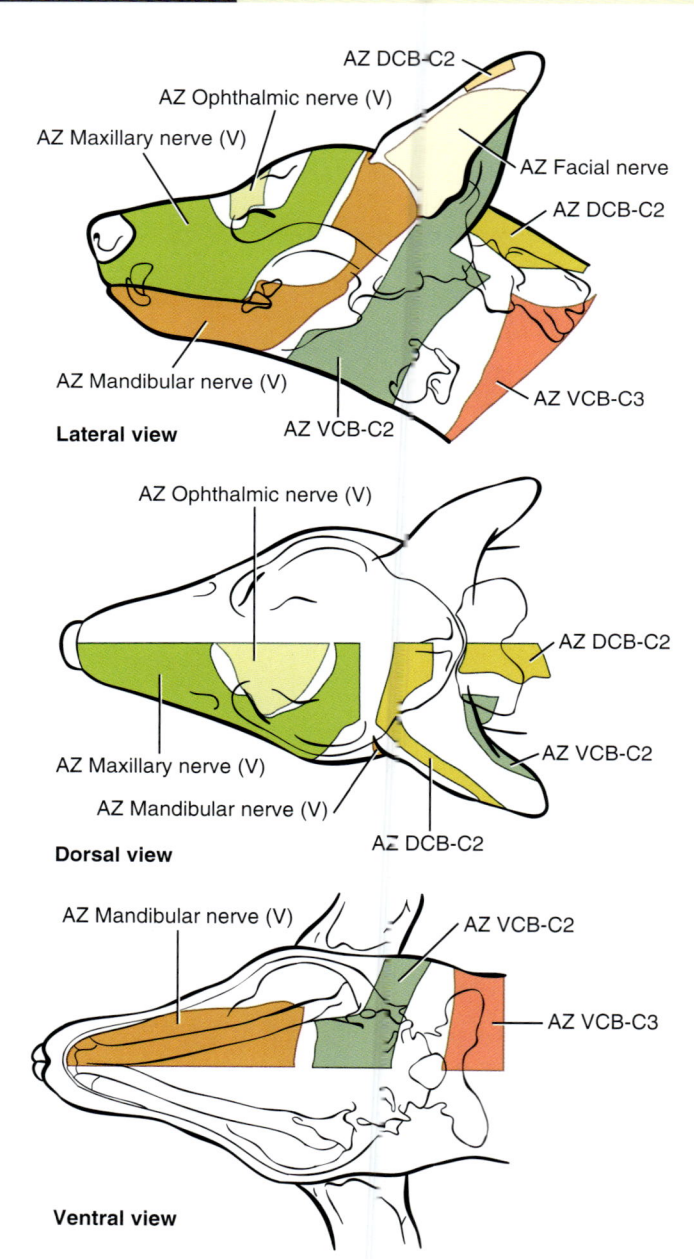

Fig. 19.11 Autonomous zones (AZ) of the head of the dog. The clear areas are zones of overlap between adjacent cutaneous areas. Dorsal cervical branch (DCB), ventral cervical branch (VCB). (Modified with permission from Whalen LR, Kitchell RL: Electrophysiologic studies of the cutaneous nerves of the head of the dog, Am J Vet Res 44:615–627, 1983a.)

of the temporalis muscle cranial to the external ear (Fig. 19.14). It overlaps the cutaneous area of the frontal nerve, dorsal to the lateral canthus of the eye. The lateral canthus of the eye is in the overlap zone of the frontal (ophthalmic V) and of the zygomaticofacial (maxillary V) nerves (Figs. 19.13 and 19.14).

The **pterygopalatine nerve** (*n. pterygopalatinus*) arises from the deep surface of the maxillary nerve on the dorsal surface of the medial pterygoid muscle (Figs. 19.15 and 19.16). The pterygopalatine ganglion (discussed with the facial nerve) lies dorsal to the pterygopalatine nerve and gives off postganglionic parasympathetic axons that join the lacrimal branch of the ophthalmic (V) and zygomaticotemporal nerve (maxillary V) to supply the lacrimal gland (Fig. 19.8). Other branches from the pterygopalatine ganglion go to the following nerves to convey postganglionic parasympathetic axons to the nasal and palatine glands. The **minor palatine nerve** (*n. palatinus minor*) arises from the pterygopalatine nerve and curls around the rostral border of the medial pterygoid muscle (Figs. 19.15 and 19.16) to reach the soft palate. In addition to supplying general visceral afferent axons to the soft palate, this nerve contains the postganglionic parasympathetic axons referred to previously and special visceral afferent axons for taste that have their cell bodies in the geniculate ganglion of the facial nerve (discussed with the facial nerve). These taste buds are in the mucosa of the ventral surface of the soft palate. Their special visceral afferent axons travel to the geniculate ganglion through the pterygopalatine ganglion and the major petrosal nerve. The **major palatine nerve** (*n. palatinus major*) arises from the pterygopalatine nerve distal to the minor palatine nerve (Figs. 19.5 and 19.16). The major palatine nerve gives off an **accessory palatine nerve** (*n. palatinus accessorius*), which supplies the caudal part of the hard palate (Fig. 19.2). The major palatine nerve provides a branch to the caudal nasal nerve and continues rostrally to enter the palatine canal via the caudal palatine foramen. It emerges on the hard palate from the major palatine foramen and supplies most of the mucosa of the hard palate (Fig. 19.2). The **caudal nasal nerve** (*n. nasalis caudalis*) is the continuation of the pterygopalatine nerve. It lies dorsal to the major palatine nerve in the pterygopalatine fossa (Figs. 19.2, 19.15, and 19.16). The caudal nasal nerve leaves the fossa via the sphenopalatine foramen to enter the nasal cavity (Figs. 19.1 and 19.2). It gives off a small branch to supply the maxillary recess (Fig. 19.2), then the major part of the nerve continues to run rostrally to give sensory innervation to the nasal mucosa surrounding the ventral meatus of the nasal cavity. In addition, it contains postganglionic parasympathetic axons from cell bodies located in the pterygopalatine ganglion (Fig. 19.7). These axons supply the nasal glands.

The **infraorbital nerve** (*n. infraorbitalis*) is a direct continuation of the maxillary nerve after the caudal nasal nerve separates from the maxillary (Fig. 19.16). In the pterygopalatine fossa, the infraorbital nerve gives off the **caudal superior alveolar branches** (*rami alveolares superiores caudalis*) (Figs. 19.15 and 19.16). These arise from the ventral aspect of the infraorbital nerve and run rostroventrally to enter the alveolar canals via the alveolar foramina of the maxilla to supply the caudal superior cheek teeth. An alveolar canal leads to the tip of each alveolus to enter the root of each tooth. After the caudal superior alveolar branches are given off, the infraorbital nerve enters the infraorbital canal by passing through the maxillary foramen. Once within the canal, the infraorbital nerve gives off from its ventral border, the **middle superior alveolar branches** (*rami alveolares superiores medi*), which enter alveolar canals

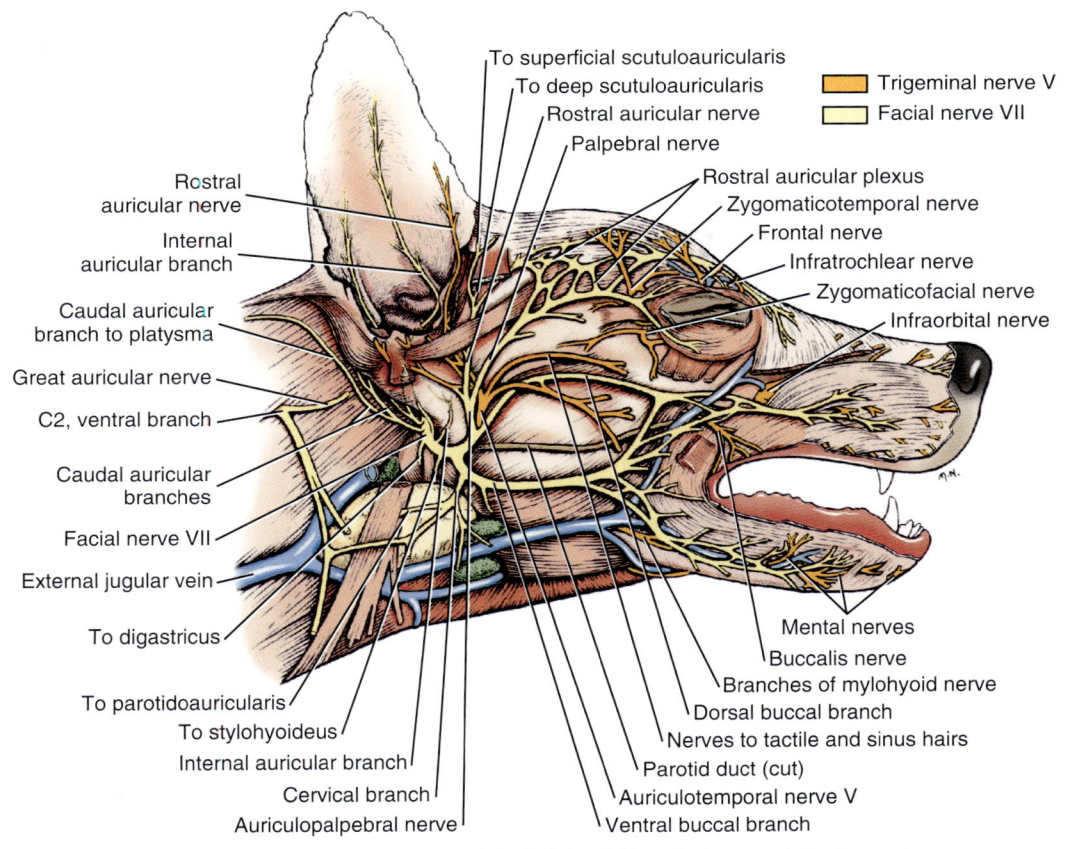

- **Fig. 19.12** Superficial branches of the facial and trigeminal nerves, lateral aspect.

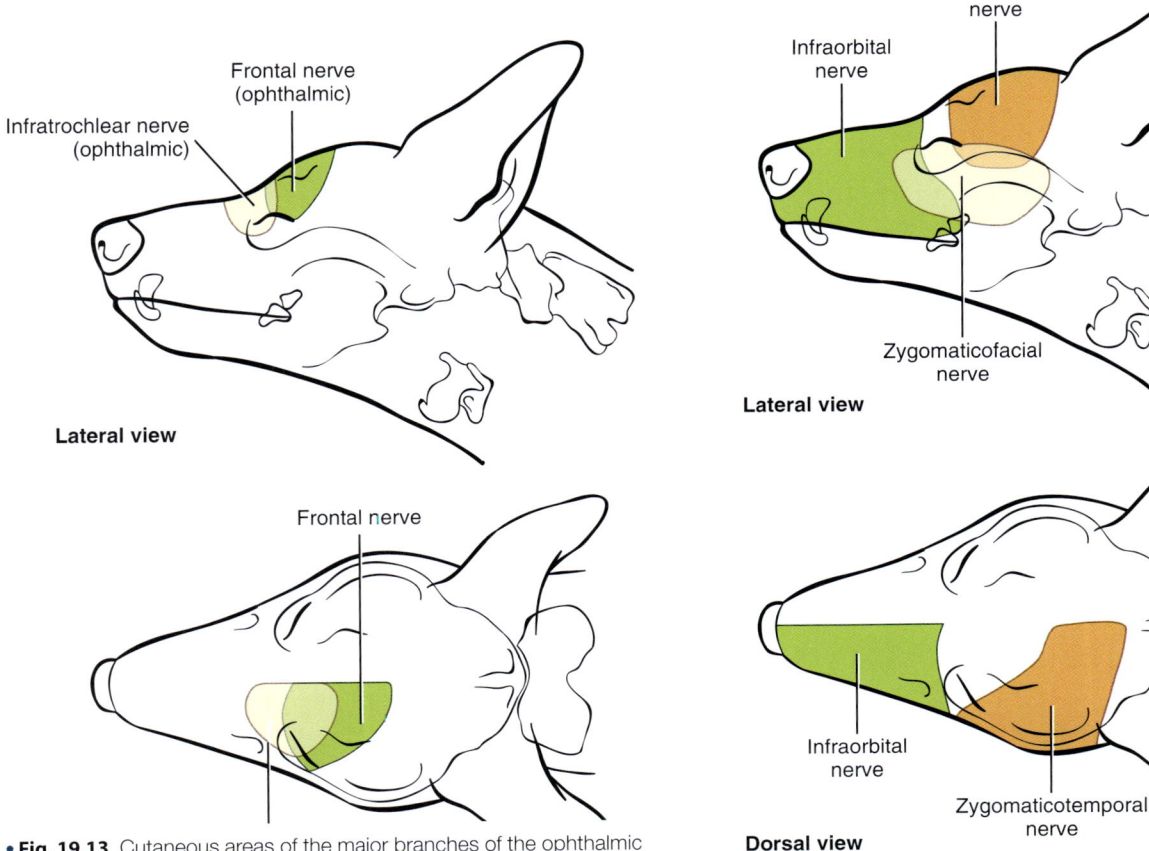

- **Fig. 19.13** Cutaneous areas of the major branches of the ophthalmic nerve (V). The *clear* areas are zones of overlap between adjacent cutaneous areas. (Modified with permission from Whalen LR, Kitchell RL: Electrophysiologic studies of the cutaneous nerves of the head of the dog, *Am J Vet Res* 44:615–627, 1983a.)

- **Fig. 19.14** Cutaneous areas of the major branches of the maxillary nerve (V). The *clear* areas are zones of overlap between adjacent cutaneous areas. (Modified with permission from Whalen LR, Kitchell RL: Electrophysiologic studies of the cutaneous nerves of the head of the dog, *Am J Vet Res* 44:615–627, 1983a.)

824 CHAPTER 19 Cranial Nerves

• **Fig. 19.15** The pterygopalatine ganglion, lateral aspect.

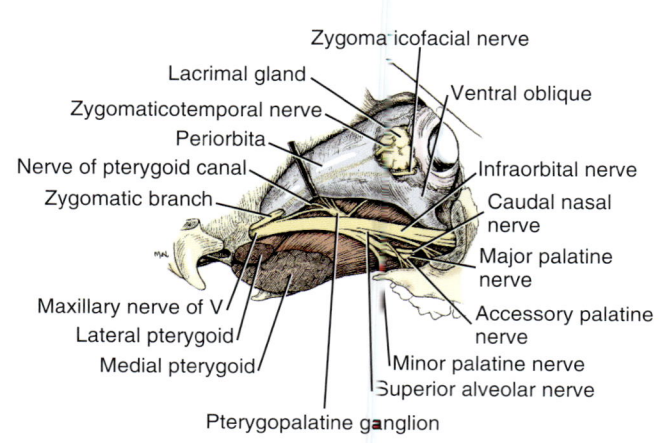

• **Fig. 19.16** Maxillary nerve from the trigeminal nerve, lateral aspect.

via alveolar foramina to supply the superior cheek teeth. Just before the infraorbital nerve exits from the infraorbital canal through the infraorbital foramen, it gives off from its ventral surface the **rostral superior alveolar branches** (*rami alveolares superiores medii*) (Fig. 19.10). These branches enter the incisivomaxillary canals to supply the superior canine and incisor teeth. External to the infraorbital foramen, the infraorbital nerve divides into a number of fasciculi, which are named **external nasal branches** (*rami nasales externi*), **internal nasal branches** (*rami nasales interni*), or **superior labial branches** (*rami labiales superioris*), depending on the area supplied (Fig. 19.12). The cutaneous area for the infraorbital nerve is shown in Fig. 19.14. It is overlapped by other branches of the maxillary nerve (Fig. 19.14) and by the infratrochlear nerve (ophthalmic V) ventral to the medial canthus of the eye (Fig. 19.13).

The Mandibular Nerve

The **mandibular nerve** (*n. mandibularis*) is both motor and sensory. It is motor to the muscles that move the mandibles and change the size of the oral cavity thus controlling biting, prehension (using the teeth only), and mastication. These muscles include the masseter, temporalis, medial and lateral

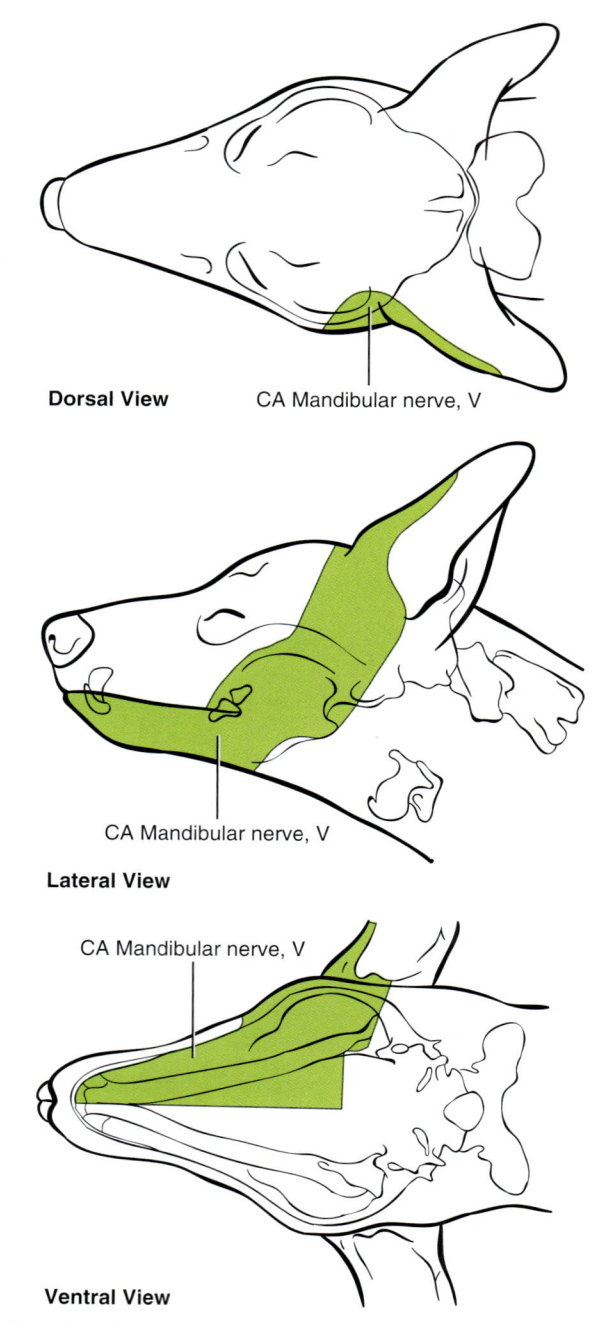

• **Fig. 19.17** Cutaneous area of the mandibular nerve (V). For the cutaneous areas of the major branches of the mandibular nerve (V), see Figs. 19.18 and 19.22. (Modified with permission from Whalen LR, Kitchell RL: Electrophysiologic studies of the cutaneous nerves of the head of the dog, Am J Vet Res 44:615–627, 1983a.)

pterygoids, rostral digastricus, and mylohyoideus. The mandibular nerve is sensory to the cheek and inferior labium, tongue, teeth of the mandible, and the skin of the head, in part (Fig. 19.17), and skin of the intraosseous part of the external ear canal (Fig. 19.18).

The cell bodies of the somatic efferent neurons of this nerve are located in the **motor nucleus of the trigeminal nerve** (*nucleus motorius n. trigemini*), which lies in the lateral reticular formation of the pons at the level of

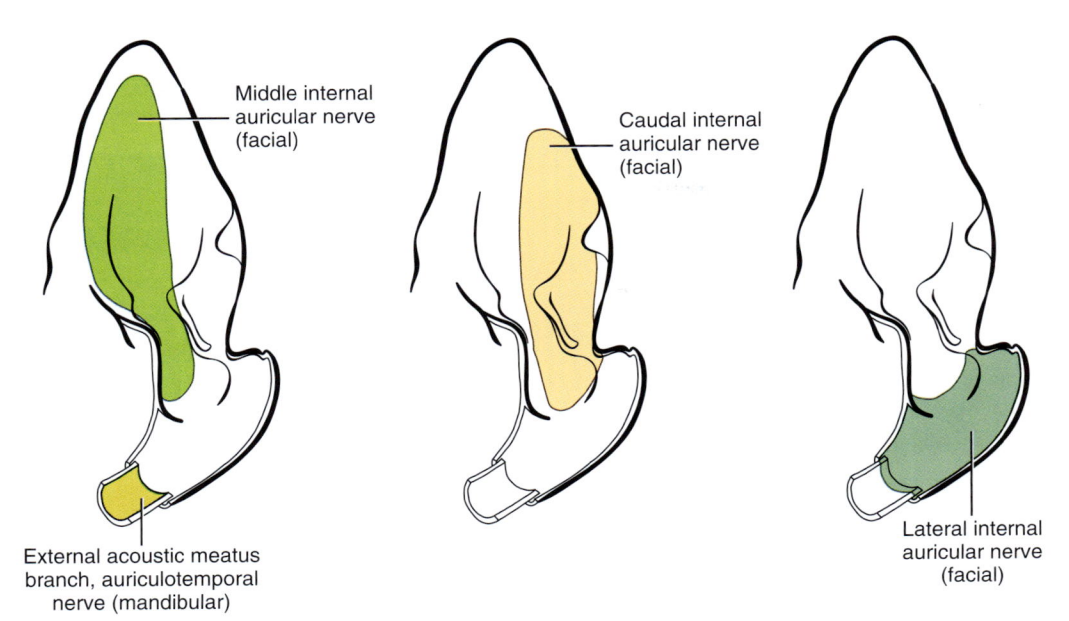

• **Fig. 19.18** Cutaneous areas of the rostral concave surface of the external ear. For the cutaneous areas of the caudal convex surface of the external ear see Figs. 19.17 and 19.30. (Modified with permission from Whalen LR, Kitchell RL: Electrophysiologic and behavioral studies of the cutaneous nerves of the concave surface of the pinna and the external ear canal of the dog, *Am J Vet Res* 44:628–634, 1983b.)

the rostral cerebellar peduncle. The axons of these motor neurons pass laterally through the pons to form the **minor root** (*radix minor*) of the trigeminal nerve that joins the **major root** (*radix major*) that contains the sensory neurons of the trigeminal nerve entering from the trigeminal ganglion (Figs. 19.3 and 19.4).

The trigeminal motor neurons pass through the ventral part of the trigeminal ganglion in the trigeminal canal of the petrosal part of the temporal bone and join the mandibular nerve, which leaves the cranial cavity through the oval foramen (Fig. 19.5). Primary branches of the mandibular nerve include the masticatory nerve, lateral and medial pterygoid nerves, tensor tympani nerve, tensor veli palatini nerve, buccal nerve, auriculotemporal nerve, lingual nerve, inferior alveolar nerve, and the mylohyoid nerve (Fig. 19.10).

The **masticatory nerve** (*n. masticatorius*) of trigeminal V has a digastric ramus to the rostral belly of the digastricus muscle, which in concert with the caudal belly of the digastricus muscle (innervated by facial nerve VII) opens the mouth. A **masseteric nerve** (*n. massetericus*) to the masseter muscle (Fig. 19.20) and **deep temporal nerves** (*nn. temporalis profundi*) to the temporalis muscle (Fig. 19.9) initiate forceful closing of the mouth.

The **lateral** and **medial pterygoid nerves** (*n. pterygoideus lateralis et medialis*) innervate the small lateral pterygoid muscle and the larger medial pterygoid muscle (Figs. 19.9 and 19.20), both of which function to raise the mandible when chewing. These muscles do not result in rotational (grinding) movements of the mandibles in the dog as they do in some other species.

The **tensor tympani nerve** (*n. tensoris tympani*) is motor to the tensor tympani muscle of the malleus (Fig. 19.20). Because the malleus was derived phylogenetically from the articular bone of the mandible and the muscles associated with the articular joint were first branchial arch muscles, they retain their innervation from the trigeminal nerve. The tensor tympani muscle plays an active role in modulating the movements of the malleus, thus affecting the movement of the ossicular chain in the middle ear (Chapter 20). This muscle reflexively contracts and tightens the tympanic membrane following loud sounds and prevents large excursions of the malleus.

The **tensor veli palatini nerve** (*n. tensoris veli palatini*) is motor to the thin muscle of the same name in the soft palate (Fig. 19.20). Contraction of this muscle, in concert with the levator veli palatini muscle (innervated by the facial nerve), tends to keep the pharyngeal orifice of the auditory tube open.

The **buccal nerve** (*n. buccalis*) is sensory to the mucosa and skin of the cheek (Figs. 19.9, 19.10, 19.12, 19.20, and 19.21). It crosses the pterygoid muscles, curls around the rostral border of the masseter muscle, and enters the cheek lateral to the zygomatic salivary gland. (The term *rami buccales* designates the motor branches of the facial nerve to the muscles of the cheeks, lips, and nose). The buccal nerve supplies a cutaneous area on and ventral to the zygomatic arch, dorsal and caudal to the commissure of the mouth (Fig. 19.22).

The **auriculotemporal nerve** (*n. auriculotemporalis*) leaves the mandibular nerve at the oval foramen (Fig. 19.9), passes medial and caudal to the retroarticular process of the

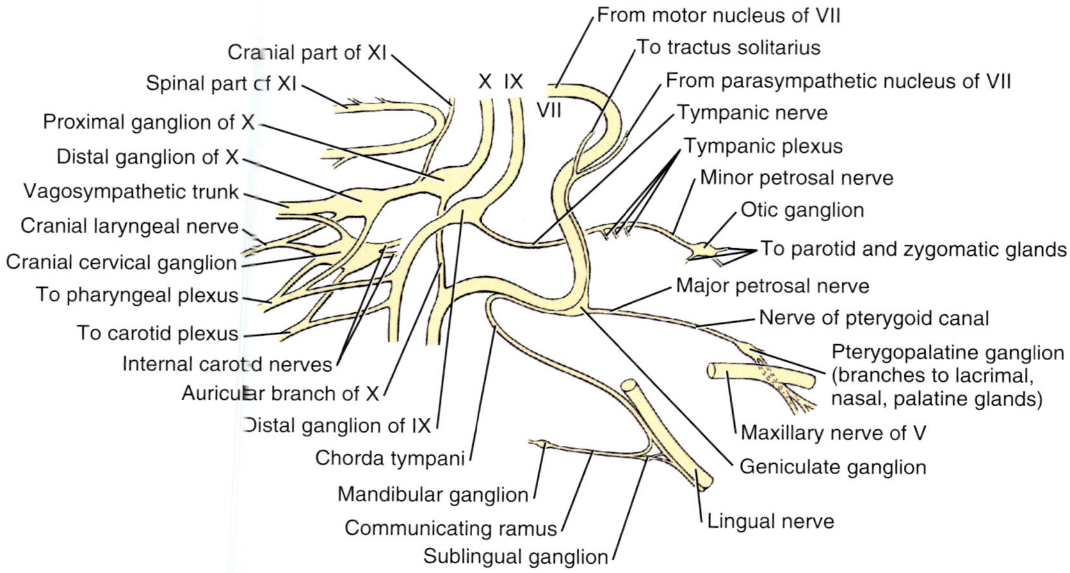

Fig. 19.19 Schema of cranial nerves VII, IX, X, and XI, and autonomic interconnections.

temporal bone (Figs. 19.10 and 19.21), and emerges between the base of the auricular cartilage caudally and the masseter muscle rostrally. It gives off the **external acoustic meatus nerve** (*n. meatus acustici externi*), which is sensory to the skin of the external acoustic meatus near the tympanic membrane (Fig. 19.18) and a **ramus to the tympanic membrane** (*ramus membranae tympani*). As the auriculotemporal nerve passes rostral to the parotid salivary glands it gives **off parotid branches** (*rami parotidei*) to that gland (Fig. 19.10). These branches contain postganglionic parasympathetic axons from the otic ganglion (Figs. 19.7, 19.9, and 19.19) (discussed with the glossopharyngeal nerve). Farther distally, the auriculotemporal nerve gives off **rostral auricular nerves** (*nn. auriculares rostrales*) (Figs. 19.10 and 19.12), which supply the skin over the lateral aspect of the tragus, a small portion of the medioventral part of the pinna's (auricle's) rostral (concave) surface, the medial border of the pinna, the skin over the ventral aspects of the temporalis muscle, and ventrally over the zygomatic arch (Fig. 19.22). The auriculotemporal nerve turns dorsorostrally and gives off a **transverse facial branch** (*ramus transversus faciei*) (labeled as branches to tactile hairs and skin, Figs. 19.10 and 19.12), which supplies an area of skin extending dorsal and ventral from the zygomatic arch (Fig. 19.22), including the tactile hairs of the cheek, and **communicating branches to the facial nerve** (*rami communicantes cum n. faciali*), which join the dorsal buccal branch of the facial nerve to innervate the skin over the surface of the masseter muscle, ventral to the zygomatic arch (Fig. 19.22). The cutaneous area of the transverse facial nerve overlaps with the cutaneous areas of the rostral auricular and the communicating branches (Fig. 19.22).

The **inferior alveolar nerve** (*n. alveolaris inferior*), formerly *mandibular alveolar nerve*, arises from the mandibular nerve on the lateral aspect of the medial pterygoid muscle (Fig. 19.21). In most dogs, the mylohyoid nerve arises immediately from the inferior alveolar nerve, but in some dogs the mylohyoid nerve arises more proximally from the mandibular (Figs. 19.20 and 19.21). The inferior alveolar nerve enters the mandibular foramen on the medial side of the ramus of the mandible. It passes through the mandibular canal of the mandible supplying caudal, middle, and rostral alveolar sensory nerves to the teeth. Near the rostral end of the mandible terminal extensions of this nerve exit from mental foramina as **mental nerves** (*nn. mentales*), which are sensory to the inferior lip and to the rostral intermandibular region (Figs. 19.10, 19.12, and 19.22).

The **mylohyoid nerve** (*n. mylohyoideus*) is usually a branch of the inferior alveolar nerve, although it may arise separately from the mandibular nerve (Figs. 19.21 and 19.22). It runs distally medial to the ramus of the mandible. It gives off a muscular branch to the rostral belly of the digastricus muscle, which opens the mouth then gives off a proximal cutaneous branch, which passes rostrally along the lateral aspect of the mandible to join the ventral buccal branch of the facial nerve to supply a cutaneous area of the inferior lip and the cheek, caudal to the cutaneous area of the mental branches (Fig. 19.22). The mylohyoid nerve then divides into a branch that supplies the sheetlike mylohyoideus muscle, which raises the floor of the oral cavity and pulls the basihyoid rostrally, and the distal cutaneous branch of the mylohyoid nerve, which innervates a cutaneous area of the intermandibular region caudal to the area supplied by the proximal branch (Fig. 19.22).

The **lingual nerve** (*n. lingualis*) (Figs. 19.20, 19.21, 19.23 to 19.25) is sensory to the rostral two-thirds of the tongue and conveys tactile, noxious, and thermal sensations as well as taste. The fibers conveying taste impulses from taste buds located in fungiform papillae on the rostral two-thirds of the tongue have their cell bodies in the geniculate ganglion of the facial nerve (VII). These special visceral afferents course centrally in the lingual nerve and leave via

CHAPTER 19 Cranial Nerves 827

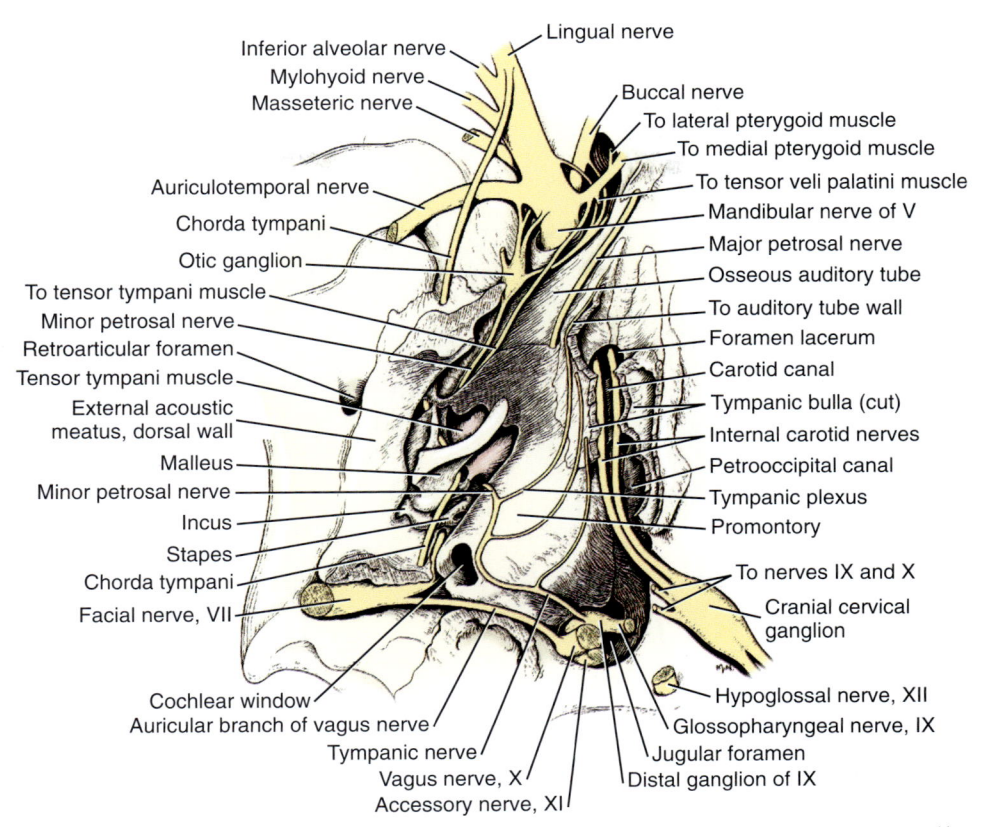

- Fig. 19.20 Nerves in the region of the middle ear, ventral aspect. (The tympanic bulla is removed.)

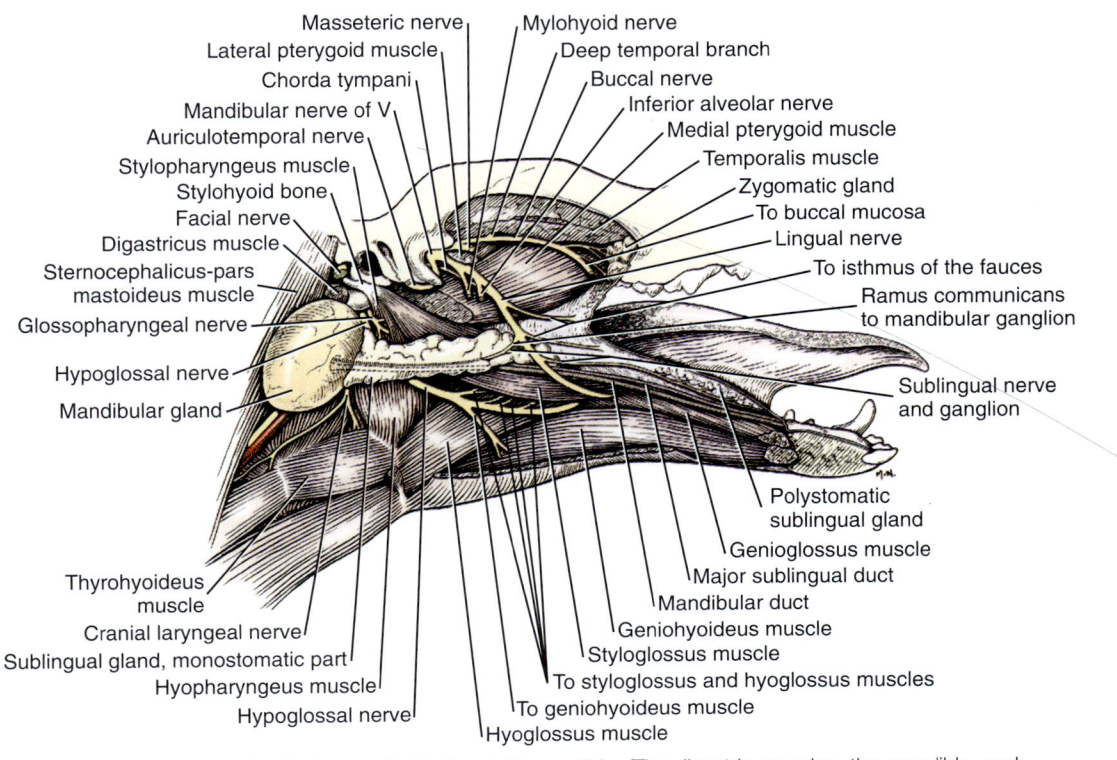

- Fig. 19.21 Nerve distribution medial to the right mandible. (The digastric muscles, the mandible, and structures lateral to it have been removed.)

828 CHAPTER 19 Cranial Nerves

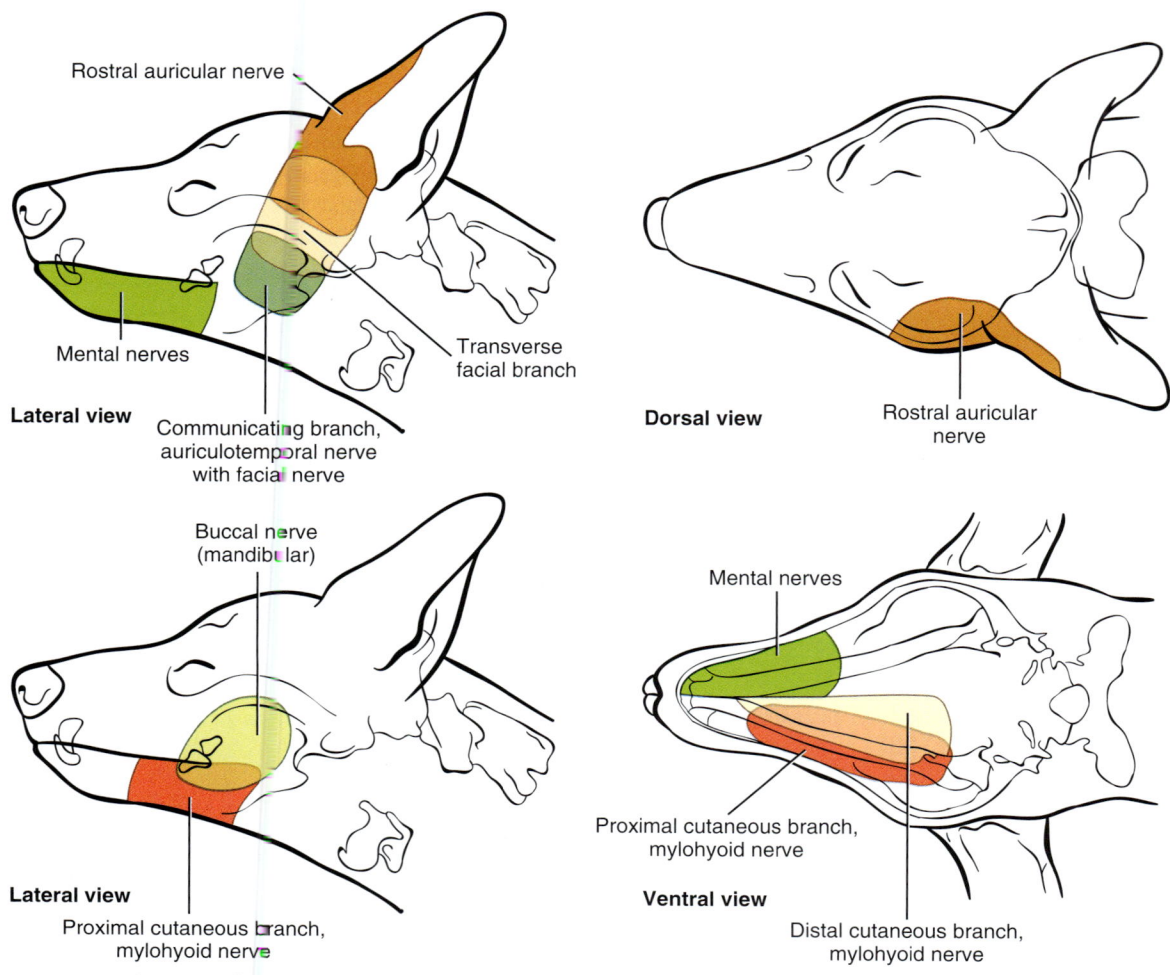

• **Fig. 19.22** Cutaneous areas of the major branches of the mandibular nerve (V). The clear areas are zones of overlap between adjacent cutaneous areas. For the cutaneous area of the external acoustic meatus branch of the auriculotemporal nerve see Fig. 19.18. For the cutaneous area of the entire mandibular nerve, see Fig. 19.17. (Modified with permission from Whalen LR, Kitchell RL: Electrophysiologic studies of the cutaneous nerves of the head of the dog, Am J Vet Res 44:615–627, 1983a.)

the chorda tympani to join the facial nerve at the geniculate ganglion within the petrous part of the temporal bone. The chorda tympani joins the lingual nerve on the dorsolateral surface of the medial pterygoid muscle just distal to where the inferior alveolar nerve branches from the mandibular (Figs. 19.20, 19.21, and 19.23). The lingual nerve of the mandibular is a large nerve that crosses the pterygoid muscles, gives off branches to the buccal mucosa of the isthmus of the fauces (Fig. 19.21), and passes between the styloglossus and mylohyoideus muscles. It gives off caudally communicating branches to the mandibular ganglion (Fig. 19.21), which are preganglionic parasympathetic axons that reach the lingual nerve via the chorda tympani (facial VII) (Figs. 19.7, 19.19, and 19.20). Synapse occurs on the neuronal cell bodies in the mandibular ganglion, which provide postganglionic parasympathetic axons that innervate the mandibular gland. At the base of the tongue, the lingual nerve gives off the **sublingual nerve** (*n. sublingualis*) (Fig. 19.21), which innervates the sublingual mucosa and gives off communicating branches that are preganglionic parasympathetic axons that reached the lingual via the chorda tympani of the facial nerve (Fig. 19.19). These preganglionic parasympathetic axons synapse with neuronal cell bodies of postganglionic axons located in the sublingual ganglion (Fig. 19.21). The postganglionic axons from this ganglion supply the sublingual salivary glands. The lingual nerve has communicating branches with the hypoglossal nerve (Fig. 19.24) just proximal to where the lingual nerve subdivides into a number of lingual branches that enter the base of the tongue (Fig. 19.24).

Abducent Nerve (Cranial Nerve VI)

The **abducent nerve** (*n. abducens*), or sixth cranial nerve, contains general somatic efferent axons that innervate the lateral rectus and retractor bulbi muscles of the eyeball. The cell bodies that form the abducent nucleus lie in the rostral medulla at the level of the trapezoid body. The genu of the facial nerve passes dorsal to the abducent nucleus. The axons from the abducent nucleus pass ventrally through the reticular formation and emerge from the brainstem through the trapezoid body, lateral to the pyramid (Fig. 19.3). The small abducent nerve courses rostrally through the middle cranial fossa beside the hypophysis and dorsal to the cavernous sinus and exits from the cranial cavity through the orbital fissure. It enters the periorbita, and innervates the lateral rectus muscle and the retractor bulbi (Figs. 19.5 and 19.6). The nerve enters the dorsal border of the lateral rectus deep in the orbit (Fig. 19.8).

Facial Nerve (Cranial Nerve VII)

The **facial nerve** (*n. facialis; n. intermediofacialis*), or seventh cranial nerve, provides general somatic efferent innervation for all of the superficial muscles of the head, face, and external ear (mimetic muscles) as well as the caudal belly of the digastricus, the stapedius, stylohyoideus, and the platysma of the neck. It also contains special visceral afferent neurons for taste that innervate taste buds of the palate and the rostral two-thirds of the tongue, general somatic afferents from receptors in the surface of the tongue and preganglionic parasympathetic general visceral efferent axons that synapse in ganglia that send postganglionic axons to the lacrimal gland; the dorsal buccal, mandibular, and sublingual salivary glands; and glands of the nasal, buccal, and lingual mucosa (Fig. 19.19).

The somatic efferent axons in the facial nerve have their cell bodies located in the motor nucleus of the facial nerve in the ventrolateral part of the rostral medulla oblongata. The intramedullary axons from the nucleus run dorsally, slightly medially, and rostrally to curve medially and dorsally just deep to the fourth ventricle where they loop laterally around the abducent nucleus. The axons then are directed caudally and ventrolaterally to emerge from the medulla through the trapezoid body just medial to the

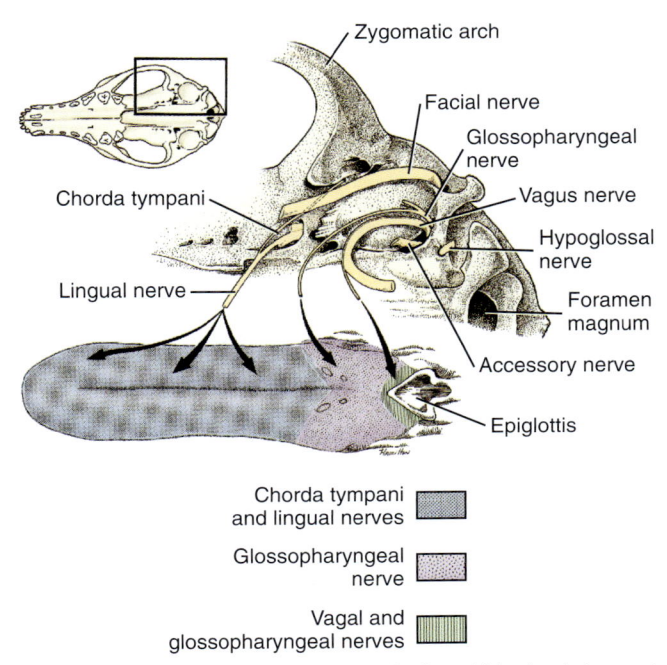

• **Fig. 19.23** Innervation of the tongue by the lingual (V), chorda tympani (VII), glossopharyngeal (IX), vagus (X), and hypoglossal (XII) nerves. (With permission from Chibuzo GA: *Locations of primary motor and sensory cell bodies that innervate the dog's tongue*, Ph.D. Thesis, Ithaca, NY, 1979, Cornell University.)

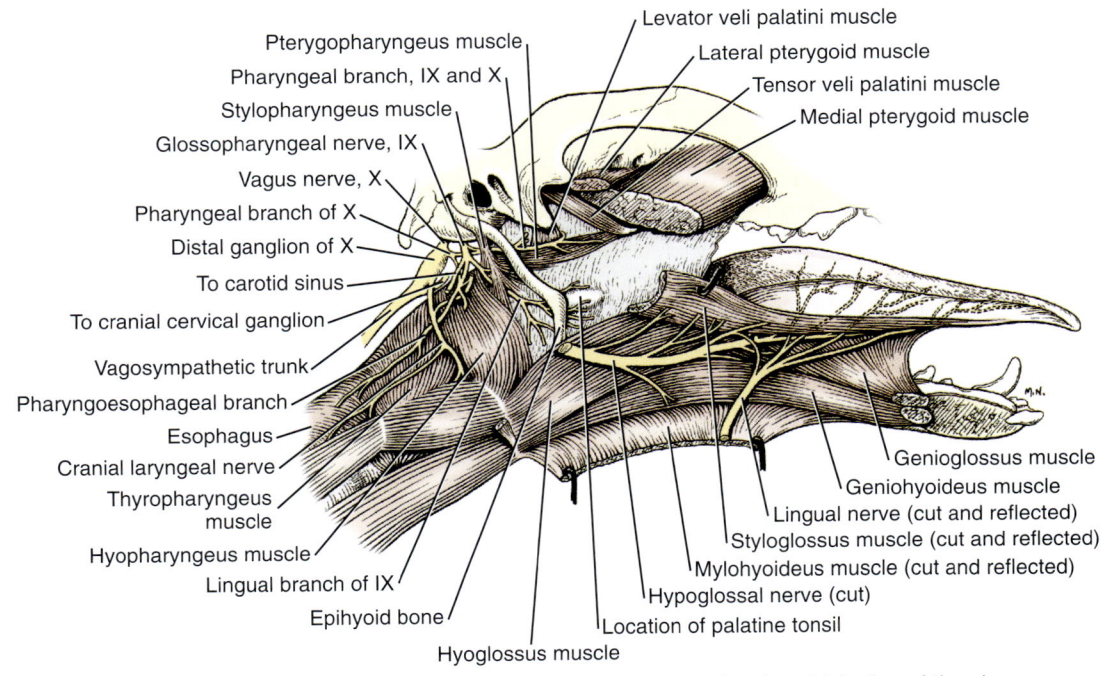

• **Fig. 19.24** Deep dissection of the pharyngeal region and tongue, showing distribution of the glossopharyngeal, hypoglossal, and lingual nerves.

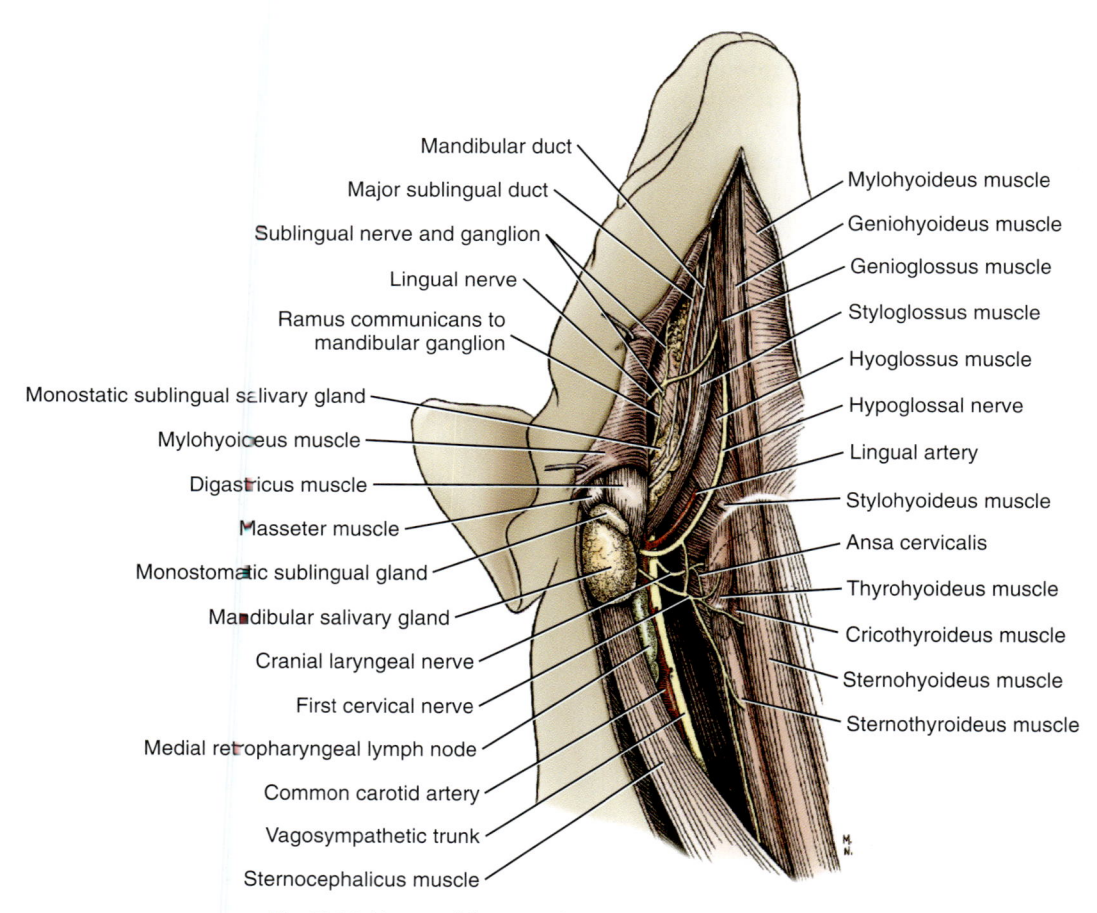

Fig. 19.25 Nerves of the ventral surface of the head and neck.

Labels (clockwise from top left):
- Mandibular duct
- Major sublingual duct
- Sublingual nerve and ganglion
- Lingual nerve
- Ramus communicans to mandibular ganglion
- Monostatic sublingual salivary gland
- Mylohyoideus muscle
- Digastricus muscle
- Masseter muscle
- Monostomatic sublingual gland
- Mandibular salivary gland
- Cranial laryngeal nerve
- First cervical nerve
- Medial retropharyngeal lymph node
- Common carotid artery
- Vagosympathetic trunk
- Sternocephalicus muscle
- Mylohyoideus muscle
- Geniohyoideus muscle
- Genioglossus muscle
- Styloglossus muscle
- Hyoglossus muscle
- Hypoglossal nerve
- Lingual artery
- Stylohyoideus muscle
- Ansa cervicalis
- Thyrohyoideus muscle
- Cricothyroideus muscle
- Sternohyoideus muscle
- Sternothyroideus muscle

---

cochlear nuclei (Figs. 19.3, 19.4, and Chapter 18: plates 5 and 6). The **intermediate nerve** (*n. intermedius*) is the afferent and preganglionic parasympathetic efferent root of the facial nerve. The preganglionic parasympathetic general visceral efferent axons in the intermediate nerve have their cell bodies in the parasympathetic nucleus of the facial nerve in the medulla, dorsal and rostral to the somatic efferent nucleus. The intermediate nerve and the somatic motor root join just distal to their emergence from the brainstem. The facial nerve leaves the cranial cavity via the internal acoustic meatus accompanied by the vestibular and cochlear nerves (Fig. 19.9). Blauch and Strafuss (1974) note that the facial and vestibulocochlear nerves are enclosed in a common sheath of dura as they enter the internal acoustic meatus. Within the meatus the vestibular nerve divides into a superior and inferior division. The superior part remains in contact with the facial nerve as they traverse the dorsal part of the internal acoustic meatus and enter the facial canal together. After a short distance in the meatus, the facial nerve enters the facial canal of the petrous part of the temporal bone. After running a short distance in the canal, near the tensor tympani muscle, the facial nerve bends to form the genu of the facial nerve. At this point there is an indistinct enlargement, the **geniculate ganglion** (*ganglion geniculi*) (Fig. 19.9). The **major petrosal nerve** (*n. petrosal major*) branches rostrally from the nerve at this point and runs rostroventrad in the small petrosal canal in the rostral wall of the petrous part of the temporal bone. The major petrosal nerve emerges from the petrosal canal adjacent to foramen lacerum where it is joined by the **deep petrosal nerve** (*n. petrosus profundus*), which contains postganglionic sympathetic axons from the internal carotid plexus. The union of the major petrosal and deep petrosal nerves forms the **nerve of the pterygoid canal** (*n. canalis pterygoidei*). This canal is dorsomedial to the alar canal in the pterygoid process of the basisphenoid bone. The nerve of the pterygoid canal traverses this canal and emerges from this canal on the dorsal surface of the medial pterygoid muscle. The preganglionic parasympathetic axons in this nerve synapse in the pterygopalatine ganglion (Figs. 19.15, 19.16, and 19.19) for distribution to the lacrimal glands and the glands in the nasal and palatine mucosa.

The facial nerve continues in the facial canal, which straightens after the first turn and opens into the cavity of the middle ear near the vestibular window. The nerve continues in the S-shaped facial canal and gives off the **stapedial nerve** (*n. stapedius*) to the stapedius muscle. (The stapedius is probably the smallest striated muscle in the body. It contracts reflexively, almost simultaneously with the tensor tympani, when the ear receives sound. This reflex contraction is a protective mechanism to prevent loud sounds from causing excessive movements of the ossicles.) The facial nerve within the facial canal then gives off the **chorda tympani** (Figs. 19.9, 19.19, and 19.20), which runs in the *canaliculus chordae tympani*. This canal carries the chorda tympani to the middle ear cavity (Fig. 19.20), where the nerve crosses the medial surface of the handle of the malleus, passes across the medial surface of the tympanic membrane and through a small canal in the rostrodorsal wall of the tympanic bulla, and emerges through the petrotympanic fissure (Figs. 19.20 and 19.23) to join the lingual branch of the mandibular nerve (V). The chorda tympani was found to contain myelinated axons that range from 2 to 12 μm (Kitchell, 1963) with the majority of the axons from 6 to 8 μm. The median total number of axons in the chorda tympani of the dog was 2854, compared with 1555 in the cat and 5735 in the horse (Kitchell, 1963). Large numbers of nonmyelinated axons were also present. The chorda tympani contains mechanoreceptor and thermal afferent axons (Iriuchijima & Zotterman, 1961) as well as taste axons from the fungiform papillae on the rostral two-thirds of the tongue (Andersson et al., 1950; Kitchell, 1963, 1978). When the chorda tympani is cut the taste buds degenerate (Olmsted, 1922). Taste axons responding selectively to distilled water, salt, bitter, sweet, or acid solutions have been studied by Andersson et al. (1950) and Kitchell (1963, 1978). Preganglionic parasympathetic axons destined for the mandibular and sublingual ganglia via various branches of the lingual nerve are also found in the chorda tympani (Fig. 19.19). These preganglionic parasympathetic axons are motor to the salivary glands and are secretory and vasodilator to the glands of the tongue (Gomez, 1961).

For experimental purposes, Chibuzo et al. (1979b) described a surgical procedure to expose the small chorda tympani, prior to its union with the lingual nerve, by a ventral approach to the pharynx that required section and reflection of the medial pterygoid muscle.

After the facial nerve emerges from the stylomastoid foramen it greatly increases in size owing to more epineurium. Shortly after emerging, the facial nerve is joined by the auricular branch of the vagus nerve (Figs. 19.20 and 19.26). The axons from this nerve are quite likely distributed to the external ear canal via the internal auricular branches of the facial (see later discussion). As the large facial nerve emerges between muscles caudal to the base of the ear it sends muscular branches to the caudal auricular muscles and the **caudal auricular nerve** (*n. auricularis caudalis*), formerly *retroauricular nerve*, to the platysma on the dorsum of the neck (Fig. 19.12). This nerve courses caudally close to the dorsal midline of the neck. The facial nerve curves ventrally and rostrally around the annular cartilage and gives off a **digastric branch** (*ramus digastricus*) to the caudal belly of the digastricus muscle and a **stylohyoideus branch** (*rami stylohyoideus*) to the stylohyoid muscle (Fig. 19.12). The next branches to arise from the facial contain general somatic afferents to the skin of the ear, the **internal auricular branches** (*rami auriculaeis interni*) (Fig. 19.12). These branches supply the skin of the medial and lateral parts of the rostral (concave) surface of the auricle (Fig. 19.18) (Whalen & Kitchell, 1983b). Facial nerve branches also supply axons to the nonosseous part of the external ear canal (Fig. 19.18).

The facial nerve curves around the caudal border of the mandible on the surface of the masseter muscle and divides

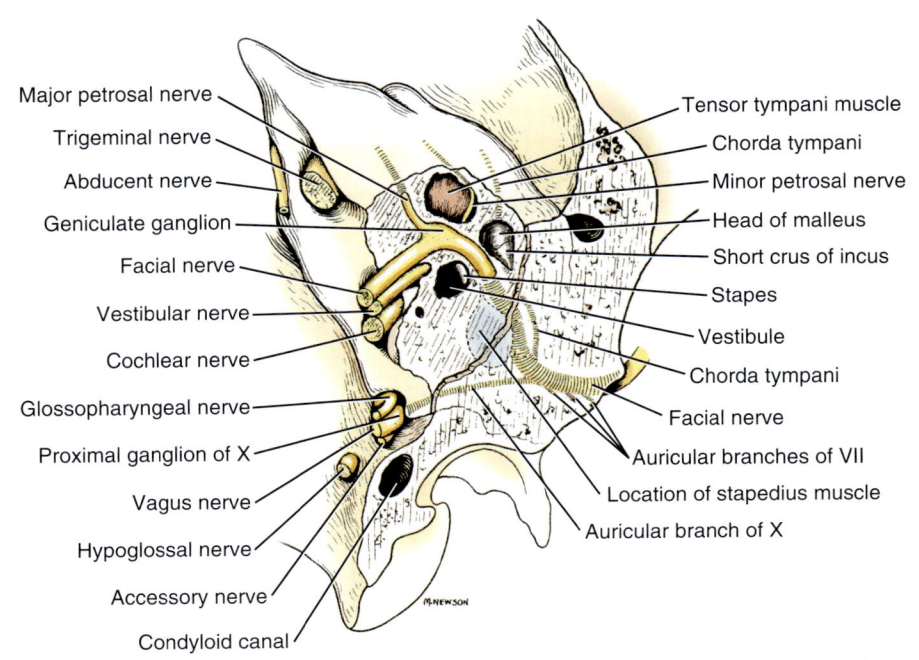

• **Fig. 19.26** The petrous temporal bone sculptured to show the path of the facial nerve, dorsal aspect.

into the cervical, buccal, and auriculopalpebral branches (Fig. 19.12).

The **cervical branch** (*ramus colli*) passes superficial to the mandibular salivary gland and innervates the parotidoauricularis and sphincter colli muscles before joining a ventral branch of the second cervical nerve.

Two **buccal branches** (*rami buccales*), a dorsal and a ventral, turn rostrally over the masseter muscle (Fig. 19.12) to innervate muscles of the cheek (buccinator muscle), the superior and inferior lip (orbicularis oris), and the lateral surface of the nose (nasolabial muscles). The dorsal buccal branch receives a communication from the auriculotemporal nerve from the mandibular nerve (V), which is sensory to the skin ventral to the zygomatic arch on the caudal aspect of the cheek (Fig. 19.22).

The **auriculopalpebral nerve** (*n. auriculopalpebralis*) courses dorsally from the base of the ear and divides into palpebral and rostral auricular branches (Fig. 19.12). The **palpebral branches** (*rami palpebrales*) form a rostral auricular plexus between the eye and the ear. From this plexus several superficial facial muscles, such as the rostral auricular, nasolabialis, and orbicularis oculi, are innervated. The terminal portion of the **rostral auricular branches** (*rami auriculars rostrales*) innervates the superficial and deep scutuloauricularis muscles.

Vestibulocochlear Nerve (Cranial Nerve VIII)

The **vestibulocochlear nerve** (*n. vestibulocochlearis*), or eighth cranial nerve, is composed of two roots. The **vestibular root** (*radix vestibularis*) innervates hair cells in the cristae ampullarae and macula utriculi and sacculi of the membranous labyrinth with their cell bodies in the vestibular ganglion within the petrous part of the temporal bone. The **cochlear root** (*radix cochlearis*) consists of axons whose cell bodies are located in the spiral ganglion within the osseous modiolus of the cochlea. The peripheral processes (dendritic zones) of these spiral ganglion neurons end by synapsing with hair cells of the spiral organ in the cochlear duct (see Chapter 20). The vestibular nerve transmits afferent impulses to the brain that relate to the position of the head relative to the pull of gravity and to linear and angular acceleration. The cochlear nerve transmits impulses perceived as sound.

The vestibulocochlear nerve never leaves the skull because it originates in the inner ear of the petrosal part of the temporal bone. The nerve leaves this bone via the internal acoustic meatus, along with the facial nerve (VII) and courses to the adjacent medulla of the brainstem (Figs. 19.9 and 19.26).

The combined vestibulocochlear nerve, formerly *auditory, acoustic*, or *statoacoustic*, enters the medulla at the ventrolateral margin of the trapezoid body (Figs. 19.3 and 19.4). The eighth nerve lies adjacent (dorsal) to the seventh nerve and directly caudal to the superficial origin of the trigeminal nerve from the caudal part of the pons (Figs. 19.3 and 19.4). The axons of the vestibular nerve penetrate the side of the medulla to terminate in the vestibular nuclei or course into the cerebellum via the caudal cerebellar peduncle. The axons in the cochlear nerve all synapse in the cochlear nuclei located on the lateral wall of the medulla just caudal to where the caudal cerebellar peduncle enters the cerebellum. Axons from neuronal cell bodies in the cochlear nuclei continue into the medulla via two routes: the acoustic stria that crosses the dorsal surface of the caudal cerebellar peduncle or the trapezoid body that crosses the ventral surface of the entire medulla.

Glossopharyngeal Nerve (Cranial Nerve IX)

The **glossopharyngeal nerve** (*n. glossopharyngeus*), or ninth cranial nerve, is both sensory and motor. It carries general visceral afferent fibers (visceral sensory) from the caudal portion of the tongue, the pharyngeal mucosa, and the carotid sinus (Adams, 1958). It also contains special visceral afferent axons for taste from the taste buds in the foliate and vallate papillae of the caudal third of the tongue. The glossopharyngeal nerve contains somatic efferent axons from cell bodies in the rostral portion of nucleus ambiguus and preganglionic parasympathetic general visceral efferent axons, which have their cell bodies located in the parasympathetic nucleus of the glossopharyngeal nerve (Fig. 19.7).

The glossopharyngeal nerve emerges from the central region of the lateral aspect of the medulla oblongata just caudal to the vestibulocochlear nerve (Fig. 19.4). The axons of the glossopharyngeal nerve leave the cranial cavity by traversing the jugular foramen and the tympanooccipital fissure along with those of the vagus and accessory nerves (Figs. 19.20 and 19.26). As the glossopharyngeal nerve leaves the cranial cavity, the **tympanic nerve** (*n. tympanicus*) arises within the space between the jugular foramen and tympanooccipital fissure. This nerve contains the preganglionic parasympathetic axons. The tympanic nerve enters the adjacent tympanic cavity and forms the tympanic plexus on the surface of the promontory (Fig. 19.20). Branches leaving the plexus form the **minor petrosal nerve** (*n. petrosus minor*) (Figs. 19.9 and 19.20), which synapses in the **otic ganglion** (*ganglion oticum*) that is adjacent to the oval foramen. Postganglionic axons leave this ganglion and join the auriculotemporal nerve, a branch of the mandibular nerve from the trigeminal, to course to the parotid and zygomatic salivary glands (Figs. 19.19 and 19.20). Chibuzo et al. (1979a, b) demonstrated that the innervation of serous and mucous glands of the tongue was via axons that reach the tongue in the chorda tympani and glossopharyngeal nerves (Fig. 19.23). Holmberg (1971) concluded that a large number of postganglionic axons from the otic ganglion also run in the adventitia of the maxillary artery, and a small number of axons run in the facial nerve. The glossopharyngeal nerve is also motor

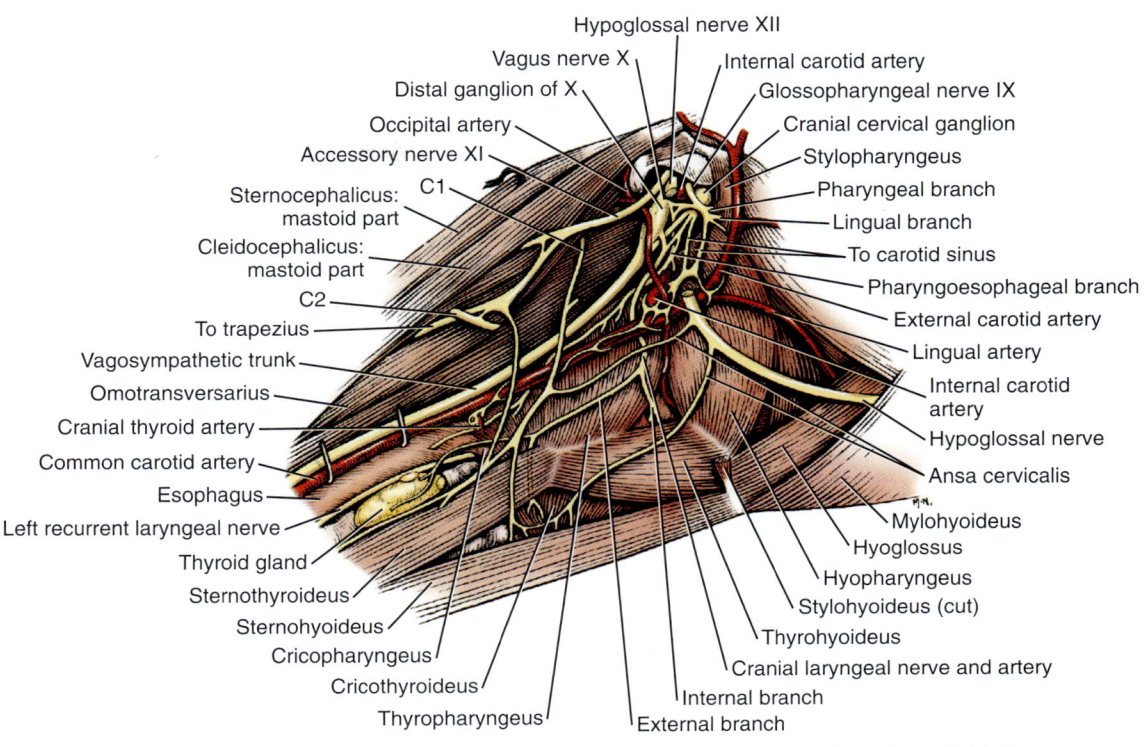

• Fig. 19.27 Nerves of the pharyngeal region, lateral aspect. (The digastric muscle and superficial structures have been removed.)

to the stylopharyngeus and jointly with the vagus (X) supplies other pharyngeal muscles.

External to the tympanooccipital fissure, the glossopharyngeal nerve crosses the medial side of the cranial cervical sympathetic ganglion and gives off a **branch to the carotid sinus** (*ramus sinus carotici*) (Figs. 19.24 and 19.27), which supplies baroreceptors in the wall of the carotid bulb and chemoreceptors in the carotid body. A small **stylopharyngeal branch** (*n. ramus m stylopharyngeus caudalis*) is given off to innervate the stylopharyngeus muscle (Fig. 19.24) and tonsillar branches (*rami tonsillares*) to the palatine tonsil. The glossopharyngeal nerve terminates by dividing into **lingual** (*rami linguales*) and **pharyngeal** (*ramus pharyngeus*) **branches** (Figs. 19.24 and 19.27). The lingual branch runs rostroventrad to enter the base of the tongue medial to the epihyoid bone. The lingual branches supply general visceral afferents to mechanoreceptor, temperature, and nociceptive receptors in the mucosa of the caudal third of the tongue and special visceral afferents for taste to taste buds located in the wall of the moat surrounding the vallate papillae and the grooves in the foliate papillae. The cell bodies for these sensory axons are located in the distal ganglion of the glossopharyngeal nerve where it passes between the jugular foramen and tympanooccipital fissure. Kitchell (1963, 1978) recorded electrophysiologic responses from the lingual branch of the glossopharyngeal nerve and determined that, although responses were present to all modalities of taste in the glossopharyngeal nerve, the responses to quinine (bitter taste) were relatively greater in the glossopharyngeal than in the chorda tympani, suggesting that bitter taste in the dog was more acute on the caudal one-third of the tongue. Kitchell (1963) also reported that in order for substances to reach these taste buds, the papillae had to be moved mechanically to open the moats or grooves. The lingual nerve also supplies parasympathetic axons to the glands of the tongue. The pharyngeal branch of the glossopharyngeal nerve joins with pharyngeal branches of the vagus (X) to form the **pharyngeal plexus** (*plexus pharyngeus*), which also receives hypoglossal nerve branches and postganglionic sympathetic axons from the adjacent cranial cervical ganglion (Fig. 19.20). The pharyngeal musculature is jointly supplied by the vagus and glossopharyngeal nerves. Somatic efferent fibers to the pharyngeal musculature from both cranial nerves have their cell bodies located in the nucleus ambiguus of the caudal medulla oblongata. Both the glossopharyngeal nerve and the vagus supply sensory fibers to the pharynx, which function as the sensory limb of the gag reflex. Their cell bodies are in the distal ganglia of these two cranial nerves.

Cranial nerves IX, X, and XI emerge close to one another and have some communications for purposes of distribution. The dog does not have separate proximal and distal glossopharyngeal ganglia (Chibuzo, 1979).

Vagus Nerve (Cranial Nerve X)

The **vagus nerve** (*n. vagus*), or tenth cranial nerve, formerly the *pneumogastric nerve*, is both sensory and motor to the palate, pharynx, larynx, trachea, and esophagus as well as to thoracic and abdominal organs. In Latin, *vagus* means "wandering, rambling, unfixed," and is an apt term, considering the wide distribution and frequent variations of this nerve and its branches. The vagus nerve contains mostly general visceral afferent axons (80%), which are visceral sensory from the pharynx, larynx, trachea, esophagus, and thoracic and abdominal viscera. These afferent axons are related to digestive, respiratory, and cardiovascular functions with very few axons related to nociception. There are numerous general visceral efferent preganglionic parasympathetic axons and some somatic efferents to the striated musculature of the pharynx, larynx, and esophagus in the vagus nerve. In addition there are a small number of special visceral afferent axons for taste from the epiglottis and a few general somatic afferent axons from the skin of the external ear canal.

The efferent axons in the vagus arise from two nuclei located in the medulla oblongata. The somatic efferent fibers have their cell bodies in the nucleus ambiguus from which the glossopharyngeal nerve (IX) arises rostrally and the cranial root of the accessory nerve (XI) arises caudally. These fibers supply the striated muscles of the pharynx, larynx, and esophagus. The parasympathetic cell bodies of preganglionic axons are located in the parasympathetic nucleus of the vagus (*n. parasympatheticus n. vagi*), formerly *dorsal motor nucleus of the vagus*. Preganglionic axons from this nucleus supply cardiac muscle and smooth muscle and glands of the digestive tract as far caudally as the left colic flexure. Kitchell et al. (1977), using a study of the axon reaction of neuronal cell bodies following transection of their axons, determined that the preganglionic neurons of the parasympathetic nucleus of the vagus are topographically organized. The majority of neurons in the rostral region of the nucleus supply abdominal viscera, the majority of neurons in the middle region supply abdominal and thoracic regions, and the majority of cells in the caudal region of the nucleus supply cervical viscera. Two-thirds of the total number of cell bodies in the nucleus are found in the rostral half of the nucleus.

The vagus arises by many small rootlets from the medulla in line with the rootlets of the glossopharyngeal nerve (IX) and cranial roots of the accessory nerves (XI) (Fig. 19.4). Some of the vagal axons are so closely associated with the cranial portion of the accessory nerve that several workers have described these vagal axons as the "bulbar," cranial, or internal root of the accessory nerve. Chase and Ranson (1914) concluded that a true cranial root of the accessory nerve does not exist in the dog. The vagus nerve leaves the lateral surface of the medulla and passes through the jugular foramen (Fig. 19.26) and tympanooccipital fissure (Fig. 19.20) along with the glossopharyngeal and accessory nerves (Fig. 19.26). The **auricular branch** (*ramus auricularis*) leaves the vagus near the jugular foramen and runs laterally through the petrous part of the temporal bone to join the facial nerve (VII) in the facial canal (Figs. 19.20 and 19.26). The auricular branch, via the facial, innervates the mucosa of the nonosseous part of the external acoustic meatus and rostral surface of the pinna (Fig. 19.18).

The vagus has two sensory ganglia associated with it. The **proximal ganglion** (*ganglion proximale*) (formerly *g. jugulare* according to the *Nomina Anatomica Veterinaria* [NAV], 2005) of the vagus lies within the jugular foramen and the **distal ganglion** (*ganglion distale*) (formerly the *g. nodosum*) lies external to the tympanooccipital fissure ventral and medial to the tympanic bulla (Figs. 19.20, 19.24, 19.27, and 19.28). These ganglia are composed of sensory cell bodies of neurons that have their receptors located in the viscera. The cell bodies of the general somatic afferent axons in the auricular branch are located in the proximal ganglion. Cell bodies of the visceral afferents are located in the distal vagal ganglion. Caudal to the distal ganglion, the vagus is bound in a common epineurium with the sympathetic trunk and with it courses caudally in the neck within the carotid sheath. The vagus is one fascicle in the common epineurium and the sympathetic trunk is bound by perineurium as a separate fascicle. The vagus separates from the sympathetic trunk at the level of the thoracic inlet just caudal to where it passes through the middle cervical ganglion of the sympathetic trunk.

Chase and Ranson (1914) reported on the myelinated and nonmyelinated structure of the roots, trunk, and branches of the vagus nerve in the dog at various points along its course. They illustrated and discussed the roots of the vagus and the accessory nerve and the relationship of the sympathetic trunk to these nerves. Although the vagus and accessory nerves form a common trunk at the level of the proximal ganglion, Chase and Ranson were able, histologically, to distinguish three areas corresponding to the spinal root of the accessory, the cranial roots of the accessory, and the roots of the vagus. The great preponderance of nonmyelinated axons in the vagus as it passed through the diaphragm puzzled them because the prevailing view at the time was that the vagus contained mostly efferent parasympathetic preganglionic axons. They remarked that "it does not seem at all probable that all of the non-medullated axons are afferent in function, otherwise the abdominal vagus would be almost wholly an afferent nerve." As we now know, the vagal trunk in the neck of the dog is approximately 80% afferent and 20% efferent, so, indeed, it is largely an afferent nerve.

Pharyngeal branches (*ramii pharyngeui*) leave the vagus just rostral to the distal vagal ganglion and are soon joined by a **communicating ramus from the glossopharyngeal nerve** (*ramus communicans cum n. glossopharyngeo*) to form the **pharyngeal plexus** (*plexus pharyngeus*) (Figs. 19.24, 19.27, and 19.28), which innervates the caudal pharyngeal muscles and the cranial esophagus. The cranial cervical ganglion sends postganglionic sympathetic axons to the pharyngeal plexus for distribution to visceral structures in the pharynx, larynx, and cervical esophagus. The pharyngeal rami of the vagus continue into the pharynx and branch to innervate the cricopharyngeal muscle and a cervical portion

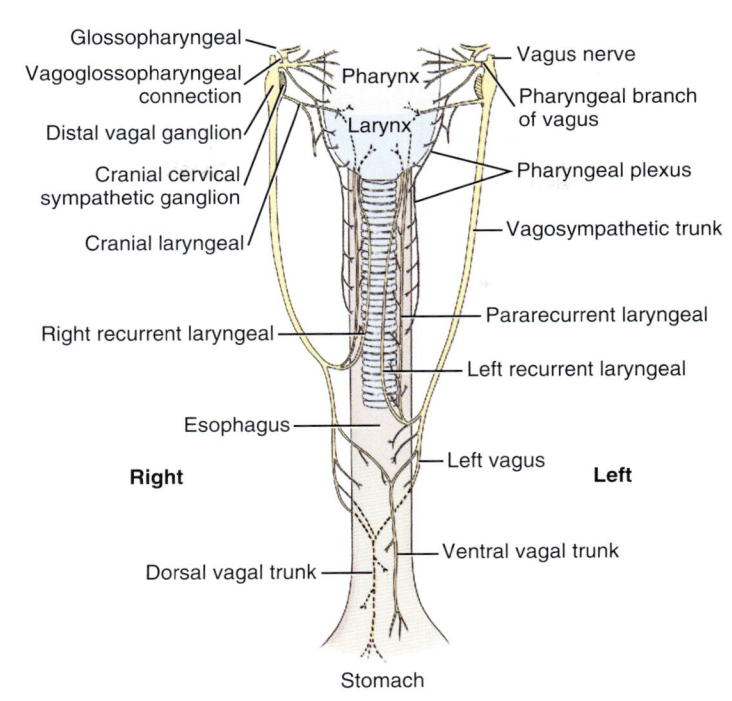

• **Fig. 19.28** The pharynx, larynx, and esophagus are innervated by the glossopharyngeal and vagus nerves. (With permission from Watson AG: *Some aspects of the vagal innervation of the canine esophagus, an anatomical study,* Master's Thesis, New Zealand, 1974, Massey University.)

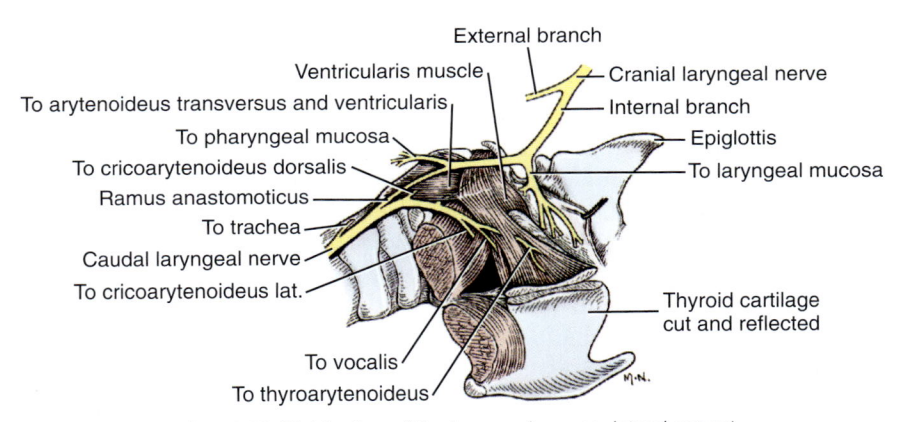

• **Fig. 19.29** Distribution of the laryngeal nerves, lateral aspect.

of the esophagus (Hwang et al., 1948). The vagal innervation of the cranial portion of the esophagus in the dog, as shown by Watson (1974), consists of right and left pharyngoesophageal nerves, right and left recurrent laryngeal nerves, and right and left pararecurrent laryngeal nerves (Fig. 19.28). The latter nerves, named by Lemere (1932) but not recognized by the NAV, are branches of the right and left recurrent laryngeal nerves (considered as tracheal and esophageal branches of the recurrent laryngeal nerves by the NAV [1983]).

The **cranial laryngeal nerve** (*n. laryngeus craniales*) leaves the vagus at the distal ganglion and passes ventrally to the larynx where it divides into an external ramus and an internal ramus (Fig. 19.29). The **external ramus** (*ramus externus*) innervates the cricothyroideus muscle and ends by supplying the pharyngeal mucosa. The **internal ramus** (*ramus internus*) supplies no muscles. It supplies the laryngeal mucosa and carries special visceral afferent axons to taste buds located on the epiglottis, which are important in reflexively closing the glottis when stimulated by water and other solutions. The cranial laryngeal nerve is important in being the afferent limb of the cough reflex when substances irritate the laryngeal or cervical tracheal mucosa. The internal ramus sends a communicating branch (*ramus communucans cum n. laryngeo caudali*) to the caudal laryngeal nerve (Fig. 19.29). This communication does not degenerate when the vagosympathetic trunk is surgically severed (Kitchell et al., 1977), suggesting that it is not a motor nerve but is largely a sensory projection from the cranial laryngeal nerve to the caudal laryngeal nerve. It may contain axons that supply baroreceptors in the aortic arch and chemoreceptors in the aortic bodies (part of the depressor nerve). The **depressor nerve** (*n. depressor*) arises from the vagus or the adjacent origin of the cranial laryngeal nerve. This small nerve rejoins the vagus to course caudally and within the cranial mediastinum is distributed to the baroreceptors in the aortic arch and chemoreceptors in the aortic bodies

At the thoracic inlet the vagus separates from the sympathetic trunk and innervates the heart via **cardiac branches** (*rami cardiaci*) (cardiovagal branches). These branches contain preganglionic parasympathetic axons and general visceral afferent axons from baroreceptors in the aorta, chemoreceptors from aortic bodies near the aortic arch, and volume receptors from the cranial and caudal vena cava. The left vagus gives rise to the left **recurrent laryngeal nerve** (*n. laryngeus recurrens*), which arches around the ligamentum arteriosum and aorta, courses cranially along the trachea, and gives off branches to the trachea and esophagus referred to by Watson (1974) as pararecurrent laryngeal nerves, and terminates as the left **caudal laryngeal nerve** (*n. laryngeus caudalis*), which innervates all of the muscles of the left side of the larynx except the left cricothyroideus. The right vagus gives rise to the right recurrent laryngeal nerve, which turns around the right subclavian artery and courses cranially along the trachea to end as the right caudal laryngeal nerve to supply all the muscles of the right side of the larynx except the right cricothyroideus muscle. The right recurrent laryngeal nerve also gives off branches; in other words, pararecurrent laryngeal nerve branches supply the trachea and the esophagus (Fig. 19.28). Braund et al. (1988) reported on morphologic and morphometric studies of the vagus and recurrent laryngeal nerves in normal dogs.

Within the thorax, at the hilus of the lung, the vagus supplies branches to the bronchi and passes onto the esophagus where the right and left vagal nerves each divide into a dorsal and a ventral vagal branch on the sides of the esophagus (Fig. 19.28). Just caudal to the heart, the left and right vagal ventral branches join to form a **ventral vagal trunk** (*truncus vagalis ventralis*). At approximately the level of the diaphragm the left and right vagal dorsal branches join to form the **dorsal vagal trunk** (*truncus vagalis dorsalis*). This recombination of right and left dorsal and ventral vagal nerves as dorsal and ventral trunks takes place at slightly different levels on the esophagus within the thorax. The result is that half of each left and right vagus nerve is recombined with its counterpart from the opposite side of the esophagus, at the level of the diaphragm, as one dorsal and one ventral vagal trunk on the esophagus.

On reaching the stomach, the dorsal vagal trunk courses through the celiacomesenteric plexus (without synapsing) so that its axons may follow blood vessels to the viscera where each axon will synapse with a cell body with a short postganglionic axon in the wall of the gastrointestinal tract. In their course along these blood vessels the preganglionic parasympathetic axons from the dorsal vagal trunk are accompanied by postganglionic sympathetic axons from the various abdominal sympathetic ganglia. The ventral vagal trunk innervates the lesser curvature of the stomach and the liver. The vagal branches supply the digestive tract as far caudally as the left colic flexure. The descending colon and rectum receive their parasympathetic supply from the sacral region of the spinal cord via pelvic splanchnic nerves.

Accessory Nerve (Cranial Nerve XI)

The **accessory nerve** (*n. accessorius*), or eleventh cranial nerve, formerly the *spinal accessory nerve,* has its origin in the medulla oblongata and also in the cervical spinal cord. The **cranial roots** (*radices craniales*) have their cell bodies in the caudal portion of the nucleus ambiguus of the medulla oblongata. Lateral to the medulla, they join the axons of the **spinal roots** (*radices spinales*), which enter the cranial cavity via the foramen magnum. This union forms the accessory nerve, which is short, entirely intracranial, and divides into internal and external branches. The **internal branch** (*ramus internus*) of the accessory nerve joins the vagus nerve within the space between the jugular foramen and the tympanooccipital fissure (Figs. 19.19 and 19.26). The somatic efferent axons of the internal branch are thought to carry the axons of the cranial roots that innervate the muscles of the larynx and esophagus by way of the recurrent laryngeal nerve (Fig. 19.28).

The somatic efferent neuronal cell bodies of axons that form the spinal roots and then the **external branch** (*ramus externus*) of the accessory nerve are located in the motor nucleus of the accessory nerve in the lateral portion of the ventral gray column from the first to the seventh cervical spinal cord segment. The spinal roots emerge laterally from the spinal cord midway between the dorsal and ventral roots of the cervical spinal nerves and consecutively join the more caudal roots as the spinal part of the nerve runs cranially between the dorsal and ventral roots of the cervical nerves to enter the cranial cavity via the foramen magnum (Figs. 16.3 and 16.4). Within the cranial cavity the spinal part of the accessory nerve lies on the ventrolateral surface of the medulla before joining the cranial roots to form the accessory nerve. The axons in the spinal roots are contained in the external branch of the accessory nerve, which leaves the cranial cavity with the vagus and glossopharyngeal nerves through the jugular foramen and tympanooccipital fissure (Fig. 19.26). The external branch of the accessory nerve courses caudally in the neck at first ventral to, then dorsal to, the transverse processes of the cervical vertebrae (Fig. 19.27). The accessory nerve intermingles with the ventral branches of the cervical nerves as it traverses the cervical region. The accessory nerve innervates the trapezius and cleidocephalicus by a dorsal branch (*ramus dorsalis*). A ventral branch (*ramus ventralis*) innervates the sternocephalicus. The morphologic phenomenon of a cranial nerve innervating muscles of the scapula and neck came about as a result of the phylogenetic envelopment of spinal nerves XI and XII by the developing skull of higher vertebrates.

Hypoglossal Nerve (Cranial Nerve XII)

The **hypoglossal nerve** (*n. hypoglossus*), or twelfth cranial nerve, is a somatic efferent nerve that innervates both intrinsic and extrinsic muscles of the tongue. The latter include the hyoglossus, genioglossus, and styloglossus muscles (Chibuzo, 1979). The geniohyoideus, passing from the intermandibular articulation to the basihyoid bone, is also innervated by this nerve. Chibuzo and Cummings (1982) have shown that each genioglossus muscle is innervated by axons originating from both hypoglossal nuclei; thus there is bilateral innervation.

The cell bodies of the hypoglossal axons form the hypoglossal nucleus of the caudal medulla, which is located adjacent to the midline in the floor of the fourth ventricle (Figs. 18.5 and 18.9). The hypoglossal axons pass ventrolaterally through the reticular formation and olivary nucleus and emerge from the medulla oblongata lateral to the pyramid as a longitudinal series of small rootlets on the ventral surface of the medulla (Fig. 19.3). The rootlets of the hypoglossal nerve are on the same sagittal axis as the third and sixth cranial nerve rootlets rostrally and the ventral rootlets of the spinal nerves caudally. The hypoglossal rootlets form the hypoglossal nerve, which exits from the cranial cavity via the hypoglossal canal on each side (Figs. 19.20 and 19.26). The nerve appears much larger after emerging from the skull because of its expansion by myelination and a connective tissue sheath. It courses ventrorostrally lateral to the external carotid artery. Ventral to the external carotid artery, the hypoglossal nerve has two communications with the ventral branch of the first cervical nerve to form the **cervical loop** (*ansa cervicalis*) (Figs. 19.25 and 19.27). Variations in the cervical loop are common (Benson & Fletcher, 1971). According to Benson and Fletcher, the branches of the loop that innervate the sternothyroid and sternohyoid muscles are largely from the hypoglossal nerve. As the hypoglossal nerve courses ventrally and rostrally, it passes medial to the mandibular salivary gland (Fig. 19.21). The hypoglossal nerve lies close to the lingual artery as it enters the tongue. On each side of the tongue, a lateral division of the hypoglossal nerve connects with one or two branches of the lingual nerve (FitzGerald & Law, 1958), all bundles of which enter the styloglossus muscle (Fig. 19.24).

Chibuzo (1979) demonstrated that some sensory nerve axons from the cranial cervical spinal ganglia reach the muscles of the dog's tongue via the hypoglossal nerve (perhaps via the cervical loop). Nerve fibers innervating the lyssa of the tongue may act as stretch receptors.

Cutaneous Innervation of the Head by Noncranial Nerves

The cutaneous areas of the head caudal to the areas innervated by branches of the trigeminal, vagus, or facial nerves (Fig. 19.11) are innervated by cutaneous branches of the second cervical nerve. (The first cervical nerve does not have any cutaneous branches [Whalen & Kitchell, 1983a]). The second cervical nerve has three cutaneous branches: the greater occipital nerve (*n. occipitalis major*), which arises from the dorsal branch of the second cervical nerve; the transverse cervical nerve (*n. transversus colli*); and the great auricular nerve (*n. auricularis magnus*) (Fig. 19.12), which arises from the ventral branch of the second cervical nerve. The cutaneous areas innervated by each of these nerves are shown in Fig. 19.30. Their areas of overlap with cutaneous areas of the cranial nerves are shown in Fig. 19.11. This plethora of sources of cutaneous innervation of the ear prevents its use for testing trigeminofacial reflexes. This overlap is seen in Figs. 19.11 and 19.30.

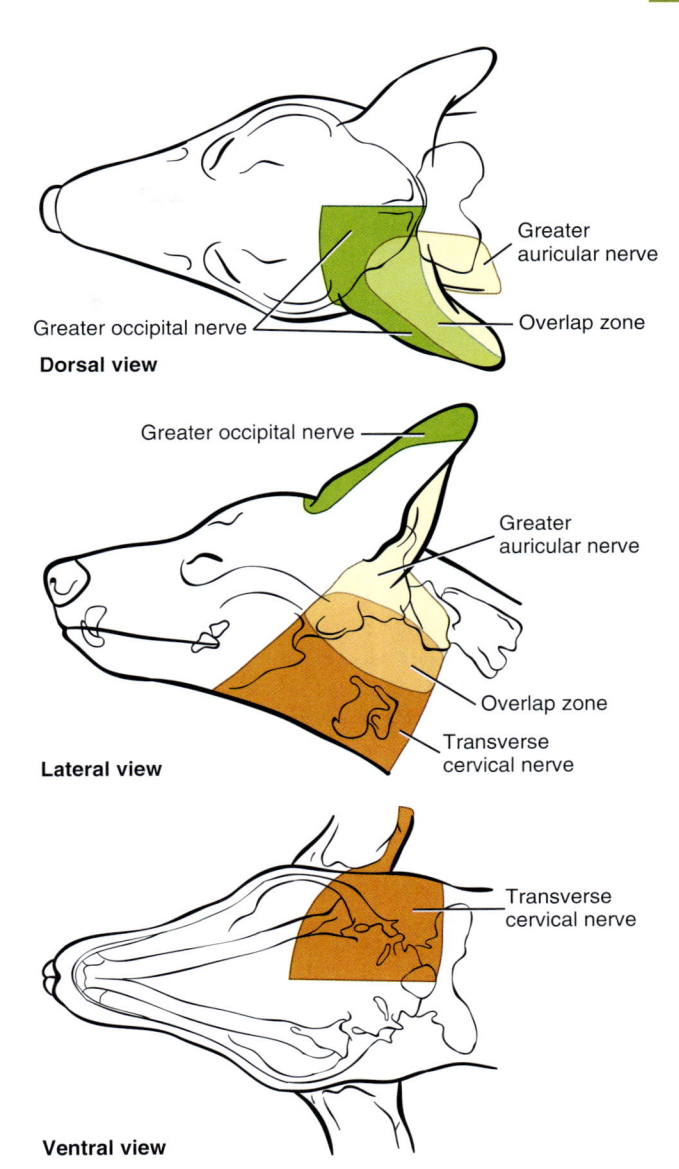

• **Fig. 19.30** Cutaneous areas of the major branches of the second cervical nerve (C2) supplying the head. The greater occipital nerve is a branch of the dorsal branch of C2. The other branches shown are peripheral branches of the ventral branch of C2. The *clear* areas are zones of overlap between adjacent cutaneous areas. (Modified with permission from Whalen LR, Kitchell RL: Electrophysiologic studies of the cutaneous nerves of the head of the dog, *Am J Vet Res* 44:615–627, 1983a.)

Bibliography

Adams, W. E. (1958). *The comparative morphology of the carotid body and carotid sinus.* Springfield, IL: Charles C Thomas.

Andersson, B., Landgren, S., Olsson, S., et al. (1950). The sweet taste fibers of the dog. *Acta Physiol Scand, 21,* 105–119.

Barone, R., Lombard, M., & Morand, M. (1966). Organe de Jacobson, nerf vomero-nasal et nerf terminal du chien. *Bull Soc Vet Med Comp Lyon, 68,* 257–270.

Benson, R. O., & Fletcher, T. F. (1971). Variability of the ansa cervicalis in dogs. *Am J Vet Res, 32,* 1163–1168.

Blauch, B., & Strafuss, A. C. (1974). Histologic relationship of the facial (7th) and vestibulocochlear (8th) cranial nerves within the petrous temporal bone in the dog. *Am J Vet Res, 35,* 481–486.

Braund, K. G., Steiss, J. E., Marshall, A. E., et al. (1988). Morphologic and morphometric studies of the vagus and recurrent laryngeal nerves in clinically normal adult dogs. *Am J Vet Res, 49,* 2111–2116.

Brookover, C. (1914). The nervus terminalis in adult man. *J Comp Neurol, 24,* 131–135.

Chase, M. R., & Ranson, S. W. (1914). The structure of the roots, trunk and branches of the vagus nerve. *J Comp Neurol, 24,* 31–60.

Chibuzo, G. A. (1979). *Locations of primary motor and sensory cell bodies that innervate the dog's tongue.* Ph.D. Thesis, Ithaca, NY: Cornell University.

Chibuzo, G. A., & Cummings, J. F. (1982). An enzyme tracer study of the organization of the somatic motor center for the innervation of different muscles of the tongue: Evidence for two sources. *J Comp Neurol, 205,* 273–281.

Chibuzo, G. A., Cummings, J. F., & Evans, H. E. (1979a). Experimental investigation of the salivatory centers in the dog: Evidence for trigeminal innervation. *Anat Rec, 193,* 162.

Chibuzo, G. A., Cummings, J. F., & Evans, H. E. (1979b). Surgical procedure for exposure of the chorda tympani in dogs: A ventral approach. *Cornell Vet, 69,* 295–301.

de Lahunta, A., Glass, E., & Kent, M. (2015). *Veterinary neuroanatomy and clinical neurology* (4th ed.). Philadelphia: Elsevier.

FitzGerald, M. J. T., & Law, M. E. (1958). The peripheral connexions between the lingual and hypoglossal nerves. *J Anat, 92,* 178–188.

Gomez, H. (1961). The innervation of lingual salivary glands. *Anat Rec, 139,* 69–76.

Goslow, G. E., Jr., & Hildebrand, M. (2001). *Analysis of vertebrate structure* (5th ed.). New York: John Wiley.

Holmberg, J. (1971). The secretory nerves of the parotid gland of the dog. *J Physiol (Lond), 219,* 463–476.

Hwang, K., Grossman, M. I., & Ivy, A. C. (1948). Nervous control of the cervical portion of the esophagus. *Am J Physiol, 154,* 343–357.

Iriuchijima, J., & Zotterman, Y. (1961). Conduction rates of afferent fibres to the anterior tongue of the dog. *Acta Physiol Scand, 51,* 283–289.

Jenkins, T. W. (1972). *Functional mammalian neuroanatomy with emphasis on the dog and cat including an atlas of dog central nervous system.* Philadelphia: Lea & Febiger.

Johnston, J. B. (1914). The nervus terminalis in man and mammals. *Anat Rec, 8,* 185–198.

Kappers, C. U. A., Huber, G. C., & Crosby, E. C. (1936). *The comparative anatomy of the nervous system of vertebrates including man.* New York: Macmillan.

Kitchell, R. L. (1963). *Comparative anatomical and physiological studies of gustatory mechanisms.* Wenner-Gren Centennial Symposium Series. New York: Pergamon Press.

Kitchell, R. L. (1978). Taste perception and discrimination by the dog. *Adv Vet Sci Comp Med, 22,* 287–314.

Kitchell, R. L., Stromberg, M. W., & Davis, L. H. (1977). Comparative study of the dorsal motor nucleus of the vagus nerve. *Am J Vet Res, 38,* 37–49.

Larsell, O. (1920). Studies on the nervus terminalis of mammals. *J Comp Neurol, 30,* 3–68.

Lemere, F. (1932). Innervation of the larynx. I. innervation of laryngeal muscles. *Am J Anat, 51,* 417–437.

Locy, W. A. (1899). New facts regarding the development of the olfactory nerve. *Anat Anz, 16,* 273–290.

McCotter, R. E. (1912). The connection of the vomeronasal nerves with the accessory olfactory bulb in the opossum and other mammals. *Anat Rec, 6,* 299–318.

McCotter, R. E. (1913). The nervus terminalis in the adult dog and cat. *J Comp Neurol, 23,* 145–152.

Meyer, H. (1979). The brain. In H. E. Evans & G. C. Christensen (Eds.), *Miller's anatomy of the dog.* Philadelphia: Saunders.

Nomina anatomica veterinaria (NAV), 5th ed. International Committee on Veterinary Anatomical Nomenclature (ICVGAN) of World Association of Veterinary Anatomists (WAVA). 2005.

Noden, D. M., & de Lahunta, A. (1985). *The embryology of domestic animals: Developmental mechanisms and malformations.* Baltimore, MD: Williams & Wilkins.

Olmsted, J. M. D. (1922). Taste fibers and the chorda tympani nerve. *J Comp Neurol, 34,* 337–342.

Read, E. A. (1908). A contribution to the knowledge of the olfactory apparatus in dog, cat, and man. *Am J Anat, 8,* 17–47.

Romer, A. S., & Parsons, T. S. (1986). *The vertebrate body* (6th ed.). Philadelphia: Saunders.

Scalia, F., & Winans, S. S. (1976). New perspectives on the morphology of the olfactory system: Olfactory and vomeronasal pathways in mammals. In R. L. Doty (Ed.), *Mammalian olfaction, reproductive processes and behaviour.* New York: Academic Press.

Warwick, R. (1953). Representation of the extra-ocular muscles in the oculomotor nuclei of the monkey. *J Comp Neurol, 98,* 449–503.

Watson, A. G. *Some aspects of the vagal innervation of the canine esophagus, an anatomical study.* Master's Thesis, New Zealand: Massey University, 1974.

Whalen, L. R., & Kitchell, R. L. (1983a). Electrophysiologic studies of the cutaneous nerves of the head of the dog. *Am J Vet Res, 44,* 615–627.

Whalen, L. R., & Kitchell, R. L. (1983b). Electrophysiologic and behavioral studies of the cutaneous nerves of the concave surface of the pinna and the external ear canal of the dog. *Am J Vet Res, 44,* 628–634.

20
The Ear

The **ear** (*organum vestibulocochleare* [*auris*]) evolved as an organ of balance and hearing in vertebrates. The most primitive part is the **internal ear** (*auris interna*), which in all vertebrates consists of a membranous labyrinth within a bony labyrinth and functions for both balance and hearing. Fish have only an internal ear, whereas amphibians and reptiles developed an additional chamber, the **middle ear** (*auris media*), formed by a **tympanic cavity** (*cavum tympani*) that is an extension of the pharynx. The tympanic cavity connects with the pharynx via the auditory tube, (formerly *eustachian* or *pharyngotympanic tube*), which is closed to the outside by a tympanic membrane, or eardrum. A portion of the hyomandibular bone from the second branchial arch develops into a sound-conducting ossicle, the **columella**, which transmits vibrations from the tympanic membrane, across the air-filled tympanic cavity, to the internal ear. In mammals two more bones, the malleus and incus, are added to the middle ear, and the columella becomes a stapes, making a chain of three bones from the tympanic membrane to the internal ear. Although lizards and birds have an **external ear** (auris externa) it consists only of an auditory meatus and a short canal. To protect the entrance to the canal and help direct sound into it, lizards sometimes have specialized scales, and birds have specialized feathers and a cutaneous muscle for pulling a skin flap across the opening. Only mammals (except cetaceans and a few others) have a well-defined external ear formed by a cartilaginous **auricle** (auricula) or pinna covered by skin and moved by muscles.

The three major components of the dog ear will be considered here in developmental sequence, which is similar to their phylogenetic evolution: (1) the internal ear, (2) the middle ear, and (3) the external ear (Fig. 20.1).

The receptor for special proprioception, the vestibular system, develops in conjunction with the receptor for the auditory system (special somatic afferent system). They are derived from ectoderm but are contained in a mesodermally derived structure. Together these receptors are the components of the internal ear. The ectodermal component arises as a proliferation of ectodermal epithelial cells on the surface of the embryo adjacent to the developing rhombencephalon. This structure is the **otic placode**, which subsequently invaginates to form an **otic pit** and **otic vesicle** (otocyst) that breaks away from its attachment to the surface ectoderm. This saccular structure undergoes extensive modification of its shape but always retains its fluid-filled lumen (endolymph) and surrounding thin epithelial wall as it becomes the **membranous labyrinth** of the internal ear. Special modifications of its epithelial surface at predetermined sites form the receptor organs for the vestibular and auditory systems.

Corresponding developmental modifications occur in the surrounding paraxial mesoderm to provide a supporting capsule for the membranous labyrinth. This fluid-filled (perilymph) ossified structure is the **bony labyrinth** contained within the developing petrous portion of the temporal bone (Fig. 20.1).

These membranous and bony labyrinths are formed adjacent to the first and second branchial arches and their corresponding first pharyngeal pouch and first branchial groove. The first branchial groove gives rise to the external ear canal. The first pharyngeal pouch forms the auditory tube and the mucosa of the middle-ear cavity. The intervening tissue forms the tympanum. The ear ossicles are derived from the neural crest of branchial arches 1 (malleus and incus) and 2 (stapes). These ossicles become components of the middle ear associated laterally with the tympanum (malleus) and medially with the vestibular window of the bony labyrinth of the internal ear (stapes).

The Internal Ear

Bony Labyrinth

Anatomically, the **bony labyrinth** in the petrous part of the temporal bone consists of three continuous fluid-filled portions. These areas are the large **vestibule** and the three **semicircular canals** and the **cochlea**, which arise from the vestibule. All three continuous bony components contain **perilymph**, a fluid similar to cerebrospinal fluid (CSF), from which it may be at least partly derived.

Vestibule

The **vestibule** is an irregular, oval space, approximately 3 mm in diameter, that communicates with the cochlea rostrally and with the semicircular canals caudally. The walls of the vestibule are marked by depressions and ridges that correspond to the various portions of the enclosed membranous labyrinth. The medial wall contains two depressions: caudodorsal is the **elliptical recess**, which contains the

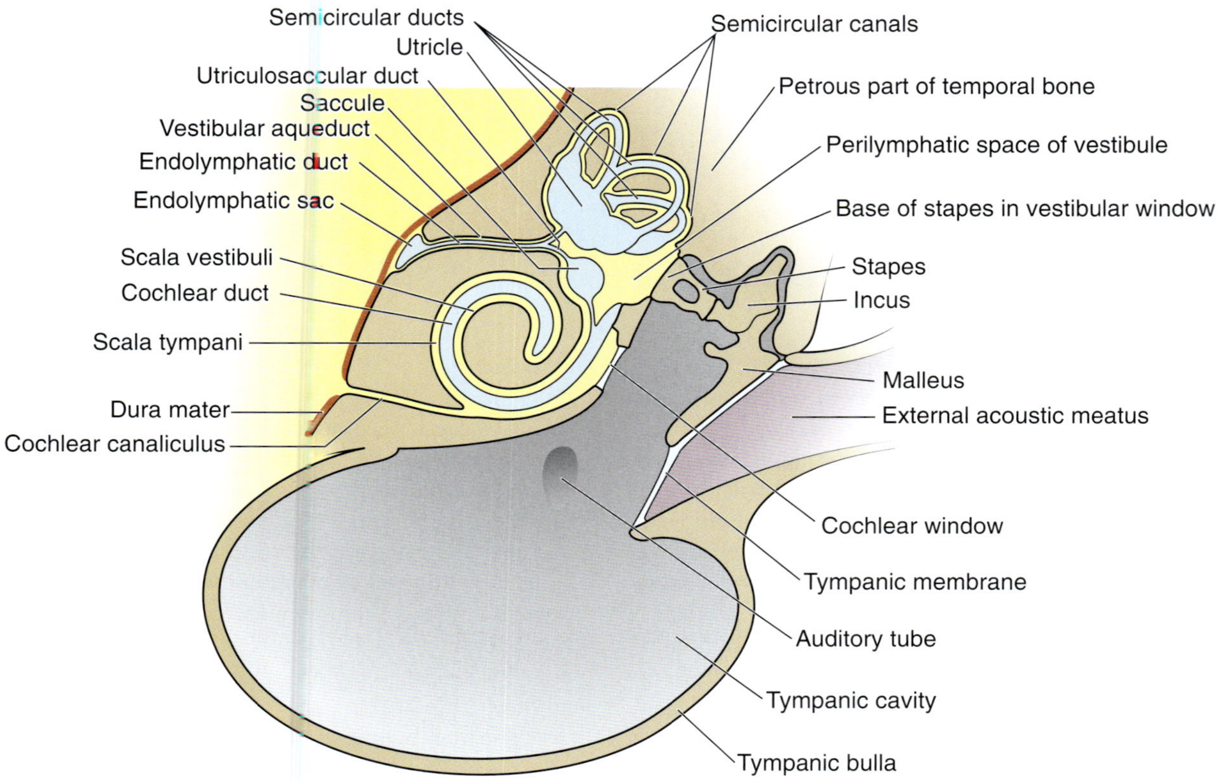

Fig. 20.1 Schematic section through the internal ear, middle ear, and external acoustic meatus of a dog.

utricle, and rostroventral to it is the **spherical recess** for the saccule. The **vestibular crus** separates the two recesses. Several groups of small openings that accommodate the nerves of this region occur near the recesses. These tiny groups of foramina are called **maculae cribrosae**. In the vestibule are two openings: the more dorsal **vestibular window** in which is inserted the foot plate of the stapes and the more ventrorostral **cochlear window**, which is closed by a membrane and is located at the end of the cochlea where perilymph vibrations can be dampened into the tympanic cavity.

Semicircular Canals

There are three semicircular canals, an anterior, a posterior, and a lateral canal (Figs. 20.2 and 20.3). They lie caudal and slightly dorsal to the vestibule. Each canal describes approximately two-thirds of a circle in a single plane, and each is approximately at a 90-degree angle to the other two. The segment of the canal that communicates with the vestibule is called the **crus**. Each canal has two crura that communicate with the vestibule (with the exception of the common crus, to be noted later). One crus of each canal has a dilation, the **osseous ampulla** (*ampullae osseae*) near the junction with the vestibule. The lumen diameter of the canals averages roughly 0.5 mm, the ampulla being approximately twice as large.

The anterior canal of one ear is roughly parallel with the posterior canal of the opposite ear. The lateral canal of each side occupies a nearly horizontal plane. The anterior canal is the longest. The arc it forms measures approximately 6 mm across at the widest part. The lateral canal forms an arc that measures approximately 4.5 mm, while the arc of the posterior semicircular canal is the smallest, measuring only 3.5 mm in medium-sized dogs. These measurements vary with the size of the dog. The **common crus** is formed by the nonampullated ends of the posterior and anterior canals. In sculptured specimens the anterior semicircular canal is seen to surround the floccular fossa, a small but deep depression on the medial side of the petrous part of the temporal bone. This depression is occupied by the paraflocculus of the cerebellum. The ampullated end of the posterior canal and the nonampullated end of the lateral canal are united for a short distance caudal to the vestibule.

Cochlea

The cochlea is the bony shell that surrounds the cochlear duct in a spiral of three and one-quarter turns around a central hollow core of bone, the **modiolus**, which contains the cochlear nerve and blood vessels. The cochlea points ventrorostrally and slightly laterally within the promontory of the petrous part of the temporal bone (Fig. 20.4). The osseous **spiral lamina** that winds around the modiolus, much like the thread of a screw, nearly bisects the lumen of the cochlea into two portions, called the *scala tympani* and *scala vestibuli* (Fig. 20.5). The osseous spiral lamina begins within the vestibule and ends at the apex in a free

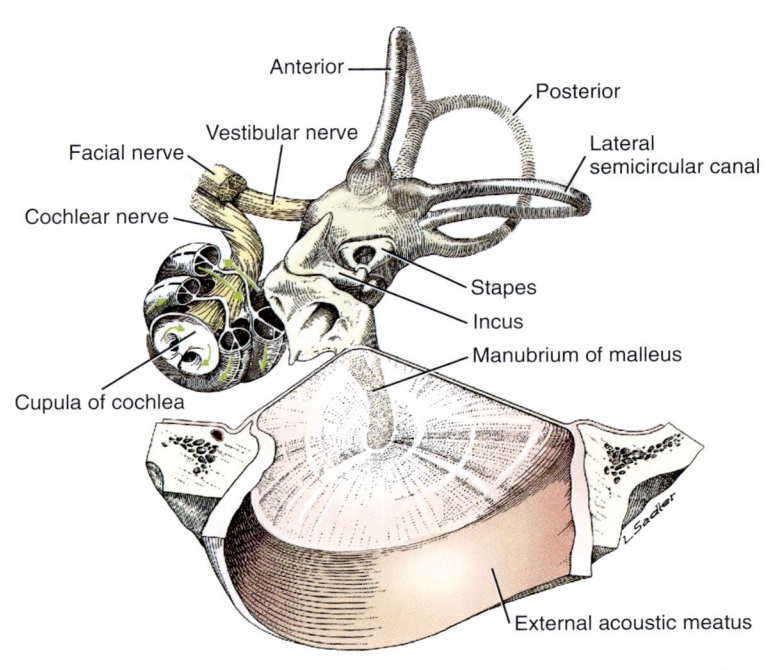

• **Fig. 20.2** Schematic of the tympanic membrane, middle ear ossicles, and internal ear. The cochlea has been opened to expose the scalae and cochlear duct, shown in greater detail in Fig. 20.5.

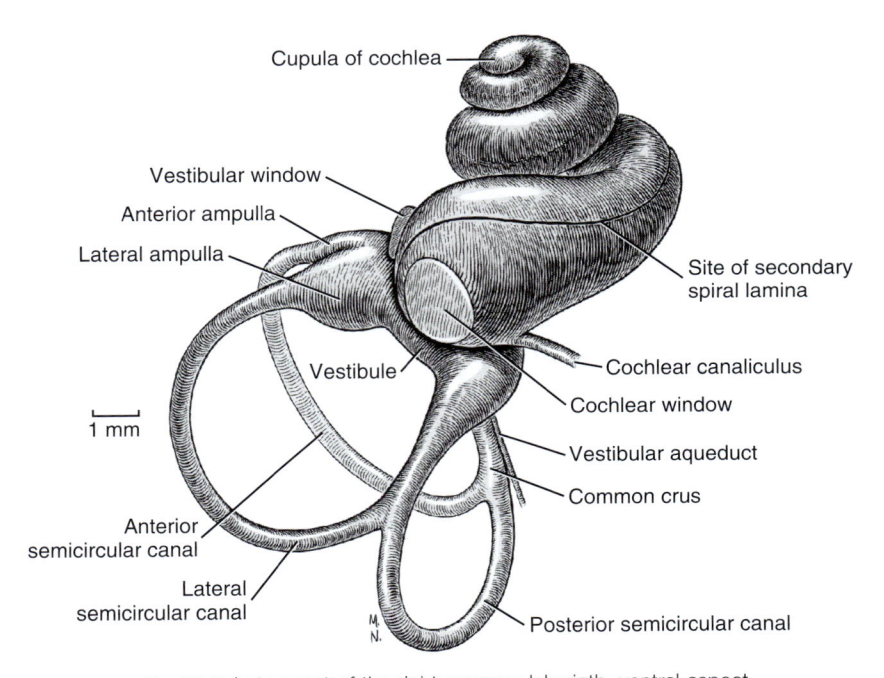

• **Fig. 20.3** Latex cast of the right osseous labyrinth, ventral aspect.

hooklike process, the **hamulus**. The scala vestibuli communicates with the vestibule, and hence the perilymph within it is acted on by the vibrations of the base of the stapes in the vestibular window. The cochlear window (see Figs. 20.1 and 20.3) is an opening situated near the rostral end of the vestibule by which the scala tympani communicates with the tympanic cavity. A **secondary tympanic membrane closes** this cochlear window. The membranous cochlear duct, formerly *scala media*, completes the separation of the two scalae. The scalae communicate at the apex of the modiolus by a small opening, the **helicotrema**, formed at the free border of the hamulus. The basal turn of the cochlea is approximately 4 mm in diameter and lies close to the medial side of the vestibule. The total height of the cochlea measures approximately 7 mm. **Longitudinal modiolar canals** and a spiral modiolar canal serve for the distribution of both blood vessels and nerves to the cochlea. The source of perilymph may depend on its location. One source is CSF from the subarachnoid space that gains entrance to the scala tympani of the cochlea via the **perilymphatic duct** (*ductus*

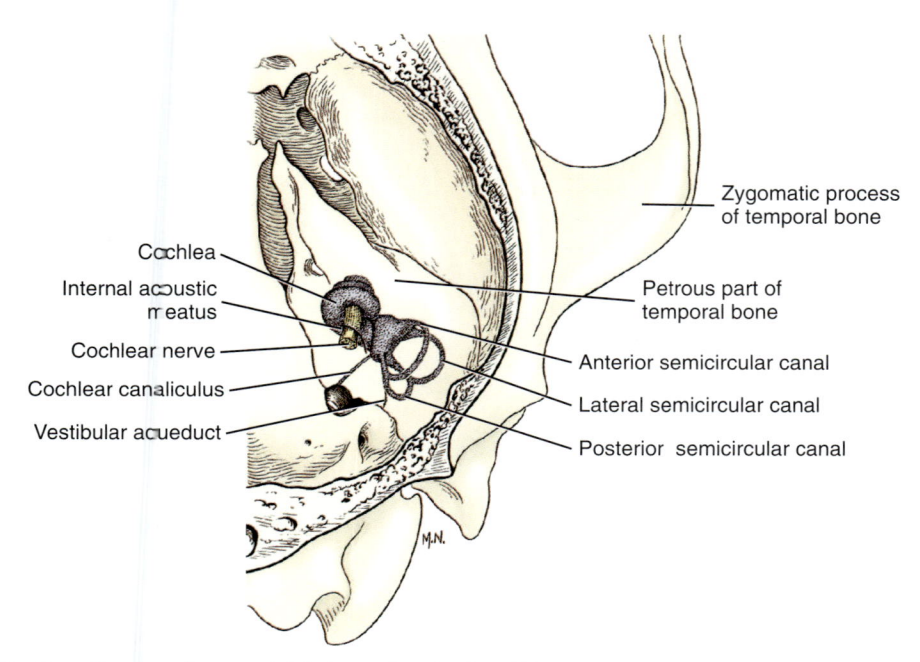

• **Fig. 20.4** Phantom diagram of right internal ear in situ within the petrous temporal bone, dorsal aspect.

perilymphaticus) (not part of the membranous labyrinth) in the small **cochlear canaliculus** (*canaliculus cochleae*). This small canal courses directly ventrad from a point on the ventral wall of the scala tympani near its origin to communicate with the subarachnoid space (see Fig. 20.1). The other source is as an ultrafiltrate from the cochlear blood vessels in the modiolus into the scala vestibuli.

Membranous Labyrinth

The ectodermally derived **membranous labyrinth** consists of four fluid-filled compartments, all of which communicate. These compartments are contained within the components of the bony labyrinth and include the **saccule** and **utriculus** within the bony vestibule connected by the **utriculosaccular duct**, the three **semicircular ducts** within the bony semicircular canals that connect to the utriculus, and a **cochlear duct** within the bony cochlea that is connected to the saccule by the **ductus reuniens**. The **endolymphatic duct** is an extension from the utriculosaccular duct through the bony **vestibular aqueduct** to the intracranial dura where the duct expands into an **endolymphatic sac**. The endolymphatic sac is often described as a simple terminus of the endolymphatic system; however, some researchers have demonstrated that this "sac" may exhibit a complex arrangement of small tubules arranged in a tree-like structure in humans (Antunez et al., 1980; Friberg et al., 1984). Blockage in the normal flow of endolymph, which may occur in the ductus reuniens or in the endolymphatic duct of humans, may cause Ménère's disease, which may result in vertigo and hearing loss (Shimizu et al., 2011). The **endolymph** contained within the membranous labyrinth is thought to be derived from the blood vessels and epithelium of the **stria vascularis** along the peripheral wall of the cochlear duct and is absorbed back into the blood through the blood vessels surrounding the endolymphatic sac (see Guild, 1927, based on study of the guinea pig). Some authors have postulated an immunologic function within the endolymphatic sac in response to presentation of antigens in the inner ear (Tomiyama & Harris, 1986). The labyrinth artery, a branch of the basilar artery, provides blood to internal ear and the stria vascularis. The three **semicircular ducts** are the anterior (vertical), posterior (vertical), and lateral (horizontal). Each semicircular duct is oriented at right angles to the others. Thus, rotation of the head around any plane causes endolymph to flow within one or more of the ducts. Each semicircular duct connects at both ends with the utriculus (Fig. 20.6).

Crista Ampullaris

The crista ampullaris is the receptor organ associated with each semicircular duct. At one end of each membranous semicircular duct is a dilation called the ***ampulla***. On one side of the membranous ampulla, a proliferation of connective tissue forms a transverse ridge called the ***crista ampullaris***. It is lined on its internal surface by columnar neuroepithelial cells. On the surface of the crista is a gelatinous structure that is composed of a protein-polysaccharide material called the ***cupula***, which extends across the lumen of the ampulla. This neuroepithelium is composed of two basic cell types: hair cells and supporting cells. The dendritic zones of the vestibular neurons are in synaptic contact with the base of the hair cells. These hair cells have on their luminal surface 40 to 80 *hairs*, or modified microvilli (stereocilia), and a single modified cilium (kinocilium). These structures project into the overlying cupula. Movement of fluid in the semicircular ducts causes deflection of the cupula, which is oriented transversely to the direction of

Bony labyrinth—cochlea—from mesoderm

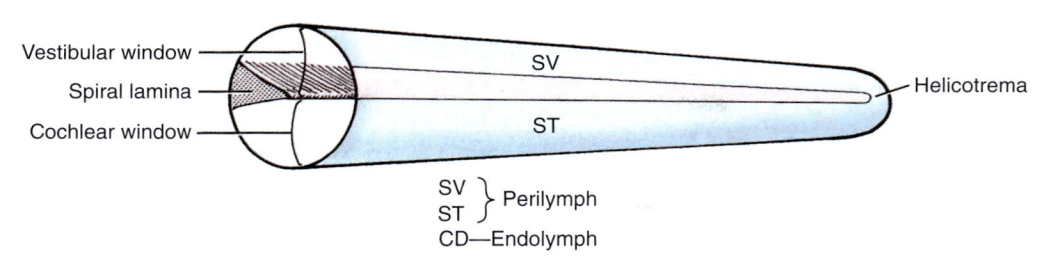

Vestibular window — SV — Helicotrema
Spiral lamina
Cochlear window — ST

SV } Perilymph
ST
CD—Endolymph

Membranous labyrinth—cochlear duct and the spiral organ—from estoderm (otic placode and cyst)

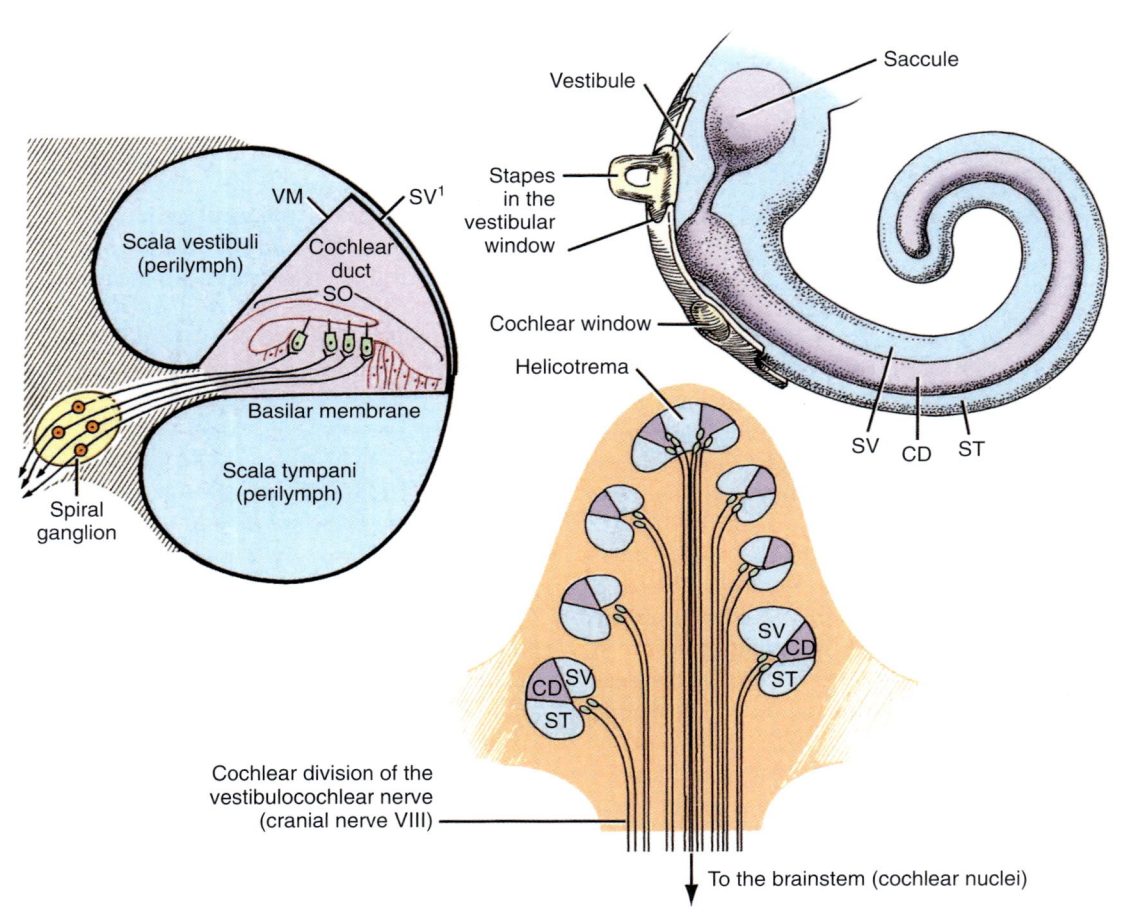

- **Fig. 20.5** Schematic transection of a cochlea and cochlear duct. The scala vestibuli and scala tympani are filled with perilymph, and the cochlear duct with endolymph. Transduction of hearing takes place in the spiral organ. (From de Lahunta A, Glass E & Kent M: *Veterinary Neuroanatomy and Clinical Neurology*, ed 4, St. Louis, 2015, Elsevier.)

flow of the endolymph. This deflection bends the stereocilia, which is the source of the stimulus by way of the hair cells to the dendritic zone of the vestibular neuron that is in synaptic relationship with the plasmalemma of the hair cell. In one end of each semicircular duct is one membranous ampulla with its crista ampullaris. Because the three semicircular ducts are all at right angles to each other, movement of the head in any plane or angular rotation affects a crista ampullaris and stimulates vestibular neurons. These cristae function in dynamic equilibrium. The numbers of and the structure of hair cells in the spiral ganglion vary among mammals studied (Nadol, 1988).

Macula

The **macula** is the receptor organ found in the utriculus and saccule, which are located in the bony vestibule (Fig. 20.7). These maculae are on one surface of each of these saclike structures. Each macula is an oval-shaped plaque in which the membranous labyrinth has proliferated. The surface of the macula consists of columnar epithelial cells. This

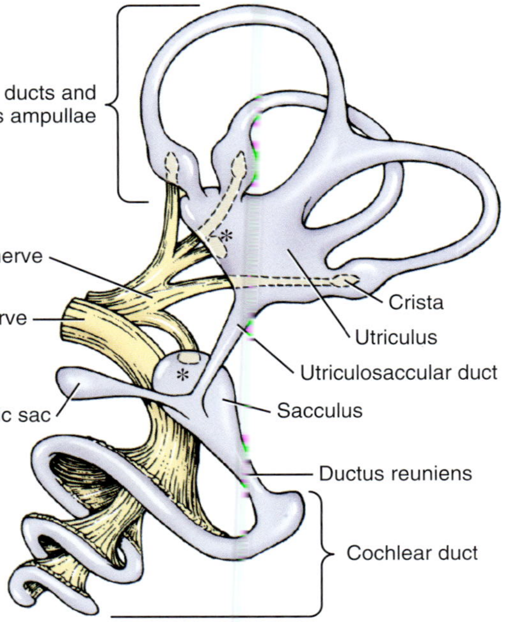

Fig. 20.6 The membranous labyrinth of the internal ear of a dog. (Note a sensory macula [*] in the utriculus and in the sacculus. This structure lies within the osseous labyrinth shown as Fig. 20.8.)

neuroepithelium is composed of hair cells and supporting cells. Covering the neuroepithelium is a gelatinous material, the *statoconiorum* (**otolithic**) **membrane**. On the surface of this membrane are calcareous crystalline bodies known as *statoconia* (*otoliths*). Similar to the hair cells of the cristae, the macular hair cells have projections of their luminal cell membranes—stereocilia and kinocilia—into the overlying statoconiorum membrane. Movement of the statoconia away from these cells is the initiating factor in bending the stereocilia to stimulate an impulse in the dendritic zones of the vestibular neurons that are in synaptic relationship with the base of the hair cells. The macula of the saccule is oriented in a vertical direction (sagittal plane), whereas the macula of the utriculus is in a horizontal direction (dorsal plane). Thus, gravitational forces continually affect the position of the statoconia relative to the hair cells. These structures are responsible for the sensation of the static position of the head and linear acceleration or deceleration. They function in static equilibrium. The macula of the utriculus may be more important as a receptor for sensing changes in head posture, whereas the macula of the saccule may be more sensitive to vibrational stimuli and loud sounds.

Vestibular Nerve

The dendritic zone of the vestibular portion of cranial nerve VIII is in a synaptic relationship with the hair cells of each crista ampullaris and the macula utriculi and macula sacculi. The axons course through the internal acoustic meatus with those of the cochlear nerve. The cell bodies of these bipolar-type sensory neurons are inserted along the course of the axons within the petrous portion of the temporal bone, where they form the **vestibular ganglion** (Giene & Kuder, 1983). The vestibular nerve axons pass to the lateral surface of the rostral medulla where they enter the medulla and terminate in telodendria at one of two sites. The majority terminate in the vestibular nuclei in the medulla and pons. A few course directly into the cerebellum by way of the caudal cerebellar peduncle.

Cochlear Duct-Spiral Organ

The most highly developed and differentiated portion of the membranous labyrinth is the **cochlear duct** (Figs. 20.5 and 20.6). This duct has a triangular shape with its base, the **stria vascularis** adjacent to the peripheral wall of the cochlea. A thin **vestibular membrane** forms the roof of the cochlear duct and a thicker **basilar membrane** forms the floor of the duct. The **spiral organ** (*organum spirale*), formerly organ of Corti, is a collection of hair cells and supporting cells that rests on the basilar membrane. These structures are involved in the transduction and transmission of sound impulses via the cochlear nerve to the brain. Special somatic afferent axons in the cochlear nerve make synaptic contact with these hair cells. Their neuronal cell bodies are centrally located in the attachment of the spiral lamina to the modiolus. The axons leave the internal ear through the internal acoustic meatus accompanied by the vestibular nerve and synapse in the cochlear nuclei on the lateral side of the medulla oblongata. The **basilar membrane** separates the endolymph of the cochlear duct from the perilymph of the **scala tympani**, which is a part of the cochlea. The thin **vestibular membrane** separates the endolymph of the cochlear duct from the perilymph in the **scala vestibuli** of the cochlea. Thus the membranous cochlear duct filled with endolymph is enclosed within the bony cochlea (scala tympani-scala vestibuli), which is filled with perilymph. These fluids have different chemical compositions and are not in open communication with each other. Likewise, the membranous semicircular ducts containing endolymph are enclosed within the semicircular canals that contain perilymph. The distinction between the osseous (Fig. 20.8) and the membranous labyrinth (see Fig. 20.6) is sometimes blurred in textbooks by the carefree use of *canal* for *duct* and *cochlea* for *cochlear duct*. To understand the structural and functional relationships of the labyrinths to each other, the terminology must be kept clear and consistent.

Hearing depends on the ability of sound waves in the external gaseous environment reaching the tympanic membrane via a patent external acoustic meatus. Here the oscillations in the air are converted to oscillations in the three auditory ossicles in the tympanic cavity. At the vestibular window the bony oscillations are converted to oscillations of the perilymphatic fluid, which in turn affects the spiral organ by oscillations of the basilar membrane in the cochlear duct. Any interruption of this pathway can result in loss of hearing. Most deafness is related to disorders of the spiral organ. There is no regenerative capacity in the hair cell population of the adult mammalian cochlea although some regeneration was possible in neonatal mice (Oshima et al., 2007;

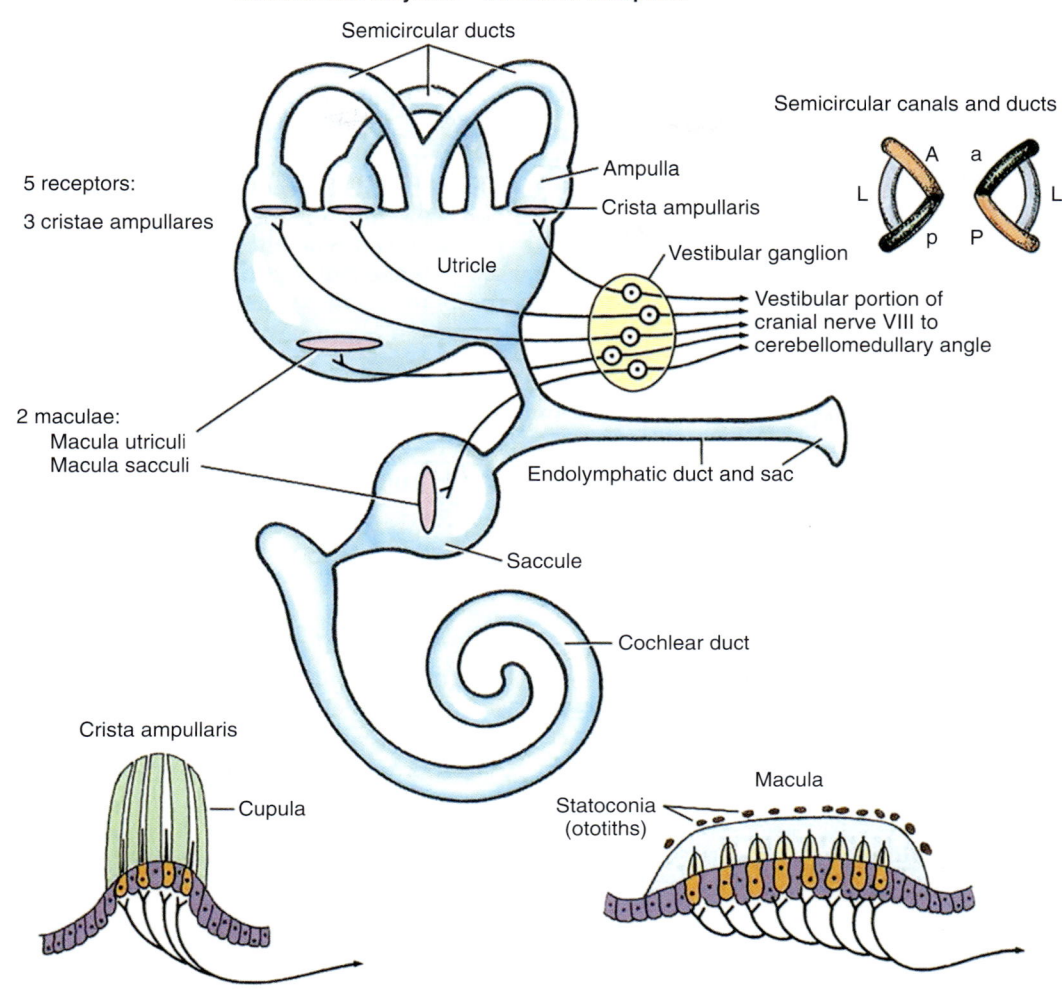

• **Fig. 20.7** Schematic of the anatomy underlying special proprioception, or the vestibular system, in the internal ear. There is a crista ampullaris in the dilated portion of each semicircular duct containing neuroepithelial receptor or hair cells. The cupula is a gelatinous structure surrounding the hair cells and their microvilli. This cupula is deflected by movement of the endolymph, bending and stimulating the hair cells. The macula is found in the utriculus and in the saccule. Macular hair cells extend into a gelatinous matrix that is deflected by movement of otoliths (statoconia) overlying the statoconiorum membrane. While crista ampullaris assess dynamic equilibrium of head position, the macular and saccular maculae may assess static head position. (From de Lahunta A, Glass E, and Kent M: *Veterinary neuroanatomy and clinical neurology*, 4th ed., St Louis, 2015, Elsevier.)

Xu et al., 2017). Foss and Flottorp (1974) found that hearing in puppies first occurred as a functional modality at 14 days after birth (on average), which coincides with the opening of the eyelids. Congenital inherited sensorineural deafness is very common in many breeds of dogs and is usually present shortly after birth. Johnsson et al. (1973) and Branis & Burda (1985) studied deafness and pathology of the cochlear in Dalmatian dogs. Rouse et al. (1984) considered abnormal otoconia and calcification of the labyrinth in deaf Dalmatian dogs. Albinotic and abiotrophic forms are recognized and can be diagnosed in puppies using brainstem auditory response testing (de Lahunta, Glass & Kent, 2015.)

Shambaugh (1923) injected the vessels of the dog labyrinth and found that the arterial supply was from a single labyrinthine artery that entered through the internal acoustic meatus. In some specimens a small artery came along the cochlear canaliculus and was distributed to a small area of periosteum along the scala tympani. The first branch to be given off from the labyrinthine artery was the anterior vestibular artery, a vessel that supplied the macula of the utriculus and the cristae of the lateral and anterior semicircular ducts. The second branch of the labyrinthine artery supplied the crista of the posterior duct, the posterior crura of the posterior and horizontal canals and ducts and the crus commune. The venous drainage from the labyrinth was collected by two trunks, the larger one leaving along the cochlear canaliculus collected all of the blood from the cochlea as well as most of the blood from the capillaries

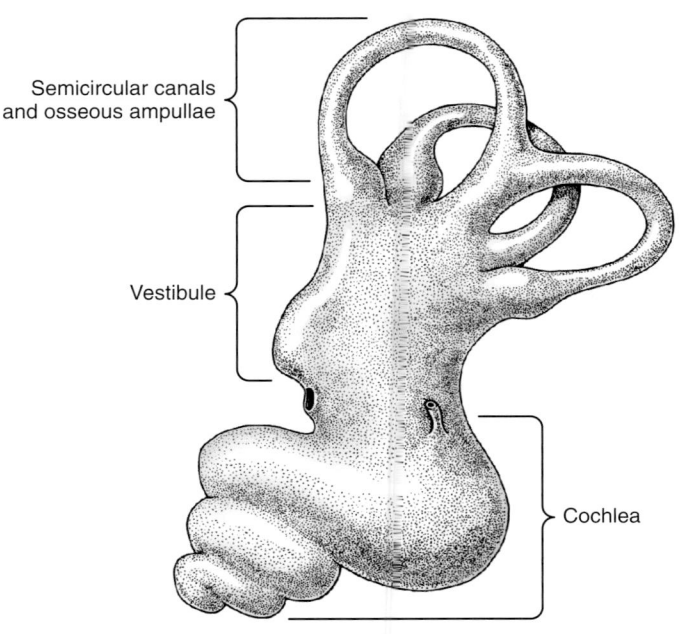

• Fig. 20.8 The osseous labyrinth of the internal ear encloses the membranous labyrinth.

supplied by the anterior and posterior vestibular arteries. The lesser vein leaving along the vestibular aqueduct drained the remainder of the labyrinth.

The Middle Ear

The **middle ear** consists of an air-filled **tympanic cavity** (*cavum tympani*) (see Figs. 20.1 and 20.10) connected with the nasopharynx via the **auditory tube** (*tuba auditiva*) and closed to the outside by the **tympanic membrane** (*membrana tympani*) at the level of the external acoustic meatus. The tympanic cavity has a small, dorsal **epitympanic recess** and a large, ventral **tympanic bulla** (*bulla tympanica*). There is an incomplete septum bulla that is composed of trabecular bone and that partially extends inside of the tympanic (Njaa & Sula, 2012). The middle portion of the tympanic cavity contains the three auditory ossicles—malleus, incus, and stapes—and the two muscles associated with them—the tensor tympani on the malleus and the stapedius on the stapes. (Getty et al., 1956).

Tympanic Membrane

The eardrum, or **tympanic membrane** (*membrana tympani*) (Fig. 20.1), covers the entrance to the tympanic cavity and separates the middle ear cavity from the external acoustic meatus. It is a thin, semitransparent, three-layered membrane somewhat oval in shape and concave when viewed externally. The inner epithelium is of pharyngeal pouch origin, the central layer is fibrous connective tissue of the pharyngeal wall, and the outer stratified squamous epithelium is derived from the ectoderm of the first branchial groove.

The tympanic membrane may be divided into two parts: the ***pars flaccida*** and the ***pars tensa***. The pars flaccida is a small dorsal triangular portion that lies between the short lateral process of the malleus and the margins of the tympanic incisure. The *pars flaccida* contains loose collagen fibers, some mast cells, and a few elastin fibers, which contrasts with the human ear in which the *pars flaccida* has abundant elastin (Njaa, 2017). The pars tensa constitutes the remainder of the membrane (see Fig. 20.11) that attaches peripherally to the fibrocartilaginous anulus. Wakuri et al. (1988) examined the connective tissue layer of the dog tympanum and found outer radial and inner circular fibers in the pars tensa.

The external aspect of the tympanic membrane is somewhat concave, owing to traction on the medial surface by the manubrium of the malleus (see Fig. 20.2). The most depressed point, which is opposite the distal end of the manubrium, is termed the **umbo membranae tympani**. A light-colored streak, **stria mallearis**, may be seen running dorsocaudally from the umbo toward the pars flaccida when viewed from the external side. This is caused by the manubrium being partly visible through the tympanic membrane along its attachment. The manubrium is embedded in the tunica propria and is covered with the epithelium of the tympanic cavity that lines the membrane. The epithelium on the external surface of the tympanic membrane originates around the site of attachment of the manubrium of the malleus to the membrane. From this site (Alberti, 1964; Michaels & Soucek, 1989) at the umbo of the tympanic membrane in humans, there is continuous mitotic proliferation and migration across the membrane, radiating in all directions. This migration cleanses the membrane of keratinized debris by moving it first to the periphery, and then into the external acoustic meatus, where it builds up and is shed via the external ear canal. Epithelial migration and regeneration was studied in dogs by Tabacca et al. (2011) who measured approximately 96 μm/day and 225 μm/day movement rates of the *tensa* and *pars flaccida* portions, respectively, of the tympanic membrane. When injured or perforated the tympanic membrane is repaired in the same manner. Stem cell–like properties have been described for epidermal cells of the rat tympanic membrane tissues (Liew et al., 2018). Within the ear canal there are sebaceous glands often associated with hair follicles and deeper tubular glands that produce cerumen, or earwax.

Maher (1988) injected and cleared the tympanic membranes and adnexa of neonatal dogs to study microangiology relative to surgical procedures. He found the structure and arterial supply of the dog tympanic membrane to be very similar to that of the human. There was a dual source of arterial supply: extrinsic sources from the stylomastoid branch of the caudal auricular artery and intrinsic sources from deep auricular and rostral tympanic branches of the maxillary artery. More specifically, the tympanic membrane was supplied centrally by ramifications from the malleus periosteal network and circumferentially by ramifications from the annulus perichondrial network. The origin of the

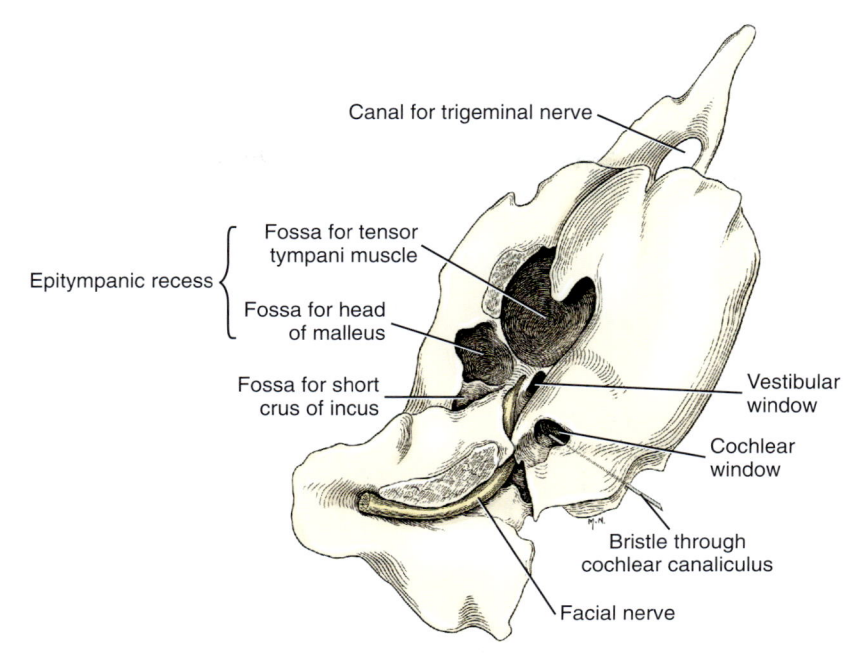

• **Fig. 20.9** Petrous part of temporal bone and middle ear cavity, ventral aspect. Tympanic bulla and auditory ossicles removed.

tympanic membrane venous plexus was from an extensive capillary bed that ultimately formed two distinct venous pathways. The principal route extended into the middle ear via the pars flaccida and joined the middle ear venous plexus. Minor routes joined cutaneous veins of the external acoustic meatus at the tympanic membrane junction. The exit portals for veins were not the same as the entrance portals for arteries.

Tympanic Cavity

The **tympanic cavity** (*cavum tympani*) is the oblique space between the petrosal and tympanic parts of the temporal bone. It contains the three auditory ossicles that transmit vibrations of the tympanic membrane to the perilymphatic space of the vestibule of the internal ear and numerous nerves cross through the tympanic cavity. The epitympanic recess is dorsal to a dorsal plane through the osseous external acoustic meatus. It is a small portion of the tympanic cavity occupied almost entirely by the head of the malleus and the incus at their articulation.

The tympanic cavity adjacent to the tympanic membrane is irregularly quadrangular in shape, being flattened laterally by the tympanic membrane that forms its lateral wall. In the caudal portion, but facing rostrally, is the secondary tympanic membrane closing the **cochlear window** (*fenestra cochleae*), formerly round window (see Fig. 20.1). Just within the cochlear window is the cochlear canaliculus (Figs. 20.1, 20.3, and 20.9).

On the medial wall of the tympanic cavity is a bony eminence, the **promontory** (Figs. 20.11 and 20.13), that houses the cochlea; it lies opposite the tympanic membrane medial to the epitympanic recess. The **vestibular window** (*fenestra vestibuli*), formerly oval window (see Figs. 20.1 and 20.9), is occupied by the base of the stapes. It is located on the dorsolateral surface of the promontory just medial to the pars flaccida. The **ostium of the auditory tube** (*ostium tympanicum tubae auditivae*) is the rostral extremity of the tympanic cavity proper. The tendon of the m. tensor tympani (Fig. 20.10) descends ventrolaterally through an arch in a thin lamina of bone that overlies the muscle. It inserts on the muscular process of the malleus. The ossicles form a short chain across the dorsal part of the tympanic cavity.

Nerves that are found coursing through the tympanic cavity include the *chorda tympani* (see Fig. 20.10), from the nerve that passes through the tympanic cavity medial to the malleus to join the lingual nerve. The tympanic plexus arising from the tympanic nerve (*n. tympanicus*) of the glossopharyngeal nerve lies on the promontory and supplies the tympanic mucosa and the minor petrosal nerve to the otic ganglion (see Fig. 19.20). The caroticotympanic (*nn. carotidotympanici*) nerves from the internal carotid plexus also contribute to this tympanic plexus.

The facial nerve courses within the facial canal of the petrous temporal bone near the vestibular window. Near the tendon of the stapedius muscle, the bone encasing the facial canal is incomplete, essentially forming a facial foramen (Njaa, 2017), which allows direct contact of the facial nerve with contents of the tympanic cavity. Infection or masses within the middle ear can directly impact the facial nerve at this point resulting in facial nerve dysfunction (Njaa, 2017).

The **auditory tube** (*tuba auditiva*), formerly Eustachian tube, is a short canal that extends from the nasopharynx to the rostral portion of the tympanic cavity. Its short bony wall is formed rostrally by the squamous part of the temporal

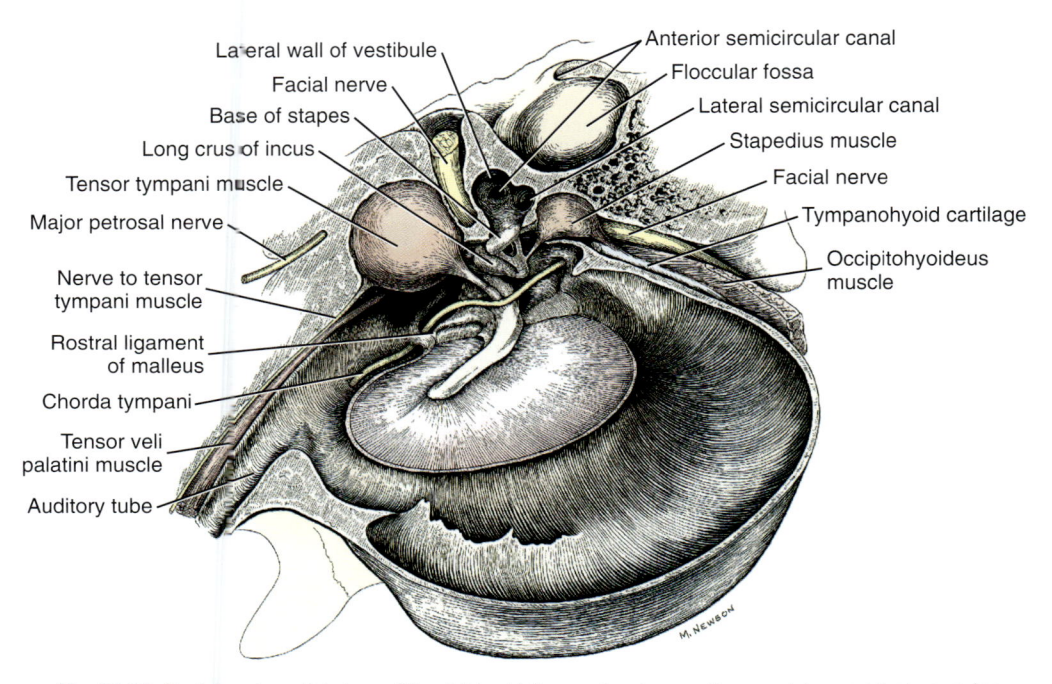

• **Fig. 20.10** Sculptured medial view of the right middle ear showing auditory ossicles and their muscles.

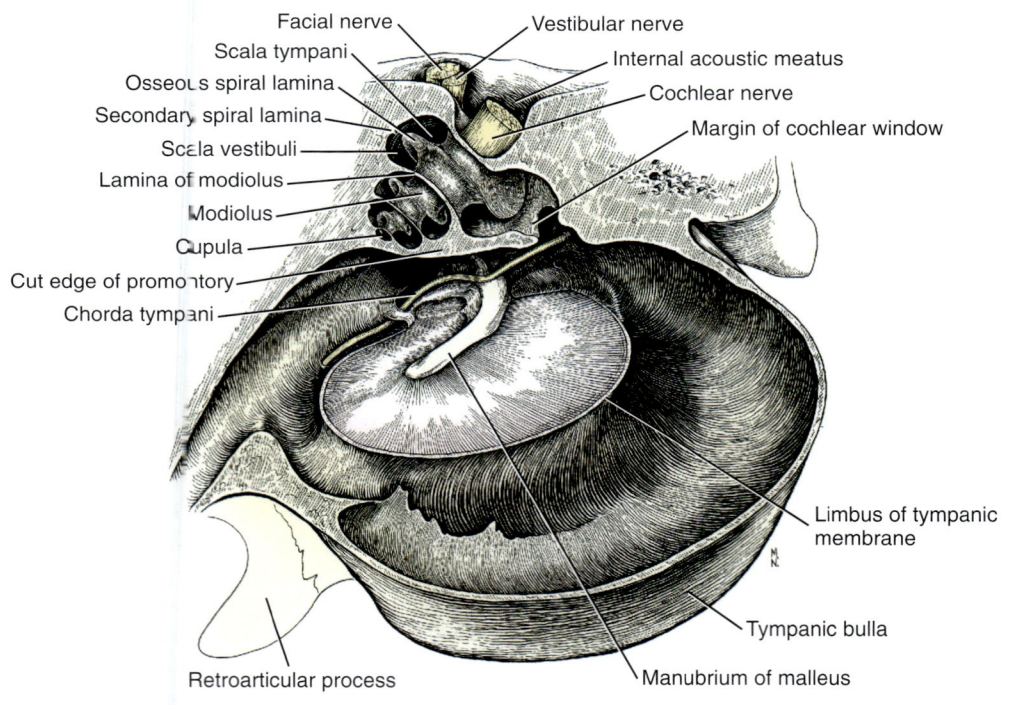

• **Fig. 20.11** Sculptured medial view of the right middle ear and cochlea.

bone, and ventrally its floor is formed by the tympanic part of the temporal bone. The lateral wall, which is approximately 8 mm long, is nearly twice the length of the medial wall. The tube is oval in cross-section, with its greater diameter 1.5 mm. The medial wall of the membranous part of the tube is supported by a plate of hyaline cartilage, the rostral end of which curves medially to form a short hook.

The m. tensor veli palatini (see Fig. 20.10) arises in the groove of the petrous part of the temporal bone ventrolateral to the m. tensor tympani. It supports the lateral wall of the auditory tube. The branch of the fifth cranial nerve that supplies the m. tensor tympani enters the tympanic cavity in association with the tendon of origin of the m. tensor veli palatini.

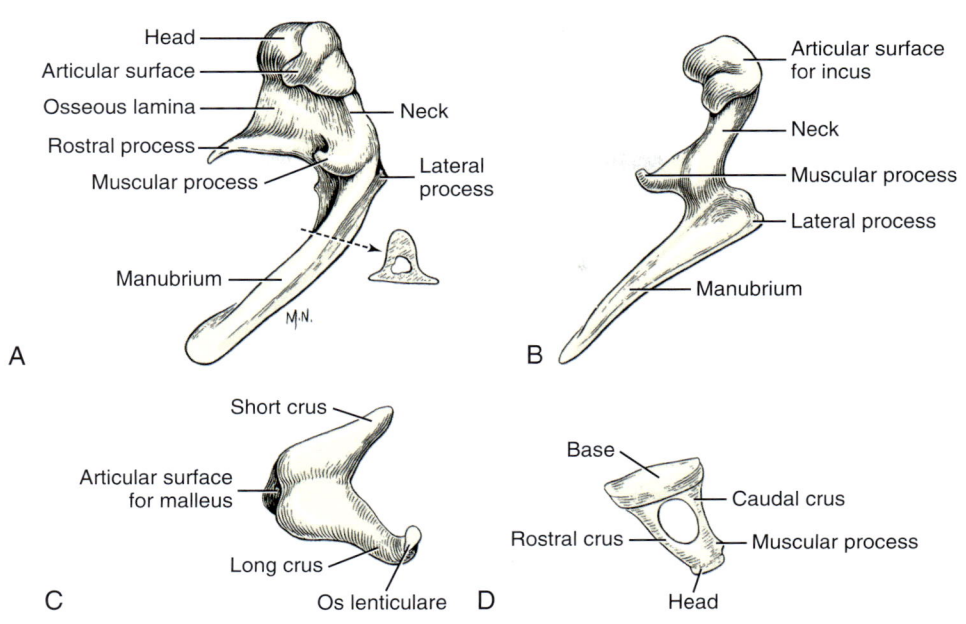

Fig. 20.12 Auditory ossicles of right ear. **A,** Malleus, medial aspect and cross-section. **B,** Malleus, caudal aspect. **C,** Incus, medial rostral aspect. **D,** Stapes, medial caudal aspect.

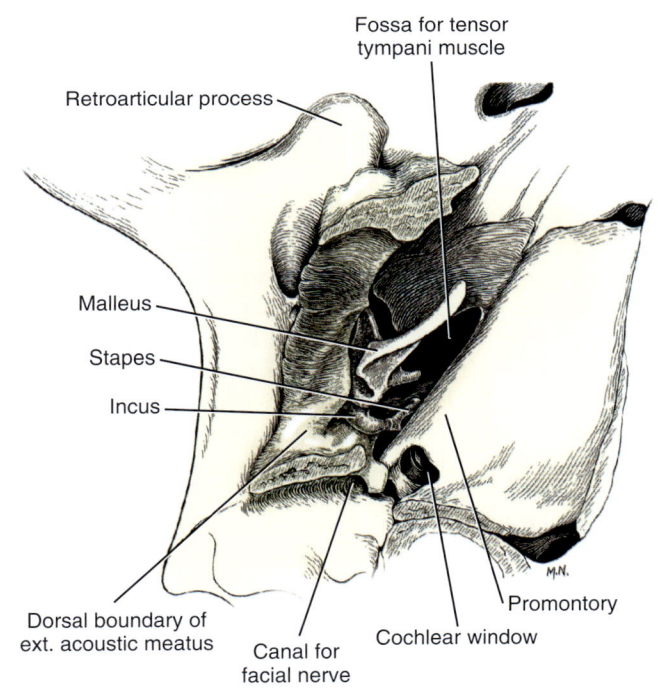

Fig. 20.13 Auditory ossicles of right ear, ventral aspect. Tympanic bulla removed.

Bones and Articulations of the Middle Ear

The **auditory ossicles** (*ossicula auditus*) (Figs. 20.1, 20.2, 20.12, and 20.13) are three small bones that transmit air vibrations from the tympanic membrane across the cavity of the middle ear to the internal ear. The most lateral and largest of the three bones is the malleus (see Figs. 20.1 and 20.12). The three-ossicle system of the mammalian middle ear transmits higher sound frequencies more effectively than would occur in a single-ossicle middle ear, as seen in mammalian ancestors (Manley, 2010; Vater & Kössl, 2011).

The **malleus** consists of a head; a wide, thin neck; and a manubrium, or handle. The **manubrium** is three-sided in cross-section. The side embedded in the substance of the tympanic membrane is wider and smoother than the other two; it is also slightly concave longitudinally. At the base of the manubrium, extending medially and slightly rostrally, is the **muscular process** of the malleus. This is provided with a tiny hook at its end, to which the m. tensor tympani attaches. The **rostral process** (Fig. 20.12A), or long process, is largely embedded in the tympanic membrane. It extends directly rostral from the neck of the malleus, arising at the same level as the muscular process. Opposite the muscular process at an angle of approximately 90 degrees with the rostral process is the short, **lateral process**. This is the most dorsal attachment of the manubrium to the tympanic membrane. The head of the malleus articulates with the body of the incus in the epitympanic recess, the most dorsal portion of the tympanic cavity.

The **incus** (Fig. 20.12C), measuring approximately 4 mm long and 3 mm high, is much smaller than the malleus. Its shape has often been likened to a human bicuspid tooth with divergent roots. The incus consists of a body, two crura, and a process. It lies caudal to the malleus in the epitympanic recess where the head of the malleus articulates with the **body** of the incus. The crura are located on each side of a transverse ridge that forms the caudal limit of the recess. The **short crus** points caudally into the fossa incudis dorsal to this ridge. The **long crus** is also directed caudally but presents a small bone, the **os lenticularis**, which is in the articulation between the incus and the stapes. It extends rostrally and somewhat medially from the distal end of the incus. In some instances this connection ossifies to form the **processus lenticularis**.

The **stapes** (Fig. 20.12D) consists of a head, two crura, a base, and a muscular process. It lies in a horizontal plane, the base facing medially. The **head** articulates with the incus via the os lenticulare or lenticular process. The **base** articulates with the fibrocartilaginous ring that covers the edge of the vestibular window. The stapes is the innermost ossicle and is the smallest bone in the body, being approximately 2 mm in length. The **rostral** and **caudal crura** are hollowed on their concave or opposed sides. A cross-section of a single crus appears as a narrow semicircle of bone. There is a thin **stapedial membrane** (*membrana stapedis*) that connects one crus to the other. In many mammals, there is an artery passing between the crura. The rostral crus is slightly longer than the caudal crus. Arising from the caudal crus near the head is a minute **muscular process** that provides attachment for the stapedius muscle (Figs. 20.10 and 20.12D).

Ligaments of the Ossicles

Several ligaments that attach the ossicles to the wall of the tympanic cavity were described by Getty et al. (1956) (*ligg. ossiculorum auditus*). A short but fairly well-defined **lateral ligament of the malleus** connects the lateral process of the malleus to the margins of the tympanic notch. The **dorsal ligament of the malleus** is a somewhat diffuse mass of ligamentous tissue that joins the head of the malleus to a small area on the roof of the epitympanic recess. The **rostral ligament of the malleus** (Fig. 20.10) is a short ligament attaching the rostral process of the malleus to the osseous tympanic ring just ventral to the canal by which the chorda tympani leaves the tympanic cavity. The body of the incus is attached to the roof of the epitympanic recess by the **dorsal ligament of the incus**. The **caudal ligament of the incus** attaches the short crus of the incus to the fossa incudis. An **anular ligament** (*lig. anulare stapedis*) attaches the base of the stapes to the cartilage that lines the vestibular window.

Muscles of the Ossicles

Two tiny muscles (Fig. 20.10) are associated with two of the ossicles. The *m. tensor tympani* is spherical, with its base in the fossa tensor tympani. The short tendon of insertion is attached to the hook on the apex of the muscular process of the malleus. Contraction of this muscle tends to draw the handle of the malleus medially, tensing the tympanic membrane and placing tension on the auditory ossicles (Njaa, 2017). Innervation is by a branch from the mandibular nerve from the trigeminal nerve (cranial nerve V). The *m. stapedius* is the smallest skeletal muscle in the body, and its origin is in the fossa musculae stapedis. The body of the muscle lies largely medial to the facial nerve. Its tendon of insertion passes through the facial nerve foramen and attaches to the muscular process of the stapes (see Fig. 20.10). Contraction of the stapedius muscle moves the rostral end of the base of the stapes caudolaterally and tenses the ossicle to reduce movement. Stapedius muscle action attenuates sound transmission to protect the receptor organs of the internal ear. This muscle is innervated by the stapedial branch of the facial nerve (cranial nerve VII).

The External Ear

The **external ear** of mammals consists of the auricle and external acoustic meatus. It varies greatly in size and shape between species and within domestic breeds. The external ear evolved as a sound-gathering structure, although its morphologic features in some breeds of domestic dogs appear to impede rather than enhance its function (Fig. 20.14). The ears, when erect, can be directed independently to localize and collect sound. Sound is conducted via the external acoustic meatus to the tympanic membrane deep in the external acoustic meatus.

External Acoustic Meatus

The **external acoustic meatus** (*meatus acousticus externus*) is the canal from the base of the auricle to the tympanic membrane surrounded by annular cartilage and the tubular portion of the auricular cartilage. The latter is the rolled up proximal part of the auricular cartilage.

Auricle

The **auricle** (*auricula*), pinna, is the externally visible part of the ear. The size and shape of the nontubular part of the **auricular cartilage** (*cartilago auriculae*) determines the appearance of the auricle, which may be upright or pendulous. In some breeds, such as the Boxer, it is often surgically trimmed (Fig. 20.14) The auricle is covered by skin and is moved by muscles. The auricular cartilage is pierced by many foramina that permit the passage of blood vessels and nerves from the convex surface to the concave surface (Miller & Witter, 1942). When the ear is traumatized and blood vessels rupture, large hematomas may develop between the skin and the cartilage; in such cases surgical intervention is often required.

With the ear (auricle) erect, the concave surface of the auricle is directed rostrally and the convex surface caudally. The **conchal cavity** (*cavum conchae*) is the proximal portion of the auricle where it is funnel-shaped at the entrance into the external acoustic meatus. The **anthelix** is a transverse fold of cartilage on the concave surface of the auricle. It is adjacent to the distal portion of the conchal cavity and separates the conchal cavity from the *scapha*, which is the large flat concave internal side of the auricle. The proximal portion of the auricular concha that surrounds the conchal cavity is rolled into a tube to enclose the external acoustic meatus. This opening faces dorsally. The tubular external acoustic meatus extends ventrally and then bends medially until it meets the small **anular cartilage** (*cartilago anularis*)

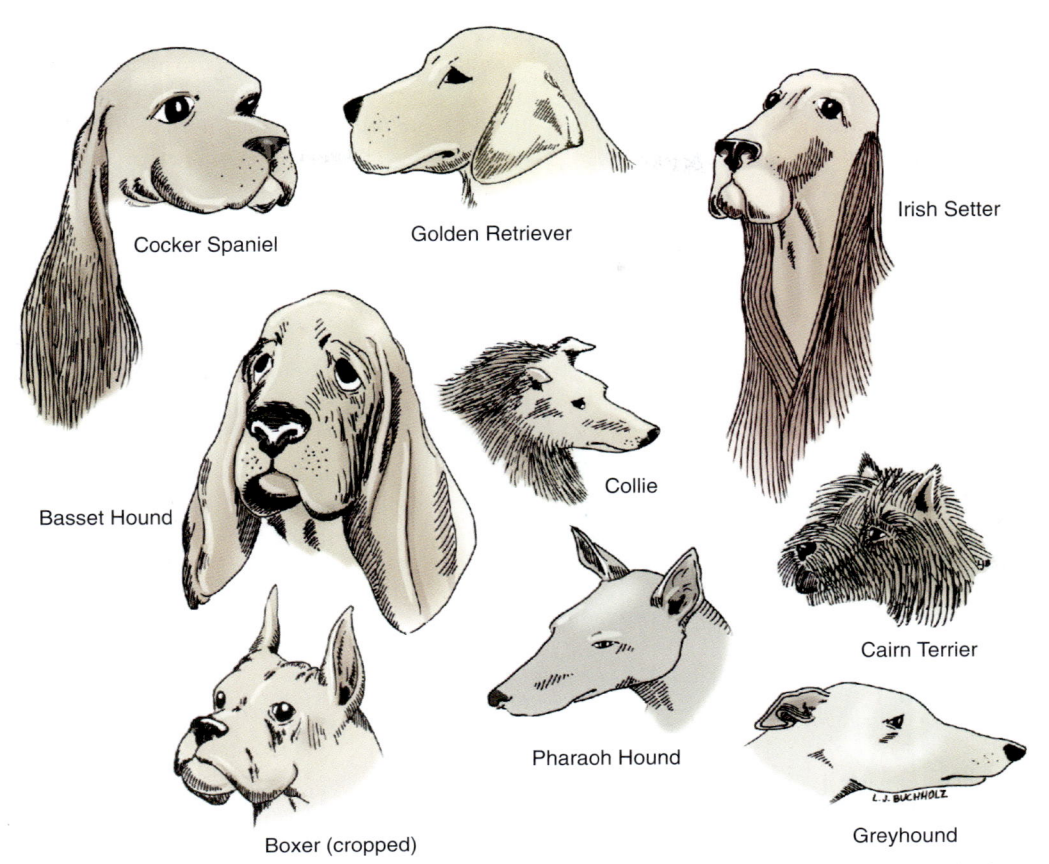

Fig. 20.14 The external ear varies greatly in size and shape. The bend in the auricle of lop-eared animals occurs distal to the anthelix in the scapha. The skin lining the scapha and concha shows pigmentation characteristic of the breed. It has, in most specimens, a decreasing amount of hair from the distal to the proximal parts. A few very fine hairs are found at the entrance of the cartilaginous external acoustic meatus. The rather prominent transverse ridges, as well as the longitudinal ridges, are simple skin folds that frequently continue toward the apex of the ear. Cartilage is not discernible in them on histologic section. The protective hair of the skin becomes fine and scanty in the conchal cavity.

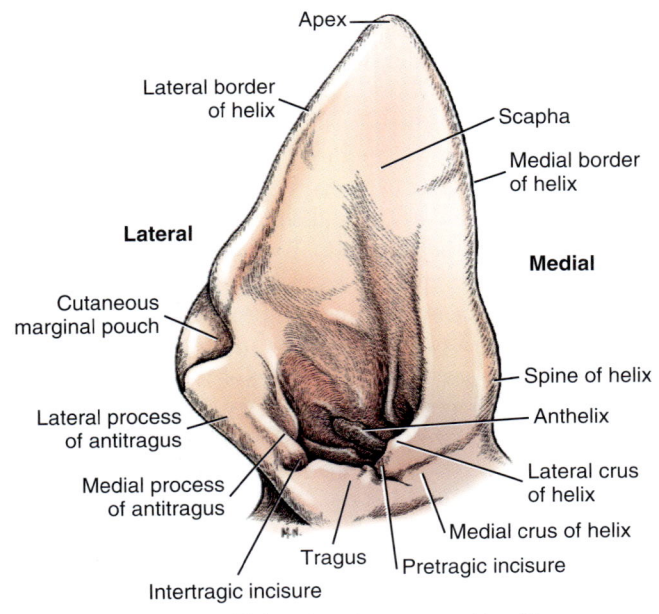

Fig. 20.15 Right external ear covered by skin.

that fits into the proximal portion of the tubular cartilage of the external acoustic meatus. The anular cartilage is approximately 2 cm long in the average size dog (see Fig. 20.16). The proximal portion of the anular cartilage overlaps and attaches to the osseous portion of the external acoustic meatus. This arrangement of a separate cartilaginous "joining ring" connecting these two portions of the external acoustic meatus by fibrous tissue gives the external ear flexibility.

The auricular cartilage is elastic, thin, and pliable. It thickens proximally where it rolls into a tube. The entire free margin of the auricle and passing over the apex is the **helix**. The **spine of the helix** (*spina helicis*) is a medial projection on the proximal part of the helix medially. On the proximal lateral portion of the helix is a fold of skin partly supported by cartilage known as the **marginal cutaneous sac** (*saccus cutaneus marginalis*) or pouch.

A number of cartilaginous projections are found at the entrance into the external acoustic meatus where the conchal portion of the auricular cartilage is rolled into a tube. The

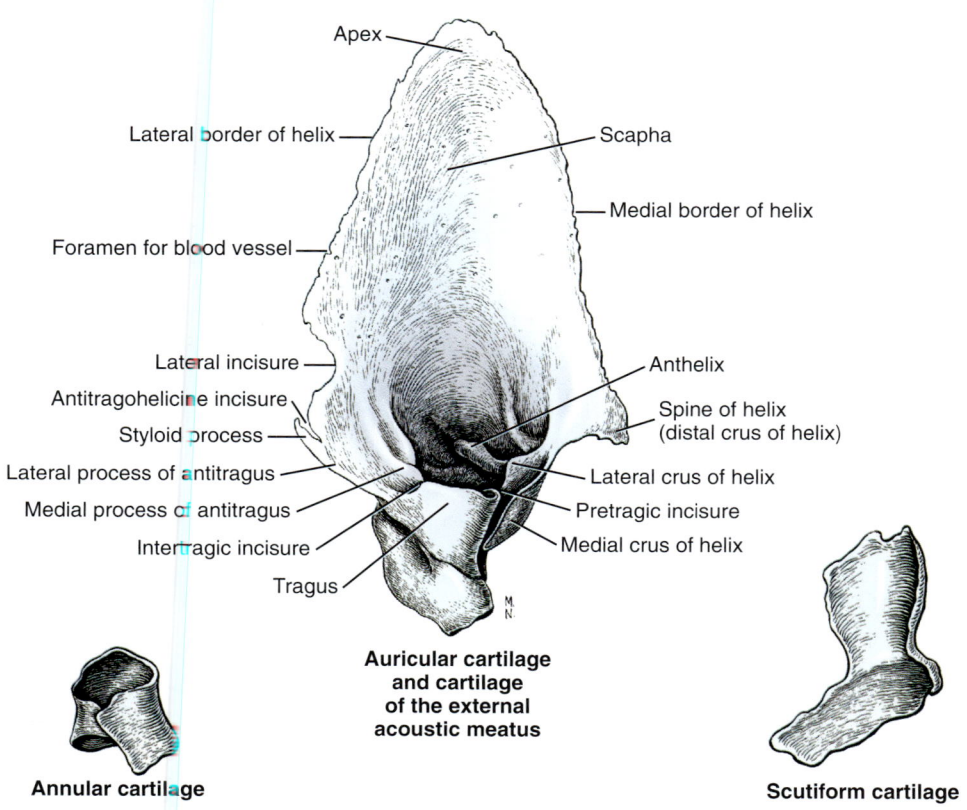

Fig. 20.16 Cartilages of the right external ear.

tragus is a thick blunt irregularly quadrangular plate of cartilage that projects from the rostral border of this entrance. Lateral to the tragus on this rostral border is a thin elongate projection of cartilage, the **antitragus**. The antitragus is separated from the tragus by a notch, the **intertragic incisure** (*incisura intertragica*). The antitragus consists of medial and lateral processes that project laterally. The apex of the lateral process ends in a sharp point laterally called the **styloid process** (*processus styloideus*). This process is separated from the lateral portion of the helix by the **antitragicohelicine incisure** (*incisura antitragicohelicina*). The marginal cutaneous sac is just distal to this incisure. Medial to the tragus on this rostral border are two crura formed from the medial portion of the helix. These **medial** and **lateral crura** (*crus helicis mediale and laterale*) project laterally and are separated from the tragus by the **pretragic incisure** (*incisura pretragica*). The lateral crus of the helix is close to the opening of the external acoustic meatus and caudal to the medial crus of the helix, which borders the pretragic incisure.

Muscles of the Ear

The facial muscles of mammals are very complex and variable. Even though the dog does not have the same range of facial expression as that seen in humans, the muscles of the dog's face are well developed. They consist of several layers and numerous slips that may differ in size or insertion from one individual to another. Their innervation, however, by the nervus facialis is constant.

Ernst Huber, assistant in the Anatomical Institute at the University of Zurich, set himself the task of investigating the facial musculature and its innervation in carnivores. His well-illustrated publications (Huber, 1918, 1922, 1923) are the most detailed findings available on the muscles of the face and ear of carnivores.

The difficulty in distinguishing one facial muscle from another muscle results from their lack of distinct connective tissue sheaths or fascia between the delaminated layers and slips. Thus, adjacent layers and slips often join each other in various ways, or slips may become independent and constitute separate muscles deserving of a name. Variations of this sort, which make neat classifications difficult, often show the relations of one muscle to another and clarify the ontogenetic and phylogenetic history of the slip or muscle. (A similar situation was encountered by Evans [1959] with the digastric and hyoid muscles of the dog [see Figs. 6.24 and 6.25].)

Scutiform Cartilage

A small, boot-shaped cartilaginous plate, the **scutiform cartilage** (*cartilago scutiformis*) (Figs. 20.16 and 20.19), is located in the rostroauricular muscles medial to the ear. Several muscles that move the ear attach to the scutiform cartilage. In addition to some short auricular muscles, the broad m. interscutularis passes from its attachment on the medial dorsal border of one scutiform cartilage to the other and, in so doing, blends with the m. frontalis. The scutiform cartilage is thought to be a detached portion of the conchal spina helicis that separates at birth or shortly afterward, so it should be considered a part of the external ear. Deep to the scutiform cartilage there is a fatty cushion, the **corpus adiposum auriculare**, that extends over a portion of the temporal muscle and around the base of the ear, giving the overlying muscle mass more mobility. Huber (1922) found many individual variations in auricular and facial muscles of dogs caused by delaminations, divisions, and fusions. Frequently, shared muscle fibers indicated common origins and shared relationships. Many of these variations were shown by Huber (1922, 1923) and reproduced by Leahy (1949). A few examples are reproduced here (Figs. 20.17 to 20.20).

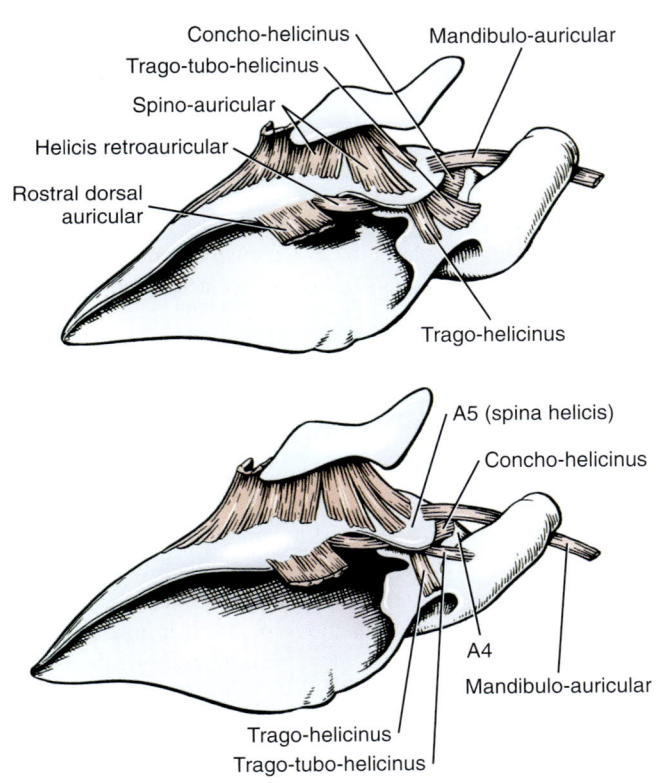

- **Fig. 20.17** The proper auricular muscles of the convex surface of the right ear. Note the variation in size of the m. trago-helicinus, m. trago-tubo-helicinus, and m. concho-helicinus. All these muscles are derived from a sheet of muscle that bridges the gap between the tragus and the spina helicis. (From Leahy JR: *Muscles of the head, neck, shoulder, and forelimb of the dog*, Thesis, Ithaca, NY, 1949, Cornell University. Modified from Huber E: Über das Muskelgebiet des Nervus facialis beim Hund, nebst allgemeinen Betrachtungen über die Facialis-Muskulatur. I, *Teil Morph Jahrb* 52:1–110, 1922.)

Because the external ears of mammals vary so much in shape, it is difficult to homologize the parts in different species. Huber (1922, 1923), in his two-part, well-illustrated monograph on the facial muscles of the dog, calls attention to the work of Boas (1912), who devised a method for studying and describing the auricular cartilage. Boas introduced a uniform nomenclature that allowed comparisons between the ears of mammals regardless of the contour of the ear in life. Anatomic preparation consists of macerating the ear to remove the skin and rolling it open to lie flat. Leahy's redrawing of Huber's illustration of the flattened dog ear (after Boas [1912]) is reproduced here with modified labels as Fig. 20.21. When the auricular cartilage is flattened, each margin (anterior = *Nomina Anatomica Veterinaria* [NAV] medial; posterior = NAV lateral) can be said to bear seven lobulations or projections. These are numbered A1 to A7 and P1 to P7. For the details of muscle attachment to these processes or how they relate to each other when the ear cartilage is rolled into its normal position, see Boas (1912), Huber (1922, 1923), or the translation from Leahy (1949).

The borders of the auricular cartilage were named *anterior* and *posterior* for a long time, and these were the terms used by Boas (1912) and Huber (1922, 1923) in naming the parts of the auricle. The anterior and posterior auricular muscles of these authors are now rostral and caudal auricular muscles (NAV, 2005), with added designations of dorsal and ventral auricular muscles. Miller (1948) designated the rostral muscles as preauricular and the caudal muscles as postauricular in early editions of his dissection guide. Because the external muscles of the ear develop by splitting and delamination of muscle sheets or bundles, there may be superficial and deep layers, each of which may be further delaminated and given a Roman numeral.

Because various directional terms have been used for the ear, and these required different terms for muscles, vessels, and nerves, the application of these terms in the literature is not always consistent. Directional terms for structures of the internal and external ear as given in the NAV (2005) include the following:

Internal ear: Anterior, posterior, or lateral for semicircular ducts, canals, and ampullae; superior or inferior for the area vestibularis
Middle ear: Rostral or caudal on the tympanic membrane; medial or lateral in the auditory tube; rostral or lateral for the processes of the malleus; rostral or caudal in the cavum tympani
External ear: Directional terms apply to the ear with the concave surface of the auricle facing rostrally. Thus the concave surface is the rostral surface and the convex surface is the caudal surface and there are medial and lateral borders. There are rostral and caudal auricular nerves. The caudal auricular artery has lateral, intermediate, and medial branches.

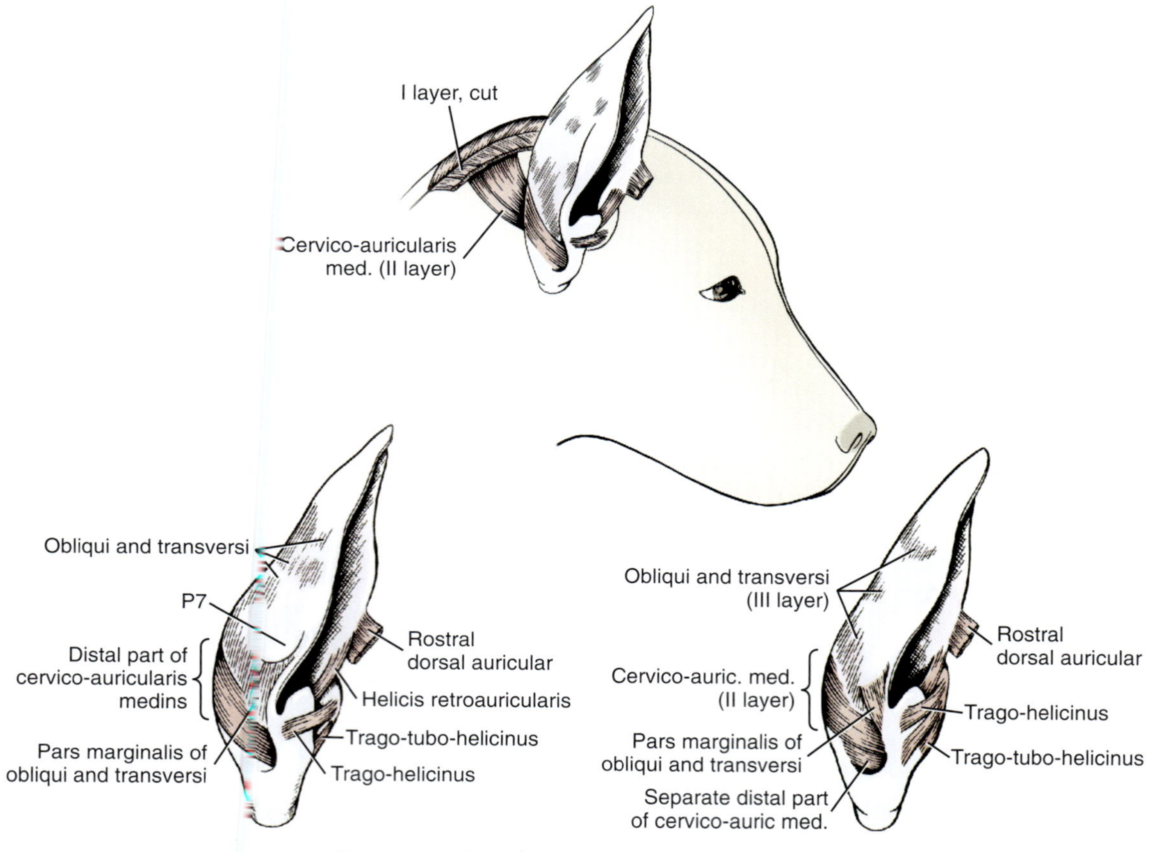

Proper muscles of the base of the right ear

• **Fig. 20.18** The cervicoauricular muscles represent the most cranial portion of the cervical platysma. Layer I is the superficial cervico-auriculo-occipitalis of Huber (1922). Layer II is the cervico-auricularis medius, a uniform muscle plate that is continuous with the second leaf of the cervical platysma. It attaches to the concha. (From Leahy JR: *Muscles of the head, neck, shoulder, and forelimb of the dog,* Thesis, Ithaca, NY, 1949, Cornell University. Modified from Huber E: Über das Muskelgebiet des Nervus facialis beim Hund, nebst allgemeinen Betrachtungen über die Facialis-Muskulatur. I, *Teil Morph Jahrb* 52:1–110, 1922.)

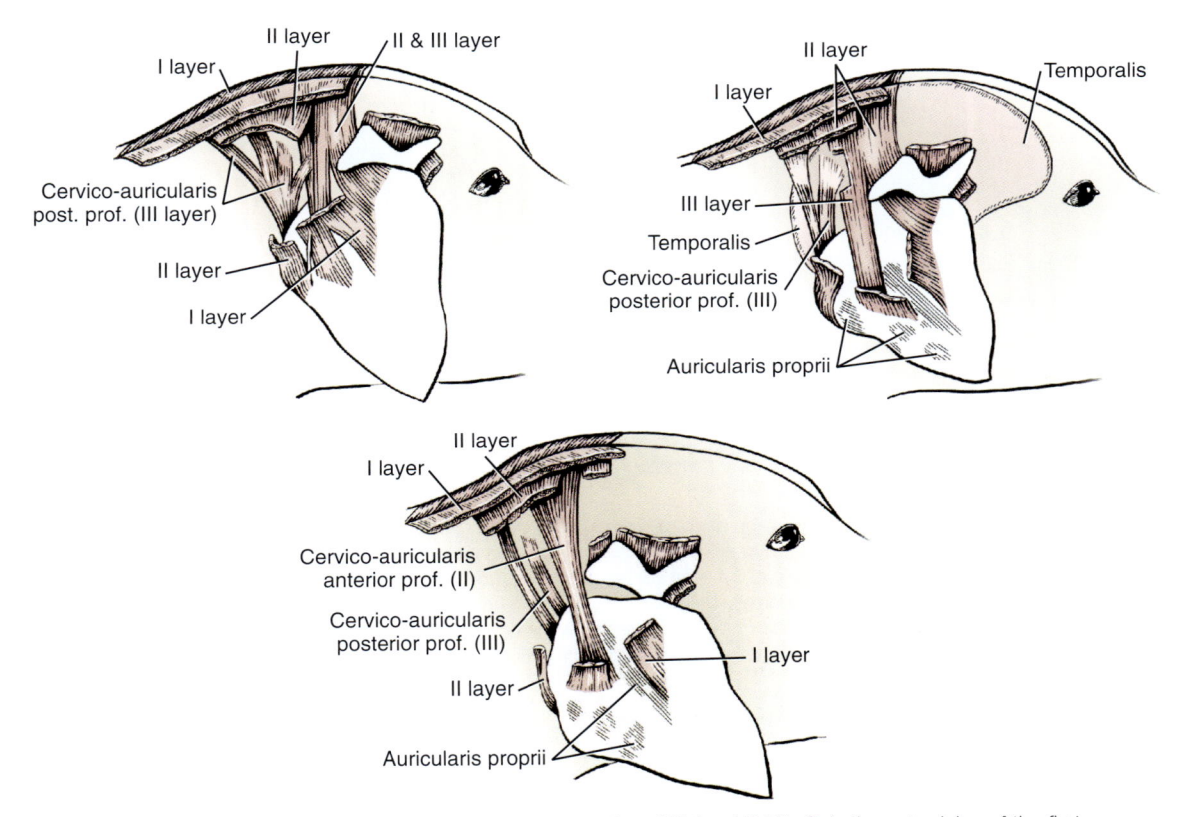

• **Fig. 20.19** The third layer of the retroauricular muscles of Huber (1922). Only the cut origins of the first and second layers are shown. This drawing illustrates the great variation that can be seen in three random dogs. There are differences in the origin, degree of development, number of crura, and insertion of muscles. (From Leahy JR: *Muscles of the head, neck, shoulder, and forelimb of the dog,* Thesis, Ithaca, NY, 1949, Cornell University. Modified from Huber E: Über das Muskelgebiet des Nervus facialis beim Hund, nebst allgemeinen Betrachtungen über die Facialis-Muskulatur. I, *Teil Morph Jahrb* 52:1–110, 1922.)

856 CHAPTER 20 The Ear

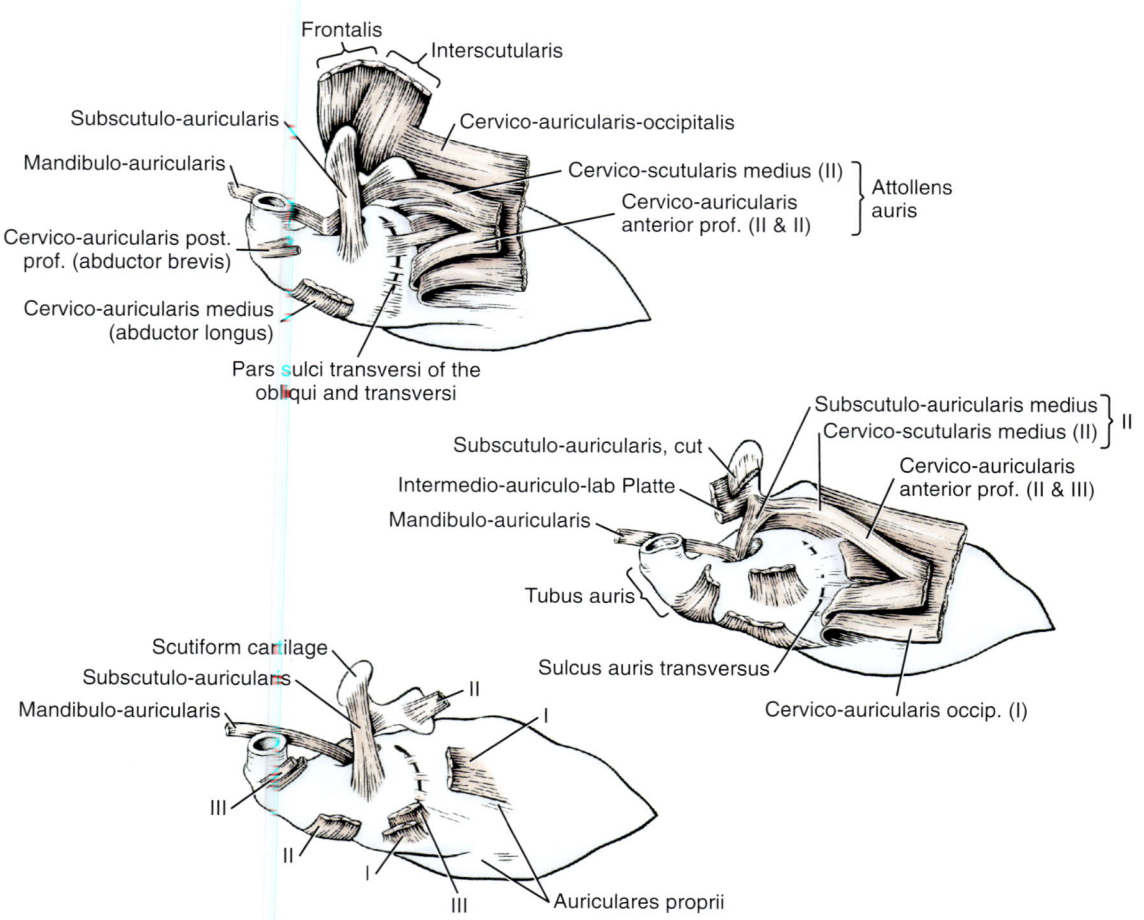

• **Fig. 20.20** Ear removed to show the deep muscles on the convex surface of the right auricular cartilage and on the scutiform cartilage. The cervicoauricular muscles have been reflected to expose the deeper muscles. This is another example of random variations that can be seen in three dogs. (From Leahy JR: *Muscles of the head, neck, shoulder, and forelimb of the dog*, Thesis, Ithaca, NY, 1949, Cornell University. Modified from Huber E: Über das Muskelgebiet des Nervus facialis beim Hund, nebst allgemeinen Betrachtungen über die Facialis-Muskulatur. I, Teil *Morph Jahrb* 52:1–110, 1922.)

• **Fig. 20.21** The auricular cartilage of the dog. **A**, The unrolled and flattened cartilage, showing the seven marginal projections, or lobes, described by Boas, some of which serve for muscle attachment. A1 to A7 are on the medial border, and P1 to P7 on the lateral border. A1 and P1 constitute the free ends of the annular cartilage. **B**, The rolled auricular cartilage, showing its normal topography. In life P4 and A6 are joined by connective tissue and form a cone, or concha, that narrows to enter the tuba, or cartilaginous auditory tube. (Modified from Boas JEV: *Uber den Ohrknorpel und das aussere Ohr der Saugetiere*, Copenhagen, 1912; Huber E: Über das Muskelgebiet des Nervus facialis beim Hund, nebst allgemeinen Betrachtungen über die Facialis-Muskulatur. I, Teil *Morph Jahrb* 52:1–110, 1922; and Leahy JR: *Muscles of the head, neck, shoulder, and forelimb of the dog*, Thesis, Ithaca, NY, 1949, Cornell University.)

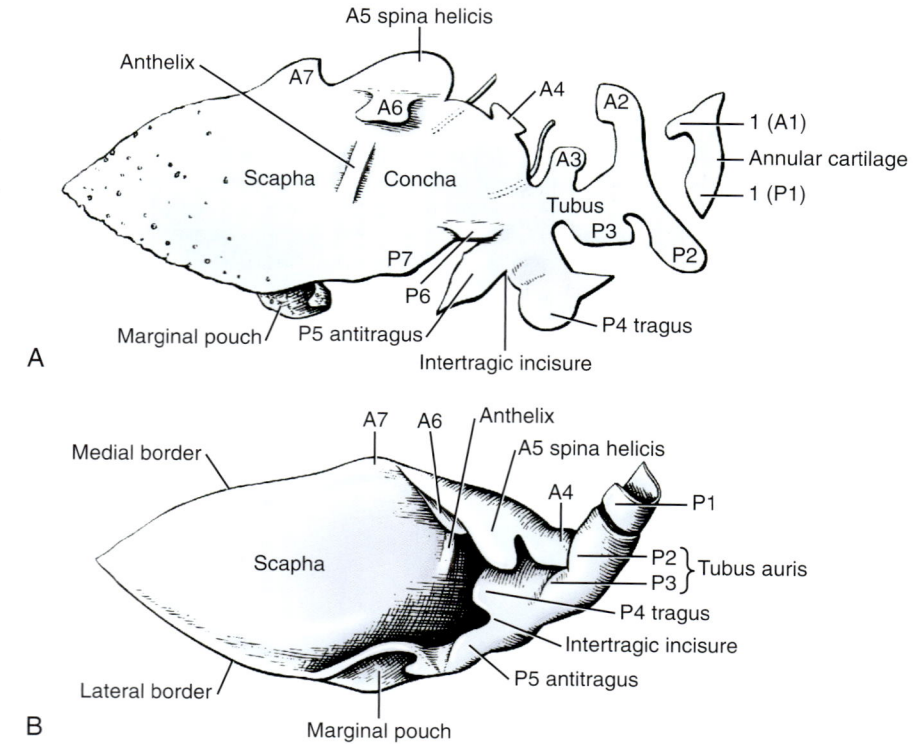

Bibliography

Alberti, P. W. (1964). Epithelial migration on the tympanic membrane. *J Laryngol Otol, 74*, 808–830.

Antunez, J.-C. M., Galey, F. R., Linthicum, F. H., et al. (1980). Computer-aided and graphic reconstruction of the human endolymphatic duct and sac: A method for comparing Meniere's and non-Meniere's disease cases. *Ann Otol Rhinol Laryngol, 89*(Suppl. 76), 23–32.

Boas, J. E. V. (1912). *Uber den ohrknorpel und das aussere ohr der saugetiere.* Copenhagen.

Branis, M., & Burda, H. (1985). Inner ear structure in the deaf and normally hearing Dalmatian dog. *J Comp Pathol, 95*, 295–299.

de Lahunta, A., Glass, E., & Kent, M. (2015). *Veterinary neuroanatomy and clinical neurology* (4th ed.). St Louis, MO: Elsevier.

Evans, H. E. (1959). Hyoid muscle anomalies in the dog (*Canis familiaris*). *Anat Rec, 133*, 145–162.

Foss, I., & Flottorp, G. (1974). A comparative study of the development of hearing and vision in various species commonly used in experiments. *Acta Otolaryngol, 77*, 202–214.

Friberg, U., Rask-Andersen, H., & Bagger-Sjöbäck, D. (1984). Human endolymphatic duct: An ultrastructure study. *Arch Otolaryngol, 110*, 421–428.

Getty, R. H., Foust, L., Presley, E. T., & Miller, M. E. (1956). Macroscopic anatomy of the ear of the dog. *Am J Vet Res, 17*, 364–375.

Gienc, J., & Kuder, T. (1983). Otic ganglion in dog. Topography and macroscopic structure. *Folia Morphol, 42*, 31–40.

Guild, S. R. (1927). The circulation of the endolymph. *Am J Anat, 39*, 57–81.

Huber, E. (1918). Über das muskelgebiet des n. facialis bei katze und hund nebst allgemeinen betrachtungen über die facialis-muskulatur der säuger. *Anat Anz, 51*, 1–17.

Huber, E. (1922). Über das muskelgebiet des nervus facialis beim hund, nebst allgemeinen betrachtungen über die facialis-muskulatur. I. *Teil Morph Jahrb, 52*, 1–110.

Huber, E. (1923). Über das muskelgebiet des nervus facialis beim hund, nebst allgemeinen betrachtungen über die facialis-muskulatur. II. *Teil Morph Jahrb, 52*, 353–414.

Johnsson, L. G., Hawkins, J. E., Jr., Muraski, A. A., et al. (1973). Vascular anatomy and pathology of the cochlea in Dalmatian dogs. In A. J. D. DeLorenzo (Ed.), *Vascular disorders and hearing defects.* Baltimore, MD: University Park Press.

Leahy, J. R. (1949). *Muscles of the head, neck, shoulder, and forelimb of the dog.* Thesis. Ithaca, NY: Cornell University.

Liew, L. J., Chen, L. Q., Wang, A. Y., et al. (2018). Tympanic membrane derived stem cell-like cultures for tissue regeneration. *Stem Cells Dev*, doi:10.1089/scd.2018.002.

Maher, W. P. (1988). Microvascular networks in tympanic membrane, malleus periosteum, and annulus perichondrium of neonatal mongrel dog: A vasculoanatomic model for surgical considerations. *Am J Anat, 183*, 294–302.

Manley, G. A. (2010). An evolutionary perspective on middle ears. *Hear Res, 263*, 3–8. doi:10.1016/j.heares.2009.09.004.

Michaels, L., & Soucek, S. (1989). Development of the stratified squamous epithelium of the human tympanic membrane and external ear canal: The origin of auditory epithelial migration. *Am J Anat, 184*, 334–344.

Miller, M. E. (1948). *Guide to the dissection of the dog.* Ann Arbor, MI: Edwards Brothers.

Miller, M. E., & Witter, R. (1942). Applied anatomy of the external ear of the dog. *Cornell Vet, 32*, 64–86.

Nadol, J. B., Jr. (1988). Comparative anatomy of the cochlea and auditory nerve in mammals. *Hear Res, 34*, 253–266.

Njaa, B. L. (2017). The ear. In J. F. Zachary (Ed.), *Pathologic basis of veterinary disease* (6th ed.). St. Louis, MO: Elsevier.

Njaa, B. L., & Sula, J. M. (2012). Collection and preparation of dog and cat ears for histologic examination. *Vet Clin North Am Small Anim Pract, 42*, 1127–1135.

NAV (2005). *Nomina anatomica veterinaria* (NAV) (5th ed.). NY: World Association of Veterinary Anatomists.

Oshima, K., Grimm, C. M., Corrales, C. E., et al. (2007). Differential distribution of stem cells in the auditory and vestibular organs of the inner ear. *J Assoc Res Otolaryngol, 8*, 18–31. doi:10.1007/s10162-006-58-3.

Rouse, R. C., Johnsson, L. G., Wright, C. G., & Hawkins, J. E. (1984). Abnormal otoconia and calcification in the labyrinth of deaf Dalmatian dogs. *Acta Otolaryngol, 98*, 61–71.

Shambaugh, G. E. (1923). Blood stream in the labyrinth of the ear of dog and man. *Am J Anat, 32*, 189–198.

Shimizu, S., Cureoglu, S., Yoda, S., et al. (2011). Blockage of longitudinal flow in Meniere's disease: A human temporal bone study. *Acta Otolaryngol, 131*, 263–268. doi:10.3109/00016489.2010.532155.

Tabacca, N. E., Cole, L. K., Hillier, A., & Rajala-Schultz, P. J. (2011). Epithelial migration on the canine tympanic membrane. *Vet Dermatol, 22*, 502–510. doi:10.1111/j.1365-3164.2011.00982.x.

Tomiyama, S., & Harris, J. P. (1986). The endolymphatic sac: Its importance in inner ear immune responses. *Laryngoscope, 96*, 685–691.

Vater, M., & Kössl, M. (2011). Comparative aspects of cochlear functional organization in mammals. *Hear Res, 273*, 89–99. doi:10.1016//j.heares.2010.05.018.

Wakuri, H., Mori, S., Mutoh, K., et al. (1988). Fiber arrangement in the canine tympanic membrane. *Okajimas Folia Anat Jpn, 65*(1), 11–18.

Xu, J., Ueno, H., Xu, C. Y., et al. (2017). Identification of mouse cochlear progenitors that develop hair and supporting cells in the organ of Corti. *Nat Commun, 8*, 15046. doi:10.1038/ncomms15046.

21
The Eye

CHRISTOPHER J. MURPHY AND J. CLAUDIO GUTIERREZ

The **eye** (*organum visus*) (Fig. 21.1) develops as a neuroectodermal outgrowth of the embryonic prosencephalon that contacts surface ectoderm and is enveloped by induced mesodermal and neural crest mesenchyme. The definitive eye and its adnexa are contained within an orbit that is only partly bony. Associated with the bulb of the eye are extraocular muscles that move it; periorbital fascia and fat that surround and cushion it; eyelids and conjunctivae that protect it; and a lacrimal apparatus that keeps its surface moist, provides the first barrier to infection, and helps to nourish the cornea.

As a consequence of its dual origin, the eye has both central and peripheral neural elements. The optic nerve is a central nervous system structure with myelin formed by oligodendroglial cells, whereas the nerves of the extraocular muscles and iris are peripheral nervous system structures with lemmocyte (Schwann cell) sheaths for myelin. The vascular and fibrous tunics surrounding the optic nerve are homologous to the meninges surrounding the brain and spinal cord. The intervaginal space of the optic nerve is continuous with the subarachnoid space of the brain and contains cerebrospinal fluid.

There is considerable variation between breeds in regard to the position of the eyes, the size of the orbit, and the size and shape of the palpebral opening.

Development

Aguirre et al. (1972) studied the early development of the dog's eye and its adnexa from day 15 to functional maturity using serially sectioned embryos in the Cornell University Collection (Evans & Sack, 1973). Subsequent studies involved histologic examination of fetuses removed from the uterus 25, 28, 30, 33, and 35 days post coitum (Boevé et al., 1988; Boevé et al., 1989). Johnston et al. (1979) described the relative contributions of mesoderm and neural crest cells to the developing eye.

The first indication of the formation of the eye is seen as an **optic sulcus** on the neural fold rostral to the notochord on each side. The neuroectoderm surrounding this sulcus proliferates rostrolaterally to form the optic vesicle, a hollow diverticulum of the prosencephalon. As the optic vesicle forms, its caudal surface is contacted by mesodermal mesenchyme and its peripheral surface is surrounded by superficial ectoderm (Fig. 21.2A). Shortly thereafter, migrating neural crest cells contribute to the forming vesicle and future orbital tissues. The anterior portion of the vesicle invaginates to form an **optic cup** with the concomitant formation of the lens placode in the adjacent surface ectoderm. The optic cup assumes a rounded appearance by day 30. There is an optic fissure along the ventral meridian where the lateral and medial folds of the optic cup meet and eventually fuse (Fig. 21.2B). The occurrence of the fissure allows for the penetration of the vascular mesoderm. Failure of the fissure to close results in defects of one or more of the tunics of the eye (colobomata). Such defects are common in the Collie breed as part of the heritable Collie eye syndrome.

The connection of the optic cup to the brainstem lengthens and attenuates as growth proceeds, forming the **optic stalk**, which will later become the optic nerve. Anteriorly, the **optic vesicle** induces the overlying surface ectoderm to proliferate, forming the **lens placode**, which is present by gestational day 15. As the optic vesicle invaginates, the placode also invaginates into the optic cup. By day 25, it pinches off from the surface ectoderm to form the **lens vesicle**, the anlage of the crystalline lens (see Fig. 21.2B). The first anlage of the lens capsule is evident by day 25 (Boevé et al., 1988). The remaining surface ectoderm becomes the epithelium of the cornea. The deeper stromal and posterior epithelial layers of the cornea are derived from neural crest mesenchymal cells.

The **hyaloid artery** (*a. hyaloidea*) is present at day 25, arising from the mesenchyme surrounding the optic cup. It enters the posterior end of the optic fissure to supply the inner surface of the cup and the mesenchyme filling the optic cup becomes the primary vitreous (see Fig. 21.2B). The hyaloid artery grows anteriorly and reaches the posterior lens surface by day 28, where it branches extensively to form the posterior portion of the *tunica vasculosa lentis*, a plexus of vessels derived from the anterior ciliary vessels that completely surrounds the lens by day 30. Secondary vitreous, secreted by the glial component consisting of Müller cells within the inner layer of the optic cup, surrounds

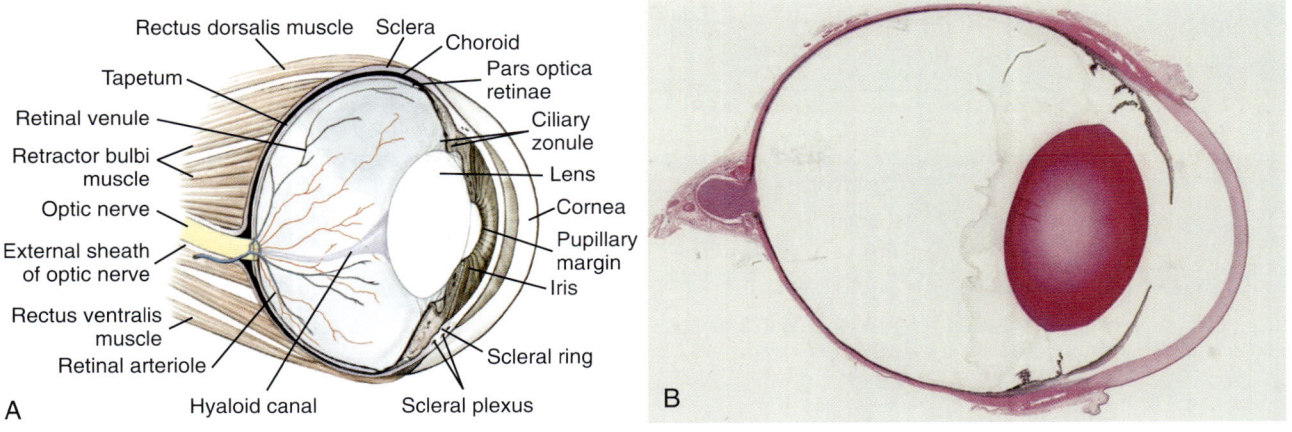

• Fig. 21.1 Bulbus oculi. A, Sagittal section of the dog eye with associated musculature. B, Low-magnification view of a parasagittal histologic section of the canine eye.

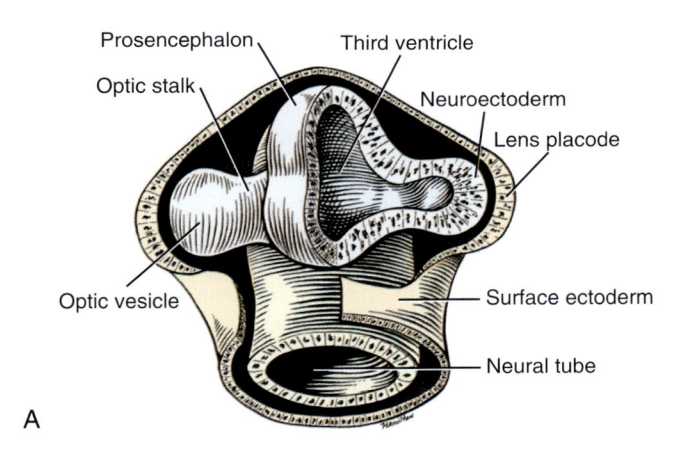

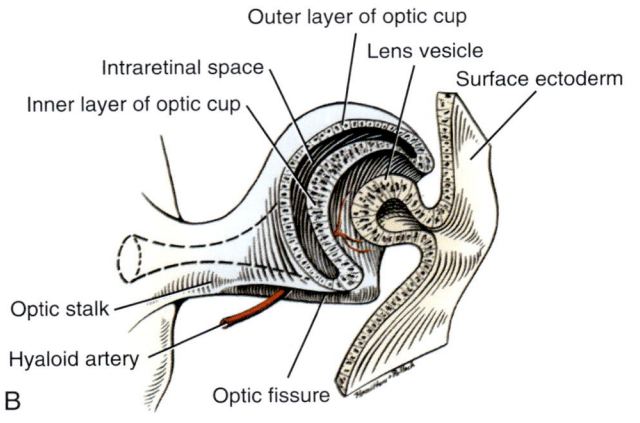

• Fig. 21.2 Development of the eye. A, Optic vesicle (4-mm embryo). B, Optic cup (7-mm embryo).

the primary vitreous beginning at approximately gestational day 26. With the growth of the eyeball, the secondary vitreous continues to elaborate, and the primary vitreous becomes reduced to a narrow funnel (hyaloid or cloquet canal or *canalis hyaloideus*) between the optic nerve and posterior lens surface (Fig. 21.1). The hyaloid vessels between the optic disc and lens begin to atrophy at approximately day 45, with remnants commonly present until 10 or 11 days after birth. The retinal arteries of the adult are derived from the portion of the hyaloid vasculature that supplied the inner layer of the optic cup. Normal retinal vascular development is mediated, at least in part, by vascular endothelial growth factor (Lutty et al., 2010)

The anterior face of the lens and primordial iris are supplied by the anterior portion of the tunica vasculosa lentis. The portion of the vascular tunic supplying the lens also atrophies late in gestation so that the lens is normally avascular at birth and in adult life.

The cavity of the optic vesicle, originally continuous with the third ventricle of the brain, is obliterated on approximately day 33, when the inner and outer walls of the optic cup fuse. The outer layer becomes the retinal pigment epithelium. The inner layer proliferates to form all layers of the neurosensory retina. Axons from the ganglion cells of the innermost layer grow toward the optic stalk, which they invade on approximately gestational day 30, and follow toward the brainstem. Maturation of the retina proceeds from central to peripheral and is not complete until 8 weeks after birth (Gum et al., 1984; Shively et al., 1971).

By day 25, the primary vitreous body contains amorphous fibrillar material and no cellular components except for vascular elements. By day 30, the vitreous body consists of randomly oriented fibrillar structures and some loose cells with cytologic characteristics of fibroblasts. Subsequently, the primitive vitreous body becomes increasingly more confined to the central part of the vitreal space. By day 33, the vitreous body is avascular at the periphery, becoming the definitive or secondary vitreous body. At day 35 the primary vitreous body is an empty space with few hyalocytes and almost no hyaloid vasculature.

The epithelia of the ciliary body and the posterior surface of the iris are also derived from the neuroectoderm of the inner layer of the optic cup, but are nonvisual (*pars ceca retinae*). The richly vascular mesenchyme surrounding the anterior tunica vasculosa lentis forms the stroma of the iris. The central area of the iris (pupillary membrane) is thin and normally completely atrophies by 14 days after birth, forming the pupil. Incomplete atrophy, resulting in

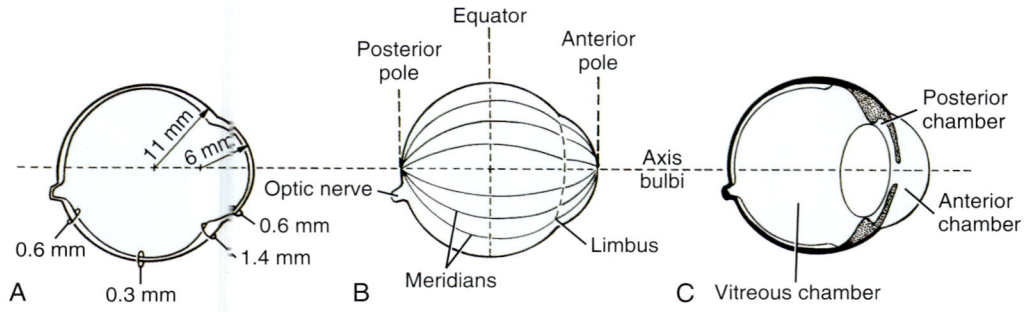

Fig. 21.3 Bulbus oculi. **A,** Average dimensions of sclera and cornea. **B,** Directional terminology. **C,** Chambers of the eyeball.

persistent pupillary membranes, has been observed as a heritable defect in Basenji dogs (Roberts & Bistner, 1968). The dilator and sphincter muscles of the iris differentiate from the neuroectodermal *pars iridica retinae.*

Rarefaction of the mesenchyme between that which forms the stroma of the iris and that which forms the substantia propria and posterior epithelium of the cornea is evident by day 45. Progressive rarefaction forms a cavity that fills with aqueous humor to become the **anterior chamber** (*Camera anterior bulbi*) of the adult eye (Fig. 21.3).

The mesenchyme (much of which is neural crest in origin) adjacent to the optic cup is induced by the outer layer of the cup to form the richly vascular *tunica vasculosa bulbi*. This vascular tunic comprises the iris, ciliary body, and choroid. At the periphery of the lens, the vascular mesenchyme proliferates into the folds, ciliary processes, of the ciliary body. Fibers form from the nonpigmented epithelium of the ciliary body and extend to the lens equator. These elongate as the globe increases in size to form the definitive *zonula ciliaris,* the suspensory ligament of the lens. Neural crest cells form the ciliary muscle fibers of the ciliary body. Contraction of these muscles is thought to relax tension on the zonula fibers, allowing the lens to become rounder, increasing its refractive power for near vision (accommodation). As the anterior optic cup develops in unison with the mesenchyme to create the iris, ciliary body, and suspensory ligament of the lens, the **posterior chamber** (*Camera posterior bulbi*) is formed (Fig. 21.3C).

External to the vascular tunic, the mesenchyme (primarily of neural crest origin) condenses to form the fibrous sclera, which is homologous to the dura mater of the brain. Neural crest cells are the source of the posterior corneal epithelial cells of the cornea as well as stromal fibroblasts (keratocytes). The extraocular muscles are derived from somitomere mesoderm caudal to the developing eye vesicle. Although the myofibers of these muscles are mesodermal, the connective tissues associated with them are of neural crest origin. Gilbert (1947) demonstrated that the extrinsic ocular muscles of the cat arise from three distinct but closely approximated anlagen that are homologous with the premandibular, mandibular, and hyoid head cavities of lower vertebrates. The same is probably true for the dog.

The **eyelids** appear as folds superior and inferior to the eye on approximately day 25 of gestation. These enlarge, grow over the cornea, and narrow the palpebral fissure by approximately half on day 35. The eyelids completely cover the cornea and fuse by day 40 (Evans, 1974). The superficial musculature of the lids, the *m. orbicularis oculi,* forms from the platysma sheet and is recognizable by approximately day 40. Huber (1922) has described the postnatal development of the platysma derivatives.

Dogs are born with the lid margins still adherent to one another. Final maturation of the eye occurs after birth; most notable are changes in the retina, iridocorneal angle, corneal epithelium, and tapetum. The fused lids normally separate approximately 2 weeks postpartum, and the palpebral fissure is able to be opened. Premature separation of the lids results in severe ophthalmitis, apparently as a result of the immaturity of the lacrimal apparatus (Aguirre & Rubin, 1970). During the first weeks after birth both the intraocular pressure and tear production increase (da Silva et al. 2013; Verboven et al., 2014).

The retina of the dog, as in many precocial species, is not fully developed at birth. Differentiation of the multicellular inner layer of the optic cup into inner (marginal) and outer (nucleated) layers to form the precursor of the sensory retina does not occur until embryonic days 25 to 28. Intracellular pigment granules may be observed at the periphery of the outer layer near the ora serrata, which will later form the pigment epithelium. By day 30, the anterior part of the pigment epithelium consists of cells arranged in pseudostratified columnar fashion and the nerve fiber layer may be observed at the posterior pole of the retina. The inner and outer neuroblastic layers of the retina may be distinguished posterior to the equator by day 30. In the posterior region, the nerve fiber layer becomes prominent and the axons join to form the optic nerve. By day 35, the retinal pigment epithelium becomes pigmented posterior to the equator of the optic cup. The photoreceptors are not developed until approximately 16 to 35 days after birth (Aguirre et al., 1972; Miller et al., 1989; Perry, 1940; Shively et al., 1971; Whiteley & Young, 1985). This lag in photoreceptor maturation is reflected by the electrical activity of the retina in response to photic stimulation (Gum et al., 1984). Vascularization of the retina occurs postnatally (Flower et al., 1985).

The Eyeball

The **eyeball** (*bulbus oculi*) is formed by three concentric coats: the **fibrous tunic** (*tunica fibrosa bulbi*), the **middle vascular tunic** (*tunica vasculosa bulbi*), and the **inner nervous tunic** (*tunica interna bulbi*). In the dog, the eyeball is nearly spherical, differing little in its sagittal, transverse, and vertical diameters. The size of the eyeball varies among breeds, but the diameter is usually approximately 20 to 22 mm (Table 21.1). In one study, the radius of the canine eye varied across breeds from 9.56 to 11.57 mm and was correlated with the width and length of the skull (McGreevy et al., 2004).

The transparent cornea forms the anterior one-fourth of the eyeball, and because it has a smaller radius of curvature (approximately 8.5 to 9 mm) than the rest of the eye, it bulges anteriorly (see Fig. 21.3). The vertex of the cornea is designated the ***anterior pole*** of the eye (*polus anterior*). The point directly opposite this is the **posterior pole** (*polus posterior*). The latter is a geometric point and does not correspond to the exit point of the optic nerve, which lies ventrolateral to the posterior pole. The line connecting the anterior and posterior poles and passing through the center of the lens is the ***axis bulbi*** (Fig. 21.3). In the mesaticephalic dog the axis forms an angle of approximately 30 degrees with the median plane. The angle is greater in the brachycephalic breeds (see Fig. 21.22).

Lines connecting the anterior and posterior poles of the eye on the surface of the globe are designated **meridians** (*meridiani*). The **equator** (*aequator*) of the globe is its maximum circumference located midway between the poles (Fig. 21.3). Because the eye is essentially spherical, the common anatomic terms of direction are not applicable for certain structures, such as the retinal layers. In such cases, the terms *inner* and *outer* are used with reference to the center of the bulb.

Fibrous Tunic

The **fibrous outer tunic** (*tunica fibrosa bulbi*) of the eye is responsible for the shape of the eye, protection from the external environment, and conduction with refraction (bending) of light rays via the cornea. Additionally, the sclera is the site for insertion of the extraocular muscles. The fibrous tunic is composed of two parts: the opaque sclera, which encloses approximately the posterior three fourths of the globe, and the transparent cornea anteriorly. The junction of the cornea and the sclera is designated the **limbus** (*limbus corneae*).

Sclera

The **sclera** consists of a dense network of collagen and elastic fibers and their attendant fibrocytes. It varies in thickness, being greatest in the region just posterior to the corneoscleral junction, where it receives the insertions of the rectus and oblique muscles and contains the scleral venous plexus. The ciliary muscle is attached to a small ridge of fibrous tissue that forms a ring (*anulus sclerae*) on the inner surface of the sclera posterior to the iridocorneal angle (Fig. 21.14).

The mean scleral surface area of canine eyes is reported to be 12.87 (±2.24) cm^2 (Gilger et al., 2005). The thickness of the sclera is only 0.34 (±0.13) mm near the equator (Gilger et al., 2005). It becomes thicker again on the posterior aspect of the globe. Where the optic nerve leaves the eyeball, the sclera is sievelike (*area cribrosa sclerae*). Here the collagen, elastic, and reticular fiber bundles of the sclera form a net through the interstices of which the optic nerve myelinated axons pass. The trabeculae of the area cribrosa continue caudally as the prominent connective tissue septae of the optic nerve. The dura mater surrounding the optic nerve (*vagina externa n. optici*) is continuous with the outer layers of the sclera at the periphery of the area cribrosa and with the periorbita and dura mater encephali at the optic canal.

The ciliary nerves and the short posterior ciliary vessels enter the eyeball through foramina in the sclera at the periphery of the area cribrosa.

Cornea

The **cornea** forms the anterior segment of the fibrous tunic. The normally transparent cornea contains 80% (±2%) water (Scott & Bosworth, 1990). The mean full thickness of the adult canine cornea is approximately 600 μm. In one study, central corneal thickness was reported to be 585 (±79) μm. In dogs less than 1 year of age it was 555 (±64) μm, whereas in older dogs it was 606 (±85) μm (Kafarnik et al., 2007) (see Table 21.1). Its thickness increases with age (Gwin et al., 1982). In another study the mean central corneal thickness of 43 dogs was found to be 611 μm (Lynch & Brinkis, 2006). Measurements made with optical and ultrasonic pachymeters in vivo show the cornea to be uniformly thinner axially than at the limbus (see Fig. 21.3 and Table 21.1). The radius of curvature of the living dog cornea is approximately 8.5 to 9.0 mm (Gaiddon et al., 1991; Murphy et al., 1992). Large-breed dogs have been shown to have a slightly flatter cornea (a larger radius of curvature) than small or medium-sized breeds (Gaiddon et al., 1991). The cornea of the dog is very slightly oval; the mediolateral dimension is usually approximately 10% greater than the dorsoventral dimension, which is typically 16 to 18 mm in an average-sized dog.

The canine cornea consists of 4 distinct layers: the anterior epithelium, the substantia propria, the posterior limiting lamina (Descemet's membrane), and the posterior epithelium (endothelium). A fifth layer, the anterior limiting lamina (Bowman's layer) is characteristic of primates, birds and selected other vertebrate species but is not evident by light microscopy in the dog (Nautscher et al., 2015). Shively and Epling (1970), in a study of the fine structure of the canine cornea, were unable to demonstrate a distinct layer comparable to the anterior limiting lamina. This was confirmed by Morrin et al. (1982), who described the ultrastructure of the Beagle cornea. They did describe, however,

TABLE 21.1 Ocular Dimensions of the Dog Eye[a]

Parameter	N	Measurement/(SD)	Source[b]
Globe axial length	124	20.43/(1.48) mm	1
	32	21.6/(0.77) mm	2
	20	21.6/(0.6) mm	3
	98	21.92/(0.54) mm	4
	57	22.12 mm	5
	22	20.9/(1.4) mm	6
Globe equatorial diameter	20	22.0/(0.8) mm	3
	22	20.9/(1.0) mm	6
Globe volume	22	4,646/(767) mm^3	6
Corneal thickness			
(Axial)	59	620/(SE = 9) μm	3
	37	585/(79) μm	7
	20	607/(39) μm	8
	133	497/(30) μm (FD-OCT)	9
		555/(17) μm (ultrasound)	
		595/(33) μm (TD-OCT)	
(Peripheral)	59	670/(SE = 10) μm	3
	133	618/(33) μm (ultrasound)	9
		646/(60) μm (FD-OCT)	
	100	535 μm (range 500 to 620 μm)	10
Anterior corneal curvature	124	8.46/(0.55) mm	1
	98	9.20/(0.67) mm	4
	57	9.13 mm	5
Anterior chamber depth	32	4.95/(0.45) mm	2
	57	4.27 mm	5
	22	4.0/(0.5) mm	6
Anterior chamber volume	6	770/(240) μL	11
Lens: axial length	6	7.83/(0.45) mm	12
	57	7.83 mm	5
	32	7.14/(0.3) mm	2
	22	7.4/(0.5) mm	6
Equatorial diameter	6	11.33/(0.79) mm	12
	22	11.5/(0.8) mm	6
Lens volume	22	434/(124) mm^3	6
Anterior curvature	6	7.29/(0.89) mm	12
	57	7.65 mm	5
Posterior curvature	6	−6.72/(0.75) mm	12
		−8.20 mm	5
Vitreous chamber depth	32	9.51/(0.31) mm	2
	57	10.02 mm	5
	22	9.6/(0.6) mm	6
Vitreous chamber volume	6	1.7/(0.86) mL	11
Scleral thickness			
(Limbus)	approx14	0.80/(0.19) mm	11
(Equator)	approx14	0.34/(0.13) mm	11
(Optic nerve)	approx14	0.55/(0.18) mm	11

SD, Standard deviation.

[a]These values are taken from the literature and are based on measurements made in vivo or from freshly excised tissues. A summary of the older literature pertaining to ocular dimensions, commonly made from fixed specimens, is available in Bayer (1914).

[b]1, Gaiddon et al., 1991; 2, Schiffer et al., 1982; 3, Gwin et al., 1982; 4, Murphy et al., 1992 (from adult German Shepherd Dogs); 5, Mutti et al., 1999 (from adult Labrador Retrievers); 6, Salguero et al., 2015 (computed tomography measurements of differing ages and breeds); 7, Kafarnik et al., 2007; 8, Alario and Pirie 2013 (Measured by optical coherence tomography [OCT]); 9, Strom et al., 2016 (ultrasound pachymetry as well as spectral domain OCT [SD-OCT] and time domain OCT [TD-OCT]); 10, Famose 2014; 11, Gilger et al., 2005 (average of multiple modes of measurement); 12, Kreuzer and Sivak, 1985.

the subepithelial stroma (for a thickness of approximately 9 μm) as being hypocellular and to contain randomly oriented collagen bundles.

The anterior epithelium of the dog comprises slightly more than 10% of the total corneal thickness (Fig. 21.4A). There is a single layer of basal cells with multiple overlying layers of polygonal wing cells and superficial squamous cells (Fig. 21.4B). Basal cells have a much smaller cell diameter (approx. 4.5 μm) compared to the superficial squamous cells (approx. 43 μm) (Strom et al., 2016a) that are in direct contact with the precorneal tear film. The thickness of the central corneal epithelium measured in vivo in laboratory Beagles is approximately 52 μm (Strom et al., 2016b). Dendritic cells, considered to be the main antigen-presenting cells of the ocular surface, have been identified among the basal and wing cell layers of the anterior corneal epithelium of the dog (Killian et al., 2013). The single layer of columnar basal cells attaches to the underlying stroma via hemidesmosomes through a specialization of the extracellular matrix, the anterior corneal basement membrane.

The anterior corneal basement membrane of the dog has been documented to possess a rich three-dimensional "felt-like" topographic architecture composed of nanoscale to submicron intertwining fibers, pores, and elevations (Abrams et al., 2002a). The surface topographic features as well as the intrinsic compliance (relative stiffness) of basement membranes have been shown to profoundly modulate a wide menu of corneal epithelial cell behaviors (Abrams et al., 2002b; Last et al., 2009). Over the basal cell layer are approximately three layers of polygonal wing cells. The superficial layers are composed of flattened squamous cells.

The most superficial layer of squamous cells is in direct contact with the precorneal tear film and has a microplicated surface. The rugae of this surface are thought to be important in anchoring the precorneal tear film and may also play a role in transport processes by amplification of the membrane surface. Both the anterior and posterior corneal epithelia, but especially the latter, regulate the degree of the hydration of the substantia propria by an active transport mechanism. Disruption of either epithelium results in corneal edema with more severe edema developing with involvement of the posterior epithelium.

The canine corneal epithelium contains carbonic anhydrase, which may facilitate the elimination of metabolic carbon dioxide against small concentration gradients via catalytic conversion to bicarbonate (HCO_3^-) (Conroy et al., 1992). The opioid growth factor peptide [met^5]enkephalin and its corresponding receptor are found in the canine cornea where they may play a role in homeostasis and repair of the corneal epithelium (Robertson & Andrew, 2003). Toll-like receptor 4, which is important for recognizing highly conserved molecular patterns of pathogens, is expressed in the canine cornea (Wassef et al., 2004). The nucleotide-binding oligomerization domain (NOD) proteins NOD1 and NOD2 are also expressed in the canine corneal anterior and posterior epithelia where they serve as signaling receptors of the innate immune system (Scurrell et al., 2009). NOD1 and NOD2 are also found in the conjunctival and nonpigmented iridal epithelium. Interleukin 11, a cytokine that has multiple effects on inflammation and cellular responses, is expressed in the epithelial and stromal cells of the normal dog cornea

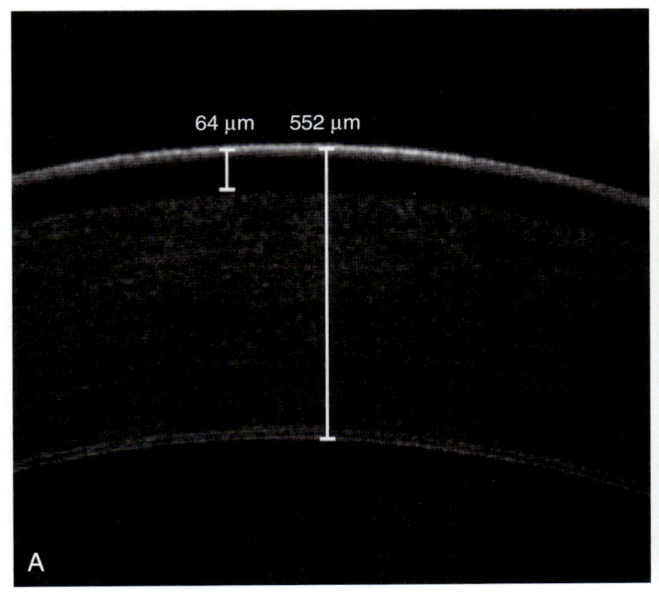

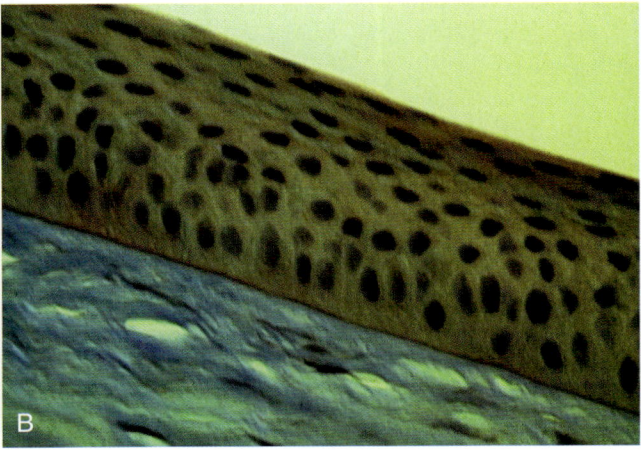

• **Fig. 21.4** Central cornea of the dog. **A**, Spectral domain optical coherence tomographic image of the central cornea of the dog. Note that the anterior corneal epithelium comprises slightly more than 10% of the total corneal thickness (From Strom et al., 2016). **B**, Hematoxylin and eosin stained photomicrograph of the anterior corneal epithelium. A single layer of basal cells, polygonal wing cells, and superficial squamous cells can be clearly identified. The most superficial aspect of the squamous cell layer would be in direct contact with the precorneal tear film.

(Richards et al., 2014). Cholestyramine, a highly nonpolar dehydration product of cholesterol, is present in normal dog corneas where it accounts for 20% to 25% of the total steroid-sterol present (Cenedella et al., 1992). Striatin, a desmosomal protein, has been documented in the anterior corneal epithelium of the dog (Stern et al., 2015).

The limbus is considered to be the site of the stem cells of the corneal epithelium. In dogs, invagination of the limbal epithelial cells can be observed (Patruno et al., 2017). Cells generated here migrate centripetally toward the vertex of the cornea. Extensive damage to the limbal region can result in chronic corneal surface disease as the generation of new cells must be adequate to replace the loss of superficial squamous cells that continually desquamate into the precorneal tear film (Patruno et al., 2017; Sanchez & Daniels, 2016; Thoft & Friend, 1983). The course of migration is not normally evident but is thought to be curvilinear in response to weak electromagnetic fields, and the path of migration can become visible with drug and/or pigment deposition and in conditions that promote high epithelial turnover (Kim et al., 2018). While a consensus has not been reached as to the constellation of definitive biomarkers that identify limbal stem cells, the putative biomarker ABCG2 has been localized to limbal epithelial cells in the dog whereas p63 was more promiscuous in its expression throughout the anterior corneal epithelium (Morita et al., 2015).

The transparency of the cornea remains incompletely understood. There are three elements thought to participate in achieving and maintaining corneal transparency: (1) uniform sizing and spatial distribution of the collagen fibrils that compose the extracellular matrix of the stroma, (2) the distribution of media of differing refractive indices within the stroma, and (3) the expression of crystallins by the stromal cells of the cornea (Jester, 2008). Other factors that contribute to corneal transparency are the lack of pigment, vessels, and large myelinated nerve fibers. Any disruption of the highly ordered structure of the collagen fibers, such as by edema or by scar tissue, results in a loss of transparency.

The cornea, normally avascular, is nourished by the capillary loops at the corneoscleral junction (limbus), the precorneal tear film, and the aqueous humor. It has been suggested that the avascularity of the cornea is due to the expression of soluble vascular endothelial growth factor (VEGF) receptor-1 within corneal tissues. This receptor serves as a "trap," binding available VEGF and preventing it from inciting vessel formation (Ambati et al., 2006).

The substantia propria is composed of highly ordered collagen fibrils with interspersed cellular elements. These fibrils are of uniform small diameter and are arranged in distinct lamellae. The cornea is easily dissected along these lamellar planes. The majority of fibrils within a lamella run parallel to each other and to the corneal surface, although the fibrils in each lamella run at an angle to those in the other layers. Additionally, recent work in the human cornea using second-harmonic imaging demonstrates a high degree of lamellar interweaving especially in the anterior stroma (Morishige et al., 2007). Ongoing work in the dog suggests that the degree of interweaving is less than that observed in humans but more than in other species such as the rabbit (Thomasy et al., 2014; Winkler et al., 2015). The fibrocytes of the cornea (keratocytes) are flattened between the lamellae. Keratocyte density is greater in the anterior stroma (approx. 993/mm^2) compared to the posterior stroma (approx. 789/mm^2) as measured by in vivo confocal biomicroscopy (Strom et al., 2016).

The posterior limiting lamina (Descemet's membrane) is the exaggerated basement membrane of the posterior epithelium of the cornea. It is approximately two times thicker in the dog than in humans (Engerman & Colquhoun, 1982). The posterior epithelium of the cornea is composed of a simple cuboidal epithelium, individual cells of which are mostly hexagonal in outline with a mean cell area of 395 ($\pm$36) μm^2 (Pigatto et al., 2006). The mean endothelial cell density of the canine cornea has been reported as 3175 ($\pm$776)/mm^2 (Kafarnik et al., 2007) and 2555 ($\pm$240) cells/mm^2 (Pigatto et al., 2006). In dogs less than 1 year of age it has been reported to be 3641 ($\pm$752)/mm^2, whereas in older dogs it is 2851 ($\pm$634)/mm^2 (Kafarnik et al., 2007). The density of these cells has been shown to decrease with age and following intraocular surgery (Gwin et al., 1982, 1983; Yee et al., 1987). The morphologic characteristics of these cells have also been shown to be altered in some disease states such as diabetes (Yee et al., 1985). The ability of this layer to regenerate is species variable and thought to be limited in the dog. Severe trauma to this layer of cells frequently results in chronic corneal edema.

The cornea is innervated by branches of the ciliary nerves that arise from the ophthalmic nerve, a branch of the trigeminal nerve. Nerve branches to the cornea enter the anterior layers of the stroma at the limbus and soon lose their myelin sheaths as they converge toward the vertex. The corneal nerve plexus is formed by thick-, medium-, and thin-diameter nerve bundles. The mean nerve bundle length in 1 mm^2 of cornea is 10.32 ($\pm$0.11) mm in adult dogs, which is significantly higher than the 9.42 ($\pm$0.02) mm and 7.75 ($\pm$0.14) mm in young and old dogs, respectively (Lasys et al., 2003). In mesocephalic dogs, the mean density of subepithelial and subbasal nerve fibers is 12.39 ($\pm$5.25) mm/mm^2 and 14.87 ($\pm$3.08) mm/mm^2, respectively. These values are significantly higher than the corresponding values in brachycephalic dogs of 10.34 ($\pm$4.71) mm/mm^2 and 11.80 ($\pm$3.73) mm/mm^2, respectively (Kafarnik et al., 2008).

The limbal plexus is a 0.8 to 1 mm network of superficial nerves around the peripheral cornea (Marfurt et al., 2001). The numerous origins of the limbal fibers include collateral branches of stromal and subconjunctival fibers in passage to the cornea, recurrent collaterals from the peripheral corneal plexus, and perivascular fibers associated with the rich limbal vasculature. The limbal plexus is morphologically subdivided into outer periscleral and inner pericorneal zones. The periscleral zone contains largely perivascular nerve fascicles and a stromal plexus with axons extending randomly through the limbal stroma. The pericorneal zone is a much denser meshwork of highly branched and anastomotic axons and small-diameter fascicles. Many inner zone fibers are intimately associated with vascular elements of the superficial limbal arcade, and others travel through the corneoscleral transition zone and anastomose with axons in the peripheral anterior stromal plexus. The limbal and conjunctival epithelia contain modest numbers of short, wavy, beaded, and mostly radially oriented axons.

Most nerve fibers enter the peripheral cornea at the corneoscleral limbus in a series of 14 to 18 prominent, radially directed, superficial stromal nerve bundles containing 30 to 40 axons (Marfurt et al., 2001). These are located at regular intervals around the limbal circumference. Smaller nerve fascicles enter the peripheral cornea between and slightly superficial to the main bundles. Subsequently, the main stromal bundles undergo extensive dichotomous branching to form elaborate axonal trees. The distal branches of these trees are extensively joined at angular junctions to form a dense, anatomically complex stromal plexus that extends uninterrupted to all areas of the cornea. The latter plexus occupies approximately the anterior 0.4 to 0.5 mm half of the corneal stroma and can be further subdivided into posterior and anterior levels. The posterior level contains modest numbers of primarily small- to medium-diameter bundles and scattered individual axons. The anterior level is much more densely innervated and morphologically complex. A very fine meshwork of thin, preterminal axons occupies the region immediately beneath the epithelial basement membrane. In contrast to the highly innervated anterior stroma, the posterior corneal stroma of the dog is largely noninnervated.

After entering the basal epithelial cell layer, most intraepithelial axons form preterminal arborizations known as *epithelial leashes* (Marfurt et al., 2001). Each epithelial leash comprises 2 to 6 axons attached to a single subepithelial fiber. Individual axons course horizontally to the surface and roughly parallel to each other through the basal epithelial cell layer tangential to the corneal for 1 to 1.4 mm. Most axons are less than 2.5 µm in diameter but range from 1.2 to 3.5 µm. As they travel horizontally through the basal epithelium they give rise to an abundance of thin, ascending branches that divide extensively to form irregular clusters of short terminal branches ending throughout the basal, wing, and squamous epithelial layers. Most axonal endings consist of single large bulbous terminal expansions.

Trigeminal nerve innervation of the cornea is essential to maintaining homeostasis. Loss of sensory innervation apparently disrupts a trophic influence normally supplied by the ciliary nerves. Corneal denervation results in corneal ulceration, edema, and loss of stromal tissue (neurotrophic keratitis), even though eyelid function is unimpaired (Scott & Bistner, 1973). There is some evidence to suggest that the neuropeptide, substance P, associated with the corneal terminations of the trigeminal nerve, is the neuronal factor necessary to the maintenance of normal corneal health (Marfurt et al., 2001; Murphy et al., 1990; Murphy et al., 2001). The cornea also receives sympathetic innervation, and the anterior corneal epithelium of the dog, apparently independent of a neuronal source, is rich in acetylcholine (Gwin et al., 1979). An extensive review of corneal innervation including the dog is provided by Muller et al. (2003).

At the corneoscleral junction, the anterior corneal epithelium is continuous with the bulbar conjunctiva (see later section on conjunctiva). The collagen fibers of the substantia propria become abruptly less ordered as they approach the sclera, with a resulting loss of transparency. The corneoscleral junction is oblique; with the scleral elements of the limbus externally overlapping the corneal elements of the limbus (Fig. 21.5 B and C). Immediately peripheral to the limbus, the posterior corneal epithelium reflects onto the anterior face of the iris, forming the iridocorneal (filtration) angle.

The **iridocorneal angle** is a regional term that includes the most anterior internal aspect of the sclera, the most posterior internal aspect of the cornea, the most anterior external aspect of the ciliary body, the root of the iris, and all intervening tissue associated with these structures (Fig. 21.6). In the embryo the iridocorneal angle is a smooth, unfenestrated fornix. Late in gestation and continuing in the early postnatal period, the tissue in this area undergoes progressive rarefaction until a long cleft extends the anterior chamber posteriorly between the base of the iris and the sclera (Aguirre et al., 1972; Martin, 1975; Samuelson & Gelatt, 1984a,b). Examination of 23 normal dogs (46 eyes) that were 5 (±2.73) years of age revealed a mean iridocorneal angle of 12.6 (±5.3) degrees (range, 5 to 29) and mean angle opening distance of 273.4 (±88.9) µm (range, 107 to 557) (Rose et al., 2008). This cleft is bridged by a network of fine collagenous pillars that in aggregate form the **pectinate ligament** (*lig. pectinatum anguli iridocornealis*). The heavily pigmented strands of the canine pectinate ligament exhibit large variations in size and thickness. They exist primarily as single strands but may fuse with adjacent strands or ramify into a characteristic branching pattern prior to inserting obliquely onto the corneal limbus (Simones et al., 1996). Because the strands are relatively slender and few in number, there are wide intertrabecular spaces. The iridocorneal angle is further divided into corneoscleral trabeculae and deeper uveal trabeculae.

The region of the iridocorneal angle contains Schwalbe line cells, which possess secretory and epithelial characteristics that are associated with the nonfiltering portion of the corneoscleral trabecular meshwork and are considered to be a subpopulation of trabecular cells (Samuelson et al., 2001). The number of Schwalbe line cells declines gradually with age in normal dogs but more rapidly in dogs with glaucoma.

The trabecular cells can actively phagocytose small particulate matter (Samuelson et al., 1984). Samuelson and Gelatt (1984a, b) and Bedford and Grierson (1986) have provided detailed anatomic descriptions of the aqueous outflow pathway in the dog. In many cases, the various reports concerning this region have conflicting findings

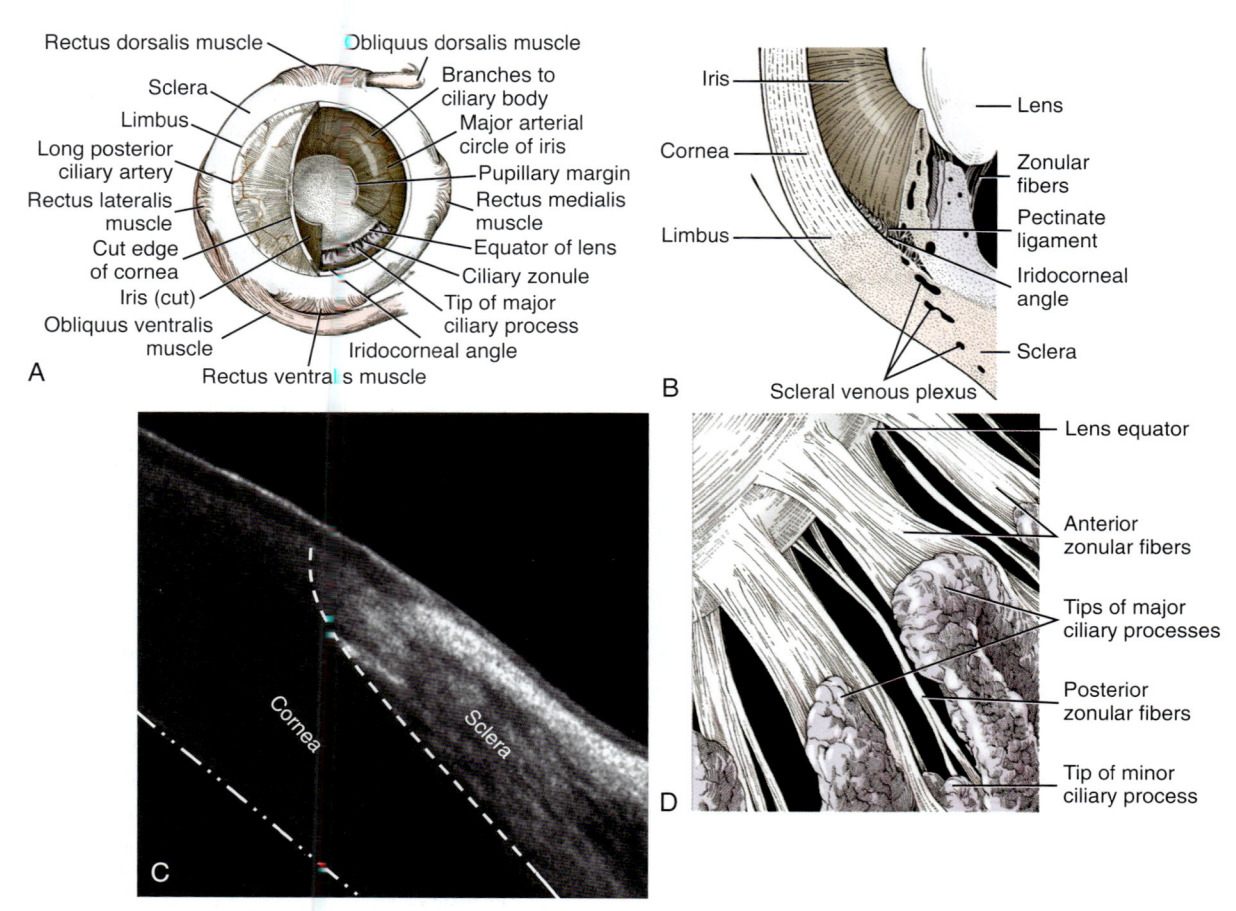

• **Fig. 21.5** Bulbus oculi. **A**, Anterior aspect of right eyeball, cornea, and iris partially removed. **B**, Detail of limbal region. **C**, Spectral domain OCT image of the limbal region of the dog. Note that the more hyperreflective elements of the sclera externally overlap the less reflective elements of the corneal elements of the limbal region (modified from Strom et al., 2016). **D**, Detail of anterior aspect of ciliary zonule.

and the terminology lacks uniformity (Samuelson, 1996). Bedford (1977) has described the clinical appearance of the iridocorneal angle using a goniolens. The appearance of the iridocorneal angle in the living dog as viewed by use of a goniolens is depicted in Fig. 21.7. The aqueous humor leaves the eye by filtering through the spaces between the corneoscleral trabeculae to aqueous collector vessels, the angular aqueous plexus, that join the scleral venous plexus, which, in turn, is drained by the anterior ciliary and vorticose veins (Samuelson & Gelatt, 1984b; Van Buskirk, 1979). The outermost corneoscleral trabeculae appear to contribute to the canine aqueous outflow barrier by compartmentalizing the glycosaminoglycans in the intervening spaces between trabeculae (Gum et al., 1993). They also prevent widening of the angle and hold the initial filtration structures in a relatively compressed state (Morrison & Van Buskirk, 1982). Dilation of the pupil (mydriasis) impedes the outflow of aqueous humor; the iridocorneal angle is narrowed by the increased thickness of the peripheral iris. Constriction of the pupil (miosis) opens the spaces of the iridocorneal angle and facilitates drainage (Mark, 2003).

In certain breeds, notably the Basset Hound, the corneoscleral angle is dysplastic. The pectinate ligament is sheetlike with few openings (Martin, 1975), which impedes the outflow of the aqueous humor. Animals with this condition are thought to be predisposed to developing glaucoma. A positive relationship between pectinate ligament dysplasia and narrowing of the iridocorneal angle with the development of glaucoma has been demonstrated in English Springer Spaniels (Bjerkås et al., 2002).

Vascular Tunic

The **vascular tunic** (*tunica vasculosa bulbi*) is the thick middle coat of the eye, interposed between the retina and the sclera. It is commonly referred to as the *uvea* or *uveal tract*. The vascular tunic includes three contiguous parts, which, from posterior to anterior, are the choroid, the ciliary body, and the iris (Fig. 21.1). Its functions are numerous and include regulating the amount of light entering the eye through the pupil; producing the aqueous humor, which maintains the intraocular pressure and bathes the structures of the anterior segment; suspending the lens via

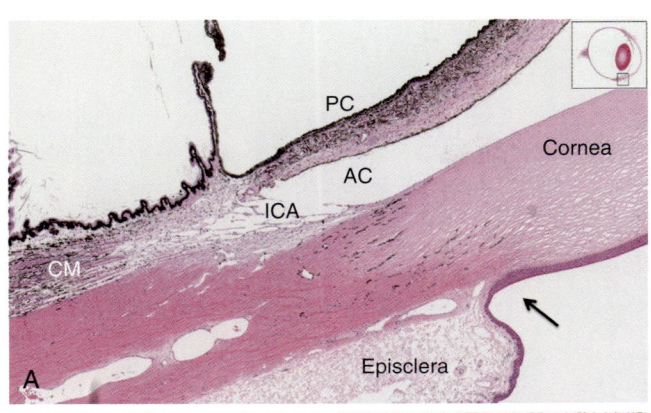

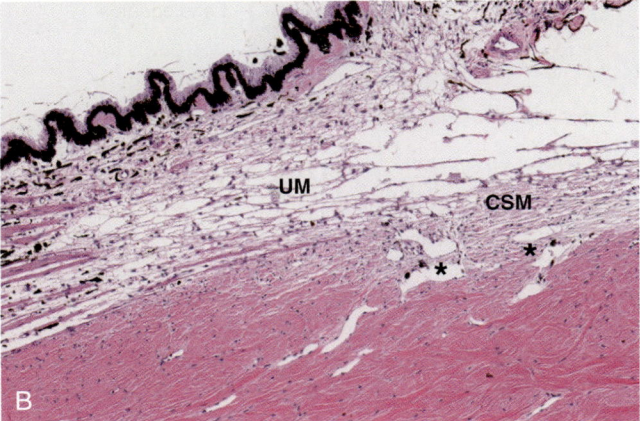

• **Fig. 21.6** Iridocorneal angle of the normal beagle. **A,** Low-magnification photomicrograph depicting the structures associated with the iridocorneal angle. *AC* = anterior chamber, *ICA* = iridocorneal angle, *PC* = posterior chamber, *CM* = ciliary muscle; *arrow* indicates region of the limbus. **B,** Higher magnification of the normal iridocorneal angle of the beagle. *CSM* = corneoscleral meshwork, *UM* = Uveal meshwork, * indicate channels of the angular aqueous plexus.

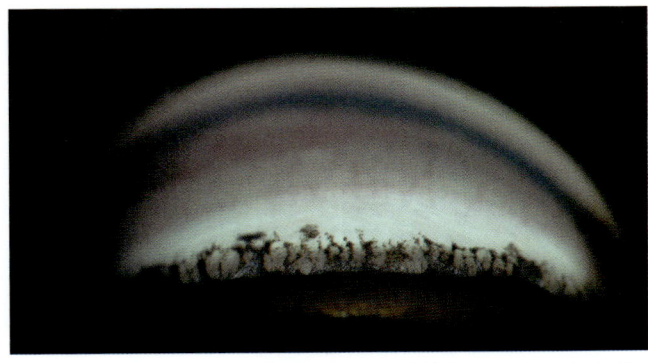

• **Fig. 21.7** Goniophotograph of the normal iridocorneal angle in the living dog. A goniolens allows direct visualization of the iridocorneal angle. Note the trabeculae of the pectinate ligament that traverse the iridocorneal angle. Aqueous humor passes through the iridocorneal angle to exit the eye.

zonula fibers; changing the visual focus via the ciliary body muscle; limiting the amount of scattered light within the eye (inner pigmented portion of uvea); increasing the photic stimulation of the retina under low light levels (tapetum lucidum of the choroid); and providing nutrition to structures within the eye (ciliary body and choroid).

Choroid

The **choroid** is a pigmented vascular layer. It is continuous with the ciliary body anteriorly and completely envelops the posterior hemisphere of the eyeball, except in the region of the area cribrosa (region of the optic nerve head), where it is absent.

The choroid is further divided into layers, which, from the outermost inward, are the **suprachoroid** (*lamina suprachoroidea*), the **vascular layer** (*lamina vasculosa*), the **reflective layer** (*tapetum lucidum*), the **choriocapillary layer** (*lamina choroidocapillaris*), and the **basal lamina** (*lamina basalis*). The last is poorly developed in the dog.

The **tapetum** is a specialized reflective layer of the choroid (Fig. 21.8). It is thought to increase the ability of the retina to function under low light levels. In addition to the reflection of incident light back through the overlying photoreceptor layer, it is also thought to increase photoreceptor stimulation by intrinsic fluorescence of its structure when stimulated by incident light (Bellhorn, 1990; Elliott & Futterman, 1963). A tapetum is present in all domestic mammals except the pig. In almost all mammals it is located within the middle-sized vessel layer of the choroid, interposed between the choriocapillaris and the large-sized vessel layer. It is cellular (*tapetum lucidum cellulosum*) in all carnivores, whereas it is collagenous (*tapetum lucidum fibrosum*) in all herbivores (Ollivier et al., 2004). It occupies approximately one-third of the superior area of the choroid. Central areas of the canine tapetum have been reported to contain 9 to 20 layers of tapetal cells (Lesiuk & Braekvelt, 1983; Wen et al., 1985; Yamaue et al., 2014; 2015). The thickest part of the tapetum is reported to be dorsotemporal to the optic disc with a mean thickness (measured in histologic sections) of 53 μm (±17 μm) (Yamaue et al., 2014). Cell numbers diminish to a single layer peripherally and next to the optic nerve. The cells are layered in a step-wise manner that form a brick-wall appearance. The zinc- and cysteine-rich tapetal cells are packed with highly refractive, membrane-bound tapetal rodlets. These rodlets are oriented parallel to the retina and are thought to be responsible for the tapetum's reflectivity (Hebel, 1969, 1971). The unique structure of the tapetum makes it exquisitely sensitive to the toxic effects of a beta adrenergic blocking agent that may have no toxic effects whatsoever in Beagles that inherit an aplasia of the tapetum (Massa et al., 1984; Schiavo et al., 1984). Penetrating vessels are oriented radially and connect the choriocapillaris with the stromal vessels (Fig. 21.8). The radial orientation of these penetrating vessels minimizes their potential interference on tapetal function.

In dogs, the tapetum is in roughly the shape of a rounded right triangle with the hypotenuse resting on a dorsal plane and the right angle situated dorsally (Fig. 21.8). The medial angle is more acute than the lateral. In large breeds of dogs, the hypotenuse (inferior border) is usually inferior to the optic disc. In small breeds of dogs, the tapetum is relatively smaller and does not extend inferiorly to include the optic disc. In some toy breeds, the tapetum may be

868 CHAPTER 21 The Eye

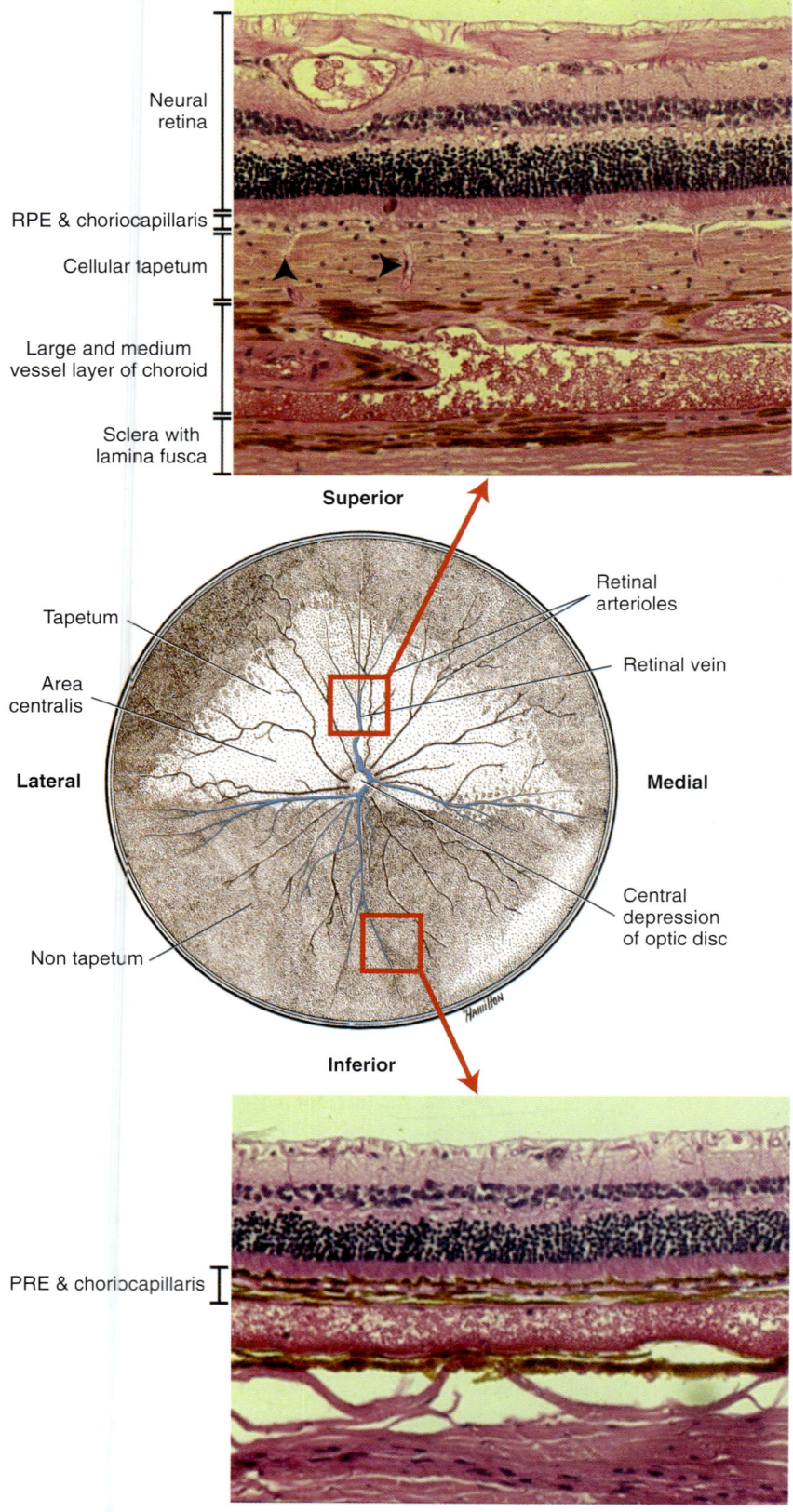

• **Fig. 21.8** Ocular fundus of the right eye depicting tapetal and nontapetal regions and corresponding histologic photomicrographs. Upper photomicrograph of tapetal region; note the absence of pigment in the retinal pigmented epithelium (*RPE*). Penetrating vessels (*arrowheads*) pass through the tapetum from the larger vessel layer and the choroid to the choriocapillaris that lies immediately external to the retinal pigmented epithelium. Lower photomicrograph of nontapetal region; note presence of pigment in the RPE.

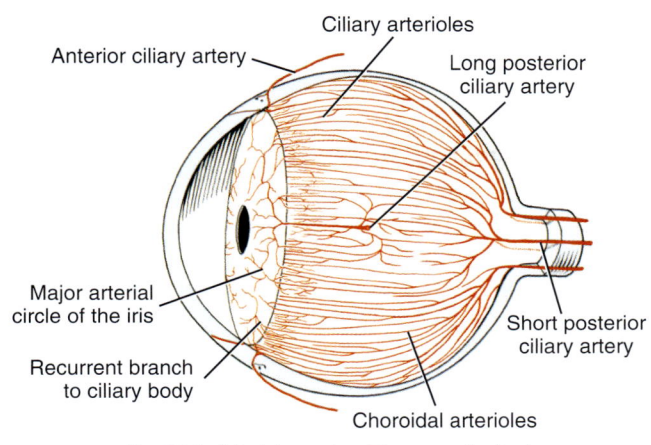

Fig. 21.9 Arterial supply of the vascular tunic.

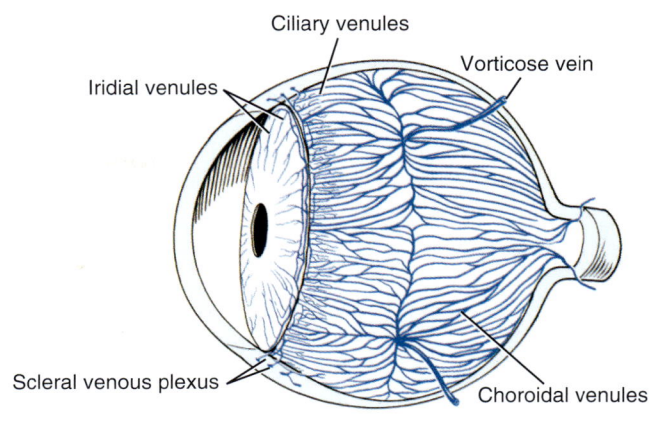

Fig. 21.10 Veins of the vascular tunic.

greatly diminished in area or may be entirely absent as a normal variation. A heritable lack of the tapetum has been described in the Beagle, in which tapetal cells are initially present but fail to develop normal tapetal rodlets (Bellhorn et al., 1975; Burns et al., 1988a; Burns et al., 1988b).

The tapetum develops after birth. As the dog matures, the color of the tapetum changes from a slate gray to violet to red-orange at approximately 4 months of age (Rubin, 1974). The color is generally uniform except at the junction of the tapetal and nontapetal choroid, which may be quite irregular and demonstrate considerable pleochroism. The distinctive coloration of the tapetum is due to the optical phenomenon of thin film interference rather than the presence of specific pigments. In other words, tapetal coloration is structural rather than pigmentary. Tapetal coloration as well as the degree of pigmentation present in the nontapetal region of the fundus is correlated with coat color (Granar et al. 2011). Generally, dogs with brown and red coat colors had a more orange-tinted tapetal color while dogs with white or gray coats more often had a green-colored tapetal region. This same study reported tapetal size was in some cases correlated with breed with the smaller breeds such as the Papillon often having proportionally smaller areas of the fundus occupied by tapetum. The tapetum can be lacking as a normal variation in dogs with approximately 5% of Labradors reported to lack an identifiable tapetum on ophthalmoscopic exam.

The **vascular layer** of the choroid is a plexus of arteries, arterioles, veins, and venules supported by a collagenous and elastic stroma and traditionally subdivided into an outer large-sized vessel layer and an inner middle-sized vessel layer. The outer large-sized vessel layer is the terminal branches of the ciliary arteries and the vorticose veins. Most of the large choroidal vessels run parallel to the meridians and to one another with the choroidal veins fanning outward from the point at which the vorticose veins penetrate the sclera (Figs. 21.9 and 21.10). Branches of these vessels form the middle-sized vessel layer, which leads to and empties the choroidal capillary layer, which in turn nourishes the outer layers of the retina.

In the majority of dogs, the vascular layer of the choroid and the retinal pigment layer are darkly pigmented. The choroid-RPE complex has been reported to be more densely pigmented peripherally than centrally (Durairaj et al., 2012). The nontapetal region in these dogs appears dark brown or black. In dogs with amber, blue, or heterochromic irides, however, the choroid and retinal pigment layers are unpigmented or nearly so. In these animals, the vessels of the choroid can be visualized with the ophthalmoscope, and the nontapetal fundus appears red or striped (so-called tigroid fundus). The absence of a tapetum lucidum or choroidal pigment or both is considered a normal variation that apparently does not affect the dog's vision. Focal areas of choroidal hypoplasia, however, are serious ocular defects. They are a common manifestation of the Collie eye syndrome, a serious and widespread heritable defect in the Collie and Sheltie breeds.

Ciliary Body

The **ciliary body** (*corpus ciliare*) is the thickened middle segment of the vascular tunic, between the iris and choroid (Figs. 21.11 through 21.14). The ciliary body consists of a ciliary ring and ciliary crown. The **ciliary ring** (*orbicularis ciliaris*) is the posterior flat portion of the ciliary body adjacent to the anterior border of the pars optica retina and continuous with the choroid. The **ciliary crown** (*corona ciliaris*) is the raised portion of the ciliary body anterior to the ciliary ring and adjacent to the iris. The ciliary processes are developed on the ciliary crown. Many texts refer to the ciliary ring as the pars plana and the ciliary crown as the pars plicata (Fig. 21.12A). The *ora ciliaris retinae* is the line that demarcates the boundary between the *pars ciliaris retinae* and the *pars optica retinae* as well as separating the choroid from the ciliary body. Anterior to the *ora ciliaris retinae*, at the ciliary crown, is the elevation of the ciliary body into approximately 100 small, flat, parallel, regular processes. These increase rapidly in height and coalesce as they pass anteriorly along the meridians, forming tall, thin folds rising up from the base plate of the ciliary body (Figs. 21.11 and 21.12). At the root of the iris (*margo ciliaris*),

870 CHAPTER 21 **The Eye**

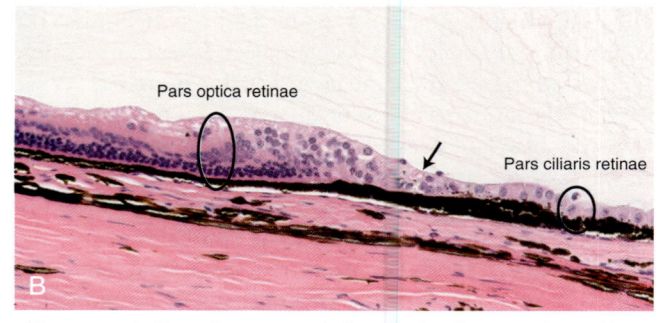

• **Fig. 21.11** A, Posterior aspect of ciliary body, ciliary zonule, and lens. B, Ora ciliaris retinae (*arrow*). Note that the pars optica retinae to the left includes the external pigmented epithelium and the internal photoreceptor and neural elements. To the right, the pars ciliaris retina consists of the inner nonpigmented and the outer pigmented epithelium of the ciliary body.

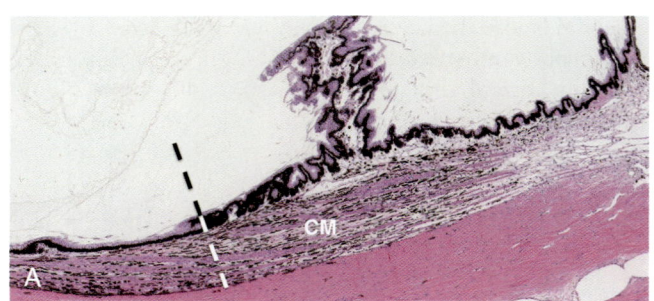

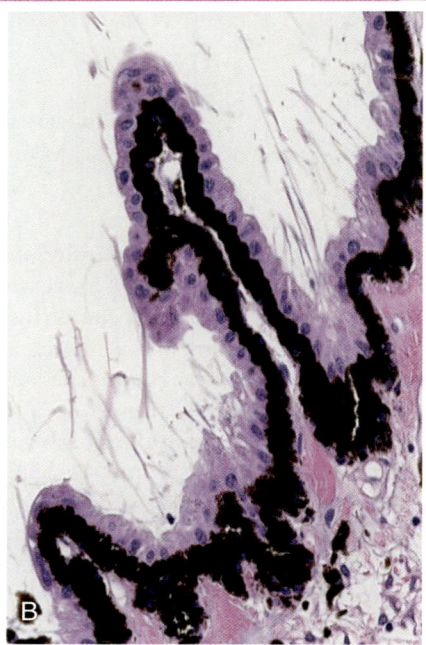

• **Fig. 21.12** Photomicrographs of the ciliary body of the beagle. A, *CM* = ciliary muscle, dashed line indicates junction between the pars plan (to the left) and the pars plicata (to the right) of the ciliary body. B, Higher magnification view of a single ciliary process in the pars plicata. Note the bilayered epithelium consisting of inner non-pigmented and outer pigmented cells. Also note the multiple fine fragmented zonular fibers extending toward the lens.

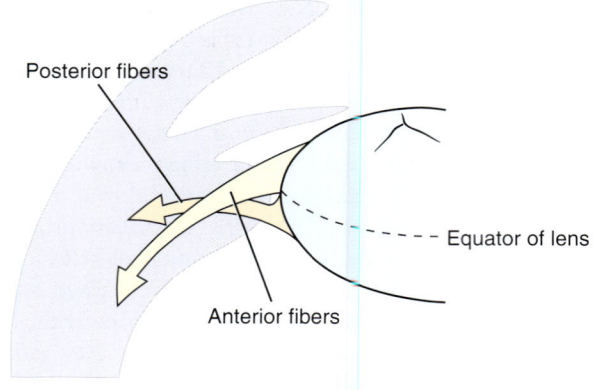

• **Fig. 21.13** Schema of zonular fibers.

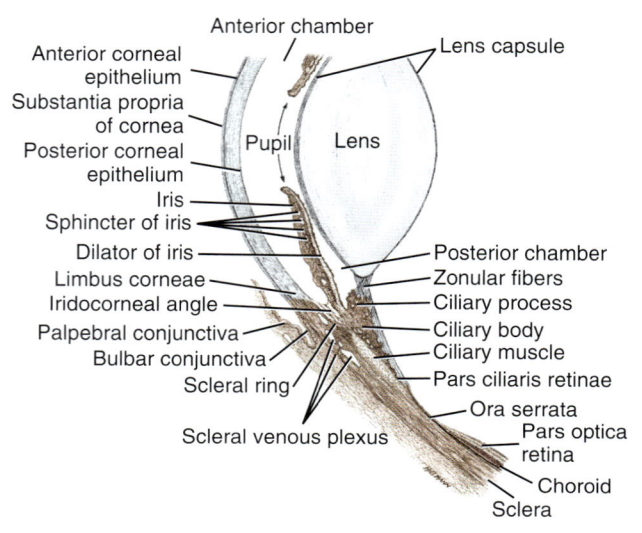

• **Fig. 21.14** Anterior segment of eyeball.

these folds lose their outer attachment to the sclera via the ciliary body musculature and iridocorneal angle and arc centrally toward the lens as the short, blunt, free **ciliary processes** (*processus ciliaris*). There are approximately 76 major processes in the canine eye, which vary from 2 to 4 mm in length (Tanimura, 1977; Samuelson, 2007). Minor ciliary folds and processes are interposed between the major processes, although this relationship is not constant; two major processes may occur together without an intervening minor process. The minor processes are neither as tall nor do they approximate the lens as closely as the major processes (Fig. 21.5D). The posterior surface of the ciliary processes is almost entirely covered by fibers of the ciliary zonule (Fig. 21.11). The major and minor processes together form the ciliary crown. The width of the ciliary body from the tips of the ciliary processes to the *ora ciliaris retinae* is greater on the lateral aspect of the globe

Like the choroid, the ciliary body is highly vascular. Radial ciliary arteries branch directly from the posterior margin of the greater arterial circle of the iris (see Fig. 21.5). Initially, these arteries pass through the peripheral iris for 0.1 to 1 mm. At the anterior margin of the ciliary processes branches are given off that course inward to the anterior edge of the processes (Sharpnack et al., 1984). Each ciliary process is supplied by a single arteriole traveling posteriorly throughout its length and sending capillary arcades to its margin from where they drain outward into venous sinuses at the base of the process (Morrison et al., 1987). After giving off branches to the processes, the ciliary arteries pass posteriorly to supply a dense network of capillaries associated with the ciliary muscle fibers, and finally collateralize with the choroidal vasculature (Sharpnack et al., 1984). The blood flow from the radial ciliary arteries thus has four possible destinations. It can branch anteriorly to become a radial iris artery; it can branch interiorly to become an afferent arteriole supplying a ciliary process; it can supply the fine capillary network of the ciliary muscle; or it can shunt through the region of the ciliary body and ramify with the choroidal vasculature. The ciliary body is drained by the choroidal and vorticose veins.

The inner nonpigmented and outer pigmented epithelia of the two-cell-thick pars ciliaris retinae produce the aqueous humor (Fig. 21.12B). The production of aqueous involves active transport processes. The canine ciliary body receives both adrenergic and cholinergic innervation, which is thought to play a role in the regulation of aqueous production and outflow (Gwin et al., 1979). The topical application of a β-adrenergic antagonist inhibits the aqueous humor formation (Kurata et al., 1998).

The **ciliary body muscle** (*m. ciliaris*) consists of numerous meridionally oriented smooth muscle fascicles located in the outer portions of the ciliary body (Fig. 21.12A). Both **circumferential fibers** (*fibrae circulares*) and **meridional fibers** (*fibrae meridionales*) are present in primates (which possess an extensive accommodative range), whereas only meridional fibers are present in the dog. The meridional fibers originate from the **scleral ring** (*annulus sclerae*) on the inner surface of the sclera posterior to the iridocorneal angle (Figs. 21.12A and 21.14). The anterior-most muscle fibers form tendinous endings with the posterior uveal trabeculae of the iridocorneal angle. The meridional fibers insert in the stroma of the ciliary body near the *ora ciliaris retinae*. In blue-eyed dogs, contraction of the ciliary body muscles occurs following stimulation of M_5 muscarinic receptors, whereas contraction of the ciliary muscle in brown-eyed dogs may require activation of M_5 and M_3 receptors (Choppin & Eglen, 2001). The ciliary body muscles lack functional adrenoreceptors (Yoshitomi & Ito, 1986). Exogenous norepinephrine inhibits contracture of the ciliary body muscle via activation of alpha$_2$-adrenoreceptors of parasympathetic axons, which in turn inhibit release of acetylcholine. When the fibers of the ciliary body muscle contract on parasympathetic stimulation, they decrease tension on the zonular fibers supporting the lens. With the release in tension, the lens becomes more spherical as a result of the inherent elasticity of its capsule. The more spherical lens has a shorter focal distance, and close objects are now brought into critical focus on the retina, a process called *accommodation*. It is not known whether the ora ciliaris retinae actually moves anteriorly during this process, or whether the zonule fibers are relaxed because of a sphincterlike action of the ciliary body muscle that decreases the diameter of the ciliary body at the ciliary crown. The extent of the accommodative ability of the dog is much less than that of primates, in which the ciliary muscle is far better developed. Accommodation in dogs has been reported to be only 1 to 3 diopters (Duke-Elder, 1958), which has been verified using the technique of videoretinoscopy (Murphy & Howland, unpublished observations).

Zonule

The lens is fixed in position by a delicate suspensory apparatus, the **zonula ciliaris** (Fig. 21.5D). The zonule is composed of a highly ordered array of **zonular fibers** (*fibrae zonulares*) that are aggregates of fibrils 10 nm in diameter, similar to those described in elastic tissue by Greenlee et al. (1966). The zonule lies posterior to the iris and ciliary body and separates the posterior chamber from the vitreous body. It is not visible in the intact eye unless the iris is very widely dilated or the lens is subluxated.

The majority of the zonular fibers originate from the pars ciliaris retinae just anterior to the ora serrata. They pass anteriorly, closely adherent to the surface of the ciliary body. Small auxiliary fibers arise from the epithelium of the ciliary folds and serve to anchor the main fiber bundles. As the small folds of the ciliary body unite to form the major ciliary folds, the zonule fibers also converge until they completely cover the sides of each major ciliary process (Fig. 21.11). These fibers continue centrally beyond the apices of the processes, span the circumlental space, and insert primarily on the anterior lens capsule near the equator (Fig. 21.13). They are thus designated the **anterior zonular fibers** (Pollock, 1978).

The zonular attachments to the posterior lens capsule are not as well developed. Two subsets of fibers compose the **posterior fiber group**. Where a minor ciliary fold is present, fibers arise from its surface and the surrounding epithelium and insert on the posterior lens capsule. Fibers also originate from the valleys between ciliary folds. These arc toward the major ciliary processes, cross the face of the anterior fibers obliquely, and insert on the posterior lens capsule.

The anterior face of the vitreous body bulges forward between the ciliary folds and into the spaces between the zonular fiber bundles (*spatia zonularia*) (Fig. 21.18). The zonular fibers are described as being under tension when the ciliary muscle is relaxed.

Iris

The **iris** is the most anterior segment of the vascular tunic. It is a thin circular diaphragm, which rests against the anterior surface of the lens (Fig. 21.5). The central opening in the iris, the **pupil** (*pupilla*), is circular in the dog. The size of the pupil is variable and serves to regulate the amount of light reaching the retina. The diameter of the pupil is smallest when the intensity of illumination is greatest. The periphery of the iris (*margo ciliaris*) is continuous with the ciliary body and trabeculae of the iridocorneal angle (Fig. 21.5B).

In the fetus, the iris is not fenestrated and thus completely covers the anterior surface of the lens. The central portion of the iridial anlage (*membrana pupillaris*) contains vessels that nourish the growing lens (see section on development). Normally the **pupillary membrane** atrophies so that only remnants of these vessels are present when the eyelids open at approximately 2 weeks of age. Remnants commonly persist, especially on the dorsal pupillary margin, until the age of 4 to 5 weeks. Abnormal persistence of the pupillary membrane into adult life is a heritable condition in Basenji dogs (Roberts & Bistner, 1968).

The anterior surface of the iris is lined by a discontinuous layer of flat fibrocytes (Donovan et al., 1974; Samuelson, 2007). Large intercellular spaces are evident, and communication between the anterior chamber and the underlying stroma can be traced (Shively & Epling, 1969). The stroma (*stroma iridis*) contains fibroblasts, collagen, myelinated and unmyelinated axons, smooth muscle fibers, melanocytes, and blood vessels. Mast cells have also been reported to normally reside within the anterior uveal stroma of the canine eye (Louden et al., 1990). Melanin is the only identified pigment in the dog iris. Blue-eyed dogs have a paucity of pigment restricted to the posterior pigmented epithelium of the pars iridica retinae of the iris (Newkirk et al., 2010). The blue color is caused by the differential absorption and selective reflection of light by the iris tissue itself and the posteriorly located melanin. In darkly pigmented irides there is an accumulation of pigment-laden melanocytes within the anterior iris stroma.

Two antagonistic muscles regulate the diameter of the pupil: the *m. sphincter pupillae* and the *m. dilator pupillae* (Fig. 21.14). Both are derived from the outer layer of neuroepithelium of the pars iridica retinae. They both receive parasympathetic and sympathetic innervation. The **sphincter muscle** is a sheet of circumferentially arranged smooth muscle fibers near the pupillary margin. It is the larger of the two muscles. The **dilator of the pupil** is composed of radially arranged smooth muscle fibers that form a meshwork through which the collagen bundles of the iris stroma are looped. The dilator is posterior to the sphincter muscle. Both muscles are well-developed in the dog when compared with other domestic species.

The sphincter is innervated by postganglionic parasympathetic axons whose cell bodies are located in the ciliary ganglion. Preganglionic axons reach the ciliary ganglion via the oculomotor nerve (Fig. 21.15). Postganglionic axons reach the iris via short ciliary nerves (branches of the nasociliary nerve). Parasympathetic activity is mediated by the activation of adenylate cyclase via M_3 muscarinic receptors (Tachado et al., 1994). An accessory ciliary ganglion has been described in a variety of mammalian species including the dog. This ganglion is located on a short ciliary nerve, has been shown to carry parasympathetic axons in the cat, and has been postulated to mediate pupillary constriction in association with convergence and accommodation of the eyes (Kuchiiwa et al., 1989). The sphincter fibers also receive sympathetic innervation, which inhibits contraction of the muscle fibers. Recent evidence suggests that prostaglandins may also contribute to the tonus of the sphincter muscle (and to a lesser degree the dilator muscle) in the dog. The prostaglandins apparently act directly on these muscles rather than through the release of cholinergic neurotransmitters (Yoshitomi & Ito, 1988). The neuropeptide substance P is variably effective in inducing miosis in many mammals, but it does not induce contraction of the iris sphincter in the dog (Tachado et al.,

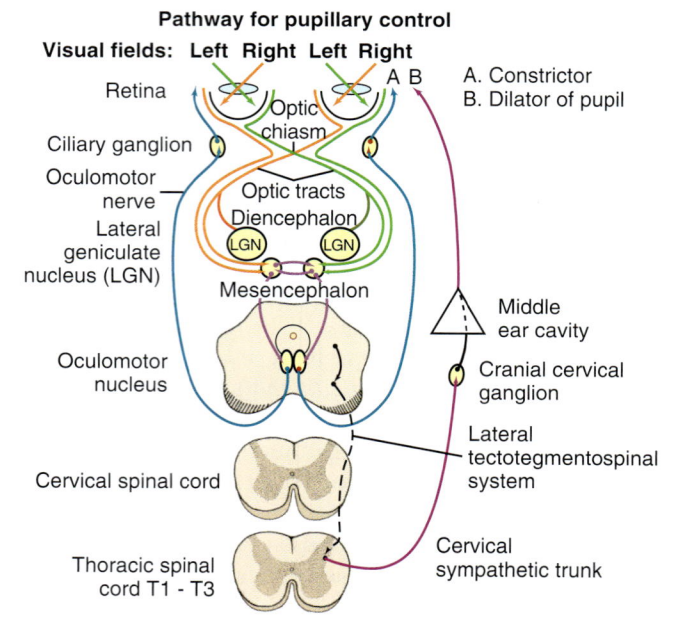

• **Fig. 21.15** Neuroanatomic pathway for pupillary control.

1991; Unger & Tighe, 1984). Interestingly, substance P is inactivated by aqueous humor (Igić, 1993).

The **dilator muscle** is innervated by sympathetic and parasympathetic axons. The preganglionic sympathetic neuronal cell bodies are located in the intermediate gray column of the first three thoracic spinal cord segments (Fig. 21.15). Their axons course cranially in the vagosympathetic trunk to synapse on cell bodies of postganglionic axons located in the cranial cervical ganglion. From the ganglion, the postganglionic axons pass rostrally through the tympanooccipital fissure with the internal carotid artery. They enter the cranial cavity through the foramen lacerum and join the ophthalmic nerve on the ventral surface of the trigeminal ganglion. They are distributed with the ciliary branches of the ophthalmic nerve. Sympathetic stimulation causes contraction of these fibers, causing pupillary dilation, and parasympathetic stimulation inhibits contraction. Other endogenous compounds, such as prostaglandins, also have been shown to play a role in regulating the state of pupillary dilation, typically in concert with the reduction of intraocular pressure (Abdel-Latif, 1989; Gelatt et al., 2004; Yoshitomi & Ito, 1988). This may be why dogs exposed to a natural photoperiod exhibit significant circadian rhythms of intraocular pressure, which peaks during diurnal hours (Giannetto et al., 2009; Piccione et al., 2010). This circadian rhythm disappears under conditions of constant light (Piccione et al., 2010).

The blood supply of the iris arises primarily from the two long posterior ciliary arteries (Figs. 21.5A and 21.9). These arteries follow the medial and lateral meridians from the area cribrosa to the iris. They are visible in the episcleral space from the optic nerve to approximately the equator of the eyeball and are useful landmarks for orienting an isolated eyeball to the horizontal plane. At the equator, the long posterior ciliary arteries pass deep to the sclera and continue anteriorly to the base of the iris. Some branches may be given to the choroid, where they anastomose with the choroidal arterioles. In the ciliary margin of the iris, the medial and lateral posterior arteries each divide into superior and inferior branches. This bifurcation may occur 2 to 3 mm posterior to the base of the iris (Sharpnack et al., 1984). The branches run circumferentially in the iris, forming the undulating **greater arterial circle of the iris** (*circulus arteriosus iridis major*) (Fig. 21.5A). The position of the circle approximates that of the equator of the lens. The circle is not directly completed at the superior and inferior points. In most specimens, however, a smaller vessel completes the circle near the base of the iris (Purtscher, 1961; Sharpnack et al., 1984). The formation of the greater arterial circle of the iris in the dog is similar to that in humans but differs significantly in that the greater arterial circle of humans is within the ciliary body. In the dog, the greater arterial circle of the iris is often visible (especially in blue irides) and commonly protrudes slightly from the anterior iridial surface (Bedford, 1977).

Fine radial arterioles originate from the arterial circle. These originate either directly from the circle or from radial ciliary arteries at a point close to where they branched from the major arterial circle and started posteriorly (Sharpnack et al., 1984). Arterioles run either centrally toward the pupil to supply the iris stroma and musculature or peripherally to anastomose with the ciliary vessels supplying the ciliary processes (Anderson & Anderson, 1977) (see Fig. 21.9). A lesser arterial circle near the pupil is not present in the dog. Venules begin blindly at the pupillary margin and course posteriorly to pass deep to the major arterial circle and into the ciliary vasculature (Sharpnack et al., 1984). Incision of the iris in the dog results in profuse hemorrhage.

Internal Tunic

The innermost tunic of the eye (*tunica interna bulbi*) consists of the **retina** with its pigmented epithelium. It is often referred to as the *nervous coat*. The internal tunic develops from an outgrowth of the diencephalon, the optic vesicle (Fig. 21.2). The optic nerve is therefore actually a tract of the central nervous system and has the characteristics of central nervous tissue. The meninges of the brain are continued along the optic nerve to the eyeball as the **internal** and **external sheaths of the optic nerve** (*vaginae n. optici interna et externa*.).

At approximately 17 days of gestation, the optic vesicle invaginates to form the optic cup, which folds into a hemisphere (Fig. 21.2B). The inner and outer walls of the cup are opposed to each other and together form the definitive retina. The outer wall of the cup becomes a single layer of retinal pigment epithelium that is directly apposed to the choroid. The inner layer of the cup differentiates into the three layers of neurons that form the photoreceptor and synaptic layers of the *pars optica retinae*. The interphotoreceptor matrix is largely composed of hyaluronan, which may serve to provide structural support for macromolecules (Hollyfield et al., 1998). In traumatic retinal detachment, or in postmortem material, the retina usually separates along the line of the embryonic neural canal, leaving the pigment epithelium adhering to the choroid.

There are three distinct areas of the retina, which, from anterior to posterior, are the *pars iridica retinae,* the *pars ciliaris retinae,* and the *pars optica retinae*. Only the last is photosensitive (visual retina). The pars iridica and pars ciliaris together constitute the nonvisual, or blind, retina (*pars ceca retinae*), which consists of two layers of epithelial cells.

The ***pars iridica retinae*** is a bilayered epithelium that covers the posterior surface of the iris. The pupillary margin is the anterior limit of tissue of neuroectodermal origin in the eye. The anterior face of the iris is covered by epithelium derived from mesoderm. The outer layer of the pars iridica retinae gives rise to the muscles of the iris. The inner layer, adjacent to the lens, is a heavily pigmented epithelium that has prominent radial striations in most dogs.

At the ciliary margin of the iris, the pars iridica retinae reflects onto the ciliary body to become the ***pars ciliaris retinae***. This bilayered cuboidal epithelium produces the aqueous humor. The outer layer is heavily pigmented; the inner layer is unpigmented. The zonular fibers that support the lens originate in the interstices between the cells of the epithelium (Raviola, 1971).

The **ora ciliaris retinae** is the demarcation between the visual and nonvisual retina (see Fig. 21.11A and B). The term *ora serrata* is used to define this junction in humans, but in the dog (and other domestic species) this junction lacks a markedly serrated appearance. The pars optica retinae, posterior to the ora, is three to four times as thick as the pars ciliaris retinae. Intraretinal cysts adjacent to the ora serrata are a common finding in older dogs (Heywood et al., 1976; Rubin, 1974). The **pars optica retinae** is responsible for the transduction of photic energy into chemical energy and finally into electrical energy transmitted as an action potential along the optic nerve to the visual centers of the brain. The optic retina is classically described as having 10 layers. In general terms, these 10 layers represent various components of 4 cellular layers: an externally situated epithelium and 3 internally situated neuronal cell layers. The retinal pigmented epithelium, which develops from the outer layer of the optic cup, forms the outermost layer immediately internal to the choriocapillaris of the choroid. This layer phagocytoses the effete portions of the outer segments of the photoreceptors. The inner layer of the optic cup develops into the neuronal elements of the retina: photoreceptors, interneurons, and ganglion cells with associated astrocytes (Müller cells). The use of the term *ganglion cell* is an exception to the rule that ganglia are collections of neuronal cell bodies within the peripheral nervous system.

In normal dogs, the mean thickness of the retinal nerve fiber layer is 141.69 (±18) μm ranging from 148.03 (±8.5) to 141.06 (±8.73) μm in the superior and inferior retinal quadrants, respectively (García-Sánchez et al., 2007).

The canine retina contains a range of ganglion cell types, including alpha cells with large somata and large, densely branched dendritic trees; beta cells with medium-sized somata and small densely branched dendritic trees; and other types of ganglia with smaller somata and varying dendritic branching patterns and field sizes (Peichl, 1992a). Alpha and beta cell dendritic trees are stratified in a single layer on either the inner or outer part of the inner plexiform layer, suggesting an on-off response to light. The dendritic field size of alpha cells increases from a diameter of 160 to 200 μm in the central area to approximately 1100 μm in the peripheral retina. The dendritic field size of beta cells increases from a diameter of 25 μm in the central area to approximately 360 μm in the peripheral retina (Peichl, 1992b).

The topographical distribution of retinal ganglion cells in the dog retina is variable, documenting the presence of a moderate to pronounced area centralis. Estimates of total ganglion cell number range from approximately 115,000 (Peichl, 1992b) to 148,303 (Albrecht May, 2008). Ganglion cell density is greatest in the area centralis but ranges from 6,400 to 14,400/mm^2, suggesting individual differences in visual acuity. Depending on their location, alpha cells make up 3% to 14% of all retinal ganglia (Hebel, 1976; Peichl,

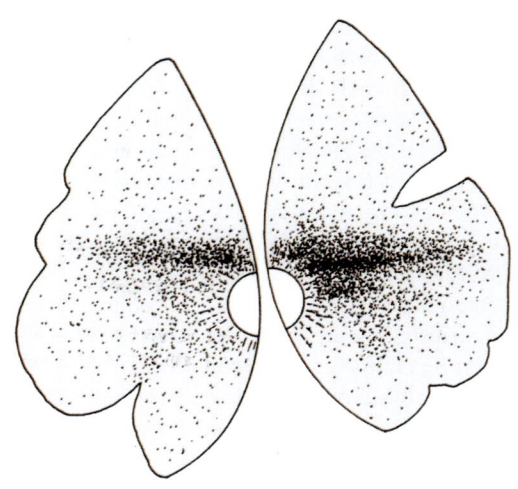

• **Fig. 21.16** Ganglion cell density of the retina of the left eye of the dog. The greatest concentration of ganglion cells is associated with the area centralis. (Redrawn after Hebel R: Distribution of retinal ganglion cells in five mammalian species [pig, sheep, ox, horse, dog], *Anat Embryol* 150:45–51, 1976.)

1992b) (Fig. 21.16). In this region, the ganglion cell density may exceed 7000 cells per mm^2. This area of most acute vision is poorly developed in the dog as compared with humans and higher primates. The area is not clearly defined either grossly or by means of the ophthalmoscope. There is no thinning of the inner retinal layers and therefore no fovea. Histologically, an increase in the number of cones and ganglion cells is noted, although the area centralis in the dog does not consist exclusively of cones, as does the foveal region in humans.

In the German Shepherd Dog, the distribution of ganglion cells ranges from 530 to 13,000 cells/mm^2 in the densely packed central area, decreasing to 1000 cells/mm^2 or less in the periphery (Gonzalez-Soriano et al., 1995); however, the distribution of retinal ganglion cells depends on the shape of the skull. Among dogs with cephalic indices ranging from 41.5 to 93.5, the distribution of ganglion cells shows considerable variation, ranging from a strong horizontal visual streak of 880 cells/mm^2 to a weaker streak of 160 cells/mm^2 and with peak cell densities in the area centralis ranging from 880 to 2640 cells/mm^2 (McGreevy et al., 2004). There is a positive correlation between skull length and width and the total number of retinal ganglion cells and a positive correlation between skull length and peak cell density in the streak; however, skull length was negatively correlated with peak cell density in the area centralis. The morphologic features of canine retinal ganglion cells are unaffected by age (Coli & Marroni, 1996). Major retinal blood vessels do not cross the area centralis but curve superior or inferior to it (Fig. 21.17).

Astrocyte density varies according to retinal topography, with an increased number around retinal blood vessels and in the peripapillary retina (Albrecht May, 2008). Large numbers of astrocytes are found in the region of the temporal raphe and over the area centralis. Astrocyte processes are oriented along axon bundles and across blood vessels

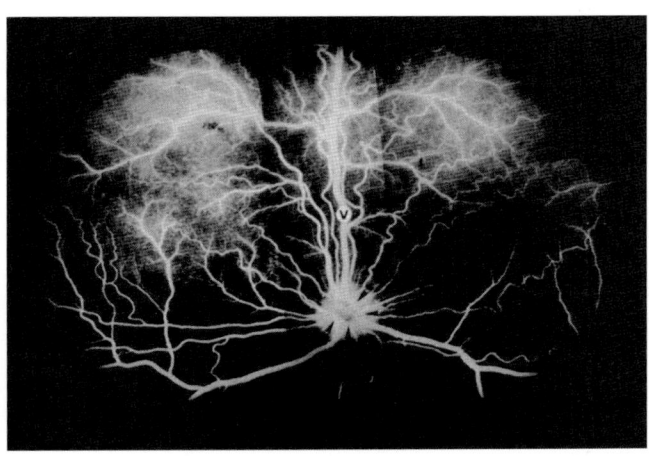

• **Fig. 21.17** Angiogram of the fundus of the left eye. Fluorescein was injected intravenously, and sequential photographs were taken. At the phase shown above, both arteries and veins are visible. *v*, Retinal vein; *arrows* indicate a venous anastomotic ring on the surface of the disc. (Courtesy Professor Dr. Paul Simoens, Ghent.)

(Chan-Ling & Stone, 1991). Microglia are resident immune cells found throughout the retina and central nervous system and have been isolated from the dog retina (Genini et al., 2014).

Catecholamine-containing amacrine cells are characterized by large somata (≈14 μm diameter) and large, moderately branched dendritic trees (Peichl, 1991) with somata located in the inner portion of the inner nuclear layer (normal amacrines) or in the ganglion cell layer (displaced amacrines). Most dendrites are stratified in a narrow band in the inner plexiform layer close to the inner nuclear layer where they form a dense plexus with a characteristic dendritic ring pattern. The displaced cells have some of their dendrites in a proximal stratum of the inner plexiform layer. A few processes are found in the outer plexiform layer (interplexiform processes). The mean cell density of amacrine cells in dogs is 21/mm^2 but varies from less than 1/mm^2 in the periphery to 40 to 55/mm^2 in central retina (Peichl, 1991). The total proportion of displaced amacrines is approximately 41% but varies locally from 10% to 85%.

The photoreceptor segments of the rods and cones are situated outward, adjacent to the pigment epithelium. There are no specialized morphologic junctions uniting the photoreceptors to the retinal pigmented epithelium. The adhesion of these two layers is predominantly physiologic in nature, and pathologic separation between these two layers results in retinal detachment. Light must pass through the retinal nerve fibers, the various synaptic cells of the retina, and the cell bodies of the rods and cones themselves before it reaches the photosensitive layer. Light passing through the photoreceptors is absorbed by the pigment of the pigment epithelium and choroid. In the area of the tapetum lucidum, the pigment epithelium of the retina lacks melanosomes, and the light is reflected by the tapetum back through the pigment epithelial layer, giving the photoreceptors two chances to capture a given quantum of light. This is presumably an adaptation for improved vision in low levels of illumination.

The rods and cones are not evenly distributed throughout the retina (Koch & Rubin, 1972). The area centralis is the site of maximal rod and cone photoreceptor cell density (Mowat et al., 2008). Based on the mean cone density distribution, the area centralis appears to be located at a point 1.5 mm temporal and 0.6 mm superior to the optic disc. Funduscopically, this represents 1.2 disc diameters temporal and 0.4 disc diameters superior to the optic disc. Recently, a unique fovea-like bouquet of cones has been identified within the area centralis of the dog (Beltran et al., 2014). In the dog approximately 95% of the photoreceptors are rods. It has been demonstrated, however, that the dog retina possesses two classes of cone photopigment (spectral peaks of approximately 429 nm and 555 nm), and dichromatic color vision has been verified (Neitz et al., 1989). A dichromat, such as the dog, is able to distinguish between stimuli having predominantly short and long wavelengths (blues from greens, yellows, and reds) and can distinguish narrow spectral energy stimuli from those with broad spectral energy (discriminates blues, yellows, or browns from grays or whites); however, the dog cannot discriminate between subtle differences in middle and long wavelength stimuli. Small differences among yellows, greens, and reds that are quite obvious to animals with trichromatic vision (such as humans and higher primates) are unseen by the dog. Using 30 shades of gray ranging from white to black, the ability to discriminate differences in brightness resulted in a calculated Weber fraction of 0.22 for one German Shepherd Dog and 0.27 for two Belgian Shepherds, suggesting the brightness discrimination in dogs is approximately one-half as good as humans (Pretterer et al., 2004).

The synaptic pathway of the visual impulse initially passes inward toward the vitreous. The photoreceptors synapse with the adjacent horizontal and bipolar cells. These synapse with the still more interior amacrine and ganglion cells. The unmyelinated axons of the ganglion cell layer arc toward the optic disc. Here they become myelinated, turn, and pass through the area cribrosa of the sclera to form the optic nerve. A multilayered area cribrosa with a diameter of 1592 μm and having three-dimensional similarities to the primate lamina cribrosa has been described in the dog eye (Albrecht May, 2008; May, 2008). The intraocular myelinated portion of the nerve forms the **optic disc** (see Figs. 21.1; 21.8; 21.16 and 21.17). The morphologic features of the disc vary greatly among dogs. It may be round to oval or triangular to quadrilateral. It is commonly pink or white but may contain pigment. A ring of pigmentation or hyperreflectivity may surround the disc. Myelin may extend along the axons onto the retina for a variable distance, giving the disc a large and ragged appearance. The optic disc commonly contains a **central depression** (physiologic cup), the *excavatio disci*, although in some dogs the disc is level with the surrounding retina or slightly elevated above it. There are no photoreceptors overlying the disc, and hence the optic disc represents a "blind spot" in the eye. The normal disc is 1 to 2 mm in diameter (Wyman & Donovan, 1965). It is located inferiolateral to the posterior pole of the eyeball. Retinal blood vessels are readily visualized with the ophthalmoscope, and their examination represents an important part of the ophthalmic examination (Magrane, 1977). The part of the retina and all associated structures that are visible with the ophthalmoscope are referred to as the *ocular fundus* clinically (Figs. 21.8 and 21.17).

The **retinal arteries** originate from the short posterior ciliary arteries, where the latter penetrate the sclera at the periphery of the area cribrosa. The retinal arteries pass into the eyeball closely applied to the surface of the optic nerve. There is no central artery or vein in the dog (Engerman et al., 1966; Wyman & Donovan, 1965). The retinal arteries appear at the periphery of the optic disc and branch into 15 to 20 arterioles that radiate toward the periphery (Fig. 21.17). The region of the area centralis is relatively avascular; the retinal vessels curve around it. Except for the area centralis, the retina of the dog is uniformly vascularized and, as such, is said to be a holoangiotic retina. The canine retina thus receives a dual nutritional supply; the retinal vessels supply nourishment to the internal aspect of the retina, and the choriocapillaris supplies the external layers of the retina. In a comparative survey of retinal vascular patterns, Chase (1982) found that animals that lack a robust retinal vascular supply have thinner retinas owing to the inability of the choriocapillaris to meet the metabolic needs of retinal tissue in excess of 143 μm thick (the theoretical oxygen diffusion maximum). A vascular retina also appears to be a prerequisite to the possession of a choroidal tapetum.

The primary **retinal veins** are three or four and occasionally five in number. Veins directed superiorly, inferiomedially, and inferiolaterally are constant. A fourth vein, running inferiorly, is present in approximately 80% of dogs. The retinal veins form a variable anastomosis on, or just below, the surface of the optic disc. This anastomosis may be in the form of a complete circle or any portion thereof. The veins are easily recognized ophthalmoscopically, being two to four times the diameter of the arterioles and a darker red in color. They project very slightly from the retinal surface and indent the vitreous body

Lens

The **lens** of the eye is a soft, transparent, protein-rich, biconvex structure suspended in contact with the posterior face of the iris and the anterior face of the vitreous body (Fig. 21.1). Its function is to bring images into critical focus on the photoreceptor layer of the retina. The crystallins, the major structural proteins of the lens, are considered organ-specific, have been characterized in the dog (Daniel et al., 1984), and are known to exist as α-crystallin, β-crystallin, and γ-crystallin subunits (Denis et al., 2003). Zeta crystalline, an inactivated form of DAD(H)P/quinine dehydrogenase has also been described in the dog and some other mammalian species (Gagna et al., 2001). Other major components of the canine lens are phospholipids including ethanolamine plasmalogen, phosphatidylethanolamine, phosphatidylserine, sphingomyelin, and phosphatidylcholine (Iwata et al., 1995).

In an assessment of lens morphologic examination using ultrasonography, Williams (2004) reported the following mean intraocular measures ($N = 50$): globe diameter 20 (±1.6) mm, axial lens thickness 6.7 (±1.0) mm, axial lens thickness/globe diameter ratio 0.33 (±0.1).

Images are focused on the retina by the combined refraction of the cornea, aqueous, lens, and vitreous. Most refraction occurs at the anterior face of the cornea. The lens actually alters the path of the light rays only slightly, but it is the only structure in the dog eye capable of altering its refractive power. It therefore is solely responsible for changing visual focus (accommodation) in the dog eye. The focal length of the lens is altered by changes in its shape brought about by the action of the ciliary muscle, zonular fibers, and lens capsule. The lens has an extraordinarily high protein content giving it a refractive index substantially higher than the surrounding fluid media and allowing it to refract light effectively. The dog lens has been shown to exhibit negative spherical aberration (Sivak, 1985; Sivak & Kreuzer, 1983). In a spherical lens of uniform refractive index, the light rays that pass through the most peripheral aspect of the lens will be brought to a point focus in front of rays that pass through the paraxial region of the lens. This is referred to as *positive spherical aberration*. In the canine lens, peripheral rays are brought to a point focus at a distance farther from the lens than rays passing through the paraxial region (negative spherical aberration). This occurs because the lens possesses a gradient of refractive indices. In the dog, the more peripheral cortical regions of the lens have a lower refractive index than the more centrally located nuclear regions. The canine lens has also been shown to possess chromatic aberration (Kreuzer & Sivak, 1985). Longitudinal chromatic aberration arises when longer wavelengths of light (reds) are refracted less by the lens than shorter wavelengths (blues). Red wavelengths would therefore be focused behind blue wavelengths. The percentage of chromatic aberration with respect to focal length (or power) found for the dog lens is quite high compared with other vertebrates.

The lens contributes significantly to the overall refractive power of the eye. When it is surgically removed during cataract surgery, the eye becomes significantly hyperopic (focused behind infinity). The aphakic canine eye is approximately 14 diopters hyperopic relative to infinity (Davidson et al., 1993). Intraocular lenses are currently being implanted by many veterinary ophthalmic cataract surgeons to replace the optical power lost by lens removal.

An anterior and posterior pole and equator are described for the lens in a manner analogous to that for the eyeball as a whole. The equator demarcates the anterior and posterior faces.

The lens is circular in transverse section but slightly ellipsoidal in sagittal or dorsal section. The superior-inferior and mediolateral diameters average approximately 11 mm, whereas the anteroposterior length along the axis bulbi is approximately 4 mm less (Table 21.1). The posterior face is

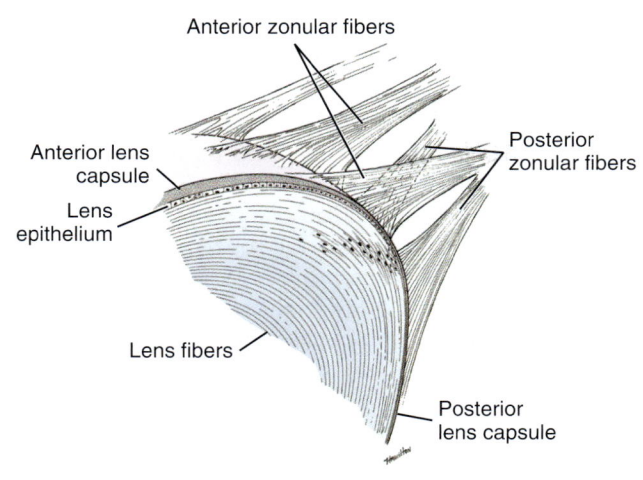

• **Fig. 21.18** Detail of lens equator in section.

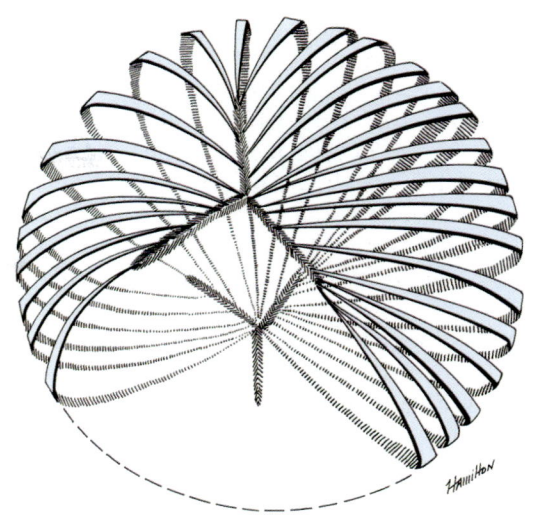

• **Fig. 21.19** Schema of lens fibers, posterior view.

more convex than the anterior. The posterior pole of the lens approximates the equatorial plane of the eyeball as a whole.

The lens is ectodermal, originating from an invagination of the surface epithelium overlying the optic cup (Fig. 21.2B), which pinches off to form the lens vesicle by approximately 27 days of gestation (Andersen & Shultz, 1958). The cells forming the posterior wall elongate until they reach the anterior epithelium obliterating the cavity of the vesicle. These cells then lose their nuclei to become the primary lens fibers of the embryonal nucleus. As a result, there is a cuboidal lenticular epithelium only on the anterior face of the lens at birth. This simple epithelium gradually becomes squamous in the adult (Monaco et al., 1985) (Fig. 21.18).

Throughout life the epithelium continues to proliferate slowly near the anterior equatorial margin. Cells at the equator elongate along the meridians until their apices approach the poles. In section, the nuclei of these elongating cells form an arc, the so-called lens bow, from the equator toward the deeper portions of the lens (Fig. 21.18). As successive layers of cells accumulate, the deeper cells lose their nuclei but remain viable as secondary **lens fibers**. This manner of growth results in a lens that is distinctly lamellar, resembling an onion in cross-section. In dogs older than 1 year of age, an embryonal, fetal, and adult nucleus and an adult cortex are recognized (Martin, 1969).

For the normal lenses, the thickness of the anterior lens capsule increases linearly with age by 5 to 8 μm/year (Bernays & Peiffer, 2000; Paunksnis et al., 2001). Because the continued epithelial proliferation is unaccompanied by cell loss, the weight of the lens also increases with age. The increase in weight is most rapid during the first few months of life but continues at a slow rate throughout life. Because individual variation of the growth rate of the lens within a species is usually slight, there is a direct correlation between age and dry lens weight. This method for age determination has been used for several wild carnivores (Lord, 1961).

The nuclear portion of the lens undergoes progressive dehydration and condensation (nuclear sclerosis). In adults, this shrinkage occurs at a rate roughly equal to the rate of growth at the periphery, so that the lens does not continually increase in size. The progressive nuclear sclerosis results in a much firmer and less elastic lens in older individuals. The development of sclerosis in older dogs has been associated with a myopic shift in resting refractive state (Murphy et al., 1992). Nuclear sclerosis causes the deeper portions of the lens to appear blue-gray and hazy. This normal age change should not be confused with cataracts, which are pathologic lenticular opacities.

The apices of the lens fibers do not all meet at a single point at each pole, like sections of an orange. Rather, the junctions form distinct linear markings known as the **lens sutures** (Fig. 21.19). On the anterior face, the lens sutures form an upright letter Y. On the posterior face the Y is inverted. Lens fibers that begin at the tip of one of the arms of the Y on the anterior face end in the crotch between the arms of the Y on the posterior face (Fig. 21.19). This pattern is most obvious in the adult nuclear region. The prominence of the sutures increases with age, beginning at approximately the third year (Heywood et al., 1976). In the cortex the lens sutures are more stellate in form. The lens sutures are easily visualized in the living dog with a slit lamp and are frequently the site of cataracts. With suitable illumination, a small white dot (Mittendorf dot), a remnant of the hyaloid artery, can be seen in the center of the posterior lens face (Martin, 1969).

The entire lens is enveloped by the **lens capsule** (Fig. 21.18). The capsule is a basement membrane secreted by the cells of the lenticular epithelium. It is highly refractile and elastic. The elasticity of the capsule aids in cataract surgery when a prosthetic lens is introduced through a relatively small opening in the anterior capsule. The posterior epithelium is present only in the early fetal period and the posterior capsule remains thin, approximately 4 μm throughout life (Monaco et al., 1985). The anterior capsule in the dog is approximately 82 μm in thickness, roughly eight times thicker than in humans. Its thickness, which may increase in diabetic patients, reduces anterior

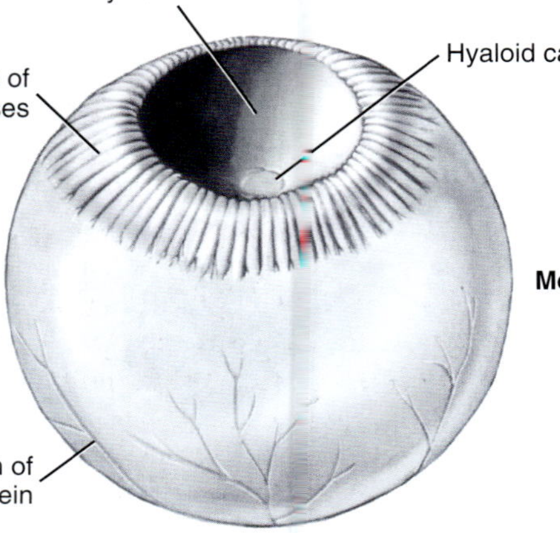

Fig. 21.20 Dorsal view of isolated vitreous of left eye.

rounding of the lens during accommodation (Engerman & Colquhoun, 1982).

The zonular fibers, which suspend the lens, insert into the superficial layers of the lens capsule. More and larger fibers insert in the thicker anterior capsule than on the posterior surface (see section on zonule). The lens rests in a depression in the vitreous, the **hyaloid fossa** (Fig. 21.20). The vitreous is tightly adherent to the posterior capsule.

In the adult, the lens, although active metabolically, is avascular. Nutrition is received from, and wastes are eliminated into, the aqueous and vitreous humors. Disease processes, for example diabetes mellitus, that affect lenticular metabolism result in a loss of transparency (cataract).

Chambers of the Eye

Within the eyeball are three chambers: the **anterior chamber** (*camera anterior bulbi*), the **posterior chamber** (*camera posterior bulbi*), and the **vitreous chamber** (*camera vitrea bulbi*) (Fig. 21.3C).

The anterior chamber is the space bounded by the cornea anteriorly and the iris and anterior lens surface posteriorly. It is filled with the aqueous humor. The anterior chamber is in direct communication with the posterior chamber through the aperture of the iris. The periphery of the chamber is continuous with the spaces of the iridocorneal angle.

The posterior chamber is smaller than the anterior chamber, being approximately 50% of the latter in volume (Gum et al., 2007). It is bounded anteriorly by the iris, posteriorly by the lens capsule and anterior face of the vitreous, and peripherally by the zonule and ciliary epithelium.

Aqueous humor fills the anterior and posterior chambers. The humor is produced by an active secretory process from the epithelium (*pars ciliaris retinae*) of the richly vascular ciliary body. The mean volume of aqueous humor is 1.7 (±0.86) mL in the dog (Gilger et al., 2005). The aqueous is normally clear and colorless. It is very low in protein compared with blood plasma and more closely resembles the cerebrospinal fluid in composition than any other fluid formed in the body. Normally the aqueous humor is maintained at an intraocular pressure of approximately 17 to 21 mm Hg in the dog (Giannetto et al., 2009). This pressure is essential to maintain the normal shape and firmness of the eyeball. When the intraocular pressure is lost postmortem or as a result of the escape of aqueous humor through a corneal laceration, the eye becomes soft and deformed.

The conventional pathway for aqueous outflow in the dog has been described by Samuelson and Gelatt (1984a, b). The aqueous humor flows from its site of production, the epithelium of the ciliary processes, into the posterior chamber, through the pupil into the anterior chamber and peripherally to the intertrabecular spaces of the iridocorneal angle. Here it is resorbed into the blood stream by the angular aqueous plexus. A second, unconventional, uveoscleral pathway for aqueous drainage has recently been described in a variety of species (Sedacca et al., 2011). In the uveoscleral route, aqueous humor leaves the anterior chamber, passes caudally through the uveal trabecular meshwork and tendinous attachments of the anterior ciliary body musculature, percolates through the meridional ciliary body muscle, and enters the supraciliary and suprachoroidal spaces (Samuelson et al., 2001). The fluid is then absorbed by the choroidal and scleral circulation (Barrie et al., 1985a). This route has been shown to account for approximately 15% of total aqueous outflow in the normal dog and to be markedly diminished, accounting for only 3% of total outflow, in glaucomatous Beagles (Barrie et al., 1985b) because of morphological changes associated with the outflow pathways (Samuelson & Streit, 2012). The trabecular meshwork and aqueous outflow channels are innervated with sympathetic axons, suggesting a neural influence on aqueous dynamics (Gwin et al., 1979). The trabecular meshwork cells within the iridocorneal angle contain smooth muscle actin and contraction is likely to alter aqueous outflow (Hassel et al., 2007). A delicate balance between production and resorption maintains the normal intraocular pressure. The production of aqueous humor is not regulated by the intraocular pressure. Canine uveoscleral tissue demonstrates high succinic dehydrogenase and lactic dehydrogenase activity (Cavallotti et al., 1998). Although this may suggest greater metabolic activity in this tissue, the importance of these enzymes for the outflow of aqueous humor is unknown. Occlusion of the primary outflow pathway, either at the pupil or iridocorneal angle, results in an increase in intraocular pressure (glaucoma) leading to optic neuropathy, retinal atrophy, and blindness.

Elevated levels of endothelin-1, nitric oxide, and glutamate are associated with various forms of glaucoma. The mean concentration of endothelin-1, nitric oxide, and glutamate in the aqueous humor of normal dogs is 3.05 pg/mL, 4.12 μm, and 2.35 μm, respectively (Källberg et al., 2007).

The topical application of angiotensin-converting enzyme inhibitors decreases intraocular pressure (Abrams et al., 1991); however, the role of angiotensin-converting enzyme in the normal canine eye remains unclear. Age-related vitreous degeneration, especially mild vitreal syneresis, is not an uncommon finding in normal dogs (Labruyère et al., 2008).

Vitreous

The **vitreous chamber** is the largest of the three chambers of the eye, accounting for approximately 80% of the volume of the eyeball. The zonule and posterior lens capsule form the anterior limit of the chamber. The retina encloses the remainder.

The **vitreous body** occupies the vitreous chamber. The vitreous body is a soft, clear gel, which conforms to the shape of the cavity it occupies (Fig. 21.20). Thus the anterior face of the vitreous is indented (*fossa hyaloidea*) by the posterior face of the lens. Similarly, the surface of the vitreous is fluted where it projects anteriorly between the ciliary processes.

The vitreous body is almost entirely acellular. The bulk of the vitreous is formed by the liquid component (*humor vitreus*), a solution of mucopolysaccharides rich in hyaluronic acid (Balazs, 1973). The vitreous body is composed of approximately 98% water and 2% solids. Among the solids, proteins are the major constituents (88%) followed by lipids (9%) and carbohydrates (4%) (Swann et al., 1975). Although the canine vitreous body is classically considered to be an inert structure, recent studies have documented that it is metabolically active (Reddy et al., 1986). The structure of the vitreous is reinforced by fibers of vitrein (*stroma vitreum*), which consists of collagen type II and are essential to its gel characteristics (Ayad & Weiss, 1984; Balazs, 1973). Vitrein fibers are especially numerous near the ora ciliaris retinae but do not lend sufficient rigidity to maintain the shape of the vitreous after its removal from the eye. Fine and Yanoff (1972) have aptly described the vitreous as the "most delicate of all the connective tissue in the body."

The anterior face of the vitreous is limited by the membrana vitrea. This is not a discretely demonstrable membrane in the ordinary sense but rather a local condensation of the filamentous framework found throughout the vitreous (Fine & Yanoff, 1972). In humans it is of sufficient strength to contain the vitreous after removal of the lens and lens capsule via the hyaloid-lenticular ligament. In the dog, intracapsular lens removal is impractical because the vitreous membrane is thin and tightly adherent to the posterior lens capsule. Attempts to remove the lens within its capsule usually result in tearing of the vitreous face with subsequent loss of the vitreous body (Bistner et al., 1977).

The vitreous body is also tightly adherent to the pars ciliaris retinae at the ora ciliaris retinae and to the optic disc, as well as to the posterior lens capsule. In the adult dog it is easily separated from the retina except at these points.

Elevated levels of endothelin-1, nitric oxide, and glutamate are associated with various forms of glaucoma. The concentration of endothelin-1, nitric oxide, and glutamate in the vitreous of normal dogs is 1.83 pg/mL, 4.86 μm and 1.37 μm, respectively (Källberg et al., 2007).

The **hyaloid canal** (*canalis hyaloideus*) traverses the vitreous from the optic disc to the posterior face of the lens (Fig. 21.1). It is the funnel-shaped remnant of the primary (embryologic) vitreous. As the secondary or definitive vitreous is elaborated by the retina, the primary vitreous is compressed centrally. At the same time, the primary vitreous is attenuated by being stretched as the globe increases in size. The hyaloid canal is broadest anteriorly, where it is attached to the posterior surface of the lens. The attachment to the lens can be visualized with the biomicroscope as a thin, white circle approximately 3 mm in diameter surrounding the posterior pole of the lens (Martin, 1969). The canal tapers posteriorly toward the optic disc and usually exhibits an inferior sag between its points of attachment (Fig. 21.1); the hyaloid canal is concave superiorly in most dogs. The primary vitreous is normally of the same optical clarity as the rest of the vitreous body and can be distinguished only by a slight difference in optical refractivity resulting from local differences in the vitreous stroma (Balazs, 1973). With the appropriate illumination, a line of demarcation can be detected at the interface of the primary and secondary vitreous (the "wall" of the canal). Occasionally, hemorrhage into the vitreous spreads along the interface, clearly outlining the canal (Fine & Yanoff, 1972).

In the embryo, the **hyaloid artery** courses through the hyaloid canal from the optic disc to the lens to supply the posterior surface of the growing lens. This artery normally atrophies completely by the time the eyelids open; a small white dot on the posterior pole of the lens marks its site of attachment (Martin, 1969). The multilayered fenestrated sheaths peculiar to the fine structure of the primary vitreous probably derive from the tunica media of the hyaloid vessels (Balazs, 1973). Remnants of the artery itself are occasionally seen ophthalmoscopically, especially in very young dogs. Rarely, persistent hyaloid arteries occur and result in posterior lenticular cataracts (Boevé et al., 1990; Rebhun, 1976). The vitreous degenerates with age, and its breakdown can be detected more effectively by ultrasonography than by ophthalmoscopy (Labruyère et al., 2008).

The Eye as an Optical Device

A primary function of the eye is to form a crisply focused image on the retina. The optical components through which light travels to reach the retina are the cornea, aqueous humor, lens, and vitreous body. For proper image formation these components must remain transparent and maintain precise relationships to one another. One of the exciting areas of ongoing research is attempting to define the mechanisms whereby these relationships are maintained during growth of the eye.

A point source of light located at the visual horizon emits rays that are convergent, divergent, and parallel relative to the eye. At a great distance only rays that are essentially parallel will enter the pupil of the dog. Divergent and convergent rays will pass peripheral to the pupillary aperture. If the eye is focused at infinity (is emmetropic), parallel rays will be refracted and imaged as a point on the dog's retina. If the dog's eye is ametropic (either myopic or hyperopic), the rays will not be properly imaged on the retina and will form a blurred circle. As an object is brought closer and closer to the dog's eye, the percentage of divergent rays entering the pupil will increase, requiring an increase in refractive power of the eye to properly image the object on the retinal plane. This is accomplished in the dog by increasing the optical power of the lens (accommodation).

The eye can be considered to consist of several optical surfaces, the combined action of which accurately focus images on the retina. The refractive power of an optical component is determined by its refractive index, thickness, and surface curvature. Refraction is greater in structures with more highly curved surfaces (i.e., having a smaller radius of curvature). The refractive power of an optical component is influenced by the difference in refractive indices between it and the surrounding media; the greater the difference, the greater the refractive power. It is primarily for this reason that the cornea is the most powerful refractive component of the eye. The difference in refractive indices encountered by a light ray en route to the retina is greatest at the air-cornea interface (the refractive index of air is 1 and the refractive index of the cornea is 1.3745). Although the lens has the highest refractive index of any of the optical components (approximately 1.53), it is surrounded by media with similar refractive indices (aqueous refractive index is 1.3364; vitreous refractive index is 1.3359).

The lens is the only structure capable of changing its refractive power. The most widely espoused paradigm for mammals is as follows: In the resting state, the lens is maintained in a relatively flattened configuration by the intrinsic elastic tension exerted on its equator by the ciliary body acting through the zonular fibers. To focus on near objects (accommodate), the ciliary muscles contract, counteracting this elastic force, allowing the lens to "round up" (decrease its radius of curvature) thereby increasing its refractive power. The lens rounds up because of the intrinsic elasticity of the lens capsule. It has not been proven, however, that this is the mechanism of accommodation in the dog. The raccoon has been shown to accommodate through linear translocation of the lens (lens moves forward) (Rohen et al., 1989). The anatomy of the ciliary muscle in the dog (muscle fibers having a merional orientation) suggests that a similar mechanism for changing refractive state is possible

The mean refractive state in 1,440 dogs across a large number of dog breeds ($N = 90$) was found to be emmetropic at -0.05 (± 1.36) D but varied widely (range, -6.00 to $+6.00$ D) (Kubai et al., 2008). Breeds with a mean myopic (≤ -0.5 D) refractive state include Rottweiler, Collie, Miniature Schnauzer, and Toy Poodle (Murphy et al., 1992). Similar to humans, myopia in the Labrador Retriever is caused by an elongated vitreous chamber (Mutti et al., 1999). Approximately 8% to 15% of Labrador Retrievers are reported to have myopia (nearsightedness), which may have a significant genetic component (Black et al., 2008; Mutti et al., 1999). Refractive myopia (excessive optical power in the lens) rather than elongation of the globe has been reported as the underlying cause of myopia in Miniature Poodles, Collies, and English Springer Spaniels (Williams et al., 2011). Data suggest a heritable component to refractive myopia reported in English Springer Spaniels (Kubai et al., 2013). Breeds with a mean hyperopic ($\geq +0.5$ D) refractive state include Australian Shepherd, Alaskan Malamute, and Bouvier des Flandres. For all breeds the length of the vitreous chamber (Paunksnis et al., 2001) and the degree of myopia increases with age (Kubai et al., 2008; Maehara et al., 2011; Hernandez et al. 2016). The induction of myopia in trained field trial dogs was shown to significantly impair performance (Ofri et al., 2012).

The accommodative range of the canine eye is approximately 2 to 3 diopters. Because a diopter is a term that expresses the refractive power of an optical system in reciprocal meters, this means that most dogs can accurately focus objects to within one-half to one-third of a meter of the eye. Myopic individuals cannot accurately focus objects in the distance.

A schematic eye for the dog has been published (Coile & O'Keefe, 1988). A schematic eye is an internally consistent mathematical model that approximates the normal static optical behavior of the eye for a given species. The optics of an individual animal's eye affect on the appearance of the fundus as viewed by direct and indirect ophthalmoscopy (Murphy & Howland, 1987). Owing to the intrinsic optical properties of the eye, which are related to the axial length of the globe, the ophthalmoscopic features of a small eye (such as the rat) will be perceived as much more magnified than that of the dog. By direct ophthalmoscopy (using a standard direct ophthalmoscope) the canine fundus will appear approximately 17 times more magnified in lateral extent relative to its actual dimensions.

The value for axial magnification, which is related to the square of lateral magnification, is approximately 400 times greater for the dog's eye. *Axial magnification* refers to the apparent displacement of an object along the optical pathway, either in front of or behind a reference plane. Similarly, the millimeter equivalent of a one diopter change in ophthalmoscopic focus is directly proportional to the axial length of the globe and is approximately 0.275 mm in the dog. In other words, a one diopter shift in ophthalmoscopic focus will shift the focal plane of the ophthalmoscope 0.275 mm anterior or posterior to the original plane of focus.

It has been suggested that morphological differences, such as nose length and placement of the eyes, limit or aid certain dogs when perceiving their surroundings. These morphological differences do not directly affect cognitive ability. However, in certain cognitive tasks, some breeds and morphological types perform better than others (Byosiere et al., 2017).

Orbit

The **orbit** (*orbita*) is the conical cavity that contains the eyeball and the ocular adnexa. The orbital margin outlines the base of the cone, which is directed rostrolaterally. The shape of the base approximates a rounded trapezoid more than a true circle (Fig. 21.21). The axis of the orbit, a line passing from the center of the base to the apex at the optic canal, is directed obliquely caudal and ventral. In mesaticephalic dogs, the axis of the orbit forms an angle of approximately 30 degrees with a median plane and 30 degrees with a dorsal plane. In the foreshortened skulls of the brachycephalic breeds, the axis of the orbit deviates as much as 50 degrees from the median plane (Fig. 21.22). A recent report found brachycephalic breeds to be 20 times more likely to develop corneal ulceration than nonbrachycephalic breeds (Packer et al., 2015). The eyeball occupies the base of the orbit and projects a variable distance rostral to the orbital margin. The average dog's visual field encompasses approximately 250 degrees of arc. Binocular vision is confined to the central 60 degrees (Sherman et al., 1975).

The **orbital margin** (*margo orbitale*) is bony for approximately four-fifths of its circumference. The bony orbital margin contains a supraorbital and an infraorbital border (*margo supraorbitalis and margo infraorbitalis*). The caudolateral one-fifth of the margin is completed by the **orbital ligament** (*ligamentum orbitale*). In the brachycephalic dog the ligament forms a larger proportion of the circumference. The ligament is a thick fibrous band that unites the zygomatic process of the frontal bone with the frontal process of the zygomatic bone (Figs. 21.21 and 21.23). The ligament serves as the lateral attachment of the m. orbicularis oculi and the lateral **palpebral ligament** (*ligamentum palpebrale laterale*). The dorsal and medial segments of the orbital margin are formed by the frontal bone. In most dogs, the lacrimal bone forms a small portion of the ventromedial orbital margin. In some brachycephalic skulls, however, the lacrimal bone is confined to the medial orbital wall and does not contribute to the orbital margin. In these cases only, the medioventral orbital margin is formed by the maxillary bone. The ventrolateral orbital margin is the orbital border of the zygomatic bone.

In humans the confines of the orbit are entirely bony and readily discernible from a study of the skull. In the dog, only the medial wall and part of the roof of the orbit are osseous. The lateral wall and floor are formed by soft tissue (Figs. 21.21, 21.23, and 21.24). Consequently, the orbit of the dog cannot be properly appreciated solely from study of a skeletal preparation. The anatomic difference between the orbit of the dog and that of the human is manifested by marked differences in diseases that affect the orbit and in surgical approaches to this area.

The medial wall of the orbit is formed primarily by the orbital part of the frontal bone (see Fig. 21.21). The **wing** of the sphenoid complex forms the caudal part of the medial wall and contains the optic canal. The lacrimal bone contributes to a small portion of the rostroventral medial wall and contains the fossa for the lacrimal sac and the caudal orifice of the nasolacrimal canal.

Five foramina are found in the medial wall of the orbit (see Chapter 4). At the apex of the orbit are the optic canal and orbital fissure. The optic nerve and internal ophthalmic artery leave the cranial cavity through the optic canal. The

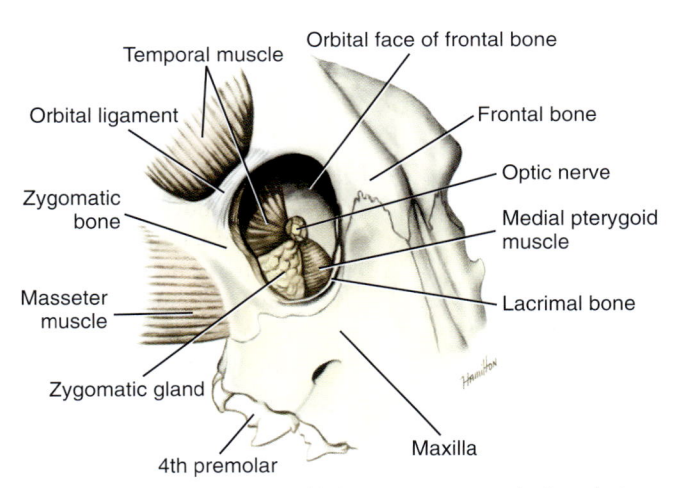

• **Fig. 21.21** The right orbit, orbital contents removed, viewed along orbital axis.

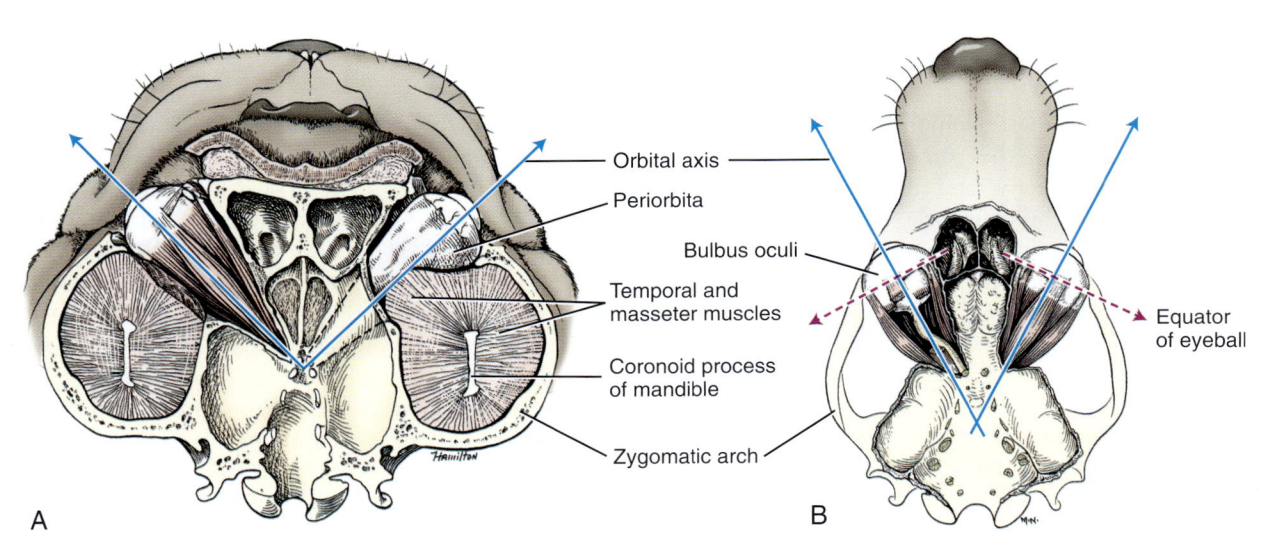

• **Fig. 21.22** Orbital axes of a brachycephalic (**A**) versus mesocephalic (**B**) dog.

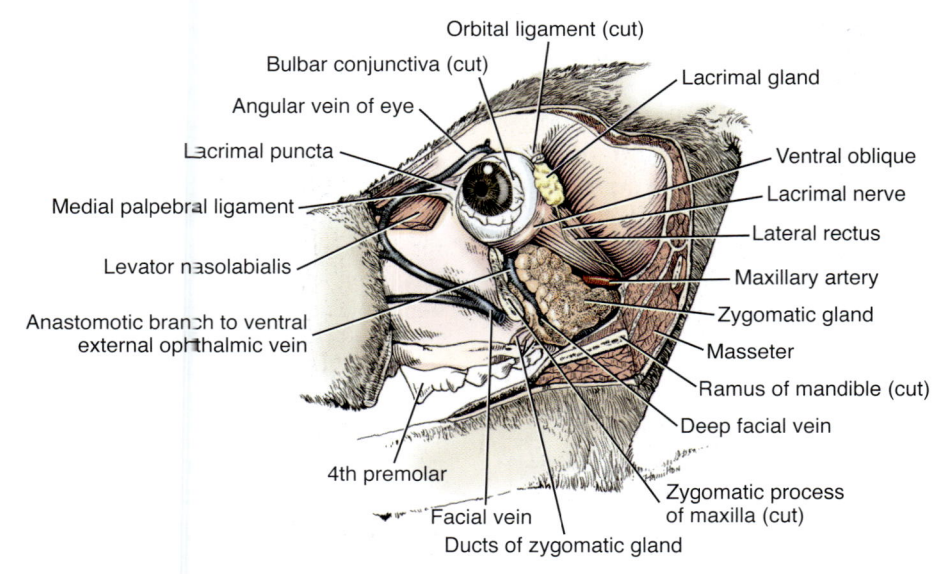

Fig. 21.23 Lateral aspect of orbit; zygomatic arch, ramus of mandible, and temporal and masseter muscles partly removed.

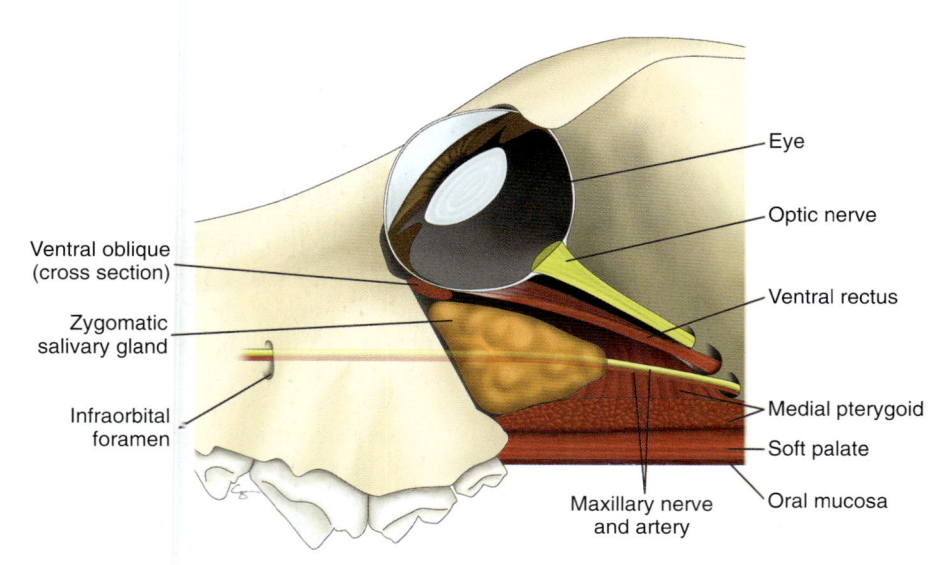

Fig. 21.24 Soft tissue components of the orbital floor.

orbital fissure between the basisphenoid and presphenoid bones gives passage to the oculomotor, trochlear, abducent, and ophthalmic nerves, the anastomotic branch of the external ophthalmic artery, and the ophthalmic venous plexus. The retractor bulbi muscle originates within the orbital fissure. Rostrodorsal to the orbital fissure are the two small ethmoidal foramina that transmit the external ethmoidal artery and the ethmoidal nerve. Rostrally the **fossa for the lacrimal sac** (*fossa sacci lacrimalis*) occupies the center of the orbital face of the lacrimal bone. This fossa is continued rostromedially as the lacrimal canal, which contains the **nasolacrimal duct** (*ductus nasolacrimalis*).

The dorsally convex **ventral orbital crest** (*crista orbitalis ventralis*) of the frontal bone demarcates the boundary between the orbit dorsally and the more ventral pterygopalatine fossa. The crest is not prominent, and in unfleshed skulls the orbit appears to extend much farther ventrally than is actually the case. The ventral orbital crest is the dorsal boundary of the origin of the medial pterygoid muscle, which forms the medial third of the orbital floor (Fig. 21.21). The zygomatic salivary gland rests on the dorsolateral surface of the medial pterygoid muscle. Its dorsal surface forms most of the floor of the orbit, from the orbital margin to nearly the optic canal. The maxillary artery and nerve cross the floor of the orbit near its apex. The pterygopalatine ganglion is just dorsal to the maxillary nerve on the dorsal surface of this muscle.

The medial aspect of the roof of the orbit is formed by the zygomatic process of the frontal bone. A very small foramen is often found in the midorbital face of the process, through which a small artery passes dorsally. In some skulls a palpable depression, the **fossa for the lacrimal gland**

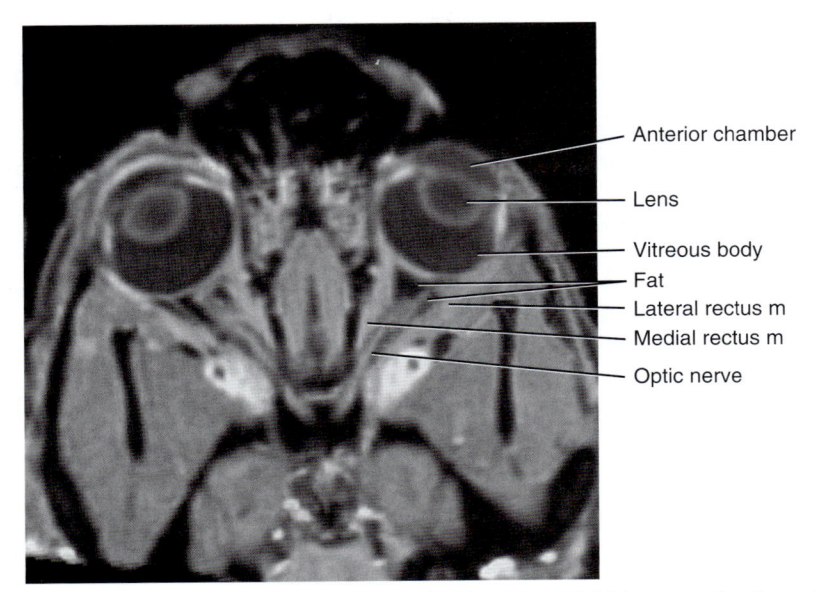

- **Fig. 21.25** Magnetic resonance image of the head showing intraorbital fat surrounding the optic nerve and muscle cone. (Courtesy Dr. Allison Zwingenberger, Department of Veterinary Surgical and Radiological Sciences, School of Veterinary Medicine, University of California–Davis.)

(*fossa glandulae lacrimalis*), is present on the ventral surface of the zygomatic process of the frontal bone at the origin of the orbital ligament.

The orbit is bounded dorsolaterally and laterally by the medial surface of the temporal muscle (temporalis) and the orbital ligament (Fig. 21.21). The ramus of the mandible is embedded in the masseter and temporal muscles immediately caudal to the orbit (Fig. 21.23). When the mouth is opened, the dorsal aspect of the ramus of the mandible moves rostrally, compressing the orbital contents. Thus pain on opening the mouth is a cardinal sign of retrobulbar abscesses. Denervation atrophy of the masseter and temporal muscles effectively enlarges the orbit, and a sinking of the eye into the orbit (enophthalmos) results. Conversely, swelling of the muscles of mastication, as in masticatory myositis, results in exophthalmos. Periorbital fat cushions the globe within the orbit (Fig. 21.25). In this regard, dynamic exophthalmos and strabismus secondary to myositis affecting a small area of the masseter muscle has been reported in the dog (Czerwinski et al., 2015).

Because the floor of the orbit is composed entirely of soft tissue, a retroorbital abscess can be drained into the oral cavity by blunt dissection caudal to the last molar tooth (Magrane, 1977). Similarly, the lateral aspect of the orbit can be explored surgically without osseous resection.

The relationship of the orbit to surrounding structures is well illustrated in Hamon's *Atlas of the Head of the Dog* (1977). This relationship is important when investigating clinical orbital disease (Fig. 21.26). Bone defects of the orbit can occur as a result of facial trauma, tumor invasion, congenital malformation, or inflammatory disease and often lead to impairment of visual function and deformity of facial appearance. A fractured orbital wall can lead to infection and can result in the distortion of facial appearance

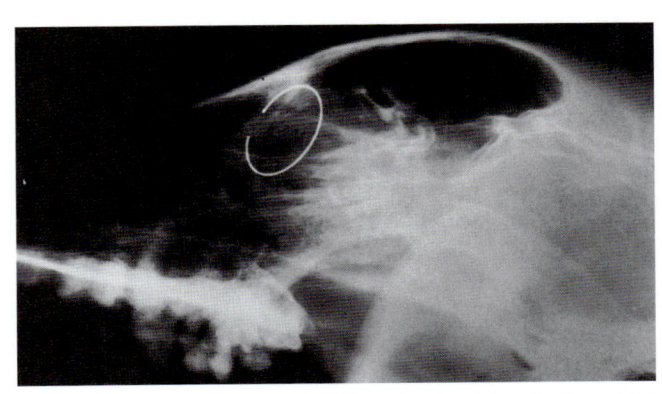

- **Fig. 21.26** Lateral radiograph with a ring to delineate the orbital margin.

including enophthalmos, eyeball dislocation, and ptosis. Because bone fractures allow communication of the orbit with the paranasal sinuses, infection can spread through the defect in the bony wall to the orbit and brain (Zhou et al., 2013). Such defects usually arise at the inferior and medial orbital walls because of their thickness of only 0.3 to 0.9 mm and cannot heal spontaneously since the orbital contents occupy the defect area and herniate into the paranasal sinus through the defect. Consequently orbital bone defects often need proper and precise repair and reconstruction. Grafts of enriched autologous bone marrow stromal cells have been reported as an option for such treatment (Betbeze, 2015; Wang et al., 2014).

Zygomatic Gland

The **zygomatic salivary gland** (*glandula zygomatica*, formerly the orbital or dorsal buccal gland) forms the lateral two-thirds of the floor of the orbit (Fig. 21.21; 21.23 and

21.24). When diseased (Knecht, 1970) it may produce ocular manifestations.

The zygomatic gland lies dorsal and lateral to the pterygoid muscles and ventral to the periorbita and the ventral orbital margin. Rostrally and laterally it is bounded by the orbital surface of the zygomatic bone. The gland extends caudally almost to the optic canal. It is roughly pyramidal, tapering caudomedially. The surface of the gland is lobulated and covered by a thin capsule and a layer of fat.

Exophthalmos, protrusion of the third eyelid and soft tissue swelling ventral to the globe, can be a sign of zygomatic sialolithiasis or zygomatic mucocele. Even though zygomatic gland disease is rare in dogs, it should be considered in any dog presenting with these symptoms. In a condition like this, computed tomography (CT) imaging and low-field magnetic resonance imaging (MRI) are very useful tools, providing information about characteristics of the lesion and invasiveness into surrounding tissues, and they are particularly helpful in planning a surgical approach and results (Boland et al., 2013; Cirla et al., 2017; Lee et al., 2014).

Orbital Fasciae (*Fasciae Orbitales*)

There are three important fascial structures of the orbit: the **muscular fasciae** (*fasciae musculares*), the **vagina bulbi** also known as *bulbar sheath* or *Tenon capsule*, and the **periorbita**.

The muscular fasciae are within the periorbita and can be divided into superficial, middle, and deep components (Constantinescu & McClure, 1990). The **superficial muscular fascia** inserts rostrally on the orbital septum and ventrally is associated with the base of the third eyelid. The orbital septum is the fibrous membrane that extends from the margin of the orbit to the tarsi of the eyelids. The lacrimal gland is located on the superficial surface of the superficial fascia. The fascia is thickest at the level of the eyeball and thins considerably near the orbital apex. It sends fibrous septa between the extraocular rectus muscles. The **middle muscular fascia** originates from the limbus, covers the eyeball, and is thinner ventrally. It gives off intermuscular septa that unite with the deep fascia. At the lateral commissure, the middle fascia divides into superficial and deep sheets. The deep sheet inserts on the lateral angle of the third eyelid and acts as a supportive ligament. The **deep muscular fascia** originates near the limbus, caudal to the middle fascia. Anteriorly, it is intimately associated with the more deeply residing vagina bulbi. The *vagina bulbi* is a thin fibrous capsule that envelops the eyeball from the limbus to the optic nerve (Fig. 21.27). It is separated from the sclera by the **episcleral space** (*spatium espisclerale*). Delicate fibrous trabeculae bridge this space and anchor the sheath to the eyeball. Anteriorly, the sheath ends in the subconjunctival and episcleral tissues at the limbus. It is well developed in the dog and complicates certain ophthalmologic surgical procedures. Medicants may be injected either superficial or deep to the sheath of the vagina bulbi into the subconjunctival or episcleral tissues. The pharmacokinetics of the spaces are distinctly different (Severin, 1976).

Near the equator of the globe the vagina bulbi reflects onto the tendinous insertions of the extraocular muscles as the insertions continue on to fuse with the sclera (Figs. 21.27 and 21.28). The vagina bulbi is continuous with the muscular fasciae at these points. Posteriorly, the sheath is continuous with the fascia binding the ciliary vessels and nerves to the dura mater of the optic nerve.

The thickest and most easily demonstrated fascial structure of the orbit is the **periorbita**, which is the conical fibrous sheet surrounding the eyeball and its associated muscles, nerves, and vessels. In humans, in whom the orbit is entirely osseous, the periorbita and periosteum of the orbit are one and the same. In the dog, the periorbita is a double layer structure (superficial and deep), which encloses the eyeball and extraocular structures (Constantinescu & McClure, 1990). The medial aspect of the orbital ligament fuses with the periorbita via thick fibrous bands. The periorbita is in contact with the medial pterygoid and temporal muscles and the zygomatic salivary gland. In the dog the periorbita and orbital periosteum are typically distinct and separate. Medioventrally, fibrous bands may be observed uniting the superficial layer of the periorbita with the periosteum.

The apex of the periorbita is firmly attached to the margins of the orbital fissure and the optic canal. At these sites the

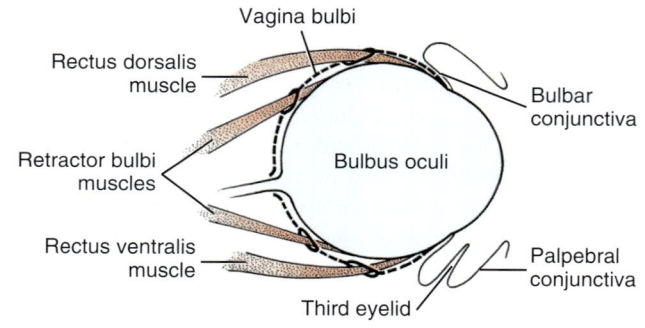

• **Fig. 21.27** Schema of vagina bulbi in section.

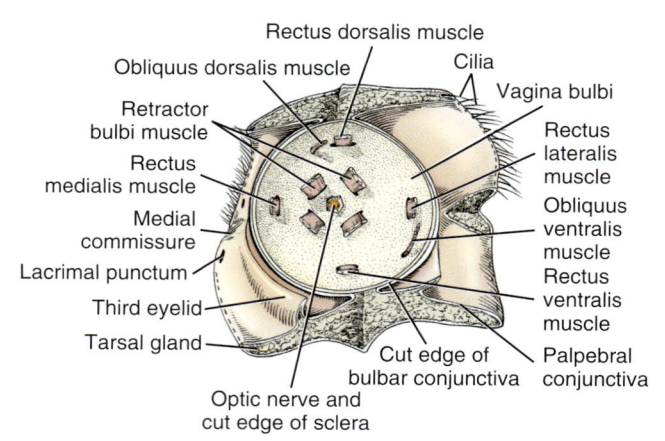

• **Fig. 21.28** Left eyeball removed to show anterior aspect of vagina bulbi with entering extraocular muscles.

periorbita is continuous with the intracranial dura mater and the external sheath of the optic nerve. All the extraocular muscles originate from the periorbita adjacent to the orbital fissure except the ventral oblique muscle. The cranial nerves to the eye and the internal and external ophthalmic vessels enter the periorbital cone at its apex. The base of the periorbital cone is the orbital margin. At the orbital margin, the periorbita reflects onto the face to become the periosteum of the facial bones. A sheet of connective tissue, the **orbital septum** (*septum orbitale*), extends from the periorbita at the orbital margin to blend with the tarsi of the lids. The orbital septum is the anterior limit of the orbit.

In the dog, the periorbita contains numerous circular, smooth muscle fibers that belong to the orbitalis muscle and normally exhibit a degree of tonus. This tonus acts to squeeze the eyeball out of the orbit and causes the normal prominence of the globe as it projects beyond the orbital margin. Sympathetic stimulation causes marked exophthalmos (Code & Essex, 1935). The **superior** and **inferior tarsal muscles** (*mm. tarsalis dorsalis et ventralis*) are smooth muscle fibers, also derived from the periorbita and are components of the orbitalis muscle, which insert in the eyelids and help to maintain their retracted positions when the palpebral fissure is open (Nicholas, 1914). It is occasionally referred to as Mueller's muscle in the literature and contracts in response to sympathetic α_{1A} stimulation (Yano et al., 2010). Smooth muscle fibers from the periorbita also insert on the base of the cartilage of the third eyelid and help to maintain it in its normal retracted position. Innervation of these smooth muscle cells is derived from the **cranial cervical ganglion** (*ganglion cervicale craniale*). Lesions resulting in denervation cause a sinking of the globe into the orbit (enophthalmos), protrusion of the third eyelid, and a narrowing of the palpebral fissure (de Lahunta, 1983).

The **orbital fat body** (*corpus adiposum orbitae*) cushions the contents of the orbit and, being easily deformable, permits the rotation and retraction of the eyeball. The orbital fat is found both within the periorbita (*corpus adiposum intraperiorbitale*) and between the periorbita and the surrounding structures (*corpus adiposum extraperiorbitale*). Adipose tissue commonly separates the periorbita from the adjacent bony orbit.

A well-developed intraperiorbital fat pad is present near the posterior pole of the eyeball. It is in the shape of a hollow cone, surrounding the optic nerve and filling the space between it and the diverging extraocular muscles. Thin sheets of intraperiorbital fat are present between the retractor bulbi and the rectus muscles (Fig. 21.25). An island of extraperiorbital adipose tissue is situated on the medial aspect of the zygomatic bone in contact with the zygomatic salivary gland. Extraperiorbital fat is lacking in the region of the orbital ligament. Extraorbital fat deposits may be extensive ventral and lateral to the periorbita, especially in obese animals. A prominent fat body is a constant finding caudal to the ventral orbital margin. Hibernomas are rare benign neoplasms of brown adipose tissue. In a recent study, the presence of orbital hibernomas has been reported in the adult dog with no breed predilection (Ravi et al., 2014). Though not described, this report suggests that brown fat remnants may be resident in the normal canine orbit.

Recent biometric studies of the canine skull and periorbita reveal a mathematical relationship between cranial length and periorbital length. The results of these studies propose the use of canine cranial length as a parameter for the calculus of the volume to be injected during intraconal regional ocular anesthesia and to establish a better method than using the patient's body weight (Klaumann et al., 2017).

Eyelids

The **eyelids** (*palpebrae*) are mobile folds of skin that can be drawn over the anterior aspect of the eyeball to occlude light and protect the cornea.

The opening, palpebral fissure, between the lids (*rima palpebrarum*) is variable in size. This fissure also varies considerably in orientation and is located more frontally in smaller breeds and more laterally in larger breeds (McGreevy et al., 2004). The width of the opening is controlled by opposing groups of muscles. The superior lid (*palpebra superior*) is slightly greater in extent and somewhat more mobile than the inferior (*palpebra inferior*). The m. orbicularis oculi acts to close the palpebral fissure. The levator palpebrae superioris, the pars palpebralis of the m. sphincter colli profundus, and smooth muscles derived from the periorbita (*mm. tarsales*) widen the fissure. The dog blinks approximately 14 times per minute with two-thirds of the blink excursions being incomplete. It has been shown that dogs with a higher complete blink rate frequently have a thinner lipid layer of the precorneal tear film (Carrington et al., 1987).

The superior and inferior lids join at the medial and lateral commissures (*commissura palpebrarum medialis et lateralis*) (Fig. 21.29). The angles formed by the lids at the commissures are the medial and lateral angles (canthi) of the eye (*anguli oculi medialis et lateralis*). The lateral is slightly more acute. A triangular prominence, the **lacrimal caruncle**, lies in the medial angle (Fig. 21.29). Small, fine hairs project from the lacrimal caruncle, and sebaceous glands, similar to the tarsal glands but smaller, are present (*glandulae carunculae lacrimalis*). The caruncle may or may not be pigmented. The superior and inferior lacrimal puncta, through which the tear film drains, open onto the bulbar surfaces of the lid margins 2 to 5 mm from the medial commissure (Fig. 21.30).

The skin of the face continues onto the anterior surface of the lids with little alteration. The typical hair and glandular structure of the skin can be identified in sections of the lids (Fig. 21.30).

Long hairs (*cilia*) project from the superior lid margin. Cilia are not present on the inferior lid in dogs. At the level of the dorsal medial orbital margin, there is a tuft of long tactile hairs (*pili supraorbitales*) that corresponds to the eyebrows in humans (Fig. 21.29). In many dogs, the region of the pili supraorbitales contrasts in color to the

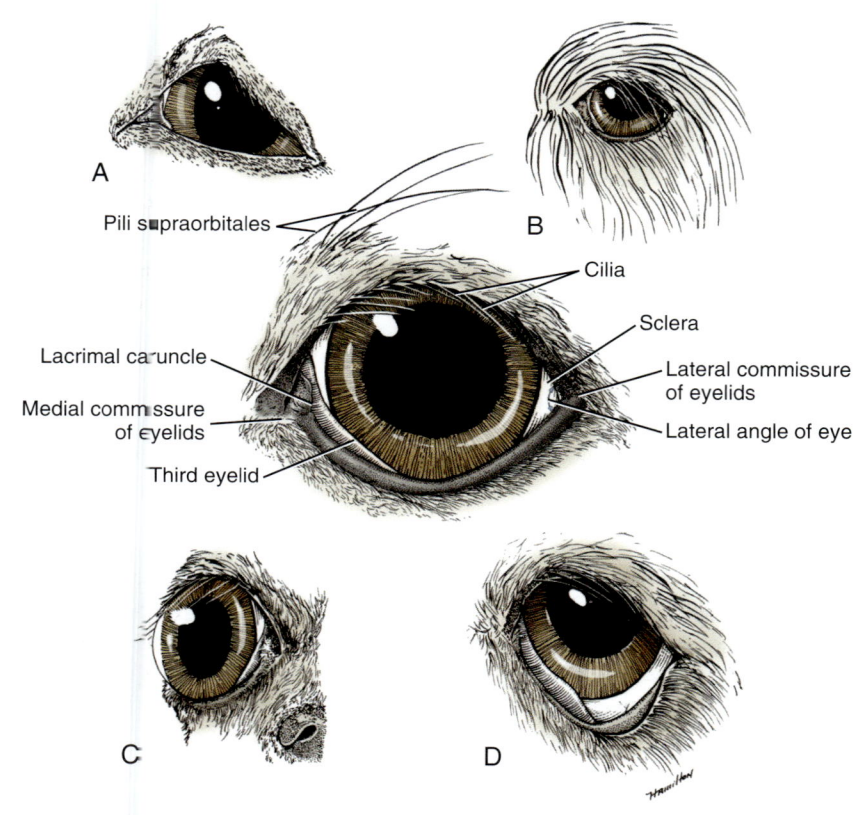

Fig. 21.29 The eyelids. **A,** Bull Terrier. **B,** English Sheepdog. **C,** Boston Terrier. **D,** St. Bernard.

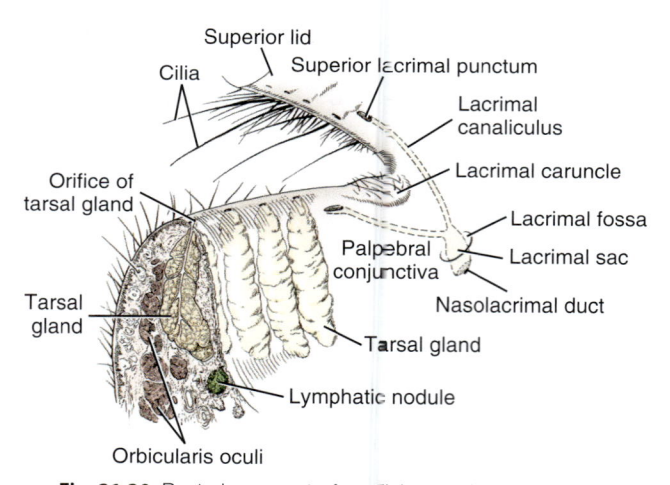

Fig. 21.30 Posterior aspect of medial commissure of eyelids.

rest of the face. Such dogs achieve particularly animated facial expressions.

Although similar to glands found elsewhere in the skin, the glands of the lid margin have received special designations. **Sebaceous glands** (*glandulae sebaceae*) open into the follicles of the cilia on the superior lid. **Ciliary glands** (*glandulae ciliares*) are coiled, tubular, apocrine sweat glands that secrete into hair follicles or sebaceous glands or directly onto the lid margin (Riis, 1976). At the palpebral margin, the epidermis changes abruptly from pigmented, keratinized, stratified squamous epithelium typical of skin to the unpigmented, nonkeratinized, stratified squamous epithelium of the conjunctiva (see section on conjunctiva).

Specially modified compound sebaceous glands, the **tarsal glands** (Meibomian glands) (*glandulae tarsales*), are present in both eyelids. The openings of the ducts of the tarsal glands lie in a shallow furrow immediately posterior to the mucocutaneous junction of the palpebral margin of each lid (Fig. 21.30). They are easily visualized when the lid is everted slightly. The glands themselves are usually visible through the conjunctiva as white or yellow columnar structures (3 mm long) that run at right angles to the palpebral margin. There are 20 to 40 glands in each eyelid. They are usually better developed on the superior lid. The oily superficial layer of the tear film is produced by the tarsal glands. It is common to find very fine hairs originating from some of these glands. This condition (distichiasis), if severe, may lead to corneal irritation and ulceration (Bedford, 1971).

Surrounding the tarsal glands in the human is a thickening of the palpebral fibrous tissue, the **tarsus**, which helps to stiffen the lid margin. In contrast to the human and some other domestic animals, the tarsus of the dog is much less developed or essentially absent.

The commissures of the lids are stabilized by the medial and lateral palpebral ligaments. The **lateral palpebral ligament** (*ligamentum palpebrale laterale*) is a poorly defined thickening of the orbital septum deep to the retractor anguli oculi lateralis muscle. The lateral ligament originates from the zygomatic arch and ventral end of the orbital ligament and inserts by blending with the fibers of the superior and inferior tarsi.

The medial commissure is much more firmly anchored than the lateral. The **medial palpebral ligament** (*Ligamentum palpebrae mediale*)(Fig. 21.23) is a distinct fibrous band originating from the periosteum of the frontal bone near the nasomaxillary suture. A small oval area of roughening at the site of origin is observed on most skulls. From its origin, the ligament passes laterally deep to the angular vein of the eye, then superficial to the origin of the levator nasolabialis to blend with the tarsi at the medial commissure. The orbicularis oculi muscle both originates and inserts on the medial palpebral ligament (see section on muscles). The palpebral ligaments and retractor anguli oculi lateralis muscle prevent the palpebral fissure from becoming circular when the sphincterlike orbicularis oculi muscle contracts.

Conjunctiva

The inner aspect of the eyelids is lined by a special mucous membrane, the **palpebral conjunctiva**. At the level of the orbital rim, the palpebral conjunctiva reflects onto the surface of the globe to become the **bulbar conjunctiva** (Fig. 21.14). The point of reflection is the **conjunctival fornix** Superiorly, there is only a single fornix, however, in the region of the third eyelid there are two fornices; at the base of its palpebral surface (reflecting from the palpebral conjunctiva onto the palpebral surface of the third eyelid) and at the base of its bulbar surface (reflecting from the third eyelid onto the surface of the sclera). The **conjunctival sac** is the potential space between the lid and the eyeball that normally contains a thread of mucus and fluid tears

The normal conjunctiva of the dog has been described by Riis (1976). Near the palpebral margin the conjunctival epithelium is stratified squamous. Toward the fornices, the epithelium thins, and the surface cells become cuboidal. The corneal epithelium is thicker than the epithelium of the bulbar conjunctiva (Strom et al., 2016). Moore et al. (1987) have described the distribution and density of the goblet cells in the dog. They found the greatest density of goblet cells in the inferior medial and middle fornix, and inferior medial palpebral regions. Goblet cells are essentially absent from the bulbar conjunctival epithelium. The bulbar conjunctival epithelium is very thin and is continuous with the limbal epithelium (Fig. 21.14). Goblet cells are absent in the perilimbal region, where the epithelium again becomes squamous. There are no perilimbal glands (glands of Manz) in the dog. With regard to the conjunctival lining of the third eyelid, numerous goblet cells reside on the palpebral side, being much less populated on its bulbar side (Umeda et al., 2010). The $P2Y_2$ receptor, involved in transport and secretory function has been reported to be associated with epithelial cells and goblet cells of the conjunctiva of the dog (Terakado et al., 2014).

The conjunctival epithelium rests on a loose connective tissue stroma rich in fibrocytes, mast cells, plasma cells, lymphocytes, and macrophages. It is very mobile, permitting extensive excursions of the eyeball and eyelids. Multiple small folds of conjunctiva are formed in the fornix when the lids are open.

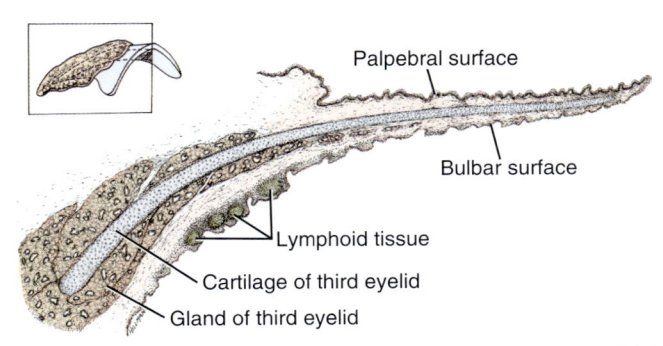

• **Fig. 21.31** Section of the third eyelid. *Inset,* Cartilage and superficial gland of third eyelid showing plane of section.

The conjunctiva is richly vascular. It is supplied by branches of the dorsal and ventral palpebral and malar arteries as well as by terminal small branches from the anterior ciliary arteries. Deep and superficial components of the conjunctival vasculature have been recognized. These react differently to inflammation of various segments of the eyeball and may be distinguished by biomicroscopy or topically applied vasoconstrictor pharmaceuticals (Riis, 1976). The conjunctiva is well innervated by branches of the long ciliary, zygomaticofacial, zygomaticotemporal, infratrochlear, and frontal nerves (see section on innervation). Corneal or conjunctival irritation results in reflex lacrimation.

Lymphatic tissue within the conjunctiva is both diffuse and nodular. Numerous **lymphatic nodules** are found throughout the conjunctiva (Fig. 21.30). Their number, size, and location vary with the age of the dog and the degree of antigenic stimulation. They are especially prominent on the bulbar surface of the third eyelid (Fig. 21.31), where they may greatly enlarge in chronically infected or irritated eyes. When enlarged, they may protrude from posterior to the third eyelid into the palpebral fissure. These lymphatic nodules are distinct from, and more superficial than, the superficial gland of the third eyelid, with which they have often been confused. The lymphatic drainage from the conjunctiva in the dog empties into the parotid lymph nodes (Wenzel-Hora et al., 1982).

Third Eyelid

The third eyelid (*palpebra tertia*), or **semilunar fold of the conjunctiva** (*plica semilunaris conjunctivae*), is well developed in the dog (Fig. 21.31). The third eyelid arises as a fold from the ventromedial aspect of the conjunctiva. The free edge of the fold is concave and faces superiolaterally to accommodate the shape of the eyeball and is usually darkly pigmented in contrast to the rest of the conjunctiva. The third eyelid is highly mobile and sufficient in extent to cover the entire anterior face of the cornea. When the eye is in its normal position in the live dog, the bulk of the third eyelid is hidden within the orbit; only the free edge is visible in the ventromedial aspect of the palpebral fissure being covered in part by the lacrimal caruncle.

The body of the third eyelid of the dog is reinforced by a T-shaped hyaline cartilage plate (*cartilago plica semilunaris conjunctivae*) (Fig. 21.31). The column of the T curves around the inferiomedial aspect of the globe. The concave crossbar of the T stiffens the free edge of the fold. The length of the cartilaginous column is surrounded by the **superficial gland of the third eyelid**. The gland is a pink, tear-drop-shaped, mixed seromucous gland. Numerous microscopic ducts empty the secretion of the gland into the inferior conjunctival fornix. The gland contributes significantly to the production of the tear film (see section on lacrimal apparatus). Consequently, surgical removal of the third eyelid results in morphologic changes in the corneal epithelium including decreased bright cells (as assessed by scanning electron microscopy), cell exfoliation, intercellular detachment of superficial cell layers, and hemidesmosome detachment of basal cell layers (Saito et al., 2004).

The superficial and deep muscular fasciae of the orbit (see section on orbital fasciae) are associated with the base of the third eyelid. A portion of the middle muscular fasciae inserts at the lateral angle of the third eyelid, forming a supportive ligament (Constantinescu & McClure, 1990).

When the eyeball is retracted into the orbit, the column of the cartilage, surrounded by its bulky gland, is displaced anteriorly, and the third eyelid sweeps across the cornea from inferiomedial to superiolateral. The motion of the third eyelid is passive, the result of displacement by the globe's being pulled into the orbit by the retractor bulbi and rectus muscles (de Lahunta & Habel, 1986). Consequently, the third eyelid may be exposed for examination by manual displacement of the globe into the orbit. The dog has no specific muscle that draws the third eyelid across the globe such as is present in the cat. Smooth muscle cells derived from the periorbital orbitalis muscle attach to the fascia of the base of the third eyelid and help to maintain its retracted position. Loss of sympathetic innervation to the orbitalis muscle results in partial protrusion of the third eyelid.

Lacrimal Apparatus

The **precorneal tear film** is essential to maintain the normal transparent state of the cornea. The tear film consists of a superficial oily layer, a central aqueous (serous) layer, and a thin mucous (glycoproteinaceous) layer covering the cornea (Yañez-Soto et al. 2014) (Fig. 21.32). The oily layer, produced by the modified sebaceous glands of the lid margin (tarsal or Meibomian glands), provides lubrication, prevents overflow of tears from the lid margins, and retards evaporation of the underlying aqueous layer. The thickness of this lipid layer varies from 0.013 to 0.586 µm in the normal dog (Carrington et al., 1987). Expressed as equivalents of lauryl laurate, lipid levels in canine tears ranged between 3.51 (±0.8) and 3.41 (±0.68) g/mm^2 eyelid margin surface

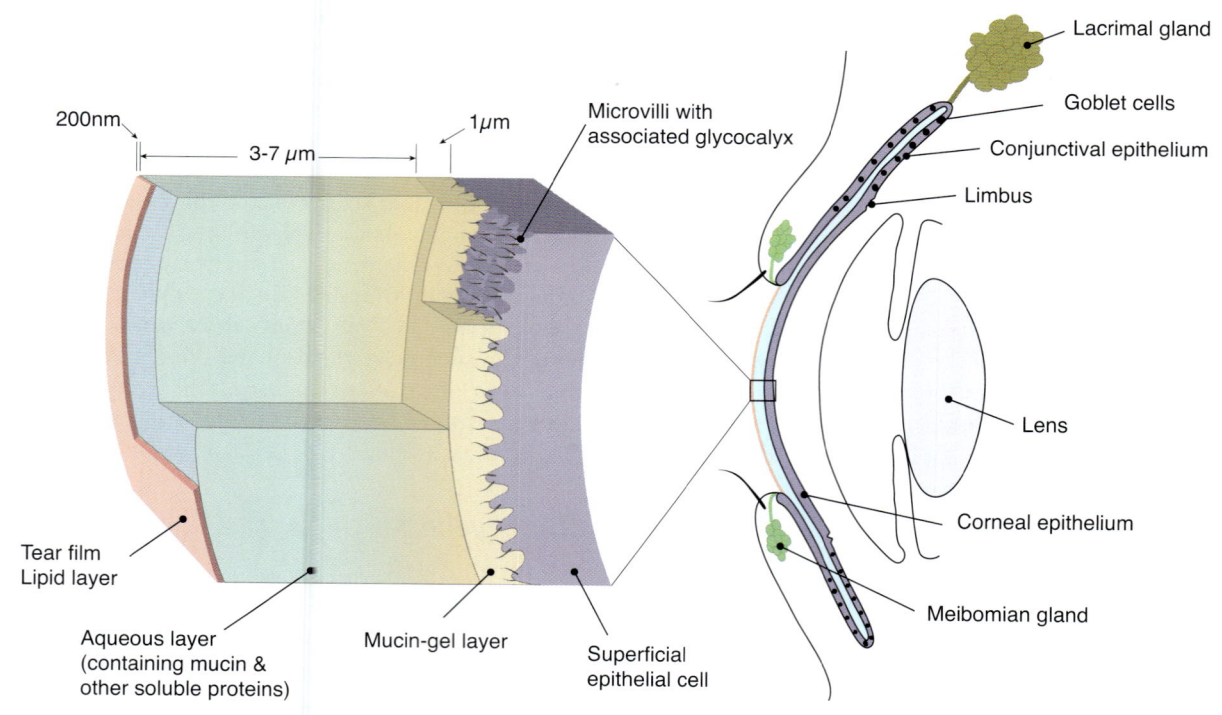

• **Fig. 21.32** The precorneal tear film of the dog has lipid, aqueous, and mucin constituents arising from different anatomic sites. The lipid layer arises from the Meibomian (tarsal) glands, the aqueous layer from the lacrimal gland and gland of the third eyelid, and the soluble mucin components from the goblet cells associated with the conjunctiva. (Permission from Yañez-Soto B, Mannis MJ, Schwab IR, et al: Interfacial phenomena and the ocular surface. *Ocular Surface* 12(3):178–201, 2014. https://doi.org/10.1016/j.jtos.2014.01.004.)

(Benz et al., 2008). The lipidome of the secretions of the canine tarsal gland has been reported (Butovich et al., 2012). In this report dogs and mice were found to share attributes with humans while rabbits were found to be vastly different. The aqueous layer is the major component of the precorneal tear film and is understood to mix readily with the subjacent mucous later. It is produced by the lacrimal gland and the superficial gland of the third eyelid and contains a variety of factors necessary for maintaining corneal health. Total protein content in the dog has been reported to range from 5.6 to 14.6 mg/mL (Sebbag et al., 2018), with another investigative team reporting canine tear protein values up to 54 mg/mL (Farias et al., 2013). Both publications report significant differences in the values obtained depending on the collection method used. The proteome of the canine tear film has also been recently reported with 125 distinct proteins being identified (Winiarczyk et al., 2015). It has been proposed that the proteome of the canine tear film could serve as a tool for identifying biomarkers of systemic cancer (de Freitas Campos et al., 2008). The aqueous layer also contains antimicrobial compounds such as transferrin and the immunoglobulin (Ig) A (the predominant immunoglobulin), IgG, and IgM. Lysozyme, another nonspecific antimicrobial compound, is absent in the dog.

Nerve growth factor is found in normal dog tears, corneal epithelium, third eyelid gland, and lacrimal gland at concentrations of 15.4 (±4.6) ng/mL, 33.5 (±12.3) ng/mL, 52.4 (±17.4) ng/mL, and 48.8 (±9.4) ng/mL, respectively (Woo et al., 2005). Although the concentration of nerve growth factor increases following corneal injury, it does not appear to facilitate wound healing in the dog. Additionally, the neuropeptide substance P has been measured in canine tears and has been implicated in the development of spontaneous chronic corneal epithelial defects in dogs (Murphy et al., 2001).

The deepest layer of the precorneal tear film is the glycoproteinaceous or mucous layer, which is intimately associated with the surface of the superficial squamous cells of the anterior corneal epithelium. This layer, a product of the conjunctival goblet cells, is thought to assist in adherence of the precorneal tear film to the corneal surface by decreasing the surface tension of the tears. A deficiency in the mucous layer will result in a decreased tear breakup time. The glycoprotein associated with mucus contains high levels of sialic acids, which mediate a variety of events including those associated with immunity (Corfield et al., 2005). Normal canine ocular mucin contains neutral O-linked glycans consisting mainly of di-, tri-, or tetrasaccharides terminating in α 1-2 fucose or α 1-3 N-acetylgalactosamines (Royle et al., 2008). Mucins with different subunit structures, one of which may be complexed with lipid, and two membrane-bound mucins have also been described (Hicks et al., 1997). A recent report found mucin 16 to be the most prevalent cell associated mucin transcript of the anterior corneal epithelium in dogs and humans (Leonard et al., 2016).

The lacrimal apparatus includes those structures responsible for the production, dispersal, and disposal of the tears. The lacrimal gland, tarsal glands, conjunctival goblet cells, and the superficial gland of the third eyelid contribute to the tear film. It has been established that the canine drainage system is very similar to its human equivalent (Hirt et al., 2012).

Lacrimal fluid flows across the cornea, aided by blinking, to the lacrimal puncta at the medial commissure of the lids and thence through the lacrimal canaliculi and nasolacrimal duct to the nasal vestibule. Three-dimensional reconstruction of the lacrimal drainage pathway in the dog based on CT imaging has been reported (Rached et al., 2011). The upper and lower canaliculi leave the eye 0.5 to 1 cm medially from the medial palpebral fissure. The canaliculi are lined by a multiple-layered squamous epithelium. External to the basement membrane there is a layer of connective tissue that is several millimeters thick. Bundles of skeletal muscle (from the orbicularis oculi muscle) are present up to 1 cm away from the duct. At the entrance to the lacrimal sac the epithelial layer changes into a two-layered columnar epithelium. The lacrimal sac and the nasolacrimal duct are lined by the same two-layered epithelium (Hirt et al., 2012).

A deficiency in the aqueous layer of the tear film resulting from a defect in the lacrimal apparatus may result in corneal lesions or chronic conditions such as keratoconjunctivitis sicca (dry eye) (Corfield et al., 2005; Ofri et al., 2009).

When exposed to a natural photoperiod, dogs exhibit significant circadian rhythms of tear production, which peaks during nocturnal hours (Giannetto et al., 2009; Piccione et al., 2009). This circadian rhythm disappears during periods of constant light but not during constant darkness (Piccione et al., 2009). Changes in the protein composition of the tear film may indicate the presence of systemic disease such as cancer.

Lacrimal Gland

The **lacrimal gland** (*glandula lacrimalis*) is a pink, oval, lobated gland that lies deep to the periorbita on the superiolateral aspect of the eyeball (Figs. 21.23 and 21.32). The gland is flattened between the eyeball and the orbital ligament and zygomatic process of the frontal bone (Zwingenberger et al., 2014). A shallow fossa for the lacrimal gland may be present in the orbital face of the frontal bone. A thin sheet of fascia separates the gland from the underlying dorsal and lateral rectus muscles. The shape of the lacrimal gland ranges from round, triangular, or oval to heart- or dumbbell-shaped. Some differences in breed have been reported for the dimensions of the lacrimal gland. In Beagles, the length and width of the lacrimal gland are significantly smaller than those in Pit Bull terriers and Pointer mixed dogs. In Pit Bull terriers, the lacrimal gland is significantly thicker than those in Beagles and Pointer mixed dogs (Park et al., 2016).

The seromucous secretion of the gland empties into the dorsolateral conjunctival fornix through three to five microscopic secretory ducts (Michel, 1955). Removal of the lacrimal gland results in only a minor decrease in tear production, probably as a result of a compensatory increase in production by the superficial gland of the third eyelid (Helper, 1970).

The lacrimal gland is innervated by the lacrimal nerve, a small branch of the ophthalmic nerve from the trigeminal nerve (Figs. 21.40 through 21.42). Parasympathetic postganglionic axons from the pterygopalatine ganglion enter the periorbita in orbital rami and are distributed to the gland with the lacrimal or zygomaticotemporal nerves. Parasympathomimetic drugs increase the rate of glandular secretion. Tear production can also be stimulated by the topical application of nerve growth factor (Coassin et al., 2005). The blood supply is derived from the muscular branches of the external ophthalmic artery (Fig. 21.43). The lacrimal vein drains the gland into the dorsal external ophthalmic vein (Fig. 21.45).

Superficial Gland of the Third Eyelid

The superficial gland of the third eyelid (*glandula superficialis plica semilunaris conjunctivae*) in the dog is an accessory lacrimal gland that normally produces a significant proportion of the aqueous component of the tear film (Helper et al., 1974). The gland surrounds the column of the cartilage of the third eyelid in the inferiomedial aspect of the eyeball (Fig. 21.31). The gland is mixed in the dog; both mucous and serous acini are seen microscopically. The secretions of this gland flow through numerous microscopic ductules into the conjunctival sac. By breed, pit bull terriers have significantly wider third eye lid glands compared to the pointer mixed-breed dogs (Park et al., 2016). The dimensional values of the canine gland of the third eyelid as measured by CT have been recently reported (Zwingenberger et al., 2014). There is no deep, lipid-producing (Harder) gland of the third eyelid in the dog.

Water channel protein, aquaporin isoform 5 (AQP5), is normally present in the lacrimal and third eyelid glands of the dog. AQP5 tends to show a stronger localization at the apical site of the membrane of acinar epithelial cells than in the membrane of ductal epithelial cells. However, AQP5 has not been detected by immunohistochemistry in dogs affected by keratoconjunctivitis sicca (KCS). This correlates with the deficiency in tear secretion in clinical cases of KCS (Terakado et al., 2012).

Conjunctiva

The soluble glycoprotein component of the tear film is produced mostly by the goblet cells of the conjunctivae. These cells are especially numerous in the regions of the fornices and contribute significantly to the tears. The soluble mucins as well as the cell-associated mucins play critical roles in the interfacial properties of the ocular surface as well as in tear film dynamics (Leonard et al., 2016; Yañez-Soto et al., 2014). The dog does not have isolated accessory lacrimal glands throughout the conjunctiva corresponding to the several types bearing eponyms in humans. The tarsal glands (see section on eyelids) produce the oily superficial layer of the tear film. Tears accumulate in the **lacrimal lake** (*lacus lacrimalis*), which is the shallow cleft between the third eyelid and inferior palpebral conjunctiva just lateral to the medial commissure. Blinking both facilitates tear secretion and spreads the tear film over the cornea. This action is essential to its health. Inability to close the lids, as a result of facial nerve lesions, allows the cornea to dry and results in marked pathologic alterations (neuroparalytic keratitis) (Bistner, 1978). The lacrimal fluid produced in excess of that which evaporates from the surface of the cornea drains into the nasal cavity through the nasolacrimal duct system.

Nasolacrimal Duct System

The outflow pathway of excess lacrimation includes the puncta, the lacrimal canaliculi, the lacrimal sac, and the nasolacrimal duct. The **lacrimal puncta** (*puncta lacrimalia*) are located on the deep surface of the superior and inferior lid margins 2 to 5 mm from the medial commissure (Fig. 21.30). The puncta are the oval openings of the **lacrimal canaliculi** (*canaliculi lacrimale*) and measure approximately 0.7 by 0.3 mm. The long axis of each punctum is parallel to the lid margin. The puncta are distinguished from the openings of the tarsal glands by their larger size and greater distance from the lid margin. In some dogs, one or both puncta may be smaller than normal or absent. Spilling of tears onto the face (epiphora) results.

The superior lacrimal canaliculus runs medially parallel to the lid margin for 3 to 7 mm from the superior punctum, and then turns ventrally medial to the commissure of the lids to enter the **lacrimal sac** (*saccus lacrimalis*) (see Fig. 21.30). The inferior lacrimal canaliculus arcs inferiomedially from its punctum to join the superior duct at the lacrimal sac. The canaliculi are easily cannulated if the instrument is directed medially, parallel to the lid margin. Radiopaque contrast material can be introduced into the nasolacrimal duct system through the canaliculi to outline the duct system radiographically (Fig. 21.32A and B) (Yakely & Alexander, 1971).

The lacrimal sac is the dilated origin of the nasolacrimal duct. It is not as prominent in the dog as in humans, leading some authors to conclude that it is not present (Yakely & Alexander, 1971). The sac occupies a depression (*fossa sacci lacrimalis*) in the center of the orbital surface of the lacrimal bone, medial and ventral to the medial commissure.

The **nasolacrimal duct** (*ductus nasolacrimalis*) forms an arch, which is concave dorsally as it passes rostrally from the lacrimal sac through the lacrimal canal of the lacrimal bone and maxilla (Fig. 21.33). Rostral to the conchal crest, the duct is no longer covered by bone but continues rostrally deep to the nasal mucosa on the nasal face of the maxilla. In approximately 50% of dogs, the nasolacrimal duct has two openings. At the level of the root of the canine tooth, there is an inconstant communication of the duct with the nasal extraocular muscles, and the palpebral muscles. The intraocular muscles are those that lie entirely internal to the sclera and act to regulate pupillary diameter and the shape of the lens. The extraocular muscles insert on the sclera and effect rotation and retraction of the eyeball as a whole. The palpebral muscle group includes a number of muscles of the lids and head that regulate the shape and position of the palpebral fissure.

Intraocular Muscles

The **dilator** and **sphincter muscles of the iris** and the **ciliary muscles** lie entirely within the eyeball (Figs. 21.12 and 21.14). They are composed of smooth muscle fibers. The iris musculature acts reflexly to regulate the amount of light that reaches the retina. The ciliary muscle accomplishes visual accommodation (focusing) by altering the tension of the zonular fibers and possibly by anterior-posterior translocation of the lens. These muscles are described in detail under the headings "Iris" and "Ciliary Body," of which they are integral parts.

Extraocular Muscles

The **extraocular muscles**, or *musculi bulbi*, are striated muscles: the dorsal, medial, ventral, and lateral rectus muscles; the dorsal and ventral oblique muscles; and the retractor bulbi muscle. The expression of myosin heavy chain type-2B is restricted to extraocular muscles such as the rectus lateralis and retractor bulbi muscles (Toniolo et al., 2007).

The extraocular muscles rotate the globe around three mutually perpendicular axes passing through the center of the globe (Fig. 21.34). The dorsal and ventral rectus muscles rotate the globe around a medial to lateral axis. The medial and lateral rectus muscles rotate the globe about a superior to inferior axis, and the oblique muscles rotate the eyeball around the axis bulbi. In addition, the eyeball can be retracted into the orbit along the optic axis by the retractor bulbi muscle as well as the recti muscles functioning as a group. Contraction of two or more muscles simultaneously accomplishes oblique movements. The dog is able to rotate the eye through approximately 90 degrees of arc in the dorsal plane and 60 degrees in a sagittal plane. The rotation produced by the oblique muscles is more limited, amounting to only approximately 30 degrees. The oblique muscles also help fix the eye against the posterior pull of the rectus muscles because the pull of their tendons includes an anterior vector. Classical proprioceptors such as Golgi tendon organs and muscle spindles are absent in the extraocular muscles of many mammals, including the dog (Maier et al., 1974). In the dog, the sense of proprioception in the extraocular muscles is recognized by palisade endings located at the proximal and distal muscle tendon junction (Rungaldier et al., 2009). Depending on the affected muscle, myositis with associated swelling may result in ventral, ventromedial, or medial strabismus (Allgoewer et al., 2000).

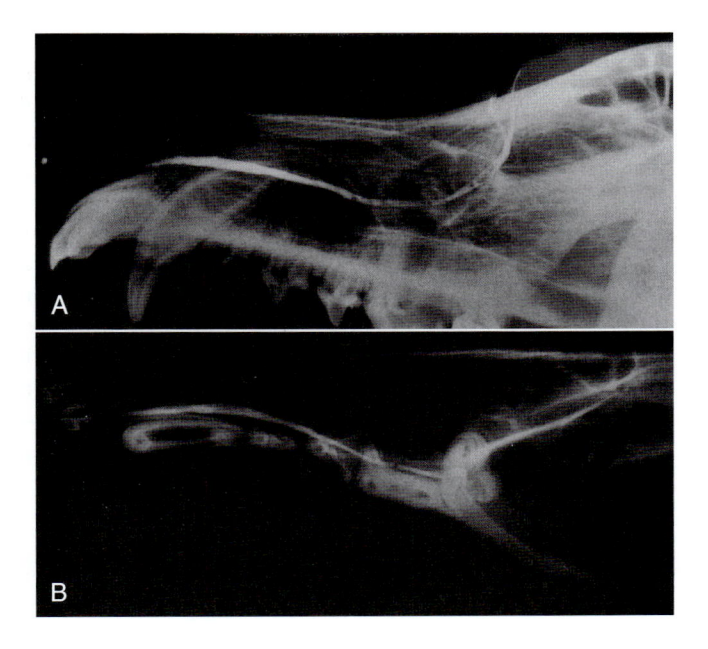

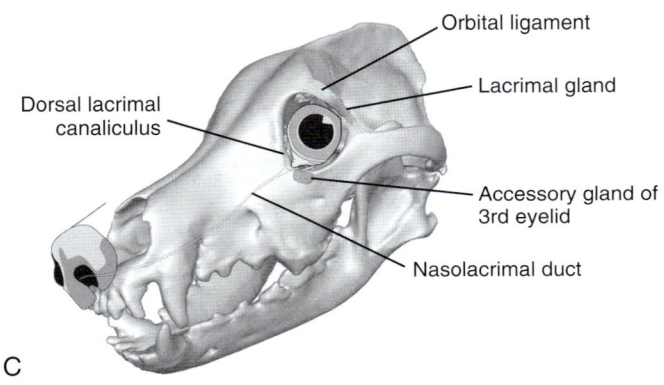

• **Fig. 21.33** **A**, Lateral radiograph showing the nasolacrimal duct. **B**, Dorsoventral radiograph showing the course of the nasolacrimal duct. **C**, Lacrimal gland, gland of the third eyelid and lacrimal drainage apparatus of the dog. (**B**, Courtesy of V. Rendano, Cornell University. **C**, Courtesy of John Doval and Dr. Allison Zwingenberger. Department of Veterinary Surgical and Radiological Sciences, School of Veterinary Medicine, University of California–Davis.)

cavity ventral to the ventral nasal concha (Michel, 1955). Rostrally the duct passes medial to the ventral lateral nasal cartilage and ends by opening onto the ventrolateral floor of the nasal vestibule ventral to the alar fold. The rostral opening cannot be visualized without a speculum in the living dog. In a recent report, the nasal opening of the duct was noted to have variable placement, and stenosis of the opening was observed in a number of dogs with insufficient drainage of tears (Strom et al., in press 2018).

The nasolacrimal duct is supplied by a small branch of the malar artery.

Muscles

The muscles important to the function of the visual apparatus constitute three groups: the intraocular muscles, the

892 CHAPTER 21 The Eye

• Fig. 21.34 Schema of motion produced by extraocular muscles.

The **m. retractor bulbi** is a striated muscle, derived from the lateral rectus that originates from the periosteum within the orbital fissure, lateral to the optic nerve (Figs. 21.34 through 21.37). The retractor bulbi passes laterally between the dorsal and lateral rectus muscles and divides into dorsal and ventral components that come to lie dorsal and ventral to the optic nerve. Each component again bifurcates, forming four flat fasciculi. These diverge as they run anteriorly deep to the rectus muscles to insert on the equator of the eyeball approximately 1 cm posterior to the corneoscleral junction. The fasciculi are very broad and thin at their insertions, and in some specimens, adjacent fasciculi nearly meet to form a complete muscular cone around the posterior aspect of the eyeball. The conical space between the diverging fasciculi of the retractor bulbi and the optic nerve is filled with intraperiorbital fat (see Fig. 21.25).

The primary action of the retractor bulbi muscle is to pull the eyeball deeper into the orbit (see Figs. 21.34 and 21.35). This displaces the base of the cartilage of the third

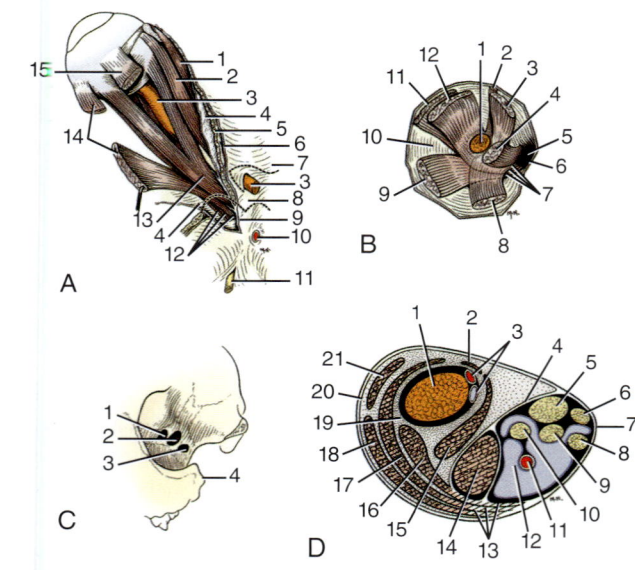

A, Dorsal aspect. (Dotted lines are internal borders of optic canal and orbital fissure.)
1. M. obliquus dorsalis
2. M. rectus medialis
3. Optic nerve
4. Periorbita
5. Frontal bone
6. Dura mater
7. Jugum of presphenoid
8. Rostral clinoid process
9. Orbital fissure
10. Internal carotid artery
11. Oculomotor nerve
12. Tendons of mm. rectus lateralis, rectus medialis, and rectus ventralis originating ventrally in orbital fissure
13. M. retractor bulbi
14. M. rectus lateralis
15. M. rectus dorsalis

B, Origin of extraocular muscles, rostral lateral aspect.
1. Optic nerve
2. M. levator palpebrae superioris
3. M. rectus dorsalis
4. M. retractor bulbi
5. Orbital fissure
6. Cut edge of periorbita
7. Tendons of mm. rectus lateralis, rectus medialis, and rectus ventralis originating ventrally in orbital fissure
8. M. rectus lateralis
9. M. rectus ventralis
10. Periorbita
11. M. obliquus dorsalis

12. M. rectus medialis
C, Foramina in caudal orbit.
1. Optic canal
2. Orbital fissure
3. Rostral alar foramen
4. Zygomatic arch (cut)
D, Schematic transection of structures within the apex of the periorbita, rostral aspect.
1. Optic nerve in optic canal
2. M. levator palpebrae superioris
3. Internal ophthalmic artery and vein
4. Cut edge of dura lining orbital fissure
5. Oculomotor nerve in orbital fissure
6. Trochlear nerve
7. Cut edge of periorbita (dura)

8. Frontal nerve (V)
9. Nasociliary nerve (V)
10. Abducent nerve
11. Anastomotic artery
12. Emissary vein of orbital fissure
13. Tendons of mm. rectus lateralis, rectus medialis, and rectus ventralis
14. M. retractor bulbi in orbital fissure
15. M. rectus dorsalis
16. M. rectus lateralis
17. M. rectus medialis
18. M. rectus ventralis
19. Intraperiorbital fat
20. Cut edge of periorbita
21. M. obliquus dorsalis

• Fig. 21.35 Schema of muscle attachments in orbital fissure and relationship of dura to periorbita. A, Dorsal aspect. B, Origin of extraocular muscles. C, Left orbit, rostrolateral aspect of caudal foramina. D, Schematic transection of structures within the apex of the periorbita.

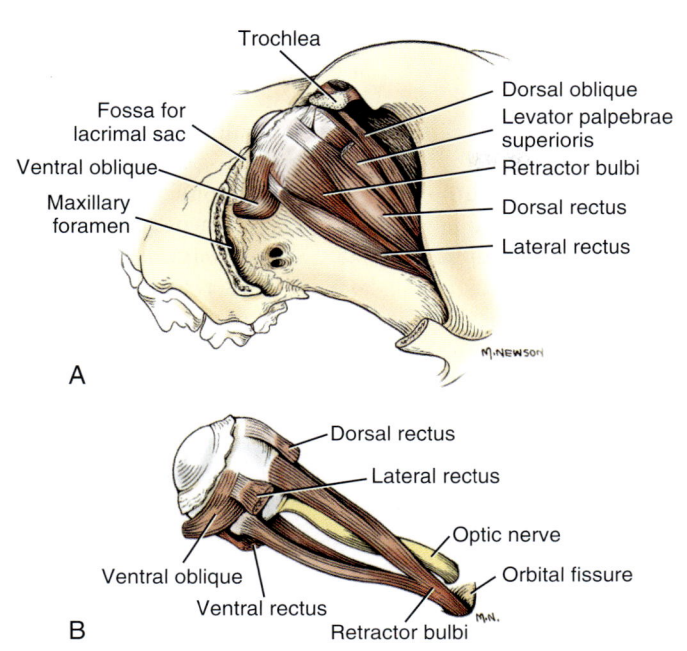

Fig. 21.36 Extrinsic muscles of the eye. **A**, Caudolateral aspect. (The eye is displaced slightly lateral.) **B**, The m. retractor bulbi, lateral aspect.

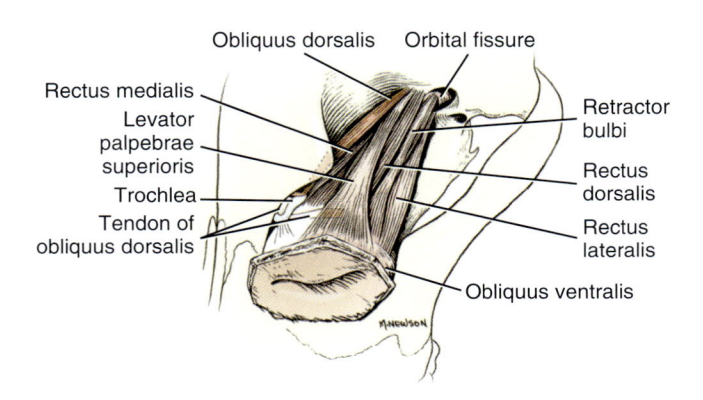

Fig. 21.37 Extrinsic muscles of the eye, dorsolateral aspect.

21.36). The dorsal rectus originates between the optic canal and the orbital fissure. The lateral, medial, and ventral recti originate ventral to the orbital fissure in order from dorsal to ventral. From their origin they diverge toward their insertions on the dorsal, lateral, medial, and ventral aspects of the eyeball. Over most of their course, the rectus muscles are deep to the periorbita and superficial to the fascicles of the retractor bulbi. Dorsally the m. levator palpebrae superioris is interposed between the dorsal rectus and the periorbita (Fig. 21.37).

The global and orbital layers of canine rectus muscles have different passive viscoelastic properties. The mean elastic modulus (stiffness) of the global layer is approximately 35% greater than the orbital layer, and the mean elastic modulus of both layers of dog rectus muscles is significantly greater than that of fast- and slow-twitch skeletal muscles (Reiser et al., 2005). In the same regard, myosin heavy chain isoform expression patterns differ between and along global and orbital layers and among individual fibers of the canine rectus muscles. These variations on gene expression can be used to quantitatively assess differences in patterns during pathophysiological states (Bicer & Reiser, 2009). The global and orbital layers are predominantly fast, as reflected in the abundant expression of multiple fast-type MHC isoforms. Regarding tropomyosin and troponin T isoform composition of global and orbital fibers, an elaborate diversity in contractile protein isoform expression in canine extraocular muscle fibers suggests that major differences in calcium-activation properties exist among these fibers based on isoform expression patterns (Bicer & Reiser, 2013).

The muscle bellies of the rectus muscles are oval in transverse section, measuring approximately 9 mm wide by 2 mm thick at their broadest point. The medial rectus is slightly larger than the other recti, which are comparable in size. At approximately the equator of the globe, the muscles form flat tendons that insert on the sclera anterior to the insertion of the m. retractor bulbi, 3 to 7 mm posterior to the corneoscleral junction. Anterior to the equator of the lens, the dorsal rectus passes dorsal to the tendon of insertion of the dorsal oblique muscle (Figs. 21.5A and 21.36). The tendon of the ventral rectus passes deep to the ventral oblique muscle. The actual distal locations of insertion of the tendons of the extraocular muscles vary among breeds at least perinatally. Klećkowska et al. (2006) found that the tendons of the dorsal, ventral, and lateral recti muscles of American Staffordshire terriers insert further from the limbus than those of the dogs of Bordeaux. On the other hand, the muscular funiculi of the retractor bulbi of the dogs of Bordeaux were overall more posteriorly attached than those of the American Staffordshire terriers.

The action of the rectus muscles has been described (Fig. 21.34). The oculomotor nerve is motor to the dorsal, medial, and ventral recti. The abducent nerve innervates the lateral rectus. The rectus muscles are supplied by the muscular branches of the external ophthalmic artery. Venous return is by means of muscular branches of the external ophthalmic veins.

eyelid with its encircling gland, causing the free edge of the third eyelid to sweep across the cornea (see section on the third eyelid). The retractor bulbi may also play a part in the rotatory movements of the eye. Watrous and Olmsted (1941) reported that following excision of all other extrinsic muscles in the dog, the retractor bulbi was eventually capable of moving the eye in all directions. Blood supply to the retractor muscle is derived from the muscular branches of the external ophthalmic artery. The abducent nerve supplies general somatic efferent axons to the retractor muscle. It has also been reported that the ventral ramus of the oculomotor nerve sends branches that partially supply two fasciculi of the retractor bulbi muscle of the dog (Shimokawa et al., 2002).

The four **mm. recti** are named for the position of their insertion on the globe. They originate in proximity to one another at the apex of the periorbital cone (Figs. 21.35 and

The ***m. obliquus dorsalis*** arises at the dorsomedial margin of the optic canal closely associated with the origin of the other extraocular muscles (Fig. 21.35). It runs anteriorly within the periorbita between the dorsal and medial recti. At approximately the posterior pole of the eyeball, the muscle gives rise to a thin, round tendon that passes over a small cartilaginous trochlea located at the phylogenetic origin of the muscle on the medial wall of the orbit near the medial angle of the eye (Fig. 21.36).

The **trochlea** is a small, oval plate of hyaline cartilage in the periorbita. It is firmly anchored to the medial orbital wall by three ligamentous thickenings of the periorbita. The longest of these runs from the anterior end of the trochlea to the periosteum at the medial commissure of the eyelids. A short ligament anchors the trochlea to the dorsal orbital margin, and a third runs from the posterior aspect to the periosteum of the zygomatic process of the frontal bone.

The tendon of the dorsal oblique muscle runs through a groove in the trochlea formed by a prominence on its medial face near the anterior end. A synovial sheath (*vagina synovialis m. obliqui dorsalis*) is present at this point. As the tendon passes over the trochlea, it turns through an angle of approximately 135 degrees to the muscle belly to run obliquely caudodorsolaterally to its insertion on the sclera deep to the tendon of the dorsal rectus muscle (Fig. 21.36A).

The dorsal oblique muscle consists of central and peripheral layers made up of type I (dark) and type 2 (light) muscle fibers. The mean total area of the dorsal oblique muscle ($N = 6$) is 9.95 (±4.01) mm^2 of which 44.8% (±4.4) corresponds to the central layer (Vivo et al., 2004). The dorsal oblique muscle is the only structure innervated by the fourth cranial nerve (n. trochlearis).

The ***m. obliquus ventralis*** is the only extraocular muscle that arises from a site remote from the apex of the orbit (Fig. 21.36A). The ventral oblique originates from a small depression in the palatine bone near the junction of the palatomaxillary and palatolacrimal sutures. In prepared skulls this site may appear as a foramen because the attachment plate is thin and easily lost. The muscle courses dorsolaterally, passing ventral to the insertion of the ventral rectus. It is fusiform in shape and roughly circular in transverse section. At the ventrolateral aspect of the orbit, it gives rise to two short tendons. The shorter tendon inserts deep to the insertion of the lateral rectus. The superficial portion passes lateral to the lateral rectus to insert on the superiolateral aspect of the eyeball (Figs. 21.5 and 21.36B). The ventral oblique is supplied by branches of the malar artery. The muscle is innervated by the oculomotor nerve.

Christiansen et al. (1992) studied the effect of cranial nerve III denervation on the canine extraocular musculature. This study suggested a variable response to denervation depending on the muscle fiber type and influenced by whether the individual muscle fibers were singly or multiply innervated. They found significant, persistent atrophy of the singly innervated fibers of extraocular muscle. The multiinnervated fibers were predominantly spared from denervation atrophy. These results suggest a relative neurotrophic independence of multiinnervated fibers in canine extraocular muscle.

Palpebral

The muscles that alter the size or position of the palpebral fissure include the m. orbicularis oculi, the m. levator palpebrae superioris, m. levator anguli oculi medialis, m. retractor anguli oculi lateralis, mm. tarsalis inferior et superior, and the pars palpebralis of the m. sphincter colli profundus (Figs. 21.37 to 21.39).

The ***m. orbicularis oculi*** is the most important muscle that acts to close the palpebral fissure. It is composed of two parts: the pars orbitalis and the pars palpebralis. The division between the parts is not distinct in the dog. The *pars palpebralis* is composed of fibers that run in the substance of the lids themselves. These fibers originate from the medial palpebral ligament, encircle the palpebral fissure, and insert again on the ligament. The muscle is wedge-shaped in transverse section, tapering toward the lid margin. Fibers of the pars palpebralis lie anterior to the tarsus and tarsal glands and closely approach the lid margin; some fibers are found almost to the level of the opening of the tarsal glands (Fig. 21.30). The pars palpebralis is better developed in the superior lid.

The *pars orbitalis* of the orbicularis oculi surrounds the pars palpebralis. It consists of dorsal and ventral components that originate from the medial palpebral ligament and follow the curve of the orbital margin laterally. At the lateral commissure of the lids, some of the peripheral fibers of the ventral component fan out caudally and dorsally on the superficial surface of the frontalis muscle (Figs. 21.38 and 21.39). Fibers of the dorsal pars orbitalis decussate with the ventral fibers caudal to the lateral commissure, forming the lateral **palpebral raphe** (*raphe palpebralis lateralis*). No pars lacrimalis could be identified in the dog.

The orbicularis oculi muscle exerts a sphincterlike action to close the palpebral fissure. The medial and lateral palpebral ligaments and the retractor anguli oculi lateralis muscle stabilize the commissures of the lids and prevent the fissure from becoming circular when the muscle contracts. Constant corneal irritation results in hypertrophy of the orbicularis oculi muscle, which, if pronounced, will actually roll the haired anterior surface of the lid posteriorly against the cornea (spastic entropion). Motor innervation is supplied by the palpebral branches of the auriculopalpebral nerve, a branch of the facial nerve. A prominent sign of facial nerve palsy is therefore the inability to close the palpebral fissure (de Lahunta, 1983). Blood supply to the orbicularis oculi is derived from the malar artery medially and the superior and inferior lateral palpebral arteries laterally.

The ***m. levator palpebrae superioris*** (Fig. 21.37) is the most important muscle that acts to retract the superior eyelid. The muscle originates deep within the orbit, dorsal to the optic canal between the origins of the dorsal rectus and dorsal oblique muscles. The levator courses rostrally deep to the periorbita on the dorsomedial aspect of the

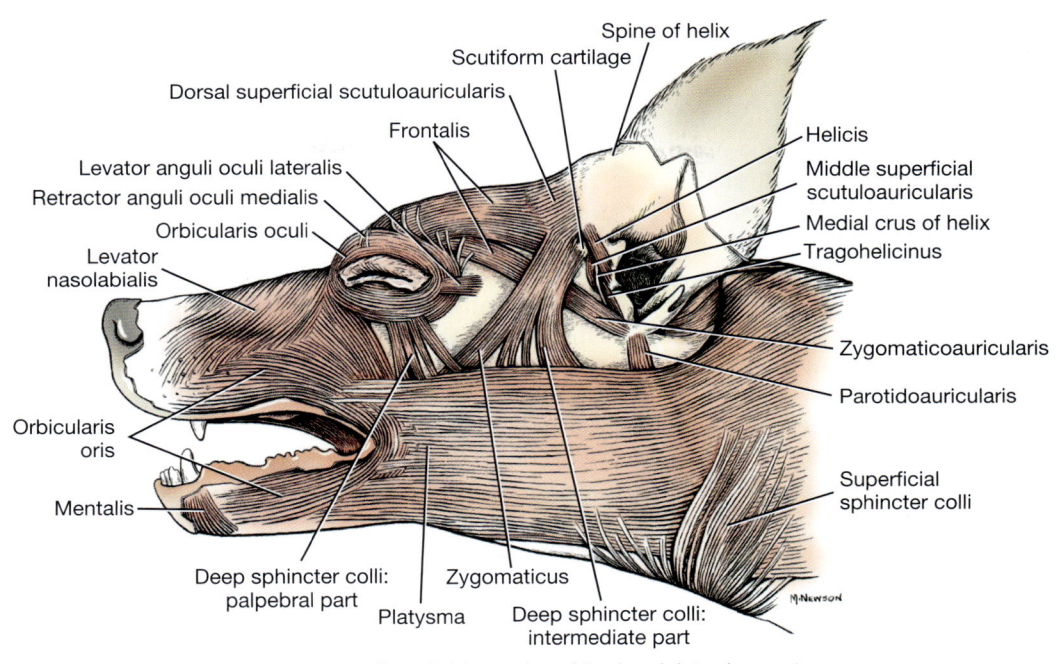

• **Fig. 21.38** Superficial muscles of the head, lateral aspect.

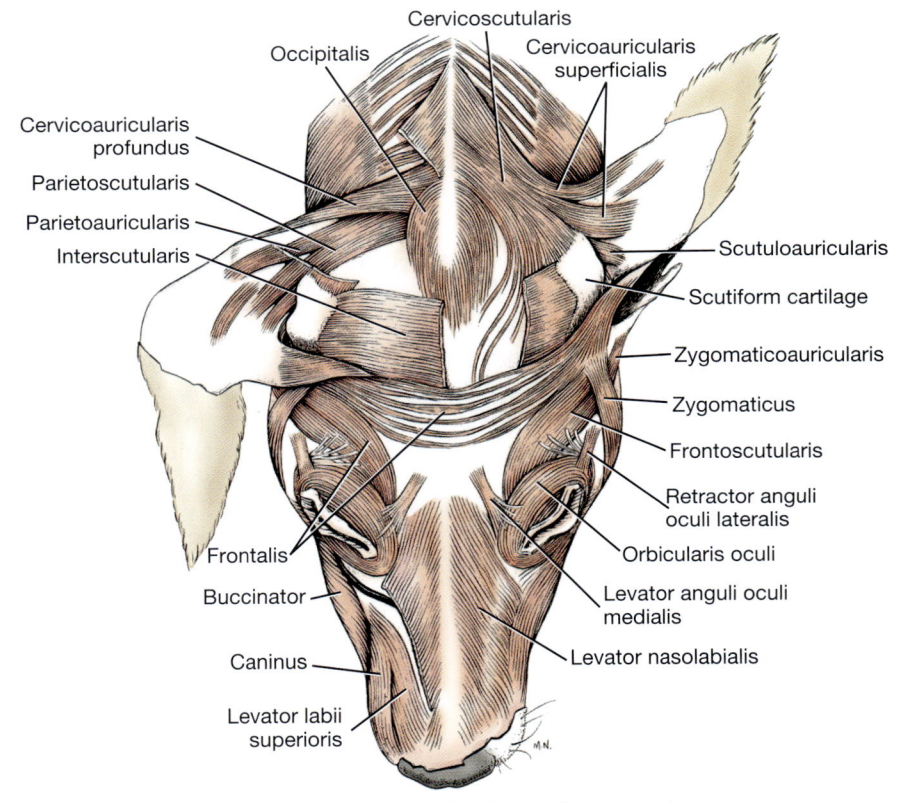

• **Fig. 21.39** Muscles of the head, dorsal aspect.

dorsal rectus muscle toward its insertion in the superior eyelid. The muscle becomes progressively wider and flatter anteriorly. Anterior to the equator of the eyeball, a broad aponeurosis continues the muscle into the superior lid, where it inserts on the palpebral connective tissue among the fibers of the orbicularis oculi muscle. The m. levator palpebrae superioris is innervated by the oculomotor nerve. Blood is supplied by the muscular branches of the external ophthalmic artery.

The ***m. retractor anguli oculi lateralis*** is a small, flat muscle that arises from the temporal fascia near the temporozygomatic suture (Figs. 21.38 and 21.39). The muscle is parallel and superficial to the lateral palpebral ligament. It passes rostrally superficial to the orbital part of the orbicularis oculi muscle and inserts by blending with fascicles of the palpebral part at the lateral commissure of the lid. The lateral retractor draws the lateral canthus posteriorly and thus has some action in closing the palpebral fissure. The retractor is innervated by the zygomatic branch of the auriculopalpebral nerve, and is supplied by branches of the lateral ventral palpebral artery.

Superior and inferior tarsal muscles, consisting of smooth muscle fibers, are derived from the periorbital orbitalis muscle and help maintain lid position. These muscles are innervated by sympathetic nerves. One of the signs of ocular sympathetic denervation (Horner syndrome) is the narrowing of the palpebral fissure.

The **pars palpebralis** of the *m. sphincter colli profundus* acts as a depressor of the inferior lid (Fig. 21.38). It consists of several delicate straps of muscle that originate near the ventral midline. These course dorsally caudal to the angle of the mouth to insert on the inferior tarsus. The ventral portion of these muscular straps is deep to the platysma. The dorsal portion is subcutaneous and closely applied to the skin. The muscle is innervated by the buccal branches of the facial nerve.

Innervation

The eye and its adnexa are innervated by cranial nerves II, III, IV, V, VI, and VII (see Chapter 19 on cranial nerves).

Optic Nerve

The **optic nerve** (*n. opticus*), or cranial nerve II, is considered as a component of the special somatic afferent system but it is not a nerve based on its structure. It is equivalent to a central nervous system tract because the ganglion cell layer of the retina is a development of the optic vesicle from the neural tube. The axons from the neuronal cell bodies in the ganglion cell layer of the retina invade the hollow stalk of the original neuroectodermal outpouching that forms the optic vesicle. Centripetal growth of the ganglion cell axons begins at approximately day 32 of gestation and is not completed until after birth.

Because the eye forms as an outgrowth of the brainstem (see section on development), the myelin of the optic nerve is of the central nervous system type, being formed by oligodendrocytes. Ganglion cell axons are unmyelinated in the nerve fiber layer of the retina. They become myelinated as they turn from the nerve fiber layer into the optic nerve. The intraocular myelinated portion is the white or gray optic disc seen grossly. Myelin may extend a variable distance from the optic nerve head onto the retina, giving the disc a large and ragged appearance. The size and shape of the optic disc varies widely among dogs (see section on the retina).

The optic nerve is surrounded by outer and inner sheaths (*vagina externa et vagina interna n. optici*), which are continuations of the dura mater, and the arachnoid and pia mater of the brain, respectively. The space within the vagina interna (between the arachnoid and pia) is continuous with the intracranial subarachnoid space and contains cerebrospinal fluid, and a linear relationship between pressure in the cerebrospinal fluid and optic nerve subarachnoid space has been demonstrated (Morgan et al., 1995). This space serves as a conduit for spread of infection between the eyeball and the brain. Optic neuritis is a form of encephalitis. The ciliary vessels and nerves are closely applied to the outer surface of the external sheath. Radicles of the internal ophthalmic and ciliary vessels supply the intraorbital portion of the optic nerve.

Brooks and colleagues (1995) reported a mean ($N = 4$) of 24,610 (±8791) myelinated axons (range 16,035 to 37,246) representing 16.6% of the total axons in the optic nerve. The mean total area of the individual axons per optic nerve was 43,466 (±10,807) μm^2 (range 38,081 to 59,267). This was estimated to represent a mean axonal diameter of 1.49 μm (range 0.4 to 23). Axons greater than 2 μm in diameter represented approximately 12.7% of axonal optic nerve fibers. The mean cross-sectional area of the entire optic nerve was 2.93 (±0.81) mm^2 (range 2.03 to 3.99). The total number of optic nerve axons for the normal dog was estimated to be 148,303 (±58,865) (range 95,755 to 232,690). Overall, the axon density was 51,725 axons/mm^2.

Using MRI, Boroffka et al. (2008) reported the following mean measurement of the optic nerve and related structures ($N = 5$): optic disk width 5.2 (±0.17) mm (range 5 to 5.5), intraorbital diameter of the optic nerve sheath complex 3.7 (±0.27) mm (range 3.6 to 3.8), optic nerve 1.7 (±0.06) mm (range 1.6 to 1.8), intracanalicular and intracranial diameter of the optic nerve 2.2 (±0.15) mm (range 2 to 2.5), optic chiasm height 2.1 (±0.08) mm (range 2.1 to 2.4), and optic chiasm width 4.8 (±0.16) mm (range 4.4 to 5).

The optic nerve follows an undulating course from its origin lateral and inferior to the posterior pole of the eyeball to the optic canal of the presphenoid bone. The nerve traverses the optic canal to the rostroventral floor of the middle cranial fossa, where fibers are exchanged with the opposing optic nerve at the **optic chiasm**. In the dog, approximately 75% of the optic nerve axons cross to join the contralateral optic tract caudal to the chiasm (de Lahunta & Cummings, 1967). The crossing axons are derived from the central and medial retinal areas; axons from the lateral retina join the ipsilateral optic tract (Fig. 21.15). Abnormal eye movements (pendular nystagmus) are observed in dogs with congenital mutations involving absent or malformed optic chiasms (Dell'Osso et al., 1998).

Each optic nerve is composed of approximately 150,000 axons, all of which are myelinated (Bruesch & Arey, 1942). There is a correlation between the size of the eyeball and the number of axons, but larger eyes have fewer axons relative to retinal surface area (Arey et al., 1942).

In humans and cats, centrifugal axons, as well as the centripetal ganglion cell axons, have been identified in the optic nerve. It is probable that centrifugal axons also occur in the dog. Their function has not yet been elucidated.

Within the orbit, the optic nerve occupies the center of the cone formed by the extraocular muscles. A well-developed intraperiorbital fat body lies between the nerve and the muscle cone.

The optic nerve is longer than the straight-line distance from the posterior pole of the eyeball to the optic canal of the presphenoid bone to allow for the rotation of the eyeball. The degree of undulation in the nerve depends on the position of the eyeball and the degree of retraction or protrusion. In dolichocephalic and mesaticephalic dogs, the eyeball can be almost completely retracted into the orbit. In the dog, the optic nerve is sufficiently long that proptosis can occur without rupture of the nerve.

Oculomotor Nerve

The **oculomotor nerve** (*n. oculomotorius*), or cranial nerve III, as its name implies, is the primary general somatic efferent innervation to the muscles of the eye. The oculomotor nerve is motor to the dorsal, medial, and ventral rectus muscles, the ventral oblique, and the levator palpebrae superioris muscle. It also contains parasympathetic preganglionic general visceral efferent axons that synapse in the ciliary ganglion (Figs. 21.15 and 21.40). The mean diameter of myelinated and unmyelinated fibers in the oculomotor nerve ($N = 6$) is 10.23 (±0.68) μm and 0.43 (±0.21) μm, respectively (Vivo et al., 2006). Postganglionic axons from the ciliary ganglion innervate the m. sphincter pupillae of the iris and the ciliary muscle. The parasympathetic axons are located medially at the origin of the nerve and, as such, are vulnerable to pressure damage when there is compression by a neoplasm in the middle cranial fossa. This causes a dilated pupil (mydriasis) prior to strabismus or ptosis.

The oculomotor nerve first becomes visible grossly where it leaves the ventral aspect of the mesencephalon on the medial aspect of the crus cerebri. The nerve runs laterally a short distance, then turns rostrally to pass beside the hypophysial stalk on the dorsal surface of the cavernous sinus, which it follows rostrally a short distance. It leaves the cranial cavity through the orbital fissure. Within the orbit the nerve divides into a small dorsal and larger ventral branch. The dorsal branch innervates the dorsal rectus and levator palpebrae muscles. The ventral ramus travels rostrally deep to the lateral rectus, sending branches to the medial and ventral rectus and to the ventral oblique. A short branch containing the parasympathetic axons enters the **ciliary ganglion**. The ganglion is located midway between the eyeball and the orbital fissure, closely applied to the ventrolateral surface of the optic nerve (Hara et al., 1982). **Short ciliary nerves** (*nn. ciliares breves*) leave the rostral surface of the ganglion and are distributed to the eyeball. The ciliary nerves demonstrate intense cholinergic activity (Hara et al., 1982). A communicating branch from the ganglion often joins the nasociliary nerve or long ciliary nerve (Fig. 21.40). Lesions of the oculomotor nerve result in a ventrolateral strabismus because of the unopposed tension in the lateral rectus. The pupil is dilated and there

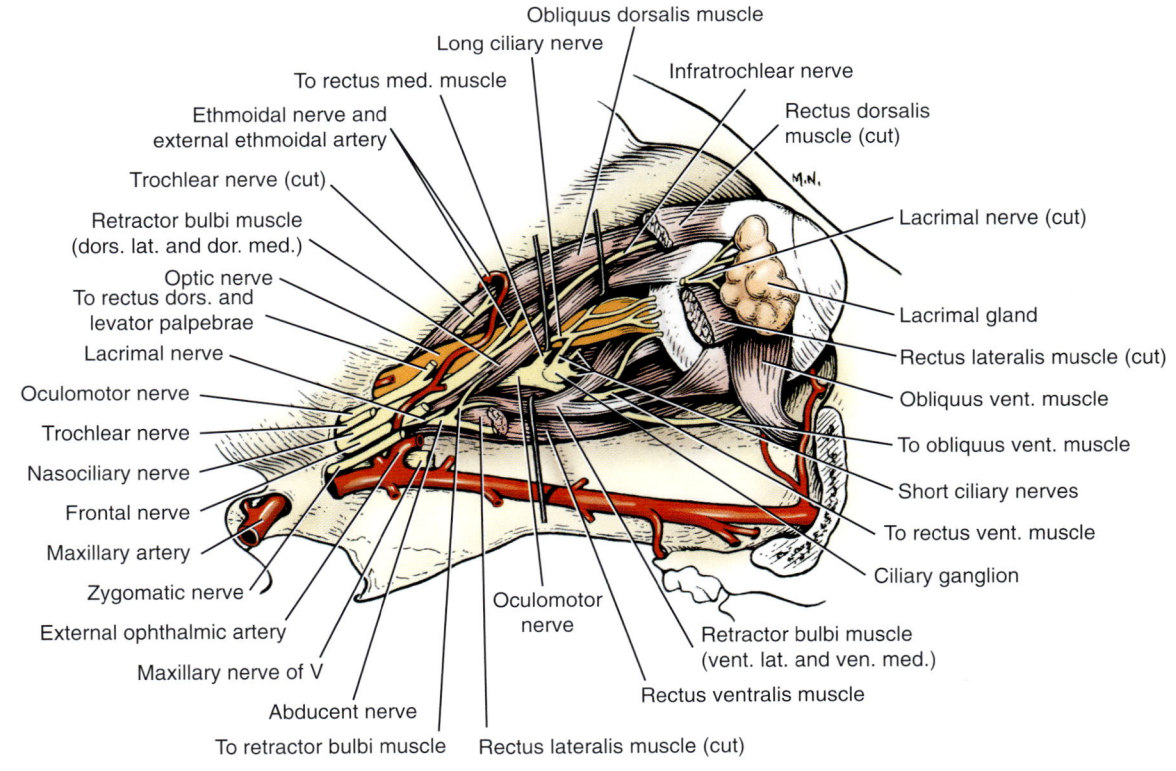

• **Fig. 21.40** Nerves of the eye and orbit, lateral aspect.

is ptosis caused by paralysis of the levator palpebrae superioris muscle.

Trochlear Nerve

The **trochlear nerve** (*n. trochlearis*, or cranial nerve IV, is unique among the cranial nerves in that it leaves the dorsal surface of the brainstem. It is the smallest of the cranial nerves and difficult to preserve in anatomic preparations. The mean diameter of myelinated and unmyelinated fibers in the trochlear nerve ($N = 6$) is 10.53 (±0.55) μm and 0.33 (±0.04) μm, respectively (Vivo et al., 2006). In adult Beagles, the average number of myelinated and unmyelinated fibers is 1476 (±260.71) and 284 (±101.82), respectively (Vivo et al., 2012). Trochlear nerve axons course dorsocaudally from their nuclear neuronal cell bodies to leave the dorsal surface of the mesencephalon immediately caudal to the caudal colliculus. The axons cross in the rostral medullary velum. It is the only nerve in the body in which all axons supply muscles on the contralateral side of the body (i.e., axons from cell bodies on the left side decussate in the rostral medullary velum and supply motor units on the right side of the body). The nerves arc ventrally between the cerebrum and cerebellum along the tentorium cerebelli and spine of the petrous part of the temporal bone. The nerve reaches the orbit by passing through the orbital fissure lateral to the oculomotor nerve (see Fig. 21.41). On emerging from the fissure, the nerve turns dorsomedially to enter the dorsal oblique muscle, the only structure it innervates.

The strabismus caused by a lesion in the trochlear nerve would not be visible on external examination of the eyeball.

Ophthalmoscopic examination would show a lateral deviation of the superior retinal vein indicating extorsion of the eyeball from the unopposed tension in the ventral oblique muscle.

Trigeminal Nerve

The eye and orbit are richly supplied by branches of the **trigeminal nerve** (*n. trigeminus*), or cranial nerve V. Although the nerve contains both general somatic afferent and somatic efferent axons, all of the axons distributed to the eye are general somatic afferent in nature.

The trigeminal nerve is the largest of the cranial nerves. The nerve leaves the brain at the juncture of the pons and trapezoid body. It passes through a canal in the rostral part of the petrous portion of the temporal bone. Here the **trigeminal ganglion** rests in the *cavum trigeminale* of the dura mater. The ganglion contains the cell bodies of the general somatic afferent neurons of the trigeminal nerve. Immediately distal to the ganglion the nerve divides into its three major divisions, the ophthalmic, the maxillary, and the mandibular nerves (Fig. 21.41). The ophthalmic nerve is the principal sensory innervation of the eye and orbit. The ophthalmic nerve also mediates the oculorespiratory cardiac reflex in response to manual pressure on the eye (Joffe & Gay, 1966). Branches of the maxillary nerve innervate a part of the superficial structure of the eyelids. The mandibular

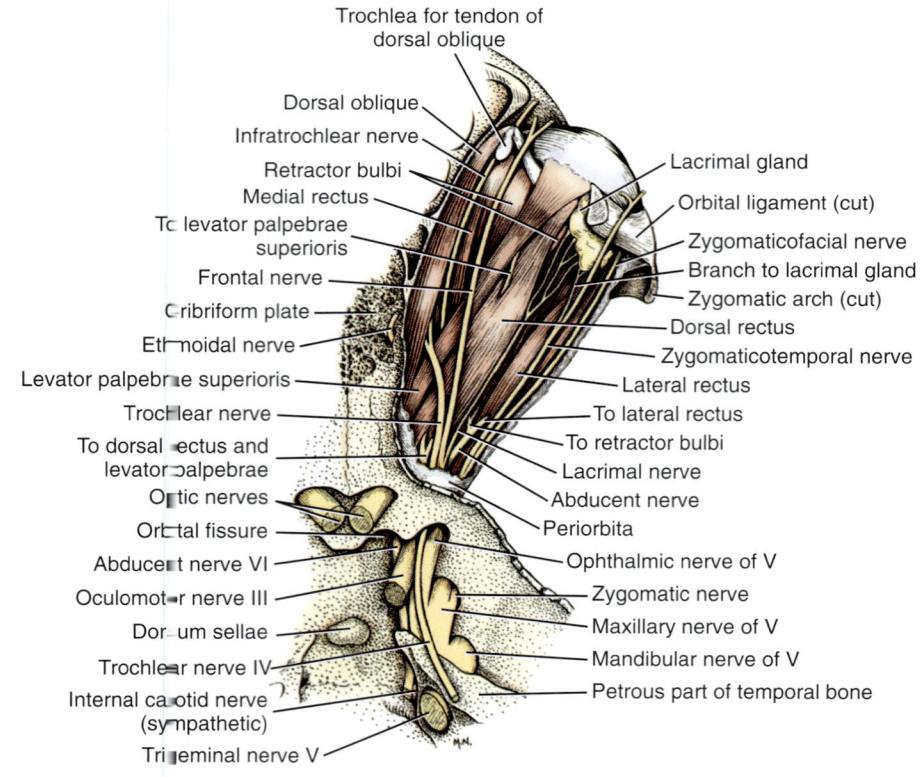

• **Fig. 21.41** Schema of the optic, oculomotor, trochlear, trigeminal (ophthalmic branch), and abducent nerves, dorsal aspect.

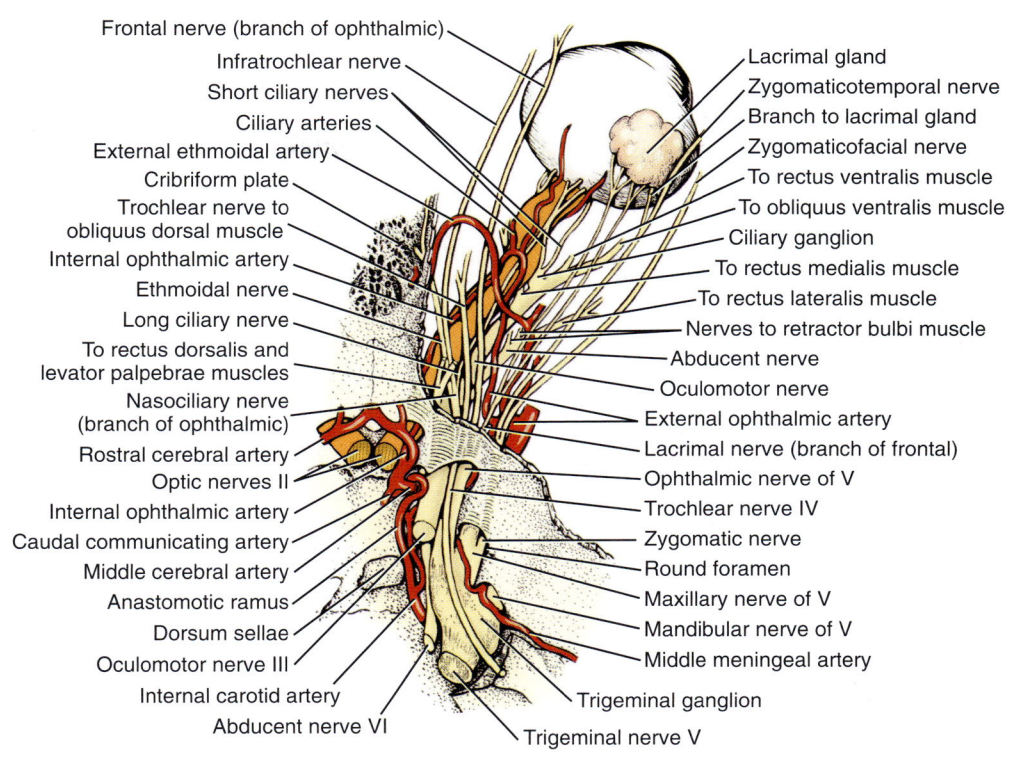

Fig. 21.42 Superficial distribution of the nerves of the eye, dorsal aspect.

nerve innervates structures of the ventral face and does not play a role in the innervation of ocular structures.

Ophthalmic Nerve

The **ophthalmic nerve** (*n. ophthalmicus*) arises from the rostromedial aspect of the trigeminal ganglion and arcs rostromedially into the orbital fissure to join cranial nerves III, IV, and VI. Sympathetic postganglionic axons from the internal carotid plexus join the ophthalmic nerve at its origin. Within, or immediately rostral to, the orbital fissure, the ophthalmic nerve divides into three branches, the frontal, lacrimal, and nasociliary nerves (Figs. 21.41 and 21.42).

The **frontal nerve** (*n. frontalis*) is a small nerve that is sensory to most of the skin of the superior eyelid and medially to the dorsal midline (Whalen & Kitchell, 1983). From the orbital fissure it passes rostrodorsally between the periorbita and dorsal rectus muscles to the superior lid (Fig. 21.42).

The **lacrimal nerve** (*n. lacrimalis*) is a very small branch of the ophthalmic nerve that travels along the lateral edge of the dorsal rectus to innervate the lacrimal gland (Fig. 21.42). Diesem (1975) found the lacrimal nerve occasionally originating from the maxillary nerve. He was also able to trace branches of the lacrimal, presumably sensory, to the lateral portion of the superior eyelid. The lacrimal nerve receives orbital branches from the pterygopalatine ganglion and supplies these parasympathetic postganglionic axons to the lacrimal gland.

The **nasociliary nerve** (*n. nasociliaris*) continues the ophthalmic into the orbit. It passes rostromedially between the dorsal and ventral rami of the oculomotor nerve to the dorsal surface of the optic nerve. Here it divides into the long ciliary nerves and the infratrochlear and ethmoidal nerves.

The **long ciliary nerves** (*nn. ciliares longi*) continue rostrally closely applied to the optic nerve. There are variable communications with the short ciliary nerves and a communicating branch to the ciliary ganglion is usually present (*ramus communicans cum ganglio ciliari*). The long and short ciliary nerves enter the globe adjacent to the optic nerve. According to Prince et al. (1960), the ciliary nerves continue anteriorly in the suprachoroidea, supplying sensory innervation to the choroid, ciliary body, iris, cornea, and bulbar conjunctiva. Axons enter the cornea at the limbus throughout its circumference and run toward the center, branching dichotomously. They may be visualized in the live dog with the biomicroscope (Martin, 1969). The sensory innervation of the cornea apparently exerts a trophic influence essential to its normal state (see Cornea). Sympathetic postganglionic axons in the long ciliary nerves are motor to the dilator muscle of the pupil.

The **infratrochlear nerve** (*n. infratrochlearis*) passes rostrodorsally along the medial edge of the dorsal rectus (Fig. 21.41). The nerve passes ventral to the trochlea, as its name implies, and ramifies in the tissues and skin associated with the medial commissure of the lids (Whalen & Kitchell, 1983).

The **ethmoidal nerve** (*n. ethmoidalis*) accompanies the external ethmoidal artery as it curves rostrally and medially dorsal to the extraocular muscles to leave the orbit through an ethmoidal foramen. It innervates part of the nasal mucosa and skin of the muzzle.

Maxillary Nerve

The **zygomatic nerve** (*n. zygomaticus*), a branch of the maxillary nerve, may enter the orbit either through the rostral alar foramen with the maxillary nerve or through a separate foramen (McClure, 1960). The nerve enters the periorbita at its apex and divides into the zygomaticofacial and zygomaticotemporal nerves (see Fig. 21.42). The **zygomaticotemporal nerve** courses rostrodorsally deep to the lateral aspect of the periorbita to the region of the orbital ligament, where it ramifies in the lateral superior eyelid and skin over the temporalis muscle to reach the dorsal midline (Whalen & Kitchell, 1983). As the nerve passes the lacrimal gland, branches may communicate with the lacrimal nerve, possibly supplying it with parasympathetic innervation derived from the pterygopalatine ganglion (see Fig. 21.40).

The **zygomaticofacial nerve** is ventral to the zygomaticotemporal and parallel to it over most of its course within the periorbita (see Fig. 21.42). Near the orbital margin it turns ventrally and ramifies in the inferior eyelid and the skin overlying the zygomatic arch (Whalen & Kitchell, 1983).

Abducent Nerve

The **abducent nerve** (*n. abducens*), or cranial nerve VI, supplies general somatic efferent axons to the lateral rectus and retractor bulbi muscles. The neuronal cell bodies are located in the rostrodorsal medulla adjacent to the midline. The abducent axons pass ventral to emerge through the trapezoid body immediately lateral to the pyramids of the medulla. The mean diameter of myelinated and unmyelinated fibers in the abducent nerve ($N = 6$) is and 10.45 (± 1.27) µm and 0.47 (± 0.09) µm, respectively (Vivo et al., 2006). The nerve runs rostrally in the subarachnoid space medial to the trigeminal ganglion and leaves the cranial cavity through the orbital fissure, closely applied to its medial wall (Figs. 21.40 and 21.41). One to two centimeters rostral to the orbital fissure, the abducent nerve gives a branch to the retractor bulbi, which further divides to supply the four fasciculi of the muscle. The abducent continues rostrally and laterally to reach the dorsal surface of the lateral rectus muscle. Lesions of the abducent nucleus or nerve result in medial strabismus because of paralysis of the lateral rectus muscle. The resultant decrease in eyeball retraction is difficult to assess.

Facial Nerve

The **facial nerve** (*n. facialis*), or cranial nerve VII, supplies somatic efferent innervation to the muscles of the eyelids and parasympathetic innervation to the lacrimal gland by way of the major petrosal nerve and pterygopalatine ganglion. It is also sensory to the concave surface of the auricle (Whalen & Kitchell, 1983).

The facial nerve emerges from the medulla through the lateral aspect of the trapezoid body. The nerve courses laterally through the internal acoustic meatus with the vestibulocochlear nerve. The facial nerve enters the facial canal and turns caudally, forming the *geniculum n. facialis*. The cell bodies of the afferent axons of the facial nerve form the **geniculate ganglion** (*ganglion geniculi*), where the nerve makes its turn.

Parasympathetic preganglionic axons leave the facial nerve just distal to the genu as the major petrosal nerve. This joins the deep petrosal nerve to form the **nerve of the pterygoid canal**, which traverses a small canal in the basisphenoid bone. The nerve ends at the **pterygopalatine ganglion**, which lies ventral to the periorbita on the dorsal surface of the medial pterygoid muscle. Postganglionic axons from the pterygopalatine ganglion innervate the lacrimal gland via the lacrimal or zygomaticotemporal nerve or both.

The facial nerve leaves the facial canal and emerges on the caudolateral aspect of the skull through the stylomastoid foramen, caudal to the external acoustic meatus. The facial nerve gives rise to the caudal auricular nerves, the digastricus branch, the internal auricular branch, and the stylohyoid branch. The continuation of the facial nerve curves ventrally around the anular cartilage of the external acoustic meatus, gives origin to the dorsal and ventral buccal branches, and continues as the **auriculopalpebral nerve** (*n. auriculopalpebralis*). The auriculopalpebral nerve turns dorsally along the rostral aspect of the cartilage of the external acoustic meatus. Throughout this course the facial nerve is especially liable to damage in surgical manipulations for diseases of the external ear canal.

At the level of the origin of the zygomatic process from the temporal bone, the auriculopalpebral nerve divides to form the rostral auricular branches and the zygomatic branch. The **zygomatic branch** (*ramus zygomaticus*) curves rostrally along the dorsal margin of the zygomatic arch. Numerous branches join in the formation of the extensive rostral auricular plexus. Dorsocaudal to the lateral commissure, the zygomatic branch gives rise to the dorsal and ventral **palpebral branches** (*rami palpebrales*), which innervate the dorsal and ventral portions of the orbicularis oculi muscle. The retractor anguli oculi lateralis and the levator anguli oculi medialis are also supplied by rami of the zygomatic and palpebral branches. The dorsal palpebral branch continues medial to the eyelids to innervate the levator nasolabialis.

Injury to the facial nerve or to its palpebral branches paralyzes the orbicularis oculi muscle and is manifested as an inability to close the palpebral fissure. Such paralysis prevents distribution of the tear film that normally occurs during blinking and results in desiccation of the cornea. Severing only the ventral palpebral branch, as in lateral exploration of the orbit, does not interfere with normal eyelid function (Bistner et al., 1977).

Roberts et al. (1974) have described a technique for blocking nerve transmission in the auriculopalpebral nerve, where it crosses the zygomatic arch, to paralyze the orbicularis oculi muscle and facilitate ocular examination or the replacement of a proptosed eyeball. It is important to remember that this does not interfere with any sensory innervation of the eye.

Vasculature

Branches of the external carotid artery are the primary source of blood supply to the eye and its adnexa. Venous blood leaves the orbit through the angular vein of the eye, the deep facial vein, and the ophthalmic veins. The retinal vascular pattern is unique to each animal, does not change with age (Gionfriddo et al., 2006), and may someday serve as a means of identification.

Arteries

The major blood supply to the eye in the dog is from the external carotid artery via the maxillary and external ophthalmic arteries. Rostral to the base of the ear, the external carotid terminates by branching to become the superficial temporal and maxillary arteries. The **superficial temporal artery** (*a. temporalis superficialis*) courses dorsally, supplying branches to adjacent structures, and terminates as the superior and inferior lateral palpebral arteries, which supply the lateral aspect of the eyelids and conjunctiva.

The corresponding superior and inferior medial palpebral arteries that supply the conjunctiva and eyelids adjacent to the medial commissure arise from the **malar artery** (*a. malaris*), a branch of the infraorbital artery. The malar also sends branches to the third eyelid, to the ventral oblique muscle, and to the nasolacrimal duct.

The **maxillary artery** (*a. maxillaris*), gives rise to the inferior alveolar, caudal deep temporal, rostral tympanic, pterygoid, and middle meningeal arteries before entering the caudal alar foramen. The maxillary artery traverses the alar canal and emerges through the rostral alar foramen on the lateral aspect of the maxillary nerve. A few millimeters rostral to the rostral alar foramen, the maxillary artery gives rise to the **external ophthalmic artery** (*a. ophthalmica externa*), which passes dorsally to enter the apex of the periorbita (Fig. 21.43). Within the periorbita an anastomotic branch leaves the external ophthalmic and passes caudally through the orbital fissure to unite with the internal carotid artery (*ramus anastomoticus cum a. carotis interna*) at the level of the sella turcica. A similar branch anastomoses with the middle meningeal artery (*ramus anastomoticus cum a. meningea media*) (Fig. 21.43). These anastomotic branches may arise independently from the external ophthalmic, but more commonly arise from a single trunk that divides within the orbital fissure.

The **external ethmoidal artery** (*a. ethmoidalis externa*) arises from the external ophthalmic artery distal to these anastomotic branches and curves dorsomedially over the extraocular muscles to enter an ethmoidal foramen on the medial orbital wall (Figs. 21.43 and 21.44). There are usually two muscular branches of the external ethmoidal artery, although they may arise from a single trunk or from the external ophthalmic directly. A ventral **muscular branch** runs rostrally toward the eyeball between the ventral and lateral rectus muscles, supplying these muscles as well as the medial rectus, the ventral fasciculi of the retractor bulbi, and the superficial gland of the third eyelid (Fig. 21.43). The blood flow (milliliter per minute per gram) to the extraocular muscles of the dog (0.33 ± 0.06) is significantly higher than that determined for other skeletal muscle (Wilcox et al., 1981). The muscular branches are continued as the **anterior ciliary arteries** (*aa. ciliares anteriores*), which follow the tendons of the rectus muscles to their insertions anterior to the equator of the eyeball. Ciliary vessels course anteriorly to the limbal region where they pierce the sclera posterior to the scleral venous plexus and divide into lateral and medial branches (Sharpnack et al., 1984). These branches run circumferentially through the sclera just anterior to the scleral venous plexus forming a complete circle. Along the course of this circle, numerous arteriolar branches are given off, which pass anteriorly to supply the capillaries

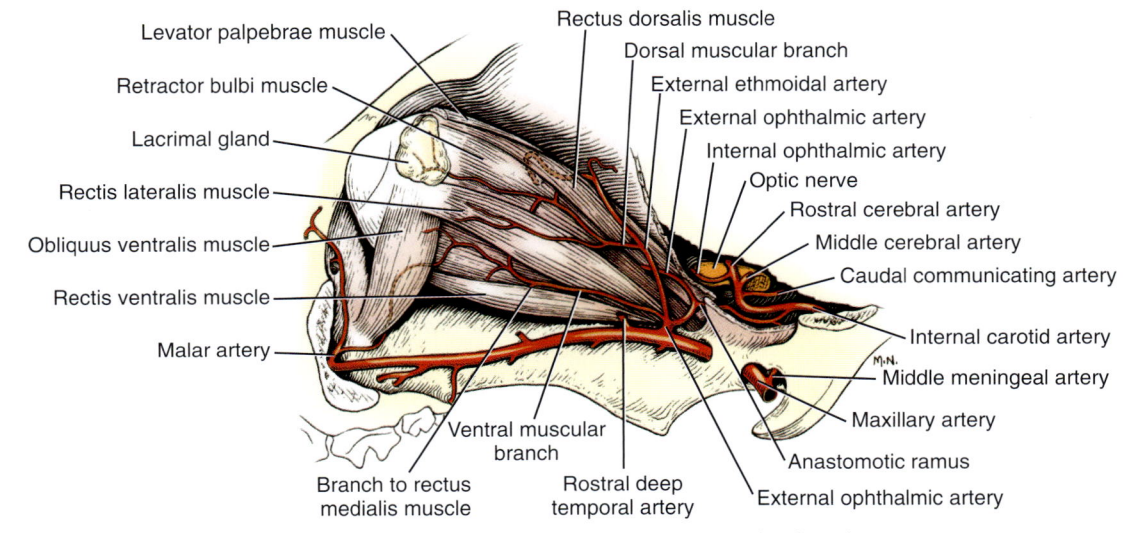

• **Fig. 21.43** Arteries of the orbit and extrinsic ocular muscles, lateral aspect.

of the limbal region. From this arterial net fine arterioles also pass inward to anastomose with terminal branches of the posterior ciliary arteries supplying the ciliary body and iris. Terminal branches of the muscular branches also contribute to the capillary loops of the bulbar conjunctiva (*aa. conjunctivales posteriores*) at the limbus and to the deeper episcleral vessels (*aa. episclerales*).

A dorsal **muscular branch** crosses over the lateral rectus to run rostrally between the lateral and dorsal recti (Fig. 21.43). It supplies branches to the lateral and dorsal rectus muscles, the dorsal fascicles of the retractor bulbi, the dorsal oblique and the levator palpebrae superioris muscles. At the equator of the eyeball, the dorsal muscular branch terminates as anterior ciliary, episcleral, and posterior conjunctival vessels analogous to those of the ventral branch. A distinct **lacrimal artery** (*a. lacrimalis*) usually arises from a muscular branch dorsally but may originate independently from the external ethmoidal or external ophthalmic arteries. It runs rostrally on the lateral edge of the dorsal rectus to supply the lacrimal gland (Fig. 21.43).

The external ophthalmic artery continues rostrally and medially to the center of the periorbital cone, where it comes to lie on the external sheath of the optic nerve. The course of the artery along the optic nerve is sinuous. Approximately midway between the optic canal and the posterior pole of the eyeball, there is a large anastomosis between the external and internal ophthalmic arteries (*ramus anastomoticus cum a. ophthalmica interna*) (Figs. 21.42 to 21.44). The **internal ophthalmic artery** (*a. ophthalmica interna*) is a small artery that arises from the rostral cerebral artery at the level of the optic chiasm. The internal ophthalmic artery passes through the optic canal on the dorsal surface of the optic nerve and runs rostrally on the nerve to anastomose with the external ophthalmic.

The internal ophthalmic artery is smaller than the external ophthalmic and is distributed almost exclusively to the eyeball itself.

From the anastomosis between the internal and external ophthalmic arteries, two **long posterior ciliary arteries** (*aa. ciliares posteriores longae*) arise, which supply most of the blood to the anterior segment of the dog eye (Keough et al., 1980). Initially, the long posterior ciliary arteries run rostrally, closely applied to the optic nerve (see Fig. 21.44). At the posterior aspect of the eyeball, the long posterior ciliary arteries give rise to a variable number of **short posterior ciliary arteries** (*aa. ciliares posteriores breves*). The short posterior ciliary arteries form a ring of 6 to 10 pillars around the optic nerve in the region of the lamina cribrosa. The laminar region of the optic nerve is also supplied by cilioretinal arteries and longitudinal pial vessels (Brooks et al., 1989b). Pathologic findings associated with the vessels of this region have been reported in dogs with glaucoma (Brooks et al., 1989a). The short posterior ciliary arteries pass through the sclera adjacent to the optic nerve and ramify in the choroid. These choroidal arterioles follow primarily in a meridional course to the ciliary body and ciliary margin of the iris (Fig. 21.9). Here they form variable anastomoses with branches of the anterior and long posterior ciliary arteries. In dogs with poorly pigmented ocular fundi, the course of the choroidal vessels may be visible with the ophthalmoscope. The choroidal blood flow of the canine eye has been estimated to be approximately 250 mL per min per 100 g (of tissue). This flow has been shown to decrease with an elevation in intraocular pressure (Yu et al., 1988). A defect in the choroidal vasculature in the lateral quadrant of the fundus is the most common manifestation of Collie eye syndrome (Latshaw et al., 1969). The resistance to blood flow within the posterior ciliary artery

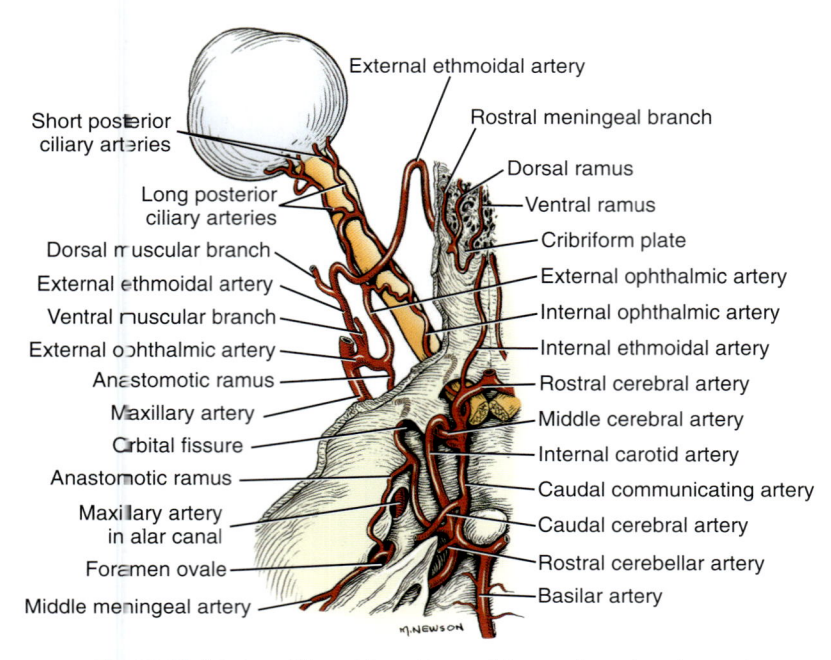

• **Fig. 21.44** Arteries of the orbit and base of the cranium, dorsal aspect.

expressed as the mean resistive index and the pulsatility index are 0.63 (±0.06) and 1.15 (±0.21), respectively (Novellas et al., 2007). Although these values provide an indirect measure of arterial resistance, they are not correlated with systolic blood pressure or pulse rate.

The **retinal arteries** are derived from the short posterior ciliary arteries as they pass through the sclera at the periphery of the optic nerve (Hetkamp, 1972). The retinal arteries continue anteriorly through the choroid and retina and emerge in the periphery of the optic disc, where they are visible ophthalmoscopically (Figs. 21.8 and 21.17). The number of retinal arterioles is variable, but there are usually approximately 15 where they first become visible at the periphery of the optic disc. They divide repeatedly toward the periphery; secondary and tertiary branches are visible in the normal eye. The retinal arterioles are distinguished from the retinal veins by their greater tortuosity, finer caliber, and brighter red color (Wyman & Donovan, 1965). The arterioles have been reported to undergo a degree of sclerosis associated with aging (Slatter et al., 1979).

Dogs possess a holangiotic retina with the presence of a circulus arteriosus around the optic nerve forming several choroidoretinal arteries (Albrecht May, 2008). From these vessels, up to six branches enter the optic nerve head at the level of the sclera and run laterally to the optic nerve head toward the retina. There is no single central retinal artery but retinal veins drain blood toward the center of the optic nerve head, forming a single central retinal vein that leaves the eye through the area of the lamina cribrosa. Because dogs possess several branches derived from a plexus of cilioretinal arteries instead of a single central retinal artery, the pial vessels are in direct contact with the cilioretinal vascular plexus from choroidal vessels of the same source. The central retinal arteries are not involved in the supply of the optic nerve head (Albrecht May, 2008).

The long posterior ciliary arteries continue anteriorly in the episcleral tissues along the medial and lateral meridians of the eyeball to its equator. Here they disappear from view, passing deep to the sclera into the suprachoroidea where they continue anteriorly to the ciliary margin of the iris. A few branches may be given off that anastomose with choroidal arterioles from the short posterior ciliary arteries (Fig. 21.9). In the periphery of the iris, each long posterior ciliary artery bifurcates into dorsal and ventral branches that run circumferentially, forming the **major arterial circle of the iris** (Fig. 21.9). The circle is incomplete dorsally and ventrally; however, in most specimens a smaller vessel completes the circle near the base of the iris (Sharpnack et al., 1984). Small corkscrew-shaped branches leave the circle to supply the pupillary region or to anastomose with arteries in the ciliary region (see Vascular Tunic).

Angiostatin is a natural component of the canine cornea and retina where this serves to inhibit unwanted angiogenesis (Pearce et al., 2007).

Veins

Blood leaves the orbit through one of three routes: (1) by way of the angular vein of the eye to the facial vein, (2) from the ophthalmic plexus to the cavernous sinus and maxillary vein, or (3) through an anastomosis of the ventral external ophthalmic vein with the deep facial vein (Fig. 21.45). These three drainage pathways are interconnected and all are filled in orbital venography.

The **angular vein of the eye** (*v. angularis oculi*) continues the facial vein dorsally and caudally. It originates where the dorsal nasal vein joins the facial vein rostral to the medial commissure of the eyelids. The angular vein passes caudally over the superficial surface of the medial palpebral ligament and passes caudodorsally medial to the commissure of the lids (Fig. 21.45). From the medial commissure the angular vein follows the dorsal orbital margin for approximately one-half the length of the zygomatic process of the frontal bone. It then turns caudally and enters the orbit. A small

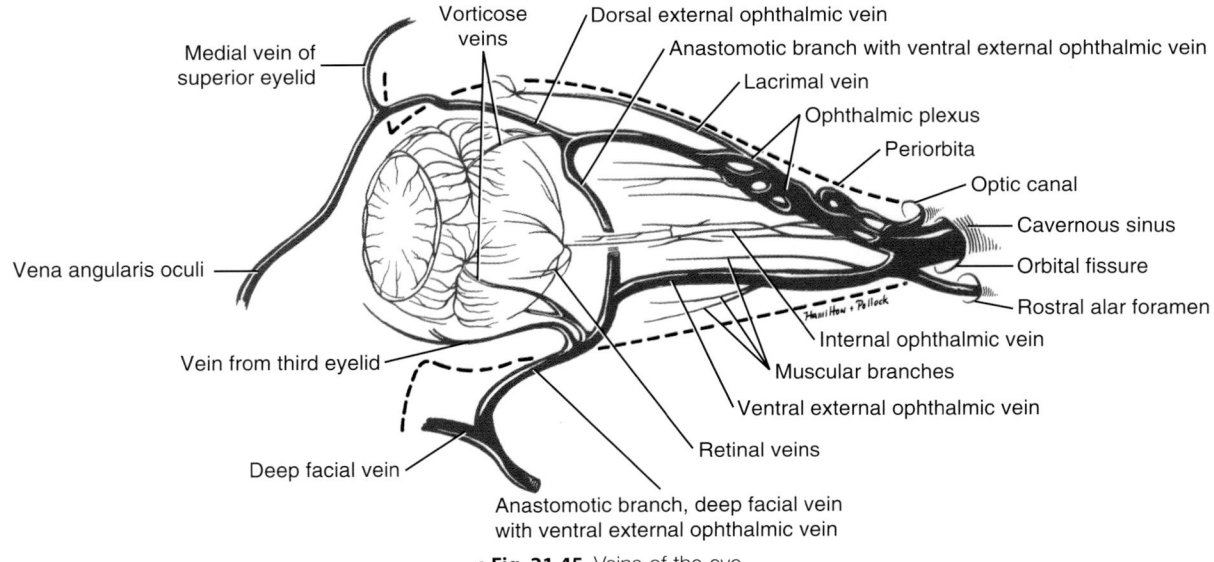

• **Fig. 21.45** Veins of the eye.

vein from the medial superior eyelid (*v. palpebralis superior medialis*) joins the angular vein where it turns to enter the orbit. At approximately the level of the equator of the eyeball, the angular vein passes into the periorbita to anastomose with the dorsal external ophthalmic vein. As the angular vein lacks valves, blood may flow through it either from the orbit into the facial vein or from the facial vein into the ophthalmic vessels.

The **dorsal external ophthalmic vein** (*v. ophthalmica externa dorsalis*) is the largest intraorbital vein. After its anastomosis with the angular vein of the eye, the dorsal external ophthalmic courses caudally along the dorsomedial orbital wall. At the posterior aspect of the eyeball, a large **anastomotic branch** (*ramus anastomoticus cum v. ophthalmica externa ventrali*) passes medially deep to the dorsal oblique muscle and winds down the medial orbital wall to join the ventral external ophthalmic vein (Fig. 21.45).

The dorsal pair of vorticose veins usually join the dorsal external ophthalmic near this anastomosis, or they may enter the anastomotic branch itself. Caudal to the anastomosis, the dorsal external ophthalmic begins to dilate markedly and assumes a more dorsal position. Numerous small muscular branches and the external ethmoidal vein enter the dilated caudal portion of the dorsal ophthalmic (Fig. 21.45). The **lacrimal vein** (*v. lacrimalis*), which drains the lacrimal gland, joins the dorsal external ophthalmic near the apex of the orbit. At the apex of the orbit, the dorsal external ophthalmic is massively dilated and envelops the other vessels and nerves entering the orbit, forming the so-called **ophthalmic plexus** (*plexus ophthalmicus*). From the ophthalmic plexus the small internal ophthalmic vein enters the optic canal with the optic nerve to anastomose with its fellow from the contralateral side on the floor of the middle cranial fossa.

The dorsal external ophthalmic vein and ophthalmic plexus joins the ventral external ophthalmic vein ventral to the optic canal. The bulk of the blood from this union leaves the orbit as the **emissary vein of the orbital fissure** to join the cavernous sinus in the middle cranial fossa. One or more small branches enter the rostral alar foramen to anastomose with the maxillary vein.

The **ventral external ophthalmic vein** (*v. ophthalmica externa ventralis*) lies within the periorbita on the floor of the orbit between the extraocular muscles and the medial pterygoid muscle. Caudally it receives numerous muscular branches and joins the dorsal external ophthalmic in the ophthalmic plexus. Rostrally it receives the large anastomotic branch from the dorsal ophthalmic and drainage from the ventral pair of vorticose veins. A large branch draining the base of the third eyelid joins the ventral external ophthalmic near or in common with the vorticose veins (Fig. 21.45). Caudal to the ventral orbital margin, a large anastomotic branch unites the ventral external ophthalmic to the deep facial vein (*ramus anastomoticus cum v. ophthalmica externa ventrali*) on the lateral surface of the zygomatic gland.

The eyeball drains into the ophthalmic vessels through the retinal, ciliary, and vorticose veins. The intraocular course of the retinal veins has already been described (see section on the retina). **Ciliary veins** (*vv. ciliares*) accompany the several ciliary arteries as satellite veins. **Retinal veins** join the posterior ciliary veins at the periphery of the area cribrosa to form the internal ophthalmic vein. There is no central retinal vein in the dog. The **internal ophthalmic vein** comprises a number of interanastomosing vessels that are closely adherent to the external sheath of the optic nerve and that receive fine radicles from the internal sheath. The internal ophthalmic runs caudally to join in the formation of the ophthalmic plexus.

The major drainage of the vascular tunic of the eye, however, is via the **vorticose veins** (*vv. vorticosae*), which have no accompanying arteries (Fig. 21.45). The vorticose veins are usually four in number and penetrate the sclera near the equator between the insertions of the four rectus muscles. The intraocular branches of the vorticose veins, the choroidal venules, radiate outward at the point of scleral penetration (Fig. 21.10). Anastomotic branches unite the vorticose veins with terminal branches of the ciliary veins and the scleral venous plexus (Van Buskirk, 1979).

Comparative Ophthalmology

Major works in comparative ophthalmology include Walls (1942), Rochon-Duvigneaud (1943), Polyak (1957), Prince (1956), Duke-Elder (1958), Prince et al. (1960), Smythe (1961), Crescitelli (1977), and Cronly-Dillon and Gregory (1991), and Schwab (2011). A full-color atlas of comparative ophthalmoscopy is also available (Rubin, 1974), and an expanding number of color atlases of veterinary ophthalmology have been published (e.g., Barnett, 1990; Walde et al., 1990). Ocular histology and fine structure are superbly treated in the text by Hogan et al. (1971).

Bibliography

Abrams, G. A., Bentley, E., Nealey, P. F., et al. (2002a). Electron microscopy of the canine corneal basement membranes. *Cell Tissues Organs, 170*, 251–257.

Abrams, G. A., Teixeira, A. I., Nealey, P. F., & Murphy, C. (2002b). The effects of substratum topography on cell behavior. In A. K. Dillow & A. Lowman (Eds.), *Biomimetic materials and design* (pp. 91–137). New York and Basel: Marcel Dekker.

Abrams, K. L., Brooks, D. E., Laratta, L. J., et al. (1991). Angiotensin converting enzyme system in the normal canine eye: pharmacological and physiological aspects. *J Ocul Pharmacol, 7*, 41–51.

Abdel-Latif, A. A. (1989). Regulation of arachidonate release, prostaglandin synthesis, and sphincter constriction in the mammalian iris-ciliary body. *Prog Clin Biol Res, 312*, 53–72.

Aguirre, G. D., & Rubin, L. F. (1970). Ophthalmitis secondary to congenitally open eyelids in a dog. *J Am Vet Med Assoc, 156*, 70–72.

Aguirre, G. D., Rubin, L. F., & Bistner, S. I. (1972). Development of the canine eye. *Am J Vet Res, 33*, 2399–2414.

Alario, A. F., & Pirie, C. G. (2013). A spectral-domain optical coherence tomography device provides reliable corneal pachymetry measurements in canine eyes. *Vet Rec, 172*, 605–608.

Albrecht May, C. (2008). Comparative anatomy of the optic nerve head and inner retina in non-primate animal models used for glaucoma research. *Open Ophthalmol J, 2*, 94–101.

Allgoewer, I., Blair, M., Basher, T., et al. (2000). Extraocular muscle myositis and restrictive strabismus in 10 dogs. *Vet Ophthalmol, 3*, 21–26.

Ambati, B. L., Nozaki, M., Singh, N., et al. (2006). Corneal avascularity is due to soluble VEGF receptor-1. *Nature, 443*, 993–997.

Andersen, A. C., & Shultz, F. T. (1958). Inherited (congenital) cataract in the dog. *Am J Pathol, 34*, 965–975.

Anderson, B. G., & Anderson, W. D. (1977). Vasculature of the equine and canine iris. *Am J Vet Res, 38*, 1791–1799.

Arey, L. B., Bruesch, S. R., & Castanares, S. (1942). The relation between eyeball size and the number of optic nerve fibers in the dog. *J Comp Neurol, 76*, 417–422.

Ayad, S., & Weiss, J. B. (1984). A new look at vitreous-humour collagen. *Biochem J, 218*, 835–840.

Balazs, E. A. (1973). The vitreous. *Int Ophthalmol Clin, 13*, 169–187.

Barnett, K. C. (1990). *Color atlas of veterinary ophthalmology*. Baltimore, MD: Williams & Wilkins.

Barrie, K. P., Gum, G. G., Samuelson, D. A., et al. (1985a). Morphologic studies of uveoscleral outflow in normotensive and glaucomatous beagles with fluorescein-labelled dextran. *Am J Vet Res, 46*, 89–97.

Barrie, K. P., Gum, G. G., Samuelson, D. A., et al. (1985b). Quantitation of uveoscleral outflow in normotensive and glaucomatous beagles by ³H-labelled dextrans. *Am J Vet Res, 46*, 84–88.

Bayer, J. (1914). *Augenheilkunde*. Wein: Braumuller.

Bedford, P. G. C. (1971). Eyelashes and adventitious cilia as causes of corneal irritation. *J Small Anim Pract, 12*, 11–17.

Bedford, P. G. C. (1977). Gonioscopy in the dog. *J Small Anim Pract, 18*, 615–629.

Bedford, P. G. C., & Grierson, I. (1986). Aqueous drainage in the dog. *Res Vet Sci, 41*, 172–186.

Beltran, W. A., Cideciyan, A. V., Guziewicz, K. E., et al. (2014). Canine retina has a primate fovea-like boquet of photoreceptors which is affected by inherited macular degenerations. *PLoS ONE, 9*(3), e90390. doi:10.1371/journal.pone.0090390.

Bellhorn, R. W. (1990). A fluorescent microscopic study of tapetal tissue, *Proc Am Coll Vet Ophthalmol* 64–70.

Bellhorn, R. W., Burns, M. B., Swarm, R. L., et al. (1975). Hereditary tapetal abnormality in the beagle. *Ophthalmic Res, 7*, 250–260.

Benz, P., Tichy, A., & Nell, B. (2008). Review of the measuring precision of the new meibometer MB550 through repeated measurements in dogs. *Vet Ophthalmol, 11*, 368–374.

Bernays, M. E., & Peiffer, R. L. (2000). Morphologic alterations in the anterior lens capsule of canine eyes with cataracts. *Am J Vet Res, 61*, 1517–1519.

Betbeze, C. (2015). Management of orbital disease. *Top Compan Anim Med, 30*, 107–117.

Bicer, S., & Reiser, P. J. (2009). Myosin isoform expression in dog rectus muscles: patterns in global and orbital layers and among single fibbers. *Invest Ophthalmol Vis Sci, 50*, 157–167.

Bicer, S., & Reiser, P. J. (2013). Complex tropomyosin and troponin T isoform expression patterns in orbital and global fibers of adult dog and rat extraocular muscles. *J Muscle Res Cell Motil, 34*, 211–231.

Bistner, S. I. (1978). Neuro-ophthalmology. In B. F. Hoerlein (Ed.), *Canine neurology: diagnosis and treatment* (3rd ed.). Philadelphia: Saunders.

Bistner, S. I., Aguirre, G. D., & Batik, G. (1977). *Atlas of veterinary ophthalmic surgery*. Philadelphia: Saunders.

Bjerkås, E., Ekesten, B., & Farstad, W. (2002). Pectinate ligament dysplasia and narrowing of the iridocorneal angle associated with glaucoma in the English springer spaniel. *Vet Ophthalmol, 5*, 49–54.

Black, J., Browning, S. R., Collins, A. V., et al. (2008). A canine model of inherited myopia: familial aggregation of refractive error in labrador retrievers. *Invest Ophthalmol Vis Sci, 49*, 4784–4789.

Boevé, M. H., van der Linde-Sipman, J. S., & Stades, F. C. (1988). Early morphogenesis of the canine lens, hyaloid system, and vitreous body. *Anat Rec, 220*(4), 435–441.

Boevé, M. H., van der Linde-Sipman, J. S., & Stades, F. C. (1989). Early morphogenesis of the canine lens capsule, tunica vasculosa lentis posterior, and anterior vitreous body: a transmission electron microscopic study. *Graefes Arch Clin Exp Ophthalmol, 227*, 589–594.

Boevé, M. H., van der Linde-Sipman, J. S., Stades, F. C., et al. (1990). Early morphogenesis of persistent hyperplastic tunica vasculosa lentis and primary vitreous: a transmission electron-microscopic study. *Invest Ophthalmol Vis Sci, 31*, 1886–1894.

Boland, L., Gomes, E., Payen, G., et al. (2013). Zygomatic salivary gland diseases in the dog: three cases diagnosed by MRI. *J Am Anim Hosp Assoc, 49*(5), 333–337.

Boroffka, S. A., Görig, C., Auriemma, E., et al. (2008). Magnetic resonance imaging of the canine optic nerve. *Vet Radiol Ultrasound, 49*, 540–544.

Brooks, D. E., Samuelson, D. A., & Gelatt, K. N. (1989a). Ultrastructural changes in laminar optic nerve capillaries of beagles with primary open-angle glaucoma. *Am J Vet Res, 50*, 929–935.

Brooks, D. E., Samuelson, D. A., Gelatt, K. N., et al. (1989b). Scanning electron microscopy of corrosion casts of the optic nerve microcirculation in dogs. *Am J Vet Res, 50*, 908–914.

Brooks, D. E., Strubbe, D. T., Kubilis, P. S., et al. (1995). Histomorphometry of the optic nerves of normal dogs and dogs with hereditary glaucoma. *Exp Eye Res, 60*, 71–89.

Bruesch, S. R., & Arey, L. B. (1942). The number of myelinated and unmyelinated fibers in the optic nerve of vertebrates. *J Comp Neurol, 77*, 631–665.

Burns, M. S., Bellhorn, R. W., Impellizzeri, C. W., et al. (1988a). Development of hereditary tapetal degeneration in the beagle dog. *Curr Eye Res, 7*, 103–114.

Burns, M. S., Tyler, N. K., & Bellhorn, R. W. (1988b). Melanosome abnormalities of ocular pigmented epithelial cells in beagle dogs with hereditary tapetal degeneration. *Curr Eye Res, 7*, 115–123.

Butovich, I. A., Lu, H., McMahon, A., & Eule, J. C. (2012). Toward an animal model of the human tear film: biochemical comparison of the mouse, canine, rabbit, and human meibomian lipidomes. *Invest Ophthalmol Vis Sci, 53*, 6881–6896.

Byosiere, S. E., Chouinard, P. A., Howell, T. J., & Bennett, P. C. (2017). What do dogs (Canis familiaris) see? *A review of vision in dogs and implications for cognition research, Psychol Bull Rev*, https://doi.org/10.3758/s13423-017-1404-7.

Carrington, S. D., Bedford, P. G. C., Guillon, J. P., et al. (1987). Polarized light biomicroscopic observations on the pre-corneal tear film. 1. The normal tear film of the dog. *J Small Anim Pract, 28*, 605–622.

Cavallotti, C., Pescosolido, N., Artico, M., et al. (1998). Uveoscleral outflow in dog's eye: role of several enzymes. *Int Ophthalmol, 22*, 233–238.

Cenedella, R. J., Linton, L. L., & Moore, C. P. (1992). Cholesterylene, a newly recognized tissue lipid, found at high levels in the cornea. *Biochem Biophys Res Commun, 186*, 1647–1655.

Chan-Ling, T., & Stone, J. (1991). Factors determining the migration of astrocytes into the developing retina: migration does not depend on intact axons or patent vessels. *J Comp Neurol, 303,* 375–386.

Chase, J. (1982). The evolution of retinal vascularization in mammals: a comparison of vascular and avascular retinae. *Ophthalmology, 89,* 1518–1525.

Choppin, A., & Eglen, R. M. (2001). Pharmacological characterization of muscarinic receptors in dog isolated ciliary and urinary bladder smooth muscle. *Br J Pharmacol, 132,* 835–842.

Christiansen, S. P., Baker, R. S., Madhat, M., et al. (1992). Type-specific changes in fiber morphometry following denervation of canine extraocular muscle. *Exp Mol Pathol, 56,* 87–95.

Cirla, A., Rondena, M., Bertolini, G., et al. (2017). Exophthalmos associated to orbital zygomatic mucocele and complex maxillary malformation in a puppy. *Open Vet J, 7*(3), 229–234.

Coassin, M., Lambiase, A., Costa, N., et al. (2005). Efficacy of topical nerve growth factor treatment in dogs affected by dry eye. *Graefes Arch Clin Exp Ophthalmol, 243,* 151–155.

Code, C. F., & Essex, H. E. (1935). The mechanism involved in the production of exophthalmos in the dog by vago-sympathetic stimulation. *Am J Physiol, 113,* 29.

Coile, D. C., & O'Keefe, L. P. (1988). Schematic eyes for domestic animals. *Ophthalmic Physiol Opt, 8,* 215–220.

Coli, A., & Marroni, P. (1996). Dog retinal ganglion cells: a morphological and morphometrical study in aging. *Anat Histol Embryol, 25,* 127–130.

Conroy, C. W., Buck, R. H., & Maren, T. H. (1992). The microchemical detection of carbonic anhydrase in corneal epithelia. *Exp Eye Res, 55,* 637–640.

Constantinescu, G. M., & Schaller, O. (Eds.), (2012). *Illustrated veterinary anatomical nomenclature* (3rd ed.). Germany: Enke-Verlag. rev.

Corfield, A. P., Donapaty, S. R., Carrington, S. D., et al. (2005). Identification of 9-O-acetyl-N-acetylneuraminic acid in normal canine pre-ocular tear film secreted mucins and its depletion in keratoconjunctivitis sicca. *Glycoconj J, 22,* 409–416.

Crescitelli, F. (Ed.), (1977). *The visual system in vertebrates.* New York: Springer-Verlag.

Cronly-Dillon, J. R., & Gregory, R. L. (Eds.), (1991). *Evolution of the eye and visual system.* Boca Raton, FL: CRC Press.

Czerwinski, S. L., Plummer, C. E., Greenberg, S. M., et al. (2015). Dynamic exophthalmos and lateral strabismus in a dog caused by masticatory muscle myositis. *Vet Ophthalmol, 18*(6), 515–520.

Daniel, W. A., Noonan, N. E., & Gelatt, K. N. (1984). Isolation and characterization of the crystallins of the normal and cataractous canine lens. *Curr Eye Res, 3,* 911–922.

Davidson, M. G., Murphy, C. J., Nasisse, M. P., et al. (1993). Refractive state of aphakic and pseudophakic eyes of dogs. *Am J Vet Res, 45,* 174–177.

da Silva, E. G., Sandmeyer, L. S., & Gionfriddo, J. R. (2013). Montiani-ferreira F: tear production in canine neonates-evaluation using a modified Schirmer tear test. *Vet Ophthalmol, 16,* 175–179.

de Freitas Campos, C., Cole, N., Van Dyk, D., et al. (2008). Proteomic analysis of dog tears for potential cancer markers. *Res Vet Sci, 85,* 349–352.

de Lahunta, A. (1983). *Veterinary neuroanatomy and clinical neurology.* Philadelphia: Saunders.

de Lahunta, A., & Cummings, J. (1967). Neuroophthalmologic lesions as a cause of visual deficit in dogs and horses. *J Am Vet Med Assoc, 150,* 994–1011.

de Lahunta, A., & Habel, R. E. (1986). *Applied veterinary anatomy.* Philadelphia: Saunders.

Dell'Osso, L. F., Williams, R. W., Jacobs, J. B., & Erchel, D. M. (1998). The congenital and see-saw nystagmus in the prototypical achiasma of canines: comparison to the human achiasmatic prototype. *Vision Res, 38,* 1629–1641.

Denis, H. M., Brooks, D. E., Alleman, A. R., et al. (2003). Detection of anti-lens crystallin antibody in dogs with and without cataracts. *Vet Ophthalmol, 6,* 321–327.

Diesem, C. (1975). Organ of vision. In R. Getty (Ed.), *Sisson and Grossman's the anatomy of the domestic animals.* Philadelphia: Saunders.

Donovan, R. H., Carpenter, R. L., Schepens, C. L., et al. (1974). Histology of the normal collie eye. II. Uvea. *Ann Ophthalmol, 6,* 1175–1189.

Duke-Elder, W. S. (1958). *System of ophthalmology* (Vol. I). The eye in evolution. London: Henry Kimpton.

Durairaj, C., Chastain, J. E., & Kompella, U. B. (2012). Intraocular distribution of melanin in human, monkey, rabbit, minipig and dog eyes. *Exp Eye Res, 98,* 23–27.

Elliott, J., & Futterman, S. (1963). Fluorescence in the tapetum of the cat's eye. *Arch Ophthalmol, 70,* 531–534.

Engerman, R. L., & Colquhoun, P. J. (1982). Epithelial and mesothelial basement membranes in diabetic patients and dogs. *Diabetologia, 23,* 521–524.

Engerman, R. L., Molitor, D. L., & Bloodworth, J. M. B. (1966). Vascular system of the dog retina: light and electron microscopic studies. *Exp Eye Res, 5,* 296–301.

Evans, H. E. (1974). *Prenatal development of the dog.* Ithaca, NY: Twenty-fourth Gaines Veterinary Symposium.

Evans, H. E., & Sack, W. (1973). Prenatal development of domestic and laboratory mammals. *Anat Histol Embryol, 2,* 11–45.

Famose, F. (2014). Assessment of the use of spectral domain optical coherence tomography (SD-OCT) for evaluation of the healthy and pathological cornea in dogs and cats. *Vet Ophthalmol, 17,* 12–22.

Farias, E., Yasunaga, K. L., Peixoto, R. V. R., et al. (2013). Comparison of two methods of tear sampling for protein quantification by Bradford method. *Presquisa Vet Brasil, 33,* 261–264.

Fine, B. S., & Yanoff, M. (1972). *Ocular histology: a text and atlas.* New York: Harper & Row.

Flower, R. W., McLeod, D. S., Lutty, G. A., Goldberg, B., & Wajer, S. D. (1985). Postnatal retinal vascular development of the puppy. *Invest Ophthalmol Vis Sci, 26,* 957–968.

Gagna, C. E., Kuo, H. R., Agostino, N., et al. (2001). Novel use of bovine zeta-crystallin as a conformational DNA probe to characterize a phase transition zone and terminally differentiating fiber cells in the adult canine ocular lens. *Arch Histol Cytol, 64,* 379–391.

Gaiddon, J., Rosolen, S. G., Steru, L., et al. (1991). Use of biometry and keratometry for determining optimal power for intraocular lens implants in dogs. *Am J Vet Res, 52,* 781–783.

García-Sánchez, G. A., Gil-Carrasco, F., Román, J. J., et al. (2007). Measurement of retinal nerve fiber layer thickness in normal and glaucomatous cocker spaniels by scanning laser polarimetry. *Vet Ophthalmol, 10*(Suppl. 1), 78–87.

Gelatt, K. N., & MacKay, E. O. (2004). Effect of different dose schedules of travoprost on intraocular pressure and pupil size in the glaucomatous beagle. *Vet Ophthalmol, 7,* 53–57.

Genini, S., Beltran, W. A., & Aguirre, G. D. (2014). Isolation and ex vivo characterization of the immunotype and function of microglia/macrophage populations in normal dog retina. In J. D. Ash, et al. (Eds.), *Retinal degenerative diseases, advances in experimental medicine and biology* (pp. 339–345). Springer Science + Business Media, LLC. Chapt 43.

Giannetto, C., Piccione, G., & Giudice, E. (2009). Daytime profile of the intraocular pressure and tear production in normal dog. *Vet Ophthalmol, 12,* 302–305.

Gilbert, P. W. (1947). The origin and development of the extrinsic ocular muscles in the domestic cat. *J Morphol, 81,* 151–194.

Gilger, B. C., Reeves, K. A., & Salmon, J. H. (2005). Ocular parameters related to drug delivery in the canine and equine eye: aqueous and vitreous humor volume and scleral surface area and thickness. *Vet Ophthalmol, 8,* 265–269.

Gionfriddo, J. R., Lee, A. C., Precht, T. A., et al. (2006). Evaluation of retinal images for identifying individual dogs. *Am J Vet Res, 67,* 2042–2045.

Gonzalez-Soriano, J., Rodriguez-Veiga, E., Martinez-Sainz, P., et al. (1995). A quantitative study of ganglion cells in the German shepherd dog retina. *Anat Histol Embryol, 24,* 61–65.

Granar, M. I. K. S., Nilsson, B. R., & Hamberg-Nystrom, H. L. (2011). Normal color variations of the canine ocular fundus, a retrospective study in Swedish dogs. *Acta Vet Scand, 53,* 13–22.

Greenlee, T. K., Ross, R., & Hartman, J. L. (1966). The fine structure of elastic fibers. *J Cell Biol, 30,* 59–71.

Gum, G. G., Gelatt, K. N., & Esson, D. W. (2007). Physiology of the eye. In K. N. Gelatt (Ed.), *Veterinary ophthalmology* (4th ed.). Lea & Febiger: Philadelphia.

Gum, G. G., Gelatt, K. N., & Knepper, P. A. (1993). Histochemical localization of glycosaminoglycans in the aqueous outflow pathways in normal beagles and beagles with inherited glaucoma. *Prog Vet Comp Ophthalmol, 3,* 52–57.

Gum, G. G., Gelatt, K. N., & Samuelson, D. A. (1984). Maturation of the retina of the canine neonate as determined by electroretinography and histology. *Am J Vet Res, 45,* 1166–1171.

Gwin, R. M., Gelatt, K. N., & Chiou, C. Y. (1979). Adrenergic and cholinergic innervation of the anterior segment of the normal and glaucomatous dog. *Invest Ophthalmol Vis Sci, 18,* 674–682.

Gwin, R. M., Lerner, I., Warren, J. K., et al. (1982). Decrease in canine endothelial cell density and increase in corneal thickness with age. *Invest Ophthalmol Vis Sci, 22,* 267–271.

Gwin, R. M., Warren, J. K., Samuelson, D. A., et al. (1983). Effects of phacoemulsification and extracapsular lens removal on corneal thickness and endothelial cell density in the dog. *Invest Ophthalmol Vis Sci, 24,* 227–236.

Hamon, M. A. (1977). *Atlas de la tete du chien.* These, L'Univ. Paul Sabatier de Toulouse.

Hara, H., Kobayashi, S., Sugita, K., et al. (1982). Innervation of dog ciliary ganglion. *Histochemistry, 76,* 295–301.

Hassel, B., Samuelson, D. A., Lewis, P. A., et al. (2007). Immunocytochemical localization of smooth muscle actin-containing cells in the trabecular meshwork of glaucomatous and nonglaucomatous dogs. *Vet Ophthalmol, 10*(Suppl. 1), 38–45.

Hebel, R. (1969). Licht-und elektronen-mikroskopische untersuchunger an den zellen des tapetum lucidum des hundes. *Z Anat Entwickl-Gesch, 129,* 274–284.

Hebel, R. (1971). Entwicklung und struktur der retina und des tapetum lucidum des hundes. *Ergeb Anat Entwicklungsgesch, 45,* 7–92.

Hebel, R. (1976). Distribution of retinal ganglion cells in five mammalian species (pig, sheep, ox, horse, dog). *Anat Embryol, 150,* 45–51.

Helper, L. C. (1970). The effect of lacrimal gland removal on the conjunctiva and cornea of the dog. *J Am Vet Med Assoc, 157,* 72–75.

Helper, L. C., Magrane, W. G., Koehm, J., et al. (1974). Surgical induction of keratoconjunctivitis sicca in the dog. *J Am Vet Med Assoc, 165,* 172–174.

Hernandez, J., Moore, C., Si, X., et al. (2016). Aging dogs manifest myopia as measured by autorefractor. *PLoS ONE, 11*(2), e0148436. doi:10.1371/journal.pone.0148436.

Hetkamp, D. (1972). *Korrosionsanatomische untersuchungen der blutgefässe des auges des haushundes (canis fam. L.) unter besonderer bericksichtigung des kapilarsystems.* Vet Diss: Giessen.

Heywood, R., Hepworth, P. L., & van Abbe, N. J. (1976). Age changes in the eyes of the beagle dog. *J Small Anim Pract, 17,* 171–177.

Hicks, S. J., Carrington, S. D., Kaswan, R. L., et al. (1997). Demonstration of discrete secreted and membrane-bound ocular mucins in the dog. *Exp Eye Res, 64,* 597–607.

Hirt, R., Tektas, O. Y., Carrington, S. D., et al. (2012). Comparative anatomy of the human and canine efferent tear duct system: impact of mucin MUC5AC on lacrimal drainage. *Curr Eye Res, 37*(11), 961–970.

Hogan, M. J., Alvarado, J. A., & Weddel, J. E. (1971). *Histology of the human eye: an atlas and textbook.* Philadelphia: Saunders.

Hollyfield, J. G., Rayborn, M. E., Tammi, M., et al. (1998). Hyaluronan in the interphotoreceptor matrix of the eye: species differences in content, distribution, ligand binding and degradation. *Exp Eye Res, 66,* 241–248.

Huber, E. (1922). Über das muskelgebiet des n. facialis beim hund, nebst allgemeinen betrachtungen über die fascialis-muskulatur. *Morph Jahrb, 52,* 1–110, 354–414.

Igić, R. (1993). Substance P inactivation by aqueous humor. *Exp Eye Res, 57,* 415–417.

Iwata, J. L., Bardygula-Nonn, L. G., Glonek, T., et al. (1995). Interspecies comparisons of lens phospholipids. *Curr Eye Res, 14,* 937–941.

Jester, J. V. (2008). Corneal crystallins and the development of cellular transparency. *Sem Cell Devel Biol, 19,* 82–93.

Joffe, W. S., & Gay, A. J. (1966). The oculorespiratory cardiac reflex in the dog. *Invest Ophthalmol, 5,* 550–554.

Johnston, M. C., Noden, D. M., Hazelton, R. D., et al. (1979). Origins of avian ocular and periocular tissues. *Exp Eye Res, 29,* 27–43.

Kafarnik, C., Fritsche, J., & Reese, S. (2007). In vivo confocal microscopy in the normal corneas of cats, dogs and birds. *Vet Ophthalmol, 10,* 222–230.

Kafarnik, C., Fritsche, J., & Reese, S. (2008). Corneal innervation in mesocephalic and brachycephalic dogs and cats: assessment using in vivo confocal microscopy. *Vet Ophthalmol, 11,* 363–367.

Källberg, M. E., Brooks, D. E., Gelatt, K. N., et al. (2007). Endothelin-1, nitric oxide, and glutamate in the normal and glaucomatous dog eye. *Vet Ophthalmol, 10*(Suppl. 1), 46–52.

Keough, E. M., Wilcox, L. M., Conally, R. J., et al. (1980). The effect of complete tenotomy on blood flow to the anterior segment of the canine eye. *Invest Ophthalmol Vis Sci, 19,* 1355–1359.

Killian, D., Reichard, M., Knueppel, A., et al. (2013). Distribution changes of epithelial dendritic cells in canine cornea and mucous membranes relate to hematopoietic stem cell transplantation. *In Vivo, 27,* 761–772.

Kim, S., Thomasy, S. M., Ramsey, D., Zhao, M., Mannis, M. J., & Murphy, C. J. (2018). Whorl pattern keratopathies in veterinary and human patients. *Vet Ophthalmol, 00,* 1–7.

Klaumann, P. R., & Moreno, J. C. (2017). Montiani-ferreira f: a morphometric study of the canine skull and periorbita and its implications for regional ocular anesthesia. *Vet Ophthalmol, 21,* 19–26. doi:10.1111/vop.12471.

Klećkowska, J., Janeczek, M., Wojnar, M., et al. (2006). Morphological examination of the intraorbital muscles (musculi bulbi) in dogs in the perinatal period. *Anat Histol Embryol, 35*, 279–783.

Knecht, C. D. (1970). Treatment of diseases of the zygomatic salivary gland. *J Am Anim Hosp Assoc, 6*, 13–19.

Koch, S. A., & Rubin, L. F. (1972). Distribution of cones in retina of the normal dog. *Am J Vet Res, 33*, 361–363.

Kreuzer, R. O., & Sivak, J. G. (1985). Chromatic aberration of the vertebrate lens. *Ophthalmic Physiol Opt, 5*, 33–41.

Kubai, M. A., Bentley, E., Miller, P. E., et al. (2008). Refractive states of eyes and association between ametropia and breed in dogs. *Am J Vet Res, 69*, 946–951.

Kubai, M. A., Labelle, A. L., Hamor, R. E., et al. (2013). Heritability of lenticular myopia in English springer spaniels. *Invest Ophthalmol Vis Sci, 54*, 7324–7328.

Kuchiiwa, S., Kuchiiwa, T., & Suzuki, T. (1989). Comparative anatomy of the accessory ciliary ganglion in mammals. *Anat Embryol (Berl), 180*, 199–205.

Kurata, K., Fujimoto, H., Tsukuda, R., et al. (1998). Aqueous humor dynamics in beagle dogs with caffeine-induced ocular hypertension. *J Vet Med Sci, 60*, 737–739.

Labruyère, J. J., Hartley, C., Rogers, K., et al. (2008). Ultrasonographic evaluation of vitreous degeneration in normal dogs. *Vet Radiol Ultrasound, 49*, 165–171.

Last, J., Liliensiek, S. J., Nealey, P. F., et al. (2009). Determining the mechanical properties of human corneal basement membranes with atomic force microscopy. *J Struct Biol, 167*, 19–24.

Lasys, V., Stanevicius, E., & Zamokas, G. (2003). Evaluation of peculiarities of the acetylcholinesterase positive nerve plexus and its length in the cornea. *Medicina (Kaunas), 39*, 955–959.

Latshaw, W. K., Wyman, M., & Venzke, W. G. (1969). Embryologic development of an anomaly of the ocular fundus in the collie dog. *Am J Vet Res, 30*, 211–217.

Lesiuk, T. P. (1983). Braekvelt CR: fine structure of the canine tapetum lucidum. *J Anat, 136*, 157–164.

Lee, N., Choi, M., Keh, S., Kim, T., Kim, H., & Yoon, J. (2014). Zygomatic sialolithiasis diagnosed with computed tomography in a dog. *J Vet Med Sci, 76*(10), 1389–1391.

Lord, R. D. (1961). The lens as an indication of age in the grey fox. *J Mammal, 42*, 109–110.

Leonard, B. C., Yanez-Soto, B., Raghunathan, V. K., et al. (2016). Species variation and spatial differences in mucin expression from corneal epithelial cells. *Exp Eye Res, 152*, 43–48.

Lutty, G. A., McLeod, D. S., Bhutto, I., & Wiegand, S. J. (2010). Effect of VEGF trap on normal retinal vascular development and oxygen-induced retinopathy in the dog. *Invest Ophthalmol Vis Sci, 51*, 4039–4047.

Louden, C., Render, J. A., & Carlton, W. W. (1990). Mast cell numbers in normal and glaucomatous canine eyes. *Am J Vet Res, 51*, 818–819.

Lynch, G. L. (2006). Brinkis JL: the effect of elective phacofragmentation on central corneal thickness in the dog. *Vet Ophthalmol, 9*, 303–310.

Maehara, S., Itoh, Y., Higashinozono, K., et al. (2011). Evaluation of refractive value by skiascopy in healthy beagles. *J Vet Med Sci, 73*, 927–929.

Magrane, W. G. (1977). *Canine ophthalmology* (3rd ed.). Philadelphia: Lea & Febiger.

Maier, A., DeSantis, M., & Eldred, E. (1974). The occurrence of muscle spindles in extraocular muscles of various vertebrates. *J Morphol, 143*, 397–408.

Marfurt, C. F., Murphy, C. J., & Florczak, J. L. (2001). Morphology and neurochemistry of canine corneal innervation. *Invest Ophthalmol Vis Sci, 42*, 2242–2251.

Mark, H. H. (2003). Aqueous humor dynamics and the iris. *Med Hypotheses, 60*, 305–308.

Martin, C. L. (1969). Slit-lamp examination of the normal canine anterior ocular segment. Part II. Description. *J Small Anim Pract, 10*, 151–162.

Martin, C. L. (1975). Scanning electron microscopic examination of selected canine iridocorneal angle abnormalities. *J Am Anim Hosp Assoc, 11*, 300–306.

Massa, T., Davis, G. J., Schiavo, D., et al. (1984). Tapetal changes in beagle dogs. II. Ocular changes after the administration of a macrolide antibiotic-rosaraniicin. *Toxicol Appl Pharmacol, 72*, 195–200.

May, C. A. (2008). Comparative anatomy of the optic nerve head and inner retina in non-primate animal models used in glaucoma. *Open Ophthalmol J, 2*, 94–101.

McClure, R. C. (1960). Occurrence of the zygomatic groove and canal in the sphenoid bone of the dog skull (*Canis familiaris*). *Anat Rec, 138*, 136. (abstr).

McGreevy, P., Grassi, T. D., & Harman, A. M. (2004). A strong correlation exists between the distribution of retinal ganglion cells and nose length in the dog. *Brain Behav Evol, 63*, 13–22.

Michel, G. (1955). Beitrag zur anatomie der tranenorgane von hunde und katze. *Dtsch Tierarztl Wochenschr, 62*, 347–349.

Miller, W. W., Albert, R. A., Boosinger, T. R., et al. (1989). Postnatal development of the photoreceptor inner segment of the retina in dogs. *Am J Vet Res, 50*, 2089–2092.

Monaco, M. A., Samuelson, D. A., & Gelatt, K. N. (1985). Morphology and postnatal development of the normal lens in the dog and congenital cataract in the miniature schnauzer. *Lens Res, 2*, 393–433.

Moore, C. P., Wilsman, N., Nordheim, E. V., et al. (1987). Density and distribution of canine conjunctival goblet cells. *Invest Ophthalmol Vis Sci, 28*, 1925–1932.

Morgan, W. H., Yu, D. Y., Cooper, R. L., et al. (1995). The influence of cerebrospinal fluid pressure on the lamina cribrosa tissue pressure gradient. *Invest Ophthalmol Vis Sci, 36*, 1163–1172.

Morishige, N., Wahlert, A. J., Kenney, M. A., et al. (2007). Second-harmonic imaging microscopy of normal human and keratoconus cornea. *Invest Ophthalmol Vis Sci, 48*, 1087–1094.

Morrin, L. A., Waring, G. O., & Spangler, W. (1982). Oval lipid corned opacities in beagles: ultrastructure of the normal beagle cornea. *Am J Vet Res, 43*, 443–453.

Morrison, J. C., & Van Buskirk, E. M. (1982). The canine eye: pectinate ligaments and aqueous outflow resistance. *Invest Ophthalmol Vis Sci, 23*, 726–732.

Morrison, J. C., DeFrank, M. P., & Van Buskirk, E. M. (1987). Comparative microvascular anatomy of mammalian ciliary processes. *Invest Ophthalmol Vis Sci, 28*, 1325–1340.

Morita, M., Fujita, N., Takahashi, A., et al. (2015). Evaluation of ABCG2 and p63 expression in canine cornea and cultivated corneal epithelial cells. *Vet Ophthalmol, 18*, 59–68.

Mowat, F. M., Petersen-Jones, S. M., Williamson, H., et al. (2008). Topographical characterization of cone photoreceptors and the area centralis of the canine retina. *Mol Vis, 14*, 2518–2527.

Muller, L. J., Marfurt, C. F., Kruse, F., et al. (2003). Corneal nerves: structure, contents and function. *Exp Eye Res, 76*, 521–542.

Murphy, C. J., & Howland, H. C. (1987). The optics of comparative ophthalmoscopy. *Vis Res, 27*, 599–607.

Murphy, C. J., Mannis, M. J., Malfroy, B., et al. (1990). Neuropeptide depletion impairs corneal epithelial wound healing. *Invest Ophthalmol Vis Sci, 31*, 55. (Suppl).

Murphy, C. J., Marfurt, C. F., McDermott, A., et al. (2001). Spontaneous chronic corneal epithelial defects (SCCED) in dogs: clinical features, innervation, and effect of topical SP, with or without IGF-1. *Invest Ophthalmol Vis Sci, 42*, 2252–2261.

Murphy, C. J., Zadnik, K., & Mannis, M. (1992). Myopia and refractive error in dogs. *Invest Ophthalmol Vis Sci, 33*, 2459–2463.

Mutti, D. O., Zadnik, K., & Murphy, C. J. (1999). Naturally occurring vitreous chamber-based myopia in the labrador retriever. *Invest Ophthalmol Vis Sci, 40*, 1577–1584.

Nautscher, N., Bauer, A., Steffl, M., & Amselgruber, W. M. (2015). Comparative morphological evaluation of domestic animal cornea. *Vet Ophthalmol, 19*, 297–304.

Neitz, J., Geist, T., & Jacobs, G. H. (1989). Color vision in the dog. *Vis Neurosci, 3*, 119–125.

Newkirk, K. M., Haines, D. K., Calvarese, S. T., et al. (2010). Distribution and amount of pigment within the ciliary body and iris of dogs with blue and brown irides. *Vet Ophthalmol, 13*, 76–80.

Nicholas, E. (1914). *Veterinary and comparative ophthalmology*. Gray H., translator. London: H&W Brown.

Novellas, R., Espada, Y., & Ruiz de Gopegui, R. (2007). Doppler ultrasonographic estimation of renal and ocular resistive and pulsatility indices in normal dogs and cats. *Vet Radiol Ultrasound, 48*, 69–73.

Ofri, R., Lambrou, G. N., Allgoewer, I., et al. (2009). Clinical evaluation of pimecrolimus eye drops for treatment of canine keratoconjunctivitis sicca: a comparison with cyclosporine A. *Vet J, 179*, 70–77.

Ofri, R., Hollingsworth, S. R., Groth, A., et al. (2012). Effect of optical defocus on performance of dogs involved in field trial competition. *Am J Vet Res, 73*, 546–550.

Ollivier, F. J., Samuelson, D. A., Brooks, D. E., et al. (2004). Comparative morphology of the tapetum lucidum (among selected species). *Vet Ophthalmol, 7*, 11–22.

Packer, R. M. A., Hendricks, A., & Burn, C. C. (2015). Impact of facial conformation on canine health: corneal ulceration. *PLoS ONE, 10*(5), e0123827.

Park, S. A., Taylor, K. T., Zwingenberger, A. L., et al. (2016). Gross anatomy and morphometric evaluation of the canine lacrimal and third eyelid glands. *Vet Ophthalmol, 19*(3), 230–236.

Patruno, M., Perazzi, A., Martinello, T., Blaseotto, A., & Di Iorio, E. (2017). Iacopetti I: morphological description of limbal epithelium: searching for stem cells crypts in the dog, cat, pig, cow, sheep and horse. *Vet Res Commun, 41*, 169–173.

Paunksnis, A., Svaldeniené, E., Paunksniené, M., et al. (2001). Ultrasonographic evaluation of the eye parameters in dogs of different age. *Ultragarsas, 2*, 1–4.

Pearce, J. W., Janardhan, K. S., Caldwell, S., et al. (2007). Angiostatin and integrin αvβ3 in the feline, bovine, canine, equine, porcine and murine retina and cornea. *Vet Ophthalmol, 10*, 313–319.

Peichl, L. (1991). Catecholaminergic amacrine cells in the dog and wolf retina. *Vis Neurosci, 7*, 575–587.

Peichl, L. (1992a). Morphological types of ganglion cells in the dog and wolf retina. *J Comp Neurol, 324*, 590–602.

Peichl, L. (1992b). Topography of ganglion cells in the dog and wolf retina. *J Comp Neurol, 324*, 603–620.

Perry, H. (1940). Degenerations of the dog retina. I. structure and development of the normal dog. *Br J Ophthalmol, 37*, 385–393.

Piccione, G., Giannetto, C., Fazio, F., et al. (2009). Daily rhythm of tear production in normal dog maintained under different light/dark cycles. *Res Vet Sci, 86*, 521–524.

Piccione, G., Giannetto, C., Fazio, E., et al. (2010). Influence of different artificial lighting regimes on intraocular pressure circadian profile in the dog (*Canis familiaris*). *Exp Anim, 59*, 215–223.

Pigatto, J. A. T., Abib, F. C., Pereira, G. T., et al. (2006). Density of corneal endothelial cells in eyes of dogs using specular microscopy. *Braz J Vet Res Anim Sci (São Paulo), 43*, 476–480.

Pollock, R. V. H. (1978). The zonula ciliaris of the dog. *Proc Can Assoc Vet Anat, 3*, 11.

Polyak, S. (1957). *The vertebrate visual system*. Chicago: University of Chicago Press.

Pretterer, G., Bubna-Littitz, H., Windischbauer, G., et al. (2004). Brightness discrimination in the dog. *J Vis, 4*, 241–249.

Prince, J. H. (1956). *Comparative anatomy of the eye*. Springfield, IL: Charles C Thomas.

Prince, J. H., Diesem, C. D., Eglitis, I., et al. (1960). *Anatomy and histology of the eye and orbit in domestic animals*. Springfield, IL: Charles C Thomas.

Purtscher, E. (1961). Die grossen isiarterien beim hunde. *Berl Munch Tierarztl Wochenschr, 74*, 436–438.

Rached, P. A., Canola, J. C., Schlutter, C., et al. (2011). Computed tomographic-dacryocystography (CT_DCG) of the normal canine nasolacrimal drainage system with three-dimensional reconstruction. *Vet Ophthalmol, 14*, 174–179.

Ravi, M., Schobert, C. S., Kiupel, M., et al. (2014). Clinical, morphologic and immunohistochemical features of canine orbital hibernomas. *Vet Pathol, 5*(3), 563–568.

Raviola, G. (1971). The fine structure of the ciliary zonule and ciliary epithelium. *Invest Ophthalmol, 10*, 851–869.

Rebhun, W. C. (1976). Persistent hyperplastic primary vitreous in a dog. *J Am Vet Med Assoc, 169*, 620–622.

Reddy, T. S., Birkle, D. L., Packer, A. J., et al. (1986). Fatty acid composition and arachidonic acid metabolism in vitreous lipids from canine and human eyes. *Curr Eye Res, 5*(6), 441–447.

Reiser, P. J., Gentry, D. G., Bicer, S., et al. (2005). Passive viscoelastic properties of global and orbital layers of dog rectus muscles. *Invest Ophthalmol Vis Sci, 46*, 5719.

Riis, R. C. (1976). *The normal canine conjunctiva*. Thesis, Ithaca, NY: Cornell University.

Richards, T. R., Mortlock, J. M. H., Pinard, C. L., et al. (2014). Interleukin 11 expression in normal canine eyes. *Vet Ophthalmol, 17*, 46–56.

Roberts, S. R., & Bistner, S. I. (1968). Persistent pupillary membrane in basenji dogs. *J Am Vet Med Assoc, 153*, 533–542.

Roberts, S. R., Vierheller, R. C., & Lennox, W. J. (1974). Eyes. In J. Archibald (Ed.), *Canine surgery*. Santa Barbara, CA: American Veterinary Publications.

Robertson, S. A., & Andrew, S. E. (2003). Presence of opioid growth factor and its receptor in the normal dog, cat and horse cornea. *Vet Ophthalmol, 6*, 131–134.

Rochon-Duvigneaud, A. (1943). *Les yeux et la vision des vertebres*. Paris: Masson.

Rohen, J. W., Kaufman, P. L., Eichhorn, M., et al. (1989). Functional anatomy of accommodation in the raccoon. *Exp Eye Res, 48*, 523–537.

Rose, M. D., Mattoon, J. S., Gemensky-Metzler, A. J., et al. (2008). Ultrasound biomicroscopy of the iridocorneal angle of the eye before and after phacoemulsification and intraocular lens implantation in dogs. *Am J Vet Res, 69*, 279–288.

Royle, L., Matthews, E., Corfield, A., et al. (2008). Glycan structures of ocular surface mucins in man, rabbit and dog display species differences. *Glycoconj J, 25,* 763–773.

Rubin, L. F. (1974). *Atlas of veterinary ophthalmoscopy.* Philadelphia: Lea & Febiger.

Rungaldier, S., Pomikal, C., Streicher, J., et al. (2009). Palisade endings are present in canine extraocular muscles and have a cholinergic phenotype. *Neurosci Lett, 465,* 199–203.

Saito, A., Watanabe, Y., & Kotani, T. (2004). Morphologic changes of the anterior corneal epithelium caused by third eyelid removal in dogs. *Vet Ophthalmol, 7,* 113–119.

Salguero, S., Johnson, V., Williams, D., et al. (2015). CT dimensions, volumes and densities of normal canine eyes. *Vet Rec, 176,* 386–390.

Samuelson, D. A. (1996). A reevaluation of the comparative anatomy of the eutherian iridocorneal angle and associated ciliary body musculature. *Vet Comp Ophthalmol, 6,* 153–172.

Samuelson, D. A. (2007). Ophthalmic anatomy. In K. N. Gelatt (Ed.), *Veterinary ophthalmology* (4th ed.). Philadelphia: Lea & Febiger.

Samuelson, D. A., & Streit, A. (2012). Microanatomy of the anterior uveoscleral outflow pathway in normal and primary open-angle glaucomatous dogs. *Vet Ophthalmol, 5,* 47–53.

Samuelson, D. A., & Gelatt, K. N. (1984a). Aqueous outflow in the beagle. I. postnatal morphologic development of the iridocorneal angle: pectinate ligament and uveal trabecular meshwork. *Curr Eye Res, 3,* 783–794.

Samuelson, D. A., & Gelatt, K. N. (1984b). Aqueous outflow in the beagle. II. Postnatal development of the iridocorneal angle: corneo-scleral trabecular meshwork and angular aqueous plexus. *Curr Eye Res, 3,* 795–807.

Samuelson, D. A., Gelatt, K. N., & Gum, G. G. (1984). Kinetics of phagocytosis in the normal canine iridocorneal angle. *Am J Vet Res, 45,* 2359–2366.

Samuelson, D., Plummer, C., Lewis, P., et al. (2001). Schwalbe line's cell in the normal and glaucomatous dog. *Vet Ophthalmol, 4,* 47–53.

Sanchez, R. F., & Daniels, J. T. (2016). Limbal stem cells deficiency in companion animals: time to give something back? *Curr Eye Res, 41,* 425–432.

Schiavo, D. M., Sinha, D. P., Black, H. E., et al. (1984). Tapetal changes in beagle dogs. I. ocular changes after oral administration of a beta-adrenergic blocking agent-SCH 19927. *Toxicol Appl Pharmacol, 72,* 187–194.

Schiffer, S. P., Rantanen, N. W., Leary, G. A., et al. (1982). Biometric study of the canine eye, using A-mode ultrasonography. *Am J Vet Res, 43,* 826–830.

Schwab, I. R. (2011). *Evolution's witness: how eyes evolved.* New York: Oxford Univ. Press.

Scott, D. W., & Bistner, S. I. (1973). Neurotrophic keratitis in a dog. *Vet Med Small Anim Clin, 68,* 1120–1122.

Scott, J. E., & Bosworth, T. R. (1990). A comparative biochemical and ultrastructural study of proteoglycan-collagen interactions in corneal stroma: functional and metabolic implications. *Biochem J, 270,* 491–497.

Scurrell, E., Stanley, R., & Schöniger, S. (2009). Immunohistochemical detection of NOD1 and NOD2 in the healthy murine and canine eye. *Vet Ophthalmol, 12,* 269–275.

Sebbag, L., McDowell, E. M., Hepner, P. M., & Mochel, J. P. (2018). Effect of tear collection on lacrimal total protein content in dogs and cats: a comparison between Schirmer strips and ophthalmic sponges. *BMC Vet Res, 14,* 61. http://doi.org/10.1186/s12917-018-1390-7.

Sedacca, K. K., Samuelson, D. A., & Lewis, P. A. (2011). Examination of the anterior uveoscleral pathway in domestic species. *Vet Ophthalmol, 15,* 1–7.

Severin, G. A. (1976). *Veterinary ophthalmology notes* (2nd ed.). Fort Collins, CO: Colorado State University.

Sharpnack, D. P., Wyman, M., Anderson, B. G., et al. (1984). Vascular pathways of the anterior segment of the canine eye. *Am J Vet Res, 45,* 1287–1294.

Sherman, S. M., & Wilson, J. R. (1975). Behavioral and morphological evidence for binocular competition in the postnatal development of the dog's visual system. *J Comp Neurol, 161,* 183–196.

Shimokawa, T., Akita, K., Sato, T., Ru, F., Yi, S.-Q., & Tanaka, S. (2002). Comparative anatomical study of m. retractor bulbi with special reference to the nerve innervations in rabbits and dogs. *Okajimas Folia Anat Jpn, 78*(6), 235–244.

Shively, J. N., & Epling, G. P. (1969). Fine structure of the canine eye: iris. *Am J Vet Res, 30,* 13–25.

Shively, J. N., & Epling, G. P. (1970). Fine structure of the canine eye: cornea. *Am J Vet Res, 31,* 713–722.

Shively, J., Epling, G., & Jensen, R. (1971). Fine structure of the postnatal development of the canine retina. *Am J Vet Res, 32,* 383–392.

Simones, P., De Geest, J. P., & Lauwers, H. (1996). Comparative morphology of the pectinate ligaments of domestic mammals, as observed under the dissecting microscope and the scanning electron microscope. *J Vet Med Sci, 58,* 977–982.

Sivak, J. G. (1985). Optics of the crystalline lens. *Am J Optom Physiol Opt, 62,* 299–308.

Sivak, J. G., & Kreuzer, R. O. (1983). Spherical aberration of the crystalline lens. *Vis Res, 23,* 59–70.

Slatter, D. H., Nelson, A. W., Young, S., et al. (1979). Retinal vessels of canine eyes at different ages-a qualitative and quantitative study. *Exp Eye Res, 28,* 369–379.

Smythe, R. H. (1961). *Animal vision: what animals see.* Springfield, IL: Charles C Thomas.

Stern, J. A., Lahmers, S., & Meurs, K. M. (2015). Identification of striatin, a desmosomal protein, in the canine corneal epithelium. *Re Vet Sci, 102,* 182–183.

Strom, A. R., Cortés, D. E., Rasmussen, C. A., et al. (2016a). In vivo evaluation of the cornea and conjunctiva of the normal laboratory beagle using time- and Fourier-domain optical coherence tomography and ultrasound pachymetry. *Vet Ophthalmol, 19,* 50–56.

Strom, A. R., Cortés, D. E., Thomasy, S. M., Kass, P. H., Mannis, M. J., & Murphy, C. J. (2016b). In vivo ocular imaging of the cornea of the normal female laboratory beagle using confocal microscopy. *Vet Ophthalmol, 19,* 63–67.

Strom, A. R., Culp, W. T. N., Leonard, B. C., et al. (2018). A multidisciplinary, minimally invasive approach combining lacrimoscopy and fluoroscopically-guided stenting for management of nasolacrimal apparatus obstruction in dogs. *J Am Vet Med Assoc, 252,* 1527–1537.

Swann, D. A., Constable, I. J., & Caulfield, J. B. (1975). Vitreous structure. IV. Chemical composition of the insoluble residual protein fraction from the rabbit vitreous. *Invest Ophthalmol Vis Sci, 14,* 613–616.

Tachado, S. D., Akhtar, R. A., Yousufzai, S. Y., et al. (1991). Species differences in the effects of substance P on inositol triphosphate accumulation and cyclic AMP formation, and on contraction in isolated iris sphincter of the mammalian eye: differences in receptor density. *Exp Eye Res, 53,* 729–739.

Tachado, S. D., Virdee, K., Akhtar, R. A., et al. (1994). M_3 muscarinic receptors mediate an increase in both inositol triphosphate production and cyclic AMP formation in dog iris sphincter smooth muscle. *J Ocul Pharmacol, 10,* 137–147.

Tanimura, I. (1977). Comparative morphology of the bulbus oculi of the domestic animals revealed by scanning electron microscopy. *Jpn J Vet Sci, 39,* 643–656.

Terakado, K., Yogo, T., Kohara, Y., et al. (2012). Marked depletion of the water-channel protein, AQP5, in the canine nictitating membrane glands might contribute to the development of KCS. *Vet Pathol, 50*(4), 664–667.

Terakado, K., Yogo, T., Kohara, Y., et al. (2014). Conjunctival expression of the P2Y$_2$ receptor and the effects of 3% diquafosal ophthalmic solution in dogs. *Vet J, 202,* 48–52.

Thoft, R. A., & Friend, J. (1983). The x, y, z hypothesis of corneal epithelial maintenance. *Invest Ophthalmol Vis Sci, 24,* 1442–1443.

Thomasy, S. M., Raghunathan, V. K., Winkler, M., et al. (2014). Elastic modulus and collagen organization of the rabbit cornea: epithelium to endothelium. *Acta Biomater, 10,* 785–791.

Toniolo, L., Maccatrozzo, L., Patruno, M., et al. (2007). Fiber types in canine muscles: myosin isoform expression and functional characterization. *Am J Physiol Cell Physiol, 292,* C1915–C1926.

Umeda, Y., Nakamura, S., Fujiki, K., et al. (2010). Distribution of goblet cells and MUC5AC mRNA in the canine nictitating membrane. *Exp Eye Res, 91,* 721–726.

Unger, W. G., & Tighe, J. (1984). The response of isolated iris sphincter muscle of various mammalian species to substance P. *Exp Eye Res, 39,* 677–684.

Van Buskirk, E. M. (1979). The canine eye: the vessels of aqueous drainage. *Invest Ophthalmol Vis Sci, 18,* 223–230.

Verboven, C. A. P. M., Djajadiningrat-Laanen, S. C., Teske, E., & Boeve, M. H. (2014). Development of tear production and intraocular pressure in healthy canine neonates. *Vet Ophthalmol, 17,* 426–431.

Vivo, J., Morales, J. L., Diz, A., et al. (2004). Intracranial portion of the trochlear nerve and dorsal oblique muscle composition in dog: a structural and ultrastructural study. *J Morphol, 262,* 708–713.

Vivo, J., Morales, J. L., Díz, A., et al. (2006). Structural and ultrastructural study of the intracranial portion of the oculomotor, trochlear and abducent nerves in dog. *Anat Histol Embryol, 35,* 184–189.

Vivo, J., Galisteo, A. M., Miro, F., et al. (2012). Morphometric changes in the dog trochlear nerve with growth. *Anat Histol Embryol, 42,* 183–190.

Walde, I., Schaffer, E. H., & Kostlin, R. G. (1990). *Atlas of ophthalmology in dogs and cats.* Philadelphia: BC Decker.

Walls, G. L. (1942). *The vertebrate eye and its adaptive radiation.* Bloomfield Hills, MI: Cranbrook Institute of Science.

Wassef, A., Janardhan, K., Pearce, J. W., et al. (2004). Toll-like receptor 4 in normal and inflamed lungs and other organs of pig, dog and cattle. *Histol Histopathol, 19,* 1201–1208.

Watrous, W. G., & Olmsted, J. M. D. (1941). Reflex studies alter muscle transplantation. *Am J Physiol, 132,* 607–611.

Wang, Y., Bi, X., Zhou, H., et al. (2014). Repair of orbital bone defects in canines using grafts of enriched autologous bone marrow stromal cells. *J Transl Med, 12,* 123. doi:10.1186/1479-5876-12-123.

Wen, G. Y., Sturman, J. A., & Shek, J. E. (1985). A comparative study of the tapetum, retina, and skull of the ferret, dog, and cat. *Lab Anim Sci, 35,* 200–210.

Wenzel-Hora, B. I., Seifert, H. M., & Grüntzig, J. (1982). Animal experimental studies of indirect lymphography of the eye, face, and neck regions using iotasul. *Lymphology, 15,* 32–35.

Whalen, L. R., & Kitchell, R. L. (1983). Electrophysiological studies of the cutaneous nerves of the head of the dog. *Am J Vet Res, 44,* 615–627.

Whiteley, H. E., & Young, S. (1985). Cilia in the fetal and neonatal canine retina. *Tissue Cell, 17,* 335–340.

Wilcox, L. M., Keough, E. M., Connolly, R. J., et al. (1981). Comparative extraocular muscle blood flow. *J Exp Zool, 215,* 87–90.

Williams, D. L. (2004). Lens morphometry determined by B-mode ultrasonography of the normal and cataractous canine lens. *Vet Ophthalmol, 7,* 91–95.

Williams, L. A., Kubai, M. A., Murphy, C. J., et al. (2011). Ocular components in three breeds of dogs with high prevalence of myopia. *Opthamol Vis Sci, 88,* 269–274.

Winiarczyk, M., Winiarczyk, D., Banach, T., et al. (2015). Dog tear film proteome in-depth analysis. *PLoS ONE, 10,* e0144242. https://doi.org/10.1371/journal.pone.0144242.

Winkler, M., Shoa, G., Tran, S. T., et al. (2015). A comparative study of vertebrate corneal structure: the evolution of a refractive lens. *Invest Ophthalmol Vis Sci, 56,* 2764–2772.

Woo, H. M., Bentley, E., Campbell, S. F., et al. (2005). Nerve growth factor and corneal wound healing in dogs. *Exp Eye Res, 80,* 633–642.

Wyman, M., & Donovan, E. F. (1965). The ocular fundus of the normal dog. *J Am Vet Med Assoc, 147,* 17–26.

Yakely, W. L., & Alexander, J. E. (1971). Dacryocystorhinography in the dog. *J Am Vet Med Assoc, 159,* 1417–1421.

Yamaue, Y., Hosaka, Y. Z., & Uehara, M. (2014). Macroscopic and histologic variations in the cellular tapetum in dogs. *J Vet Med Sci, 76,* 1099–1103.

Yamaue, Y., Hosaka, Y. Z., & Uehara, M. (2015). Spatial relationships among the cellular tapetum, visual streak and rod density in dogs. *J Vet Med Sci, 77,* 175–179.

Yañez-Soto, B., Mannis, M. J., Schwab, I. R., et al. (2014). Interfacial phenomena and the ocular surface. *Ocul Surf, 12,* 178–201.

Yano, S., Hirose, M., Nakada, T., et al. (2010). Selective α1A-adrenoceptor stimulation induces Mueller's smooth muscle contraction in an isolated canine upper eyelid preparation. *Curr Eye Res, 35,* 363–369.

Yee, R. W., Matsuda, M., Kern, T. S., et al. (1985). Corneal endothelial changes in diabetic dogs. *Curr Eye Res, 4,* 759–766.

Yee, R. W., Edelhauser, H. F., & Stern, M. E. (1987). Specular microscopy of the vertebrate corneal endothelium: a comparative study. *Exp Eye Res, 44,* 703–714.

Yoshitomi, T., & Ito, Y. (1986). Pre-synaptic actions of noradrenaline on the dog ciliary muscle tissue. *Exp Eye Res, 43,* 119–127.

Yoshitomi, T., & Ito, Y. (1988). Effects of indomethacin and prostaglandins on the dog iris sphincter and dilator muscles. *Invest Ophthalmol Vis Sci, 29,* 127–132.

Yu, D., Adler, V. A., Cringle, S. J., et al. (1988). Choroidal blood flow measured in the dog eye in vivo and in vitro by local hydrogen clearance polarography: validation of a technique and response to raised intraocular pressure. *Exp Eye Res, 46,* 289–303.

Zhou, H., Deng, Y., Bi, X., et al. (2013). Orbital wall repair in canines with beta tri-calcium phosphate and induced bone marrow stromal cells. *J Biomed Mater Res B Appl Biomater, 101*(8), 1340–1349.

Zwingenberger, A. L., Park, S. A., Murphy, C. J., et al. (2014). Computed tomographic imaging characteristics of the normal canine lacrimal glands. *BMC Vet Res, 10,* 116. http://www.biomedcentral.com/1746-6148/10/116.

Index

A

Abdomen, 319–387, 352f, 361f, 368f–369f, 425f
  autonomic plexuses of, 674t
  regions of, 349–353, 353f
  relations of organs in, 353
  superficial vessels of, 563f
  viscera of, 354f
Abdominal aorta, 551–578
  branches of, 552f
Abdominal cavity, 351, 635f
Abdominal ostium, 450
Abdominal region, sympathetic distribution in, 668f–669f, 673–675, 674t
Abdominal walls
  lymph nodes and vessels of, 633–636
  muscles of, 252–258, 253f–255f
Abducent nerve (cranial nerve VI), 818f, 828–829, 898f, 900
  motor nucleus of, 766
Abduction, 179, 212
Accessory cephalic vein, 583f
Accessory nerve (cranial nerve XI), 709f, 836
  autonomic interconnections, 826f
  external branch of, 836
  internal branch of, 836
  motor nucleus of, 687, 764
  spinal root of, 681–682
Accessory palatine nerve, 822
Accessory structures
  axillary lymph node, 618f, 627f, 628
  cartilage, 389f, 390
  cephalic vein, 584f, 591
  interosseous artery, 545
  lobe of right lung, 410f, 411
  pancreas, 381–382
  pancreatic duct, 382
  parotid glands, 342

Page numbers followed by "f" indicate figures, "t" indicate tables, and "b" indicate boxes.

Accessory structures *(Continued)*
  process of vertebrae, 132f, 133–134, 134f–135f
  right coronary artery, 506
Accommodation, 871
Accumbens nucleus, 790
Acervulus cerebri, 482
Acetabular fossa, 156–158, 158f–160f
Acetabular ligament, transverse, 197, 197f
Acetabular lips, 197
Acetabular notch, 156–158
Acetabulum, 156–158, 160f
Achilles tendon, 294, 308
Achondroplasia, 4
Acidophilic endocrine cells, 474
Acoustic meatus
  external, 93f, 94, 102f–103f, 105, 118f–120f, 840f, 850
  internal, 102f, 103, 122f, 123
Acoustic radiation, 775, 788
Acoustic stria, 765
Acoustic tubercle, 765
Acromion, 141f, 142, 144f
Active movements, 179
Acute margin, of lung, 408–409
Adam's apple, 399
Adduction, 179, 212
Adhesio interthalamica, 772–773
Adipose capsule, 416–418
Aditus laryngis, 400
Adrenal (suprarenal) arteries, 559
Adrenal capsule, 484
Adrenal gland(s), 482–486, 560f
  developmental anatomy, 483–484
  innervation, 486, 486f
  macroscopic features, 482–483, 483f
  mesoscopic features, 483f–484f, 484–485
  microscopic features, 485–486
  vascularization, 483f, 486, 486f
Adrenal veins, 597
Adrenergic system, 661, 663
Adult cortex, 483–484
Adventitia, 347
Aequator, 861

Afferent arterioles, 420
Afferent axons, 688
  primary, 656f
Afferent ganglion cell, 651f
Afferent lymph vessels, 621
Afferent neurons, 651f
  primary, 651f, 654–655
Age
  changes of dermis with, 65–66
  of embryo, 21–26, 24f–25f, 24t
Aggregated lymph nodules, 367, 620–621
Agonist, 212–213
Ala nasi, 391
Ala ossis ilii, 158
Ala ossis sacri, 136
Alae atlantis, 127–130
Alae vomeris, 114, 114f
Alar canal, 101–102, 119–120
Alar fold, 112, 390–391
Alar foramen
  of atlas, 127–130
  caudal, 101–102, 118f–119f
  rostral, 101–102, 118, 118f–119f
Alar ligaments, 183, 183f
Albumin immunologic distance, 2
Alimentary canal, 346–375
Allantois, 20, 20f
Alpha motor neurons, 685
Alpha neuron, 652f
Alveolar bone, 329
Alveolar canals, 110–111
Alveolar ducts, 388, 403
Alveolar foramina, 110–111, 110f, 122f
Alveolar juga, 110–111, 118
Alveolar process, 110–111, 110f
  of maxilla, 111
Alveolar sacs, 388, 403
Alveoli, 110–111, 388
Alveoli dentales, 109–111, 115
Alveoli pulmonis, 403
Amnion, 18, 19f
Amniotic folds, 18, 18f–19f
Amphiarthroses, 177
Ampulla, 437, 842–843
Ampulla ductus deferentis, 437
Ampullae osseae, 840

912

Amygdala, 776, 784
Anagen, 69, 75–76, 76f
Anal canal, 370f, 371–373
    nerves of, 373
    special muscles of, 372–373
    vessels of, 373
    zones of, 371
Anal columns, 371–372
Anal glands, 372
Anal region, 428f
Anal sacs, 80–81
Anal sinuses, 371–372
Anal sphincter
    external, 371f, 372–373
    internal, 371f, 372–374
Anconeal process, 192
Anconeus muscle, 717f
Anestrum, 448
Anestrus, 449
Angle
    caudal, of scapula, 141f, 142
    cranial, of scapula, 141f, 142
    of mandible, 115–116
    medial, of ischiatic tuberosity, 160f
    of rib, 139f, 140
    ventral, of scapula, 141f, 142
Angular artery, of mouth, 516–517
Angular cusps, 504
Angular incisure, 361–362
Angular process, 115–116, 115f, 120f
Angular vein
    of eye, 586, 903–904
    of mouth, 587
Angularis oculi vein, 99f, 583f, 587f
Angularis oris vein, 586f, 587
Anguli oculi medialis et lateralis, 885
Angulus caudalis, 142
Angulus costae, 140
Angulus cranialis, 142
Angulus mandibulae, 115–116
Angulus oris, 319
Angulus ventralis, 142
Annular fold, 345
Annular ligaments
    of radius, 190–191, 190f
    of trachea, 402
Annulospiral endings, 695–696
Anocutaneous line, 371
Anomalies
    dental, 329
    of kidney, 420
    of male urethra, 444
    of ovary, 450
    of prepuce, 445
    of testes, 431–432
    of tongue, 339–340
    of ureters, 421

Anomalies (Continued)
    of urinary bladder, 423
    of uterine tube, 451
Anorectal line, 371–372
Ansa cervicalis, 705f, 708–709, 837
Antagonist, 212–213
Antebrachiocarpal joint, 152f, 192
Antebrachium (forearm)
    interosseous ligament, 192
    interosseous nerve of, 722
    muscles of, 273–285
        caudal, 268f, 270f–271f, 274f, 278–285, 723t
        craniolateral, 270f, 273–278, 273f–276f, 280f–282f
        synovial apparatus of, 282f, 284
    right, nerves of, 718f
    veins of, 592f
Anterior ciliary arteries, 523, 901–902
Anterior zonular fibers, 871
Anterograde, 653–654
Anthelix, 850–851
Anticlinal vertebra, 131–132, 132f, 134f
Antidromic conduction, 653–654, 653f
Antitragicohelicine incisure, 851–852
Antitragus, 851–852
Antrum pyloricum, 362
Anular cartilage, 850–851
Anular ligament, 850
Anuli fibrosi atrioventriculares, 501
Anulus fibrosus
    of heart, 500
    of vertebral column, 125–126, 185, 185f
Anulus fibrosus aorticus, 500
Anulus fibrosus pulmonalis, 500–501
Anulus inguinalis superficialis, 257
Anulus sclerae, 861, 871
Anulus tympanicus, 105
Anus, 371, 371f
    glands of, 80–81
Aorta, 510, 511f, 574f, 729f, 740f
    abdominal, 551–578
        branches of, 552f, 561f
        parietal branches of, 559–562
        unpaired visceral branches of, 552–559
    ascending, 510
    descending, 510, 534f
    lymph vessels of, 629f
    parietal branches of, 549f, 550–551
    thoracic, 548–551
    visceral branches of, 552f
Aorta abdominalis, 510, 551–552
Aorta descendens, 510
Aorta thoracica, 510, 548–549

Aortic arch, 510–548, 511f, 631f
Aortic bulb, 505
Aortic fibrous ring, 500
Aortic hiatus, 351
Aortic ostium, 503
Aortic plexus, 450–451
Aortic sinuses, 505
Aortic thoracic nodes, 630
Aortic valve, 500, 501f
Aorticorenal ganglia, 420
Apertura externa aqueductus vestibuli, 103
Apertura externa canaliculi cochleae, 103
Apertura nasi ossea, 109–110, 123, 388
Apertura pelvis caudalis, 156–158, 352–353
Apertura pelvis cranialis, 156–158, 352–353
Apertura sinus frontalis, 124–125
Apertura thoracis cranialis, 405
Aperturae laterales, 763
Aperture
    nasal, 109–110, 121
    pelvic, 156–158
        caudal, 352–353
        cranial, 352–353
Apex
    of bladder, 421
    of epiglottic cartilage, 397–398
    of heart, 495–496
    of large intestine, 368–369
    of lungs, 408
    of nose, 388
    of orbit, 892f
    of os penis, 439
    petrosal, 102–103
    of pyramid, 103f
    of sacrum, 136–137, 136f
    of tongue, 330
    of tooth, 323–324
Apex ceci, 368–369
Apex cordis, 495–496, 499
Apex cuspidis, 323–324
Apex linguae, 330
Apex nasi, 388
Apex ossis sacri, 136–137, 136f
Apex partis petrosae, 102–103
Apex pulmonis, 408
Apex radicis dentis, 323–324
Apex vesicae, 421
Apical delta, 326–327
Apical ligament, 183, 183f
Apical lobe, 410
Apical tooth, 327
Aponeurosis, palatine, 322

Apparatus digestorius, 319
Apparatus hyoideus, 116
　bones of, 116–117, 116f
　development of, 33, 39f, 44f
　muscle of, 227f, 233f–235f, 264f
Apparatus respiratorius, 388
Apparatus urogenitalis, 416
Appendicular skeleton, 87t. see also Pelvic limb; Thoracic limb
Appendix fibrosa hepatis, 377–378
Appendix testis, 463
Aqueduct
　mesencephalic, 758t, 767
　vestibular, 102f, 104
Aqueductus mesencephali, 700–701, 767
Aqueous humor, 878
Arachnoid membrane, 679, 680f–681f, 699, 700f
Arachnoid trabeculae, 699
Arachnoid villi, 700f, 701, 702f
Arachnoidea encephali, 699
Arachnoidea spinalis, 699
Arbor bronchialis, 402–403
Arch(es)
　arterial
　　deep palmar, 546
　　deep plantar, 569–570
　　superficial palmar, 548
　costal, 139
　of cricoid cartilage, 399
　dental, 325
　dorsal, of atlas, 127–130
　hemal, 137f, 138
　inguinal, 254f, 256
　ischiatic, 157f, 160f
　lumbocostal, 250f, 251
　neural, 44, 47f–49f
　palatoglossal, 321f, 322
　palatopharyngeal, 322
　palmar, deep, 548
　venous
　　deep palmar, 592f, 594–595
　　deep plantar, 605f
　　digital, 605, 605f
　　dorsal deep, 606
　　hyoid, 586f, 588–589
　　superficial palmar, 591, 592f, 594
　　superficial plantar, 605f, 606
　ventral, of atlas, 127–130
　vertebral, 126
　　of caudal vertebrae, 137f–138
　　of third cervical vertebrae, 130f
　zygomatic, 105, 112, 117–118
Archicortex (archipallium), 779
Arcuate arteries, 420, 569–570, 569f, 751f

Arcuate fibers, 788
　deep, 761
Arcuate line, 156–160
Arcuate veins, 420
Arcus alveolaris, 115
Arcus aortae, 510
Arcus cartilaginis cricoideae, 399
Arcus costalis, 139
Arcus dentalis inferior, 325
Arcus dorsalis, 127–130
Arcus dorsalis profundus, 606
Arcus dorsalis superficialis, 605–606
Arcus hemales, 138
Arcus hyoideus, 588–589
Arcus inguinalis, 254f, 256
Arcus ischiadicus, 160–161
Arcus lumbocostalis, 250f, 251
Arcus palatoglossus, 322, 344–345
Arcus palatopharyngeus, 322
Arcus palmaris profundus, 546, 548, 594–595
Arcus palmaris superficialis, 546, 548, 591, 594
Arcus plantaris profundus, 569–570, 606
Arcus plantaris superficialis, 606
Arcus venosus digitales, 594
Arcus ventralis, 127–130
Arcus vertebralis, 126
Arcus zygomaticus, 105, 112, 117–118
Area
　cutaneous, 660, 660f
　intercondyloid, 165f–166f
　for origin of the rectus femoris, 158–160
Area cochleae, 103
Area cribrosa, 418–419
Area cribrosa sclerae, 861
Area intercondylaris caudalis, 165–167
Area intercondylaris cranialis, 165–167
Area nuda, 377
Area postrema, 763
Area vestibularis inferior, 103
Area vestibularis superior, 103
Areae gastricae, 363
Arm. see Brachium
Arrector pili muscles, 78f–79f, 79
Arteria (A.)/Arteriae (Aa.). see Artery(ies); specific arteries
A. abdominalis caudalis, 564–565
A. abdominalis cranialis, 561
A. alveolaris inferior, 520–522
A. angularis oris, 516–517
A. antebrachialis profunda, 546

A. antebrachialis superficialis cranialis, 542–543
A. arcuata, 569–570
A. auricularis magna, 517
A. auricularis profunda, 517
A. auricularis rostralis, 518
A. axillaris, 538
A. basilaris, 531–533
A. bicipitalis, 541
A. brachialis, 541
A. brachialis profunda, 541
A. brachialis superficialis, 541–542
A. bronchoesophagea, 549–550
A. buccalis, 524
A. bulbi penis, 576
A. bulbi vestibuli, 576
A. carotis communis dextra, 510–511
A. carotis communis sinistra, 510
A. carotis externa, 513
A. carotis interna, 526–527
A. caudalis femoris distalis, 568
A. caudalis femoris media, 568
A. caudalis femoris proximalis, 567–568
A. caudalis lateralis, 578
A. caudalis mediana, 578–579
A. caudalis ventralis, 579
A. cecalis, 557
A. celiaca, 552–554
A. cerebelli caudalis, 531–533
A. cerebelli rostralis, 531
A. cerebri caudalis, 530–531
A. cerebri media, 527–528
A. cerebri rostralis, 528
A. cervicalis profunda, 534
A. cervicalis superficialis, 536–537
A. choroidea rostralis, 527–528
A. ciliares anteriores, 523
A. ciliares posteriores breves, 524
A. circumflexa femoris lateralis, 567
A. circumflexa humeri caudalis, 539
A. circumflexa ilium profunda, 561
A. circumflexa ilium superficialis, 567
A. clitoridis, 576
A. colica dextra, 557
A. colica media, 557
A. colica sinistra, 558
A. collateralis radialis, 539
A. collateralis ulnaris, 541
A. comitans n. ischiadicus, 578
A. communicans caudalis, 527
A. communicans rostralis, 528
A. condylaris, 513
A. conjunctivalis posterioris, 523
A. coronaria dextra, 506
A. coronaria dextra accessoria, 506
A. coronaria sinistra, 506

A. costoabdominalis dorsalis, 550–551
A. cremasterica, 564–565
A. cystica, 554
A. digitales plantares propriae, 573
A. digitalis dorsalis communis, 542–543
A. digitalis dorsalis V abaxialis, 545
A. digitalis palmaris communis, 548
A. digitalis palmaris V abaxialis, 548
A. dorsalis nasi caudalis, 518
A. dorsalis nasi rostralis, 526
A. dorsalis pedis, 569–570
A. dorsalis penis, 576
A. ductus deferentis, 437–438, 575
A. epigastrica caudalis, 562
A. epigastrica cranialis, 536
A. epigastrica cranialis superficialis, 536
A. epigastrica superficialis caudalis, 562–563
A. ethmoidalis externa, 523–524, 901–902
A. ethmoidalis interna, 530
A. facialis, 516
A. femoralis, 565–567
A. gastrica dextra, 554
A. gastrica sinistra, 556
A. gastroduodenalis, 554
A. gastroepiploica dextra, 554–555
A. gastroepiploica sinistra, 555
A. genus descendens, 568
A. genus distalis lateralis, 569
A. genus distalis medialis, 569
A. genus media, 569
A. genus proximalis lateralis, 569
A. genus proximalis medialis, 569
A. glutea caudalis, 576
A. glutea cranialis, 577–578
A. hepatica, 554
A. ilei, 558
A. ileocolica, 557
A. iliaca externa, 562
A. iliaca interna, 573
A. iliolumbalis, 576–577
A. infraorbitalis, 526
A. intercarotica caudalis, 527
A. intercostalis dorsalis I, 535
A. intercostalis suprema, 534–535
A. interossea caudalis, 545–546
A. interossea communis, 544–545
A. interossea cranialis, 546
A. labialis inferior, 516
A. labialis superior, 517
A. labyrinthi, 531–533
A. lacrimalis, 523, 902
A. laryngea cranialis, 514–515
A. lateralis nasi, 526

A. lienalis, 555
A. lingualis, 338, 515–516
A. lumbales, 551
A. malaris, 526, 901
A. masseterica, 522
A. maxillaris, 518, 901
A. mediana, 546
A. meningea caudalis, 514
A. meningea media, 522
A. meningea rostralis, 523–524
A. mesenterica caudalis, 558
A. mesenterica cranialis, 556–557
A. metatarseae dorsalis II, 569–570
A. musculophrenica, 536
A. nutricia humeri, 539
A. nutricia tibiae, 517–518
A. nutriciae tibiae, 569
A. occipitalis, 513
A. ophthalmica externa, 523, 901
A. ophthalmica interna, 530, 902
A. ovarica, 559
A. palatina ascendens, 515–516
A. palatina descendens, 525
A. palatina major, 525
A. palatina minor, 524–525
A. palpebrae tertiae, 526
A. palpebralis inferior lateralis, 518
A. palpebralis inferior medialis, 526
A. palpebralis superior lateralis, 518
A. palpebralis superior medialis, 526
A. pancreaticoduodenalis caudalis, 557–558
A. pancreaticoduodenalis cranialis, 555
A. parotis, 517–518
A. penis, 576
A. pericardiacophrenica, 535
A. perinealis dorsalis, 578
A. perinealis ventralis, 576
A. pharyngea ascendens, 322, 515
A. phrenica caudalis, 561
A. poplitea, 569
A. profunda femoris, 562
A. profunda linguae, 515–516
A. profunda penis, 576
A. prostatica, 437–438, 575
A. pudenda externa, 562
A. pudenda interna, 573–575
A. pulmonalis dextra, 412, 509
A. pulmonalis sinistra, 412, 509
A. radiales superficiales, 541–542
A. radialis, 546
A. rectalis caudalis, 575–576
A. rectalis cranialis, 558
A. rectalis media, 438, 575
A. recurrens tibialis cranialis, 569
A. recurrens ulnaris, 517, 543–544
A. renis, 420

A. sacralis mediana, 578
A. saphena, 568
A. scapularis dorsalis, 534
A. sphenopalatine, 525
A. spinalis ventralis, 531–533
A. stylomastoidea, 517
A. subclavia, 531
A. sublingualis, 338, 516
A. submentalis, 516
A. subscapularis, 539
A. suprascapularis, 537
A. tarsea lateralis, 569–570
A. tarsea medialis, 569–570
A. temporalis profunda caudalis, 522
A. temporalis profunda rostralis, 524
A. temporalis superficialis, 518, 901
A. testicularis, 559
A. thoracica externa, 538
A. thoracica interna, 535
A. thoracica lateralis, 538–539
A. thoracodorsalis, 539
A. thyroidea caudalis, 511–512
A. tibialis caudalis, 569
A. tibialis cranialis, 569
A. transversa cubiti, 543
A. transversa faciei, 518
A. tympanica rostralis, 522
A. ulnaris, 545
A. umbilicalis, 573
A. uterina, 575
A. uterina media, 559
A. vaginalis, 575
A. vertebralis, 531
A. vertebralis thoracica, 534–535
A. vesicales craniales, 573
A. vesicalis caudalis, 437–438, 575
Aa. adrenales, 559
Aa. arcuatae, 420
Aa. carotides communes, 510
Aa. caudales dorsolaterales, 579
Aa. caudales ventrolaterales, 579
Aa. ciliares anteriores, 901–902
Aa. ciliares posteriores breves, 902
Aa. ciliares posteriores longae, 523, 902
Aa. ciliaris posteriores breves, 523
Aa. conjunctivales posteriores, 901–902
Aa. digitales communes, 570
Aa. digitales dorsales communes, 547–548, 570–571
Aa. digitales dorsales propriae, 570–571
Aa. digitales palmares communes, 546
Aa. digitales palmares propriae axialis, 548

Aa. digitales plantares communes, 572–573
Aa. digitales propriae, 570
Aa. digitalis palmares communes II-IV, 548
Aa. episclerales, 523, 901–902
Aa. gastricae breves, 555
Aa. hepaticae, 378
Aa. intercostales dorsales, 550–551
Aa. interlobares renis, 420
Aa. interlobulares, 420
Aa. jejunales, 558
Aa. lumbales, 559–560
Aa. metacarpeae dorsales, 546
Aa. metacarpeae palmares, 548
Aa. metatarseae, 569–570
Aa. metatarseae dorsales, 571–572
Aa. metatarseae plantares, 573
Aa. nasales caudales, 525
Aa. nasales laterales, 525
Aa. nasales septales, 525
Aa. nasales septales caudales, 523–524
Aa. palatinae majores, 322
Aa. palatinae minores, 322
Aa. plantaris lateralis, 572–573
Aa. plantaris medialis, 572–573
Aa. renales, 558–559
Aa. surales, 569
Arteriae meningeae mediae, 99
Arterial arch
  palmar, superficial, 546
  plantar, deep, 541–542
Arterial circle, of brain, 527
Arteries
  of bone, 90–91
  nutrient, 90–91
  periosteal, 90–91
Arteriola glomerularis afferens, 420
Arteriola glomerularis efferens, 420
Artery(ies). *see also specific arteries*
  of base of cranium, 902f
  of base of skull, 528f
  of brachium, 538f–540f, 542f–544f
  bronchial, 412
  of bulb, 441, 444
    of penis, 444
  of cervical spinal cord, 533f
  of clitoris, 576
  coronary, 506–508
  of ductus deferens, 436–438, 573f
  of eye, 901–903
  of female pelvis, 574f
  of female perineum, 745f
  of forepaw, 545f, 546–548
  of gluteal region, 576f
  of head, 510–548, 514f
  of hindpaw, 569–573

Artery(ies) *(Continued)*
  interlobar, 420
  interlobular, 420
  of leg, 749f
  of male pelvic viscera, 573f
  of male perineum, 574f, 747f
  minor palatine, 524–525
  of nasal septum, 393f
  of neck, 510–548
  of orbit, 520f, 901f–902f
  palatine, 346
    major, 322
  of pelvic limb, 562–569
  of penis, 440–441, 573f
  of popliteal region, 567f
  pulmonary, 509
  retinal, 876, 903
  of right shoulder joint, 716f
  of sacrum, 577f
  scrotal, 428
  of skin, 81, 81f
  of skull, 528f
  systemic, 510–579
  of tail, 577f
  of thigh, 564f–566f
  of thoracic limb, 531–538
  of thoracic wall, 550f
  of thorax, 510–548, 532f–533f
  of thymus gland, 535f
  urethral, 444
  vaginal, 575
  of vascular tunic, 869f
  of vestibular bulb, 574f, 602f–603f
Arthrology, 176–206
  general, 176–179
Articular capsule. *see* Joint capsule
Articular cartilage, 177–178
Articular circumference
  of radius, 147, 147f
  of ulna, 149–151
Articular disc, 179
Articular fovea, of radius, 147
Articular muscles, 212–213
Articular process
  of atlas, 127–130
  of mandible, 115–116
  of vertebrae, 126
    caudal, 137–138
    lumbar, 134, 134f–135f
    sacral, 135–136, 136f, 157f
    thoracic, 132f, 133
Articular surface
  of atlas, 126f, 127–130
  of axis, 127f, 130
  of calcaneus, 169–170
  of fibula, 168
  of larynx, 400

Articular surface *(Continued)*
  of patella, 164
  of rib, 139–140
  of talus, 170–171
  of tibia, 165–167
Articulatio antebrachiocarpea, 192
Articulatio atlantoaxialis, 182–183, 182f–183f
Articulatio atlantooccipitalis, 182, 182f
Articulatio calcaneoquartalis, 202–203
Articulatio capitis costae, 186
Articulatio centrodistalis, 202–203
Articulatio condylaris, 179
Articulatio costotransversaria, 186
Articulatio coxae, 197
Articulatio cricoarytenoidea, 400
Articulatio cubiti, 189
Articulatio dentoalveolaris, 176
Articulatio ellipsoidea, 179
Articulatio femoropatellaris, 198–199
Articulatio femorotibialis, 198–199
Articulatio genus. *see* Stifle joint
Articulatio humeri, 188–189, 188f
Articulatio humeroradialis, 189
Articulatio incudomallearis, 180
Articulatio incudostapedia, 180
Articulatio intermandibularis, 180
Articulatio mediocarpea, 192
Articulatio plana, 179
Articulatio radioulnaris distalis, 192
Articulatio radioulnaris proximalis, 189, 191–192
Articulatio sacroiliaca, 196
Articulatio sellaris, 179
Articulatio spheroidea, 179
Articulatio talocalcaneocentralis, 202–203
Articulatio tarsocruralis, 202–203
Articulatio temporohyoidea, 180
Articulatio temporomandibularis, 105, 179
Articulatio tibiofibularis distalis, 202
Articulatio tibiofibularis proximalis, 202
Articulatio trochoidea, 179
Articulationes carpi, 192, 192f–195f
Articulationes carpometacarpeae, 192
Articulationes cinguli membri pelvinae, 196–197
Articulationes costochondrales, 188
Articulationes costovertebrales, 183–184, 186
Articulationes intercarpeae, 192
Articulationes intermetacarpeae, 195
Articulationes interphalangeae proximales, 195–196

Articulationes manus, 192–196, 192f–195f
Articulationes metacarpophalangeae, 195
Articulationes ossiculorum auditus, 180
Articulationes pedis, 202–205
Articulationes sternocostales, 187, 187f–188f
Articulationes synoviales, 177. see also Joint(s), synovial
Articulationes tarsi, 202–203
Articulationes tarsometatarseae, 202–203
Articulations. see Joint(s)
Articulations processuum articularum, 183–184
Aryepiglottic fold, 345f, 400
Arytenoid cartilage, 397f, 399
Arytenoideus transversus, 398f
Ascending aorta, 510
Ascending colon, 369
Ascending mesocolon, 369–370
Ascending palatine artery, 515–516
Ascending pathways, 655
Ascending pharyngeal arteries, 322, 346, 515–516
  palatine branches, 515
  pharyngeal branches, 515
Ascending pharyngeal vein, 589
Astrocytus, 657
Atlantal fossae, 127–130
Atlantal ligament, transverse, 183, 183f
Atlantoaxial articulation, 182–183, 182f–183f
  subluxation of, 183
Atlantoaxial joint, 129f
Atlantoaxial membrane, dorsal, 182–183
Atlantooccipital articulation, 181–182, 182f
Atlantooccipital joint, 182, 182f
Atlantooccipital membrane
  dorsal, 182
  ventral, 182
Atlantooccipital space, 183f
Atlas, 126f, 127–130, 128f, 182, 182f–183f
  development/ossification of, 37, 47f, 126f, 131
  lateral mass of, 127–130
  ligaments of, 182, 183f
Atrichial sweat glands, 79, 80f
Atrioventricular bundle, 505–506
Atrioventricular fibrous rings, 501
Atrioventricular node, 505–506
Atrioventricular orifice, 499

Atrioventricular ostium, 501–502
Atrioventricular valves, 504–505
Atrium (atria), 499–500
  left, 495–496, 500
  of middle meatus, 394
  right, 495–496, 499, 499f
Atrium dextrum, 495–496, 499
Atrium meatus nasi medius, 394
Atrium sinistrum, 495–496, 500
Auditory area, 789
Auditory meatus. see Acoustic meatus
Auditory neurons, 650–651
Auditory ossicles, 848f–849f, 849
  joints of, 180
  ligaments of, 180, 850
  muscles of, 850
Auditory tube, 101–102, 396, 847–848
  ostium of, 847
  pharyngeal opening of, 344, 396
  sulcus for, 101–102
Auricle (auricula), 839, 850–852
  left, 500
  right, 499
Auricula dextra, 499
Auricula sinistra, 500
Auricular branch, 713f, 748–749
Auricular cartilage, 850, 856f
Auricular nerve, 837
Auricular surface
  of heart, 497f, 499
  of iliac wing, 158–161, 158f–159f
Auricular veins
  caudal, 342, 589–590
  deep, 589–590
  intermediate, 589–590
  lateral, 589–590
  medial, 589
  rostral, 589
Auriculopalpebral nerve, 832, 900
Auriculotemporal nerve, 342, 825–826
  parotid branches, 825–826
  transverse facial branch, 825–826
Auris externa, 839
Auris interna, 839
Auris media, 839
Autonomic nervous system, 663–678
Autonomous zone (AZ), 660
Axial magnification, 880
Axial skeleton, 87t, 91–140. see also Axial skeleton; Skull; Sternum; Vertebra(e); Vertebral column
Axillary artery, 511f, 538–541, 538f, 584f, 593f, 713f–714f, 716f
Axillary lymph center, 628
Axillary lymph node, 618f, 627f, 628

Axillary nerve, 705f, 713f–717f, 715–716
Axillary region, 593f
Axillary vein, 593–594
Axillobrachial vein, 583f–584f, 591f, 593, 593f
Axis, 127f–128f, 130, 182f–183f
  development/ossification of, 37, 47f, 127f, 130
  ligaments of, 183f
Axis bulbi, 861
Axon(s), 650, 651f, 653
  afferent, primary, 656f
  preganglionic, 661f
Axon hillock, 651–653
Azygos veins, 348, 582, 583f, 590f, 613f, 729f
  continuation of caudal vena cava, 596–597
  right, 590

B

Back-crosses, 4
Ball-and-socket joint, 179
Band, green, 20–21
Basal lamina, 867
Basal margin, of lung, 408–409
Basal nuclei, 778–779, 789–791, 791f–792f
Base
  of heart, 495–496, 498f, 499, 501f
  of lungs, 408
  of metacarpals, 153f, 154, 155f
  of metatarsal bones, 171f
  of phalanges, 155–156, 155f
  of sacrum, 136–137, 136f
  of skull, 528f
  of stapes, 850
Basicranial centers, 29–32, 40f–43f
Basihyoid, 116, 116f
Basihyoid cartilage, 33
Basihyoideum, 116, 116f
Basilar artery, 527f, 531–533, 902f
  pontine branches, 531–533
Basilar membrane, 844
Basilar sinus, 607f
Basioccipital bone, 96f, 117f, 119f–120f
  development of, 29–32, 38f, 40f
Basion, 93f, 94
Basipharyngeal canal, 119
Basis cordis, 495–496, 499
Basis ossis sacri, 136–137
Basis pulmonis, 408
Basisphenoid bone, 92f, 96f, 100f–101f, 101–102, 117f, 120f
  development of, 29–32, 38f, 40f

Basivertebral veins, 613, 613f
Basophilic endocrine cells, 474
Beta motor neurons, 685
Biceps tendon, 188f
Bicipital artery, 538f, 541, 593f
Bicipital vein, 593f
Bicuspid valve, 504–505
Bifurcatio tracheae, 402
Bile ducts, 379, 380f
   common bile duct, 357f
   intramural course of, 380f
Bile passages, 379–381
Biliary ductules, 379
Bipolar cells, 650–651
Bipolar neurons, 650–651
Bird tongue, 339, 339f
Biventer cervicis muscle, 710f
Bladder, urinary, 416, 420f–421f, 421–423, 427f
   anomalies of, 423
   fixation of, 422–423
   lymph vessels of, 642f
   nerves of, 423
   structure of, 421–422
   vessels of, 423
Blastocyst, 15–17, 16f–17f, 16t
"Blind spot," 875–876
Blood supply, of spleen, 555f
Blood vessels. *see also* Artery(ies); Vein(s); *specific vessels*
   of anal canal, 373
   of axillary region, 593f
   bronchial, 412–413
   of ductus deferens, 436
   of esophagus, 348
   of eye, 901–904
   of female external genitalia, urethra, 457
   of heart, 506–509
   of hypophysis, 521f
   of kidneys, 419–420, 419f
   of liver, 378–379
   of male urethra, 444
   of mammary gland, 461–462, 461f
   of os penis, 440–442
   of ovary, 449–450
   palatine, 322
   of pancreas, 382–383
   of prepuce, 444–445, 602f–603f
   of prostate gland, 437–438
   pulmonary, 411–412
   of scrotum, 428
   of small intestine, 367
   of spleen, 644
   of stomach, 364
   of testes, 430–431
   of thymus gland, 535f

Blood vessels *(Continued)*
   of tongue, 338
   of ureters, 421
   of urinary bladder, 423
   of uterine tube, 450–451
   of uterus, 453
   of veins, 602f–603f
Body
   of atlas, 126f, 127–130
   of axis, 127f
   of basisphenoid bone, 101
   of bladder, 421
   of brain, 757
   of caudal vertebrae, 137, 137f
   of cervical vertebrae, 129f
   of clitoris, 455
   of epididymis, 435
   of femur, 162f–163f, 163–164
   of fibula, 168
   of fifth cervical vertebra, 128f
   of gallbladder, 379
   of humerus, 143, 143f, 145
   of ilium, 157f, 158
   of incisive bone, 109–110
   incus, 849–850
   of ischium, 160–161
   of large intestine, 368–369
   of lumbar vertebra, 134f
   of mandible, 115, 115f, 120f
   of metacarpals, 153f, 154
   of metatarsal, 169–170, 169f
   of pancreas, 381
   of penis, 438
   of perineum, 374
   of phalanges, 155–156, 155f
   of presphenoid bone, 101, 121
   of pubis, 161
   of radius, 147–148, 147f, 149f
   of rib, 139f, 140
   of sacrum, 136f, 157f
   of stomach, 362
   of talus, 169–170, 170f
   of tarsal bones, 168f
   of thoracic vertebra, 131–132, 132f
   of tibia, 166f, 167
   of tongue, 330
   of ulna, 149f, 151
   of uterus, 451–452
   of vertebra, 125–126
   vitreous, 879
Bone(s). *see also specific bones and at* Os
   alveolar, 329
   basihyoid, 116, 116f
   basioccipital, 96f, 117f, 119f–120f
      development of, 29–32, 38f, 40f

Bone(s) *(Continued)*
   basisphenoid, 92f, 96f, 100f–101f, 101–102, 117f, 120f
      development of, 29–32, 38f, 40f
   calcium phosphate of, 90
   carpal. *see* Carpal bone(s)
   cartilage, 89
   ceratohyoid, 116–117, 116f
   compact, 89–90
   cranial, 95–109. *see also* Skull
   dentary, 28, 45f
   development of, 88–89
   epihyoid, 116f, 117, 227f–228f, 344f
   ethmoid, 96f, 99f, 106–109, 106f–108f, 117f, 120f
      development of, 29–32
   exoccipital, 120f
   of face, 91f, 109–116
   flat, 88
   frontal, 91f–92f, 96f, 99–100, 116f–117f
   function of, 91
   heterotopic, 86
   hip, 156–158, 157f
   hydroxyapatite of, 90
   incisive, 91f–92f, 96f, 109–110, 109f, 116f–117f, 120f
   interparietal, 28–29, 39f, 92f, 96f
   irregular, 88
   lacrimal, 91f–92f, 113–114, 114f, 116f–117f
   long, 87
   maxilla, 91f–92f, 96f, 107f–108f, 110–111, 110f, 116f–117f, 120f
   membrane, 89
   metacarpal. *see* Metacarpal bones
   metatarsal. *see* Metatarsal bones
   of middle ear, 849–850
   nasal, 91f–92f, 96f, 107f–108f, 110, 110f, 116f–117f, 120f
   nutrient arteries of, 90–91
   nutrient vein of, 90–91
   occipital. *see* Occipital bone
   orbitosphenoid, development of, 29–32, 40f–41f
   palatine, 91f–92f, 96f, 112–113, 116f–117f, 120f
   parietal, 91f–92f, 98–99, 98f, 116f
   of pelvic limb, 156–172
   physical properties of, 90
   pneumatic, 88
   presphenoid, 92f, 96f, 100f–101f, 101, 117f, 120f, 122f
      development of, 29–32, 41f–42f
   pterygoid, 91f–92f, 96f, 114, 114f, 117f, 120f

Bone(s) *(Continued)*
  sesamoid. *see* Sesamoid bone(s)
  shape of, 86–88
  short, 88
  skull. *see* Skull, bones of
  sphenoid, 91*f*, 100–102, 100*f*–101*f*
  spongy, 90
  structure of, 89–90
  stylohyoid, 116*f*, 117, 227*f*–228*f*
  supraoccipital, 28–29, 39*f*–40*f*, 96*f*, 117*f*
  surface contour of, 90
  tarsal. *see* Tarsal bones
  temporal. *see* Temporal bone
  thoracic. *see* Rib(s); Sternum
  of thoracic limb, 140–156
  thyrohyoid, 116, 116*f*
  vertebral. *see* Vertebra(e)
  vessels and nerves of, 90–91
  vomer, 92*f*, 96*f*, 106*f*, 108*f*, 114–115, 114*f*, 117*f*, 120*f*
  zygomatic, 91*f*–92*f*, 112, 112*f*, 116*f*–117*f*, 120*f*
Bone marrow, 90
Bony labyrinth, 839–842
Bony nasal aperture, 109–110, 388
Bony plaques, 433*f*
Border(s)
  interosseous
    of fibula, 168
    of radius, 147*f*
    of ulna, 151
  of mandible, 115, 115*f*
  of parotid gland, 340–341
  of pubis, 156–158
  of scapula, 141*f*
  of tibia, 165–167, 165*f*–167*f*
Brachial artery, 538*f*, 541–546, 713*f*–714*f*, 718*f*–720*f*
  superficial, 541–542
Brachial plexus, 705*f*, 706–707, 708*f*, 712–728, 713*f*–715*f*
  nerves of
    that supply extrinsic muscles, of thoracic limb, 727–728
    that supply intrinsic muscles, of thoracic limb, 715–723, 716*f*
Brachial vein, 583*f*–584*f*
Brachialis tendon, 190*f*
Brachiocephalic nerve, 715*f*, 727–728
  cutaneous branch of, 727–728
Brachiocephalic trunk, 510–531, 511*f*, 584*f*
Brachiocephalic vein, left, 584*f*

Brachium
  arteries of, 538*f*
  bone of, 143, 143*f*–145*f*
  muscles of, 269–273
Brachium pontis, 794
Brachycephalic, definition of, 94, 94*t*, 125*f*
Brachygnathic, definition of, 94
Brain, 650, 657, 757–813, 817*f*
  arterial circle of, 527*f*
  definitive cavities of, 758*t*
  dorsal plane section of, 806*f*
  embryonic, 758*f*, 758*t*
  forebrain, 757, 758*t*
  hindbrain, 757, 758*t*
  horizontal section of, 796*f*
  juncture with spinal cord, 762*f*
  lateral view of, 769*f*, 781*f*–783*f*, 785*f*
  major parts of, 658, 658*f*
  median view of, 772*f*
  midbrain, 757, 758*t*
  sagittal section of, 805*f*
  transverse section of, 796*f*–804*f*
  veins of, 609*f*, 610–611
  ventral view of, 759*f*
  ventricles of, 696–701, 700*f*
Brain atlas, 796
Brainstem, 658, 658*f*, 757–778, 758*f*–759*f*
  axonal connections between cerebral hemisphere and, 783*f*
  neurons involved with visceral regulation, 762*f*
"Breed quality" of bone, 5
Breeds, 5–9, 7*f*
  behavior of, 2
  herding of, 11*f*
  hound, 8*f*
  miscellaneous class, 8
  non-sporting, 10*f*
  sporting, 7*f*
  terrier, 9*f*
  toy, 10*f*
  working, 9*f*
Bregma, 93, 93*f*
Broad ligaments
  of female genital organs, 445
  of peritoneum, 355
  of uterus, 422–423, 452
Bronchi, 402–404, 402*f*–403*f*
  lobar, 388, 402–403
  principal, 388, 402–403
  secondary, 402–403
  segmental, 388, 402–403
  tertiary, 402–403
Bronchi lobares, 402–403
Bronchi segmentales, 402–403

Bronchial arteries, 412
Bronchial lymph center, 631–633
Bronchial lymph nodes, 348, 634*f*
Bronchial tree, 402–403, 402*f*–404*f*
Bronchial veins, 413
Bronchial vessels, 412–413
Bronchioles, 388
  respiratory, 403
Bronchioli respiratorii, 403
Bronchoesophageal artery, 348, 549–550
Bronchoesophageal vein, 591
Bronchopulmonary segments, 402–403
Bronchus principalis dexter, 402–403
Bronchus principalis sinister, 402–403
Buccae, 320
Buccal artery, 524
Buccal lymph nodes, 625
Buccal nerve, 825
Bulb
  of aorta, 510
  artery of, 602*f*–603*f*
  of penis, 438–439
Bulbar conjunctiva, 887
Bulbar sheath, 884
Bulbospongiosus muscle, 438, 747*f*
Bulbus aortae, 505, 510
Bulbus glandis, 432*f*–433*f*, 439
Bulbus oculi, 860*f*, 861, 866*f*
Bulbus penis, 438–439
Bulbus vestibuli, 455
Bulla, tympanic (bulla tympanica), 105, 119*f*, 846
Bulldog, French, 7, 7*f*
Bundle, atrioventricular, 505–506
Bursa(e), 213
  omental, 356–359, 358*f*
  ovarian, 445, 446*f*, 447, 450
  testicular, 435
Bursa omentalis, 356–358
Bursa ovarica, 445, 450
Bursa testicularis, 435

C

CA (cutaneous area), 660, 660*f*
Calcaneal tuber, 168*f*, 170*f*–171*f*
Calcanean sulcus, 170–171
Calcanean (Achilles) tendon, 294, 308
Calcaneocentral ligament, 205
Calcaneoquartal joint, 202–203
Calcaneoquartal ligaments, 205
Calcaneus, 166*f*, 168*f*–169*f*, 170–171
Caliculus gustatorius, 333
Calvaria, 121. *see also* Skull
  development of, 28–29, 36*f*–39*f*

Index

Camera anterior bulbi, 878
Camera posterior bulbi, 878
Camera vitrea bulbi, 878
Canal(s)
    alar, 101–102, 119–120
    alveolar, 110–111
    basipharyngeal, 119
    carotid, 102f, 105, 123
    condyloid, 96f, 97, 122f, 123
        ventral opening of, 96f
    craniopharyngeal, 101
    facial, 104, 119f
    for facial nerve, 102f–103f
    hyaloid, 879
    hypoglossal, 96f, 97, 119f, 122f, 123
        internal opening of, 96f
    incisivomaxillary, 110–111
    infraorbital, 110–111, 110f
    inguinal, 254f, 257
    interincisive, 109–110, 121
    lacrimal, 111, 113–114, 114f, 118
    for major petrosal nerve, 104
    mandibular, 115–116
    for minor petrosal nerve, 104
    musculotubal, 102f, 105, 119f
    nasolacrimal, 110f
    optic, 100f–101f, 101, 118, 118f–119f, 122f
    palatine, 108f, 112–113
    petrooccipital, 97–98, 102f, 105, 123
    for petrosal nerve, major superficial, 102f
    pterygoid, 101–102, 114, 119f
        rostral opening of, 101f, 118f
    sacral, 136–137, 136f
    semicircular, 104
    temporal, 105
    transverse, 97, 122f
    for transverse sinus, 123
    for trigeminal nerve, 102f, 103, 122f, 123
    vertebral, 126, 138
    for vestibulocochlear nerve, 102f
Canales alveolares, 110–111
Canales optici, 101
Canales semicirculares ossei, 104
Canaliculi lacrimale, 890
Canaliculus, cochlear, 840–842
Canaliculus bilifer, 379
Canaliculus chordae tympani, 104, 830–831
Canaliculus cochleae, 840–842
Canalis alaris, 101–102
Canalis analis, 371
Canalis caroticus, 105
Canalis carpi, 193
Canalis centralis, 679
Canalis condylaris, 97
Canalis craniopharyngeus, 101
Canalis facialis, 104
Canalis hyaloideus, 879
Canalis infraorbitalis, 110–111
Canalis inguinalis, 254f, 257
Canalis interincisivus, 109–110
Canalis lacrimalis, 111, 113–114, 114f
Canalis mandibulae, 115–116
Canalis maxilloincisivus, 110–111
Canalis musculotubarius, 105
Canalis n. hypoglossi, 97
Canalis n. petrosi minoris, 104
Canalis nutricius, 90
Canalis palatinus, 112–113
Canalis petrooccipitalis, 97–98, 105
Canalis petrosi majoris, 104
Canalis pterygoideus, 101–102, 114
Canalis pyloricus, 362
Canalis radicis dentis, 327
Canalis sacralis, 136–137
Canalis transversus, 97
Canalis trigemini, 103
Canalis vaginalis, 424
Canidae, 2–5
Caniformia, 2
Canine lumbosacral plexuses, 737f
Canine teeth, 107f, 120f, 326f, 327. see also Teeth
    eruption of, 325t
    permanent, 110f
Canis familiaris, 1
Capacitation, 435
Capilli, 64
Capitulum humeri, 143f, 146
Capsula, 643
Capsula adiposa, 416–418
Capsula articularis, 177, 183–184, 188–189
Capsula externa, 788
Capsula extrema, 788
Capsula fibrosa, 416–418
Capsula fibrosa perivascularis, 377
Capsula glomeruli, 419
Capsula interna, 771–772, 788
Capsula prostatae, 437
Capsule
    adipose, 416–418
    joint. see Joint capsule
    prostate, 437
    spleen, 643
Caput, 435
Caput costae, 139–140
Caput fibulae, 168
Caput humeri, 143
Caput radii, 147
Caput tali, 169–170
Cardia, 359–361
Cardiac. see Heart
Cardiac conduction fibers, 505
Cardiac glands, 364
Cardiac impression, 408, 411
Cardiac incisure, 362
Cardiac lobe, 410
Cardiac notch, 411
    of right lung, 408, 411
"Cardiac skeleton," 500
Cardiac sphincter, 363
Cardiac veins, 509
    great, 508–509
    middle, 509
    oblique vein of the left atrium, 508–509
    right, 509
Carina, 388
Carina tracheae, 402
Carnassial teeth, 327–328
Carnivora, 1–2, 3f
Caroticotympanic nerves, 847
Carotid artery, branches of, 512f
Carotid body, 526–527
Carotid canal, 102f, 105, 123
Carotid foramen
    caudal, 102f, 105
    external, 105
    internal, 105
Carotid incisure, 102
Carotid notch, 103f
Carotid sheath, 510–511
Carotid sinus, 526–527
    branch to, 833
Carotid sulcus, 100f
Carpal bone(s), 152–153, 153f, 155f
    accessory, 152f–153f, 154, 155f
    first, 152f, 154, 155f
    fourth, 154
    intermedioradial, 152f–153f, 153, 155f
    second, 152f, 154, 155f
    third, 152f, 154, 155f
    ulnar, 152f, 153–154, 155f
Carpal canal, 193
Carpal joints, 192–195, 192f–195f
    middle, 192
Carpometacarpal joints, 152f, 192
Carpus
    bones of, 150f–152f, 152–154, 155f
    development of, 51
Cartilage, 89
    accessory, 389f, 390
    anular, 850–851
    articular, 177–178

Cartilage *(Continued)*
 arytenoid, 397f, 399
 auricular, 850, 856f
 costal, 139, 139f
 cricoid, 116f, 397f, 399
 epiglottic, 397–398
 epiphyseal, 87–88
 of external ear, 852f
 growth distortion, 4
 interarytenoid, 397f
 intersternebral, 139f, 140
 laryngeal, 397, 397f–398f
 of nasal septum, 107f–108f
 of nose, 388–390, 389f
 physeal, 87
 scapular, 142
 scutiform, 852–853
 septal, of nose, 389
 sesamoid, 397f, 400
 thyroid, 116f, 397f, 398
 tracheal, 402
 tympanohyoid, 116f, 117
 vomeronasal, 107f
 xiphoid, 139f, 140
Cartilage bone, 89
Cartilagines laryngis, 397
Cartilagines nasi, 388
Cartilagines tracheales, 402
Cartilaginous joints, 176–177
Cartilago accessoria, 390
Cartilago anularis, 850–851
Cartilago articularis, 177
Cartilago arytenoidea, 399
Cartilago auriculae, 850
Cartilago costalis, 139
Cartilago cricoidea, 399
Cartilago epiglottica, 397–398
Cartilago epiphysialis, 87–88
Cartilago interarytenoidea, 400
Cartilago intersternebralis, 139f, 140
Cartilago nasi lateralis dorsalis, 389–390
Cartilago nasi lateralis ventralis, 390
Cartilago parapatellaris mediale et lateralis, 202
Cartilago plica semilunaris conjunctivae, 888
Cartilago scapulae, 142
Cartilago scutiformis, 852–853
Cartilago septi nasi, 389, 391
Cartilago sesamoidea, 400
Cartilago thyroidea, 398
Cartilago tympanohyoideum, 116f
Cartilago vomeronasalis, 390
Cartilago xiphoidea, 140
Caruncula sublingualis, 320–321, 343

Catagen, 69, 76, 76f
Cauda epididymidis, 435
Cauda equina, 683, 704, 731–732
Caudal alar foramen, 101–102, 101f, 118f–119f
Caudal angle, 141f, 142
Caudal arteries
 abdominal, 564–565, 740f
 auricular, 342–343, 517
 cerebellar, 531–533
 circumflex humeral, 538f, 539, 714f, 716f
 communicating, 527, 901f–902f
 deep temporal, 522
 dorsal alveolar, 526
 epigastric, 562, 740f
 genicular, 742f
 gluteal, 371f, 573f, 576, 603, 744f–745f, 747f
 hypophyseal, 476, 527
 intercarotid, 527
 interosseous, 545–546, 719f, 725f
  branch of, 717f
 mesenteric, 558, 573f
 nasal septal, 523–524
 pancreaticoduodenal, 367, 382, 557–558
 phrenic, 561
 rectal, 371f, 373, 573f, 575–576, 745f, 747f
  left, 373
  right, 373
 superficial epigastric, 562–563, 740f
 thyroid, 511–512
 tibial, 567f, 569, 742f
 ventrolateral, 579
 vesical, 423, 437–438, 573f, 575
  branches, 575
Caudal clinoid process, 100f, 101, 121–123
Caudal colliculus, 768
Caudal commissure, 769
Caudal cornua, 398
Caudal crura, 850
Caudal crural abductor muscle, 300f, 744f
Caudal ligament, of incus, 850
Caudal longitudinal sulcus or groove, 498–499
Caudal mediastinum, 406–407
Caudal medullary velum, 763
Caudal nerves, 754, 754f
 1st, 741f
  communication with, 734f
 auricular, 709f, 831
 cervical, cutaneous areas of, 712f

Caudal nerves *(Continued)*
 clunial, 733–734, 739f, 746
 cutaneous antebrachial, 713f, 717f–720f, 722, 723f
  overlap zone, 727f
 cutaneous femoral, 730f, 732f, 734f–737f, 741f, 745f, 746, 747f
 cutaneous sural, 576f, 732f, 742f, 744f, 749f, 751f, 753f
 gluteal, 732f, 734f, 737f, 741f, 744f–745f, 745–746
 iliohypogastric, 730f, 732f–733f
  lateral cutaneous branch, 739f
 laryngeal, 401–402, 836
 lateral brachial cutaneous, 718–720
 nasal, 815–816, 822
 pectoral, 715f, 728
 rectal, 734f, 737f, 745f, 746, 747f
Caudal process, 126
Caudal projecting tract, 695f
Caudal superior alveolar branches, 822–824
Caudal tactile dermatomes, 738f
Caudal tibial muscle. *see* M. tibialis caudalis, 749f
Caudal veins, 613f
 abdominal, 602–603, 740f
 auricular, 342, 589–590
 epigastric, 602–603, 740f
 gluteal, 371f, 583f, 602f–603f, 603
 lateral, 583f, 604
 mesenteric, 373, 583f, 595f, 598–599
 pancreaticoduodenal, 382–383, 598
 phrenic, 597
 rectal, 373, 604
 thyroid, 584f–585f, 585
 vesicle, 604
Caudal vena cava, 584f, 740f
Caudal vertebrae. *see* Vertebra(e), caudal
Caudate nucleus, 790
Caudate process, 377
Cava nasi, 391
Caval foramen, 351
Cavernous sinus, 607f
Cavitas glenoidalis, 142
Cavity(ies)
 abdominal, 351
 cranial, 91, 121–123, 122f
 glenoid, 141f, 142, 145f
 infraglottic, 401
 joint, 177
 of larynx, 400

Cavity(ies) *(Continued)*
  lesser peritoneal, 356–357
  medullary, 90
  for molar, 110*f*
  nasal, 107*f*, 123–124, 388, 391–396, 392*f*–393*f*, 395*f*
  of the nose, 91
  oral, 319–344
  pelvic, 156–158, 352–353
    male, 428*f*
  pericardial, 495
  peritoneal, 351
  pleural, 407
  preputial, 444
  pulp, 327
  thoracic, 404–405, 404*f*
  tympanic, 102–105
  for zygomatic articulation, 110*f*
Cavum abdominis, 351
Cavum articulare, 177
Cavum conchae, 850–851
Cavum coronale dentis, 326–327
Cavum cranii, 91, 121, 122*f*
Cavum dentis, 327
Cavum epidurale, 699
Cavum infraglotticum, 401
Cavum laryngis, 400
Cavum mediastini serosum, 356–357, 407
Cavum medullare, 90
Cavum nasi, 91, 123, 388
Cavum oris, 319
Cavum oris proprium, 320
Cavum pelvis, 352–353
Cavum pericardii, 495
Cavum peritonei, 351
Cavum pharyngis, 344
Cavum pleurae, 407
Cavum subarachnoideale, 699
Cavum thoracis, 404
Cavum trigeminale, 898–899
Cavum tympani, 104–105, 839, 847
Cavum vaginale, 424
Cecal artery, 367, 557
Cecal sphincter, 368–369
Cecal vein, 598
Cecocolic orifice, 368–369
Cecum, 366*f*, 368*f*
Celiac artery, 357*f*, 382, 553*f*
Celiac ganglia, 379
Celiac lymph center, 637–639
Celiac plexus, 364, 367–368, 383
Celiac trunk, 640
Celiacomesenteric plexus, 364
Cell body, 650
  segments, of neurons, 652

Cell columns, 660–661
Cementum, 326, 329
Central canal, 679, 681*f*, 700*f*
Central conductile segment, 653
Central depression, 875–876
Central intermediate substance, 679, 681*f*
Central nervous system (CNS), 650, 657–659
  lymph drainage of, 618
  supporting cells, 657
  veins of, 606–614
Central tegmental tract, 770
Central veins, of liver, 378
Centrodistal joint, 202–203
Centrodistal ligament, 204–205
  plantar, 205
Centrum, 127*f*, 130
Centrum semiovale, 781
Centrum tendineum perinei, 374–375
Cephalic vein, 583*f*–584*f*, 591
  brachiocephalic vein, 584*f*–585*f*, 585
  proximal communicating vein of, 593
Ceratohyoid bones, 116–117, 116*f*
Ceratohyoid cartilage, 33
Ceratohyoideum, 116–117, 116*f*
Ceratohyoideus, 344*f*
Cerebellar cortex, 795–796
  layers of, 796*f*
Cerebellar fossa, 102*f*, 103, 122*f*, 123
Cerebellar peduncles, 794–795
  caudal, 763*f*, 794, 794*f*
  middle, 794, 794*f*
  rostral, 794–795, 794*f*–795*f*
Cerebellar projection nuclei, 759
Cerebellomedullary cistern, 700*f*
Cerebellum, 757, 758*f*, 792–796, 793*f*–794*f*
  arteries of, 530*f*
  descriptive and numerical nomenclature of lobules of, 793*t*
  lateral or hemispheric zone of, 794
  major axonal input to, 795*f*
  nuclei of, 792–794
  paravermis zone of, 794
  peduncles of, 794–795
  vermis zone of, 794
Cerebral artery, 531*f*, 901*f*–902*f*
Cerebral cortex
  functional areas of, 788*f*
  neocortex, 787–789
    functional regions of, 788–789, 790*f*

Cerebral cortex *(Continued)*
  horizontal layers of, 787*f*
  white matter related, 787–788
Cerebral hemisphere, 778–781
Cerebral juga, 99*f*, 100
Cerebral veins
  dorsal, 609*f*, 610
  great, 607*f*, 610
  internal, 609*f*, 610–611
Cerebrospinal fluid, 696–701
  drainage, 701, 702*f*
  flow, 701
Cerebrum, 757, 758*f*, 778–789
  arteries of, 530*f*
  dorsolateral view of, 778*f*
  external capsule, 788
  extreme capsule, 788
  internal capsule, 771–772, 788
  longitudinal fissure, 778
  medial view of, 782*f*
  transverse fissure, 778
  ventral view of, 779*f*
Cerumen, 80
Cervical artery, superficial, 536–537
  branches of, 537*f*
Cervical cardiac nerve, 667–668
Cervical enlargement, 682
Cervical loop, 708–709, 837
Cervical lymph center
  deep, 627–628
  superficial, 627
Cervical lymph nodes
  deep, 348, 627, 627*f*
  superficial, 618*f*, 627, 627*f*
Cervical nerves, 705*f*, 708–711
  2 through 5, ventral branches of, 711
  3 through 7
    dorsal branches of, 710
    medial branches of, 711
  dorsal branches of, 710*f*, 730*f*
  dorsal cutaneous branches of, 711
  first, 708
    dorsal branch of, 708
    ventral branch of, 708–709
  second, 709
    dorsal branch of, 709
    ventral branch of, 709
  transverse, 709–710
Cervical plexus, 708
Cervical rib, 131
Cervical spinal cord, arteries of, 529*f*
Cervical veins
  superficial, 586
  vertebral, 612*f*
Cervical vertebrae. *see* Atlas; Axis; Vertebra(e), cervical

Cervicoauricular muscles, 854f
Cervicoauricularis superficialis muscle, 710f, 895f
Cervicointerscutularis of Huber, 217f–218f, 221
Cervicoscutularis muscle, 710f, 895f
Cervix, 452
Cervix dentis, 323–324
Cervix uteri, 451
Cervix vesicae, 421
Chambers, of eye, 878–879
Cheek teeth, 327
Cheeks, 320
Chiasma opticum, 757
Choanae, 394
Cholinergic system, 661, 663–664
Chondrocranium, 27–28, 33f–36f
Chorda tympani, 338–339, 338f, 830–831
Chordae tendineae, 503
Chorioallantoic membrane, 20, 20f
Choriocapillary layer, 867
Chorion, 19f–20f, 20
Choriovitelline membrane, 18, 19f–20f
Choroid, 867–869
  basal lamina, 867
  layers, 867
Choroid arteries, 524
Choroid plexus, 700f, 701, 763
Choroidal vein, 610–611
Chromophobic cells, 474
Chromosomes, 13
Chyme, 362
Cilia (eyelashes), 64, 885–886
Ciliary artery, anterior, 523, 901–902
Ciliary body, 869–871, 870f
  muscle, 871
Ciliary crown, 869–871
Ciliary ganglion, 665, 816–817, 897–898
  communicating branch to, 819
Ciliary glands, 886
Ciliary processes, 869–871
Ciliary ring, 869–871
Ciliary veins, 904
Ciliary zonule, 866f, 869–871
Cingulate gyrus, 786–787
Cingulum, 327, 788
Circular layer, 363
Circulatory system, lymph drainage of, 619
Circulus arteriosus cerebri, 527, 527f
Circulus arteriosus iridis major, 523, 873
Circulus articularis vasculosus, 177
Circumanal glands, 80, 372

Circumduction, 179, 212
Circumferentia articularis
  of radius, 147
  of ulna, 151
Circumferential fibers, 871
Circumflex arteries
  femoral, 563
  humeral, 541
  scapular, 539f, 541
Circumflex veins
  humeral, 593–594, 593f
  iliac
    deep, 597
    superficial, 601
Circumflexa humeri cranialis, 593–594
Circumvallate, 333
Cisterna cerebellomedullaris, 699
Cisterna chyli, 622–623
Cisterna magna, 699
Clarke column, 687
Classification, 1
Classification of Mammals above the Species Level, 1–2
Claustrum, 791
Clavicle, 140–141, 141f
  development of, 47, 53f
  fascial connections of, 189
Clavicula, 140–141
Claws, 64, 82–83, 82f–83f
Cleft
  of glottis, 401
  vestibular, 400–401
Cleidobrachialis muscle, 717f
Cleidocephalicus pars cervicalis, 709f
Cleidocephalicus pars mastoideus, 709f
Clinoid processes
  caudal, 100f, 101, 121–123
  development of, 29–32
  rostral, 100f, 101
Clitoris, 445, 455–456, 455f–456f
  artery of, 576
  dorsal nerve of, 745f, 747
  vein of, 602f–603f, 604
Coats
  of esophagus, 347–348
  fibrous, 347
  hair. *see* Hair coat
  of large intestine, 373–374
  mucous. *see* Mucous coat
  muscular. *see* Muscular coat
  nervous, 873
  of small intestine, 367
  of stomach, 362–363
  submucous. *see* Submucous coat
Coccygeal roots, 681

Cochlea, 840–842, 843f, 848f
Cochlea tibiae, 167
Cochlear canaliculus, 102f–103f, 103, 840–842
Cochlear duct, 842, 843f, 844–846
Cochlear root, 832
Cochlear window, 103f, 104, 839–840, 847
Cochlea-tarsocrural joint, 166f
Colic flexures, 369
Colic lymph nodes, 367, 638f, 639
Colic trunk, 640
Colic vein, 598
Collagen fibers, 65–66
Collateral ligaments, 177–178
Collateral radial artery, 539, 540f, 716f–717f, 719f
Collateral ulnar artery, 713f, 717f–720f
Collecting tubules, 463
Colliculus, 757
Colliculus axonis, 651–652
Colliculus caudalis, 768
Colliculus rostralis, 768
Colliculus seminalis, 437, 443–444
Collum costae, 139–140
Collum femoris, 163
Collum humeri, 145
Collum radii, 147
Collum tali, 169–170
Collum vesicae felleae, 379
Colon, 366f, 368f, 369–370. *see also* Large intestine
  ascending, 369
  descending, 369
  mesentery of, 369–370
  transverse, 369
Colon ascendens, 369
Colon descendens, 369
Colon transversum, 369
Columella, 839
Column(s)
  anal, 371–372
  cell, 660–661
  gray, 658, 658f
  vertebral. *see* Vertebra(e); Vertebral column
Columna vertebralis, 125
Columnae anales, 371–372
Columnar zone, 371–372
Commissura alba, 680
Commissura caudalis, 769
Commissura grisea, 679
Commissura habenularum, 777–778
Commissura palpebrarum medialis et lateralis, 885
Commissura rostralis, 784–785

Commissures, 455
Commissuura labiorum dorsalis, 455
Commissuura labiorum ventralis, 455
Common bile duct, 357f
Common carotid artery, 510–513, 584f
  bicarotid trunk, 510
  branches of, 510b, 512f, 515f
  dorsal, 570–571, 570f
  left, 510, 512f
  plantar, 571f
  right, 510–511, 512f
Common crus, 840
Common fibular nerve, 602f–603f, 732f, 742f, 744f, 749, 749f
Common iliac vein, 561f, 583f, 602–603, 605, 613f
Common interosseous artery, 542f, 544–545, 718f–719f
Common interosseous vein, 594–595
Common nasal meatus, 106, 107f–108f, 112, 392f, 394
Common peroneal nerve, 749
Common trunk, 597
Communicating branch, 704, 705f–706f, 713f, 716–718
Compact bone, 89–90
Comparative ophthalmology, 904
Compartment, neuromuscular, 212
Complexus muscles, 243f, 710f
Concha(e)
  ethmoidal, 391f, 393
  nasal, 388, 391f, 392–393
    dorsal, 107–112, 107f–108f, 122f, 391f, 392
    middle, 392–393
    ventral, 107–109, 108f, 112, 391f, 392
Concha nasalis dorsalis, 110–112, 123, 392
Concha nasalis media, 392–393
Concha nasalis ventralis, 123–124, 392
Conchae ethmoidales, 393
Conchae nasales, 392
Conchal cavity, 850–851
Conchal crest, 108f, 110f, 111, 123–124, 392
Conductile segments, of neurons, 653–654
Conduction system, of heart, 505–506
Condylar joint, 179
Condyles
  of femur, 162f–163f, 164
  of humerus, 143f, 146
  occipital, 96f, 97, 118–119, 118f–119f, 128f–129f
  of tibia, 165–167, 166f

Condyloid artery, 513
Condyloid canal, 96f, 97, 122f, 123
  ventral opening of, 96f
Condyloid vein, 610
Condylus humeri, 146
Condylus lateralis et medialis, of tibia, 165–167
Confluence of the sinuses, 608
Confluens sinuum, 607f, 608
Conical papillae, 334
Conjugata, 156–158
Conjunctiva, 887, 890
  bulbar, 887
  palpebral, 887
  semilunar fold of, 887–888
Conjunctival fornix, 887
Conjunctival sac, 887
Connecting peritoneum, 354, 357f
Connective tissue, 213
Constrictor muscles
  of female anus, 457f
  of female genitalia, 457f–458f
  vestibular, 456
Constrictor vestibuli muscle, 434f, 745f
Constrictor vulvae muscle, 456, 745f
Contact surface, of tooth, 327
Conus arteriosus, 497f–499f, 501–502
Conus medullaris, 682
Convoluted seminiferous tubules, 428
Copulation, 434f
Cor, 495–496
Coracoid process, 141f, 142–143
Cornea, 861–866, 863f
Corniculate process, 400
Corniculate tubercle, 345f–346f, 400
Cornu caudalis, 398
Cornu dorsale, 679
Cornu laterale, 679
Cornu rostralis, 398
Cornu ventrale, 679
Cornua uteri dextrum, 451
Cornua uteri sinistrum, 451
Corona ciliaris, 869–871
Corona dentis, 323–324
Corona glandis, 439
Corona radiata, 781
Coronal tooth, 327
Coronary arteries, 506–508
  branches, 506
  left, 506, 507f, 584f
  right, 506, 583f
Coronary groove, 498–499
Coronary ligament, 357f, 377
Coronary sinus, 499
Corpora bulboidei, 652
Corpora caudalia, 579

Corpora neurona, 650
Corpora tacti, 652
Corpus, 435
Corpus adiposum auriculare, 852–853
Corpus adiposum extraperiorbitale, 885
Corpus adiposum infrapatellare, 199–201
Corpus adiposum intraperiorbitale, 885
Corpus adiposum orbitae, 885
Corpus albicans, 447
Corpus callosum, 700f, 779–781
Corpus ceci, 368–369
Corpus ciliare, 869–871
Corpus clitoridis, 455
Corpus costae, 140
Corpus femoris, 163–164
Corpus geniculatum laterale, 775
Corpus geniculatum mediale, 775
Corpus hemorrhagicum, 447
Corpus humeri, 145
Corpus linguae, 330
Corpus luteum, 447
Corpus mamillare, 777
Corpus mandibulae, 115, 115f
Corpus neurona, 650
Corpus ossis incisivum, 109–110
Corpus ossis ischii, 160–161
Corpus ossis pubis, 161
Corpus pancreatis, 381
Corpus penis, 438–439
Corpus radii, 147–148
Corpus spongiosum, 432f, 439
Corpus tibiae, 167
Corpus trapezoideum, 765
Corpus uteri, 451
Corpus ventriculi, 362
Corpus vertebrae, 125–126
Corpus vesicae, 421
Corpus vesicae felleae, 379
Corpuscle, renal, 419
Corpusculi nervosi capsulata, 652
Corpusculum renale, 419
Cortex
  cerebellar, 794–795
    layers of, 796f
  cerebral neocortex, 787–789
    functional regions of, 788–789
    horizontal layers of, 787f
    white matter related, 787–788
  of lymph node, 621
  renal, 418, 447
Cortex ovarii (zona parenchymentosa), 447
Cortex renis, 418
Corti, organ of, 844

Corticopontine tract, 766
Corticospinal axons, 694
Corticospinal tract
  lateral, 760–761
  ventral, 760–761
Costae. see Rib(s)
Costal arch, 139, 353f
Costal cartilage, 139, 139f
Costal fovea, 131–132
Costal groove, 140
Costal pleura, 407
Costal surface, of lungs, 408
Costal surface, of scapula, 141f, 142
Costoabdominal nerve, 731
Costocervical trunk, 534, 584f
Costocervical vein, 582–583, 584f
  left, 584f
Costochondral joints, 188
Costodiaphragmatic recess, 251–252, 407
Costomediastinal recess, 407
Costotransverse foramen, 139–140
Costotransverse ligament, 184f, 186, 186f–187f
Costovertebral joints, 186
Costovertebral ligament, 187f
Costoxiphoid ligaments, 187, 188f
Cranial abdominal connecting peritoneum, 356
Cranial angle, 141f, 142
Cranial arteries, 367
  abdominal, 561
  branches of, 529f, 557f
  circumflex femoral, 743f
  circumflex humeral, 538f, 541, 713f–714f, 716f
  epigastric, 536
  gluteal, 573f–574f, 744f–745f
  hemorrhoidal, 558
  interosseous, 544f, 546, 717f, 719f
  laryngeal, 344f, 514–515
  mesenteric, 357f, 553f, 556–557, 556f
  pancreaticoduodenal, 367, 382, 555
  rectal, 373, 558
  superficial antebrachial, 542–543
    lateral branch, 543, 726–727
    median branch, 542–543
  thyroid
    branches of, 512, 512f
    pharyngeal branches of, 346
  tibial, 569, 569f, 742f, 749f, 751f
    branches, 569
  vesical, 423, 573, 574f
Cranial articular fovea, 127–130, 128f
Cranial cavity, 91, 121–123, 122f
Cranial cervical ganglion, 672, 885

Cranial cervical sympathetic ganglion, 351f
Cranial cutaneous antebrachial branch, 720f
Cranial dura mater, 699
  venous sinuses of, 606–610
Cranial fossa
  caudal, 123
  middle, 121–123
  rostral, 121
Cranial index, 95t
Cranial interlobar fissure, 409, 411
Cranial longitudinal sulcus or groove, 498–499
Cranial mediastinum, 405
Cranial nerve I. see Olfactory nerve
Cranial nerve II. see Optic nerve
Cranial nerve III. see Oculomotor nerve
Cranial nerve IV. see Trochlear nerve
Cranial nerve V. see Trigeminal nerve
Cranial nerve VI. see Abducent nerve
Cranial nerve VII. see Facial nerve
Cranial nerve VIII. see Vestibulocochlear nerve
Cranial nerve IX. see Glossopharyngeal nerve
Cranial nerve X. see Vagus nerve
Cranial nerve XI, Accessory nerve
Cranial nerve XII. see Hypoglossal nerve
Cranial nerves, 650, 733–734, 814–838, 815b, 817f. see also specific nerves
  clunial, 733–734
  cutaneous antebrachial, 716, 717f
  cutaneous innervation of head by, 837
  gluteal, 732f, 734f, 737f, 741f, 744–745, 744f–745f
  iliohypogastric, 730f, 732f–733f, 734
    lateral cutaneous branch, 735f
  laryngeal, 351f, 401, 667, 835–836
    external ramus of, 835–836
  lateral cutaneous brachial, 716, 716f–717f, 730f
  lumbar
    cutaneous areas, 731f
    cutaneous branches of, 730f
  nuclei of, 757–758, 760f
  pectoral, 715f, 728
  thoracic, cutaneous areas of, 712f
Cranial process, 126
Cranial projecting tract, 695f
Cranial roots, 836
Cranial spinocerebellar tract, 691f, 693

Cranial tibial muscle, 749f
Cranial veins
  abdominal, 597
  circumflex humeral, 593f
  cranial, 598
  epigastric, superficial, 563f
  gluteal, 601f–603f, 604
  laryngeal, 585f–586f, 589
  mesenteric, 583f, 595f
  pancreaticoduodenal, 599
  phrenic, 598
  rectal, 373
  thyroid, 585–586, 585f–586f, 588f
  tibial, 583f, 600, 601f, 605f
  ureteric, 597
Cranial vena cava, 584f
Craniometry, 93–94, 93f
Craniopharyngeal canal, 101
Craniosacral system, 663
Craniospinal (afferent) ganglia, 654–655
Cranium. see Skull
Cremaster muscle, 424, 428
Cremasteric artery, 564–565
Crest
  conchal, 108f, 110f, 111, 123–124, 392
  condyloid, 115f
  coronoid, 115f
  ethmoidal, 110, 110f, 113, 113f, 392
  frontal, internal, 100
  of greater tubercle, 143f, 145–146
  iliac, 158, 158f–161f
  of ilium, 157f
  intertrochanteric, 161f–162f, 163
  of lesser tubercle, 146
  median, 399
  nasal, 112–113
  nuchal, 92f, 96–97, 96f, 103f, 105, 121
  occipital
    external, 96–97, 121
    internal, 96f, 97, 123
  orbital, 118, 118f
  orbitosphenoidal, 100f, 101
  orbitotemporal, 99f
  petrosal, 102–103, 102f, 122f, 123
  sacral, 135–136, 136f, 157f
  sagittal
    of cranial cavity, 123
    external, 96–97
    internal, 96–97
    of metacarpal bone, 153f, 154
    of occipital bone, 92f
  sphenoidal, 121

Index

Crest (Continued)
supracondylar, lateral, 143f–144f, 146
supramastoid, 105
transverse, 103
for uncinate process, 110f
ungual, 155f, 156
urethral, 437, 443–444
ventral ethmoidal, 110f
Cribriform foramina, 107, 121
Cribriform plate, 106f, 107, 109, 120f, 121
Cricoarytenoid articulation, 400
Cricoesophageal muscle, 347
Cricoid articular surface, 399
Cricoid cartilage, 116f, 344f–345f, 397f, 399
Cricothyroid ligament, 399
Crista ampullaris, 842–843
Crista capitis costae, 139–140
Crista conchalis, 111, 123–124, 352
Crista condyloidea, 115f
Crista coronoidea, 115f
Crista ethmoidalis, 110, 113, 392
Crista frontalis interna, 100
Crista galli, 107, 121
Crista iliaca, 158
Crista intertrochanterica, 163
Crista mediana, 399
Crista nasalis, 112–113
Crista nuchae, 96–97
Crista occipitalis externa, 97
Crista occipitalis interna, 97
Crista orbitalis, 118
Crista orbitalis ventralis, 118, 882
Crista orbitosphenoidalis, 101
Crista petrosa, 102–103, 123
Crista renalis, 418–419
Crista sacralis intermedia, 135–136
Crista sacralis lateralis, 136
Crista sacralis mediana, 135–136
Crista sagittalis externa, 96–97
Crista sagittalis interna, 96–97, 123
Crista supracondylaris lateralis, 146
Crista supramastoidea, 105
Crista supraventricularis, 501–502
Crista terminalis, 500
Crista transversa, 103
Crista tuberculi majoris, 145–146
Crista tuberculi minoris, 146
Crista unguicularis, 156
Crista urethralis, 437, 443–444
Cristae sagittales, 154
Crown, 323–324
Crown-rump (C-R) length, 15, 24t, 26f, 27t
Crura clitoridis, 455

Crural extensor retinaculum, 204–205
Crus (crura)
caudal, 190f, 850
common, 840
cranial, 190f
lateral, 851–852
long, 849–850
medial, 851–852
of penis, 438
rostral, 850
of semicircular canals, 840
short, 849–850
Crus (leg), muscles of, 303–311
caudal, 291f, 299f–300f, 303f–306f, 308–311, 310f
craniolateral, 291f, 299f–300f, 303–308, 303f–307f, 310f
Crus cerebri, 757, 769–770
Crus helicis laterale, 851–852
Crus helicis mediale, 851–852
Crus laterale, 253
Crus mediale, 253
Crus penis, 438
Cubital vein, median, 592, 592f
Cuneiform process, 400
Cuneiform tubercle, 345f
Cupula, 842–843
Cupula pleurae, 405, 407
Curvatura ventriculi major, 361
Curvatura ventriculi minor, 361–362
Cusp(s), 323–324
angular, 504
of atrioventricular valve, 501–502
parietal, 504
semilunar, septal, 505
septal, 504
Cuspis parietalis, 504
Cuspis septalis, 504
Cutaneous afferents, 650–651
Cutaneous area, 660, 660f
Cutaneous innervation, 708f
Cutaneous nerves, 660, 660f
of head, cranial, 837
Cutaneous plexus, 81, 81f
Cutaneous trunci muscle, 79
Cutaneous trunci reflex, 696
Cutaneous zone, 371
Cutis. see Skin
Cystic artery, 554
Cystic duct, 379, 380f

D

Dachshund-Pekingese hybrids, 4f–6f, 5
DaDa gene, 131
Deciduous dentition, 328
Deciduous teeth, 323–324, 324f

Decussatio nervorum trochlearium, 818
Decussatio pyramidum, 759–760
Deep antebrachial artery, 718f, 720f
Deep arcuate fibers, 761
Deep arteries
antebrachial, 538f, 544f, 546
auricular, 517
brachial, 538f, 541, 714f
cervical, 534
circumflex iliac, 567, 740f
femoral, 567, 740f, 743f
forepaw, 547f
of hindpaw, 572f
lingual, 515–516
palmar arch, 546
of penis, 441
plantar arch, 569–570
Deep branch, 720, 725f, 726
Deep fascia, muscular, 884
Deep nerves
fibular, 732f, 736f, 742f, 749f, 750, 751f
petrosal, 829–830
temporal, 825
Deep palmar arterial arch, 725f, 726–727
Deep pectoral muscle, 705f, 713f, 729f
Deep pectoral nerve, 713f
Deep perineal fascia, 374
Deep ramus, 717f
Deep veins
auricular, 589–590
cervical, 583
circumflex iliac, 583f, 597, 740f
femoral, 583f, 595f, 740f
of glans, 431f, 441
intercostal, 583
of penis, 602f–603f, 604
scapular, 583
Deferent ducts, 423, 435
Deltoideus muscle, 713f, 717f
nerve to, 716f
Dendrites, 650, 653
Dendriti, 650
Dendritic zone, 652
Dens, 126f–129f, 127–130
fracture, 130–131
Dens sectorius, 327–328
Dental alveoli. see Alveoli dentales
Dental anomalies, 329
Dental arches, 325, 326f
Dental formulae, 328
Dental lamina, 33–34
Dental nomenclature, 328–329
Dentary bone, 28, 45f
Dentes, 323–324. see also Teeth

Dentes canini, 327
Dentes incisivi, 327
Dentes molares, 328
Dentes permanentes, 324
Dentes premolares, 327
Denticulate ligaments, 679, 681f, 700
Dentin, 325–326
Dentinum, 325
Dentition. see Teeth
Depressor nerve, 835–836
Dermatome, 707
Dermis, 64–65
    of claw, 83
    nasal, 67, 67f
    structure of, changes with age and, 65–66
Descending aorta, 510, 534f
Descending colon, 369
Descending genicular artery, 742f
Descending mesocolon, 355, 370
Descending palatine artery, 525
Descending pathways, 655
Desmocranium, 27–28, 35f
Development, prenatal. see Prenatal development
Dewclaw, 86, 155, 168, 172
    in-grown, 83f
Diagonal gyrus, 783–784
Diameter obliqua, 156–158
Diameter transversa, 156–158
Diaphragm (diaphragma), 250–252, 250f, 357f
    lymph vessels of, 629f, 633f, 641f
    nerves to, 711–712
    pleural surface of, 630f
Diaphragma pelvis, 374
Diaphragma sellae, 699
Diaphragmatic lobe, 410–411
Diaphragmatic pleura, 407
Diaphragmatic surface
    of liver, 375
    of lungs, 408
Diaphysis, 87
Diencephalic caudal projecting axons, 694
Diencephalic fibers, 691f
Diencephalon, 658, 757, 758f, 758t, 771–778, 772f, 774f
Diestrus, 448–449
Digastricus, 340f
Digestive apparatus, 319–387
Digestive system, 319
Digestive tract, lymph drainage of, 619
Digit(s). see Phalanx (phalanges)
Digital arteries
    common, 546
    proper, 546–547, 571–572, 571f

Digital cushion, 68
Digital fascia, 196
Digital footpad
    IV, 726–727
    nerves to, 725f, 753f
Digital pads, 66–69, 68f, 82f
Dilator muscle, 873
Dingo, 1, 6
Diploë, 88, 90
Diploic veins, 611
Directional terminology
    for along teeth, 327
    for eye, 860f
    for structures of internal and external ear, 853
Disc, 178
    articular, 179
    intervertebral, 184f, 185–186, 186f, 197f
Disci intervertebrales, 184f, 185, 197f
Discus articularis, 178–179
Distal caudal cutaneous sural nerve, 735f–736f, 748–749
Distal caudal femoral artery, 742f, 749f
Distal interphalangeal joints, 196
Distal intertarsal joint, 202–203
Distal muscular branch, 716–718, 729f
Distal surface, of tooth, 327
Distal tibiofibular joints, 202
Distal vagal ganglia, 667
DNA hybridization, 2
Dog, relatives of, 1–12
Dolichocephalic, definition of, 94, 94t, 125f
Domestication, 1
Dorsal arteries
    costoabdominal, 550–551
    intercostal, 348, 535, 550–551
    lateral caudal, 573f
    metacarpal, 546
    metacarpal III, 726–727
    pedal, 569–570, 570f, 751f
    of penis, 441, 444
    perineal, 574f, 578
    scapular, 534
    scrotal, 576
Dorsal branches, 704, 705f–706f, 717f, 725–726, 729f
    of lumbar nerves, 733
    of sacral nerves, 743–744
Dorsal carpal branch, 725f
Dorsal carpal rete, 546
Dorsal caudal plexus, 754, 754f
Dorsal column post-synaptic path, 691f
Dorsal column post-synaptic tract, 691f, 692

Dorsal condyloid fossa, 96f, 97, 118f
Dorsal corticospinal tract, 694
Dorsal cutaneous branches, 707, 708f
Dorsal digital arteries
    common, 542–543, 548, 751f
    III, 726–727
    proper, axial
        III, 726–727
        IV, 726–727
Dorsal digital nerves
    abaxial, 723–724
    common, 751f
        I, 723–724
        II, 724
        III, 724, 726–727, 750
        IV, 724, 750
    proper, abaxial
        II, 723–724, 751f
        III, 751f
        IV, 724, 750, 751f
        V, 725–726, 750, 751f
    proper, axial, 751f
        II, 724
        III, 724, 726–727
        IV, 724, 726–727
        V, 750
Dorsal digital veins
    common, 591–592, 594, 605–606
    proper, 605
Dorsal ethmoidal crest, 110f
Dorsal funiculus, 680, 681f, 690–692
    projection pathways in, 690b
Dorsal horn, 679, 681f
    nuclei, 687
Dorsal interbasilar sinus, 610
Dorsal intermediate septum, 680–681, 681f
Dorsal intermediate sulcus, 680–681, 681f
Dorsal ligament
    of incus, 850
    of malleus, 850
Dorsal longitudinal fasciculus, 776
Dorsal margin, of lung, 408–409
Dorsal median fissure, 680
Dorsal median septum, 680, 681f
Dorsal median sulcus, 680, 681f
Dorsal mediastinum, 406
Dorsal nasal meatus, 108f, 110
Dorsal nerves
    metatarsal, 750–751, 751f
    of penis, 442, 444–445
    scrotal, 746–747
    thoracic, 715f
Dorsal petrosal sinus, 607f
Dorsal rete of the carpus, 542–543

Dorsal sagittal sinus, 583f, 606–603, 607f–609f, 700f
Dorsal sagittal sinus, foramen for, 96f, 97, 123
Dorsal spinocerebellar tract, 691f, 692–693
  nucleus of, 687
Dorsal surface
  of pancreas, 381
  of penis, 438
Dorsal vagal trunk, 669
Dorsal veins
  cerebellar, 609f, 611
  of clitoris, 458
  common, 591–592, 592f
  costoabdominal, 590
  external ophthalmic, 586f, 587, 904
  intercostal, 590
  metacarpal, 594
  of penis, 433f, 441, 444, 602f–603f, 604
  perineal, 603
  scrotal, 604
Dorsal venous rete of the carpus, 592f, 594
Dorsolateral fasciculus, 691f
Dorsolateral nasal cartilage, 389–390
Dorsolateral spinothalamic tract, 692
Dorsolateral sulcus, 680–681, 681f, 695f
Dorsolateral tract, 692
Dorsomarginal nucleus, 687
Dorsomedial hypothalamic nucleus, 777
Dorsomedial thalamic nucleus, 774
Dorsum linguae, 330
Dorsum penis, 438
Dorsum sellae, 100f, 101, 121–123, 122f
Duct(s)
  alveolar, 388, 403
  bile, 379, 380f
  cochlear, 842, 843f, 844–846
  cystic, 379, 380f
  endolymphatic, 842
  hepatic, 379, 379f–380f
  incisive, 390–391, 390f
  of lateral nasal gland, 107f
  mandibular, 341f, 342
  mesonephric, 462–463
  nasolacrimal, 107f, 391–392, 391f–392f, 395, 890–891, 891f
  pancreatic, 380f, 382
  papillary, 418–419, 460, 463

Duct(s) (Continued)
  parotid, 340f–341f, 341–342
  perilymphatic, 104, 840–842
  pronephric, 462–463
  semicircular, 842
  sphincters of, 461
  utriculosaccular, 842
Ductuli alveolares, 403
Ductuli biliferi, 379
Ductuli efferentes testis, 428–430
Ductuli hepaticae, 379
Ductuli interlobularis bilifer, 379
Ductus choledochus, 379–380
Ductus cystica, 379
Ductus cysticus, 379–380
Ductus deferens, 435–436, 463
  artery of, 430–431, 436–438
  nerves of, 436
  structure of, 436
  vein of, 436
  vessels of, 436
Ductus deferens, artery of, 573f
Ductus deferens, vein of, 604
Ductus incisivus, 321, 390–391
Ductus lymphaticus dexter, 622, 624
Ductus mandibularis, 342
Ductus nasolacrimalis, 391–392, 395, 890–891
Ductus pancreaticus, 382
Ductus pancreaticus accessorius, 382
Ductus papillares, 418–419, 460
Ductus parotideus, 341–342
Ductus perilymphaticus, 104, 840–842
Ductus reuniens, 842
Ductus sublingualis major, 343
Ductus thoracicus, 622
Ductus venosus, 378, 598
Duodenal bulb, 365
Duodenal cap, 365
Duodenal flexure
  caudal, 365
  cranial, 365
Duodenal fossa, 365
Duodenal glands, 367
Duodenal impression, 376
Duodenal lymph nodes, 383
Duodenal papilla
  major, 380
  minor, 380
Duodenocolic fold, 365
Duodenocolic ligament, 357f
Duodenojejunal flexure, 365
Duodenum, 360f, 365, 366f
  lymph vessels of, 638f

Dura mater, 679, 680f–681f, 696–699, 700f
  venous sinuses of, 606
  confluence of, 608
Dura mater encephali, 699
Dura mater spinalis, 699

E

Ear(s), 839–857
  external, 839, 840f, 850–853, 851f
    cartilages of, 852f
    directional terms for, 853
    muscles of, 216f–218f, 219–221
  internal, 839–846, 840f, 842f
    development of, 33, 38f, 43f
    directional terms for, 853
  middle, 840f, 846–850
    articulations of, 849–850
    bones of, 849–850
    development of, 28, 33, 36f–38f
    muscles of, 221–222, 222f
    nerves of, 827f
  muscles of, 216f, 219–222, 220f, 222f, 852–853, 853f–856f
  tympanic cavity, 839, 847–848
Ear canal, glands of, 80
Eccrine glands, 68
Ectoturbinalia, 107–109
Ectoturbinates, 106f, 107–109, 124
Efferent arterioles, 420
Efferent axons, 688
Efferent ductules, 428–430, 463
Efferent lymph vessels, 621
Efferent neurons, 651f
  spinal cord, 685
Elbow, 189–191, 190f–191f
  contact areas in, 192
  development of, 150
  right, nerves and arteries of, 719f
Ellipsoidal joint, 179
Elliptical recess, 839–840
EMBARK, 1
Embryo, 17–21, 18f–20f, 29f. see also Fetus; Prenatal development
  age of, 21–26, 24f–25f, 24t
  amniotic folds and, 18, 18f–19f
  crown-rump (C-R) length of, 15, 24t, 26f, 27t
  death of, 17, 20
  genital tubercle of, 27, 29f
  weight of, 23, 25f
Embryonic brain, 758f, 758t
Embryonic vesicles, 758t
Eminence
  iliopubic, 156–158, 157f–160f, 161
  intercondylar, 165–167, 167f
Eminentia iliopubica, 161

Emissary veins
  of carotid canal, 609
  of hypoglossal canal, 608–609
  of orbital fissure, 904
  from oval foramen, 589
  from retroarticular foramen, 589
  of retroarticular foramen, 588f, 589
  of round foramen, 589
Enamel, 325
Enamelum, 325
Encephalon, 650, 657, 757
Endocardium, 500
Endocrine system, 469–494
  adrenal gland, 482–486
  endocrine tissues of kidney, 489
  endocrine tissues of ovary, 488
  endocrine tissues of testis, 489
  enteroendocrine cells, 488
  fetal membrane endocrine tissues, 488–489
  general features of, 469–470
  hypophysis, 470–476, 471f–473f
  lymph drainage of, 618
  parathyroid glands, 480–481
  pars endocrina pancreatis, 487–488
  pineal gland, 481–482
  thyroid gland, 476–480, 477f–478f
Endocrinocytus parafollicularis, 479
Endocrinology, 469
Endolymph, 842
Endolymphatic duct, 842
Endolymphatic sac, 842
Endometrium, 452–453
Endomysium, 210
Endopeduncular nucleus, 790–791
Endoplasmic reticulum, 650–652
Endosteum, 90
Endothoracic fascia, 404
Endoturbinates, 107–109, 108f, 124
  first, 108f
English Bulldog, 95
Enteric nervous system, 661, 675–676
Enteroendocrine cells, 488
Ependymocytus, 657
Epicardium, 495
Epicondyle, 90
  of femur, 162f, 164
  of humerus, 143f–144f, 146, 149f
Epicondylus lateralis, 146
Epicondylus medialis, 146–147
Epidermal papillae, 78, 78f
Epidermis, 64–65
  of digital pad, 68–69
  histologic characteristics of, 78–79
  nasal, 67

Epididymides, 423
Epididymis, 435, 463
  structure of, 435
  tail of, 435
    ligament of, 436
Epidural space, 699
Epiglottic cartilage, 397–398
Epiglottis, 116f, 345f, 396f–397f, 397–398
Epihyoid bones, 116f, 117, 227f–228f, 344f
Epihyoid cartilage, 33
Epihyoideum, 116f, 117
Epimysium, 210
Epiphyseal cartilage, 87–88
Epiphysis, 87
  of axis, 127f
  of radius, 194f
Epiploic foramen, 356–358
Epiploon, 353, 354f
Episcleral arteries, 523
Episcleral space, 884
Epithalamus, 758t, 777–778
Epithelioidocyti tacti, 652
Epithelium
  germinal, 447
  soft palate, 322
  superficial, of ovary, 447
Epitrichial sweat glands, 79–80, 80f
Epitympanic recess, 103f, 104–105, 846–847
Epoophoron, 451, 463
Equator, 861
Erection, 434f, 442–443
Erector spinae muscles, 242–245
Esophageal glands, 348
Esophageal hiatus, 351
Esophageal vein, 591
Esophagus, 346–349, 357f, 584f, 714f
  abdominal portion of, 347
  cervical portion of, 346
  coats of, 347–348
  drainage from, 349f
  lymph vessels of, 629f
  musculature of, 346f
  nerves of, 348–349, 351f, 835f
  thoracic portion of, 346–347
  vessels of, 348
Estrous cycle, 447–449
Estrum, 448
Estrus, 13, 14f, 447–448
Ethmoid bone, 96f, 99f, 106–109, 106f–108f, 117f, 120f
  development of, 29–32
Ethmoid crest, 392
Ethmoid incisure, 100

Ethmoidal arteries
  external, 523–524, 901–902, 901f–902f
  internal, 529f, 530
Ethmoidal conchae, 391f, 393
Ethmoidal crest, 110, 110f, 113, 113f
Ethmoidal foramina, 99–100, 99f, 106f, 107, 118, 122f
Ethmoidal fossa, 110, 110f
Ethmoidal incisure, 99f
Ethmoidal labyrinths, 107–109, 120f, 124
Ethmoidal nerve, 815–816, 819, 898f, 899
Ethmoidal vein, external, 587
Ethmoidomaxillary suture, 109, 111
Ethmoturbinalia, 107–109
Ethmoturbinates, 107–109, 108f, 124, 392–393
Eustachian tube, 839
Excavatio disci, 875–876
Excavatio pubovesicalis, 355, 422–423
Excavatio rectogenitalis, 355, 422–423
Excavatio vesicogenitalis, 355
Exoccipital bones, 96f, 120f
Exostoses, 90
Extension, 179
External acoustic meatus, 840f, 850
  nerve, 825–826
External anal sphincter muscle, 745f, 747f
External capsule, 788
External carotid artery, branches of, 512f, 513–526
External carotid nerves, 672
External ethmoidal artery, 523–524, 901–902, 901f–902f
External genitalia
  development of, 463
  female, 455–457
External iliac artery, 561f, 562–565, 740f, 743f
External iliac vein, 561f, 583f, 595f, 602–603, 613f
External jugular vein, 583f–584f, 586, 588f, 591, 709f, 714f
External nares, 388
External nasal branches, 815–816, 819, 822–824
External ophthalmic artery, 523, 901, 901f–902f
External pudendal artery, 424f–425f, 428, 440–441, 444, 457, 562, 562f, 740f
External pudendal veins, 425f, 441, 444, 740f

External thoracic artery, 538, 593f
External vertebral venous plexus
  dorsal, 614
  ventral, 614
Extradural segment, 704
Extraocular muscles, 891–894, 892f
Extreme capsule, 788
Extremitas dorsalis, 643
Extremitas ventralis, 643
Extrinsic muscles
  of eye, 893f
  of tongue, 334–335
Eye(s), 858–911
  anterior chamber, 860, 878
  anterior pole, 861
  chambers of, 878–879
  development of, 858–860, 859f
  fibrous tunic, 861–866
  innervation of, 896–901, 897f–899f
  internal tunic, 873–876
  lens, 877f
  muscles of, 891–896
    extraocular, 891–894, 892f
    extrinsic, 520f, 893f
    intraocular, 891
    palpebral, 894–896
  nerves of, 587f, 818f, 820f
  ocular dimensions of, 862t
  as optical device, 879–880
  posterior chamber, 860, 878
  posterior pole, 861
  vascular tunic, 866–873
    arterial supply of, 869f
    veins of, 869f
  vasculature of, 901–904
  vitreous, 878f, 879
  vitreous chamber, 879
Eyeball, 861–879, 870f
  extrinsic muscles of, 215b, 225–227, 226f
Eyelashes, 64
Eyelid(s), 860, 885–888, 886f
  muscles of, 216f–218f, 219–222, 226f
  third, 887–888
    gland of, 887f
    superficial gland of, 890

F

Fabellae. see Sesamoid bone(s)
Face
  bones of, 91f, 109–116
    dorsal nasal concha, 107–112, 107f–108f, 122f, 123
    incisive, 91f–92f, 96f, 109–110, 109f, 116f–117f, 120f

Face (Continued)
    lacrimal, 91f–92f, 113–114, 114f, 116f–117f
    mandible, 115–116, 115f–116f, 120f
    maxilla, 91f–92f, 96f, 107f–108f, 110–111, 110f, 116f–117f, 120f
    nasal, 91f–92f, 96f, 108f, 110, 110f, 116f–117f, 120f
    palatine, 91f–92f, 96f, 112–113, 116f–117f, 120f
    pterygoid, 91f–92f, 96f, 114, 114f, 117f, 120f
    ventral nasal concha, 107–109, 108f, 112, 122f, 123–124
    vomer, 92f, 96f, 106f, 108f, 114–115, 114f, 117f, 120f
    zygomatic, 91f–92f, 112, 112f, 116f–117f, 120f
  muscles of, 214–222, 215b. see also specific muscles
    deep, 216–219, 217f–218f
    ear, 216f–218f, 219–222, 220f, 222f
    eyelid, 216f–218f, 219–222, 226f
    forehead, 216f–218f, 219–222
    lip, 216–219, 216f–218f
    nose, 216–219
    superficial, 214–216, 216f
Facial artery, 342–343, 516
  branches of, 520f
  transverse, 518
Facial canal, 104
Facial expression: muscles of, 214–222, 215b, 216f–218f
Facial nerve (cranial nerve VII), 665, 829–832, 900–901
  autonomic interconnections, 826f
  buccal branches, 832
  canal for, 102f–103f
  cervical branch, 832
  communicating branches to, 825–826
  digastric branch, 831
  genu of, 764
  internal auricular branches, 831
  motor nucleus of, 764
  palpebral branches, 832, 900
  parasympathetic nucleus of, 665, 763–764
  superficial branches of, 823f
  zygomatic branch, 900
Facial nucleus, level of, 764–765

Facial vein, 342–343, 583f, 586, 587f–588f
  deep, 903f
  transverse, 589
Facies articularis, 400
Facies articularis arytenoidea, 399
Facies articularis calcanea, 169–170
Facies articularis capitis fibulae, 168
Facies articularis carpea, 149–150
Facies articularis cricoidea, 399
Facies articularis cuboidea, 168
Facies articularis hyoidea, 399
Facies articularis malleoli
  of fibula, 168
  of tibia, 167
Facies articularis navicularis, 169–170
Facies articularis proximalis, 165–167
Facies articularis talaris, 168
Facies articularis thyroidea, 399
Facies articularis tuberculi costae, 139–140
Facies atrialis, 499
Facies auricularis
  of heart, 499
  of iliac wing, 158–160
  of sacrum, 136
Facies buccalis, 115
Facies caudalis
  of humerus, 144f, 146
  of radius, 149
  of tibia, 167
Facies cerebralis, 101
Facies contactus, 327
Facies costalis
  of lungs, 408
  of scapula, 142
Facies cranialis
  of humerus, 146
  of radius, 147–148, 147f–148f
  of ulna, 151
Facies diaphragmatica, 375, 408
Facies dorsalis
  of pancreas, 381
  of sacrum, 135–136
Facies externa, 110
  of parietal bone, 98–99
Facies facialis
  of lacrimal bone, 113–114, 114f
  of maxilla, 110–111
Facies gastrica, 643
Facies glutea, 158–160
Facies interlobares, 409
Facies interna
  of frontal bone, 100
  of nasal bone, 110
  of parietal bone, 99

Facies intestinalis, 643
Facies labialis, 115
Facies laryngea, 397–398
Facies lateralis
　of fibula, 168
　of humerus, 143f, 145
　of scapula, 142
　of tibia, 167
　of zygomatic bone, 112
Facies lingualis, 397–398
　of mandible, 115
　of tooth, 327
Facies lunata, 156–158
Facies maxillaris, of palatine bone, 113
Facies medialis, 146
　of fibula, 168
　of lung, 408
　of tibia, 167
Facies nasalis, 112–113
　of lacrimal bone, 113–114
　of maxilla, 111
　of palatine bone, 113
Facies occlusalis, 327
Facies orbitalis
　of lacrimal bone, 113–114, 114f
　of zygomatic bone, 112
Facies palatina, 112–113
　of maxilla, 111
Facies parietalis, 361, 643
Facies pelvina, 136
Facies poplitea, 163–164
Facies renalis, 643
Facies sacropelvina, 158–160
Facies serrata, 142
Facies temporalis, 105
　of basisphenoid bone, 101
　of frontal bone, 100
　of temporal bone, 105
Facies urethralis, 438
Facies ventralis, 381
Facies ventralis linguae, 330
Facies vestibularis, 327
Facies visceralis, 361, 376, 643
Falciform ligament, 357f, 378
Falx cerebri, 699
Fascia(e), 213
　of antebrachium, 286–287
　of brachium, 286
　crural, 312–313
　deep, 213
　deep perineal, 374
　diaphragmatic, 353
　endothoracic, 404
　femoral, 312–313
　gluteal, 371f
　of head, 236–237
　iliac, 353

Fascia(e) (Continued)
　muscular, 884
　of neck, 240–241
　orbital, 884–885
　pelvic, 353
　of pelvic limb, 287–313
　of pelvis, 287–302
　perineal, 374
　spermatic, 353, 424
　　external, 437
　　internal, 437
　of stifle joint, 312–313
　superficial, 213
　superficial caudal, 312
　superficial perineal, 374
　of tail, 262–263
　of thigh, 287–302, 312
　of thoracic limb, 286–287
　transversalis, 424
　of trunk, 262–263, 263f
Fascia antebrachii, 286–287
Fascia axillaris, 286–287
Fascia brachii, 286–287
Fascia caudae, 263
Fascia cruris, 312–313
Fascia digitii, 196
Fascia dorsalis pedis, 312–313
Fascia endothoracica, 240, 252, 262, 404
Fascia genus, 312–313
Fascia iliaca, 262
Fascia lata, 312–313
Fascia manus, 286–287
Fascia masseterica profunda, 236–237
Fascia palmaris, 196
Fascia parotidea profunda, 236
Fascia pelvis, 262
Fascia perinei, 374
Fascia perinei profunda, 374
Fascia perinei superficialis, 374
Fascia thoracolumbalis, 262–263, 263f
Fascia transversalis, 256, 262, 353
Fascia trunci superficialis, 262
Fasciae musculares, 884
Fasciculi, 658f
Fasciculus atrioventricularis, 505–506
Fasciculus cuneatus, 690–692, 691f, 761
Fasciculus gracilis, 690, 691f, 761
Fasciculus longitudinalis dorsalis, 776
Fasciculus longitudinalis inferior, 788
Fasciculus longitudinalis superior, 788
Fasciculus medialis telencephali, 776
Fasciculus of Lissauer, 692
Fasciculus proprii, 689
Fasciculus retroflexus, 778

Fat
　intraperiorbital, 883f, 885
　subcutis, 66
Fat body, orbital, 885
Fauces, 344–345
Feliformia, 2
Female genital organs, 434f, 445–458, 446f, 451f, 458f
　external genitalia
　　muscles of, 456–457
　　structure of, 456
　　vessels and nerves of, 457–458
　lymph vessels of, 642f
Female pelvic viscera, 454f
Female pelvis, 574f
Female perineum, 745f
Female pseudohermaphroditism, 432
Female urethra, 457–458
　vessels and nerves of, 457–458
Female urogenital system, 417f
Females: heart weight to body weight ratios, 498
Femoral artery, 563f, 565–568, 740f, 742f–743f, 745f
　circumflex, 563
　cranial, 567
　deep, 562
Femoral fascia, 312–313
Femoral lymph node, 640
Femoral nerves, 732f, 734f, 736f–737f, 740–741, 740f–741f
　caudal cutaneous, 602f–603f
Femoral region, 602f–603f
Femoral triangle, 565–567
Femoral vein, 583f, 595f, 600, 600f, 740f
　cranial, 602
　deep, 583f, 595f, 602–603
　lateral circumflex, 602
Femoropatellar joint, 198–199
Femorotibial joint, 198–199, 201
Femur, 161–164, 162f–163f, 742f, 745f
　development of, 51, 54f–56f
　head of, ligaments of, 197, 197f, 199f
Fenestra cochleae, 104, 847
Fenestra vestibuli, 104, 180, 847
Fertilization, 13, 15–16
Fetal cortex, 483–484
Fetal membrane endocrine tissues, 488–489
Fetus, 26–51
　carpus of, 51
　claw of, 82f
　crown-rump (C-R) length of, 15, 24t, 26f, 27t

Fetus (Continued)
　　external features of, 27, 29f–32f, 59f–60f
　　external genitalia of, 30f–32f
　　girdles of, 44–51, 52f–56f
　　hair follicles of, 69–70
　　limbs of, 44–51, 54f–56f
　　measurements and growth plots of, 23–24, 26f, 27t
　　ossification in, 27, 32f, 89
　　phalanges of, 47–51, 53f–57f
　　ribs of, 44, 60f
　　size index of, 26, 28f
　　skull of, 27–35, 33f–36f, 44f–45f
　　　　basicranial centers of, 29–32, 40f–43f
　　　　calvarial centers of, 28–29, 36f–39f
　　　　hyoid apparatus of, 33, 39f, 44f
　　　　interparietal bone of, 28–29, 39f
　　　　otic centers of, 33, 38f
　　　　teeth of, 33–35, 34f, 45f
　　sternum of, 44, 49f–51f
　　vertebral column of, 35–44, 46f
　　　　atlas, 47f
　　　　axis, 47f
　　　　caudal, 37–44, 46f–47f, 49f
　　　　centra of, 37–44, 46f–49f
　　　　cervical, 46f, 48f
　　　　lumbar, 37, 46f, 48f
　　　　neural arches of, 44, 47f–49f
　　　　sacral, 37, 46f, 49f
　　　　thoracic, 46f, 48f
　　weight of, 23, 25f
Fibrae arcuatae cerebri, 788
Fibrae arcuatae profundae, 761
Fibrae circulares, 871
Fibrae intercrurales, 253–254
Fibrae longitudinales profundae, 336–337
Fibrae longitudinales superficiales, 336
Fibrae meridionales, 871
Fibrae obliquae, 363
Fibrae perpendiculares, 337
Fibrae pontis transversae, 766
Fibrae transversae, 337
Fibrae zonulares, 871
Fibroblast nuclei, in dermis, 66
Fibrocartilage
　　medial and lateral, 202
　　palmar carpal, 192f, 193–195
Fibrocartilago carpometacarpeum palmare, 192f
Fibrous appendix, of liver, 377–378
Fibrous base, of heart, 500–501
Fibrous capsule, 377, 416–418
Fibrous coat, 347

Fibrous joint, 176
Fibrous membrane, 177–178
Fibrous pericardium, 495
Fibrous rings, 185, 500
Fibrous trigones, 500
Fibrous tunic, of eye, 861–866
Fibula, 165f–166f, 167–168, 171f, 742f
　　development of, 51, 54f–56f
Fila radicularia, 681, 704
Filament(s)
　　myofilaments, 207
　　spinal dura mater, 682–683
　　terminal, 682–683
Filiform papillae, 331–332, 331f
Filum durae matris spinalis, 682–683, 699
Filum terminale, 682–683
Fimbriae, of infundibulum, 450
Fissura interlobalis caudalis, 409
Fissura interlobalis cranialis, 411
Fissura interlobaris cranialis, 409
Fissura lig. teretis, 376
Fissura longitudinalis cerebri, 778
Fissura mediana ventralis, 680
Fissura orbitalis, 101
Fissura palatina, 109–111
Fissura petrooccipitalis, 105–106, 123
Fissura petrotympanica, 104
Fissura thyroidea, 399
Fissura transversa cerebri, 778
Fissura tympanooccipitalis, 105–106
Fissura uvulonodularis, 792
Fissure
　　caudal, caudal edge, 110f
　　caudal interlobar, 409
　　cranial interlobar, 409
　　dorsal median, 680
　　oral, 319
　　orbital, 101, 101f, 118, 118f–119f, 121–123, 122f
　　　　emissary vein of, 904
　　　　muscle attachments in, 892f
　　　　notch of, 100f
　　palatine, 92f, 109–111, 109f, 119f, 121, 122f
　　petrooccipital, 105–106, 123
　　petrotympanic, 102f, 104, 119f
　　for round ligament, 376
　　thyroid, 399
　　tympanooccipital, 105–106
　　ventral median, 680
Fixation muscle, 212–213
Flat bones, 88
Flehmen, 390–391
Flexion, 179
Flexor retinaculum, 192f, 193, 282f
Flexura coli dextra, 369

Flexura coli sinistra, 369
Flexura dudeni caudalis, 365
Flexura duodeni cranialis, 365
Flexura duodenojejunalis, 365
Flexure
　　colic, 369
　　duodenal
　　　　caudal, 365
　　　　cranial, 365
　　duodenojejunal, 365
Flocculonodular lobe, 792
Fluid
　　cerebrospinal, 696–701
　　follicular, 447
　　synovial, 177–178
Fold(s)
　　alar, 112, 390
　　aryepiglottic, 400
　　duodenocolic, 365
　　gastropancreatic, 359
　　genital, 422–423, 435–436, 452
　　hepatopancreatic, 359
　　ileocecal, 366, 368–369
　　of lank, 350–351
　　preputial, 642f
　　semilunar, of conjunctiva, 887–888
　　synovial, 177
　　tonsillar, 344–345
　　of uterus, 452
　　vestibular, 397f, 400–401
　　vocal, 397f, 401
Foliate papillae, 334
Foliate suture, 176
Folium, 757
　　cerebellar, 796f
Follicle(s)
　　hair. see Hair follicles
　　primary, 447
　　primordial, 447
　　tertiary, 447
　　vesicular, 447
Folliculae thyroideae, 479
Follicular endocrine cells, 479
Folliculus ovaricus primarius, 447
Folliculus ovaricus tertiarius (vesiculosus), 447
Foramen
　　alar
　　　　of atlas, 127–130
　　　　caudal, 101–102, 101f, 118f–119f
　　　　rostral, 101–102, 101f, 118f–119f
　　alveolar, 110–111, 110f, 122f
　　carotid, caudal, 102f
　　costotransverse, 139–140
　　cribriform, 107, 121

Foramen *(Continued)*
   for dorsal sagittal sinus, 96f, 97, 123
   ethmoidal, 99–100, 99f, 106f, 107, 118, 122f
   frontal, 119f
   infraorbital, 92f, 118, 118f, 122f
   intervertebral, 126, 132f–133f
      lumbar, 134f–135f
   jugular, 103, 122f, 123
   mandibular, 115f
   mastoid, 98, 104–105, 121, 122f
   maxillary, 110–111, 122f
   mental, 115–116, 115f
   nutrient, 90–91, 146, 147f
   obturator, 156–158, 157f–160f
   oval, 92f, 101–102, 118–119, 119f, 121–123, 122f
   palatine
      caudal, 118, 118f
      major, 111–113, 119f, 121
      minor, 112–113, 119f, 121
   retroarticular, 103f, 105, 118f–119f
   round, 101–102, 121–123, 122f
   sacral, 135–136, 136f
   sphenopalatine, 108f, 113, 113f, 118, 118f, 122f, 124
   spinous, 119f
   stylomastoid, 103f, 104–105, 118f–119f
   supratrochlear, 143f, 146
   transverse, 126
      of atlas, 128f
      of axis, 127f–128f
      of cervical vertebra, 128f, 131
   vertebral
      of atlas, 126, 126f, 128f
      of axis, 128f–129f
      of cervical vertebrae, 129f–130f
   for zygomatic nerve, 101f
Foramen alare, 127–130
Foramen alare parvum, 101–102
Foramen alare rostralis, 101–102
Foramen apices dentis, 326–327
Foramen caroticum caudalis, 105
Foramen caroticum internum, 105
Foramen epiploicum, 358
Foramen infraorbitale, 110–111, 118
Foramen interventriculare, 772–773, 781
Foramen ischiadicum minus, 197
Foramen jugulare, 103
Foramen lacerum, 101–102, 105, 118–119, 119f, 526–527
Foramen magnum, 91, 95–98, 96f, 118f–119f, 121, 123, 183f
   keyhole notch in, 95–96, 97f

Foramen mandibulae, 115f
Foramen mastoideum, 98, 104–105
Foramen maxillare, 110–111
Foramen mentale, 115–116, 115f
Foramen nutricium, 90
Foramen obturatum, 156–158
Foramen omentale- epiploicum, 356–357
Foramen ovale, 100f, 101–102, 118–119, 119f, 122f
Foramen ovale (heart), 499–500
Foramen palatinum caudalis, 113
Foramen palatinum majus, 111–113
Foramen retroarticulare, 105
Foramen rotundum, 100f, 101–102
Foramen sinus sagittalis dorsalis, 96f, 97, 123
Foramen sphenopalatinum, 113, 124
Foramen spinosum, 101–102, 522
Foramen stylomastoideum, 104–105
Foramen supratrochleare, 146
Foramen transversarium, 126
   of atlas, 126f
   of axis, 127f
Foramen vertebrale, 126
Foramen vertebrale laterale, 127–130
Foramina alveolaria, 110–111, 122f
Foramina ethmoidalia, 99–100, 107
Foramina intervertebralia, 126
Foramina laminae cribrosae, 107
Foramina papillaria, 418–419
Foramina sacralia dorsalia, 135–136
Foramina sacralia pelvina, 136
Forearm. *see* Antebrachium
Forebrain, 757
   derived brain structures and definitive brain cavities, 758t
   origin, 694
Forepaw (manus)
   arteries of, 545f, 546–548, 547f, 724f
   bones of, 150f–153f, 151–156
   cutaneous innervation of, 727f
   fasciae of, 286–287
   muscles of, 276f–283f
   nerves of, 723–727, 724f–726f
   superficial arteries of, 545f, 547f
   veins of, 592f, 594–595
Formatio reticularis, 688, 757–759
Fornix, 776
   conjunctival, 887
   of hippocampus, 700f
   of penis, 444
Fossa
   acetabular, 156–158, 158f–160f
   atlantal, 127–130
   cerebellar, 102f, 103, 122f, 123
   dorsal condyloid, 96f, 97, 118f

Fossa *(Continued)*
   ethmoidal, 110, 110f
   extensor, of femur, 162f, 164
   frontal, 117
   for gallbladder, 376–377
   hypophyseal, 100f, 101, 121–123, 122f
   infraspinous, of scapula, 141f, 142
   intercondylar, of femur, 164, 167f
   for lacrimal gland, 99f
   for lacrimal sac, 92f, 113–114, 114f, 118, 122f
   mandibular, 102f–103f, 105, 119f
   masseteric, 115–116, 115f
   olecranon, 144f, 146
   piriform, 101
   pterygoid, 114
   pterygopalatine, 110f, 111, 113, 118
   radial, 143f, 146, 146f
   sesamoid, 152f–153f, 154
   sphenoidal, 106f
   for stapedius muscle, 104
   subscapular, 141f, 142
   supraspinous, 141f, 142
   temporal, 98–99
   for tensor tympani, 104, 119f
   trochanteric, 162f–163f, 163
   ventral condyloid, 96f
Fossa acetabuli, 156–158
Fossa cerebellaris, 103
Fossa clitoridis, 455
Fossa condylaris dorsalis, 97
Fossa condylaris ventralis, 97
Fossa cranii caudalis, 123
Fossa cranii media, 121–123
Fossa cranii rostralis, 121
Fossa extensoria, 164
Fossa frontalis, 117
Fossa hyaloidea, 879
Fossa hypophysialis, 101
Fossa infraspinata, 142
Fossa intercondylaris, 164
Fossa ischiorectalis, 374
Fossa m. stapedius, 104
Fossa m. tensor tympani, 104
Fossa mandibularis, 105
Fossa masseterica, 115–116, 115f
Fossa olecrani, 146
Fossa ovalis, 499–500
Fossa paralumbalis, 350–351
Fossa pararectalis, 370–371
Fossa piriformis, 101
Fossa pterygoidea, 114
Fossa pterygopalatina, 111
Fossa radialis, 146
Fossa rhomboidea, 757, 763

Fossa sacci lacrimalis, 113–114, 114f, 881–882
Fossa sesamoidalis, 172
Fossa subscapularis, 142
Fossa supraspinata, 142
Fossa temporalis, 98–99
Fossa tonsillaris, 344–345
Fossa trochanterica, 163
Fossa vesicae felleae, 376–377
Fossae atlantis, 127–130
Fourth ventricle, 700–701, 700f, 758t, 763
　choroid plexuses of, 763
　lateral aperture of, 700f
　lateral recess, 700f
　roof of, 763
　tenia of, 763
Fovea
　articular
　　caudal, 126f, 127–130
　　cranial, 127–130, 128f
　　of radius, 147, 147f
　of dens, 126f, 127–130
　of femur, 162f, 163
Fovea articularis caudalis, 126f, 127–130
Fovea articularis cranialis, 127–130
Fovea capitis radii, 147
Fovea costalis cranialis et caudalis, 131–132
Fovea dentis, 127–130
Foveae costales transversales, 132
Foveolae gastricae, 363
Fracture, of dens, 130–131
French Bulldog, 7, 7f
Frenulum, 340f
Frenulum linguae, 331
Frontal bone, 91f–92f, 96f, 99–100, 116f–117f
　inner table of, 106f
　orbital part of, 99–100
　outer table of, 106f
　temporal surface of, 100
　zygomatic process of, 92f, 99–100, 99f, 118f–120f
Frontal diploic vein, 587, 609f, 611
Frontal fossa, 117
Frontal nerve, 587f, 898f, 899
Frontal process
　of lacrimal bone, 113–114, 114f
　of maxilla, 110f, 111
　of nasal bone, 110, 110f
　of zygomatic bone, 92f, 99f, 112, 112f
Frontal sinus, 99, 107–109, 108f, 120f, 122f, 124–125, 125f
　aperture to, 100

Frontal sinus *(Continued)*
　lateral part, 106f, 124–125
　medial part, 124–125
　rostral part, 124–125
　septum of, 99f
Frontal squama, 100
Frontal suture, 100
Frontoethmoidal suture, 100, 109
Frontolacrimal suture, 100, 114
Frontomaxillary suture, 99–100, 111
Frontonasal suture, 100, 110
Frontopalatine suture, 100
Frontoparietal suture, 100
Functional segments, of neurons, 652–654
Fundus
　of gallbladder, 379
　ocular, 875–876, 875f
　of stomach, 362
Fundus ventriculi, 362
Fundus vesicae felleae, 379
Fungiform papillae, 331–333, 331f
Funiculus
　dorsal, 680
　lateral, 680
　ventral, 680
Funiculus dorsalis, 680
Funiculus lateralis, 680
Funiculus spermaticus, 436
Funiculus ventralis, 680
Furcation, 327–328
Fusi neuromusculari, 652
Fusi neurotendini, 652

G

Gallbladder, 357f, 379–381, 379f
Gamma motor neurons, 685
Ganglia aorticorenalia, 420
Ganglia spinalia, 704
Ganglia trunci sympathici, 671
Ganglion (ganglia), 650
　aorticorenal, 420
　caudal mesenteric, 423
　celiac, 379
　cervical sympathetic, 351f
　ciliary, 816–817, 897–898
　cranial cervical, 351f
　craniospinal (afferent), 654–655
　dorsal root, 704, 705f
　geniculate, 829–830
　mandibular, 342–343
　otic, 821f, 832–833
　pelvic plexus, 423
　pterygopalatine, 824f
　spinal, 680f
　sublingual, 343
　trigeminal, 818–819, 898–899

Ganglion (ganglia) *(Continued)*
　vagal
　　distal, 351f
　　proximal, 667
　vestibular, 844
Ganglion cell, 874, 874f
Ganglion cervicale craniale, 885
Ganglion ciliare, 665, 816–817
Ganglion distale, 834
Ganglion distale n. vagi, 667
Ganglion geniculi, 829–830, 900
Ganglion impar, 675
Ganglion mandibulare, 665
Ganglion oticum, 832–833
Ganglion proximale, 834
Ganglion proximale n. vagi, 667
Ganglion pterygopalatinum, 665
Ganglion spinale, 704
Ganglion sublinguale, 665
Ganglion trigeminale, 818–819
Gaster, 359–361
Gastric artery, 364, 556
　left, 348
Gastric glands, 363–364
Gastric glands proper, 364
Gastric groove, 362
Gastric impression, 376
Gastric lymph nodes, 639
Gastric vein, 364, 599
Gastroduodenal artery, 382, 554, 554f
Gastroduodenal vein, 583f, 599
Gastroepiploic artery, 364, 554–555
Gastroepiploic vein, 364, 599
Gastropancreatic fold, 359
Gastrophrenic ligament, 357, 358f
Gastrosplenic ligament, 357, 643
General visceral efferent (GVE) system, 663–675, 665f, 820f
Genicular artery, 569
　descending, 565f, 568
Genicular vein
　descending, 566f
　medial, 600
Geniculate body, 775
Geniculate ganglion, 829–830, 900
Geniculum canalis facialis, 104
Genioglossus muscle, 335f–336f, 336
　oblique bundle of, 336
　straight bundle of, 336
　vertical bundle of, 336
Geniohyoideus, 344f
Genital fold, 422–423, 435–436, 452
Genital organs
　embryonic indifferent stage, 458f, 461f

Genital organs *(Continued)*
   female, 434f, 445–458, 446f, 451f, 458f
      external genitalia, 455–457
      lymph vessels of, 642f
      lymph nodes and vessels of, 636–637
   male, 423–445, 424f–427f
      lymph vessels of, 642f
Genital rami, 428
Genital ridge, 463
Genital system, lymph drainage of, 619
Genital tubercle, 463
Genitofemoral nerve, 731f–734f, 736f–737f, 739–740, 740f–741f
   cutaneous area of, 741f
Genu, of facial canal, 104
Genu n. facialis, 764
Germinal epithelium, 447
Gestation, 13–15. *see also* Prenatal development
Gestational age, 21–26, 24f–25f, 24t
Gigantocellular reticular nucleus, 759
Gingiva, 323–324, 329
Ginglymus, 179
Girdles, development of, 44–51, 52f–56f
Glabella, 117
Gland(s)
   adrenal, 560f
   anal, 373
   of anus, 80–81, 372
   apocrine, 80–81
   atrichial, 79
   cardiac, 364
   ciliary, 886
   circumanal, 80, 372
   duodenal, 367
   of ear canal, 80
   eccrine, 68
   epitrichial, 79–80
   esophageal, 348
   gastric, 363–364
   gustatory, serous, 334, 338
   intestinal, 367, 373–374
   lacrimal, 889–890
   mammary, 64, 458–459, 459f
   mandibular, 340f–341f, 342–343
   Meibomian (tarsal), 80
   of nose, 395
   orbital, 343
   palatine, 322, 340f
   paranal sinus, 372
   parotid, 340–342, 340f–341f
   pyloric, 364
   salivary, 320f, 338, 340–344, 340f

Gland(s) *(Continued)*
   sebaceous, 80, 80f, 886
   of skin, 79–81
   of stomach, 363–364
   sublingual, 340f, 343
   superficial, of third eyelid, 890
   tail, 80f, 81
   tarsal, 80, 884f, 886f
   tarsal (Meibomian), 886
   of third eyelid, 887f
   thymus, 644–646, 645f
   tongue, 338
   urethral, 444
   von Ebner's, 334
   zygomatic, 340f–341f, 343–344, 625f, 883–884
Gland sinus, 461
Glandula esophageae, 348
Glandula lacrimalis, 889
Glandula mammaria, 64, 458–460
Glandula mandibularis, 342
Glandula nasalis lateralis, 395
Glandula parotis, 340
Glandula pinealis, 777
Glandula sublinguali monostomatica, 343
Glandula sublinguali polystomatica, 343
Glandula superficialis plica semilunaris conjunctivae, 890
Glandula zygomatica, 320, 343, 883–884
Glandulae anales, 372
Glandulae cardiacae, 364
Glandulae carunculae lacrimalis, 885
Glandulae caudae, 80f, 81
Glandulae ciliares, 886
Glandulae circumanales, 80, 372
Glandulae duodenales, 367
Glandulae gastricae, 363–364
Glandulae gustatoriae, 334, 338
Glandulae intestinales, 367, 373–374
Glandulae linguales, 338
Glandulae oris, 340
Glandulae palatinae, 322
Glandulae parotis accessoria, 342
Glandulae pyloricae, 364
Glandulae salivariae majores, 340
Glandulae salivariae minores, 340
Glandulae sebaceae, 80, 886
Glandulae sine ductibus, 469
Glandulae sinus paranalis, 80–81, 80f, 372
Glandulae sudorifera apocrina, 79–80
Glandulae sudorifera merocrina, 79
Glandulae tarsales, 886
Glandular vein, 586

Glans, 439
   of clitoris, 455
   of penis, 438
Glans clitoridis, 455
Glans penis, 438
Glenohumeral ligaments, 188–189, 188f
Glenoid cavity, 141f, 145f
Glenoid lips, 178, 188–189
Gliocyti centrales, 475
Glisson's capsule, 377
Globus pallidus or pallidum, 790–791
Glomerulus, 419
Glomus caroticum, 526–527
Glossopharyngeal nerve, 322, 338f, 339, 348, 351f
Glossopharyngeal nerve, parasympathetic nucleus of, 763–764
Glossopharyngeal nerve (cranial nerve IX), 666, 829f, 832–833, 835f
   autonomic interconnections, 826f
   communicating ramus from, 834–835
   lingual branch, 833
   parasympathetic nucleus of, 666
   pharyngeal branch, 833
Glottis, 401
Gluteal fascia, 312, 371f
Gluteal region
   arteries and veins of, 576f
   deep structures of, 602f–603f
Golgi tendon organs, 177
Gomphosis, 176
Gracilis muscle, 740f–741f
   nerve to, 743f
Granulationes arachnoideales, 701
Gray columns, 658, 658f
Gray commissure, 679
Gray matter, 679, 681f, 757
   laminae, 687–688
   nuclei, 687
   nucleus, 757
   organization of, 686–687
   periaqueductal, 767–768
   of spinal cord, 658f, 685–688, 686f
Great auricular nerve, 705f, 709–710, 709f
Great cardiac vein, 508–509
Great cerebral vein, 607f, 608, 700f
Great coronary vein, 584f
Great occipital nerve, 705f
Great vessels, 511f, 584f
Greater auricular nerve, 711f
Greater curvature, 361
Greater occipital nerve, 709, 710f–711f, 837

Index

Greater tubercle, 716f
Green band, 20–21
Groove(s)
   for abductor digiti I longus, 148f
   brachialis, 143f, 145–146
   coronary, 498–499
   costal, 140
   cranial longitudinal, 498–499
   extensor, of tibia, 165–167
   for extensor carpi radialis, 148f
   for extensor digitalis communis, 148f
   gastric, 362
   interarytenoid, 400
   intertubercular, 143, 143f
   interventricular, 495–496
   of lateral malleolus, 166f
   median, alveolar, 330
   middle meningeal artery, 122f
   for middle meningeal artery, 100f
   paraconal interventricular, 495–496
   pterygoid, 101–102, 119–120
   for sphenopalatine artery, 113f
   transverse sinus, 123
   urethral, 439
   vascular, 123
Gubernaculum testis, 436
Gums, 323–324, 329
Gustatory (taste) area, 788
Gustatory glands, 338
   serous, 334
Gyri, 757, 779, 780f
Gyri cerebri, 779
Gyri insulae, 788
Gyrus diagonalis, 783–784
Gyrus olfactorius lateralis, 784
Gyrus parahippocampalis, 784
Gyrus paraterminalis, 784

H

Haarscheiben, 78, 78f
Habenula, 777–778
Habenular commissure, 777–778
Habenular stria, 778
Hair cells, 844
Hair coat, 64
   color of, 74–75
   variability in, 74
Hair follicles, 65f, 69
   complex, 72f–73f, 73–74
   cycle of, 75–76, 76f–77f
   development of, 71–72
   seasonal shedding of, 75–76
Hair shaft, 69, 69f
   embryology of, 69–71, 72f
   growth rate of, 69, 70f–71f

Hairs
   bristle, 74
   bristled wavy, 74
   cover, 64
   fine wavy, 74
   implantation of, 75
   large wavy, 74
   length of, 75
   regrowth of, 69
   straight, 74
   tactile, 64
   tylotrich, 78, 78f
   types of, 74, 74f
   wavy bristle, 74
   wool, 64
Hamulus, 840–842
Hamulus pterygoideus, 114, 114f
Hard palate, 108f, 111–113, 113f, 120–121, 321, 321f
   nerves of, 816f
   vascular plexus of, 107f
Head (anatomic part)
   of epididymis, 435
   of femur, 161f, 163, 163f
   of fibula, 168
   of humerus, 143, 143f
   of metacarpals, 152f–153f, 154, 155f
   of metatarsals, 169f–170f, 172
   of phalanges, 155–156, 155f
   of radius, 147, 147f, 149f
   of rib, 139–140, 139f
   of stapes, 850
   of talus, 169–170
   of tarsus, 170f
Head (body part). see also Skull
   artery of, 510–548, 514f
   autonomous zones (AZ) of, 822f
   fasciae of, 236–237
   lymph nodes and vessels of, 624–628
   muscles of, 214–237, 895f. see also Muscle(s), of head
   nerves of, 830f, 837f
      cutaneous, noncranial, 837
      sympathetic distribution of, 666f–667f, 672–673
   shapes of, 93–94
   veins of, 586f, 588f
Heart, 495–509, 496f–498f, 584f. see also under Cardiac
   apex of, 495–496
   base of, 495–496, 498f
      fibrous, 499–500
   blood vessels of, 506–509
   conduction system of, 505–506
   innervation of, 505–506
   lymph vessels of, 634f

Heart *(Continued)*
   orientation of, 496–498
   size of, 498
   surfaces of
      auricular, 497f
      tomography of, 497f, 498–499
   weight of, 498
Heart rate, 498
Heart weight to body weight ratios, 498
Helicine arteries, 441
Helicotrema, 840–842
Helix, 851
   spine of, 851
Hemal nodes, 621
Hematomata, gestational, 20–21
Hemiazygos vein, 590–591
Hemophagous organs, 20–21
Hepar, 375. see also Liver
Hepatic arteries, 357f, 378, 382, 554, 554f
Hepatic ducts, 379, 380f
Hepatic lobes
   left, 376
      lateral, 376
      medial, 376
   right, 377
      lateral, 377
      medial, 377
Hepatic lobules, 378
Hepatic lymph nodes, 364, 367, 378–379, 383, 637–638, 638f
Hepatic veins, 373, 378, 583f–584f, 595f–596f, 597–598
Hepatoduodenal ligament, 358
Hepatogastric ligament, 358
Hepatopancreatic fold, 359
Hepatorenal ligament, 357f, 378
Herding, of breeds, 11f
Hermaphroditism, true, 432
Heterotopic skeleton, 87t
Hiatus aorticus, 250f, 251
Hiatus esophageus, 250f, 251
High innervation ratio, 212
High-resolution G-banding of karyotypes, 2
Hilus
   of kidney, 416, 417f
   of lung, 409
   of lymph node, 621
   of spleen, 643
Hilus lienis, 643
Hilus pulmonis, 409
Hilus renalis, 418
Hind limb, 600f
Hindbrain, 757
   derived brain structures and definitive brain cavities, 758t

Hindpaw
  arteries of, 569–573, 570f–572f, 751f, 753f
    deep, 572f
    superficial, 571f
  bones of, 168–172, 168f–171f
  dorsal surface of, 751f
  muscles of, 303–311, 306f–307f, 310f
  nerves of, 751f, 753f
  phalanges of, 172
  plantar surface of, 752f
    nerves of, 752–754
Hinge joint, 178–179
Hip, 197
  arteries of, 743f–745f
  dysplasia of, 197
  muscles of, 289–294, 291f–293f, 744f
  nerves of, 743f–745f
Hip bone, 156–158, 157f–159f
Hippocampal formation, 784f, 785–786
Hippocampus, 776
  fornix of, 700f
Homeostasis, 663
Hormones, 469
Horns
  of spinal cord, 658f, 679
  of uterus, 451
Horny claw, 82–83
Hound breeds, 8f
Humeral retinaculum, transverse, 188–189, 188f
Humeroradial joint, 189
Humeroulnar joints, 189
Humerus, 143–147, 143f–145f, 190f, 716f
  development of, 47–51, 53f
  head of, 143f
  neck of, 143f, 145
  nutrient artery of, 719f
  physis of, 144f, 149f
Humor vitreus, 879
Hyaloid artery, 858–859, 879
Hyaloid canal, 879
Hyaloid fossa, 878
Hybrids, 2–5, 4f–6f
  Dachshund-Pekingese, 4f–6f, 5
  digits in, 172
  jaw in, 94
Hyoepiglotticus, 344f
Hyoglossus muscle, 335, 335f, 344f
Hyoid apparatus, 397f–398f
  bones of, 116–117, 116f
  development of, 33, 39f, 44f
  joints of, 180
  muscles of, 227f, 233f–235f, 264f

Hyoid articular surface, 399
Hyoid venous arch, 586f, 588–589
Hyopharyngeus, 344f
Hypochondriac regions, 350–351, 353f
Hypodermis, 64–65
Hypogastric lymph nodes, 423, 436, 453, 635
Hypogastric nerve, 373, 423, 436, 438, 441–442, 458
Hypogastric nerves, 675
Hypoglossal canal, 96f, 97, 119f, 122f, 123
  emissary veins of, 608–609
  internal opening of, 96f
Hypoglossal nerve (cranial nerve XII), 335f, 339, 829f, 837
  motor nucleus of, 763
Hypophyseal cavity, 473
Hypophyseal fossa, 100f, 101, 121–123, 122f
Hypophyseal portal vessels, 475–476
Hypophysis, 344f, 470–476, 471f–473f, 700f
  arterial supply of, 521f
  developmental anatomy, 473–474
  innervation, 476
  mesoscopic features, 471f–473f, 473
  microscopic features, 474–475
  vascularization, 473f, 475–476
Hypothalamic nuclei, 776f
Hypothalamus, 758t, 775–777
  superficial arterial supply of, 527f

I
Ileal arteries, 558
Ileal orifice, 365–366
Ileal papilla, 365–366
Ileal vein, 598
Ileocecal fold, 366, 368–369
Ileocolic artery, 367, 557
Ileocolic vein, 598
Ileum, 365–366, 366f
Iliac arteries
  external, 562–565
  internal, 601f
  superficial circumflex, 567
Iliac crest, 158, 158f–159f, 161f
Iliac fascia, 262, 353
Iliac lymph nodes, 438
  external, 635, 641
  internal, 635, 641f
  medial, 373, 436, 635, 635f
Iliac spine, 158, 158f–159f
Iliac tuberosity, 158–160, 160f
Iliac vein
  common, 583f, 602–603, 605
  external, 561f, 595f, 602–603, 613f

Iliac vein (Continued)
  internal, 583f, 603
  superficial circumflex, 601
Iliocostalis dorsi muscle, 729f
Iliocostalis lumborum, 733f
Iliofemoral ligament, 197
Iliofemoral lymph center, 640–641
Ilioinguinal nerve, 730f, 732f–734f, 736, 736f–737f, 740f–741f
  lateral cutaneous branch, 739f
Iliolumbar artery, 573f, 576–577, 602f–603f, 744f
Iliolumbar vein, 602f–603f, 604–605
Iliopsoas nerve, 737f
Iliopubic eminence, 156–158, 157f–160f, 161
Iliosacral lymph center, 635–636
Ilium, 158, 158f–159f, 371f, 745f
Impressio cardiaca, 408
Impressio cardiaca pulmonis dextri, 411
Impressio duodenalis, 376
Impressio esophagea, 375
Impressio gastrica, 376
Impressio medullaris, 97–98
Impressio pontina, 97–98
Impressio renalis, 376
Impressio vermialis, 96–97
Impression
  cardiac, 408, 411
  duodenal, 376
  gastric, 376
  renal, 376
Impressiones digitatae, 97
Impressions
  digital, 99–100, 123
  pontine, 96f
  sesamoid, 154
  vermiform, 96f, 97, 121, 123
Incisive bone, 91f–92f, 96f, 109–110, 109f, 116f–117f, 120f
Incisive duct, 321, 390–391, 390f
Incisive papilla, 321
Incisivomaxillary canal, 110–111
Incisivomaxillary suture, 109–110, 110f
Incisor teeth, 109f, 326f, 327
  eruption of, 325t
Incisura acetabuli, 156–158
Incisura alaris, 127–130
Incisura angularis, 361–362
Incisura antitragicohelicina, 851–852
Incisura cardiaca, 362
Incisura cardiaca pulmonis dextri, 408, 411
Incisura carotica, 101–102
Incisura ethmoidalis, 100

Incisura interarytenoidea, 400
Incisura intercondyloidea, 97–98
Incisura intertragica, 851–852
Incisura ischiadica major, 158
Incisura ischiadica minor, 160–161
Incisura mandibulae, 115–116, 115f
Incisura poplitea, 165–167
Incisura pretragica, 851–852
Incisura radialis, 150
Incisura scapulae, 142
Incisura tentorii, 699
Incisura thyroidea caudalis, 399
Incisura trochlearis, 150
Incisura ulnaris, 149–150
Incisura uncinata, 106–107
Incisura vertebralis caudalis, 126
Incisura vertebralis cranialis, 126
Incisure
　antitragicohelicine, 851–852
　carotid, 101–102
　ethmoid, 99f, 100
　intertragic, 851–852
　jugular, 102f
　pretragic, 851–852
Incudomallear joint, 180
Incudostapedial joint, 180
Incus, 849–850, 849f
　ligaments of, 850
Inferior alveolar artery, 520–522
Inferior alveolar nerve, 826
Inferior alveolar vein, 588f, 589
Inferior dental arch, 325
Inferior labial artery, 516
Inferior labial vein, 588, 588f
Inferior longitudinal fasciculus, 738
Inferior palpebral artery, lateral, 518
Inferior palpebral vein, 587
Inferior tarsal muscle, 885
Infraglenoid tubercle, 141f, 142, 144f
Infraglottic cavity, 401
Inframammillary recess, 773
Infraorbital artery, 343–344, 520, 526
Infraorbital canal, 110–111, 110f
Infraorbital foramen, 92f, 110–111, 118, 118f, 122f
Infraorbital margin, 99–100, 112, 112f
Infraorbital nerve, 822–824
Infraorbital vein, 587, 587f
Infrapatellar fat body, 199–201
Infraspinatus muscle, nerve to, 716f
Infraspinous fossa, 141f, 142
Infratrochlear nerve, 818f, 819, 899
Infundibular or arcuate nucleus, 777

Infundibular recess, 700f
Infundibulum, 450, 473
Infundibulum tubae uterinae, 450
In-grown claw, 83f
Inguinal canal, 254f, 257, 436
Inguinal ligament, 254f, 256
Inguinal lymph nodes, superficial, 641
Inguinal mammae, 459f
Inguinal mammary gland, 740f
Inguinal regions, of abdomen, 350–351, 353f
Inguinal ring, 253, 425f, 436
Inguinofemoral lymph center, 641–642
Inion, 93, 93f
Inlet
　laryngeal, 400
　pelvic, 136–137, 156–158
　thoracic, 405
Inner nervous tunic, 861
Insula gyrus, 788
Integument, 64–85. see also Hair; Skin
Integumentary papillae, 78, 78f
Interalveolar margin, 110–111, 115
Interalveolar septa, 109–111, 115
Interarcuate space, 126
Interarcuate veins, 614
Interarytenoid cartilage, 344f, 397f, 400
Interarytenoid groove, 400
Interatrial septum, 499–500
Interbasilar sinus, 607f
Intercapital ligament, 184f, 186, 186f
Intercarpal joints, 192
Intercartilaginous part, 401
Intercavernous sinuses, 609–610
Intercondylar eminence, 165–167, 167f
Intercondylar fossa, of femur, 164, 167f
Intercondylar tubercles, 165–167
Intercondyloid area, of tibia, 165f–166f
Intercondyloid notch, 96f, 97–98
Intercostal arteries
　6th, 729f
　dorsal, 348, 535, 550–551
Intercostal lymph nodes, 633f
Intercostal lymph trunks, 633f
Intercostal nerves, 728–729
　1st, 705f
　2nd, 705f, 714f, 731
　　lateral cutaneous, 717f, 731
　3rd, 714f, 731
　4th, 714f
　6th, 729f
　7th, 729f

Intercostal nerves (Continued)
　lateral cutaneous branches of, 730f
　ventral cutaneous branches of, 730f
Intercostal space, 139, 139f
Intercostal vein, 583f, 612f
Intercostobrachial nerve, 705f, 730f
　II, 731f
　III, 731f
Interdental spaces, 110–111
Interdigital vein, 592f
Interincisive canal, 109–110, 121
Interincisive suture, 109–110
Interlobar arteries, 420
Interlobar fissure, caudal, 409
Interlobar surfaces, of lung, 409
Interlobar veins, 420
Interlobular arteries, 420
Interlobular ductules, 379
Interlobular veins, 378, 420
Intermandibular joint, 180
Intermandibular suture, 115–116
Intermediate lobe, 411
Intermediate nerve, 665, 829–830
　parasympathetic nucleus of, 665
Intermediate olfactory tract, 783
Intermediate substance nuclei, 687
Intermediate zone, of canal, 371
Intermediolateral nucleus, 687
Intermediomedial nucleus, 687
Intermembranous part, 401
Intermetacarpal joints, 195
Internal abdominal oblique muscle, 733f
Internal capsule, 771–772, 788
Internal carotid artery, 521f, 526–531
Internal carotid nerve, 672
Internal cerebral veins, 609f, 610–611
Internal ethmoidal artery, 529f, 530
Internal iliac artery, 573–578
Internal iliac vein, 561f, 583f, 603, 613f
Internal intercostal muscles, 729f
Internal jugular vein, 583f–584f
Internal nasal branches, 822–824
Internal obturator nerve, 737f
Internal ophthalmic artery, 529f, 530, 901f–902f, 902
Internal ophthalmic vein, 903f
Internal pudendal artery, 440–441, 457, 573–575, 602f–603f, 745f, 747f
Internal pudendal vein, 373, 424f, 441, 458, 583f, 602f–603f
Internal ramus of cranial laryngeal nerve, 835–836
Internal spermatic artery, 559

Internal thoracic artery, 534f–535f, 535, 584f, 729f
Internal thoracic trunk, 585f
Internal thoracic vein, 583f–584f, 729f
Internal tunic, of eye, 873–876
Internal vertebral venous plexus, 583f
　interarcuate branches, 614
　ventral, 610, 612–613
Internasal suture, 93f, 110
Interneurons, 650–651, 655
　spinal cord, 685
Interosseous antebrachial nerve, 719f
Interosseous border
　of fibula, 168
　of radius, 147f
　of ulna, 151
Interosseous ligament, of the antebrachium, 191f, 192
Interosseous membrane
　of the antebrachium, 191f, 192
　of crus, 202
Interosseous nerve, 713f, 718f
　of antebrachium, 722
Interosseous ramus, 545–546
Interosseous spaces
　branch to, 717f, 719f
　of fibula and tibia, 165f
　of metacarpus, 195
Interparietal bone, 28–29, 39f, 92f, 96f
Interparietal process, 96–97
Interparietoauricularis, 217f–218f, 221
Interparietoscutularis, 217f–218f, 221
Interpeduncular cistern, 700f
Interpeduncular nucleus, 770
Interphalangeal joints
　distal, 196
　proximal, 195–196
Interradicular septa, 110–111
Intersegmental reflex, 696
Intersphenoidal synchondrosis, 43f, 102
Interspinal muscles, 246f, 247
Interspinalis muscle, 729f
Interspinous ligaments, 184f, 185, 187f
Interspinous vein, 614
Intersternebral cartilage, 139f, 140
Intertarsal joint, 171f
　distal, 202–203
　proximal, 202–203
Interthalamic adhesion, 700f
Intertragic incisure, 851–852
Intertransverse ligaments, 185
Intertransverse muscles, 246f, 247–248

Intertrochanteric crest, 161f–162f, 163
Intertubercular groove, 143, 143f
Intervenous tubercle, 499–500
Interventricular foramen, 700f, 772–773, 781
Interventricular grooves, 498–499
Interventricular septum, 495–496, 504
Intervertebral disc(s), 125–126, 185–186, 186f, 197f
　cervical, 129f–130f
　lumbar, 133f–135f, 185f
　lumbosacral, 135f
　thoracic, 132f, 184f
　width of, 185
Intervertebral foramina, 126, 132f–133f, 706
　lumbar, 134f–135f
Intervertebral vein, 583, 583f, 612–614
Intestinal glands, 367, 373–374
Intestinal lymph trunk, 635f, 637f, 639–640
Intestinal villi, 367
Intestines. see Large intestine; Small intestine
Intestinum crassum, 368
Intestinum tenue, 364–365
Intradural segment, 704
Intrafusal fibers, 655–656
Intramural nervous system, 661
Intraocular muscles, 891
Intraperiorbital fat, 883f, 885
Intrapharyngeal opening, 344
Intrapharyngeal ostium, 119, 396
Intrinsic muscle, of tongue, 334–335
Intumescentia cervicalis, 682
Intumescentia lumbalis, 682
Involuntary muscle, 207
Iridocorneal angle, 865, 867f
Iris, 869–873
　greater arterial circle of, 873
　sphincter muscles of, 872
Irregular bones, 88
Ischial symphysis, 196
Ischiatic arch, 157f, 160f
Ischiatic nerve, 371f, 576f, 732f, 737f, 742f, 745f, 747f, 748
Ischiatic notch
　greater, 157f, 158, 160f
　lesser, 157f–159f
Ischiatic spine, 158, 158f–160f, 160–161, 743f
Ischiatic table, 157f–159f, 160–161
Ischiatic tuberosity, 157f–160f, 163f
Ischiocavernosus muscle, 438, 457, 745f, 747f

Ischiofemoral ligament, 197
Ischiorectal fossa, 374
Ischiourethralis muscles, 438, 456–457, 745f, 747f
Ischium, 160, 161f
Isthmus faucium, 321, 344–345
Isthmus of the fauces, 321, 344–345
Ix nerve, 344f

J

Jacobson's organ, 390
Jaw. see Mandible; Maxilla
Jejunal arteries, 367, 558
Jejunal lymph nodes, 348, 367, 383, 635f, 637f, 639
Jejunal vein, 583f, 598
Jejunum, 365–366
Joint(s). see also specific joints
　antebrachiocarpal, 152f, 192
　atlantoaxial, 129f, 182–183, 183f
　of auditory ossicles, 180
　ball-and-socket, 179
　calcaneoquartal, 202–203
　carpal, 192–195, 192f–195f
　　middle, 152f, 192
　carpometacarpal, 152f, 192
　cartilaginous, 176–177
　centrodistal, 202–203
　cochlea-tarsocrural, 166f
　condylar, 179
　costochondral, 188
　costovertebral, 186
　elbow. see Elbow
　ellipsoidal, 179
　femoropatellar, 198–199
　femorotibial, 198–199, 201
　fibrocartilaginous, 177
　fibrous, 176
　hinge, 178–179
　hip. see Hip
　humeroradial, 189
　humeroulnar, 189
　hyaline cartilage, 176–177
　of hyoid apparatus, 180
　incudomallear, 180
　incudostapedial, 180
　intercarpal, 192
　intermandibular, 180
　intermetacarpal, 195
　interphalangeal, proximal, 195–196
　intertarsal, 171f, 202–203
　metacarpal, 192–196
　metacarpophalangeal, 195
　metatarsal, 205
　occipitotympanic, 98
　of pelvic girdle, 196–197
　of pelvic limb, 196–205

Joint(s) *(Continued)*
  phalangeal, 192–196, 205
  plane, 179
  proximal radioulnar, 189, 191–192
  radiohumeral, 149f
  radioulnar, 191–192
  of ribs, 186–188
  sacroiliac, 161f, 196–197
  saddle, 179
  scapulohumeral, 144f
  shoulder, 188–189
  of skull, 179–181. *see also* Suture(s); Synchondrosis(es)
  sphenooccipital, 98
  sternocostal, 187, 187f–188f
  of sternum, 186–188
  stifle. *see* Stifle joint
  synovial, 176–179
    blood supply of, 177
    classification of, 178–179
    lymphatic vessels of, 177
    movements of, 179
    nerve supply of, 177
    pathologic conditions of, 178
    structure of, 177–178
    of vertebral column, 183–184
  talocalcaneal central, 202–203
  tarsal, 202–205, 203f
  tarsocrural, 171f, 202–203
  tarsometatarsal, 171f, 202–203
  temporomandibular, 105
  tibiofibular, 202
    distal, 202
    proximal, 202
  trochoid, 179
  of vertebral column, 181–186. *see also* Intervertebral disc(s)
Joint capsule, 177, 186, 197f, 716f, 719f, 742f–743f
  artery to, 745f
  of atlantoaxial joint, 182–183, 183f
  of atlantooccipital joint, 182, 133f
  branch to, 716f, 719f
  of elbow joint, 189–190, 190f–191f
  of hip bone, 197
  of metacarpophalangeal joints, 195
  nerve to, 716f
  of phalangeal joint, 195–196
  of sacroiliac joint, 196
  of shoulder joint, 188–189, 183f
  of stifle joint, 199–201, 199f
  tarsal, 203–204
  of temporomandibular joint, 179–180
Juga
  alveolar, 110–111, 118
  cerebral, 99f, 100

Juga alveolaria, 110–111
Juga cerebralia et cerebellaria, 97
Jugular foramen, 103, 122f, 123
Jugular incisure, 102f
Jugular vein, external, 583f–584f, 586, 588f, 591f
Jugum sphenoidale, 100f, 101
Junctura cartilaginea, 176
Junctura fibrosa, 176
Junctura synovialis, 176. *see also* Joint(s), synovial
Juncturae zygapophyseales, 183–184

K
Kidney(s), 416–420, 417f, 560f. *see also under* Renal
  anomalies, 420
  endocrine tissues of, 489
  fixation of, 416–418
  left, 417f–418f
  lymph vessels of, 641f
  nerves of, 419–420
  position of, 418
  relations of, 418
  right, 417f
  structure of, 418–419, 418f
  vessels of, 419–420, 419f
Knee. *see* Stifle joint
Kneecap. *see* Patella
Krinein, 469

L
Labia glenoidalia, 178
Labia oris, 319
Labial artery
  inferior, 516
  superior, 517
Labial veins
  dorsal, 604
  inferior, 588, 588f
  superior, 587, 587f
Labii, 455
Labium inferius, 319
Labium mediate et laterale, 163–164
Labium pudendi, 455
Labium superius, 319
Labrum acetabulare, 197
Labrum glenoidale, 188–189
Labyrinth arteries, 531–533
Labyrinthine artery, 529f
Labyrinths
  ethmoidal, 107–109, 120f, 124
  osseous, 104
Labyrinthus ethmoidalis, 107–109, 124, 393
Lacrimal apparatus, 888–891
Lacrimal artery, 523, 902

Lacrimal bone, 91f–92f, 113–114, 114f, 116f
Lacrimal canaliculi, 890
Lacrimal canals, 111, 114f, 118
Lacrimal caruncle, 885
Lacrimal gland, 340f, 889–890
  fossa for, 99f
Lacrimal lake, 890
Lacrimal nerve, 818f, 819, 898f, 899
Lacrimal puncta, 890
Lacrimal sac, fossa for, 92f, 113–114, 114f, 118, 122f, 881–882
Lacrimal vein, 903f, 904
Lacrimoethmoidal suture, 109
Lacrimomaxillary suture, 114
Lacrimozygomatic suture, 112, 114
Lacteals, 616
Lactiferous sinus, 459f, 460–461
Lacus lacrimalis, 890
Lambdoid suture, 98
Lamina(e), 113
  basal, 867
  of cervical vertebra, 129f
  of cricoid cartilage, 399
  dental, 33–34
  external, 444
  internal, 444
  of larynx, 397f, 398
  lateral, 108f
  orbital, 106f, 124
  of palatine bone, 113f
  sphenoethmoid, 113
  spiral, 840–842
  tectorial, 106f
  of thoracic vertebra, 131–132
  of vertebral arch, 126
Lamina I, 687–688
Lamina II, 688
Lamina III, 688
Lamina IV, 688
Lamina V, 688
Lamina VI, 688
Lamina VII, 688
Lamina VIII, 688
Lamina X, 688
Lamina XI, 688
Lamina basalis, 106–107, 867
Lamina cartilaginis cricoideae, 399
Lamina choroidocapillaris, 867
Lamina cribrosa, 107
Lamina dextra, 398
Lamina externa
  of prepuce, 444
  of rectus abdominis, 253–254
  of rectus sheath, 256–257
Lamina horizontalis, 112–113, 113f

Lamina interna
   of prepuce, 444
   of rectus sheath, 256–257
Lamina medullaris lateralis, 790–791
Lamina medullaris medialis, 790–791
Lamina muscularis mucosae, 348, 367, 373–374
Lamina orbitalis, 106–107
Lamina parietalis, 495
Lamina perpendicularis
   of ethmoid bone, 106
   of palatine bone, 113, 113*f*
Lamina pretrachealis, 240
Lamina prevertebralis, 240
Lamina sinistra, 398
Lamina sphenoethmoidalis, 113
Lamina suprachoroidea, 867
Lamina tectoria, 106–107
Lamina terminalis, 773, 778
Lamina terminalis grisea, 773
Lamina vasculosa, 867
Lamina ventralis, 131
Lamina visceralis, 495
Laminae arcus vertebrae, 126
Large intestine, 368–374
   apex of, 368–369
   body of, 368–369
   coats of, 373–374
   lymph vessels and lymph nodes of, 638*f*
Laryngeal inlet, 400
Laryngeal mucosa, 400–401
Laryngeal nerves, 399*f*, 835*f*
   pararecurrent, 351*f*
   recurrent, 351*f*, 836
Laryngeal prominence, 399
Laryngeal surface, 397–398
Laryngeal ventricle, 401
Laryngeal vestibule, 400
Laryngopharyngeus muscles, 346
Laryngopharynx, 344*f*–345*f*, 345
Larynx, 388, 396–402, 397*f*–399*f*
   cartilages of, 397–400, 397*f*–398*f*
   cavity of, 400–401
   innervation of, 401–402
   lymph vessels of, 625*f*, 627*f*
   muscles of, 230*f*–231*f*, 231–233, 398*f*
   nerve of, 835*f*
Lateral aperture, 763
Lateral branches, 720–721, 725*f*, 729*f*
   of lumbar nerves, 733, 735
   of superficial radial nerve, 721*f*
   of thoracic nerves, 728
Lateral calcaneal branch, 748–749

Lateral caudal artery, 574*f*, 578, 745*f*, 747*f*
Lateral caudal nucleus, 774
Lateral cervical nucleus, 687
Lateral circumflex femoral artery, 743*f*–745*f*
Lateral collateral ligament, 719*f*
Lateral corticospinal tract, 691*f*, 760–761
Lateral cricoarytenoideus muscle, 398*f*
Lateral crura, 851–852
Lateral cutaneous antebrachial nerve, 717*f*, 720–721, 720*f*–721*f*
Lateral cutaneous brachial nerve, 713*f*
Lateral cutaneous branches, 707, 708*f*, 717*f*, 729*f*, 730
   of lumbar nerve, 733, 733*f*, 735–736
   of thoracic nerves, 728
Lateral cutaneous femoral nerve, 730*f*, 732*f*–734*f*, 736–739, 736*f*–737*f*, 740*f*
Lateral cutaneous sural nerve, 730*f*, 732*f*, 736*f*, 739*f*, 744*f*, 748, 749*f*
Lateral dorsal nucleus, 774
Lateral funiculus, 680, 681*f*, 692–693
   projection pathways in, 690*b*
Lateral geniculate body, 775
Lateral geniculate nucleus, 775
Lateral horn, 679, 681*f*
Lateral hypothalamic nucleus, 777
Lateral intermediate substance, 679, 681*f*
Lateral lamina, 108*f*
Lateral lemniscus, 765
   nuclei of, 765
Lateral ligament
   of bladder, 422–423
   of malleus, 850
   of temporomandibular joint, 179–180
Lateral mammary branches, 730
Lateral medullary lamina, 790–791
Lateral motor nuclei, 687, 688*f*
Lateral nasal branch, 815–816, 819
Lateral nasal gland, 391–392, 391*f*–392*f*, 395, 395*f*
   duct of, 107*f*
Lateral olfactory gyrus, 784
Lateral olfactory tract, 783
Lateral palpebral ligament, 881, 886–887
Lateral palpebral raphe, 894
Lateral plantar artery, 753*f*
Lateral plantar nerve, 732*f*, 752–753, 752*f*–753*f*
Lateral process, 849

Lateral pterygoid nerve, 825
Lateral recess, 700*f*, 763
Lateral regions, of abdomen, 350–351, 353*f*
Lateral reticular nucleus, 764
Lateral (medullary) reticulospinal tract, 759
Lateral rhinal sulcus, 781
Lateral tectotegmentospinal tract, 691*f*, 694
Lateral thalamic nuclei, 774
Lateral thoracic nerve, 705*f*, 713*f*–715*f*, 728, 730*f*
Lateral thoracic vein, 593–594
Lateral tuberal nuclei, 777
Lateral ventricles, 700–701, 700*f*, 758*t*, 778–779, 781
   caudal horn, 700*f*
   choroid plexus in, 700*f*
   rostral horn, 700*f*
   ventral horn (temporal), 700*f*
Lateral vestibulospinal tract, 691*f*, 694–695
Latissimus dorsi muscle, 713*f*–714*f*, 729*f*
Left uterine horn, 740*f*
Leg, nerves, arteries, and muscles of, 749*f*
Lemniscus
   lateral, 765
   medial, 761
Lemniscus lateralis, 765
Lemniscus medialis, 761
Lens, 876–878, 877*f*
Lens capsule, 877–878
Lens fibers, 877
Lens placode, 858
Lens sutures, 877
Lens vesicle, 858
Leptomeninges, 699–700
Lesser curvature, 361–362
Lien, 642–643. *see also* Spleen
Ligament(s)
   accessory metacarpal, 195
   annular, of the radius, 190–191, 190*f*
   anular, 190*f*
   atlantoaxial, 183*f*
   of auditory ossicles, 180
   calcaneocentral, 205
   calcaneoquartal, 205
   caudal, 198*f*
      of auditory ossicles, 180
      of femoral head, 202
      of fibular head, 198*f*
   centrodistal, 204–205
   of cervical vertebrae, 184*f*

Ligament(s) (Continued)
　collateral
　　of carpal joint, 193f–194f
　　of distal interphalangeal joint, 193f–194f
　　of elbow, 190, 191f
　　metacarpophalangeal joint, 193f–194f
　　of metacarpophalangeal joints, 195
　　of phalangeal joints, 195–196
　　of stifle joint, 199f–200f, 201
　　of synovial joint, 177–178
　　of tarsal joint, 204
　of conus, 500–501
　costotransverse, 184f, 186, 186f–187f
　costovertebral, 187f
　cranial, of femoral head, 199f, 202
　cruciate
　　of sesamoid bones, 194f
　　of stifle joint, 198f, 200f, 201
　deep transverse metacarpal, 196
　defined, 178
　dorsal
　　of auditory ossicles, 180
　　of phalangeal joint, 196
　　radiocarpal, 195
　　sacroiliac, 196–197, 197f
　duodenocolic, 357f
　elastic, of phalangeal joints, 193f–194f
　femoral, of lateral meniscus, 201
　of femoral head, 197, 197f
　of the femoral head, 163
　femoropatellar, of stifle joint, 202
　of forepaw, 193f–194f
　glenohumeral, 188–189
　of the head, 186
　iliofemoral, 197
　inguinal, 254f, 256
　intercapital, 184f, 186, 186f
　interosseous, 191f, 192
　　metacarpal, 195
　intersesamoidean, 195
　interspinous, 184f, 185, 187f
　intertransverse, 185
　intraarticular head, 186
　ischiofemoral, 197
　lateral
　　of atlantooccipital joint, 182
　　of auditory ossicles, 180
　　of temporomandibular joint, 179–180
　long, of vertebral column, 184
　longitudinal
　　dorsal, 184, 186f
　　ventral, 184, 184f

Ligament(s) (Continued)
　meniscofemoral, 198f, 200f
　of nose, 391
　nuchal, 184f, 185, 187f
　oblique, of elbow, 190f, 191
　olecranon, 191, 191f
　orbital, 112, 118, 183f
　of ossicles, 850
　of ovaries, 447
　palmar, 194f, 195
　patellar, 199f–200f
　　of stifle joint, 198f, 202
　of the pelvic limb, 196–205
　periodontal, 176
　peritoneal, 354
　plantar, of tarsus, 205
　radiate, 184f
　radiating head, 186
　radiocarpal, palmar, 195
　of ribs, 186–188, 186f
　rostral, of auditory ossicles, 180
　sacrotuberous, 197, 197f, 292f
　of the sesamoid bones, 195
　sesamoidean, 194f, 195
　　short, 195
　short, of vertebral column, 185–186
　of the skull, 179–181
　special, of the carpus, 193–195
　sternocostal radiate, 187, 187f
　of sternum, 186–188, 188f
　of stifle joint, 198f–199f, 201–202
　supraspinous, 184, 184f, 187f
　of tail of epididymis, 430, 435–436
　of tarsus, 203f
　of thoracic limb, 188–196
　tibial
　　of lateral meniscus, 201
　　of medial meniscus, 200f, 201
　tibiofibular, 202
　transverse
　　acetabular, 197, 197f
　　of stifle joint, 198f, 201
　ulnocarpal, palmar, 194f, 195
　urogenital, of male, 422f
　ventral, sacroiliac, 196, 197f
　of vertebral column, 181–186
　yellow, 184f, 185–186, 197f
Ligamentum, 178
Lig. accessoriometacarpeum, 195
Lig. annulare stapedis, 180
Lig. anulare radii, 190–191
Lig. anulare stapedis, 850
Lig. apicis dentis, 183, 183f
Lig. arteriosum, 509, 584f
Lig. calcaneocentralis, 205
Lig. calcaneoquartale, 205

Lig. capitis costae intraarticulare, 186
Lig. capitis costae intraarticularis, 186, 187f
Lig. capitis costae radiatum, 186
Lig. capitis femoris, 197, 197f
Lig. capitis fibulae caudale, 202
Lig. capitis fibulae craniale, 202
Lig. caudae epididymidis, 430
Lig. collaterale carpi laterale, 195
Lig. collaterale carpi mediale, 195
Lig. collaterale cubiti laterale, 190, 190f
Lig. collaterale cubiti mediale, 190
Lig. collaterale laterale, 201, 204
Lig. collaterale mediale, 201, 204
Lig. coronarium hepatis, 377
Lig. costotransversarium, 186, 187f
Lig. cricothyroideum, 399
Lig. cruciatum caudale, 201
Lig. cruciatum craniale, 201
Lig. denticulatum, 700
Lig. falciforme hepatis, 378
Lig. gastrophrenicum, 357
Lig. gastrolienale, 357, 643
Lig. hepatoduodenale, 358
Lig. hepatogastricum, 358
Lig. hepatorenale, 378
Lig. iliofemorale, 197
Lig. inguinale, 254f, 256
Lig. intercapitale, 186
Lig. interossei antebrachii, 192
Lig. ischiofemorale, 197
Lig. laterale
　of atlantooccipital joint, 182
　of temporomandibular joint, 179–180, 179f–180f
Lig. latum uteri, 355, 445, 452
Lig. longitudinale dorsale, 184, 186f
Lig. longitudinale ventrale, 184, 184f
Lig. mallei, 180
Lig. meniscofemorale, 201
Lig. metacarpeum transversum profundum, 196
Lig. nasale dorsale, 391
Lig. nasale laterale, 391
Lig. nuchae, 184f, 185
Lig. olecrani, 191
Ligamentum orbitale, 881
Lig. ovarii proprium, 447
Lig. palmaria, 195
Lig. palpebrae mediale, 887
Lig. palpebrale laterale, 881, 886–887
Lig. patellae, 202
Lig. pectinatum anguli iridocornealis, 865
Lig. phrenicolienale, 357, 643
Lig. phrenicopericardiacum, 405, 495
Lig. *plantare longuum*, 205

Lig. pulmonale, 407–408
Lig. radiocarpeum dorsale, 195
Lig. radioulnare, 192
Lig. sacroiliacum ventrale, 196, 197f
Lig. sacrotuberale, 197, 197f
Lig. scroti, 430
Lig. sesamoideum breve, 195
Lig. supraspinale, 184, 184f, 187f
Lig. suspensorium ovarii, 447
Lig. teres vesicae, 422–423, 573
Lig. testis proprium, 430
Lig. transversum acetabuli, 197
Lig. transversum atlantis, 183, 183f
Lig. transversum perinei, 438
Lig. triangulare dextrum, 377
Lig. triangulare sinistrum, 377–378
Lig. ulnocarpeum palmare, 195
Lig. venosum, 378, 598
Lig. vesicae laterales, 422–423
Lig. vesicae medianum, 422
Lig. vocale, 401
Ligg. alaria, 183, 183f
Ligg. anularia (trachelia), 402
Ligg. collateralia, 177–178
Ligg. costoxiphoidea, 187, 188f
Ligg. cruciata genus, 201
Ligg. femoropatellare mediale et laterale, 202
Ligg. flava, 184f, 185–186
Ligg. glenohumeralia medialis et lateralis, 188–189
Ligg. interspinalia, 184f, 185, 187f
Ligg. intertransversaria, 185
Ligg. metacarpea interossea, 195
Ligg. ossiculorum auditus, 180
Ligg. sacroiliacum dorsale breve et longum, 196–197, 197f
Ligg. sesamoidea collateralia laterale et mediale, 195
Ligg. sesamoidea cruciata, 195
Ligg. sternocostalia radiata, 187
Ligg. ossiculorum auditus, 850
Limbic system, 786–787, 786f–787f
Limbs
    development of, 44–51, 54f–56f
    pelvic. see Pelvic limb
    thoracic. see Thoracic limb
Limbus, 861
Limbus corneae, 861
Limbus fossae ovalis, 499–500
Limen pharyngoesophageum, 345
Line(s)
    anocutaneous, 371
    anorectal, 371–372
    arcuate, 156–160
    massetric, 115f
    mylohyoid, 115, 115f

Line(s) (Continued)
    oblique, 398
    popliteal, 167
    temporal, 92f, 98–100
    terminal, 156–158, 352–353
    transverse, 136
    tricipital, 143f, 145
    of vastus lateralis, 162f
    of vastus medialis, 162f
Linea alba, 253f, 255f, 257
    median raphe of, 64
Linea anocutanea, 371
Linea arcuata, 156–158
Linea m. tricipitis, 145
Linea mylohyoidea, 115, 115f
Linea obliqua, 398
Linea rectalis, 371–372
Linea terminalis, 156–158, 352–353
Lineae temporales, 98–99
Lineae transversae, 136
Lingua, 329
Lingual artery, 338, 515–516, 516f
Lingual frenulum, 331
Lingual mucosa, 331
Lingual muscles, proper, 336
Lingual nerve, 338, 338f, 826–828, 829f
Lingual surface
    of epiglottis, 397–398
    of mandible, 115
    of tooth, 327
Lingual tonsil, 345
Lingual vein, 338, 342–343, 585f–586f, 588, 588f
Linguofacial vein, 583f, 586, 588f
Lip(s), 107f, 319
    acetabular, 197
    of femur, 162f, 163–164
    glenoid, 178, 188–189
    muscles of, 216–219, 216f–218f
Lip-curl, 390
Liquor cerebrospinalis, 701
Liquor follicularis, 447
Liquor pericardii, 495
Liver, 357f, 375–381, 375f. see also Hepatic
    blood vessels of, 378–379
    lobes and processes of, 376–377
    lymph vessels of, 378–379, 638f
    nerves of, 379
    peritoneal attachments and fixation in, 377–378
    physical characteristics of, 375
    structure of, 378
    surfaces, borders, and relations of, 375–376
Lobar bronchi, 388, 402–403

Lobe(s)
    of brain, 757
    caudate, 377
    cerebral, 779
    intermediate, 411
    of lungs, 409–411
    quadrate, 376–377
Lobi dexter et sinister, 646
Lobuli hepatis, 378
Lobuli testes, 428
Lobuli thymi, 646
Lobus accessorius, 411
Lobus caudalis, 410–411
Lobus caudatus, 377
Lobus cranialis, 410–411
Lobus flocculonodularis, 792
Lobus hepatis dexter, 377
Lobus hepatis dexter lateralis, 377
Lobus hepatis dexter medialis, 377
Lobus hepatis sinister, 376
Lobus hepatis sinister lateralis, 376
Lobus hepatis sinister medialis, 376
Lobus medius, 411
Lobus pancreatis dexter, 381
Lobus pancreatis sinister, 381
Lobus piriformis, 784
Lobus quadratus, 376–377
Lobus thoracicus, 645–646
Locomotor system, lymph drainage of, 617–618
Locus ceruleus, 695
    fibers, 691f
Long ciliary nerves, 818f, 819, 899
Long crus, 849–850
Long posterior ciliary arteries, 902
Long thoracic nerve, 705f, 728
Longitudinal modiolar canals, 840–842
Lower motor neurons (LMNs), 650–652, 652f, 655–656, 656f, 658–659, 659f, 685
    alpha neuron, 652f
    kinds of, 655–656, 657f
Lumbar arteries, 551, 559–560, 573f
Lumbar dermatomes, 738f
Lumbar (lumbosacral) enlargement, 682
Lumbar lymph center, 633–634
Lumbar lymph nodes, 423, 449–451, 453, 641f
Lumbar lymph trunks, 622–623
Lumbar nerves, 731–743, 732f
    2nd, 735
    7th, 734f
        ventral branch of, 741f
    first four, arrangement of, 733f
Lumbar plexus, 735

Lumbar splanchnic nerve, 674–675
Lumbar veins, 590, 597
Lumbar vertebrae. see Vertebra(e), lumbar
Lumbodiaphragmatic recess, 251–252
Lumbosacral plexus, 706–707, 734–735, 734f
  nerves of, 736f
Lumbosacral trunk, 744, 744f–745f
Lung(s), 404f, 408–413, 409f. see also under Pulmonary
  accessory lobe of, 410f, 411
  bronchial vessels of, 412–413
  cardiac impression of, 411
  cardiac notch of, 408, 411
  caudal lobe of, 410–411
  cranial lobe of, 410–411, 410f
  interlobar surfaces of, 409–411
  left, 409f–410f, 410–411
  lobes of, 409–411
  lymph nodes and vessels of, 634f
  margins of, 408–409, 410f
  mediastinal part of, 408
  middle lobe of, 411
  pulmonary vessels of, 411–412
  relationship to other organs, 411
  right, 410f, 411
  root of, 409
  surfaces of, 408, 410f
  vertebral part of, 408
Lunulae, 505
Lunulae valvularum semilunarium, 505
Luxations, of synovial joint, 178
Lymph
  primary, 621–622
  secondary, 621–622
Lymph channels, 631f
Lymph drainage, 617–619
Lymph nodes, 617f, 621
  of abdominal cavity, 635f
  of abdominal viscera, 637–640
  of abdominal walls, 633–636
  axillary, 628
  bronchial, 348, 634f
  buccal, 625
  cervical
    deep, 348, 627, 627f
    superficial, 618f, 627, 627f
  colic, 367
  duodenal, 383, 638f
  gastric, 348
  of genital organs, 636–637
  of head and neck, 624–628
  hepatic, 367, 378–379, 383
  hypogastric, 423, 436, 453
  iliac, 438
    medial, 373, 436, 635, 635f

Lymph nodes (Continued)
  inguinal, superficial, 442, 444–445, 602f–603f
  innervation of, 620
  jejunal, 348, 367, 383
  of large intestine, 638f
  lumbar, 423, 449–451, 453, 641f
  lumbar aortic, 633–634, 635f, 638f, 642f
  of lungs, 634f
  mandibular, 618f, 624, 625f
  mesenteric, cranial, 639–640
  of neck, 627f
  of pancreas, 638f
  pancreaticoduodenal, 367
  parotid, 342, 618f, 624, 625f
  of pelvic limb, 640–642
  of pelvic viscera, 636–640
  of pelvic walls, 633–636
  popliteal, 618f, 636f, 640
  portal, 348
  regional, 621–622
  retropharyngeal
    lateral, 626–627, 626f
    medial, 322, 342–343, 345, 348, 625–626, 625f–627f
  sacral, 373, 635–636, 635f
  of salivary glands, 626f
  splenic, 348, 378–379, 383, 638f
  of stomach, 638f
  of thoracic limb, 628
  of thorax, 628–633
  tracheobronchial, 413
  ventral to aorta, 641f
Lymph nodules, 620–621
  aggregated, 367, 620–621
  solitary, 370–371, 620–621
Lymph trunks, 622–623
Lymph vessels, 619–620
  of abdominal cavity, 635f
  of abdominal viscera, 637–640
  of abdominal walls, 633–636
  afferent, 621
  of aorta, 629f
  of diaphragm, 629f
  efferent, 621
  of esophagus, 629f
  of female genital organs, 642f
  of genital organs, 636–637
  of head and neck, 624–628
  innervation of, 620
  of kidney, 641f
  large, 622–624
  of large intestine, 638f
  of larynx, 625f, 627f
  of left side of the heart, 634f
  of liver, 378–379, 638f

Lymph vessels (Continued)
  of lungs, 634f
  of male genital organs, 642f
  of mammary glands, 629f
  of mediastinum, 629f
  of neck, 624–628, 627f
  of omentum, 637f
  of pancreas, 382–383, 638f
  of pelvic limb, 640–642
  of pelvic viscera, 636–640
  of pelvic walls, 633–636
  of pericardium, 629f
  of periosteum, 90–91
  from peritoneal cavity, 630f–631f, 633f
  of pleura, 633f
  of preputial folds, 642f
  of rectum, 638f
  of salivary glands, 626f
  of small intestine, 637f
  of soft palate, 625f
  of spleen, 638f
  of stomach, 638f
  superficial, 640
  of testicles, 642f
  of thoracic limb, 628
  of thorax, 628–633
  of tongue, 625f
  of urethra, 642f
  of urinary organs, 642f
Lymphatic duct, 622, 624
Lymphatic nodules, in conjunctiva, 887
Lymphatic system, 616–649
  general considerations for, 616
  ontogenesis of, 616–617
  regional anatomy of, 621–646
Lymphocentrum, 621
Lymphocentrum axillare, 628
Lymphocentrum bronchale, 631
Lymphocentrum celiacum, 637
Lymphocentrum cervicale profundum, 627
Lymphocentrum cervicale superficiale, 627
Lymphocentrum iliofemorale, 640
Lymphocentrum iliosacrale, 635
Lymphocentrum inguinofemorale, 641
Lymphocentrum lumbale, 633
Lymphocentrum mandibulare, 624
Lymphocentrum mediastinale, 631
Lymphocentrum mesentericum craniale, 639
Lymphocentrum parotideum, 624
Lymphocentrum popliteum, 640
Lymphocentrum retropharyngeum, 625

Lymphocentrum thoracicum dorsale, 630
Lymphocentrum thoracicum ventrale, 628
Lymphoglandular complexes, 639
Lymphoid tissue, 620–621
Lymphonodi buccales, 625
Lymphonodi cervicales profundi, 627
Lymphonodi cervicales profundi caudales, 627–628
Lymphonodi cervicales profundi craniales, 627–628
Lymphonodi cervicales profundi medii, 627–628
Lymphonodi cervicales superficiales, 627
Lymphonodi colici, 639
Lymphonodi gastrici, 639
Lymphonodi hepatici, 637–638
Lymphonodi iliaci interni, 635
Lymphonodi iliaci mediales, 635
Lymphonodi inguinales superficiales, 641
Lymphonodi intercostales, 630
Lymphonodi jejunales, 639
Lymphonodi lienales, 639
Lymphonodi lumbales aortici, 633–634
Lymphonodi mammarii, 641
Lymphonodi mandibulares, 624
Lymphonodi mediastinales craniales, 631
Lymphonodi pancreaticoduodenales, 639
Lymphonodi parotidei superficiales, 624
Lymphonodi pulmonales, 631
Lymphonodi renales, 634
Lymphonodi retropharyngei laterales, 626–627
Lymphonodi retropharyngei mediales, 625–626
Lymphonodi sacrales, 635–636
Lymphonodi scrotales, 641
Lymphonodi sternales craniales, 628
Lymphonodi tracheobronchales dextri, 631–632
Lymphonodi tracheobronchales dextri et sinistri, 631–632
Lymphonodi tracheobronchales medii, 632
Lymphonodi tracheobronchiales, 631
Lymphonoduli lienales, 644
Lymphonoduli solitarii, 370–371
Lymphonodus(i), 621
Lymphonodus axillaris accessorius, 628
Lymphonodus axillaris proprius, 628
Lymphonodus femoralis distalis, 640
Lymphonodus hemalis, 621
Lymphonodus iliaci externi, 641
Lymphonodus popliteus superficiales, 640
Lyssa, 336f–337f, 337–338
Lytta, 337–338

M

Macula, 843–844
Maculae cribrosae, 839–840
Major arterial circle of iris, 523, 903
Major palatine artery, 322, 525
Major palatine nerve, 822
Major palatine vein, 587–588
Major petrosal nerve, 665, 829–830
Major salivary glands, 340
Major splanchnic nerve, 673–674
Major sublingual duct, 343
Malar artery, 526, 587f, 901
Malar bone. see Zygomatic bone
Malar vein, 587
Male genital organs, 423–445, 424f–427f. see also specific organs
  lymph vessels of, 642f
  superficial vessels of, 562f
Male pelvic viscera, 573f
Male perineum, 428f, 747f
Male pseudohermaphroditism, 432
Male urethra, 443–444
  anomalies and variations of, 444
  vessels and nerves of, 444
Males: heart weight to body weight ratios, 498
Malformation, 4
Malleolus
  lateral, 166f, 168
  medial, 165f, 167, 171f
Malleus, 849, 849f
  ligaments of, 850
  manubrium, 103f, 849
Mamelons, 327
Mamillary body, 777
Mamillary peduncle, 777
Mamillary process, of vertebrae, 132–133
  caudal, 137–138, 137f
  lumbar, 134, 134f–135f
Mamillotegmental tract, 777
Mamillothalamic tract, 777
Mammae masculina, 459
Mammalian Species of the World, 2
Mammary glands (mammae), 458–462, 459f
  glandular part of, 460–461
  nerves of, 461–462

Mammary glands (mammae) *(Continued)*
  papillary part of, 460–461
  structure of, 460–461
  vessels of, 461–462, 461f
Mammary lymph nodes, 641
Mammary ridge, 459, 459f
Mandible, 115–116, 115f–116f, 120f
  border of, 115
  brachygnathic, 94
  development of, 28, 45f
  nerve distribution medial to, 828f
Mandibular alveolar artery, 519f
  branches of, 519f
Mandibular alveolar nerve, 826
Mandibular canals, 115–116
Mandibular duct, 341f, 342
Mandibular foramen, 115f
Mandibular fossa, 102f–103f, 105, 119f
Mandibular ganglion, 342–343, 665
Mandibular gland, 340f–341f, 342–343, 586f, 709f
Mandibular lymph center, 624–625
Mandibular lymph nodes, 618f, 624, 625f
Mandibular nerve, 824–828, 824f, 827f–828f, 898–899
Mandibular notch, 115–116, 115f
Mandibular teeth, 325
Mandibular vein, 589
Manica flexoria, 280f
Mantle plexus, 475
Manubrium
  of malleus, 103f, 849
  of sternum, 139f, 140
Manus. see Forepaw
Margin(s)
  infraorbital, 99–100, 112, 112f
  interalveolar, 110–111, 115
  of lung, 408–409
  masseteric, 112f
  of tongue, 330–331
Marginal cutaneous sac, 851
Marginal nucleus, 687
Marginal (dorsomarginal) nucleus (zone), 687–688
Marginal papillae, 332f, 334
Margo acutus, 408–409
Margo alveolaris, 110–111
Margo basalis, 408–409
Margo caudalis
  of scapula, 141f, 142
  of spleen, 643
  of ulna, 151
Margo ciliaris, 869–872

Margo cranialis
  of scapula, 141f, 142
  of spleen, 643
  of tibia, 165–167
Margo dexter, 376
Margo dorsalis, 82–83
  of liver, 376
  of lung, 408–409
  of scapula, 141f, 142
Margo frontalis, 99
Margo infraorbitalis, 99–100, 112
Margo interalveolaris, 115
Margo interosseous
  of fibula, 168
  of ulna, 151
Margo lateralis
  of tibia, 167
  of ulna, 151
Margo linguae, 330–331
Margo medialis, 151
Margo occipitalis, 99
Margo orbitale, 881
Margo sagittalis, 99
Margo squamosus, 99
Margo ventralis
  of liver, 376
  of lung, 408–409
  of mandible, 115
Margo ventricularis dexter, 499
Margo ventricularis sinister, 499
Massa lateralis, 127–130
Masseteric artery, 522
Masseteric fossa, 115–116, 115f
Masseteric line, 115f
Masseteric margin, 112f
Masseteric nerve, 825
Masseteric vein, 589
Mast cells, 66
Mastication: muscles of, 222f–224f
Masticatory nerve, 825
Mastoid foramen, 98, 104–105, 121, 122f
Mastoid process, 102f–103f, 104–105
Maxilla, 91f–92f, 96f, 107f–108f, 110–111, 110f, 116f–117f, 120f
Maxillary artery, 518, 901
  branches of, 519f
    first part or mandibular portion, 518–520
    second part or pterygoid portion of, 522
    third part or pterygopalatine portion of, 522–523
Maxillary foramen, 110–111, 122f
Maxillary nerve, 322, 819–824, 823f–824f, 827f, 900
Maxillary process, 99f

Maxillary recess, 106–107, 108f, 110f, 111, 113, 124, 125f
Maxillary sinus, 124
Maxillary teeth, 325
Maxillary tuberosity, 110f, 111
Maxillary vein, 342–343, 583f, 589
Maxilloincisive suture, 111
Maxilloturbinate, 111–112, 389–390, 392
Meatus(es)
  acoustic/auditory, 388
  nasal, 388
  nasopharyngeal, 124, 394
  temporal, 123
Meatus acusticus externus, 105, 850
Meatus acusticus internus, 103
Meatus nasi communis, 106, 124, 394
Meatus nasi dorsalis, 110, 124, 393–394
Meatus nasi medius, 112, 124, 394
Meatus nasi ventralis, 112, 124, 394
Meatus nasopharyngeus, 394
Meatus temporalis, 123
Mechanical motion detectors, 652
Medial branches, 707, 720–721, 725f, 729f
  in longissimus lumborum, 733
  of lumbar nerve, 735
  of superficial radial nerve, 721f
  of thoracic nerves, 728
Medial circumflex femoral artery, 743f
  branch of, 745f
Medial collateral ligament, 742f
  nerve to, 719f
Medial crura, 851–852
Medial cuneate nucleus, 761
Medial cutaneous antebrachial nerve, 713f, 716–718, 718f–720f, 727f
Medial cutaneous branches, 708f, 729f
  of lumbar nerve, 733, 733f
  of thoracic nerves, 728
Medial cutaneous tarsal nerve, 751f
Medial digital flexor muscle, 749f
Medial forebrain bundle, 776
Medial genicular artery, 742f
Medial geniculate body, 775
Medial geniculate nucleus, 775
Medial lemniscus, 761
Medial mammary branches, 730
Medial medullary lamina, 790–791
Medial motor nucleus, 687
Medial nasal branch, 815–816, 819
Medial nerve, 721–722
Medial olfactory tract, 783
Medial palpebral ligament, 887
Medial plantar artery, 753f

Medial plantar nerve, 732f, 752, 752f–753f
Medial pterygoid nerve, 825
Medial (pontine) reticulospinal tract, 759
Medial rhinal sulcus, 781
Medial surface, of lung, 408
Medial tarsal cutaneous nerves, 752f
Medial tectospinal tract, 691f, 694
Medial vestibulospinal tract, 691f, 695
Median artery, 193f, 538f, 546, 718f, 720f, 725f
Median caudal artery, 578–579
Median crest, 399
Median cubital vein, 584f
Median fixed plexus, 736
Median groove, 330
Median ligament, of bladder, 422
Median nerve, 705f, 713f–715f, 718f–720f, 725f
  communicating branch musculocutaneous to, 720f
  palmar branches of, 725f
Median palatine suture, 111
Median sacral artery, 561f, 566f, 573f–574f, 578–579
Median sacral vein, 583f, 605
Median sulcus, 763
Median tongue bud, 329, 330f
Median vein, 583f
Mediastinal lymph center, 631
Mediastinal lymph nodes, cranial, 631, 632f
Mediastinal pleura, 407
Mediastinal recess, 406–408
Mediastinal serous cavity, 407
Mediastinum, 405–407, 406f
  lymph vessels of, 629f
Mediastinum caudale, 406–407
Mediastinum craniale, 405
Mediastinum dorsale, 406
Mediastinum medium, 405–406
Mediastinum testis, 428
Mediastinum ventrale, 405
Medulla
  of kidney, 418
  of lymph node, 621
  of ovary, 447
  parasympathetic general visceral efferent in, 665f, 820f
Medulla oblongata, 757, 758t, 759–766, 764f–765f
  caudal half of, 761–764, 763f
  rostral end of, 765–766
Medulla ossium flava, 90
Medulla ossium rubra, 90
Medulla ovarii, 447

Medulla renis, 418
Medulla spinalis, 650, 657, 757
Medullary cavity, 90
Medullary reticulospinal tract, 691f, 695
Medullary vein, 611
Medullary velum
  caudal, 763
  rostral, 763
Meibomian glands, 886
Melanoblasts, 66
Melanocytes, 66
Membrana atlantooccipitalis dorsalis, 182
Membrana atlantooccipitalis ventralis, 182
Membrana fibrosa, of joint, 177–178
Membrana interossea antebrachii, 191f, 192
Membrana interossea cruris, 202
Membrana pupillaris, 872
Membrana stapedis, 850
Membrana sterni, 187
Membrana synovialis, 177
Membrana tectoria, 182–183
Membrana thyrohyoidea, 399
Membrana tympani, 105, 846
Membrane
  arachnoid, 679
  atlantoaxial, 182–183
  atlantooccipital
    dorsal, 182
    ventral, 182
  basilar, 844
  chorioallantoic, 20, 20f
  choriovitelline, 18, 19f–20f
  fibrous, 177–178
  interosseous
    of antebrachium, 191f, 192
    of crus, 202
  otolithic, 843–844
  pupillary, 872
  stapedial, 850
  statoconiorum, 843–844
  sternal, 187, 188f
  synovial, 177
  thyrohyoid, 399
  tympanic, 105, 841f, 846–847
    secondary, 840–842
  vestibular, 844
Membrane bone, 89
Membranous labyrinth, 839, 842–846, 844f
  development of, 33, 38f
Membrum pelvinum. see Pelvic limb
Membrum thoracicum. see Thoracic limb

Meninges, 679–703, 681f
  schema of, 700f
Meningeal arteries, 518–520
  middle, 522, 901f–902f
Meningeal branch, 704, 706f
Meningeal veins, 611
Meningovertebral ligament, 184
Meniscus, 178, 198–199
  lateral, 165–167
  lateral and medial, 201
  medial, 165–167
Meniscus articularis, 178
Meniscus lateralis, 198–199, 201
Meniscus medialis, 198–199, 201
Meniscus medialis et lateralis, 165–167
Mental foramen, 115–116, 115f
Mental nerves, 826
Meridians (meridiani), 861
Meridional fibers, 871
Mesaticephalic, definition of, 94, 94t, 125f
Mesencephalic aqueduct, 700–701, 700f, 758t, 767
Mesencephalic caudal projecting axons, 694
Mesencephalic tract of trigeminal nerve, 768
  nucleus of, 758, 768
Mesencephalon, 658, 757, 758f, 758t, 767
Mesenteric ganglion, caudal, 423
Mesenteric lymph center, 639–640
Mesenterium, 354, 366–367
Mesenterium dorsale, 355
Mesentery, 354
  of colon, 369–370
  root of, 366–367
Mesethmoid. see Perpendicular plate
Mesial surface, of tooth, 327
Mesocolon, 355, 357f, 369–370
  ascending, 369–370
  descending, 355, 370
  transverse, 370
Mesocolon ascendens, 369–370
Mesocolon descendens, 355, 370
Mesocolon transversum, 370
Mesoductus deferens, 435–436
Mesoduodenum, 355, 357f, 365
Mesofuniculus, 436
Mesogastrium, 355
  dorsal, 357f
  ventral, 378
Mesojejunoileum, 355, 357f
Mesometrium, 422–423, 445, 452
Mesonephric duct, 462–463
Mesonephric tubules, 462–463

Mesorchium, 431, 436
  distal, 435
  proximal, 435–436, 559, 597
Mesorchium distale, 435, 559
Mesorchium proximale, 435, 559, 597
Mesorectum, 355, 370–371
Mesosalpinx, 445, 452
Mesotendon, 213
Mesovarium, 445, 452
Metacarpal bones, 150f, 151–152, 152f–153f, 155f, 196
  development of, 47–51, 53f
  I, 150f–153f, 154
  II to V, 150f, 152f–153f, 154
Metacarpal foot pad, 726–727
  nerves to, 725f
Metacarpal joints, 192–196
Metacarpus, 153f, 154–155, 155f
Metanephros, 463
Metaphysis, 87–88, 167f
Metapodials, 155
  development of, 51, 57f
Metatarsal arteries
  dorsal, 569–572, 751f
  plantar, 573
Metatarsal bones, 172
  fourth, 172
  second, 172
  third, 172
Metatarsal footpad, nerves to, 753f
Metatarsal joints, 205
Metatarsal veins
  dorsal, 605f, 606
  plantar, 605f, 606
Metatarsus, 172
Metathalamus, 758t, 775
  lateral geniculate nucleus, 775
  medial geniculate nucleus, 775
Metencephalon, 658, 757, 758f, 758t
Metestrum, 448
Metestrus, 14–15, 14f, 448–449
  early, 448f
Microfilamentae, 652
Microglia, 657
Midbrain, 757, 767–771, 768f–770f
  derived brain structures and definitive brain cavities, 758t
Midbrain tegmentum, 770
Middle cerebral artery, 527–528, 529f–530f, 901f–902f
Middle clunial nerves, 733–734, 743–744, 743f
Middle colic artery, 557
Middle colic vein, 598
Middle fascia, muscular, 884

Middle mediastinum, 405–406
Middle meningeal artery, 522, 901f–902f
 groove for, 100f
 sulcus for, 101–102
Middle meningeal vein, 589, 611
Middle nasal meatus, 107f–108f, 111–112
Middle rectal artery, 438, 575
Middle rectal vein, 604
Middle septal artery, 525–526
Middle superior alveolar branches, 822–824
Middle thyroid vein, 585–586
Middle uterine artery, 559, 575
Middle vascular tunic, 861
Minor palatine arteries, 322, 346
Minor palatine artery, 524–525
Minor palatine nerve, 822
Minor petrosal nerve, 832–833
Minor salivary glands, 340
Minor splanchnic nerve, 673–674
Miscellaneous class, breeds and, 8
Mitochondria, 652
Mitral valve, 504–505
Mixed nerve, 704
Modified Triadan System, 324f, 328
Modiolar canals, longitudinal, 840–842
Modiolus, 840–842
Molar teeth, 323–324, 323f, 328
 cavity for, 110f
 development of, 108f, 119f
 eruption of, 325t
Mongrel, 1, 9
Motor neurons
 alpha, 652f
 lower, 650–652, 652f, 655–656, 656f–657f, 658–659, 659f
 upper, 654
Motor nuclei, 687
Motor unit, 212, 685
Mouth, 319
Movements
 of muscles, 212
 of synovial joint, 179
 of vertebral column, 138
Mucoperiosteum, 90
Mucosa
 laryngeal, 400–401
 lingual, 331
 muscular layer of, 348
 nasal, 393f, 394–395
 ureteral, 421
Mucous coat
 of esophagus, 348
 of large intestine, 373–374

Mucous coat *(Continued)*
 of small intestine, 367
 of stomach, 363
Mucous glands, 345f
Multipolar cells, 650
Muscle(s), 207–318. *see also* Musculus (M.)/Musculi (Mm.); *specific muscles*
 of abdominal wall, 252–258, 253f–255f
 accessory structures of, 213
 agonist, 212–213
 of anal canal, 372–373
 of anal region, 261f, 289f, 298f
 antagonist, 212–213
 antebrachial, 273–285
  caudal, 268f, 271f, 274f, 276f–282f, 278–285
  craniolateral, 270f, 273–278, 273f–276f, 280f–282f
  synovial apparatus of, 282f, 284
 aponeurosis of, 211–212
 articular, 212–213
 belly of, 212
 bipennate, 212
 blood supply of, 213–214
 brachial, 265f, 268f–270f, 269–273, 276f
 of cervical vertebrae, 215b, 235–236, 240f, 244f
 connective tissue of, 213
 contraction of, 212
 of crus, 291f, 299f–300f, 303–311, 303f–307f, 310f
 diaphragm as, 250–252, 250f
 of dorsum, 241–248
 of ears, 215b, 216f–218f, 219–222, 220f, 852–853, 853f–856f
 of esophagus, 346f
 extensor, 212
 of eye, 891–896
  extraocular, 891–894, 892f
  extrinsic, 520f, 893f
  intraocular, 891
 of eyeball, 215b, 225–227, 226f
 of eyelid, 215b, 216f–218f, 219–222, 226f
 of facial expression, 214–222, 215b, 216f–218f
 of female perineum, 745f
 fixation, 212–213
 flexor, 212
 of forehead, 216f–218f, 219–222
 of forepaw, 276f–283f, 285–286
 function of, 212–213
 of head, 212, 215b
  external ear, 216f–218f, 219–221, 220f

Muscle(s) *(Continued)*
 eyeball, 215b, 225–227, 226f
 eyelid, 216f–218f, 219–222, 226f
 facial, 214–222, 216f–218f
 hyoid apparatus, 227f, 233–235, 233f–235f, 264f
 laryngeal, 230f, 231–233
 masticatory, 222–225, 222f–224f, 233f
 palatal, 229f–230f
 pharyngeal, 228f–231f, 229–230
 superficial, 895f
 tongue, 227–229, 227f–229f, 232f
 of hindpaw, 306f–307f, 310f
 of hip, 289–294, 291f–293f
 of hyoid apparatus, 215b, 227f, 233–235, 233f–235f, 264f
 innervation ratio of, 212
 insertion of, 211–212
 involuntary, 207
 of larynx, 215b, 230f, 231–233, 398f
 of leg, 749f
 of lip, 216–219, 216f–218f
 during locomotion, 212–213
 of male perineum, 747f
 of mastication, 215b, 222–225, 222f–224f, 233f
 motor units of, 212
 movements of, 212
 of Müller, 219
 multipennate, 212
 of neck, 232f, 237–241, 239f–240f, 244f, 264f
 nerve supply of, 213–214
 of nose, 215b, 216–219
 origin of, 211–212
 of ossicles, 850
 palatine, 322, 323f
 palpebral, 894–896
 papillary, 502–504
 of pelvic limb, 287–313
  crus, 299f–300f, 303–311, 303f–307f, 310f
  hindpaw, 303–311, 306f–307f, 310f
  lumbar hypaxial, 287–289, 288f–289f
  pelvis, 289–294, 289f, 291f–293f, 300f
  thigh, 287–302, 290f–292f, 295f–296f, 298f, 305f, 310f
 of penis, 438
 pennate, 212
 of pes, 306f–307f, 310f, 311–312

Muscle(s) *(Continued)*
  of pharynx, 215*b*, 228*f*–231*f*, 229–230
  as prime movers, 212–213
  of rectum, 372–373
  red, 207–209
  regeneration of, 214
  of scapula, 265–267, 265*f*, 268*f*–269*f*
  shapes of, 210
  size range, 210
  skeletal, 210–214
  of the skin, 79
  slips of, 212
  smooth, 207
  of soft palate, 228*f*–230*f*, 230–231
  somatic, 207
  of stomach, 361*f*
  striated, 207
  synergist, 212–213
  of tail, 258–262, 259*f*–261*f*
  of thigh, 287–302
    caudal, 290*f*–292*f*, 294–297, 296*f*, 299*f*–301*f*, 305*f*, 310*f*
    cranial, 290*f*–292*f*, 295*f*–296*f*, 297–298, 298*f*–301*f*
    medial, 290*f*–292*f*, 295*f*, 298*f*–301*f*, 299–302
  of thoracic limb, 263–287
    antebrachial, 270*f*–271*f*, 273–285, 273*f*–282*f*
    brachial, 265*f*, 269–273
    extrinsic, 239*f*, 241–242, 248*f*, 263–265, 264*f*–268*f*, 270*f*
    forepaw, 276*f*–283*f*, 285–286
    intrinsic, 265–269, 265*f*–269*f*
    scapula, 265–267, 265*f*
  of thoracic wall, 239*f*, 248–252, 248*f*–250*f*
  of tongue, 215*b*, 227–229, 227*f*–229*f*, 232*f*, 334–337, 335*f*–336*f*, 625*f*
  tracheal, 402
  of trunk, 262–263
    abdominal wall, 252–258, 253*f*–255*f*
    diaphragm as, 250–252, 250*f*
    neck, 232*f*, 237–241, 239*f*–240*f*, 264*f*
    spinal epaxial, 239*f*, 242–245, 243*f*–244*f*, 246*f*
    thoracic wall, 239*f*, 248–252, 248*f*–250*f*
  unipennate, 212
  unstriated, 207
  of vertebral column, 242–245

Muscle(s) *(Continued)*
  cervical, 215*b*, 235–236, 240*f*, 244*f*
  erector spinae, 242–245, 243*f*
  interspinal, 246*f*, 247
  intertransverse, 246*f*, 247–248
  transversospinal, 239*f*, 243*f*–244*f*, 245–247, 246*f*, 259*f*
  voluntary, 207
  white, 207–209
Muscle fibers, 207. *see also specific muscles*
  cardiac, 207
  classification of, 207, 208*t*, 209*f*
  length of, 210
  red, 207–209
  skeletal, 207
  smooth, 207
  type 1, 207–209, 209*f*, 211*f*
  type IIa, 207–209, 210*f*
  type IIM, 209–210
  type IIX, 207–209
  white, 207–209
Muscle layer, of urethra, 444
Muscle spindles, 650–651, 658
Muscular branches, 722, 725*f*, 726, 729*f*, 741–742
  of caudal nerve, 754
  of plantar nerve, 753
  of sciatic nerve, 748
  of ventral sacral nerves, 747–748
Muscular coat
  of esophagus, 347
  of large intestine, 374
  of small intestine, 367
  of stomach, 363
Muscular fasciae, 884
Muscular layer, of mucosa, of esophagus, 348
Muscular process, 102*f*, 119*f*, 400, 849
Muscular ramus, 750
Muscular tubercles, 97–98, 118–119
Musculi linguae, 334–335
Musculocutaneous nerve, 705*f*, 713*f*–715*f*, 716–718, 718*f*–720*f*, 727*f*
  communicating branch of, 718*f*
Musculophrenic artery, 536
Musculotubal canal, 102*f*, 105, 119*f*
Musculus (M.)/Musculi (Mm.), 207–318
M. abductor cruris caudalis, 295, 300*f*–301*f*, 303*f*, 744*f*
M. abductor digiti I (pollicis) brevis, 276*f*–279*f*, 285–286
M. abductor digiti I (pollicis) longus, 273*f*–276*f*, 280*f*–282*f*

M. abductor digiti V (pelvic limb), 306*f*, 310*f*, 312
M. abductor digiti V (thoracic limb), 280*f*, 282*f*, 286
M. adductor digiti I (pollicis) brevis, 280*f*, 282*f*, 286
M. adductor digiti II, 280*f*, 282*f*, 286
M. adductor digiti quinti, 193*f*
M. adductor digiti secundi, 193*f*
M. adductor digiti V (thoracic limb), 280*f*, 282*f*, 286
M. adductor longus, 298*f*, 302, 743*f*
M. adductor magnus et brevis, 298*f*, 302, 743*f*
M. anconeus, 266*f*–268*f*, 271*f*, 272
M. articularis coxae, 289*f*, 291*f*–292*f*, 298
M. articularis genus, 291*f*, 298
M. arytenoideus transversus, 230*f*–231*f*, 232
M. biceps brachii, 264*f*, 269*f*–270*f*, 270, 276*f*
  nerve to, 713*f*–714*f*, 718*f*, 720*f*
M. biceps femoris, 289*f*–290*f*, 294, 299*f*, 301*f*, 303*f*, 305*f*, 310*f*, 744*f*–745*f*
M. biventer cervicis, 243*f*, 245–246
M. brachialis, 264*f*, 266*f*–270*f*, 271, 276*f*
  nerve to, 716–718, 719*f*
M. brachiocephalicus, 232*f*, 237, 264*f*, 266*f*–267*f*
M. brachioradialis, 268*f*, 270*f*, 273–274, 273*f*–274*f*
M. buccinator, 216*f*–218*f*, 218
M. caninus, 216*f*–218*f*, 218
M. ceratohyoideus, 228*f*–229*f*, 234
M. cervicis, 243*f*
M. cervicoauricularis medius (cervicoauricularis profundus major), 217*f*–218*f*, 220*f*, 221
M. cervicoauricularis profundus (cervicoauricularis profundus minor), 216*f*–218*f*, 220*f*
M. cervicoauricularis superficialis, 217*f*–218*f*, 221
M. ciliaris, 871
M. cleidobrachialis, 237, 264*f*, 266*f*–268*f*, 270*f*
M. cleidocephalicus
  pars cervicalis, 232*f*, 237, 264*f*, 266*f*–267*f*
  pars mastoideus, 237
M. coccygeus, 260–261, 260*f*–261*f*, 289*f*, 300*f*, 371*f*, 734*f*, 737*f*, 741*f*
M. complexus, 243*f*, 710*f*

M. concho-helicinus, 853f
M. constrictor vestibuli, 261f, 456, 945f
M. constrictor vulvae, 261f, 455–456, 745f
M. coracobrachialis, 266f–269f, 271, 705f, 713f–714f
M. cricoarytenoideus dorsalis, 230f–231f, 231
M. cricoarytenoideus lateralis, 230f–231f, 231
M. cricopharyngeus, 228f, 230, 346f
M. cricothyroideus, 228f, 230f, 231, 264f, 340f, 346f, 398f
M. cutaneous trunci, 257, 266f–267f
M. deltoideus, 264f–268f, 266–267
M. deltoideus pars acromialis, 266–267
M. deltoideus pars scapularis, 266–267
M. depressor auriculae, 340–341
M. digastricus, 222f, 225, 233f–235f, 264f
M. dilator pupillae, 872
M. erector spinae, 242
M. esophageus longitudinalis dorsalis, 347
M. esophageus longitudinalis lateralis, 347–348
M. esophageus longitudinalis ventralis, 347–348
M. extensor carpi radialis, 268f, 273f–276f, 281f
M. extensor carpi ulnaris, 273f–274f, 276–277, 279f, 281f–282f
M. extensor digiti I et II, 271f, 273f, 275f–277f, 277–278, 279f, 281f
M. extensor digiti I (hallucis) longus, 299f, 303f–304f, 307f
M. extensor digitorum brevis (pelvic limb), 307f, 310f, 311
M. extensor digitorum communis (thoracic limb), 268f, 273f–275f, 275, 280f–282f, 713f, 717f
M. extensor digitorum lateralis (pelvic limb), 299f–300f, 303f–307f, 307
M. extensor digitorum lateralis (thoracic limb), 273f–276f, 276–277
M. extensor digitorum longus (pelvic limb), 300f, 303f–304f, 304–305, 307f
M. extensor pollicis longus et indicis proprius, 282f
M. fibularis (peroneus) brevis, 299f–300f, 304f, 306f, 308, 310f
M. fibularis (peroneus) longus, 299f–300f, 303f–306f, 306–307, 310f

M. flexor carpi radialis, 274f, 276f–280f, 279–280
M. flexor carpi ulnaris, 270f, 274f, 276f–279f, 281
M. flexor digiti I brevis, 280f, 282f, 286, 312
M. flexor digiti V, 280f, 282f, 286
M. flexor digitorum brevis, 280f
M. flexor digitorum lateralis (pelvic limb), 299f–300f, 303f–306f, 309, 310f
M. flexor digitorum medialis (pelvic limb), 299f, 305f–306f, 309–311, 310f
M. flexor digitorum profundus (pelvic limb), 309
M. flexor digitorum profundus (thoracic limb), 270f–271f, 274f, 276f–280f
  nerve to, 718f–720f
M. flexor digitorum superficialis (pelvic limb), 300f, 303f–306f, 309
M. flexor digitorum superficialis (thoracic limb), 274f, 276f–280f, 280–281
  nerve to, 718f, 720f
M. frontalis, 216f–218f, 220
M. frontoscutularis, 217f, 220
M. gastrocnemius, 300f, 303f–306f, 308, 310f
  nerve to, 742f, 749f
M. genioglossus, 227f–228f, 229, 264f, 335f–336f, 336
M. geniohyoideus, 222f, 232f–233f, 234, 264f
M. gluteus medius, 290f, 292f, 300f
M. gluteus profundus, 260f, 289f, 291f–293f, 292–293, 300f
M. gluteus superficialis, 290f–291f, 291
M. gracilis, 289f, 295f, 299f, 301–302, 301f, 310f
M. helicis, 216f, 219–220
M. hyoepiglotticus, 232–233
M. hyoglossus, 222f, 227f–228f, 228, 232f, 264f, 335
M. hyopharyngeus, 228f, 229–230, 232f
M. iliacus, 289, 289f
M. iliocostalis, 239f, 242, 244f, 248f
M. iliocostalis cervicis, 242–243
M. iliocostalis lumborum, 239f, 243f, 288f
M. iliocostalis thoracis, 239f, 242–243, 243f
M. iliopsoas, 289, 298f
M. infraspinatus, 265f–269f, 266
M. intercostalis externus, 248f

M. interflexorius, 280f, 285
M. interscutularis, 217f–218f, 220–221
M. interspinales, 239f, 246f, 247
M. intertransversarius, 300f
M. intertransversarius dorsales caudae, 260, 260f
M. intertransversarius ventrales caudae, 260, 260f
M. ischiocavernosus, 261f
M. ischiourethralis, 261f
M. latissimus dorsi, 241, 264f, 266f–268f, 270f
M. levator anguli oculi medialis, 217f–218f, 219
M. levator ani, 260f, 261, 289f, 300f
M. levator labii superioris, 216f–218f
M. levator nasolabialis, 216f–218f, 218–219
M. levator palpebrae superioris, 219, 226f, 894–895
M. levator veli palatini, 228f–230f, 230–231
M. levator costae, 249f
M. lingualis proprius, 336
M. longissimus, 239f, 243, 243f–244f, 259f
M. longissimus atlantis, 245
M. longissimus capitis, 239f, 243f–244f, 245
M. longissimus cervicis, 239f, 243f–244f, 244–245
M. longissimus lumborum, 239f
M. longissimus thoracis, 239f, 243f–244f, 244, 248f
M. longus capitis, 238, 240f, 264f
M. longus colli, 238, 240f
M. masseter, 222f–224f, 264f
M. mentalis, 216f–218f, 218
M. multifidus, 239f, 244f, 246, 259f, 729f
M. mylohyoideus, 232f–233f, 233–234, 264f
M. obliquus capitis caudalis, 244f
M. obliquus capitis cranialis, 236, 244f
M. obliquus dorsalis, 225, 226f, 894
M. obliquus externus abdominis, 248f, 253, 253f
M. obliquus internus abdominis, 248f, 253f–255f, 254
M. obliquus ventralis, 225, 226f, 894
M. obturator externus, 289f, 291f–293f, 293
M. obturator internus, 289f, 291f–293f, 293
  nerve to, 744f–745f

M. occipitalis, 217f–218f, 219
M. occipitohyoideus, 233f, 235
M. omotransversarius, 237, 244f, 264f–267f
M. orbicularis oculi, 216f–218f, 219, 860, 894
M. orbicularis oris, 216, 216f
M. palatinus, 222f, 231
M. palatopharyngeus, 228f–230f, 230, 322
M. papillaris subatrialis, 503–504
M. papillaris subauricularis, 503–504
M. pectineus, 289f, 291f, 295f, 298f, 301f, 302
M. pectorales profunda, 264–265, 264f, 268f
  nerve to, 714f
M. pectoralis superficialis, 264f
M. piriformis, 291f–292f, 292
  nerve to, 734f, 741f, 744f–745f
M. popliteus, 291f, 295f, 299f, 303f, 305f, 311
M. preputialis, 257
M. pronator quadratus, 270f, 274f, 279f, 285
M. pronator teres, 268f, 270f–271f, 274f, 276f–279f, 279
M. propria linguae, 229
M. psoas major, 288f, 289, 291f
M. psoas minor, 287–289, 288f–289f
M. pterygoideus lateralis, 222f–224f, 224
M. pterygoideus medialis, 222f–224f, 224, 232f
M. pterygopharyngeus, 222f, 228f–230f, 230
M. quadratus femoris, 289f, 291f–292f, 293–294, 298f
  nerves to, 732f, 734f, 744f–745f
M. quadratus lumborum, 288f–289f, 289
  nerve to, 740f
M. quadratus plantae, 306f, 310f, 312
M. quadriceps femoris, 289f–291f, 295f–296f, 297, 298f–301f
M. rectococcygeus, 261–262, 261f, 373
M. rectus abdominis, 239f, 248f, 253f–255f, 256
  nerves to, 729f, 733f, 740f
M. rectus capitis dorsalis major, 235, 244f
M. rectus capitis dorsalis minor, 236
M. rectus capitis lateralis, 236, 240f
M. rectus capitis ventralis, 235, 240f
M. rectus femoris, 295f–296f, 297, 300f
  nerves to, 741f, 744f

M. rectus thoracis, 244f, 248f, 249
M. retractor anguli oculi lateralis, 217f–218f, 219, 895–896
M. retractor bulbi, 226f, 227, 892
M. retractor clitoridis, 261f, 262, 373
M. retractor costae, 249, 250f, 288f
M. retractor penis, 261f, 262
M. rhomboideus, 239f, 265f–267f
M. rhomboideus capitis, 242
M. rhomboideus cervicis, 242
M. rhomboideus thoracis, 242
M. rotatores, 239f, 246f, 247
M. sacrocaudalis dorsalis lateralis, 258, 259f
M. sacrocaudalis dorsalis medialis, 259f
M. sacrocaudalis ventralis lateralis, 258, 260f–261f
M. sartorius, 253f–254f, 289f–290f, 295f, 299, 299f–301f
  nerves to, 733f, 740f–741f, 744f
M. scalenus, 238, 239f–240f, 244f, 264f
M. scalenus dorsalis, 248f
M. scalenus medius, 238
M. scalenus ventralis, 238
M. scutuloauricularis profundus, 220, 220f
M. scutuloauricularis superficialis, 216f–218f
M. semimembranosus, 289f–291f, 295f–296f, 296–297, 299f–301f
M. semispinalis, 239f, 248f
M. semispinalis capitis, 243f–244f, 245
M. semispinalis cervicis, 245
M. semispinalis thoracis, 245
M. semitendinosus, 289f–290f, 295f–296f, 295f, 299f–301f, 310f
M. serratus dorsalis, 239f, 242, 248f
M. serratus dorsalis caudalis, 242, 248f
M. serratus dorsalis cranialis, 239f, 242, 248f
M. serratus ventralis, 264f, 266f–267f
M. serratus ventralis cervicis, 238–240, 239f, 244f, 266f–267f
M. serratus ventralis thoracis, 239f, 265, 265f–267f, 729f
M. sphincter ampullae hepatopancreaticae, 380
M. sphincter ani externus, 261f, 262, 372–373
M. sphincter ani internus, 261f, 262, 372–373
M. sphincter cardiae, 363
M. sphincter ceci, 368–369
M. sphincter colli profundus, 896
M. sphincter colli superficialis, 214–215, 216f

M. sphincter ductus choledochi, 380
M. sphincter ilex, 365–366
M. sphincter papillae, 461
M. sphincter pupillae, 872
M. sphincter pylori, 363
M. spinalis, 239f, 244f, 245, 248f
M. spinalis et semispinalis cervicis, 243f, 245
M. spinalis et semispinalis thoracis, 239f, 243f, 245
M. splenius, 239f
M. splenius capitis, 237–238, 239f
M. stapedius, 221–222, 222f, 850
M. sternocephalicus, 237, 239f, 266f–267f
  pars mastoideus, 232f, 237
  pars occipitalis, 232f, 237, 264f
M. sternohyoideus, 228f, 232f, 233, 234f–235f
M. sternothyroideus, 228f, 232f, 233, 239f, 264f
M. styloauricularis (mandibuloauricularis), 220f, 221, 222f
M. styloglossus, 227, 228f, 232f, 264f, 335
M. stylohyoideus, 233f–235f, 234–235
M. stylopharyngeus, 228f–229f, 230, 232f
M. subscapularis, 264f–265f, 267–268, 268f
M. supinator, 268f, 270f–271f, 276f, 277
M. supramammaricus, 257–258
M. supraspinatus, 265–266, 265f, 269f
M. temporalis, 222f–224f, 223–224
M. tensor fasciae antebrachii, 268f, 270f, 272–273
M. tensor fasciae latae, 289–291, 289f–290f, 295f
M. tensor tympani, 222, 850
M. tensor veli palatini, 230, 848
M. teres major, 265f–268f
M. teres minor, 265f, 266, 268f–269f
M. thyroarytenoideus, 230f–231f, 232
M. thyrohyoideus, 228f, 232f, 233, 264f
M. thyropharyngeus, 228f, 230, 232f
M. tibialis caudalis, 299f, 303f, 305f, 311, 749f
M. tibialis cranialis, 299f–300f, 303f–305f, 307f
M. trachealis, 402
M. tragicus, 216f, 221
M. trago-helicinus, 853f

M. trago-tubo-helicinus, 853*f*
M. transversospinalis, 243*f*–244*f*, 245–247, 246*f*, 259*f*
M. transversus abdominis, 253*f*–255*f*, 255, 288*f*
M. transversus thoracis, 249–250, 250*f*
M. trapezius, 265*f*–267*f*
　pars cervicalis, 241
　pars thoracica, 241
M. triceps brachii, 270*f*–271*f*, 271, 713*f*, 718*f*
M. ulnaris lateralis. *see* M. extensor carpi ulnaris
M. urethralis, 444
M. vastus intermedius, 296*f*, 297–298, 301*f*
M. vastus lateralis, 296*f*, 297, 300*f*–301*f*
M. vastus medialis, 296*f*, 297, 301*f*
M. ventricularis, 230*f*–231*f*, 232
M. vocalis, 230*f*–231*f*, 232
M. zygomaticoauricularis, 216*f*–218*f*, 220
M. zygomaticus, 216, 216*f*–218*f*
Mm. adductores, 289*f*–292*f*, 295*f*–296*f*, 298*f*, 300*f*–301*f*, 302
Mm. adductores digiti II et V, 310*f*, 312
Mm. arrectores pilorum, 78*f*–79*f*, 79
Mm. caudae, 258–262, 259*f*–261*f*, 300*f*
Mm. gemelli, 289*f*–293*f*, 293, 300*f*
Mm. incisivus superioris et inferioris, 218
Mm. intercostales externi, 248, 248*f*–249*f*, 253*f*–254*f*
Mm. intercostales interni, 249, 249*f*, 253*f*–254*f*
Mm. interflexorii, 310*f*, 312
Mm. interossei, 278*f*, 280*f*, 282*f*, 285
Mm. intertransversarii, 239*f*, 244*f*, 246*f*, 247–248
Mm. intertransversarii dorsales cervicis, 244*f*, 246*f*, 247–248
Mm. intertransversarii lumborum, 239*f*, 247–248
Mm. intertransversarii medii cervicis, 247–248
Mm. intertransversarii thoracis, 247–248
Mm. intertransversarii ventrales cervicis, 244*f*, 246*f*
Mm. levatores costarum, 248–249, 249*f*
Mm. lumbricales (pelvic limb), 310*f*, 312
Mm. lumbricales (thoracic limb), 279*f*–281*f*, 285
Mm. palatini, 322
Mm. papillares, 503–504

Mm. pectinati, 500
Mm. pectorales superficiales, 264, 264*f*, 268*f*
Mm. recti, 226*f*, 227, 893
Mm. subcostales, 249
Mm. tarsalis dorsalis et ventralis, 885
Muzzle, 388
Myelencephalon, 658, 757, 758*f*, 758*t*
Myenteric plexus, 670
Mylohyoid line, 115, 115*f*
Mylohyoid nerve, 826
Mylohyoideus, 340*f*, 344*f*
Myocardium, 495–496, 504
Myofibers, 207
Myofibra conducens cardiaca, 505
Myofibrils, 207
Myofilaments, 207
Myometrium, 452
Myotatic reflex, 695–696
Myotome, 707, 736

N

Nares, 391
　external, 388
Nasal aperture, bony, 109–110, 121
Nasal arteries
　lateral, 526
　septal, 525
Nasal bone, 91*f*–92*f*, 96*f*, 108*f*, 110, 110*f*, 116*f*, 120*f*
Nasal cartilage, 388, 389*f*
Nasal cavity, 107*f*, 123–124, 388, 391–396, 392*f*–393*f*, 395*f*
Nasal conchae, 391*f*, 392–393
　dorsal, 107–112, 107*f*–108*f*, 122*f*, 123, 391*f*, 392
　middle, 392–393
　ventral, 107–109, 108*f*, 112, 122*f*, 123–124, 391*f*, 392
Nasal crest, 112–113
Nasal epidermis, 67
Nasal glands, lateral, 391–392, 391*f*–392*f*, 395, 395*f*
Nasal ligaments, 391
　dorsal, 391
　nasal, 391
Nasal meatus, 393–394
　common, 106, 107*f*–108*f*, 112, 124, 392*f*, 394
　dorsal, 108*f*, 110, 124, 392*f*, 393–394
　middle, 107*f*–108*f*, 111–112, 124, 394
　atrium of, 394
　ventral, 107*f*–108*f*, 112, 124, 394
Nasal mucosa, 394–395
　nerves on, 393*f*, 394

Nasal nerve, caudal, 815–816, 822
Nasal opening, 123
Nasal pharynx, 344, 345*f*
Nasal plane, 388
Nasal portion, of pharynx, 396
Nasal process, 99*f*, 109–110, 110*f*
　of frontal bone, 100
　of incisive bone, 107*f*, 109*f*
Nasal septum, 108*f*, 120*f*, 123, 389*f*, 391
　arteries of, 393*f*, 521*f*
　cartilage of, 107*f*–108*f*
　membranous, 389
Nasal skin, 67, 67*f*
Nasal spine, 112–113, 121
　of palatine bone, 119*f*
Nasal turbinate, 107–109, 111–112
Nasal vein
　dorsal, 586, 587*f*
　lateral, 587, 587*f*
Nasal vestibule, 389, 391–392
Nasal wall
　arteries of, 521*f*
　nerves of, 816*f*
Nasion, 93, 93*f*
Nasociliary nerve, 818*f*, 819, 899
Nasoethmoidal suture, 109–110
Nasofrontal opening, 124–125
　location of, 106*f*, 108*f*
Nasoincisive suture, 109–110
Nasolacrimal canal, 110*f*
Nasolacrimal duct, 107*f*, 391–392, 391*f*, 395
　system, 890–891, 891*f*
Nasomaxillary suture, 111
Nasopalatine duct, 390–391
Nasopalatine nerve, 815–816
Nasopharyngeal meatus, 394
Nasopharynx, 108*f*, 344*f*, 396
Nasoturbinate, dorsal, 392
Nasus, 388. *see also* Nose
Nasus externus, 388
Neck
　artery of, 510–548
　of bladder, 421
　fasciae of, 240–241
　of femur, 163*f*
　of fibula, 168
　of gallbladder, 379
　of humerus, 143*f*, 145
　lymph nodes and vessels of, 624–628, 627*f*
　muscles of, 232*f*, 237–241, 239*f*–240*f*, 244*f*, 264*f*
　nerves of, 830*f*
　　cutaneous, 730*f*
　　superficial, 709*f*

Neck *(Continued)*
    sympathetic distribution of, 666f–667f, 672–673
    of radius, 147, 147f
    of rib, 139–140, 139f
    of talus, 169–170, 170f
    of tooth, 323–324
    of uterus, 451
    veins of, 584f–585f, 588f
Neocortex (neopallium), 779
Nephron, 419, 419f, 463
Nephronum, 419
Nephros, 416
Nerve(s), 650, 659. *see also specific nerves*
    of anal canal, 373
    base of skull, 528f
    of bone, 90–91
    cranial, 650, 814–838
    to diaphragm, 711–712
    of ductus deferens, 436
    of esophagus, 348–349, 351f
    of eye, 818f, 820f, 897f–899f
    of female external genitalia, urethra, 457
    of female perineum, 745f
    of forepaw (manus), 723–727, 726f
    functional components of, 657f, 659–661
    of kidneys, 419–420
    of larynx, 399f, 835f
    of leg, 749f
    of liver, 379
    of male perineum, 747f
    of male urethra, 444
    to mandible, 828f
    of middle ear, 827f
    of muscles, 213–214
    of nasal wall, 816f
    olfactory, 393, 393f
    of orbit, 818f, 897f
    of os penis, 440–442
    of ovary, 449–450
    palatine, 322
    of pancreas, 383
    of pharyngeal region, 666f, 833f
    of pharynx, 835f
    of prepuce, 444–445
    of prostate gland, 437–438
    of pupil, 872f
    of right antebrachium, 718f
    of right shoulder joint, 716f
    of right thoracic limb, 713f
    of scrotum, 428
    on septal mucosa, 815f
    of skin, 653f
    of skull, 529f

Nerve(s) *(Continued)*
    of small intestine, 367–368
    of stomach, 364, 367–368
    of testes, 430–431
    of tongue, 338–340, 338f
    of ureters, 421
    of urinary bladder, 423
    of uterine tube, 450–451
    of uterus, 453
Nerve fibers. *see* Axon(s)
Nerve supply, to skin, 82
Nervi craniales, 659, 757
Nervi spinales, 659, 704
Nervous coat, 873
Nervous system, 650–662. *see also* Nerve(s)
    autonomic, 663–678
    cells in, 650
    central, 650, 657–659
    enteric, 661
    general, 650–659
    intramural, 661
    parasympathetic, 661f, 664–670, 664f–665f, 820f
    peripheral, 650, 657, 659, 660t
    supporting cells, 657
    sympathetic, 661f, 664f, 671–675
Nervus, 650
Nervus (N.)/Nervi (Nn.),. *see* Nerve(s); *specific nerves*
N. abducens, 828–829, 900
N. accessorius, 836
N. alveolaris inferior, 826
N. auricularis caudalis, 831
N. auricularis magnus, 710, 837
N. auriculopalpebralis, 832, 900
N. auriculotemporalis, 825–826
N. axillaris, 715–716
N. brachiocephalicus, 727–728
N. buccalis, 825
N. canalis pterygoidei, 665, 829–830
N. cardiacus cervicalis, 667–668
N. cervicalis
    I, 708
    II, 709
N. costoabdominalis, 731
N. cutaneus, 727–728
N. cutaneus antebrachii caudalis, 722
N. cutaneus antebrachii cranialis, 716
N. cutaneus antebrachii lateralis, 720–721
N. cutaneus antebrachii medialis, 716–718
N. cutaneus brachii lateralis caudalis, 718–720
N. cutaneus brachii lateralis cranialis, 716

N. cutaneus colli, 709–710
N. cutaneus femoralis lateralis, 736–739
N. cutaneus femoris caudalis, 746
N. cutaneus surae caudalis distalis, 748–749
N. cutaneus surae caudalis proximalis, 748
N. cutaneus surae lateralis, 748
N. depressor, 835–836
N. digitalis dorsali I abaxialis, 723–724
N. digitalis dorsalis communis I, 723–724
N. digitalis dorsalis proprius II abaxialis, 723–724
N. digitalis dorsalis proprius IV abaxialis, 750
N. digitalis dorsalis proprius V axialis, 750
N. digitalis palmaris communis
    I, 724
    II, 724
    III, 724
    IV, 726
N. digitalis palmaris I abaxialis, 724
N. digitalis palmaris proprius I axialis, 724
N. digitalis palmaris proprius II abaxialis, 724
N. digitalis plantaris abaxialis V, 752–753
N. digitalis propius dorsalis V abaxialis, 750
N. digitalis proprii dorsalis V abaxialis, 725–726
N. digitalis proprii palmaris V abaxialis, 726
N. dorsalis clitoridis, 747
N. dorsalis penis, 747
N. ethmoidalis, 815–816, 819, 899
N. facialis, 829, 900
N. femoralis, 740–741
N. fibularis communis, 749
N. fibularis profundus, 750
N. fibularis superficialis, 749–750
N. frontalis, 819, 899
N. genitofemoralis, 739–740
N. glossopharyngeus, 322, 339, 832
N. gluteus caudalis, 745–746
N. gluteus cranialis, 744–745
N. hypogastricus, 675
N. hypoglossus, 335, 339, 837
N. ilioinguinalis, 736
N. infraorbitalis, 822–824
N. infratrochlearis, 819, 899

N. intercostalis, 728–729
  II, 731
N. intercostobrachialis
  II, 731
  III, 731
N. intermediofacialis, 829
N. intermedius, 665, 829–830
N. interosseus antebrachii, 722
N. ischiadicus, 748
N. lacrimalis, 819, 899
N. laryngeus caudalis, 836
N. laryngeus craniales, 835–836
N. laryngeus cranialis, 667
N. laryngeus recurrens, 667–668, 836
N. lingualis, 338, 826–828
N. mandibularis, 824
N. massetericus, 825
N. masticatorius, 825
N. maxillaris, 322, 819
N. meatus acustici externi, 825–826
N. medianus, 721–722
N. metatarseus dorsalis II, 750–751
N. musculocutaneus, 716–718
N. mylohyoideus, 826
N. nasalis caudalis, 815–816, 822
N. nasociliaris, 819, 899
N. nasopalatinus, 815–816
N. obturatorius, 742–743
N. occipitalis major, 709, 837
N. oculomotorius, 816, 897
N. ophthalmicus, 819, 899
N. opticus, 775, 816, 896
N. palatinus accessorius, 822
N. palatinus major, 822
N. palatinus minor, 822
N. parasympatheticus n. vagi, 834
N. perinealis profundus, 746–747
N. perinealis superficialis, 746–747
N. petrosal major, 829–830
N. petrosus major, 665
N. petrosus minor, 832–833
N. petrosus profundus, 829–830
N. phrenicus, 711
N. plantaris lateralis, 752–753
N. plantaris medialis, 752
N. pterygoideus lateralis et medialis, 825
N. pterygopalatinus, 822
N. pudendus, 746
N. radialis, 718–720
N. radius manus, 723
N. ramus m stylopharyngeus caudalis, 833
N. rectalis caudalis, 746
N. saphenus, 741–742
N. splanchnicus major, 673–674
N. stapedius, 830–831

N. sublingualis, 826–828
N. suboccipitalis, 708
N. subscapularis, 715
N. supraorbitalis, 819
N. suprascapularis, 715
N. supratrochlearis, 819
N. tensoris tympani, 825
N. tensoris veli palatini, 825
N. terminalis, 815–816
N. thoracicus lateralis, 728
N. thoracicus longus, 728
N. thoracodorsalis, 728
N. tibialis, 751–752
N. transversus colli, 837
N. trigeminus, 322, 818–819, 898
N. trochlearis, 817, 898
N. tympanicus, 832–833, 847
N. ulnaris, 722
N. vagus, 322, 833–834
N. vestibulocochlearis, 832
N. vomeronasalis, 815
N. zygomaticus, 819–822, 900
Nn. auriculares rostrales, 825–826
Nn. carotidotympanici, 847
Nn. caudales, 754
Nn. cervicales, 708
Nn. ciliares breves, 897–898
Nn. ciliares longi, 819, 899
Nn. clunii, 733–734
Nn. clunii caudales, 733–734
Nn. clunii craniales, 733–734
Nn. clunii medii, 733–734
Nn. clunium caudales, 746
Nn. clunium craniales, 733
Nn. clunium medii, 743–744
Nn. digitales, 723
Nn. digitales communes, 723
Nn. digitales proprii, 723
Nn. digitales proprii palmares axiales et abaxiales, 726–727
Nn. digitalis dorsalis communis III et IV, 750
Nn. digiti plantares propii, 752
Nn. iliohypogastrici craniales et caudales, 734
Nn. intercostales, 728–729
Nn. lumbales, 731–732
Nn. mentales, 826
Nn. metacarpal palmares, 726
Nn. metacarpei, 723
Nn. metatarsei, 723
Nn. olfactorii, 815–816
Nn. pectorales caudales, 728
Nn. pectorales craniales, 728
Nn. pelvini, 670, 746
Nn. perinei, 746–747
Nn. sacrales, 743

Nn. scrotales dorsales, 746–747
Nn. splanchncius minor, 673–674
Nn. splanchnici lumbales, 674–675
Nn. supraclaviculares, 711
Nn. temporalis profundi, 825
Nn. thoracici, 728
Neural arches, 44, 47f–49f
Neural lobe, 473
Neuritum, 650
Neurocranium, 117
Neurocytus, 650
Neurofilamenta, 652
Neuroglia, 657
Neurohypophyseal (infundibular) recess, 773
Neurohypophysis, 775
Neurolemmocytus, 657
Neuromodulation, overview, 767, 767f
Neuromuscular compartment, 212
Neuron(s)
  afferent, 651f, 654–655
  auditory, 650–651
  efferent, 651f
    spinal cord, 685
  groups of, 654–656
  interneurons, 650–651, 655
    spinal cord, 685
  motor
    alpha, 685
    beta, 685
    gamma, 685
    lower, 650–652, 652f, 655–656, 656f–657f, 658–659, 659f, 685
    upper, 654
  olfactory, 650–651
  peripheral, 660t
  preganglionic, 659
  projection, 655
    spinal cord, 685
  segments of
    cell body, 652
    conductile, 653–654
    functional, 652–654
    receptive, 652
    transmissive, 654
  structure of, 650–652
  trigger zone of, 653
Neurona, 650
Neuronal fiber, 653
Neuronum autonomicum, 655–656
Neuronum bipolare, 650
Neuronum fusi neuromuscularis, 655–656
Neuronum multipolare, 650
Neuronum pseudounipolare, 650
Neuronum somaticum, 655–656

Neuronum unipolare, 650
Nipples, 459
Nissl bodies, 651–652
Nissl substance, 651–652
Node(s)
  aortic thoracic, 630
  atrioventricular, 505–506
  lymph. see Lymph nodes
  sinoatrial, 505
Nodules
  in aortic valve, 505
  lymph, 620–621
    aggregated, 367, 620–621
    in conjunctiva, 887
    solitary, 370–371, 620–621
Noduli lymphatici aggregati, 367
Noduli lymphatici aggregati, 620–621
Noduli valvularum semilunarium, 505
Nodulus lymphaticus, 620–621
Nodulus lymphaticus solitarius, 620–621
Nodulus primarius, 620–621
Nodulus secondarius, 620–621
Nodus atrioventricularis, 505–506
Nodus sinuatrialis, 505
Nomenclature
  dental, 328–329
  directional terminology
    for along teeth, 328–329
    eye, 860f
    for structures of internal and external ear, 853
Non-sporting breeds, 10f
Nose, 388, 389f, 815f. see also under Nasal
  arteries of lateral nasal wall, 521f
  cartilage of, 388–390, 389f
  cavity of, 91
  external, 388–391, 389f
  functional considerations of, 395–396
  glands of, 395
  ligaments of, 391
  movable portion of, 388
  sagittal section of, 389f
  skin of, 67, 67f
Nostrils, 388, 391
Notch
  acetabular, 156–158
  alar, 126f, 127–130
  cardiac, 411
    of right lung, 408, 411
  carotid, 103f
  caudal thyroid, 399
  for caudal vena cava, 411
  intercondyloid, 96f
  ischiatic

Notch (Continued)
  greater, 157f, 158, 160f
  lesser, 157f–159f, 160–161
  mandibular, 115–116, 115f
  popliteal, 165–167, 166f
  radial, 147f, 150
  scapular, 141f, 142
  thyroid, caudal, 399
  trochlear, 147f, 150
  ulnar, 147f, 149–150
  vertebral, 126
Nuchal crest, 92f, 96–97, 96f, 103f, 105, 121
Nuchal ligament, 184f, 185, 187f, 710f
Nuchal tubercles, 96f, 97–98, 119f
Nuclei, 658f, 660–661, 686
Nuclei habenulares, 777–778
Nuclei laterales thalami, 774
Nuclei parasympathici n. oculomotorii, 771
Nuclei paraventriculares thalami, 774
Nuclei pontis, 766
Nuclei raphe, 758–759
Nuclei rostrales thalami, 774
Nuclei septi, 784
Nuclei tuberis laterales, 777
Nuclei ventrales corporis trapezoidei, 765
Nuclei vestibulares, 765
Nucleus
  basal, 778–779, 789–791, 791f–792f
  cerebellar, 792–794
  gray matter, 757
  habenular, 777–778
  of mesencephalic tract of trigeminal nerve, 758, 768
  red, 771, 771f
  of solitary tract, 757–758, 764
  of spinal tract of trigeminal nerve, 758, 761
  subthalamic, 778
Nucleus accumbens, 790
Nucleus ambiguus, 764
Nucleus caudatus, 790
Nucleus cervicalis lateralis, 687
Nucleus cuneatus medialis, 761
Nucleus dorsalis, 687
Nucleus dorsalis corporis trapezoidei, 765
Nucleus dorsomedialis thalami, 774
Nucleus endopeduncularis, 790–791
Nucleus geniculatus lateralis, 775
Nucleus geniculatus medialis, 775
Nucleus gracilis, 761
Nucleus hypothalamicus dorsomedialis, 777

Nucleus hypothalamicus lateralis, 777
Nucleus hypothalamicus rostralis, 776
Nucleus hypothalamicus ventromedialis, 777
Nucleus infundibularis, 777
Nucleus intercalatus, 764
Nucleus interpeduncularis, 770
Nucleus lateralis caudalis, 774
Nucleus lateralis dorsalis, 774
Nucleus menisci lateralis, 765
Nucleus motorius n. abducentis, 766
Nucleus motorius n. accessorii, 687, 764
Nucleus motorius n. facialis, 764
Nucleus motorius n. hypoglossi, 763
Nucleus motorius n. oculomotorii, 771
Nucleus motorius n. trigemini, 824–825
Nucleus motorius n. trochlearis, 770–771
Nucleus olivaris, 761
Nucleus parasympatheticus n. facialis, 665, 763–764
Nucleus parasympatheticus n. glossopharyngei, 763–764
Nucleus parasympatheticus n. intermedii, 665
Nucleus parasympatheticus n. vagi, 666, 763–764
Nucleus paraventricularis, 776
Nucleus pulposus, 125–126, 184f–185f, 185
Nucleus pulvinaris, 774
Nucleus raphe magnus, 758–759
Nucleus reticularis lateralis, 764
Nucleus ruber, 771
Nucleus sensibilis pontinus n. trigemini, 758
Nucleus subthalamicus, 778
Nucleus suprachiasmaticus, 776
Nucleus supraopticus, 776
Nucleus thoracicus, 687
Nucleus tractus mesencephalici n. trigemini, 758, 768
Nucleus tractus solitarii, 757–758, 764
Nucleus tractus spinalis n. trigemini, 758, 761
Nucleus ventralis caudalis, 774
Nucleus ventralis lateralis, 774
Nucleus ventralis medialis, 774
Nucleus ventralis rostralis, 774
Nucleus Z, 761
Nutrient arteries, 90–91
  of humerus, 539, 540f
  of ilium, 576–577
  of radius, 545–546

Nutrient arteries *(Continued)*
  of tibia, 569
  of ulna, 545–546
Nutrient canal, 90
Nutrient foramen, 90–91, 146, 147f.
  see also specific bones
Nutrient vein, 90–91

O
Obex, 763
Oblique diameter, of pelvic cavity, 156–158
Oblique fibers, 363
Oblique ligament, 190f, 191
Oblique line, 398
Obliquus capitis caudalis muscle, 710f
Obturator externus muscle, nerve to, 743f
Obturator foramen, 156–158, 157f–160f, 743f
Obturator nerves, 732f, 736f–737f, 740f–741f, 742–743, 743f
Occipital artery, 513
Occipital bone, 91f–92f, 95–98, 96f, 116f
  basilar part of, 97–98
  squamous part of, 96–97
  variations in, 97f–98f, 98
Occipital condyles, 96f, 97, 118–119, 118f–119f, 128f–129f
Occipital crest
  external, 96–97, 121
  internal, 96f, 97, 123
Occipital diploic vein, 607f, 611
Occipital emissary vein, 607f, 608
Occipital protuberance
  external, 92f, 96–97, 96f, 118f, 121
  internal, 96f, 97
Occipitomastoid suture, 98
Occipitosquamous suture, 98
Occipitotympanic joint, 98
Occlusal surface, of tooth, 327
Ocular fundus, 875–876, 875f
Oculomotor nerve (cranial nerve III), 665, 816, 818f, 897–898, 898f
  motor nucleus of, 771
  parasympathetic nucleus of, 771
Olecranon, 147f, 149f
Olecranon fossa, 144f, 146
Olecranon ligament, 191, 191f
Olecranon tuber, 149f
Olfactory bulb, cavity of, 700f
Olfactory nerve (cranial nerve I), 393, 393f, 815–816, 815f–816f
Olfactory neurons, 650–651
Olfactory pathways, 783–785
Olfactory reflex, 390

Olfactory tubercle, 783
Oligodendrocytus, 657
Olivary nucleus, 761
Omenta, 354
Omental bursa, 356–359, 358f
  caudal recess of, 359
  dorsal recess of, 358
  splenic recess of, 359
Omental tuber, 376
Omental veil, 357–358
Omentum
  greater, 353, 354f, 356–358, 357f
  lesser, 357f–358f, 358, 378
  lymph vessels of, 637f
Omentum majus, 356
Omentum minus, 358, 378
Omobrachial vein, 583f–584f
Omocervical trunk, 536–537
Omphalopleure, bilaminar, 18
Oocytes, 445
Ophthalmic artery
  external, 523, 901, 901f–902f
  internal, 529f, 530, 901f–902f, 902
Ophthalmic nerve, 818f, 819, 823f, 898f, 899
Ophthalmic plexus, 586f, 587, 588f, 607f, 903f, 904
Ophthalmic vein, 588f
Ophthalmology, comparative, 904
Optic canal, 100f–101f, 101, 118f–119f, 122f
Optic chiasm, 757, 896
Optic cup, 858, 859f
Optic disc, 875–876
Optic nerve (cranial nerve II), 700f, 775, 816, 818f, 896–897, 898f
  sheath of, 873
Optic radiation, 775, 788
Optic recess, 700f, 773
Optic stalk, 858
Optic sulcus, 858
Optic tract, 775
Optic vesicle, 858, 859f
Ora ciliaris retinae, 869–871, 874
Ora serrata, 874
Oral cavity, 319–344
Oral cavity proper, 319–344
Oral fissure, 319
Oral glands, 340
Oral pharynx, 344–345
Oral surface, 397–398
Orbicular zone, 197
Orbicularis ciliaris, 869–871
Orbit, 118, 880–885, 881f–883f
  apex of, 892f
  arteries of, 520f, 523, 901f–902f
  nerves of, 818f, 897f

Orbital crest, 118, 118f
Orbital fasciae, 884–885, 884f
Orbital fat body, 885
Orbital fissure, 101, 101f, 118, 118f–119f, 121–123, 122f
  emissary vein of, 904
  muscle attachments in, 892f
  notch of, 100f
Orbital gland, 343
Orbital lamina, 106f, 124
Orbital ligament, 112, 118, 183f, 340f, 881
Orbital margin, 881
Orbital process, 113
Orbital septum, 884–885
Orbital wing, 100f–101f
Orbitosphenoid bone, 29–32, 40f–41f
Orbitosphenoidal crest, 100f, 101
Orbitotemporal crest, 99f
Organ of Corti, 844
Organa genitalia feminina, 445
Organa genitalia masculina, 423
Organa urinaria, 416
Organum spirale, 844
Organum subcommissurale, 773
Organum subfornicale, 773
Organum vestibulocochleare (auris), 839
Organum visus, 858
Organum vomeronasale, 390
Orifice
  atrioventricular, 499
  cecocolic, 368–369
  external, 452
    urethral, 454–455
  ileal, 365–366
  internal, 452
  laryngeal, 345f
  of major zygomatic duct, 340f
  of mandibular duct, 340f
  of parotid duct, 340f
  preputial, 444
  of sublingual duct, 340f
Oropharynx, 344–345, 344f
Orthodromic conduction, 653–654, 653f
Os carpale primum, 154
Os carpale quartum, 154
Os carpale secundum, 154
Os carpale tertium, 154
Os carpi accessorium, 154
Os carpi intermedioradiale, 153
Os carpi ulnare, 153–154
Os clitoridis, 439–440, 455, 456f
Os clitoris, 86
Os conchae nasalis ventralis, 111–112
Os coxae, 88, 156–161, 157f–161f
Os ethmoidale, 106

Os femoris, 161–163
Os frontale, 99
Os genitale, 439–440
Os ilium, 158
Os incisivum, 109–110
Os interparietale, 96–97
Os ischii, 160
Os lacrimale, 113–114, 114f, 116f
Os lenticularis, 849–850
Os metatarsale
  I, 172
  II, 172
  III, 172
  IV, 172
Os nasale, 110
Os oris, 319
Os palatinum, 112–113
Os penis, 86, 431f, 439–442
  development of, 432f, 440
  nerves of, 440–442
  vessels of, 440–442
Os priapi, 439–440
Os pterygoideum, 114, 114f
Os pubis, 161
Os tarsale
  I, 171
  II, 171
  III, 171
  IV, 171–172
Os tarsi centrale, 171
Os temporale, 102, 116f
Os zygomaticum, 112, 116f
Ossa brevis, 88
Ossa carpi, 152–153
Ossa digitorum manus, 155
Ossa irregulata, 88
Ossa longa, 87
Ossa metacarpalia, 154
Ossa metatarsalia, 172
Ossa plana, 88
Ossa pneumatica, 88
Ossa sesamoidea, 88
Ossa sphenoidales, 100–101
Ossa tarsi, 169
Osseous ampulla, 840
Osseous labyrinth, 104, 841f, 846f
Osseous nasal septum, 106
Ossicles, auditory, 848f–849f, 849
  joints of, 180
  ligaments of, 850
  muscles of, 850
Ossicula auditus, 849
Ossification
  in fetal skeleton, 89
  in fetus, 27, 32f. see also Prenatal development
  intramembranous, 89

Osteoblasts, 89
Osteoclasts, 89
Osteoid, 88–89
Ostia venarum pulmonalium, 500
Ostium
  of auditory tube, 847
  intrapharyngeal, 119
Ostium abdominale tubae uterinae, 450
Ostium aortae, 503
Ostium atrioventriculare dextrum, 499, 501–502
Ostium atrioventriculare sinistrum, 503
Ostium cecocolicum, 368–369
Ostium ileale, 365–366
Ostium intrapharyngeum, 119, 344, 396
Ostium pharyngeum tubae auditivae, 344, 396
Ostium preputiale, 444
Ostium pyloricum, 362
Ostium trunci pulmonalis, 501–502
Ostium tympanicum tubae auditivae, 847
Ostium urethrae externum, 454–455
Ostium uteri externum, 452
Ostium uteri internum, 452
Ostium uterinum tubae, 450
Otic capsule, 33, 102–103
Otic ganglion, 821f, 832–833
Otic pit, 839
Otic placode, 839
Otic vesicle (otocyst), 839
Otolithic membrane, 843–844
Otoliths, 843–844
Oudenodon, 155
Outlet, pelvic, 156–158, 352–353
Oval foramen, 92f, 101–102, 118–119, 119f, 121–123, 122f
Ovarian artery, 449–451, 453, 559
Ovarian bursa, 445, 446f, 447, 450
Ovarian veins, 449–450, 453, 583f, 597
Ovary, 445–450, 447f
  anomalies and variations of, 450
  endocrine tissues of, 488
  ligaments of, 447
  nerves of, 449–450
  relations of, 446f
  structure of, 447
  vessels of, 449–450
Overlap zone, 660, 660f
Oviduct, 450
Ovocytes, 445
Ovulation, 13, 14f

P
Pachymeninx, 696–698
Pads, digital, 66–69, 68f, 82f
Palatal index, 95t
Palate, 321–322, 321f
  hard, 108f, 111–113, 113f, 120–121, 321, 321f
    nerves of, 816f
  soft, 228f–230f, 230–231, 321, 321f, 344f, 396f
    epithelium of, 322
    lymph vessels of, 625f
    structure of, 322
Palatine aponeurosis, 322
Palatine arteries
  ascending, 515–516
  descending, 525
  major, 322
  minor, 322, 346, 524–525
Palatine bone, 91f–92f, 96f, 112–113, 116f–117f, 120f
  perpendicular plate, 106f
Palatine canal, 108f, 112–113
Palatine fissure, 121
  caudal edge, 110f
  of incisive bone, 92f, 109–111, 109f, 119f, 122f
Palatine foramen
  caudal, 113, 118, 118f
  major, 111–113, 119f, 121
  minor, 112–113, 119f, 121
Palatine glands, 322, 340f
Palatine muscles, 322, 323f
Palatine nerves, 322, 822
Palatine plexus, 322, 345, 586f, 588f
Palatine process, 110f
  of incisive bone, 107f, 109–110, 109f, 119f
  of maxilla, 107f, 111, 119f
Palatine sulcus, 111, 119f
Palatine suture, 121
  median, 113
  transverse, 113
Palatine tonsil, 340f, 344–345
Palatine veil, 322
Palatine vessels, 322
Palatoethmoidal suture, 109, 113
Palatoglossal arch, 321f, 322
Palatolacrimal suture, 114
Palatomaxillary suture, 111
Palatopharyngeal arch, 322
Palatopharyngeal muscle, 322, 323f
Palatopharyngeus, 344f
Palatum, 321. *see also* Palate
Palatum durum, 321
Palatum molle, 321–322
Palatum osseum, 111–113

Paleocortex (paleopallium), 779
Palmar branch, 717f, 726
Palmar carpal branch, 725f
Palmar carpal fibrocartilage, 192f, 193–195
Palmar digital arteries
 common, III, 726–727
 proper, axial
  III, 726–727
  IV, 726–727
Palmar digital nerves
 common
  I, 724
  II, 724, 725f
  III, 724, 725f, 726–727
  IV, 725f, 726
 proper, abaxial
  II, 724, 725f, 726–727
  III, 725f, 726–727
  IV, 725f, 726–727
  V, 725f, 726
 proper, axial
  I, 724, 725f
  II, 725f, 726–727
  III, 725f, 726–727
  IV, 725f, 726–727
  V, 725f
Palmar digital veins
 common, 591–592, 592f, 594
 proper, 594
Palmar fascia, 196
Palmar metacarpal artery III, 726–727
Palmar metacarpal nerve
 I, 725f, 726
 II, 725f, 726
 III, 725f, 726–727
 IV, 725f, 726
Palmar ulnocarpal ligaments, 194f, 195
Palmar veins, metacarpal, 592f, 594
Palpebra inferior, 885
Palpebra superior, 885
Palpebra tertia, 887–888
Palpebrae, 885
Palpebral artery, lateral superior, 518
Palpebral branches, 900
Palpebral conjunctiva, 887
Palpebral ligament
 lateral, 881, 886–887
 medial, 887
Palpebral muscles, 894–896
Palpebral nerve, 587f
Palpebral raphe, lateral, 894
Palpebral vein, inferior, 587
Pampiniform plexus, 430–431, 597
Pancreas, 357f, 381–383
 accessory, 381–382
 blood vessels of, 382–383

Pancreas (Continued)
 dorsal surface of, 381
 ducts of, 382
 left lobe of, 381
 lobes and relations of, 381–382
 lymph vessels of, 382–383, 638f
 nerves of, 383
 right lobe of, 381
 ventral surface of, 381
Pancreas accessorium, 381–382
Pancreatic angle, 381
Pancreatic duct, 380f, 382
 accessory, 382
Pancreatic veins, 599
Pancreaticoduodenal lymph nodes, 367, 637f, 639
Papilla duodeni major, 380
Papilla duodeni minor, 380
Papilla ilealis, 365–366
Papilla incisiva, 321
Papilla mammae, 459
Papilla parotidea, 319
Papilla renalis, 418–419
Papillae
 conical, 334
 duodenal
  major, 380
  minor, 380
 epidermal, 78, 78f
 filiform, 331–332, 331f
 foliate, 334
 fungiform, 331–333, 331f
 ileal, 365–366
 incisive, 321
 integumentary, 78, 78f
 marginal, 332f, 334
 vallate, 330, 331f–332f
Papillae conicae, 334
Papillae filiformes, 331–332
Papillae foliatae, 334
Papillae fungiformes, 332–333
Papillae marginales, 334
Papillae vallatae, 330, 333
Papillary ducts, 418–419, 460, 463
Papillary foraminae, 418–419
Papillary muscles, 502–503
Papillary ostium, 459f
Papillary process, 376–377
Paraconal interventricular branch, 584f
Paraconal interventricular groove, 495–496, 498–499
Paracondylar process, 96f, 97, 119f
Parahippocampal gyrus, 784, 786–787
Parahypophysis, 474
Parallel, 658
Paralumbar fossa, 350–351

Paramesonephric duct, 463
Paranal sinus glands, 372
Paranal sinuses, 372
Paranalis sinuses, 80–81
Paranasal sinuses, 88, 124–125, 125f, 394
Pararectal fossa, 370–371, 371f
Pararecurrent laryngeal nerve, 348, 351f
Parasympathetic nervous system, 664–670, 664f–665f
 GVE nuclear column, 820f
 preganglionic axons of, 661f
Paraterminal gyrus, 784
Parathyroid glands, 480–481
 developmental anatomy, 481
 mesoscopic features, 477f–478f, 480–481
 microscopic anatomy, 481
 vascularization and innervation, 481
Paraventricular nucleus, 776
Paraventricular thalamic nuclei, 774
Paraventriculohypophyseal tract, 776
Parenchyma, 643
Paries profundus, 356
Paries superficialis, 356
Parietal bone, 91f–92f, 98–99, 98f, 116f
 internal surface of, 99
Parietal cusp, 504
Parietal diploic veins, 609f
Parietal peritoneum, 354, 357f
Parietal surface
 of spleen, 643
 of stomach, 361
Parietoauricularis muscle, 710f
Parietointerparietal suture, 99
Parietosphenoidal suture, 99
Paroophoron, 451, 463
Parotid artery, 342, 517–518
Parotid duct, 340f–341f, 341–342
Parotid gland, 340–342, 340f–341f, 709f
 accessory, 342
 borders of, 340–341
 deep portion, 340
 superficial portion, 340
 superficial surface of, 340–341
 three angles of, 340–341
Parotid lymph center, 624
Parotid lymph nodes, 618f, 624, 625f
Parotid papilla, 319
Parotideoauricularis, 216f–217f
Parotidoauricularis, 709f
Pars abdominalis, 347
Pars analis, 373
Pars analis m. retractor clitoridis, 373

Pars analis m. retractor penis, 373
Pars ascendens, 365
Pars basilaris, 97–98
Pars buccalis, 218
Pars cardiaca, 362
Pars caudalis, 410
Pars ceca retinae, 859–860, 873
Pars cervicalis, 346
Pars ciliaris retinae, 873, 878
Pars clitoridae, 373
Pars costalis, 250f, 251
Pars cranialis, 365, 410
Pars descendens, 365
Pars distalis adenohypophysis, 473–474
Pars endocrina pancreatis, 487–488
  developmental and mesoscopic anatomy, 487
  microscopic features, 487–488
Pars flaccida, 846
Pars glandularis, 460–461
Pars intercartilaginea, 401
Pars intermedia adenohypophysis, 473, 475
Pars intermembranacea, 401
Pars intestinum tenue mesenteriale, 365–366
Pars iridica retinae, 859–860, 873
Pars laryngea pharyngis, 345
Pars lateralis, of sacrum, 136
Pars longa glandis, 439
Pars lumbalis, 250f, 251
Pars mediastinalis, 408
Pars membranacea, 504
Pars membranacea septi nasi, 389
Pars mobilis nasi, 388
Pars molaris, 218
Pars muscularis, 504
Pars nasalis, 99f, 100
Pars nasalis pharyngis, 344, 396
Pars occipitalis, 709f
Pars optica retinae, 869–871, 874
Pars oralis pharyngis, 344–345
Pars orbitalis, of frontal bone, 99–100, 99f
Pars orbitalis, of orbicularis oculi, 894
Pars palpebralis, 896
Pars papillaris, 460–461
Pars parasympathica, 661
Pars pelvina, 443
Pars penina, 443
Pars petrosa, 102–103
Pars profunda, 340
Pars prostatica, 443–444
Pars pylorica, 362
Pars rectalis, 373
Pars reticulata, 770

Pars squamosa, 102f, 105
Pars sternalis, 250f, 251
Pars superficialis, 340
Pars sympathica, 661
Pars tensa, 846
Pars thoracica, 346–347
Pars transversa (pars caudalis), 365
Pars tuberalis adenohypophysis, 475
Pars tympanica, 105
Pars vertebralis, 408
Partes laterales, 97
Passive movements, 179
Patella, 162f–163f, 164, 167f, 742f
Patellar ligament, 742f
Patent ductus arteriosus, 502f
Paw. see Forepaw; Hindpaw
Pecten, of pubic bone, 156–158, 158f–160f, 161
Pectinate ligament, 865
Pedicles, of vertebra, 126, 131–132
Pediculi arcus vertebrae, 126
Peduncle, 757
Peduncles, cerebellar, 794–795
Pedunculopontine nucleus, 770
Pedunculus cerebellaris caudalis, 794
Pedunculus cerebellaris medius, 794
Pedunculus cerebellaris rostralis, 794–795
Pedunculus mamillaris, 777
Pelvic aperture, 156–158
  caudal, 352–353
  cranial, 352–353
Pelvic axis, 156–158
Pelvic cavity, 156–158, 352–353, 428f
Pelvic diaphragm, 374
Pelvic fascia, 353
Pelvic girdle. see also Pelvis
  development of, 44–51, 52f–56f
  joints of, 196–197
Pelvic inlet, 136–137, 156–158
Pelvic limb
  artery of, 562–569
  bones of, 156–172
  cutaneous nerves of, 735f, 739f–740f, 743f
  deep veins of, 600–603, 601f
  development of, 44–51, 54f–56f
  fasciae of, 312–313
  lymph nodes and vessels of, 640–642
  muscles of, 287–313
Pelvic nerves, 373, 423, 438, 441–442, 458, 670, 732f, 734f, 737f, 741f, 746
Pelvic outlet, 156–158, 352–353
Pelvic peritoneal excavations, 355

Pelvic plexus, 373, 423, 438, 441–442, 444, 451
Pelvic plexus ganglia, 423
Pelvic region, sympathetic distribution in, 675
Pelvic splanchnic nerves, 746
Pelvic structures
  male, 429f
  relations of, 424f
Pelvic symphysis, 156–158, 157f, 196–197
Pelvic tendon, 253, 253f
Pelvic walls, 633–636
Pelvis. see also Pelvic girdle
  artery of, 566f
  bony, 156, 157f
  measurement of, 156–158
  muscles of, 288f–289f, 289–294, 291f–293f, 300f
  renal, 416–418, 463
  veins of, 603–605
Pelvis renalis, 416–418
Penis, 423, 438–439
  artery of, 576, 602f–603f
  circulatory pathways of, 433f
  dorsal artery of, 576, 747f
  dorsal nerve of, 736f, 747, 747f
  extrinsic muscles of, 438
  glans, 431f, 434f, 439
  internal morphologic characteristics of, 429f
  median section of, 429f
  os, 431f–432f, 439–442
  proximal half of, 430f
  relations of, 424f
  root of, 428f, 438
  semidiagrammatic view of, 430f
  ventral surface of, 438
  vessels of, 602f–603f
Periaqueductal gray, 767–768
Pericardiacophrenic artery, 535
Pericardial cavity, 495
Pericardial sac, 496f
Pericardium, 495
  parietal layer of, 495
  visceral layer of, 495
Pericardium, lymph vessels of, 629f
Pericardium fibrosum, 495
Pericardium serosum, 495
Perichondrium, 90
Perikaryon, 652
Perilymph, 839
Perilymphatic duct, 104, 840–842
Perineal arteries, 371f, 440–441, 602f–603f, 740f, 745f, 747f
  ventral, 576
Perineal body, 374–375

Perineal fascia, 374
Perineal nerves, 732f, 734f, 740f–741f, 745f, 746–747, 747f
Perineal vein, 371f, 373, 740f
  ventral, 604
Perineum, 374–375
  arteries of, male, 574f
Periodontal ligament, 176, 329
Periodontal membrane, 329
Periodontium, 176, 326f, 329
Periorbita, 884, 892f
Periosteal arteries, 90–91
Periosteal veins, 90–91
Periosteum, 90
Peripheral branches segment, 706f
Peripheral conductile segment, 653
Peripheral nervous system (PNS), 650, 657, 659, 660t
  functional classification of neurons, 660t
  supporting cells, 657
Peritoneal cavity, 351
  lesser, 356–357
Peritoneum, 353–355, 357f–358f
  connecting, 354, 357f
  parietal, 354, 357f
  pelvic excavations, 355
  visceral, 354
Peritoneum parietale, 354
Peritoneum viscerale, 354
Periventricular nuclei, 777
Permanent dentition, 328
Perpendicular fibers, 336f–337f, 337
Perpendicular plate
  of ethmoid bone, 96f
  of palatine bone, 106f
Pes, 605
Petiolus epiglottidis, 398
Petrooccipital canal, 97–98, 102f, 105, 123
Petrooccipital fissure, 105–106, 123
Petrooccipital suture, 98
Petrooccipital synchondrosis, 105–106
Petrosal apex, 102–103
Petrosal crest, 102–103, 102f, 122f, 123
Petrosal nerve, canal for, 104
Petrotympanic fissure, 104, 119f
  for chorda tympani, 102f
Phalangeal joints, 192–196, 205
Phalanx (phalanges), 155–156, 155f
  development of, 47–51, 53f–57f
  of forepaw, 155
  of hindpaw, 172
  muscles of, 278–285, 280f–281f
Phalanx distalis, 156

Phalanx media, 155–156
Phalanx proximalis, 155
Pharyngeal artery, ascending, 346, 515–516
  palatine branches, 515
  pharyngeal branches, 515
Pharyngeal chiasma, 344
Pharyngeal isthmus, 344, 396
Pharyngeal muscles, 345f
Pharyngeal plexus, 348, 833–835
Pharyngeal region, 833f
Pharyngeal region, nerves of, 666f
Pharyngeal tubercle, 97–98
Pharyngeal vein, ascending, 589
Pharyngoesophageal limen, 345f
Pharyngoesophageal nerve, 351f
Pharyngotympanic tube, 839
Pharynx, 344–346, 344f, 388
  laryngeal, 345–346, 345f
  muscles of, 228f–229f, 229–230
  nasal, 344, 345f, 396
  nerves of, 835f
  oral, 344–345
  relation to esophagus and trachea of, 396f
Philtrum, 319, 388
Phrenic nerve, 705f, 711, 713f–714f
Phrenicoabdominal trunk, 560
Phrenicopericardial ligament, 405
Phrenicosplenic ligament, 357, 643
Physeal cartilage, 87
Physis
  of humerus, 144f, 149f
  of olecranon tuber, 149f
  of radius, 149f, 152f
Pia mater, 679, 680f–681f, 699–700, 700f
Pigmentation
  of hair, 74–75
  of skin, 66–67
Pili, 64
Pili lanei, 64
Pili supraorbitales, 885–886
Pili tactiles, 319
Pili tactiles labiales superiores, 64
Pili tactiles supraorbitales, 64
Pineal gland, 481–482, 481f, 777
  developmental anatomy, 482
  mesoscopic features, 481–482
  microscopic anatomy, 482
  vascularization and innervation, 482
Pinna, 850
Piriform fossa, 101
Piriform lobe, 784
Piriform recess, 345f, 400
Placenta, 20, 20f

Plane joint, 179
Plane suture, 176
Plantar arteries
  lateral, 569–570
  medial, 569–572
Plantar centrodistal ligament, 205
Plantar digital arteries, common, 753f
Plantar digital nerves
  common, 752, 753f
  proper, 752
    abaxial, 752–753, 753f
    axial, 753f
Plantar digital veins, common, 599f–600f, 606
Plantar metatarsal arteries, 753f
Plantar metatarsal nerves, 753–754, 753f
Plantar veins, metatarsal, 605, 605f
Planum nasale, 67, 67f, 388
Plates
  cribriform, 106f, 107, 120f, 121
    of ethmoid, 96f, 109
  perpendicular
    of ethmoid bone, 96f
    of palatine bone, 106f
Platysma, 79, 215–216, 709f–710f
Pleura(e), 404–408, 729f
  costal, 407
  diaphragmatic, 407
  lymph vessels of, 633f
  mediastinal, 407
  parietal, 407
  pulmonary, 407
Pleura costalis, 407
Pleura diaphragmatica, 407
Pleura mediastinalis, 407
Pleura parietalis, 407
Pleura pulmonalis, 407
Pleural cavity, 407
Pleural cupula, 407
Pleurapophyses, 131
Plexus
  aortic, 450–451
  celiac, 364, 367–368, 379, 383
  cranial mesenteric, 367–368, 383
  cutaneous, 81, 81f
  of hard palate, 107f
  mesenteric, cranial, 367–368, 383
  ophthalmic, 586f, 587, 588f, 607f
  palatine, 322, 345
  pampiniform, 430–431, 597
  pelvic, 373, 423, 438, 441–442, 444, 451
  pharyngeal, 348
  prostatic, 438
  pterygoid, 586f

Plexus *(Continued)*
  renal, 420, 450–451
  subcutaneous, 81, 81*f*
  subpapillary, 81–82
  testicular, 431
  venous
    palatine, 589
    rectal, 604
    urethral, 604
    vaginal, 604
    vertebral, 612–613
  vestibular, 604
Plexus brachialis, 706–707, 712–714
Plexus cervicalis, 708
Plexus choroideus ventriculi quarti, 763
Plexus lumbalis, 735
Plexus lumbosacralis, 706–707, 734–735
Plexus myentericus, 670
Plexus ophthalmicus, 587, 904
Plexus pampiniformis, 430–431
Plexus pharyngeus, 833–835
Plexus renalis, 420
Plexus sacralis, 735, 743–744
Plexus venosus palatinus, 589
Plexus vertebralis externus dorsalis, 614
Plexus vertebralis externus ventralis, 614
Plexus vertebralis internus ventralis, 610, 612–613
Plica alaris, 390–391
Plica aryepiglottica, 400
Plica duodenocolica, 365
Plica gastropancreatica, 359
Plica genitalia, 452
Plica genitalis, 422–423, 435–436
Plica hepatopancreatica, 359
Plica ileocecalis, 366, 368–369
Plica pterygomandibularis, 344–345
Plica semilunaris, 344–345
Plica semilunaris conjunctivae, 887–888
Plica sublingualis, 321
Plica synovialis, 177
Plica venae cavae, 406–408
Plica vestibularis, 400–401
Plica vocali, 401
Plicae gastricae, 363
Plicae villosae, 363
Pneumatic bones, 88
Pneumogastric nerve, 833–834
Pogonion, 94
Polus anterior, 861
Polus posterior, 861
Polystomatic sublingual gland, 343

Pons, 757, 758*t*, 766–767, 766*f*
Pontine impression, 96*f*
Pontine nuclei, 766
Pontine reticulospinal tract, 691*f*, 695
Pontine tegmentum, 766
Pontine vein, 611
Popliteal artery, 569, 742*f*, 749*f*
Popliteal line, 167
Popliteal lymph center, 640
Popliteal lymph nodes, 618*f*, 636*f*, 640
Popliteal notch, 165–167, 166*f*
Popliteus muscle, 749*f*
  nerve to, 742*f*
  tendon of, 742*f*
Porta hepatis, 376
Porta of the liver, 376
Portal lymph nodes, 348
Portal vein, 357*f*, 373, 378, 583*f*, 595*f*, 598–599
Porus acusticus internus, 103
Porus gustatorius, 333
Posterior fiber group, 872
Postfixed plexus, 736
Postganglionic axons, 672
Pouch
  pubovesical, 355, 422–423
  rectogenital, 355, 422–423, 452–453
  vesicogenital, 355, 452–453
Precava, 582
Precorneal tear film, 888–889, 888*f*
Prefixed plexus, 736
Prefrontal association cortex, 789
Preganglionic axons, 661*f*, 672
Preganglionic neurons, 659
Premolar teeth, 327
  development of, 107*f*–108*f*, 120*f*
  eruption of, 325*t*
Prenatal development, 13–63. *see also* Embryo; Fetus
  of carpus, 51, 53*f*
  fertilization in, 15–16
  first trimester of, 17*b*
  gestation length in, 13–15, 14*f*, 16*t*
  of girdles, 44–51
  implantation in, 17, 17*f*
  of pelvic limb, 44–51, 54*f*–56*f*
  periods of, 15, 16*f*
  of ribs, 44, 60*f*
  second trimester of, 21, 21*t*, 22*f*–23*f*
  of skull, 27–35, 33*f*–45*f*
  of sternum, 44, 49*f*–51*f*
  third trimester of, 51, 58*t*–59*t*, 59*f*–61*f*
  of thoracic limb, 44–47, 52*f*–53*f*

Prenatal development *(Continued)*
  ultrasonography of, 15
  of vertebral column, 35–44, 46*f*–49*f*
Preoptic nuclei, 776
Prepuce, 444–445
  anomalies and variations of, 445
  nerves of, 444–445
  vessels of, 444–445, 602*f*–603*f*
Preputial cavity, 444
Preputial folds, 642*f*
Preputial muscle, 444
Preputial orifice, 444
Preputium, 444
Preputium clitoridis, 455
Presphenoid bone, 92*f*, 96*f*, 100*f*–101*f*, 101, 117*f*, 120*f*, 122*f*
  development of, 29–32, 41*f*–42*f*
Pretragic incisure, 851–852
Primary afferent axon, 656*f*
Primary afferent neurons, 651*f*, 654–655
Primary blood capillary network, 475–476
Primary branches segment, 706*f*
Primary follicle, 447
Primary germ cells, 463
Primary lymph, 621–622
Primary macroglossia, 339*f*
Prime movers, 212–213
Primordial follicle, 447
Proatlas, 127*f*, 130–131
Process
  accessory, of vertebrae, 132*f*, 133–134, 134*f*–135*f*
  alveolar, 109–111, 110*f*
    of maxilla, 111
  anconeal, 149*f*, 150
  angular, of mandible, 115–116, 115*f*, 120*f*
  articular, 126
    of atlas, 127–130
    of caudal vertebrae, 137–138
    of lumbar vertebrae, 134, 134*f*–135*f*
    of mandible, 115–116
    of sacral vertebrae, 135–136, 136*f*, 157*f*
    of thoracic vertebrae, 132*f*, 133
  of calcaneal tuber, 168*f*
  caudal, of vertebrae, 126
  clinoid
    caudal, 100*f*, 101, 121–123
    rostral, 100*f*, 101
  condylar, of mandible, 115–116, 115*f*, 120*f*
  coracoid, of scapula, 141*f*, 142–143

Process *(Continued)*
  coronoid
    of mandible, 115–116, 115*f*, 120*f*
    of ulna, 147*f*, 149*f*
  cranial, of vertebra, 126
  frontal
    of lacrimal bone, 113–114, 114*f*
    of maxilla, 110*f*, 111
    of nasal bone, 110, 110*f*
    of zygomatic bone, 92*f*, 112, 112*f*
  hemal, 134*f*, 137*f*, 138
  mamillary, of vertebrae, 132–133
    caudal, 137–138, 137*f*
    lumbar, 134, 134*f*–135*f*
  mastoid, 102*f*–103*f*, 104–105
  muscular, 102*f*
  nasal, 110, 110*f*
    of frontal bone, 100
    of incisive bone, 107*f*, 109–110, 109*f*
  orbital, 113
  palatine, 110*f*
    of incisive bone, 107*f*, 109–110, 109*f*, 119*f*
    of maxilla, 107*f*, 111, 119*f*
  paracondylar, of occipital bone, 96*f*, 97, 119*f*
  plantar, 168*f*
  pterygoid, 100*f*–101*f*, 101–102
  retroarticular, 102*f*–103*f*, 105, 118*f*
  septal, 110*f*
  sphenoidal, 113, 113*f*
  spinous, 126
    of axis, 127*f*, 129*f*, 130
    of caudal vertebrae, 137*f*
    of cervical vertebrae, 129*f*, 131
    of lumbar vertebrae, 133*f*–135*f*
    of sacral vertebrae, 136*f*
    of thoracic vertebrae, 131–132, 132*f*–133*f*
  styloid
    of radius, 147*f*, 149–150
    of ulna, 151
  temporal, of zygomatic bone, 112, 112*f*
  tentorial, of parietal bone, 98*f*, 99
  transverse, 126
    of atlas, 127–130, 128*f*–129*f*
    of axis, 127*f*–129*f*
    of caudal vertebrae, 137*f*
    of cervical vertebrae, 128*f*–130*f*, 131
    of lumbar vertebrae, 134, 134*f*–135*f*

Process *(Continued)*
    of sacral vertebrae, 136*f*
    of thoracic vertebrae, 132
  uncinate, 106–107, 106*f*
    crest for, 110*f*
  ungual, 152*f*, 155*f*
  xiphoid, 139*f*, 140
  zygomatic, 105
    of frontal bone, 99–100, 118*f*–120*f*
    of maxilla, 111
    of temporal bone, 92*f*, 102*f*–103*f*, 120*f*
Process muscularis, 400
Processi pterygoidei, 102
Processus alveolaris, 109–111
Processus anconeus, 150
Processus angularis, 115–116, 115*f*
Processus articularis caudalis, 126
Processus articularis cranialis, 126
Processus caudatus, 377
Processus ciliaris, 869–871
Processus clinoideus, 101
Processus clinoideus rostralis, 101
Processus condylaris, 115–116, 115*f*
Processus coracoideus, 142–143
Processus corniculatus, 400
Processus coronoideus, of mandible, 115–116, 115*f*
Processus cuneiformis, 400
Processus frontalis
  of lacrimal bone, 113–114, 114*f*
  of maxilla, 110*f*, 111
  of nasal bone, 110, 110*f*
  of zygomatic bone, 92*f*, 112
Processus lateralis tali, 169–170
Processus lenticularis, 849–850
Processus mamillaris, of vertebrae, 132–133
Processus mastoideus, 104–105
Processus nasalis, 109–110
Processus orbitalis, 113
Processus palatinus, of maxilla, 111
Processus papillaris, 376–377
Processus paracondylaris, 97
Processus pterygoideus, 101–102
Processus retroarticulare, 105
Processus sphenoidalis, 113
Processus styloideus, 149–151
  of ear, 851–852
Processus temporalis, of zygomatic bone, 112
Processus tentoricus, 99
Processus transversus, 126
Processus uncinatus, 106–107
Processus unguicularis, 156
Processus vocalis, 400

Processus xiphoideus, 140
Processus zygomaticus, 99–100, 105, 111
Proestrum, 448
Proestrus, 448, 448*f*
Prognathism, 94
Projection neurons, 655
Projection neurons, spinal cord, 685
Prominentia laryngea, 399
Promontorium, 104
Promontory, 104, 847
  of pyramid, 103*f*
  of sacrum, 136–137, 136*f*, 156–158, 157*f*
  of temporal bone, 119*f*
Pronephric duct, 462–463
Pronephros, 462–463
Proper digital veins, 592*f*
Proper ligament
  of ovary, 447
  of testis, 430
Proper lingual muscles, 336
Proprioception, 845*f*
Prosencephalon, 757
Prostata, 437
Prostate gland, 420*f*, 423, 437–438
  nerves of, 437–438
  pathologic conditions of, 438
  vessels of, 437–438
Prostatic artery, 371*f*, 421, 437–438, 444, 575
Prostatic plexus, 438
Prostatic utricle, 443–444, 463
Prostatic vein, 371*f*, 438, 583*f*, 604
Prosthion, 93, 93*f*
Protein electrophoresis, 2
Protractor preputii, 444
Protuberance, occipital
  external, 92*f*, 96–97, 96*f*, 118*f*, 121
  internal, 96*f*, 97
Protuberantia occipitalis externa, 96–97
Protuberantia occipitalis internus, 96–97
Proximal caudal cutaneous sural nerve, 740*f*, 748
Proximal interphalangeal joints, 195–196
Proximal intertarsal joint, 202–203
Proximal muscular branch, 716–718, 729*f*
Proximal radioulnar joint, 189
Proximal tibiofibular joints, 202
Proximal vagal ganglion, 667
Pseudounipolar cells, 650–651, 651*f*
Pterygoid bone, 91*f*–92*f*, 96*f*, 114, 114*f*, 117*f*, 120*f*

Pterygoid canal, 101–102, 119f, 900
  rostral opening of, 101f, 118f
Pterygoid canal, nerve of, 665, 829–830
Pterygoid fossa, 114
Pterygoid groove, 101–102, 119–120
Pterygoid hamulus, 114, 114f
Pterygoid nerves, lateral and medial, 825
Pterygoid plexus, 586f
Pterygoid process, 100f–101f, 101–102
Pterygoideus medius, 344f
Pterygomandibular fold, 344–345
Pterygopalatine fossa, 110f, 111, 113, 118
Pterygopalatine ganglion, 665, 824f, 900
Pterygopalatine nerve, 822
Pterygopalatine suture, 114
Pterygopharyngeal muscle, 322, 323f
Pterygopharyngeus, 344f
Pterygosphenoid suture, 102, 114
Pubic region, 350–351, 353f
Pubic tubercle, 160f, 161
Pubis, 161, 161f
Pubovesical pouch, 355, 422–423
Pudendal artery
  external, 424f, 428, 440–441, 444, 457, 562, 562f
  internal, 440–441, 457, 575
Pudendal nerve, 373, 423, 441–442, 732f, 734f, 737f, 741f, 745f, 746, 747f
  branch to, 745f
Pudendal veins
  external, 425f, 441, 444, 602–603, 602f–603f
  internal, 373, 424f, 441, 458, 602f–603f
Pudendoepigastric trunk, 562, 583f, 740f, 743f
Pudendoepigastric vein, 602–603
Pudendum femininum, 445, 455
Pulmo, 408
Pulmo dexter, 408, 411
Pulmo sinister, 408, 410–411
Pulmo sinistra, 410
Pulmonary alveoli, 403
Pulmonary arteries
  left, 410f, 411–412, 509, 584f
  right, 412, 509
Pulmonary fibrous ring, 500–501
Pulmonary ligament, 407–408
Pulmonary lymph nodes, 631, 634f
Pulmonary lymphatics, 413

Pulmonary pleura, 407
Pulmonary trunk, 412, 497f, 584f
Pulmonary trunk ostium, 501–502
Pulmonary valve, 501f, 505
Pulmonary veins, 410f, 412, 509–510, 584f
Pulp, 326–327
Pulp cavity, 326–327
Pulp chamber, 326–327
Pulpa dentis, 326–327
Pulpa lienis rubra et alba, 643
Pulpy nucleus, 184f–185f, 185
Pulvinar nucleus, 774
Puncta lacrimalia, 890
Pupil (pupilla), 872
  dilator of, 872
  neuroanatomic pathway for, 872f
Pupillary membrane, 872
Purkinje fibers, 505
Putamen, 790
Pyloric antrum, 362
Pyloric canal, 362
Pyloric glands, 364
Pyloric sphincter, 363
Pylorus, 359–362
Pyramidal decussation, 759–760, 762f
Pyramidal tract, 766
Pyramides renales, 418–419
Pyramids, 757
  of temporal bone, 102–103, 103f
  of white matter, 757, 760–761

Q

Quadrate lobe, 376–377
Quadrigeminal cistern, 700f

R

Radial artery, 546, 718f, 720f, 725f
  collateral, 539, 540f
  distal, 543
Radial fossa, 143f, 146, 146f
Radial nerve, 705f, 713f–715f, 717f, 718–720, 719f
  deep branch of, 719f
  of forepaw, 723
  superficial branch of, 719f, 730f
Radial notch, 147f, 150
Radial tuberosity, 147, 147f
Radial vein, 591–592, 592f
Radiate ligament, 184f
Radiatio acustica, 775
Radiatio optica, 775
Radices craniales, 836
Radices plexus, 715
Radices spinales, 836
Radices spinales n. accessorius, 681–682

Radiohumeral joint, 149f
Radioulnar joints, 191–192
  distal, 192
  proximal, 189, 191–192
Radioulnar ligament, 192
Radius, 147–150, 147f–150f, 190f. see also Elbow
  development of, 47–51, 53f
Radix cochlearis, 832
Radix dentis, 323–324
Radix dorsalis, 681, 704
Radix lateralis, 721–722
Radix linguae, 330
Radix major, of trigeminal nerve, 824–825
Radix medialis, 721–722
Radix mesenterii, 366–367
Radix minor, of trigeminal nerve, 824–825
Radix penis, 438
Radix pulmonis, 409
Radix ventralis, 681, 704
Ramus
  of mandible, 115–116, 115f
  of pubis, 160–161
Ramus externus
  of accessory nerve, 836
  of cranial laryngeal nerve, 835–836
Ramus internus
  of accessory nerve, 836
  of cranial laryngeal nerve, 835–836
R. acetabularis, 563–564
R. acromialis, 537
R. adrenales caudales, 558–559
R. adrenales craniales, 559
R. amus communicans cum ganglio ciliari, 819, 899
R. anastomoticus cum a. carotide interna, 523
R. anastomoticus cum a. carotis interna, 901
R. anastomoticus cum a. meningea media, 901
R. anastomoticus cum v. ophthalmica externa ventrali, 904
R. articularis, 748–749
R. articularis genus, 568
R. articularis temporomandibularis, 520
R. ascendens, 537, 563–564
R. auricularis, 834
R. auricularis intermedia, 517
R. auricularis lateralis, 517
R. auricularis medialis, 517
R. calcanei lateralis, 748–749
R. carpeus dorsalis, 545–546
R. carpeus palmaris, 546

R. caudalis, 568, 606
R. caudalis ossis pubis, 160–161
R. circumflexus, 506–507
R. colici, 557
R. colicus, 557, 598
R. colli, 832
R. communicans, 586f, 588f, 680f, 704, 729f
R. communicans cum n. glossopharyngeo, 834–835
R. communicans cum n. laryngeo caudali, 835–836
R. communicans cum n. mediano, 716–718
R. cranialis, 568, 600, 605–606
R. cranialis ossis pubis, 160–161
R. cranialis v. saphenae latera, 605–606
R. cricothyroideus, 513
R. cutaneous lateralis, 560
R. cutaneous medialis, 551, 560
R. cutaneus, 741–742
R. cutaneus lateralis, 728, 730, 735–736
R. cutaneus medialis, 728
R. cutaneus ventralis, 730
R. deltoideus, 537
R. descendens, 567
R. dexter lateralis, 554
R. dexter medialis, 554
R. digastricus, 831
R. dorsales, 551
R. dorsalis, 545, 560, 578, 704, 725–726
  lateral branch of, 710–711
R. dorsalis n. cervicalis I, 708
R. dorsalis n. cervicalis II, 709
R. glandularis, 516
R. glandularis zygomaticus, 524
R. ilei antimesenterialis, 367, 557
R. ilei mesenterialis, 557
R. interarcuales, 614
R. interosseus, 545–546
R. interventricularis paraconalis, 507
R. interventricularis subsinuosus, 507
R. labialis dorsalis, 576
R. labialis ventralis, 562
R. laryngeus, 507
R. laryngeus caudalis, 513
R. lateralis, 543, 720–721, 735
R. lateralis n. radialis superficialis, 724
R. lobi caudalis, 509
R. lobi cranialis, 509
R. lobi medii, 509
R. mandibulae, 115–116, 115f
R. marginalis dextra, 506
R. marginalis sinister, 507

R. medialis, 542–543, 720–721, 735
R. medialis n. radialis superficialis, 723–724
R. membranae tympani, 825–826
R. meningeus, 704
R. muscularis, 741–742, 748, 750, 753
R. muscularis distalis, 716–718
R. muscularis proximalis, 716–718
R. mylohyoideus, 520–522
R. nasalis lateralis, 815–816, 819
R. nasalis medialis, 815–816, 819
R. obturatorius, 563–564
R. occipitalis, 514, 517
R. ossis ischii, 160–161
R. palmaris, 545–546, 726
R. parotideus, 517
R. perforans distalis, 548
R. perforans proximalis, 548
R. perforans proximalis II, 569–570
R. pericardiaci, 550
R. pharyngeus, 513, 833
R. preputiales, 562–563
R. prescapularis, 537–538
R. profundus, 545–546, 563–564, 720
R. pterygoideus, 524
R. scrotalis dorsalis, 576
R. scrotalis ventralis, 562
R. septalis, 508
R. sinister, 554
R. sinistri laterales, 554
R. sinus carotici, 833
R. spinalis, 551, 560, 578
R. sternocleidomastoideus, 513, 517
R. submentalis, 588–589
R. superficialis, 545–546, 569, 720–721
R. transversus, 563–564, 567
R. transversus faciei, 825–826
R. tubarius, 559
R. uretericus, 437–438, 558–559
R. urethralis, 437–438
R. uterinus, 559
R. ventralis, 704
R. ventralis cervicalis II, 709
R. ventralis n. cervicalis I, 708–709
R. ventriculares dextri, 508
R. zygomaticus, 900
Rr. ad pontem, 531–533
Rr. alveolares superiores caudalis, 822–824
Rr. alveolares superiores medi, 822–824
Rr. alveolares superiores medii, 822–824
Rr. auricularis interni, 831

Rr. auriculars rostrales, 832
Rr. bronchiales, 549–550
Rr. buccales, 832
Rr. cardiaci, 836
Rr. centrales, 527–528
Rr. collaterales, 551
Rr. communicantes cum n. faciali, 825–826
Rr. corticales, 527–528
Rr. cutanei medialis et lateralis, 733
Rr. cutaneus dorsales, 707, 711
Rr. cutaneus medialis et lateralis, 707
Rr. cutaneus ventrales, 707
Rr. dentales, 520–522, 526
Rr. dorsales, 733, 743–744
Rr. dorsales nn. cervicales III-VII, 710
Rr. esophagei, 549–550, 556
Rr. intercostales ventrales, 536
Rr. labiales superioris, 822–824
Rr. laterales, 728, 733
Rr. lienales, 644
Rr. linguales, 833
Rr. lobi cranialis, 509
Rr. mammarii, 536, 551
Rr. mammarii laterales, 730
Rr. mammarii mediales, 730
Rr. mediales, 711, 728, 733
Rr. mediastinales, 535–536, 550
Rr. mentales, 520–522
Rr. musculares, 523, 722–723, 726, 747–748, 754
Rr. nasales externi, 815–816, 819, 822–824
Rr. nasales interni, 822–824
Rr. palatini, 515
Rr. palpebrales, 832, 900
Rr. pancreatici, 555
Rr. parotidei, 589–590, 825–826
Rr. perforantes, 536
Rr. perihyoidei, 515–516
Rr. pharyngei, 515
Rr. pharyngeui, 834–835
Rr. pterygoidei, 522
Rr. sacrales, 578
Rr. spinales, 531–533
Rr. sternales, 536
Rr. striati, 527–528
Rr. stylohyoideus, 831
Rr. thymici, 535
Rr. thyroidei, 512
Rr. tonsillares, 833
Rr. urethrales, 575
Rr. ventralis, 728–729
Raphe descending fibers, 691f
Raphe nuclei, 695
Raphe palati, 322
Raphe palpebralis lateralis, 894

Raphe reticular nuclei, 758–759
Receptive segments, of neurons, 652
Receptori, 652
Receptors
  of neurons, 652
  Pacinian-like, 177
  Ruffini-like, 177
  sensory, 653f–654f
Recess(es)
  caudal duodenal, 365
  costodiaphragmatic, 251–252, 407
  costomediastinal, 407
  elliptical, 839–840
  epitympanic, 103f
  epitympanic, 104–105, 846–847
  maxillary, 106–107, 108f, 110f, 111, 124, 125f
  mediastinal, 406–408
  of omental bursa
    caudal, 359
    dorsal, 358
    splenic, 359
  pelvic, 418–419
  piriform, 345f, 400
  spherical, 839–840
Recesses inframammillaris, 773
Recessus caudalis omentalis, 356, 359
Recessus costodiaphragmatici, 407
Recessus costodiaphragmaticus, 251–252
Recessus costomediastinales, 407
Recessus costomediastinalis, 407
Recessus dorsalis omentalis, 358–359
Recessus duodenali caudalis, 365
Recessus epitympanicus, 104–105
Recessus lateralis, 763
Recessus lienalis, 359
Recessus lumbodiaphragmaticus, 251–252
Recessus maxillaris, 106–107, 111
Recessus mediastini, 406–408
Recessus neurohypophysis, 773
Recessus opticus, 773
Recessus pelvis, 418
Recessus piriformis, 400
Rectal arteries
  caudal, 371f, 373, 573f, 575–576, 745f, 747f
    left, 373
    right, 373
  cranial, 373, 558
  middle, 438, 575
Rectal veins
  caudal, 373, 604
  cranial, 373, 598–599
  middle of, 604
Rectal venous plexus, 604

Rectogenital pouch, 355, 422–423, 452–453
Rectum, 370–371, 370f
  lymph vessels of, 638f
  special muscles of, 372–373
Rectus femoris muscle, 741f, 744f
Recurrent collateral, 658
Recurrent cranial tibial artery, 569
Recurrent laryngeal nerve, 667–668, 836
  left, 351f
  right, 351f
Recurrent ulnar artery, 718f
Red bone marrow, 90
Red nucleus, 771, 771f
Red splenic pulp, 643
Reflective layer, 867
Reflex, olfactory, 390
Reflex arcs, 658, 659f
Reflexes, 661–662
Regeneration, of muscles, 214
Regio hypochondriaca dextra, 350–351
Regio hypochondriaca sinistra, 350–351
Regio inguinalis dextra, 350–351
Regio inguinalis sinistra, 350–351
Regio lateralis dextra, 350–351
Regio lateralis sinistra, 350–351
Regio plicae lateris, 350–351
Regio pubica, 350–351
Regio umbilicalis, 350–351
Regio xiphoidea, 350–351
Regional lymph nodes, 621–622
Regiones abdominis, 351
Relay nuclei for sensory pathways, 759
Ren, 416. see also Kidney(s)
Renal arteries, 558–559
Renal artery, 420–421
Renal corpuscle, 419
Renal cortex, 418, 447
Renal crest, 418–419
Renal hilus, 418
Renal impression, 376
Renal lymph nodes, 634
Renal medulla, 418, 447
Renal papillae, 418–419
Renal pelvis, 416–418, 463
Renal plexus, 420, 450–451
Renal pyramids, 418–419
Renal sinus, 416
Renal vein, 420, 583f, 597
Reproductive organs, 423–462
Respiratory bronchioles, 403
Respiratory system, 388–415
  lymph drainage of, 619

Ret. transversum humerale, 188–189
Rete articulare cubiti, 541
Rete carpi dorsale, 542–543, 594
Rete testis, 428–430
Reticular formation, of brain, 757–759, 761f
Reticular nucleus, lateral, 764
Reticulospinal fibers, 695
Reticulospinal tract
  lateral (medullary), 759
  medial (pontine), 759
Reticulum endoplasmicum, 651–652
Retina, 775, 873
Retinaculum, flexor, 286–287
Retinaculum, transverse humeral, 188–189, 188f
Retinaculum flexorum, 193
Retinal arteries, 876, 903
Retinal veins, 876, 904
Retractor anguli oculi lateralis, 587f
Retractor clitoridis muscle, 373
Retractor penis muscle, 373, 438, 747f
Retroarticular foramen, 103f, 105, 118f–119f
Retroarticular process, 102f–103f, 105, 118f
Retroauricular muscles of Huber, 855f
Retroauricular nerve, 831
Retropharyngeal lymph center, 625–627
Retropharyngeal lymph nodes, 342
  lateral, 626–627, 626f
  medial, 322, 342–343, 345, 348, 625–626, 625f–627f
Rhinencephalon, 778–779, 781–783
Rhinos, 388
Rhombencephalic caudal projecting axons, 694–695
Rhombencephalon, 757
Rhomboid fossa, 757, 763
Rib(s), 139–140
  1st, 130f, 714f
  6th, 729f
  7th, 729f
  asternal, 139
  cervical, 131
  development of, 44, 60f
  floating, 139, 139f
  sacral, 136
  sternal, 139
Rima glottidis, 401
Rima oris, 319
Rima palpebrarum, 885
Rima pudendi, 455
Rima vestibuli, 400–401

Ring(s)
  ciliary, 869–871
  fibrous
    aortic, 500
    atrioventricular, 501
    of heart, 500
    pulmonary, 500–501
    of vertebral body, 185
  inguinal, 253
    deep, 436
    superficial, 253, 425f, 436
  scleral, 861, 871
  superficial, 436
  vaginal, 436
Root
  of clitoris, 455
  of lung, 409
  of mesentery, 366–367
  of penis, 428f, 438
  spinal, 681, 683f
  of tongue, 330
  of tooth, 323–324
Root canal, 327
Root filaments, 704
Root segment, 706f
Rootlets, 681, 704
Rostral alar foramen, 101f, 118, 118f–119f
Rostral arteries
  auricular, 518
  cerebellar, 530f
  choroidal, 527–528
  communicating, 475
  deep temporal, 524, 901f
  hypophyseal, 475–476, 527
  intercarotid, 475, 526–527
  tympanic, 522
Rostral auricular branches, 832
Rostral auricular nerves, 825–826
Rostral clinoid process, 100f, 101
Rostral colliculus, 768
Rostral commissure, 784–785
Rostral cornua, 398
Rostral crura, 850
Rostral hypothalamic nucleus, 776
Rostral intercavernous sinus, 608f
Rostral ligament, of malleus, 850
Rostral medullary velum, 763
Rostral process, 849
Rostral superior alveolar branches, 822–824
Rostral thalamic nuclei, 774
Rostrum sphenoidale, 101
Rotation, 179, 212
Rotatores muscle, 729f
Round foramen, 101–102, 121–123, 122f

Round ligaments
  of bladder, 422–423
  of uterus, 452
Rubrospinal tract, 691f, 694, 771
Ruffini endings, 177
Rugae palatinae, 321

S

Sac(s)
  anal, 80–81
  conjunctival, 887
  endolymphatic, 842
  lacrimal, fossa for, 92f, 113–114, 114f, 118, 122f
  marginal cutaneous, 851
  pericardial, 496f
  yolk, 18, 19f, 22f, 59f
Saccule, 842
Sacculi alveolares, 403
Sacculus infundibuli, 473–474
Saccus adenohypophysialis, 473–474
Saccus cutaneus marginalis, 851
Saccus lacrimalis, 890
Saccus medialis et lateralis, 199–201
Sacral artery, median, 578–579
Sacral canal, 136–137, 136f
Sacral crest, 135–136, 136f, 157f
Sacral dermatomes, 738f
Sacral foramina, 135–136, 136f
Sacral lymph nodes, 373, 635–636, 635f, 641f
Sacral nerves, 732f, 743–754
  1st, 734f
    ventral branch of, 741f
  3rd, 754f
Sacral parasympathetic nucleus, 687
Sacral parasympathetics, 670, 671f
Sacral plexus, 735, 743–744
Sacral rib, 136
Sacral vein, median, 595f, 613f
Sacral vertebrae. *see* Vertebra(e), sacral
Sacroiliac joints, 135f, 161f, 196–197
Sacroiliac ligament
  dorsal, 196–197, 197f
  ventral, 196, 197f
Sacroiliac synchondrosis, 196
Sacrotuberous ligament, 197, 197f, 292f, 371f, 745f
Sacrum, 745f. *see also* Vertebra(e), sacral
Saddle joint, 179
Sagittal crest
  of cranial cavity, 123
  external, 96–97
  internal, 96–97
  of metacarpal bone, 153f, 154
  of occipital bone, 92f

Sagittal suture, 99
Salivary glands, 320f, 338, 340–344, 340f
  lymph vessels and nodes associated with, 626f
  monostomatic sublingual, 341f, 343
Saphenous artery, 568, 742f, 751f, 753f
Saphenous nerve, 732f, 741–742, 741f–743f, 751f
Saphenous vein
  lateral, 583f, 606
  medial, 583f, 606
Sarcolemma, 210
Sarcopenia, 212
Satellite artery of the ischiatic nerve, 578
Satellite veins, 582
Scala media, 840–842
Scala tympani, 840–842
Scala vestibuli, 840–842
Scapha, 850–851
Scapula, 141–143, 141f, 716f
  development of, 47, 53f
  muscles of, 265–267, 265f, 268f–269f
  spine to, 716f
  superficial structures of, 591f
Scapular artery, circumflex, 539f, 541
Scapular cartilage, 142
Scapular notch, 141f, 142
Scapular spine, 141f, 142
Scapulohumeral joint, 144f
Schindylesis, 176
Sciatic nerve, 602f–603f, 734f, 736f, 741f, 744f–745f, 748, 749f
Sclera, 859f, 861
Scleral ring, 861, 871
Scrotal arteries, 428
Scrotal ligament, 430
Scrotal lymph nodes, 641
Scrotal septum, 424
Scrotum, 423–428, 426f
  nerves of, 428
  vessels of, 428
Scutiform cartilage, 710f, 852–853
Sebaceous glands, 80, 80f, 886
Secondary blood capillary network, 475–476
Secondary lymph, 621–622
Sectorial teeth, 327–328
Segmenta bronchopulmonalia, 402–403
Segmental bronchi, 388, 402–403
Sella turcica, 101, 121–123
Semicircular canals, 104, 840
Semicircular ducts, 842

Semilunar cusps, septal, 505
Semimembranosus muscle, 744f–745f, 747f, 749f
Seminal colliculus, 437
Seminal hillock, 443–444
Semispinalis dorsi muscle, 729f
Semispinalis muscle, 729f
Semitendinosus muscle, 744f–745f, 747f, 749f
Sensory pathways, relay nuclei for, 759
Sensory receptors, 653f–654f
Septa interalveolaria, 109–111, 115
Septa interradicularia, 110–111
Septal cartilage, of nose, 389
Septal cusp, 504
Septal mucosa, 393f, 815f
Septal nasal arteries, 525
Septal nuclei, 784
Septal olfactory organ, 394
Septal process, 110f
Septula testis, 428
Septum(a), 784–785
  dorsal intermediate, 680–681, 681f
  dorsal median, 680, 681f
  frontal sinus, 100
  interalveolar, 109–111, 115
  interatrial, 495–496, 500
  interventricular, 495–496
  nasal, 120f, 123, 389f, 391
  orbital, 884–885
  radicular, 110–111
  scrotal, 424
Septum corticomedullae, 484
Septum interatriale, 495–496, 500
Septum intermedium, 680–681
Septum interventriculare, 495–496, 504
Septum medianum dorsale, 680
Septum nasi osseum, 106, 391
Septum orbitale, 884–885
Septum pellucidum, cut edge of, 700f
Septum scroti, 424
Septum sinuum frontalium, 100
Septum sinuum sphenoidalis, 101
Serous coat
  of large intestine, 374
  of liver, 377
  of small intestine, 367
  of stomach, 362–363
Serous gustatory glands, 334
Serous membranes, 353
  lymph drainage of, 618–619
Serous pericardium, 495
Serrated suture, 176
Serratus dorsalis muscle, 239f, 242, 248f
  nerve branches to, 729f

Serratus ventralis muscle. *see* Mm. serratus ventralis cervicis and serratus ventralis thoracis
Sesamoid bone(s), 86, 88, 164–165, 213
  of abductor digiti 1 longus, 152f, 155f
  of forepaw, 151–152, 156, 281f
  of gastrocnemius muscle, 167f
  of stifle joint, 167f
  of supinator muscle tendon, 146f
Sesamoid cartilage, 397f, 400
Sesamoid impressions, 154
Sesamoidean ligaments, 194f, 195
Sex index, 95
Shearing teeth, 326f
Sheath
  bulbar, 884
  carotid, 510–511
  of optic nerve, 873
  of rectus abdominis muscle, 253–254, 253f–255f
  tendon, 213
Short bones, 88
Short ciliary nerves, 818f, 897
Short crus, 849–850
Short gastric arteries, 364, 555
Short posterior ciliary arteries, 902
Shoulder, 188–189, 188f–189f
  nerves and arteries of, 716f
  stability of, 189
  veins of, 584f
Sigmoid sinus, 607f, 608–609
Simpson, George G., 1–2
Sinoatrial node, 505
Sinus(es)
  anal, 371–372
  aortic, 505
  basilar, 607f
  carotid, 526–527
  cavernous, 609–610
  coronary, 499, 508
  dorsal interbasilar, 610
  dorsal petrosal, 609
  dorsal sagittal, 606–608
  dorsal sagittal, foramen for, 96f, 97, 123
  frontal, 99, 107–109, 108f, 120f, 122f, 124–125, 125f
    aperture to, 100
    lateral part of, 106f
    septum of, 99f, 100
  gland, 461
  intercavernous, 609–610
  lactiferous, 460–461
  maxillary, 124
  paranalis, 80–81

Sinus(es) *(Continued)*
  paranasal, 88, 124–125, 125f, 371f, 372, 394
  renal, 416, 418
  sphenoidal, 100f–101f, 107–109, 124–125
  tarsal, 170–171
  temporal, 608
  transverse, 607f, 608
    of pericardium, 495
  urogenital, 463
  venous, of spleen, 644
  ventral interbasilar, 610
  ventral occipital, 610
  ventral petrosal, 609
Sinus anales, 371–372
Sinus aortae, 505, 510
Sinus basilaris, 608–609
Sinus caroticus, 526–527
Sinus cavernosus, 609–610
Sinus coronarius, 508
Sinus frontalis, 99
Sinus interbasilaris dorsalis, 610
Sinus interbasilaris ventralis, 610
Sinus intercavernosi, 609–610
Sinus lactifer, 460
Sinus lienis, 644
Sinus paranalis, 372
Sinus petrosus dorsalis, 609
Sinus petrosus ventralis, 609
Sinus rectus, 608
Sinus renalis, 418
Sinus sagittalis dorsalis, 606–608
Sinus sigmoideus, 608–609
Sinus sphenoidalis, 107–109, 125
Sinus tarsi, 170–171
Sinus temporalis, 608
Sinus transversus, 608
Sinus transversus pericardii, 495
Sinus venarum cavarum, 499
Sinus vertebrales, 612–613
Size index, 26, 28f
Skeletal muscle fibers, 207
Skeletal muscles, 210–214. *see also specific muscles*
Skeleton, 86–175, 87f–88f, 87t. *see also* Bone(s)
  appendicular, 87t
  axial, 87t, 91–140
  cardiac, 500
  classification of, 86–91
  development of
    of carpus, 51, 53f
    of girdles, 44–51
    of pelvic limb, 44–51, 54f–56f
    of ribs, 44, 60f
    of skull, 27–35, 33f–45f

Skeleton (Continued)
    of sternum, 44, 49f–51f
    of thoracic limb, 44–47, 52f–53f
    of vertebral column, 35–44, 46f–49f
  fetal, 89
  heterotopic, 87t
Skin, 64
  blood supply to, 81–82, 81f
  dermis of, 64–65
    structure of, changes with age and, 65–66
  digital pads, 66–69, 68f
  epidermis of, 64–65
  function of, 64
  glands of, 79–81
  grafting of, 82
  hairy, 69–79, 69f
    surface contour of, 78–79, 80f
  immunosurveillance potential of, 64
  lymph drainage of, 618
  muscles of, 79
  nasal, 67, 67f
  nerve supply to, 82, 653f
  pigmentation of, 66–67
  senile changes in, 66
  subcutis of, 64–65
  tension lines of, 65–66, 66f
Skull, 91–125
  apex of, 121
  arteries of, 528f
  base of, 528f
  bones of, 96b
    basisphenoid, 29–32, 38f, 40f, 92f, 96f, 100f–101f, 101–102, 117f, 120f
    craniometry of, 93–94, 93f
    dorsal aspect of, 92f
    ethmoid, 106–109, 106f–108f, 117f, 120f
    frontal, 91f–92f, 96f, 99–100, 116f–117f
    incisive, 91f–92f, 96f, 109–110, 109f, 116f–117f, 120f
    lacrimal, 91f–92f, 113–114, 114f, 116f–117f
    lateral aspect, 91f, 118f
    lateral surface of, 117–118
    maxilla, 91f–92f, 96f, 107f–108f, 110–111, 110f, 116f–117f, 120f
    nasal, 91f–92f, 96f, 108f, 110, 110f, 116f–117f, 120f
    occipital, 91f–92f, 95–98, 96f, 116f
    palatine, 91f–92f, 96f, 112–113, 116f–117f, 120f

Skull (Continued)
    parietal, 91f–92f, 98–99, 98f, 116f
    pterygoid, 91f–92f, 96f, 114, 114f, 117f, 120f
    sphenoid, 91f, 100–102, 100f–101f
    temporal, 91f–92f, 102–106, 102f–103f, 116f–117f, 120f
    ventral aspect of, 92f, 119f
    vomer, 92f, 96f, 106f, 108f, 114–115, 114f, 117f, 120f
    zygomatic, 91f–92f, 112, 112f, 116f–117f, 120f
  capacity of, 95
  caudal surface of, 121
  cavities of, 121–125
    cranial, 121–123, 122f
    nasal, 107f, 123–124
    paranasal sinuses, 88, 124–125, 125f
  development of, 27–35, 33f–45f
  dorsal surface of, 117
    cranial part of, 117
    facial part of, 117
  indices for, 95, 95t
  joints of, 179–181, 179f–180f, 182f–183f
  lateral surface of
    cranial part of, 117–118
    facial part of, 118
  ligaments of, 179–181
  nerves of, 528f
  sutures of, 181
  synchondroses of, 180–181
  ventral surface of, 118–121
    cranial part of, 118–120
Slips, of muscle, 212
Small intestine, 360f, 364–368
  ascending portion of, 365
  attachments and peritoneal relations, 365
  coats of, 367
  cranial portion of, 365
  descending portion of, 365
  lymph vessels of, 637f
  mesentery of, 366–367
  nerves of, 367–368
  position of, 366
  transverse portion of, 365
  vessels of, 367
Small median vein, 593
Smooth muscle fibers, 207
Smooth muscles, 207
Smooth-Haired Dachshund, 8
Snout index, 95t

Soft palate, 228f–230f, 230–231, 321, 321f, 344f, 396f
  epithelium, 322
  lymph vessels of, 625f
  structure of, 322
Solitary lymph nodules, 370–371, 620–621
Solitary tract, 757–758, 764
Somatic muscle, 207
Somatic plexuses, 660, 706–707
Somatosensory area, 788
Spaces
  episcleral, 884
  interarcuate, of vertebra, 126
  intercostal, 139, 139f
  interdental, 110–111
  interosseous
    of fibula and tibia, 165f
    of metacarpus, 195
Spatia interossea metacarpi, 195
Spatia zonularia, 872
Spatium episclerale, 884
Spatium interarcuale, 126
Spatium interarcuale atlantooccipitale, 127–130
Spatium intercostale, 139
Special visceral efferent, 758
Spermatic cord, 423, 436–437
Spermatic fascia, 424
  external, 437
  internal, 437
Spermatozoa, 13
Sphenoethmoid lamina, 113
Sphenoethmoidal suture, 102, 109
Sphenofrontal suture, 100–102
Sphenoid bone, 91f, 100–102, 100f–101f
Sphenoid sinus, 125
Sphenoidal crest, 121
Sphenoidal fossa, 106f
Sphenoidal process, 113, 113f
Sphenoidal septum, longitudinal, 101
Sphenoidal sinus, 100f–101f, 107–109, 124
Sphenoidal spine, 100f, 101–102
Sphenooccipital joint, 98
Sphenooccipital synchondrosis, 32, 43f, 102
Sphenopalatine artery, 525
Sphenopalatine foramen, 108f, 113, 113f, 118, 118f, 122f, 124
Sphenopalatine suture, 101–102
Sphenopalatine vein, 586f
Sphenoparietal suture, 101
Sphenosquamosal suture, 105–106
Sphenosquamous suture, 102
Spherical recess, 839–840

Sphincter
- anal
  - external, 371f, 372–373
  - internal, 371f, 372–374
- cardiac, 363
- cecal, 368–369
- muscles, of iris, 872
- pyloric, 363

Sphincter ampullae
- hepatopancreaticae, 380

Sphincter ceci, 368–369
Sphincter colli profundus, 79, 216
Sphincter colli superficialis, 79
Sphincteric muscle, 365–366
Sphincters, of ducts, 461
Spina alaris, 158
Spina helicis, 851
Spina iliaca dorsalis caudalis, 158
Spina iliaca dorsalis cranialis, 158
Spina iliaca ventralis cranialis, 158
Spina ischiadica, 160–161
Spina ossis sphenoidalis, 101–102
Spina scapulae, 142
Spinal accessory nerve, 836
Spinal artery, ventral, 531–533
Spinal cord, 650, 657, 679–703, 680f, 706f, 729f
- caudal projecting tracts, 693–695
- cranial projecting tracts, 689–693, 690b, 691f, 692b
- dura mater, 699
- efferent neurons of, 685
- embryonic, 758f
- general functions of, 679
- gray matter of, 658f, 685–688, 686f
- interneurons of, 685
- juncture with brain, 762f
- morphologic features of, 679–681, 680f–681f
- projection neurons of, 685
- regions, 683
- reticular formation, 688
- segment and root length, 684f
- segmental relationships to vertebrae, 683, 684f
- segments of, 681–683, 682f–683f, 759f
- terminal, 683f
- transected segments, 697f
- transverse sections of, 696
- veins of, 611–614
- white matter of, 658f, 688–695, 689f

Spinal dura mater filament, 682–683
Spinal ganglia, 680f, 704, 705f–706f

Spinal nerves, 650, 680f, 704–756, 705f
- cutaneous branches
  - dorsal, 705f
  - ventral, 705f
- dorsal branches of, 707f
- dorsal root, 680f, 704, 705f–706f, 729f
- dorsal rootlets, 680f, 689f, 706f
- general features of, 706–707
- initial or primary branches of, 705–706
- lateral branches of, 707f
- longitudinal segments of, 706f
- peripheral branches of, 662
- trunks, 706f
- ventral branches of, 707f
- ventral root, 680f, 704, 705f–706f, 729f
- ventral rootlets, 680f, 706f

Spinal reflexes, 695–696, 695f
Spinal roots, 681, 683f, 836
- length of, 684f

Spinal tract, of trigeminal nerve, 758, 761, 762f
- nucleus of, 758, 761

Spinalis cervicis muscle, 710f
Spinalis muscle, 729f
Spine
- alar, 158
- of helix, 851
- iliac, 158, 158f–159f
- ischiatic, 158, 158f–160f, 160–161
- nasal
  - caudal, 112–113, 119f
  - of palatine bone, 119f
- scapular, 141f, 142, 145f
- sphenoidal, 100f, 101–102

Spinocervicothalamic tract, 691f, 692
Spinocuneocerebellar pathway, 692
Spinomedullary junction, 759–761
Spinomedullary tract, 691f, 693
Spinomesencephalic tract, 691f, 693
Spinoolivary tract axons, 693
Spinopontine axons, 693
Spinopontine fibers, 691f
Spinoreticular tract, 691f, 693
Spinotectal tract, 693
Spinothalamic tract, 691f, 692
Spinous foramen, 119f
Spinous process, 126
- of axis, 127f, 129f, 130
- of caudal vertebrae, 137f
- of cervical vertebrae, 129f, 131
- of lumbar vertebrae, 133f–135f
- of sacral vertebrae, 136f
- of thoracic vertebrae, 131–132, 132f–133f

Spinovestibular tract, 693
Spiral cribriform tract, 103
Spiral decussation, 346f
Spiral lamina, 840–842
Spiral organ, 844–846
Splanchnic nerves, 367–368, 379
Spleen, 357f, 642–644
- blood supply in, 555f, 643f
- borders of, 643
- dorsal extremity of, 643
- functions of, 644

Splenic artery, 382, 555
Splenic lymph nodes, 348, 378–379, 383, 635f, 638f, 639
Splenic vein, 583f, 599
Splenius muscle, 710f
Spongy bone, 90
Sporting breeds, 7f
Squama frontalis, 100
Squama occipitalis, 96–97
Squamosal suture, 101, 105–106
Squamous suture, 176
Stalk
- of epiglottis, 397–398
- optic, 858

Stapedial membrane, 850
Stapedial nerve, 830–831
Stapes, 849f, 850
Statoconia, 843–844
Statoconiorum membrane, 843–844
Stellate veins, 420
Stensen canal, 390–391
Sternal lymph nodes, cranial, 628
Sternal membrane, 187, 188f
Sternebrae, 140
Sternocephalicus, 340f, 709f
Sternocostal joints, 187, 187f–188f
Sternocostal radiate ligaments, 187, 187f–188f
Sternum, 139f, 140, 729f
- development of, 44, 49f–51f
- manubrium of, 139f, 140

Stifle joint, 164–165, 198–202, 198f–200f
- fascia of, 312–313
- ligaments of, 201–202
- nerves and arteries of, 742f
- sesamoid bones of, 167f

Stockard, Charles R., 4
Stomach, 359–364, 359f–360f
- cardiac part of, 362
- circular layer of, 363
- coats of, 362–363
- curvatures of, 361–362
- glands of, 363–364
- longitudinal layer of, 363
- lymph vessels of, 638f

Stomach (Continued)
   musculature of, 361f
   nerves of, 364
   pyloric part of, 360f–361f, 362
   regions of, 362
   shape, position, and capacity of, 362
   vessels of, 364
Stop, 117
Straight seminiferous tubules, 428–430
Straight sinus, 608, 700f
Stratum basale
   of digital pads, 68–69, 83
   of hairy skin, 78–79
Stratum circulare, 363, 367, 374
Stratum corneum
   of digital pads, 68–69
   of hairy skin, 78–79
Stratum granulosum
   of digital pads, 68–69, 83
   of hairy skin, 78–79
Stratum longitudinale, 363, 367, 374
Stratum lucidum
   of digital pads, 83
   of hairy skin, 78–79
Stratum lucidum, of digital pads, 68–69
Stratum spinosum
   of digital pads, 68–69
   of hairy skin, 78–79
Stratum spongiosum, 444
Stria acustica, 765
Stria habenularis thalami, 778
Stria mallearis, 846
Stria terminalis, 776, 784
Stria vascularis, 842
Striated muscle, 207
Stroma (stroma iridis), 872
Stroma vitreum, 879
Styloglossus muscle, 335, 335f, 344f
Stylohyoid bone, 116f, 117, 227f–228f
Stylohyoid cartilage, 33, 39f, 44f
Stylohyoideum, 116f, 117
Stylohyoideus branch, 831
Styloid process
   of ear, 851–852
   of radius, 147f, 149–150
   of ulna, 151
Stylomastoid artery, 517
Stylomastoid foramen, 103f, 104–105, 118f–119f
Stylopharyngeal branch, 833
Subarachnoid space, 681f, 699, 700f
Subatrial papillary muscle, 503–504
Subauricular papillary muscle, 503–504

Subcallosal fasciculus, 788
Subclavian artery, 531–538
   left, 531, 584f
Subclavian vein, 584f
Subcommissural organ, 773
Subcutaneous plexus, 81, 81f
Subcutis, 64–65
Subfornical organ, 773
Sublingual artery, 338, 343, 516, 516f
Sublingual caruncle, 320–321, 343
Sublingual fold, 321
Sublingual ganglion, 343, 665
Sublingual glands, 340f, 343
Sublingual nerve, 826–828
Sublingual vein, 588
Subluxations, of synovial joint, 178
Submental artery, 516
Submental vein, 588
Submucous coat
   of esophagus, 348
   of large intestine, 374
   of small intestine, 367
   of stomach, 363
Suboccipital nerve, 708
Subpapillary plexus, 81–82
Subscapular artery, 538f, 539, 714f, 716f
Subscapular fossa, 141f, 142
Subscapular nerve, 705f, 713f–715f, 715
Subscapular vein, 584f
Subscapularis muscle. see M. subscapularis
   nerve to, 713f–714f, 716f
Subserosal lymph vessels, 634f, 638f
Subsinuosal interventricular groove, 495–496
Substantia alba, 679, 757
Substantia chromatophilia, 651–652
Substantia compacta, 89–90
Substantia corticalis, 89–90
Substantia gelatinosa, 687–688
Substantia grisea, 679, 757
Substantia grisea centralis, 767–768
Substantia intermedia centralis, 679
Substantia intermedia lateralis, 679
Substantia nigra, 770
Substantia spongiosa, 90
Subthalamic nucleus, 778
Subthalamus, 758t, 778
Sulci cerebri, 779
Sulcus, 779, 780f
   calcanean, 170–171
   carotid, 100f
   dorsal, 109–110
   dorsal intermediate, 680–681, 681f
   dorsal median, 680

Sulcus (Continued)
   dorsolateral, 680–681
   for middle meningeal artery, 99, 101–102
   optic, 858
   palatine, 111, 119f
   for short auditory tube, 101–102
   transverse, 97, 99
   for transverse sinus, 96f, 97
   for ventral petrosal sinus, 96f, 97–98
Sulcus arteriae meningeae mediae, 101–102
Sulcus calcanei, 170–171
Sulcus chiasmatis, 100f, 101, 121, 122f
Sulcus coronarius, 498
Sulcus costae, 140
Sulcus extensorius, 165–167
Sulcus intermedius dorsalis, 680–681
Sulcus intertubercularis, 143
Sulcus interventricularis paraconalis, 495–496, 498–499
Sulcus interventricularis subsinuosus, 495–496, 498–499
Sulcus lateralis dorsalis, 680–681
Sulcus lateralis ventralis, 680–681
Sulcus limitans, 763
Sulcus m. brachialis, 145–146
Sulcus medianus, 763
Sulcus medianus dorsalis, 680
Sulcus medianus linguae, 330
Sulcus palatinus, 111
Sulcus rhinalis lateralis, 781
Sulcus rhinalis medialis, 781
Sulcus septi nasi, 109–110
Sulcus sinus petrosi ventralis, 97–98
Sulcus sinus transversi, 97, 123
Sulcus tendinum mm. extensoris digitorum lateralis et fibularis brevis, 168
Sulcus terminalis, 500
Sulcus tubae auditivae, 101–102
Sulcus urethrae, 439
Sulcus venae cavae, 375
Sulcus venae cavae caudalis, 411
Sulcus ventriculi, 362
Sulcus vomeris, 114
Superficial arteries
   brachial, 538f, 591f, 713f, 717f–720f
   cervical, 584f, 714f
   of forepaw, 547f
   of hindpaw, 571f
   palmar arch, 546
   radial, 541–542
   temporal, 518, 901

Superficial branch, 720–721, 725f, 726
Superficial cervico-auriculo-occipitalis of Huber, 854f
Superficial digital flexor muscle. *see* M. flexor digitorum superficialis
Superficial epithelium, of ovary, 447
Superficial fascia
   muscular, 884
   perineal, 374
Superficial gland of third eyelid, 890
Superficial gluteus muscle, 741f, 744f–745f, 747f
Superficial inguinal lymph node, 740f
Superficial inguinal ring, 740f
Superficial lymph nodes
   cervical, 618f, 627, 627f
   inguinal, 442, 444–445, 602f–603f, 641, 641f
   popliteal, 640
Superficial lymph vessels, 618f, 640
Superficial nerves
   fibular, 732f, 736f, 739f, 742f, 749–750, 749f, 751f
   of neck, 709f
   perineal, 428, 737f, 740f
   radial
     lateral branch, 713f, 724
     medial branch, 713f, 718f, 720f, 723–724, 727f
Superficial palmar arterial arch, 725f
Superficial pectoral muscle, 705f, 713f
Superficial ramus
   lateral branch, 717f
   medial branch, 717f
Superficial veins
   brachial, 592f, 593
   cervical, 584f
   circumflex iliac, 600–601
   dorsal arch, 605–606
   of glans, 441, 444, 602f–603f
   of head, 586f
   of hind limb, 599f
   palmar arch, 591
   of pelvic limb, 599–600
   temporal, 583f, 588f, 589
   of thoracic limb, 591–593
Superior dental arch, 325
Superior labial artery, 517
Superior labial branches, 822–824
Superior labial veins, 587, 587f
Superior longitudinal fasciculus, 788
Superior palpebral artery, lateral, 518
Superior tarsal muscle, 885
Supinator muscle, 713f, 717f
   nerve to, 719f
Suprachiasmatic nucleus, 776

Suprachoroid, 867
Supraclavicular nerves, 711
Supracondylar crest, lateral, 143f–144f, 146
Supracondylar tuberosity, of femur, 162f, 164
Supraglenoid tubercle, 141f, 144f
Supraglenoid tuberosity, 142–143
Supramastoid crest, 105
Supraoccipital bone, 28–29, 39f–40f, 96f, 117f
Supraoptic nucleus, 776
Supraopticohypophyseal tract, 776
Supraorbital nerve, 819
Suprapineal recess, III ventricle, 700f
Suprascapular artery, 537, 593f, 716f
Suprascapular nerve, 705f, 713f–716f, 715
Supraspinatus muscle, 265–266, 269f
   nerve to, 713f–714f, 716f
Supraspinous fossa, 141f, 142
Supraspinous ligament, 184, 184f, 187f
Supratrochlear foramen, 143f, 146
Supratrochlear nerve, 819
Supraventricular crest, 501–502
Supreme intercostal vein, 583
Sural arteries, 569
Surface(s)
   of acetabulum, 156–158
   of atlas, 127–130, 127f
   of axis, 127f
   buccal, 115
   of calcaneus, 169–170
   of femur, 163–164
   of fibula, 168
   of hip, 156–158
   of humerus, 143f, 145
   of iliac wing, 158–160
   of ilium, 127f, 157f, 158–160
   of lacrimal bone, 114, 114f
   laryngeal, 397–398
   of mandible, 115
   of radius, 147–148, 147f–148f
   of sacrum, 131, 136f, 141, 141f
   of the skull
     dorsal, 117
     lateral, 117–118
     ventral, 118–121
   of tibia, 165–167
   of ulna, 151
Suspensory ligament, of ovary, 447
Sustentaculum tali, 168f, 170–171, 170f–171f
Sutura, 176
Sutura coronalis, 99
Sutura ethmoidomaxillaris, 109, 111
Sutura foliata, 176

Sutura frontoethmoidalis, 100, 109
Sutura frontolacrimalis, 100, 114
Sutura frontomaxillaris, 99–100, 111
Sutura frontonasalis, 100, 110
Sutura frontopalatina, 100
Sutura incisivomaxillaris, 109–110
Sutura interfrontalis, 100
Sutura interincisiva, 109–110
Sutura intermandibularis, 115–116, 180
Sutura internasalis, 110
Sutura lacrimoethmoidalis, 109
Sutura lacrimomaxillaris, 111, 114
Sutura lacrimozygomatica, 112, 114
Sutura lambdoidea, 98
Sutura maxilloincisiva, 111
Sutura nasoethmoidalis, 109–110
Sutura nasoincisiva, 109–110
Sutura nasomaxillaris, 110–111
Sutura occipitomastoidea, 98
Sutura occipitoparietalis, 99
Sutura occipitosquamosa, 98
Sutura occipitotympanica, 98
Sutura palatina mediana, 111, 113
Sutura palatina transversa, 113
Sutura palatoethmoidalis, 109
Sutura palatolacrimalis, 114
Sutura palatomaxillaris, 111
Sutura parietointerparietalis, 99
Sutura parietosphenoidalis, 99
Sutura petrooccipitalis, 98
Sutura plana, 176
Sutura pterygopalatina, 114
Sutura pterygosphenoidalis, 102, 114
Sutura sagittalis, 99
Sutura serrata, 176
Sutura sphenoethmoidalis, 102, 109
Sutura sphenofrontalis, 100–102
Sutura sphenopalatina, 101–102
Sutura sphenoparietalis, 101–102
Sutura sphenosquamosa, 102, 105–106
Sutura squamosa, 99, 101, 105–106, 176
Sutura temporozygomatica, 105–106, 112
Sutura vomeroethmoidalis, 109, 114–115
Sutura vomeroincisiva, 109–110, 114–115
Sutura vomeromaxillaris, 111, 114–115
Sutura vomeropalatina dorsalis, 114–115
Sutura vomeropalatina ventralis, 114–115
Sutura vomerosphenoidalis, 102, 114–115

Sutura zygomaticomaxillaris, 111–112
Suturae capitis, 181
Suture(s), 176
  ethmoidomaxillary, 109, 111
  foliate, 176
  frontal, 100
  frontoethmoidal, 109
  frontolacrimal, 100, 114
  frontomaxillary, 99–100, 111
  frontonasal, 100, 110
  frontopalatine, 100
  frontoparietal, 100
  incisivomaxillary, 109–110, 110f
  interincisive, 109–110
  intermandibular, 115–116
  internasal, 110
  lacrimoethmoidal, 109
  lacrimomaxillary, 111, 114
  lacrimozygomatic, 112, 114
  lambdoid, 98
  maxilloincisive, 111
  median palatine, 111
  nasoethmoidal, 109–110
  nasoincisive, 109–110
  nasomaxillary, 110–111
  occipitomastoid, 98
  occipitosquamous, 98
  palatine, 121
    median, 113
    transverse, 113
  palatoethmoid, 109
  palatolacrimal, 114
  palatomaxillary, 111
  parietointerparietal, 99
  parietosphenoidal, 99
  petrooccipital, 98
  plane, 176
  pterygopalatine, 114
  pterygosphenoid, 102, 114
  sagittal, 99
  serrated, 176
  of skull, 181
  sphenoethmoidal, 102, 109
  sphenofrontal, 100–102
  sphenopalatine, 101–102
  sphenoparietal, 101–102
  sphenosquamosal, 105–106
  sphenosquamous, 102
  squamous, 99, 101, 105–106, 76
  temporozygomatic, 105–106, 112
  vomeroethmoid, 109, 114–115
  vomeroincisive, 109–110, 114–115
  vomeromaxillary, 111, 114–115
  vomeropalatine
    dorsal, 114–115
    ventral, 114–115

Suture(s) *(Continued)*
  vomerosphenoid, 102, 114–115
  zygomaticomaxillary, 111–112
Sweat glands
  atrichial, 79, 80f
  epitrichial, 79–80, 80f
Swellings, of tongue
  lateral, 329, 330f
  median proximal, 329
Sympathetic ganglion, 729f
Sympathetic nervous system, 664f, 671–675
Sympathetic trunk, 671, 705f–706f
Sympathetic trunk ganglia, 671, 680f
Symphysis
  ischial, 196
  pelvic, 156–158, 157f, 196
  pubis, 156–158, 157f
Symphysis ischiadica, 196
Symphysis ischii, 156–158, 157f
Symphysis pelvis, 156–158, 196, 743f
Symphysis pubica, 196
Symphysis pubis, 156–158
Synapses, 655f
Synarthrosis, 176
Synchondroses cranii, 180–181
Synchondrosis(es), 176
  intersphenoidal, 43f, 102
  petrooccipital, 105–106
  sacroiliac, 196
  sphenooccipital, 32, 43f, 102
Synchondrosis intersphenoidalis, 102
Synchondrosis intraoccipitalis basilateralis, 97–98
Synchondrosis intraoccipitalis squamolateralis, 97
Synchondrosis petrooccipitalis, 98, 105–106
Synchondrosis sacroiliaca, 196
Synchondrosis sphenooccipitalis, 98, 102
Syndesmosis, 176
Syndesmosis tympanostapedia, 180
Synergists, 212–213
Synostosis, 176–177
Synovia, 177–178
Synovial fluid, 177–178
Synovial fold, 177
Synovial membrane, 177
Synovial sheath, 894
Synovial tendon sheaths, 213
Synovial villi, 177
Systema nervosum, 650
Systema nervosum centrale, 650
Systema nervosum periphericum, 650

T

Tabula ossis ischii, 160–161
Tactile hairs, 319
Taenia choroidea, 701
Tail (anatomic part), of epididymis, 435
Tail (body part)
  arteries of, 577f
  fasciae of, 262–263
  glands of, 80f, 81
  muscles of, 258–262, 259f–260f
Talocalcaneal central joints, 202–203
Talus, 169–170, 169f
Tapetum, 867, 868f
Tapetum lucidum, 867
Tapetum lucidum cellulosum, 867
Tapetum lucidum fibrosum, 867
Tarsal arteries, 569–570
Tarsal bones
  central, 169f, 171
  first, 169f, 171
  fourth, 169f, 171–172
  second, 169f, 171
  third, 169f, 171
Tarsal extensor retinaculum, 204–205
Tarsal glands, 80, 886
Tarsal joints, 202–205, 203f–204f
Tarsal sinus, 170–171
Tarsal vein, 606
Tarsocrural joints, 171f, 202–203
Tarsometatarsal joints, 171f, 202–203
Tarsus, 169–172
  eyelid, 886–887
Taste buds, 331f, 333
Tectonuclear tract, 768
Tectorial lamina, 106f
Tectum, 758t, 768
Teeth, 323–329, 323f
  anomalies, 329
  canine, 107f, 120f, 326f, 327
    permanent, 110f
  carnassial, 327–328
  cheek, 327
  deciduous, 323–324, 324f
    formula for, 328
  development of, 33–35, 34f, 45f
  direction along, 327
  eruption of, 325t
  groupings of, 327–328
  incisor, 109f, 326f, 327
    eruption of, 325t
  molar, 323f, 328
    development of, 108f, 119f
    eruption of, 325t
  permanent, 324, 324f
    formula for, 328

Teeth (Continued)
    premolar, 327
        development of, 107f–108f, 120f
        eruption of, 325t
    sectorial, 327–328
    shearing, 326f
    structure of, 325–327
    supernumerary, 329
    surfaces of, 327
Tegmen ventriculi quarti, 763
Tegmentum mesencephali, 770
Tegmentum pontis, 766
Tela choroidea, 701, 763, 773
Tela choroidea ventriculi quarti, 763
Tela choroidea ventriculi tertii, 773
Tela subcutanea, 64–65
Tela submucosa, 348, 363, 367, 374
Tela subserosa, 362–363, 377
Telencephalic caudal projection axons, 694
Telencephalon, 658, 757, 758f, 758t, 777f, 779f
Telodendron, 650
Telogen, 69, 76, 76f
Temporal arteries
    caudal deep, 522
    rostral deep, 524, 901f
    superficial, 518, 587f, 901
        masseteric branch, 518
Temporal bone, 91f–92f, 102–106, 102f–103f, 116f–117f, 120f
    petrosal part of, 102–103, 102f, 831f, 847f
    squamous part of, 102f–103f, 106
    tympanic part of, 102f, 105
    zygomatic process of, 92f, 102f–103f, 120f
Temporal canal, 105
Temporal fossa, 98–99
Temporal lines, 92f, 98–100
Temporal meatus, 123
Temporal process, of zygomatic bone, 112, 112f
Temporal sinus, 607f
Temporal vein
    superficial, 342, 583f, 588f, 589
    temporal, 342
Temporal wing, 100f–101f
Temporomandibular joint, 105, 179–180, 179f–180f
Temporozygomatic suture, 105–106, 112
Tendo calcaneus, 294, 308
Tendo cricoesophageus, 347
Tendo prepubicus, 253f–254f, 254

Tendon(s), 211–212
    abdominal, 252–258, 253f–254f
    of abductor digit I longus, 194f
    biceps, 188f
    calcanean (Achilles), 294, 308
    central, of diaphragm, 250
    cricoesophageal, 347
    of long digital extensor, 199f
    pelvic, 253, 253f–254f
    of popliteus, 199f
    prepubic, 253f–254f, 254
    of quadriceps, 199f
Tendon sheath, 213
Tenia ventriculi quarti, 763
Tenon capsule, 884
Tension lines, 65–66, 66f
Tensor fasciae antebrachii muscle, 713f–714f, 718f, 720f
Tensor fasciae latae muscle, 744f
Tensor tympani nerve, 825
Tensor veli palatini, 322, 323f
Tensor veli palatini nerve, 825
Tentorium cerebelli, 699
Tentorium cerebelli membranaceum, 699
Tentoriumcerebelli osseum, 99
Teres major muscle, 265f–268f, 713f–714f
    nerve to, 716f
Teres minor muscle, 265f–266f, 713f
    nerve to, 716f
Terminal filament, 682–683
Terminal line, 156–158, 352–353
Terminal spinal cord, 683f
Terminal ventricle, 679
Terminationes folliculi pili, 652
Terminationes nervi libera, 652
Terminationes neuromusculi, 654
Terrier breeds, 9f
Testes, 423, 428–435
    anomalies of, 431–432
    attachments to, 430
    descent of, 433–435
    endocrine tissues of, 489
    nerves of, 430–431
    structure of, 426f
    vessels of, 430–431
Testicles, lymph vessels of, 642f
Testicular artery, 430–431, 559
Testicular bursa, 435
Testicular plexus, 431
Testicular tumors, 431–432
Testicular veins, 430–431, 583f
    left, 597
    right, 597
Thalamic adhesion, 772–773

Thalamostriate vein, 610–611
Thalamus, 758t, 773–774, 773f
Thebesian veins, 509
Thigh
    arteries and veins of, 564f
    muscles of, 287–302, 310f
        caudal, 290f–292f, 294–297, 296f, 299f–301f, 305f
        cranial, 290f–292f, 296f, 297–298, 298f–301f
        medial, 290f–292f, 295f, 298f–301f, 299–302
Third eyelid, 887–888
    gland of, 887f
    superficial gland of, 890
Third ventricle, 700–701, 700f, 758t, 772–773
    suprapineal recess, 700f
Thoracic aorta, 548–551, 584f
    branches of, 549–550
Thoracic arteries
    internal, 534f–535f, 535
    lateral, 593f
Thoracic cage, 404f, 409f
Thoracic cavity, 404–405, 404f, 633f
Thoracic duct, 584f, 622–623, 622f–623f
Thoracic girdle, development of, 44–47, 52f–53f
Thoracic inlet, 405
Thoracic limb, 140–156
    arteries of, 531–538
    brachial plexus
        that supply extrinsic muscles of, nerves of, 727–728
        that supply intrinsic muscles of, nerves of, 715–723
    development of, 44–47, 52f–53f
    fasciae of, 286–287
    joints of, 188–196
    ligaments of, 188–196
    lymph nodes and vessels of, 628
    muscles of, 241–242, 263–287
        antebrachial, 270f–271f, 273–285, 273f–282f
        brachial, 269–273
        extrinsic, 239f, 241–242, 248f, 263–265, 270f
        intrinsic, 265–269, 265f–269f
    right, nerves of, 713f
    veins of, 591–595
        deep, 593–594
        superficial, 591–593
Thoracic lymph center, dorsal, 630–631
Thoracic muscle, 729f

Thoracic nerves, 728–731
  cutaneous areas, 731*f*
  cutaneous branches of, 730*f*
  distribution of, 729*f*
  lateral cutaneous branches of, 730*f*
  medial cutaneous branches of, 730*f*
  sixth, 729*f*
  thirteenth, ventral branch, 732*f*
Thoracic region, sympathetic distribution of, 667*f*, 673
Thoracic vertebrae. *see* Vertebra(e), thoracic
Thoracic vertebral artery, 534–535
Thoracic vertebral vein, 612*f*
Thoracic wall
  fascia of, 252
  muscles of, 239*f*, 248–252, 248*f*–250*f*
Thoracodorsal artery, 538*f*, 539, 543*f*, 716*f*
Thoracodorsal nerve, 705*f*, 713*f*–714*f*, 728
Thoracodorsal vein, 593*f*
Thoracolumbar system, 663
Thorax, 405*f*–406*f*, 410*f*
  arteries of, 510–548, 532*f*–533*f*
  cranial, 405*f*
  lymph nodes and vessels of, 628–633
  muscles of, 239*f*, 248–252, 248*f*–250*f*
  skeleton in, 139–140
Thymocyte, 646
Thymus gland, 644–646, 645*f*
  arterial supply of, 535*f*
  left lobe of, 646
  right lobe of, 646
Thyroarytenoideus, 398*f*
Thyroglossal duct, 478
Thyrohyoid bone, 116, 116*f*, 227*f*–228*f*
Thyrohyoid cartilage, 33
Thyrohyoideus, 340*f*
Thyroid arteries, 348
Thyroid cartilage, 116*f*, 345*f*–346*f*, 397*f*, 398
Thyroid diverticulum, 478
Thyroid fissure, 399
Thyroid gland, 476–480, 477*f*–478*f*
  developmental anatomy, 478–479
  innervation, 480
  macroscopic features, 476–477, 477*f*–478*f*
  mesoscopic features, 477–478, 477*f*–478*f*
  microscopic features, 479
  vascularization, 477*f*–478*f*, 479–480

Thyroid notch, caudal, 399
Thyroid veins
  caudal, 584*f*–585*f*, 585
  cranial, 585–586, 585*f*, 588*f*
  middle, 585–586, 585*f*
Tibia, 165–167, 165*f*–167*f*, 742*f*
  development of, 51, 54*f*–56*f*
Tibial ligament
  of lateral meniscus, 201
  of medial meniscus, 200*f*, 201
Tibial nerve, 602*f*–603*f*, 732*f*, 742*f*, 744*f*, 749*f*, 751–752, 751*f*, 753*f*
  superficial branch, 753*f*
Tibial tuberosity, 165*f*–167*f*
Tibialis caudalis muscle, nerve to, 742*f*
Tibialis cranialis muscle, nerve to, 742*f*
Tibiofibular joints, 202
  distal, 202
  proximal, 202
Tissue(s)
  adipose, subcutis, 66
  connective, 213
  lymphoid, 620–621
Tongue, 329–340, 330*f*–332*f*, 335*f*, 337*f*
  anomalies of, 339–340
  apex of, 330, 337*f*
  bird tongue, 339, 339*f*
  blood vessels of, 338
  body of, 330
  glands of, 338
  innervation of, 829*f*
  lymph vessels of, 625*f*
  margin of, 330–331
  muscle fibers of
    deep, 336–337, 336*f*–337*f*
    superficial, 336, 337*f*
  muscles of, 227–229, 227*f*–229*f*, 232*f*, 334–337, 335*f*–336*f*
  nerves supply of, 338–340, 338*f*
  oversized, 339–340, 339*f*
  papillae of
    conical, 334
    filiform, 331–332, 331*f*
    foliate, 334
    fungiform, 331–333, 331*f*
    marginal, 332*f*, 334
    vallate, 330, 331*f*–332*f*
  parts of, 329, 330*f*
  root of, 330, 337*f*
  swellings of
    lateral, 329, 330*f*
    median proximal, 329
Tongue bud, median, 329, 330*f*
Tonsil
  lingual, 345
  palatine, 340*f*, 344–345

Tonsilla lingualis, 345
Tonsilla palatina, 344–345
Tonsillar artery, 344*f*, 345
Tonsillar branches, 833
Tonsillar fold, 344–345
Tonsillar fossa, 344–345
Tooth. *see* Teeth
Toruli tactiles, 78, 78*f*, 652
Torus digitalis, 67–68, 68*f*
Touch spots, 78, 78*f*
Toy breeds, 10*f*
Trabecula septomarginalis dextra, 503
Trabeculae, 643
Trabeculae carneae, 503
Trabeculae lienis, 643
Trabeculum septomarginalis sinistrae, 503–504
Trachea, 116*f*, 345*f*, 388, 396*f*–397*f*, 402, 584*f*
  bifurcation of, 402
Tracheal carina, 402
Tracheal cartilages, 402
Tracheal muscle, 402
Tracheal trunk
  left, 584*f*, 624
  right, 624
Tracheobronchial lymph nodes, 413, 631, 632*f*, 634*f*
Tract, 658*f*
  corticopontine, 766
  corticospinal, 760–761
  mamillotegmental, 777
  mamillothalamic, 777
  mesencephalic, of trigeminal nerve, 768
    nucleus of, 758, 768
  paraventriculohypophyseal, 776
  reticulospinal, 759
  solitary, 757–758, 764
  spinal, of trigeminal nerve, 758, 761, 762*f*
    nucleus of, 758, 761
  supraopticohypophyseal, 776
  uveal, 866–867
  white matter, 757
Tractus corticopontinus, 766
Tractus dorsolateralis, 689, 692
Tractus mamillotegmentalis, 777
Tractus mamillothalamicus, 777
Tractus olfactorius intermedius, 783
Tractus olfactorius lateralis, 783
Tractus olfactorius medialis, 783
Tractus opticus, 775
Tractus paraventriculohypophysialis, 776
Tractus pyramidalis, 766
Tractus pyramidalis lateralis, 694

Index

Tractus pyramidalis ventralis, 694
Tractus reticulospinalis lateralis, 695, 759
Tractus rubrospinalis, 694, 771
Tractus solitarius, 757–758, 764
Tractus spinalis n. trigemini, 758, 761
Tractus spinocerebellaris dorsalis, 692–693
Tractus spinocerebellaris ventralis, 693
Tractus spinoolivaris, 693
Tractus spinotectalis, 693
Tractus spinothalamicus, 692
Tractus spiralis foraminosus, 103
Tractus supraopticohypophysialis, 776
Tractus tectonucleares, 768
Tractus tectospinalis, 694
Tractus tectospinalis lateralis, 694
Tractus tegmenti centralis, 770
Tragus, 851–852
Transmissive segments, of neurons, 654
Transversalis fascia, 353, 424
Transverse abdominal oblique muscle, 740f
Transverse acetabular ligament, 197, 197f
Transverse atlantal ligament, 183, 183f
Transverse cervical nerve, 837
Transverse cervical nerves, 705f, 709–710, 709f, 711f
Transverse colli, 583
Transverse crest, 103
Transverse cubital artery, 542f, 543, 719f
Transverse fibers, 337, 337f
Transverse foramen, 126
    of atlas, 128f
    of axis, 128f
    of cervical vertebra, 128f, 131
Transverse humeral ligament, 716f
Transverse humeral retinaculum, 188–189, 188f
Transverse line, of sacrum, 136
Transverse palatine suture, 113
Transverse palmar carpal ligament, 193
Transverse pontine fibers, 766
Transverse process, 126
    of atlas, 127–130, 128f–129f
    of axis, 127f–129f
    of caudal vertebrae, 137f
    of cervical vertebrae, 128f–130f, 131
    of lumbar vertebrae, 134, 134f–135f
    of sacral vertebrae, 136f
    of thoracic vertebrae, 132

Transverse sinus, 607f, 608, 700f
    intraosseous part of, 609f
    of pericardium, 495
    sulcus for, 96f, 97
Transverse sulcus, 97
Transversospinalis muscle, 245–247
Transversus thoracis muscle, 729f
Trapezius muscle, 709f–710f, 729f
Trapezoid body, 765
    dorsal nucleus of, 765
    ventral nuclei of, 765
Triadan System, modified, 324f, 328
Triangular ligaments, 357f
    left, 377–378
    right, 377
Triceps brachii muscle. see M. triceps brachii
Tricipital line, 143f, 145
Tricuspid valve, 504
Trigeminal ganglion, 818–819, 898–899
Trigeminal nerve (cranial nerve V), 322, 766–767, 818–828, 821f–822f, 898–900, 898f
    canal for, 102f, 103, 122f, 123
    mesencephalic tract of, 768
        nucleus of, 758, 768
    motor nucleus of, 824–825
    pontine sensory nucleus of, 758
    roots of, 824–825
    spinal tract of, 758, 761, 762f
    superficial branches of, 823f
Trigone
    of bladder, 421–422
    fibrous, 500
Trigonum femorale, 565–567
Trigonum fibrosum dextrum, 500
Trigonum fibrosum sinistrum, 500
Trigonum vesicae, 421–422
Trochanter
    greater, 161f–163f, 163
    lesser, 160–161, 163, 163f
    third, 162f, 163–164
Trochanter major, 163
Trochanter minor, 163
Trochanter tertius, 163–164
Trochanteric fossa, 162f–163f, 163
Trochlea, 894
    of femur, 162f, 164
    of humerus, 143f, 146
    of radius, 147f, 149–150
    of talus, 169–170, 169f
Trochlea humeri, 146
Trochlea ossis femoris, 164
Trochlea talis, 169–170
Trochlear decussation, 818

Trochlear nerve (cranial nerve IV), 817–818, 818f, 898, 898f
    motor nucleus of, 770–771
Trochlear radii, 149–150
Trochoid joint, 179
Trunci lumbales, 622–623
Trunci plexus, 714–715
Truncus bicaroticus, 510
Truncus brachiocephalicus, 510
Truncus celiacus, 640
Truncus colicus, 640
Truncus costocervicalis, 534
Truncus intestinalis, 639–640
Truncus lumbosacralis, 744
Truncus phrenicoabdominalis, 560
Truncus pudendoepigastricus, 562
Truncus pulmonalis, 412, 509
Truncus sympathicus, 671
Truncus trachealis, 624
Truncus vagalis dorsalis, 836
Truncus vagalis ventralis, 836
Truncus visceralis, 622–623, 640
Trunk
    cutaneous nerves of, 730f
    fasciae of, 262–263, 263f
    muscles of, 262–263
        abdominal wall, 252–258, 253f–255f
        diaphragm as, 250–252, 250f
        neck, 232f, 237–241, 239f–240f, 244f, 264f
        thoracic wall, 239f, 248–252, 248f–250f
    superficial arteries of, 550f
Tuba auditiva, 101–102, 396, 847–848
Tuba uterina, 450
Tuber
    calcaneal, 168f, 170f–171f
    olecranon, 149f
    omental, 376
Tuber calcanei, 169f, 170–171
Tuber cinereum, 473
Tuber coxae, 158, 158f–159f, 561
Tuber ischiadicum, 160–161
Tuber maxillae, 111
Tuber omentale, 376
Tuber sacrale, 158
Tubercles
    of atlas, 127–130, 128f
    corniculate, 345f, 400
    cuneiform, 345f, 400
    genital, 463
    of humerus
        greater, 143–145, 143f
        lesser, 143–145, 143f–144f

Tubercles (Continued)
  infraglenoid, 141f, 142, 144f
  intercondylar, 165–167
  muscular, 97–98, 118–119
  nuchal, 97–98, 119f
  pharyngeal, 97–98
  plantar, 169f
  pubic, 158f–160f, 161
  of rib, 139–140, 139f
  supraglenoid, 141f, 144f
  urethral, 454–455
Tubercula muscularia, 97–98
Tubercula nuchalia, 97–98
Tuberculum acousticum, 765
Tuberculum corniculatum, 400
Tuberculum costae, 139–140
Tuberculum cuneiforme, 400
Tuberculum dorsale, 127–130
Tuberculum infraglenoidale, 142
Tuberculum intercondylare mediale et alterale, 165–167
Tuberculum intervenosum, 499–500
Tuberculum linguale laterale, 329
Tuberculum linguale proximale (copula), 329
Tuberculum lingulae medium, 329
Tuberculum majus, 143–145
Tuberculum minus, 143–145
Tuberculum olfactorium, 783
Tuberculum pharyngeum, 97–98
Tuberculum pubicum, 161
Tuberculum pubicum ventrale, 161
Tuberculum sellae, 100f, 101
Tuberculum supraglenoidale, 142–143
Tuberculum ventrale, 127–130
Tuberositas deltoides, 145
Tuberositas iliaca, 158–160
Tuberositas radii, 147
Tuberositas teres major, 146
Tuberositas tibiae, 165–167
Tuberosity
  deltoid, 143f, 145
  iliac, 158–160, 160f
  ischiatic, 157f–160f, 163f
  maxillary, 110f, 111
  radial, 147, 147f
  supracondylar, 162f, 164
  supraglenoid, 142–143
  for teres major, 143f–144f, 146
  for teres minor, 143f
  tibial, 165f–167f
  ulnar, 147f, 151
Tubules
  collecting, 463
  mesonephric, 462–463

Tubules (Continued)
  renal, 419f
  seminiferous
    convoluted, 428
    straight, 428–430
  uterine, 463
Tubuli seminiferi contorti, 428
Tubuli seminiferi recti, 428–430
Tunica adventitia
  of ductus deferens, 436
  of esophagus, 347
Tunica albuginea, 428, 439
Tunica dartos, 424
Tunica fibrosa, of liver, 377
Tunica fibrosa bulbi, 861
Tunica interna bulbi, 861, 873
Tunica mucosa, 421, 452–453
  of esophagus, 348
  of large intestine, 373–374
  of small intestine, 367
  of stomach, 363
Tunica mucosa linguae, 331
Tunica muscularis
  of bile duct, 380
  of large intestine, 374
  of liver, 347
  of small intestine, 367
  of stomach, 363
  of urethra, 444
  of uterus, 452
  of vagina, 453–454
Tunica serosa
  of large intestine, 374
  of liver, 377
  of peritoneum, 353
  of small intestine, 367
  of stomach, 362–363
  of uterine tube, 450
Tunica vaginalis, 424
Tunica vasculosa bulbi, 860–861, 866–867
Tunica vasculosa lentis, 858–859
Turbinates, 388
Twins, 21
Tylotrich hair, 78, 78f
Tympanic bulla, 102f–103f, 119f, 846
Tympanic cavity, 102–105, 847–848
Tympanic membrane, 105, 841f, 846–847
  ramus to, 825–826
  secondary, 840–842
Tympanic nerve, 832–833, 847
Tympanic ring, 105
Tympanicum, 105
Tympanohyoid cartilage, 33, 116f, 117
  areas of attachment of, 103f
Tympanooccipital fissure, 105–106

U

Ulna, 147f–149f, 150–151, 190f. see also Elbow
  development of, 47–51, 53f
Ulnar artery, 545, 719f–720f
  collateral, 538f, 541, 542f, 593f
  dorsal branch, 545
  recurrent, 542f, 543–544
Ulnar nerve, 705f, 713f–715f, 717f–720f, 722
  distal branch, 723f, 727f
  dorsal branch, 713f, 723f, 725f, 727f
  of forepaw, 725
  palmar branch, 723f, 725f
  proximal branch, 723f, 727f
Ulnar notch, 147f, 149–150
Ulnar tuberosity, 147f, 151
Ulnar vein, 583f, 592f, 593
Ulnaris lateralis muscle, nerve to, 717f
Umbilical artery, 573
Umbilical region, 350–351, 353f
Umbo membranae tympani, 846
Uncinate notch, 106–107
Uncinate process, 106–107, 106f
  crest for, 110f
Ungual process, 152f, 155f
Unguicula, 64, 82–83
Unipolar neurons, 650–651
Upper motor neurons, 654
Ureteral mucosa, 421
Ureteric bud, 463
Ureteric veins, right cranial, 597
Ureters, 416, 417f, 420–421, 420f, 463
  anomalies of, 421
  nerves of, 421
  structure of, 421
  vessels of, 421
Urethra, 416, 423, 427f
  female, 457–458
  lymph vessels of, 642f
  male, 443–444
    penile part of, 444
    prostatic portion of, 443–444
Urethra feminina, 416, 457
Urethra masculina, 416, 443
Urethral arteries, 444, 575, 602f–603f
Urethral crest, 437, 443–444
Urethral gland, 444
Urethral groove, 439
Urethral surface, of penis, 438
Urethral tubercle, 454–455
Urethral vein, 438, 444
Urethral venous plexus, 604
Urethralis muscle, 423

Urinary organs, 416–423. *see also specific organs*
Urinary system. *see also* Reproductive organs; Urinary organs
  lymph drainage of, 619, 642*f*
Urogenital ligaments, 422*f*
Urogenital sinus, 463
Urogenital system, 416–468. *see also* Urinary organs
  embryologic characteristics of, 460*f*–461*f*, 462–464, 463*b*
  female, 417*f*
Urogenital veins, 604
Uterine artery, 449–451, 453
Uterine horns, 451–452
Uterine ostium, 450
Uterine tube, 445, 450–451
  anomalies and variations of, 451
  nerves of, 450–451
  structure of, 450
  vessels of, 450–451
Uterine tubules, 463
Uterine vein, 449–450, 453, 604
Uterine velum, 452
Utero-ovarian artery, 559
Uterus, 445, 451–453, 463
  body of, 452
  nerves of, 453
  round ligament of, 740*f*
  spaces and folds of, 452
  structure of, 452–453
  vessels of, 453
Uterus masculinus, 443–444, 463
Utriculosaccular duct, 842
Utriculus, 842
Utriculus prostaticus, 443–444
Uvea, 866–867
Uveal tract, 866–867
Uvulonodular fissure, 792

V

Vagal ganglion
  distal, 351*f*
  proximal, 667
Vagal nerves, 348, 351*f*
  dorsal trunk, 351*f*
  left, 351*f*
  ventral trunk, 351*f*
Vagina, 445, 453–454
  cranial, 463
  nerves of, 454
  relations of, 453
  structure of, 453–454
  vessels of, 454
Vagina bulbi, 884
Vagina carotica, 510–511
Vagina externa n. optici, 861, 873, 896
Vagina interna n. optici, 873, 896
Vagina m. recti abdominis, 253–254, 253*f*, 255*f*, 256–257
Vagina synovialis m. obliqui dorsalis, 894
Vaginal artery, 421, 457
Vaginal process, 426*f*, 445
Vaginal ring, 436
Vaginal tunic, 424, 425*f*–426*f*, 436
Vaginal vein, 583*f*, 604
Vaginal venous plexus, 604
Vagosympathetic trunk, 351*f*
Vagus nerve, 322, 338*f*, 364, 367–368
Vagus nerve, parasympathetic nucleus of, 763–764
Vagus nerve (cranial nerve X), 666–670, 668*f*–669*f*, 833–836, 835*f*
  auricular branch, 834
  autonomic interconnections, 826*f*
  cardiac branches, 836
  distal ganglion, 834
  dorsal vagal trunk, 836
  parasympathetic nucleus of, 834
  parasympathetic nucleus of the, 666
  pharyngeal branch, 585*f*
  pharyngeal branches, 834–835
  proximal ganglion, 834
  ventral vagal trunk, 836
Vallate papillae, 330, 331*f*–332*f*
  complex, 333–334
Vallecula, 397–398
Vallecula epiglottica, 397–398
Valva aortae, 505
Valva atrioventricularis dextra, 504
Valva atrioventricularis sinistra, 504–505
Valva trunci pulmonalis, 505
Valvae atrioventriculares, 504
Valve(s)
  aortic, 500, 501*f*, 505
  atrioventricular, 504–505
  bicuspid, 504–505
  mitral, 504–505
  pulmonary, 505
  of pulmonary trunk, 505
  tricuspid, 504
Valvula sinus coronarii, 508
Valvulae semilunares dextra, 505
Valvulae semilunares intermedia, 505
Valvulae semilunares septales, 505
Vasa lymphatica, 619. *see also* Lymph vessels
Vasa lymphatica afferentia, 621
Vasa lymphatica efferentia, 621
Vasa recti, 367, 558

Vascular layer, 867
Vascular plexus, of hard palate, 107*f*
Vascular tunic, of eye, 866–873
  arterial supply of, 869*f*
  veins of, 869*f*
Vasculature, somatic, sympathetic distribution in, 675
Vastus lateralis muscle, 744*f*, 749*f*
Vastus medialis nerve, 741*f*
Veil
  omental, 357–358
  palatine, 322
Vein(s), 582–615. *see also specific veins*
  arcuate, 420
  of bone, 90–91
  of brain, 609*f*, 610–611
  bronchial, 413
  of bulb, 441
  cardiac, 508–509
  of central nervous system, 606–614
  of clitoris, 602*f*–603*f*, 604
  of corpus callosum, 607*f*, 608, 610
  of Diploë, 611
  of ductus deferens, 436, 604
  of eye, 903–904, 903*f*
  of forepaw, 592*f*, 594–595
  general considerations of, 582
  of head, 586*f*, 588*f*
  of hindpaw, 605–606, 605*f*
  interlobar, 420
  interlobular, 420
  of muscles, 213
  of neck, 584*f*–585*f*, 588*f*
  nutrient, 90–91
  of pelvis, 603–605
  of penis, 604
  periosteal, 90–91
  portal, 378, 598
  pulmonary, 509–510
  retinal, 876, 904
  of shoulder, 584*f*
  of spinal cord, 611–614
  stellate, 420
  Thebesian, 509
  of thigh, 565*f*
  of thoracic limb, 591–595
  of vascular tunic, 869*f*
  of vertebrae, 611–614
  of vestibular bulb, 604
Velum medullare caudale, 763
Velum medullare rostrale, 763
Velum omentale, 357–358
Velum palatinum, 321–322
Velum uteri, 452
Vena cava
  caudal, 357*f*, 373, 498*f*, 499, 595–598, 595*f*

Vena cava (Continued)
  cranial, 498f, 502f, 582–591, 583f–584f
  plica, 406–408
Vena cava caudalis, 499
Vena (V.)/Venae (Vv.). see Vein(s); specific veins
V. abdominalis caudalis, 602–603
V. alveolaris inferior, 589
V. angularis oculi, 586f, 587, 903–904, 903f
V. auricularis caudalis, 589–590
V. auricularis lateralis, 589–590
V. auricularis medialis, 589–590
V. auricularis profunda, 589–590
V. auricularis rostralis, 589
V. axillaries, 593–594
V. axillobrachialis, 593
V. azygos, 348, 582, 583f, 590f, 613f, 729f
V. azygos dextra, 590
V. bicipitalis, 593
V. brachialis superficialis, 593
V. bronchoesophageae, 591
V. bulbi penis, 604
V. bulbi vestibuli, 604
V. caudalis femoralis distalis, 600
V. caudalis femoralis proximalis, 601
V. caudalis femoris media, 601
V. caudalis lateralis, 604
V. cava caudalis, 595–596
V. cava cranialis, 582–583
V. cecalis, 598
V. centrales, 378
V. cephalica, 591
V. cephalica accessoria, 591–592, 594
V. cerebri magna, 608
V. cerebri ventralis, 610
V. cervicalis profunda, 583
V. cervicalis superficialis, 586
V. choroidea, 610–611
V. circumflexa femoris lateralis, 602
V. circumflexa femoris medialis, 602–603
V. circumflexa humeri caudalis, 593–594
V. circumflexa ilium profunda, 597, 600
V. circumflexa ilium superficialis, 601
V. clitoridis, 604
V. colica dextra, 598
V. colica media, 598
V. colica sinistra, 598–599
V. collateralis ulnaris, 593
V. cordis magna, 508–509
V. cordis media, 509
V. corporis callosi, 608, 610
V. costocervicalis, 582–583

V. digitalis dorsalis communis I, 591–592, 594
V. digitalis dorsalis communis III, 605–606
V. diploica frontalis, 587, 611
V. diploica occipitalis, 611
V. diploica parietalis, 611
V. dorsalis penis, 604
V. dorsalis ventriculi sinistri, 508–509
V. ductus deferentis, 604
V. emissaria canalis carotici, 609
V. emissaria canalis n. hypoglossi, 608–609
V. emissaria foraminis laceri, 589
V. emissaria foraminis ovalis, 589
V. emissaria foraminis retroarticularis, 105, 589, 608
V. emissaria foraminis rotundi, 587, 589
V. emissaria occipitalis, 608
V. epigastrica caudalis, 602–603
V. esophageae, 591
V. ethmoidalis externa, 587
V. facialis, 586
V. faciei profunda, 587
V. femoralis, 600
V. femoris profunda, 602–603
V. gastrica dextra, 599
V. gastrica sinistra, 599
V. gastroduodenalis, 599
V. gastroepiploica dextra, 599
V. gastroepiploica sinistra, 599
V. glandularis, 586
V. glutea caudalis, 603
V. glutea cranialis, 604
V. ileocolica, 598
V. iliaca communis, 605
V. iliaca externa, 602–603
V. iliaca interna, 603
V. iliolumbalis, 604–605
V. infraorbitalis, 587
V. intercostalis dorsalis, 583
V. intercostalis suprema, 583
V. interossea communis, 593
V. jejunales, 598
V. jugularis externa, 586
V. jugularis interna, 585–586
V. labialis dorsalis, 604
V. labialis inferior, 588
V. labialis superior, 587
V. lacrimalis, 904
V. laryngea cranialis, 589
V. laryngea impar, 588–589
V. lateralis nasi, 587
V. lienalis, 599
V. lingualis, 588
V. linguofacialis, 586

V. malaris, 587
V. masseterica, 589
V. maxillaris, 589
V. mediana, 593
V. mediana cubiti, 592
V. meningea media, 589
V. mesenterica caudalis, 598–599
V. mesenterica cranialis, 598
V. nasalis dorsalis, 586
V. obliqua atrii sinistri, 508–509
V. omobrachialis, 593
V. ophthalmica externa dorsalis, 587, 904
V. ophthalmica externa ventralis, 587, 904
V. ovarica dextra, 597
V. ovarica sinistra, 597
V. palpebralis inferior, 587
V. palpebralis superior medialis, 903–904
V. pancreaticoduodenalis caudalis, 598
V. pancreaticoduodenalis cranialis, 599
V. penis, 604
V. pharyngeal ascendens, 589
V. phrenica caudalis, 597
V. poplitea, 600
V. portae, 378, 598
V. profunda antebrachii, 593
V. profunda brachii, 593
V. prostatica, 604
V. radialis, 593
V. rectalis cranialis, 598–599
V. rectalis media, 604
V. renis, 420
V. sacralis mediana, 605
V. saphena lateralis, 599–600
V. saphena medialis, 600
V. scapularis dorsalis, 583
V. sublingualis, 588
V. submentalis, 588
V. subscapularis, 593–594
V. tarsea lateralis, 606
V. tarsea medialis, 606
V. temporalis superficialis, 589
V. testicularis dextra, 597
V. testicularis sinistra, 597
V. thalamostriata, 610–611
V. thoracica externa, 593–594
V. thoracica lateralis, 593–594
V. thoracodorsalis, 593–594
V. thyroidea caudalis, 585
V. thyroidea cranialis, 585–586
V. thyroidea ima, 585
V. thyroidea media, 585–586
V. tibialis caudalis, 600
V. tibialis cranialis, 600
V. transversa cubiti, 593

V. transversa faciei, 589
V. ulnaris, 593
V. uterina, 604
V. vaginalis, 604
V. vertebralis, 583–585
V. vesicalis caudalis, 604
Vv. adrenales, 597
Vv. arcuatae, 420
Vv. basivertebrales, 613
Vv. cerebellii ventralis, 611
Vv. cerebri dorsales, 610
Vv. cerebri internae, 610–611
Vv. ciliares, 904
Vv. comitantes, 582
Vv. cordis, 508
Vv. cordis dextrae, 509
Vv. costoabdominales dorsales, 590
Vv. digitales dorsales communes, 591–592, 594, 605–606
Vv. digitales palmares communes, 591, 594
Vv. digitales palmares propriae, 594
Vv. digitales plantares communes, 606
Vv. digitales plantares propriae, 606
Vv. diploicae, 611
Vv. genus, 600
Vv. hepaticae, 378, 597–598
Vv. ilei, 598
Vv. intercostales dorsales, 590
Vv. interlobares, 420
Vv. interlobulares, 378, 420
Vv. intervertebrales, 583, 613–614
Vv. lumbales, 590, 597
Vv. metacarpeae dorsales, 594
Vv. metacarpeae palmares, 594
Vv. metatarseae dorsales, 606
Vv. metatarseae plantares, 606
Vv. pancreaticae, 599
Vv. pulmonales, 412, 509–510
Vv. pulmonales dextrae, 509–510
Vv. pulmonales sinistrae, 509–510
Vv. renales, 597
Vv. vorticosae, 904
Venous angle, 622
Venous arch
    deep palmar, 594–595
    deep plantar, 606
    digital, 605f
    hyoid, 586f, 588–589
    superficial palmar, 594
    superficial plantar, 605f, 606
Venous plexus
    palatine, 589
    vaginal, 604
    vertebral, ventral internal, 680f
Venous sinuses, of spleen, 644
Ventral angle, 141f, 142

Ventral arteries
    caudal, 579
    perineal, 574f, 576
    spinal, 531–533
Ventral branches, 704, 705f–706f, 729f
    of lumbar nerves, 734
    of sacral nerves, 744
    scrotal, 562
    of thoracic nerve, 728–729
Ventral buccal branch, 709f
Ventral caudal nerve trunk, 737f
Ventral caudal nucleus, 774
Ventral caudal plexus, 754, 754f
Ventral cerebellar veins, 611
Ventral condyloid fossa, 96f, 97
Ventral corticospinal tract, 691f, 760–761
Ventral cutaneous branch, 707, 708f, 729f, 730
    of lumbar nerve, 733f
Ventral ethmoidal crest, 110f
Ventral external ophthalmic vein, 587, 904
    anastomotic branch with, 903f
Ventral funiculus, 680, 681f, 693
    projection pathways in, 690b
Ventral horn, 679, 681f
    lateral ventricle, 700f
    nuclei, 687
Ventral interbasilar sinus, 610
Ventral internal vertebral venous plexus, 680f
Ventral intraoccipital synchondrosis, 97–98
Ventral lateral nucleus, 774
Ventral margin, of lung, 408–409
Ventral medial nucleus, 774
Ventral median fissure, 680, 681f
Ventral mediastinum, 405
Ventral metencephalon, 757, 766–767
Ventral nasal meatus, 107f–108f, 112
Ventral occipital sinus, 610
Ventral orbital crest, 882
Ventral petrosal sinus, 609
    sulcus for, 96f
Ventral plexus, 754
Ventral rostral nucleus, 774
Ventral sacroiliac ligament, 196, 197f
Ventral scrotal branch, 428
Ventral spinocerebellar tract, 691f, 693
Ventral thoracic lymph center, 628–630
Ventral vagal trunk, 669

Ventricle(s)
    of brain, 700f
        fourth, 700–701, 700f, 758t, 763
        lateral, 700–701, 700f, 758t, 778–779, 781
        third, 700–701, 700f, 758t, 772–773
    of heart
        left, 495–496, 497f, 501f, 503, 503f, 584f
        right, 495–496, 501, 501f–502f, 507f, 584f
    laryngeal, 401
    schema of, 700f
    terminal, of spinal cord, 679
Ventricular margin, 499
Ventricular system, 700–701, 700f
Ventriculus, 359–361
Ventriculus dexter, 495–496, 501
Ventriculus laryngis, 401
Ventriculus lateralis, 700–701, 781
Ventriculus quartus, 700–701
Ventriculus sinister, 495–496, 503
Ventriculus terminalis, 679
Ventriculus tertius, 700–701, 772–773
Ventrolateral nasal cartilage, 390
Ventrolateral sulcus, 680–681, 681f
Ventromedial hypothalamic nucleus, 777
Venulae stellatae, 420
Vermiform impression, 96f, 97
Vertebra(e), 88
    anticlinal, 131–132, 132f, 134f
    body of, 125–126
    caudal, 125, 137–138, 137f, 138t
        development of, 37–44, 46f–47f, 49f
    cervical, 125–131, 126f–129f, 138t
        development of, 46f, 48f
        fifth, 128f, 131
        fourth, 129f–130f, 131
        muscles of, 235–236, 240f, 244f
        seventh, 129f–130f, 131
        sixth, 129f–130f, 131
        third, 129f–130f, 131
    development of, 35–44, 46f
    lumbar, 125, 133–134, 134f–135f, 138t
        development of, 37, 46f, 48f
    sacral, 125, 135–137, 136f, 138t
    segmental relationships to, 683, 684f
    thoracic, 125, 131–133, 132f–133f, 138t
        development of, 46f, 48f
        second, 710f
    veins of, 611–614

Vertebra anticlinalis, 131–132
Vertebrae cervicales, 126–131
Vertebral arch, 126
  of caudal vertebrae, 137–138
  of cervical vertebra, 130f
Vertebral artery, 533f, 584f
  muscular branches, 531
  spinal branches, 531–533
Vertebral canal, 126, 138, 680f
Vertebral column, 125–139. see also
  Vertebra(e)
  deformity of, 138–139
  development of, 35–44, 46f
  functions of, 138
  joints of, 181–186
    synovial, 183–184
  lateral radiograph of, 698f
  length of, 138, 138t
  long ligaments of, 181–186
  short ligaments of, 185–186
Vertebral foramen
  of atlas, 126, 126f, 128f
  of axis, 128f–129f
  of cervical vertebrae, 129f–130f
Vertebral notch, 126
Vertebral vein, 583–585, 583f, 588f, 607f, 612f
  thoracic, 612f
Vesica fellea, 379
Vesica urinaria, 416, 421. see also
  Bladder, urinary
Vesicogenital pouch, 355, 452–453
Vesicula synaptica, 654
Vesicular follicle, 447
Vestibular aqueduct, 102f, 104, 842
Vestibular area, 789
  of temporal bone, 103
Vestibular bulb, 455
  artery of, 576
Vestibular cleft, 400–401
Vestibular constrictor muscle, 456
Vestibular crus, 839–840
Vestibular fold, 397f, 400–401
Vestibular ganglion, 844
Vestibular lamina, 33–34
Vestibular membrane, 844
Vestibular nerve, 844
Vestibular neurons, 650–651
Vestibular nuclei, 765
Vestibular surface, of tooth, 327
Vestibular window, 103f, 104, 839–840, 847
Vestibule
  bony, 107f
  bony labyrinth, 839–840
  laryngeal, 400
  nasal, 389, 391–392

Vestibule *(Continued)*
  of omental bursa, 358
  of oral cavity, 319
  vaginal, 445, 454–455
Vestibulocochlear nerve (cranial nerve VIII), 765, 832
  canal for, 102f
Vestibulum, 104
Vestibulum bursae omentalis, 358
Vestibulum laryngis, 400
Vestibulum nasi, 391–392
Vestibulum oris, 319
Vestibulum vaginae, 454–455
Vestigial ductus deferens, 463
Village dogs, 1
Villi, synovial, 177
Villi intestinales, 367
Villi synoviales, 177
Viscera, 352f, 354f, 359f
  abdominal, lymph nodes and vessels of, 637–640
Visceral lymph trunks, 622–623
Visceral muscle, 207
Visceral peritoneum, 354
Visceral piston hypothesis, 251–252
Visceral plexuses, 660, 706–707
Visceral surface
  of liver, 376
  of spleen, 643
  of stomach, 361
Visceral trunk, 640
Visceral vaginal tunic, 428
Viscerocranium, 27–28, 36f
Visual area, 788–789
Vitreous, 878f, 879
Vitreous body, 879
Vitreous chamber, 878–879
Vocal fold, 397f, 401
Vocal ligament, 401
Vocal process, 400
Vocalis muscle, 232, 398f
Voluntary muscle, 207
Vomer, 92f, 96f, 106f, 108f, 114–115, 114f, 120f
Vomeroethmoid suture, 109, 114–115
Vomeroincisive suture, 109–110, 114–115
Vomeromaxillary suture, 111, 114–115
Vomeronasal cartilage, 107f
Vomeronasal nerve, 815
Vomeronasal organ, 390–391, 390f, 393f
  distribution of nerves to, 815f
Vomeropalatine sutures, dorsal, 114–115

Vomerosphenoid suture, 102, 114–115
von Ebner's glands, 334
Vorticose veins, 904
Vulva, 445, 455

W
Wall
  abdominal, 252–258, 253f–255f
  nasal
    arteries of, 521f
    nerves of, 816f
  thoracic
    arteries of, 550f
    fascia of, 252
    muscles of, 239f, 248–252, 248f–250f
Weight, prenatal, 23, 25f
White commissure, 680, 681f
White matter, 679
  of brain, 757
  cerebral, 778–779
  related cerebral neocortex, 787–788
  of spinal cord, 658f
White splenic pulp, 643
Window
  cochlear, 103f, 104, 119f, 839–840, 847
  vestibular, 103f, 104, 839–840, 847
Wing(s)
  of atlas, 126f, 127–130
  of ilium, 158
  of nostril, 391
  orbital, 100f–101f
  of sacrum, 136, 136f, 734f
  temporal, 100f–101f
  of vomer, 114, 114f
WISDOM Panel MX of Mars Veterinary, Inc., 1
Withdrawal reflex, 696
Working breeds, 9f

X
Xiphoid cartilage, 139f, 140
Xiphoid process, 139f, 140
Xiphoid region, 350–351, 353f

Y
Yellow bone marrow, 90
Yellow ligaments, 184f, 185–186, 197f
Yoke, of presphenoid bone, 101
Yolk sac, 18, 19f, 22f, 59f

Z
Zona arcuata, 484
Zona columnaris, 371–372
Zona cutanea, 371

Zona fasciculata, 484–485
Zona glomerulosa, 485
Zona incerta, 778
Zona intermedia, 371
Zona intermedia corticalis, 485
Zona orbicularis, 197
Zona reticularis, 484
Zone(s)
    of anal canal, 371
    autonomous, 660
    dendritic, 652
    overlap, 660, 660f
Zonula ciliaris, 860, 871

Zonular fibers, 870f, 871
Zonule, 871–872
Zygomatic arch, 105, 112, 117–118, 340f
Zygomatic artery, 523
Zygomatic articulation, cavity for, 110f
Zygomatic bone, 91f–92f, 112, 112f, 116f–117f, 120f
    frontal process of, 92f
Zygomatic branch, 900
Zygomatic gland, 320, 340f–341f, 343–344, 625f, 883–884

Zygomatic nerve, 818f, 819–822, 900
    foramen for, 101f
Zygomatic process, 105
    of frontal bone, 92f, 99f, 118f–120f
    of maxilla, 111
    of temporal bone, 92f, 102f–103f, 120f
Zygomaticofacial nerve, 587f, 898f, 900
Zygomaticomaxillary suture, 111–112
Zygomaticotemporal nerve, 587f, 898f, 900